CLINICAL
DIALYSIS

Notice

Medicine is an ever-changing science. As new research and clinical experience broaden our knowledge, changes in treatment and drug therapy are required. The editors and the publisher of this work have checked with sources believed to be reliable in their efforts to provide information that is complete and generally in accord with the standards accepted at the time of publication. However, in view of the possibility of human error or changes in medical sciences, neither the editors nor the publisher nor any other party who has been involved in the preparation or publication of this work warrants that the information contained herein is in every respect accurate or complete, and they disclaim all responsibility for any errors or omissions or for the results obtained from use of the information contained in this work. Readers are encouraged to confirm the information contained herein with other sources. For example and in particular, readers are advised to check the product information sheet included in the package of each drug they plan to administer to be certain that the information contained in this work is accurate and that changes have not been made in the recommended dose or in the contraindications for administration. This recommendation is of particular importance in connection with new or infrequently used drugs.

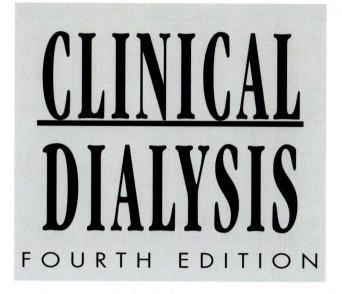

CLINICAL DIALYSIS

FOURTH EDITION

Editors

Allen R. Nissenson, MD, FACP, FASN
Professor of Medicine
Director, Dialysis Program
David Geffen School of
Medicine at the
University of California, Los Angeles
Los Angeles, California

Richard N. Fine, MD
Chairman
Department of Pediatrics
State University of New York
Stony Brook University Hospital
Stony Brook, New York

McGraw-Hill
Medical Publishing Division

New York   Chicago   San Francisco   Lisbon   London   Madrid   Mexico City
Milan   Seoul   New Delhi   San Juan   Singapore   Sydney   Toronto

*The **McGraw·Hill** Companies*

Clinical Dialysis, Fourth Edition

1234567890 CCW/CCW098765

ISBN: 0-07-141939-X

This book was set in Times Roman by Pine Tree Composition, Inc.
The editors were James Shanahan, Michelle Watt, and Lester A. Sheinis.
The production supervisor was Sherri Souffrance.
The cover designer was Mary McKeon.
The indexer was Alexandra Nickerson.
Courier Westford was printer and binder.

This book is printed on acid-free paper.

Library of Congress Cataloging-in-Publication Data

Clinical dialysis / edited by Allen R. Nissenson, Richard N. Fine.—4th ed.
    p.; cm.
  Originally published: New York: Appleton & Lange, © 1990.
  Includes bibliographical references and index.
  ISBN 0-07-141939-X
  1. Hemodialysis. 2. Peritoneal dialysis. 3. Continuous ambulatory peritoneal dialysis. I.
Nissenson, Allen R. II. Fine, Richard N.
  [DNLM: 1. Kidney Failure, Chronic—therapy. 2. Renal Dialysis. 3. Peritoneal Dialysis.
WJ 378 C641 2005]
RC901.7.H45C55 2005
614.4´ 61059—dc22

                                            2004045912

This book is dedicated to the memory of James Shinaberger and Jack Coburn. These two outstanding physicians and researchers worked tirelessly to improve the care and the lives of countless patients with kidney disease. Their contributions are greatly appreciated and will long be remembered.

Contents

Contributors

Rajiv Agarwal, MD
Associate Professor of Clinical Medicine
Division of Nephrology
Indiana University School of Medicine
Indianapolis, Indiana
Chapter 27B

Mohammad Akmal, MD
Professor of Medicine
Medical Director
University of Southern California Kidney Center
Department of Nephrology
Los Angeles, California
Chapter 29

Ziyad Al Aly, MD
Division of Nephrology
Saint Louis University
St. Louis, Missouri
Chapter 30

Walter S. Andrews, MD
Director of Pediatric Transplant
Children's Mercy Hospital
Kansas City, Missouri
Chapters 44, 45

Stephen R. Ash, MD, FACP
Medical Director
HemoCleanse Inc.
Director of Dialysis
St. Elizabeth Hospital
Lafayette, Indiana
Chapter 13

William M. Bennett MD
Director of Solid and Cellular Transplantation
Legacy Good Samaritan Hospital
Portland, Oregon
Chapter 33

Michael S. Berkoben, MD
Associate Professor of Medicine
Duke University Medical Center
Durham, North Carolina
Medical Director
Gambro Healthcare Dialysis Unit
Henderson, North Carolina
Chapter 2

Anatole Besarab, MD
Senior Staff
Division of Nephrology and Hypertension
Henry Ford Hospital
Detroit, Michigan
Chapter 26

Stefano Biasioli, MD
Chief
Department of Nephrology and Dialysis
Legnago Hospital
Legnago (Verona), Italy
Chapter 31

Jason Biederman, MD
Pediatric Psychopharmacology Unit
Massachusetts General Hospital
Boston, Massachusetts
Chapter 26

Patrick D. Brophy, MD, FAAP, FRCPC
Pediatric Nephrology, Dialysis and Transplantation
Co-Director, Pediatric Hypertension Program
University of Michigan
CS Mott Children's Hospital
Ann Arbor, Michigan
Chapter 40

Timothy Bunchman, MD
Professor, Pediatric Nephrology & Transplantation
DeVos Children's Hospital
Grand Rapids, Michigan
Chapters 40, 42

Suphamai Bunnapradist, MD
Medical Director
Kidney-Pancreas Transplant Program
Cedars-Sinai Medical Center
Los Angeles, California
Chapter 24

Bernard Canaud, MD
University of Montpellier
Lapeyronie Hospital
Department of Nephrology
Montpellier
Renal Research and Training Institute
Montpellier, France
Chapter 36

David J. Carr, MSChe
HemoCleanse Inc.
Lafayette, Indiana
Chapter 13

Christopher T. Chan, MD, FRCPC
Assistant Professor of Medicine
University of Toronto
Toronto, Ontario, Canada
Chapter 44

M. K. Chan, MD FRCP
Formerly Reader
Department of Medicine
University of Hong Kong, Queen Mary Hospital
Pokfulam Road
Hong Kong, China
Chapter 28

T. M. Chan, MD, FRCP
Professor, Department of Medicine
University of Hong Kong
Queen Mary Hospital, Hong Kong
Pokfulam Road
Hong Kong, China
Chapter 28

David N. Churchill, MD, FRCPC
Professor of Medicine
Faculty of Health Sciences
McMaster University
Hamilton, Ontario, Canada
Chapter 34

William R. Clark, MD
Clinical Assistant, Professor of Medicine
Indiana University School of Medicine
Indianapolis, Indiana
Chapter 4

Richard A. Cohn, MD
Medical Director
Kidney Transplantation
Children's Memorial Hospital–Chicago
Professor of Pediatrics
Northwestern University
Feinberg School of Medicine
Chicago, Illinois
Chapter 42

John H. Crabtree, MD, FACS
Assistant Chief of Surgery
Kaiser Permanente
Bellflower Medical Center
Bellflower, California
Chapter 13

Angelo M. deMattos MD
Associate Professor of Medicine
Division of Nephrology and Hypertension
Portland, Oregon
Chapter 33

Thomas A. Depner, MD
Professor of Medicine
University of California–Davis
Sacramento, California
Chapter 9

Annemiere Dhondt, MD
University Hospital–Gent
Department of Internal Medicine
Nephrology Division
De Pintelaan
Gent, Belgium
Chapter 18

Jose A. Diaz-Buxo, MD, FACP
Senior Vice President
Home Therapies
Fresenius Medical Care
Lexington, Massachusetts
Clinical Professor of Medicine
University of North Carolina
Charlotte, North Carolina
Chapters 13, 16

Alberto Edefonti, MD
Nephrology and Dialysis Unit
Clinica Pediatrica G. e D. De Marchi
Milano, Italy
Chapter 22

Pedram Enayati, MD
Department of Medicine
Cedars Sinai Medical Center
Los Angeles, California
Chapter 25

Fabrizio Fabrizi, MD
Nephrology and Dialysis Division
Azienda Ospedale di Lecco
Lecco, Italy
Chapter 24

Harold I. Feldman, MD MSCE
Director
Clinical Epidemiology Unit
Center for Clinical Epidemiology and Biostatistics
Associate Professor of Medicine and Epidemiology
Renal-Electrolyte and Hypertension Division
University of Pennsylvania School of Medicine
Philadelphia, Pennsylvania
Chapter 11

Richard N. Fine, MD
Chairman
Department of Pediatrics
State University of New York
Stony Brook University Hospital
Stony Brook, New York
Chapter 23

Robert N. Foley, MD
Assistant Professor
Department of Medicine
University of Minnesota School of Medicine
Minneapolis, Minnesota
Chapter 27A

Linda F. Fried, MD, MPH
Assistant Professor of Medicine
University of Pittsburgh School of Medicine
Veterans Administration Pittsburgh Healthcare System
Pittsburgh, Pennsylvania
Chapter 17

Esther A. González, MD
Associate Professor of Internal Medicine
Division of Nephrology
Saint Louis University School of Medicine
St. Louis, Missouri
Chapter 30

Frank Gotch, MD
Associate Clinical Professor of Medicine
University of California, San Francisco
San Francisco, California
Chapters 7, 15

Larry A. Greenbaum, MD
Associate Professor of Pediatrics
University of Wisconsin Medical School
Madison, Wisconsin
Chapter 7

Jennifer Abbott Hollon, MD
Fellow in Nephrology
Kidney Disease Program
University of Louisville School of Medicine
Louisville, Kentucky
Chapter 20

Walter H. Hörl, MD
Division of Nephrology
Department of Medicine
University of Vienna
Vienna, Austria
Chapter 5

Rome Jutabha, MD
Director
UCLA Center for Small Bowel Diseases
Associate Professor of Medicine
University of California at Los Angeles Medical Center
Los Angeles, California
Chapter 25

Charoen Kaitwatcharachai, MD
Research Fellow, Nephrology
Renal Research Institute
Beth Israel Medical Center
New York, New York
Chapter 10

Elaine M. Kaptein, MD
Professor of Medicine
University of Southern California School of Medicine
Los Angeles, California
Chapter 29

Marcia Keen, PhD
Amgen Inc.
Thousand Oaks, California
Chapters 7, 15

Stefan G. Kiessling, MD
Associate Professor of Pediatrics
Division of Pediatric Nephrology
University of Kentucky School of Medicine
Lexington, Kentucky
Chapter 12

Sidney M. Kobrin, MD
Associate Professor of Medicine
Renal-Electrolyte and Hypertension Division
University of Pennsylvania School of Medicine
Philadelphia, Pennsylvania
Chapter 11

Detlef H. Krieter, MD
Department of Nephrology
Montpellier University Renal Research
    and Training Institute
Montpellier, France
Chapter 36

Victoria A. Kumar, MD
Assistant Professor of Medicine
University of California Davis Medical Center
Davis, California
The Permanente Medical Group, Inc.
Sacramento, California
Chapter 9

Nathan W. Levin, MD
Medical and Research Director
Renal Research Institute
Beth Israel Medical Center
New York, New York
Chapter 10

Hilary Lloyd, MD
Department of Child and Adolescent Psychiatry
CAMHS Directorate
Royal Manchester Children's Hospital
Pendlebury, Manchester, England
Chapter 35

Mariana S. Markell, MD
Associate Professor of Medicine
Director, Transplant Nephrology
State University of New York
Downstate Medical Center
Brooklyn, New York
Chapter 32

Kevin J. Martin, MB, BCh, FACP
Professor of Internal Medicine
Saint Louis University
St. Louis, Missouri
Chapter 30

Paul Martin, MD
Medical Director
Liver Transplant Program
Center for Liver and Kidney Diseases and Transplantation
Cedars-Sinai Medical Center
University of California at Los Angeles School of Medicine
Los Angeles, California
Chapter 24

Patrick T. McBride, MD*
Director of Renal Development
McGaw Inc.
Irvine, California
Chapter 1

Phil McFarlane, MD, FRCPC
Medical Director, Home Dialysis
St. Michael's Hospital
Toronto, Ontario, Canada
Chapter 43

Allen R. Nissenson, MD, FACP, FASN†
Professor of Medicine
Director, Dialysis Program
David Geffen School of Medicine
    at the University of California, Los Angeles
Los Angeles, California

Ali J. Olyaei, PharmD, BCPS
Associate Professor of Medicine
Division of Nephrology and Hypertension
Oregon Health Sciences University
Portland, Oregon
Chapter 33

Fabio Paglialonga, MD
Nephrology and Dialysis Unit
De Marchi Pediatric Clinic
Milan, Italy
Chapter 22

Paul M. Palevsky, MD
Professor of Medicine
Chief, Renal Section
Veterans Administration Pittsburgh Healthcare System
Pittsburgh, Pennsylvania
Chapter 39

Marina Picca, MD
Nephrology and Dialysis Unit
De Marchi Pediatric Clinic
Milan, Italy
Chapter 22

Andreas Pierratos, MD, FRCPC
Associate Professor of Medicine
Humber River Regional Hospital
University of Toronto
Toronto, Ontario, Canada
Chapter 43

Beth Piraino, MD
Professor of Medicine
Director of Peritoneal Dialysis
University of Pittsburgh School of Medicine
Pittsburgh, Pennsylvania
Chapter 17

Robert J. Postlethwaite, MD
Department of Child and Adolescent Psychiatry
CAMHS Directorate
Royal Manchester Children's Hospital
Pendlebury, Manchester, England
Chapter 35

Bruce M. Robinson, MD
Research Associate
Renal-Electrolyte and Hypertension Division
University of Pennsylvania School of Medicine
Philadelphia, Pennsylvania
Chapter 11

Claudio Ronco, MD
Director
Department of Nephrology
St. Bortolo Hospital
Vicenza, Italy
Chapter 4

Cheryl P. Sanchez, MD
Assistant Professor
Department of Pediatrics
University of Wisconsin Medical School
Madison, Wisconsin
Chapter 46

Shubho R Sarkar, MD
Resident, Internal Medicine
Renal Research Institute
Beth Israel Medical Center
New York, New York
Chapter 10

Sabine Schmaldienst, MD
Division of Nephrology
Department of Medicine
University of Vienna
Vienna, Austria
Chapter 5

*Deceased.
†Dr. Nissenson is supported in part by the Richard Rosenthal Dialysis Fund.

Daniel Schneditz, PhD
Department of Systems Physiology
Medical University–Graz
Graz, Austria
Chapter 3

Cornelis H. Schröder, MD
Department of Pediatric
    Nephrology and Dialysis
University Hospital Utrecht
Wilhelmina Children's Hospital
Utrecht, The Netherlands
Chapter 19

Steve J. Schwab, MD
Regents Professor and Chairman
Department of Medicine
Medical College of Georgia
Augusta, Georgia
Chapter 2

Warren B. Shapiro, MD
Associate Professor of Clinical Medicine
State University of New York Health Sciences
    Center at Brooklyn
Co-Chief Division of Nephrology and Hypertension
Brookdale University Hospital and Medical Center
Brooklyn, New York
Chapter 38

Michael J. G. Somers, MD
Director, Clinical Services
Division of Nephrology
Children's Hospital
Assistant in Medicine
Harvard Medical School
Boston, Massachusetts
Chapter 12

Donald Stablein, MD
The Emmes Corporation
Rockville, Maryland
Chapter 41

Lynya Talley, PhD
Medical Statistics Section
Department of Medicine
University of Alabama at Birmingham
Birmingham, Alabama
Chapter 41

Burkhard Tönshoff, MD, PhD
Professor of Pediatrics and Pediatric Nephrology
Department of Pediatrics I
University Children's Hospital
Heidelberg, Germany
Chapter 25

Tam Tran, MD
Department of Medicine
UCLA Medical Center
Los Angeles, California
Chapter 25

Zbylut J. Twardowski, MD
Professor Emeritus of Medicine
Division of Nephrology
University of Missouri School of Medicine
Columbia, Missouri
Chapter 14

Raymond Vanholder, MD
Nephrology Section
Department of Internal Medicine
University Hospital–Gent
Gent, Belgium
Chapter 18

Bradley A. Warady, MD
Professor of Pediatrics
University of Missouri-Kansas City School of Medicine
Chief, Section of Pediatric Nephrology
Director, Dialysis and Transplantation
The Children's Mercy Hospital
Kansas City, Missouri
Chapter 8

David M. Ward, MD
Professor of Medicine
University of California, San Diego School of Medicine
San Diego, California
Chapter 6

Richard A. Ward, PhD
Professor of Medicine
University of Louisville
Louisville, Kentucky
Chapter 20

Jay B. Wish, MD
Professor of Medicine
Case Western Reserve University School of Medicine
Division of Nephrology
University Hospitals of Cleveland
Cleveland, Ohio
Chapter 37

Frieda Wolf, MD
Assistant Professor of Medicine
State University of New York
Downstate Medical Center
Brooklyn, New York
Chapter 32

Marsha Wolfson, MD, FACP
Clinical Professor of Medicine
Division of Nephrology
Oregon Health Sciences University
Portland, Oregon
Chapter 21

Preface

In the 1980's, we collaborated with our talented, now deceased, colleague and friend Dominick E. Gentile in editing the first edition of *Clinical Dialysis*, which was published in 1984 and contained 29 chapters. The focus of the text at that time was to provide updated information for pediatric and adult nephrologists involved in the clinical care of dialysis patients, as well as nephrology fellows in training and house staff. At the time of publication of the first edition over 70,000 patients were undergoing chronic dialysis in the United States and continuous ambulatory peritoneal dialysis (CAPD) was emerging as a viable chronic dialytic therapy.

The second edition was published in 1990 with a similar focus as the first. The variants of CAPD—CCPD, APD, TPD—however, had been developed in the interim to address clinical needs for patients with end-stage renal disease (ESRD), and the management of acute renal failure had markedly changed with the development and refinement of continuous forms of renal replacement therapy including CAVH, CVVH, and CAVHD. These newer techniques, in addition to the sophisticated improvements in the delivery of dialysis therapy, dictated an increase in the number of chapters in the text to 38. At the time of publication, there were over 125,000 patients receiving chronic dialysis in the United States.

As the fifth decade of renal replacement therapy approached, the third edition of the text was published in 1995. The chronic dialysis population continued to expand with increasing numbers of diabetic and geriatric patients developing ESRD and initiating chronic dialysis. Quality of care as judged by adequacy of dialysis was reemerging as a critical goal of the delivery of chronic dialytic therapy at that time. The focus and intent of the text remained consistent; however, it required an increase in the number of chapters to 44 to adequately address the additional technical and clinical information.

It has been a decade since the last edition of *Clinical Dialysis*. At the time we commenced work on this new edition there were approximately 430,000 patients with ESRD in the United States and one million patients undergoing renal replacement therapy worldwide, 80 percent of whom are receiving a form of dialysis, while less than 20 percent have a functioning kidney transplant. In the time since publication of the third edition of *Clinical Dialysis* there have been dramatic advances in multiple areas related to the delivery of acute and chronic renal replacement therapy. For example, there have been marked changes in the management of anemia, renal osteodystrophy, and cardiovascular disease associated with chronic kidney disease. Precise guidelines (KDOQI) have been promulgated to assist the clinician in improving outcomes of patients with ESRD requiring chronic dialytic therapy. In addition, important new epidemiologic and clinical developments in pediatric renal replacement therapy have been reflected and expanded upon in this latest edition.

The focus of this edition remains unchanged from previous editions, with our ongoing effort to provide the latest information to those involved in the clinical care of patients requiring dialytic therapy as the major objective. As with each successive edition, the content has expanded, and the fourth edition now contains 48 chapters to adequately include the relevant materials.

As previously, we are exceedingly grateful to the many contributors who made the fourth edition of *Clinical Dialysis* a reality. The individuals who took time to provide a contribution to this text have many commitments, and we are exceedingly appreciative that they were willing to join us in accomplishing this latest edition of the text. Their only reward is the knowledge that the information contained in this edition of the text will undoubtedly benefit patients requiring clinical dialytic therapy. The editors would like to make special mention of the many contributions of Dr. Patrick McBride, who died while this edition was in preparation.

Allen R. Nissenson, MD

Richard N. Fine, MD

The Development of Hemodialysis and Peritoneal Dialysis

*Patrick T. McBride**

RENAL CARE PIONEERS

This chapter tells the story of those who had the vision and courage to risk everything in search of effective treatment for renal failure. In doing so, it develops a critical-path analysis of how the various components of renal care were brought together and evolved into the treatment techniques used today. It is striking that the most dramatic progress has been made in recent times and that many of the critical investigators are still among us, actively providing this vital care to more than 350,000 patients worldwide.

THE FIRST STEPS

As early as 3000 B.C., the Egyptians made note of the peritoneal cavity and other parts of the mammalian anatomy.[1] Their interest lay in understanding the body's functions so that they could keep it free of toxic substances. They used many medicinal aids to promote evacuation and diuresis and thus achieve "cleansing."

THE FIRST INVESTIGATORS

Sir William Harvey, who described the circulatory system in 1600, stimulated others to look at the relationship between disease and the blood.[2] Just a few decades later, in 1658, Christopher Wren—the noted architect, astronomer, and mathematician—injected dogs intravenously with blood, using a duck's quill securely fastened to the animal's neck.[3] Because the injected blood was incompatible with that of the animal, the experiment failed, but it did excite the interest of others in gaining access to blood. The difficulties of transporting blood from one patient or animal to another became obvious. Various methods were therefore developed, such as using the blood vessel of one patient to transport the blood to another. Defibrinating blood and lining the surface of the conduit (e.g., a silver tube) with paraf-

---

*Deceased.

fin were other methods used to prevent clotting outside the body. Richard Lower, an English physiologist, was the first to successfully administer blood from one patient to another using a silver tube and high flow rates.[3]

These early physicians became acutely aware of clotting in extracorporeal circuits as well as the danger of allowing air to enter the patient's bloodstream. Two particularly interesting devices for blood administration and removal were the Blundell gravitator[3] and the Higginson syringe. The Blundell gravitator was nothing more than a funnel elevated above a patient's open blood vessel; this permitted a rapid flow of blood and therefore helped to prevent clotting. The Higginson syringe[4] provided the physician with a method of adding fluid to the bloodstream or removing blood from the patient. This device was used as early as 1823 by Dr. Latta, who, working in London, successfully treated patients suffering from cholera by administering intravenous fluid directly into a blood vessel.[5]

As outlined above, from 1600 to 1800, techniques for entering the blood vessels were being refined slowly but surely. The dangers of air embolization and clotting were well recognized. Physicians at this time may or may not have been university-trained.[6] Those who were not served apprenticeships to learn how to treat the four liquid humors—blood, phlegm, yellow bile, and black bile—and how to keep these in balance.

The traditional method of treating renal insufficiency was by applying heat, immersing the patient in warm baths, bloodletting, or administering diaphoretic mixtures with nitric acid in alcohol and antimonial wine.[6] This last medication, it was hoped, would correct the problem within 24 hours. Prior to 1850, there were no other treatments for the management of patients in renal failure except these very crude, conservative procedures. It is interesting to note that bloodletting and diaphoresis therapy were common treatments for renal failure as late as the 1950s. These methods may still be in use in less developed parts of the world.

THE FIRST DIALYZER

In 1854, Thomas Graham, a Scottish chemist, presented a paper called "Osmotic Force," which described for the first time a process whereby colloids and crystalloids could be separated.[7]

Graham was appointed professor of chemistry at Andersonian University in 1830.[8] His classes were filled with both aspiring chemists and physicians because training in both disciplines was quite similar. At that time, a university professor would rent his lecture hall from the university and charge the students a fee for attendance. Because of Graham's dynamic approach in teaching chemistry and encouraging independent study, his classes were well attended and he prospered. Later he would become a fellow of the Royal Society in London. He developed close relationships with others in his field, such as the famous chemist Baron Justus von Liebig in Giessen, Germany.

Graham became well known throughout the scientific world. His paper "Osmotic Force" is of primary importance to the development of dialysis. It makes the first reference to the process of separating substances by using a semipermeable membrane. He noted that urea diffuses as fast as sodium chloride, and he was also the first to use a treated parchment membrane to separate colloids and crystalloids. His definition and experimental proofs of the laws of diffusion and osmosis are classics on which the very essence of dialysis rests.

It appears that Thomas Graham was held in high esteem not only by chemists but by doctors of medicine. This may have been the reason that his work was adapted not only as an analytic tool but later as a technique for treating uremic patients.

Besides designing the "hoop" type of dialyzer, Graham also suggested that animal tissue could be used as a functioning semipermeable membrane (Fig. 1–1). In addition, he described in very specific terms the relationship of solute diffusion rate to molecular size, showing that the larger the molecule, the slower the rate of diffusion. These principles are used by every dialysis practitioner today.

OTHER MEMBRANE RESEARCHERS

A. Fick

Fick was the first to point out that collodion had application as a diffusion membrane. He recognized the selectivity of this material and also described the technical difficulties in utilizing it.[9]

W. Schumacher

Schumacher developed a successful method for making small tubes or sacks of collodion; this allowed him to do a variety of experiments to verify the selective porosity of this material.[9]

Baranetzky

In 1872, Baranetzky described a method for controlling water permeability during the manufacture of collodion membrane. He stated that he was able to control the pore size of the membrane by adjusting the rinsing solution during the membrane's manufacture. This clear and concise description of Baranetzky's procedure was likely noticed by later investigators, who used collodion membranes in their prototype dialyzers.[9]

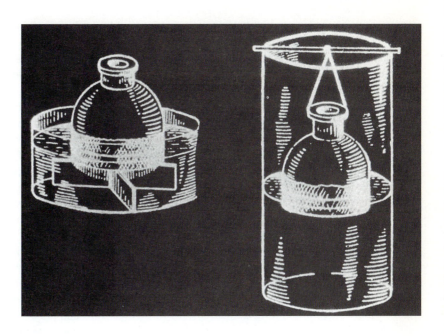

Figure 1–1. The Graham dialyzer.

B. W. Richardson

Richardson is credited with having been the first to suggest that animal blood could be dialyzed by utilizing a colloidal tube surrounded by a saline solution.[10]

Bigelow and Gemberling

In 1907, Bigelow and Gemberling reviewed the earlier technologic development of several membranes, including parchment paper, gold-beater's skin, and collodion. They reviewed in detail the advantages and disadvantages of the various materials and made reference to the dialytic properties of these membranes. Their work was so complete that they were able to compare and measure the relative merits of the three membranes for effecting diffusion by dialysis. They found that gold-beater's skin was the best, followed by collodion and parchment paper. They described the effects of temperature, membrane thickness, membrane support, and the varying permeabilities of different collodion preparations and the associated rates of diffusion. These experiments were carried out at the University of Michigan. Later investigators from the same institution may have utilized this information in taking the next critical steps in the development of the first dialyzers.[11]

VIVIDIFFUSION

One of the key turning points in the development of an efficient dialysis system has been credited to Dr. John Jacob Abel. There was, however, more to Abel's work than just the development of what we would today call the artificial kidney. Dr. Abel—who was educated in the United States

and Europe at such illustrious universities as Leipzig, Strasbourg, Heidelberg, Berne, Vienna, Berlin, and Paris—developed a keen interest in pharmacology[12] and understood the unique value of research in the practice of medicine. After completion of his studies, Abel returned to the United States and accepted a position at the University of Michigan for 2 years; then, in 1893, he proceeded to Johns Hopkins University School of Medicine, where he set up and directed the first department of pharmacology. His interest lay in teaching physiologic chemistry. His research in basic endocrine principles led to the isolation of epinephrine derivatives as well as the identification of the activities of the pituitary gland. While reviewing the secretions of the skin of various frogs, he discovered bufagin, a known poison, which, when properly utilized, served as a powerful cardiac stimulant that could be used in the treatment of heart failure.

Together with his colleagues Rowntree and Turner, Abel looked at ways of extracting solutes from the blood of animals.[13] Because of the work of earlier investigators, the diffusive properties of collodion membrane were known to these men. Abel made his own anticoagulant, called hirudin, which was obtained by crushing leech heads. His classic paper describes how he purchased and manufactured this very vital ingredient, which prevented blood from clotting in his dialysis device. His colleagues had developed their own skills in producing glass manifolds, which allowed them to make a device of relatively large surface area employing collodion membrane tubing. The procedure of setting up an experiment was extremely tedious because the membrane had to be manufactured by the Abel group and attached to the glass manifolds. The entire cylinder had to be filled with physiologic solution before the device was finally attached to the experimental animal; fractionalized dialysis began once the hirudin was introduced proximal to the dialyzer. Abel's contribution was to describe the first extracorporeal device that permitted the diffusion of substances from blood and to develop methods of quantitating this diffusion. These principles are in many respects the same as those used today in treating patients. Abel first presented his findings in London and then in Groningen, Holland, in 1913. It appears that his work was not forgotten by those who attended the sessions, because a development would later occur in a nearby Dutch city that would prove once and for all that dialysis was possible with humans. Abel did not apply his procedure to humans because of the antigenic properties of hirudin.

Abel's most outstanding contribution to medicine was the crystallization of insulin, a discovery that is not often attributed to him.[14] He first isolated this substance in December 1925, and some of these early crystals are still available for viewing.

THE HIGH-FLOW DIALYZER

Another investigative group, headed by Hess and McGuigan, proposed a system that allowed for the study of glucose in the blood.[15] These investigators used the same collodion membrane tubing as Abel had done in a system very similar to Abel's. The primary feature of their system was the absence of an anticoagulant. They felt that high blood flows would overcome the tendency of blood to clot in the extracorporeal circuit. The purpose of their experiments was to produce glucose equalization between blood and dialysate, and they were able to accomplish this without using an anticoagulant. Instead, they utilized a very interesting concept of pulsations in the blood compartment, which inhibited clotting in the device.

OTHER MEMBRANE RESEARCH

An important observation by George Stanley Walpole in 1915 related to the merits of sheet versus tubular membrane and the difference in ultrafiltration produced by those configurations.[16] Walpole not only demonstrated the varying porosity of different types of membrane but also proposed various devices that could best utilize the properties of these membranes.

An experiment devised by Alice Rohde in the same year was designed to demonstrate the diffusion rate of ammonia from blood.[17] She used a modified Abel device to reduce the priming volume and demonstrate the diffusive properties of the membrane. She showed that the level of ammonia in the dialysate was equivalent to the level in the blood, which again demonstrated the diffusive capabilities of the collodion membrane.

THE FIRST PLATE DIALYZER

Heinrich Necheles, a German-born physician, became aware of the problems associated with renal failure during the First World War, when he was assigned to care for injured German soldiers. He noticed the despair of these patients once their kidneys failed. Necheles stated that he began to look for ways of removing enough urea from the blood to allow the patients to recover. In his paper "A Method of Vividiffusion,"[18] Necheles makes note of a person referred to only as "Love," who employed the membrane of chicken intestines, and of "Heyde and Morris," who used fish-bladder tissue to develop a membrane material that could permit the diffusion of toxic substances. Necheles used flattened tubes of gold-beater's skin impregnated with gelatin bichromate. This shape permitted maximal surface exposure with a minimal volume of blood. He pressed the gold-beater's tubing between screening that provided for both low blood volume and turbulent flow through the device. His experiments were conducted in animals because he was using hirudin as an anticoagulant. What is extremely interesting about his device is that, for the first time, multiple stacked blood paths, manifolded together to minimize blood volume and maximize surface area, were used. It appears that Necheles was the first to devise a continuous blood-flow system in which the blood entered one end of an extracorporeal device and exited the other in separate tubes connected by latex rubber. He included for the first time a bubble trap and an entry port for infusing saline during the experiment. His blood circuit is the forerunner of the standard arterial and venous blood lines used today. Necheles's dialyzer work is of fundamental importance in that it addresses some of the shortcomings of the Abel device and for the first time introduces the concept of the flat-plate dialyzer using external screening for rigidity and to produce a well-mixed flow of blood. Necheles presented his work at the University of Hamburg. Later, he continued his study of the artificial kidney in cooperation with R. K. S. Lim at Peking Union Medical College in Peking, China.[19] Necheles did not take his studies beyond animal experimentation.

THE FIRST CLINICAL DIALYSIS

George Haas

According to Haas's personal records, reviewed by Jost Benedum at the University of Giessen,[20] Haas began his studies of hemodialysis in animals in 1914–1915. The results of this early investigation were not satisfactory and were interrupted when Haas was called to serve in the German army, where he remained until January 1919. After the war, he returned to the University of Giessen and continued his research with a device that looked like a modified Abel kidney.

Haas still faced the problem of obtaining an adequate anticoagulant. He worked with various membrane materials—such as reed tubing, sheep peritoneum, and paper membrane. However, none of these was satisfactory, and they brought him complete disappointment. Haas refers to the work of Pregl[21] on the use of collodion tubes, which were similar to the material that Abel had employed in his device. Haas used collodion and had a device that would function satisfactorily for diffusion. Nevertheless, he still had the problem of obtaining an adequate anticoagulant.

It must be noted that Haas's primary intent in this research was to treat patients with severely diseased kidneys. In 1923, Haas visited with Heinrich Necheles to review his work and again took up the challenge of developing a system that could be used to treat patients in renal failure.[22] Haas also communicated with the Johns Hopkins group. It appears that Haas carried out all of his investigation or early experimentation independently and without being aware of the work of Dr. Abel and others.

Haas performed his first clinical dialysis in mid-October 1924; he must, therefore, be credited with being the first to perform dialysis on a uremic human (Fig. 1–2). The second dialysis he performed lasted approximately 30 minutes; cannulation was made via the radial and carotid arteries and the portal vein, and the blood passed through three dialyzer cells or tubes. The anticoagulant used was a refined form of hirudin that did not allow for long-term dialysis. An addi-tional "first" credited to Haas was his use of a blood pump in his fourth dialysis.

In 1918, W. H. Howell and L. E. Holt, two Americans from Johns Hopkins, presented a paper that called attention to the use of heparin as an anticoagulant. Haas was fascinated by their discovery; after many failures, he was able to produce his first batch of heparin in 1925. He found it to be very effective in his animal experimentation. In 1927, Haas used heparin for the first time in treating a human patient on hemodialysis. He had now finally brought all the pieces together. He had developed a large-surface-area dialyzer, found a workable membrane with adequate blood distribution, and used a blood pump; finally, he had been able to employ a purified form of heparin, thus avoiding the previous problems with allergic reactions to hirudin. These early technical successes in treating patients in renal failure would remain unnoticed until the later work of Willem Kolff again proved that dialysis was a viable form of therapy for patients in renal failure.

THE EMERGENCE OF MANUFACTURED MEMBRANES

In 1927, H. F. Pierce of Columbia University reviewed the state of the art on cellulose membranes and how the permeability, manufacture, and use of these membranes could be quantified.[23] He referred to the early work of Fick (1855)

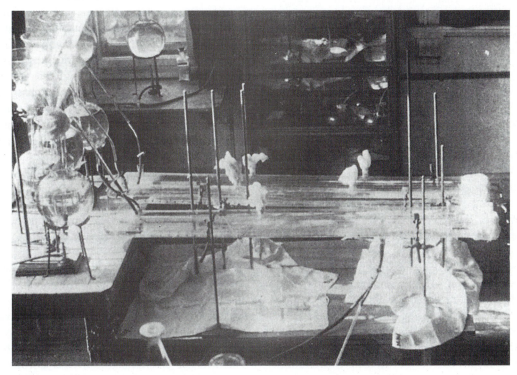

Figure 1–2. The Haas kidney in Giessen, Germany. *(Courtesy of J. Benedum, MD.)*

and to Baranetzky and Bechhold to complete his presentation. It is interesting to note that he changed the terminology from *collodion* to *nitro-cellulose* or, as we know it today, *cellulose*. Pierce for the first time consulted with an industrial supplier of nitro-cellulose to better understand the process of controlling the permeability characteristics of membranes. Later, it would become obvious that a joint venture between medicine and industry would be necessary to make dialysis practical for the treatment of renal failure.

Further evidence of the ability to control ultrafiltration with the use of manufactured membranes was presented by J. W. McBain and S. S. Kistler,[24] whose primary interest lay in adapting cellophane to the filtration of various solutes. These researchers made direct reference to cellophane, and they noted its utility as a molecular sieve.

Alexander Geiger also performed membrane experimentation with manufactured membrane.[25] He wished to examine blood without removing it from the vascular system. Of particular interest is that he used a microcapillary tube of collodion membrane placed inside a device that allowed the blood to enter and exit using a coil-type configuration.

The First Use of Cellophane for Dialysis

William Thalhimer had been Abel's student at Johns Hopkins School of Medicine, where Thalhimer developed a keen interest in Abel's work with the artificial kidney. Thalhimer identified the membrane as the weakest component of the Abel device. It appears that during his stay in Chicago, at Michael Reese Hospital, he was able to obtain for his experimentation some of the tubing made of cellulose acetate membrane that was being used in the manufacture of sausages.[26] This material was made by the Visking Corporation in Chicago. Thalhimer became aware of the work of previous investigators by his frequent correspondence with Abel (personal correspondence, 1937, courtesy of Johns Hopkins University School of Medicine). Furthermore, he had worked in Toronto with Dr. C. H. Best, who had experimented with a purified form of heparin. Thalhimer would use this heparin to prevent clotting in his primitive dialyzer. The hypothesis tested by Thalhimer was that the urea level and water concentration in blood could be reduced. Thalhimer used a device similar to the Abel kidney to conduct these experiments. He not only proved that cellulose acetate membrane was a strong, reliable material but also that it was relatively inexpensive, readily available, and safer than previous membrane materials. He also suggested that this membrane and these dialyzer devices might possibly be used in the treatment of human patients.[26]

Professor C. H. Best of Toronto, Canada, pursued some of these clinical applications and may have stimulated others to finalize the dialyzer designs eventually used in the treatment of patients.

Although Howell and Holt first isolated a substance that they called heparin in 1918, it appears that a purified form other than the Haas heparin was not readily available until 1933, when it was prepared by Charles and Scott in Toronto. It is apparent that a collaborative team was evolving that included Best, Thalhimer, and, a little later, Gordon Murray. Thalhimer may have initiated interest in developing a practical and useful artificial kidney at Toronto General Hospital.

James McBain and R. F. Stuewer observed as early as 1935 that commercial cellophane membrane had selective properties that allowed small molecules to pass through the membrane while larger molecules, such as colloids, were partially or wholly held back.[27] It is obvious from the number of studies on membrane porosity published by that time that the properties of membranes were well known throughout the scientific world by the 1930s; it then took a foresighted scientist like William Thalhimer to define an application for this membrane material in the treatment of uremia.

THE KOLFF ERA

Willem Kolff, a young physician of the department of medicine at the University of Groningen in the Netherlands, dreamt of preventing the death of those of his patients who were suffering from renal failure; he proposed to do this by removing just 20 g of urea from their blood.[28] Dr. R. Brinkman, a biochemist, introduced Kolff to the use of cellophane as a membrane that would allow him to accomplish his goal. Brinkman, like Thalhimer, had used cellophane to concentrate blood plasma and had built several dialyzers for this purpose. Kolff then built several devices and attempted to do dialysis with them. However, this work was interrupted by the German invasion of Holland in May 1940. Kolff's work on dialysis ceased and he opened a blood bank, which proved useful in helping him understand how to handle blood outside a patient's body. A short time later, Kolff was assigned a position in Kampen, and, with the help of H. Berk, a director of an enamel factory, began building a revised version of his artificial kidney that included many of the principles of the previous ones but also increased its efficiency by some very subtle modifications. Many of the materials—such as cellophane tubing, rubber blood tubing, and the various cannula connections—had to be reused because of the scarcity of these materials during the war. From March 17, 1943, to July 27, 1944, a total of 15 patients were treated with dialysis by Kolff; only 1 survived. It was not until September 11, 1945, that Kolff was able to show that his device (Fig. 1–3) could be effectively used to treat a patient in acute renal failure. This patient, who was suffering from acute renal failure, was presented to Kolff after her condition had deteriorated to the point where she was comatose. Kolff treated her with the artificial kidney and

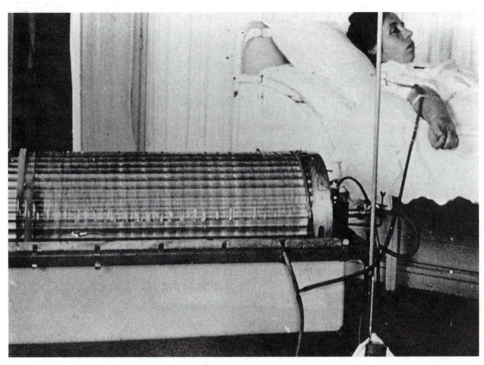

Figure 1–3. Clinical dialysis utilizing the original Kolff rotating drum. *(Courtesy of Willem Kolff, MD.)*

brought her out of the coma. Her renal function improved and she survived. This was a critical milestone in the development of the artificial kidney because, for the first time, its lifesaving potential was realized.

Kolff published his classic *New Ways of Treating Uremia* in 1946.[29] In it, he describes all the requirements of an artificial kidney and clearly shows the proper method for managing a patient who is undergoing this treatment. The principles detailed in this book are used by all clinicians today. This appears to be the first manual for the treatment of patients undergoing hemodialysis. Kolff, along with P. S. M. Kop, one of his associates, also included some very interesting data on peritoneal lavage using a system that was also manufactured by Berk Enamel Company in Kampen, Holland.

Kolff must be credited with starting many dialysis teams throughout the world at the close of World War II. Among them was one headed by Russell Palmer, a young Canadian physician, who had invited Kolff to present his dialysis experience to a number of Canadian military physicians during the war.[30] Kolff offered him one of his devices, but because of his military obligations, Palmer was unable to accept it. He he did, however, take a set of Kolff's plans and, on returning to Vancouver, had his brother build a replica of the original kidney machine. Palmer subsequently performed dialysis in Vancouver using the Kolff rotating-drum kidney.

Kolff and Berk produced additional machines and sent them to centers throughout the world, which, in turn, began

treating patients with hemodialysis for the first time. Machines were sent to London, Montreal, New York City, and Krakow, Poland.

THE FIRST DIALYSIS IN THE UNITED STATES

Dr. I. Snapper, who had visited Holland, was fascinated by Kolff's work. He invited Kolff to bring one of his machines to Mt. Sinai Hospital in New York City to set up a dialysis program. Drs. Irving Kroop and Alfred Fishman were selected to operate the device. They treated their first patient on January 26, 1948, and used the artificial kidney on a number of occasions before they left Mt. Sinai to pursue other interests.[31]

DEVELOPMENT OF THE KOLFF-BRIGHAM KIDNEY

In 1948, Drs. George Thorne and John Merrill, from the Peter Bent Brigham Hospital in Boston, visited Mt. Sinai Hospital to see the Kolff device in operation. They were interested in the application of this device for patients who required the removal of potassium and fluid. As a result of this visit, Dr. Kolff was invited to Boston, and because he did not have additional artificial kidneys available, he met with Dr. Carl Walter of the Peter Bent Brigham Hospital and Edward Olson, a machinist, to build one. These men sketched out their ideas for a modified rotating-drum kidney.[32] The Kolff-Brigham kidney was to gain worldwide acceptance and to become the device that would be used to train many future renal teams in the operation of the artificial kidney. On June 11, 1948, this device was used for the first time in Boston on a patient in renal failure.[33] This appears to have been the first operation of a hemodialysis machine manufactured in the United States.

The Brigham group would concentrate on the use of the artificial kidney in support of renal transplantation. They performed the first kidney transplant under the direction of John Merrill in 1954.[34]

OTHER DEVELOPERS OF ARTIFICIAL KIDNEYS

A number of groups began developing artificial kidney devices and programs between 1945 and 1950. Because it is

difficult to write about them in chronological order, a description of each group is presented here.

Nils Alwall

As early as 1945, a group in Sweden headed by Nils Alwall began dialyzing with a vertical-drum-type kidney.[34] The initial device developed by Alwall was called the Ultrafilterer. Its operation was similar to that of the Kolff device, but it employed some unique engineering concepts. Alwall used a drum, which he placed in the vertical position (Fig. 1–4), and an outer jacket to compress the membrane tubing and prevent it from bulging. This "sandwiching" effect is very similar to the principle described by Necheles 23 years earlier. The device was designed so that dialyzing fluid would circulate around the vertical drum and not vice versa, as was the case in the Kolff device. The internal core was placed inside a large glass or metal container, and a

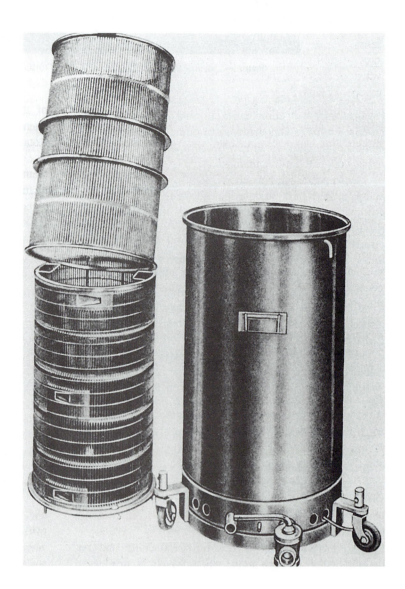

Figure 1–4. The large-surface-area Alwall dialyzer. *(Courtesy of Nils Alwall, MD.)*

dialysate agitator was used to better control the solute concentration gradient. A heater rod was incorporated to help maintain the temperature at the desired level. The advantage of this system was that it allowed ultrafiltration to be performed by positive pressure. This was accomplished by pumping the blood into the device and constricting the outflow blood tubing with a clamp.

This system overcame many of the problems of the Kolff system with its rotating drum. The Alwall system obviated the need for the split coupling used to prevent rotation of the blood lines going into and out of the dialyzer. It also minimized the blood volume outside the patient's body. Clinical dialysis was begun in Sweden in 1946 using a larger, modified vertical-drum kidney that was hermetically sealed, thus allowing negative pressure to be applied on the dialysate side.[35] As a result, ultrafiltration could be achieved by either positive or negative pressure for the first time. With the help of the Swedish Air Force, Alwall's patients were brought to his center from all over Sweden, since there were a limited number of these devices available for treating patients in renal failure.

A modification of the Alwall system allowed for a number of units to be connected to a large central dialyzing fluid system.[35]

Another important aspect of Alwall's work in 1948 was his use of indwelling catheters.[36] His experiments with more than 2000 rabbits demonstrated that vessel access was possible using a long-term shunt-type arrangement. This rabbit work involved cannulation of the carotid artery and the jugular vein. The vessel tips were made of glass, and cellophane was used to connect the two segments in order to permit a continuous flow of blood through the shunt. Alwall noted the limited patency of these devices and the constant need for heparin. He abandoned this vessel access procedure because of local infection and difficulty with clotting. He appears to be the first to have described the arteriovenous (AV) shunt technique, although the choice of materials was not adequate for long-term patency.

Alwall would continue his work by developing a lower-resistance dialyzer; later, he would develop the Alwall Plate Dialyzer, utilizing sheets of membrane sandwiched between polyethylene plates.

Gordon Murray

Murray developed a vertical-drum-type kidney similar to the Alwall system but with some very distinct differences.[37] He used smaller-diameter tubing and eliminated the outer jacket. The kidney housing was quite compact, which did not allow for a large membrane surface. Murray was very familiar with the use of anticoagulants because of his association with C. H. Best in Toronto. He also looked at a number of ways of pumping blood through the device because he knew that flow rates were critical for adequate perfor-

mance. A few of his devices were built and sent throughout North America. Acceptance was limited, however, because the efficiency of these devices was much less than that of other artificial kidneys at the time. It is important to note that Murray's system again pointed out the advantages of the vertical-drum, stationary-type kidney, which had a relatively low priming volume.

Leonard Skeggs and Jack Leonards

Jack Leonards, who had received a doctorate in nutrition at Case Western Reserve University, operated a chemistry laboratory and became fascinated by references in the literature to removing toxic substances from the blood. In a personal interview with Dr. Leonards, he stated that he had obtained a copy of Kolff's *New Ways of Treating Uremia* in 1946 and felt that he could improve on the basic design of the Kolff kidney. Leonards developed a flat-plate type of dialyzer using sheets of membrane encased in a grid-type press.

Leonards' dialyzer appears to be somewhat similar to the Geiger system, previously described. This device used a rubber coating to make the seals around the outer edge, so that blood leaks would not occur. However, Leonards found that both the blood and dialysate distribution were inadequate for achieving the desired results. He was able to obtain the help of Leonard Skeggs, who also had a doctorate from Case Western Reserve University, and they began work on developing a large-surface-area "multichanneled" dialyzer that would not require the use of a blood pump.[38] Along with engineering support from the Seiberling Rubber Company, they were able to obtain the key elements of their system, which were the rubber grooved pads that would compress the sheets of membrane and the compression plates. After Skeggs worked out the appropriate blood and dialysate manifold problems, animal studies began in earnest in 1947.[39]

These studies were continued until 1949, when, at the urging of Willem Kolff, Skeggs and Leonards began clinical dialysis with their device. Skeggs notes that when a large surface area was required, two units were used and a blood pump was employed to ensure distribution of blood throughout the kidney (Fig. 1–5). Skeggs commented that slight oozing of blood from the various blood paths was quite common and to be expected. Skeggs and Leonards were very familiar with chemical solute determinations, and Skeggs notes that routine blood chemistries were done every 15 to 30 minutes on the patients to assure adequate dialysis.

These investigators did not limit their efforts to the artificial kidney. Leonards, now a physician, developed Glucola, a glucose indicator for use in diabetes treatment, and also became an expert on the use of high doses of aspirin for patients with gout and arthritis. Skeggs continued his work with diffusion devices and developed the Auto Analyzer, which is considered a state-of-the-art device in blood analysis today.

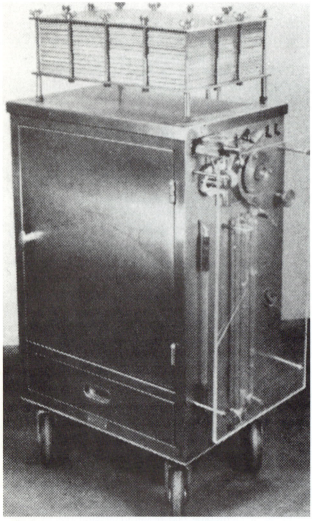

Figure 1–5. The Skeggs-Leonards dialyzer with blood pump. *(Courtesy of Jack Leonards, MD.)*

Stephen Rosenak

After Fishman and Kroop had left Mt. Sinai Hospital in New York City, Stephen Rosenak continued the use of the rotating-drum kidney.[40]

Rosenak, a very inventive physician, first suggested the use of a peritoneal catheter in 1923. He treated one of his friends, who was in renal failure, with peritoneal dialysis in 1933, but the treatment was not successful.

In 1950, Rosenak developed a parallel-flow type of dialyzer utilizing membrane tubing. With this device, Rosenak and Sherman Kupfer, a colleague, provided the first known mobile dialysis service in the United States. They would prepare the dialyzer and go to the hospital where their services were required. Kupfer noted that at times their equipment would be transported by a fire truck or whatever other vehicle happened to be available.

A number of treatments were performed throughout the area, but neither the device nor the technique was generally accepted by the medical community.

The Malinow-Korzon Dialyzer

In 1948, a group at Michael Reese Hospital in Chicago developed a unique concept for a dialyzer system. Using multiple-plate technology and cellophane tubing, they put together a system for ultrafiltration only. Employing a Debakey-type pump, blood was pumped under pressure through the dialyzer and ultrafiltrate produced. In analyzing the solute concentration of the ultrafiltrate, they found that it was similar to the solute concentration in the patient's blood. This concept was proposed as an alternative to the drawing of blood for determining blood chemistry values.[41]

The Von Garrelts Kidney

Also in 1948, Dr. Bodo Von Garrelts from Stockholm developed a very unique adaptation of the vertical-drum concept.[42] He constructed his artificial kidney using concentrically wrapped membrane tubing separated by a number of pins, so that the volume of blood in the membrane tubing could be controlled (Fig. 1–6) and good distribution of the dialyzing fluid could be achieved. According to Von Garrelts, this device weighed more than 150 pounds, and only one was ever built. Its unique construction would lead later investigators to study the concentric wrap concept, which would be used in coil-type dialyzers and would eventually allow for low-cost, disposable devices.

The MacNeill-Collins Dialyzer

Arthur MacNeill, in early 1942, designed several types of membrane oxygenators to demonstrate the principles of the diffusion of blood across a membrane.[43] Later, in 1948, one of these designs was revived for use as a dialyzer.

MacNeill's approach was to construct a compact, self-contained autoclavable device, which had multiple blood paths with low resistance to blood flow and a minimal blood priming volume.[44] It also had a relatively low pressure drop and utilized cellulose acetate tubing. The key elements of this device were the blood manifolding and the nylon screening necessary to separate the various blood paths. MacNeill recognized that in order to prevent clotting within the dialyzer at the manifold junctions, Teflon was the material of choice. He included a flowmeter and a pulsatile blood pump to complete his circuit. The devices were manufactured by the Warren E. Collins Company in Boston, and several were used by the U.S. Army and other medical groups around the country. The primary investigators with this device were Drs. Sidney and Roland Anthone at Buffalo General Hospital in Buffalo, New York.[45]

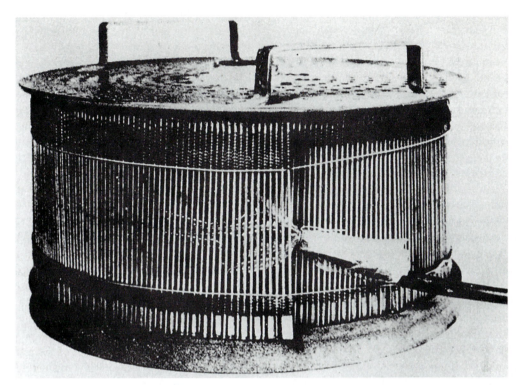

Figure 1–6. The Von Garrelts kidney. *(Courtesy of B. Von Garrelts, MD.)*

Muirhead and Reed

The 1950s produced a number of innovative diffusion-based devices and procedures for treating uremia. A resin kidney developed by Muirhead and Reed in Dallas used a different principle.[46] Their device contained two levels of resin beds, one called amberlite and the other deacidite. These resins adsorbed urea and other solutes. One of the difficulties with this system was that it could not be autoclaved and had to be rinsed with alcohol. Some adverse reactions were noted, but the experiments showed that resin-bed dialyzers could be considered for possible use as an alternative form of therapy.

The Kirwin-Lowsley Group

Two rather unique dialyzers were developed by the group headed by Oswald Lowsley and Thomas J. Kirwin of New York City.[47] Using many of the principles previously described, the Kirwin-Lowsley investigators produced two types of dialyzers that employed blood pumps and cellophane-sheet membranes. The first was a parallel-countercurrent-flow dialyzer and the second comprised a series of cells in a countercurrent-flow configuration. Again, it appears that the Geiger design for membrane permeability testing was adapted for the hemodialyzer system. These devices were manufactured by the American Cystoscope Company and were used on a limited basis in a clinical setting. They were assembled the day before use and were

sterilized by soaking in a cold sterilization solution for 16 hours. Apparently the series dialyzer, because of its increased surface area, was more efficient than the single-unit countercurrent-flow dialyzer. It is of interest to note that the series dialyzer contained a relatively small amount of blood, 300 mL, considering the state of the art at that time. The device itself was quite compact; contained its own dialyzing fluid, blood pump, and dialyzer; and could be wheeled directly to the patient's bedside. It appears that the two initial units were the only ones ever manufactured.

In 1950, there were very few operating hemodialysis centers anywhere. In order to follow the growth and development of hemodialysis, the following text traces the distribution of the various dialysis devices themselves. We begin with the Kolff-Brigham rotating drum.

Kolff-Brigham Kidney

After the meeting with Drs. Kolff and Walter in 1947, Edward Olson, the engineer involved in the production of the Kolff-Brigham kidney, made some very innovative changes in the basic Kolff design.[48] Among these were a bath heating mechanism and a Plexiglass hood, which would allow for control of temperature. He also devised a method of automatically lowering the bath so that the drum portion would not have to be removed when the bath was mixed or changed. He developed a plastic connector system so that the blood line could be connected to the membrane and the drum could rotate independently of the blood line without twisting either segment. This also prevented blood leaks at this connection site. Some other features were lights in the bath, which allowed the operator to view the mixing procedure, and lights over the hood, to prevent condensation, so that the operator could observe the flow of blood through the dialyzer. Additional ancilliary items that were included were the sterilizing container for the membrane and a reel for rapid placement of this membrane on the device. Olson made a number of these devices, which sold for about $5000 to $6000 each and were at that time considered very expensive. One of the first was shipped to Dr. Paul Doolan at Georgetown University. He would later turn it over to Dr. George Schreiner, who subsequently established Georgetown as one of the leading teaching centers using the artificial kidney.

Another of these devices was ordered for the Walter Reed Medical Center in Bethesda, Maryland, and an additional unit would later be shipped to Korea to be operated by Dr. Paul Teschan and his group.

One must keep in mind that at this time these devices were used for acute dialysis only and, as a result, an individual center would usually have no more than one device available for treating patients. The total number of patients treated per year was therefore very small.

KOREA, 1952

Colonel Paul Teschan reported on the use of the Kolff-Brigham rotating-drum kidney for treating severely injured troops who were being rapidly evacuated from the front lines. Teschan stated that one of the problems he encountered was that the troops were often being given massive amounts of blood replacement and that their potassium levels were therefore greatly elevated. One of the primary goals in using the artificial kidney was to reduce potassium levels so patients would not die of hyperkalemia and would have an opportunity to survive their injuries. Teschan was quite successful at this. The secondary result of this treatment was that a number of physicians became aware of the artificial kidney and were trained in its operation.

THE SKEGGS-LEONARDS DIALYZER IN NORWAY

One of the Skeggs-Leonards dialyzers was sent to the University Clinic in Oslo, Norway (a list noting where different models of the Skeggs-Leonards dialyzers were either shipped or constructed was obtained from Jack Leonards, 1960). The dialyzer had been purchased by a women's group in hopes that it could be used to treat patients in renal failure. Unknown to them, no one at the hospital was trained in its operation. It therefore sat unused until the arrival of Dr. Fred Kiil. According to Dr. Kiil, the device was difficult to assemble and operate and constantly oozed blood during its operation. Kiil began to modify the device and developed what is known today as the Kiil dialyzer (Fig. 1–7). The Kiil provided a larger surface area with fewer stacked blood compartments than the Skeggs-Leonards kidney. The primary differences between the Kiil and the Skeggs-Leonards devices were that the Kiil was more efficient and easier to handle; moreover, it did not require the use of a blood pump. It appears that Dr. Kiil was the first to employ Cuprophan membrane in place of cellulose acetate to increase the efficiency of the device.

THE SEATTLE ARTIFICIAL KIDNEY PROGRAM

Dr. Belding Scribner began his use of the artificial kidney at the VA Hospital in Seattle (Belding Scribner, personal communication, 1982). Dr. John Merrill had suggested to him that dialysis did indeed have a place in the care of acutely ill patients. Scribner used the coil system initially, but he was concerned about its high priming volume and the use of the blood pump. He also used the Skeggs-Leonards dialyzer and, along with the engineering group at the University of Washington, modified it so that it could be assembled more quickly and operated without excessive blood loss. Scribner also refers to a visit to Europe, where he came across one of the Kiil dialyzers with a Cuprophan membrane and was able to purchase it for under $1000. He returned to Seattle with the device and, along with a local manufacturer, attempted to make additional dialyzers. However, it was not easy to duplicate the fine engineering techniques developed by Dr. Kiil. It took more than 6 months to produce the first Kiil dialyzer that did not leak or shunt blood from one blood path to another.

DEVELOPMENT OF DIALYZING FLUIDS

Kolff had previously described the need for a buffering solution in the dialyzing fluid.[29] He chose to use sodium bicarbonate and also to bubble carbon dioxide through the bath to control the pH. If this was not done, the calcium and magnesium would combine with the bicarbonate and precipitate. Also, he found that if he made a large quantity of this solution and kept it at body temperature, the chance of bacterial contamination was very high. This problem would continue to plague dialysis teams and prevent them from expanding the treatment to more than one patient at a time.

The Seattle group along with Wayne Quinton devised a method of batching the dialyzing fluid with a modified refrigeration system (Wayne Quinton, personal communication, 1982). By keeping the dialyzing fluid cold, they could

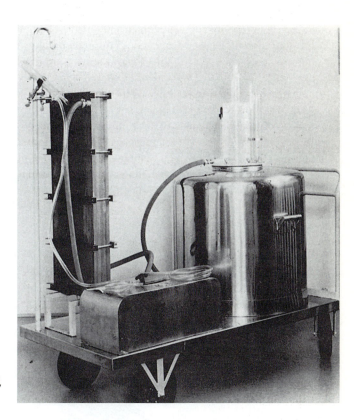

Figure 1–7. The Kiil dialyzer and fluid delivery system. *(Courtesy of F. Kiil, MD.)*

minimize bacterial growth. The problem with this system was that it also lowered the temperature of the blood in the extracorporeal circuit; therefore a secondary blood warmer had to be included, but this increased the amount of blood outside the patient's body during dialysis.

OTHER ARTIFICIAL KIDNEY DEVELOPMENTS IN THE 1950s

The Guarino Kidney

The Guarino kidney was one of the most unique kidneys developed up to this time.[49] Its basic geometry was totally different from that of any other kidney design. The device was constructed so that no blood pump was required. The dialyzing fluid flowed inside the membrane tubing and the blood cascaded on the outside. The purpose of this design was to offer low resistance to blood flow, provide a very thin blood film, and minimize the priming volume within the device itself. There was complete visibility, and the membrane was supported by the use of metal tubing on the inside. Guarino made note of the fact that the rate of ultrafiltration could be monitored visually and that, in more than 40 uses, there were no blood leaks. Others who critiqued this device expressed concern over the possibility of dialysate leaking into blood; as a result, this dialyzer was used on only a limited basis.

Inouye-Engelberg Kidney

A group at the University of Pennsylvania headed by Dr. Louis Bluemle began an experimental program in the early 1950s utilizing a Skeggs-Leonards dialyzer. Like other groups using this device, they identified some of the physical shortcomings of the dialyzer and modified it.

William Inouye, a young physician working with the Bluemle group, developed a unique dialyzer for use clinically.[50] It is called the Inouye-Engelberg "pressure cooker" kidney (Fig. 1–8). It used a concentrically wrapped membrane with layers separated by fiberglass screening. The center core was a stainless steel graduated cylinder and the entire coil configuration was placed inside a hermetically sealed pressure cooker commercially available from the Presto Pressure Cooker Company. This system allowed blood to enter and exit from the top of the pressure cooker and dialyzing fluid to enter and exit from the bottom. It was connected to a closed system, so diffusion or ultrafiltration could be controlled separately. A key point in this closed system was that the amount of ultrafiltration could be monitored. This device was used in more than 30 dialyses, and it appears that both the Inouye-Engelberg kidney and the previously described Von Garrelts kidney were the forerunners of other coil developments in the early 1950s.

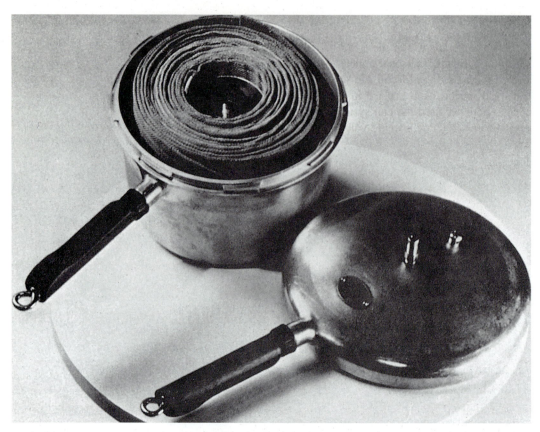

Figure 1–8. The Inouye-Engelberg kidney.

Kolff Twin-Coil Kidney

Willem Kolff accepted a position at the Cleveland Clinic in 1950. There, he continued to pursue his interest in the development of a more practical artificial kidney device. Along with the help of Drs. Victor Vertes and Bruno Watschinger, a modification of the previously described coil-type dialyzer emerged.

Kolff and Watschinger developed the "orange juice" kidney, which was a concentrically wrapped coil kidney using an orange juice can as the core.[51] They used two lengths of cellulose acetate tubing in order to reduce the pressure drop across the device. As a result, the term *twin-coil* evolved. Kolff made these devices in his own laboratory using a winding machine. He then placed them in a polyethyelene bag and sterilized them. He now had a ready-to-use, disposable artificial kidney.

To perform dialysis with this device, the bag with the dialyzer in it was elevated on an intravenous infusion pole, and blood and dialyzing fluid were pumped up to the coil. This technique was later abandoned because of the loss of heat and the amount of blood priming required. Armed with this device and with the experience in its application, Kolff approached three companies to get a commercial model manufactured. Two of the companies felt that there was no

market for this type of device and declined to help him. Fortunately, Kolff convinced Bill Graham of Baxter Laboratories, a chemistry-trained patent lawyer, to manufacture the device. The first disposable presterilized artificial kidney was made available for sale in 1956 by Baxter Laboratories.

Other industrial firms, such as Allis Chalmers, developed a version of Kolff's original rotating drum, but they discontinued its production after six devices were manufactured.[52] The cost of this device between 1952 and 1954 was in excess of $6000.

Another version of the vertical-drum kidney was developed by the Westinghouse Corporation. Three of these devices were produced before Westinghouse decided that the demand was not great enough to warrant the manufacture of additional units.[53]

The First Artificial Kidney System

The first twin-coil system became commercially available in 1956. It included a 100-L stainless steel tank with a finger-type blood pump and a disposable artificial kidney that included blood lines. The disposable portion cost approximately $60. A number of these systems were purchased and shipped to hospitals throughout the world for acute care. Many of the devices were never uncrated or used because there was no one to operate them. In 1959, renewed cooperation between the Cleveland Clinic and Baxter Laboratories was initiated, which allowed for training in the operation of the artificial kidney at the clinic. A number of physicians throughout the United States attended these training sessions and returned to their own units to begin their acute care programs.

PROPHYLACTIC DIALYSIS

In 1958, a very interesting indication for dialysis was suggested by Dr. Paul Teschan, who had been assigned to Brook Army Hospital in Texas after his return from Korea. Dr. Teschan was involved in the treatment of acutely ill burn patients who were receiving massive amounts of antibiotics to prevent infection and who subsequently developed renal failure. Teschan proposed a form of "prophylactic dialysis,"[54] in which cannulas were placed in the patient's arm and were irrigated and accessed periodically for dialysis in order to maintain near-normal renal function.

He suggested that long-term hemodialysis was possible if blood access could be maintained. His cannulation techniques did not allow for continuous blood flow from one vessel to another, but his experience did suggest that a permanent indwelling catheter, as opposed to acute intermittent blood access, was needed.

1960: THE BEGINNING OF CHRONIC DIALYSIS

The story of Clyde Shields has been told many times, but it is important to note that Mr. Shields's life was saved by the expertise not only of physicians but also of farsighted scientists and businesspeople in the academic and industrial worlds. By 1960, Dr. Belding Scribner had established a small dialysis center for acute care at the University of Washington (Belding Scribner, personal communication,

1982). A patient presented with progressive renal failure. Scribner hypothesized that if he could obtain continuous access to the patient's bloodstream he might be able to dialyze him chronically and keep him alive. With the help of Wayne Quinton, an engineer, and after a chance observation by an electrician about the properties of Teflon, Teflon tubing (then being used as electrical conduit) was selected to carry the patient's blood outside the body and through the artificial kidney. Quinton explored the properties of Teflon and worked with the material until he developed a smooth cannula intima that would help prevent blood components from accumulating on its surface.

Scribner eventually found that Teflon's "nonsticking" feature was the key in keeping the shunt patent. After much effort, Quinton was able to develop the shunt (Fig. 1–9), and it did indeed exhibit the desired characteristics. As a result of this work, Clyde Shields had a shunt inserted and became the first person to be chronically treated with an artificial kidney. The problem with the initial access device was that it had very rigid tips and external segments, which caused irritation to the patient's vessels, although it did allow for continuous access.

Others would adopt the Scribner access technique and would note the same irritation problems when using straight Teflon. Quinton then modified the shunt by including segments of silicone rubber, which acted as shock absorbers between the vessel tip and the exit site on the skin. This solved the irritation problem, and later shunt designs included Teflon tips and silicone rubber. The manufacturer of the silicone stated that it could not be extruded to the required tolerance. After a number of failures, however, Quinton was able to extrude the tubing successfully himself.

Seattle, 1964

Scribner had a growing chronic dialysis population and he had exhausted his capacity for treating additional patients. His thought was that if he could dialyze patients at their homes, he would be able to expand his patient population

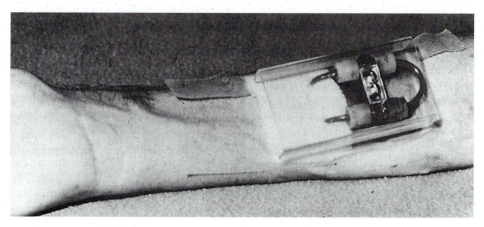

Figure 1–9. The all-Teflon shunt. *(Courtesy of Belding Scribner, MD.)*

and reduce the cost of dialysis. There were still some significant technical issues, as far as equipment was concerned, that had to be overcome before this type of care could be attempted.

Albert Babb

Albert Babb, a biomedical engineer at the University of Washington, was asked by Scribner to help refine a number of aspects of the artificial kidney system.[55] The first problem presented to him was how to overcome the shortcomings of the large-batch system, in which large quantities of dialyzing fluid were made up and then chilled to prevent bacterial growth. Babb and his group proposed that a continuous proportioning system might work. This would be accomplished by synchronizing three pumps to deliver a properly proportioned amount of water, electrolytes, and bicarbonate. The question of how much dialyzing fluid would be necessary was of concern. In the last, 2L/min had been used. Babb pointed out that 500 mL/min provided the same efficiency as a dialysate flow rate of 2000 mL/min, and that this would be cheaper and easier to manage.

Another concern noted by Babb was that the bicarbonate buffer caused significant problems because of the potential for the precipitation of calcium carbonate. His group proposed that if a buffer were necessary, acetate could be substituted for bicarbonate, and acetate could be premixed in the electrolyte concentrate. An additional advantage of this approach was that one pump in the system could be eliminated.

Finally, Babb proposed a 34:1 mixture of water and concentrate, which greatly facilitated the preparation of the dialyzing fluid. The development of proportioning systems provided for a more efficient and easy-to-use dialysis system.

Babb developed the first central delivery system that automatically took 34 parts of water and 1 part of concentrate and mixed them on a continuous basis. The device also contained a bicarbonate pump, which was later abandoned. Now for the first time, a number of patients could be dialyzed from the same dialysis solution source without the need for cooling tanks, blood warmers, or tedious batch preparation.

The First Seattle Home Patient

A young college student presented with deteriorating renal function. Scribner notes that she was not a candidate for the in-center program because of her age and the lack of available space. He again called on the Babb group to develop a fail-safe proportioning machine that could be used at the patient's home for self-administered overnight dialysis. His group began work on miniaturizing their original design and providing all of the various monitors necessary to safely operate this device for overnight unattended dialysis. As a result, in 1964, Scribner's group was credited with

having achieved the first overnight, unattended home dialysis with the help of a nonmedically trained aid. Other investigators, including Stanley Shaldon in England and John Merrill in Boston, would shortly utilize this procedure successfully as well.

James Cimino, 1964

One of the most important advances in the development of chronic dialysis was made by Dr. James Cimino of the Bronx VA in New York City. Dr. Cimino, who had been working in the blood bank, hypothesized that access to the bloodstream could be achieved through arterialized veins in the patient's arm or leg by using a blood cuff.[56] He was able to distend the vessel, gain access with a needle, and dialyze the patient using this approach. In 1964, with the help of Dr. Kenneth Appel, a surgeon, and James Abooty, he performed the first dialysis using an arterialized vein.[57] This was accomplished by opening a small window between an artery and a vein and suturing them together. As a result, the vein distended. Cimino used a blood-donor needle for access. Adequate blood flow could be obtained for dialysis, and the needles could be removed at the end of the procedure. Scribner and others noted that this procedure was extremely innovative and helped to expand interest in chronic dialysis because it overcame the problems of infection and disconnection previously experienced with the shunt. The dialysis community had now solved some of the major technologic barriers to making dialysis relatively simple and efficient.

Dialyzing fluid delivery systems became smaller and easier to use, dialyzer designs were simplified and made more compact, and a better understanding of the physiology of the patient treated with the artificial kidney was acquired. Calcium depletion, bone disease, neuropathy, dietary management, and anemia were now being looked at closely to better determine how much dialysis was required to be considered adequate. The technical issues—such as miniaturization of the artificial kidney and the delivery system and emphasis on self-care—continue to preoccupy many investigators and clinicians today.

THE HOLLOW-FIBER KIDNEY

As early as 1956, Dr. Richard Stewart, a young physician at the University of Michigan, began looking at medical applications for a recently developed hollow-fiber material made of cellulose diacetate.[58] This fiber appeared to be very permeable not only to gas but also to solutes. Stewart began work on applying this technology to medical needs. Because the internal lumen of this fiber was so small, the high blood flow required for oxygenators negated its use in that setting. Stewart, therefore, looked for other applications that would require lower flow rates and eventually adapted this technology for use in artificial kidneys (Fig. 1–10).

Stewart worked for more than 11 years before the first clinical units were available for testing. The first treatment of a patient with a hollow-fiber kidney took place at the University of Michigan. Later, the project would be moved to Milwaukee, Wisconsin, where additional patients would be dialyzed using these devices. The objective of this research was to develop a compact, noncompliant artificial kidney that would at least equal the performance of the existing coil-type dialyzers but overcome some of the shortcomings of the coil, such as high blood volume and high internal resistance. These hollow-fiber dialyzers became available in 1970 and today are by far the most widely used artificial kidneys.

The years 1967 and 1969 saw the introduction of more compact, easy-to-use dialysis delivery systems, such as the coil batch Recirculating Single Pass (RSP) and proportioning systems, which allowed for installation in the patient's home. Also, various types of dialyzers were being miniaturized and their price was being reduced. It was possible to purchase a complete delivery system for under $2000 and to acquire disposable products for less than $25 per treatment. Home programs began to appear at various VA hospitals throughout the United States and in a few private hospitals. The non-VA programs did not expand rapidly because funds for care of these patients were not available. Many of the existing programs in operation at that time were funded by the Hartford Foundation, the National Institutes of Health, the Rockefeller Foundation, and other charitable groups. The insurance industry at that time was very reluctant to allow coverage for this type of care because the prognosis and ultimate cost were not known. As a result, care was denied to many patients because of a lack of adequate funding.

Intense pressure began to emerge from groups such as the National Kidney Foundation to develop legislation that would cover the cost of care for patients with end-stage renal disease. As a result of intense lobbying, legislation was enacted in 1973 that provided payment through the Social Security system for the care of dialysis patients. With the advent of adequate funding, centers began to expand and open throughout the United States. In addition, other countries became aware of this advanced medical technology and began to adopt programs similar to the one established in the United States.

DIALYSIS, A MATURING TECHNIQUE

In the latter part of the 1970s, a shift to totally automated systems as well as emphasis on negative-pressure dialysis had a major impact in moving the dialysis community from coil to hollow-fiber dialyzers. As this occurred, other needs became more apparent. There were some patients who did not tolerate hemodialysis well, including infants, children, geriatric patients, and diabetics, as well as patients who had been subjected to traumatic injuries. As a result, the nephrology community began to look toward peritoneal dialysis and automated peritoneal dialysis delivery systems. The complexity and length of time required for this procedure, however, limited its widespread application. Most recently, the ability to easily deliver bicarbonate-containing dialyzing fluid for hemodialysis without major equipment modification and increased understanding of the causes of poor tolerance to hemodialysis have led to fewer symptoms during treatment for many patients.

Development of Peritoneal Dialysis

The earliest reference to diffusion across the peritoneal membrane is credited to Wegner,[59] who in 1876 reported the increase of effluent fluid volume after first infusing saline solutions and later glycerine into the peritoneal cavity. In 1895, Orlow may have provided the stimulus for other in-

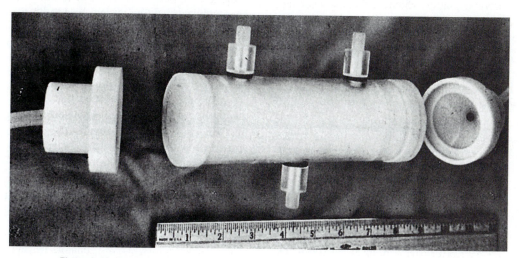

Figure 1–10. The first clinical model of the hollow-fiber kidney. *(Courtesy of Richard Stewart, MD.)*

vestigators to look at the peritoneal cavity as an alternative for removing toxins from the bloodstream.[60] Orlow's work is very clear in distinguishing between the concentration of solute in the blood and in the peritoneal cavity. Other investigators around this time included Starling and Tubby[61] as well as Putnam.[62] While at Johns Hopkins University, Putnam made extensive reference to the peritoneum as a viable membrane for transferring solutes from blood into the peritoneal cavity. His experiments were performed on animals but did suggest that clinical application was possible.

In Germany in 1923, Dr. G. Ganter was also very concerned about the failing kidney.[63] One must assume that he was aware of the work of other investigators and saw the obvious problems with anticoagulants needed for hemodialysis. He therefore sought a different method for removing toxins from the patient's blood. In 1918 at the Clinic in Greiswald, Germany, Ganter experimented with controlling toxin levels in the blood of a uremic patient with peritoneal dialysis. His method was to instill a physiologic solution into the patient's peritoneal cavity and then drain it. When he did this, there was a definite improvement in the patient's clinical condition. After the urea level dropped, he sent the patient home. The patient died a few days later because Ganter was unaware that nitrogenous wastes would reaccumulate. He continued his experimentation with animals, noting that the rise and fall of the animals' appetite and activity level was directly related to the exchange phases. Ganter made a very important observation in that he found that humans tolerated high toxin levels much better than animals. He suggested that studies in animals should not be used as the sole criterion for determining a course of treatment for humans using peritoneal dialysis. It appears that Ganter was also the first to publish on the problems of peritonitis associated with peritoneal contamination. He also made note of the importance of draining the peritoneal solution once equilibration had been attained, observing that if the fluid is left in the abdomen too long, it may be absorbed.

Because Ganter's research was limited in quantity, he felt it impossible to obtain conclusive judgments of the practicability of peritoneal dialysis. Peritoneal dialysis as a treatment for kidney failure lay dormant until the mid-1940s. At that time a group of physicians—Frank, Seligman, and Fine at Beth Israel Hospital in Boston—became involved in a government-sponsored project looking at the scientific needs of the United States in order to win World War II. The Fine group was instructed to look for ways of treating renal failure. They developed a system (Fig. 1–11) for preparing sterile solutions and instilling them into the peritoneal cavity in order to reduce the toxin levels in the patient's blood.[64] Their system was first used successfully in 1945 on a patient suffering from antibiotic-induced acute renal failure. The Fine group's work in establishing the proper constituents of the dialysis solution and in develop-

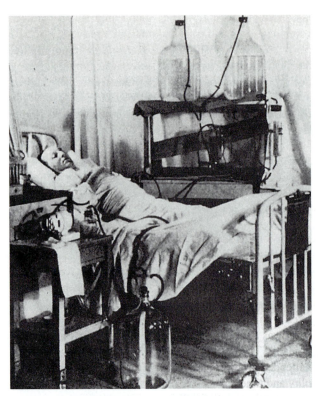

Figure 1–11. The Frank, Seligman, and Fine peritoneal dialysis system. *(Courtesy of Howard Frank, MD.)*

ing a closed dialysis system was unique and became the standard for peritoneal dialysis. Two very prominent physicians, Arthur Grollman from Southwestern Medical School and Morton H. Maxwell of The University of California, Los Angeles, appear to have provided the bridge between the work of Seligman, Frank, Fine, and Fred Boen. In 1951, Grollman performed peritoneal dialysis on patients using a polyethylene catheter and a trocar.[65] He used a closed intermittent method for solution infusion. In 1959, Maxwell used commercially prepared peritoneal dialysis solutions.[66] He employed a closed system by instilling 2 L of solution into the abdomen and then draining it out into the same bottle after a period of 2 hours. He used disposable tubing and a semirigid nylon catheter.

Fred Boen

Fred Boen, an Indonesian physician working in Holland, was invited by Dr. Scribner to visit Seattle and develop a system for home peritoneal dialysis. Boen had written a thesis on the kinetics of peritoneal dialysis, and Scribner saw an application for patients who could not receive in-center hemodialysis care.[67] Boen's system was similar to the one developed by Seligman and Frank in 1946 and allowed the patient to be chronically dialyzed using peritoneal dialysis without a permanent catheter. Scribner saw this system as an opportunity to do overnight unattended dialysis at home, which would allow him to expand the number of patients he could treat. Because access to the peritoneal cavity was still a problem, Boen developed "the intermittent paracentesis method." This involved placing a catheter in the abdomen for each successive dialysis. At the end of the dialysis, it would be removed. As a result, Boen overcame the problem of peritonitis, which was seen when catheters were left in place for more than 48 hours. The procedure was not readily accepted by the medical community, however, because of the bulky equipment, the length of time of the dialysis, and the difficulty with the periodic cannulation.

Russell Palmer

Russell Palmer, the first to do clinical hemodialysis in North America, was also looking for ways to treat renal patients without the use of the anticoagulants required for hemodialysis. His interest in peritoneal dialysis had been stimulated by the work of the Seattle group, and with the help of Wayne Quinton, he developed the first silicone rubber catheter (Fig. 1–12), utilizing a very unique coiled design, in 1964.[68]

THE COMING OF AGE OF PERITONEAL DIALYSIS

Various groups throughout the United States had worked with peritoneal dialysis, but the full implication of its use did not come until late in the 1970s.

Harold McDonald

McDonald, who first became interested in dialysis at Peter Bent Brigham Hospital in Boston in 1960, went to the University of Michigan and developed a technique for teaching patients how to do peritoneal dialysis by themselves either at the hospital or at home. It appears that he may have trained the first patient for self-care peritoneal dialysis at home as early as 1962 (McDonald, personal communication, 1982).

Later at the University of Michigan and also at the University of Washington, McDonald developed methods for inserting peritoneal catheters using a trocar. His interest in peritoneal dialysis led him to treat pediatric patients and to develop automated delivery systems for peritoneal dialysis.[69] He also evaluated various types of silicone catheters that could be implanted on a long-term basis.

Henry Tenckhoff

The home peritoneal dialysis program at the University of Washington grew at a very slow rate because of the complexity of the equipment being used at the time. Henry Tenckhoff, who had developed an interest in dialysis in Boston, took over the home peritoneal dialysis program in the early 1960s. He continued to use the intermittent catheter insertion method in the patient's home that was initiated by Fred Boen, even though it was a labor-intensive procedure.

As time passed, it became apparent that the patients needed more dialysis. They were now requiring two dialyses a week in order to control their uremia. This forced Tenckhoff to seek an alternate peritoneal dialysis system (Fig. 1–13). With the help of George Shilipetar, he constructed a miniature still that could be installed in the home to purify the incoming water. This distilled water was mixed with a peritoneal dialysate concentrate at a 19:1 ratio, which was then pumped in and out of the peritoneum automatically. The patient was now able to dialyze overnight unattended. The problems with this system were that it was bulky and time-consuming. Commercial versions were con-

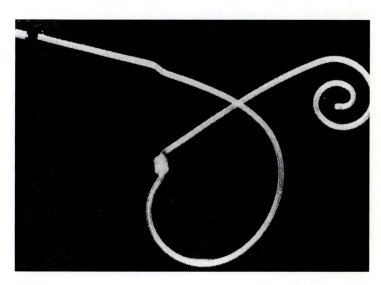

Figure 1–12. The first silicone catheter for peritoneal dialysis. *(Courtesy of Russell Palmer, MD.)*

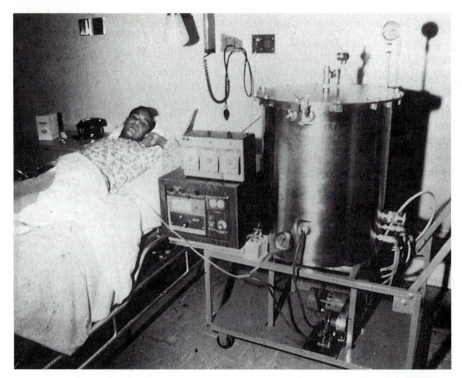

Figure 1–13. The first machine for batch peritoneal dialysis. *(Courtesy of Henry Tenckhoff, MD.)*

structed, but they were not widely used because they were unable to overcome these drawbacks.

With the introduction of reverse-osmosis water treatment, Tenckhoff[70] and his group were able to construct a more compact system that was more efficient and easier for the patient to use.

The only other obstacle to self-sufficient home peritoneal dialysis was the access problem. Tenckhoff[71] modified the Palmer catheter by shortening its length and adding Dacron cuffs to seal the exit site. He also refined the trocar, thus facilitating catheter insertion. The system was now complete, and it was adopted by a number of hospitals for in-center and home use. The straight and curled Tenckhoff catheters would become the standard for peritoneal access.

Norman Lasker

Dialysis in 1961 was restricted to a very few centers because of its cost and the lack of funding. As a result, there was a shortage of systems for treatment, and dialysis was often complicated and difficult to manage.

Lasker, who had trained at Georgetown University School of Medicine, looked for ways to expand dialysis availability. He had visited Tenckhoff's program in Seattle, and he was very impressed with the potential of peritoneal dialysis. He felt that the automated systems he saw in Seattle would have to be made simpler if peritoneal dialysis were to be applied more widely.

Fortunately, he was approached by the Gottscho Foundation in 1961. This organization was set up to honor the memory of Mr. Ira Gottscho's daughter, who had died of kidney disease. Lasker proposed that the foundation help him develop a gravity-fed peritoneal dialysis system that would be easy for any practitioner to use. He felt that this type of system would be ideal for home dialysis. With the help of Mark Schachter,[72] an engineer with the Gottscho Company, he developed a machine that used 2-L bottles of dialysate and a disposable tubing set. It allowed the practitioner to operate the device for a prolonged period or for overnight unattended peritoneal dialysis (Fig. 1–14).

Lasker moved to Thomas Jefferson School of Medicine in 1967 and continued his work with the peritoneal dialysis "cycler." Funding at that time in Pennsylvania would only allow for home dialysis. He began sending patients home on this peritoneal dialysis system.

Dimitrios Oreopoulos

In 1969, Oreopoulos accepted a position at the Toronto General Hospital to manage a four-bed intermittent peritoneal dialysis program. The program began to grow despite the shortcomings experienced with peritoneal access. Stanley Fenton, another Canadian, had visited the University of Washington's chronic peritoneal dialysis program and was very impressed with the progress being made with the Tenckhoff catheter. On his return to Toronto, he met with

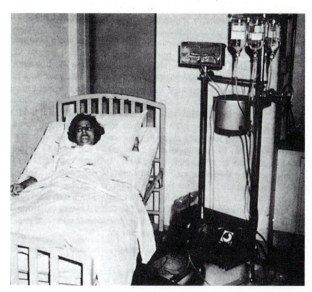

Figure 1–14. Lasker peritoneal dialysis machine. *(Courtesy of Norman Lasker, MD.)*

Oreopoulos and introduced him to the Tenckhoff access system. Oreopoulos was so impressed with the catheter that he adopted it for his program. He began sending patients home on reverse osmosis machines like those developed by Tenckhoff.

Oreopoulos continued to look for simpler systems for his growing home patient population. He visited Philadelphia and saw the Lasker cycler; he was so impressed that he ordered a number of them for his home patients. The patient population grew rapidly.

Jack Moncrief and Robert Popovich

The passage of legislation in 1972 and its enactment in 1973 provided funding for all patients in the United States who required dialysis treatment and who were otherwise eligible for Social Security benefits. This milestone allowed physicians to treat patients who were previously not considered candidates for dialysis. During this period, Jack Moncrief finished a residency in nephrology at Georgetown University School of Medicine and set up his practice in Austin, Texas. In 1970, Moncrief received a grant from the Texas Rehabilitation Foundation to open an in-center dialysis program. The patient population grew very rapidly in those early days, and it was evident that the community's needs were not being met. A new facility was built at the Austin Diagnostic Clinic in 1973 to accommodate the increased number of patients now eligible for hemodialysis treatment.

In 1975, Peter Pilcher was accepted for chronic dialysis care at the Austin Diagnostic Clinic. A standard AV fistula was created, and his dialysis was attempted. The fistula clotted during the first treatment. This was corrected, and

again dialysis was attempted with the same results. The fistula would not function. It became obvious that Pilcher was not a candidate for hemodialysis.

It was then suggested that Pilcher move to Dallas, where there was an intermittent peritoneal dialysis (IPD) program. This form of dialysis would require over 60 hours of treatment per week in order to adequately control uremia. Pilcher, however, refused to move to Dallas.

Pilcher's case was reviewed at the next research meeting at the Austin Diagnostic Clinic. It was pointed out that there was no hope for him because peritoneal dialysis was not available in Austin at the time. One of the research associates said that they could not let the patient die—that there must be a way to treat him with peritoneal dialysis.

Robert Popovich, a Ph.D. member of the research group, worked out the kinetics of "long-dwell equilibrated peritoneal dialysis," which was proposed for treating this patient.

The technique was based on the work of Fred Boen, who pointed out that if dialysis solution was left in the peritoneal cavity for longer than 2 hours, the urea level in the blood would equal the level of urea in the solution. It was also determined that it would take five exchanges of 2 L of dialysate per day to achieve the desired control of the blood chemistries, and that 12 L of equilibrated solution had to be removed from the patient per day to achieve this.

The method utilized consisted of a standard 2-L bottle of peritoneal dialysate attached to a simple piece of tubing and a Tenckhoff catheter. The fluid would be instilled and left in the abdomen for a period of 4 hours and then drained out. This procedure would be repeated up to five times per day. The Austin group called the procedure continuous ambulatory peritoneal dialysis (CAPD) and found that they were able to control Pilcher's chemistries and fluid removal with this simple technique. Its only shortcomings were that infection and protein loss were potential complications. The investigators then submitted an article on CAPD to a leading publication, but it was rejected. Undaunted, they continued to work with the procedure and tried to perfect their technique.

Pilcher was trained to do the exchanges by himself once Moncrief had been able to determine that the solution could be left in the peritoneum overnight without compromise. Pilcher dialyzed with this system for over 2 months and was then transplanted.

Moncrief notes that large amounts of peritoneal protein were lost very early in the treatment series. Because of this, it became evident that the patient's diet would have to be supplemented with protein and that other dietary restrictions could be relaxed. They were impressed with the results, and because CAPD was not covered by Medicare, they requested a grant from the National Institutes of Health so that they could continue dialyzing patients with this method.

Karl Nolph was notified of the progress with CAPD, and the National Institutes of Health asked him to join the investigative group to evaluate its clinical value. Nolph had an interest in the kinetics and transport of the peritoneum that had been stimulated by the work of Boen and his collaboration with Popovich on peritoneal dialysis. Nolph's group began to treat patients with CAPD as early as January 1977.[73] They were able to publish their results, which included the Moncrief experience, in 1978. The results were promising but the high incidence of peritonitis continued to plague them.

Oreopoulos was very skeptical of the clinical application of CAPD. Fortunately, Jack Rubin, a former rotating resident of the Toronto Western Hospital, had worked with the University of Missouri on the CAPD program. On a visit to Toronto, he told Oreopoulos of the results of the CAPD program at the University of Missouri and noted the therapeutic benefit of CAPD. He also pointed out the problems they were having with peritonitis that appeared to be related to the use of bottled dialysate.

Oreopoulos's First Patient

Another milestone in the development of CAPD occurred in 1977. One of Oreopoulos's patients, who had been trained in reverse-osmosis (R/O) peritoneal dialysis, was readmitted into the hospital to be trained on the cycler because she was deteriorating clinically. The patient had an unfortunate fall in the hospital, and the staff decided to perform manual peritoneal dialysis on her. Fortunately, in Canada, the 2-L collapsible container of peritoneal dialysis solution was being used prior to the incident. They used a standard "Y" set with the 2-L containers and began to perform the usual CAPD procedure. The empty bag was used to collect the spent solution and the procedure was repeated every 4 hours. The patient's condition improved so dramatically she was able to ambulate safely.

Oreopoulos consulted with Ron Hamade, his local Baxter salesman, and asked him to find a piece of tubing that had a spike on one end and a male fitting on the other. Hamade suggested that they use a piece of the tubing that was used on the R/O set. It worked perfectly.

It was fortunate that Oreopoulos had over 70 patients on peritoneal dialysis. He was able to convert the IPD patients quite rapidly to CAPD and could evaluate the results on a broad-based patient population very quickly. He had the opportunity to evaluate the advantages of using the peritoneal solution in the flexible container and observe the ease of use and success of the system as compared with the bottle method in controlling infection (Fig. 1–15). The interest in CAPD continued to grow, but it became apparent that if peritonitis could not be controlled, CAPD did not have a future.

The focus on CAPD development was now centered on gaining approval for the 2-L flexible container so that the advantages of the closed system could be used. The container was approved by the U.S. Food and Drug Administration (FDA) in 1978. Once approval was obtained, CAPD began to elicit wide interest and acceptance. Shortly thereafter, the treatment was approved for reimbursement by Medicare.

TREATING THE DIABETIC PATIENT

The first reference to adding insulin to the peritoneal dialysis solution was made by Carl Kjellstrand,[74] who was treating patients with intermittent peritoneal dialysis. He

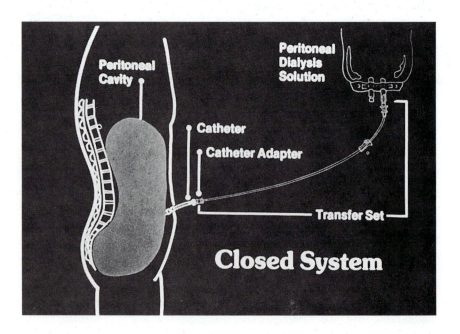

Figure 1–15. CAPD closed system.

observed that insulin diffused very slowly into the bloodstream and that large amounts of insulin were required to control the blood sugar because the short dwell time of 30 minutes was not long enough to allow the insulin to diffuse into the blood adequately.

C. T. Flynn

Another important innovation in peritoneal dialysis treatment was proposed by C. T. Flynn,[75] who was the first to publish that diabetic dialysis patients may do better on CAPD.

Flynn noted that the long dwell time of the dialysis fluid in the peritoneal cavity during CAPD could be used as a method for insulin administration. Due to the large molecular size of insulin (5000 MW), it is slowly absorbed from the peritoneal cavity. With this technique, he was able to maintain blood sugars in the acceptable range required for good patient management.

Prior to 1972, diabetics were often excluded from dialysis. Currently, over 30 percent of the patients on peritoneal dialysis are diabetics.

Intraperitoneal insulin administration has become an important technique in treating the myriad complications of the diabetic who has renal disease.

THE GROWTH OF HOME CARE

The Medicare legislation of 1983 provided for the same reimbursement regardless of whether treatment is at home or in-center, hemodialysis or peritoneal dialysis. This stimulated the use of CAPD for home training programs.

OTHER ADVANCES

The basic CAPD procedure was further modified to help control peritonitis. Ultraviolet treatment of the bag/spike junction helped to prevent contamination during the exchange procedure. Modifications of the container size and formulations further expanded the usefulness of CAPD. Automated cyclers were developed to accommodate the needs of the pediatric patient and others who could not perform the normal CAPD procedure (Fig. 1–16).

Recent developments in technology have allowed the patient to remove the container between exchanges in order to accommodate his or her lifestyle requirements.

THE FUTURE

The goal of the medical community and industry is to provide the quality of care that will minimize the burden that must be borne by those afflicted with renal disease. Future efforts will be directed at understanding the causes of progressive renal failure and how it can be prevented. No one can be satisfied until the consequences of renal disease can be controlled or eliminated.

REFERENCES

1. Cunningham RS. The physiology of the serous membranes. *Physiol Rev* 1926;6:242.
2. DeGowan R, Hardin A, Alsener. *Blood Transfusion*. Philadelphia: Saunders, 1949.
3. Walter CW. Development of blood banks. *Hygiene* 1964; 544–545.

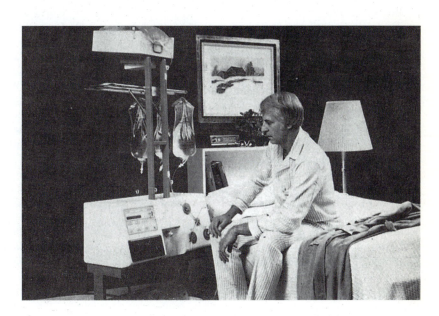

Figure 1–16. Automated cycler machine.

4. Higginson A. *Liverpool Med Chir J* 1857;1:102–110.

5. Latta I. Malignant cholera. *Lancet* 1832;22:274–281.

6. Estes JW. Practice of medicine in 18th-century Massachusetts. *N Engl J Med* 1981;5:1040.

7. Graham T. Osmotic force. *Philos Trans R Soc Lond* 1854;144:177–228.

8. Odling W. *Weekly Evening Meeting Proceedings Royal Institute, Great Britain,* January 28, 1870, pp 15–53.

9. Ferry J. Ultrafilter membranes and ultrafiltration. *Chem Rev* 1936;18:3.

10. Richardson BW. Practical studies in animal dialysis. *Asclepiad* 1889;6:331–332.

11. Bigelow G. Collodion membranes. *J Am Chem Soc* 1907;29:1576–1589.

12. Talalay P. *Notes on the History of the Department, Research and Educational Program, 1963–1971.* Baltimore, MD: Johns Hopkins University Press.

13. Abel J, Rowntree L, Turner B. On the removal of diffusible substances from the circulating blood of living animals by dialysis. *J Pharmacol Exp Ther* 1914;5:275–316.

14. Murnaghan A, Talalay J. John Jacob and the crystallization of insulin. *Perspect Biol Med* 1967;10:334–376.

15. Hess J, McGuigan W. The condition of the sugar in the blood. *Pharmacology* 1914;6:45–55.

16. Walpole GS. Notes on collodion membranes for ultrafiltration and pressure dialysis. *Biol Chem* 1915;9:284–297.

17. Rohde A. Vividiffusion experiments on the ammonia of the circulating blood. *J Biol Chem* 1915;21:325–330.

18. Necheles H. A method of vivi dialysis. *Clin Physiol* 1926;1:69–80.

19. Necheles H. Demonstration of a gastric secretory excitant in circulating blood by vivi dialysis. *Proc Soc Exp Biol Med* 1926;24:197–198.

20. Benedum J. Pioneer of dialysis, George Haas (1886–1971). *Med Hist* 1979;14:196–217.

21. Haas G. Blood cleansing. *MMWR Morb Mortal Wkly Rep* 1923;70:1–13.

22. Haas G. Dialysis of the flowing blood in the patient. *Klin Wochenschr* 1923;70:1888.

23. Pierce HF. Nitrocellulose membranes of graded permeability. *J Biol Chem* 1927;75:795–815.

24. McBain J, Kistler S. Membranes for ultrafiltration of graduated fineness down to molecular sieves. *J Gen Physiol* 1928;12:187–200.

25. Geiger AA. A method of ultrafiltration in vivo. *J Physiol* 1931;71:111–120.

26. Thalhimer W. Experimental exchange transfusions for reducing azotemia. *Proc Soc Exp Biol Med* 1938;37:643.

27. McBain J, Stuewer R. Ultrafiltration through cellophane of porosity adjusted between collodial and molecular dimensions. *J Physiol Chem* 1936;40:1157–1168.

28. Kolff W. First clinical experience with the artificial kidney. *Intern Med* 1965;63.

29. Kolff W. *New Ways of Treating Uremia.* London: Churchill, 1946.

30. Palmer R, Rutherford P. Kidney substitutes in uremia. The use of Kolff's dialyzer in two cases. *Can Med Assoc J* 1949;60:261–266.

31. Fishman A, Kroop I, Leijer H, Hyman A. Experiences with the Kolff artificial kidney. *Am J Med* 1949;7:15–34.

32. Merrill J, Thorne G, Walter C, et al. The use of the artificial kidney. *J Clin Invest* 1950;29:412–424.

33. Focus. *Harvard Medical Area,* September 6, 1979, pp 1–2.

34. Alwall N. On the artificial kidney. *Acta Med Scand* 1947;78:128.

35. Alwall N. *Therapeutic and Diagnostic Problems in Severe Renal Failure.* Stockholm: Scandinavian University Books, 1963:2, 11.

36. Alwall N. On the artificial kidney. *Acta Med Scand* 1949;133:397–398.

37. Murray G. Development of an artificial kidney. *Arch Surg* 1947;55:505–522.

38. Skeggs I, Leonards J. Studies on the artificial kidney. *Science* 1948;108:212–213.

39. Skeggs L, Leonards J, Heisler C. Artificial kidney II. *Proc Soc Exp Biol Med* 1949;72:539.

40. Rosenak S, Saltzman A. A new dialyzer for use as an artificial kidney. *Proc Soc Exp Biol Med* 1951;76:471–475.

41. Malinow M, Korzon W. An experimental method for obtaining an ultrafiltrate of the blood. *J Lab Clin Med* 1947;32: 461–471.

42. Von Garrelts B. *Twenty-Third Meeting of Northern Surgical Association. Stockholm, Sweden. 1947.* Copenhagen: Menkogaard, 1948:423.

43. MacNeill A. Synthetic organ mechanism, medical instrumentation. Session II. *ISA Proc* 1953;8:306.

44. MacNeill AE, Doyle JE, Anthone R, Anthone S. Technique with a parallel flow, straight tube blood dialyzer. *NY State J Med* 1959;59:4137–4149.

45. Doyle JE, Anthone R, Anthone S, MacNeill AE. Treatment of renal failure with a parallel flow, straight tube blood dialyzer. *NY State J Med* 1959;59:4149–4170.

46. Muirhead E, Reed A. A resin artificial kidney. *J Lab Clin Med* 1948;33:841–844.

47. Lowsley C, Kirwin T. Artificial kidney—preliminary report. *J Urol* 1951;65:163–176.

48. Merrill J, Thorne G, Walter C, et al. The use of the artificial kidney. *J Clin Invest* 1950;29:412–424.

49. Guarino J, Guarino L. An artificial kidney—a simplified apparatus. *Science* 1952;115:285–288.

50. Inouye W, Engelberg J. A simplified artificial dialyzer and ultrafilter. *Surg Forum* 1953;4:438–443.

51. Kolff W, Watschinger B, Vertes V. Results in patients treated with the coil kidney. *JAMA* 1956;161:1433–1437.

52. Product brochure from Allis Chalmers Manufacturing Co., Milwaukee, WI.

53. Development reports, artificial kidney project, Westinghouse Electric Corporation, East Pittsburgh Works, Pittsburgh, PA, 1950. Provided by George Jernstedt.

54. Teschan P, Baxter C, O'Brien T, et al. Prophylactic hemodialysis in the treatment of acute renal failure. *Ann Intern Med* 1960:53.

55. Babb A, Grimsrud L, Bell R, Layno S. Engineering aspects of artificial kidney streams. *Chemical Engineering in Medicine and Biology.* New York: Plenum Press, 1967:389–331.

56. Cimino J, Bescia M, Alvrdy R. Simpler venipunture for hemodialysis. *N Engl J Med* 1967;276:609–609.

57. Comments. *ASAIO J* 1966;12:227.
58. Stewart R, Cerny J, Henry M. The capillary "kidney": preliminary report. *U Mich Med Ctr J* 1964;30:116–118.
59. Wegner G. Surgical comments on peritoneal cavity with special emphasis on ovariotomy. *Arch Klin Chir* 1877;20:106.
60. Orlow R. Some studies of the absorption of the abdominal cavity. *Arch Physiol* 1895;59:170.
61. Starling J, Tubby W. *J Physiol* 1894;46:140.
62. Putnam T. The living peritoneum as a dialyzing membrane. *Am J Physiol* 1923;3:548–565.
63. Ganter G. About the elimination of poisonous substances from the blood by dialysis. *Munch Med Wochnschr* 1950;1478–1480.
64. Frank H, Seligman A, Fine J. Treatment of uremia after acute renal failure by peritoneal irrigation. *JAMA* 1946;130:703–705.
65. Grollman A, Turner LB, McLean JA. Intermittent peritoneal lavage in nephrectomized dogs and its application to the human being. *Arch Intern Med* 1951;87:379–390.
66. Maxwell MH, Rockney RE, Kleeman CR, Twiss MR. Peritoneal dialysis: techniques and applications. *JAMA* 1959;170:917–924.
67. Boen ST. Kinetics of peritoneal dialysis. *Medicine* 1961;40:243–287.
68. Palmer R, Quinton W, Gray J. Prolonged peritoneal dialysis for chronic renal failure. *Lancet* 1964;1:700–702.
69. McDonald H. Mechanical approach to peritoneal dialysis. *Med World News,* April 30, 1965, pp 23–24.
70. Tenckhoff H, Shilipetar G, Van Paaschen WH, Swanson E. A home peritoneal dialysis delivery system. *ASAIO Trans* 1969;15:103.
71. Tenckhoff H, Schechter H. A bacterial safe peritoneal access device. *ASAIO Trans* 1968;15:181.
72. Lasker N, McCaukey EP, Passarotti CT. Chronic peritoneal dialysis. *ASAIO Trans* 1966;12:94–105.
73. Popovich RP, Nolph KD, Ghods AJ, Twardowski ZJ. *Ann Intern Org* 1979;4:114–117.
74. Crossley K, Kjellstrand CM. Intraperitoneal insulin for control of blood sugar in diabetic patients during peritoneal dialysis. *Br Med J* 1971;1:269–270.
75. Flynn CT, Nanson JA. Intraperitoneal insulin with CAPD-artificial pancreas. *ASAIO Trans* 1979;25:114–117.

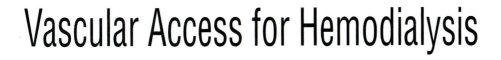

Vascular Access for Hemodialysis

Michael S. Berkoben
Steve J. Schwab

Hemodialysis is required in three general situations: acute renal failure, poisonings, and end-stage renal disease. Successful hemodialysis in any of these settings requires access to large blood vessels capable of supporting rapid extracorporeal blood flow. In acute renal failure and in poisonings, immediate and perhaps only temporary access to the circulation is required. These requirements are best met by the percutaneous insertion of dual-lumen hemodialysis catheters into large central veins. In end-stage renal disease, reliable long-term access to the circulation is essential for adequate dialytic therapy. Long-term access to the circulation is best accomplished by the construction of an endogenous arteriovenous fistula. Less desirable is the construction of a synthetic arteriovenous fistula.

ACUTE VASCULAR ACCESS

External Arteriovenous Fistulas

The external arteriovenous fistula, introduced by Scribner and Quinton in 1960, was the first acceptable device for vascular access in hemodialysis and expanded the clinical application of both acute and chronic hemodialysis.[1] Scribner shunts are constructed by placing Silastic tubes fitted with appropriately sized Teflon tips into the radial artery and cephalic vein at the wrist or into the posterior tibial artery and saphenous vein at the ankle. The cannulated vessels are ligated distally. When the shunt is in use, the Silastic tubes are connected directly to the blood tubing and thus to the dialysis machine; when the device is not in use, the tubes are joined by a Teflon connector.

Scribner shunts provide high rates of extracorporeal blood flow and can be placed in intensive care units under local anesthesia. Several inherent disadvantages, however, argue against their routine use for acute or chronic vascular access. The requirement for surgical support may lead to delays in shunt placement. Ligation of the artery and vein sacrifices potential permanent vascular access sites. Thrombosis rates are high for Scribner shunts, and accidental dislodgment and hemorrhages may occur. Because of these disadvantages, Scribner shunts are now very rarely used for acute or chronic hemodialysis.

Double-Lumen Hemodialysis Catheters

Double-lumen central venous catheters are the preferred vascular access device for acute hemodialysis. These catheters are composed of polyurethane, polyethylene, or polytetrafluoroethylene. Their advantages are many. Central venous catheters can be quickly inserted at the bedside using the Seldinger technique and provide extracorporeal blood flow rates in excess of 300 mL/min. Separation of the arterial and venous ports minimizes recirculation of the blood (Fig. 2–1). Central venous catheters may be used for conventional hemodialysis and for continuous renal replacement therapy.

Catheter Insertion Sites. Double-lumen hemodialysis catheters may be inserted into the femoral, subclavian, or internal jugular veins. Each insertion site has associated advantages and disadvantages.

Femoral Vein. Femoral vein catheters are inserted by cannulating the femoral vein immediately below the inguinal ligament. Femoral vein cannulation requires less skill than subclavian or internal jugular vein cannulation and generally provides more rapid access to the circulation. Because femoral vein cannulation may be performed with the patient in the semirecumbent position, it is the preferred technique for patients with pulmonary edema. Complications include ileofemoral venous thrombosis, arteriovenous fistula, retroperitoneal hemorrhage from venous perforation, and hemorrhage from inadvertent puncture of the femoral artery. Life-threatening complications, however, occur less frequently with femoral vein cannulation than with cannulation of other central veins. Patients with femoral vein catheters must remain at bed rest and in the hospital. Because of a high rate of infection, femoral vein catheters should generally stay in place no longer than 7 days. One additional

problem with femoral vein catheters should be noted: significant blood recirculation occurs in 15-cm femoral vein catheters but not in 24-cm catheters.[2] If the blood flow rate is increased, recirculation increases and dialytic efficiency is not increased. Femoral catheters should be at least 19-cm long, so that the catheter tip resides in the inferior vena cava.

Subclavian Vein. The subclavian vein is cannulated by passing the cannula directly beneath the midpoint of the clavicle and aiming at the suprasternal notch. Subclavian vein catheters provide the most comfortable and secure means of temporary vascular access and do not require that the patient remain in the hospital. Because of low infection rates, they may be left in place for weeks. Subclavian vein cannulation requires considerably more skill than femoral vein cannulation, however, and is associated with more serious complications, such as pneumothorax. Subclavian vein catheterization is associated with subsequent subclavian vein stenosis, which may preclude permanent vascular access placement in the ipsilateral arm (see below). Because of this potential complication, subclavian vein catheters should be avoided in patients who will ultimately require fistula creation for chronic hemodialysis.

Internal Jugular Vein. The anterior approach to cannulation of the internal jugular vein is most commonly used. The cannula enters the skin at a 20-degree angle from the sagittal plane, two finger breadths above the clavicle, between the sternal and clavicular heads of the sternocleidomastoid muscle; it is aimed at the ipsilateral nipple. Internal jugular catheters offer perhaps the best balance of comfort and safety. Like subclavian catheters, internal jugular vein catheters may be left in place for weeks and do not require that the patient remain in hospital. Internal jugular vein can-

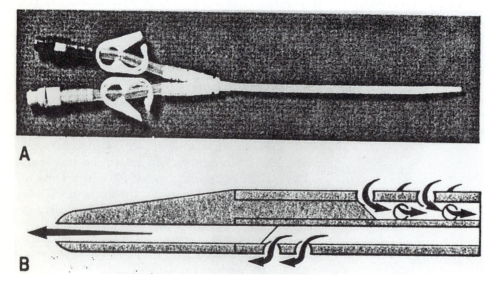

Figure 2–1. *A.* Temporary hemodialysis catheter. *B.* Separation of arterial and venous lumens minimizes recirculation of blood. (*Reprinted with permission from Schwab SJ. Hemodialysis vascular access. In: Jacobson HR, Striker GE, Klahr S, eds.* The Principles and Practice of Nephrology. *Philadelphia: Decker, 1991:766–772. Catheter courtesy of Quinton Instrument Co., Seattle, WA.*)

nulation entails less risk of pneumothorax than does subclavian vein cannulation, and prolonged catheterization is much less likely to cause central vein thrombosis. The introduction of looped port extensions has increased patient comfort, but internal jugular vein catheters are generally less comfortable and secure than are subclavian vein catheters. Because it entails a lower risk of pneumothorax and central vein stenosis, however, internal jugular vein cannulation is, in our opinion, the preferred technique.

Complications of Central Vein Cannulation

Insertion Complications. The types and frequencies of insertion complications depend on the insertion site and on the experience of the operator.[3] Table 2–1 lists the most common insertion complications.

Atrial arrhythmias caused by endocardial irritation by the guidewire or catheter may complicate up to 40 percent of subclavian and internal jugular vein cannulations but are generally unrecognized,[4] Ventricular arrhythmias occur in approximately 20 percent, but antiarrhythmic medications and cardioversion are rarely required.[5]

Inadvertent arterial puncture is another common complication. Punctures of the femoral and carotid arteries are successfully managed by the application of manual pressure; significant hematomata rarely result, even in patients with bleeding diatheses.[6] It is more difficult to apply direct pressure to the subclavian artery, yet serious hemorrhage complicates less than 1 percent of subclavian vein catheterization attempts.[7,8] Because of the risk of inadvertent subclavian artery puncture, attempts at subclavian vein cannulation should be avoided in patients with coagulopathies or thrombocytopenia.

Pneumothorax complicates 1 to 5 percent of subclavian vein cannulations[3,7,8] but less than 0.1 percent of internal jugular vein cannulations.[3,8] In order to reduce the likelihood of fatal pneumothorax, two rules should be followed: One should never attempt to cannulate the subclavian vein ipsilateral to the only healthy lung. Also, because an unsuccessful attempt at subclavian vein catheterization does not preclude a pneumothorax having been caused, a chest radiograph should be obtained before cannulation of the contralateral subclavian vein is attempted. Clinically significant air embolism is a rare complication of central vein catheterization.[8] Care must be taken to avoid the inadvertent introduction of air through the introducer needle, dilator, or catheter.

Perforations of the superior vena cava or of a cardiac chamber with resultant hemothorax, mediastinal hemorrhage, or pericardial tamponade are rare but life-threatening complications.[8] The subclavian approach carries a greater risk of these complications than does the internal jugular, presumably because of the curved path that the subclavian catheter must follow. To reduce the likelihood of perforation during insertion, the catheter should never be advanced unless it is protected by a J-tipped guidewire.[9] Following insertion, a chest radiograph must be obtained to confirm that the catheter is positioned within a central vein. The catheter tip should not be allowed to protrude into the right atrium, as right atrial perforation may result. Because prolonged catheterization may cause vascular erosion and delayed perforation of the superior vena cava, pericardial tamponade should be suspected in any hypotensive hemodialysis patient with a central venous dialysis catheter.

Injuries to the brachial plexus,[10] trachea,[11] and recurrent laryngeal nerve[12] have also been reported as complications of central vein cannulation.

At our institution, handheld ultrasound devices are commonly used to guide central vein cannulation. Before cannulation is attempted, ultrasonography is used to demonstrate the patency of the target vein. The introducer needle is then inserted under direct visualization. Fewer needle passes are required for successful cannulation when this technique is employed.[13] It is hoped that this practice will decrease the incidence of insertion complications.

Infection. Catheter-related infection remains a major problem for patients with central venous hemodialysis catheters. Gram-positive bacteria, particularly *Staphylococcus aureus*, are the most common culprits. Infection typically results from migration of microorganisms from the patient's skin through the catheter insertion site and down the outer surface of the catheter, or from contamination of the catheter lumen during the hemodialysis procedure.[14] Less commonly, infection results from the infusion of infected solutions.[14]

The risk of bacteremia from temporary hemodialysis catheters increases with the duration of catheterization.[7,14–16] This risk has recently been quantified.[16] For

---

TABLE 2–1. ACUTE COMPLICATIONS OF HEMODIALYSIS CATHETER INSERTION

Atrial and ventricular dysrhythmias
Arterial puncture
Hemothorax
Pneumothorax
Air embolism
Perforation of central vein or cardiac chamber
Pericardial tamponade

femoral catheters, the risk of bacteremia is 3.1 percent up to 1 week of catheterization, but it increases to 10.7 percent by 2 weeks. Femoral catheters should therefore be removed after 1 week. For internal jugular catheters, the risk of bacteremia is 5.4 percent up to 3 weeks, but it increases to 10.3 percent by 4 weeks. It has been recommended that internal jugular vein catheters be removed after 3 weeks. In each case, however, we believe that the risk of bacteremia from prolonged catheterization should be weighed against the risk of repeated catheter insertion. Catheters should be removed if there are signs of exit-site infection, even if there is no evidence of systemic infection. Exit-site infection leads quickly to bacteremia, presumably because the absence of a cuff allows migration of bacteria along the tunnel and outer surface of the catheter.[16]

Several steps may be taken to help prevent catheter-related infection (Table 2–2). Hemodialysis catheters should be used only for hemodialysis and not for infusions or phlebotomy. Disinfection with 2% aqueous chlorhexidine at the time of insertion appears to be superior to disinfection with povidone-iodine or isopropyl alcohol.[17] Bacterial resistance to chlorhexidine is rare, and minimal inhibitory concentrations are low in relation to its concentrations in topical solutions. Chlorhexidine's antibacterial effects persist for hours; povidone-iodine's effects are brief. Application of povidone-iodine ointment or mupirocin ointment to the catheter insertion site at the time of each dressing change is another measure that will reduce infection rates.[18] Finally, the use of dry gauze rather than occlusive dressings appears to reduce catheter infection rates.[19]

Catheter-related bacteremia should be the presumptive diagnosis in the febrile hemodialysis patient with a central venous catheter if the history, physical examination, and initial laboratory and radiologic evaluation reveal no other site of infection. Blood cultures should be obtained, the catheter removed, and antibiotics administered. If hemodialysis is scheduled within a few hours, the catheter may be left in place until the treatment has been completed. Antibiotic therapy should be continued for 2 to 3 weeks; if there is evidence of metastatic infection, a longer course of antibiotic therapy is required. The management of *S. aureus* bacteremia is discussed in detail in the section on cuffed catheter–related bacteremia, below.

Thrombosis. Intracatheter clots are easily detected, as they impede extracorporeal blood flow. These clots can usually be lysed by instilling alteplase (recombinant human tissue plasminogen activator) reconstituted to a concentration of 1 mg/mL in volumes sufficient to fill the catheter lumens for 30 to 120 minutes.[20] This procedure can be repeated if impaired blood flow persists. In the event of refractory occlusion, a J-tipped guidewire should be inserted through the clotted catheter, the clotted catheter removed, and a new catheter threaded over the guidewire.

Mural thrombus occurs less commonly than intracatheter clotting but is a much more serious complication.[21] Arm or leg edema is the usual presenting sign. Treatment consists of catheter removal and systemic anticoagulation. The thrombosed vein is usually permanently occluded, however, and placement of acute or permanent vascular access in the involved arm is permanently precluded.

Central Vein Stenosis. Central vein stenosis, particularly subclavian vein stenosis, is associated with antecedent placement of subclavian dialysis catheters,[22–24] but this complication is less common after internal jugular vein cannulation.[25,26] Arm edema may be the presenting complaint, but it may become evident only after placement of an ipsilateral arteriovenous fistula.[27] It is not clear whether fistulas, by increasing blood flow to the ipsilateral limb, simply unmask clinically silent stenoses or are essential to their development. In regard to this question, two phenomena should be noted. Central vein stenosis has been reported to develop in the absence of antecedent catheterization. In addition, central vein stenosis may become clinically evident months after placement of an ipsilateral arteriovenous fistula. These phenomena suggest that ipsilateral fistulas may initiate or at least accelerate the development of central vein stenoses. The treatment of central vein stenoses is discussed later in this chapter.

PERMANENT VASCULAR ACCESS

Successful maintenance hemodialysis requires repetitive access to large vessels capable of supporting rapid extracorporeal blood flow. The establishment and maintenance of ade-

---

TABLE 2–2. PREVENTION OF ACUTE HEMODIALYSIS CATHETER INFECTION

Skin disinfection with 2% aqueous chlorhexidine at the time of insertion
Sound insertion technique
Skin disinfection with chlorhexidine or povidone-iodine solution at each hemodialysis treatment
Application of povidone-iodine ointment or mupirocin ointment to the catheter insertion site at each dressing change
Dry gauze dressings
Use of face shield or surgical mask by patients and nurses during connection and disconnection procedures
Limited duration of catheterization (1 week for femoral vein catheters, 3 weeks for internal jugular vein catheters)

quate vascular access, however, remain the Achilles' heel of maintenance hemodialysis. Vascular access that provides insufficient blood flow or that is beset with complications is costly to both the patient and society. The failure of vascular access is the most frequent reason for hospitalization of patients with end-stage renal disease.

Types of Chronic Vascular Access (Table 2–3)

Primary Arteriovenous Fistulas. The primary arteriovenous fistula, first described by Cimino and Brescia in 1961, remains the preferred form of vascular access for maintenance hemodialysis.[28] These fistulas are typically created by an end-to-side vein-to-artery anastomosis of the cephalic vein and radial artery and generally require 2 to 6 months to mature. Other primary fistulas include brachiocephalic fistulas at the elbow and transposed brachiobasilic fistulas. Transposed brachiobasilic fistulas are created by making an incision from the forearm to the axilla along the route of the basilic vein, dividing the basilic vein where it becomes too small to use, and mobilizing the vein toward the axilla, where it is anastomosed to the brachial artery.

Once mature, endogenous fistulas have excellent long-term patency rates and are rarely beset with infectious complications. In the authors' experience, it is not unheard of for primary arteriovenous fistulas to provide adequate vascular access for 20 years. As the proportion of elderly and diabetic patients entering maintenance hemodialysis programs has increased, however, the proportion of patients with arterial and venous anatomy suitable for endogenous fistula construction has decreased. Injudicious use of cephalic veins for phlebotomy or intravenous cannulation can also preclude the successful creation of a primary fistula. Even with careful planning, however, 24 to 27 percent of native fistulas fail to mature; such fistulas clot in the early postoperative period or never achieve sufficient caliber to allow cannulation.[29,30] A minority of patients in most dialysis centers have functional primary arteriovenous fistulas.

Synthetic Arteriovenous Grafts. Synthetic fistulas are composed of polytetrafluoroethylene (PTFE). Initial PTFE graft placement is in the forearm or upper arm (brachial artery to proximal basilic vein) (Fig. 2–2). Forearm grafts may have either a loop (brachial artery to basilic vein) or straight (distal radial artery to basilic vein) configuration. Maturation usually requires 3 weeks; fibrous tissue will anchor the graft in its subdermal tunnel and promote hemostasis at needle puncture sites. PTFE is durable and will withstand multiple thrombectomies and revisions. However, PTFE grafts are more prone to thrombosis and infection than are primary arteriovenous fistulas, and, by 3 years, most grafts have been lost to thrombosis or infection. Following forearm or upper arm graft loss, new PTFE grafts may be placed in the chest wall (axillary artery to axillary vein or axillary artery to jugular vein) or thigh (femoral artery to femoral vein).

Tunneled Cuffed Catheters. Double-lumen Silastic or silicone catheters with felt cuffs (Fig. 2–3) can provide temporary

TABLE 2–3. TYPES OF PERMANENT VASCULAR ACCESS

Type of Access	Patency Rates	Advantages	Disadvantages
Primary arteriovenous fistula	60–70% at 1 year 50–65% at 2–4 years	Low thrombosis and infection rates May provide complication-free access for many years (few if any interventions required to maintain patency)	May require 6 months or more to mature during which time tunneled cuffed catheter may be required 24–27% fail to mature (primary failure rate may be even higher if determined efforts are made to increase likelihood of primary fistula creation)
PTFE[a] graft	62–83% at 1 year 50–77% at 2 years < 50% at 3 years	May be cannulated 3 weeks after placement	Thrombosis and infection rates higher than those for primary fistulas (many interventions required to maintain patency)
Tunneled cuffed catheter	30–74% at 1 year	May be used immediately No risk of arterial steal Morbidity of insertion and removal low No needle puncture required for hemodialysis	High rate of catheter-related bacteremia and metastatic infection Persistently low blood-flow rates may lead to inadequate hemodialysis
Subcutaneous ports attached to catheters	Device survival as high as 90% at 6 months [40]	May have longer survival rates and lower infection rates than tunneled cuffed catheters	More difficult to remove than tunneled cuffed catheters

[a]Polytetrafluoroethylene.

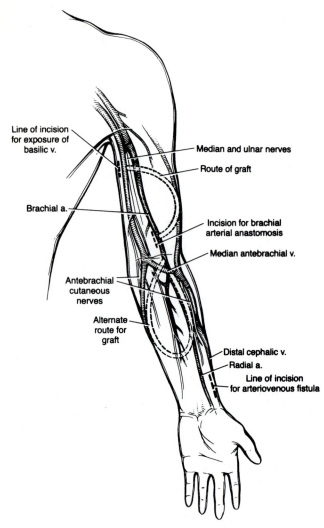

Line of incision for exposure of basilic v.

Median and ulnar nerves

Route of graft

Brachial a.

Incision for brachial arterial anastomosis

Median antebrachial v.

Antebrachial cutaneous nerves

Alternate route for graft

Distal cephalic v.

Radial a.

Line of incision for arteriovenous fistula

Figure 2–2. Upper arm graft and forearm graft in loop configuration. *(Reprinted with permission from Stickel DL. Renal dialysis access procedures. In: Sabiston DC Jr, ed.* Atlas of General Surgery. *Philadelphia: Saunders, 1994:90–98.)*

access[31] in those patients whose primary or synthetic fistulas have not yet matured and permanent access[32–34] in patients who have exhausted all available access sites, in patients in whom peripheral vascular disease precludes fistula placement, and in those who cannot tolerate the increase in cardiac output associated with the placement of a primary or synthetic fistula. These catheters are typically inserted through a subcutaneous tunnel under fluoroscopic guidance into an internal jugular vein, external jugular vein, subclavian vein, or, if necessary, femoral vein. The internal jugular vein is the preferred insertion site, and the right internal jugular vein is preferred to the left. The approach via the right internal jugular vein offers a less curved route to the superior vena cava, a lower risk of complications,[25,26,35] and a lower rate of central vein stenosis and thrombosis.[33,35] To enhance the likelihood of high blood flow rates, the catheter

tip should reside at the junction of the superior vena cava and right atrium or in the right atrium.

Tunneled cuffed catheters may be used immediately after insertion. There is no risk of arterial steal, and needle puncture is not required for hemodialysis. Intracatheter thrombosis is very common but is successfully treated in the great majority of cases by instilling alteplase. In spite of these advantages, tunneled cuffed catheters are the least desirable form of permanent vascular access. Catheter-related infection is much more common than primary or synthetic fistula infection. In addition, intracatheter clotting and fibrin sheath formation on the outer surface of the catheter often impede extracorporeal blood flow. In our experience, only 73 percent of catheters consistently provided extracorporeal blood flow rates of 400 mL/min, in spite of prompt lytic therapy for catheter thrombosis and prompt mechanical removal of fibrin sheaths.[36] The use of tunneled cuffed catheters should be restricted to those patients in whom primary or synthetic fistula creation is not possible.

Subcutaneous Ports with Catheters. The LifeSite Hemodialysis Access System (Vasca, Inc., Tewksbury, MA) consists of two subcutaneous ports implanted beneath the clavicle.[37] Each port is attached to a catheter tunneled to the right internal jugular vein. Each port is accessed transcutaneously with a dialysis needle. Compared to tunneled cuffed catheters, the LifeSite device, when used with 70% isopropyl alcohol as the disinfectant, provided higher blood flow rates, had a lower infection rate, and had a higher device survival rate.[38]

The Dialock (Biolink Corporation, Middleboro, MA) consists of a single subcutaneous port attached to two catheters.[39] The port is accessed transcutaneously with two dialysis needles. Use of this system may also lead to a lower infection rate than that reported for tunneled cuffed catheters.[40]

Preparation for Vascular Access Placement

As noted above, a primary arteriovenous fistula created by an anastomosis of the radial artery and cephalic vein near the wrist of the nondominant arm is the preferred form of vascular access for maintenance hemodialysis. Careful planning will maximize the chance of successful fistula maturation. The patient and the primary care physician should be instructed that the patient's morbidity on maintenance hemodialysis will in large part be determined by the ability of the nephrologist and vascular surgeon to establish and maintain adequate vascular access.[41] The patient should be taught to protect the vasculature of the nondominant arm; placement of radial artery catheters and cephalic vein catheters should be scrupulously avoided. If possible, venipuncture should be avoided in the nondominant arm. The patient should be referred to the vascular surgeon

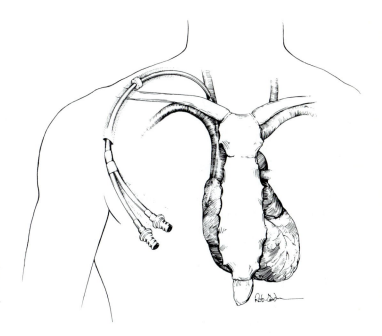

Figure 2–3. Cuffed double-lumen Silastic catheter inserted through a subcutaneous tunnel into the right internal jugular vein. *(Reprinted with permission from Schwab SJ, Buller GL, McCann RL, et al. Prospective evaluation of a Dacron cuffed hemodialysis catheter for prolonged use. Am J Kidney Dis 1988;11:166–169.)*

months before the anticipated need for hemodialysis. Venography should be requested if there is a history of subclavian vein catheterization or current or previous transvenous pacemaker placement ipsilateral to the planned access site. Subclavian vein stenosis or occlusion precludes ipsilateral access placement. The primary arteriovenous fistula should be constructed 6 to 8 months prior to the anticipated need for hemodialysis. If an anastomosis of the radial artery and cephalic vein is not possible, then brachiocephalic fistula creation at the elbow is the next best option.[42]

In recent years, some nephrologists and vascular surgeons have undertaken measures to enhance the likelihood of primary arteriovenous fistula creation. Allon and colleagues have described the effect of preoperative sonographic vascular mapping on vascular access outcomes.[43] Sonographic evaluation was used to identify arteries and veins of sufficient caliber for access construction. Criteria for minimum vessel diameter were developed jointly by nephrologists, radiologists, and vascular surgeons. The minimum arterial diameter for graft and fistula construction was 2 mm. The minimum vein diameter was 2.5 mm for fistula construction and 4 mm for graft construction. The investigators discovered that many patients were found to have large veins that were too deep to be identified by routine visual inspection. Sonographic evaluation was also used to exclude stenosis or thrombosis of the proposed draining vein up to the medial subclavian vein. Using this approach, the investigators doubled the proportion of patients in their dialysis units who had a usable primary arteriovenous fistula. The primary failure rate of these fistulas was substantial (46.4 percent) and exceeded that of grafts. However, the long-term failure rates for these fistulas was lower than that for grafts, and many fewer interventions

were necessary to maintain their patency. Another group of investigators has demonstrated that it is possible to create usable primary ateriovenous fistulas in a majority of Veterans Administration patients undergoing maintenance hemodialysis and that these fistulas have higher patency rates and require fewer interventions than do synthetic grafts.[44]

If radiocephalic or brachiocephalic fistula creation is not possible, a synthetic graft or transposed brachiobasilic primary fistula should be placed in the nondominant arm.[42] In some hands, transposed brachiobasilic fistulas are less likely to thrombose than are upper arm grafts.[45] The surgeon's experience and the patient's vascular anatomy, however, should be the main determinants of the type of operation. The synthetic graft may be placed in either the forearm (loop configuration preferred) or the upper arm. While an upper arm graft may be expected to have a higher blood flow rate and longer patency, forearm graft placement will preserve access sites in the proximal limb. Following loss of vascular access in the arms, a synthetic graft may be placed in the chest wall or in the thigh.

Tunneled cuffed catheters may be placed in patients whose primary or synthetic fistulas have not yet matured and in those in whom primary or synthetic fistula placement is not possible.

Vascular Access Blood Flow and Patency

The chief determinant of the adequacy and patency of vascular access is access blood flow. Insufficient blood flow results in recirculation of blood within the access and decreases dialytic efficiency. More importantly, low access blood flow rates lead to access thrombosis and subsequent access loss.

Access blood flow depends on the type, age, and location of the access. Initial blood flows in primary arteriovenous fistulas are 200 to 300 mL/min,[46] but they increase with time as the venous runoff system dilates. Blood flow rates in mature fistulas may reach 2000 mL/min; more typically, they are 800 to 1200 mL/min. In contrast, blood flows in synthetic fistulas are high initially[47,48] but appear to decrease over time, presumably because of progressive neointimal hyperplasia in the venous outflow tract. Investigators have demonstrated that synthetic fistulas with low blood flow rates are more likely to clot; these findings are described in more detail later in this chapter. Grafts constructed from proximal arteries appear to have higher blood flows rates[46,48] and may have higher patency rates. The cumulative patency rate is defined as the percentage of accesses that remain patent at a given time regardless of the need for intervention. Table 2–3 lists published patency rates for the three types of permanent vascular access. The cumulative patency rate for primary arteriovenous fistulas has been estimated to be 60 to 70 percent at 1 year and 50 to 65 percent at 2 to 4 years.[29,49] Cumulative patency rates for PTFE grafts are approximately 62 to 83 percent at 1 year and 50 to 77 percent at 2 years; fewer than 50 percent of synthetic fistulas survive beyond 3 years.[29,30,49–53] The lower patency rates for endogenous fistulas are due chiefly to early failure; roughly 24 to 27 percent of primary fistulas fail to mature. Patency rates for primary fistulas are higher than those for synthetic fistulas after correction for early primary fistula failure.[29,30,49] At our institution, thrombosis ultimately accounts for 80 percent of vascular access loss, infection for 20 percent, and arterial steal for a small percentage of vascular access loss.

Tunneled cuffed catheters and subcutaneous ports attached to catheters are best used for temporary vascular access in those patients awaiting fistula maturation. When tunneled cuffed catheters are used for permanent vascular access, the access survival rate is 30 to 74 percent at 1 year.[32–34,36,54] Infection is the leading cause of catheter loss. We await long-term studies of subcutaneous ports attached to catheters.

COMPLICATIONS OF VASCULAR ACCESS

Thrombosis

Thrombosis is the leading cause of the loss of vascular access. Thrombosis that occurs within 1 month of vascular access placement is due to technical errors in fistula construction or premature use of the access. After the first month, the thrombosis rate is approximately 0.5 to 0.8 episodes per patient-year.[55] Access type greatly affects thrombosis rates; synthetic grafts clot much more frequently than do native fistulas.

About 90 percent of thromboses of PTFE grafts are due to venous stenosis.[29,56–58] The majority of venous stenoses develop at or within 2 to 3 cm of the vein-graft anastomosis[59] and are due to progressive neointimal hyperplasia.[29,60] Stenoses also occur in more proximal veins, including central veins, or in the graft itself.[60,61] Subclavian vein lesions are associated with previous subclavian vein cannulation and with the presence of cardiac pacemaker wires.[22,27,62]

The pathogenesis of neointimal hyperplasia is only beginning to be understood. An excellent descriptive study of tissue samples of vein-graft anastomoses from stenosed PTFE grafts has recently been published.[63] Factors that appear to play a role in the pathogenesis of neointimal hyperplasia include neoangiogenesis within the neointima and adventitia of upstream graft and downstream vein, the proliferation of smooth muscle cells within the neointima, attraction of activated macrophages to the lesion, and secretion by these macrophages (or by smooth muscle cells or endothelial cells) of platelet-derived growth factor, basic fibroblast growth factor, and vascular endothelial growth factor. This study suggests that interventions directed against any of these biologic processes could prevent neointimal hyperplasia and graft thrombosis.

A small percentage of graft thromboses occur in the absence of an identifiable anatomic lesion. Hypotension, intravascular volume depletion, and prolonged compression of the fistula during sleep may lead to markedly decreased graft flow and subsequent thombosis. Excessive graft compression by patients or dialysis staff attempting to achieve hemostasis after dialysis may also lead to graft thrombosis.

Malfunction of tunneled cuffed hemodialysis catheters is very common. The most common cause of malfunction is intracatheter clotting; instillation of alteplase will reestablish patency in the majority of cases. In the event of refractory malfunction, radiocontrast should be injected to detect fibrin sheath formation or catheter malposition. To strip a fibrin sheath from the catheter, a gooseneck snare is passed through a common femoral vein sheath into the right atrium.[36] The snare encircles the catheter and strips away the fibrin sheath as it is retracted (Fig. 2–4). Fibrin sheath formation may also be treated by replacement of the catheter over a guidewire. In these cases, the sheath must be broken and embolized or care must be taken to avoid reentry of the sheath. A malpositioned catheter may be repositioned or may be replaced over a guidewire.

Infection of Primary and Synthetic Fistulas

Primary fistula infections are uncommon, are usually localized, and can often be treated successfully with antibiotic therapy alone.[29] Because of the endovascular nature of these infections, however, it has been recommended that they be treated with a 6-week course of antibiotic therapy.[64]

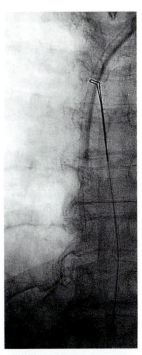

Figure 2–4. A gooseneck snare encircles a cuffed catheter in order to strip a fibrin sheath from it. *(Reprinted with permission from Suhocki PV, Conlon PJ, Knelson MH, et al. Silastic cuffed catheters for hemodialysis vascular access: thrombolytic and mechanical correction of malfunction. Am J Kidney Dis 1996;28:379–386.)*

PTFE graft infections are common; they are the second leading cause of graft loss.[29,50,65] The great majority of graft infections are caused by gram-positive cocci—*S. aureus* and, less commonly, *Staphylococcus epidermidis* and other gram-positive organisms. Gram-negative organisms account for approximately 15 percent of episodes of bacteremia in hemodialysis patients.[66–69]

Many of the factors that predispose patients to graft infections are beyond the nephrologist's control. Intravenous drug use,[29] dermatitis overlying the graft, excessive scratching of needle insertion sites, and poor personal hygiene[69] all have been reported to increase the likelihood of graft infection. Femoral grafts appear to have a high rate of infection, presumably because of the proximity of the graft to the perineum.[70,71] Nevertheless, we do believe that two preventive measures should be undertaken. We recommend that patients wash the skin overlying their grafts with soap and water before each hemodialysis treatment. This practice may reduce the likelihood of the introduction of bacteria into the bloodstream during graft cannulation. In addition, we recommend monitoring of graft cannulation and infection records. Such monitoring may allow the nephrologist to identify a staff member who demonstrates poor needle insertion technique.

Bacteremic hemodialysis patients typically present with fever and chills. Symptoms and signs of graft infection are often absent. If the history, physical examination, and initial investigations do not reveal a source of infection, it should be presumed, until proved otherwise, that the febrile patient with a synthetic fistula has graft-associated bacteremia. Blood cultures should be obtained. At our institution, we administer loading doses of vancomycin (20 mg/kg) and either gentamicin (2 mg/kg) or tobramycin (2 mg/kg). Because methicillin-resistant *S. aureus* (MRSA) and coagulase-negative staphylococci are common isolates, we do not recommend that a beta-lactam antibiotic be used as an empiric agent. If blood cultures yield staphylococci that are susceptible to beta-lactam antibiotics, a beta-lactam antibiotic should be substituted for vancomycin unless the patient has a beta-lactam allergy.

Bacteremic patients who defervesce promptly in response to antimicrobial therapy and whose grafts have no associated pustule or abscess can often be treated successfully with antibiotic therapy alone. Because extensive graft infection may be present even when the physical examination is unremarkable, strong consideration should be given to graft excision if fever or bacteremia persists. Staphylococcal bacteremia has a propensity to cause metastatic infections, including endocarditis, osteomyelitis, septic pulmonary emboli, empyema, septic arthritis, and meningitis. Therefore persistent *S. aureus* bacteremia should prompt the nephrologist to look for evidence of metastatic infection. This search should include transesophageal echocardiography to exclude infective endocarditis. If fever and bacteremia promptly remit and there is no evidence of metastatic infection, a 3-week course of antibiotic therapy should be prescribed. Otherwise, a 6-week or longer course of antibiotic therapy should be prescribed. In either case, blood cultures should be obtained after completion of therapy to ensure that the infection has been eradicated. For gram-negative infections, a 2- to 3-week course of antibiotic therapy should suffice.

Regardless of the pathogen, evaluation by a vascular surgeon is necessary if a pustule or abscess overlies the graft. The surgical procedure that is required depends on the extent of the infection; simple incision and drainage, partial graft excision with bypass grafting, or total graft excision may be necessary. PTFE grafts placed within the preceding month should be completely excised. Recently placed grafts are incompletely incorporated into surrounding tissue, and the infection is unlikely to be localized.[72] Finally, it should be noted that the initial manifestation of a synthetic graft infection may be bleeding through an area of eroded skin overlying the graft. A "herald bleed" mandates surgical evaluation.

Cuffed Catheter–Related Infection

Catheter-related bacteremia is common. Studies have demonstrated a frequency of catheter-related bacteremia of 0.7 to 1.5 episodes per patient per year.[54,73–76] In a study from our institution, 64 percent of episodes were due to gram-positive cocci, 29 percent to gram-negative bacilli, and 5 percent to both gram-positive and gram-negative organisms.[75] The most common culprit was *S. aureus.*

Catheter-related bacteremia should be the presumptive diagnosis in the febrile hemodialysis patient with a tunneled cuffed catheter unless there is strong evidence to the contrary. It is our practice to administer loading doses of vancomycin and either tobramycin or gentamicin after blood cultures are obtained. A standard practice has been to remove the catheter and reinsert another at a new central venous site after eradication of bacteremia. If fever or bacteremia persists after catheter removal, a search for metastatic infection should be undertaken. For those patients with persistent *S. aureus* bacteremia, transesophageal echocardiography should be performed.[77,78] If there is no evidence of metastatic infection, a 3-week course of antibiotic therapy should suffice. While effective, this approach has several disadvantages. A several-day hospital stay may be required. One or more hemodialysis treatments via a temporary femoral vein catheter may be required. Finally, placement of a new tunneled cuffed catheter leads to use (and eventual loss) of another central venous access site. Because of these drawbacks, other approaches have been tried.

Antibiotic therapy without catheter removal (catheter salvage) is an approach that is not recommended. A study from our institution described the results of attempted catheter salvage in 38 instances.[75] This approach failed in 26 instances; catheter removal was ultimately necessary in these instances because of persistent infection. Attempted catheter salvage did not, however, increase the risk of complications.

Catheter exchange over a guidewire can be recommended for the treatment of catheter-related bacteremia if there is no associated exit-site or tunnel infection. Shaffer has demonstrated the efficacy of catheter exchange over a guidewire using the same venous insertion site with creation of a new tunnel and exit site.[79] Beathard has demonstrated the efficacy of catheter exchange over a guidewire in patients with mild symptoms and no exit-site or tunnel infection using the same venous insertion site, tunnel, and exit site.[76] This approach was successful in 87.8 percent of cases. In those patients with mild symptoms but with exit-site or tunnel infection, catheter exchange over a guidewire (after resolution of fever and chills) with creation of a new tunnel and exit site was successful in 75 percent of cases. Other investigators have compared catheter exchange over a guidewire to catheter removal followed by delayed catheter replacement in bacteremic hemodialysis patients and have reported similar outcomes in the two groups.[73] Catheter removal is mandatory, however, in patients with severe symptoms and in those in whom symptoms of infection persist after 36 hours of antibiotic therapy.[80]

A newer approach has been to salvage the catheter with a 3-week course of parenteral antibiotic therapy along with antibiotic lock solution at the end of each hemodialysis treatment. Biofilms coat the luminal surfaces of catheters within days of placement and may lead to persistent or recurrent bacteremia if the catheter is not removed. Instillation of highly concentrated antibiotic solutions (roughly 100-fold higher than therapeutic plasma concentrations) into catheter lumens at the end of each hemodialysis treatment may eradicate these biofilms. A recent study described success in 51 percent of patients treated with this approach.[81] However, only two infections in this study were due to *S. aureus.* This approach cannot yet be recommended for the treatment of *S. aureus* bacteremia.

S. aureus bacteremia has a propensity to cause complications. A study from our institution reported complications in 9 of 41 bacteremic patients: osteomyelitis in 6, septic arthritis in 1, infective endocarditis in 4, and death in 2.[75] All 9 patients with complications had gram-positive bacteremia. We have also described several cases of epidural abscess associated with catheter-related staphylococcal bacteremia.[82] The only consistent presenting complaint was excruciating back pain. Severe back pain in a hemodialysis patient with current or recent staphylococcal bacteremia should prompt magnetic resonance imaging of the spine.[83]

Efforts should be undertaken to prevent catheter-related bacteremia. The exit site should be examined at each hemodialysis treatment. Recent studies have demonstrated that topical application of mupirocin ointment[84] or Polysporin Triple Ointment (bacitracin, gramicidin, and polymyxin B)[85] to the exit sites of tunneled cuffed hemodialysis catheters at each hemodialysis treatment dramatically reduces the risk of bacteremia. A dry gauze dressing should be applied over the ointment, but occlusive dressings should be avoided[19]; they trap drainage and create a moist environment at the exit site.

Exit-site infections (erythema, crusting, scant drainage) and tunnel infections may be treated without catheter removal if there are no signs of systemic infection and if blood cultures are negative. Exit-site infections may be treated with topical antibiotic therapy. Tunnel infections, however, should be treated with parenteral antibiotic therapy. If there is no response, the catheter should be removed.

Antibiotic Dosing. Empiric antibiotic therapy for the febrile hemodialysis patient consists of vancomycin 20 mg/kg and gentamicin 2 mg/kg or tobramycin 2 mg/kg. Vancomycin therapy should be continued if blood cultures yield MRSA. Subsequent doses of 500 mg after each hemodialysis treatment maintain prehemodialysis serum levels of vancomycin above 10μg/mL in the great majority of patients.[86] If the aminoglycoside is to be continued, subsequent doses of 1 mg/kg should be administered. Because of the risk of otovestibulotoxicity, we discourage the prolonged use of an aminoglycoside in combination with vancomycin.

If the blood culture isolate is susceptible to cefazolin and the patient has no allergy to beta-lactam antibiotics, we recommend that cefazolin be prescribed. Recommended dosing strategies include 20 mg/kg (rounded to the nearest 500-mg increment) administered after each hemodialysis treatment or 2 g administered after each hemodialysis treatment.[87] It is hoped that use of cefazolin for susceptible strains of *S. aureus* will limit the emergence of vancomycin resistance. In 1999, strains of *S. aureus* with intermediate resistance to vancomycin were reported in two patients on chronic dialysis.[88,89] Both were treated with a prolonged course of vancomycin therapy for MRSA infections. It was hypothesized that prolonged exposure to vancomycin in the presence of prosthetic material led to the emergence of vancomycin resistance.

Congestive Heart Failure

High-output congestive heart failure may develop in patients with underlying ventricular dysfunction if fistular flow exceeds 20 percent of cardiac output.[90] Reduction of fistular flow by banding or interposition of a tapered synthetic segment[91–93] may be of benefit; ligation should be performed if heart failure is intractable.

Hand Ischemia

Hand ischemia following native or synthetic fistula placement may be due to either arterial insufficiency or venous hypertension. Arterial insufficiency is due to direct shunting of arterial blood through the low-resistance conduit and to vascular steal, in which blood flows retrograde from the palmar arch through the radial artery into the fistula.[94] Ischemic symptoms generally lessen in severity in the weeks following access placement; a period of careful observation and conservative management is warranted. Reduction of fistular blood flow by banding or interposition of a tapered synthetic graft[91–93] is occasionally effective in the treatment of severe symptoms, such as coldness or weakness of the hand. In addition, the distal revascularization-interval ligation (DRIL) technique can be effective in alleviating hand ischemia.[95,96] Fistula takedown should be performed if symptoms are intractable or if limb viability is threatened.

Venous hypertension occurs when the pressure in the venous system of the hand approaches the arterial pressure.[94,97] A proximal venous stenosis or occlusion may result in retrograde flow and arterialization of the distal venous system. Such a phenomenon typically occurs with a side-to-side anastomosis of the radial artery and cephalic vein. Ligation of the distal vein combined with excision of the venous stenosis may allow preservation of the fistula.

Aneurysms and Pseudoaneurysms

True aneurysms of primary fistulas are common and generally cause no problems. Surgical intervention is required if there is compromise of the arterial anastomosis, infection, embolism, or rupture.[98,99] Because wall stress increases with increasing diameter of the aneurysm (law of Laplace), the nephrologist should request surgical evaluation of expanding aneurysms.

Pseudoaneurysms may complicate the life of a PTFE graft because of progressive damage to the graft material and the resultant difficulty in sealing needle puncture sites. Pseudoaneurysms may expand rapidly or threaten the integrity of the overlying skin. In these cases, surgical intervention may prevent hemorrhage. Surgical treatment consists of excision of the involved graft segment followed by placement of an interposition graft.

Prospective Identification of Venous Stenoses

Venous stenoses increase intraaccess pressure and decrease access blood flow. Ultimately, the access may fail. Roughly 90 percent of access thromboses are associated with venous stenoses.[29,56–58] Prospective detection of venous stenoses followed by either percutaneous transluminal angioplasty (PTA) or surgical revision decreases access thrombosis rates and prolongs access survival.[57,59,100–104] The methods by which one may prospectively identify venous stenoses are described below. Many areas of uncertainty remain, however. Published studies have yielded conflicting results, and many studies lack proper controls. The optimal surveillance program for the prospective detection of venous stenoses has not yet been identified.

Physical Evidence. Arm edema is a common sign of subclavian stenosis; difficult cannulation of a synthetic graft may indicate intragraft stenosis.[62] Prolonged bleeding after hemodialysis may indicate venous stenosis. Physical examination may be used to estimate access blood flow.[105] A thrill at the arterial, midgraft, and venous segments is associated with an access blood flow rate greater than 450 mL/min. A pulse without a thrill is associated with a lower access blood flow rate.

Dynamic Venous Dialysis Pressure. Dynamic venous dialysis pressure denotes venous dialysis pressure in the presence of extracorporeal blood flow. The measurement of dynamic venous dialysis pressure costs nothing and may be performed during each hemodialysis treatment. Ideally, an elevated dynamic venous dialysis pressure would simply reflect elevated intraaccess pressure from outflow obstruction. In reality, dynamic venous dialysis pressure also depends on needle gauge and the extracorporeal blood flow rate. These factors must therefore be held constant. It is recommended that dynamic venous dialysis pressure be measured through 15-gauge needles at an extracorporeal blood-flow rate of 200 mL/min within the first 5 minutes of the hemodialysis treatment. Because different hemodialysis machines have different pressure monitors and different types and lengths of tubing, each hemodialysis unit must establish its own threshold pressure.

Threshold dynamic venous dialysis pressures range from 125 to 150 mmHg.[106] Dynamic venous dialysis pressure should be measured during each hemodialysis treatment. If the dynamic venous dialysis pressure exceeds the threshold during three consecutive treatments or if it is clearly increasing, fistulography should be performed and any venous stenosis should be treated. The efficacy of this strategy in prolonging graft patency has been confirmed by numerous investigators.[57–59,101,107]

Static Venous Dialysis Pressure. Static venous dialysis pressure denotes venous dialysis pressure in the absence of extracorporeal blood flow. It may be measured by inserting a stopcock-transducer system between the venous needle and the venous blood line. Besarab and colleagues measured static venous dialysis pressure in this manner and requested fistulography if static venous dialysis pressure/systolic blood pressure was > 0.4.[100] Angioplasty was performed if the stenosis reduced the luminal diameter by more than 50 percent. As this approach evolved, the angioplasty rate at their institution increased 13-fold, the thrombosis rate increased 70 percent, and the access replacement rate decreased 79 percent. A drawback of static venous dialysis pressure monitoring is that special equipment is required. Some investigators have found surveillance programs using static venous dialysis pressure monitoring to be ineffective.[108] A new static intraaccess pressure surveillance is detailed in the most recent *Clinical Practice Guidelines for Vascular Access.*[109]

Access Blood Flow. The chief determinant of vascular access patency is access blood flow. Sequential measurement of access blood flow has therefore been proposed as the preferred method for monitoring vascular accesses. Doppler evaluation, magnetic resonance imaging, and ultrasound dilution are techniques that may be used to measure access blood flow rates.

In synthetic grafts, Doppler blood flow <450 mL/min had a sensitivity of 83 percent and a specificity of 75 percent for the occurrence of graft thrombosis with 2 to 6 weeks.[110] Other investigators reported a mean blood flow rate of 307 mL/min in synthetic grafts that thrombosed within 2 weeks and mean blood flow rate of 849 mL/min in grafts that remained patent.[48] Unfortunately, Doppler blood-flow monitoring has several drawbacks that have precluded its widespread use: *interobserver* variability of measurements is considerable; measurements cannot be performed during the hemodialysis treatment because of interference from the hemodialysis needles. Magnetic resonance measurements of access flow[111] are accurate but expensive, therefore this technique is not in widespread use.

Access blood flow may also be measured by ultrasound dilution, conductance dilution, or thermal dilution. The ultrasound dilution technique has been used by numerous investigators. This technique is performed as follows[112,113]: The hemodialysis blood lines are reversed, the blood pump is set at a rate of 300 mL/min, and ultrafiltration is turned off. A bolus of isotonic saline is injected into the venous port. The velocity of ultrasound in blood is determined chiefly by the blood protein concentration. The isotonic saline bolus dilutes blood protein and changes the sound velocity in proportion to the concentration of injected saline in the blood. An ultrasound flow sensor on the arterial line permits measurement of the extracorporeal blood flow rate by a transit-time method. In addition, this sensor detects saline dilution of the blood by measuring the velocity of an ultrasound beam. These measurements permit calculation of access blood flow. The ultrasound dilution technique may be performed during the hemodialysis treatment.

Recent studies have demonstrated the efficacy of access blood-flow monitoring using the ultrasound dilution technique. At our institution, access blood flow measurements are performed monthly.[114] Fistulography is performed if access blood flow is <600 mL/min or access blood flow falls by 20 percent and is <1000 mL/min. Using this protocol, all patients who agreed to fistulography were found to have significant access stenosis. PTA increased access blood flow by at least 20 percent in 80 percent of cases. The thrombosis rate for patients in this study was lower than that for historical controls. There were 10 episodes of access thrombosis during the study; 8 occurred in patients who refused fistulography or surgical revision following unsuccessful PTA. Another group of investigators reported that monitoring of vascular access blood flow using a similar protocol reduced thrombosis rates for both synthetic grafts and primary arteriovenous fistulas.[115] These investigators also found that the access blood-flow monitoring program—by reducing hospitalizations, missed hemodialysis treatments, catheter placements, and surgical interventions—substantially reduced the cost of care. In this study, access blood flow monitoring was superior to dynamic venous dialysis pressure monitoring. Other investigators, however, have reported that access surveillance using blood-flow monitoring, when compared to surveillance using dynamic venous dialysis pressure monitoring, increases the detection of venous stenoses but does not prolong access patency.[116] These investigators suggest that better treatment of venous stenoses is necessary if the full potential of access surveillance using blood-flow monitoring is to be realized.

Treatment of Venous Stenoses and Access Thrombosis

PTA is an effective treatment for venous stenoses (Fig. 2–5). Dilatation of hemodynamically significant venous stenoses prolongs access survival.[57,59,100,101] Hospitalization is not required, and hemodialysis may be performed immediately after the procedure. PTA is more effective when

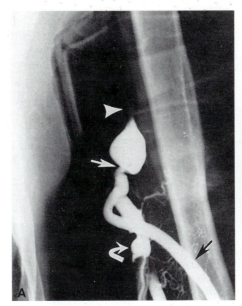
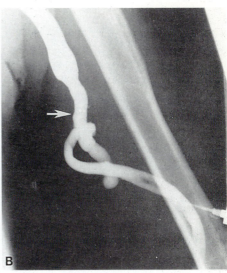

Figure 2–5. Stenosis at vein-graft anastomosis *(A)* before and *(B)* after percutaneous transluminal angioplasty. *(Reprinted with permission from Schwab SJ, Saeed M, Sussman SK, et al. Transluminal angioplasty of venous stenoses in polytetrafluoroethylene vascular access grafts.* Kidney Int *1987;32:395–398.)*

combined with an access surveillance program; patency rates are far higher for stenotic accesses angioplastied before thrombosis than for accesses angioplastied at the time of thrombolysis.[57,117–119] Surgical revision is also an effective treatment for venous stenoses. This approach, however, requires hospitalization and, by extending the access up the arm, may sacrifice a segment of vein suitable for future access construction. Studies comparing PTA and surgical revision have yielded conflicting results.[120,121]

PTA may be employed for vein-graft anastomotic lesions, proximal vein lesions, central vein lesions (Fig. 2–6), and intragraft lesions. Long (6- to 40-cm) venous stenoses and complete venous occlusions are also amenable to angioplasty.[62] Initial technical success is achieved in 82 to 94 percent of cases. In a large and carefully studied series, a successful treatment was defined as one that maintained graft patency and did not have to be repeated; success rates were 61 percent at 6 months and 38 percent at 1 year.[62] Success rates for repeat treatments were no different than success rates for initial treatments. Other investigators have reported similar results.[57,59,122–127]

Percutaneously placed endovascular stents may be used in combination with PTA for the treatment of venous stenoses. A randomized trial comparing PTA with PTA plus endovascular stenting for the treatment of vein-graft anastomotic lesions demonstrated that stenting offered no benefit.[128] Endovascular stenting should be reserved for elastic stenoses. A study performed at our institution examined the use of stents in the treatment of central venous stenoses.[129] Endovascular stenting delayed recurrence of elastic stenoses but was not helpful in the treatment of nonelastic lesions.

Once access thrombosis occurs, surgical thrombectomy, pharmacomechanical thrombolysis, or mechanical

thrombolysis may be performed. These approaches are more effective in the treatment of thrombosed synthetic grafts than in the treatment of thrombosed endogenous fistulas.[130] Regardless of the approach, treatment of the venous stenosis is necessary. Palder and colleagues demonstrated that surgical thrombectomy combined with bypass of the venous stenosis (Fig. 2–7) produced significantly longer patency than did simple thrombectomy or patch an-

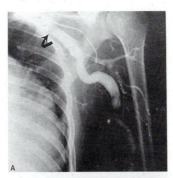
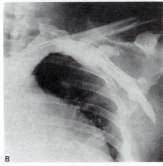

Figure 2–6. Subclavian vein stenosis *(A)* before and *(B)* after percutaneous transluminal angioplasty. *(Reprinted with permission from Schwab SJ, Quarles LD, Middleton JP, et al. Hemodialysis-associated subclavian vein stenosis.* Kidney Int *1988;33:1156–1159.)*

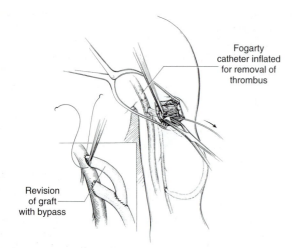

Fogarty
catheter inflated
for removal of
thrombus

Revision
of graft
with bypass

Figure 2–7. Thrombectomy of PTFE graft and bypass of venous stenosis. *(Reprinted with permission from Stickel DL. Renal dialysis access procedures. In: Sabiston DC Jr, ed.* Atlas of General Surgery. *Philadelphia: Saunders, 1994:90–98.)*

gioplasty.[29] Others have reported that surgical thrombectomy combined with PTA is as effective as surgical thrombectomy combined with surgical revision.[131]

In the technique of pharmacomechanical thrombolysis (pulse-spray thrombolysis),[118,132] angiography is performed to determine the extent of the thrombus and to image the graft and draining veins. Two catheters with closely spaced side holes are inserted into the midportion of the graft in a crossed manner, and a thrombolytic agent is "sprayed" into the clot under high pressure. Thrombolysis is achieved by both pharmacologic and mechanical means. An angioplasty balloon is then used to macerate residual thrombus and dilate the venous stenosis. In the technique of mechanical thrombolysis,[118] no thrombolytic agent is used; thrombolysis is achieved by mechanical means. Saline is injected through a pulse-spray catheter to macerate the thrombus, and an angioplasty balloon is then used to macerate residual thrombus and to dilate the venous stenosis. These techniques may be performed in 1 to 2 hours, and the graft may be used immediately for hemodialysis. These techniques appear to be equally effective. Initial success rates are excellent and 90-day unassisted patency rates are roughly 30 to 48 percent.[118,132–135]

Surgical thrombectomy and revision may produce a similar patency rate,[136,137] but surgical treatment may entail delays, hospitalization, and extension of the access up the extremity. The decision as to whether an individual patient should be treated by surgical thrombectomy or by a percutaneous technique should be guided by the expertise of the institution's vascular surgeons and vascular radiologists. No one technique can be recommended over the others.

Pharmacologic Methods for the Prevention of Access Thrombosis. Pharmacologic prevention of access thrombosis has heretofore been disappointing. Two studies have found that the antiplatelet agent ticlopidine reduces thrombosis rates of native arteriovenous fistulas in the first postoperative month.[138,139] A prospective, randomized study suggested that dipyridamole decreases the thrombosis rate for new synthetic grafts but that aspirin does not.[140] In a small randomized trial, fish oil at a dose of 4000 mg daily increased the patency rate for PTFE grafts.[141] Proposed mechanisms of action for fish oil include inhibition of cyclooxygenase and of neointimal hyperplasia. In a retrospective study of synthetic graft survival, it was found that therapy with an angiotensin-converting enzyme (ACE) inhibitor was associated with a higher graft survival rate.[142] In animal models, angiotensin II induces smooth muscle proliferation; by reducing smooth muscle proliferation, ACE inhibitors may inhibit neointimal hyperplasia. A recent study comparing aspirin plus clopidogrel to placebo in patients with synthetic grafts was halted because of an increased risk of bleeding in those receiving clopidogrel and aspirin.[143] Large, randomized controlled trials are under way which will assess the efficacy of clopidogrel in maintaining primary fistula patency and the efficacy of dipyridamole/aspirin in maintaining synthetic graft patency.

SUMMARY

Double-lumen central venous catheters are the preferred vascular access devices for acute hemodialysis. Insertion complications become much less likely as the operator gains experience. Although catheter-related infection remains a major problem, measures may be undertaken that will decrease its likelihood. Catheter thrombosis is a very frequent complication but may be successfully managed by the instillation of human tissue plasminogen activator into the catheter lumens or by replacement of the catheter over a guidewire. Because of the association of subclavian vein catheterization with subsequent subclavian vein stenosis, subclavian vein catheterization should be avoided in those patients in whom native fistula or synthetic graft placement is anticipated.

The morbidity of a maintenance hemodialysis patient is in large part determined by the ability of the nephrologists, vascular surgeon, and vascular radiologist to establish and maintain adequate vascular access. Primary arteriovenous fistulas are the preferred form of vascular access because they are the more likely to provide long-term complication-free hemodialysis access. Careful planning months before the anticipated need for hemodialysis will maximize the chance for successful primary arteriovenous fistula creation. If an endogenous fistula cannot be created, a synthetic graft should be placed. The use of tunneled cuffed catheters are permanent vascular access should be avoided if possible.

Once vascular access is established, maintaining its patency is a challenge. Thrombosis is the leading cause of vascular access loss, and venous stenoses are the leading cause of vascular access thrombosis. Prospective detection of venous outflow obstruction may be accomplished by serial measurements of venous dialysis pressures or by serial measurements of access blood flow rates. Correction of venous stenoses detected in this manner will prolong access patency. We await a safe and effective approach to the pharmacologic prevention of venous stenosis.

REFERENCES

1. Quinton W, Dillard D, Scribner BH. Cannulation of blood vessels for prolonged hemodialysis. *ASAIO Trans* 1960;6:104.
2. Kelber J, Delmez JA, Windus DW. Factors affecting the delivery of high-efficiency dialysis using temporary vascular access. *Am J Kidney Dis* 1993;22:24–29.
3. Sznajder JI, Zveibil FR, Bitterman H, et al. Central vein catheterization: failure and complication rates by three percutaneous approaches. *Arch Intern Med* 1986;146:259–261.
4. Stuart RK, Shikora SA, Akerman P, et al. Incidence of arrhythmia with central venous catheter insertion and exchange. *JPEN* 1990;14:152–155.
5. Brothers TE, Von Moll LK, Neiderhuber JE, et al. Experience with subcutaneous infusion ports in three hundred patients. *Surg Gynecol Obstet* 1988;166:295–301.
6. Goldfarb G, Lebrec D. Percutaneous cannulation of the internal jugular vein in patients with coagulopathies: an experience based on 1,000 attempts. *Anesthesiology* 1982;56:321–323.
7. Vanholder R, Hoenich N, Ringoir S. Morbidity and mortality of central venous catheter hemodialysis: a review of 10 years' experience. *Nephron* 1987;47:274–279.
8. Vanherweghem JL, Cabolet P, Dhaene M, et al. Complications related to subclavian catheters for hemodialysis. *Am J Nephrol* 1986;6:339–345.
9. Uldall PR. Temporary vascular access for hemodialysis. In: Nissenson AR, Fine RN, eds. *Dialysis Therapy*. 2d ed. Philadelphia: Hanley & Belfus, 1993:5–10.
10. Briscoe CE, Bushman JA, McDonald WI. Extensive neurological damage after cannulation of the internal jugular vein. *Br Med J* 1984;288:1195–1196.
11. Blitt CD, Wright WA. An unusual complication of percutaneous internal jugular vein cannulation: puncture of an endotracheal cuff. *Anesthesiology* 1974;40:306–307.
12. Butsch JL, Butsch WL, Derosa JFT. Bilateral vocal cord paralysis: a complication of percutaneous cannulation of the internal jugular vein. *Arch Surg* 1976;111:828–829.
13. Hartle E, Conlon P, Carstens R, Schwab SJ. Ultrasound guided cannulation of the femoral vein for acute hemodialysis access (abstr). *J Am Soc Nephrol* 1993;4:352.
14. Cheesbrough JS, Finch RG, Burden RP. A prospective study of the mechanisms of infection associated with hemodialysis catheters. *J Infect Dis* 1986;154:579–589.
15. Maki DG, Weise CE, Sarafin HW. A semiquantitative culture method for identifying intravenous-catheter-related infection. *N Engl J Med* 1977;296:1305–1309.
16. Oliver MJ, Callery SM, Thorpe KE, et al. Risk of bacteremia from temporary hemodialysis catheters by site of insertion and duration of use: a prospective study. *Kidney Int* 2000;58:2543–2545.
17. Maki DG, Ringer M, Alvarado CJ. Prospective randomized trial of povidone-iodine, alcohol, and chlorhexidine for prevention of infection associated with central venous and arterial catheters. *Lancet* 1991;338:339–343.
18. Levin A, Mason AJ, Jindal KK, et al. Prevention of hemodialysis subclavian vein catheter infection by topical povidone-iodine. *Kidney Int* 1991;40:934–938.
19. Conly JM, Grieves K, Peters B. A prospective, randomized study comparing transparent and dry gauze dressings for central venous catheters. *J Infect Dis* 1989;159:310–319.
20. Ponec D, Irwin D, Haire WD, et al, for the COOL Investigators. Recombinant tissue plasminogen activator (alteplase) for restoration of flow in occluded central venous access devices—a double-blind placebo-controlled trial: the Cardiovascular thrombolytic to Open Occluded Lines (COOL) efficacy trial. *J Vasc Intervent Radiol* 2001;12:951–955.
21. Brismar B, Hardstedt C, Jacobson S. Diagnosis of thrombosis by catheter phlebography after prolonged central venous catheterization. *Ann Surg* 1981;194:779–783.
22. Davis D, Petersen J, Feldman R, et al. Subclavian venous stenosis: a complication of subclavian dialysis. *JAMA* 1984;252:3404–3406.
23. Fant GF, Dennis VW, Quarles LD. Late vascular complication of the subclavian dialysis catheter. *Am J Kidney Dis* 1986;3:225–228.
24. Barrett N, Spencer S, McIvor J, Brown EA. Subclavian stenosis: a major complication of subclavian dialysis catheters. *Nephrol Dial Transplant* 1988;3:423–425.
25. Cimochowski GE, Worley E, Rutherford WE, et al. Superiority of the internal jugular over the subclavian access for temporary dialysis. *Nephron* 1990;54:154–161.
26. Schillinger F, Schillinger D, Montagnac R, Milcent T. Postcatheterisation vein stenosis in haemodialysis: comparative angiographic study of 50 subclavian and 50 internal jugular accesses. *Nephrol Dial Transplant* 1991;6:722–724.
27. Schwab SJ, Quarles LD, Middleton JP, et al. Hemodialysis-associated subclavian vein stenosis. *Kidney Int* 1988;33:1156–1159.
28. Brescia MJ, Cimino JE, Appel K, Hurwich BJ. Chronic hemodialysis using venipuncture and a surgically created arteriovenous fistula. *N Engl J Med* 1966;275:1089–1092.
29. Palder SB, Kirkman RL, Wittemore AD, et al. Vascular access for hemodialysis: patency rates and results of revision. *Ann Surg* 1985;202:235-239.
30. Winsett OE, Wolma FJ. Complications of vascular access for hemodialysis. *South Med J* 1985;78:513–517.
31. Schwab SJ, Buller GL, McCann RL, et al. Prospective evaluation of a Dacron cuffed hemodialysis catheter for prolonged use. *Am J Kidney Dis* 1988;11:166–169.
32. Shusterman NH, Kloss K, Mullen JL. Successful use of double-lumen, silicone rubber catheters for permanent hemodialysis access. *Kidney Int* 1989;35:887–890.

33. Moss AH, Vasilakis C, Holley JL, et al. Use of a silicone dual-lumen catheter with a Dacron cuff as a long-term vascular access for hemodialysis patients. *Am J Kidney Dis* 1990;16:211-215.

34. Gibson SP, Mosquera D. Five years experience with Quinton Permcath for vascular access. *Nephrol Dial Transplant* 1991;6:269–274.

35. DeMeester J, Vanholder R, Ringole S. Factors affecting catheter and technique survival in permanent silicone single lumen dialysis catheters (abstr). *J Am Soc Nephrol* 1992;3:361.

36. Suhocki P, Conlon P, Knelson M, et al. Silastic cuffed catheters for hemodialysis vascular access: thrombolytic and mechanical correction of malfunction. *Am J Kidney Dis* 1996;28:379–386.

37. Beathard GA, Posen GA. Initial clinical results with the LifeSite Hemodialysis Access System. *Kidney Int* 2000;58:2221–2227.

38. Schwab SJ, Weiss MA, Rushton F, et al. Multicenter clinic trial results with the LifeSite hemodialysis access system. *Kidney Int* 2002;62:1026–1033.

39. Levin NW, Yang PM, Hatch DA, et al. Initial results of a new access device for hemodialysis. *Kidney Int* 1998;54:1739–1745.

40. Canaud B, My H, Morena M, et al. Dialock: a new vascular access device for extracorporeal renal replacement therapy. Preliminary clinical results. *Nephrol Dial Transplant* 1999;14:692–698.

41. Stone WJ, Hakim RM. Therapeutic options in the management of end-stage renal disease. In: Jacobson HR, Striker GE, Klahr S, eds. *The Principles and Practice of Nephrology.* Philadelphia: Decker, 1991:736–739.

42. *NKF-K/DOQI Clinical Practice Guidelines for Vascular Access.* New York: National Kidney Foundation, 2001:24–27.

43. Allon M, Lockhart ME, Lilly RZ, et al. Effect of preoperative sonographic mapping on vascular access outcomes in hemodialysis patients. *Kidney Int* 2001;60:2013–2020.

44. Gibson KD, Caps MT, Kohler TR, et al. Assessment of a policy to reduce placement of prosthetic hemodialysis access. *Kidney Int* 2001;59:2335–2345.

45. Oliver MJ, McCann RL, Indridason OS, et al. Comparison of transposed brachiobasilic fistulas to upper arm grafts and brachiocephalic fistulas. *Kidney Int* 2001;60:1532–1539.

46. Anderson CB, Etheredge EE, Harter HR, et al. Blood flow measurements in arteriovenous dialysis fistulas. *Surgery* 1977;81:459–461.

47. Burdick JF, Scott W, Cosimi AB. Experience with Dacron graft arteriovenous fistulas for dialysis access. *Ann Surg* 1978;187:262–266.

48. Rittgers SE, Garcia-Valdez C, McCormick JT, Posner MP. Noninvasive blood flow measurement in expanded polytetrafluoroethylene grafts for hemodialysis access. *J Vasc Surg* 1986;3:635–642.

49. Kherlakian GM, Roedersheimer LR, Arbaugh JJ, et al. Comparison of autogenous fistula versus expanded polytetrafluoroethylene graft fistula for angioaccess in hemodialysis. *Am J Surg* 1986;152:238–243.

50. Munda R, First MR, Alexander JW, et al. Polytetrafluoroethylene graft survival in hemodialysis. *JAMA* 1983;249:219–222.

51. Tordoir JHM, Herman JMMPH, Kwan TS, Diderich PM. Long-term follow-up of the polytetrafluoroethylene (PTFE) prosthesis as an arteriovenous fistula for haemodialysis. *Eur J Vasc Surg* 1987;2:3–7.

52. Raju S. PTFE grafts for hemodialysis access: techniques for insertion and management of complications. *Ann Surg* 1987;206:666–673.

53. Tellis VA, Kohlberg WI, Bhat DJ, et al. Expanded polytetrafluoroethylene graft fistula for chronic hemodialysis. *Ann Surg* 1979;189:101–105.

54. Lund GB, Trerotola SO, Scheel PF, et al. Outcome of tunneled hemodialysis catheters placed by radiologists. *Radiology* 1996;198:467–472.

55. Schwab SJ. Hemodialysis vascular access. In: Jacobson HR, Striker GE, Klahr S, eds. *The Principles and Practices of Nephrology.* Philadelphia: Decker, 1991:766–772.

56. Etheredge EE, Haid SD, Maeser MN, et al. Salvage operations for malfunctioning polytetrafluoroethylene hemodialysis access grafts. *Surgery* 1983;94:464–470.

57. Beathard GA. Percutaneous angioplasty for the treatment of venous stenosis: a nephrologist's view. *Semin Dial* 1995;8:166–170.

58. Beathard GA. Percutaneous therapy of vascular access dysfunction: optimal management of access stenosis and thrombosis. *Semin Dial* 1994;7:165–167.

59. Schwab SJ, Raymond JR, Saeed M, et al. Prevention of hemodialysis fistula thrombosis. Early detection of venous stenoses. *Kidney Int* 1989;36:707–711.

60. Bone GE, Pomajzl MJ. Management of dialysis fistula thrombosis. *Am J Surg* 1979;138:901–906.

61. Carty GA, Davis VH. Mid-graft stenosis in expanded polytetrafluoroethylene hemodialysis conduits. *Dial Transplant* 1990;19:486–489.

62. Beathard GA. Percutaneous transvenous angioplasty in the treatment of vascular access stenosis. *Kidney Int* 1992;42:1390–1397.

63. Roy-Chaudhury P, Kelly BS, Miller MA, et al. Venous neointimal hyperplasia in polytetrafluoroethylene dialysis grafts. *Kidney Int* 2001;59:2325–2334.

64. *NKF-K/DOQI Clinical Practice Guidelines for Vascular Access.* New York: National Kidney Foundation, 2001:70.

65. Bhat DJ, Tellis VA, Kohlberg WI, et al. Management of sepsis involving expanded polytetrafluoroethylene grafts for hemodialysis access. *Surgery* 1980;87:445–450.

66. Keane WF, Shapiro FL, Raji L. Incidence and type of infections occurring in 445 chronic hemodialysis patients. *ASAIO Trans* 1977;23:41–46.

67. Dobkin JF, Miller MH, Steigbigel NH. Septicemia in patients on chronic hemodialysis. Ann Intern Med 1987;88:28–33.

68. Higgins RM. Infections in a renal unit. *Q J Med* 1989;70:41–51.

69. Kaplowitz LG, Comstock JA, Landwehr DM, et al. A prospective study of infections in hemodialysis patients: pa-

tient hygiene and other risk factors for infection. *Infect Control Hosp Epidemiol* 1988;9:534-541.

70. O'Brien TF. Infection in dialysis and transplant patients. In: Tilney NL, Lazarus JM, eds. *Surgical Care of the Patient with Renal Failure*. Philadelphia: Saunders, 1982:67–97.

71. Morgan AP, Knight DC, Tilney NL, Lazarus JM. Femoral triangle sepsis in dialysis patients. *Ann Surg* 1980;191: 460–464.

72. *NKF-K/DOQI Clinic Practice Guidelines for Vascular Access*. New York: National Kidney Foundation, 2001:69.

73. Tanriover B, Carlton D, Saddekni S, et al. Bacteremia associated with tunneled dialysis catheters: comparison of two treatment strategies. *Kidney Int* 2000;57:2151–2155.

74. Swartz RD, Messana JM, Boyer CJ, et al. Successful use of cuffed central venous hemodialysis catheters inserted percutaneously. *J Am Soc Nephrol* 1994;4:1719–1725.

75. Marr KA, Sexton DJ, Conlon PJ, et al. Catheter-related bacteremia and outcome of attempted catheter salvage in patients undergoing hemodialysis. *Ann Intern Med* 1997;127: 275–280.

76. Beathard GA. Management of bacteremia associated with tunneled-cuffed hemodialysis catheters. *J Am Soc Nephrol* 1999;10:1045–1049.

77. Robinson DL, Fowler VG, Sexton DJ, et al. Bacterial endocarditis in hemodialysis patients. *Am J Kidney Dis* 1997;30:521–524.

78. Rosen AB, Fowler VG, Corey GR, et al. Cost-effectiveness of transesophageal echocardiography to determine the duration of therapy for intravascular catheter-associated *Staphylococcus aureus* bacteremia. *Ann Intern Med* 1999;130: 810–820.

79. Shaffer D. Catheter-related sepis complicating long-term, tunneled central venous dialysis catheters: management by guidewire exchange. *Am J Kidney Dis* 1995;25:593–596.

80. *NKF-K/DOQI Clinical Practice Guidelines for Vascular Access*. New York: National Kidney Foundation, 2001:71–72.

81. Krishnasami Z, Carlton D, Bimbo L, et al. Management of hemodialysis catheter-related bacteremia with an adjunctive antibiotic lock solution. *Kidney Int* 2002;61:1136–1142.

82. Kovalik EC, Raymond JR, Albers FJ, et al. A clustering of epidural abscesses in chronic hemodialysis patients: risks of salvaging access catheters in cases of infection. *J Am Soc Nephrol* 1996;7:2264–2267.

83. Berkoben M, Provenzale J. A hemodialysis patient with excruciating back pain. *Semin Dial* 1996;286–288.

84. Johnson DW, MacGinley R, Kay TD, et al. A randomized controlled trial of topical exit site mupirocin application in patients with tunneled, cuffed haemodialysis catheters. *Nephrol Dial Transplant* 2002;17:1802–1807.

85. Lok CE, Stanley KE, Hux JE, et al. Hemodialysis infection prevention polysporin ointment. *J Am Soc Nephrol* 2003;13: 169–179.

86. Barth RH, DeVincenzo N. Use of vancomycin in high-flux hemodialysis: experience with 130 courses of therapy. *Kidney Int* 1996;50:929–936.

87. Marx MA, Frye RF, Matzke GR, Golper TA. Cefazolin as empiric therapy in hemodialysis-related infections: efficacy

and blood concentrations. *Am J Kidney Dis* 1998;32: 410–414.

88. Smith TL, Pearson ML, Wilcox KR, et al. Emergence of vancomycin resistance in *Staphylococcus aureus*. *N Engl J Med* 1999;340:493–501.

89. Sieradzki K, Roberts RB, Haber SW, Tomasz A. The development of vancomycin resistance in a patient with methicillin-resistant Staphylococcus aureus infection. *N Engl J Med* 1999;340:517–523.

90. Anderson CB, Codd JR, Graff RA, et al. Cardiac failure and upper extremity arteriovenous dialysis fistulas. *Arch Intern Med* 1976;136:292–297.

91. West JC, Bertsch DJ, Petersen SL, et al. Arterial insufficiency in hemodialysis access procedures: correction by "banding" technique. *Trans Proc* 1991;23:1838–1840.

92. Rivers SP, Scher LA, Veith FJ. Correction of steal syndrome secondary to hemodialysis access fistulas: a simplified quantitative technique. *Surgery* 1992;112:593–597.

93. Kirkman RL. Technique for flow reduction in dialysis access fistulas. *Surg Gynecol Obstet* 1991;172:231–233.

94. Tawa NE, Tilney NL. Angioaccess in the renal failure patient. In: Maher JF, ed. *Replacement of Renal Function by Dialysis*. 3d ed. Boston, MA: Kluwer, 1989:218–228.

95. Schanzer H, Schwartz M, Harrington E, Haimov M. Treatment of ischaemia due to "steal" by arteriovenous fistula with distal artery ligation and revascularization. *J Vasc Surg* 1998; 7:770–773.

96. Knox RC, Berman SS, Hughes JD, et al. Distal revascularization-interval ligation: a durable and effective treatment for ischemic steal syndrome after hemodialysis access. *J Vasc Surg* 2002;36:250–256.

97. Bell PRF, Veitch PS. Vascular access for hemodialysis. In: Nissenson AR, Fine RN, Gentile DE, eds. *Clinical Dialysis*, 2d ed. Norwalk, CT: Appleton & Lange, 1990:26–44.

98. *NKF-K/DOQI Clinical Practice Guidelines for Vascular Access*. New York: National Kidney Foundation, 2001:74.

99. Konner K, Nonnast-Daniel B, Ritz E. The arteriovenous fistula. *J Am Soc Nephrol* 2003;14: 1669–1680.

100. Besarab A, Sullivan KL, Ross RP, Moritz MJ. Utility of intra-access pressure monitoring in detecting and correcting venous outlet stenoses prior to thrombosis. *Kidney Int* 1995;47:1364–1373.

101. Burger H, Zijlstra JJ, Kluchert SA, et al. Percutaneous transluminal angioplasty improves longevity in fistulae and shunts for hemodialysis. *Nephrol Dial Transplant* 1990;5: 608–611.

102. Todoir JHM, Hoeneveld H, Eikelboom BC, Kitslaar PJEHM. The correlation between clinical and duplex ultrasound parameters and the development of complications in arteriovenous fistulae for hemodialysis. *Eur J Vasc Surg* 1990;4:179–184.

103. Sands JJ, Miranda CL. Prolongation of hemodialysis access survival with elective revision. *Clin Nephrol* 1995;44: 329–333.

104. Anderson CB, Gilula LA, Harter HR, Etheredge EE. Venous angiography and surgical management of subcutaneous hemodialysis fistulas. *Ann Surg* 1978;187:194–204.

105. Trerotola SO, Scheel PJ, Powe NR, et al. Screening for access graft malfunctions: comparison of physical examination with US. *J Vasc Intervent Radiol* 1996;7:15–20.

106. *NKF-K/DOQI Clinical Practice Guidelines for Vascular Access.* New York: National Kidney Foundation, 2001:41.

107. Safa AA, Valji K, Roberts AC, et al. Detection and treatment of dysfunctional hemodialysis access grafts: effects of a surveillance program on graft patency and the incidence of thrombosis. *Radiology* 1996;199:653–657.

108. Dember LM, Holmberg EF, Kaufman JS. Valve of static venous pressure for predicting arteriovenous graft thrombosis. *Kidney Int* 2002;61:1899–1904.

109. *NKF-K/DOQI Clinical Practice Guidelines for Vascular Access.* New York: National Kidney Foundation, 2001:39–40.

110. Shackleton CR, Taylor DC, Buckley AR, et al. Predicting failure in polytetrafluoroethylene vascular access grafts for hemodialysis: a pilot study. *Can J Surg* 1987;30:442-444.

111. Oudenhoven LFIJ, Pattynama PMT, DeRoos A, et al. Magnetic resonance, a new method for measuring blood flow in hemodialysis fistulae. *Kidney Int* 1994;45:884–889.

112. Krivitsky NM. Theory and validation of access flow measurement by dilution technique during hemodialysis. *Kidney Int* 1995;48:244–250.

113. Depner TA, Krivitsky NM. Clinical measurement of blood flow in hemodialysis access fistulae and grafts by ultrasound dilution. *ASAIO J* 1995;41:M745–M749.

114. Schwab SJ, Oliver MJ, Suhocki P, McCann R. Hemodialysis arteriovenous access: detection of stenosis and response to treatment by vascular access blood flow. *Kidney Int* 2001;59:358–362.

115. McCarley P, Wingard RL, Shyr Y, et al. Vascular access blood flow monitoring reduces access morbidity and costs. *Kidney Int* 2001;60:1164–1172.

116. Moist LM, Churchill DN, House AA, et al. Regular monitoring of access flow compared with monitoring of venous pressure fails to improve graft survival. *J Am Soc Nephrol* 2003;14:2645–2653.

117. Katz SG, Kohl RD. The percutaneous treatment of angioaccess graft complications. *Am J Surg* 1995;170:238–242.

118. Beathard GA. The treatment of vascular access graft dysfunction: a nephrologist's view and experience. *Adv Ren Replace Ther* 1994;1:131–147.

119. Trerotola SO. Pulse-spray thrombolysis of hemodialysis grafts: not the final word. *Am J Roentgenol* 1995;164:1501–1503.

120. Brooks JL, Sigley RD, May KJ Jr, Mack RM. Transluminal angioplasty versus surgical repair for stenosis of hemodialysis grafts. A randomized study. *Am J Surg* 1987;153:530–531.

121. Dapunt O, Feurstein M, Rendl KH, Prenner K. Transluminal angioplasty versus surgical conventional operation in the treatment of hemodialysis fistula stenosis: results from a 5-year study. *Br J Surg* 1987;74:1004–1005.

122. Kanterman RY, Vesely TM, Pilgram TK, et al. Dialysis access grafts: anatomic location of venous stenosis and results of angioplasty. *Radiology* 1995;195:135–139.

123. Glanz S, Gordon DH, Butt KMH, et al. The role of percutaneous angioplasty in the management of chronic hemodialysis fistulas. *Ann Surg* 1987;206:777–781.

124. Glanz S, Gordon D, Butt KMH, et al. Dialysis access fistulas: treatment of stenoses by transluminal angioplasty. *Radiology* 1984;152:637–642.

125. Mori Y, Horikawa K, Sato K, et al. Stenotic lesions in vascular access: treatment with transluminal angioplasty using high-pressure balloons. *Intern Med* 1994;33:284–827.

126. Gmelin E, Winterhoff R, Rinast E. Insufficient hemodialysis access fistulas: late results of treatment with percutaneous balloon angioplasty. *Radiology* 1989;171:657–660.

127. Turmel-Rodrigues L, Pengloan J, Blanchier D, et al. Insufficient dialysis shunts: improved long-term patency rates with close hemodynamic monitoring, repeated percutaneous balloon angioplasty, and stent placement. *Radiology* 1993;187:273–278.

128. Beathard GA. Gianturco self-expanding stent in the treatment of stenosis in dialysis access grafts. *Kidney Int* 1993;43:872–877.

129. Kovalik EC, Newman GE, Suhocki P, et al. Correction of central venous stenoses: use of angioplasty and vascular Wallstents. *Kidney Int* 1994;45:1171–1181.

130. *NKF-K/DOQI Clinical Practice Guidelines for Vascular Access.* New York: National Kidney Foundation, 2001:66.

131. Schwartz CI, McBrayer CV, Sloan JH, et al. Thrombosed dialysis grafts: comparisons of treatment with transluminal angioplasty and surgical revision. *Radiology* 1995;194:337–341.

132. Valji K, Bookstein JJ, Roberts AC, Davis GB. Pharmacomechanical thrombolysis and angioplasty in the management of clotted hemodialysis grafts: early and late clinical results. *Radiology* 1991;178:243–247.

133. Beathard GA. Mechanical versus pharmacomechanical thrombolysis for the treatment of thrombosed dialysis access grafts. *Kidney Int* 1994;45:1401–1406.

134. Trerotola SO, Lund GB, Scheel PJ, et al. Thrombosed dialysis access grafts: percutaneous mechanical declotting without urokinase. *Radiology* 1995;191:721–726.

135. Middlebrook MR, Amygdalos MA, Soulen MC, et al. Thrombosed hemodialysis grafts: percutaneous mechanical balloon declotting versus thrombolysis. *Radiology* 1995;196:73–77.

136. Summers S, Drazan K, Gomes A. Urokinase therapy for thrombosed hemodialysis access grafts. *Surg Gynecol Obstet* 1993;176:534–538.

137. Beathard GA. Thrombolysis versus surgery for the treatment of thrombosed dialysis access grafts. *J Am Soc Nephrol* 1995;6:1619–1624.

138. Grontoft K, Mulec H, Gutierrez A, Olander R. Thromboprophylactic effect of ticlopidine in arteriovenous fistulas for hemodialysis. *Scand J Urol Nephrol* 1985;19:55–57.

139. Fiskerstrand CE, Thompson IW, Burnet ME, et al. Double-blind randomized trial of the effect of ticlopidine in arteriovenous fistulas for hemodialysis. *Artif Organs* 1985;9:61–63.

140. Sreedhara R, Himmelfarb J, Lazarus JM, Hakim RM. Antiplatelet therapy in graft thrombosis: results of a prospective randomized double blind study. *Kidney Int* 1994;45:1477–1483.

141. Schmitz PG, McCloud LK, Reikes ST, et al. Prophylaxis of hemodialysis graft thrombosis with fish oil: double-blind,

randomized, prospective trial. *J Am Soc Nephrol* 2002;13:184–190.

142. Gradzki R, Dhingra RK, Port FK, et al. Use of ACE inhibitors is associated with prolonged survival of arteriovenous grafts. *Am J Kidney Dis* 2001;38:1240–1244.

143. Kaufman JS, O'Connor TZ, Zhang JH, et al, for the Veterans Affairs Cooperative Study Group on Hemodialysis Access Graft Thrombosis. Randomized controlled trial of clopidogrel plus aspirin to prevent hemodialysis access graft thrombosis. *J Am Nephrol* 2003;14:2313–2321.

Technologic Aspects of Hemodialysis and Peritoneal Dialysis

Daniel Schneditz

Replacement of kidney function by a technical device is now possible for extended periods of time. There is no doubt that the quality and precision of the machines and techniques involved in this process importantly contribute to this success. A review of the progress in dialysis technology achieved during the last few years shows two major lines of development. Some ideas conceived in the early period of dialysis, such as on-line production of ultrapure dialysate, have finally reached the market. Major improvements have also been made in the control of both hemodialysis and peritoneal dialysis treatments. In this regard, the important question of whether the prescribed dose of dialysis is indeed delivered with every treatment can now be addressed with technology developed in the past few years. This will help to reduce treatment variability and system failure and improve patient and staff compliance. Other developments have expanded the concepts of feedback control present in the dialysis machine to the control of treatment delivery within the limitations presented by the individual patient.

The following presentation focuses on technical aspects related to the delivery of dialysis as well as to the measurement of effects resulting from the perturbations caused by the treatment. With so much interest in measuring treatment and patient variables and identifying the state of the patient, the extracorporeal blood circulation and the management of dialysate are described in some detail. While these components are essential for dialysis, they also provide a unique access to patient-specific information. This information, together with the definition of a treatment goal, is the basis for the feedback control in hemodialysis that is likely to guide future technical development and to involve even more aspects of dialysis treatment.

EXTRACORPOREAL CIRCULATION

The components of a dialysis apparatus consist of an extracorporeal circuit, a dialyzer where mass exchange occurs, a system to prepare and/or deliver the dialysate, a system to move the blood, safety and control mechanisms, input and output systems, and interfaces to database systems.

The extracorporeal circulation serves to move the blood between the patient's circulation and the dialyzer in a safe and efficient fashion (Fig. 3–1). The extracorporeal circulation consists of tubing of various diameters, special components such as a pump segment and drip chambers, and T-segments to connect transducers and infusions. Recently, new components have been added to measure changes in patient variables in response to treatment.

Blood Flow

In conventional and high-efficiency hemodialysis, blood is pumped from the patient via an access at a preset flow rate; it is then passed through the extracorporeal circuit, where it is processed in the dialyzer and returned to the access. The blood flow (Q_b) as well as the duration of treatment are important factors in determining the efficiency (the rate of dialysis) of the treatment and the delivered treatment dose.

The blood flow in the extracorporeal circuit is usually controlled by rotary peristaltic pumps that are operated by two or more rollers on the rotor that press against a short, flexible pumping segment within the rotor housing. With rotation, the rollers push fluid from the pump inflow to the pump outflow. During operation, at least one of the rollers completely occludes the tube at all times, preventing uncontrolled flow from the patient into the extracorporeal circuit as well as backflow of blood from the extracorporeal circulation and the dialyzer when the pump is stopped. Thus, when blood flow is stopped, the rotor in the arterial line segment acts as an arterial clamp.

With one full revolution of the rotor, two (or more) stroke volumes are pushed toward the dialyzer in a pulsatile

manner. In a simple approach, the volume flow per minute is given by the number of revolutions per minute multiplied by the stroke volumes released into the circuit, where the stroke volume is determined by the geometry of the pump and the diameter of the blood line. The diameter of most pump segments is 8 mm. With this diameter, pumps are designed to produce a unidirectional flow of up to 700 mL · min^{-1}.

The actual volume flow generated by the peristaltic pump is not independent of pressures at both the inflow and outflow sides of the pump. The actual volume flow is particularly dependent on the arterial inflow pressure, which determines the elastic recoil of the flexible tube segment following occlusion of the moving rollers. If the recoil is incomplete and the tube does not attain a circular cross section because of excessive negative pressure in the arterial inflow, the filling of the segment is reduced, along with the stroke volume. At a given tube circumference, the maximum stroke volume is obtained with a circular cross section of the tube. Any deviation from the circular shape at the same circumference reduces the cross-sectional area, the stroke volume, and the effective blood flow.[1]

A review of the laws of fluid dynamics shows that a low prepump pressure is likely to develop with a high blood flow and high resistance in the upstream parts of the arterial blood line, especially in the arterial cannula. Thus the discrepancy between set and actual delivered blood flow is more likely to develop in the high-efficiency environment, which requires high blood flows. However, since the dimensional changes in the elastic recoil of the flexible pump segment depend on arterial line pressures in a predictable fashion, it is possible to compute a corrected blood flow from the actual arterial pressure and the number of revolutions of the pump rotor. Some dialysis machines offer a correction to consider the effect caused by a reduced arterial line pressure and display a so-called effective blood flow.

On the other hand, the pressure in the outflow is determined by the resistance of downstream segments, by the force with which the rollers occlude the flexible pump segment, and by the power of the pump. The occlusion force of the rollers is usually controlled by springs, and when outflow pressure increases, the rollers will be lifted and no longer completely occlude the pump segment. In this case there is backflow of stroke volume back past the incomplete occlusion at very high shear rates, considerably enhancing the mechanical stress to all blood constituents.

A pump operating against a low inflow and high outflow pressure makes a characteristic smacking noise, probably caused by retrograde flow from the pressurized downstream line segment into the incompletely filled stroke volume (because of low arterial pressure). This indicates that the pump is no longer operating in its linear range. Whether this situation causes increased hemolysis has not been investigated.

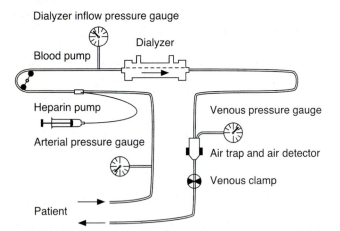

Figure 3–1. Extracorporeal circuit. The extracorporeal circuit basically consists of arterial and venous lines that include line segments for arterial and venous pressure measurements, a pump segment to be inserted into the blood pump, an infusion line for the heparin pump, special connectors for the dialyzer, and a venous drip chamber for the detection of air.

Given these limitations, the accuracy of extracorporeal pumps is in the range of ±5 percent at best. This error is important and significant when it comes to measuring clearance or quantifying the dose of the delivered treatment.

Resistance

The resistance (R, in Pa · s · m^{-3}) is described by the pressure gradient ($\Delta p = p_1 - p_2$, in Pa) required to generate a given flow (Q, in m^3 · s^{-1}):

$$R = \frac{p_1 - p_2}{Q} \qquad (1)$$

where p_1 and p_2 refer to the pressures at the inflow and outflow of the tubing section under investigation. The resistance is governed by characteristics of the fluid (material constants such as viscosity), flow profile (laminar or turbulent, and the inflow length), and characteristics of the conduit (geometry).

Material Constants. The viscosity (η) of blood is not constant. Blood exhibits viscoelastic behavior that is attributed to the reversible aggregation, deformation, and orientation of red blood cells in shear flow.[2] The viscosity of blood is high at low shear rates (= deformation rate γ, in s^{-1}) and decreases as shear rate increases, which is also known as shear thinning. Beyond a shear rate of approximately 100 s^{-1}, the viscosity of blood can be assumed as constant.

In a cylindrical tube perfused by the volume flow (Q) and with laminar flow, the shear rate is determined as the gradient of the flow velocity (v) over the radius (r):

$$\dot{\gamma} = \frac{dv}{dr} = \frac{4Q}{r^3 \pi} \qquad (2)$$

With an inner diameter of approximately 4.5 mm and blood flows larger than 100 mL · min^{-1}, shear rate is above 100 s^{-1} almost throughout all parts of the extracorporeal blood lines, so that, for the resistance in this circuit, blood may be considered as a fluid with a constant viscosity. Shear rates will be lower in the wide drip chambers. However, since drip chambers are short, an increased viscosity in these parts of the circulation is unlikely to contribute significantly to overall flow resistance.

The viscosity of whole blood depends on the characteristics of its two main components, the red blood cells and the plasma, and decreases with increasing temperature. At high shear rates, the red blood cells are quite deformable and behave almost like fluid drops.[3] Taylor's constant (T_{bl}) describes the relative importance of the circulation of the concentrated hemoglobin solution within the red blood cells as follows:

$$T_{bl} = \frac{\eta_{RBC} + 0.4\eta_{pl}}{\eta_{RBC} + \eta_{pl}} \qquad (3)$$

where η_{RBC} and η_{pl} refer to internal cell viscosity and plasma viscosity, respectively.[4]

The effect of volume concentration of disaggregated red blood cells at shear rates well above 40 s^{-1} on blood viscosity has been described by the following relationship[5]:

$$\eta_{bl} = \frac{\eta_{pl}}{(1 - Hct T_{bl})^{2.5}} \qquad (4)$$

where Hct refers to the hematocrit of the sample. This relationship models the exponential increase in whole blood viscosity as the volume concentration of red blood cells increases. Thus, with an internal viscosity of red blood cells (η_{RBC}) in the range of 3 mPa · s, a plasma viscosity (η_{pl}) around 1 mPa · s, and with a hematocrit (Hct) in the range of 30 to 40 percent, the viscosity of blood at 37°C and at shear rates beyond 100 s^{-1} is in the range of 3 to 4 mPa · s.

At 37°C, normal plasma viscosity is in the range of 1.16 to 1.35 mPa · s and primarily depends on the concentration of large proteins such as fibrinogen.[6] Unlike whole blood, plasma behaves like a Newtonian fluid. The viscosity of plasma is important for processes that occur close to the vessel wall, where marginal plasma skimming lowers frictional energy losses. Wall effects become more important as the diameter of the conduit decreases below approximately 200 μm, where whole-blood viscosity decreases because of more pronounced two-phase flow (Fahraeus-Lindqvist effect). Such effects are likely to be of importance in dialyzer fibers.

Flow Profile. The flow profile in tubes may be laminar or turbulent. The difference between these flow types is important with regard to both flow resistance and transport characteristics. The flow profile is laminar when viscous forces are prevailing, while inertial effects govern in turbulent flow. The Reynolds number (Re) defines the threshold for the transition from laminar (Re <2300) to turbulent flow (Re >2300):

$$Re = \frac{vd\rho}{\eta} \qquad (5)$$

where v is the velocity, ρ and η refer to the density and viscosity of the fluid, and d is the characteristic length, which in this case is the tube diameter.

With the mean velocity $v = Q \cdot A^{-1}$, where A is the cross-sectional area of the vessel, with a blood viscosity of 3 mPa · s and a blood density of 1040 kg · m^{-3}, Re stays below 2300 throughout the extracorporeal circulation even at the highest possible blood flows of 600 mL/min. This holds for the normal tube (d = 4.5 mm, Re=981) as well as for the small-bore cannula (d = 2 mm; Re=2207). Why is it then, that flow in the cannula is assumed to be turbulent?

Inflow Length. The lumen of the extracorporeal system changes at several locations—for example, at the connection between the tube and the cannula. This change in cross-sectional area has an important effect on the flow profile. At the edge of this diameter change, the laminar flow entering the needle picks up vorticity and a boundary layer forms inside the needle, with a thickness that increases with distance from the needle's entry. A dwindling core of liquid, which is virtually vorticity-free, survives over what is called the inlet length (L_i). Within this length, it is inertia that matters, as is the case with turbulent flow.[7] The magnitude of the input length depends on Re and can be estimated from the following relationship:

$$L_i \approx 0.03 \text{Re} d \qquad (6)$$

Thus, with a needle diameter of $d = 2$ mm (≈ 14 gauge) and Re = 1000, the inflow length is about 60 mm, which is much longer than the length of common dialysis cannulas. Thus, even though developed flow would be laminar in dialysis cannulas, the cannulas are too short for laminar flow to develop after the transition from the large to the narrow bore.

Geometric Factors. With laminar flow, the pressure drop of a Newtonian fluid flowing through a cylindrical tube of length (L) and radius (r) is proportional to the flow rate (Q), as described by the Hagen-Poiseuille law, where

$$\Delta p = \frac{8 \eta L}{r^4 \pi} Q \qquad (7)$$

The flow resistance can then be calculated using Eq. (1). The relationship given by Eq. (7) is a good approximation for established blood flow more or less throughout the extracorporeal circulation.

The situation is dramatically different for turbulent flow, where the pressure drop is proportional to the square of the flow rate:

$$\Delta p = \lambda \frac{\rho L}{4r} \left(\frac{Q}{r^2 \pi} \right) \qquad (8)$$

and where the frictional coefficient (λ) is a function of Re.[8] This relationship may help to explain the resistance to undeveloped laminar flow in dialysis cannulas, where a doubling in viscosity does not result in a doubling of the resistance, as would be expected with laminar flow.[9]

Pressure

Pressures in the extracorporeal circulation are generally measured at two or at most three locations: in the arterial line preceding the blood pump (p_{art}), in the venous line before blood is returned to the patient (p_{ven}), and—in some systems—in the line connecting the pump to the dialyzer.

Pressures are measured relative to ambient atmospheric pressure. Line pressures are in the first place measured for safety reasons. Sudden changes in arterial or venous line pressures exceeding the allowable limits of a properly set pressure monitor will trigger an alarm, stop the blood pump, and close the venous clamp. A rapid pressure increase may occur with infiltration of the cannula or with line kinks, while a pressure drop will be found with needle displacements and line separations. On the other hand, there are slow and predictable pressure changes within the extracorporeal circulation that are not related to connection problems and therefore should be recognized as harmless so as to avoid unnecessary nuisance alarms. Slow changes in arterial and venous line pressures are expected to occur with increasing blood viscosity, because of ultrafiltration-induced hemoconcentration, or with decreasing intra-access pressure, because of ultrafiltration-induced hypovolemia. Rapid pressure changes are also expected to occur when the extracorporeal blood flow is changed. New-generation pressure monitors do not trigger an alarm in these situations.

In the arterial and upstream part of the extracorporeal circuit connected to the patient access, the peristaltic pump lowers the arterial line pressure (p_{art}), thus increasing the pressure gradient and pulling blood from the vascular access into the extracorporeal circuit. The minimal arterial pressure accepted by current dialysis machines is in the range of -300 mmHg. The entire pressure gradient driving blood from the access into the arterial line depends not only on the negative arterial line pressure measured by the machine but also on the pressure within the access. Since intra-access pressure (p_{iac}) may vary from a few millimeters of mercury in central-venous accesses to more than about 25 mmHg for arteriovenous fistulas and approximately 50 mmHg for arteriovenous grafts,[10,11] the same arterial line pressure of, for example, -200 mmHg produces a pressure gradient of 200 mmHg in the central venous access, compared to 250 mmHg in the arteriovenous graft. Thus the driving force is increased by 25 percent when a peripheral arteriovenous graft is used, and almost one-fourth of the overall driving force is supplied by the patient, partly explaining why high-efficiency dialysis utilizing high blood flows is more easily carried out with arteriovenous grafts. With a hematocrit of 35 percent and using a 16-gauge needle at the same arterial pressure, blood flow would increase from 250 to about 320 mL/min when switching from a central venous access to an arteriovenous graft.[12] The effective pressure drop in the arterial line caused by the cannula can be estimated from the mean of arterial and venous line pressures [see also Eq. (9)].[13]

It is evident that the major resistance to the pull of the blood pump is due to the cannula. Even if blood flow through the cannula is controlled by inertial effects, as described above, both an increase in cannula diameter (or a reduction in needle gauge) as well as a decrease in cannula length [Eq. (8)] will reduce the flow resistance of the cannula.

The change in pressures and the action of the blood pump may lead to the formation of microbubbles. Such microembolic signals were recorded in the drainage vein from arteriovenous fistulas in patients as soon as hemodialysis and extracorporeal blood flow was started.[14] From in vitro experiments, the authors assumed that microembolic signals were formed by the blood pump without being removed by the air trap. Microbubbles may lead to activation of platelets and cause microemboli. While the formation of microemboli by means of the extracorporeal circulation has been confirmed, its exact nature and origin is not known.[15] The reduction of microembolic signals by technical improvements of the extracorporeal circulation in cardiac surgery has led to a decrease of neuropsychological deficits in humans, strongly suggesting that microembolic signals are harmful.[16]

Downstream of the pump segment, the pressure is raised to the level needed to drive flow through the downstream series of resistances represented by the dialyzer, the venous tubing, and the venous needle. Note that the pressure between the pump and the dialyzer is about 100 to 150 mmHg higher than the pressure measured in the venous line and that it is usually not measured by hemodialysis devices. In some machines, this pressure is monitored to control ultrafiltration and detect fiber clotting in the dialyzer, which may lead to high pressures in this part of the extracorporeal circuit. In any case, extracorporeal blood lines are tested for a transmural pressure of 2 bar. To avoid the risk of a bursting line without measuring the postpump pressure, some blood pumps are limited in their power output and will stop rotating at an increased flow resistance.[17]

Flow and Pressure Modeling

With given geometries of cannulas, blood lines, and dialyzers and with the known physical characteristics of blood, the pressure and flow relationships in the extracorporeal circulation have been modeled in order to describe the filtration/backfiltration characteristics in the dialyzer.[18,19] Backfiltration in downstream sections of dialyzers has been discussed as a potential source of bacterial contamination; however, with new synthetic membranes adsorbing bacterial residues and with ultrapure dialysate, this concern is no longer an issue.

More recently, extracorporeal flow and pressure modeling has focused on extracting information about the access and about the patient from extracorporeal flow and pressure measurements. Even though arterial and venous line pressures are in direct contact with the access, these pressures do not precisely reflect the pressure within the access, nor do they represent the full pressure gradient driving the blood flow. Under static conditions (i.e., when flow is stopped), the lines of the extracorporeal circulation take on the function of catheters and can be used for intraaccess pressure measurements. The placement of the needle tip within the access—whether facing or following the direction of access flow—will affect the pressure reading because of dynamic pressure effects at the cannula, and this may cause an error in estimation of intraaccess pressure as great as 10 mmHg.[13] The measurements must also be corrected for the height of the fluid column between the access and the pressure transducer (a 10 cm blood column = 7.4 mmHg). As soon as blood flow is established through the blood lines, arterial line pressures will drop and venous line pressures will increase. Assuming symmetry of flow resistances in arterial and venous line segments, the changes in pressures are more or less symmetrical around the mean access pressure.[20] With symmetrical lines, the pressure drop in the extracorporeal blood line is then given as

$$\Delta p = (p_{ven} - p_{art})/2 \qquad (9)$$

so that the intraaccess pressure at the arterial and venous cannulas ($p_{ac,art}$ and $p_{ac,ven}$) can be derived as

$$p_{ac,art} = p_{art} - \Delta p$$
$$p_{ac,ven} = p_{ven} - \Delta p \qquad (10)$$

respectively.

Static and dynamic line pressures have been used to detect low intra-access pressures to identify accesses at risk for future thrombosis.[12,21,22] The continuous measurement of access pressure is one of the goals in this field of research.

Intraaccess pressure varies with the arterial pulse, and the oscillations caused by the pulse are transmitted to the extracorporeal circulation. However, the pressure measured in the arterial line segment also varies because of the cyclic action of the blood pump, which is close to the arterial pulse in its frequency. If the signals are adequately processed, spectral analysis of the arterial line pressure can provide a continuous measurement of heart rate.[23] Pressure pulses can also be measured by piezoelectric transducers directly mounted to the extracorporeal circulation.[24] Whether this noninvasive technique can be used to detect the patient's pulse remains to be investigated.

Flow Control

Blood flow is one of the important treatment variables in hemodialysis, so that the pump is usually set and manually controlled by the operator to deliver the prescribed blood flow. The situation can be understood from a historical perspective, when it was assumed that blood flow alone determined clearance and there was no way to measure the delivery of dialysis with every treatment.

Currently the pump is set at a prescribed flow and the arterial and venous pressures result from that set flow. If the limits of the pressure monitor are surpassed, the pump stops and the operator has to adjust the blood flow. With a difficult access, such as a central venous access, this procedure may lead to frequent interruptions in flow during treatment. It is, however possible to smooth out such a treatment by using a feedback control of the pump flow based on the range of line pressures to be attained during a treatment.

Sometimes the sole focus on blood flow causes more harm than good, as blood flow may be increased at the cost of access recirculation. It is well known that effective clearance decreases as soon as access recirculation develops and that the patient would have received more clearance if blood flow had not been increased above the point where access recirculation began.[25] For the operator focusing on blood flow and extracorporeal line pressure alone, there is no way to know when an increment in flow in fact causes a decrease in effective clearance. With systems that also measure effective clearance with every treatment, blood flow can also be under the control of the clearance monitor.

The direction of the pump rotations is fixed. Thus, the direction of blood flow in the extracorporeal circulation depends on the orientation of the pump segment inserted into the pump housing. However, for special applications that require a reversal of blood flow in the extracorporeal circulation, as for the measurement of access flow by the various indicator dilution techniques (see below) it may be useful to have the direction of blood flow reversed for a short period of time. This, however, will need special safety adaptations in the extracorporeal circulation.

Thermal Energy Flow

The importance of temperature in hemodialysis has long been known. Even though most studies were focused on the effects of dialysate temperature, a mere reduction or control of dialysate temperature alone does not properly address the issue of thermal balance during hemodialysis. Dialysate temperature is only one of the variables involved in this issue.

Temperatures in the extracorporeal circulation are important for two reasons. First, the reaction of specific blood components is likely to depend on actual temperature. Second, arteriovenous temperature gradients measured at the fistula will lead to considerable flows of thermal energy from or to the patient.

The direct thermal effect of extracorporeal treatments depends on the amount of thermal energy (in joules) removed from (negative sign) or delivered to (positive sign) the patient through the extracorporeal circulation per unit time (in seconds). The extracorporeal heat flux J_{ex} has the dimension of a power and is measured in watts (W). J_{ex} is determined by the following relationship[26,27]:

$$J_{ex} = -cp(T_{art} - T_{ven})(Q_b - UFR) \qquad (11)$$

where the product cp (3.81, in $J \cdot °C^{-1} \cdot cm^{-3}$) refers to material constants of blood, T_{art} and T_{ven} refer to the arterial and venous line temperatures determined at the fistula, Q_b is the extracorporeal blood flow (Q_b, in $mL \cdot s^{-1}$), and UFR is the ultrafiltration rate (UFR, in $mL \cdot s^{-1}$). In reality, both c and ρ depend on hematocrit and the product $(c \cdot \rho)$ decreases from approximately 3.9 to 3.8 $J \cdot °C^{-1} \cdot cm^{-3}$ when the hematocrit increases from 30 to 50 percent.[9]

What is the magnitude of J_{ex}? For example, at a blood flow of 400 $mL \cdot min^{-1}$ (= 6.67 $mL \cdot s^{-1}$) and a UFR of 1.5 L $\cdot h^{-1}$ (= 0.42 $mL \cdot s^{-1}$), an arteriovenous temperature gradient of 0.5°C will lead to an extracorporeal heat flux of 11.9 W. It is instructive to compare J_{ex} to the patient's overall energy expenditure. The resting energy expenditure for the average adult is in the range of 75 W and can be estimated from anthropometric data using the Harris-Benedict equation.[28] The example shows that an arteriovenous temperature gradient of only half a degree in a high-efficiency treatment will lead to an extracorporeal heat flux in the range of 15 percent of estimated resting energy expenditure. The arteriovenous gradients may be much larger than assumed in the example above. But how do arteriovenous temperature gradients develop?

Temperature Effects

As blood flows from the access to the dialyzer, the temperature of the arterial line blood falls because this section of the extracorporeal blood line is exposed to the cooler environment. The degree of cooling in the arterial blood line depends on several factors, such as environmental temperatures (T_{env}), the length (L, in meters) and the thermal conductivity (α, in $mL \cdot min^{-1} \cdot m^{-1}$) of the blood line as well as on the duration of the exposure to the cooler environment, which is determined by blood flow Q_b. The following simplified relationship may be assumed to estimate the temperature drop from a point upstream (T_{up}) to a point downstream (T_{down}) of a typical line segment exposed to the environment at a given temperature (T_{env}) in still air[29]:

$$T_{up} - T_{down} = (T_{up} - T_{env}) \cdot \left(1 - e^{\frac{L \cdot \alpha}{Q_b}}\right) \qquad (12)$$

The temperature drop in the line will be small if either one or both expressions in parentheses on the right side of Eq. (12) become small. If the temperature of the environment is identical to T_{up}, so that $(T_{up} - T_{env}) = 0$, there will be no thermal loss in the blood line, so that $T_{up} = T_{down}$. On the other hand, with a high Q_b, the exposure of blood to the environment is short, so that the expression $[1 - e^{\wedge}(-L\alpha/Q_b)] \approx 0$ and the temperature drop $(T_{up} - T_{down} \approx 0)$ will be small as well. If, however, $T_{env} < T_{up}$, as in most cases, there will be thermal energy loss depending on Q_b, T_{env}, and L, and the temperature drop in the blood line may be significant (Fig. 3–2).

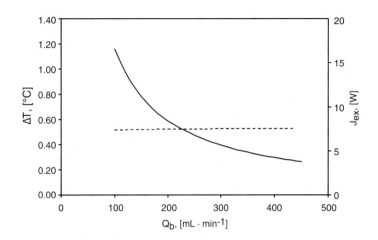

Figure 3–2. Temperature and thermal energy flow. The drop in blood temperature ($\Delta T = T_{in} - T_{out}$, full line) and of thermal energy flow (J_{ex}, broken line) as a function of blood flow (Q_b) calculated for a blood-line segment with length 1.5 m and thermal conductivity $\alpha = 5$ mL · min^{-1} · m^{-1}, based on Eqs. (11) and (12).

At the end of the arterial line segment, blood enters the dialyzer, which acts like an almost perfect heat exchanger, so that blood exiting from the dialyzer will have equilibrated with the temperature of the dialysate. Notice that the dialysate temperature is measured within the dialysis machine and that the dialysate will cool on its way from the machine to the dialyzer in a flow-dependent fashion. If there is no correction for flow-dependent temperature losses along the dialysate lines, the actual dialysate temperature will be somewhat lower than that displayed on the machine. Thus the temperature of blood leaving the dialyzer will also be lower than shown on the monitor of the dialysis machine.

On its way through the venous segment and back to the patient, blood is again exposed to the cooler environment and comparable temperature changes to those described above are expected to occur in the venous line. With low Q_b, the temperature of blood flowing from the dialyzer to the access may drop by as much as 1°C, and the temperature of blood returned to the patient may be significantly different from the temperature set at the monitor. The temperature drop in the venous blood line cannot be avoided with current dialysis techniques. Even wrapping the line with thermal insulation cannot entirely prevent venous line cooling. Thus, to return blood to the patient at a given temperature, the dialysate temperature must be increased by the magnitude of the temperature gradient to be expected in the venous blood line. If blood were to be returned to the patient at the same temperature as it was removed through the arterial line (no arteriovenous gradient for so-called isothermic dialysis) the actual dialysate temperature would have to be increased above body temperature. The exact magnitude of this offset depends on the parameters described in Eq. (12) (Fig. 3–2). It follows from these considerations that, for isothermic dialysis, the temperature in the dialyzer must be higher than in any other part of the extracorporeal circulation and also must be higher than the core temperature. Such an increase above body temperature may cause unfavorable humoral and cellular activation at the dialyzer membrane.

Whereas the temperature in the venous line importantly depends on the length of time for which blood is exposed to the cooler environment and thus on blood flow, the amount of thermal energy exchanged (J_{ex}) with the environment is not as sensitive to changes in Q_b. This is because the energy flow is proportional to Q_b as well as to the temperature gradient between up- and downstream temperatures. Whereas the energy flow increases with increasing blood flow [Eq. (11)] the temperature gradient decreases with increasing Q_b [Eq. (12)] so that the two effects almost compensate. In contrast to temperature gradients, thermal energy flow is almost constant and independent of blood flow (Fig. 3–2).

Standard Components

New processor-controlled syringe pumps permit time-programmed dosing of anticoagulant and the administration of a bolus into the arterial segment of the extracorporeal blood line. Drip chambers are used wherever needed to prevent air from entering the downstream section of the extracorporeal circulation. Drip chambers in the arterial line prevent air from entering the dialyzer, which may obstruct fibers and increase fiber clotting. Drip chambers in the venous line are mandatory and are used to prevent air from entering the patient. Drip-chamber levels are monitored by optical, acoustic, or capacitative means. Often the levels are automatically adjusted by clamping the venous outflow and venting the drip chamber while the blood pump is running.

Blood Line Sensors

The latest development in dialysis technology utilizes the extracorporeal circulation as an extension to the patient's circulation to measure patient variables, which can be used to control and optimize the extracorporeal treatment. With proper sensors attached to the extracorporeal circulation, it is possible to gain important invasive information by noninvasive means.

Blood Flow. As discussed above, blood flow in the extracorporeal system may be largely overestimated if it is calculated from the revolutions of the blood pump alone. Blood flow is easily measured by ultrasonic means.

The transit time of acoustic pulses transmitted through blood is a function of the velocity of ultrasound in blood and of the conduit holding the blood, i.e., the material and the wall thickness of the tube. Sound velocity (v) is a function of blood composition and temperature. Depending on the intersection of the sound beam relative to the direction of blood flow, the sound wave in the moving sample travels with or against flow, so that the transit time is either shortened or lengthened when compared to the situation with a resting sample or with illumination perpendicular to the direction of flow. The shift in ultrasonic transit times together with the known inclination of the sound beam can then be used to measure the flow velocity in the sample.

Bypass Flowmeter. This approach is applied in the HT110 Bypass Flowmeter and HXL Flowsensors (Transonic Systems Inc., Ithaca, New York), providing noninvasive and reliable measurements of extracorporeal blood flow. The transducers are mounted to the blood line and give readouts of flows in the arterial and venous lines.

The measuring principle in these transducers is based on intersecting illumination of the extracorporeal tube's lumen (Fig. 3–3). The times of flight are determined for a pair of acoustic pulses transmitted in upstream and downstream flow directions. With complete illumination of the tube's lumen and sampling of the whole flow profile, the difference between down- and upstream transit times becomes a measure of blood flow.[30] The system must be calibrated for tubing material, tube wall thickness, ultrasound velocity of the liquid flowing through the tube, and temperature.

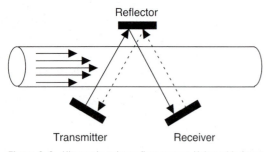

Figure 3–3. Ultrasonic volume flow sensor. Using wide-beam illumination, two transducers pass ultrasonic signals back and forth alternately intersecting the flowing blood in upstream and downstream directions. The difference signal provides information on blood flow, the averaged signal provides information on the composition of blood.

Temperature. The temperature reading on a temperature probe attached to the outside of the extracorporeal blood line is determined by the temperature of the tubing and the temperature of the environment of the temperature probe. Unlike a probe inserted into the bloodstream, such a probe is seeing two temperatures, and its reading will lie between these. However, if the temperature gradient between the blood and the environment can be eliminated by adjusting the temperature of the environment, the temperature measured by the probe will eventually reflect the temperature within the blood line.[31] The response of such a system depends on the control algorithm and the gains to adjust the temperature of the environment, the thermal conductivity of the blood line, and the thermal inertance of the components.

Blood Temperature Monitor. The measurement of blood temperatures without inserting a thermistor probe into the bloodstream is solved by the Blood Temperature Monitor (BTM, Fresenius Medical Care, Bad Homburg, Germany). Short sections of the extracorporeal blood line are inserted into arterial and venous measuring heads mounted on the module, which is equipped with sensors to measure arterial and venous blood temperatures at the sensor site. The measuring heads are housed in small boxes to control the temperature of the sensor environment, so that the temperature measured by the sensor touching the outside of the blood line accurately reflects the temperature of the blood within the blood line. The distance of the sensors from the access is approximately 1.5 m. Because of temperature drops in the lines leading to the access, arterial line temperature will be lower than that at the access, whereas the venous blood temperature will be higher than the actual temperature of blood entering the access. If temperature is measured at the same distance from the access, the magnitude of the temperature drop will be comparable; the sign of the drop, however will be different for arterial and venous lines. Thus, the arteriovenous gradient measured at the sensor site is not the same as that at the access. To measure the full arteriovenous gradient from the point where blood leaves the access to the point where it returns to the access, the temperatures at the access must be calculated for given insulation and environmental conditions using the extracorporeal blood flow measured by the dialysis machine. The precision of the temperature measurement is better than $0.1°C$ for blood flows above 120 mL/min. T_{art} and T_{ven} are measured with a sampling period of 15 s.

Optical Density. With hemoglobin routinely measured by photometric methods, the utility of optical techniques to measure hemoconcentration seems self-evident. However, the optical properties of whole blood are very complex and do not follow Lambert-Beer's law. In whole blood, photons undergo multiple scatterings and reflections on interacting with red blood cells, which actually lengthens the path through the sample and increases the chance of photons being absorbed. This "path-lengthening" effect accounts for the distinct nonlinearities in optical density with varying hematocrit. In fact, within the physiologic hematocrit range, scattering contributes significantly more to total optical density than absorbency. Thus the optical density of whole blood is more a measure of red blood cell (RBC) concentration than of hemoglobin.[32] Scattering is determined by intrinsic sample properties, such as the shape and the ratio of refractive indexes of the RBCs and the plasma.[33] Factors that affect the shape—such as blood flow, osmolarity, [Na$^+$]—or the refractive index of the components—plasma protein and mean cellular hemoglobin concentration—importantly affect optical density. A considerable compensation for the variability of intrinsic effects is obtained by measuring the ratio of optical densities at different wavelengths, similar to the ratiometric measurement of oxygen saturation at a pair of isosbestic (i.e., 505, 547, or 568 nm) and nonisosbestic (i.e., 600, 577, or 470 nm) wavelengths. The explanation for taking the ratio of optical densities at two wavelengths is that changes in intrinsic properties should affect the two signals similarly, so that the ratio remains unchanged. The scattering effect in whole blood is eliminated when hemoglobin concentration is measured in hemolyzed and diluted blood samples.[34]

Optical properties of whole and hemolyzed blood have been used for a variety of experimental devices.[34-38] Today, two systems are commercially available. Both make use of specially designed, disposable measuring cells that are inserted into or part of the arterial section of the extracorporeal circulation.

Crit-Line. The Crit-Line instrument (Crit-Line III, Hemametrics, Kaysville, Utah) is a multiple-wavelength device that utilizes the ratiometric approach to correct for nonlinearities between optical density and hematocrit.[39] The hematocrit reading is derived from an internal calibration curve and thus is a relative measure. The Crit-Line instrument is designed as stand-alone monitor.

Hemoscan. The Hemoscan (Hospal-Dasco, Medolla, Italy) measures at an isosbestic wavelength to eliminate the effect of varying oxygen saturation.[40] The Hemoscan is part of the dialysis machine, which opens the possibility for automatic control of ultrafiltration rates and dialysate conductivities.

Sound Velocity. At a given temperature the velocity of sound in blood depends on sample density (ρ) and compressibility (κ), both of which are linear functions of hematocrit, hemoglobin, plasma protein, total protein concentrations, or water concentration.[41-44] The relationship between sound velocity, density, and compressibility is given as

$$v = \sqrt{\frac{1}{\rho\kappa}} \qquad (13)$$

Density increases and compressibility decreases with increasing hematocrit. If density and compressibility are linear functions of hematocrit, it follows from [Eq. (13)] that v will be a nonlinear function of hematocrit; however, in the range of hematocrits between 20 to 80 percent, there is an almost perfect linear relationship between the two, since sound velocity increases as hematocrit increases.

Blood density is most accurately measured by the mechanical oscillator technique.[45] A variety of high-resolution density-measuring devices are available for research purposes (A. Paar KG, Graz, Austria), but their everyday use in a clinical situation is difficult because of the unique measuring cell. However, if sound velocity (v) is measured, a disposable measuring cell can be used for continuous monitoring of total protein concentration (TPC) in extracorporeal blood lines.[46] Although sound is scattered by RBCs, sound velocity is not affected by multiple scattering. Both density and sound velocity depend on sample temperature, which must be measured to compensate for temperature effects. The measurement of sound velocity in extracorporeal blood has two major applications focusing on long- and short-term measurements.

Fresenius BVM. The measurement of sound velocity over the course of an entire dialysis treatment can be used to track hemoconcentration caused by ultrafiltration and vascular refilling.[46] This application requires enhanced stability of the measuring system and continuous correction for temperature-related changes in sound velocity. This approach has been realized in the blood volume monitor (BVM, Fresenius Medical Care, Bad Homburg, Germany). In this device, the time of flight of short acoustic pulses transmitted across the sample volume perpendicular to the direction of blood flow is evaluated and corrected for temperature effects. The blood lines to be used with the device are equipped with a special measuring cell introduced into the prepump segment of the arterial line. This acoustic cuvette is inserted into the measuring head of the blood-volume monitor. The system is factory calibrated, but, for enhanced accuracy, it may be recalibrated during the priming process of the extracorporeal blood lines. From the change in hemoconcentration measured with a maximum sampling period of 1.2 seconds, the relative change in blood volume is determined assuming a single blood-volume compartment. The module fits current Fresenius dialysis machines. It is one of the elements used for feedback control of relative blood-volume changes during dialysis and ultrafiltration.

Transonic HD02. When down- and upstream transit times measured in the ultrasonic transit-time sensors are averaged instead of subtracted, the effect of blood flow on ultrasonic transit time is eliminated (Fig. 3–3). When calibrated for tubing material, tube wall thickness, and temperature, the transit time becomes a function of the velocity of sound in blood.

The measurement of short and transient changes in sound velocity is realized in the HD02 (Transonic Systems Inc., Ithaca, New York). The main application of this device is in the measurement of transient changes in hemoconcentration caused by the injection of indicator into the extracorporeal blood line. The HD02 brings classic indicator dilution technique to diagnostic testing in hemodialysis using isotonic saline as an indicator. Injection of isotonic saline into the venous blood line leads to a delayed and dispersed dilution of blood, which is measured by the downstream sensors at high sampling rates. Variables of interest—such as cardiac output, central blood volume, access recirculation, and access flow—can be measured with different configurations of the experimental setup.

Urea Concentration. The process of paired filtration and dialysis opens the possibility for on-line measurement of plasma components such as urea.[47] Ultrafiltrate obtained upstream from the dialyzer reflects the urea concentrations in arterial blood entering the dialyzer. Plasma concentrations, even when measured before the dialyzer, are not independent of the efficiency of dialysis, as access and cardiopulmonary recirculation of cleared blood will lead to a systematic reduction in these concentrations in arterial line blood.

Multimat. The Multimat (Bellco SNIA Group, Mirandola, Italy) is equipped with a sensor for continuous measurement of urea in ultrafiltrate by the urease technique. The ultrafiltrate recovered from the extracorporeal blood in a convective step preceding the diffusive hemodialysis step is passed through a urease column, and conductivity cells before and after the urease column measure the conductivity increase caused by the formation of NH_4^+ and HCO_3^- from neutral urea. The advantage of this setup compared to the other urea techniques (see below) is that it gives a direct measurement of blood urea concentration, so that all the methods developed for dose estimation based on laboratory values for blood urea concentration can be directly applied. Using the continuous nature of the measurements, more sophisticated models can easily be incorporated.[48,49]

Indicator Dilution

The sensors discussed in this chapter can be used to measure access recirculation (R) and access flow (Q_a), important variables modifying hemodialysis delivery, by the indicator dilution technique. This technique is based on the addition of a known amount of a substance, the indicator, to the bloodstream, and on the measurement of its dispersion caused by different transport phenomena.[50] The indicator dilution technique becomes the method of choice when direct access to blood flow is impossible. The injection of an indicator into the bloodstream changes characteristic physical properties of blood, such as temperature or optical density, in a dose-related manner, so that the measurement of the altered blood properties by one of the extracorporeal line sensors provides information on indicator concentration. This information can be obtained at high sampling rates. Because hemodialysis is associated with the controlled exchange of water, solutes, and thermal energy in the extracorporeal circulation, the indicator dilution technique is inherent to the technology of hemodialysis and has therefore attracted most interest in the quantification of transport phenomena such as the measurement of access flow and access recirculation. An important variant of classic indicator dilution is offered by the controlled removal of indicators such as urea or ultrafiltrate by the process of hemodialysis and ultrafiltration, so that urea concentration or measures of hemoconcentration can also be used to detect and quantify recirculation.[51] The measurement of access flow and access recirculation ideally requires two sensors to be mounted to the extracorporeal circulation and a defined injection of the indicator into the extracorporeal blood line.

Recirculation. To measure recirculation, indicator is added to the venous bloodstream returning to the patient's access. The indicator is diluted by extracorporeal blood flow, enters the access, and—in the case of access recirculation—reappears in the arterial blood line with a delay of only a few seconds.[20,52,53]

The magnitude of access recirculation is determined by the amount of indicator retrieved in the arterial line (m_{art}) during its first transit relative to the amount of indicator delivered to the access using the venous line (m_{ven}):

$$R = \frac{m_{art}}{m_{ven}} = \frac{AUC_{art}Q_{b,art}}{AUC_{ven}Q_{b,ven}} \qquad (14)$$

where AUC is the area under the indicator concentration-vs.-time curve. The technique requires two sensors, one on the arterial and one on the venous blood line, to measure AUC_{ven} and AUC_{art}, respectively. The difference between venous ($Q_{b,ven}$) and arterial line blood flows ($Q_{b,art}$) caused by ultrafiltration is usually small, so that the measurement of recirculation reduces to a measurement of concentrations. Important differences between techniques, however, relate to the measurement of the first transient and to the important separation of access and cardiopulmonary recirculation.[54]

Access recirculation is measured by the Hemodialysis Monitor (HDM01, Transonic Systems, Inc., Ithaca, New York),[52] which utilizes changes in ultrasound velocity caused by the dilution of blood with isotonic saline. The technique is often improperly referred to as *ultrasound dilu-*

tion. Ultrasound is not diluted but, rather, used to detect dilution.

The decrease in optical density caused by the dilution of blood with isotonic saline can also be used to detect and quantitate access recirculation using the Crit-Line Monitor (Crit-Line III, HemaMetrics, Kaysville, Utah).[39,55] Since only one measuring cell is available in this system, the measurement of the venous transient entering the access [the denominator in Eq. (14)] is substituted by an additional and identical injection of indicator into the arterial line before the actual recirculation test is done. This approach—of performing a combination of arterial and venous injections when only one arterial sensor is available—is also realized in other systems.

The change in blood conductivity (Λ) caused by the dilution with hypertonic saline can be measured noninvasively by utilizing electromagnetic sensors. Such sensors are used by the Hemodynamic Monitor (HDM, Gambro Healthcare, Lakewood, Colorado). In this device, a sensor measuring the difference between arterial and venous blood conductivities ($\Delta\Lambda = \Lambda_{ven} - \Lambda_{art}$) is clamped around both the venous and arterial lines. The sensor requires a modification of the blood lines, which must contain closed loops (toroids) that are placed around the electromagnetic excitation and sensing cores of the measuring head. The requirement to utilize dedicated disposable blood lines probably explains why this technique remained at the prototype level.

The transient of hypertonic saline can also be measured by conductivity cells originally designed for on-line measurement of blood urea concentration, as in the Multimat (Bellco SNIA Group, Mirandola, Italy).[56] However, because of delays and dead spaces, the technique appears to be sensitive to effects caused by cardiopulmonary recirculation as well.

In the blood-temperature monitor (BTM, Fresenius Medical Care, Bad Homburg, Germany) the temperature of venous blood returning to the access is changed by changing the dialysate temperature without changing Q_b and without affecting the flow and recirculation conditions in the vascular access. Recirculation is derived from the change in arterial temperatures (ΔA) caused by a change in venous line temperatures (ΔV)[57]:

$$R = \frac{\Delta A}{\Delta V} \qquad (15)$$

Because of the duration of the test, the result includes a component related to cardiopulmonary recirculation.[58]

Access Flow. The techniques described to measure access recirculation can also be used to measure access flow. One of the basic requirements, however, is the reversal of extracorporeal blood flow in at least part of the extracorporeal circulation. This is usually done by switching the blood lines manually at the connections to the arterial and venous

needles so that blood is drawn from the venous puncture site at the downstream section of the access and returned through the arterial needle at the upstream section of the arteriovenous access. This configuration produces so-called forced recirculation (R_x), which is a function of access flow and can be used to measure it (Q_a)[59]:

$$Q_a = \frac{1 - R_x}{R_x}(Q_{b,x} - \text{UFR}) \qquad (16)$$

where $Q_{b,x}$ relates to blood flow with reversed placement of blood lines.

Again, the measurement of access flow requires separation of forced recirculation occurring in the access from cardiopulmonary recirculation (CPR), which is present with any peripheral arteriovenous access.[60]

If the effects of cardiopulmonary recirculation cannot be separated from recirculation (R_x) measured with reversed placement of blood lines, access flow (Q_a) calculated from the original formula will be erroneously low because R_x is inflated by the combined effects of forced access recirculation and cardiopulmonary recirculation. The resulting underestimation of access flow was shown to be proportional to the term 1-CPR.[58] Since CPR can reach up to 50 percent, the error introduced by not accounting for CPR is significant.[61] These considerations are especially important for techniques in which the dilution and/or detection of indicator resembles a constant infusion rather than a bolus technique.

However, when two recirculation measurements are taken with both correct and reversed placement of blood lines and with the assumption that the fraction of Q_a/CO (= CPR) does not change when switching blood lines, then the effect of constant cardiopulmonary recirculation can be eliminated. The approach of taking two measurements with correct and reversed placement of blood lines has been termed the *double recirculation technique,* and it is the basis to measure access flow either by thermodilution, on-line clearance, or ultrafiltration techniques.[51,58,62,63]

The procedure to reverse the blood flow in the access needles for the purpose of performing an access flow measurement during hemodialysis is greatly facilitated by special line segments whereby flow reversal is possible without disconnecting and reconnecting the extracorporeal circulation (Bloodline Twister, Fresenius Medical Care, Lexington, Massachusetts; Reverso Flow Reversing Interconnector, Medisystems Corporation, Elizabeth, Colorado).

DIALYSATE

The typical dialysate is prepared by diluting a fluid concentrate with warm, degassed, ultrapure water. The typical concentrations accepted today for the different components of a standard dialysate are given in Table 3–1. Concentrates are provided in containers of different sizes, ranging from bags to tanks. While fluid concentrates are still the most widely used, dry salt mixtures for the on-line production of dialysate offer significant advantages and their use is likely to expand.

Acetate, Bicarbonate

To correct the metabolic acidosis associated with chronic kidney disease, the dialysate must contain a base to be delivered to the patient during hemodialysis. The major difference between various dialysates relates to the type of base used. While the base of choice would be HCO_3^-, the simultaneous delivery of HCO_3^- together with Ca^{2+} causes technical difficulties, as both components cannot be maintained in a stable solution at the required concentrations. Depending on the concentration of each component, HCO_3^- and Ca^{2+} react to form insoluble $CaCO_3$, which precipitates from the solution. Therefore, when a single concentrate is used, HCO_3^- must be replaced by other bases that do not form insoluble salts when mixed for dialysate. Conjugated bases of weak acids—such as L-lactate or acetate, which are normally produced by the metabolism in large quantities— are prime candidates for this purpose. L-lactate has been used successfully as the sole buffer base in hemodialysis solutions, with only minor, transient intradialytic elevations of plasma levels of the anion and without any obvious adverse effects.[64] L-lactate is also used in peritoneal dialysis solutions.[65] However, for economic reasons, acetate is chosen for most applications. With the consumption of one proton, acetate is metabolized to CO_2 and H_2O:

$$CH_3COO^- + H^+ \leftrightarrow CH_3COOH$$
$$CH_3COOH + 2O_2 \rightarrow 2CO_2 + 2H_2O \quad (17)$$

While acetate dialysis requires only a single fluid concentrate or solid-phase salt mixture, bicarbonate dialysis requires two types of concentrates or solid-phase salt mixtures. The A component (color-coded red) is also termed the *acid* (A) component, as it usually contains small amounts of acetic acid, leading to an acidic pH of the solution (pH ≈ 3.4). Usually this component also contains the majority of electrolytes. The B component (color-coded blue) is also termed the *base* (B) component, as it contains the bicarbonate, leading to a slightly alkaline pH of the solution because of hydrolysis (pH ≈ 7.8). The majority of the NaCl and all divalent cation salts are usually contained in the A component. However, since the operation of conductivity-controlled proportioning systems requires a distinct change in conductivity, the accuracy of such systems is improved if the NaCl is split between A and B components.

While the problem of precipitating $CaCO_3$ is eliminated in concentrates when the components are separated, precipitation of $CaCO_3$ may still occur in the diluted dialysate. $CaHCO_3$ is soluble, but its solubility depends on the pH value and the CO_2 tension of the volatile anhydride, which is difficult to control in an open system:

$$Ca(HCO_3)_2 \leftrightarrow H_2O + CO_2 \uparrow + CaCO_3 \downarrow \quad (18)$$

The formation of $CaCO_3$ precipitates interferes with the mechanical function of valves and pumps in the hydraulic system of the dialysis machine, so that maintaining a dialysate flow and immediate rinsing after every treatment increases the lifetime of the hydraulic components.

Solid-Phase Mixtures

The components of acetate and bicarbonate dialysis are also available in the form of solid-phase mixtures. However, on-line production of dialysate from dry salt mixtures is available only with newer hemodialysis machines.

Dry salt mixtures were first developed for the B component used for bicarbonate dialysis in the form of car-

TABLE 3–1. ELECTOLYTES IN PLASMA, PLASMA WATER, AND DIALYSATE

Component	Bicarbonate-based [mmol · L⁻¹]	Acetate-based [mmol · L⁻¹]	Plasma [mmol · L⁻¹]	Plasma water [mmol · L⁻¹]	Ultrafiltrate [mmol · L⁻¹]	Λ^0 [S · cm² · mol⁻¹]
Na⁺	137–144	132–145	142	153	145	50.9
K⁺	0–4	0–4	4.3	4.6	4.4	74.5
Ca²⁺	1.25–2.0	1.5–2.0	1.3	1.4	1.25	120
Mg²⁺	0.25–1	0.5–1.0	0.7	0.8	0.7	107.8
Cl⁻	98–112	99–110	104	112	118	75.5
HCO₃⁻	27–38	-	24	26	27.5	43.5
CH₃COO⁻	2.5–10	31–45	<0.1	<0.1	<0.1	40.1
Glucose	0–11	0–11	4.5	4.8	4.8	-

[a]Electrolyte concentrations and limiting equivalent conductivities (Λ^0) of separate ions at 25°C. Electrolyte concentrations in dialysate are taken from Grassmann et al.[167] Plasma water concentrations are calculated for a plasma water fraction of 93 percent. The concentrations in ultrafiltrate in equilibrium with plasma are calculated using a Donnan factor of 0.95, 0.90, and 1.05 for univalent cations, divalent cations, and univalent anions, respectively.

tridges (BiCart, Gambro AB, Lund, Sweden; Altracart II by Baxter Althin Medical, Inc., Deerfield, Illinois; SOLU-CART by Baxter, Deerfield, Illinois; SmartCar, Fresenius Medical Care, Bad Homburg, Germany) or bags (bibag, Fresenius Medical Care, Bad Homburg, Germany). Since the composition of a saturated solution in equilibrium with undissolved material at a given temperature is determined by the solubility product, a well-defined concentrate can be prepared by means of solvent percolating through the solid matrix of the salt mixture at a well-defined temperature. The saturated concentrate is then used for further dilution to obtain the final dialysate, similarly to the dilution of fluid concentrates. Difficulties to be overcome reside with the formulation of a loose powder or granule to optimize flow and dissolution and to reach saturation of the liquid concentrate. The formulation of a dry A component in the form of a loose powder or granule is more difficult because of its liquid (acetic acid) and hygroscopic (KCl, $MgCl_2$) components. Therefore, the A component has been split into a solid component for a cartridge (SelectCart, Gambro Lundia AB, Lund, Sweden) or bag (sobag, Fresenius Medical Care, Bad Homburg, Germany) just containing crystalline NaCl and a fluid component containing acetic acid, KCl, and the divalent electrolytes with (indibag, Fresenius Medical Care, Bad Homburg, Germany) or without glucose (Select-bag, Gambro Lundia AB, Lund, Sweden). The separation within the A component increases the technical complexity but opens the possibility of separately adjusting the concentration of Na^+ (contained in the dry component) and the other electrolytes (K^+, Ca^{2+}, Mg^{2+}) contained in the liquid component. An alternative to splitting the A component is to replace fluid acetic acid by solid lactic or citric acid.[66] A unique dry A component using solid citric acid has been developed and is available commercially as DRYalysate (Advanced Renal Technologies, Kirkland, Washington). With this concentrate, the citric acid content is only 0.8 mmol · L^{-1} in the final dialysate, well below the 2.3 to 5 mmol · L^{-1} threshold required for true anticoagulation. Citric acid adds anticlotting attributes to the dialysate, which may help to keep the dialyzer cleaner and might explain improved clearance observed with citrate dialysis.[67]

Electrical Conductivity

Measurement of the electrical conductivity of the final dialysate plays an important role in controlling its composition and preventing exposure of blood to potentially hazardous dialysate mixtures. Other physical measures have been employed, but the measurement of conductivity combines reliability and cost-effectiveness. The electrical conductivity is easily measured by flow-through cells positioned in the dialysate inflow to the dialyzer.

The electrical conductivity (λ, in S · cm^{-1}) of a solution (when the geometry of the measuring chamber and the elec-

trodes and the temperature is given) depends on the type and concentration of solutes and their dissociation into ions. More specifically, the electrical conductivity of an ion is determined by its mobility in the solution, which depends on the electrical charge and the radius of the hydrated ion.

With recent developments, especially the measurement of on-line clearance or Na^+ modeling, electrical conductivity has become a surrogate for the concentration of Na^+; it is therefore important to remember the relationships between conductivity and concentration.

Molar Conductivities. Electrical conductivity represents a bulk property and thus reflects the sum effect of all ionic components present in the solution. Since electrical conductivity primarily depends on the nature of the ion, it is helpful to normalize the measured conductivity for molecular weight and define the molar conductivity (Λ, in S · cm^2 · mol^{-1}). The molar conductivity thus compares the conductivity of solutions with the same number of ions. At a given concentration, the magnitude of the molar conductivity is also affected by other ions and counter-ions in the solution, which interfere with the electrical mobility of the studied solute. Therefore, to really compare the characteristics of different ionic species, molar conductivities are extrapolated to infinite dilution to yield the so-called limiting molar conductivities (Λ^0, in S · cm^2 · mol^{-1})[68] (Table 3–1).

When the limiting molar conductivities for each component are known it is possible to obtain a rough estimate of the contribution of the different components to the overall conductivity of the solution. Even though Na^+ presents with the least limiting molar conductivity among the cations present in dialysate (Table 3–1), the major contribution to overall dialysate conductivity originates from Na^+, because of its high concentration in dialysate. The contributions of K^+, Ca^{2+}, and Mg^{2+} are much lower, but deviations from the normal concentration of these substances are much more important. Unfortunately, the overall conductivity of the solution cannot simply be calculated from concentrations and limiting molar conductivities, because at higher concentrations the relationships between conductivity and concentration become nonlinear. This nonlinearity is due to interactions between ions and counter-ions. Temperature also has a major effect, which must be measured together with electrical conductivity. Measured conductivities are usually compensated for a constant temperature of 25°C. The conductivity of the dialysate displayed on the dialysis monitor at this temperature will be in the range of 13 to 15 mS · cm^{-1}.

Sodium Concentration

Even though the major contribution to overall dialysate conductivity originates from Na^+ and Cl^- concentrations, dialysate conductivity cannot be taken as a surrogate for Na^+ concentration—an important factor in dialysis. A substitution of Na^+ concentration for solute conductivity is permissible only with well-defined systems. For example, the drop in K^+ concentration throughout hemodialysis will cause a parallel drop in effluent dialysate conductivity. However, without information on the composition of effluent dialysate, it is not possible to distinguish whether this drop was actually due to a drop in effluent $[K^+]$ or $[Na^+]$. Even if NaCl is responsible for 90 percent of dialysate conductivity, a change in dialysate conductivity does not mean that any change is 90 percent attributable to NaCl. The change might be caused by the change of a single ionic species such as K^+ and not be related to NaCl at all. This is even more important, as the limiting molar conductivity for K^+ is about 50 percent higher than that for Na^+ (Table 3–1). Thus, unless solutes are measured by specific means, such as ion-selective electrodes, the composition of the effluent dialysate cannot be derived from conductivity measurements alone. Control algorithms based on measurement of the conductivity of effluent dialysate may therefore lead to potentially dangerous situations.

Temperature

The temperature of dialysate entering the dialyzer is usually kept between 36 and 38°C and can be adjusted to individual needs. The set value is controlled within the limits of ±0.5 to 1.5°C. The control systems of the machine ensure that the temperature of the dialysate in contact with blood will not exceed the limits between 34 and 40°C.

Filtration

If contaminants are present in the dialysis fluid, they may cross the dialysis membrane and enter the blood by back-transport. Backtransport is the transport of water or solutes from the dialysis fluid to the blood across the membrane. Backtransport cannot be totally prevented even when back-filtration in the dialyzer is suppressed because of concomitant diffusion.[69,70] But with the use of ultrapure and pyrogen-free dialysate, backtransport—whether convective or diffusive—will not be harmful to the patient. Therefore, in new dialysis machines such as the AK 200 ULTRA S (Gambro Lundia AB, Lund, Sweden), all dialysate is filtered before it is brought into contact with the dialyzer, which removes bacterial contaminants as well as endotoxin and provides an ultrapure solution equivalent to the standards set for parenteral solutions.

Dialysate Delivery

Dialysate can be provided by batch systems, which have advantages when it comes to the control of volume balance and ultrafiltration, or it can be provided by the single pass of fresh dialysate through the dialyzer, which has certain advantages when it comes to the delivery of high-efficiency dialysis.

Batch Systems. In batch systems, a given dialysate volume of up to 100 L is circulated through the dialyzer and returned to the reservoir. In the original batch systems, the increase in solute concentration in the dialyzer bath caused an exponential decrease in the concentration driving force, thereby reducing the efficiency of the treatment with the progress of treatment time. The recirculation of spent dialysate also set the stage for bacterial contamination. Batch systems were used at the beginning of the development of hemodialysis and have been largely replaced by single-pass systems; however, two variants of the closed batch system have gained interest because they can be operated with much reduced technologic requirements.

The issues of efficiency and contamination were most elegantly addressed in a system developed by the late B. Terstegen, leading to a revival and increased interest in batch systems (Fig. 3–4).[71,72] The core of the system consists of a cylindrical, well-insulated container filled with the ready-made, warm dialysate. Fresh dialysate is removed from the top of this container, circulated through the dialyzer, and returned to the bottom of the container. The procedure makes use of the small, albeit important, difference between fresh and spent dialysate densities. Spent dialysate contains more solutes and is somewhat cooler than fresh dialysate, so that it has a higher density. Thus, if it is gently returned to the bottom of the container, the spent dialysate will stay below the fresh dialysate and maintain a more or less sharp separation layer of not more than 2 cm between spent and fresh dialysate. At the same time as spent dialysate enters the bottom of the container, fresh and uncontaminated dialysate is displaced from the top of the container. The system is commercially available as the GENIUS Therapy System (Fresenius Medical Care, Bad Homburg, Germany).

The Aksys PHD System (Aksys Ltd., Lincolnshire, Illinois) employs a variant of the batch system described above. The separation in the 50-L tank is also based on density differences between fresh and spent dialysate. However, in the Aksys PHD System, the fresh dialysate is kept at 29 to 30°C and the solution has a high density to begin with. The fresh dialysate with the high density is therefore removed from the bottom instead of the top of the tank, warmed to the temperature required for hemodialysis, and returned to the tank on top of the fresh dialysate, where it forms a separation layer because the warm dialysate has a reduced density. As with the GENIUS Therapy System, the Aksys PHD System is designed to reuse all components of the extracorporeal circulation.

Single-Pass Systems. In single-pass systems, the continuous production of dialysate is achieved by proportioning systems that exactly measure the required amounts of concentrates to be mixed with water. The number of proportioning systems depends on the number of concentrates used; for

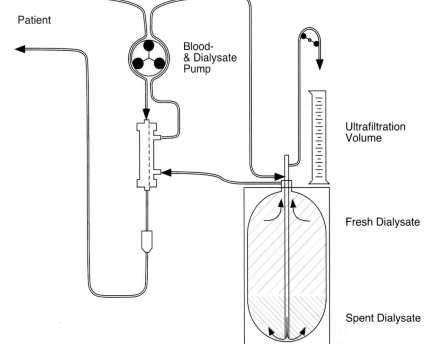

Figure 3–4. Batch dialysate delivery. The closed system of the dialysis tank allows for simple volume control. The ultrafiltration volume refers to the volume removed from the closed system. It is measured in the graduated cylinder. Fresh and spent dialysate are separated by the effect of different densities. In the system shown (Genius, Fresenius Medical Care, Bad Homburg, Germany) fresh dialysate has a lower density and thus remains on top of the spent dialysate which is cooler and loaded with solutes.

example, two systems are used for the two components required for bicarbonate dialysate. Current technology utilizes either volumetric or conductometric measuring principles (Fig 3–5).

Volumetric Mixing. This procedure is based on additivity of volumes of a mixture. In a mixture, the total volume (V_t) is assumed to be the sum of the volumes of the components (ΣV_i). Hence the volume fraction of a component is given as the volume of that component relative to the entire volume of the mixture (V_i/V_t). Thus the volume fraction of component A in a bicarbonate dialysate, described as 1 + 1.225 + 32.775, is 1/35 (or 2.857 vol%), whereas the volume fraction of component B in the same dialysate is 1.225/35 (or 3.5 vol%). When the volume of water (component C in the example above) is given as in most dialysis machines, the corresponding volumes of components A and B are added to reach the final dialysate concentration. The final concentration is measured by conductivity as the correct mix of solutes producing a defined conductivity provided that the proper concentrates are used. The use of independent variables (volume and conductivity) to control and prepare the final dialysate adds to the safety of the method.

Conductometric Mixing. This procedure is based on adjusting the conductivity of the mixture by feedback control of the concentrate delivery pump for each mixing step. However, without measuring the actual concentrate volume, the correct conductivity can also be obtained by using a wrong concentrate. The actual concentrate volume can be derived

from the feedback control; however, this does not provide independent information on the proper dilution, as both the measured conductivity and the controlled volume depend on the function of the same component of the system. Thus, the actual dilution is best checked by an independent variable—for example, by the pH value of the dilution.

Electrolyte Measurement. Today electrolytes are measured by ion-selective electrodes that measure the activity of the ion in the solvent—i.e., plasma water or dialysate water. In fact, this is the relevant concentration to be considered for electrolyte balance between extra- and intracellular spaces and also to determine the concentration gradient at the dialyzer or in the native kidney glomerulus. Unfortunately, this concentration is converted to fit the concentrations obtained by flame photometry, which does not consider the fraction of solvent (i.e., water) in the solution but relates the amount of solute to the bulk of the solution, which in the case of plasma contains a significant amount of nonwater components, mostly proteins (Table 3–1).

What is the dialysate sodium concentration in equilibrium with plasma sodium concentration?

The equilibrium sodium concentrations in plasma and dialysate are different from each other for analytic and physicochemical reasons. In plasma, the sodium concentration is measured in reference to plasma volume, which includes the nonaqueous components, mostly protein and lipid. Thus, in a given plasma sample with the same total amount of sodium (Na^+), the concentration of sodium is larger when related to plasma water volume (index pw) than

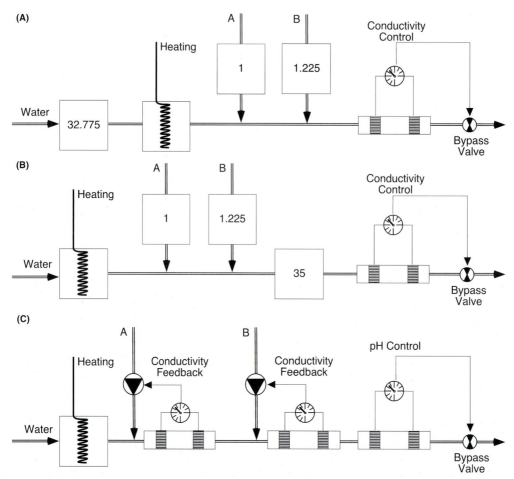

Figure 3–5. Mixing of dialysate. *A.* Volumetric mixing based on a defined water inflow. A and B components are added to yield the specified dialysate composition. *B.* Volumetric mixing based on defined dialysate outflow. Volumes of A and B components are defined, and water is added to yield the specified dialysate composition. In both panels, the numbers refer to volume parts of the components. The composition of the fresh dialysate is controlled by temperature compensated conductivity monitors. *C.* Conductometric mixing with pH control. Components are mixed and the resulting conductivities are used to control the concentrate pumps. The final composition of the dialysate is controlled by a temperature compensated pH measuring cell. *(Adapted from Grassman et al.)*[166]

when related to the whole plasma volume (index p), which includes a significant volume of proteins:

$$\left(\frac{Na^+}{H_2O}\right)_{pw} = \frac{1}{PWC} \cdot \left(\frac{Na^+}{H_2O + protein}\right)_p \qquad (19)$$

The factor to correct for the contribution of nonaqueous components is given by the plasma water concentration (PWC, in g H_2O per 100 g plasma). This factor depends on the protein and lipid content of the plasma and is in the range of 93 percent.[73] The sodium concentration in plasma water is 153 mmol $\cdot$ L^{-1}, the corresponding plasma sodium concentration, however, is only 153 mmol $\cdot$ L^{-1} $\cdot$ 0.93 = 142.3 mmol $\cdot$ L^{-1} (Table 3–1).

When the solvent, such as water, is separated from an electrolyte solution by a membrane that is not permeable to

some of the ions, the other permeable ions are also affected in their distribution across the membrane because of the Donnan effect. This is the case with dialysis membranes that are impermeable to the negatively charged proteins. The Donnan equilibrium in blood/dialysate systems is characterized by a higher concentration in anions—[Cl$^-$], [HCO$_3^-$]—and by a lower concentration in cations—[Na$^+$], [K$^+$]—in the dialysate (indexed) when compared to the corresponding plasma water concentrations:

$$\left[Na^+\right]_d = {}^f Donnan \cdot \left[Na^+\right]_{pw} \qquad (20)$$

where f_{Donnan} is the so-called Donnan factor. At normal protein concentrations for univalent ions, f_{Donnan} is in the range of 0.95.

Thus, when plasma sodium is measured as plasma water concentration, the equilibrium concentration in dialysate can be calculated from the Donnan equilibrium and dialysate sodium concentration has to be much lower than plasma sodium concentration. For example, if plasma water sodium is 153 mmol $\cdot$ L^{-1}, dialysate sodium would have to be 145 mmol $\cdot$ L^{-1} (Table 3–1). The difference of 8 mmol $\cdot$ L^{-1} is not trivial.

If plasma sodium is measured as plasma concentration, the equilibrium concentration can be found by combining Eqs. (19) and (20):

$$[Na^+]_d = \frac{{}^f Donnan}{PWC} \cdot [Na^+]_p \qquad (21)$$

The combined factor f_{Donnan}/PWC is in the range of 1.02 and the dialysate sodium concentration must be higher to be in equilibrium with a given plasma sodium concentration. For example, if plasma sodium concentration is 142 mmol $\cdot$ L^{-1}, dialysate sodium concentration would have to be 145 mmol $\cdot$ L^{-1} (Table 3–1).

To summarize, under the assumption of a normal plasma protein concentration, a dialysate sodium concentration of 145 mmol $\cdot$ L^{-1} is in equilibrium with a plasma water sodium concentration of 153 mmol $\cdot$ L^{-1} and with a plasma sodium concentration of 142 mmol $\cdot$ L^{-1}. These relationships have to be kept in mind in considering sodium balance, especially in view of recent interest in sodium modeling and the emphasis on maintaining neutral sodium balance in dialysis patients. One can also see that manual sodium measurements and individual adjustments of dialysate sodium concentration are essentially futile, because the exact sodium balance depends on many factors, such as plasma water concentration (PWC), which change in the extracorporeal circulation and also changes throughout dialysis because of hemoconcentration.

Volume Balance. This is more complicated with single-pass systems than is generally appreciated, because large volumes have to be measured with high accuracy. A typical high-efficiency dialysis treatment requires approximately 100 L of dialysate to pass by the highly permeable dialysis membrane. However, to limit the overall balance error during that treatment to the magnitude of ±100 mL, flows have to be measured and balanced with an accuracy of ±0.1 percent. This accuracy exceeds that of typical flowmeters. The problem has been solved by either matching timed volumes in the dialysate inflow and outflow using so-called balance chambers or by measuring the inflow and outflow rates by electrical or mechanical techniques (Fig 3–6).[74]

Accuracy. Errors in the delivery of the prescribed sodium concentration are often blamed on the accuracy of the machine's mixing procedure. However, there are other important sources of error to be considered. The concentrations in fluid concentrates are specified with an error of ±2.5 percent. Thus, with a declared concentration of 140 mmol $\cdot$ L^{-1},

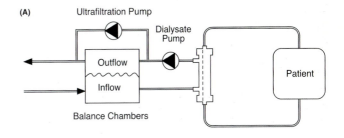

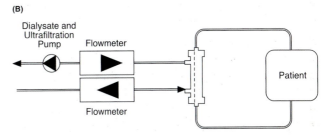

Figure 3–6. Open dialysate delivery. Open systems require tight control of the dialysate flows. *A.* Dialysate flow can be controlled by matching timed inflow and outflow volumes using balance chambers. In this system, ultrafiltrate must be removed from the dialysate flow before matching the volumes. *B.* Volume balance can also be maintained by controlling the dialysate inflow and outflow rates using dedicated flowmeters and by increasing the outflow above the inflow rate to achieve a controlled ultrafiltration.

the concentration may range from 136.5 to 143.5 mmol $\cdot$ L^{-1}. The error of proportioning systems can also be in the range of ±2 percent of the prescribed value. Thus, the overall error can be in the range of ±5 mmol $\cdot$ L^{-1} of [Na$^+$]. This error is difficult to control even with individual plasma and dialysate measurements under optimal conditions.

Clearance and Dialysis Quantification

The outcome of dialysis is determined by the dose of dialysis delivered with every treatment. One measure of dialysis dose is the *Kt/V* urea index obtained from urea kinetic modeling, where *K* refers to urea clearance, *t* to treatment time, and *V* to the volume of urea distribution which is related to the size of the patient.[75] Urea kinetic modeling provides a convenient tool for measuring and assessing the efficacy of dialysis. It also facilitates quality assurance in a dialysis unit through assessment of the actual delivered dose of dialysis relative to the prescribed dose. Substantial differences between the prescribed and delivered dose suggest problems with the delivery of dialysis. These include vascular access patency, calibration of the blood pump, nonattainment of desired dialysate flow rate, and loss of dialysis time due either to frequent alarms or to the patient being late to go on dialysis or early to come off it.[76] Despite these benefits derived from urea kinetic modeling, the technique is underutilized because of its perceived mathematical complexity, requiring several blood samples, measurements of blood and dialysate flow rates and treatment time, and the need for specialized software as well as a computer system. Technologic developments in the accurate and automatic measurement of clearance and/or urea concentration have facilitated the development of systems that provide on-line urea kinetics.

Clearance Measurements. The clearance of a solute found both in blood and dialysate is called dialysance (D) and is given as

$$D = Q_d \frac{d_o - d_i}{b_i - d_i} \tag{22}$$

where Q_d is dialysate flow, d_i and d_o refer to dialysate inflow and outflow concentrations, respectively, and b_i refers to blood inflow concentration. The measurement of clearance thus requires the measurement of four variables, three of which (d_i, d_o, Q_d) are easily available in the dialysis machine. The measurement of the fourth variable, the concentration in blood (b_i), however, causes a problem and is approached in the following way.

Step Techniques. Measurement of the blood concentrations (b_i) can be avoided by a special procedure.[77-79] If a pair of postdialysate concentrations (d_{o1} and d_{o2}) are measured at two different levels of inlet dialysate concentrations (d_{i1} and d_{i2}), and with the assumption that b_i remains unchanged, Eq. (22) can be solved to eliminate b_i and give the following relationship:

$$D = Q_d \left(1 - \frac{\Delta d_o}{\Delta d_i}\right) \tag{23}$$

In this relationship, the problem reduces to the measurement of a change in dialyzer outlet concentrations ($\Delta d_o = d_{o2} - d_{o1}$) when applying a step-change in dialyzer inlet concentration ($\Delta d_i = d_{i2} - d_{i1}$). Notice the similarity of [Eq. (15)] to that established for the measurement of recirculation Eq. (23). However, the assumption that the blood concentration (b_i) does not change with the step change in dialysate inflow concentration (Δd_i) is not really valid. This assumption is violated because of recirculation and a finite pool size. A given dialysate concentration will result in a certain blood concentration leaving the dialyzer and returning to the vascular access. When this concentration recirculates through the access because of access recirculation and through the cardiopulmonary loop when using a peripheral arteriovenous access within a short period of time, this concentration will affect the blood inflow concentration to the dialyzer (Fig 3–7). Thus, when dialysate concentration is increased by a step function, the concentration in dialyzer blood inflow also increases by a factor determined by the magnitude of both access and cardiopulmonary recirculation. This increase reduces the gradient between dialysate

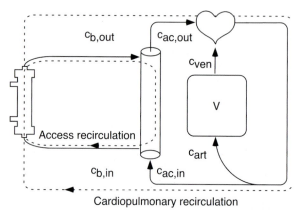

Figure 3–7. Recirculation with a peripheral access. The efficiency of extracorporeal clearance is reduced by access and cardiopulmonary recirculation. Access recirculation leads to a reduction of $c_{b,in}$ relative to c_{art}. Cardiopulmonary recirculation leads to a reduction of c_{art} relative to c_{ven}. $c_{b,in}$ and $c_{b,out}$ refer to extracorporeal blood inflow and outflow concentrations. $c_{ac,in}$ and $c_{ac,out}$ refer to access blood inflow and outflow concentrations. c_{art} and c_{ven} refer to arterial and mixed venous blood concentrations. V refers to the systemic volume compartments to be cleared during hemodialysis.

and blood and hence reduces the mass transfer across the dialyzer, thereby increasing the concentration remaining in the dialysate outflow. If the numerator in Eq. (23) is erroneously high, the computed dialysance (D) will be lower than that measured in a situation without recirculation. Interestingly, the effect of both access and cardiopulmonary recirculation on clearance turns out to be an advantage of the technique, as the dialysance measured by this approach refers to effective dialysance delivered to the patient and not to extracorporeal dialysance, which is not always delivered as prescribed.

Bolus Techniques. Instead of applying a step change in dialyzer inflow concentrations, the transport characteristics of the dialyzer can also be measured by a bolus technique:

$$D = Q_d \left(1 - \frac{\int \Delta d_o \, dt}{\int \Delta d_i \, dt}\right) \tag{24}$$

where the integrals refer to the area under the inlet and outlet dialysate concentration curves. In this approach, it is not required to reach a steady state in the dialysate concentrations, so that the duration of the bolus can be significantly reduced. Again, the interpretation of D depends on the duration of the bolus relative to the time constants for access and/or cardiopulmonary recirculation. If the duration is long enough to incorporate effects caused by both access and cardiopulmonary recirculation, D refers to effective dialysance. Notice the similarity of Eq. (24) to that established for the measurement of recirculation [Eq. (14)].

Electrolyte Dialysance. Dialyzer clearance can be measured with a variety of solutes using different sensors.[80] However, for practical reasons in everyday dialysis, the solutes of choice are the electrolytes present in the dialysate. The concentration of these electrolytes is best measured by electrical conductivity. Based on the observation that dialysance of ionized sodium is almost identical to urea clearance and that dialysate conductivity over the range of clinical conductivities (12 to 18 S · cm^{-1}) is a fairly linear function of dialysate sodium, the on-line measurement of conductivities is now used in several dialysis machines to determine a surrogate for urea clearance without additional equipment and without blood sampling (Diascan Quality Control Monitor in the Phoenix Dialysis System, Gambro Renal Products, Lakewood, Colorado; OLC for the 4008K Dialysis System, Fresenius Medical Care, Lexington, Massachusetts; OCM for 4008S and H Dialysis Systems, Fresenius Medical Care, Bad Homburg, Germany).

The measurement of so-called on-line clearance is based on conductivity measurements done at the inlet and outlet of the dialyzer. To eliminate the concentration measurement on the blood side (b_i), either the step or the bolus technique mentioned above is used. Even though the bolus technique has the potential to eliminate effects caused by access and/or cardiopulmonary recirculation, the application of the bolus, the delay, and the dispersion of the bolus in the dialysate lines and in the dialyzer takes too much time, so that the conductivity measured in the dialysate outflow overlaps with effects caused by recirculation. Thus, the clearance obtained by either approach refers to effective urea clearance.

There is, however, an important difference with both approaches regarding loading effects. The step techniques must reach a steady state with their inflow and outflow sodium concentrations, which is usually achieved after only a few minutes. During this time, significant amounts of sodium may be transferred into the patient. Therefore a second step with decreased dialysate sodium concentrations is made to follow the high dialysate concentration phase. During this phase, sodium will be removed from the blood and from the patient. Neutral sodium balance is achieved by matching the amplitudes and durations of the high/low sodium phases. The duration of the dialysate bolus is much shorter when using the bolus technique, so that the net sodium flux into the patient is reduced and sodium balance is less affected.

Other variations relate to the technical layout of the clearance measurement. For example, instead of using two separate conductivity cells for simultaneous measurement of dialysate inflow and outflow conductivities, a single conductivity cell can be used for subsequent measurements of these conductivities. However, using the same component to measure both fresh and spent dialysate may cause contamination of fresh dialysate and sections of the dialysis hydraulics that are upstream of the dialyzer.

The measurement of clearance by conductivity-based techniques is inexpensive and requires only one or two conductivity cells added to the dialysate circuit. These conductivity cells are very accurate and rugged, and the device requires little maintenance. To monitor the delivered dose of dialysis, the on-line clearance measurement is enabled at the start of dialysis and a series of equally spaced clearance measurements is automatically programmed. The software calculates the time-averaged value of the effective clearance for the entire treatment. The calculation of dialysis dose measured as *Kt/V*, however, requires information on *V* that is not accessible through on-line clearance measurements alone and must be entered into the program either using anthropometric estimates or, preferably, from monthly formal urea kinetic modeling data. With this information on patient volume (*V*) and time the software computes the dose of dialysis either as single pool or equilibrated *Kt/V* and projects estimated values of these parameters for the end of dialysis.

Dialysate Urea Measurements. In the past few years, several devices have been developed that can measure urea more or less continuously in a flow of fluid from the dialyzer. A surrogate for blood urea concentration is obtained by analyzing pure ultrafiltrate obtained from paired filtration dialysis. Alternatively, urea can be measured in the spent dialysate. Traditionally, blood concentrations have been used to quantitate the presence of urea in the body, and the concentration change has been used in calculations of dialysis dose. The dialysate-side concentration itself is usually of no interest and will always be an indirect measure of the blood concentration, requiring knowledge of both clearance and dialysate flow for the conversion.

On the other hand, the dialysate concentration multiplied by the dialysate flow rate will give a urea removal rate. The total mass of urea removed can then be obtained by integration over the entire treatment. In addition, the collection of all dialysate is the most straightforward approach to determining the total amount of solute removed from the body. These calculations would be much more difficult to obtain using blood-side measurements. Total dialysate collection leads to large volumes of dilute solutions difficult to handle in everyday dialysis. One approach is to split the dialyzer outlet flow and collect only a fraction of the spent dialysate.[81] However, partial dialysate collection as well as continuous dialysate sampling, utilizing the devices described below, has to be able to recognize and exclude phases in which the dialyzer is in bypass.

With continuous blood-side urea measurements, all the theory developed for dose quantification based on urea kinetic modeling can be applied directly, using, for example, the formulas of Daugirdas.[82] These equations cover both single-pool Kt/V and, in addition, the deviations from single-pool behavior using the equilibrated Kt/V.[83] The continuous flow of data obtained by blood-side measurements also makes it possible to predict the final outcome of a single treatment after about 90 minutes of hemodialysis.[84]

From dialysate-side measurements, the same calculations of dialysis dose can be performed. Equating the urea removal rate from blood, as quantified by clearance (K), to the urea appearance rate in dialysate (D), one obtains

$$K \cdot c_b = D \cdot c_d \qquad (25)$$

Here, c_b and c_d are the urea concentrations in blood and dialysate, respectively. Provided that K and D remain constant during the treatment, the blood and dialysate concentrations of urea will thus be proportional to one another. Because the measures of dialysate dose given as either Kt/V or urea reduction ratio (URR) depend only on the ratio of urea concentrations before and after the treatment, it is possible to use dialysate concentrations instead of blood concentrations to obtain them. This approach is used in the Baxter and Gambro devices.

The measurement of urea in spent dialysate avoids the need for blood sampling. Random measurement errors can be minimized using serial measurements, and a whole range of important treatment and patient parameters can be calculated from these continuous measurements. Finally these new devices may be coupled on line to a central database so that measured and calculated values can be recorded without manual intervention, providing almost instant information of clinical value in patient management. Eventually this input side can be connected via feedback that will control the time of the dialysis session to ensure that a prescribed dialysis dose is actually delivered.

The basis of urea measurement in all the devices is the action of the enzyme urease on urea, which leads to the formation of ammonia and bicarbonate:

$$\left(NH_2\right)_2 CO + 2H_2O \xrightarrow{\text{Urease}} NH_3 + NH_4^+ + HCO_3^- \qquad (26)$$

The formation of ammonia causes an increase in pH, while the formation of charged particles from the uncharged precursor leads to an increase in electrical conductivity, both of which can be measured by appropriate techniques. The concentration of ammonia can also be measured by photometric techniques, which are more difficult to carry out than continuous measurements. In any case, it is important to have enough urease to avoid saturation effects and to convert all of the urea to ammonia. A more detailed discussion of the various techniques can be found elsewhere.[85]

Biostat 1000. The Biostat (Baxter Healthcare Corporation, McGaw Park, Illinois) was one of the first on-line systems to reach the clinician. Unfortunately this device is no longer available. However, the results obtained with the Biostat 1000 led to the development of other systems. The Biostat 1000 monitored urea nitrogen concentration in effluent dialysate at intervals of up to 5 minutes and determined urea kinetic parameters, such as Kt/V and urea removal, from the dialysate concentration-time profile.[86,87] No blood sampling was required, since all measurements were made on effluent dialysate. In order to provide additional information, such as distinct measurements of K and V, the Biostat 1000 had an equilibration mode for deducing the predialysis blood urea nitrogen (BUN) by allowing dialysate in the dialysate compartment of the dialyzer to come into equilibrium with blood, dialysate flow bypassing the dialyzer. The Biostat 1000 used an ion-specific ammonium electrode with a membrane cap, which had immobilized urease on the membrane surface to catalyze the breakdown of urea to ammonia. The technique required daily quality control and frequent calibrations using standard solutions, as well as replacement of the urease cap after 20 treatments.

Biotrack. The Biotrack (BioCare Corp., Hsinchu, Taiwan) uses an ammonium-sensitive electrode and is placed in the dialysate line immediately after the dialyzer; it can calculate approximately the same set of parameters and requires the same kind of care with regard to calibration as the Biostat 1000.

DQM 200. The Gambro Dialysis Quality Monitor, DQM 200, is used together with an AK100, AK 200, or an AK200S dialysis machine (Gambro Lundia AB, Lund, Sweden). Urea concentration in the spent dialysate is measured continuously throughout the treatment. A fraction of the dialysate is diverted from the main flow and drawn into two fluid paths, the reference path and a reaction path. The reference path leads to a conductivity cell that measures the baseline conductivity of the dialysate. In the reaction path, the dialysate is first carbonated, then run through a column containing immobilized urease to a conductivity cell, where conductivity is measured. In passing through the urease column, urea is completely converted into ammonia and bicarbonate ions, which increases the conductivity of the dialysate. The increase in conductivity relative to the conductivity measured in the reference path is proportional to the concentration of urea in the spent dialysate. The result is a linear and accurate response over a large measuring range. The conductivity cells are temperature-controlled to a tolerance of approximately $0.001°C$ difference. To ensure complete conversion of urea into ammonium ions, the solution must be maintained below a pH of 7.3, which is achieved by adding gaseous CO_2 upstream of the urea conversion column. Calibration is carried out automatically before monitoring starts. Positioned in the spent dialysate path, it is difficult to obtain a predialysis blood urea value using isolated ultrafiltration at the start of the treatment, since the ultrafiltrate is diluted in the machine by unused dialysis fluid. Otherwise the same parameters can be obtained as in the Biostat 1000.

MODES OF DELIVERY

Purity

Contamination of dialysate and infusate with chemical or biological impurities may seriously harm the patient. Thus the quality of water and of dialysate is strictly defined by regulatory agencies. It is also important to realize the peculiarities of a biological contaminant. It is not sufficient to merely lower the concentration of bacteria to a level that seems safe at a certain moment, because growth will restore the numbers to previous magnitudes within a short time. Even though water is the major component of dialysate and the medium for bacterial growth, it is not sufficient to control the purity of the water alone. Contamination may occur throughout the process of preparing the dialysis fluid, and the control of dialysate purity includes several steps and measures. The last step in controlling the purity of the dialysate is the ultrafiltration of the mixed dialysate through special filters immediately before the dialysate is brought into contact with the dialyzer or infused into the extracorporeal circulation in one of the new on-line hemodiafiltration (HDF) techniques (Fig. 3–8).[88]

The quality of effluent produced by ultrafiltration depends on the membrane characteristics—such as the sieving coefficients and adsorption characteristics and the physical integrity of the membrane—as well as on the level of contamination in the inflow fluid. The membranes should be highly permeable to water and solutes up to a molecular weight of 30 to 40 kDa but impermeable to intact bacteria and large cell wall components. Solutes such as lipopolysaccharides triggering pyrogenic reactions are removed from the solution by the process of adsorption.[89] The adsorptive capacity of the membrane depends on the choice of the polymer blend, in which hydrophobic components are important for the retention of similarly hydrophobic bacterial products. Many pyrogenic bacterial products are smaller than the pores, so that the adsorptive capacity is vital for the preparation of nonpyrogenic fluids.[90] High hydraulic permeability facilitates operation at low transmembrane pressures, thereby minimizing the risk of fiber ruptures. As there is currently no way of measuring bacterial contamination on-line, membrane integrity must be repeatedly tested by pressure-holding tests.

The arrangement of ultrafilters in a generalized on-line system is shown in Fig. 3–8. The first filter is a water filter, which makes it possible to use standard water for dialysis. The second filter prepares ultrapure dialysis fluid. Both of these filters are integrated into the flow path and can be used for a certain time, usually 2 to 3 months, depending on the operating conditions.

Convective Treatment Modes

Convective techniques such as hemofiltration and hemodiafiltration are based on augmented ultrafiltration in the dialyzer far above the requirements to adjust the fluid balance in the dialysis patient (Fig 3–9). In hemofiltration there is ultrafiltration in the dialyzer without dialysate. The volume loss is compensated by infusion of replacement fluid into the bloodstream in pre- or postdilution mode before or after the dialyzer or in a combination of both. The major limitation of hemofiltration to achieve a high clearance within the usual treatment time of 4 hours is the ultrafiltration rate, which is determined by the plasma flow and the maximum filtration fraction to be attained in the filter. A high degree of hemoconcentration in the dialyzer can reduce both the permeability and life of the filter. Experience shows that the filtration fraction—i.e., the percentage of plasma water flow filtered per specified time interval—should not exceed 25 percent. Machines will provide a warning when hemofiltration is approaching this critical filtration fraction. Plasma water flow (Q_{pw}) is proportional to blood flow, hematocrit, and plasma water concentration:

$$Q_{pw} = Q_b(1 - \text{hct}) \cdot 0.93 \qquad (27)$$

Thus, even in a high-efficiency system using high blood flows, such as 400 mL $\cdot$ min^{-1} and with a hematocrit of 35 percent, the plasma water flow is 242 mL $\cdot$ min^{-1} and

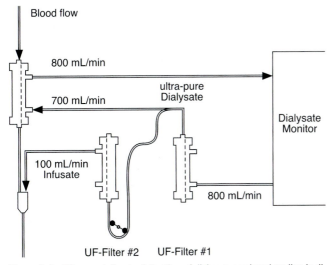

Figure 3–8. Ultrapure infusate. A fraction of dialysate produced on-line is diverted from the normal dialysate path and passed over a second filter. In the case shown, the infusate is infused into the venous line in postdilution mode.

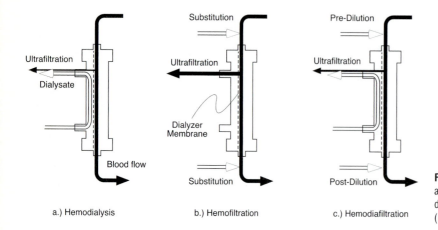

Figure 3–9. Diffusive and convective modes. Ultrapure and volume-balanced dialysate can be used for high-flux dialysis (*A*), as replacement fluid in pure hemofiltration (*B*), and as infusate in hemodiafiltration (*C*).

the maximum clearance to be attained by hemofiltration at a filtration fraction of 25 percent will be in the range of only 60 mL · min⁻¹. This is insufficient for an intermittent, thrice weekly hemodialysis regime. This limitation can be addressed by combining both convective and diffusive transport processes in hemodiafiltration. Hemodiafiltration appears to be the most effective therapy combining the benefits of both hemodialysis and hemofiltration.[91] By increasing the convective flux across the dialyzer membrane to rates of 100 mL · min⁻¹ and more, the removal of large molecules with small diffusion coefficients, such as β_2-microglobulin, is significantly enhanced, thereby improving clinical outcomes.[92,93] Still, to maintain fluid balance, the fluid volume removed by ultrafiltration must be replaced by a physiologic solution. Hemofiltration and hemodiafiltration require handling of large volumes of sterile infusate and matching of infusion to ultrafiltration, which used to be done by weighing the ultrafiltrate and infusate volumes. This is much more difficult than with pure dialysis and is one of the factors that prevented the widespread application of this approach. The situation changed with the on-line production of infusate.

Today it is possible to use systems that continuously prepare, in practically unlimited quantities, high-quality fluids for dialysis, ultrapure dialysis fluids, and sterile solutions for substitution and rinsing. This has led to a widespread acceptance of convective treatment modes. Although on-line production of pyrogen-free infusion fluid was first described almost 25 years ago, a series of technical challenges and regulatory issues had to be resolved before this technique could be applied for everyday use.[94,95] Essential steps in this process were the preparation of ultrapure dialysate from solid concentrates and the development of synthetic high-flux membranes with high adsorptive capacity and reliable mechanical integrity.[96]

Today's hemodiafiltration is based on hemodialysis using on-line production of ultrapure dialysate and volumetric control of dialysate inflows and outflows (Fig. 3–8).

However, for the purpose of hemodiafiltration, a fraction of the total dialysate is diverted from its usual path to the dialyzer and serves as infusion flow (Fig. 3–9). The fraction of dialysate flow bypassing the dialyzer is determined by the flow rate set at the infusion pump of the hemodiafiltration module. Also, before being added to the bloodstream in either pre- or postdilution modes, the ultrapure infusate is passed through an additional ultrafiltration filter. Thus, the dialysate entering the bloodstream passes an additional membrane, comparable to dialysate passing a high-flux membrane in the presence of backfiltration.

As a consequence of splitting the dialysate flow in the on-line hemodiafiltration module, the remaining dialysate flow entering the dialyzer is reduced by a magnitude equal to the infusion flow (Fig. 3–8). Since a significant amount of dialysate is used for infusion and thus bypasses the dialyzer, unbalanced dialysate outflow would be much smaller than total dialysate flow before the split. The dialysate outflow, however, is matched to the sum of dialysate inflow and infusion flow by additional ultrafiltration in the dialyzer. Because the entire dialysate circuit is designed as a closed system using flow or volume control (Fig. 3–6), any diversion of dialysate from the dialyzer inflow used for infusion is automatically balanced by a mandatory increase in dialyzer outflow caused by ultrafiltration in the dialyzer.

There are, however, differences in the details of the available commercial systems. In the ONLINEplus system (Fresenius Medical Care, Bad Homburg, Germany) developed for Fresenius 4008 dialysis machines, the ultrafiltration filter may be reused for as many as 100 treatments for a period of up to 12 weeks. Repeated pressure-holding tests throughout the treatment ensure filter integrity. Thus, there is no need for a single-use filter in the infusion line, which, by means of special connectors (ON-Line Lock System), ensures a safe and aseptic connection to the ports, which are sterilized between treatments.

Whether on-line HDF provides the same hemodynamic benefit as standard HDF remains to be clarified, as standard HDF may have been associated with previously underrecognized side effects.

Temperature and Cooling. The amount of cooling observed with standard HDF covers 30 to 50 percent of estimated energy expenditure. This insight has been helpful in clarifying the hemodynamic benefits of convective vs. diffusive treatments.[97] Without hemodialysis and with convective treatment modes such as isolated ultrafiltration, there is no heat exchange in the dialyzer and the entire length of the extracorporeal circulation is exposed to the lower temperature of the environment. With regard to the model presented in Eq. (12), these differences have two major implications. The length (L) of the extracorporeal system to be considered for heat exchange doubles and the inflow temperature to the extracorporeal circulation is given by T_{art} ($T_{in} = T_{art}$) instead of T_{dia}. With the same thermal conductivity of the blood line and doubling the effective length exposed to the environment, the drop in blood temperature from the arterial sampling to the venous return site will be in the range of 1 to 2°C, depending on the blood flow. The magnitude of extracorporeal heat flow will be between −15 and −30 W, depending on the insulation characteristics of the blood lines, and, again, combined arterial and venous line cooling will be largely independent of blood flow. For example, assuming a thermal conductivity $\alpha = 9.3$ mL · min^{-1} · m^{-1} and a total length of 3 m for the extracorporeal circuit, the extracorporeal heat flow with isolated ultrafiltration calculated from and when $T_{art} = 36.5$°C, $T_{env} = 22$°C, and $Q_b = 250$ mL · min^{-1} is predicted to be −24 W. The actual average heat flow measured under these conditions was −27 W.[98]

In terms of extracorporeal cooling, there should be no difference between hemodialysis and predilution HDF, because all blood passes the dialyzer so that all blood is controlled by the dialysate temperature. The situation is different with postdilution HDF. It was recently shown that even when the infusion fluid is taken from dialysate with on-line HDF, the postdilution mode provides additional cooling. This can be explained by the additional infusion line, which increases the exposure surface, and the reduced blood flow from the dialyzer to the infusion port. The exact amount of cooling provided by postdilution on-line HDF clearly depends on the ratio of blood flows to infusion flows.

Donnan Effect. Note that the infusion of dialysate into the bloodstream without a membrane interface abolishes the transmembrane gradients caused by the Donnan effect. This may have an immediate effect on electrolyte balance, as direct infusion of dialysate reduces the plasma water sodium concentration.[99] In predilution mode, this effect will lead to reduced sodium removal in the dialyzer and subsequently to sodium accumulation. This accumulation of Na$^+$ may contribute to the improved hemodynamic stability seen with convective treatment modes.[97]

Profiled Dialysis

The classic delivery of hemodialysis is based on setting the treatment variables—such as the blood and dialysate flows, the ultrafiltration rate, dialysate composition, and dialysate temperature—before or at the beginning of the treatment and maintaining these settings up to the end of dialysis. Indeed, most hemodialysis treatments are still done using constant settings for the different treatment variables. However, the objective of reducing hemodialysis-related side effects, such as hypotension, cramps, or nausea, inspired investigators to look for a more refined way of controlling the treatment variables. The observation that hemodialysis-related side effects using constant treatment variables are not evenly distributed throughout the entire treatment indicates that the same perturbation has a different impact on patient stability when applied at different stages of the dialysis treatment. Therefore, to optimize patient stability, it would be advisable to adjust the perturbation to the relative susceptibility of the patient to particular treatment effects at different treatment stages. This rationale is most clearly understood for ultrafiltration, which is accepted as one of the main causes for hemodialysis-related hypotension.[100] Hypotensive events most often occur late in dialysis, so that it appears justified to shift the major part of overall fluid removal to early treatment phases, where excessive fluid volume is abundant, and to reduce ultrafiltration rates during later stages of the treatment, when the patient is close to the target weight and the risk of ultrafiltration-induced hypovolemia increases. It was therefore suggested that degressive ultrafiltration rates could be beneficial in decreasing ultrafiltration-induced side effects.

The use of variable treatment settings has become known as *profiled hemodialysis,* for which there are two distinct approaches. One approach is based on the predetermined setting of the treatment variable without feedback control, and the other is based on feedback control of this variable.

Fixed Profiles. Profiled dialysis must meet boundary conditions determined by the treatment goal and the time prescribed to reach that goal. For example, the ultrafiltration volume and the electrolyte balance achieved with a profiled treatment must be equal to that achieved with a treatment utilizing constant treatment settings. While the boundary conditions are easily met with profiled ultrafiltration rates, the same electrolyte balance may not always be attained using so-called Na$^+$ profiles. The reason for the discrepancy lies in the differences in the control of removal rates. With ultrafiltration, removal rate is exclusively controlled by the dialysis machine. With electrolyte balance, however, the actual solute transfer depends not only on variables controlled by the machine but also on patient variables, such as plasma sodium and potassium concentrations, which change during hemodialysis and can also be affected by changes in recirculation and electrolyte distribution volume.

Fixed profiles are available for variations of ultrafiltration rate and for dialysate conductivity as a surrogate for dialysate Na$^+$ concentration. They can be used separately or in combination (Fig. 3–10).

Continuous Profiles. The linear decrease in ultrafiltration rates represents the most common continuous profile. The boundary condition to reach the same ultrafiltration volume as with a constant ultrafiltration rate requires that initial ultrafiltration rates be increased above the level required for constant ultrafiltration. Similar considerations apply to the use of linear Na$^+$ profiles. For example, the profile for dialysate conductivity can be defined by the average conductivity used without profile and by the amplitude of the change in conductivities delivered between the start and the end of the treatment. Exponentially decreasing treatment variables can be seen as a variant of continuously degressive profiles.

Step Profiles. A modification of the continuous profile is obtained by a stepwise change of the treatment variable. Apart from the "roughness" introduced by the step change, the effect of the staircase profile can be assumed to resemble the continuous profile, especially with increasing numbers of steps.

Intermittent Profiles. Intermittent profiles have been very useful in analyzing the kinetics and dynamics of the physiologic system. A pulsed perturbation allows for analysis of the perturbation and return of the system to the equilibrated state. The best example for this approach is the analysis of

postdialysis urea rebound resulting from a step change in extracorporeal urea clearance, which reveals the two-compartment behavior of urea and can be used to estimate the intercompartmental urea transfer rate.[60,101] The same approach has been used to study the dynamics of vascular refilling, where a pulsed perturbation allows for analysis of the perturbation and the return of the system to the equilibrated state.[102] Intermittent ultrafiltration and dialysate conductivity profiles provide a number of pulses with high ultrafiltration rates and/or dialysate conductivities separated by phases without ultrafiltration and/or low dialysate conductivity. The number and height of successive pulses can be chosen within the limits of the boundary conditions.

Discussion of Profiles. A detailed discussion of the motivation and of the benefits of profiled dialysis may be found elsewhere.[103] There is good justification for degressive ultrafiltration profiles, especially since these ultrafiltration profiles develop naturally with feedback control of relative blood volume changes (see "*Hemoconcentration Control,*" *below*).[104,105] The benefit of Na$^+$ profiles is very much in debate, and a detailed discussion of this topic is beyond the scope of this chapter.[103] But the use of pulsed profiles has no justification at all. As much as intermittent urea clearance would be wasting valuable treatment time (the time between pulses), intermittent ultrafiltration wastes valuable time for fluid removal, especially with an interruption of ultrafiltration early in the treatment. When ultrafiltration phases are interrupted by phases without ultrafiltration, the treatment is in fact split into short segments, where the perturbation during each ultrafiltration phase must be increased, because of the boundary condition, to remove all of the excess body water. With a two-compartment system, such a procedure can be expected to greatly enhance compartment effects.[83] A pulsed treatment splits the treatment into even shorter segments and reduces effective treatment time. In view of the current impetus to increase treatment frequency and/or treatment time, the use of pulsed profiles is to be discouraged.

With two concentrates to mix, the opportunity to adjust the various components in dialysate is rather limited, as any change in the mixing ratio will proportionally affect all other components. However, to independently adjust the HCO$_3^-$, Na$^+$, K$^+$, and Ca^{2+} levels, these components must be available in separate concentrates and must be added to the dialysate by individual pumps. Some dialysis machines, such as the Integra (Hospal Dasco, Mirandola, Italy), offer profiles for individual dialysate ions such as K$^+$.

Finally, the use of predetermined profiles is based on the assumption that the physiologic system reacts in a predetermined way. This is certainly not always the case, especially with more complex and unusual patient reactions. A number of patients can be expected to benefit from the use

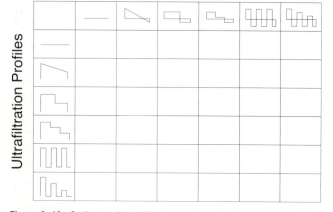

Figure 3–10. Sodium and ultrafiltration profiles. Example of the choice of profiles for separate and combined application of treatment variables.

of continuous and step profiles, but for complex treatments other approaches must be sought.

FEEDBACK CONTROL

Hemodynamic instability remains a key issue in current hemodialysis.[100] The system that must be controlled to ensure hemodynamic stability is complex and includes a number of variables—such as heart rate, arterial pressure, blood volume, central venous pressure, cardiac output, extracellular volume, total body water, hematocrit, and concentrations of various solutes—to name but a few. Which of these variables should be used as a measure to control for hemodynamic stability?

At first glance it seems that one should control for a desired blood pressure, similar to the physiologic barocontrol mechanism.[106,107] But this approach is not feasible. First, a continuous, reliable, and comfortable technique for the noninvasive measurement of arterial blood pressure during hemodialysis is not available. Second, hemodialysis has no direct means of driving heart rate, cardiac contractility, and peripheral vasoconstriction, which represent the powerful actuators of physiologic barocontrol. When the automatic administration of pharmacologic compounds is excluded, the only actuators to be driven by a controller incorporated into a current hemodialysis machine are composition, temperature, and flow of dialysate as well as blood flow and ultrafiltration rate. Therefore, to establish a feedback control system, it is necessary to measure variables that are directly affected by the dialysis process and exert an indirect effect on hemodynamic stability.

The choice of variables to be measured is also determined by practical considerations. The measurement of the variable must be noninvasive and continuous and the preferred location to measure it is in the extracorporeal system, either in the extracorporeal circulation, as for blood temperature, or in the dialysis machine, as for plasma water conductivity.[108]

Feedback control requires on-line monitoring of output variables with high accuracy and resolution and short response times, requiring special sensors. For ease of handling and minimal discomfort and because of the repeated nature of hemodialysis, sensors must be noninvasive. The extracorporeal system offers many locations for placement of sensors, providing well-defined measuring conditions that ensure proper sensor performance. Sensors should be placed as close to the patient as possible so as to minimize the delay between the actual system output and the measured sensor output, which may affect the stability of the control system. With a low blood flow and a remote sensor, the delayed actions of the control system have the potential to drive the output variable and the system into sustained oscillations and eventual instability.

Temperature Control

Patient temperature was one of the first physiologic variables to be automatically controlled during hemodialysis by the T-control mode offered by the Blood Temperature Monitor (BTM). The BTM automatically adjusts for confounding factors of thermal balance in hemodialysis patients, such as variable blood flows, variable patient, and variable dialysate temperatures.

The T-control mode is used to control body temperature. Mixed venous blood temperature draining from all tissues can be considered a good representative of core temperature. However, the temperature of blood drawn from the patient's access does not necessarily reflect mixed venous blood temperature, because of possible access and cardiopulmonary recirculation. The effects of recirculation on arterial line temperature are comparable to the effects of recirculation on arterial line urea concentration during dialysis and depend on the type and function of the access used. Thus, to determine mixed venous temperature as a surrogate for body temperature (T_b), arterial blood temperature (T_{art}) must be corrected for the combined effects of access and cardiopulmonary recirculation (R) and the temperature of venous blood returning to the patient (T_{ven}):[109]

$$T_b = T_{art} \frac{1}{1-R} - T_{ven} \frac{R}{1-R} \qquad (28)$$

The T-control mode requires the prescription of an hourly change in body temperature—for example, $-0.10°C \cdot h^{-1}$ for a desired decrease in body temperature of $0.4°C$ within a 4-hour dialysis treatment. Accordingly, to control for a constant body temperature throughout a treatment (a so-called isothermic treatment) one would have to prescribe a temperature change rate of $±0.00°C$. A proportional-integral controller uses the error signal between desired and actual change in temperature to actuate a bounded change in dialysate temperature, which changes the temperature of the venous blood returning to the patient, thereby changing the extracorporeal heat flow. The measurement of body temperature by the BTM is affected by delays determined by intra- and extracorporeal transport characteristics, the response characteristics of the sensor, and external influences. Since delays may destabilize a control system, the controller gain is kept low in order to provide stability. Although physiologic thermoregulation does not rely on the measurement of core temperature alone, both BTM feedback control and physiologic thermoregulation measure the same system output: i.e., arterial or mixed venous temperature. The BTM can also be operated in an E-control mode, which controls for the rate of thermal energy removal (dE/dt, in $kJ \cdot h^{-1}$). Even if this type of control affects patient temperature, it actually controls thermal flow rate, which is not a physiologic variable. Therefore it is not typical for a physiologic feedback control.

Thermoneutral Dialysis. Based on the concept of minimal perturbance of the physiologic system, it appears straightforward neither to remove nor add thermal energy through the extracorporeal circulation ($J_{ex} = 0$ W). Such a treatment is called *extracorporeally thermoneutral*. Since blood temperatures tend to fall in the venous line, because blood leaving the dialyzer is exposed to the cool environment, extracorporeally thermoneutral treatments usually require dialysate temperatures in the range of 37 to 37.5°C. This approach has been followed in a few studies, with the result that patient temperatures increased by approximately 0.5°C throughout dialysis.[110–112] Since an increase in body temperature is expected to increase cutaneous blood flow and to decrease total peripheral resistance,[113] thermoneutral hemodialysis may indeed favor hypotensive episodes and do more harm than good.

Isothermic Dialysis. The other major approach would be to adjust the removal of thermal energy so that there is no heat accumulation in the patient.[114] This goal can be achieved by controlling for a constant body temperature (T_b = const). Such a treatment is called *isothermic* ($\Delta T_b = 0$°C).

The clear hemodynamic benefits of isothermic compared to thermoneutral dialysis have been documented in a multicenter study carried out in 95 hypotension-prone dialysis patients.[115] In this field, this work stands out for the number of patients studied and for the approach, which eliminated the influence of confounding individual variables such as absolute body temperatures, blood flows, and dialysate temperatures.

As expected, body temperatures increased by 0.47 ± 0.24°C with thermoneutral treatments, and the 50 percent incidence of intradialytic morbid events was not affected when compared to the control period. However, with isothermic treatment modes ($\Delta T_b = 0.01 \pm 0.16$°C), thermal energy was removed from patients at a mean rate of -0.90 ± 0.35 kJ $\cdot$ kg^{-1} $\cdot$ h^{-1}, amounting to 24 percent of estimated energy expenditure. While this occurred, the incidence of intradialytic morbid events fell to 25 percent.

Isothermic treatments involved considerable cooling but did not affect the dose of delivered dialysis measured by Kt/V_{urea}, as might be expected from the alterations in regional blood-flow distribution.[116] This is in accordance with results of previous studies and can be explained by the reduction in hypotensive episodes, which are in themselves known to augment compartment effects and reduce Kt/V_{urea}.[111,117,118]

One aspect of this work deserves special attention. Isothermic treatments required a drop in dialysate temperatures, but the drop developed gradually throughout dialysis and the minimum dialysate temperature of 35.7°C never reached the lower levels used in many previous studies. This probably explains the excellent patient tolerance of the treatment. Is this an indicator of optimal care for this aspect

of dialysis? One can think of treatment modes where extracorporeal cooling exceeds the requirements for an isothermic treatment, so that body temperature will eventually fall. The BTM used in this study can indeed be set to prescribe an hourly change in body temperature. It is not known whether there are any benefits to be expected from such a prescription. However, a control to merely lower body temperature abandons the concept of physiologic feedback control, as under these circumstances the extracorporeal control system is working against physiologic temperature control. Unless there is a resetting in the hypothalamic thermostat during hemodialysis, which might be linked to the removal of uremic toxins or to other aspects of the dialysis procedure, the attempt to lower body temperature by the extracorporeal device can be expected to be counterregulated by the much more powerful internal temperature-control mechanisms. Patients can be expected to start shivering and feel uncomfortable, which is likely to defeat one of the objectives of an optimal dialysis—that is, to minimize perturbation of the dialysis patient.

In conclusion, when there is concern about hemodynamic stability, it is probably best to prevent an increase in body temperature during hemodialysis. Since a decrease in body temperature is likely to elicit powerful compensatory mechanisms, such as an increase in metabolic rate, maintaining body temperature at a constant level where feasible, is probably the best approach.

Hemoconcentration Control

Most of the fluid accumulated in the interdialytic period distributes in the extravascular space; however, its removal by ultrafiltration must occur via the intravascular space. While removal of fluid from the blood by ultrafiltration is limited only by technical factors, the fluid shift between extra- and intravascular compartments, also termed *vascular refilling*, is limited by physiologic factors such as the hydraulic conductivity of the microvascular wall.[102,119] If the vascular refilling rate does not match the ultrafiltration rate, blood volume will drop, and a drop in blood volume elicits a cascade of compensatory mechanisms.[120] Failure to compensate for a critically low blood volume eventually leads to symptomatic hypotension, which requires immediate attention.

Given that the patient has to be brought from an equilibrated state at the beginning of the treatment to a new equilibrated state at the end of ultrafiltration, the optimal trajectory of this transition is critical. So far, however, there is no clear guidance for this because of the compartmentalization of water in the body, the constraints given by the volume to be removed within the allocated time, and the lack of studies utilizing different trajectories.

Critical Blood Volume. The concept of a critical blood volume and of threshold values emerged from one of the earliest studies done in this field.[121] The authors studied 22 treatments, where 7 out of 9 hypotensive episodes occurred with absolute blood volumes below 2800 mL, which corresponded to a specific blood volume of less than 50 mL · kg^{-1}. Blood volume decreased by 24 ± 5 percent in hypotensive patients compared to 20 ± 9 percent in stable treatments. It is of note that one patient became hypotensive in spite of a blood volume of 3800 mL (57 mL · kg^{-1}) and where blood volume was reduced by only 18 percent. This "outlier" provides important information. A drop in blood volume is of little consequence to arterial blood pressure as long as the loss does not reflect a significant drop in central venous and right arterial pressures.

Critical Hemoconcentration. The concept of relative blood volume or hematocrit thresholds is attractive, as it eliminates the need to measure absolute blood volume. Because RBC mass remains essentially constant during hemodialysis, changes in hematocrit are inversely related to changes in blood volume. As a consequence, the critical blood volume could be identified by a critical hemoconcentration measured as a critical hematocrit.

There are reports that support the value of a relative blood-volume threshold and others that do not find a relationship between the relative blood volume and the onset of hypotension.[122–124] These discrepancies could be due to variations in overhydration and fluid distribution at the beginning of ultrafiltration, which would affect the calculation of relative blood changes as well as the relative blood-volume threshold but would not affect the hematocrit measured at the critical blood volume. Indeed, 12 of 16 patients studied during 93 dialysis sessions exhibited recurrent intradialytic morbid events when the hematocrit reached a patient-specific threshold.[125] The concept of a hematocrit threshold is not fully compatible with the concept of a relative blood-volume threshold. If RBC mass is really constant, then the hematocrit at the critical blood volume is also constant. However, variable degrees of overhydration and fluid distribution at the beginning of hemodialysis will lead to variations in the initial hematocrit, so that the change in hematocrit (and the corresponding change in blood volume) may be quite variable in reaching the same and constant threshold hematocrit. A major practical concern of this concept is, however, whether the threshold can be determined with sufficient consistency. The basic assumption of a constant RBC mass may be violated because of erythropoietin therapy or bleeding. Another problem with these thresholds is that they may not represent equilibrated states, which is essential if they are in fact to be used as true thresholds.

Slope of the Relative Blood-Volume Curve. In the ideal system with a constant ultrafiltration rate, the transition from over- to euhydration is associated with a blood-volume curve that is expected to be concave. The slope is large and negative at the beginning and continually flattens toward the end of dialysis. Based on this consideration, it has been hypothesized that a sudden decrease in slope despite constant ultrafiltration indicates reduced vascular refilling and an increased risk of intradialytic complications. It has been demonstrated that blood volume decreases more rapidly in hemodialysis sessions with hypotensive events than in sessions without hypotension.[122] This observation was confirmed in a study done in 16 patients, where the rate of blood-volume changes during sessions without morbidity was half that preceding intradialytic morbid events in other sessions (5.6 ± 3.6 vs. 12.2 ± 5.5%/h).[125] However, this criterion could not predict the onset of complications.

Blood-Volume Trajectory. It is generally assumed that the risk of hemodynamic instability increases during the second half and toward the end of the ultrafiltration treatment. One explanation is that this is due to the excessive drop in blood volume observed at the end of treatment carried out at a constant ultrafiltration rate. It was therefore suggested that one stimulate vascular refilling at the beginning of the treatment with the potential to prevent the excessive drop in blood volume toward the end of ultrafiltration.[126] One approach to increasing vascular refilling is to increase the ultrafiltration rate. High initial ultrafiltration rates will lead to a more rapid increase in colloid osmotic pressure gradient and higher vascular refilling rates at the beginning of the treatment.[127] With the goal of removing the same ultrafiltration volume, ultrafiltration rates can then be lowered during later phases of the treatment. Thus both enhanced refilling early during ultrafiltration as well as reduced fluid removal late during ultrafiltration are expected to prevent an excessive decrease in blood volume, especially late during dialysis.

A variety of feedback control algorithms covering the wide range from simple on-off techniques[128] to more complex fuzzy logic controllers have been proposed,[129] but only two systems are commercially available today, the Hospal and the Fresenius system.

The Hospal System. This system (Hemocontrol, Hospal-Dasco, Mirandola, Italy) is designed to control the trajectory of relative blood-volume changes by adjusting the dialysate composition and the ultrafiltration rate of the hemodialysis and ultrafiltration process.[130] The control system requires the definition of a target for the three variables incorporated into this control, i.e., weight reduction, dialysate conductivity, and blood-volume change (ΔBV). The rationale for inclusion of dialysate conductivity is based on the effects of sodium concentration on extracellular volume, vascular refilling, and blood-volume preservation.[131,132] Thus, in this system vascular refilling early during dialysis is enhanced by both a high ultrafiltration rate and a high dialysate sodium concentration. Based on the target values for weight change and treatment duration, the system determines a trajectory for intradialytic blood-volume changes, which are to be followed with a certain tolerance. Ultrafiltration rate is limited by a maximum rate of $2 \text{ L} \cdot \text{h}^{-1}$. Dialysate conductivity is controlled by the goal of providing the same sodium mass balance as a comparable treatment with constant dialysate conductivity. Calculations are based on the conductivity of the dialysate bath and on a sodium kinetic model. The control algorithm does not have access to a direct on-line measurement of plasma sodium concentration, so there is no feedback control of this system variable. Upper and lower bounds of 13.5 and $16 \text{ mS} \cdot \text{cm}^{-1}$ respectively limit dialysate conductivities. Failure to remain within the bounded region leads to specific alarms informing the operator when the control goal cannot be met. The system utilizes exponential blood-volume trajectories derived from the considerations outlined above. Ultrafiltration profiles obtained with this control system are anything but smooth. However, there is a trend toward declining ultrafiltration rates, as expected in controlling for exponential blood-volume trajectories. Ultrafiltration rates are higher than average at the beginning of the treatment and gradually decrease toward the end of the treatment (see also Fixed Profiles, this chapter, p. 69).

The Fresenius System. This control system is based on the definition of a critical relative blood volume (RBV_{crit}) and on declining ultrafiltration rates.[104] However, the system does not track a predefined blood-volume trajectory and does not aim to reach a target blood-volume reduction. Controlled fluid removal is achieved by a continuous determination of ultrafiltration rate according to the following rules: (1) volume must be removed within the treatment time; (2) initial ultrafiltration rate is set at twice the constant ultrafiltration rate; and (3) if relative blood volume drops more than half of the distance between the current (= 100 percent) and the critical relative blood volume, ultrafiltration rate is linearly decreased. Thus, in a treatment without a drop of relative blood volume below half the distance between current and critical relative blood volume, the algorithm provides a linear decrease in ultrafiltration rates, with ultrafiltration starting at twice the constant ultrafiltration rate and reaching zero ultrafiltration at the end of the treatment. However, when relative blood volume falls below half the distance between current and critical relative blood volume, ultrafiltration rate is further reduced, as defined by rule 2, with the consequence that ultrafiltration at the end of the treatment can no longer be zero. The system does not include a control of dialysate conductivity; however, it can be operated in combination with the T-control system offered by the BTM.

Comparison of Systems. Although both systems are based on measuring the same system output, i.e., relative blood-volume changes, there are important differences between the Hospal and the Fresenius concepts. A trivial difference relates to using a different representation of the calculated blood-volume change. A relative blood volume (RBV) of 85 percent measured by the Fresenius system corresponds to a RBV change (ΔBV) of -15 percent in the Hospal system. The two values are easily converted into each other. More importantly, the target volume reduction used in the Hospal system is not the same as the critical relative blood volume in the Fresenius system, and these values must not be mixed up. In the Hospal system, the relative volume reduction is used as a target, which the system will try to reach; whereas in the Fresenius system, the critical RBV serves as a threshold not to be reached. A use of Fresenius thresholds in the Hospal system is likely to enhance hemodynamic instability.

Clinical Studies. The first prospective study done for two periods of 1 month in 8 hypotensive patients showed that the pre- to postdialysis arterial blood pressure changes (-12.4 vs. -17.5 percent), number of severe hypotensive episodes (3 vs. 16), overall incidence of patient complaints (especially of muscle cramps), and need for therapeutically administered saline in each session (60 vs. 95 mL) were significantly reduced in controlled treatments using the Hospal system.[130] The target value for the change in RBV at the end of the treatment was deliberately kept lower with controlled ultrafiltration compared to treatments without volume control (-10.6 vs. -12.5 percent). Using the same system in 12 hypotension-prone patients in a short-term prospective crossover design, a significant reduction in the occurrence and severity of hypotensive episodes by 60 and 70 percent, respectively, was observed, as well as a 9 percent increase in equilibrated Kt/V in treatments performed with automatic feedback control of RBV changes.[133] The results show that cardiovascular stability also provides a positive effect on urea kinetics, most likely because of an adequate blood-flow distribution to all organ systems. In another study using the same system in 19 hypotension-prone patients for a duration of 14 to 30 months, the overall occurrence of symptomatic hypotension and muscle cramps decreased by 34 and 40 percent, respectively.[134]

Remaining Problems. Although the clinical studies using feedback control of RBV show an impressive reduction in intradialytic morbid events, one would expect optimal control to prevent all treatment complications. Whether failure to reach this goal is related to uncertainties of the measured output variables, such as RBV, to the missing control of other variables, or to the constraints determined by the prescription of targets to be reached within a given time, or whether this is related to other conceptual shortcomings remains to be investigated.

Could it be that RBV is not the relevant variable to be controlled during ultrafiltration? Current techniques to monitor RBV changes assume that blood volume behaves like a single compartment. Arterial, venous, and microcirculatory volumes, not to mention the blood volumes contained in the different organ systems, are lumped into one single blood volume. Thus a measured decline in blood volume cannot indicate which of these volumes really decreases. However, to defend against a decline in blood pressure and ensure diastolic filling, it is important to maintain a high central venous pressure, probably by means of a high central blood volume. It has been shown that the drop in central blood volume was larger in treatments accompanied by intradialytic morbid events (22 ± 12 vs. 14 ± 13 percent) even when absolute central blood volumes were comparable at the end of the treatment (1120 ± 500 vs. 1130 ± 440 mL).[135] The question of whether absolute volumes or relative changes of central blood volume determine hemodynamic stability is difficult to answer without the possibility of continuous measurements.

The variability in RBV changes in the same patient under identical treatment conditions from one treatment to another and the failure to identify useful blood-volume thresholds could be related to variations in initial blood volumes. The possibility of such variations is probably underestimated. Assume a patient with a critical blood volume of 4.5 L. On treatment A, the patient presents with an initial blood volume of 5 L, so that the RBV at the end of the treatment will be 90 percent (ΔBV = −10 percent). On treatment B, the patient presents with a blood volume of 5.25 L (only a 5 percent difference compared to treatment A). To reach the same critical blood volume of 4.5 L, the RBV at the end will have to be 85.7 percent (ΔBV −14.3 percent). It can be seen that a small change in initial blood volume compatible with the same weight gain and the same target weight makes a big difference for the actual RBV (and ΔBV) achieved at the critical blood volume. The measurement of absolute blood volume could be of help in identifying absolute volume thresholds.

Optimal Control

The systems discussed in this chapter control for one or two patient variables at best. However, to achieve increased benefits of feedback control, the systems would have to integrate all aspects of a controlled perturbation, such as ultrafiltration, dialysate composition, and dialysate temperature. But even such a system will be far from exhibiting the full benefits of feedback control. Take ultrafiltration as an example. Current systems still require an input regarding the ultrafiltration volume, the RBV limit, or the desired target volume reduction. However, the ultimate goal of ultrafiltration is to normalize blood pressure and the intrinsic blood pressure control system with the fewest complications in

the shortest time possible. Thus, an integrated feedback system must be able to identify the amount of fluid to be removed from the patient, depending on the degree of overhydration and under the constraints of the patient's level of hemodynamic stability. One can envision a future system that will measure overhydration, for example, by bioimpedance, set an ultrafiltration volume, and perform a controlled removal of this volume within an optimal time using information on blood volume, blood pressure, heart rate, cardiac output, and the physiologic control characteristics of the patient.

PERITONEAL DIALYSIS

The requirements to perform peritoneal dialysis (PD) are a catheter for instillation of dialysate into the peritoneal cavity, a system to connect the catheter to the source of the dialysate, the peritoneal dialysate, and a delivery system for the preparation or the delivery of dialysate into the peritoneal cavity.

Peritoneal dialysate delivery systems may be subdivided into on-line proportioning systems and cycler devices. With proportioning systems, a peritoneal dialysate concentrate is used with on-line blending of the concentrate and purified water comparable to the procedure in a hemodialysis machine. The composition and temperature of the resulting dialysate are controlled and monitored, and means are provided for safe instillation of this dialysate into the peritoneal cavity. In both on-line systems and cyclers, means are provided for timing and sequencing the various phases of the peritoneal dialysis cycle, namely the fill, dwell, and drain phases (Fig. 3–11).

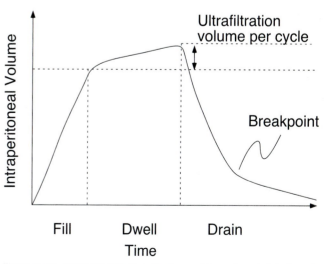

Figure 3–11. Peritoneal dialysis cycle. A complete peritoneal dialysis cycle consists of fill, dwell, and drain phases.

Dialysate

Dialysate Volume and Flow. The capacity of peritoneal dialysis is highly dependent on the transport characteristics of the peritoneal membrane. The three-pore model of the peritoneal membrane describes transport of water, small solutes, and large solutes through aquaporins, small, and large pores.[136] A fill volume of 2 L is the most commonly prescribed volume in the adult patient. This volume may, however, have to be adapted to the patient's body surface area to reach the peak normalized mass transfer area coefficient (MTAC).[137] The fill volume must be adapted to the size of the patient and should be as close to the maximal value, so as to use all of the functional peritoneum while generating an intraperitoneal pressure below 18 cmH_2O. One exchange, which is also referred to as a *cycle* in automated PD, consists of three phases: the fill, dwell, and drain phases (Fig. 3–11).

The fill phase usually provides a constant flow rate. This depends on the pressure gradient, the size and position of the peritoneal catheter, and the patient's posture. Fluid administration in PD cyclers can be controlled for pressure or flow rate.[138] The drain phase is characterized by an initially high flow rate followed by an abrupt transition to a very low flow rate. The transition is also referred to as the breakpoint.[139] More than 50 percent of the drain time may be spent on draining less than 20 percent of the total fluid volume. The higher the number of cycles used in automated PD, the more important it is to reduce the time spent on draining and filling. This is particularly important when performing tidal PD, where only part of the fill volume is exchanged at each cycle. The higher the fill volume, the more solutes can be removed in a given time. On the other hand, the intraperitoneal pressure will increase with increasing fill volume, thereby reducing ultrafiltration as well as convective solute removal.

Dialysate Composition. The typical dialysate used for peritoneal dialysis has a high osmotic pressure for the purpose of ultrafiltration. The ideal osmotic agent is characterized by a high reflection coefficient (of 1), so that it will not be absorbed[140]; it exerts a dose-dependent effect on ultrafiltration, does not accumulation in the body, has a neutral pH, and is inexpensive. Glucose fulfills most of these requirements but causes problems with regard to the stability of the dialysate solutions, the high caloric load, and its reactions with proteins and other biological material.

The typical concentration of glucose in peritoneal dialysate is in the range of 2.5 to 4 wt%. At the molecular weight of glucose ($180 g \cdot mol^{-1}$), this corresponds to an increment in osmolarity in the range of 135 to 220 mOsmol $\cdot$ L^{-1}. When used in a typical continuous ambulatory PD regimen with four exchanges per day, the high glucose concentration in the dialysate and the absorption of glucose into the blood will lead to a glucose load between 150 and 300 g

$\cdot$ day^{-1}, depending on the type of concentrate used. This glucose load corresponds to 3000 to 6000 kJ $\cdot$ day^{-1}, a significant fraction of energy expenditure. On the other hand, there is a considerable loss of protein across the peritoneal membrane, in the range of 5 to 15 g $\cdot$ day^{-1}. The negative nitrogen balance can be improved by replacing the glucose in the PD solutions by amino acids. The ultrafiltration effect of a 1.1 wt% amino acid solution is comparable to that of a 1.5% glucose solution.[141]

The rate of glucose resorption can be slowed by replacing glucose with glucose polymers, such as icodextrin. Icodextrin consists of 4 to 30 glucose units per molecule and has a mean molecular weight of 16800 g $\cdot$ mol^{-1}. A 7.5% solution of icodextrin exerts an osmotic pressure of only 280 mOsmol $\cdot$ L^{-1} and is isoosmolar to plasma. The osmotic action of icodextrin, however, is based on the high reflection coefficient of the glucose polymer. Thus, there is colloid-osmotic pressure-driven ultrafiltration even with a solution of the same or even lower osmotic pressure than plasma.[142]

The standard base in PD solutions is lactate. The use of bicarbonate-based PD fluids requires a bag material that is impermeable to CO_2 and separation of the Ca^{+2} and HCO_3^- components to avoid precipitation of insoluble $CaCO_3$. The use of bicarbonate as base is possible with two or more compartment bags, where one compartment contains the bicarbonate and the other compartment contains the glucose in a strongly acidic environment. The components are mixed just before use to yield a neutral dialysate solution. Separation of the components has an additional benefit, as the degradation of traces of glucose into aggressive and toxic aldehydes during heat sterilization and storage is inhibited by the acidic environment.[143]

Delivery Systems

In automated peritoneal dialysis (APD), the exchange of fresh and spent dialysate is controlled by the PD machine, the PD cycler, according to a preprogrammed schedule. The dialysate is commercially prepared according to the desired formulation and is contained in bags or bottles ready for use. The cycler is usually provided with a heating device for bringing the dialysate temperature into the physiologic range. The treatment takes place during the night, while the patient is asleep and connected to the cycler. A number of variable treatment parameters—such as fill volumes, dwell times, fill and drain times, and the number of cycles, all of which affect the outcome of the APD procedure—can be controlled by the machine (Fig. 3–12). Means are also provided for monitoring the outflow to ensure that the volume drained is at least equal to that instilled.

Cyclers were first developed for intermittent peritoneal dialysis typically performed three times per week during the patient's visit to the outpatient center.[144,145] Recognizing that treatment frequency and/or treatment duration had to be

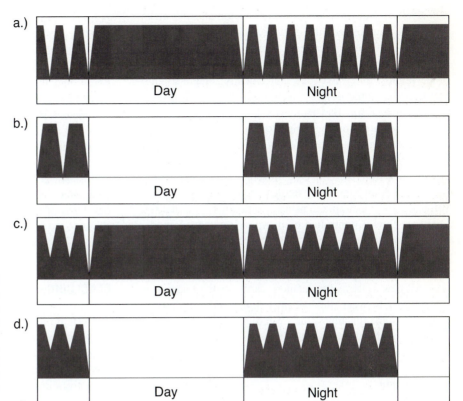

Figure 3–12. Modes for automated peritoneal dialysis. *A.* Continuous-cycling peritoneal dialysis (CCPD) with eight exchanges during the night and the peritoneal cavity filled during the day (=wet day). *B.* Nightly intermittent peritoneal dialysis (NIPD) with five exchanges during the night and the peritoneal cavity drained during the day (=dry day). *C.* Tidal peritoneal dialysis (TPD) with a wet day. *D.* TPD with a dry day.

increased to provide sufficient clearance, continuous ambulatory peritoneal dialysis (CAPD) was developed.[146] In CAPD, the total fill volume is administered via four to five exchanges during the day and a filled peritoneal cavity is maintained during the night. However, because the exchanges occur during the entire day, the use of automatic cyclers is not convenient for CAPD.

Automated Peritoneal Dialysis. Automated peritoneal dialysis (APD) requires that the patient remain connected to the system and that the components such as the dialysate and all the required equipment can stay in one place. Thus, automated PD is best done during the night. The administration of dialysate in APD differs depending on the selected regimen (Fig. 3–12). A difference in APD modes relates to the state of the peritoneal cavity during the day. In continuous cycling peritoneal dialysis (CCPD), four to eight exchanges are performed during the night and the abdominal cavity is filled during the day (also known as wet day APD).[147,148] In nightly intermittent peritoneal dialysis (NIPD), five to ten exchanges are performed during the night and the abdominal cavity remains empty during the day (also known as dry day APD).

Tidal PD (TPD) was introduced with the aim to enhance the performance of peritoneal dialysis. Both forms of cycler APD (NIPD and CCPD) can also be performed in the tidal mode (Fig. 3–12). An initial fill volume is instilled but only part of this (50 to 80 percent) is drained out and replaced with each cycle. More frequent exchanges and larger volumes are normally required than with other regimens. TPD can be combined with a wet or a dry day. Clinical studies, however, have shown that tidal modes do not lead to an improved dialysis.[149–151]

The efficiency of PD can also be enhanced by a continuous flow of dialysate through the peritoneal cavity, where the spent dialysate is cleared by an extracorporeal system and returned to the peritoneal cavity. Continuous-flow peritoneal dialysis (CFPD) revisits the concept of peritoneal extracorporeal recirculation dialysis (RPD).[152] Clearance of small molecules was tripled utilizing perfusion volumes of up to $18 \text{ L} \cdot \text{h}^{-1}$.[153] This treatment mode could be an option when targets of adequacy for PD recommended by the NKF-DOQI guidelines are difficult to reach. To perform CFPD, a two-way access must be available in order to allow for the continuous inflow and outflow of the dialysate. This is also the most important concern with CFPD. A feasible two-way access is most likely achieved with a double-lumen peritoneal catheter. The double-lumen design does not necessarily increase the size of the tube or discomfort to the patient. The real challenge is to minimize recirculation and mixing of the inflow and outflow dialysate. The development of special double-lumen catheters (Medcomp, Medical Components, Inc., Harleysville, Pennsylvania) has led to increasing interest in this technique.[154–156]

ADP Cyclers. New-generation cyclers automatically make the connection between the peritoneal catheter and the machine and perform the treatment as programmed into the cycler or downloaded from a memory card. Connectors, membrane pumps, and valves are conveniently integrated into one cassette. Some devices, such as the SleepSafe (Fresenius Medical Care, Bad Homburg, Germany), utilize barcoded information on the connectors of the different bags. The proper bags are recognized by the cycler program and the PD mode is performed according to the prescription downloaded from the chip card. Several systems to connect the fill and drain bags under sterile conditions have been developed—for example, using ultraviolet irradiation. Dialysate flow is controlled by membrane pumps. A modified membrane pump is used by the Serena system (Gambro Lundia AB, Lund, Sweden), where the entire fill bag is placed in a flow-control chamber to produce a steady flow.

All new systems use memory cards for the transfer of information between the patient's home and the dialysis center. In some machines, the fresh dialysate is warmed by a flow-through cell, so that the dialysate bags do not have to be preheated.

Telemedicine

Typically, APD is performed at home, and the physician has little control over it. Recent technical developments aim at improving this situation.[157] The new generation of APD devices is equipped with memory cards to improve the transfer of information between the PD cycler located at the patient's home and the physician. At the dialysis unit, memory cards such as the HomeChoice Pro Card (Baxter Inc., Deerfield, IL), the SleepSafe Patient Card (Fresenius Medical Care, Bad Homburg, Germany), and the Serena Patient Card (Gambro Lundia AB, Lund, Sweden) can be used to save the prescribed dialysis schedule. At home, the program is downloaded to the cycler by the patient.[158] The memory cards can also be used to save all relevant aspects of a series of treatments. At regular intervals, the memory cards are brought to the center, where all treatments can be analyzed with a computer program. This approach facilitates identification of treatment problems such as ultrafiltration failures. Other developments allow a data connection by phone and modem for on-line control of remote treatments.

Control and Quantification

The standardized peritoneal equilibration test provides information on the rate of transport by measuring the dialysate-to-plasma ratio (D/P) for creatinine and the dialysate to 0-hour dialysate ratio (D/D_0) for glucose at given intervals during a 4-hour dwell.[159,160] The patient is then characterized as having a low, low average, high average, or high transport rate. A number of computer programs using different models for data collection and calculation of peritoneal transport characteristics are available.[161–163] The PDC program (Gambro Lundia AB, Lund, Sweden) uses data collected during actual treatments in either CAPD or APD modes.[164,165] Data are sampled over a period of 24 hours, and the greater the quantity of data collected, the more accurate the identified model parameters. The PDC parameters provide information on the effective surface area and on the ultrafiltration coefficient of the peritoneal membrane compared to the characteristics of a dialyzer. The actual creatinine clearance and Kt/V for a given PD regime are also calculated. By knowing the patient's PDC parameters, it is possible to simulate a PD regime to best fit the needs of the patient, whether in the CAPD or the APD mode.

CONCLUDING REMARKS

There is no doubt that the quality and the precision of the machines involved in renal replacement therapy have a major impact on the quality of life and on overall patient survival. It is also clear that the current technical approach is far from perfect in many respects—for example, with regard to patient mobility and rehabilitation, which must consider the conflicting issues of treatment duration and treatment frequency. With the current focus on molecular and genetic engineering, expectations for "classic" technical solutions are declining, even though there is ample room for real technical improvement. There also is a general feeling that there has been a lack of major breakthroughs in dialysis technology, as the gains made in patient outcomes over the past two decades appear to be small. This may be one of the reasons why the field is so conservative. Several recent products were conceived decades ago but made it to the market only within the last few years. With only dinosaurs left in the ecosystem, the field is likely to become more conservative. One can only speculate about the nature and consequences of the next substantial breakthrough in the technical delivery of dialysis.

REFERENCES

1. Depner TA, Rizwan S, Stasi TA. Pressure effects on roller pump blood flow during hemodialysis. *ASAIO Trans* 1990;36:M456–M459.
2. Schneditz D, Rainer F, Kenner T. Viscoelastic properties of whole blood; influence of fast sedimenting red blood cell aggregates. *Biorheology* 1987;24:13–22.
3. Schmid-Schönbein H, Wells R. Fluid drop-like transition of erythrocytes under shear. *Science* 1969;165:288–291.
4. Taylor GI. The viscosity of a fluid containing small drops of another fluid. *Proc R Soc (London)* 1932;138A:41–45.

5. Dintenfass L. Internal viscosity of the red cell and a blood viscosity equation. *Nature* 1968;219:956–957.

6. Harkness J. The viscosity of human blood plasma; its measurement in health and disease. *Biorheology* 1971;8:171–193.

7. Faber TE. *Fluid Dynamics for Physicists.* Cambridge, UK: Cambridge University Press, 1995.

8. Prandtl L, Oswatitsch K, Wieghardt K. *Führer durch die Strömungslehre.* Braunschweig/Wiesbaden: Vieweg, 1984.

9. Polaschegg HD. Pressure and flow in the extracorporeal circuit. *Clin Nephrol* 2000;53:S50–S55.

10. Besarab A, Dorrell S, Moritz M, et al. Determinants of measured dialysis venous pressure and its relationship to true intra-access venous pressure. *ASAIO Trans* 1991;37:M270–M271.

11. Besarab A, al-Saghir F, Alnabhan N, Lubkowski T, Frinak S. Simplified measurement of intra-access pressure. *ASAIO J* 1996;42:M682–M687.

12. Besarab A, Sullivan KL, Ross RP, Moritz MJ. Utility of intra-access pressure monitoring in detecting and correcting venous outlet stenoses prior to thrombosis. *Kidney Int* 1995;47:1364–1373.

13. Polaschegg HD. Access physics. *Semin Dial* 1999;12:S33–S40.

14. Rolle F, Pengloan J, Abazza M, et al. Identification of microemboli during haemodialysis using Doppler ultrasound. *Nephrol Dial Transplant* 2000;15:1420–1424.

15. Droste DW, Beyna T, Frye B, et al. Reduction of circulating microemboli in the subclavian vein of patients undergoing haemodialysis using pre-filled instead of dry dialysers. *Nephrol Dial Transplant* 2003;18:2377–2381.

16. Borger MA, Feindel CM. Cerebral emboli during cardiopulmonary bypass: effect of perfusionist interventions and aortic cannulas. *J Extracorp Technol* 2002;34:29–33.

17. Kleinekofort W, Kleiner N, Krämer M. Non-invasive measurement of postpump arterial pressure (abstr). *ASAIO J* 2003;49:A191.

18. Stiller S, Mann H, Brunner H. Backfiltration in hemodialysis with highly permeable membranes. *Contrib Nephrol* 1985;46:23–32.

19. Pallone TL, Hyver SW, Petersen J. A model of the volumetrically-controlled hemodialysis circuit. *Kidney Int* 1992;41:1366–1373.

20. Aldridge C, Greenwood RN, Cattell WR, Barrett RV. The assessment of arteriovenous fistulae created for haemodialysis from pressure and thermal dilution measurements. *J Med Eng Technol* 1984;8:118–124.

21. Schwab SJ, Raymond JR, Saled M, et al. Prevention of hemodialysis fistula thrombosis. Early detection of venous stenoses. *Kidney Int* 1989;36:707–711.

22. Van Stone JC, Jones M, Van Stone J. Detection of hemodialysis access outlet stenosis by measuring outlet resistance. *Am J Kidney Dis* 1994;23:562–568.

23. Moissl U, Wabel P, Leonhardt S, et al. Continuous observation and analysis of heart rate during hemodialysis treatment. *Med Biol Eng Comput* 1999;37:S558–S559.

24. Polaschegg HD. Pressure pulses measured non-invasively in the extracoproreal circuit (abstr). *Int J Artif Organs* 2003;26:646.

25. Collins AJ, Hanson G, Berkseth R, Keshaviah PR. Recirculation and effective clearances (abstr). *Kidney Int* 1988;33:219.

26. Rosales LM, Schneditz D, Morris AT, et al. Isothermic hemodialysis and ultrafiltration. *Am J Kidney Dis* 2000;36:353–361.

27. Schneditz D, Rosales L, Kaufman AM, et al. Heat accumulation with relative blood volume decrease. *Am J Kidney Dis* 2002;40:777–782.

28. Svirbely JR, Sriram MG. The Medical Algorithms Project. http://www.medal.org, 2003.

29. Schneditz D. Temperature and thermal balance in hemodialysis. *Semin Dial* 2001;14:357–364.

30. Drost CJ. Vessel diameter-independent volume flow measurements using ultrasound. *Proc San Diego Biomed Symp* 1978;17:299–302.

31. Krämer M, Steil H, Polaschegg HD. Optimization of a sensor head for blood temperature measurement during hemodialysis. *Proc IEEE EMBS* 1992;14:1610–1611.

32. Steinke JM, Shepherd AP. Role of light scattering in spectrophotometric measurements of arteriovenous oxygen difference. *IEEE Trans Biomed Eng* 1986;33:729–734.

33. Twersky V. Absorption and multiple scattering by biological suspensions. *J Opt Soc Am* 1970;60:1084–1093.

34. Schallenberg U, Stiller S, Mann H. A new continuous haemoglobinometric measurement of blood volume during haemodialysis. *Life Support Systems* 1987; 5: 293–305

35. Oppenheimer L, Richardson WN, Bilan D, Hoppensack M. Colorimetric device for measurement of transvascular fluid flux in blood-perfused organs. *J Appl Physiol* 1987;62:364–372.

36. Wilkinson JS, Fleming SJ, Greenwood RN, et al. Continuous measurement of blood hydration during ultrafiltration using optical methods. *Med Biol Eng Comput* 1987;25:317–323.

37. McMahon MP, Campbell SB, Shannon GF, et al. A noninvasive continuous method of measuring blood volume during haemodialysis using optical techniques. *Med Eng Phys* 1996;18(2):105–109.

38. de Vries JPPM, Olthof CG, Visser V, et al. Continuous measurement of blood volume using light reflection: method and validation. *Med Biol Eng Comput* 1993;31:412–415.

39. Steuer RR, Harris DH, Conis JM. A new optical technique for monitoring hematocrit and circulating blood volume: its application in renal dialysis. *Dial Transplant* 1993; 22:260–265.

40. Paolini F, Mancini E, Bosetto A, Santoro A. Hemoscan: a dialysis machine-integrated blood volume monitor. *Int J Artif Organs* 1995;18:487–494.

41. Urick RJ. A sound velocity method for determining the compressibility of finely divided substances. *J Appl Phys* 1947;18:983–987.

42. Kenner T, Hinghofer-Szalkay H, Leopold H, Pogglitsch H. Verhalten der Blutdichte in Relation zum Blutdruck im Tierversuch und bei Hämodialyse von Patienten. *Z Kardiol* 1977;66:399–401.

43. Schneditz D, Heimel H, Stabinger H. Sound speed, density and total protein concentration of blood. *J Clin Chem Clin Biochem* 1989;27:803–806.

44. Wang SH, Lee LP, Lee JS. A linear relation between the compressibility and density of blood. *J Acoust Soc Am* 2001;109:390–396.

45. Kenner T. The measurement of blood density and its meaning. *Basic Res Cardiol* 1989;84:111–124.

46. Schneditz D, Pogglitsch H, Horina JH, Binswanger U. A blood protein monitor for the continuous measurement of blood volume changes during hemodialysis. *Kidney Int* 1990;38:342–346.

47. Ghezzi PM, Frigato G, Fantini GF, et al. Theoretical model and first clinical results of the paired filtration-dialysis (PFD). *Life Support Syst* 1983:1(suppl 1), 5271–5274.

48. Santoro A, Tetta C, Mandolfo S, et al. On-line urea kinetics in haemodiafiltration. *Nephrol Dial Transplant* 1996;11: 1084–1092.

49. Canaud B, Bosc JY, Cabrol L, et al. Urea as a marker of adequacy in hemodialysis: lesson from in vivo urea dynamics monitoring. *Kidney Int Suppl* 2000;76:S28–S40.

50. Lassen NA, Henriksen O, Sejrsen P. Indicator methods for measurement of organ and tissue blood flow. In: Shepherd JT, Abboud FM, eds. *Handbook of Physiology. Section 2: The Cardiovascular System.* Vol 3. Bethesda, MD: American Physiological Society, 1983:21–63.

51. Yarar D, Cheung AK, Sakiewicz P, et al. Ultrafiltration method for measuring vascular access flow rates during hemodialysis. *Kidney Int* 1999;56:1129–1135.

52. Depner TA, Krivitski NM, MacGibbon D. Hemodialysis access recirculation measured by ultrasound dilution. *ASAIO J* 1995;41:M749–M753.

53. Lindsay RM, Burbank J, Brugger J, et al. A device and a method for rapid and accurate measurement of access recirculation during hemodialysis. *Kidney Int* 1996;49: 1152–1160.

54. Schneditz D, Krivitski NM. Vascular access recirculation: measurement and clinical implications. *Contrib Nephrol* 2004; 142:254–268.

55. Hester RL, Ashcraft D, Curry E, Bower J. Non-invasive determination of recirculation in the patient on dialysis. *ASAIO J* 1992;38:M190–M193.

56. Bosc JY, Leblanc M, Garred LJ, et al. Direct determination of blood recirculation rate in hemodialysis by a conductivity method. *ASAIO J* 1998;44:68–73.

57. Kaufman AM, Krämer M, Godmere RO, et al. Hemodialysis access recirculation (R) measurement by blood temperature monitoring (BTM)–a new technique (abstr). *J Am Soc Nephrol* 1991;2:324.

58. Schneditz D, Fan Z, Kaufman AM, Levin NW. Measurement of access flow during hemodialysis using the constant infusion approach. *ASAIO J* 1998;44:74–81.

59. Krivitski NM. Theory and validation of access flow measurement by dilution technique during hemodialysis. *Kidney Int* 1995;48:244–250.

60. Schneditz D, Kaufman AM, Polaschegg HD, et al. Cardiopulmonary recirculation during hemodialysis. *Kidney Int* 1992;42:1450–1456.

61. Schneditz D, Wang E, Levin NW. Validation of hemodialysis recirculation and access blood flow measured by thermodilution. *Nephrol Dial Transplant* 1999;14:376–383.

62. Mercadal L, Hamani A, Bene B, Petitclerc T. Determination of access blood flow from ionic dialysance: theory and validation. *Kidney Int* 1999;56:1560–1565.

63. Gotch FA, Buyaki R, Panlilio F, Folden T. Measurement of blood access flow rate during hemodialysis from conductivity dialysance. *ASAIO J* 1999;45:139–146.

64. Dalal S, Yu AW, Gupta DK, et al. L-lactate high-efficiency hemodialysis: hemodynamics, blood gas changes, potassium/phosphorus, and symptoms. *Kidney Int* 1990;38: 896–903.

65. Nolph KD, Twardowski ZJ, Khanna R, et al. Tidal peritoneal dialysis with racemic or L-lactate solutions. *Perit Dial Int* 1990;10:161–164.

66. Ing TS, Yu AW, Nagaraja V, et al. Employing L-lactic acid powder in the preparation of a dry "acid concentrate" for use in a bicarbonate-based dialysis solution-generating system: experience in hemodialysis patients. *Int J Artif Organs* 1994;17:70–73.

67. Ahmad S, Callan R, Cole JJ, Blagg CR. Dialysate made from dry chemicals using citric acid increases dialysis dose. *Am J Kidney Dis* 2000;35:493–499.

68. McInnes DA. *The Principles of Electrochemistry*. New York: Reinhold, 1939.

69. Hosoya N, Sakai K. Backdiffusion rather than backfiltration enhances endotoxin transport through highly permeable dialysis membranes. *ASAIO Trans* 1990;36:M311–M313.

70. Pereira BJ, Snodgrass BR, Hogan PJ, King AJ. Diffusive and convective transfer of cytokine-inducing bacterial products across hemodialysis membranes. *Kidney Int* 1995;47: 603–610.

71. Fassbinder W. Renaissance of the batch method? *Nephrol Dial Transplant* 1998;13:3010–3012.

72. Fassbinder W. Experience with the GENIUS hemodialysis system. *Kidney Blood Press Res* 2003;26:96–99.

73. Waugh WH. Utility of expressing serum sodium per unit of water in assessing hyponatremia. *Metabolism* 1969;18: 706–712.

74. Polaschegg HD, Levin NW. Hemodialysis machines and monitors. In: Jacobs C, Kjellstrand CM, Koch KM, Winchester JF, eds. *Replacement of Renal Function by Dialysis*. Dordrecht, The Netherlands: Kluwer, 1996:333–380.

75. Gotch FA. Evolution of the single-pool urea kinetic model. *Semin Dial* 2001;14:252–256.

76. Brimble KS, Treleaven DJ, Onge JS, Carlisle EJ. Risk factors for increased variability in dialysis delivery in haemodialysis patients. *Nephrol Dial Transplant* 2003;18: 2112–2117.

77. Petitclerc T, Bene B, Boukhlafa Z, et al. Estimation of in vivo dialysance without blood or dialysate sampling (abstr). *Blood Purif* 1992;10:84.

78. Polaschegg HD. Automatic, noninvasive intradialytic clearance measurement. *Int J Artif Organs* 1993;16:185–191.

79. Petitclerc T, Goux N, Reynier AL, Bene B. A model for noninvasive estimation of in vivo dialyzer performances and patient's conductivity during hemodialysis. *Int J Artif Organs* 1993;16:585–591.

80. Polaschegg HD. On-line clearance measurement of uremic solutes: in vitro evaluation (abstr). *Int J Artif Organs* 2003; 26:597.

81. Ing TS, Yu AW, Wong FK, et al. Collection of a representative fraction of total spent hemodialysate. *Am J Kidney Dis* 1995;25:810–812.

82. Daugirdas JT. Second generation logarithmic estimates of single-pool variable volume *Kt/V*: an analysis of error. *J Am Soc Nephrol* 1993;4:1205–1213.

83. Daugirdas JT, Schneditz D. Overestimation of hemodialysis dose depends on dialysis efficiency by regional blood flow but not by conventional two pool urea kinetic analysis. *ASAIO J* 1995;41:M719–M724.

84. Garred LJ, Canaud B, Bosc JY, Tetta C. Urea rebound and delivered *Kt/V* determination with a continuous urea sensor. *Nephrol Dial Transplant* 1997;12:535–542.

85. Sternby J. Urea sensors–a world of possibilities. *Adv Renal Replace Ther* 1999;6:265–272.

86. Keshaviah PR, Ebben JP, Emerson PF. On-line monitoring of the delivery of the hemodialysis prescription. *Pediatr Nephrol* 1995;9(suppl):S2–S8.

87. Depner TA, Keshaviah PR, Ebben JP, et al. Multicenter clinical validation of an on-line monitor of dialysis adequacy. *J Am Soc Nephrol* 1996;7:464–471.

88. Weber C, Stummvoll HK, Passon S, Falkenhagen D. Monocyte activation and humoral immune response to endotoxins in patients receiving on-line hemodiafiltration therapy. *Int J Artif Organs* 1998;21:335–340.

89. Lonnemann G, Schindler R. Ultrafiltration using the polysulfone membrane to reduce the cytokine-inducing activity of contaminated dialysate. *Clin Nephrol* 1994;42(suppl 1):S37–S43.

90. Weber C, Linsberger I, Rafiee-Tehrani M, Falkenhagen D. Permeability and adsorption capacity of dialysis membranes to lipid A. *Int J Artif Organs* 1997;20:144–152.

91. Canaud B, Bosc JY, Leray H, et al. On-line haemodiafiltration: state of the art. *Nephrol Dial Transplant* 1998;13 (suppl 5):3–11.

92. Locatelli F, Marcelli D, Conte F, et al. Comparison of mortality in ESRD patients on convective and diffusive extracorporeal treatments. The Registro Lombardo Dialisi E Trapianto. *Kidney Int* 1999;55:286–293.

93. Wizemann V, Lotz C, Techert F, Uthoff S. On-line haemodiafiltration versus low-flux haemodialysis. A prospective randomized study. *Nephrol Dial Transplant* 2000;15 (suppl 1):43–48.

94. Henderson LW, Sanfelippo ML, Beans E. "On line" preparation of sterile pyrogen-free electrolyte solution. *Trans Am Soc Artif Intern Organs* 1978;24:465–467.

95. Ledebo I. On-line preparation of solutions for dialysis: practical aspects versus safety and regulations. *J Am Soc Nephrol* 2002;13(suppl 1):S78–S83.

96. Morris AT, Schneditz D, Levin NW. Challenging an on-line hemodiafiltration system with *Pseudomonas aeruginosa* (abstr). *J Am Soc Nephrol* 1998;9:178A.

97. Maggiore Q, Pizzarelli F, Dattolo P, et al. Cardiovascular stability during haemodialysis, haemofiltration and haemodifiltration. *Nephrol Dial Transplant* 2000;15:S68–S73.

98. van der Sande FM, Gladziwa U, Kooman JP, et al. Energy transfer is the single most important factor for the difference in vascular response between isolated ultrafiltration and hemodialysis. *J Am Soc Nephrol* 2000;11:1512–1517.

99. Di Filippo S, Manzoni C, Andrulli S, et al. Sodium removal during pre-dilution haemofiltration. *Nephrol Dial Transplant* 2003;18(suppl 7):vii31–vii36; discussion vii57–vii58.

100. Daugirdas JT. Pathophysiology of dialysis hypotension: an update. *Am J Kidney Dis* 2001;38:S11–S17.

101. Pedrini LA, Zereik S, Rasmy S. Causes, kinetics and clinical implications of post-hemodialysis urea rebound. *Kidney Int* 1988;34:817–824.

102. Schneditz D, Roob JM, Oswald M,. Nature and rate of vascular refilling during hemodialysis and ultrafiltration. *Kidney Int* 1992;42:1425–1433.

103. Grassmann A, Uhlenbusch-Körwer I, Bonnie-Schorn E, Vienken J. Neuere Entwicklungen im Bereich Dialysierflüssigkeit. In: Grassmann A, Uhlenbusch-Körwer I, Bonnie-Schorn E, Vienken J, eds. *Zusammensetzung und Handhabung von Dialysierflüssigkeiten.* Lengerich, Germany: Pabst Science Publishers, 2001:276–335.

104. Krämer M. New strategies for reducing intradialytic symptoms. *Semin Dial* 1999;12:389–395.

105. Santoro A, Mancini E, Paolini F, et al. Automatic control of blood volume trends during hemodialysis. *ASAIO J* 1994;40:M419–M422.

106. Lipps BJ. Automated hemodialysis control based upon patient blood pressure and heart rate. US Patent 4718891, 1988.

107. Schmidt R, Roeher O, Hickstein H, Korth S. Prevention of haemodialysis-induced hypotension by biofeedback control of ultrafiltration and infusion. *Nephrol Dial Transplant* 2001;16:595–603.

108. Petitclerc T. Festschrift for Professor Claude Jacobs. Recent developments in conductivity monitoring of haemodialysis session. *Nephrol Dial Transplant* 1999;14:2607–2613.

109. Krämer M, Polaschegg HD. The relevance of thermal effects during hemodialysis. In: Friedman EA, Beyer MM, eds. *American Society for Artificial Internal Organs, 39th Annual Meeting.* Philadelphia: Lippincott, 1993:M84.

110. Schneditz D, Martin K, Krämer M, Kenner T, Skrabal F. Effect of controlled extracorporeal blood cooling on ultrafiltration induced blood volume changes during hemodialysis. *J Am Soc Nephrol* 1997;8:956–964.

111. Kaufman AM, Morris AT, Lavarias VA, et al. Effects of controlled blood cooling on hemodynamic stability and urea kinetics during high-efficiency hemodialysis. *J Am Soc Nephrol* 1998;9:877–883.

112. van der Sande FM, Kooman JP, Burema JH, et al. Effect of dialysate temperature on energy balance during hemodialysis: quantification of extracorporeal energy transfer. *Am J Kidney Dis* 1999;33:1115–1121.

113. Gotch FA, Keen ML, Yarian SR. An analysis of thermal regulation in hemodialysis with one and three compartment models. *ASAIO Trans* 1989;35:622–624.

114. Maggiore Q. Isothermic dialysis for hypotension-prone patients. *Semin Dial* 2002;15:187–190.

115. Maggiore Q, Pizzarelli F, Santoro A, et al. The effects of control of thermal balance on vascular stability in hemodialysis patients: results of the European randomized clinical trial. *Am J Kidney Dis* 2002;40:280–290.

116. Schneditz D, Van Stone JC, Daugirdas JT. A regional blood circulation alternative to in-series two compartment urea kinetic modeling. *ASAIO J* 1993;39:M573–M577.

117. Yu AW, Ing TS, Zabaneh RI, Daugirdas JT. Effect of dialysate temperature on central hemodynamics and urea kinetics. *Kidney Int* 1995;48:237–243.

118. Ronco C, Brendolan A, Crepaldi C, La Greca G. Ultrafiltrations—Rate und Dialyse—Hypotension. *Dialyse J* 1992; 40:8–15.

119. Chamney PW, Johner C, Aldridge C, et al. Fluid balance modelling in patients with kidney failure. *J Med Eng Technol* 1999;23:45–52.

120. Cavalcanti S, Di Marco LY. Numerical simulation of the hemodynamic response to hemodialysis-induced hypovolemia. *Artif Organs* 1999;23:1063–1073.

121. Kim KE, Neff M, Cohen B, et al. Blood volume changes and hypotension during hemodialysis. *ASAIO Trans* 1970;16:508–514.

122. de Vries JPPM, Kouw PM, van der Meer NJ, et al. Non-invasive monitoring of blood volume during hemodialysis: its relation with post-dialytic dry weight. *Kidney Int* 1993; 44:851–854.

123. Maeda K, Morita H, Shinzato T, et al. Role of hypovolemia in dialysis-induced hypotension. *Artif Organs* 1988;12: 116–121.

124. Krepel HP, Nette RW, Akcahuseyin E, et al. Variability of relative blood volume during haemodialysis. *Nephrol Dial Transplant* 2000;15:673–679.

125. Steuer RR, Leypoldt JK, Cheung AK, et al. Hematocrit as an indicator of blood volume and a predictor of intradialytic morbid events. *ASAIO J* 1994;40:M691–M696.

126. Stiller S, Wirtz D, Waterbär F, et al. Less symptomatic hypotension using blood volume controlled ultrafiltration. *ASAIO Trans* 1991;37:M139–M141.

127. Schneditz D. Fisiopatologia del "Refilling." In: D'Amico GD, Bazzi C, Colasanti G, eds. *Attualita Nefrologiche & Dialitiche*. Milan: Wichtig Editore, 1995:205–213.

128. Polaschegg HD, Knoflach A, Binswanger U. Ultrafiltrationskontrolle mittels Hämatokritmessung bei der Hämodialyse. *Biomed Technik* 1996;41:374–375.

129. Giove S, Nordio M. Proposal of an adaptive fuzzy control module for hemodialysis. In: Patterson BW, ed. *Modeling and Control in Biological Systems*. Galveston, TX: University of Texas Medical Branch and Shriners Burns Institute, 1994:212–213.

130. Santoro A, Mancini E, Paolini F, et al. Blood volume regulation during hemodialysis. *Am J Kidney Dis* 1998; 32:739–748.

131. Fleming SJ, Wilkinson JS, Greenwood RN, Aldridge C, Baker LR. Effect of dialysate composition on intercompartmental fluid shift. *Kidney Int* 1987;32:267–273.

132. Mann H, Stefanidis I, Reinhardt B, Stiller S. Prevention of haemodynamic risk by continuous blood volume measurement and control. *Nephrol Dial Transplant* 1996;11: S48–S51.

133. Ronco C, Brendolan A, Milan M, et al. Impact of biofeedback-induced cardiovascular stability on hemodialysis tolerance and efficiency. *Kidney Int* 2000;58:800–808.

134. Basile C, Giordano R, Vernaglione L, et al. Efficacy and safety of haemodialysis treatment with the Hemocontrol biofeedback system: a prospective medium-term study. *Nephrol Dial Transplant* 2001;16:328–334.

135. Krivitski NM, Depner TA. Cardiac output and central blood volume during hemodialysis: methodology. *Adv Renal Replace Ther* 1999;6:225–232.

136. Rippe B. A three-pore model of peritoneal transport. *Perit Dial Int* 1993;13(suppl 2):S35–S38.

137. Keshaviah P, Emerson PF, Vonesh EF, Brandes JC. Relationship between body size, fill volume, and mass transfer area coefficient in peritoneal dialysis. *J Am Soc Nephrol* 1994;4: 1820–1826.

138. Ronco C, Brendolan A, Zanella M. Evolution of machines for automated peritoneal dialysis. *Contrib Nephrol* 1999; 129:142–161.

139. Durand PY, Freida P, Issad B, Chanliau J. How to reach optimal creatinine clearances in automated peritoneal dialysis. *Perit Dial Int* 1996;16(suppl 1):S167–S170.

140. Staverman RJ. The theory of measurement of osmotic pressure. *Rev Trav Chim Pays-bas Belg* 1951;70:344–352.

141. Riegel W, Friedrichsohn C. The impact of bicarbonate and amino acid solutions on peritoneal dialysis treatment. *Wien Klin Wochenschr* 2000;112(suppl 5):47–50.

142. Roob JM. Possible applications of polyglucose (Icodextrin) as a peritoneal dialysis fluid. *Wien Klin Wochenschr* 2000;112(suppl 5):43–46.

143. Dawnay A, Wieslander AP, Miller DJ. In vitro advanced glycation endproducts (AGE) formation is reduced in PD fluid heat sterilized in two-compartment bag (abstr). *J Am Soc Nephrol* 1996;7:1477.

144. Boen ST, Mion CM, Curtis FK, Shilipetar G. Periodic peritoneal dialysis using the repeated puncture technique and an automatic cycling machine. *Trans Am Soc Artif Intern Organs* 1964;10:409–414.

145. Lasker N, Shalhoub R, Habibe O, Passarotti C. The management of end-stage kidney disease with intermittent peritoneal dialysis. *Ann Intern Med* 1965;62:1147–1169.

146. Popovich RP, Moncrief JW, Nolph KD, et al. Continuous ambulatory peritoneal dialysis. *Ann Intern Med* 1978;88: 449–456.

147. Diaz-Buxo JA, Walker PJ, Farmer CD, et al. Continuous cyclic peritoneal dialysis. *Trans Am Soc Artif Intern Organs* 1981;27:51–54.

148. Nakagawa D, Price C, Stinebaugh B, Suki W. Continuous cycling peritoneal dialysis: a viable option in the treatment of chronic renal failure. *Trans Am Soc Artif Intern Organs* 1981;27:55–57.

149. Piraino B, Bender F, Bernardini J. A comparison of clearances on tidal peritoneal dialysis and intermittent peritoneal dialysis. *Perit Dial Int* 1994;14:145–148.

150. Vychytil A, Lilaj T, Schneider B, et al. Tidal peritoneal dialysis for home-treated patients: should it be preferred? *Am J Kidney Dis* 1999;33:334–343.

151. Juergensen PH, Murphy AL, Pherson KA, et al. Tidal peritoneal dialysis: comparison of different tidal regimens and automated peritoneal dialysis. *Kidney Int* 2000;57: 2603–2607.

152. Shinaberger JH, Shear L, Barry KG. Increasing efficiency of peritoneal dialysis: experience with peritoneal-extracorporeal recirculation dialysis. *Trans Am Soc Artif Intern Organs* 1965;11:76–82.

153. Roberts M, Ash SR, Lee DB. Innovative peritoneal dialysis: flow-thru and dialysate regeneration. *ASAIO J* 1999;45: 372–378.

154. Mineshima M, Suzuki S, Sato Y, et al. Solute removal characteristics of continuous recirculating peritoneal dialysis in experimental and clinical studies. *ASAIO J* 2000;46:95–98.

155. Diaz-Buxo JA. Evolution of continuous flow peritoneal dialysis and the current state of the art. *Semin Dial* 2001;14: 373–377.

156. Ronco C, Wentling AG, Amerling R, et al. New catheter design for continuous flow peritoneal dialysis. *Contrib Nephrol* 2004;142:447–461.

157. Rosman J. Telemedicine in patients on automated peritoneal dialysis. *Wien Klin Wochenschr* 2000;112(suppl 5):31–34.

158. Diaz-Buxo JA, Plahey K, Walker S. Memory card: a tool to assess patient compliance with peritoneal dialysis. *Artif Organs* 1999;23:956–958.

159. Prowant BF, Schmidt LM. The peritoneal equilibration test: a nursing discussion. *ANNA J* 1991;18:361–366.

160. Schmidt LM, Prowant BF. How to do a peritoneal equilibration test. *ANNA J* 1991;18:368–370.

161. Haraldsson B. Assessing the peritoneal dialysis capacities of individual patients. *Kidney Int* 1995;47:1187–1198.

162. Vonesh EF, Keshaviah PR. Applications in kinetic modeling using PD ADEQUEST. *Perit Dial Int* 1997;17(suppl 2): S119–S125.

163. Gotch FA, Lipps BJ. Pack PD: A urea kinetic modeling computer program for peritoneal dialysis. *Perit Dial Int* 1997;17(suppl 2):S126–S130.

164. Haraldsson B. Three-pore model applied to automated peritoneal dialysis. *Contrib Nephrol* 1999;129:35–43.

165. Haraldsson B, Broms E, Johansson AC. How to evaluate and optimize peritoneal dialysis treatment. *Nephrol Dial Transplant* 1998;13(suppl 6):112–116.

Hollow-Fiber Dialyzers: Technical and Clinical Considerations

Claudio Ronco
William R. Clark

Dialyzers containing hollow-fiber membranes are now used almost exclusively for hemodialysis (HD) therapy. Relative to older devices incorporating other membrane types, such as coil and flat-sheet dialyzers, hollow-fiber dialyzers display relatively low blood-compartment resistance.[1] This characteristic enhances the efficiency of therapy because high blood-flow rates can be achieved at acceptable axial (arterial-to-venous) pressure drops.[2] Moreover, a hollow-fiber design allows high shear rates to be achieved within the annular structure, thus attenuating boundary (unstirred) layer effects. Additional benefits of the hollow-fiber artificial kidney relative to prior dialyzer designs include an enhanced ability to control transmembrane pressure and a lower extracorporeal blood volume.[3,4] In the original development of this dialyzer type in the 1960s, the membrane was unsubstituted cellulose with low water permeability. Since that time, dialyzers having numerous types of membrane material and water permeability have been developed.[5–7]

The purpose of this chapter is to provide an overview of hollow-fiber dialyzer characteristics. In the first part of the chapter, hollow-fiber membranes are discussed specifically, including the chemical composition and physical characteristics of commonly used membranes. In addition, the membrane characteristics determining solute and water permeability are reviewed. The remainder of the chapter deals with the properties of the dialyzer itself, with emphasis on the major determinants of performance characteristics.

HOLLOW-FIBER MEMBRANES: CLASSIFICATION BY MATERIAL (TABLE 4–1)

Unmodified Cellulosic Dialyzers

The constituent component of cellulosic membranes is cellobiose, a saccharide found in a number of naturally occurring substances.[8] From the perspective of blood's interac-

Table 4-1.   **Hemodialysis Membranes**

Unmodified Cellulosic	Modified Cellulosic (substitution group)	Synthetic
Cuprophan	Cellulose (di) acetate (acetate)	Polysulfone
Cuprammonium rayon	Cellulose triacetate (acetate)	Polyamide
SCE	Hemophan (tertiary amine)	Polyethersulfone
	SMC (benzyl)	PAN
	Vitamin E–bonded	PMMA

Abbreviations: SCE = saponified cellulose ester; SMC = synthetically modified cellulose; PAN = polyacrylnitrile; PMMA = polymethylacrylate.

tion with a cellulosic membrane, the most important characteristic of cellobiose is its high density of hydroxyl groups. Although the contact of blood with any artificial surface elicits activation of the alternative complement pathway, the abundance of hydroxyl groups makes this phenomenon particularly pronounced for unmodified cellulosic dialyzers. This cellulosic characteristic was deemed clinically undesirable when first reported and has contributed to the progressive decline in unmodified cellulosic use over the years. However, the relatively long duration of popularity of cellulosic membranes in general can be explained largely by their particular suitability for a diffusion-based procedure like HD. The underlying hydrogel structure of these membranes and their tensile strength allow the combination of low wall thickness (see below) and high porosity to be attained in the fiber spinning process.[9] These characteristics allow the attainment of high rates of diffusive membrane transport and efficient removal of small, water-soluble uremic solutes, such as urea and creatinine. Another characteristic feature of these membranes is symmetry with respect to composition, implying an essentially uniform resistance to mass transfer over the entire wall thickness. On the other hand, these membranes are characterized by low mean pore size and pronounced hydrophilicity, such that neither transmembrane nor adsorptive removal of middle- and larger-sized uremic toxins is typically significant.[10,11]

Modified Cellulosic Membranes

Like regenerated cellulose membranes, modified cellulosic membranes are characterized by low wall-thickness values, typically in the 6- to 15-μm range, and symmetrical structures. However, dialyzers composed of these membranes, first used for HD in the 1980s, cause less pronounced complement activation and generally have a larger mean pore size[12] than their unmodified cellulosic counterparts. This latter characteristic results in higher water permeability and middle molecule clearances relative to the unmodified cellulosic class.

The two most commonly used modified cellulosic dialyzers contain membranes in which the hydroxyl replacement mechanisms are quite different. For cellulose acetate membranes (rigorously, cellulose diacetate),[13] approximately 75 percent of the hydroxyl groups on the cellulosic backbone are replaced with an acetate group. As opposed to a hydroxyl group, an acetate group does not bind avidly to a complement C3 molecule to initiate activation of the alternate complement pathway. Consequently, complement activation is attenuated, as is the leukopenic response, in which the white blood cell (WBC) count decrease from baseline is usually in the range of 35 to 40 percent, compared to the typical reduction of 60 to 70 percent seen with unmodified cellulosic membranes. Because production of cellulose triacetate membranes involves complete hydroxyl substitution replacement, further attenuation of complement activation and leukopenia is achieved.

Along with cellulose acetate dialyzers, Hemophan dialyzers are the most commonly used products containing modified cellulosic membranes.[14] However, the substitution approach is completely different from that used for cellulose acetate. For Hemophan, only a small percentage (less than 5 percent) of the hydroxyl groups is actually replaced. However, the tertiary amine replacement group is bulky and effectively shields a significantly greater percentage of hydroxyl groups by a steric mechanism. The attenuation in the degree of complement activation and leukopenia with Hemophan dialyzers is similar to that observed with cellulose acetate dialyzers. This same approach of providing a low degree of hydroxyl substitution with a relatively bulky moiety is employed for synthetically modified cellulose (SMC), a more recently developed membrane for which the substitution group is a benzyl moiety.[15]

Synthetic Membranes

Synthetic membranes were developed essentially in response to concerns related to the narrow scope of solute removal and the pronounced complement activation associated with unmodified cellulosic dialyzers. The AN69 membrane, a copolymer of acrylonitrile and an anionic sulfonate group, was first employed in flat sheet form in a closed-loop dialysate system in the early 1970s.[5] Since that time, a number of other synthetic membranes have been developed, including polysulfone,[6] polyamide,[16] polymethylmethacrylate (PMMA),[17] polyethersulfone,[18] and polyarylethersulfone/polyamide.[19] Largely related to the interest in hemofiltration (HF) as a therapy for end-stage renal disease (ESRD) in the late 1970s and early in the following decade, coupled with the inability to use low-flux unmodified cellulosic dialyzers for this therapy, these membranes were initially formulated with high water permeability.[20] The large mean pore size and thick wall structure of these membranes made possible the high ultrafiltration rates necessary in HF to be achieved at relatively low transmembrane pressures. However, with the waning of interest in HF as a chronic dialysis therapy, dialyzers with these highly permeable membranes were used subsequently in the diffusive mode as components of high-flux dialyzers. This latter mode continues to be the most common application of these membranes, although they are increasingly being employed for chronic hemodiafiltration (HDF) as well.[21] Synthetic dialyzers with relatively low water permeability[22] are now also utilized widely in certain markets.

An obvious difference between synthetic and cellulosic membranes is chemical composition. As opposed to naturally occurring cellulose, synthetic membranes are manufactured polymers that are classified as thermoplastics. In fact, for most of the synthetic membranes, the HD market represents only a small fraction of their entire industrial utilization. As noted above, another feature differentiating cellulosic and synthetic membranes is wall thickness. Synthetic membranes have wall thickness values of at least 20 μm and may be structurally symmetrical (e.g., AN69, PMMA) or asymmetrical (e.g., polysulfone, polyamide, polyethersulfone, polyamide/polyarylethersulfone). In the latter category, a very thin "skin" (approximately 1 μm) contacting the blood compartment lumen acts primarily as the membrane's separative element with regard to solute removal. The structure of the remaining wall thickness ("stroma"), which determines a synthetic membrane's thermal, chemical, and mechanical properties, varies considerably among the various synthetic membranes.[23] For example, the stroma has a relatively homogeneous, sponge-like consistency in the Fresenius polysulfone membrane. On the other hand, the Gambro Polyflux membrane, which is actually a blend of polyamide and polyarylethersulfone, has three distinct layers. Like the Fresenius polysulfone membrane, one layer is a thin blood-contacting inner lumen, composed of polyarylethersulfone enriched with polyvinylpyrrolidone (PVP), while the outer surface is composed of relatively PVP-free polyamide. Interspersed between these two layers is a polyarylethersulfone stroma, which has a finger-like structure.[19,23] Finally, the DiaPES polyethersulfone membrane, developed by Membrana GmbH, contains both inner and outer skin layers surrounding a sponge-like stroma.[24] For this membrane, the average pore radius of the inner and outer skin layers is approxi-

mately 5 and 10 nm, respectively. Takeyama and Sakai[25] have suggested that an effective mean pore radius between 5 and 8 nm achieves the appropriate balance between β2M removal and albumin loss (see below).

Many of the synthetic polymers used in manufacturing the above membranes are hydrophobic and require the addition of a hydrophilic agent (PVP) to avoid excessive protein adsorption upon blood exposure. During membrane preparation, water-soluble PVP is blended into the hydrophobic base polymer through the formation of hydrogen bonds. This hydrogen bonding provides miscibility for the hydrophilic-hydrophobic mixture and prevents leaching of PVP during blood contact. In addition to imparting hydrophilicity, PVP also influences membrane pore-size distribution through its effects on pore surface tension; its content may vary considerably across a synthetic membrane's wall thickness.

PHYSICAL CHARACTERISTICS OF HOLLOW-FIBER MEMBRANES

Pressure/Flow Relationship and the Concept of Flow Resistance

An individual hollow fiber can be viewed as a solid cylinder from which a central region has been removed ("cored out") to form the blood compartment. The process of manufacturing ("spinning") a hollow-fiber membrane is complex, incorporating aspects of a broad array of scientific disciplines including polymer chemistry, thermodynamics, reaction kinetics, and chemical engineering.[7] Although there are clear differences among the various types of membranes (see below), a number of common features are evident. From a structural perspective, most hollow fibers have a relatively standard inner (blood compartment) diameter (approximately 180 to 220 μm) and length (approximately 20 to 24 cm). These parameters are dictated essentially by the operating conditions used during HD and result from the compromise between opposing forces. On one hand, a relatively small hollow-fiber inner diameter is desirable because it provides a short diffusive distance for solute mass transfer. At a given blood-flow rate, a lower inner diameter also provides a higher shear rate, resulting in greater attenuation of blood-side boundary layer effects.[2] However, a decrease in hollow-fiber inner diameter also has undesirable effects. Fluid flow along the length of a cylinder (i.e., the axial flow) in many situations is governed by the Hagen-Poiseuille equation[26]:

$$Q_B = \Delta P / (8 \, \mu L / \pi r^4) \qquad (1)$$

where Q_B is blood-flow rate, ΔP is axial pressure drop, μ is blood viscosity, L is fiber length, and r is hollow-fiber radius. A specific application of this equation is axial blood flow (i.e., from the arterial to the venous end) in a hollow-fiber membrane during HD. A more general form of Eq. (1) is:

$$Q_B = \Delta P / R \qquad (2)$$

From Eqs. (1) and (2), the resistance to blood flow (R) is:

$$R = 8 \, \mu L / \pi r^4 \qquad (3)$$

Due to the inverse relationship between R and r^4, a small decrease in hollow-fiber inner diameter induces a large increase in flow resistance. Equation (3) also demonstrates that increases in fiber length and hematocrit (μ) are associated with an increase in flow resistance. In turn, as indicated by Eq. (2), an increase in flow resistance results in a higher axial pressure drop requirement to generate a given blood-flow rate.

Surface Area Considerations

For a particular hollow fiber, the inner annular surface represents the nominal blood compartment surface area and is the theoretically maximal area available for blood contact. For the entire group of fibers comprising a dialyzer, total nominal surface area then depends on fiber length, inner diameter, and overall number, the latter varying generally from approximately 7000 to 14,000.

A frequently asked question relates to the manner in which membrane surface area is calculated.[27] For the inner annular region of a single hollow fiber described above, the surface area (A) is given by the equation defining the surface area of a cylinder:

$$A_{\text{fiber}} = 2\pi r L \qquad (4)$$

Based on assumed values of $r = 100 \, \mu m$ (10^{-4} m) and $L = 24$ cm (0.24 m), the surface area of an individual hollow fiber can be calculated as:

$$A_{\text{fiber}} = (2\pi)(10^{-4} \text{ m})(0.24 \text{ m})$$
$$= 1.51 \times 10^{-4} \text{ m}^2$$

For the large-surface-area dialyzers routinely used now, the total number of fibers (N) typically used is approximately 12,000. Therefore:

$$A_{\text{dialyzer}} = (A_{\text{fiber}})(N)$$
$$= (1.51 \times 10^{-4} \text{ m}^2)(12,000) \qquad (5)$$
$$= 1.81 \text{ m}^2$$

PROPERTIES OF HEMODIALYZER MEMBRANES INFLUENCING DIALYZER PERFORMANCE

Membrane Water Permeability

A hollow-fiber dialyzer membrane can be modeled as having straight cylindrical pores, all of the same radius (r) and all with a directional orientation that is perpendicular to the flow of blood and dialysate.[9] As discussed below, this model does not exactly replicate a clinical dialyzer but is useful from a quantitative perspective nevertheless. The major determinants of plasma ultrafiltrate flow rate through the pores are the number of pores (i.e., number per unit area of membrane surface area), transmembrane pressure, and pore size. Just as the Hagen-Poiseuille equation[26] can be used to model axial blood flow through an individual hollow fiber (see above), it can also be employed to assess ultrafiltrate flow through an individual pore. Thus, the rate of ultrafiltrate flow is actually dependent on the fourth power of the pore radius (i.e., r^4). As such, the membrane characteristic that most directly influences water permeability is mean pore size.

Membrane Diffusive Permeability

Membrane wall thickness is one important determinant of diffusive transport.[28] The relatively thin-walled structure of cellulosic membranes (usually 6 to 15 μm) is largely responsible for their particular suitability in the setting of diffusive HD. Another major determinant of dialyzer membrane diffusive transport is porosity, also known as pore density. Based on the cylindrical pore model described above, membrane porosity is directly proportional to both the number of pores and the square of the pore radius (r^2).[29] Therefore the smaller dependence of membrane porosity on pore size, relative to the case of water permeability, implies a relatively greater importance of pore number in determining diffusive permeability. That the major determinants of flux (r^4) and diffusive permeability (number of pores, r^2, and wall thickness) differ so significantly implies the two properties can be independent of one another for a particular hemodialysis membrane. Such is the case for cellulosic high-efficiency dialyzers, which typically have very high diffusive permeability values for small solutes but low water permeability.

Membrane Pore-size Distribution Effects

A membrane represented by the cylindrical pore model described above deviates from an actual membrane used for clinical HD in that the latter actually has a distribution of pore sizes. Ronco et al.[30] have recently discussed the manner in which pore-size distribution may differ among HD membranes and the manner in which this distribution influences a membrane's sieving properties (Fig. 4-1). The membrane represented by curve A has a large number of relatively small pores, while the membrane represented by curve B has a large number of relatively large pores. Based on the relatively narrow pore-size distributions, the solute sieving coefficient vs. molecular-weight (MW) profile for both membranes has the desirable sharp cutoff, similar to that of the native kidney. (See below for a discussion of

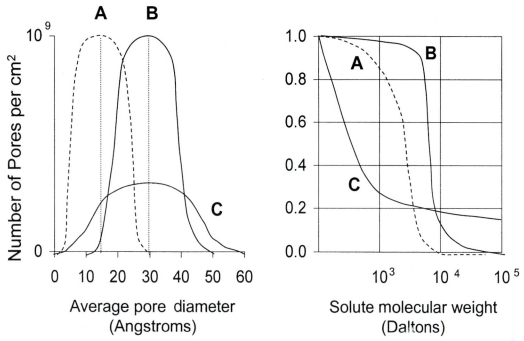

Figure 4–1. Relationship between pore-size distribution and sieving-coefficient profiles for three hypothetical membranes. *(Adapted with permission from Ronco et al.[30])*

sieving coefficient.) However, the MW cutoff for membrane A (approximately 10 kDa) is consistent with a high-efficiency membrane, while that of membrane B (approximately 60 kDa) is consistent with a high-flux membrane. In addition, primarily due to the large number of pores, both membranes would be expected to demonstrate favorable diffusive transport properties. On the other hand, membrane C exhibits a pore-size distribution that is unfavorable from the perspective of both diffusive transport and sieving. The relatively small number of pores accounts for the poor diffusive properties. In addition, the broad distribution of pores explains not only the "early" drop-off in sieving coefficient at relatively low MW but also the "tail" effect at high MW. This latter phenomenon is highly undesirable, as it may lead to unacceptably high albumin losses across the membrane.

Membrane Properties Influencing Nondiffusive Removal

The removal of relatively large compounds, such as peptides and proteins, during HD occurs primarily by nondiffusive mechanisms, namely convection and adsorption. For a specific solute, its sieving coeffient is typically used to characterize the convective removal capabilities of a membrane.[31–34] As described above, desirable features for a high-flux membrane include a large number of relatively large pores having a narrow distribution of sizes. This type of distribution leads ideally to a solute sieving coefficient vs. MW profile with a sharp cutoff at a MW just below that of albumin, similar to that of the native kidney.

In actual practice, all highly permeable membranes have measurable albumin sieving coefficient values, such that the design of this type of membrane involves striking a balance between optimized high-MW toxin removal and minimal albumin losses.[35] However, the manner in which pore sizes are reported in the literature may be confusing, as both pore diameter and radius have been used for characterization. Moreover, some studies have reported mean pore size while others have described a maximal (cutoff) pore size.[12] Irrespective of the method used to quantify pore sizes, this parameter has an impact on the degree to which albumin transport occurs across a highly permeable membrane.

Another convection-related mechanism by which large uremic toxins can be removed by high-flux dialyzers relates to fluid flow within the filter. An important distinction between dialyzers of low and high water permeability is the directionality of transmembrane fluid flow. In clinical HD, an individual patient's weight-loss requirement dictates the rate of plasma water ultrafiltration, and a specified ultrafiltration profile is achieved by providing prescriptive information (weight loss, treatment time, etc.) to the HD machine. However, it is important to recognize that this prescriptive ultrafiltration rate represents a *net* value and may or may not be equivalent to the *absolute* ultrafiltration rate in specific segments of the dialyzer. Under typical HD conditions (i.e., net ultrafiltration rate of 10 to 15 mL/min), the absolute ultrafiltration rate in the proximal (arterial) end of a high-flux dialyzer is considerably higher than the above net value. In the proximal (arterial) end of the dialyzer, because the blood compartment pressure is higher than the dialysate compartment pressure, ultrafiltrate leaves the blood compartment rapidly. This results in a significant pressure drop and, at some point along the length of the hollow fibers, the blood compartment pressure becomes less than the dialysate compartment pressure. This dialysate-to–blood pressure gradient results in a reversed ultrafiltrate flow directionality (i.e., "backfiltration") from this point to the distal (venous) end of the dialyzer. This phenomenon is a routine occurrence during high-flux HD.[36] Under most HD scenarios in which a low-K_{UF} dialyzer (< 20 mL/h/mmHg) is used, the high proximal ultrafiltration rate described above is not observed. Consequently, axial pressure drop is less pronounced and a reversed pressure gradient does not develop. As such, backfiltration is not a significant issue for dialyzers of relatively low water permeability.

Although the combination of significant backfiltration and contaminated dialysate raises many concerns (see below), this internal filtration ("Starling's flow") mechanism can significantly augment the removal of larger molecules.[32–40] In fact, attempts to accentuate this internal filtration mechanism, either through a decrease in hollow-fiber inner diameter or manipulations in dialysate compartment pressure, have recently been described.[38,39] Middle and large molecule clearance is enhanced with internal filtration due to convective removal in the proximal part of the dialyzer. At the same time, the concentrations of such molecules entering the dialysate compartment by convection from the blood are immediately and significantly reduced by the dilution effect of the oncoming fresh dialysate moving in a direction opposite to that of the blood. Consequently, the driving force for "reentry" of such solutes back into the bloodstream in the distal (i.e, backfiltration) segment of the dialyzer is very low.

Adsorption (membrane binding) is another mechanism by which hydrophobic compounds like peptides and proteins may be removed during dialysis.[11,41,42] Although adsorption during HD is a relatively poorly understood phenomenon, certain membrane characteristics play an important role. First, adsorption of hydrophobic uremic toxins primarily occurs within the pore structure of the membrane rather than at the nominal surface contacting the blood only.[40] Therefore the open pore structure of high-flux membranes affords more adsorptive potential than do low-flux counterparts. Second, synthetic membranes, many of which are fundamentally hydrophobic, generally are much more adsorptive than hydrophilic cellulosic membranes.[11] This latter characteristic of synthetic membranes renders effects related to secondary membrane formation more important for them relative to their more hydrophilic cellulosic counterparts (see below).

The adsorptivity of a membrane also appears to influence the "inflammatory" potential of a dialysis treatment.

Dialysate may contain both endotoxin-related and exotoxin-derived compounds, which have collectively been called cytokine-inducing substances (CIS), due to their ability to stimulate cytokine production by mononuclear cells in vitro. CIS transfer may play a causative role in the occurrence of both acute and chronic adverse effects in ESRD patients treated with HD.[43] The size range of these CIS is such that the majority of them have the potential to be "back-transported" by either diffusion or convection from dialysate to blood during HD. The potential for convective CIS transport from contaminated dialysate in association with backfiltration across a highly permeable dialyzer membrane has received the most attention. However, CIS backtransport from contaminated dialysate can occur across dialyzer membranes of relatively low water permeability, for which the only relevant mechanism is diffusion. Thus, mean pore size alone does not determine the extent of CIS transfer; other membrane-related factors, such as hydrophobicity and diffusive characteristics, also play important roles. Several groups have demonstrated that in vitro CIS transfer from highly contaminated dialysate is abrogated either significantly or totally by certain high-flux synthetic HD membranes.[43] This attenuation has been attributed largely to adsorptive removal of CIS by the membrane via nonspecific hydrophobic interactions.

HOW IS A HOLLOW-FIBER DIALYZER CONSTRUCTED?

In the assessment of the clinical effects of a particular dialyzer, the membrane justifiably receives the most scrutiny. Although the membrane itself is a key determinant of overall dialyzer function, the manner in which the membrane interacts with other components of the dialyzer is also very important. In Fig. 4–2, the sequence of events resulting in the conversion of polymethylmethacrylate (PMMA) hollow fibers to a dialyzer is shown.[44] After removal of glycerin (used in the hollow-fiber preparation), fibers are covered with spacer yarns, which are filaments designed to create optimal spacing between fibers.[28] Subsequently, the fibers that eventually serve as the collective membrane in the dialyzer are assembled ("bundled") and inserted in the dialyzer casing. The fiber bundle is then "potted" (encapsulated) at both ends with silicone rubber and cut. Finally, the dialyzer is placed in a pouch and the entire unit is sterilized, usually by ethylene oxide, gamma rays, or steam.

Several of these manufacturing steps may have a direct effect on dialyzer function and performance. Fiber bundle configuration and spacing have a major impact on mass transfer, as has recently been demonstrated.[45,46] One consideration is the spacing of fibers within the bundle. However, of equal or more importance is the degree to which the dialyzer jacket is "packed" with fibers. A dialyzer's packing density is the ratio of the area comprising fibers to the total

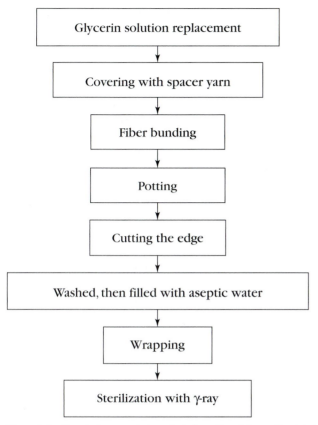

Figure 4–2. Steps in the manufacture of a hollow–fiber dialyzer. *(Reprinted with permission from Sugaya and Sakai.[44])*

area based on a transverse cut through the dialyzer. Empirically, on the one hand, packing densities of less than approximately 50 percent imply insufficient membrane surface area for an appropriate set of flow rates. On the other hand, values greater than approximately 60 percent are associated with a high risk of dialysate flow maldistribution, in which dialysate is "channeled" to the peripheral aspect of the fiber bundle at the expense of flow to the inner bundle area. Finally, sterilization technique may influence dialyzer performance through an effect on mean membrane pore size.

CHARACTERIZATION OF DIALYZER PERFORMANCE: CLEARANCE, SIEVING COEFFICIENT, AND ULTRAFILTRATION COEFFICIENT

Clearance

Whole-Blood Clearance. By definition,[47] solute clearance (K) is the ratio of mass removal rate (N) to blood solute concentration (C_B):

$$K = N / C_B \qquad (6)$$

For a hemodialyzer, mass removal rate is simply the difference between the rate of solute mass (i.e., product of flow rate and concentration) presented to the dialyzer in the arterial blood line and the rate of solute mass leaving the dialyzer in the venous blood line. This mass balance applied to the dialyzer results in the classic (i.e., arteriovenous) whole-blood dialyzer-clearance equation[15]:

$$K_B = [(Q_{Bi} \cdot C_{Bi}) - (Q_{Bo} \cdot C_{Bo})]/C_{Bi} + Q_F \cdot (C_{Bo}/C_{Bi}) \qquad (7)$$

where K_B is whole-blood clearance, Q_B is blood-flow rate, C_B is whole-blood solute concentration, and Q_F is net ultrafiltration rate. [The subscripts "i" and "o" refer to the inlet (arterial) and outlet (venous) blood lines.]

It is important to note that diffusive, convective, and possibly adsorptive solute removal occur simultaneously in HD. For a nonadsorbing solute like urea, diffusion and convection interact in such a manner that total solute removal is significantly less than what would be expected if the individual components were simply added together.[48] This phenomenon is explained in the following way. Diffusive removal results in a decrease in solute concentration in the blood compartment along the axial length of the hemodialyzer. As convective solute removal is directly proportional to the blood compartment concentration, convective solute removal decreases as a function of this axial concentration gradient. On the other hand, hemoconcentration resulting from ultrafiltration of plasma water causes a progressive increase in plasma protein concentration and hematocrit along the axial length of the dialyzer. This hemoconcentration and resultant hyperviscosity causes an increase in diffusive mass transfer resistance and a decrease in solute transport by this mechanism.

The effect of this interaction on overall solute removal has been analyzed rigorously by numerous investigators. The most useful quantification has been developed by Jaffrin[48]:

$$K_T = K_D + Q_F \cdot \text{Tr} \qquad (8)$$

where K_T is total solute clearance, K_D is diffusive clearance under conditions of no net ultrafiltration, and the final term is the convective contribution to total clearance. The latter term is a function of the ultrafiltration rate (Q_F) and an experimentally derived transmittance coefficient (Tr), such that:

$$\text{Tr} = S (1 - K_D/Q_B) \qquad (9)$$

where S is solute sieving coefficient. Thus, Tr for a particular solute is dependent on the efficiency of diffusive removal. At very low values of K_D/Q_B, diffusion has a very small impact on blood compartment concentrations and the convective component of clearance closely approximates the quantity $S \cdot Q_F$. However, with increasing efficiency of diffusive removal (i.e., increasing K_D/Q_B), blood compartment concentrations are significantly influenced. The result is a decrease in Tr and, consequently, in the convective contribution to total clearance.

Blood-water and Plasma Clearance. An implicit assumption in the determination of whole-blood clearance is that the volume from which the solute is cleared is the actual volume of blood transiting through the dialyzer at a certain time. This assumption is incorrect for two reasons. First, in both the erythron and plasma components of blood, a certain volume is composed of solids (proteins or lipids) rather than water. Second, for solutes like creatinine and phosphate, which are distributed in both the erythron and plasma water, slow mass transfer from the intracellular space to the plasma space (relative to mass transfer across the dialyzer) results in relative sequestration (compartmentalization) in the former compartment.[49-51] This reduces the effective volume of distribution from which these solutes can be cleared by the dialyzer. As such, whole-blood dialyzer clearances derived by using plasma water concentrations in conjunction with blood-flow rates, a common practice in dialyzer evaluations, results in a significant overestimation of actual solute removal. The more appropriate approach is to employ blood-water clearances, which account for the above hematocrit-dependent effects on effective intradialyzer solute distribution volume[52]:

$$Q_{BW} = 0.93 \cdot Q_B[1 - Hct + K(1 - e^{-\alpha t})Hct] \qquad (10)$$

where Q_{BW} is blood-water flow rate. In this equation, K is the RBC water/plasma water partition coefficient for a given solute, α is the transcellular rate constant (units: time^{-1}), and t is the characteristic dialyzer residence time. Estimates for these parameters have been provided by numerous prior studies and have been summarized by Shinaberger et al.[53] [The factor 0.93 in Eq. (10) corrects for the volume of plasma occupied by plasma proteins and lipids.] Finally, K_{BW} can be calculated by substituting Q_{BW} for Q_B in Eq. (7).

Although the distribution volume of many uremic solutes approximates total body water, it is much more limited for other toxins, particularly those of higher MW. For example, the distribution space of beta$_2$ microglobulin (β_2M) and many other low-MW proteins is the plasma volume. Consequently, in using Eq. (7) to determine β_2M clearance, plasma flow rates (inlet and outlet) should replace blood-flow rates in the first term of the right-hand side of the equation.

The distinction between whole-blood, blood-water, and dialysate-side clearances is very important when interpreting clinical data. However, clearances provided by dialyzer manufacturers are typically in vitro data generated from experiments in which the blood compartment fluid is an aqueous solution. Although these data provide useful information to the clinician, they overestimate the actual dialyzer performance that can be achieved clinically (under the same conditions). This overestimation is related to the inability of aqueous-based experiments to capture the effects of red blood cells (see above) and plasma proteins (see below) on solute mass transfer.

Dialysate-Side Clearance. Although blood-side measurements are typically used to determine solute mass removal rate, clearance can also be estimated from dialysate-side measurements:

$$K_D = Q_{Do} \cdot C_{Do} / C_{Bi} \qquad (11)$$

where dialysate-side solute clearance (K_D) is determined by measuring the rate of mass appearance in the effluent dialysate stream ($= Q_{Do} \cdot C_{Do}$). Dialysate-side measurements provide more accurate mass transfer information than do blood-side determinations and are generally considered the "gold standard" dialyzer evaluation technique. Relative to dialysate-side values, whole-blood clearances substantially overestimate true dialyzer performance. Blood-water clearances also moderately overestimate dialyzer performance, although the agreement between these and simultaneous dialysate-side values (for nonadsorbing solutes) is usually within 5 percent under rigorous test conditions. The major disadvantage of dialysate-based clearance techniques is the need to assay solute concentrations at very low levels. For some solutes (e.g., phosphate), these dilute concentrations may be difficult to assay with standard automated chemistry devices.

Clearance vs. Mass Removal Rate. It is important to recognize that clearance is *not* a measure of actual dialytic mass removal of a particular solute. As Eq. (6) indicates, clearance is the ratio of mass removal rate to blood concentration for a given solute. In HD, the mass removal rate of small solutes like urea is very high during the early stage of an HD treatment due to a favorable transmembrane concentration gradient for diffusion at this time. As the treatment proceeds, a proportional decrease in the blood urea nitrogen (BUN) and the urea mass removal rate, which is determined by the instantaneous BUN, occurs.[54] Equation (6) predicts that a proportional decrease in these parameters results in a constant dialyzer clearance during the treatment (provided that dialyzer function is preserved) (Fig. 4–3). For this reason, despite not being a measure of actual dialytic solute removal, clearance nevertheless remains a very reasonable parameter with which to assess dialyzer function. The discordance between solute clearance and mass removal rate described above is a much more relevant consideration when a whole-body (rather than dialyzer) clearance approach is used (see below).

Whole-Body Clearance vs. Dialyzer Clearance. The discussion to this point has focused on clearance of a solute by the dialyzer and has included the implications of solute compart-

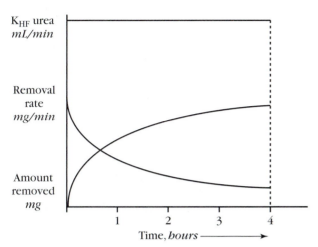

Figure 4–3. Relationship between solute clearance and mass removal in hemodialysis. *(Reprinted with permission from Henderson et al.[54])*

mentalization within the dialyzer for solutes such as creatinine and phosphate. Compartmentalization may also occur during HD within the patient's body. During HD, direct removal of a particular solute can occur only from that portion of its volume of distribution which actually perfuses the dialyzer, and sequestration of solute occurs in the remaining volume of distribution. Solute compartmentalization involves an interplay between dialyzer solute clearance and patient/solute parameters, such as compartment volumes and intercompartment mass transfer resistances.[55] Even if solute removal by the dialyzer is relatively efficient, overall (effective) solute removal may be limited by slow intercompartment mass transfer.

To account for these effects of "intracorporeal" solute compartmentalization on overall solute removal, many clinicians prefer to use whole-body rather than dialyzer clearance, as the former is felt to be a better measure of overall treatment efficacy.[56] Whole-body clearance methodologies employ blood samples obtained before and after the HD treatment. An example of a widely used whole-body clearance approach is the second-generation Daugirdas equation. In this approach, a logarithmic relationship between delivered urea *Kt/V* and the extent of the intradialytic reduction in the BUN is assumed. Two issues complicate the use of these methodologies. One is the assumed distribution volume of the solute for which the clearance is being estimated and whether or not this volume is multicompartmental. The second important consideration, incorporation of the effects of post-HD rebound, is closely tied to multicompartment kinetics.[57]

Relationship of Dialyzer Clearance and Treatment "Efficiency." Although not precisely defined, HD treatment efficiency is very closely related to a dialyzer's small solute-removal capabilities. The term "high efficiency," currently widely used, actually had its origin as a therapy, first described by

Keshaviah et al,[58] rather than a specific type of dialyzer. These investigators employed large-surface-area cellulose acetate dialyzers and relatively high blood-flow rates to achieve sufficiently high urea clearances to allow reductions in treatment time. The use of large-surface-area dialyzers capable of achieving these high urea clearances has increased to the point that a separate albeit somewhat indistinct class of high-efficiency dialyzers now exists.

Sieving Coefficient. When a dialyzer is operated as an ultrafilter (i.e., ultrafiltration with no dialysate flow), solute mass transfer occurs almost exclusively by convection. Convective solute removal during dialysis is primarily determined by membrane pore size and treatment ultrafiltration rate. Mean pore size is the major determinant of a dialyzer's ability to prevent or allow the transport of a specific solute. The sieving coefficient (*S*) represents the degree to which a particular membrane permits the passage of a specific solute[32]:

$$S = C_F / C_P \qquad (12)$$

where C_F and C_P are the solute concentrations in the ultrafiltrate and the plasma (water), respectively. (It should be noted that a sieving coefficient measurement is influenced by the ultrafiltration rate used during the determination.) Irrespective of membrane type, all dialyzers have small solute sieving-coefficient values of approximately unity, and these values are typically not reported by dialyzer manufacturers. Sieving coefficient values for solutes of higher MW are more applicable and manufacturers frequently provide data for one or more middle-molecule surrogates, such as vitamin B_{12}, inulin, cytochrome c, and myoglobin. As is the case for solute clearance in HD, the relationship between *S* and solute MW is highly dependent on membrane mean pore size (i.e., flux)[30,31](Fig. 4–1).

The data on sieving coefficient provided by manufacturers are usually derived from in vitro experimental systems in which non-protein-containing aqueous solutions are used as the blood compartment fluid. In clinical HD, nonspecific adsorption of plasma proteins to a dialyzer membrane effectively reduces the permeability of the membrane.[20,59–61] Consequently, in vivo values for sieving coefficient are typically less than those derived from aqueous experiments, sometimes by a considerable amount.

Ultrafiltration Coefficient. Currently there is considerable confusion regarding the exact meaning of "dialyzer flux." By definition, flux is the transmembrane rate of transfer of a substance normalized to membrane surface area. Thus, one may define a diffusive or convective flux for a membrane-based process with respect to solute removal as the mass removal rate normalized to membrane surface area. Likewise, the hydraulic flux of membrane is the volumetric rate (normalized to surface area) at which ultrafiltration of water occurs. Although numerous classification schemes have been proposed,[62] hemodialysis membranes are traditionally classified according to *water flux*, a term synonymous with *water permeability*. The clinical parameter used to characterize the water permeability of a dialyzer is the ultrafiltration coefficient (K_{UF}: mL/h/mmHg). The water permeability of a dialyzer is usually derived from in vitro experiments in which bovine blood is ultrafiltered at varying transmembrane pressure (TMP). The relationship between plasma ultrafiltration rate and TMP is linear at relatively low TMP values for all membranes, whereas a plateau in ultrafiltration rate occurs at relatively high TMP values.[32] Dialyzer K_{UF} is defined by the slope of the linear portion of the curve representing this ultrafiltration rate vs. TMP. As noted previously, the membrane characteristic having the largest impact on water permeability is pore size, such that ultrafiltrate flux is roughly proportional to the fourth power of the mean membrane pore radius.[9] Therefore small changes in pore size have a very large effect on water permeability.

DETERMINANTS OF DIALYTIC SOLUTE CLEARANCE

Diffusive Solute Clearance

Diffusion is the dominant mass transfer mechanism mediating small solute removal in HD. Diffusive solute removal involves sequential mass transfer from the dialyzer blood compartment, through the membrane, and into the dialysate compartment. To quantify a dialyzer's diffusive capabilities, the concept of mass transfer resistance is frequently employed[63]:

$$R_O = R_B + R_M + R_D$$

where the overall resistance to diffusive mass transfer of a particular solute (R_O) by a dialyzer has three components: blood compartment resistance (R_B), resistance due to the membrane itself (R_M), and dialysate compartment resistance (R_D). In turn, R_O is the inverse of the overall mass transfer coefficient (K_O), which is a component of the overall mass-transfer-area coefficient (K_OA), discussed below.[64] Each of resistances influencing mass transfer is also discussed below.

Blood compartment. A fundamental relationship exists between diffusive clearance and blood-flow rate for all solutes. For a given solute, a graph of clearance vs. blood-flow rate (Q_B) has two domains[65] (Fig.4–4). In the relatively low Q_B regime, an effectively linear relationship exists between these two parameters. For all solutes, the line defined by this relationship falls below the line of identity, thus indicating that dialyzer clearance can never exceed the blood-flow rate. For a given dialyzer, the slope of the line defining this flow-limited regime is inversely related to solute size. Beyond a certain Q_B, the curve defining the relationship of clearance vs. Q_B for a given solute/dialyzer combination demonstrates a plateau. This plateau defines the K_OA-limited region. For a given solute/dialyzer combination, the

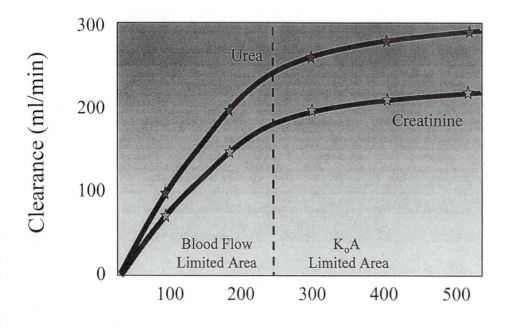

Figure 4–4. Relationship between dialyzer solute clearance and blood-flow rate.

K_OA parameter can be regarded as the maximal clearance attainable under a given set of flow conditions. Both the Q_B at which the transition from the blood flow–limited to the K_OA-limited region and the plateau clearance value are specific for a given solute/dialyzer combination. For a given solute, an increase in either diffusive permeability (K_O) or area (A) has the effect of increasing both the transition Q_B and the plateau clearance value.

Minimizing the mass transfer resistance in the blood compartment is achieved primarily by the use of relatively high flow rates (i.e., shear rates) that minimize effects related to boundary (unstirred) layers. A boundary layer can be conceptualized as a stagnant film of fluid residing on the membrane surface.[66] However, another important factor influencing blood compartment resistance is hematocrit. Blood is a complex fluid in which red blood cells (RBCs) are suspended in plasma.[67] Plasma is an aqueous solution but does have a solid component (approximately 7 percent by volume) consisting of proteins and lipids. The erythron is also primarily aqueous, with water constituting approximately 70 percent of the total erythron and the remaining solid component comprising primarily cellular membranes.[68] Although many uremic solutes are distributed in the aqueous phase of both the RBC and plasma fractions of blood, solute removal during HD can occur only from plasma water. Before actual dialytic removal of solutes with this type of distribution can be achieved, mass transfer from the RBC water to the plasma water must occur.[69] In turn, the rate at which this latter process occurs is solute-specific. Prior data[70,71] indicate that the movement of urea across the RBC membrane is relatively fast. Therefore, during HD, urea in the plasma water leaving the dialyzer is in equilibrium with urea in the RBC water, with the ratio of these concentrations (approximately 0.76) being determined by the ratio of the water fractions of the aqueous and RBC compartments.[71] On the other hand, the transcellular rate of movement for other uremic solutes, such as creatinine and phosphate, is small (or negligible) relative to the rate of dialytic removal.[49–52] For a given unit volume of whole blood, an increase in hematocrit (Hct) causes a relative increase in the distribution of solute in the RBC water, resulting in a relative sequestration of solutes with low RBC membrane diffusivity.

The application of rheologic principles to the flow of blood in a dialyzer also raises concerns that blood compartment mass transfer may be impaired by increasing Hct. For a given solute, diffusive mass transfer resistance in the blood compartment of a dialyzer is the ratio of effective diffusive path length (x) to effective solute diffusivity (D), both of which may be influenced by Hct.[72] As the volume comprised by the RBC mass per unit volume of blood increases with increasing Hct, solutes diffusing to the membrane surface are relatively more likely to encounter a RBC, causing an effective lengthening of the diffusion distance.

In addition, solute diffusivity may decrease as a function of increasing Hct due to the latter's effect on viscosity, itself a determinant of mass transfer resistance.[51]

Lim et al.[52] studied five patients in whom pre-HD Hct was raised from a mean of 22.9 to 37.8 percent with the use of erythropoietin. Whole-blood (K_B) and dialysate-side (K_D) clearances of urea, creatinine, and phosphate were measured under the following (prescribed) conditions: Q_B, 400 mL/min; dialysate flow rate (Q_D), 500 mL/min; and treatment time, 180 minutes. Dialysate-side clearance was used as the truer (gold standard) estimate of mass removal. The ratio K_D/K_B, an estimate of the degree to which whole-blood clearance overestimates mass removal, was observed to decrease significantly for both creatinine and phosphate but not for urea, as a function of Hct. In urea kinetic analyses (based on the direct dialysate quantification method), both Kt/V (1.21 vs. 1.17) and percent urea reduction (64.2 vs. 61.6 percent) decreased, but not significantly, as Hct increased.

Data from Ronco and colleagues suggest Hct may also influence flow distribution within the blood compartment of a dialyzer.[46] These investigators employed a computed tomography (CT)-based technique to measure fiber bundle perfusion of blood with varying Hct (25 to 40 percent). A centralized distribution of flow was observed. Moreover, the extent of this maldistribution was proportional to Hct. In fact, at Hct = 40 percent, the flow velocity and wall shear rate were two- to threefold higher in the central region of the bundle than in its peripheral region. For clinical correlation, these investigators also measured dialyzer urea and creatinine clearances as a function of Hct. As shown in Fig. 4–5, this study corroborated the differential effect of increasing Hct on urea and creatinine clearance reported by Lim and colleagues.

Dialysate Compartment. In recent years, enhanced efficiency of blood compartment and transmembrane small solute mass transfer has been attained through the use of high blood-flow rates and improved membrane designs, respectively. Consequently, most recent efforts have focused on dialysate-side mass transfer. Based on the K_OA concept introduced above, both the dialysate-side mass transfer coefficient and membrane surface area may influence mass transfer. The dialysate-side mass transfer coefficient is determined largely by boundary layer phenomena, as in the blood compartment. As discussed below, effective mass transfer area (A) is not necessarily equal to the manufacturer-reported (nominal) value.

Dialyzer characteristics that influence dialysate-side mass transfer include packing density, fiber undulation (also known as crimping), and the presence or absence of spacer yarns. Recent magnetic resonance imaging (MRI) and CT studies[73–76] suggest that nonoptimized packing density may

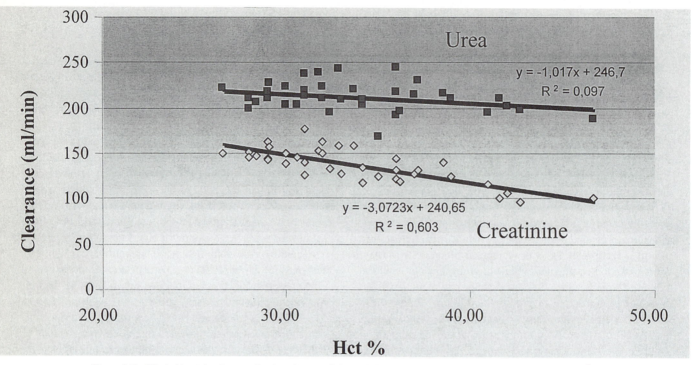

Figure 4–5. Effect of hematocrit on small solute clearance in hemodialysis. *(Reprinted with permission from Ronco et al.[46])*

be the cause of channeling of dialysate at standard flow rates. These investigations demonstrate that a large proportion of the dialysate stream may flow peripheral to the fiber bundle in dialyzers that are not optimally configured. From a physical perspective, the interior of a fiber bundle packed too tightly represents a path of relatively large resistance, while the peripheral pathway is the path of least resistance. Obviously, an inwardly situated hollow fiber cannot participate in diffusive mass exchange if it is not perfused with dialysate. Packing density values beyond the optimum may account for the recent finding that large-surface-area dialyzers (i.e., greater than 1.7 m^2) are generally associated with less efficient dialysate small solute mass transfer relative to dialyzers of smaller surface area.[77]

Another dialyzer characteristic that influences hollow-fiber perfusion with dialysate is fiber-bundle spacing. Dialysate may not be able to perfuse the area between adjacent fibers that are spatially too close. As is the case for nonoptimized packing density, this reduces the effective membrane surface area available for mass exchange. Two recently developed approaches to address this fiber spacing problem are spacer yarns and a specific fiber undulation pattern. Spacer yarns are multifilament, linear structures interspersed longitudinally in a specific spatial distribution within the fiber bundle.[28] With respect to undulation, all hollow fibers are manufactured with a relatively specific periodicity (amplitude and frequency). However, as discussed below, recent evidence suggests that specific fiber undulation approaches improve dialysate flow distribution and small solute mass transfer.[46,74]

In a recent clinical evaluation, Ronco and colleagues measured the effect of a "microcrimping" undulation and spacer yarns on both small solute removal and dialysate flow distribution.[46] The microcrimped polysulfone fibers contained in the dialyzers used in this study have a relatively low amplitude and high frequency. In comparison to conventional dialyzers (i.e., fibers with standard undulation and no spacer yarns), urea clearances were found to be significantly higher for dialyzers with both microcrimped fibers and spacer yarns. Based on a CT-based technique, these investigators also found that dialysate flow distribution was most homogenous in dialyzers with microcrimped fibers and least homogeneous in conventional dialyzers, with dialyzers having spacer yarn technology in an intermediate range. These data suggest that both of these newer approaches improve dialysate flow distribution and thus increase effective membrane surface area.

In addition to this influence on effective surface area, microcrimping may also reduce dialysate-side mass transfer resistance essentially by disrupting ("agitating") the boundary layer. These boundary-layer effects may be attenuated through creation of a turbulent flow regime at relatively high Q_D values. At a relatively common Q_B and Q_D combination of 300 and 500 mL/min, respectively, it is possible that dialysate-side mass transfer is rate-limiting under certain conditions.[78] For several high-efficiency and high-flux dialyzers, Leypoldt et al.[77] reported a mean increase of 14 percent in in vitro urea K_OA when Q_D was increased from 500 to 800 mL/min at a constant Q_B of 450 mL/min. These laboratory data have been corroborated clinically.[79,80] Interestingly, a recent investigation has also suggested the benefit of increasing Q_D on small solute clearance is relatively greater for high-flux dialyzers than high-efficiency dialyzers of comparable surface area.[81]

Two important points about Q_D-related effects on small solute mass transfer require comment. First, for Q_D to have a significant effect on K_OA, a minimal Q_B must be achieved. Specifically, if the blood-flow rate is much less than 50 percent of the dialysate flow rate at baseline, an increase in the latter is not expected to derive much benefit.[65] Second, it is important to note the beneficial effect of increasing Q_D on small solute mass transfer may also be due to a reduction in channeling with improved perfusion of the inner fiber bundle. Thus, the mass transfer benefit of both microcrimping and increased dialysate flow mechanisms may be due to dissipation of boundary layer effects, an increase in effective membrane surface area, or both.

Convective Solute Clearance

The determinants of convective solute removal differ significantly from those of diffusion. Convective solute removal is determined primarily by the sieving properties of the membrane used and the ultrafiltration rate.[30,32] The mechanism by which convection occurs is termed *solvent drag*. If the molecular dimensions of a solute are such that transmembrane passage to some extent occurs, the solute is swept ("dragged") across the membrane in association with ultrafiltered plasma water. Thus, the rate of convective solute removal can be modified by changes either in the rate of solvent (plasma water) flow or in the mean effective pore size of the membrane. As discussed below, the blood concentration of a particular solute also influences its convective removal rate.

Both the water and solute permeability of an ultrafiltration membrane are influenced by the phenomena of secondary membrane formation[20,59–61] and concentration polarization.[82] The exposure of an artificial surface to plasma results in the nonspecific, instantaneous adsorption of a layer of proteins, the composition of which generally reflects that of the plasma itself. Therefore plasma proteins such as albumin, fibrinogen, and immunoglobulins form the bulk of this secondary membrane. Moreover, the plasma total protein concentration also influences this phenomenon. This layer of proteins, by serving as an additional resistance to mass transfer, effectively reduces both the water and solute permeability of an extracorporeal membrane. Evidence of this is found in comparisons of solute sieving coefficients determined before and after exposure of a membrane to plasma or other protein-containing solution.[20,59–61]

Although concentration polarization primarily pertains to plasma proteins, it is distinct from secondary membrane formation. Concentration polarization specifically relates to ultrafiltration-based processes and applies to the kinetic behavior of an individual solute. Accumulation of a solute that is predominantly or completely rejected by a membrane used for ultrafiltration of plasma occurs at the membrane surface of the blood compartment. This surface accumulation causes the solute concentration just adjacent to the membrane surface (i.e., the submembranous concentration) to be higher than the bulk (plasma) concentration. In this manner, a submembranous (high) to bulk (low) concentration gradient is established, resulting in "backdiffusion" from the membrane surface out into the plasma. At steady state, the rate of convective transport to the membrane surface is equal to the rate of backdiffusion. The polarized layer of solute is the distance defined by the gradient between the submembranous and bulk concentrations. This distance (or thickness) of the polarized layer, which can be estimated by mass balance techniques, reflects the extent of the concentration polarization process.

By definition, concentration polarization is applicable in clinical situations where relatively high ultrafiltration rates are used. Conditions which promote the process are high ultrafiltration rate (high rate of convective transport), low blood-flow rate (low shear rate or membrane "sweeping" effect), and the use of postdilution (rather than predilution) replacement fluids (increased local solute concentrations).[83] The extent of the concentration polarization determines its effect on actual solute removal. In general, the degree to which the removal of a rejected solute is influenced is directly related to that solute's extent of rejection by a membrane. In fact, concentration polarization may actually enhance the removal of uremic toxins falling in the low-molecular-weight protein category that otherwise would have minimal convective removal.[82] This is explained by the fact that the pertinent blood compartment concentration subjected to the ultrafiltrate flux is the high submembranous concentration primarily rather than the much lower bulk concentration.

On the other hand, the use of very high ultrafiltration rates in conjunction with other conditions favorable to solute polarization may significantly impair overall membrane performance. As noted previously, the relationship between ultrafiltration rate and transmembrane pressure (TMP) is linear for relatively low ultrafiltration rates. However, as the ultrafiltration rate further increases, this curve eventually plateaus.[56] At this point, fouling of the membrane with denatured proteins may occur, followed by an irreversible decline in solute and water permeability of the membrane. Therefore the ultrafiltration rate (and associated TMP) used for a convective therapy with a specific membrane must fall on the initial (linear) portion of the UFR-vs.-TMP relationship, with avoidance of the plateau region.

Convective solute removal can be quantified in the following manner[84]:

$$N = (1 - \sigma) J_V C_M$$

In this equation, N is the convective flux (mass removal rate per unit membrane area), J_V is the ultrafiltrate flux (ultrafiltration rate normalized to membrane area), C_M is the mean intramembrane solute concentration, and σ is the reflection coefficient, a measure of solute rejection. As Werynski and Waniewski have explained,[84] the parameter $(1-\sigma)$ can be viewed as the membrane resistance to convective solute flow. If σ equals 1, no convective transport occurs, while a value of 0 implies no resistance to convective flow. Of note, C_M is the average of the filtrate-side and blood-side solute concentrations, with the latter represented by the submembranous concentration rather than the bulk-phase concentration. Therefore this parameter is significantly influenced by the effects of concentration polarization.

REFERENCES

1. Clark WR. Hemodialyzer membranes and configurations: a historical perspective. *Semin Dial* 2000;13:309–311.
2. Colton CK, Lowrie EG. Hemodialysis: Physical principles and technical considerations; in Brenner BM, Rector FC, eds. *The Kidney*, 2d ed. Philadelphia, Saunders, 1981:2425–2489.
3. Lipps B, Stewart R, Perkins H, et al. The hollow fiber artificial kidney. *Trans Am Soc Artif Intern Organs* 1967;13: 200–207.
4. Gotch FA, Lipps B, Weaver J, et al. Chronic hemodialysis with the hollow fiber artificial kidney (HFAK). *Trans Am Soc Artif Intern Organs* 1969;15:87–96.
5. Funck-Bretano J, Sausse A, Man NK, et al. A new hemodialysis treatment associating a membrane highly permeable to middle molecules with a closed circuit dialysate system. *Proc EDTA* 1972;9:55–66.
6. Streicher E, Schneider H. The development of a polysulfone membrane: a new perspective in dialysis? *Contrib Nephrol* 1985;46:1–13.
7. Strathmann H, Gohl H. Membranes for blood purification: state of the art and new developments. *Contrib Nephrol* 1990;78:119–141.
8. Lysaght MJ. Evolution of hemodialysis membranes. *Contrib Nephrol* 1995;113:1–10.
9. Lysaght MJ. Hemodialysis membranes in transition. *Contrib Nephrol* 1988;61:1–17.
10. Jindal KK, McDougall J, Woods B, et al. A study of the basic principles determining the performance of several high–flux dialyzers. *Am J Kidney Dis* 1989;14:507–511.
11. Clark WR, Macias WL, Molitoris A, Wang NHL. Plasma protein adsorption to highly permeable hemodialysis membranes. *Kidney Int* 1995;48:481–488.
12. De Vriese AS, Langlois M, Bernard D, et al. Effect of dialyzer membrane pore size on plasma homocysteine levels in haemodialysis patients. *Nephrol Dial Transplant* 2003;18: 2596–2600.
13. Hoenich N, Woffindin C, Cox P, et al. Clinical characterization of Dicea a new cellulose membrane for haemodialysis. *Clin Nephrol* 1997;48:253–259.
14. Schaefer R, Horl W, Kokot K, Heidland A. Enhanced biocompatibility with a new cellulosic membrane: Cuprophan vs Hemophan. *Blood Purif* 1987;5:262–267.
15. Clark WR, Shinaberger JH. Clinical evaluation of a new high-efficiency hemodialyzer: Polysynthane (PSN). *ASAIO J* 2000;46:288–292.
16. Gohl H, Buck R, Strathmann H. Basic features of polyamide membranes. *Contrib Nephrol* 1992;96:1–25.
17. Bonomini M, Fiederling B, Bucciarelli T, et al. A new polymethylmethacrylate membrane for hemodialysis. *Int J Artif Organs* 1996;19:232–239.
18. Jaber BL, Gonski JA, Cendoroglo M, et al. New polyethersulfone dialyzers attenuate passage of cytokine-inducing substances from *Pseudomonas aeruginosa* contaminated dialysate. *Blood Purif* 1998;16:210–219.
19. Ronco C, Crepaldi C, Brendolan A, et al. Evolution of synthetic membranes for blood purification: the case of the Polyflux family. *Nephrol Dial Transplant* 2003;18(suppl 7):vii10–vii20.
20. Rockel A, Hertel J, Fiegel P, et al. Permeability and secondary membrane formation of a high flux polysulfone hemofilter. *Kidney Int* 1986;30:429–432.
21. Ledebo I. Principles and practice of hemofiltration and hemodiafiltration. *Artif Organs* 1998;22:20–25.
22. Ward R, Buscaroli A, Schmidt B, et al. A comparison of dialysers with low–flux membranes: significant differences in spite of many similarities. *Nephrol Dial Transplant* 1997;12:965–972.
23. Mishkin GJ. What clinically important advances in understanding and improving dialyzer function have occurred recently? *Semin Dial* 2001;14:170–173.
24. Brendolan A, Tetta C, Granziero A, et al. Flow dynamic characteristics of DIAPES hemodialyzers. *Contrib Nephrol* 2003;138:27–36.
25. Takeyama T, Sakai Y. Polymethylmethacrylate: one biomaterial for a series of membrane. *Contrib Nephrol* 1998;125: 9–24.
26. Bird RB, Stewart WE, Lightfoot EN. Velocity distributions in laminar flow. In: Bird RB, Stewart WE, Lightfoot EN, eds. *Transport Phenomena*. New York: Wiley, 1960: 34–70.
27. Clark WR, Gao D. Properties of membranes used for hemodialysis therapy. *Semin Dial* 2002;15:1–5.
28. Clark WR, Hamburger RJ, Lysaght MJ. Effect of membrane composition and structure on performance and biocompatibility in hemodialysis. *Kidney Int* 1999;56:2005–2015.
29. Gao D, Kraus MA, Ronco C, Clark WR. The biology of dialysis. In: Warady B, Schaefer F, Fine RN, Alexander SR, eds. *Pediatric Dialysis*. Dortdrecht, The Netherlands: Kluwer, 2004:13–34.
30. Ronco C, Ballestri M, Gappelli G. Dialysis membranes in convective treatments. *Nephrol Dial Transplant* 2000;15 (suppl 2):31–36.
31. Clark WR, Ronco C. Determinants of hemodialyser performance and the potential effect on clinical outcome. *Nephrol Dial Transplant* 2001;16(suppl 5):56–60.
32. Henderson LW. Biophysics of ultrafiltration and hemofiltration. In: Jacobs C, Kjellstrand C, Koch K, Winchester J, eds. *Replacement of Renal Function by Dialysyis*. Dortdrecht, The Netherlands: Kluwer, 1995:114–117.

33. Leypoldt JK. Solute fluxes in different treatment modalities. *Nephrol Dial Transplant* 2000;15(suppl 1):3–9.

34. Ofsthun NJ, Zydney AL. Importance of convection in artificial kidney treatment. *Contrib Nephrol* 1994;108:53–70.

35. Krieter DH, Canaud B. High permeability of dialysis membranes: what is the limit of albumin loss? *Nephrol Dial Transplant* 2003;18:651–654.

36. Ronco C. Backfiltration: a controversial issue in modern dialysis. *Int J Artif Organs* 1988;11:69–74.

37. Clark WR, Gao D. Low-molecular-weight proteins in endstage renal disease: potential toxicity and dialytic removal mechanisms. *J Am Soc Nephrol* 2002;13:S41–S47.

38. Ronco C, Brendolan A, Lupi A, et al. Enhancement of convective transport by internal filtration in a modified experimental hemodialyzer. Kidney Int 1998;54:979–985.

39. Ronco C, Brendolan A, Lupi A, et al. Effects of a reduced inner diameter of hollow fibers in hemodialyzers. *Kidney Int* 2000;58:809–817.

40. Clark WR, Macias WL, Molitoris BA, Wang NHL. ß₂-microglobulin membrane adsorption: equilibrium and kinetic characterization. *Kidney Int* 1994;46:1140–1146.

41. Klinke B, Rockel A, Abdelhamid S, et al. Transmembrane transport and adsorption of beta₂–microglobulin during hemodialysis using polysulfone, polyacrylonitrile, polymethylmethacrylate, and cuprammonium rayon membranes. *Int J Artif Organs* 1989;12:697–702.

42. Floege J, Granolleras C, Bingel M, et al. Beta₂-microglobulin kinetics during hemodialysis and hemofiltration. *Nephrol Dial Transplant* 1987;1:223–228.

43. Lonnemann G. Chronic inflammation in hemodialysis: the role of contaminated dialysate. *Blood Purif* 2000;18:214–223.

44. Sugaya H, Sakai Y. Polymethylmethacrylate: from polymer to dialyzer. *Contrib Nephrol* 1998;125:1–8.

45. Ronco C, Scabardi M, Goldoni M, et al. Impact of spacing filaments external to hollow fibers on dialysate flow distribution and dialyzer performance. *Int J Artif Organs* 1997;20:261–266.

46. Ronco C, Brendolan A, Crepaldi C, et al. Blood and dialysate flow distributions in hollow fiber hemodialyzers analyzed by computerized helical scanning technique. *J Am Soc Nephrol* 2002;13:S53–S61.

47. Henderson LW. Why do we use clearance? *Blood Purif* 1995;13:283–288.

48. Jaffrin MY. Convective mass transfer in hemodialysis. *Artif Organs* 1995;19:1162–1171.

49. Katz M, Hull A. Transcellular creatinine disequilibrium and its significance in hemodialysis. *Nephron* 1974;12:171–177.

50. Slatsky M, Schindhelm K, Farrell P. Creatinine transfer between red blood cells and plasma: a comparison between normal and uremic subjects. *Nephron* 1978;22:514–521.

51. Schmidt B, Ward R. The impact of erythropoietin on hemodialyzer design and performance. *Artif Organs* 1989;13:35–42.

52. Lim V, Flanigan M, Fangman J. Effect of hematocrit on solute removal during high efficiency hemodialysis. *Kidney Int* 1990;37:1557–1562.

53. Shinaberger J, Miller J, Gardner P. Erythropoietin alert: risks of high hematocrit hemodialysis. *Trans Am Soc Artif Intern Organs* 1988;34:179–184.

54. Henderson L, Leypoldt JK, Lysaght M, Cheung A. Death on dialysis and the time/flux trade–off. *Blood Purif* 1997;15:1–14.

55. Clark WR, Leypoldt JK, Henderson LW, et al. Quantifying the effect of changes in the hemodialysis prescription on effective solute removal with a mathematical model. *J Am Soc Nephrol* 1999;10:601–610.

56. Clark WR, Rocco MV, Collins AJ. Quantification of hemodialysis: analysis of methods and relevance to clinical outcome. *Blood Purif* 1997;15:92–111.

57. Pedrini L, Zereik S, Rasmy S. Causes, kinetics, and clinical implications of post-hemodialysis urea rebound. *Kidney Int* 1988;34:817–824.

58. Keshaviah P, Luehmann D, Ilstrup K, Collins A. Technical requirements for rapid high efficiency therapies. *Artif Organs* 1986;110:189–194.

59. Bosch T, Schmidt B, Samtleben W, Gurland H. Effect of protein adsorption on diffusive and convective transport through polysulfone membranes. *Contrib Nephrol* 1985;46:14–22.

60. Langsdorf LJ, Zydney AL. Effect of blood contact on the transport properties of hemodialysis membranes: a two-layer model. *Blood Purif* 1994;12:292–307.

61. Morti SM, Zydney AL. Protein–membrane interactions during hemodialysis: effects on solute transport. *ASAIO J* 1998;44:319–326.

62. Akizawa T, Kinugasa E, Ideura T. Classification of dialysis membranes by performance. *Contrib Nephrol* 1995;113:25–31.

63. Huang Z, Clark WR, Gao D. Determinants of small solute clearance in hemodialysis. *Semin Dial.* In press.

64. Michaels AS. Operating parameters and performance criteria for hemodialyzers and other membrane-separation devices. *Trans Am Soc Artif Intern Organs* 1966;12:387–392.

65. Leypoldt JK, Cheung AK. Optimal use of hemodialyzers. *Contrib Nephrol* 2002;137:129–137.

66. Popovich R, Hlavinka D, Bomar J, et al. The consequences of physiological resistances of metabolite removal from the patient-artificial kidney system. *Trans Am Soc Artif Intern Organs* 1975;21:108–115.

67. Guyton AC. Partition of body fluids: osmotic equilibria between extracellular and intracellular fluids. In: Guyton AC, ed. *Textbook of Medical Physiology.* Philadelphia: Saunders, 1981.

68. Savitz D, Sidel V, Solomon A. Osmotic properties of human red cells. *J Gen Physiol* 1964;48:79–94.

69. Langsdorf L, Zydney A. Effect of uremia on the membrane transport characteristics of red blood cells. Blood 1993;81:820–827.

70. Cheung A, Alford M, Wilson M, et al. Urea movement across erythrocyte membrane. *Kidney Int* 1983;23:866–869.

71. Shinaberger J, Miller J, Gardner P. Erythropoietin alert: risks of high hematocrit hemodialysis. *Trans Am Soc Artif Intern Organs* 1988;34:179–184.

72. Colton C, Smith K, Merrill E, Friedman S. Diffusion of urea in flowing blood. *AIChE J* 1971;17:800–808.

73. Zhang J, Parker D, Leypoldt JK. Flow distributions in hollow fiber hemodialyzers using magnetic resonance Fourier velocity imaging. *ASAIO J* 1995;41:M678–M682.

74. Ronco C, Brendolan A, Crepaldi C, et al. Flow distribution and cross filtration in hollow fiber hemodialyzers. *Contrib Nephrol* 2002;137:120–128.

75. Poh CK, Hardy PA, Liao Z, et al. Effect of flow baffles on the dialysate flow distribution in hollow-fiber hemodialyzers: a non-intrusive experimental study using MRI. *J Biomech Eng* 2003;125:481–489.

76. Liao Z, Poh CK, Huang Z, et al. A numerical and experimental investigation of mass transfer in an artificial kidney. *J Biomech Eng* 2003;125:472–480.

77. Leypoldt JK, Cheung AK, Agodoa LY, et al: Hemodialyzer mass transfer-area coefficients for urea increase at high dialysate flow rates. *Kidney Int* 1997;51:2013–2017.

78. Sigdell J, Tersteegen B. Clearance of a dialyzer under varying operating conditions. *Artif Organs* 1986;10:219–225.

79. Ouseph R, Ward RA. Increasing dialysate flow rate increases dialyzer urea mass transfer-area coefficients during clinical use. *Am J Kidney Dis* 2001;37:316–320.

80. Hauk M, Kuhlmann M, Riegel W, Kohler H. In vivo effects of dialysate flow rate on Kt/V in maintenance hemodialysis patients. *Am J Kidney Dis* 2000;35:105–111.

81. Leypoldt JK, Cheung AC. Increases in mass transfer-area coefficients and urea Kt/V with increasing dialysate flow rate are greater for high-flux dialyzers. *Am J Kidney Dis* 2001;38:575–579.

82. Kim S. Characteristics of protein removal in hemodiafiltration. *Contrib Nephrol* 1994;108:23–37.

83. Henderson LW. Pre vs post dilution hemofiltration. *Clin Nephrol* 1979;11:120–124.

84. Werynski A, Waniewski J. Theoretical description of mass transport in medical membrane devices. *Artif Organs* 1995;19:420–427.

Biocompatibility

Sabine Schmaldienst
Walter H. Hörl

Biocompatibility is the ability of a material device, procedure, or system to perform without a clinically significant host response.[1]

The first dialysis membranes designed for maintenance hemodialysis (HD) were made of regenerated cellulose (cuprophan). In cuprophan-treated patients, a low permeability of larger solutes was observed; this led to the formulation of the middle-molecule hypothesis, where a discrepancy between the clearance of small molecules and uremic symptoms was found. A number of bioactive substances accumulate in uremic patients or increase during HD treatment. These factors, associated with possible long-term complications, are collagenase, angiogenin, elastase, various cytokines [interleukin-1 (IL-1), IL-6, IL-8, tumor necrosis factor alpha (TNF-α)], complement factor D, advanced glycation end products (AGEs) such as pentosidine or carboxymethyl lysine, and reactive carbonyl compounds (RCOs) such as 3-desoxyglucosone or beta$_2$ microglobulin (β2-m). Furthermore, intradialytic leukopenia was associated with the use of cuprophan.[2] Intradialytic leukopenia and the formation of anaphylatoxins (e.g., C3a and C5a) initiated the discussion of membrane biocompatibility.

The increased survival of patients on maintenance HD has enabled an improvement in the understanding of the biological phenomena that take place during dialysis therapy. Thus significant acute and long-term host responses during dialysis (complement activation, monocyte and granulocyte activation, endotoxin transfer) have an impact on long-term patient survival and should be avoided. These processes lead to hypersensitivity reactions, dialysis-related amyloidosis, accelerated loss of residual renal function, and/or lipidologic disorders. The main factor influencing the patient's intradialytic biological response seems to be the blood-membrane contact in the extracorporeal device. During 15 years of HD, for example, the blood of each patient comes into contact with 4000 m^2 of foreign surface.[3]

MEMBRANES

The central component of the HD process is the membrane, which is the ultimate determinant of the quality and success of therapy. Nowadays membranes are produced in sheet or hollow fiber form and are packed into either parallel-plate or hollow fiber hemodialyzers, with the latter now having a 90 percent share of the market.[4] The advantages of hollow fiber dialyzers include enhanced blood-flow and mass-transport capacity and lower production costs. In contrast to sheet dialyzers, they have a high mechanical stability and a lower filling volume. Each dialyzer consists of approximately 10,000 single hollow fibers with intraluminal blood flow. The dialyzers have different membrane surfaces; as a result, the treatment can be adapted to the patients' body weight and the dialysis modality (Table 5–1).

Membranes are traditionally perceived as diffusive-convective structures. Studies within the last three decades suggest a more complex function. Membranes have the ca-

pacity to activate plasma proteins, thrombocytes, leukocytes, and the enzymatic cascades of the coagulation and complement systems. Furthermore, membranes such as polyacrylonitrile or polymethylmethacrylate are able to bind significant amounts of plasma proteins, therefore having an additional function as adsorptive structures.[5] The protein layer that develops on first use of a hemodialyzer membrane is associated with the following: (1) when dialyzer membranes are reused, a reduced activation of white blood cells and complement has been observed, and (2) because of the adsorption of proteins during dialysis, pore size decreases and the clearance of larger molecules is diminished.

Membranes with a high efficiency have a high urea clearance. This can often be achieved by increasing the surface area. The term *high-flux* is used for dialyzers with a large pore size and therefore a high ultrafiltration coefficient (>20 mL/h/mmHg) and high clearance of middle molecules (e.g., for β2-m: up to 600 mg/week).

For the sake of discussion, HD membranes are often separated into cellulosic and synthetic types. Both are commercially available as low- and high-flux dialyzers.

Cellulosic Membranes

Regenerated Cellulose Membranes. Cellulosic membranes, the most commonly used dialysis membranes in the 1970s, are formed by regenerating cellulose (linear polysaccharides), using a variety of methods.[6] Such membranes are macroscopically homogeneous and contain linked anhydroglucose units that incorporate free hydroxyl groups. This feature is involved, at least partly, in the activation of the complement system via the alternate pathway. Cellulose is an extreme polar molecule with strong Van der Waals energy. Thus the membrane is a hydrophilic polymer resulting, in combination with water, in a hydrogel. The original membranes made by the cuprammonium process had high porosity but low permeability to larger solutes. Now cuprammonium membranes with high permeability to larger solutes (due to an increase in pore size) are available. Cellulosic membranes are often relatively inexpensive and can be reused extensively.

Substituted Cellulose Membranes. In the 1970s, modified (substituted) cellulose membranes were introduced; the hydroxyl groups on the surface of such membranes were diminished. This resulted in reduced activation of the complement system. Hydroxyl groups are masked either with a synthetic polymer or by acetyl substitution. By varying the degree of substitution, cellulose acetate, cellulose diacetate, and cellulose triacetate were developed. All cellulose acetate membranes are more hydrophobic than regenerated cellulose membranes and have a moderately increased pore size, yielding a slightly broader spectrum of water perme-

TABLE 5–1. PROPERTIES OF DIFFERENT MATERIALS USED FOR HEMODIALYSIS (HD) AND HEMODIAFILTRATION (HDF)

Material	Surface (m²)	Dialysis Modality	Ultrafiltration Coefficient	Producer
Cellulose acetate	0.3–2.2	HD/HDF	1.1–45.0	Althin
				Baxter
				Cobe
				Hospal
				Nipro
Cuprammonium	0.6–2.2	HD/HDF	2.5–37.0	Asahi
Cuprophan	0.7–2.0	HD	2.6–11.2	Baxter
				Bellco
				Braun
				Cobe
				Fresenius
				Gambro
				Nikkiso
Hemophan	0.2–2.0	HD	3.1–17.6	Bellco
				Braun
				Cobe
				Fresenius
				Gambro
				Hospal
				Nikkiso
Polyamide	1.1–2.1	HD/HDF	8.6–71.0	Gambro
Polyacrylonitrile	0.3–2.2	HD/HDF	16.0–65.0	Asahi
				Hospal
Polymethyl-methacrylate	0.5–2.1	HD/HDF	2.5–41.0	Toray
Ethylene vinyl alcohol	0.7–1.6	HD	4.8–14.5	Kuraray
Polysulfone	0.7–2.5	HD/HDF	1.7–103.0	Asahi
				Baxter
				Bellco
				Cobe
				Fresenius
				Hospal
				Nikkiso
				Toray

ability and solute removal. Unique and new was the development of Hemophan membranes—cuprammonium membranes derived from diethylaminoethyl groups (second cellulosic substitution mechanism) via the hydroxyl moieties. They were the first dialyzers specially developed to improve biocompatibility, although only 1 percent of the free hydroxyl groups have been substituted. Hemophan has a larger pore size and a higher transport capacity for middle molecules, as well as a higher ultrafiltration rate. Activation of the complement system is diminished, as is leukocytopenia in the initial phase of HD treatment. Hemophan membranes cause a pronounced activation of the coagulation cascade; thus these dialyzers must be prerinsed with heparin. To further improve biocompatibility, vitamin E–modified cellulosic membranes have recently been introduced.[7–9]

Synthetic Membranes

Synthetic membranes, developed in the 1970s, are hydrophobic, symmetrical or asymmetrical, and have anisotropic structures without hydroxyl groups on their surface. Synthetic membranes have thicker walls than cellulosic membranes (20 μm vs. 6 to 15 μm). Since they were primarily introduced for hemofiltration and high-flux HD, they have a significantly larger pore size, higher hydraulic permeability, and higher solute clearance. The materials have the ability to bind complement-regulating proteins such as factor B and factor D, both promotors of complement activation, or factor H, an inhibitor on exposure to blood (Fig. 5–1). Synthetic membranes have a markedly reduced ability to activate the complement pathway or other cellular elements. They are associated with a 20 percent lower mortality and are therefore considered biocompatible.[10–13] Because of their high solute clearance and biocompatibility properties, synthetic membranes have recently become more popular.

Polyacrilonitrile. Polyacrylonitrile (PAN), known under the trade name AN69, is a copolymer (acrylonitrile and sodium methalyl sulfonate) that was used in one of the first high-flux dialyzers. This symmetrical and morphologically homogeneous membrane contains negatively charged ionizable groups on its surface, similar to the glomerular basement membrane.[14] Besides excellent diffusive as well as convective properties, PAN membranes have a high adsorptive capacity, leading to a favorable reduction in β2-m levels.[15] Important in respect to biocompatibility is the adsorption of C3a, C5a, IgG, fibrinogen, and IL-1.[16–19] Due to the binding of anaphylatoxins, complement activation and intradialytic leukocytopenia is negligible.[20,21] Many features of PAN membranes are markedly distinct from those of cellulosic membranes; thus they are frequently cited in the literature. In the 1990s, anaphylactic reactions were observed during HD in patients dialyzed with the PAN membrane

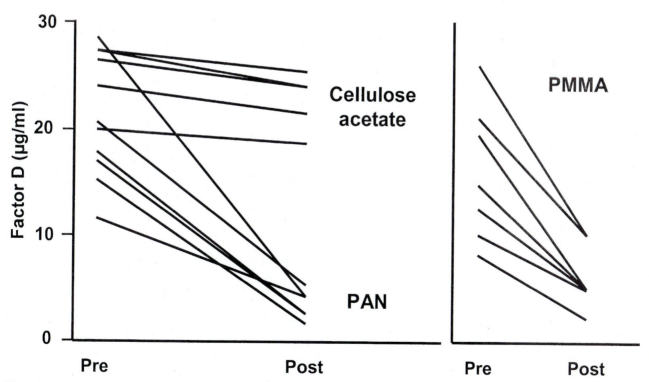

Figure 5–1. Adsorption of complement factor D onto the dialysis membrane is observed only in synthetic membranes. *(From Swinford RD, Baid S, Pascual M. Dialysis membrane adsorption during CRRT. Am J Kidney Dis 1997;30:S32–S37. With permission.)*

who were taking angiotensin-converting enzyme (ACE) inhibitors. This reaction occurs in the first 10 to 20 minutes of the dialysis session, mainly by the induction of bradykinin release (due to the negatively charged membrane) combined with the reduced degradation of bradykinin (due to ACE inhibition). Such an adverse event may occur not only in chronically uremic patients on intermittent HD but also in patients with acute renal failure during continuous extracorporeal treatment.[22] The prevalence of acute hypersensitivity reactions in patients on maintenance HD was calculated to be 1.3 percent, of which 0.25 percent were severe anaphylactoid reactions. The annual incidence of anaphylactoid reactions was 0.17 per 1000 sessions with cellulosic membranes but 4.2 per 1000 sessions with synthetic membranes. Treatment of HD patients with ACE inhibitors strongly increased the risk of anaphylactoid reactions in patients treated with PAN membranes (7.2 percent) as compared to those dialyzed with synthetic membranes (1.6 percent).[23]

Bradykinin is a mediator of anaphylactoid reactions during HD with PAN membranes, particularly in those patients taking ACE inhibitors.[24] In sheep, elevated bradykinin levels were found in arterial blood during HD with PAN membranes. Pretreatment of the animals with 10 or 20 mg of enalapril resulted in a further significant increase in bradykinin, while prekallikrein and high-molecular-weight kininogen concentrations decreased markedly. Anaphylactoid reactions in these animals were completely prevented with the bradykinin β_2-receptor antagonist icatibant.[25] In patients who developed hypersensitivity reactions during HD, a significant increase in the half-life of des-Arg9-bradykinin, but not bradykinin, was observed. Preincubation of sera with enalapril increased the half-life of both bradykinin and des-Arg9-bradykinin.[26]

Therefore the combination of negatively charged HD membranes or other biomaterials with ACE inhibitor therapy should be avoided. In a retrospective and uncontrolled study, the use of alkaline rinsing solution, by keeping the pH value above 7.5, prevented the development of hypersensitivity reactions due to inhibition of kallikrein synthesis.[27] Reduction of surface electronegativity by coating the PAN membrane with a polycationic saline solution prevented the generation of bradykinin.[28] Nevertheless, an anaphylactoid reaction has been reported in a patient during dialysis with a surface-treated AN69 membrane who received a single dose of captopril.[29]

The administration of angiotensin II receptor antagonists is thought to be safe in HD patients treated with PAN membranes with respect to hypersensitivity reactions. In patients receiving therapy with an angiotensin II receptor antagonist, no anaphylactoid reactions were observed in the course of 1188 HD sessions.[30] Nevertheless, in other reports, anaphylactoid reactions were observed in this setting.[31–33] The mechanism for such adverse reactions in these patients is unclear, since ACE inhibitors reduce angiotensin II levels and increase bradykinin, whereas angiotensin II receptor blockers are believed to augment angiotensin II without affecting bradykinin.

Polysulfone. Polysulfone (PS) was developed in the 1970s. When polyvinylpyrrolidone is added, it becomes a foam-like copolymer. It exhibits highly diffusive as well as convective properties. This membrane material induces less complement activation and leukopenia than cellulose.[34,35] Plasma levels of granulocyte elastase remain low during dialysis with PS. Therefore it can be concluded that almost no activation of neutrophil granulocytes occurs during HD with PS. Interactions between PS and ACE inhibitors are unlikely, because there is no generation of bradykinin when this membrane is used.[36] PS membranes can adsorb plasma proteins, although to a lesser extent than PAN and polymethylmethacrylate (PMMA) membranes. PS membranes are produced as high-flux (ultrafiltration coefficient >20 mL/h/mmHg) and low-flux (ultrafiltration coefficient <15 mL/h/mmHg) dialyzers.

Polyamide. Polyamide (PA) membranes, developed in the 1970s, are asymmetrical high-flux membranes with a great hydraulic permeability. PA is composed of a thin internal layer (0.1 µm) with many fine pores (diameter 5 to 10 Å) and an external layer of 30 to 40 µm with macropores (40 to 50 Å), which represents the support structure. The originally hydrophobic membrane is still in use to produce ultrapure dialysate. This is achieved because of the material's adsorptive capacity to bind bacterial endotoxins. Polyvinylpyrrolidone has been added to the primary hydrophobic material, making the surface more hydrophilic and leading to reduced interactions with plasma proteins. Because of its sponge-like structure, this membrane provides excellent diffusive and convective properties. During HD with PA, complement activation and leukopenia are diminished. There is no contact activation, therefore this material is biocompatible. The PA membrane is furthermore characterized by a low adsorption of plasma proteins and modest thrombogenicity.

Polymethylmethacrylate. Polymethylmethacrylate (PMMA) is a hydrophobic membrane with an asymmetrical structure. It is a hydrogel and contains large amounts of water. The membrane is produced by the fusion of isotactic polymethylacrylate and dimethylsulfoxide. The capillary fiber is produced by gelification and substitution of water. By varying their concentrations of the syntactic and isotactic polymers and the water content, membranes of varying composition, density, and porosity can be obtained. PMMA is used for low- and high-flux HD as well as for hemodiafiltration. The biocompatibility of the membrane is good because it has a low potential for activating the complement system, although increased degranulation of neutrophils has been observed. Beta$_2$-microglobulin levels are reduced during HD with PMMA membranes, primarily by adsorption.

Ethylene Vinyl Alcohol. Ethylene vinyl alcohol (EVAL) is a hydrophilic, symmetrical synthetic membrane. Its structure is similar to that of regenerated cellulose and other cellulosic membranes. It is produced by the polymerization of ethylene and vinyl acetate with successive alkaline saponification and extrusion. Membranes with different pore densities can be fabricated. EVAL is available only for low-flux HD. The clearance for small solutes is somewhat inferior to that of cellulosic membranes, but there is better clearance for higher-molecular-weight molecules. The membrane leads to reduced blood contact by diminished activation of substances such as factor XII, high molecular-weight-kallikrein, and prekallikrein. Thus EVAL can be used for heparin-free HD.

COMPLEMENT ACTIVATION

Biocompatibility as it relates to HD is the sum of interactions between blood and various components of the HD equipment.

Direct interaction between complement proteins and specific chemical residues on dialysis membranes results in the activation of the complement system. Cellulosic membranes have a sequence of repetitive polysaccharide units on their surface, reminiscent of bacterial and yeast wall lipopolysaccharides, that provide the basis for complement activation via the alternative pathway during dialysis with these membranes.[37,38] Anaphylatoxins (C3a and C5a) and the membrane attack complex (C5b-9) are present without detectable amounts of C4a generated from the classic pathway. This confirms that complement activation during HD proceeds by the alternative pathway.[39–41] While both anaphylatoxins cause smooth muscle contraction, particular in the respiratory tree, the leukocyte-directed activities of C5a are greater than those from C3a.[42,43] The high affinity to specific receptors on leukocytes results in relatively low C5a levels, thus C3a is the better marker for measuring complement activation. By measuring biocompatibility with respect to complement activation, it must be kept in mind that anaphylatoxins can be lost from the circulation. C3a has a low molecular weight (9 kDa) and can, therefore, diffuse across the membrane of high-flux dialyzers and enter the dialysate, as has been described for PS.[43–45] PAN membranes have a high capacity to adsorb anaphylatoxins, thus prohibiting the transport of these molecules to the dialysis compartment despite the high permeability of

this membrane.[17] Therefore the degree of complement activation is likely underestimated with high-flux dialysis membranes.[45]

C-terminal arginine is removed in plasma to form C3a$_{desArg}$ and C5a$_{desArg}$, leading to the production of C5b, and initiates the formation of the membrane attack complex (C5b-9). There is also increasing evidence that the membrane attack complex can participate in the process of cellular activation.[46,47] Among the different types of dialysis membranes, cellulosic membranes activate complement to the greatest degree, with maximum activation reached 15 minutes after blood contacts the membrane. As dialysis proceeds, complement activation decreases, mainly due to deposition of complement fragments such as C3b as well as nonspecific deposition of fibrin on the activating sites of the dialyzer membrane surface.

Newer cellulosic membranes like Hemophan and cellulose triacetate are more biocompatible than cuprophan membranes.[48] The newer synthetic membranes (i.e., PAN, PS, PMMA) do not significantly activate complement.[21,48] However, as already mentioned, PAN and PMMA have a high capacity to adsorb C3a. Despite a high permeability, only low concentrations of complement fragments are detectable in the ultrafiltrate.[17] Due to the large pores of synthetic membranes, anaphylatoxins are cleared from the circulation by transport into the dialysate.[43]

Activation of the alternative complement pathway will proceed after C3b has been covalently attached to the dialysis membrane (mainly via hydroxyl groups). On complement-activating membranes, covalently bound C3b will be protected from the physiologic inactivation by factor H and factor I (two complement-inhibitory proteins). Therefore the activation of alternative pathway can proceed in the presence of factor B and factor D. Factor D, a highly specific serine protease, cleaves factor B bound to C3b, generating the C3bBb complex and enhancing the resulting activity of C3 convertase. Thus, factor D is a rate-limiting enzyme of the alternative pathway. Its enzymatic function is not altered in uremia, but there is an accumulation of factor D in uremic patients. In patients with end-stage renal disease (ESRD), serum levels are elevated tenfold as compared to healthy controls.[49] On noncomplement activating membranes, factor H can bind to C3b on the membrane. The net result is the inactivation by factor I. The local availability of factor H in contact with C3b appears to be important in determining the complement-activation potential of a membrane (Fig. 5–2). Membranes with a high capacity to bind factor D, such as PAN and PMMA, are not complement-activating, since bound factor D is enzymatically inactive.[50–52]

In the case of complement activation, C5a and C5a$_{desArg}$ are able to induce the activation of phagocytes, including neutrophils and monocytes, through their complement receptors.[38,53] Complement activation may induce an increased responsiveness of phagocytes in the resting state,

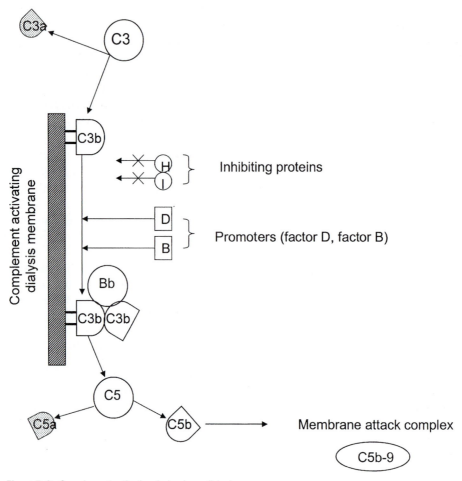

Figure 5–2. Complement activation during hemodialysis.

leading to an enhanced release of phagocytic end products. This results in a decreased responsiveness to further stimulation.[11]

ACTIVATION OF THE COAGULATION SYSTEM AND THROMBOGENICITY

The increased thrombogenicity during an extracorporeal procedure remains an unsolved problem. Only a few studies dealing with this topic are available.

When blood comes into contact with foreign surfaces, plasma proteins are adsorbed. This leads to adhesion of thrombocytes, leukocytes, and erythrocytes. Which kind of proteins will be adsorbed depends on the surface material. Negatively charged surfaces favor the binding of various components of the coagulation system—such as prekallikrein, kininogen, coagulation factor XI, and Hageman factor (factor XII)—through activation of the intrinsic coagulation pathway. By autoactivation of factor XII, large amounts of active serine protease factor XIIa will be generated. Factor XIIa cleaves prekallikrein to kallikrein,

thereby again activating factor XII and the intrinsic coagulation pathway through the generation of factor XIa. Kallikrein can cleave factor XIIa. Factor XIIa has lost its surface binding domain and will be inactivated by potent inhibitors such as C1 inhibitor. Activation of the coagulation system leads to the conversion of prothrombin to thrombin. In an ex vivo model, unchanged levels of factor XIIa during circulation of blood through cuprophan and PS dialyzers has been demonstrated, whereas a 3.5-fold increase of factor XIIa was observed with the PAN membrane.[54] An increase of the thrombin-antithrombin complex was observed in all membranes, but highest values were obtained in the case of the PAN membrane, even with respect to the release of platelet factor 4 (PF4) and platelet consumption. Up to now, contact-phase activation was thought to be the main trigger of the coagulation cascade during HD. Since thrombin-antithrombin generation occurs in the absence of factor XIIa with cuprophan and PS membranes, contact activation seems not to be important for the activation of the coagulation system during HD. How the activation works in the absence of factor XIIa remains unclear. Even in platelet-poor plasma, generation of thrombin-antithrombin occurs, thus monocytes are thought to play an important role.[55] It has been shown that an elevation of thrombin-antithrombin complexes has a direct influence on the thrombogenicity of dialyzers. During continuous hemofiltration, a short life span of the filter is accompanied by an increase of thrombin-antithrombin complexes over time.[56] In vivo studies have shown that PAN membranes induce stronger thrombocyte activation and thrombin generation but are less thrombogenic than cuprophan. In vivo studies are difficult to interpret, since removal or adsorption of activation markers such as fibrinopeptide A or platelet factor (PF) 4 occurs. Activation of the coagulation system can be observed by a decrease in the half-life of fibrinogen. This is accompanied by an increase of fibrinopeptides (fibrinopeptide A and fibrinopeptide B).[57,58] Sufficient anticoagulation with heparin prevents the cleavage of fibrinogen; thus fibrinopeptide A is not elevated.[57]

Activation of the coagulation system is counteracted by activation of the fibrinolytic system. Increased levels of tissue plasminogen activator, which lead to the activation of plasmin and plasminogen, have been observed during the first hour of cuprophan dialysis.[59] Furthermore, plasma concentrations of tissue plasminogen activator inhibitor, which is released from pulmonary endothelial cells due to injury by complement factors and proteases from granulocytes, are also diminished. This activation of the fibrinolytic system during cuprophan dialysis could help, at least in part, to prevent clotting in the dialyzer.

A comparison of low-molecular-weight heparin and standard heparin as anticoagulants during HD with PS membranes has demonstrated some differences. The use of low-molecular-weight heparin was associated with lower levels of thrombin-antithrombin complexes and fibrinopeptide A.[60]

An important side effect of heparin therapy is heparin-induced thrombocytopenia (HIT), which is associated with a significant increase in morbidity and mortality. Thrombosis is one of the major complications. The presence of HIT antibody (IgG) leads to the generation of procoagulant microparticles that generate thrombin and induce endothelial damage and activation. Furthermore, plasma from patients with HIT has been shown to induce the formation of leukocyte-platelet aggregates in a heparin-dependent manner. This interaction can be inhibited by antibody to P-selectin.[61]

CELL SYSTEMS AFFECTED BY HEMODIALYSIS

Neutrophil Granulocytes

A transient neutropenia at the beginning of treatment has been described during HD with cuprophan membranes. In vitro as well as in vivo, it could be shown that this process is induced by complement activation via the alternative pathway.[3,39] (Fig. 5–3). There is pulmonary sequestration of activated neutrophils, leading to mild pulmonary dysfunction during dialysis. This effect is pronounced if acetate-containing dialysate is used. During dialysis with cuprophan membranes, measurement of C3a levels show a significant increase 10 to 15 minutes after initiation of treatment. There is a direct correlation between complement activation and leukocytopenia.[62] Complement activation has been shown to increase the adhesiveness of granulocytes to foreign surfaces.[63] Furthermore, activated granulocytes and thrombocytes (CD63-positive platelets) have the ability to aggregate, leading to microemboli in the capillaries of the lung.[64] Biocompatible and less complement-activating membranes are associated with less leukocytopenia and hypoxemia. Reduced complement activation is observed when dialyzers are reused, because of fixation of plasma proteins on the dialyzer membrane.

Reversal of neutropenia during dialysis with cellulosic membranes is due to downregulation and internalization of C5a complement receptors on granulocytes and reduction of C5a concentrations to levels that are ineffective for further granulocyte-endothelial adhesion.[65] Since C5a receptor number does not change significantly during cuprophan dialysis, it was found that activation of the complement system is not the only mechanism leading to adhesion of granulocytes.[66] In addition, complement activation may cause an increased expression of β2-integrin receptors, thus leading to the aggregation of activated cells, which will then adhere to the pulmonary endothelium. This effect is less pro-

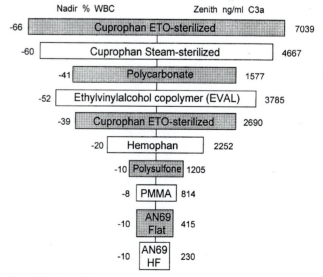

Figure 5–3. Intradialytic leukopenia and complement activation depends on the polymeric structure of the dialysis membrane. *(From Shaldon S, Vienken J. Biocompatibility: is it a relevant consideration for today´s haemodialysis?* Int J Artif Organs *1996;19:201–214. With permission.)*

nounced in synthetic membranes than in cellulosic membranes.[67]

Phagocyte function is suppressed during dialysis with cellulosic membranes, whereas neutrophil activity is not altered during dialysis with non-complement-activating membranes. Twelve weeks after the initiation of maintenance HD with cuprophan membranes, the glycolytic response and reactive oxygen production of neutrophils was significantly lower than that of cells from patients who underwent dialysis with PS membranes.[68] Thus it was concluded that complement activation suppresses the phagocytic response both acutely and chronically. In the presence of a bacterial stimulus (e.g., *Staphylococcus aureus*), production of granulocyte oxygen species was diminished during dialysis with complement-activating membranes.[53] It has been demonstrated that direct contact of granulocytes with cuprophan membranes is associated with an increased production of reactive oxygen species.[69–71] This is due mainly to the generation of platelet-neutrophil microaggregates.[71] The production of superoxide anions can cause endothelial damage. This could be of clinical interest in dialysis patients who are exposed to the elevated levels of oxygen species three times a week. In the long term, a deterioration of granulocyte function has been observed in dialysis patients, which could in part explain the immunodeficiency seen in this population. Vitamin E–coated membranes, recently introduced, lead to an improvement in granulocyte function and can diminish oxidative stress.[72,73]

Cellulosic membranes induce an increased expression of cell-specific surface receptors (CR-1 and Mac-1), whereas the expression of selectin LAM-1 and sialophorin (CD 43) is reduced. Dialysis with biocompatible membranes does not alter receptor expression significantly. Complement split products are responsible for the up- and downregulation of integrins and selectins. Selectins are responsible for the initial rolling interaction of leukocytes with the vascular endothelium, whereas firm adhesion of leukocytes to endothelial cells is dependent on the β2-integrins. The decreased ratio between L-selectin and Mac-1 can impair the host defense of HD patients, particularly when cellulosic membranes are used.[74] Degranulation of granulocytes occurs during dialysis even in the absence of complement activation.[75] HD therapy with PMMA membranes induces only mild complement activation, but neutrophil degranulation is comparable to that seen with cuprophan.[76] Reuse of cuprophan membranes reduces complement activation but has no effect on the degranulation of secondary granules. Clotting of the dialyzer leads to complement activation, but neutrophil release does not increase. Degranulation of neutrophils during HD depends on intracellular calcium concentrations. Calcium channel blockers reduce cytosolic calcium and degranulation during extracorporeal therapy (i.e., HD or aortocoronary bypass operation) even when complement activation

occurs. Regional anticoagulation with citrate induces extracorporeal calcium depletion and abolishes the release of lactoferrin and myeloperoxidase from neutrophils.[77,78] Interleukin(IL)-8 is a chemotactic factor for neutrophils. IL-8 stimulates degranulation of neutrophils as well as production of superoxide anion and leukotriene B4.[79] Regenerated cellulose and PMMA, but not PAN, dialyzers significantly increase plasma IL-8 levels and induce significant expression of IL-8 mRNA in peripheral blood mononuclear cells.[80] This suggests that the release of granulocyte elastase during HD with PMMA may be at least partially caused by IL-8 production. However, the difference in IL-8 production between PAN and PMMA dialyzers does not explain the marked lactoferrin release from neutrophils during dialysis with PAN and PMMA.

Degranulation of polymorphonuclear leukocytes is also dependent on the concentration of degranulation-inhibiting proteins (i.e., angiogenin and complement factor D). These two proteins are markedly elevated in patients with end-stage renal failure.[81] During dialysis with low-flux biocompatible membranes, plasma levels of angiogenin and complement factor D are nearly unaffected.[82] Under these conditions there is only a mild release of lactoferrin from neutrophils. Dialysis with PMMA or PAN is associated with a marked release of lactoferrin. This is explained by the fact that both dialyzers cause a marked reduction of both proteins.[83] This is a novel mechanism explaining neutrophil degranulation during dialysis, although there must be more to this process than just removal of degranulation-inhibiting proteins, otherwise there would not be degranulation with low-flux cellulose membranes.

Compared with normal neutrophils, uremic neutrophils demonstrate greater apoptosis in the presence of autologous plasma as well as 10 percent fetal calf serum. Neutrophils from healthy subjects exposed to heterologous uremic serum exhibit higher apoptosis rates, reduced production of oxygen reactive species, and a lower phagocytosis index than normal neutrophils exposed to heterologous sera.[84] The apoptosis rate depends on the dialyzer material used. Synthetic membranes are associated with less apoptosis than cellulosic membranes.[85]

Mononuclear Cells

Activation of the complement system may have an impact on mononuclear cell function. Monocytes have specific receptors for complement products and complement activation has been shown to result in increased transcription of IL-1 and tumor necrosis factor alpha (TNF-α).[86,87] Recent studies show that monocytes have a receptor that can be activated directly by cellulosic membranes. IL-1 is present in mononuclear cells of patients undergoing maintenance HD but not in mononuclear cells obtained from healthy subjects.[88] Patients undergoing regular HD with cellulosic membranes show elevated levels of IL-1 and TNF-α before a dialysis session and a further increase during the procedure. During dialysis with biocompatible membranes, cytokine genes are not activated.[89] Monocytes from dialysis patients in whole blood cultures are hyporesponsive to stimuli, which might be a further explanation for the immune defect in uremic and HD patients. This phenomenon is pronounced when bioincompatible membranes are used. Anaphylatoxins stimulate cytokine synthesis, particularly in the presence of endotoxin.[90]

Lymphocytes exposed to cellulosic membranes are unable to express the maximum number of IL-2 receptors and are therefore less responsive to immune stimuli.[10] IL-12 produced by mononuclear cells causes an increased INF-α production and enhancement of cell-mediated cytotoxicity. In unstimulated conditions, cuprophan-treated mononuclear cells show a higher IL-12 production than PMMA and controls. The release of IL-12 remained unchanged under mitogen stimulation when cells were exposed to cuprophan and was lower than in PMMA treated patients and controls.[12] INF-α production in unstimulated conditions is similar for all membrane materials. Under stimulation, INF-α production was lower in cuprophan-exposed mononuclear cells than in biocompatible membranes or controls (Fig. 5–4).[12] The altered release of these cytokines could play a further role in cell-mediated immunodeficiency in patients treated with cuprophan membranes.

ESRD patients undergoing regular HD exhibit increased mononuclear cell apoptosis. This apoptosis is directly related to the biocompatibility of the membrane. Apoptosis is activated when monocytes come in contact with the cellulosic membrane through cell surface receptors linked to G-proteins (Fig. 5–5).[91] An improvement of biocompatibility can be achieved by coating cellulosic membranes with vitamin E. The vitamin E–bonded membrane reduces IL-6 production during dialysis and is comparable to biocompatible PA dialyzers in terms of its effect on lymphocyte function.[47]

Contamination of the dialysate with endotoxins can induce IL-1 and TNF synthesis and secretion by activation of monocytes. Endotoxin transfer depends on the porosity and structure of the membrane. Synthetic membranes are a sufficient barrier because of their thickness, hydrophobic surface, and ability to adsorb pyrogens and plasma proteins (proteins coating the membrane surface).[92] Another tool for measuring biocompatibility is the IL-1 receptor antagonist (IL-1RA). In the presence of elevated IL-1 levels, the neutralizing IL-1RA is released. IL-1RA blocks the ability of IL-1 to activate cells and is therefore a regulating antibody. In dialysis patients, IL-1RA levels are significantly elevated as compared to those of healthy subjects. Since IL-1 is a proinflammatory cytokine associated with an increased risk

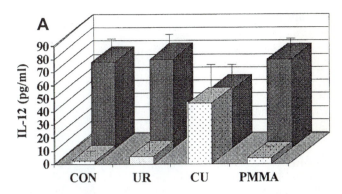

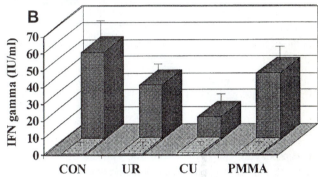

Figure 5–4. *A.* Interleukin-12 (IL-12) production after incubating both unstimulated (▫) and stimulated (■) peripheral blood mononuclear cells (PBMCs) for 24 hours. Results obtained from healthy subjects (CON), uremic nondialyzed patients (UR), patients dialyzed with either cuprophan (CU) or polymethylmethacrylate (PMMA) membrane. In unstimulated PBMCs, IL-12 production in CU is significantly higher than in CON, UR, or PMMA (*p* <0.01). Under mitogen stimulation, IL-12 production is significantly lower in CU than in CON (*p* <0.02), UR, or PMMA (*p* <0.05). In CON, UR, and PMMA, IL-12 release after mitogen stimulation is significantly greater than in the basal condition (*p* <0.01), which is not the case for CU. *B.* Interferon-gamma (INF-γ) production after incubating both unstimulated (▫) and stimulated (■) PBMCs for 24 hours. INF-γ production by stimulated PBMC is significantly lower in CU than in CON, UR, or PMMA (*p* <0.01). In all groups, the INF-γ production after stimulation is significantly greater than in the respective basal condition (*p* <0.01). *(From Memoli B, Marzano L, Bisesti V, et al. Hemodialysis-related lymphomononuclear release of interleukin-12 in patients with end-stage renal disease. J Am Soc Nephrol 1999;10:2171–2176. With permission.)*

for coronary artery disease, elevated IL-1RA levels show a positive correlation with this disease.[93] With increasing time on dialysis, a lowering of IL-1RA levels is observed, which can be interpreted as hyporesponsiveness of cells and may contribute to the increased infection rate of long-term dialysis patients.[94]

Hypotension is one of the most common adverse events during dialysis. It can be linked to membrane-associated cytokine release (IL-1 and TNF-α), and further associated with nitric oxide production. A number of acute (fever, sleeping disturbances) and chronic (anemia, impaired bone metabolism, malnutrition, immunologic dysfunction, atherosclerosis) symptoms observed in HD patients are related, at least in part, to increased cytokine production.

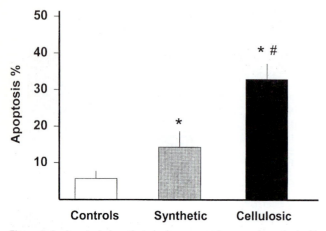

Figure 5–5. Apoptosis is activated when monocytes come in contact with the cellulosic membrane. This is mediated through cell surface receptors linked to G-proteins. *(From Carracedo J, Ramirez R, Madueno JA, et al. Cell apoptosis and hemodialysis-influenced inflammation.* Kidney Int *2002; 61:S89–S93. With permission.)*

Thrombocyte Function

Thrombocytes participate in the physiologic clotting process and are thought to play a leading role in thrombotic events during extracorporeal procedures. Platelet adhesion on artificial surfaces depends on the chemical structure of bound proteins. Albumin-coated surfaces are relatively resistant to thrombocyte adhesion. Increased thrombocyte adhesion is observed when foreign surfaces are coated with glycoproteins that contain oligosaccharide chains, such as fibrinogen and gamma globulins. Once platelets come into contact with foreign surfaces, morphologic changes occur characterized by pseudopod formation and spreading of the cytoplasm over the contact surface. A release reaction of thrombocytes has been observed due to thrombin, mechanical trauma, or humoral factors. A number of cellular products are released into the circulation, including thromboxane A_2 and adenosine diphosphate, which will further promote coagulation and the aggregation of platelets. Platelet aggregation can be blocked by acetylic salicylic acid, which is a potent inhibitor of the cyclooxygenase pathway of arachidonic acid metabolism, and by the production of thromboxane A_2. Dipyridamole increases the levels of cyclic adenosine monophosphate, which inhibits the induction of platelet aggregation by adenosine diphosphate. Prostacyclins (PGI-2 and PGE-1) are potent stimulators of adenyl cyclase and inhibitors of platelet aggregation. They have been successfully used as anticoagulants during HD and continuous hemofiltration.[95,96] PF4 and β-thromboglobulin are intracellular substances used as specific markers for thrombocyte activation. PF4 itself has an important role during extracorporeal procedures due to its ability to neutralize heparin. The administration of heparin can further increase PF4 levels by releasing this factor from endothelial cells, even without stimulation of thrombocytes. Beta-

thromboglobulin is normally cleared by the kidney, therefore elevated baseline levels are found in dialysis patients. In the case of intradialytic clotting even higher levels are observed.[97] Increased levels of PF4 and β-thromboglobulin are found during dialysis with PS, cellulose triacetate, and cuprophan membranes, although this effect is more pronounced in the case of cuprophan.[98] The increase of PF4 is comparable for PS and cellulose triacetate membranes.[99] The total amount of GPIIb/IIIa is nearly unaffected during dialysis with these two membranes, whereas the level of bound GPIIb/IIIa, a marker of platelet aggregation, increases dramatically from 1426 ± 435 to 40446 ± 2777 mol of platelets during dialysis sessions when a PS membrane is used.[99]

Two membrane-bound glycoproteins are relevant for platelet aggregation, the fibrinogen receptor and P-selectin (GMP-140, CD62). Fibrinogen binding is an early but still reversible step in platelet activation. Once thrombocytes are activated, P-selectin will be expressed on the cell surface. Increased binding of anti-CD62 and antifibrinogen has only been observed in cuprophan-treated patients and does not occur with Hemophan or PS (Fig. 5–6).[100] Consistent with these observations, elevated levels of soluble P-selectin, glycoprotein IIb/IIIa and β-thromboglobulin have been observed during cuprophan dialysis, whereas these parameters were nearly unaffected by synthetic membranes and Hemophan.[101–103] The increased expression of glycoprotein IIb/IIIa is associated with pronounced platelet-leukocyte co-aggregation during HD with cuprophan membranes. It has been shown that sodium nitroprusside has the ability to inhibit platelet activation in patients treated with coronary angioplasty.[104] In HD patients, no downregulation of P-selectin has been observed, independent of membrane type used, when sodium nitroprusside is administered.[105] When platelets are activated, there is a fusion of α-granule membranes with the platelet plasma membrane during platelet secretion. This can be detected by an anti-CD62P monoclonal antibody.[106] Conversion of the platelet glycoprotein IIb/IIIa into a functional receptor for fibrinogen can be detected with PAC-1, a monoclonal antibody that binds only after functional receptor exposure to glycoprotein IIb/IIIa.[107] It has been demonstrated that there is a relationship between increased platelet activation and failure of the recurrent vascular access. CD 62P-positive platelets (7.3 ± 3.7 vs. 3.5 ± 1.3 percent, $p<0.005$) and PAC-1-positive platelets (2.2 ± 2.1 vs. 0.9 ± 0.7 percent, $p<0.01$) were significantly higher in patients with recurrent vascular access failure compared with patients with vascular access survival greater than 5 years.[108]

Even intracellular parameters in platelets can be altered by HD. Predialytic values of di-adenosine pentaphosphate, a hydrophilic anionic substance with a low molecular weight, are comparable in patients treated with either a PAN or a PS membrane. During dialysis with PAN, a de-

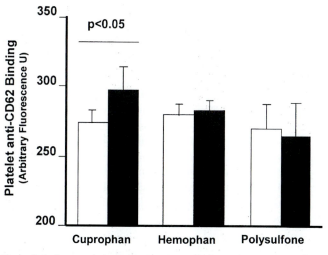
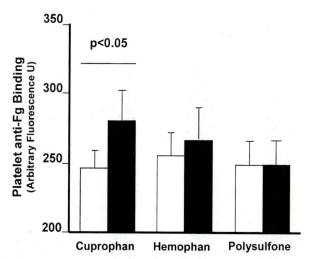

Figure 5–6. Increased platelet binding of anti-CD62 and antifibrinogen is observed only in cuprophan-treated patients. *(From Gawaz MP, Mujais SK, Schmidt B, et al. Platelet-leukocyte aggregates during hemodialysis: effect of membrane type.* Artif Organs *1999;23:29–36. With permission.)*

crease of di-adenosine pentaphosphate has been observed (93 ± 39 vs. 51 ± 18 fg per platelet, $p < 0.05$). In contrast, HD using a PS membrane was associated with significantly higher values of di-adenosine pentaphosphate compared to the values when a PAN membrane was used (250 ± 59 vs. 51 ± 18 fg per platelet, $p < 0.05$).[109]

Increased mean platelet volume has been shown to be an independent risk factor for myocardial infarction. Increased platelet size has been found in uremic patients and is correlated with coronary heart disease, even in this population.[110,111]

When platelet activation occurs due to chemical stimuli or shear stress, small particles called platelet-derived microparticles are released, which have procoagulant activity. Platelet-derived microparticles can be elevated in various conditions, such as diabetes, uremia, coronary artery disease, heparin-induced thrombocytopenia, and thrombocytopenic purpura. Platelet-derived microparticles, derived from the platelet plasma membrane, can be found when platelets are activated by collagen or in the blood of patients with intravascular platelet lysis. These particles have receptors for coagulation factor V and contribute to the acceleration of thrombin generation. The count of platelet-derived microparticles is elevated in uremic patients. Interestingly, the HD procedure itself does not affect this count, whereas erythropoietin therapy is associated with elevated levels.[112] The data on the influence of platelet-derived microparticles on thrombotic events of the vascular access are conflicting. In an investigation by Chuang et al., the levels of platelet-derived microparticles were comparable in patients with and without vascular access dysfunction, whereas Ando et al. found significantly higher levels of platelet-derived microparticles in patients with thrombotic events.[108,112] If excessive platelet activation itself causes vascular access fail-

ure or platelet activation is a coexisting phenomenon remains speculative; however, there is a clear association.

Bleeding diathesis is a major cause of morbidity and mortality in uremic patients. This can, at least in part, be related to platelet dysfunction and has been correlated with a prolonged bleeding time. Platelet adhesion depends on the interaction of the platelet glycoprotein Ib/IX complex with von Willebrand factor in the vascular wall. Proteolytic cleavage of glycoprotein Ib results in glycocalicin, which is ineffective with respect to platelet aggregation. In HD patients, increased levels of glycocalicin are observed, indicating an increased turnover of platelet glycoprotein Ib, which may contribute to thrombocyte dysfunction.[113] No differences in glycocalicin levels were measured between cellulose or PS dialysis, whereas significantly lower levels were seen in peritoneal dialysis (PD) patients. Glycoprotein Ib expression is lower in patients on maintenance HD and PD as compared to patients with mild chronic kidney disease. These findings confirm the postulated receptor defect of thrombocytes in patients with kidney disease. With respect to the receptor for von Willebrand factor (glycoprotein IIb/IIIa), PD seems to have a more favorable effect by restoring normal values of the expression of this cell membrane integrin.[114] Changes of platelet function can partly be ascribed directly to the HD procedure. Immediately after HD, bleeding time is significantly longer and response to thrombin, ristocetin, and collagen is much lower as compared to the day after dialysis.[115]

Repeated activation of thrombocytes during routine HD results in consecutive cycles of polymerization and depolymerization of the cytoskeletal proteins. This is characterized by an impairment of platelet cytoskeletal assembly and an abnormal translocation of the signaling molecules. These changes were evident 2 months after the initiation of maintenance HD. This seems to reflect the deleterious effect of repeated platelet stress during HD, since a recovery of these cohesive functions has been observed in patients switched from HD to PD.[116]

Not only platelet function but also thrombopoiesis is altered in uremic patients. A reduction of platelet count is more frequent in patients on HD and PD as compared to healthy controls. Platelet counts chronically decrease with years on HD. The cause is a decrease of megakaryocytopoiesis, measured as reticulated platelets. This is accompanied by increased thrombopoietin levels, possibly in response to reduced megakaryocytopoiesis.[117] Undialyzable myelosuppressive toxins that accumulate despite HD are thought to be involved in impaired platelet production. An autoimmune phenomenon may contribute to decreased platelet life span. Forty-two percent of HD patients have an elevation of platelet-associated IgG. In patients with positive hepatitis C virus antibody titers, increased levels of these autoantibodies are described in up to 82 percent. The occurrence of platelet antigen IgG production induces enhanced peripheral platelet destruction.[118]

Platelet-Leukocyte Aggregates

During dialysis, activation of thrombocytes and leukocytes occurs. The expression of multiple adhesion molecules on the cell surfaces leads to platelet-to-platelet (homotypic) and platelet-to-cell (heterotypic) interactions. Baseline platelet-leukocyte aggregates are lower in patients on HD than in controls, independent of the membrane used.[119] After passage of blood through the dialyzer, there is an increase of platelet-neutrophil and platelet-monocyte coaggregates during dialysis with synthetic and cellulosic membranes. This may be due to shear stress, contact activation, or agonist activation. As mentioned above, there is an increased expression of the fibrinogen receptor and P-selectin on the surface of thrombocytes during HD. On the surface of monocytes and neutrophils, Mac-1 and anti-CD62 expression is upregulated, which bind to the specific receptors on platelets.[120,121] A ligand for P-selectin on neutrophils and monocytes is the sialyl-Lewis molecule (CD15s). Monocytes express higher levels of CD62 than granulocytes but have lower levels of CD15s. The higher amount of monocyte-platelet coaggregates as compared to neutrophil-platelet coaggregates may be due to a different conformation of CD15s on monocytes, which enhances interaction with activated thrombocytes. Another possible mechanism is ligand bridging between glycoprotein IIb/IIIa on platelets and Mac-1 on granulocytes. Cuprophan membranes induce an increase in anti-CD62 (anti-P-selectin) binding, because CD62 expression is significantly increased in platelets from patients dialyzed with this membrane.[100] The complement system seems not to be involved in the platelet-leukocyte aggregation during HD, because it occurs in membranes with different complement-activating properties.[119] In vitro coaggregation can be increased by adenosine diphosphate but not by the complement factors C3a and C5a.[119]

Coaggregates induce the mechanism of cell cross talk. Thrombocytes supply free cholesterol to monocytes, which have a major role in foam cell generation in atherosclerotic plaques. Interactions between platelets and neutrophils utilize platelet-derived arachidonate to increase leukotriene and eicosanoid synthesis. Neutrophil derived cathepsin G induces further platelet aggregation. Increased levels of platelet activating factor act on thrombocytes and neutrophils and induce the amplification of cell activation and inflammatory response. The adhesion through P-selectin enhances in vitro the generation of oxygen radicals by neutrophils and monocytes.[122] Unstimulated platelets can inhibit the chemiluminescence response, superoxide anion production, and neutrophil-mediated cytolysis of activated neutrophils.[123] When platelets and neutrophils from uremic patients are isolated, the superoxide anion production of neutrophils is unaffected. The generation of platelet-neutrophil aggregates has an impact in the pathophysiology of septic shock and multisystem organ failure.[124] Neutrophils aggregated to platelets produce increased reactive oxygen species as compared to CD62-negative cells.[125] The exposure of endothelial cells to hydrogen peroxide results in endothelial cell injury and increased vascular permeability, possibly having an impact on the high incidence of atherosclerotic complications in dialysis patients. Platelet aggregation has also been implicated in the atherosclerotic process. In HD patients, a high percentage of circulating aggregated platelets has been observed.[110] Platelet activation, measured by CD62P (P-selectin) expression, and circulating platelet-monocyte aggregates, was significantly increased in HD patients compared to PD patients. The percentage of higher platelet-monocyte aggregates was associated with increased cardiovascular events.[126]

Erythrocyte Function

Hemolysis can occur during HD. This can be due to hypotonicity, contamination, or overheating of the dialysate. Another cause of hemolysis could be mechanical stress when blood passes through the blood pump. Research in the area of biocompatibility has focused on cellular functions of monocytes, neutrophils, and thrombocytes. Erythrocytes, on the other hand, have a low regenerative ability and have not been well studied in this regard. During an extracorporeal procedure, these cells are exposed to mechanical and chemical stress, which could contribute to the decreased erythrocyte life span observed in patients on maintenance HD. There are only a limited number of studies available analyzing the relationship between biocompatibility and erythrocyte function during HD.

Osmotic fragility to hypotonic lysis of erythrocytes is higher in HD patients as compared to healthy controls.[127] Acute and chronic changes in erythrocyte malonyldialdehyde content and osmotic fragility are less pronounced in patients treated with cellulose acetate or PAN as compared to cuprophan dialyzers.[128] The intracellular cholesterol content of erythrocytes is reduced by 20 percent after a single HD session with a synthetic membrane, whereas cuprophan membranes have no influence on cellular cholesterol levels. This is only an acute effect, since predialytic cellular cholesterol levels did not differ between erythrocytes of PAN- and cuprophan-treated patients. Osmotic fragility and cellular cholesterol content are markers for possible changes in erythrocyte membranes. Changes in ionic transport mechanisms have been hypothesized to be involved in altered osmotic fragility, but this thesis remains speculative.[127,128] In an in vitro experiment, less hemolysis was observed when blood came in contact with vitamin E–modified cellulose as compared to synthetic membranes.[130] Lower postdialytic membrane cholesterol content in PAN-treated patients might be due to the higher adsorptive capacity of this membrane type. The lower cholesterol content was associated with decreased osmotic fragility. This finding is unexpected, since there is good evidence that cholesterol-depleted erythrocytes are more susceptible to osmotic stress. Malonyldialdehyde, a water-soluble lipid peroxidation product, is a marker of oxidative stress and is increased by a single treatment with cuprophan or Hemophan and remains unchanged when PAN is used.[127,131] After 6 months, predialysis erythrocyte malonyldialdehyde levels were lower in PAN-treated patients. In an animal model, a reduction of malonyldialdehyde values in erythrocyte membranes was observed during dialysis with vitamin E–coated cellulosic membranes.[130] This may prove to be important, since free radical–mediated lipid peroxidation seems to play a pivotal role in the development of atherosclerotic lesions. In the pathogenesis of uremia-associated immunoinflammatory disorders, an imbalance between the antioxidant- and oxidant-generation system has been described. Glutathione is one of the major scavengers of activated oxygen species in erythrocytes. Erythrocyte glutathione levels measured before and immediately after HD with Hemophan membranes are significantly lower than in healthy controls.[131] The slight increase of glutathione levels during dialysis might be a consequence of hemoconcentration.

ANTICOAGULATION AND CELL ACTIVATION

Activation of the CD11b/CD18 receptor is responsible for the leukopenia seen during the first 30 minutes of HD. These preformed and internalized surface antigens are released from intracellular granules by a calcium-dependent process. Regional anticoagulation with citrate leads to extracorporeal calcium depletion. Expression of surface antigens (CD11b, CD11c, CD45) on neutrophil granulocytes is unaffected by citrate anticoagulation, whereas release of lactoferrin and myeloperoxidase is suppressed.[77,76,132,133] The degree of neutropenia during HD is more pronounced when unfractionated heparin (−29%) is used as compared to low-molecular-weight heparin (−175%).[134] Activation of neutrophil granulocytes, measured as elastase release, is diminished when low-molecular-weight heparin is used instead of standard heparin, whereas lactoferrin release is nearly unaffected by the mode of anticoagulation.[134] The observed platelet decrease during HD was comparable between patients treated with unfractionated heparin and patients treated with low-molecular-weight heparin. Using standard heparin during PS HD lower levels of PF4 and β-thromboglobin were observed, indicating reduced thrombocyte activation.[60] During hemofiltration, it could be shown that cellular activation can be diminished when heparin is used in combination with prostacyclin. The expression of glycoprotein IIb/IIIa and P-selectin on adenosine diphosphate–activated platelets and platelet-leukocyte aggregation is significantly lower in patients receiving an extracorporeal infusion with prostacyclin plus heparin as compared to patients given heparin only.[135] The administration of prostacyclin had no influence on the expression of CD11b on leukocytes during continuous hemofiltration.[135]

BETA₂ MICROGLOBULIN AND BIOCOMPATIBILITY

Beta₂ microglobulin is an 11.8-kDa protein necessary for the expression of HLA class I antigens on the surface of nearly all nucleated cells. The daily synthesis ranges from 2 to 4 mg/kg, with a short half-life of approximately 2.5 h. Beta₂ microglobulin is mainly eliminated by glomerular filtration (95 percent). Thus this protein is highly elevated in end-stage renal failure patients. Beta₂ microglobulin is the major constituent of dialysis-associated amyloidosis and causes carpal tunnel syndrome, arthropathy, and the formation of bone cysts leading to pathologic fractures in patients with ESRD. Advanced glycation end-product modification of β2-m occurs and induces a local inflammatory response by attracting macrophages chemotactically and stimulating these cells to produce and release proinflammatory cytokines.[136]

Low-flux biocompatible dialysis membranes and cuprophan membranes have a lower clearance for β2-m as compared to high-flux biocompatible dialysis membranes.[137] With low-flux biocompatible and cuprophan dialysis, β2-m levels were higher in patients dialyzed over 5 years than in those with a shorter duration of dialysis therapy; whereas in patients treated with high-flux biocompatible membranes, no further increase is observed over years, despite a progressive decline of residual renal function. Not only the use of low-flux dialysis membranes but also the use of bioincompatible membranes leads to a marked rise in plasma β2-m levels.[138] Routine dialysis with biocompatible low-flux membranes over a period of 18 months was not associated with a significant rise of β2-m levels, although β2-m clearance is comparable to that of bioincompatible low-flux membranes (Fig. 5–7). In vitro experiments have demonstrated an increased release of β2-m by direct contact of mononuclear cells with cellulosic membranes. This release was further increased in the presence of complement activation.[139–141] Mononuclear cells, harvested from patients who are chronically dialyzed with complement-activating membranes, have an increased release of β2-m.[142] Patients treated with vitamin E–coated cellulosic dialyzers for 6 months have a significant reduction of β2-m levels.[143] Biocompatible membranes generate less β2-m. Furthermore, PAN and PMMA have been shown to efficiently adsorb β2-m.[49,144] Oxygen-reactive species elevate β2-m levels, whereas the dialyzer sterilization method has no influence on intradialytic β2-m levels.[145]

Means to slow down the progression of β2-m–associated amyloidosis are high-flux dialysis, hemodiafiltration, and hemofiltration with synthetic membranes, which are

shown to reduce β2-m levels by approximately 20 to 30 percent. Furthermore, high-flux synthetic membranes adsorb bacterial pyrogens derived from contaminated dialysate.[136] Mononuclear cells primed with complement (as is the case during dialysis with bioincompatible membranes) and then exposed to endotoxins produce more cytokines than do mononuclear cells without contact with complement.[89] In bacterially contaminated dialysate, pyrogens of small and middle molecular sizes are found. They are able to penetrate intact dialyzer membranes and promote cytokine induction in mononuclear cells. The penetration of pyrogens is markedly higher in low-flux cuprophan membranes than in high-flux dialyzer membranes. The latter are less permeable to pyrogens, despite a larger pore size, because of their ability to adsorb substances of bacterial origin.[146] Although clinical data are scant, there are four studies showing a beneficial effect of improved dialysate quality on the incidence of carpal tunnel syndrome (Fig. 5–8).[147–150] Patients dialyzed with biocompatible membranes have a relative risk of 0.64 for the development of carpal tunnel syndrome and 0.613 for mortality compared to patients treated with cellulosic membranes.[148]

A beneficial effect on β2-m levels has been shown for daily nocturnal HD (each session lasting for 8 to 10 hours). With this approach, the removal of β2-m was twice as high

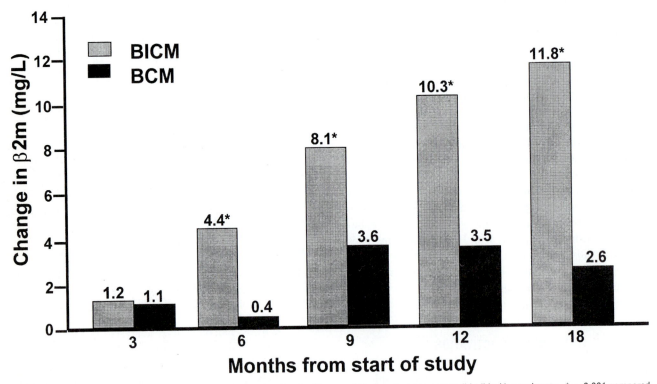

Figure 5–7. Mean change in beta₂-microglobulin levels from baseline for biocompatible (gray) and biocompatible (black) membranes. *p <0.001 compared with baseline. *(From Hakim RM, Wingard RL, Husni L, et al. The effect of membrane biocompatibility on plasma β2-microglobulin levels in chronic hemodialysis patients. J Am Soc Nephrol 1996;7:472–478. With permission.)*

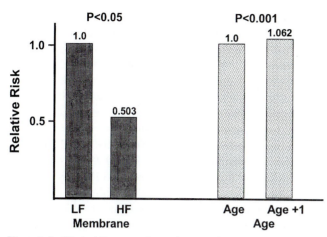

Figure 5–8. Effect of flux properties and age on the relative risk for carpal tunnel syndrome. *(From Koda Y, Nishi SI, Haginoshita S, et al. Switch from conventional to high-flux membrane reduces the risk of carpal tunnel syndrome and mortality of hemodialysis patients. Kidney Int 1997;52:1096–1101. With permission.)*

as with conventional HD, and predialysis β2-m levels decreased within the first few days on nocturnal HD.[151]

ADVANCED GLYCATION END PRODUCTS (AGES)

Irreversible nonenzymatic modification of proteins occurs in patients with chronic kidney disease. Proteins exposed to glucose or other carbohydrates form advanced AGEs by different chemical steps (Schiff reaction, generation of Amadori products, carboxymethyllysine, pentosidine, pyrroline). Diabetes mellitus and uremia are associated with elevated AGE concentrations in tissues and plasma. The implication of accumulation of AGEs in the process of aging and the pathogenesis of several diseases is still a matter of debate. In uremic patients, AGE generation occurs, even in the absence of diabetes mellitus. Pentosidine and carboxymethyllysine do not correlate with fructoselysine, suggesting that factors other than hyperglycemia are responsible for the rate of AGE formation.[152] Increased oxidative stress and impaired clearance may cause the accumulation of AGEs in patients with renal failure. Predialytic pentosidine is elevated in patients dialyzed with either cellulosic or low-flux membranes. These findings reflect inadequate removal during HD and an increased generation of these end products when bioincompatible membranes are used.[153] That flux properties of dialysis membranes are important for the elimination of AGEs has been demonstrated by Stein et al. The intradialytic reduction of AGE peptides was 62 percent in patients treated with high-flux PS membranes (ultrafiltration coefficient 40 mL/h/mmHg) as compared to an 80 percent reduction when a superflux PS membrane (ultrafiltration coefficient 60 mL/h/mmHg) was used. After a 6-month treatment period with the superflux membrane, predialytic AGE levels decreased significantly compared to values obtained in patients treated with a low-flux membrane.[154] AGEs account for a number of biological responses (i.e., accelerated atherosclerosis, dialysis-associated amyloidosis) and promote the release of cytokines, such as TNF-α and IL-1β.[24,155] AGE-modified β2-m is a major component of amyloid deposition and triggers local inflammation by increased release of TNF-α and IL-1β by macrophages, whereas normal β2-m has no effect.[153]

LIPID METABOLISM, ATHEROSCLEROSIS, AND BIOCOMPATIBILITY

HD patients have a high incidence of coronary, cerebral, and peripheral vascular diseases. One of the multiple atherogenic risk factors for these patients is hyperlipidemia, particularly the oxidatively modified low-density lipoproteins (LDL). These lipoproteins are avidly taken up by macrophages, resulting in foam cell formation, a key step in the development of the atherosclerotic lesion. Konishi et al. found enhanced gene expression of the scavenger receptor in peripheral blood monocytes obtained from patients undergoing regular HD treatment with a cuprophan dialyzer as compared to a PMMA dialyzer.[156] Mean triglyceride concentrations in patients undergoing PS dialysis decreased from 126 to 81 mg/dL ($p = 0.01$), while triglyceride concentrations showed no significant changes during saponified cellulose ester dialysis. On the other hand, mean serum cholesterol concentrations in PS patients increased from 161 to 185 mg/dL during dialysis ($p<0.02$), mainly due to a 27 percent increase in HDL cholesterol, while there was no significant change in total cholesterol in patients treated with cellulose ester dialysis.[157] Other groups have also reported an improvement in plasma lipoprotein profiles with high-flux membranes in patients on maintenance HD.[158,159] Maintenance HD patients on low-flux cuprophan membranes were either switched to high-flux PS ($n = 14$) or continued with cuprophan ($n = 14$). After 6 weeks of treatment with the high-flux membrane, fasting total triglyceride, very low density lipoprotein (VLDL), triglyceride, and VLDL cholesterol levels were significantly decreased. However, other lipid parameters and lipoprotein lipase activity did not change after switching from low-flux cuprophan to dialysis with high-flux PS membranes.[159] In contrast, PS dialysis was associated with more lipoprotein lipase activity and hepatic triglyceride lipase activity than cellulose ester dialysis.[157] The addition of serum from PS patients decreased lipoprotein lipase activity by 18 ± 4.2 percent, while serum samples from cellulose ester patients caused inhibition of lipoprotein lipase activity by 34 ± 7.8 percent. Comparing the plasma lipoprotein profiles in HD patients on high-flux vs. low-flux PS suggest that the beneficial effect of the membranes is due to the high flux rather than just the biocompatibility of the membrane.[160] It was concluded that a circulating substance, not dialyzable with cellulosic membranes, inhibits lipoprotein lipase in uremic subjects and is removed during dialysis with a PS membrane.[157] Ingram et al. conducted a blinded crossover trial of two cellulose acetate dialyzers (AN140 with a sieving coefficient at molecular weight 11,000 D; CA210 with a negligible sieving coefficient). HDL cholesterol, apo E, and apo CIII increased significantly during dialysis with AN140 but not during dialysis with CA210, while postdialysis postheparin lipase activity tended to be higher for AN140.[161] Taken together, high-flux dialyzers and membranes with good clearance of higher-molecular-weight molecules are associated with beneficial changes in plasma lipids and lipoproteins. Hepatic lipoprotein lipase was not different between diabetic and nondiabetic HD patients but significantly lower than in healthy subjects.[162] Vitamin E–bonded hemodialyzers have been developed in order to reduce the oxidative stress associated with HD therapy. Repeated use of the vitamin E–bonded membrane but not of a control dialyzer resulted

in reduced superoxide anion production by neutrophils as well as in reduced total and LDL cholesterol and oxidized LDL and malonyldialdehyde but also in increased HDL cholesterol (Fig. 5–9). It was concluded that a vitamin E–bonded hemodialyzer may be useful to reduce the incidence of cardiovascular events in patients with ESRD.[73]

Lecithin-cholesterol acetyltransferase (LCAT) catalyzes the esterification of cholesterol and circulates in association with HDL, particularly with HDL3. LCAT activity decreases with the duration of HD by 25 percent within 1 to 5 years and by 45 percent within 5 to 13 years of dialysis.[163] This decrease in LCAT activity was associated with strong alterations in HDL3 composition. The effect of biocompatible membranes on LCAT activity is yet to be determined.

BIOCOMPATIBILITY AND SERUM ALBUMIN

Low concentrations of serum albumin are associated with significantly increased risk of death in chronic HD patients. A few studies have focused on the relationship between the

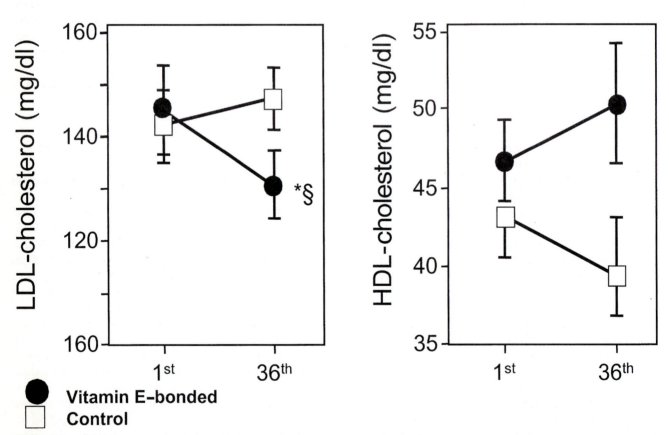

Figure 5–9. Effect of long-term use of vitamin E–bonded membranes on LDL and HDL cholesterol. *(From Tsuruoka S, Kawaguchi A, Nishiki K, et al. Vitamin E–bonded hemodialyzer improves neutrophil function and oxidative stress in patients with end-stage renal failure.* Am J Kidney Dis *2002;39:127–133. With permission.)*

type of membrane used and the serum albumin concentration.[164–166] Long-term use of biocompatible low-flux PMMA membranes resulted in greater levels of serum albumin and insulin-like growth factor 1 and significantly increased body weight as compared to those seen in patients using bioincompatible membranes.[164] Hypoalbuminemic HD patients dialyzed with cuprammonium membranes were switched to PS dialyzers. After 3 months, serum albumin levels increased significantly from 3.18 ± 0.07 to 3.33 ± 0.07 g/dL among patients with diabetes and from 3.25 ± 0.04 to 3.37 ± 0.07 g/dL in HD patients without diabetes.[165] Dialysis with low- and high-flux synthetic/semisynthetic membranes as compared to unmodified cellulose was associated with significant positive effects on baseline serum albumin. Serum albumin was higher in patients reusing dialyzers, particularly in those reusing unmodified cellulosic membranes as compared to patients not practicing reuse.[166] Memoli et al. found a significant relationship between biocompatibility of the membrane and serum albumin.[167] Serum albumin was 3.64 ± 0.07 g/dL after 6 months of dialysis with synthetically modified cellulosic membranes as compared to 3.25 ± 0.09 g/dL ($p<0.05$) during dialysis with cuprophan membranes. Interleukin-6 release by peripheral mononuclear cells and also C-reactive protein levels were lower after 6 months of dialysis with synthetically modified cellulosic membranes as compared with cuprophan membranes. Serum albumin was negatively correlated with interleukin-6 release and circulating C-reactive protein levels.[167] A detrimental effect of bioincompatible dialyzer membranes on daily protein intake has also been suggested. Lindsay and colleagues established the link between protein catabolic rate (PCR), a putative marker of dietary protein intake, and the modality and the dose of dialysis.[168,169] They also showed that the type of dialysis membrane used affects the nature of the relationship between the dose of dialysis and PCR. Patients on a high-flux biocompatible membrane had a higher PCR than patients on low-flux bioincompatible membranes for the same dose of dialysis.

In contrast, Locatelli et al. did not find any difference in serum albumin, transferrin, or PCR between HD patients treated with cuprophan, low-flux PS, or high-flux PS dialysis and patients on hemodiafiltration.[170] Unlike the studies mentioned above, patients in this study had mean serum albumin and transferrin levels within the normal range at baseline. Sham HD in healthy volunteers for 150 minutes with either a cuprophan, cellulose acetate, or PS membrane increased leg amino acid efflux by 85 percent in the cuprophan group, by 35 percent in the cellulose acetate group, and by 10 percent in the PS group.[171] In subjects exposed to cellulosic dialysis membranes, 15 to 20 g of protein were catabolized in the muscle, suggesting that reduced intake of protein may not be the only reason for low serum albumin levels.[172] This catabolic effect of dialysis membranes appears to be related to bioincompatibility.

BIOCOMPATIBILITY AND MORTALITY

Cause-specific mortality and hospitalization rates are lower for HD patients treated with synthetic membranes as compared to those dialyzed with cellulosic membranes.[13,173,174] Improved outcome could reflect improved biocompatibility or increased clearance of uremic toxins not cleared by low-flux dialyzers.[175–178] However, excellent survival rates, probably due to normalization of blood pressure, are achieved by Charra and coworkers in Tassin, France, utilizing long, slow dialysis (24 hours per week) on cuprophan membranes without significant clearance of middle molecules.[179] Woods and Nandakumar reported a surprisingly high 5-year survival of 86 percent in their HD patient population treated exclusively with PS dialyzers.[180] The 463 patients treated with high-flux PS had a lower mortality (21 vs. 36 per 1000 patient-years) than the 252 HD patients on low-flux PS. For nondiabetic patients, the 5-year probability of survival was 92 percent for high-flux patients and 69 percent for low-flux patients. The data are remarkable, since a majority of the diabetic and elderly and patients with comorbidity were allocated to the high-flux group.[180] A substantial reduction in the use of cellulosic membranes, from approximately 70 percent in 1990 to less than 20 percent in 1996, has been accompanied by a reduction in the adjusted mortality of patients with ESRD in the United States. A role for the changes in the biocompatibility of dialysis membranes in the improvement of patient mortality has been suggested.[181] In contrast, Locatelli et al. did not find any difference in morbidity and mortality between HD patients treated with cuprophan, low-flux PS, high-flux PS, or hemodiafiltration.[170]

BIOCOMPATIBILITY AND RESIDUAL RENAL FUNCTION

Residual renal function (RRF) declines over time in both PD and HD patients. Factors associated with a faster decline of residual renal function are high diastolic blood pressure, proteinuria, dialysis hypotension, and dehydration.[182] RRF declines faster in HD patients than in PD patients and faster in HD patients dialyzed with bioincompatible membranes than in those dialyzed with biocompatible dialyzers.[183] In a recent study by McKane et al., residual renal function declined in HD patients treated with biocompatible membranes and ultrapure water at a rate indistinguishable from that in patients on continuous ambulatory PD.[184] When ultrapure and conventional [up to 300 colony-forming units (CFU) per milliliter] dialysates were compared, multiple regression analysis identified the microbiologic quality of the dialysate as an independent determinant of the loss of RRF.[185] The better maintenance of RRF in HD patients treated with PS membranes as compared to cellulosic membranes is associated with higher Kt/V and increased hematocrit values.[186]

BIOCOMPATIBILITY IN ACUTE RENAL FAILURE

Factors influencing outcomes in acute renal failure (ARF) patients include the following:

Dialysis modality
Dialysis membrane type and performance
Adequacy of dialysis
Severity of the underlying illnesses
Effects of comorbidity and the response to cointerventions

A controversial issue in the management of ARF is the effect of biocompatibility of membranes, which may be an important determinant of survival and recovery of renal function in patients with ARF. Bioincompatible, complement-activating dialysis membranes lead to neutrophil activation and infiltration into the kidney. Activated neutrophils may prolong ARF by the release of vasoconstrictors and damaging oxygen radicals. Therefore, the use of bioincompatible membranes might delay recovery from ARF.[187,188] On the other hand, high-molecular-weight–clearance of the dialyzer and membrane adsorption of inflammatory mediators (e.g., cytokines and complement factors) or bacterial endotoxins can have a significant influence on the activation of blood components and patient outcome.[189]

In intensive care unit patients and ARF patients after cardiac surgery, the use of bioincompatible cuprophan membranes adversely affected survival, the occurrence of sepsis, the duration of oliguria, and the rate of renal recovery[190,191]; for example, 23 of 37 ARF patients (62 percent) undergoing HD with PMMA membranes recovered renal function, as compared to 13 of the 35 ARF patients (37 percent) dialyzed with cuprophan membranes. The median number of dialysis treatments required before the recovery of renal function was 5 in the PMMA group and 17 in the cuprophan group: 21 patients (57 percent) undergoing HD with PMMA membranes survived as compared to 13 patients (37 percent) undergoing HD with cuprophan membranes. In nonoliguric ARF patients, the survival rates were 80 percent with the PMMA membrane and 40 percent with the cuprophan membrane.[190] Schiffl et al. compared the use of PAN to cuprophan membranes in critically ill patients.[191] The survival rate of the cuprophan-treated group was found to be lower than that of the PAN-treated patients (38 percent vs. 65 percent). There was also a delayed resolution and recovery from ARF in the cuprophan-treated group. ARF patients treated with PAN membranes had a significantly lower incidence of bacterial infections and lower mortality rate due to sepsis as compared to patients treated with cuprophan membranes.[192]

Neveu et al. found a significant decline in mortality in ARF patients dialyzed with biocompatible synthetic dialysis membranes as compared to bioincompatible cellulose membranes[193]; 46 of 58 patients (79.3 percent) dialyzed with cuprophan membranes died as compared to 61 of 111

ARF patients treated with synthetic membranes (55 percent). In a prospective randomized trial of outcome from North American centers, the biocompatible membrane gave better results in terms of recovery of renal function and survival. This advantage persisted after adjustment for severity of disease but was almost entirely confined to patients who were nonoliguric at the start of dialysis.[194]

A retrospective analysis of risk factors influencing survival among patients with ARF in an intensive care unit did not confirm a beneficial effect of biocompatible membranes.[195] Similarly, Kurtal et al. found no significant differences in survival in cuprophan- vs. non-cuprophan-treated ARF patients.[196] Jörres et al. found no differences in outcome for patients with dialysis-dependent ARF between those treated with cuprophan membranes and those treated with PMMA membranes when the analysis was adjusted for age and APACHE II score: 44 ARF patients (58 percent) assigned to cuprophan membranes and 50 ARF patients (60 percent) assigned to PMMA membranes survived.[197] This study has been criticized, however, because the number of patients varied widely between centers and some centers had limited experience with dialysis-dependent ARF patients. It was further argued that APACHE II criteria do not consistently predict outcomes in patients with ARF requiring dialysis.[198] In addition, both cuprophan and PMMA membranes cause substantial complement and leukocyte activation as well as elastase and leukotriene B4 release in ARF patients.[199] Recovery from ARF may be delayed by generation of neutrophil products.[200] Further, a substantial number of the ARF patients in the study of Jörres et al.[197] received only one or two dialysis treatments,[199] while a mean of 15 dialysis treatments per ARF patient was performed in the study of Himmelfarb and colleagues.[194]

Albright et al. prospectively studied survival and the recovery of renal function in ARF patients who required intermittent HD.[201] Survival was 76 percent in patients randomized to treatment with cellulose acetate and 73 percent in patients treated with PS. Recovery of renal function at 30 days was not statistically different in the two groups. In a randomized controlled trial, ARF patients were assigned to a low-flux cellulose acetate, low-flux PS, or high-flux PS dialyzer. Neither membrane type nor flux property affected mortality or recovery of renal function.[202]

Jaber et al. performed a metanalysis of data extracted from previously published studies of controlled clinical trials to assess the impact of biocompatible membranes on mortality in patients with ARF who required intermittent HD.[203] Seven studies with a total of 722 patients met the inclusion criteria: 172 (45 percent) of 384 ARF patients died in the biocompatible membrane group as compared to 156 (46 percent) of 338 in the bioincompatible membrane group. According to Subramanian et al., eight trials including 867 ARF patients provided survival data and six trials including 641 ARF patients provided data on the recovery of renal function[204] (Fig. 5–10). The cumulative odds ratio (OR) for survival in favor of synthetic membranes was 1.37 ($p = 0.03$) and that for renal recovery was 1.23 ($p = 0.18$). It was concluded that synthetic membranes appear to confer a significant survival advantage over cellulose-based membranes. A similar benefit could not be demonstrated for recovery of renal function.

The study of Jaber et al. failed to demonstrate a dialyzer advantage (low-flux cellulose acetate vs. PS) on cytokine synthesis by peripheral blood mononuclear cells or on superoxide release by neutrophils obtained from ARF patients.[205] de Sa et al. did not observe any difference in the plasma concentrations of soluble TNF-RI (TNF-sR55), TNF-RII (TNF-sR75), interleukin-6, soluble P-selectin, and von Willebrand factor between ARF patients treated with cuprophan or PS.[206]

The use of a biocompatible dialyzer membrane had no influence on the recovery from ARF after renal transplantation.[207] The number of HD sessions required prior to the recovery of renal function, the number of oliguric days, and the number of hospital days were not different between renal transplant recipients dialyzed with cuprophan membranes and patients treated with PS membranes. However, renal biopsies were not performed systematically in this study.[208]

The effects of renal replacement therapy on outcomes of ARF is also a subject of debate. A systematic review did not find any impact of dialytic modality (intermittent HD vs. continuous renal replacement therapy) on mortality and renal recovery in critically ill adults with ARF.[209] Taken together, some clinical trials have suggested an association between the use of biocompatible dialyzer membranes and

clinical outcome in ARF. Other studies have not confirmed these findings. The biological basis underlying the benefits observed in some studies is, however, still unclear.[210]

REFERENCES

1. Gurland H, Davison A, Bonomini V. Definitions and terminology in biocompatibility. *Nephrol Dial Transplant* 1994;9:4–10.
2. Kaplow LS, Goffinet JA. Profound neutropenia during the early phase of hemodialysis. *JAMA* 1968;203:133–135.
3. Shaldon S, Vienken J. Biocompatibility: is it a relevant consideration for today´s hemodialysis? *Int J Artif Organs* 1996;19:201–204.
4. Wolffindin C, Hoenich NA, Matthews JNS. Cellulose-based haemodialysis membranes: biocompatibility and functional performance compared. *Nephrol Dial Transplant* 1992;7:340–345.
5. Cheung AK, Leypoldt JK. The hemodialysis membranes: a historical perspective, current state and future prospect. *Semin Nephrol* 1997;17:196–213.
6. Radovich JM. Composition of polymer membranes for therapy of end stage renal disease. In: Bonomini V, Berland Y, eds. *Dialysis Membranes: Structures and Predictions. Contribution to Nephrology*. Basel: Karger, 1995:11–24.
7. Galli F, Rovidati S, Chiarantini L, et al. Bioreactivity and biocompatibility of a vitamin E–modified multi-layer hemodialysis filter. *Kidney Int* 1998;54:580–589.
8. Girndt M, Lengler S, Kaul H, et al. Prospective crossover trail on the influence of vitamine E–coated dialyzer membranes on T-cell activation and cytokine induction. *Am J Kidney Dis* 2000;35:95–104.
9. Pertosa G, Grandaliano G, Soccio M, et al. Vitamin E–modified filters modulate Jun N-terminal kinase activation in peripheral blood mononuclear cells. *Kidney Int* 2002;62:602–610.
10. Hakim RM. Recent advances in the biocompatibility of haemodialysis membranes. *Nephrol Dial Transplant* 1995;10:7–11.
11. Vanholder R. Relationship between biocompatibility and neutrophil function in hemodialysis patients. *Adv Renal Replace Ther* 1996;3:312–314.
12. Memoli B, Marzano L, Bisesti V, et al. Hemodialysis-related lymphomononuclear release of interleukin-12 in patients with end-stage renal disease. *J Am Soc Nephrol* 1999;10:2171–2176.
13. Hakim RM, Held PJ, Stannard DC, et al. Effect of the dialysis membrane on mortality of chronic hemodialysis patients. *Kidney Int* 1996;50:566–570.
14. Anderson S, Garcia DL, Brenner BM. Renal and systemic manifestation of glomerular disease. In: Brenner BM, Rector FC Jr, eds. *The Kidney*, 4th ed. Philadelphia: Saunders, 1991:1831–1870.
15. Jorstad S, Smeby LC, Balstad T, Wideroe TE. Removal, generation and adsorption of b_2-microglobulin during hemofiltration with five different membranes. *Blood Purif* 1988;6:96–105.

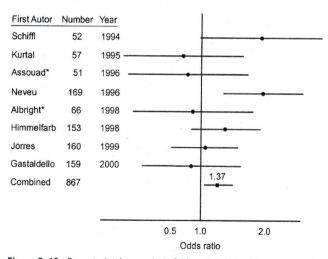

First Autor	Number	Year
Schiffl	52	1994
Kurtal	57	1995
Assouad*	51	1996
Neveu	169	1996
Albright*	66	1998
Himmelfarb	153	1998
Jörres	160	1999
Gastaldello	159	2000
Combined	867	

1.37

0.5   1.0   2.0
Odds ratio

Figure 5–10. Forrest plot for survival. Odds ratios (◆) with corresponding 95 percent CI (lines) from individual trials for survival in patients undergoing hemodialysis for acute renal failure (ARF) using synthetic vs. cellulose-based membranes. *Abstracts. *(From Subramanian S, et al. Influence of dialysis membranes on outcomes in acute renal failure: a meta-analysis. Kidney Int 2002;62:1819–1823. With permission.)*

16. Amadori A, Candi P, Sasdelli M, et al. Hemodialysis leukopenia and complement function with different dialyzers. *Kidney Int* 1983;24:775–781.

17. Cheung AK, Chenoweth DE, Otsuka D, Henderson LW. Compartmental distribution of complement activation products in artificial kidneys. *Kidney Int* 1986;30:74–80.

18. Cheung AK, Parker CJ, Wilcox L, et al. Activation of complement by hemodialysis membranes: polyacrylonitrile binds more C3a than cuprophan. *Kidney Int* 1990;37:1055–1059.

19. Lonnemann G, Koch KM, Shaldon S. Studies on the ability of hemodialysis membranes to induce, bind, and clear human interleukin-1. *J Lab Clin Med* 1988;112:76–86.

20. Kandus A, Ponikvar R, Drinovec J, et al. Anaphylatoxin C3a and C5a adsorption on acrylonitrile membranes of hollow-fiber and plate dialyzers. *Int J Artif Organs* 1990;13:176–180.

21. Ward RA, Schaefer RM, Falkenhagen D. Biocompatibility of a new high-permeability modified cellulose membrane for haemodialysis. *Nephrol Dial Transplant* 1993;8:47–53.

22. Kammerl MC, Schaefer RM, Schweda F, et al. Extracorporeal therapy with AN69 membranes in combination with ACE inhibitors causing severe anaphylactoid reactions: a current problem? *Clin Nephrol* 2000;53:486–488.

23. Simon P, Potier J, Thebaud HE. Risk factors for acute hypersensitivity reactions in hemodialysis. *Nephrologie* 1996;17:163–170.

24. Verresen L, Fink E, Lemke DH, Vanrenterghem Y. Bradykinin is a mediator of anaphylactoid reactions during hemodialysis with AN69 membranes. *Kidney Int* 1994;45:1497–1503.

25. Krieter DH, Grude M, Lemke HD, et al. Anaphylactoid reactions during hemodialysis in sheep are ACE inhibitor dose-dependent and mediated by bradykinin. *Kidney Int* 1998;53:1026–1035.

26. Blais CJ, Marc-Aurele J, Simmons WH, et al. Des-Arg9-bradykinin metabolism in patients who presented hypersensitivity reactions during hemodialysis. Role of serum ACE and aminipeptidase P. *Peptides* 1999;20:421–430.

27. Amore A, Guarnieri G, Atti M, et al. Use of alkaline rinsing solution to prevent hypersensitivity reactions during hemodialysis: data from a multicentre retrospective analysis. *J Nephrol* 1999;12:383–389.

28. Mahent H, Lacour F. Using AN69 ST membrane: a dialysis centre experience. *Nephrol Dial Transplant* 2001;16:1519–1520.

29. Peces R. Anaphylactoid reaction induced by ACEI during hemodialysis with a surface treated AN69 membrane. *Nephrol Dial Transplant* 2002;17:1859–1860.

30. Tepel M, van der Giet M, Zidek W. Efficacy and tolerability of angiotensin II type 1 receptor antagonists in dialysis patients using AN69 dialysis membrane. *Kidney Blood Press Res* 2001;24:71–74.

31. Saracho R, Martin-Malo A, Martinez I, et al. Evaluation of the losartan in haemodialysis (ELHE) study. *Kidney Int* 1998;68:S125–S129.

32. Bijin J. Anaphylactic reaction during haemodialysis on AN69 membrane in a patient receiving angiotensin II receptor antagonist. *Nephrol Dial Transplant* 2001;16:955–956.

33. Krieter DH, Canaud B. Anaphylactic reaction during haemodialysis on AN69 membrane in 9 patients receiving angiotensin II receptor antagonist. *Nephrol Dial Transplant* 2002;17:943–944.

34. Stannat S, Bahlmann J, Kiessling D, et al. Complement activation during hemodialysis: comparison of polysulfone and cuprophan membranes. *Contrib Nephrol* 1985;46:102–108.

35. Streicher E, Schneider H. The development of a new polysulfone membrane: a new perspective in dialysis? *Contrib Nephrol* 1985;46:1–13.

36. Schaefer RM, Fink E, Schaefer L, et al. Role of bradykinin in anaphylactoid reactions during hemodialysis with AN 69 dialyzers. *Am J Nephrol* 1993;13:473–477.

37. Chenoweth DE. Anaphylatoxin formation in extracorporeal circuits. *Complement* 1986;3:152–165.

38. Hakim RM, Fearon DT, Lazarus JM. Biocompatibility of membranes: effects of chronic complement activation. *Kidney Int* 1984;26:194–210.

39. Craddock PR, Fehr J, Delmasso AP, et al. Hemodialysis leukopenia: pulmonary vascular leukostasis resulting from complement activation by dialyzer cellophane membrane. *J Clin Invest* 1977;59:878–888.

40. Jacob HS. A beneficial antimicrobial mechanism that can cause disease. *Arch Intern Med* 1978;138:461–463.

41. Chenoweth DE, Cheung AK, Ward DM, Henderson LW. Anaphylatoxin formation during hemodialysis: Effects of different dialyzer membranes. *Kidney Int* 1983;24:770–774.

42. Hugli TE. The structural basis for anaphylatoxin and chemotactic functions of C3a, C4a, and C5a. *Crit Rev Immunol* 1981;2:321–366.

43. Masaki T, Gilson J, Leypoldt K, Cheung AK. Effect of permeability on indices of haemodialysis membrane biocompatibility. *Nephrol Dial Transplant* 1999;14:1176–1181.

44. Cheung AK. Quantitation of dialysis. *Blood Purif* 1994;12:42–53.

45. Cheung AK. Complement activation as index of haemodialysis membrane biocompatibility: the choice of methods and assays. *Nephrol Dial Transplant* 1994;9:96–103.

46. Deppisch R, Schmidt V, Bommer J. Fluid phase generation of the terminal complement complex C5b-9 as a novel index of biocompatibility. *Kidney Int* 1990;37:696–706.

47. Girndt M, Heisel O, Köhler H. Influence of dialysis with polyamide vs haemophan haemodialysers on monokines and complement activation during a 4-month long-term study. *Nephrol Dial Transplant* 1999;14:676–682.

48. Ward RA, Buscaroli A, Schmidt B, et al. A comparison of dialysers with low-flux membranes: significant differences in spite of many similarities. *Nephrol Dial Transplant* 1997;12:965–972.

49. Swinford RD, Baid S, Pascual M. Dialysis membrane adsorption during CRRT. *Am J Kidney Dis* 1997;30:S32–S37.

50. Pascual M, Schifferli JA. Adsorption of complement factor D by polyacrylonitrile dialysis membranes. *Kidney Int* 1993;43:903–911.

51. Pascual M, Schifferli JA, Pannatier JG, Wauters JP. Removal of complement factor D by adsorption on polymethylmethacrylate dialysis membranes. *Nephrol Dial Transplant* 1993;8:1305–1311.

52. Gasche Y, Pascual M, Suter PM, et al. Complement depletion during haemofiltration with polyacrilonitrile membranes. *Nephrol Dial Transplant* 1996;11:117–119.

53. Himmelfarb J, Lazarus M, Hakim RM. Reactive oxygen species production by monocytes and polymorphonuclear leukocytes during dialysis. *Am J Kidney Dis* 1991;3: 271–276.

54. Frank RD, Weber J, Dresbach H, et al. Role of contact system activation in hemodialyzer-induced thrombogenicity. *Kidney Int* 2001;60:1972–1981.

55. Hong J, Nilsson Ekdahl K, Reynolds H, et al. A new in vitro model to study interaction between whole blood and biomaterials. Studies of platelet and coagulation activation and the effect of aspirin. *Biomaterials* 1999;20:603–611.

56. Cardigan RA, McGloin H, Mackie IJ, et al. Activation of the tissue factor pathway occurs during continuous venovenous hemofiltration. *Kidney Int* 1999;55:1568–1574.

57. Wilhelmsson S, Asaba H, Gunnarsson B, et al. Measurement of fibrinopeptide A in the evaluation of heparin activity and fibrin formation during hemodialysis. *Clin Nephrol* 1981; 15:252–258.

58. Cheung AK, Faezi-Jenkin B, Leypoldt JK. Effect of thrombosis on complement activation and neutrophil degranulation during in vitro hemodialysis. *J Am Soc Nephrol* 1994; 5:110–115.

59. Speiser W, Wojta J, Korninger C, et al. Enhanced fibrinolysis caused by tissue plasminogen activator release in hemodialysis. *Kidney Int* 1987;32:280–283.

60. Stefoni S, Cianciolo G, Donati G, et al. Standard heparin versus low-molecular-weight heparin. A medium-term comparison in hemodialysis. *Nephron* 2002;92:589–600.

61. Reilly RF. The pathophysiology of immune-mediated heparin-induced thrombocytopenia. *Semin Dial* 2003;16: 54–60.

62. Henderson LW, Chwenoweth DE. Cellulose membranes—time for a change? *Contrib Nephrol* 1995;44:112–126.

63. Tonnesen MG, Smeldly LA, Henson PM. Neutrophil-endothelial cell interactions. Modulation of neutrophil adhesiveness by complement fragments C5a and C5a-desarg and folmyl-methionyl-leucyl-phenylalanine in vitro. *J Clin Invest* 1984;74:1582–1592.

64. Sirolli V, Ballone E, Di Stante S, et al. Cell activation and cellular-cellular interactions during hemodialysis: effect of dialyzer membrane. *Int J Artif Organs* 2002;25:529–537.

65. Craddock PR, Hammerschmidt DE. Complement mediated granulocyte activation and down-regulation during hemodialysis. *ASAIO J* 1984;7:50–56.

66. Himmelfarb J, Gerard NP, Hakim RM. Intradialytic modulation of granulocyte C5a receptors. *J Am Soc Nephrol* 1991; 2:920–926.

67. Lundahl J, Hed J, Jacobson SH. Dialysis granulocytopenia is preceded by an increased surface expression of the adhesion-promoting glycoprotein Mac-1. *Nephron* 1992;61: 163–169.

68. Vanholder R, Ringoir S. Polymorphonuclear cell function and infection in dialysis. *Kidney Int* 1992;42:S91–S95.

69. Himmelfarb J, Ault KA, Holbrook D, et al. Intradialytic granulocyte reactive oxygen species production: a prospective crossover trial. *J Am Soc Nephrol* 1993;4:178–186.

70. Rosenkranz AR, Templ E, Traindl O, et al. Reactive oxygen product formation by human neutrophils as an early marker for biocompatibility of dialysis membrane. *Clin Exp Immunol* 1994;98:300–305.

71. Bonomini M, Stuard S, Carreno MP, et al. Neutrophil reactive oxygen species production during hemodialysis: role of activated platelet adhesion to neutrophils through P-selectin. *Nephron* 1997;75:402–411.

72. Satoh M, Yamasaki Y, Nagake Y, et al. Oxidative stress is reduced by the long-term use of vitamin E–coated dialysis filters. *Kidney Int* 2001;59:1943–1950.

73. Tsuruoka S, Kawaguchi A, Nishiki K, et al. Vitamin E–bonded hemodialyzer improves neutrophil function and oxidative stress in patients with end-stage renal failure. *Am J Kidney Dis* 2002;39:127–133.

74. Thylén P, Fernvik E, Lundahl J, et al. Cell surface receptor modulation on monocytes and granulocytes during clinical and experimental hemodialysis. *Am J Nephrol* 1995;15: 392–400.

75. Hörl WH, Steinhauer HB, Schollmeyer P. Plasma levels of granulocyte elastase during hemodialysis: effects of different dialyzer membranes. *Kidney Int* 1985;28:791–796.

76. Hörl WH, Riegel W, Schollmeyer P, et al. Different compliment activation and granulocyte activation in patients dialysed with PMMA dialyzers. *Clin Nephrol* 1986;25:304–307.

77. Bos JC, Grooteman MPC, van Houte AJ, et al. Low polymorphonuclear cell degranulation during citrate anticoagulation: a comparison between citrate and heparin dialysis. *Nephrol Dial Transplant* 1997;12:1387–1393.

78. Böhler J, Schollmeyer P, Dressel B, et al. Reduction of granulocyte activation during hemodialysis with regional citrate anticoagulation: dissociation of complement activation and neutropenia from neutrophil degranulation. *J Am Soc Nephrol* 1996;7:234–241.

79. Tanaka S, Robinson EA, Yoshimura T, et al. Synthesis and biological characterization of monocyte-derived neutrophil chemotactic factor. *FEBS Lett* 1988;236:467–470.

80. Niwa T, Miyazaki T, Sato M, et al. Interleukin 8 and biocompatibility of dialysis membranes. *Am J Nephrol* 1995; 15:181–185.

81. Hörl WH. Hemodialysis membranes: interleukins, biocompatibility, and middle molecules. *J Am Soc Nephrol* 2002;13: S62–S71.

82. Schmaldienst S, Oberpichler A, Tschesche H, Hörl WH. Angiogenin: a novel inhibitor of neutrophil lactoferrin release during extracorporeal circulation. *Kidney Blood Press Res* 2003;26:107–112.

83. Schmaldienst S, Hörl WH. Degranulation of polymorphonuclear leukocytes by dialysis membranes—the mystery clears up? *Nephrol Dial Transplant* 2000;15:1909–1910.

84. Cendoroglo M, Jaber BL, Balakrishnan VS, et al. Neutrophil apoptosis and dysfunction in uremia. *J Am Soc Nephrol* 1999;10:93–100.

85. Martin-Malo A, Carracedo J, Ramirez R, et al. Effect of uremia and dialysis modality on mononuclear cell apoptosis. *J Am Soc Nephrol* 2000;11:936–942.

86. Roccatello D, Mazzucco G, Coppo R. Functional changes of monocytes due to dialysis membranes. *Kidney Int* 1989;35: 622–635.

87. Van Epps D, Chenoweth DE. Analysis of the binding of fluorescent C5a and C3a to human peripheral blood leukocyte. *J Immunol* 1984;132:2862–2867.

88. Luger A, Kovarik J, Stummvoll HK, et al. Blood-membrane interaction in hemodialysis leads to increased cytokine production. *Kidney Int* 1987;32:84–88.

89. Schindler R, Linnenweber S, Schulze M, et al. Gene expression of interleukin-1b during hemodialysis. *Kidney Int* 1993; 43:712–721.

90. Haeffner CN, Cavaillon JM, Laude M, Kazatchkine MD. C3a (C3adesArg) induces production and release of interleukin 1 by cultured human monocytes. *J Immunol* 1987; 139:794–799.

91. Carracedo J, Ramirez R, Madueno JA, et al. Cell apoptosis and hemodialysis-induced inflammation. *Kidney Int* 2002; 61(suppl 80):89–93.

92. Lonnemann G. Chronic inflammation in hemodialysis: the role of contaminated dialysate. *Blood Purif* 2000;18: 214–223.

93. Biasucci LM, Liuzzo G, Fantuzzi G, et al. Increasing levels of interleukin (IL)-1Ra and IL-6 during the first 2 days of hospitalization in unstable angina are associated with increased risk of in hospital coronary events. *Circulation* 1999;99:2079–2084.

94. Balakrishnan VS, Schmid CH, Jaber BL, et al. Interleukin-1 receptor antagonist synthesis by peripheral blood mononuclear cells: a novel predictor of morbidity among hemodialysis patients. *J Am Soc Nephrol* 2000;11:2114–2121.

95. Kozek-Langenecker SA, Kettner SC, Oismueller C, et al. Anticoagulation with prostaglandin E1 and unfractionated heparin during continuous venovenous hemofiltration. *Crit Care Med* 1998;26:1208–1212.

96. Kozek-Langenecker SA, Spiss CK, Gamsjäger T, et al. Anticoagulation with prostaglandins and unfractionated heparin during continuous venovenous haemofiltration: a randomized controlled trial. *Wien Klin Wochenschr* 2002;114: 96–101.

97. Ireland H, Lane DA, Curtis JR. Objective assessment of heparin requirements for hemodialysis in humans. *J Lab Clin Med* 1984;103:643–652.

98. De Sanctis LB, Stefoni S, Cianciolo G, et al. Effect of different dialysis membranes on platelet function. A tool for biocompatibility evaluation. *Int J Artif Organs* 1996;19: 404–410.

99. Kuragano T, Kuno T, Takahashi Y, et al. Comparison of the effect of cellulose triacetate and polysulfone membrane on GPIIb/IIIa and platelet activation. *Blood Purif* 2003;21: 176–182.

100. Gawaz MP, Mujais SK, Schmidt B, et al. Platelet-leukocyte aggregates during hemodialysis: effect of membrane type. *Artif Organs* 1999;23:29–36.

101. Kawabata K, Nagake Y, Shikata K, et al. Soluble P-selectin is released from activated platelets in vivo during hemodialysis. *Nephron* 1998;78:148–155.

102. Cases A, Reverter JC, Escolar G, et al. In vivo evaluation of platelet activation by different cellulosic membranes. *Artif Organs* 1997;21:330–334.

103. Kawabata K, Nakai S, Miwa M, et al. Platelet GPIIb/IIIa is activated and platelet-leukocyte coaggregates formed in vivo during hemodialysis. *Nephron* 2002;90:391–400.

104. Langford EJ, Brown AS, Wainwright RJ, et al. Inhibition of platelet activity by S-nitrosoglutathione during coronary angioplasty. *Lancet* 1994;344:1458–1460.

105. Jilma B, Hergovich N, Stohlawetz P, et al. Effects of sodium nitroprusside on hemodialysis-induced platelet activation. *Kidney Int* 1999;55:686–691.

106. McEver RT, Martin MN. A monoclonal antibody to a membrane glycoprotein binds only to activated platelet. *J Biol Chem* 1984;259:9799–9804.

107. Bennett JS, Vilaire G. Exposure of platelet fibrinogen receptors by ADP and epinephrine. *J Clin Invest* 1979;64: 1393–1401.

108. Chuang YC, Chen JB, Yang LC, Kuo CY. Significance of platelet activation in vascular access survival of haemodialysis patients. *Nephrol Dial Transplant* 2003;18:947–954.

109. Jankowski J, Schluter H, Henning L, et al. The AN69 hemofiltration membrane has a decreasing effect on the intracellular diadenosine pentaphosphate concentration of platelets. *Kidney Blood Press Res* 2003;26:50–54.

110. Winkler J, Fuchs J, Morduchowicz G, et al. Circulating aggregated platelets, number of platelets per aggregate and platelet size in chronic dialysis patients. *Nephron* 1997;77: 44–47.

111. Henning BF, Zidek W, Linder B, Tepel M. Mean platelet volume and coronary heart disease in hemodialysis patients. *Kidney Blood Press Res* 2002;25:103–108.

112. Ando M, Iwata A, Ozeki Y, et al. Circulating platelet-derived microparticles with procoagulant activity may be a potential cause of thrombosis in uremic patients. *Kidney Int* 2002;62: 1757–1763.

113. Himmelfarb J, Nelson S, McMonagle E, et al. Elevated plasma glycocalicin levels and decreased ristocetin-induced platelet agglutination in hemodialysis patients. *Am J Kidney Dis* 1998;32:132–138.

114. Salvati F, Liani M. Role of platelet surface receptor abnormalities in the bleeding and thrombotic diathesis of uremic patients on hemodialysis and peritoneal dialysis. *Int J Artif Organs* 2001;24:131–135.

115. Sloand JA, Sloand EM. Studies on platelet membrane glycoproteins and platelet function during hemodialysis. *J Am Soc Nephrol* 1997;8:799–803.

116. Diaz-Ricart M, Estebanell E, Cases A, et al. Abnormal platelet cytoskeletal assembly in hemodialyzed patients results in deficient tyrosine phosphorylation signaling. *Kidney Int* 2000;57:1905–1914.

117. Ando M, Iwamoto Y, Suda A, et al. New insights into the thrombopoietic status of patients on dialysis through the evaluation of megakaryocytopoiesis in bone marrow and of endogenous thrombopoietin levels. *Blood* 2001;97:915–921.

118. Kuwana M, Kaburaki J, Ikeda Y. Autoreactive T cells to platelet GPIIb-IIIa in immune thrombocytopenic purpura. Role in production of anti-platelet autoantibody. *J Clin Invest* 1998;102:1393–1402.

119. Gawaz MP, Mujais SK, Schmidt B, Gurland HJ. Platelet-leukocyte aggregation during hemodialysis. *Kidney Int* 1994;46:489–495.

120. Arnaout MA, Hakim RM, Todd RF III, et al. Increased expression of an adhesion-promoting surface glycoprotein in the granulocytopenia of hemodialysis. *N Engl J Med* 1985; 312:457–462.

121. Himmelfarb J, Zaoui P, Hakim R. Modulation of granulocyte LAM-1 and MAC-1 during dialysis—a prospective, randomized controlled trial. *Kidney Int* 1992;41:388–395.

122. Nagata K, Tsuji T, Todoroki N, et al. Activated platelets induce superoxide anion release by monocytes and neutrophils through P-selectin (CD62). *J Immunol* 1993;151: 3267–3273.

123. Moon DG, van der Zee H, Weston LK, et al. Platelet modulation of neutrophil superoxide anion production. *Thromb Haemost* 1990;63:91–96.

124. Faint RW. Platelet-neutrophil interactions: their significance. *Blood Rev* 1992;6:83–91.

125. Bonomini M, Sirolli V, Stuard S, Settefrati N. Interactions between platelets and leukocytes during hemodialysis. *Artif Organs* 1999;23:23–28.

126. Ashman N, Macey MG, Fan SL, et al. Increased platelet-monocyte aggregates and cardiovascular disease in end-stage renal failure patients. *Nephrol Dial Transplant* 2003; 10:2088–2096.

127. Martos MR, Hendry BM, Rodriguez-Puyol M, et al. Haemodialyser biocompatibility and erythrocyte structure and function. *Clin Chim Acta* 1997;265:235–246.

128. Sevillano G, Rodriguez-Puyol M, Martos R, et al. Cellulose acetate membrane improves some aspects of red blood cell function in hemodialysis patients. *Nephrol Dial Transplant* 1990;5:497–499.

129. Gambhir KK, Parui R, Agarwal V, Cruz I. The effect of hemodialysis on the transport of sodium in erythrocytes from chronic renal failure patients maintained on hemodialysis. *Life Sci* 2002;71:1615–1621.

130. Sasaki M, Hohoya N, Saruhashi M. Vitamin E modified cellulose membrane. *Artif Organs* 2000;24:779–789.

131. Ozden M, Maral H, Akaydin D, et al. Erythrocyte glutathione peroxidase activity, plasma malonyldialdehyde and erythrocyte glutathione levels in hemodialysis and CAPD patients. *Clin Biochem* 2002;35:269–273.

132. Dhondt A, Vanholder R, Waterloos MA, et al. Citrate anticoagulation does not correct cuprophan bioincompatibility as evaluated by the expression of leukocyte surface molecules. *Nephrol Dial Transplant* 1998;13:1752–1758.

133. Janssen MJFM, Deegens JK, Kapinga TH, et al. Citrate compared to low molecular weight heparin anticoagulation in chronic hemodialysis patients. *Kidney Int* 1996;49: 806–813.

134. Leitienne P, Fouque D, Rigal D, et al. Heparins and blood polymorphonuclear stimulation in haemodialysis: an expansion of the biocompatibility concept. *Nephrol Dial Transplant* 2000;15:1631–1637.

135. Kozek-Langenecker SA, Spiss CK, Michalek-Sauberer A, et al. Effect of prostacyclin on platelets, polymorphonuclear cells, and heterotypic cell aggregation during hemofiltration. *Crit Care Med* 2003;31:864–868.

136. Lonnemann G, Koch KM. Beta(2)-microglobulin amyloidosis: effects of ultrapure dialysate and type of dialyzer membrane. *J Am Soc Nephrol* 2002;13(suppl 1):S72–S77.

137. Pickett TM, Cruickshank A, Greenwood RN, et al. Membrane flux not biocompatibility determines beta-2-microglobulin levels in hemodialysis patients. *Blood Purif* 2002;20:161–166.

138. Hakim RM, Wingard RL, Husni L, et al. The effect of membrane biocompatibility on plasma b2-microglobulin levels in chronic hemodialysis patients. *J Am Soc Nephrol* 1996;7: 472–478.

139. Jahn B, Betz M, Deppisch R, et al. Stimulation of b2-m synthesis in lymphocytes after exposure to cuprophan dialyzer membranes. *Kidney Int* 1991;40:285–290.

140. Jahn B, Betz M, Deppisch R, et al. Stimulation of beta2-microglobulin synthesis in lymphocytes after exposure to cuprophan dialyzer membranes. *Kidney Int* 1991;40: 285–290.

141. Schoels M, Jahn B, Hug F, et al. Stimulation of mononuclear cells by contact with cuprophan membranes: further increase of b2-microglobulin synthesis by activated late complement components. *Am J Kidney Dis* 1993;21: 394–399.

142. Zaoui PM, Stone WJ, Hakim RM. Effects of dialysis membranes on beta2-microglobulin production and cellular expression. *Kidney Int* 1990;38:962–968.

143. Senatore M, Nicoletti A, Rizzuto G. Is the bioreactivity of vitamin E–modified dialyzer an expression of increased plasmatic vitamin E concentration? *Nephron* 2002;92: 487–489.

144. Clark WR, Macias WL, Molitoris A, Wang NHL. Plasma protein adsorption to highly permeable hemodialysis membranes. *Kidney Int* 1995;48:481–488.

145. Müller TF, Seitz M, Eckle I, et al. Biocompatibility differences with respect to the dialyzer sterilization method. *Nephron* 1998;78:139–142.

146. Lonnemann G, Behme TC, Lenzner B, et al. Permeability of dialyzer membranes to TNF alpha–inducing substances derived from water bacteria. *Kidney Int* 1992;42:61–68.

147. Schwalbe S, Holzhauer M, Schaeffer J, et al. Beta 2–microglobulin associated amyloidosis: a vanishing complication of long-term hemodialysis? *Kidney Int* 1997;52: 1077–1083.

148. Koda Y, Nishi SI, Miyazaki S, et al. Switch from conventional to high-flux membrane reduces the risk of carpal tunnel syndrome and mortality of hemodialysis patients. *Kidney Int* 1997;52:1096–1101.

149. Kleophas W, Haastert B, Backus G, et al. Long-term experience with an ultrapure individual dialysis fluid with a batch type machine. *Nephrol Dial Transplant* 1998;13:3118–3125.

150. Baz M, Durand C, Ragon A, et al. Using ultrapure water in hemodialysis delays carpal tunnel syndrome. *Int J Artif Organs* 1991;14:681–685.

151. Pierratos A, Ouwendyk M, Francoeur R, et al. Nocturnal hemodialysis: three-year experience. *J Am Soc Nephrol* 1998; 9:859–868.

152. Miyata T, Kurokawa K, Van Ypersele de Strihou C. Relevance of oxidative and carbonyl stress to long-term uremic complications. *Kidney Int* 2000;58:120–125.

153. Van Ypersele de Strihou C. Are biocompatible membranes superior for hemodialysis therapy? *Kidney Int* 1997;52: S101–S104.

154. Stein G, Franke S, Mahiout A, et al. Influence of dialysis modalities on serum AGE levels in end-stage renal disease patients. *Nephrol Dial Transplant* 2001;16:999–1008.

155. Vlassara H, Brownlee M, Manogue KR, et al. Cachectin/TNF and IL-1 induced by glucose-modified pro-

teins: role in normal tissue remodelling. *Science* 1988;240: 1546–1548.

156. Konishi Y, Okamura M, Konishi M, et al. Enhanced gene expression of scavenger receptor in peripheral blood monocytes from patients on cuprophane haemodialysis. *Nephrol Dial Transplant* 1997;12:1167–1172.

157. Seres DS, Strain GW, Hashim SA, et al. Improvement of plasma lipoprotein profiles during high-flux dialysis. *J Am Soc Nephrol* 1993;3:1409–1415.

158. Josephson MA, Fellner SK, Dasgupta A. Improved lipid profiles in patients undergoing high-flux hemodialysis. *Am J Kidney Dis* 1992;20:361–366.

159. Blankestijn PJ, Vos PF, Rabelink TJ, et al. High-flux dialysis membranes improve lipid profile in chronic hemodialysis patients. *J Am Soc Nephrol* 1995;5:1703–1708.

160. Goldberg IJ, Kaufman AM, Lavarias VA, et al. High flux dialysis membranes improve plasma lipoprotein profiles in patients with end-stage renal disease. *Nephrol Dial Transplant* 1996;11:104–107.

161. Ingram AJ, Parbtani A, Churchill DN. Effects of two low-flux cellulose acetate dialysers on plasma lipids and lipoproteins—a crossover trail. *Nephrol Dial Transplant* 1998;13: 1452–1457.

162. Gonzalez AI, Schreier L, Elbert A, et al. Lipoprotein alterations in hemodialysis: differences between diabetic and nondiabetic patients. *Metabolism* 2003;52:116–121.

163. Mekki K, Bouchenak M, Lamri M, et al. Changes in plasma lecithin: cholesterol acyltransferase activity, HDL(2), HDL(3) amounts and compositions in patients with chronic renal failure after different times of hemodialysis. *Atherosclerosis* 2002;162:409–417.

164. Parker TF, Wingard RL, Husni L, et al. Effect of the membrane biocompatibility on nutritional parameters in chronic hemodialysis patients. *Kidney Int* 1996;49:551–556.

165. Tayeb JS, Provencano R, El-Ghoroury M, et al. Effect of biocompatibility of hemodialysis membranes on serum albumin levels. *Am J Kidney Dis* 2000;35:606–610.

166. Leavey SF, Strawderman RL, Young EW, et al. Cross-sectional and longitudinal predictors of serum albumin in hemodialysis patients. *Kidney Int* 2000;58:2119–2128.

167. Memoli B, Minutolo R, Bisesti V, et al. Changes of serum albumin and C-reactive protein are related to changes of interleukin-6 release by peripheral blood mononuclear cells in hemodialysis patients treated with different membranes. *Am J Kidney Dis* 2002;39:266–273.

168. Lindsay RM, Spanner E. A hypothesis: the protein catabolic rate is dependent upon the type and amount of treatment in dialyzed uremic patients. *Am J Kidney Dis* 1989;13: 382–389.

169. Lindsay RM, Spanner E, Heidenheim AP, et al. The influence of dialysis membrane upon protein catabolic rate. *ASAIO J* 1991;37:134–135.

170. Locatelli F, Mastrangelo F, Redaelli B, et al. Effects of different membranes and dialysis technologies on patient treatment tolerance and nutritional parameters. *Kidney Int* 1996;50:1293–1302.

171. Gutierrez A, Alvestrand A, Wahren J, Bergstrom J. Effect of in vivo contact between blood and dialysis membranes on protein catabolism in humans. *Kidney Int* 1990;38:487–494.

172. Gutierrez A, Bergstrom J, Alvestrand A. Protein catabolism in sham haemodialysis: the effect of different membranes. *Clin Nephrol* 1992;38:20–29.

173. Dumler F, Stalla K, Mohini R, et al. Clinical experience with short-time hemodialysis. *Am J Kidney Dis* 1992;19:49–56.

174. Hornberger JC, Chernew M, Petersen J, Garber AM. A multivariate analysis of mortality and hospital admission with high-flux dialysis. *J Am Soc Nephrol* 1993;3:1227–1237.

175. Hakim RM. Clinical implications of hemodialysis membrane biocompatibility. *Kidney Int* 1993;44:484–494.

176. Vanholder R, De Smet R, Hsu C, et al. Uremic toxicity: the middle molecule hypothesis revisited. *Semin Nephrol* 1994; 14:205–218.

177. Leypoldt JK, Cheung AK. Removal of high-molecular-weight solutes during high-efficiency and high-flux haemodialysis. *Nephrol Dial Transplant* 1996;11:329–335.

178. Haag-Weber M, Mai B, Cohen G, Hörl WH. GIP and DIP: a new view of uraemic toxicity. *Nephrol Dial Transplant* 1994;9:346–347.

179. Charra B, Calemard E, Ruffet M, et al. Survival as an index of adequacy of dialysis. *Kidney Int* 1992;41:1286–1291.

180. Woods HF, Nandakumar M. Improved outcome for haemodialysis patients treated with high-flux membranes. *Nephrol Dial Transplant* 2000;15:36–42.

181. Hakim RM. Influence of the dialysis membrane on outcome of ESRD patients. *Am J Kidney Dis* 1998;32:S71–S75.

182. Jansen MA, Hart AA, Korevaar JC, et al. Predictors of the rate of decline of residual renal function in incident dialysis patients. *Kidney Int* 2002;62:1046–1053.

183. Lang SM, Bergner A, Töpfer M, Schiffl H. Preservation of residual renal function in dialysis patients: effects of dialysis-technique–related factors. *Perit Dial Int* 2001;21:52–57.

184. McKane W, Chandna SM, Tattersall JE, et al. Identical decline of residual renal function in high-flux biocompatible hemodialysis and CAPD. *Kidney Int* 2002;61:256–265.

185. Schiffl H, Lang SM, Fischer R. Ultrapure dialysis fluid slows loss of residual renal function in new dialysis patients. *Nephrol Dial Transplant* 2002;17:1814–1818.

186. Hartmann J, Fricke H, Schiffl H. Biocompatible membranes preserve residual renal function in patients undergoing regular hemodialysis. *Am J Kidney Dis* 1997;30:366–373.

187. Schulman G, Fogo A, Gung A, et al. Complement activation retards resolution of acute ischemic renal failure in the rat. *Kidney Int* 1991;40:1069–1074.

188. Himmelfarb J, Hakim RM. The use of biocompatible dialysis membranes in acute renal failure. *Adv Renal Replace Ther* 1997;4:72–80.

189. Modi GK, Pereira BJ, Jaber BL. Hemodialysis in acute renal failure: does the membrane matter? *Semin Dial* 2001;14: 318–321.

190. Hakim RM, Wingard RL, Parker RA. Effect of dialysis membranes in the treatment of patients with acute renal failure. *N Engl J Med* 1994;331:1338–1342.

191. Schiffl H, Lang SM, König A, et al. Biocompatible membranes in acute renal failure: prospective case-controlled study. *Lancet* 1994;344:570–572.

192. Schiffl H, Sitter T, Lang S, et al. Bioincompatible membranes place patients with acute renal failure at increased risk of infection. *ASAIO J* 1995;41:709–712.

193. Neveu H, Kleinknecht D, Brivet F, et al. Prognostic factors in acute renal failure due to sepsis. Results of a prospective multicentre study. *Nephrol Dial Transplant* 1996;11: 293–299.

194. Himmelfarb J, Tolkoff Rubin N, Chandran P, et al. A multicenter comparison of dialysis membranes in the treatment of acute renal failure requiring dialysis. *J Am Soc Nephrol* 1998;9:257–266.

195. Cosentino F, Chaff C, Piedmonte M. Risk factors influencing survival in ICU acute renal failure. *Nephrol Dial Transplant* 1994;9:179–182.

196. Kurtal H, von Herrath D, Schaefer K. Is the choice of membrane important for patients with acute renal failure requiring hemodialysis? *Artif Organs* 1995;19:391–394.

197. Jörres A, Gahl GM, Dobis C, et al. Haemodialysis-membrane biocompatibility and mortality of patients with dialysis-dependent acute renal failure: a prospective randomised multicentre trial. *Lancet* 1999;354:1337–1341.

198. Vanholder R, Lameire N. Does biocompatibility of dialysis membranes affect recovery of renal function and survival? *Lancet* 1999;354:1316–1318.

199. Schiffl H. Biocompatibility and acute renal failure. *Lancet* 2000;355:312.

200. Lauriat S, Linas SL. The role of neutrophils in acute renal failure. *Semin Nephrol* 1998;18:498–504.

201. Albright RC Jr, Smelser JM, McCarthy JT, et al. Patient survival and renal recovery in acute renal failure: randomized comparison of cellulose acetate and polysulfone membrane dialyzers. *Mayo Clin Proc* 2000;75:1141–1147.

202. Gastaldello K, Melot C, Kahn RJ, et al. Comparison of cellulose diacetate and polysulfone membranes in the outcome of acute renal failure. A prospective randomized study. *Nephrol Dial Transplant* 2000;15:224–230.

203. Jaber BL, Lau J, Schmid CH, et al. Effect of biocompatibility of hemodialysis membranes on mortality in acute renal failure: a meta-analysis. *Clin Nephrol* 2002;57:274–282.

204. Subramanian S, Venkataraman R, Kellum JA. Influence of dialysis membranes on outcomes in acute renal failure: a meta-analysis. *Kidney Int* 2002;62:1819–1823.

205. Jaber BL, Cendoroglo M, Balakrishnan VS, et al. Impact of dialyzer membrane selection on cellular responses in acute renal failure: a crossover study. *Kidney Int* 2000;57: 2107–2116.

206. de Sa HM, Freitas LA, Alves VC, et al. Leukocyte, platelet and endothelial activation in patients with acute renal failure treated by intermittent hemodialysis. *Am J Nephrol* 2001;21: 264–273.

207. Romao JE Jr, Abensur H, de Castro MC, et al. Effect of dialyser biocompatibility on recovery from acute renal failure after cadaver renal transplantation. *Nephrol Dial Transplant* 1999;14:709–712.

208. Lang SM, Schiffl H. Effect of dialyser biocompatibility on recovery from acute renal failure after cadaveric renal transplantation. *Nephrol Dial Transplant* 2000;15:134–135.

209. Tonelli M, Manns B, Feller-Kopman D. Acute renal failure in the intensive care unit: a systematic review of the impact of dialytic modality on mortality and renal recovery. *Am J Kidney Dis* 2002;40:875–885.

210. Karsou SA, Jaber BL, Pereira BJ. Impact of intermittent hemodialysis variables on clinical outcomes in acute renal failure. *Am J Kidney Dis* 2000;35:980–991.

Anticoagulation in Patients on Hemodialysis

David M. Ward

Despite continuing advances, the goal of finding a wholly satisfactory method for preventing clotting in hemodialysis circuits remains elusive. Heparin remains the standard anticoagulant for most applications, but it potentiates the risk of hemorrhage elsewhere in the patient.[1,2] When bleeding is a concern, the risk can be reduced, though not eliminated, by low-dose heparin protocols, which require careful monitoring and adjustment if they are to avoid both bleeding in the patient and clotting in the dialyzer. In patients at particularly high risk of bleeding (who are usually hospitalized), heparin may have to be avoided completely. In these circumstances hemodialysis may be performed with a "no anticoagulant" method, regional citrate anticoagulation, or other methods.[3,4] In contrast, for routine outpatient hemodialysis, heparin, by virtue of its systemic anticoagulant effect, may confer an advantage by helping prevent clot formation in the vascular access site. New anticoagulant drugs and alternative approaches continue to be developed and studied for use in hemodialysis, and some have gained a place in standard dialysis practice.[5-11]

The relative risks of bleeding and thrombosis are in general different for acute and chronic dialysis situations but have to be assessed for each individual patient. The choice of an anticoagulation prescription for hemodialysis must be based also on several other considerations, including knowledge of hemostatic mechanisms and their status in uremic patients, the pharmacology and practical aspects of each of the available methods, and the empiric results that have been achieved with respect to efficacy and complications.

COAGULATION STATUS OF PATIENTS WITH RENAL FAILURE

Hemodialysis patients are at increased risk of both hemorrhagic and thrombotic complications. Bleeding is common; the main contributing causes are the uremic platelet defect, anticoagulants used for hemodialysis or vascular access patency, traumatic and surgical sites, and the effects of uremia on various tissues (gastrointestinal tract, pericardium, etc.). Thrombotic problems are common at vascular access sites, probably reflecting disturbed vascular anatomy, measures needed to control bleeding after needle removal, and the downstream effects of procoagulant activation in the extracorporeal circuit. Systemic thrombotic events are less common and may warrant investigation to rule out other causes.

The Uremic Bleeding Diathesis

Occasional prolongation of the prothrombin time,[12] modest reductions in factors XII and IX and prothrombin levels,[13] and below-average platelet counts[14] appear to contribute little to the uremic bleeding diathesis. The prolonged bleeding time typical of the uremic patient[15] is due mainly to qualitative defects in platelet function, including impairment of adhesion, aggregation, and release reactions.[12,16,17] Partial improvement of these defects by dialysis has suggested a role for specific uremic toxins, such as phenolic acid, guanidinosuccinic acid, and other middle molecules.[18,19] Data implicating parathyroid hormone have been inconsistent.[20,21] However, other nondialyzable factors do appear responsible, including reduced production of thromboxanes by platelets and perhaps increased endothelial prostacyclin release.[16] In addition, nitric oxide (endothelium-derived relaxing factor) may exacerbate bleeding in uremia.[22] Although the issue of whether von Willebrand factor (vWF) function in uremia is normal is as yet unsettled,[16] the bleeding time in a uremic patient can be improved by augmenting vWF levels either by exogenous administration of cryoprecipitate[23] or by infusion of desmopressin [l-deamino-8-D-arginine vasopressin (DDAVP)], which releases endogenous vWF from endothelial stores.[24] Methods for treating the uremic bleeding diathesis, in addition to cryoprecipitate, DDAVP, and dialysis,[25] include administration of conjugated estrogens,[26] transfusion of red blood cells,[27] and injection of recombinant human erythropoietin (rHuEPO).[28]

Hemorrhagic Events

Bleeding in uremic patients occurs where vascular access needles or venous catheters have been placed and spontaneously in internal organs damaged by specific uremic pathology or comorbid conditions.[1] Gastrointestinal bleeding reflects a high incidence of peptic ulceration, gastritis, angiodysplasia, and rectal ulceration in renal failure patients.[29–31] Hemorrhagic pericarditis,[32] hemorrhagic pleural effusion,[33] and mediastinal,[34] retroperitoneal,[35] and subcapsular liver hemorrhage[36] also occur. Subdural and intracerebral hemorrhages are frequently fatal in hemodialysis patients,[37–39] and intraocular bleeding is of concern particularly in diabetic individuals.[40]

A quarter of a century ago, in an analysis of deaths in hospitalized patients in whom the expected risk of a fatal outcome was low, the Boston Collaborative Drug Surveillance Program concluded that "Heparin continues to be the drug responsible for a majority of deaths in patients who are reasonably healthy."[41] Heparin anticoagulation for dialysis is a common precipitating cause of serious bleeding events. Avoidance of heparin or great care in its use is necessary.[2,42–49] Swartz and Port classified bleeding risks into four degrees of severity depending on how recently the patient has suffered active bleeding, surgery, or trauma and modified by other factors such as pericarditis.[50] However, even when none of these factors is present, an excess number of serious hemorrhagic events may occur in patients with acute renal failure who are dialyzed with tightly controlled heparin.[2] This risk can be reduced substantially by "no anticoagulant" or citrate-anticoagulation methods. Complete avoidance of heparin for dialysis for all critically ill patients has been suggested.[2]

Hypercoagulability

Hemodialysis patients have some persistent abnormalities in coagulation factors that tend toward a prothrombotic state: predialysis levels of procoagulant factors VII and VIII are elevated; coagulation inhibitors such as antithrombin III, protein C, and protein S are depleted; and fibrinolysis may be impaired.[51–55] In addition, during the dialysis procedure, there is the acute release of procoagulant materials from endothelial stores, including vWF, 6-keto-prostaglandin F_1-alpha, and tissue-type plasminogen activator (t-PA).[55,56] These abnormalities in most cases may not be clinically apparent, perhaps only partially offsetting the prohemorrhagic influences.

Some hemodialysis patients, however, may present with excessive clotting at the vascular access, systemic venous thrombosis, arterial thrombosis, or even priapism[57–60]; in these patients additional pathology should be suspected. An acquired functional deficiency of protein C is a prominent feature in many instances.[55,59] Additional causes should be suspected, though they are rarely found. These would include Trousseau's syndrome, which is due to stimulation of the extrinsic coagulation pathway by tissue factor from a malignant neoplasm,[61] and heparin-induced platelet antibodies (which also cause thrombocytopenia, which is easily recognized).[62,63] The use of rHuEPO has also been implicated as a cause of increased thrombotic events.[64–67] rHuEPO has been reported to shorten the bleeding time, increase vWF and fibrinogen levels temporarily, and reduce antithrombin III and protein C activity.[64,65,68,69] A direct effect on platelets to increase their adhesion and aggregation, distinct from effects on coagulation factors or increased red cell concentration, has been documented in chronic hemodialysis patients after 20 weeks of rHuEPO therapy.[70]

The syndrome of calciphylaxis, which can cause necrosis of skin and subcutaneous tissue and digital gangrene in dialyzed patients, appears to be mediated not only by hyperparathyroidism and vessel calcification but also by an acquired functional deficiency of protein C[71,72] or protein S.[73]

Vascular Access Thrombosis

Both endogenous arteriovenous fistulas and synthetic arteriovenous grafts used for hemodialysis are at risk of recurrent thrombosis.[74] Fibrinolysis can be achieved by local injection of urokinase[75] or systemically by infusion of urokinase, streptokinase, or tissue t-PA.[76–78] When there are associated venous stenoses, these can optimally be addressed by combining pharmacomechanical thrombolysis (e.g., pulsed-spray injection of urokinase) with angioplasty.[77–82] Significant prevention of recurrent thrombosis can be achieved with aspirin or other antiplatelet agents and by warfarin.[56,83,84] Patients with functional protein C deficiency may also be helped by low-dose danazol.[85]

Experience with temporary and permanent venous catheters for hemodialysis access has shown more thrombotic and stenotic complications with subclavian than with internal jugular sites.[86–91] Heparin instilled after each usage may not suffice to maintain patency, therefore oral warfarin or aspirin is useful.[92,93] Clotted catheters can be opened by instilling low-dose urokinase (5000 IU/mL) to each limb, but frequently there is clot sheathed around the catheter that must be stripped mechanically or lysed by high-dose intravenous urokinase (250,000 IU) or streptokinase (up to 3,250,000 IU has been given in divided doses). Both thrombotic and hemorrhagic complications may occur.[91,94] Clotted catheters can also be opened by t-PA.[95] In patients intolerant of heparin because of heparin-induced thrombocytopenia, venous catheters can be kept open by instilling citrate solution or reopened by using urokinase.[96]

MECHANISMS OF THROMBOSIS IN HEMODIALYSIS CIRCUITS

Blood contact with the foreign surfaces of an extracorporeal hemodialysis circuit activates two principal mechanisms of thrombus formation. The first is the intrinsic pathway of blood coagulation, which starts with "contact activation factors" and leads through an amplifying series of enzymatic reactions to the production of thrombin and the formation of cross-linked fibrin clots. The second mechanism is platelet adhesion and activation. Note that the so-called extrinsic pathway, which is the other initiating mechanism of the coagulation cascade, is not directly implicated in extracorporeal thrombus formation; it depends on tissue factor, which is released from vessel walls by direct injury and is expressed by activated monocytes. Neither of these mechanisms has been shown to be quantitatively important in hemodialysis. However, as already mentioned, endothelial cell stimulation does occur during hemodialysis and leads among other things to the activation of a third system involved in hemostasis: the fibrinolytic system.

The Intrinsic Coagulation Pathway

Activation of the intrinsic pathway by hemodialysis has been well recognized for many years.[97] Current understanding of this complex system has been elegantly reviewed[98]; a simplified outline is given in Fig. 6–1. Nonphysiologic surfaces (e.g., dialyzer membranes) bind Hageman factor (factor XII), prekallikrein, high-molecular-weight kininogen (HMWK), and factor XI. Factor XII is activated by surface binding to XIIa, and prekallikrein is converted to kallikrein, which enhances XIIa production. XIIa then converts XI to XIa, which now can move off the activating surface to catalyze the next step. This step, which is the activation of factor IX to IXa, is common to both the intrinsic and extrinsic pathways; all subsequent reactions require the presence of calcium ions. IXa forms a complex with factor VIIIa and a phospholipid (which most often is phospholipid on the surface of platelets) and catalyzes the conversion of factor X to Xa. In similar fashion, Xa assembles with factor Va and phospholipid via various specific interactions on the platelet surface to form the prothrombin activation complex, which converts prothrombin to thrombin. Finally, thrombin cleaves fibrinogen molecules to produce fibrin monomers, which polymerize to form insoluble fibrin strands; thrombin also activates factor XIII to XIIIa, which cross-links the fibrin molecules to form a fibrin clot. Once initiated, the cascade is augmented by various positive feedback loops; for instance, thrombin is also responsible for catalyzing the production of VIIIa and Va, which are necessary for the full activity of IXa and Xa, respectively.

The coagulation cascade is regulated by several natural inhibitors, notably antithrombin III; also heparin cofactor II, protein C, and others. Antithrombin III inhibits thrombin and factors IXa and Xa; its activity is promoted when it binds to heparan sulfate (which is present on intact endothelium) or to heparin. Complexes of thrombin and antithrombin III are evidence of thrombin activation and can be measured in plasma to determine the extent of thrombin activation in hemodialysis systems.[99] Heparin cofactor II also inhibits thrombin; its activity is promoted by dermatan sulfate (which is present in extravascular tissues) and by heparin. Protein C (with its cofactor protein S) inhibits factors VIIIa and Va; protein C is activated by thrombin that has undergone alteration of its enzymatic specificity by binding to thrombomodulin on the surface of endothelial cells. The general role of all the inhibitors in vivo is to limit clot propagation. Since they are triggered mainly by factors derived from vascular and perivascular tissues, they are naturally activated in body sites but not on foreign surfaces. Hemodialysis appears to increase protein C activity acutely,

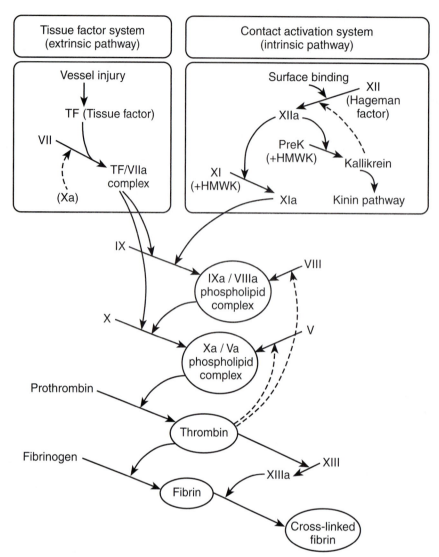

Figure 6–1. The coagulation cascade. Straight arrows show conversion of a coagulation protein from an inactive to an activated form. Curved arrows show a catalytic effect or the enzymatic action of an activated factor or complex on the next factor in the cascade. Dashed arrows show positive feedback loops. The intrinsic pathway is activated by foreign surfaces such as dialysis membranes. Heparin binds to and activates antithrombin III, which is a natural inhibitor of factors IXa, factor Xa, and thrombin. Low-molecular-weight (LMW) heparin is more active in inhibiting factor Xa and less potent against thrombin than is unfractionated heparin. Citrate is an anticoagulant because it chelates calcium ions, which are needed for the formation of all complexes shown in the figure, for the enzymatic activity of factor XIa, and for the conversion of XIII to XIIIa by thrombin. HMWK, high-molecular-weight kininogen; PreK, prekallikrein. (Adapted from Rapaport[98]. With permission.)

possibly by removing an antagonist; otherwise, as noted above, the resting levels of all these inhibitors usually remain normal to low in hemodialysis patients.[52–54,100] Their main importance for extracorporeal circuits lies in the possibility of exploiting them as anticoagulants.

Platelet Activation

Platelets at a site of vascular injury adhere to exposed collagen. This interaction is assisted by vWF, which is an adhesion protein released from endothelial cells. On dialyzer membranes, however, platelet adhesion appears not to require vWF and occurs either directly on the foreign surface or is modulated by the absorption of various plasma proteins.[102,103] Platelet adhesion sets in motion the platelet activation sequence, which can also be triggered by thrombin. The stages of platelet activation include shape change; aggregation; secretion of thromboxane B_2, which activates other platelets; release reactions that liberate the contents of alpha granules and dense granules; modification of the platelet surface membrane; and finally platelet contraction and fusion. Interactions with the coagulation cascade are numerous, including facilitation of the assembly of the proactivation complex on the platelet surface and the release of platelet factor 4, which competes with antithrombin III for binding sites and thus can neutralize heparin.[98]

Clinical observations demonstrate that platelets play a significant role in thrombus formation in hemodialysis systems. For instance, severely thrombocytopenic patients can often be hemodialyzed with no anticoagulant, and antiplatelet agents have been shown to reduce thrombus formation on dialysis membranes.[103] During hemodialysis, platelet counts fall acutely and platelet activation can be demonstrated by increased levels of thromboxane B_2 and β-thromboglobulin.[102,104,105] These effects may be related to alterative complement pathway and leukocyte activation, but it is uncertain whether they are more pronounced with cellulosic dialysis membranes than with more biocompatible membranes.[101,102,104–106] As noted above, an acute increase in vWF levels, indicating systemic release from vascular endothelium, has been demonstrated during cuprophane hemodialysis.[104]

The Fibrinolytic System

Clot lysis is achieved by the fibrinolytic system, of which the main enzyme, plasmin, is produced from plasminogen by various plasminogen activators. Plasminogen activator is neutralized in vivo by plasminogen activator inhibitor (PAI). Activated protein C, which inhibits coagulation, also promotes fibrinolysis by inhibiting PAI. Acute increases in fibrinolytic activity during hemodialysis are now known to be due to release of t-PA from endothelial storage sites.[107–109] This effect can be replicated by sham dialysis but not by heparin alone, indicating that blood contact with the dialyzer membrane provides the key stimulus.[107] Despite activation of fibrinolysis during hemodialysis, there is no evidence that it plays a significant role in limiting clotting in the dialyzer circuit.[105]

APPROACHES TO MAINTAINING THE PATENCY OF HEMODIALYSIS CIRCUITS

Although the administration of anticoagulant drugs continues to be necessary for the majority of hemodialysis procedures, research and development into less thrombogenic materials and improvements in the design of dialyzer circuits are being pursued with some success. Monitoring the anticoagulant status of the blood using appropriate tests is important. It allows the dose of anticoagulant to be minimized and helps ensure safety. The type and configuration of the extracorporeal blood circuit has implications for the choice and use of anticoagulants (Table 6–1).

Effects of Circuit Design and Operation

Modern dialyzer designs reduce clotting by better laminar-flow configurations and avoidance of stagnant areas in dialyzer headers, etc. Similar principles apply to clot and air traps and pumps inserts. Although "no-anticoagulant" protocols with saline-flush procedures are now feasible in many cases (see below), they cause clotting of the circuit in up to 9 percent of cases, even when used only in acutely ill patients, many of whom have impaired coagulation status.[2,110] Interestingly, the first signs of clotting occur much more often in the air trap than in the dialyzer itself.[110]

Thrombosis is potentiated by a high hematocrit, which is one of the potential complications of the use of rHuEPO,[64–66] though its direct effects on platelet stickiness are also implicated, as already described.[70] Large fractional filtration in hemofiltration circuits or during vigorous ultrafiltration increases the hematocrit locally and thereby promotes clotting. However, detailed studies now show that this is not just due to the rheological effects of hemoconcentration; the higher convective mass transfer of hemofiltration or hemodiafiltration, as compared to high-flux hemodialysis, is associated with increased procoagulatory activity, as shown by molecular markers in the coagulation cascade.[111]

Clotting in dialysis circuits is exacerbated when blood flow is slowed or interrupted, as occurs when vascular access or needle placement is inadequate.[110] Blood transfusion into the extracorporeal circuit upstream of the dialyzer is a common practice, but it may predispose to dialyzer clotting and certainly should be avoided during "no anticoagulant" procedures. A low dialysate pH can also exacerbate dialyzer clotting.[112]

Heparin Coating of Dialyzer Membranes

The dialysis membrane constitutes about 95 percent of the blood contact area of a typical hemodialysis circuit and is a major potential site for the initiation of clotting. Modern synthetic membranes are designed for improved biocompatibility, but no truly nonthrombogenic material has yet become available. Coating of dialyzer membranes with heparin and other anticoagulant molecules has been investigated for years, with limited success.[113–116] Attempts to covalently bond heparin to dialyzer surfaces by the Carmeda process have not been fruitful, though many other implantable vascular prosthetic materials can be modified in this way.[117]

However, attaching heparin to some dialyzer membranes by electrostatic bonding has proved feasible (see Table 6–1). Since heparin is polyanionic, it will adhere to the electropositive surface of Hemophan, rendering this dialyzer membrane less thrombogenic.[118] This can be achieved simply by running 1 L of a solution of heparin (20 IU/mL in saline) through the dialyzer for an hour before use. When dialysis is initiated, small amounts of heparin and a minor increase in aPTT are detectable in the blood at 15 minutes, but none is detectable at 1 hour or later. Clotting of the external circuit is less than when uncoated dialyzers are used with saline flushes. The systemic anticoagulant effect is minimal, much less than with low-dose heparin injec-

TABLE 6–1. CHOICE OF MODALITY AND CIRCUIT TYPE: IMPLICATIONS FOR ANTICOAGULATION

MODALITY CHOICE	IMPLICATION FOR ANTICOAGULATION (A/C)
Intermittent vs. continuous	
Intermittent (IHD, IHF)	• A/c risk to patient for only 3–4 h/day. • A/c needs only to prevent filter clotting for 3–4 h.
Slow daily (SLED)	• A/c risk to patient is present for 8+ h/day. • Slower blood flow requires good a/c.
Continuous (CRRT) (SCUF, CAVH, CAVHD, CAVHDF, CVVH, CVVHC, CVVHDF)	• A/c risk to patient is present 24 h/day. • Requirement for extended clot-free filter life implies need for more thorough a/c.
Circuit type (CRRT)	
Venovenous (CVVH, CVVHD, CVVHDF)	• Blood flow rate is slower than with IHD, therefore may require better a/c.
Arteriovenous (SCUF, CAVH, CAVHD, CAVHDF)	• Shorter tubing and better geometry of the blood flowpath may reduce a/c requirements. • Requires large-bore arterial line, which is at risk for hemorrhage or arterial embolus. • Unpredictable blood flow rate may worsen side effects (e.g., citrate)
Filtration vs. dialysis	
Convection only (IHF, SCUF, CAVH CVVH)	• Solute mass transfer less than with diffusive clearance, so may limit elimination of anticoagulant or its metabolites (e.g., citrate dose may need to be lower, or citrate accumulation is more likely).
Diffusion (IHD, CAVHD, CVVHD)	• All a/c methods feasible.
Diffusion plus convection (CAVHDF, CVVHDF)	• All a/c methods feasible.
Predilution replacement fluid (if used) (IHF, CAVH, CVVH, CAVHDF, CVVHDF)	• Reduces hemoconcentration within filter and may thus reduce a/c dose requirements.
Membrane type	
High-flux membranes	• Degree of biocompatibility affects thrombogenicity of membrane. • Higher porosity may allow removal of anticoagulant (e.g., r-hirudin) • Some high-flux membranes can be precoated with heparin (e.g., AN69-ST, Hemophan)
Unmodified cellulosic membranes	• Low flux of larger solutes promotes accumulation of some anticoagulants (e.g., r-hirudin)

KEY: IHD, intermittent hemodialysis; IHF, intermittent hemofiltration; SLED, sustained low-efficiency dialysis; CRRT, continuous renal replacement therapy; SCUF, slow continuous ultrafiltration; CAVH, continuous arteriovenous hemofiltration; CAVHD, continuous arteriovenous hemodialysis; CAVHDF, continuous arteriovenous hemodiafiltration; CVVH, continous venovenous hemofiltration; CVVHD, continuous venovenous hemodialysis; CVVHDF, continuous venovenous hemodiafiltration.

tion, and is thus more acceptable in patients at high risk of bleeding.[5]

Polyacrylonitrile membranes are electropositive; it has therefore proved possible to layer on an electronegative material and then place heparin on top of that. Thus the Hospal AN69 membrane can be treated with electronegative polyethyleneimine to create what is now designated the AN69-ST membrane. This will bind heparin when rinsed with heparinized saline before use, and the dialyzer can then be used without heparin infusion or saline flushing.[119] Twenty-eight chronic hemodialysis patients who were prone to bleeding were dialyzed repeatedly by this method, with circuit clotting in only 2 percent of runs, no bleeding complications, and a rise in systemic aPTT only transiently at 15 minutes into the run, again corresponding to some shedding of heparin from the membrane.[120]

Tests for Monitoring Anticoagulation

Heparin anticoagulation can be monitored by whole-blood clotting times, as by the Lee-White method, or more commonly by the whole-blood activated clotting time (WBACT), as with the activated clotting time (ACT) or Hemochron methods.[121] These use diatomaceous earth, kaolin, or glass particles to accelerate clotting in the test tube, which can be measured at the bedside in a desktop machine (normal ranges vary for different methods, e.g., 80 to 130 seconds).[122] The activated partial thromboplastin time (aPTT) measures thrombin inhibition and is useful for monitoring unfractionated heparin and argatroban. However, monitoring of low-molecular-weight (LMW) heparin and heparinoids like danaparoid requires measurement of anti-Xa activity, which is achieved in a chromogenic assay.[123,124]

Numerous other assays can be used for detailed assessment of anticoagulant requirements for hemodialysis.[123,125,126]

PHARMACOLOGY OF HEPARIN

Heparin remains the standard anticoagulant worldwide for intermittent hemodialysis (chronic or acute) and also for continuous hemodialysis (and hemofiltration), discussed later in this chapter. The pharmacology of heparin is discussed here. The pharmacology of other anticoagulants is discussed further on, in the sections describing their use.

Mechanisms of Action of Heparin

Heparin is a heterogeneous mixture of acidic glycosaminoglycans ranging in molecular weight from 3000 to 60,000 Da. Its main action is by binding to and activating antithrombin III, which then rapidly inhibits several of the serine proteases of the intrinsic coagulation system, particularly factors IXa and Xa and thrombin.[127] Factor Xa is inhibited by lower concentrations than is thrombin, which helps explain why small doses of heparin can prevent coagulation, whereas much larger doses are needed once thrombosis has commenced. Fractionation of heparin reveals that inhibition of factor Xa is maximal with LMW fractions, while inhibition of thrombin requires high-molecular-weight fractions (a minimum of 18 polysaccharide residues is needed). Factor Xa inhibition can prevent coagulation, whereas thrombin inhibition is more likely to cause bleeding. Thus LMW heparin (3000 to 7000 Da) should improve the therapeutic margin between desirable anticoagulation and unwanted hemorrhagic complications. Unfractionated heparin is standardized by its inhibition of clotting (1 USP unit will prevent clotting in 1 mL of recalcified sheep plasma for 1 hour). LMW heparin is standardized by its inhibition of factor Xa and is measured in anti–factor Xa units (aXa units).

Therapeutic blood concentrations of unfractionated heparin are of the order of 0.2 to 0.5 U/mL,[128] but the heparin requirement for anticoagulation in any individual is unpredictable, being higher in the presence of active thrombosis and altered by many other influences. In the intensive care unit, many patients with acute renal failure will have markedly decreased blood levels of antithrombin III (AT III) and thus will have some resistance to heparin. Replacing AT III has turned out to be of equivocal value in such cases.[129] Several commonly used drugs interfere with heparin (e.g., digitalis, antihistamines, tetracycline, nicotine, and ascorbic acid).[127] In hemodialysis patients, marked interpatient and intrapatient variability is seen in the dose of heparin needed, though the dosage and clearance of unfractionated heparin are not much altered by renal failure.[130] Unfractionated heparin has a half-life in uremic patients of between 40 and 120 minutes.[131,132] LMW heparins are eliminated more slowly than unfractionated heparin in hemodialysis patients, and dosing may therefore be more predictable.[134]

Heparin also activates heparin cofactor II, which inhibits thrombin but not Xa, though this effect is of minor importance. Heparin at high dosage also causes some inhibition of XIIa, XIa, and plasmin. However, it has no inhibitory effect on primary hemostasis by platelets; indeed, it has been known for a long time that heparin can cause platelet activation[134] and that platelet retention on dialyzer membranes is increased by heparin.[135] Elegant electron microscopy studies have shown that thrombus and cell adhesion to dialyzer membranes are worst with unfractionated heparin, somewhat less with LMW heparin, and almost negligible with citrate anticoagulation.[136]

Heparin-Induced Thrombocytopenia (HIT)

A feared complication of heparin is the severe form of heparin-induced thrombocytopenia. The mild form, type I HIT, may be nonimmunologic in origin and appears as early mild thrombocytopenia that resolves even while heparin use continues. The severe form, type II HIT, results from the interaction of a heparin-induced platelet antibody (HIPA) with a neoantigen on platelet factor 4 (PF4) that is revealed when PF4 binds heparin. Type II HIT can cause severe thrombotic and embolic complications, and thrombocytopenic bleeding.[137] Although LMW heparin may be less likely than unfractionated heparin to cause severe HIT, all forms of heparin have to be completely eliminated before the syndrome can begin to resolve.[138] Even some synthetic heparinoids can perpetuate the syndrome. Because thrombotic complications predominate, type II HIT must usually be treated with another anticoagulant (Table 6–2). The anticoagulants now preferred in the treatment of HIT are direct serine protease inhibitors such as recombinant hirudin (lepirudin) or, more often, argatroban, which has been approved specifically for this indication (see below).

Severe HIT is common in critically ill patients with acute renal failure. The diagnosis may be difficult to confirm because the antibody specificity may vary, and some commercial tests may miss some cases.[139] The overt syndrome is much less common in outpatients on maintenance hemodialysis, though cases of severe HIT are reported. Two illustrative cases were pediatric patients with end-stage renal disease (ESRD) who developed chest pain, respiratory distress, clotted dialyzers, and thrombocytopenia after several runs of heparin-anticoagulated hemodialysis; both continued to be ill after LMW heparin (dalteparin) was substituted. After they were switched to danaparoid, they got better quickly and remained well.[140] Up to 12 percent of hemodialysis patients have antibodies to the PF4-heparin complex but no overt thrombocytopenia.[141,142]

TABLE 6–2. CHOICE OF ANTICOAGULATION FOR DIALYTIC PROCEDURES IN PATIENTS WITH TYPE II HEPARIN-INDUCED THROMBOCYTOPENIA (HIT)

Anticoagulant	Mode of Action	Advantages	Disadvantages
Argatroban	Direct thrombin inhibitor (synthetic).	• Reduces HIT-induced thrombosis in the systemic circulation, as well as in the external blood circuit. • Half-life 46 min. Kinetics in dialysis similar to those of heparin (effect wears off in 2–4 h). • Can be monitored using aPTT.	• Prolonged half-life in liver failure greatly increases the risk of systemic bleeding in patients with liver failure. • No antidote except fresh frozen plasma (FFP) infusion.
Lepirudin (r-hirudin)	Direct thrombin inhibitor (recombinant form of hirudin, the naturally occurring anticoagulant in leeches).	• Reduces HIT-induced thrombosis in the systemic circulation as well as in the external blood circuit.	• Renally excreted. Long, unpredictable half-life in patients with renal failure. Drug may accumulate with prolonged risk of systemic bleeding. • No antidote except fresh frozen plasma (FFP) infusion. • Monitoring of hirudin blood levels or ecarin clotting time is recommended in addition to monitoring aPTT.
Citrate	Chelation of calcium impedes clotting in the external circuit only.	• Full-dose citrate will prevent HIT-induced thrombosis of the external blood circuit. • Does not increase the risk of systemic bleeding.	• Does not treat the risk of HIT-induced systemic thrombosis.
Saline flushes	Intermittent mechanical removal of clots from the external circuit.	• Does not increase the risk of systemic bleeding.	• May not be effective in preventing HIT-induced thrombosis of the external blood circuit. • Does not treat the risk of HIT-induced systemic thrombosis.
Danaparoid[a]	Mixture of three low-molecular-weight glycosaminoglycans; inhibits thrombin.	• Reduces HIT-induced thrombosis in the systemic circulation as well as in the external blood circuit.	• Renally excreted; long half-life in renal failure. • Monitoring requires measurement of anti–factor Xa (aXa) levels.

[a]No longer available in the United States.

Other Complications of Heparin in Dialysis Patients

Factors that place individual patients at high risk of bleeding during hemodialysis are well recognized,[42,50] but even patients who are not identifiable by these criteria may suffer an excess of serious hemorrhagic events when heparin is used.[2] Indeed, the risk of bleeding is the main motivating factor in the continued search for alternatives to heparin for hemodialysis in intensive care practice.

Problems with the chronic use of heparin for maintenance hemodialysis include hyperlipidemia associated with the release of lipoprotein lipase by heparin at each dialysis[143] and heparin-induced osteoporosis.[144] It has been suggested that both problems occur less with LMW heparin than with unfractionated heparin,[145,146] but evidence to the contrary has also been offered in each instance.[147,148] In a 44-month crossover study of 40 patients on chronic dialysis, lipid profiles were better during LMW heparin usage but bone studies were equivocal.[149] In other detailed studies during dialysis with LMW heparin compared to unfractionated heparin, circulating low-density-lipoprotein (LDL) subfractions improved with more buoyant and fewer highly atherogenic species[150] and lipid profiles were improved significantly,[145] including specifically in diabetic dialysis patients.[151] It is not

yet known whether avoidance of unfractionated heparin might improve the very high morbidity and mortality of atherosclerotic disease in hemodialyzed ESRD patients.

Among other complications of long-term heparin use for hemodialysis is aldosterone suppression, again with the possibility that the effect is less when patients use LMW heparin than unfractionated heparin.[152]

USE OF HEPARIN FOR INTERMITTENT HEMODIALYSIS

The use of heparin for anticoagulation for hemodialysis is convenient and inexpensive, and a large number of different administration strategies have been reported.[153] In chronic hemodialysis patients, dosing has to be sufficient to avoid clotting of vascular access sites and to minimize dialyzer circuit clotting, which can deplete red cells and reduce dialyzer clearances.[154] In cases of acute renal failure, the emphasis rather is on minimizing heparinization to avoid bleeding complications.[2] Thus, the needs of chronic hemodialysis patients can usually be met by standard systemic heparin methods, while critically ill or other high-risk patients are often candidates for lower-dose heparin and other alternative methods (Table 6–3).

TABLE 6–3. SELECTED REGIMENS FOR ANTICOAGULATION FOR ACUTE INTERMITTENT HEMODIALYSIS (IHD) IN CRITICALLY ILL PATIENTS

	Special Needs	Anticoagulation Regimen	Anticoagulation Monitoring
Low-dose heparin for IHD (and IHF)	• Prime circuit with heparinized saline.	• Initial heparin bolus of 11–22 U/kg (= 5–10 U/lb body weight), then infuse 22 U/kg/h (= 10 U/lb/h)[2] or • initial heparin bolus of 20–25 U/kg, then bolus 0–500 U every 30 min.[3,6]	• WBACT or aPTT every 30 to 60 min. Adjust heparin to keep at 1.5 times normal.
No anticoagulant (saline flush method) for IHD (and IHF)	• Prime circuit with heparinized saline (3000 units in 1 liter saline for 10–15 min), then flush out heparin with 1 liter saline.[6]	• Achieve maximum blood-flow rate immediately. • Flush circuit with 50–100 mL. Saline every 15–30 min.[5,6]	• WBACT or aPTT every 30–60 min. If < 1.2 times normal, consider 500-U bolus of heparin or monitor visually for venous chamber thrombus; if necessary, replace dialyzer and lines prophylactically.[108]
Citrate for IHD	• Zero calcium dialysate. Infuse calcium chloride (5%) at 30 min, then every hour: adjust calcium infusion rate if needed.[4] • Reduce dialysate sodium and bicarbonate content by setting "variable sodium" machine at minimum concentration,[4] or by making a special dialysate.[259]	• Citrate infusion as close as possible to where blood exits patient; start citrate just before blood pump is started. • Infuse 0.14 M (4%) trisodium citrate at 430 mL/h, or 0.2 molar at 300 mL/h.[4]	• Check ionized calcium every 30–60 min on postdialyzer blood; keep the value below 0.35 mmol/L by adjusting the citrate infusion rate.
Argatroban for IHD	• If liver impairment, reduce dosage to 25% of usual.	• Argatroban infusion prefilter at 0.12 mg/Kg/h[8] or • loading dose of 0.1 mg/kg, then infusion at 0.1–0.2 mg/kg/h.[203]	• Monitor aPTT hourly initially, less often on subsequent dialyses if stable. Adjust argatroban doses to keep aPTT 1.5–3.0 times normal.

KEY: WBACT, whole-blood activated clotting time; aPTT, activated partial thromboplastin time.

Standard Heparinization

Heparin for routine maintenance dialysis is best given as an intravenous loading dose followed by a continuous infusion into the predialyzer blood line. It is important to ensure that the initial bolus into the patient has 3 to 5 minutes to distribute in the circulation before blood is allowed to enter the dialyzer and that the heparin infusion solution fills the delivery line, so that the arrival of heparin at the blood does not have to wait for an initial saline prime to be cleared.[153] It is usually satisfactory to discontinue the heparin infusion 30 to 60 minutes before the end of dialysis so as to avoid excessive delay in obtaining hemostasis after the needles are withdrawn.[155] When an indwelling vascular catheter is being utilized, heparin infusion should be continued until the end of the dialysis.

The goal in outpatient hemodialysis is usually to maintain the WBACT at about two to three times the normal range.[132] Visual inspection of the extracorporeal circuit for clotting is also important. Also critical is visual monitoring for blood leaks from needle sites or line connections, which can be disastrous. Heparin dosage practice varies widely among different dialysis units.[156] Commonly the dialysis lines are primed with heparinized saline. The initial loading dose may often be 1500 to 3000 U (25 to 30 U/kg), and the

heparin infusion is given upstream of the dialyzer at perhaps 1000 to 2500 U/h (20 to 25 U/kg/h). There is wide variability in the dosage requirements among patients. That the dosing for a given individual and given dialyzer is appropriate can be ascertained by performing WBACT or other testing every hour during an initial dialysis. If the result is unsatisfactory, adjustments are made and reprofiling is repeated until satisfactory WBACTs are obtained. Confirmation thereafter can be done periodically (e.g., every 3 months).

Precise mathematical methods for modeling heparin dosage have been available since the 1970s[132] and can result in improved dialyzer clearances and increased delivered KT/V.[154] Heparin modeling techniques have been advanced by the application of neural-network computing.[157] Such work has also produced the following empirically derived formula to guide the initial dosing prescription:

$$Loading\ dose\ (units) = 1600 + [10 \times weight - 76]$$
$$- (300 \times Fd) - (100 \times Fs)$$

Continuous infusion rate (units/hours) = 1750

where **Weight** is body weight in kg, Fd indicates diabetic ($Fd = 1$) or nondiabetic ($Fd = 0$), Fs indicates smoker ($Fs = 1$) or nonsmoker ($Fs = 0$).

Using this starting formula, it took on average 3.2 readjustments to bring the ACT within 10 percent of the target, which then resulted in less dialyzer fiber-bundle volume loss and better preservation of dialyzer reuse.[158] Some patients are not predictable by this or any other current formula.

There is evidence that the use of repeated boluses instead of continuous infusion results in fluctuating levels of anticoagulation which may be less satisfactory.[159] Nevertheless, several excellent centers use a standardized single initial injection of heparin, with no further infusion or bolus, as a practical method of anticoagulation in short-duration high-efficiency dialysis (2.5 to 3.5 hours).[160]

Low-Dose or "Tight" Heparin

Low-dose or "tight" heparinization protocols have been used for 30 years for patients at increased risk of bleeding.[42,43,50,161–165] A protocol employing an initial heparin bolus of 5 to 10 U/lb body weight (11 to 22 U/kg) and a continuous infusion of 10 U/lb/h (22 U/kg/h), with variation to maintain the thrombin clotting time (TCT) at two to three times baseline, proved superior to regional heparinization in avoidance of bleeding and posed fewer technical difficulties.[50] Subsequently, in patients at high risk of bleeding, Swartz used loading doses between 11 and 22 U/kg based on a "heparin sensitivity" test performed before the dialysis, with a proportional heparin infusion rate and adjustments based on TCT results.[42] This proved satisfactory in all but actively bleeding patients. We have used a loading dose of 20 to 25 U/kg, with small hourly heparin supplements if needed to keep the WBACT in the extracorporeal circuit at only 1.5 times normal.[2] If the prehemodialysis WBACT is more than 1.2 times the upper limit of normal in a patient at high risk of bleeding, we will attempt to give no heparin, running the procedure as a "no anticoagulant" dialysis, but monitoring closely and adding small boluses of heparin (e.g., 500 U) if needed. A computer-controlled heparin infusion system has been described for hemodialysis that accurately maintains a desired ACT based on mathematical modeling and only a few actual measurements of the WBACT.[166] Limiting the dose of heparin in sustained low-efficiency dialysis (SLED) is of importance because the patient is exposed to anticoagulation for longer periods than with short intermittent dialysis procedures.[167] Constant exposure, as in continuous renal replacement therapy (CRRT) procedures, imposes the greatest rigor on the task of ensuring heparin dosing is no more than is needed (see below, under "Heparin for CRRT").

Regional Heparin with Protamine

Regional heparinization is now rarely used for intermittent hemodialysis. Heparin is infused into the arterial blood line proximal to the dialyzer, and protamine is infused into the return line at a rate designed to exactly neutralize the heparin.[50,168] Because protamine is catabolized more quickly than heparin, extra protamine may be needed a few hours after the dialysis has ended to avoid "heparin rebound." Regional heparinization is more difficult, less predictable, and no safer than low-dose systemic heparinization.[50] A variant of this approach has been to place a filter containing immobilized protamine in the venous return line.[169]

Low-Molecular-Weight (LMW) Heparins

Many different types of LMW heparin have been used for hemodialysis, including the following:

Enoxaparin (Lovonox, Clexane)[6,7,170,171]
Dalteparin (Fragmin)[6,138,172–175]
Nadroparin (Fraxiparine)[177–179]
Tinzaparin (Innohep, Logiparin)[151,180–183]
Reviparin (Clivarin)[179,184]

LMW heparins (LMWH) have half-lives about twice that of unfractionated heparin and are further prolonged in renal failure. Most dialysis regimens call for a single injection at the start of dialysis. A few give half the dose initially and the rest as an infusion.[172,173,185] Dosing depends on the brand used, the dialyzer used, and the target degree of anticoagulation, which varies in different centers. Representative results of dosing studies (single injection per dialysis) include the following:

Enoxaparin: 40 mg[6]; 0.70 mg/kg[7]; 0.68 mg/kg[171]
Dalteparin: 2500 IU[6]; 70 IU/kg[175]; 70 to 90 IU/kg[174,186]
Nadroparin: 70 IU/kg[179]; 150 to 200 IU/kg[177,187]
Tinzaparin: 3500 to 4500 IU[181]; 2186 IU average[183]; 2571, 3727, and 5020 IU for three different dialyzers[151]
Reviparin: 3300 IU[184]; 85 IU/kg[179]

Several studies comparing LMW heparins (LMWH) to unfractionated heparin (UFH) have been favorable with regard to freedom from clotting and absence of side effects.[171,181,185,188] A multicenter study in Japan reported significant shortening of the time to puncture site hemostasis after dialysis with LMWH compared to UFH.[173] Comparisons in patients at high risk of bleeding concluded that LMWH was at least as safe as low-dose UFH, in patients with acute renal failure[189] as well as in ESRD patients.[190] In contrast, other comparative studies reported that LMWH was associated with increased bleeding events or prolonged anticoagulation between dialyses.[7,170,182] There are also reports of an excessive incidence of serious bleeding complications in pre-ESRD patients treated with LMW heparins for other indications.[191] Thus it is unclear whether the known prolonged duration of the anticoagulant effect of LMW heparin is always safe.[192] Some outpatient dialysis units have used LMW heparin without measuring levels, and some reports comment on staff satisfaction because the drug requires only one injection and no monitoring. Periodic measurement of aXa levels adds safety, with recommended target levels being no more than 1.0 aXa U/mL for standard outpatient dialysis, and 0.2 to 0.4 aXa U/mL for patients at risk of hemorrhage.[185]

The evidence for improved lipid profiles in comparison with standard heparin, and other possible advantages of LMW heparin, has already been discussed (under "Other Complications of Heparin," above). Despite these advantages of LMW heparin, several factors appear to impede its more general use for hemodialysis. These factors probably include concern about bleeding, the cost of the drug in chronic dialysis, and good alternative anticoagulation choices for high-risk acute dialysis.

LMW heparins in a single dose have sufficed for dialysis of up to 5 hours in duration.[193] Their use has not yet been reported for sustained low-efficiency dialysis (SLED), but there is considerable experience of the use of LMW heparin infusion for CRRT (see further on).

Heparinoids

Danaparoid (Orgaran, Org 10172) has been discontinued in the United States; its availability elsewhere may be limited. It is a heparinoid consisting of a mixture of three nonheparin glycosaminoglycans of low molecular weight: heparan sulfate (84 percent), dermatan sulfate (12 percent), and chondroitin sulfate (4 percent). Its mode of action includes stimulation of heparin cofactor II to inhibit thrombin activity. Danaparoid has been applied successfully in both acute and chronic hemodialysis.[6,194,195] It does not cause platelet activation, and it can be used for dialysis during the treatment of heparin-induced thrombocytopenia.[196,197] It has also been used for CRRT, including during HIT (see below).

Dermatan sulfate has been studied as a single agent for anticoagulation for hemodialysis.[198–201] Sulodexide, which is a heparinoid consisting of a mixture of dermatan sulfate and LMW heparin, has also been investigated clinically as an anticoagulant for hemodialysis.[202] Depolymerized holothurian glycoaminoglycan (DHG) may soon be ready for phase I hemodialysis trials.[203]

NONHEPARIN METHODS OF ANTICOAGULATION AND THEIR USE FOR INTERMITTENT HEMODIALYSIS

Despite better dialysis and supportive care, mortality rates remain high in patients with acute renal failure. This is due largely to more frequent comorbid conditions and worsening severity of illness scores in the population of patients in whom dialysis is attempted. Many such patients are coagulopathic, which increases the chance of bleeding. Heparin, even when used regionally or in low dose, persists in the circulation and exacerbates the patient's risk of bleeding during hemodialysis. The direct thrombin inhibitors, including argatroban (a synthetic) and lepirudin (recombinant hirudin), similarly cause systemic anticoagulation, but they have a special niche because of their value in the management of heparin-induced thrombocytopenia (HIT). Other anticoagulants have short enough durations of action to be essentially regional in their action, meaning that they can be effective when given into the external circuit, with minimal spillover of the anticoagulant effect into the systemic circulation. Such drugs include prostanoids, which now are rarely used for dialysis, and serine protease inhibitors, such as nafamostat and aprotinin. Complete avoidance of any systemic anticoagulant effect can be achieved by "no anticoagulant" protocols, though at the risk of clotting of the external circuit. Citrate anticoagulation of the external circuit is also purely regional, causing no compromise of coagulation systems in the systemic blood; despite its complexities, citrate is being used increasingly for continuous therapies and for critically ill patients. The quest continues for an anticoagulation method that surpasses heparin in safety and rivals heparin in its ease of use.

Argatroban

Argatroban is a synthetic direct thrombin inhibitor that binds reversibly to the thrombin enzymatic site. Argatroban has been approved in the United States for the prophylaxis or treatment of thrombosis in patients with heparin-induced thrombocytopenia (HIT). Argatroban does not interact with PF4 and allows the syndrome to subside while providing needed anticoagulation. The pharmacokinetics of argatroban reveal a half-life of 46 minutes in normal subjects, and elimination is principally by hepatic metabolism. Though a small amount appears in the urine, the recommended dose for systemic use is the same in renally impaired patients as in normal patients (initially 2.0 µg/kg/min). In liver failure, a major reduction in dose is necessary (0.5 µg/kg/min).

Argatroban has been used successfully in several centers as an anticoagulant for hemodialysis circuits in patients with type II HIT. For intermittent hemodialysis, an infusion at the recommended dose rate (2 µg/kg/min = 0.12 mg/kg/h) has been found to be sufficient in most cases, reducing to 0.03 mg/kg/h for combined hepatic and renal failure.[8] Also satisfactory was a loading dose of 0.1 mg/kg followed by a continuous infusion of 0.1 to 0.2 mg/kg/h.[204] The earliest reports of argatroban (MD805) for intermittent hemodialysis employed higher doses, up to 0.49 mg/kg/h.[205,206] The degree of anticoagulation can be monitored readily, using the aPTT, with a target between 1.5 and 3.0 times the normal reference value (see Table 6–3). Its half-life is similar to that of unfractionated heparin in renal failure patents, so its effects disappear within 2 to 4 hours of discontinuing the drug. However, unlike heparin, there is no antidote to argatroban; its effects can be reversed only by infusing fresh frozen plasma. Thus caution and close monitoring are essential if any degree of hepatic dysfunction is suspected. Argatroban can be used also for continuous renal replacement therapies (CRRT) (see further on).

Lepirudin (Recombinant Hirudin)

Lepirudin is the recombinant form of hirudin, the anticoagulant from leeches that was used for experimental blood circuits before heparin became available around 1928.[207] Lepirudin is a direct thrombin inhibitor whose use for hemodialysis has been reported in several studies, both in acute renal failure and in chronic outpatient hemodialysis.[9,208–212] Like argatroban, lepirudin is especially useful in the management of type II HIT.

Lepirudin (r-hirudin) binds covalently with thrombin and does not need antithrombin III or other cofactors to be effective. It is cleared by the kidney[213]; in renal failure, it persists in the blood for at least 48 hours. Its long half-life allows lepirudin to be given as a single bolus at the start of each hemodialysis, usually in a dose of 0.08 to 0.17 mg/kg.[9,210–212] Its rate of disappearance depends on what type of dialyzer is employed, since it is cleared by some high-flux membranes but not others.[214,215] In a chronic dialysis study, functionally anephric patients cleared r-hirudin much more slowly than those with some residual renal function, and they needed less of the drug at subsequent dialyses.[9] The persistence of lepirudin is unpredictable also because 40 percent of patients develop antihirudin antibodies, which bind to lepirudin and prolong its presence in the bloodstream.[216]

The anticoagulant effect of lepirudin can be measured by the aPTT. However, because of the potential for accumulation, it is recommended in acute cases that r-hirudin plasma levels or the ecarin clotting time also be monitored.[217] Serious bleeding has been reported after repeated dialyses using lepirudin.[218] As with other direct thrombin inhibitors, reversal of the anticoagulant effects of lepirudin is difficult and is best approached by administration of fresh frozen plasma. Both lepirudin and argatroban have proven very valuable in the management of type II HIT. Lepirudin may be the better choice when there is concomitant liver failure, but lepirudin is more likely than argatroban to accumulate to troublesome levels in other severely ill patients. Lepirudin has been used successfully for CRRT (see further on).

A PEG (polyethylene glycol)-hirudin conjugate has been studied in 20 chronic hemodialysis patients.[219] PEG-hirudin is larger than regular r-hirudin (lepirudin), and does not pass through high-flux dialyzer membranes. It has an even longer half-life than lepirudin, such that the patient remains anticoagulated between dialyses. The merits and risks of such a strategy for maintenance dialysis need to be evaluated, though in this pilot study no serious bleeding events were encountered.

Prostanoids

Prostacyclin (PGI_2, epoprostenol) is a short-lived, powerful inhibitor of platelet aggregation. It can be used as the sole anticoagulant for hemodialysis: dosing is in the range of 2 to 5 ng/kg/min. It compares favorably with heparin with regard to hemorrhagic risk.[220–226] However, in a prospective study, activation of coagulation factors by a polysulfone dialyzer was worse with prostacyclin than with unfractionated heparin or LMW heparin.[227] Freedom from circuit clotting has usually been adequate, but circuit patency may be compromised if the dose is reduced, which is sometimes necessary because prostacyclin is vasodilatory and can cause hemodynamic instability. This risk may be avoided if lower doses are used in combination with heparin, using the heparin as a prostacyclin-sparing agent and vice versa.[228] Also, the combination of LMW heparin (nadroparin) and prostacyclin has been tried and has been compared prospectively to unfractionated heparin as the sole anticoagulant.[229] In this study, dialyzer efficiency, coagulation parameters, circuit patency, and hemodynamic stability were similar by the two methods. The use of prostanoids for hemodialytic procedures is uncommon unless other anticoagulant methods have failed[3] or in occasional cases where prostacyclin is indicated for other purposes, such as treatment of the vasoconstriction of scleroderma crisis (A. Davenport, personal communication).

Synthetic prostacyclin analogues have also been studied for hemodialysis.[230,231] Iloprost can be used in a dose of 0.5 to 1.5 ng/kg/min. Iloprost elimination is four times slower in dialysis patients than in normal.[232] Both epoprostenol and iloprost have been used for CRRT (see further on).

Nafamostat

Synthetic serine protease inhibitors, first gabexate mesylate[232] and now nafamostat mesylate,[10,234–236] have been developed in Japan. Both agents block several steps of coagulation and also complement activation. The biological half-life of nafamostat is approximately 8 minutes, so for anticoagulation of hemodialysis systems it is given as an infusion into the external circuit. The circuit may be primed with 50 mg nafamostat in 500 mL saline, and the infusion rate is often of the order of 0.5 mg/kg/h.[237] Nafamostat induces regional anticoagulation with good circuit longevity.[233,234] Its anticoagulant effects can be quantitated by the WBACT, though monitoring in the systemic blood or in the external circuit is not routinely needed. In contrast to heparin, clotting times in the systemic blood were not increased in a study of 107 patients with increased risk of bleeding; exacerbation of bleeding occurred with only 3.7

percent of dialyses, and 92 percent of active bleeding cases (Swartz group 1[50]) were dialyzed without increasing the bleeding.[10] In one reported case, conversion from heparin to nafamostat after the patient developed HIT did not completely resolve the thrombocytopenia or thrombus formation in the dialysis system until aspirin was also added.[238] Concerns with nafamostat include occasional reports of allergic reactions,[235,239,240] hypereosinophilic syndrome,[241] agranulocytosis,[242] and adsorption of the drug onto polyacrilonitrile membranes.[243] In patients with renal function nafamostat can cause hyperkalemia by aldosterone suppression, but direct inhibition of a Na-K ATPase-dependent pathway has also been implicated.[244] Nafamostat is in use in Japan routinely as an anticoagulant for intermittent hemodialysis and for CRRT (see further on).

"No Anticoagulant" Hemodialysis

The nonthrombogenic dialyzer has been an elusive "holy grail" for decades. Improved design characteristics and heparin binding to membranes have been reviewed above (under "Heparin Coating of Dialyzer Membranes"). Apart from these few, the differences between various dialyzers in terms of their thrombogenicity have not made major inroads on the general problem of anticoagulation techniques.[114] Nevertheless, the number of patients with acute renal failure who can be dialyzed without anticoagulation is burgeoning, largely because of the increasing severity of illness in such patients, with attendant thrombocytopenia and other coagulopathies. Hemodialysis with no anticoagulant is being used extensively and successfully.[2,4,44,45,110,153,245–248] The best method was evolved by Sanders et al.[44] and Schwab et al.[45] It includes priming of the circuit with heparinized saline, ensuring high blood flow rates immediately at the start of dialysis and throughout the procedure, and flushing the dialyzer every 15 minutes with 100 mL of 0.9 percent saline to detect and to deter partial clotting. However, not all protocols use saline flushes.[246] Visible signs of clotting and circuit pressures are monitored closely. WBACT results usually shorten during this procedure and may warn of imminent thrombosis.[110] Blood transfusion (and probably intradialytic parenteral nutrition) should not be given through the extracorporeal circuit because this may potentiate clotting.[45] Clotting sufficient to interrupt the treatment occurs in 2 to 9 percent of treatments.[2,45,46,110] Prophylactic conversion to heparinization or to a new dialyzer circuit accounts for an additional 7 percent to as much as 47 percent of procedures.[45,110] It is also possible to convert to citrate anticoagulation if clotting occurs and if a risk of bleeding is still present. Indeed, it is reasonable to avoid the "no anticoagulant/saline flush" method at the outset if the chances of clotting the dialyzer seem high (for instance, if the predialysis WBACT is short). Other disadvantages of this procedure are minor, but include the large saline flush volume and the higher ultrafiltration rate this imposes. Nevertheless, the "no anticoagulant" hemodialysis method is effective, safe, and widely applicable.

Citrate-Anticoagulated Hemodialysis

Citrate has been used for over 40 years to anticoagulate hemodialysis systems.[249] Citrate works by chelating calcium, which is a necessary cofactor for many of the steps of the coagulation cascade (see Fig. 6–1). In citrate-anticoagulated hemodialysis, the ionized calcium levels in the extracorporeal blood fall to about 0.30 mmol, which is low enough to arrest anticoagulation completely (normal blood ionized calcium levels are 1.1 to 1.3 mmol). When blood from the external circuit returns and mixes with central venous blood, the ionized calcium concentration is restored, and the anticoagulant effect is immediately abolished. Thus, citrate anticoagulation is necessarily regional, and it has no effect on systemic hemostasis.[250]

Methods for citrate anticoagulation for intermittent hemodialysis use either commercially available 4 percent trisodium citrate solution or ACD-A (acid citrate dextrose A solution, USP) as an infusion upstream from the dialyzer. If desired, the volume of the citrate infusion can be reduced by using hypertonic citrate instead. The citrate infusion is usually given through a side port or stopcock as close as possible to the point where the blood exits the patient, so that the proximal section of the circuit that is not anticoagulated is as short as possible. The best strategy is to use a dialysate with zero calcium and to infuse a dilute calcium solution into the blood returning to the patient to restore calcium balance.[2,47,48,251–253] Efforts in the mid-1980s to "retain simplicity" by using a dialysate that contained calcium (2.5 or 3.0 meq/L), with no calcium infusion[46,254,255] failed to ensure adequate restoration of ionized calcium levels in the systemic blood.[250] Cardiac arrests occurred[275] and serious patient injury ensued, but only when the system employed a dialysate that contained calcium. This lesson must be remembered. Maintaining adequate ionized calcium levels in the systemic circulation is absolutely essential, requires monitoring, and is easier to achieve if citrate dosing is minimized by eliminating calcium from the dialysate. Because the dialyzer membrane is the largest thrombogenic surface that has to be anticoagulated, it makes no sense to be unwittingly adding ionized calcium at that point, which occurs by diffusion if the dialysate contains calcium. Anticoagulation at the blood-membrane interface can be maintained best if there is sufficient excess citrate to chelate the calcium as it diffuses into the blood from the dialysate, which defeats the intent of restoring ionized calcium levels and increases the total dose of citrate needed. Sufficient citrate can be given in the face of a calcium-containing dialysate to effect adequate anticoagulation, and calcium levels can be monitored diligently for patient safety,[257] but the dose of citrate is higher than would otherwise be necessary. Although the risks may not be overt in a given study, if citrate is not metabolized adequately, some of the calcium in the systemic blood remains chelated, i.e., unavailable for the myriad metabolic processes for which calcium ions are necessary. Another undesired consequence results from the metabolism of excess trisodium citrate to sodium bicarbonate, which can lead to hypernatremia and alkalosis.[258] Alkalosis, in turn, exacerbates the hypocalcemia (ionized calcium levels drop as pH rises because of increased calcium binding to proteins).

Accordingly, safety and efficacy are served by employing a calcium-free dialysate and by paying close attention to ionized calcium levels. For intermittent hemodialysis using standard dialysis machines, the calcium infusion to the returning venous line can be 5 percent calcium chloride. (This can be given only while the blood pump is running and blood is flowing in the return line, because calcium solutions will severely damage veins if blood flow is insufficient to rapidly dilute the calcium solution. Alternatively, as is used with CRRT, a more dilute calcium solution can be given separately from the dialysis circuit into a deeply placed central vein catheter, where blood flow is always maintained.)

In the method used at the University of California, San Diego (UCSD) for intermittent hemodialysis (IHD), the initial infusion rate for 5 percent calcium chloride is 30 mL/h, subsequently adjusted to maintain a normal ionized calcium level in the systemic blood (sampled before the dialysis commences, again 30 minutes into dialysis, and then hourly, and drawn from a vein in an uninvolved limb or from an arterial line). If the citrate anticoagulant in use is 4 percent trisodium citrate solution (0.14 mol/L), then the starting dose is 430 mL/h (or proportionately less volume for a more concentrated solution). This is designed for a blood flow rate between 200 and 250 mL/min, since it is the ratio of citrate to incoming blood that determines the citrate concentration. The popular trend to higher blood flow rates is to be resisted in this application. Blood samples obtained from the extracorporeal circuit immediately after the dialyzer are assayed for ionized calcium (usually results can be obtained most quickly in a blood-gas laboratory). Ionized calcium levels are kept below 0.35 mmol by adjustment of the citrate infusion rate if needed. The sodium and bicarbonate load arising from the trisodium citrate infusion can be accommodated by reducing the dialysate concentrations of sodium and bicarbonate. In IHD, this is easily achieved by using a variable-sodium machine set at its lowest sodium level.[4] A logical but more labor-intensive method is to eliminate magnesium as well as calcium from the dialysate, with both being reinfused in the return line.[259,260] Since this requires a custom-made dialysate, a lower dialysate bicarbonate content can also be selected, e.g., 25 mmol/L[259] (see Table 6–3). Note that citrate anticoagulation cannot be used with the "Redy" dialysate regeneration system because citrate disrupts the urease layer.[261] Also note that citrate solu-

tions made up in the hospital pharmacy should be sterilized in polypropylene bottles, because with glass bottles aluminum contamination can occur.[260]

Citrate dialysis is suitable for acute or long-term use.[48,262] It has fulfilled its promise by reducing hemorrhagic complications in high-risk patients,[2,47,250,251,253] including in comparison to low-dose (unfractionated) heparin in a randomized trial.[46] In chronic dialysis patients, randomized trials comparing citrate to LMW heparins showed that the risk of bleeding was less with citrate than with nadroparin,[260] and that postdialysis bleeding at needle sites was shorter with citrate than with dalteparin.[263] Citrate's excellent ability to prevent clotting in the external blood circuit has been displayed by electron micrographs that show almost no cells or thrombus in hollow fiber dialyzers after citrate use, compared to extensive deposition with regular heparin and LMW heparin.[136] Citrate has also been successful in long term use in a patient with type II HIT,[264] as well as in patients with long-term bleeding risk. Experience with long-term dialysis patients shows that the required dose of citrate and calcium tends to be the same at every succeeding dialysis. Once this has been established for an individual, the extensive testing protocol can be simplified, though the systemic blood ionized calcium level near the end of dialysis should be measured at every dialysis; if it is not in the normal range, action should be taken then and arrangements made for a full reassessment at the next dialysis. Citrate toxicity due to failure to adequately metabolize citrate is rarely a clinical problem with intermittent hemodialysis by this protocol, largely because the duration of dialysis is only a few hours and any residual citrate can be metabolized after the procedure is completed. This problem is of greater concern in CRRT, and is discussed further on (under "Citrate for CRRT").

Other Anticoagulants

Defibrotide is a polydesoxyribonucleotide extract that combines antithrombotic and profibrinolytic effects with stimulation of endogenous prostacyclin; it has been investigated as an anticoagulant in chronic hemodialysis.[265,266] Several other agents have undergone limited assessment for hemodialysis.

ANTICOAGULATION FOR CONTINUOUS RENAL REPLACEMENT THERAPY (CRRT)

The terminology and abbreviations for CRRT modalities are listed in Table 6–1. CRRT circuits can be either arteriovenous (unpumped) or venovenous (pumped), the latter now being more common. The clearance technique may be purely convective (hemofiltration), principally diffusive (hemodialysis), or a combination of the two (hemodiafiltration). Differences between these techniques have implications for the choice and use of some anticoagulants (see Table 6–1). Often the choice of anticoagulant may be dictated by local expertise, but cases involving difficult complications, particularly unrelenting hemorrhage and HIT, may warrant embarking on less familiar anticoagulation strategies. Most of the methods of anticoagulation described for intermittent hemodialysis have been applied to CRRT. For each of the anticoagulants discussed below, the pharmacology and clinical attributes have already been addressed in preceding sections of this chapter. The reader is directed to those earlier sections for precautionary information.

Heparin for CRRT

Heparin remains the agent of choice in many centers for all CRRT procedures, including hemofiltration,[267–271] hemodialysis,[272] and hemodiafiltration.[49,273,274] A low-dose approach is standard because the usual candidate is a patient in the intensive care unit, with multiple medical problems and some increased risk of bleeding. A typical procedure commences with priming the circuit with heparinized saline (2400 to 10,000 U in 2 L). Published low-dose regimens then proceed with an average loading dose of 5 to 15

U/kg, and then an infusion given prefilter at a rate of 3 to 15 U/kg/h. Details are shown in Table 6–4. Monitoring with WBACT or aPTT is needed to ensure adequate but not excessive anticoagulation. Smaller children need a relatively larger dose of heparin for this purpose.[275]

Comparative data (as mentioned in each of the following sections) suggest that the incidence of bleeding complications in CRRT is greatest with low-dose systemic heparin, slightly lower with regional heparin, still lower with prostacyclin or LMW heparin, and least with no-anticoagulant/saline flush systems or citrate anticoagulation.[2,4,49,276–279] Filter patency is worst with no anticoagulant/saline flush systems, best with citrate, and intermediate with heparin. Daily platelet counts should be obtained to detect the development of heparin-induced thrombocytopenia (HIT).

Regional Heparin/Protamine for CRRT

Regional heparinization with protamine neutralization has not been used much for IHD since 1979, when Swartz et al. showed it to be inferior to low-dose heparin.[50] However, its use in CRRT procedures has been pursued successfully in the United States by Kaplan and others.[280] In Australia, Bel-

TABLE 6–4. SELECTED REGIMENS FOR ANTICOAGULATION FOR CRRT

	Special Needs	Anticoagulation Regimen	Anticoagulation Monitoring
Low-dose heparin (suitable for all CRRT modalities)[4,153]	• Prime circuit with heparinized saline (2400–10,000 U in 2 L).	• Initial heparin bolus of 5–10 U/kg, then infuse 5–10 U/kg/h, adjust as needed (range 3–15 U/kg/h).	• WBACT or aPTT initially every hour, then every 2–4 h on postdialyzer blood. Adjust heparin infusion rate to maintain in range of 1.5–2.0 times normal.
Citrate for CVVHDF[3,4,11]	• Special dialysate (no calcium or alkali; Na 117, K 4, Mg 1.5, Cl 122.5 mmol/L; dextrose 0.1– 0.5%) run at 1000 mL/h. • Calcium solution (8 g CaCl$_2$ added to 1 L saline = 1meq/10 mL.) infused to separate central venous line, initially at 40–45 mL/h. • Check ioCa of systemic blood at start, at 2 h, then every 4–12 h when stable. • Adjust calcium infusion to maintain systemic ioCa at 1.0 to 1.2 mmol/L.	• Infusion of 4% trisodium citrate (0.14 M) into blood line close to patient. Start at 170 mL/h, adjust rate to maintain postfilter ioCa between 0.25 and 0.30 mmol/L.	• Check ioCa in postfilter blood at start, at 2 h, then every 4–12 h when stable. • Check electrolytes, ABG, and total blood calcium at start, at 2 h, then every 12 h. • Modify citrate dosing if total calcium or anion gap is high (see text).
Citrate for CVVH[296]	• Prime circuit with heparinized saline (10,000 U in 2 Ls) • Calcium solution (20 g calcium gluconate in 1 L 5% dextrose) infused through separate line at 60 mL/h. • Check ioCa of systemic blood every 6 h, or more often if indicated. • Adjust calcium infusion by sliding scale based on systemic ioCa results (target 1.0–1.3 mmol/L).	• Pre filter replacement solution (Na$_3$ citrate 13.3, NaCl 100, Mg 1.5 mmol/l, and dextrose 0.2%), rate determined by fluid-balance requirements. • Flush filter with saline every 4 h.	• Check electrolytes and ABG every 6–12 h, more often if indicated. • Check total blood calcium every 24 h. • Modify regimen if systemic blood ioCa is low or total blood calcium is high (see text).

KEY: WBACT, whole-blood activated clotting time; aPTT, activated partial thromboplastin time; ABG, arterial blood gases; ioCa = ionized calcium.

lomo et al. compared it to systemic low-dose heparin and reported better filter life and possibly less hemorrhage with regional heparin.[277]

LMW Heparin for CRRT

LMW heparins have been used for two decades to anticoagulate CRRT circuits.[278,281–284] Enoxaparin can be given as a loading dose of 40 mg followed by 10 to 40 mg/h,[283] and dalteparin as a loading dose of 20 U/kg and then 10 U/kg/h.[292] In a prospective randomized controlled trial using continuous venovenous hemodialysis (CVVHDF), this fixed dosage protocol using dalteparin gave comparable results to adjusted-dose unfractionated heparin (UFH) with regard to filter life, bleeding episodes, and the incidence of HIT.[278] The extra cost of the LMW heparin method thus provided no advantage, leading the investigators to return to UFH as their standard anticoagulant for CRRT. In a study comparing two levels of dosing of dalteparin for continuous venovenous hemodiafiltration (CVVHD), all three patients in the high-dose arm of the study had mild bleeding, sufficient to discontinue in one; all seven in the low-dose arm had marked thrombus formation in the external circuit, and in two it clotted off; one patient in this group had mild bleeding.[284] Thus LMW heparin appears to offer no advantage over regular unfractionated heparin in managing the problems of clotting and bleeding in critically ill patients undergo CRRT.

Heparinoids for CRRT

Danaparoid has been used in both continuous venovenous hemofiltration (CVVH) and CVVHD, especially in severely ill patients with HIT.[285] An initial bolus of 750 U of danaparoid followed by infusion of 50 to 150 U/h has been effective, aiming for anti-Xa levels around 0.4 +/- 0.2 aXa U/mL.[195] Danaparoid has been withdrawn from use in the United States.

Argatroban for CRRT

Argatroban is especially useful in patients with HIT. Argatroban anticoagulates both the external circuit and the patient's systemic blood, and allows the HIT syndrome to subside. Argatroban has been used in several centers for CRRT. One protocol, that gave good clot-free filter duration in 11 patients undergoing CVVH, targeted an aPTT ratio of 1.8 to 2.0, and used a loading dose of 0.1 mg/kg and a maintenance infusion of 0.054 to 0.06 mg/kg/h (0.9 to 1.0 µg/kg/min).[286] Great caution is needed with hepatic failure patients, who require only about 25 percent of the usual dose.

Lepirudin (r-Hirudin) for CRRT

Lepirudin (recombinant hirudin) has been used in CVVH and in CVVHD.[287] In one case of type II HIT, lepirudin was successful for CVVH after citrate and danaparoid had both

failed due to recurrent clotting.[287] A loading dose of 0.01 mg/kg has been used, and then either intermittent boluses or an infusion starting at 0.005 to 0.01 mg/kg/h to keep the aPTT 1.5 to 2.0 times normal. Dosing is notoriously unpredictable, and it is recommended that monitoring of aPTT be supplemented by measurements of r-hirudin plasma levels or the ecarin clotting time (see above).

Prostanoids for CRRT

Prostacyclin (epoprostenol) has been used successfully for CRRT.[292] Dosing is 2 to 5 ng/kg/min, the same as for intermittent dialysis. As discussed above (see earlier discussion of prostanoids), vasodilatation and consequent hypotension may be problems. Iloprost has also been given for CRRT.[288]

Nafamostat for CRRT

Nafamostat has been used in Japan since 1990 for anticoagulation of CRRT circuits, including CVVH and CVVHDF.[237,289–292] Dosing typically includes priming the circuit with 50 mg nafamostat in 500 mL saline, then a continuous infusion of 0.5 mg/kg/h. Filter patency was good for at least 24 hours, after which clotting increasingly necessitated changing of the circuit.[237] Dosing sufficient to cause a measurable increase in systemic blood ACT is recommended, keeping the ACT at the inlet of the circuit (before the point of nafamostat infusion) at or above 130 seconds. Measuring at this site produced less random variation in results than measuring ACT in the external circuit, but the postfilter sampling site had to have an ACT of at least 150 seconds for filter patency to be adequate.[237] Thus nafamostat use does produce a measurable albeit small impairment in the coagulability of the blood in the systemic circulation. Indeed, measurement of nafamostat blood levels in CVVHDF has shown evidence of accumulation over a 24-hour period.[291] Bleeding events have not been excessive in IHD usage (see section above), but there is insufficient data for CRRT.

No-Anticoagulant (Saline-Flush Protocol) for CRRT

CRRT using no-anticoagulant (saline-flush protocol) has achieved a useful duration of filter patency in some centers,[293] but others find filter clotting to be an obstinate problem, making attempts at no-anticoagulant procedures worthwhile only in patients with the worst coagulopathies.[2,267]

Citrate for CRRT

Citrate anticoagulation for CRRT was first performed in 1989,[3,294] using CAVHDF. The same method was then applied to CVVHDF,[295] and in that form it has gained widespread acceptance. Successful application of citrate anticoagulation to CVVH (without a dialysate) was achieved in 1999,[296] and has also become established. With various modifications, citrate anticoagulated CRRT is now in use in numerous tertiary care hospitals around the world.[4,11,279,295–307]

Because citrate anticoagulates only the external circuit, it is ideal for patients at high risk of bleeding. It is being applied increasingly to CCRT in critically ill patients in the intensive care setting. The technique does not incur additional risk for the patient unless the ionized calcium or magnesium levels in the systemic blood are allowed to fall below the safe range. This can happen if they are not adequately replenished, or if citrate accumulation occurs. The key to safety is diligent monitoring of ionized calcium levels in the systemic circulation and appropriate management when variations occur. The principles of citrate chelation for anticoagulation of external blood circuits are reviewed above (in the section on citrate use in IHD). Details of two prototype methods, for CVVHDF[4] and CVVH[296] respectively, are shown in Table 6–4. CVVHDF methods,[4,11,298–307] which include diffusive clearance by a dialysate, in general can clear more citrate and therefore can tolerate higher citrate concentrations in the external circuit than the CVVH methods with only convective clearance.[279,296,297] Nevertheless filter patency is excellent with all citrate methods, better than for any other anticoagulant.[136] In a prospective randomized study in Belgium, citrate CVVH achieved filter patency for 70 hours (median duration), vs. 40 hours for CVVH using heparin.[279] Transfusion requirements were five times higher with heparin CVVH compared to citrate CVVH; one major hemorrhage occurred during heparin CVVH and one case of alkalosis with citrate CVVH. Such differences in filter patency and bleeding events had been seen previously in our retrospective comparison of heparin continuous arteriovenous hemodiafiltration (CAVHDF) vs. citrate CAVHDF in San Diego.[2] Alkalosis occurred in some cases in our UCSD experience with citrate CAVHDF, but in the decade since converting to citrate CVVHDF (pumped venovenous circuit), alkalosis is no longer encountered. This difference reflects the fact that blood flow rates in arteriovenous circuits are inherently unstable and usually not measurable, with diminished dialyzer clearance of citrate and of bicarbonate when blood flow falters.

Control of acid-base and electrolyte homeostasis with citrate CRRT has been refined. However, occasional patients fail to metabolize citrate adequately. This usually occurs when a combination of risk factors coincide, such as excessive citrate dosing (e.g., fresh frozen plasma as well as citrate CRRT), reduced metabolism (liver failure, or reduced or underperfused muscle mass), and impaired external clearance (partial filter clotting, etc.). Citrate accumulation in the patient then generates a citrate buffer system that resists attempts to increase ionized calcium concentrations to normal in the patient or to reduce them in the external circuit. The usual sliding scales make matters worse be-

cause they call for more calcium administration for low systemic ionized calcium levels and more citrate to the external circuit if postfilter ionized calciums are not low enough. Citrate accumulation can be recognized as a rising total calcium when systemic ionized calcium is falling (the "calcium gap"), usually with a rising anion gap at the same time. When this happens, it is necessary to stop or reduce citrate dosing until metabolic clearing occurs; during this time, systemic ionized calcium levels should be monitored frequently and calcium supplemented as needed.[4,308] Although its use has been published and was apparently successful,[309] utilization of a dialysate that contains calcium for CVVHDF is not favored by this author for the reasons outlined earlier in the discussion of citrate IHD.

The first-ever use of citrate CRRT was in a postoperative man with severe type II HIT who recovered and survived long term[296]; other successfully treated HIT cases are described.[310] Citrate CRRT is also very helpful in treating severe lactic acidosis.[311] It can be continued during surgical or other procedures,[2,3] and at UCSD, it is is frequently used during liver transplant operations. However, the principal importance of citrate-anticoagulated CRRT remains in preserving hemostatic competency in critically ill patients in the intensive care unit while allowing them uninterrupted dialytic therapy. Its complexity remains an impediment to wider usage. Citrate anticoagulated CRRT requires a well-trained nursing staff and well-trained nephrologists. Also, the need for nonstandard electrolyte solutions keeps hospital pharmacists busy. Several ingenious modifications have been developed to take advantage of existing fluid formulations,[297,304,307,312] but there is a need for standardization and commercial availability of the requisite dialysates and infusates.

REFERENCES

1. Lohr JW, Schwab SJ. Minimizing hemorrhagic complications in dialysis patients. *J Am Soc Nephrol* 1991;2:961–975.
2. Ward DM, Mehta RL. Extracorporeal management of acute renal failure patients at high risk of bleeding. *Kidney Int* 1993;43(suppl 41):S237–S244.
3. Mehta RL, McDonald BR, Aguilar MM, Ward DM. Regional citrate anticoagulation for continuous arteriovenous hemodialysis in critically ill patients. *Kidney Int* 1990; 38: 976–981.
4. Ward DM: The approach to anticoagulation in patients treated with extracorporeal therapy in the intensive care unit. *Adv Renal Replace Ther* 1997;4:160–173.
5. Lee KB, Kim B, Lee YH, et al. Hemodialysis using heparin-bound Hemophan in patients at risk of bleeding. *Nephron Clin Pract* 2004;97:c5–c10.
6. Polkinghorne KR, McMahon LP, Becker GJ. Pharmacokinetic studies of dalteparin (Fragmin), enoxaparin (Clexane),

and danaparoid sodium (Orgaran) in stable chronic hemodialysis patients. *Am J Kidney Dis* 2002;40:990–995.

7. Saltissi D, Morgan C, Westhuyzen J, Healy H. Comparison of low-molecular-weight heparin (enoxaparin sodium) and standard unfractionated heparin for haemodialysis anticoagulation. *Nephrol Dial Transplant* 1999;14:2698–2703.

8. Reddy BV. Argatroban use in dialysis patients. *Semin Dial* 2004;17:73.

9. Vanholder R, Camez A, Veys N, et al. Pharmacokinetics of recombinant hirudin in hemodialyzed end-stage renal failure patients. *Thromb Haemost* 1997;77:650–655.

10. Akizawa T, Koshikawa S, Ota K, et al. Nafamostat mesilate: a regional anticoagulant for hemodialysis in patients at high risk for bleeding. *Nephron* 1993;64:376–381.

11. Swartz R, Pasko D, O'Toole J, Starmann B. Improving the delivery of continuous renal replacement therapy using regional citrate anticoagulation. *Clin Nephrol* 2004;61: 134–143.

12. Jubelirer SJ. Hemostatic abnormalities in renal disease. *Am J Kidney Dis* 1985;5:219–225.

13. Vaziri ND, Toohey J, Paule P, et al. Coagulation abnormalities in patients with end-state renal disease treated with hemodialysis. *Int J Artif Organs* 1984;7:323–326.

14. Eknoyan G, Wacksman SJ, Glueck HI, et al. Platelet functions in renal failure. *N Engl J Med* 1969;280:677–681.

15. Steiner RW, Coggins C, Carvaiho ACA. Bleeding time in uremia: a useful test to assess clinical bleeding. *Am J Hematol* 1979;7:l07–l17.

16. Joist JH, Remuzzi G, Mannucci PM. Abnormal bleeding and thrombosis in renal disease. In: Colman RW, Hirsh J, Marder WJ, Salzman EW, eds. *Hemostasis and Thrombosis*, 3d ed. Philadelphia: Lippincott, 1993:921–935.

17. Livio M, Benigni A, Remuzzi G. Coagulation abnormalities in uremia. *Semin Nephrol* 1985;5:8.

18. Bazilinski N, Shayky M, Dunea G, et al. Inhibition of platelet function by uremic middle molecules. *Nephron* 1985;40:423–428.

19. Diminno G, Martinez J, McKean M-L, et al. Platelet dysfunction in uremia: multifaceted defect partially corrected by dialysis. *Am J Med* 1985;79:552–559.

20. Benigni A, Livio M, Dodesini P, et al. Inhibition of human platelet aggregation by parathyroid hormone: is cyclic AMP implicated? *Am J Nephrol* 1985;5:243–247.

21. Docci D, Turci F, Delvecchio C, et al. Lack of evidence for the role of secondary hyperparathyroidism in the pathogenesis of uremic thrombocytopathy. *Nephron* 1986;43:28–32.

22. Remuzzi G, Perico N, Zoja C, et al. Role of endothelium-derived nitric oxide in the bleeding tendency of uremia. *J Clin Invest* 1990;86:1768–1771.

23. Janson PA, Jubelirer SJ, Weinstein MJ, Deykin D. Treatment of the bleeding tendency in uremia with cryoprecipitate. *N Engl J Med* 1980;303:1318–1322.

24. Mannucci PM, Remuzzi G, Pusineri F, et al. Deamino-8-D-arginine vasopressin shortens the bleeding time in uremia. *N Engl J Med* 1983;308:8–12.

25. Lane DA, Flynn A, Ireland H, et al. On the evaluation of heparin and low molecular weight heparin in haemodialysis for chronic renal failure. *Haemostasis* 1986:16(suppl 2): 38–47.

26. Livio M, Mannucci PM, Vigano G, et al. Conjugated estrogens for the management of bleeding associated with renal failure. *N Engl J Med* 1986;315:731–735.

27. Livio M, Gott E, Marchesi D, et al. Uraemic bleeding: role of anemia and beneficial effects of red cell transfusions. *Lancet* 1982;2:1013–1015.

28. Vigano G, Benigni A, Mecca G. Recombinant human erythropoietin (r-HuEPO) to correct uremic bleeding. *J Am Soc Nephrol* 1990;1:408.

29. Zuckerman GR, Cornette GL, Clouse RE, Harter HR. Upper gastrointestinal bleeding in patients with chronic renal failure. *Ann Intern Med* 1985;102:588–592.

30. Navab F, Masters P, Subramani R, et al. Angio-dysplasia in patients with renal insufficiency. *Am J Gastroenterol* 1989; 84:1297–1301.

31. Goldberg M, Hoffman GC, Wonbolt DG. Massive hemorrhage from rectal ulcers in chronic renal failure. *Ann Intern Med* 1984;100:397.

32. Rutsky EA, Rostrand SG. Treatment of uremic pericarditis and pericardial effusion. *Am J Kidney Dis* 1987;10:2–8.

33. Galen MA, Steinberg SM, Lowrie FG. Hemorrhagic pleural effusion in patients undergoing chronic dialysis. *Ann Intern Med* 1975;82:359–361.

34. Ellison, RT, Corrao WM, Fox MI, Braman SS. Spontaneous mediastinal hemorrhage in patients on chronic hemodialysis. *Ann Intern Med* 1981;95:704–706.

35. Milutinovich I, Follette WC, Scribner BH. Spontaneous retroperitoneal bleeding in patients on chronic hemodialysis. *Ann Intern Med* 1977;86:189–192.

36. Smetana SS, David E, Pelet D, Bar-Khayim Y. Subcapsular liver hematoma in a patient on chronic hemodialysis. *Nephron* l987:45:323–324.

37. Leonard A, Shapiro FL. Subdural hematoma in regularly hemodialized patients. *Ann Intern Med* 1975; 82:650–658.

38. Onoyama K, Ibayashi S, Nanishi F, et al. Cerebral hemorrhage in patients on maintenance hemodialysis: CT analysis of 25 cases. *Eur Neurol* 1987;26:171–175.

39. Chachati A, Dechenee C, Gordon JP. Increased incidence of cerebral hemorrhage mortality in patients with analgesic nephropathy on hemodialysis. *Nephron* 1987;45:167–168.

40. Diaz-Buxo JA, Burgess WP, Greenman M, et al. Visual function in diabetic patients undergoing dialysis: comparison of peritoneal and hemodialysis. *Int J Artif Organs* 1984; 7:257–262.

41. Porter J, Jick J. Drug-related deaths among medical inpatients. *JAMA* 1977;237:879–891.

42. Swartz RD. Hemorrhage during high-risk hemodialysis using controlled heparinization. *Nephron* 1981;28:65–69.

43. Gotch FA, Keen ML. Precise control of minimal heparinization for high bleeding risk hemodialysis. *ASAIO Trans* 1977;23:168–l75.

44. Sanders PW, Taylor H, Curtis JJ. Hemodialysis without anticoagulation. *Am J Kidney Dis* 1985;5:32–35.

45. Schwab SJ, Onorato JJ, Sharar LR, Dennis PA. Hemodialysis without anticoagulation: one-year prospective trial in hospitalized patients at risk of bleeding. *Am J Med* 1987; 83:405–410.

46. Flanigan MJ, Von Brecht J, Freeman RM, Lim VS. Reducing the hemorrhagic complications of hemodialysis: a con-

trolled comparison of low-dose heparin and citrate anticoagulation. *Am J Kidney Dis* 1987;9:147–153.

47. Pinnick RV, Wiegmann TB, Diederich DA. Regional citrate anticoagulation for hemodialysis in the patient at high risk for bleeding. *N Engl J Med* 1983; 308:258–261.

48. Wiegmann TB, MacDougall ML, Diederich DA. Long-term comparisons of citrate and heparin as anticoagulants for hemodialysis. *Am J Kidney Dis* 1987;9:430–435.

49. Mehta RL, Dobos GJ, Ward DM. Anticoagulation in continuous renal replacement procedures. *Semin Dial* 1992;5: 61–68.

50. Swartz RD, Port FK. Preventing hemorrhage in high-risk hemodialysis. Regional versus low-dose heparin. *Kidney Int* 1979;16:513–518.

51. Kazuomi K, Takefumi M, Tsutomu Y, et al. Factor VII in hyperactivity in chronic dialysis patients. *Thromb Res* 1992; 67:105–113.

52. Toulon P, Jacquot C, Capron L, et al. Antithrombin III and heparin cofactor II in patients with chronic renal failure undergoing regular hemodialysis. *Thromb Haemost* 1987;57: 263–268.

53. Lai, KN, Yin JA, Yuen PMP, Li PKT. Effect of hemodialysis on proteins and antithrombin III levels. *Am J Kidney Dis* 1991;17:38–42.

54. Arik N, Ozdemir O, Akpolat T, et al. Protein C and its inhibitors during hemodialysis. *Nephron* 1992;60:488.

55. Lai KN. Protein C, protein S and antithrombin III metabolism in dialysis patients. *Int J Artif Organs* 1993;16:4–6.

56. Davenport A. The coagulation system in the critically ill patient with acute renal failure and the effect of an extracorporal circuit. *Am J Kidney Dis* 1997;30:S20–S27.

57. Harter JR, Burch J, Majerus PW, et al. Prevention of thrombosis in patients on hemodialysis by low-dose aspirin. *N Engl J Med* 1979;301:577–579.

58. Kaegi A, Pines GF, Shimuzu A, et al. Arterio-venous shunt thrombosis: prevention by sulphinpyrazone. *N Engl J Med* 1974;290:304–306.

59. Maruyama H, Gejyo F, Hanano M, Arakawa M. Acquired type II protein C deficiency in a long-term hemodialysis patient. *Nephron* 1994;66:348–350.

60. Selli C, Amato M, Salvadori M. Priapism associated with chronic hemodialysis. *Dial Transplant* 1986;15:101–102.

61. Callander N, Rapaport SI. Trousseau's Syndrome. *West J Med* 1993;158:364–371.

62. Hall AV, Clark WF, Parbtani A. Heparin-induced thrombocytopenia in renal failure. *Clin Nephrol* 1992;38:86–89.

63. Greinacher A, Potzsch B, Amiral L, et al. Heparin-associated thrombocytopenia: isolation of the antibody and characterization of a multimolecular PF4-Heparin complex as the major antigen. *Thromb Haemost* 1994;2:247–251.

64. Wirtz JJJM, van Esser JWJ, Hamulyák K, et al. The effects of recombinant human erythropoietin on hemostastis and fibrinolysis in hemodialysis patients. *Clin Nephrol* 1992;38: 277–282.

65. Taylor JE Belch IF, McLaren M, et al. Effect of erythropoietin therapy and withdrawal on blood coagulation and fibrinolysis in hemodialysis patients. *Kidney Int* 1993;44: 182–190.

66. Eschbach LW, Aquiling T, Haley NR, et al. The long-term effects of recombinant human erythropoietin on the cardiovascular system. *Clin Nephrol* l992;38(suppl 1):S98–S103.

67. Standage BA, Schuman ES, Ackerman D, et al. Does the use of erythropoietin in hemodialysis patients increase dialysis graft thrombosis rates? *Am J Surg* 1993;165:650–654.

68. Arinsoy T, Ozdemir O, Arik N, et al. Recombinant human erythropoietin treatment may induce antithrombin-III depletion. *Nephron* 1992;62:480–481.

69. Opatrny K, Opatrná S, Vit L, et al. Plasma concentrations of the thrombin-antithrombin III complex in dialysis patients during erythropoietin therapy. *Nephrol Dial Transplant* 1992;7:1072–1073.

70. Zwaginga JJ, Ijsseldijk MJ, de Groot PG, et al. Treatment of uremic anemia with recombinant erythropoietin also reduces the defects in platelet adhesion and aggregation caused by uremic plasma. *Thromb Haemost* 1991;66:638–647.

71. Mehta RL, Scott G, Sloand IA, Francis CW. Skin necrosis associated with acquired protein C deficiency in patients with renal failure and calciphylaxis. *Am J Med* 1990;88: 252–257.

72. Soundararajan R, Leehey J, Yu AW, et al. Skin necrosis and protein C deficiency associated with vitamin K depletion in a patient with renal failure. *Am J Med* 1992;93:467–470.

73. Perez-Mijares R, Guzman-Zamudio JL, Payan-Lopez J, et al. Calciphylaxis in a haemodialysis patient: functional protein S deficiency? *Nephrol Dial Transplant* 1996;11: 1856–1859.

74. Schwab SI, Raymond JR, Saeed M, et al. Prevention of hemodialysis fistula thrombosis. Early detection of venous stenoses. *Kidney Int* 1989;36:707–711.

75. Poulain F, Raynaud A, Bourquelot P, et al. Local thrombolysis and thromboaspiration in the treatment of acutely thrombosed arteriovenous hemodialysis fistulas. *Cardiovasc Intervent Radiol* 1991;14:98–101.

76. Matuszkiewicz-Rowinski J, Billip-Tomecka Z, Rowinski W, Sicinski A. Systemic streptokinase infusion for declotting hemodialysis arteriovenous fistulas. *Nephron* 1994;66: 67–70.

77. Summers S, Drazan K, Gomes A, Freischlag J. Urokinase therapy for thrombosed hemodialysis access grafts. *Surg Gynecol Obstet* 1993;176:534–538.

78. Ahmed A, Shapiro WB, Porush JG. The use of plasminogen activator to declot arteriovenous accesses in hemodialysis patients. *Am J Kidney Dis* 1993;21:38–43.

79. Valji K, Bookstein JJ, Roberts AC, Davis GB. Pharmacomechanical thrombolysis and angioplasty in the management of clotted hemodialysis grafts: early and late clinical results. *Radiology* 1991;178:243–247.

80. Roberts AC, Valji K, Bookstein JJ, Hye RJ. Pulse-spray pharmacomechanical thrombolysis for treatment of thrombosed dialysis access grafts. *Am J Surg* 1993;166:221–226.

81. Beathard GA. Mechanical versus pharmacomechanical thrombolysis for the treatment of thrombosed dialysis access grafts. *Kidney Int* 1994;45:1401–1406.

82. Kumpe DA, Cohen MAH. Angioplasty/thrombolytic treatment of falling and failed hemodialysis access sites: comparison with surgical treatment. *Prog Cardiovasc Dis* 1992; 24:263–278.

83. Domoto DT, Bauman JE, Joist JH. Combined aspirin and sulfinpyrazone in the prevention of recurrent hemodialysis vascular access thrombosis. *Thromb Res* 1991;62:737–743.

84. Uldall R. Prevention of thrombosis in arteriovenous fistulas. *Blood Purif* 1985;3:89–93.

85. Al-Momen AKM, Huraib SO. Low-dose danazol for vascular access and dialyzer thrombosis in hemodialysis patients. *Haemostasis* 1992;22:12–16.

86. Ratcliffe PJ, Oliver DO. Massive thrombosis around subclavian cannulas used for hemodialysis. *Lancet* 1982;1:1472–1473.

87. Cheung AK, Gregory MC. Subclavian vein thrombosis in hemodialysis patients. *ASAIO Trans* 1985;31:131–135.

88. Caruana RJ, Raja RM, Zeit RM, et al. Thrombotic complications of indwelling central catheters used for chronic hemodialysis. *Am J Kidney Dis* 1987;19:497–501.

89. Brady KR, Fitzcharles B, Goldberg H, et al. Diagnosis and management of subclavian vein thrombosis occurring in association with subclavian cannulation for hemodialysis. *Blood Purif* 1989;7:210–217.

90. Clark DD, Albina JE, Chazan JA. Subclavian vein stenosis and thrombosis: a potential serious complication in chronic hemodialysis patients. *Am J Kidney Dis* 1990;25:265–268.

91. Vanherweghem JL. Thromboses et stenoses des acces veineux centraux en hémodialyse. *Néphrologie* 1994;15:117–121.

92. Besley M, Thomas A, Salter S, et al. Control of oral anticoagulation in patients using long-term internal jugular catheters for hemodialysis access. *Int J Artif Organs* 1992;15:277–280.

93. Uldall R, Besley ME, Thomas A, et al. Maintaining the patency of double-lumen silastic jugular catheters for hemodialysis. *Int J Artif Organs* 1993;16:37–40.

94. Kinney TB, Valji K, Rose SC, et al. Pulmonary embolism from pulse-spray pharmacomechanical thrombolysis of clotted hemodialysis grafts: urokinase versus heparinized saline. *J Vasc Intervent Radiol* 2000;11:1143–1152.

95. Paulsen G, Reisaether A, Aasen M, Fauchald P. Use of tissue plasminogen activator for reopening of clotted dialysis catheters. *Nephron* 1993;64:468–470.

96. Purchase L, Gault MH. Hemodialysis with a Permcath kept open with streptokinase and later citrate in a heparin-sensitive patient. *Nephron* 1991;58:119–120.

97. Wardle EN, Percy DA. Studies of contact activation of blood in hemodialysis. *J Clin Pathol* 1972;25:1045–1049.

98. Rapaport SI. Hemostasis. In: West JB, ed. *Best and Taylor's Physiological Basis of Medical Practice,* 12th ed. Baltimore: William & Wilkins, 1991:385–401.

99. Schultze G, Hollmann S, Sinah P. Formation of thrombin antithrombin III complex using polyamide and Hemophan dialyzers. *Int J Artif Organs* 1992;6:370–373.

100. Sorensen PJ, Knudsen F, Nielsen AH, Dyerberg J. Protein C assays in uremia. *Thromb Res* 1989;54:301–310.

101. Sreeharan N, Crow MJ, Salter CP, et al. Membrane effect on platelet function during hemodialysis: a comparison of cuprophan and polycarbonate. *Artif Organs* 1982;6:324–327.

102. Hakim RM, Schafer AL. Hemodialysis-associated platelet activation and thrombocytopenia. *Am J Med* 1985;78:575.

103. Lindsay RM, Ferguson D, Prentice CRM, et al. Reduction of thrombus formation on dialyzer membranes by aspirin and RA233. *Lancet* 1972;2:1287.

104. Schmitt GW, Moake IL, Rudy CK, et al. Alterations in hemostatic parameters during hemodialysis with dialyzers of different membrane composition and flow design. *Am J Med* 1987; 83:411–418.

105. Sultan Y, London GM, Goldfarb B, et al. Activation of platelets, coagulation and fibrinolysis in patients on long-term hemodialysis: influence of cuprophan and polyacrylonitrile membranes. *Nephrol Dial Transplant* 1990;5: 362–368.

106. Hakim RM. Clinical implications of hemodialysis membrane biocompatibility. *Kidney Int* 1993; 44:4484–4494.

107. Opatrny K, Opatrny K, Vit L, et al. What are the factors contributing to the changes in tissue-type plasminogen activator during hemodialysis? *Nephrol Dial Transplant* 1991;6 (suppl 3):26–30.

108. Speiser W, Wojta J, Korninger C, et al. Enhanced fibrinolysis caused by tissue plasminogen activator release in hemodialysis. *Kidney Int* 1987;32:280–283.

109. Nakamura Y, Tomura S, Tachibana K, et al. Enhanced fibrinolytic activity during the course of hemodialysis. *Clin Nephrol* 1992;38:90–96.

110. Keller F, Seemann J, Preuschof L, Offermann G. Risk factors of system clotting in heparin-free hemodialysis. *Nephrol Dial Transplant* 1990;5:802–807.

111. Klingel R, Schaefer M, Schwarting A, et al. Comparative analysis of procoagulatory activity of haemodialysis, haemofiltration and haemodiafiltration with a polysulfone membrane (APS) and with different modes of enoxaparin anticoagulation. *Nephrol Dial Transplant* 2004;19:164–170.

112. Schwarzbeck A, Warner L, Squarr H-U, Strauch M. Clotting in dialyzers due to low pH of dialysis fluid. *Clin Nephrol* 1977;7:125–127.

113. Yang VC, Fu Y, Kim JS. A potential nonthrombogenic hemodialysis membrane with improved blood compatibility. *ASAIO Trans* 1991;37:M229–M232.

114. Leanza H, Rivarola G, Garcia G, et al. Heparin-free dialysis and ethylene-vinyl-alcohol (EVAL) dialyzer reuse in high-risk bleeding patients. *Transplant Proc* 1991;23:1835.

115. Olsson P, Larm O. Biologically active heparin coating in medical devices. *Int J Artif Organs* 1990;14:453–456.

116. Wright MJ, Woodrow G, Umpleby S, et al. Low thrombogenicity of polyethylene glycol–grafted cellulose membranes does not influence heparin requirements in hemodialysis. *Am J Kidney Dis* 1999;34:36–42.

117. Begovac PC, Thomson RC, Fisher JL, et al. Improvements in Gore-Tex vascular graft performance by Carmeda BioActive surface heparin immobilization. *Eur J Vasc Endovasc Surg* 2003;25:432–437.

118. Mujais SK, Chimeh H. Heparin free hemodialysis using heparin coated hemophan. *ASAIO J* 1996;42:M538–M541.

119. Lavaud S, Canivet E, Wuillai A, et al. Optimal anticoagulation strategy in haemodialysis with heparin-coated polyacrylonitrile membrane. *Nephrol Dial Transplant* 2003;18: 2097–2104.

120. Lavaud S, Maheut H, Randoux C, et al. Advantages and limits of systemic heparin-free hemodialysis in patients at risk

of bleeding using the AN69-ST membrane (abstr). *ASAIO J* 2004;50:175.

121. Uziel L, Cugno M, Cacciabue E, et al. Evaluation of tests for heparin control during long term extracorporeal circulation. *Int J Artif Organs* l986;9:111–116.

122. Hattersley PG. Heparin anticoagulation. In: Koepke JA, ed. *Laboratory Hematology*. New York: Churchill Livingstone, 1984:789–818.

123. Harenberg J, Haaf B, Schafer M, et al. Anti–factor Xa determination in blood: a new method for controlling heparin therapy. *Semin Thromb Hemost* l993;l9(suppl 1):79–85.

124. Schrader J, Stibbe W, Kandt M, et al. Low molecular weight heparin versus standard heparin: a long-term study in hemodialysis and hemofiltration patients. *ASAIO Trans* 1990; 36:28–32.

125. Ireland HA, Boisclair MD, Lane DA, et al. Hemodialysis and heparin. Alternative methods of measuring heparin and of detecting activation of coagulation. *Clin Nephrol* 1991; 35:26–34.

126. Ireland H, Lane DA, Curtis JR. Objective assessment of heparin requirements for hemodialysis in humans. *J Lab Clin Med* 1984;103:643–652.

127. Bithell TC. Thrombosis and antithrombotic therapy. In: Lee GR, Bithell TC, Forester J, et al, eds. *Wintrobe's Clinical Hematology*, 9th ed. Philadelphia: Lea & Febiger, 1993: 1524–1528.

128. Penner JA. Experience with a thrombin clotting time assay for measuring heparin activity. *Am J Clin Pathol* 1974;61: 645.

129. Nicastro MA, Plana JL, Heller MV, et al. Antithrombin III supplementation allowed hemodialysis without heparin after kidney transplantation. *Nephrol Dial Transplant* 1993;8: 1281–1282.

130. Kandrotas R, Gal P, Douglas JB, Deterding J. Pharmacokinetics and pharmacodynamics of heparin during hemodialysis: interpatient and intrapatient variability. *Pharmacotherapy* 1990;10:349–356.

131. Kandrotas R, Gal P, Douglas JB, Deterding J. Heparin pharmacokinetics during hemodialysis. *Ther Drug Monit* 1989; 11:674–679.

132. Farrell P, Ward RA, Schindhelm K, Gotch PA. Precise anticoagulation for routine hemodialysis. *J Lab Clin Med* 1978; 92:164–176.

133. Goudable C, That HT, Damani RS, et al. Low molecular weight heparin half life is prolonged in hemodialyzed patients. *Thromb Res* 1986;43:1–5.

134. Eika C. Platelet refractory state induced by heparin. *Scand J Haematol* 1972;9:665.

135. Lindsay RM, Rourke JTB, Reid BD, et al. The role of heparin on platelet retention by acrylonitrile co-polymer dialysis membranes. *J Lab Clin Med* 1977;89:4.

136. Hofbauer R, Moser D, Frass M, et al. Effect of anticoagulation on blood membrane interactions during hemodialysis. *Kidney Int* 1999;56:1578–1583.

137. Raible MD. Hematologic complications of heparin-induced thrombocytopenia. *Semin Thromb Hemost* 1999; 25(suppl 1):17–21.

138. Ramakrishna R, Manoharan A, Kwan YL, Kyle PW. Heparin-induced thrombocytopenia: cross-reactivity between standard heparin, low molecular weight heparin, dalteparin (Fragmin) and heparinoid, danaparoid (Orgaran). *Br J Haematol* 1995;91:736–738.

139. Harenberg J, Wang L, Hoffmann U, et al.: Improved laboratory confirmation of heparin-induced thrombocytopenia type II. Time course of antibodies and combination of antigenic and biologic assays. *Am J Clin Pathol* 2001;115: 432–438.

140. Neuhaus TJ, Goetschel P, Schmugge M, Leumann E. Heparin-induced thrombocytopenia type II on hemodialysis: switch to danaparoid. *Pediatr Nephrol* 2000;14:713–716.

141. Boon DMS, van Vliet HHDM, Zietse R, Kappers-Klunne MC. The presence of antibodies against a PF4-heparin complex in patients on haemodialysis. *Thromb Haemost* 1996;76:480.

142. Luzzatto G, Bertoli M, Cella G, et al. Platelet count, anti-heparin/platelet factor 4 antibodies and tissue factor pathway inhibitor plasma antigen level in chronic dialysis. *Thromb Res* 1998;89:115–122.

143. Ibels LS, Reardon MF, Nestel PJ. Plasma post-heparin lipolytic activity and triglyceride clearance in uremic and hemodialysis patients and renal allograft recipients. *J Lab Clin Med* 1976;87:648–658.

144. Dahlman TC. Osteoporotic fractures and the recurrence of thromboembolism during pregnancy and puerperium in 184 women undergoing thromboprophylaxis with heparin. *Am J Obstet Gynecol* 1993;168:1265–1270.

145. Elisaf MS, Germanos NP, Bairaktari HT, et al. Effects of conventional vs. low-molecular-weight heparin on lipid profile in hemodialysis patients. *Am J Nephrol* 1997;17: 153–157.

146. Muir JM, Hirsh J, Weitz JI, et al. A histomorphometric comparison of the effects of heparin and low-molecular-weight heparin on cancellous bone in rats. *Blood* 1997;89: 3236–3242.

147. Kronenberg F, König P, Neyer U, et al. Influence of various heparin preparations on lipoproteins in hemodialysis patients: a multicenter study. *Thromb Haemost* 1995;74: 1025–1028.

148. Sivakumaran M, Ghosh K, Zaidi Y, Hutchinson RM. Osteoporosis and vertebral collapse following low-dose, low molecular weight heparin therapy in a young patient. *Clin Lab Haematol* 1996;18:55–57.

149. Lai KN, Ho K, Cheung RC, et al. Effect of low molecular weight heparin on bone metabolism and hyperlipidemia in patients on maintenance hemodialysis. *Int J Artif Organs* 2001;24:447–455.

150. Wiemer J, Winler K, Baumstark M, et al. Influence of low molecular weight heparin compared to conventional heparin for anticoagulation during hemodialysis on low density lipoprotein subclasses. *Nephrol Dial Transplant* 2002;17: 2231–2238.

151. Yang C, Wu T, Huang C. Low molecular weight heparin reduces triglyceride, VLDL and cholesterol/HDL levels in hyperlipidemic diabetic patients on hemodialysis. *Am J Nephrol* 1998;18:384–390.

152. Hottelart C, Achard JM, Moriniere P, et al. Heparin-induced hyperkalemia in chronic hemodialysis patients: comparison

of low molecular weight and unfractionated heparin. *Artif Organs* 1998;22(7):614–617.

153. Ouseph R, Ward RA. Anticoagulation for intermittent hemodialysis. *Semin Dial* 2000;13:181–187.

154. Wei SS, Ellis PW, Magnusson MO, Paganini EP. Effect of heparin modeling on delivered hemodialysis therapy. *Am J Kidney Dis* 1994;23:389–393.

155. Wilhelmsson S, Lins L-E. Heparin elimination and hemostasis in hemodialysis *Clin Nephrol* 1984;22:303–306.

156. Ireland H, Rylance PB, Kesteven P. Heparin as an anticoagulant during extracorporeal circulation. In: Lane DA, Lindahl U, eds. *Heparin: Chemical and Biological Properties, Clinical Applications*. London: Edward Arnold, 1989:549–574.

157. Smith BP, Ward RA, Brier ME. Prediction of anticoagulation during hemodialysis by population kinetic sand an artificial neural network. *Artif Organs* 1998;22:731–739.

158. Ouseph R, Brier ME, Ward RA. Improved dialyzer reuse after use of a population pharmacodynamic model to determine heparin doses. *Am J Kidney Dis* 2000;35:89–94.

159. Mingardi G, Perico N, Pusineri F, et al. Heparin for hemodialysis: practical guidelines for administration and monitoring. *Int J Artif Organs* 1984;7:269–274.

160. Bosch JP, Ronco C. High-efficiency treatments: risks and common problems encountered in clinical application. *Contemp Issues Nephrol* 1993;27:209–224.

161. Lee JIH, Cocke TB, Gonzales FM. Regional vs. "tight" heparinization in hemodialysis. *Proc Clin Dial Transplant Forum* 1974;4:239–246.

162. Vogel GE, Kopp KF. Minimal dose heparinization for hemodialysis patients with high bleeding risk abstr. *Am Soc Nephrol* 1975;8:40.

163. Vogel GE, Kopp KF. The conflict between anticoagulation and hemostasis during hemodialysis. *Int J Artif Organs* 1978;1:181–186.

164. Williman P, Aliga I, Binswanger U. Minimal intermittent heparinization during hemodialysis. *Nephron* 1979;23:191–193.

165. Butterman G, Vogel GE, Kalinowski H, et al. Quantification of extracorporeal fibrin deposits in hemodialysis with minimal conventional heparinization. *Int J Artif Organs* 1983;6:247–254.

166. Jannett TC, Wise MG, Shanklin NH, Sanders PW. Adaptive control of anticoagulation during hemodialysis. *Kidney Int* 1994;45:912–915.

167. Marshall MR, Golper TA, Shaver MJ, et al. Sustained low-efficiency dialysis for critically ill patients requiring renal replacement therapy. *Kidney Int* 2001;60:777–785.

168. Maher JF, Lapierre L, Schreiner GE, et al. Regional heparinization for hemodialysis: technic and clinical experiences. *N Engl J Med* 1963;268:451–456.

169. Kim J-S, Vincent C, Teng C-L, et al. A novel approach to anticoagulation control. *ASAIO Trans* 1989;25:644–646.

170. Jeffrey RF, Khan AA, Douglas JT, et al. Pharmacokinetics of the low molecular weight heparin enoxaparin during 48 h after bolus administration as an anticoagulant in haemodialysis. *Nephrol Dial Transplant* 2003; 18:2348–2353.

171. Naumnik B, Borawski J, Mysliwiec M. Different effects of enoxaparin and unfractionated heparin on extrinsic blood coagulation during haemodialysis: a prospective study. *Nephrol Dial Transplant* 2003;18:1376–1382.

172. Anastassiades E, Lane DA, Ireland H, et al. A low molecular weight heparin ("fragmin") for routine hemodialysis: a crossover trial comparing three dose regimens with a standard regimen of commercial unfractionated heparin. *Clin Nephrol* 1989;32:290–296.

173. Suzuki T, Ota K, Naganuma S, et al. Clinical application of fragmin (FR-860) in hemodialysis: multicenter cooperative study in Japan. *Semin Thromb Hemost* 1990;16:46–54.

174. Ljungberg B, Jacobson SH, Lins L-E, Pejler G. Effective anticoagulation by a low molecular weight heparin (Fragmin) in hemodialysis with a highly permeable polysulfone membrane. *Clin Nephrol* 1992;38:97–100.

175. Sagedal S, Hartmann A, Sundstrom K, et al. A single dose of dalteparin effectively prevents clotting during haemodialysis. *Nephrol Dial Transplant* 1999;14:1943–1947.

176. Kerr PG, Mattingly S, Lo A, Atkins RC. The adequacy of fragmin as a single bolus dose with reused dialyzers. *Artif Organs* 1994; 18:416–419.

177. Grau F, Siguenza F, Maduell F, et al. Low molecular weight heparin (CY-216) versus unfractionated heparin in chronic hemodialysis. *Nephron* 1992;62:13–17.

178. Steinbach G, Bosc C, Caraman PL, et al. Use of hemodialysis and hemofiltration of CY 216 (fraxiparine) administered via intravenous bolus in patients with acute and chronic renal insufficiency with and without hemorrhagic risk. *Nephrologie* 1990; 11:17–21.

179. Reach I, Luong N, Chastang C, et al. Dose effect relationship of reviparin in chronic hemodialysis: a crossover study versus nadroparin. *Artif Organs* 2001; 25:591–595.

180. Hainer JW, Sherrard DJ, Swan SK, et al. Intravenous and subcutaneous weight-based dosing of the low molecular weight heparin tinzaparin (Innohep) in end-stage renal disease patients undergoing chronic hemodialysis. *Am J Kidney Dis* 2002;40:531–538.

181. Lord H, Jean N, Dumont M, et al. Comparison between tinzaparin and standard heparin for chronic hemodialysis in a Canadian center. *Am J Nephrol* 2002;22:58–66.

182. Koutsikos D, Fourtounas C, Kapetanaki A, et al. A crossover study of a new low molecular weight heparin (Logiparin) in hemodialysis. *Int J Artif Organs* 1996;19:467–471.

183. Simpson HK, Baird J, Allison M, et al. Long-term use of the low molecular weight heparin tinzaparin in hemodialysis. *Haemostasis* 1996;26:90–97.

184. Baumelou A, Singlas E, Petitclerc T, et al. Pharmacokinetics of a low molecular weight heparin (reviparine) in hemodialyzed patients. *Nephron* 1994;68:202–206.

185. Schrader J, Stibbe W, Armstrong VW, et al. Comparison of low molecular weight heparin to standard heparin in hemodialysis/hemofiltration. *Kidney Int* 1988;33:890–896.

186. Ljungberg B, Blomback M, Johnsson, Lins L-E. A single dose of low molecular weight heparin fragment for anticoagulation during hemodialysis. *Clin Nephrol* 1987;27: 31–35.

187. Nurmohamed MT, ten Cate J, Stevens P, et al. Long-term efficacy and safety of a low molecular weight heparin in chronic hemodialysis patients. *ASAIO Trans* 1991;37: M459–M461.

188. Stefoni S, Cianciolo G, Donati G, et al. Standard heparin versus low-molecular-weight heparin. A medium-term comparison in hemodialysis. *Nephron* 2002;92:589–600.

189. Hory B. Hemodialysis with low-molecular-weight heparin in high-risk hemorrhagic patients with acute renal failure. *Am J Med* 1988;84:566.

190. Leu JG, Chiang SS, Lin SM, et al. Serious adverse incidents with the usage of low molecular weight heparins in patients with chronic kidney disease. *Am J Kidney Dis* 2004; 43: 531–537.

191. Farooq V, Hegarty J, Chandrasekar T, et al. Serious adverse incidents with the usage of low molecular weight heparins in patients with chronic kidney disease. *Am J Kidney Dis* 2004; 43:531–537.

192. Cadroy Y, Pourrat J, Baladre M-F, et al. Delayed elimination of enoxaparine in patients with chronic renal insufficiency. *Thromb Res* 1991;63:385–390.

193. Lai KN, Ho K, Li M, Szeto CC. Use of single dose low-molecular-weight heparin in long hemodialysis. *Int J Artif Organs* 1998;21:196–200.

194. Ireland H, Lane DA, Flynn A, et al. The anticoagulant effect of heparinoid Org 10172 during hemodialysis: an objective assessment. *Thromb Haemost* 1986;55:271–275.

195. Lindhoff-Last E, Betz C, Bauersachs R. Use of a low-molecular-weight heparinoid (danaparoid sodium) for continuous renal replacement therapy in intensive care patients. *Clin Appl Thromb Hemost* 2001;7:300–304.

196. Rowlings PA, Mansberg R, Rozenberg MC, et al. The use of a low molecular weight heparinoid (Org 10172) for extracorporeal procedures in patients with heparin dependent thrombocytopenia and thrombosis. *Aust N Z J Med* 1991; 21:52–54.

197. Roe SD, Cassidy MJD, Haynes AP, Byrne JL. Heparin-induced thrombocytopenia (HIT) and thrombosis in a hemodialysis-dependent patient with systemic vasculitis. *Nephrol Dial Transplant* 1998;13:3226–3229.

198. Ryan KE, Lane DA, Flynn A, et al. Antithrombotic properties of dermatan sulphate (MF7O1) in hemodialysis for chronic renal failure. *Thromb Haemost* 1992;68:563–569.

199. Nurmohamed MT, Knipscheer HC, Stevens P, et al. Clinical experience with a new antithrombotic (dermatan sulfate) in chronic hemodialysis patients. *Clin Nephrol* 1993;39: 166–171.

200. Lane DA, Ryan K, Ireland H, et al. Dermatan sulphate in haemodialysis. *Lancet* 1992;339(8789):334–335.

201. Boccardo P, Melacini D, Rota S, et al. Individualized anticoagulation with dermatan sulphate for haemodialysis in chronic renal failure. *Nephrol Dial Transplant* 1997;12: 2349–2354.

202. Averna MR, Picone F, Galione A, et al. Use of 3-GS as an anticoagulant in hemodialysis: effects on serum lipoproteins. *Clin Ter [Italy]* 1982;100:35–39.

203. Minamiguchi K, Kitazato KT, Nagase H, et al. Depolymerized holothurian glycosaminoglycan (DHG), a novel alternative anticoagulant for hemodialysis, is safe and effective in a dog renal failure model. *Kidney Int* 2003;63:1548–1555.

204. Koide M, Yamamoto S, Matsuo M, et al. Anticoagulation for heparin-induced thrombocytopenia with spontaneous platelet aggregation in a patient requiring hemodialysis. *Nephrol Dial Transplant* 1995;10:2137–2140.

205. Matsuo T, Nakao K, Yamada T, Matsuo O. A new thrombin inhibitor MD805 and thrombocytopenia encountered with heparin hemodialysis. *Thromb Res* 1986;44:247–251.

206. Matsuo T, Yamada T, Yamanashi T, Ryo R. Anticoagulant therapy with MD805 of a hemodialysis patient with heparin-induced thrombocytopenia. *Thromb Res* 1990;58: 663–666.

207. George CRP. Hirudin, heparin and Heinrich Necheles. *Nephrology* 1998;4:225–228.

208. Markwardt F, Nowak G, Bucha E. Hirudin as anticoagulant in experimental hemodialysis. *Haemostasis* 1991;21(suppl l):149–155.

209. Bucha E, Markwardt F, Nowak G. Hirudin in hemodialysis. *Thromb Res* 1990;60:445–455.

210. Vanholder RC, Camez AA, Veys NM, et al. Recombinant hirudin: a specific thrombin inhibiting anticoagulant for hemodialysis. *Kidney Int* 1994;45:1754–1759.

211. Van Wyk V, Badenhorst PN, Luus HG, Kotzé HF. A comparison between the use of recombinant hirudin and heparin during hemodialysis. *Kidney Int* 1995;48:1338–1343.

212. Nowak G, Bucha E, Brauns I, Czerwinski R. Anticoagulation with r-hirudin in regular hemodialysis with heparin-induced thrombocytopenia (HIT II). *Wien Klin Wochenschr* 1997;109/110:354–358.

213. Nowak G, Bucha B, Goock T, et al. Pharmacology of r-hirudin in renal impairment. *Thromb Res* 1992;66:707–715.

214. Bucha E, Kreml R, Nowak G. In vitro study of r-hirudin permeability through membranes of different haemodialysers. *Nephrol Dial Transplant* 1999;14:2922–2926.

215. Rolf DF, Farber H, Stefanidis I, et al. Hirudin elimination by hemofiltration: a comparative in vitro study of different membranes. *Kidney Int* 2000;56(suppl):S41–S45.

216. Eichler P, Friesen HJ, Lubenow N, et al. Antihirudin antibodies in patients with heparin induced thrombocytopenia treated with lepirudin: incidence, effects on aPTT, and clinical relevance. *Blood* 2000;96:2373–2378.

217. Davenport A, Mehta S. The acute dialysis quality initiative: Part VI. access and anticoagulation in CRRT. *Adv Renal Replace Ther* 2002;9:273–281.

218. Muller A, Huhle G, Nowack R, et al. Serious bleeding in a haemodialysis patient treated with recombinant hirudin. *Nephrol Dial Transplant* 1999;14:2482–2483.

219. Pöschel KA, Bucha E, Esslinger HU, et al. Anticoagulant efficacy of PEG-hirudin in patients on maintenance hemodialysis. *Kidney Int* 2004;65:666–674.

220. Zusman RM, Rubin RH, Cato AE, et al. Hemodialysis using prostacyclin in stead of heparin as the sole antithrombotic agent. *N Engl J Med* 1981;304:934–939.

221. Swartz RD, Flamenbaum W, Dubrow A, et al. Epoprostenol (PGI$_2$ prostacyclin) during high-risk hemodialysis: preventing further bleeding complications. *J Clin Pharmacol* 1988; 28:8l8–825.

222. Miller LC, Hall JC, Crow JW, et al. Hemodialysis in heparin associated thrombocytopenia: epoprostenol as sole anticoagulant. *Dial Transplant* 1985;14:579–580.

223. Dubrow A, Flamenbaum W, Mittman N, et al. Safety and efficacy of epoprostenol (PGI$_2$ versus heparin (H) in hemodialysis (HD). *ASAIO Trans* l984;30:52–54.

224. Arze RS, Ward MK. Prostacyclin safer than heparin in hemodialysis. *Lancet* 198 1;2:50.

225. Caruana RJ, Smith MC, Clyne D, et al. Controlled study of heparin versus epoprostenol sodium (prostacyclin) as the

sole anticoagulant for chronic hemodialysis. *Blood Purif* 1991;9:296–304.

226. Hory B, Saint-Hillier Y, Perol JC. Prostacyclin as the sole antithrombotic agent for acute renal failure hemodialysis. *Nephron* 1983;33:71.

227. Novacek G, Kapiotis S, Jilma B, et al. Enhanced blood coagulation and enhanced fibrinolysis during hemodialysis with prostacyclin. *Thromb Res* 1997; 88:283–290.

228. Turney JH, Williams LC, Fewell MR, et al. Platelet protection and heparin sparing with prostacyclin during regular dialysis therapy. *Lancet* 1980;2:219–222.

229. Camici M, Giordani R, Morelli E, et al. Safety and efficacy anticoagulation in extracorporeal hemodialysis by simultaneous administration of low-dose prostacyclin and low molecular weight heparin. *Minerva Med* 1998; 89:405–409.

230. Ota K, Kawaguchi H, Takahashi K, Ito K. A new prostacyclin analogue—an anticoagulant applicable to hemodialysis. *ASAIO Trans* 1983;59:419–424.

231. Maurin N. Antithrombotic management with a stable prostacyclin analogue during extracorporeal circulation. In: Sieberth HG, Mann H, Stummvoll HK, eds. Continuous Hemofiltration. *Contrib Nephrol* 1991;93:205–209.

232. Hildebrand M, Krause W, Fabian H, et al. Pharmacokinetics of iloprost in patients with chronic renal failure and on maintenance haemodialysis. *Int J Clin Pharmacol Res* 1990; 10:285–292.

233. Taenaka N, Terada N, Takahashi H, et al. Hemodialysis using gabexate mesilate (FOY) in patients with a high bleeding risk. *Crit Care Med* 1986;14:481–483.

234. Akizawa T, Kitaoka T, Sato M, et al. Comparative clinical trial of regional anticoagulation for hemodialysis. *ASAIO Trans* 1988;34:176–178.

235. Maruyama H, Miyakawa Y, Gejyo F, Arakawa M. Anaphylactoid reaction induced by nafamostat mesilate in a hemodialysis patient. *Nephron* 1996;74:468–469.

236. Matsuo T, Matsuo M, Kario K, Koide M. Effect of an anticoagulant (heparin versus nafamostat mesilate) on the extrinsic coagulation pathway in chronic hemodialysis. *Blood Coagul Fibrinolysis* 1998;9:391–393.

237. Hu ZJ, Iwama H, Suzuki R, et al. Time course of activated coagulation time at various sites during continuous haemodiafiltration using nafamostat mesilate. *Intensive Care Med* 1999; 25:524–527.

238. Takahashi H, Muto S, Nakazawa E, et al. Combined treatment with nafamostat mesilate and aspirin prevents heparin-induced thrombocytopenia in a hemodialysis patient. *Clin Nephrol* 2003;59:458–462.

239. Yamazato M, Mano R, Oshiro-Chinen S, et al. Severe abdominal pain associated with allergic reaction to nafamostat mesilate in a chronic hemodialysis patient. *Intern Med* 2002;41:864–866.

240. Higuchi N, Yamazaki H, Kikuchi H, Gejyo F. Anaphylactoid reaction induced by a protease inhibitor, nafamostat mesilate, following nine administrations in a hemodialysis patient. *Nephron* 2000;86:400–401.

241. Nakanishi K, Kaneko T, Yano F, et al. Marked eosinophilia induced by nafamostat mesilate, an anticoagulant in a hemodialysis patient. *Nephron* 1992;62:97–99.

242. Okada H, Suzuki H, Deguchi N, Saruta T. Agranulocytosis in a haemodialysed patient induced by a proteinase inhibitor, nafamostate mesilate. *Nephrol Dial Transplant* 1992;7:980.

243. Inagaki O, Nishian Y, Iwaki R, et al. Adsorption of nafamostat mesilate by hemodialysis membranes. *Artif Organs* 1992;16:553–558.

244. Ookawara S, Tabei K, Sakurai T, et ak. Additional mechanisms of nafamostat mesilate-associated hyperkalaemia. *Eur J Clin Pharmacol* 1996;51:149–151.

245. Casati S, Moia M, Graziani G, et al. Hemodialysis without anticoagulants. *Int J Artif Organs* 1982;5:233–236.

246. Caruana RI, Raja RM, Bush JV, et al. Heparin free dialysis: comparative data and results in high risk patients. *Kidney Int* 1987;31:1351–1355.

247. Liboro R, Schwartz AB, Conroy I, et al. Heparin free hemodialysis does not cause fibrin consumptive coagulopathy and maintains alternate pathway complement activation. *ASAIO Trans* 1990;36:86–89.

248. Hathiwala S. Dialysis without coagulation. *Int J Artif Organs* 1983;6:64–66.

249. Morita Y, Johnson RW, Dorn RE, et al. Regional anticoagulation during hemodialysis using citrate. *Am J Med Sci* 1961;242:32–42.

250. Collart FE, Tielemans CL, Wens R, Dratwa M. Citrate anticoagulation for hemodialysis patients at risk of bleeding. *Am J Nephrol* 1989;9:263–264.

251. Lohr JW, Slusher S, Diederich DA. Regional citrate anticoagulation for hemodialysis following cardiovascular surgery. *Am J Nephrol* 1988;8:368–372.

252. Lohr JW, Slusher S, Diederich DA. Safety of regional citrate hemodialysis in acute renal failure. *Am J Kidney Dis* 1989; 23:104–107.

253. Collart F, Tielemans, Wens R, Dratwa M. Local experience of regional anticoagulation with sodium citrate for hemodialysis in patients at risk of bleeding. *Proc EDTA-ERA* 1985;22:325–328.

254. von Brecht JH, Flanigan M, Freeman RM, Lim VS. Regional anticoagulation: hemodialysis with hypertonic trisodium citrate. *Am J Kidney Dis* 1986;8:196–201.

255. Hocken AG, Hurst PL. Citrate regional anticoagulation in hemodialysis. *Nephron* 1987;46:7–10.

256. Charney DI, Salmond R. Cardiac arrest after hypertonic citrate anticoagulation for chronic hemodialysis. *ASAIO Trans* 1990;36:M217–M219.

257. Evenepoel P, Maes B, Vanwalleghem J, et al. Regional citrate anticoagulation for hemodialysis using a conventional calcium-containing dialysate. *Am J Kidney Dis* 2002;39: 315–323.

258. Kelleher SP, Schulman G. Severe metabolic alkalosis complicating regional citrate hemodialysis. *Am J Kidney Dis* 1987;19:235–236.

259. van der Meulen J, Janssen MJFM, Langendijk PNJ, et al. Citrate anticoagulation and dialysate with reduced buffer content in chronic hemodialysis. *Clin Nephrol* 1992;37: 36–41.

260. Janssen MJ, Deegens JK, Kapinga TH, et al. Citrate compared to low molecular weight heparin anticoagulation in chronic hemodialysis patients. *Kidney Int* 1996;49:806–813.

261. Suki WN, Boneulous RD. Yocum S, et al. Citrate for regional anticoagulation—effects of blood PO_2 ammonia, and aluminum. *ASAIO Trans* 1988;34:524–527

262. Faber LM, de Vries PMJM, Oe PL, et al. Citrate haemodialysis. *Netherlands J Med* l990;37:219–224.

263. Apsner R, Buchmayer H, Lang T, et al. Simplified citrate anticoagulation for high-flux hemodialysis. *Am J Kidney Dis* 2001;38:979–987.

264. Unver B, Sunder-Plassmann G, Horl WH, Apsner R. Long-term citrate anticoagulation for high-flux haemodialysis in a patient with heparin-induced thrombocytopenia type II. *Acta Med Austr* 2002;29:146–148.

265. Buccianti G, Valenti G, Lorenz M, et al. Kinetics of anti-Xa activity during combined defibrotide-heparin administration in hemodialysis. *Int J Artif Organs* 1990;13:416–420.

266. Filimberti B, Cinotti S, Salvadori M, et al. Hemodialysis with defibrotide: effects on coagulation parameters. *Int J Artif Organs* 1992;15:590–594.

267. Kaplan AA, Longnecker RB, Folkert VW. Continuous arteriovenous hemofiltration. *Ann Intern Med* 1984;100:358–367.

268. Lauer A, Saccaggi A, Ronco C, et al. Continuous arteriovenous hemofiltration in the critically ill patient. *Ann Intern Med* 1983;99:455–460.

269. Yagi N, Paganini EP. Acute dialysis and continuous renal replacement: the emergence of new technology involving the nephrologist in the intensive care setting. *Semin Nephrol* 1997;17:306–320.

270. Bartlett R, Bosch JP, Geronemus RO, et al. Continuous arteriovenous hemofiltration for acute renal failure: workshop summary. *ASAIO Trans* 1988;34:67–77.

271. Golper TA. Continuous arteriovenous hemofiltration in acute renal failure. *Am J Kidney Dis* 1985;6:373–386.

272. Schneider NS, Geronemus RP. Continuous arteriovenous hemodialysis. *Kidney Int* 1988;5:159–162.

273. Pattison MB, Lee SM, Ogden DA. Continuous arteriovenous hemodiafiltration: an aggressive approach to the management of acute renal failure. *Am J Kidney Dis* 1988;11:43–47.

274. Bellomo R, Parkin G, Love J, et al. Use of continuous diafiltration: an approach to the management of acute renal failure in the critically ill. *Am J Nephrol* 1992;12:240–245.

275. Ronco C, Brendolan A, Borin D, et al. Continuous arteriovenous hemofiltration in newborns. In: Siberth HG, Mann H, eds. *Continuous Arteriovenous Hemofiltration.* (Aachen International Conference.) Basel: Karger, 1985:76–79.

276. Journois D, Safran D, Castelain MH, et al. Comparing the antithrombotic effects of heparin, enoxaparin and prostacyclin during continuous hemofiltration. *Ann Fr Anest Reanius* 1990;9:331–332.

277. Bellomo R, Teede M, Boyce N. Anticoagulant regimens in acute continuous hemodiafiltration: a comparative study. *Intens Care Med* 1993;19:329–332.

278. Reeves JH, Cumming AR, Gallagher L, et al. A controlled trial of low-molecular-weight heparin (dalteparin) versus unfractionated heparin as anticoagulant during continuous venovenous hemodialysis with filtration. *Crit Care Med* 1999; 27:2224–2228.

279. Monchi M, Berghmans D, Ledoux D, et al. Citrate vs. heparin for anticoagulation in continuous venovenous hemofiltration: a prospective randomized study. *Intens Care Med* 2004;30:260–265.

280. Kaplan AA, Petrillo R. Regional heparinization for continuous arterio-venous hemofiltration. *ASAIO Trans* 1987;33:312–315.

281. Schrader J, Scheler F. Coagulation disorders in acute renal failure and anticoagulation during CAVH with standard heparin and low molecular weight heparin. In: Sieberth HG, Mann H, eds. *Continuous Arteriovenous Hemofiltration.* (Aachen International Conference.) Basel: Karger, 1985: 25–36.

282. Hory B, Cachoux A, Toulemonde F. Continuous arteriovenous hemofiltration with low-molecular-weight heparin. *Nephron* 1985;42:125.

283. Wynckel A, Bernieh B, Toupance O, et al. Guidelines to use of enoxaparin in slow continuous hemodialysis. *Contrib Nephrol* 1991;93:221–224.

284. Jeffrey RF, Khan AA, Douglas JT, et al. Anticoagulation with low molecular weight heparin (Fragmin) during continuous hemodialysis in the intensive care unit. *Artif Organs* 1993;17:717–720.

285. Davenport A. Management of heparin-induced thrombocytopenia during continuous renal replacement therapy. *Am J Kidney Dis* 1998;32:E3.

286. Reddy BV, Nahlik L, Trevino S, et al. Argatroban anticoagulation during renal replacement therapy. *Blood Purif* 2002; 20:313–314.

287. Schneider T, Heuer B, Deller A, Boesken WH. Continuous haemofiltration with r-hirudin (lepirudin) as anticoagulant in a patient with heparin induced thrombocytopenia (HIT II). *Wien Klin Wochenschr* 2000;112:552–555.

288. Brierley JK, Hutchinson A. Prolongation of filter life in contiuous arterio-venous haemodialysis. *Intens Care Med* 1991;17:187–188.

289. Ohtake Y, Hirasawa H, Sugai T, et al. Nafamostat mesylate as anticoagulant in continuous hemofiltration and continuous hemodiafiltration. *Contrib Nephrol* 1991;93:215–217.

290. Hiroma T, Nakamura T, Tamura M, et al. Continuous venovenous hemodiafiltration in neonatal onset hyperammonemia. *Am J Perinatol* 2002;19:221–224.

291. Nakae H, Tajimi K. Pharmacokinetics of nafamostat mesilate during continuous hemodiafiltration with a polyacrylonitrile membrane. *Ther Apher Dial* 2003; 7:483–485.

292. Stevens PB, Davies SP, Brown BA, et al. Continuous arteriovenous hemodialysis in critically ill patients. *Lancet* 1988; 2:150–152.

293. Paganini BP. Slow continuous hemofiltration and slow continuous ultrafiltration. *ASAIO Trans* 1988;34:63–66.

294. Ward DM, Mehta RL. Citrate anticoagulation for continuous arteriovenous hemodialysis (CAVHD)(abstr). *Kidney Int* 1990;37:323.

295. Mehta RI, Bestoso JT, Ward DM. Experience with citrate anticoagulation for continuous renal replacement therapy (CRRT). *J Am Soc Nephrol* 1993;4:368.

296. Palsson R, Niles JL. Regional citrate anticoagulation in continuous venovenous hemofiltration in critically ill patients with a high risk of bleeding. *Kidney Int* 1999;55:1991–1997.

297. Hofmann RM, Maloney C, Ward DM, Becker BN. A novel method for regional citrate anticoagulation in continuous venovenous hemofiltration (CVVHF). *Renal Failure* 2002; 24:325–335.

298. Kutsogiannis DJ, Mayers I, Chin WD, Gibney RT. Regional citrate anticoagulation in continuous venovenous hemodiafiltration. *Am J Kidney Dis* 2000;35:802–811.

299. Tolwani AJ, Campbell RC, Schenk MB, et al. Simplified citrate anticoagulation for continuous renal replacement therapy. *Kidney Int* 2001;60:370–374.

300. Gabutti L, Marone C, Colucci G, et al. Citrate anticoagulation in continuous venovenous hemodiafiltration: a metabolic challenge. *Intens Care Med* 2002;28:1419–1425.

301. Mitchell A, Daul AE, Beiderlinden M, et al. A new system for regional citrate anticoagulation in continuous venovenous hemodialysis (CVVHD). *Clin Nephrol* 2003;59: 106–114.

302. Dorval M, Madore F, Courteau S, Leblanc M. A novel citrate anticoagulation regimen for continuous venovenous hemodiafiltration. *Intensive Care Med* 2003;29:1186–1189.

303. Gong D, Ji D, Xu B, et al. Regional citrate anticoagulation in critically ill patients during continuous blood purification. *Chin Med J* (Engl) 2003;116:360–363.

304. Bunchman TE, Maxvold NJ, Brophy PD. Pediatric convective hemofiltration: Normocarb replacement fluid and citrate anticoagulation. *Am J Kidney Dis* 2003;42:1248–1252.

305. Symons JM, Brophy PD, Gregory MJ, et al. Continuous renal replacement therapy in children up to 10 kg. *Am J Kidney Dis* 2003;41:984–989.

306. Tobe SW, Aujla P, Walele AA, et al. A novel regional citrate anticoagulation protocol for CRRT using only commercially available solutions. *J Crit Care* 2003;18:121–129.

307. Cointault O, Kamar N, Bories P, et al. Regional citrate anticoagulation in continuous venovenous haemodiafiltration using commercial solutions. *Nephrol Dial Transplant* 2004; 19:171–178.

308. Maxvold NJ, Bunchman TE. Renal failure and renal replacement therapy. *Crit Care Clin* 2003;19(3):563–75.

309. Gupta M, Wadhwa NK, Bukovsky R. Regional citrate anticoagulation for continuous venovenous hemodiafiltration using calcium-containing dialysate. *Am J Kidney Dis* 2004; 43:67–73.

310. Dworschak M, Hiesmayr JM, Lassnigg A. Lifesaving citrate anticoagulation to bridge to danaparoid treatment. *Ann Thorac Surg* 2002;73:1626–1627. Erratum in *Ann Thorac Surg* 2002;74:635.

311. Kirschbaum B, Galishoff M, Reines HD. Lactic acidosis treated with continuous hemodiafiltration and regional citrate anticoagulation. *Crit Care Med* 1992; 20:349–353.

312. Davenport A. Dialysate and substitution fluids for patients treated by continuous forms of renal replacement therapy. *Contrib Nephrol* 2001;132:313–322.

Kinetic Modeling in Hemodialysis

Frank A. Gotch
Marcia L. Keen

Kinetic modeling is a widely used analytic process that describes a system from its mass balance. It is a powerful technique because it is based on the fundamental principle of conservation of matter and, hence, requires that all model parameters be rigorously defined, since the validity of the model can be directly determined from mass balance in the system. It is also a powerful system of logic for conceptualization of the clinical problem for which it has been developed. The thought processes must be highly disciplined, because a precise mathematical definition is required for each parameter in the modeled system. In this way, the relative effect of each parameter can be quantitatively assessed.

The clinical goals of modeling in dialysis therapy are to improve clinical understanding of control of the uremic syndrome by dialysis and to prescribe and deliver adequate, reproducible, and quantified doses of dialysis for a variety of solutes. The uremic syndrome is only partly responsive to adequate dialysis therapy, and there is variable ongoing morbidity, such as reduced taste and appetite, mild sensory

neuropathy, renal osteodystrophy, and other clinical entities in well-dialyzed patients. Further, the mortality rate in dialysis patients is strongly dependent on associated illnesses.[1] Because of the variable ongoing morbidity in these patients (regardless of a fully "adequate" dose of dialysis), it is difficult to reliably adjust the dose of dialysis solely from empiric observation of patient symptoms.

Calculation of the dose of dialysis is also quite complicated, both conceptually and with respect to practical details. It is useful to consider the dialysis dose in analogy with pharmacologic therapy. The size of the maintenance dose of a drug and its frequency of administration must be adequate to replace the drug loss determined by the fractional rate at which the drug is cleared from its unique volume of distribution through metabolic, hepatic, renal, and possibly other clearance pathways. In dialysis therapy, a clearance pathway is provided to remove toxic endogenous solutes; consequently, the dialysis dose is a dimensionless parameter, the fractional clearance of the volume of distribution of the specific dialyzed solute. The fractional clearance required is dependent on several interacting parameters that must be quantified: solute distribution volume (related to patient size); intercompartmental transfer coefficients if there is more than one compartment volume; solute generation rate and residual renal clearance; transport properties of the dialyzer used; blood and dialysate flow rates; ultrafiltration rate; and treatment time and dialysis frequency. Kinetic modeling provides a method for quantifying each of these components of the prescription and calculating an individualized dose of dialysis specific to the solute of interest. A major purpose of this chapter is to describe the development of several modeling techniques for a variety of solutes for clinical application. Thus, we review and describe approaches to modeling a variety of solutes—including urea, creatinine, phosphorus, and beta$_2$-microglobulin (β_2M)—that accumulate in end-stage renal disease (ESRD) patients. Clinical studies of the correlations between ongoing residual morbidity and precisely modeled doses of dialysis[2] provide a database to determine the dosage level required to minimize, if possible, the probability of any residual dialysis-dependent clinical symptomatology.

AN OVERVIEW OF UREA KINETIC MODELING

The dialysis prescription is best defined by the amount of solute transport provided relative to its distribution volume, because the rationale for this therapy is that uremia results from the retention of toxic solutes capable of removal by the dialyzer. Kinetic modeling of dialysis provides an analytic method to prescribe a quantified dose of solute removal. Rigorous clinical application of kinetic modeling in dialysis therapy would, however, require detailed knowledge of the dependence of uremic abnormalities on specific toxic solute concentrations. Unfortunately, knowledge of the molecular basis of uremia is still very incomplete. Thus, it is impossible at this time to completely model the dialysis prescription for all toxic solutes. Because dialyzer solute transport is strongly dependent on solute molecular weight, a marker solute for solutes of similar molecular weight has often been used for quantification of the dose of dialysis. In the low-molecular-weight range, urea has been extensively studied as a marker solute and its utility has been verified from correlations between the level of marker solute transport provided and control of clinical morbidity.[2] Known low-molecular-weight solutes that must be managed by dialysis to control toxicity include (among others) potassium, phosphorus, and sodium; water balance must also be controlled.

Urea has played an important historic role in biology and medicine. The unique position of biological molecules early in the nineteenth century was defined by the concept of vitalism, which was the notion that organic molecules could not be governed by physical laws alone.[3] The death knell to vitalism was the report in a letter of one of Jacob

Berzelius's students. "I must tell you that I can make urea without the use of kidneys, either man or dog." Gupta further reports:

> The year was 1828 and Friedrich Wohler, in setting out to synthesize ammonium cyanate, had obtained a white crystalline material which proved identical to urea. It was the first organic compound to be synthesized from inorganic starting materials, and the achievement knocked down one of the few meaningful tenets of vialism—that although organic chemicals could be modified in the laboratory, they could only be produced through the agency of a vital force present in living plants and animals.

We have known for many years that urea is the bulk waste product of protein catabolism, constituting about 90 percent of waste nitrogen accumulating in body water between dialyses. The net rate of urea nitrogen generation (G), in milligrams per minute, is linearly dependent on the net rate of protein catabolism; because G can be measured by urea kinetic analysis, the technique provides a precise measure of the net protein catabolic rate (PCR) in grams per day. In stable chronic dialysis patients, the dietary protein intake equals PCR, so that urea kinetic analysis provides for a quantitative measure of this important dietary constituent. In the unstable acutely ill dialysis patient, the PCR measurement provides a simple clinical method to assess nitrogen balance and optimize amino acid or whole-food protein intake in patients receiving total parenteral nutrition or tube feeding.

Although urea per se has not been established to be an important toxic solute, the dietary protein intake is an important parameter of therapy in chronic dialysis. Inadequate levels of intake may lead to protein malnutrition and increased mortality.[4–6] Excessive protein intake will be associated with high rates of mineral acid production in the body and high levels of inorganic phosphate intake.[7] The measurement of PCR in the stable patient provides the renal dietitian with a precise value for the dietary protein intake, thus permitting identification of those patients who need dietary counseling because of inadequate or excessive protein intake. The determination of protein intake and, therefore, phosphorus intake is useful in determining the phosphorus load from protein sources.

Urea kinetic analysis can also be used to measure the amount of low-molecular-weight dialyzer clearance prescribed and delivered. A wide range of dialyzers, blood and dialysate flow rates, and treatment times are readily available. These technical parameters of the prescription are all interactive, which makes it very difficult to assess the effect of changes in dialyzer flows or treatment time on the level of therapy provided. Therefore a kinetic model is useful in quantifying the relationships between these parameters.

Further, all of these technical parameters must be well controlled during delivery of the prescription, and urea modeling provides a method for technical quality assessment of delivery of the dialysis prescription in the clinical setting.

The above considerations indicate major purposes of urea modeling are to (1) quantify dialysis for individual patients, (2) assess the technical quality of therapy delivered, and (3) assess compliance with the dietary protein (phosphorus) prescription. It must be strongly emphasized that the primary purpose is not to maintain the blood urea nitrogen (BUN) at some arbitrary level. Urea is not a solute exhibiting strong concentration-dependent toxicity; as shown below, an adequate dose of dialysis may result in midweek predialysis BUN levels that vary widely as a function of the variation in PCR. The kinetics of urea accumulation in body water between dialyses and combined removal by the dialyzer and residual renal function can be modeled at variable levels of complexity. The interrelationships between these models are of great importance in optimizing clinical application of urea kinetic modeling.

APPLIED SINGLE-POOL UREA KINETIC MODELING

In Vivo Dialyzer Clearance: Effective Diffusion Volume Flow Rate

The cornerstone of dialysis therapy quantification is accurate estimation of in vivo dialyzer clearance. Determination of dialyzer clearance is a prerequisite for in vivo modeling of any solute. That, in turn, requires an understanding of the fraction of dialyzer blood water flow that is cleared of the solute during passage through the blood compartment. Clearance defines the first order solute transfer across the dialyzer as the rate of solute transfer divided by the inlet blood and dialysate concentration gradient.[8] In the case of urea, creatinine and phosphorus the inlet dialysate concentration is zero. We can write a word equation to describe clearance of these solutes as follows:

$$\text{Clearance} = \frac{\text{Rate of solute/removal from bloodstream flowing through the dialyzer } (Q_{wbi})}{\text{Dialyzer blood/inlet solute concentration}} \quad (1)$$

where Q_{wbi} refers to the flow rate of whole blood into the dialyzer.

Now we can describe the numerator in the right hand side of Eq. (1) in accordance with the following equation:

$$\begin{bmatrix} \text{Rate of solute} \\ \text{removal from blood} \end{bmatrix} = \begin{bmatrix} \text{Change in solute} \\ \text{concentration in} \\ \text{bloodstream} \end{bmatrix} \begin{bmatrix} \text{What flow rate?} \end{bmatrix} \quad (2)$$

$$J_b = \Delta C_b \times Q_e$$

The definition of the effective flow rate, Q_e, is shown as the unknown parameter in Eq. (2); that is the effective volumetric blood flow rate from which the solute diffuses from blood into dialysate. The mathematical derivation of Q_e follows from definitions of rate of solute removal from blood (J_b), as

$$J_b = (C_{pwi} - C_{pwo})Q_e + C_{pwo} \cdot Q_f \quad (3)$$

and rate of solute appearance in dialysate,

$$J_d = C_{do}(Q_{di} + Q_f) \quad (4)$$

Since J_b must equal J_d to satisfy mass balance, we can combine Eqs. (3) and (4) and solve for Q_e to show

$$Q_e = [C_{do}(Q_{di} + Q_f) - C_{pwo}(Q_f)] / [C_{pwi} - C_{pwo}] \quad (5)$$

Note in Eq. (5), that Q_e is calculated from dialysate and ultrafiltrate flow rates, plasma water inlet and outlet, and dialysate concentrations and that the derivation is independent of blood flow rate. The definition of effective blood water clearance (K_e) is simply J_b/C_{pwi}, which can be shown from Eq. (3) to be

$$K_e = [(C_{pwi} - C_{pwo})Q_e + C_{pwo} \cdot Q_f]C_{pwi} \quad (6)$$

Equation (6) shows the relationship of Q_e to blood water clearance. A recent study[9] has shown that Q_e for urea is whole blood water, while for creatinine (Cr) and phosphorus it is largely confined to the plasma flow rate. The red cell appears to be virtually impermeable to Cr and iP. The Q_e for these three solutes can be calculated as a function of Q_{bi} and Hct in accordance with

$$Q_{eu} = (0.94 - .0022 \cdot \text{Hct})(Q_{bi}) \quad (7)$$

$$Q_{ecr} = (0.94 - .0044 \cdot \text{Hct})(Q_{bi}) \quad (8)$$

$$Q_{eiP} = (0.94 - .0100 \cdot \text{Hct})(Q_{bi}) \quad (9)$$

In Vivo Dialyzer Clearance: Calculation from KoA

Clearance defines dialyzer efficiency at specific levels of dialysate and blood flow (Q_d, Q_b). A more generalized definition of dialyzer efficiency is the overall permeability (K_o), in centimeters per minute; membrane area (A), in centimeters, and product, or K_oA, in cubic centimeters per minute.[10,11] The K_oA is calculated from the clearance, blood flow, and dialysate flow in accordance with

$$K_oA = \ln[((K/Q_{di}) - 1)/((K/Q_{bi}) - 1)] \\ [Q_{bi}(1 - Q_{bi}/Q_{di})] \quad (10)$$

Correct calculation of clearance from K_oA values requires that the same flow and concentration units be used for both calculations. In the case of blood water clearance calculations, effective blood water clearance K_e and Q_e must be used to calculate KoA, so that Eq. (10) becomes

$$KoA = \ln[((K_e / Q_{di}) - 1] /$$
$$[(K_e / Q_e) - 1))(Q_e(1 - Q_e / Q_{di}))] \tag{11}$$

Once an effective K_oA is known, K_e can be calculated at any level of Q_e and Q_{di} from rearrangement of Eq. (11),

$$K_e = ((1 - \exp((K_oA / Q_e)(1 - Q_e / Q_{di})))$$
$$(Q_e / Q_{di}) - \exp((K_oA / Q_e)(1 - Q_e / Q_{di}))) \tag{12}$$

In the case with Qf, we can write

$$K_e = ((1 - \exp((K_oA / Q_e)(1 - Q_e / Q_{di}))) /$$
$$((Q_e / Q_{di}) - \exp((K_oA / Q_e)(1 - Q_e / Q_{di})))$$
$$\times (Q_e - Q_f) + Q_f \tag{13}$$

The Fixed-Volume Single-Pool (FVSP) Urea Model

This is the simplest urea model and is depicted in Fig. 7–1A. In this model, the urea distribution volume (V) is considered a single compartment approximately coextensive with total body water, and its volume is assumed to be constant over the dialysis cycle. Urea generation into V is taken to be constant (G) and removal is first-order, as represented in Fig. 7–1A by the product of urea concentration (C) and the sum of dialyzer (K) and renal (K_r) urea clearances (Ke). The model is described mathematically from rate of change in body content of urea during a dialysis treatment in accordance with

$$V(dC / dt) = G - (K_e + K_r)C \tag{14}$$

Note the rate of change in body content or urea is equal to the generation rate minus the removal rate. Integration of Eq. (14) over a complete dialysis, i.e., solution for the total change in body content of urea in an individual treatment, and solution for end dialysis BUN (C_t) results in

$$C_t = C_o \cdot \exp(-(K_e + K_r) \cdot t / V) + (G / (K_e + K_r)) /$$
$$((1 - \exp(P_b s(-(K_e + K_r) \cdot t / V)) \tag{15}$$

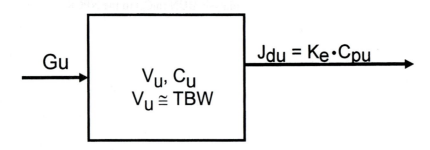

A Fixed–Volume Single–Pool (FVSP) Urea Kinetic Model

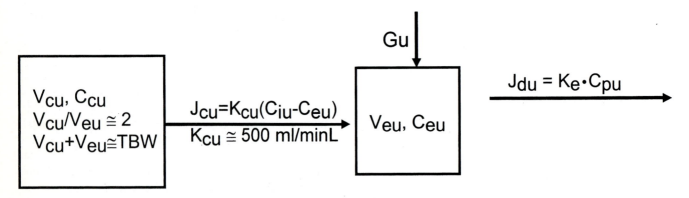

B Fixed–Volume Double–Pool (FVDP) Urea Kinetic Model

Figure 7–1. Schematic of fixed-volume double-pool urea kinetic model.

where t is treatment time. Note that if G is neglected Eq. (15) reduces to

$$C_t = C_o \cdot \exp[-((K_e + K_r) \cdot t / V)] \qquad (16)$$

The predialysis BUN (C_o) at the next dialysis is determined by the generation and removal of urea and duration of the interval (θ) between dialyses. In this case we can write Eq. (14) as

$$V(dC / d\theta) = G - K_r \cdot C \qquad (17)$$

Integration of Eq. (17) results in

$$C_o = C_t \cdot \exp(-(K_r \cdot \theta / V)) + (G / K_r) / \\ (1 - \exp((-K_r \cdot \theta / V))) \qquad (18)$$

Note that if $K_r = 0$, Eq. (18) reduces to

$$C_o = C_t + (G/V) \cdot \theta \qquad (19)$$

During dialysis, the influences of G and K_r on the C_t calculation in Eq. (15) are relatively small, and if they are neglected, Eq. (15) reduces to Eq. (16), which shows that the ratio C_t/C_o or the fractional decrease in BUN is primarily determined by the exponential term Kt/V. This is a key relationship because it demonstrates that the effectiveness of a dialysis treatment in reducing BUN (and the concentration of other solutes) can best be expressed by the magnitude of Kt/V, which is the measure of the individualized dose of dialysis prescribed with respect to urea and other low-molecular-weight solutes. As noted earlier, Kt/V is a dimensionless parameter defining the fractional clearance of the solute distribution volume.

Equation (18) shows that the rise in BUN between dialyses is determined by G, V, K_r, and the length of the interdialytic interval θ. When K_r is 0, Eq (18) reduces to Eq. (19). If a symmetrical treatment schedule is assumed so that θ is constant between each treatment, Eqs. (15) and (19) can be combined and solved for mean C_o (mC_o) in accordance with

$$mC_o = (G / V) \cdot \theta / (1 - \exp(-Kd \cdot t / V)) \qquad (20)$$

This expression illustrates a second relationship of key importance in applied urea modeling in that it shows that the predialysis BUN will increase linearly as a function of G/V when the dose of dialysis Kt/V and the interdialytic interval θ (which is determined by the number of dialyses per week) are held constant. The term G/V in Eq. (20) can also be expressed as the normalized net protein catabolic rate (NPCR). From metabolic balance studies,[12] the relationship of net PCR (PCR), in grams per day, has been shown to be

$$PCR = 9.35 \cdot G + 0.29 \cdot V \qquad (21)$$

The NPCR is defined as PCR divided by (V/0.58). The overall average value for V/body weight (BWt) is approximately 0.58, but it may vary widely from this value in individual subjects. Therefore to use NPCR, body weight (BWt) is normalized with respect to V by defining a normalized body weight (NBWt) as V/NBWt = 0.58. It is apparent now that the NPCR expression can be written as

$$NPCR = PCR / NBWt = PCR / (V / 0.58) \qquad (22)$$

Substitution of Eq. (22) in to Eq. (21) and solution for G/V results in

$$G / V = 0.185(NPCR) - 0.003 \qquad (23)$$

Equation (23) can now be substituted into Eq. (21) to show

$$mC_o[(0.185(NPCR) - .003) / (1 - \exp[-(K_t \cdot t / V)])] \cdot \theta \qquad (24)$$

Equation (24) introduces the generalized relationships between mC_o, Kt/V NPCR, and θ. The interdialytic interval θ in Eq. (24) is inversely related to the number of dialyses per week (N), so that Eq. (24) can also be written as

$$mC_o = ((0.185(NPCR) - .003)) / (1 - \exp(-(K_e \cdot t / V))) \\ \cdot ((10080 / N) - t) \qquad (25)$$

Equation (25) now shows the relationship of the mean predialysis BUN (mC_o) to the NPCR, the dose of each individual dialysis (Kt/V), and the number of dialyses per week. The concept of NBWt is similar to the commonly used expression PCR/BWt, in grams per kilogram of body weight per day. However, the distinction between PCR/BWt and PCR/NBWt is critically important in development of Eq. (25) because the latter expression, PCR/NBWt, rigorously defines PCR relative to V, whereas the relationship of PCR to V with the former expression will be quite variable; V/BWt can range from 0.30 to 0.65. The approximation expression in Eq. (25) illustrates the relationships among four basic parameters of applied urea kinetic modeling: the predialysis BUN or C_o; the dietary protein intake, expressed as NPCR, in steady state; the dose of dialysis as prescribed, Kt/V; and the number of dialyses per week (N). It shows that predialysis BUN (C_o) will be a linear function of NPCR when Kt/V and N are held constant. It must be stressed, however, that the formulation in Eq. (25) is too simplistic and inaccurate for clinical use in that it is an approximation equation based on the FVSP model. Similar but more rigorous relationships between C_o, NPCR, and Kt/V will be developed below for use in clinical application of urea kinetic modeling.

The Variable-Volume Single-Pool (VVSP) Model

This model is shown in Fig. 7–2A and is considerably more reflective of the clinical dialysis setting than the FVSP model because it includes the volume changes occurring

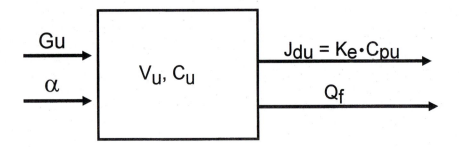

A Variable–Volume Single–Pool (VVSP) Urea Kinetic Model

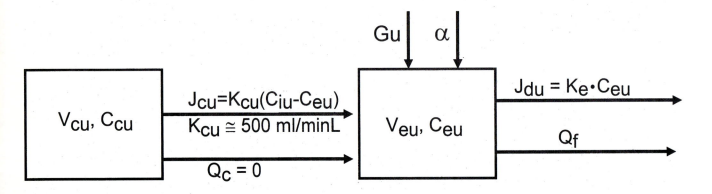

B Variable–Volume Double–Pool (VVDP) Urea Kinetic Model

Figure 7–2. Schematic of variable-volume double-pool urea kinetic model.

over the dialysis cycle. Again, V is considered to be a single pool approximately coextensive with total body water but with expansion during the interdialytic interval from fluid retention and contraction during dialysis by ultrafiltration. The defining equations for this model are

$$d(VC) / dt = G - (K_d + K_r)C \qquad (26)$$

where the changing body content is described as the change in the product of V and C, which are both changing

$$dV / dt = -Q_f; \quad V_t = V_o - Q_f \cdot t \qquad (27)$$

where the change in V during dialysis is constant at rate equal to the ultrafiltration rate

$$dV / d\theta = \alpha; \quad V_o = V_t + \alpha \cdot \theta \qquad (28)$$

$$V_o = V_t + \alpha \cdot \theta \qquad (29)$$

where interdialytic fluid accumulation is considered constant at rate α as defined in Eq. (29). Integration of Eqs. (26) and (27) over one dialysis treatment and solution for C_t results in

$$C_t = C_o[V_o - Q_f \cdot t] \wedge [(K_e + K_r - Q_f) / Q_f]$$
$$+ [G / (K_e + K_r - Q_f)][1 - [V_o - Q_f \cdot t] \wedge$$
$$\times [(K_e + K_r - Q_f) / Q_f]] \qquad (30)$$

while integration over the interdialytic interval and solution for next C_o is

$$C_o = C_t(V_t + \alpha \cdot \theta) \wedge (-(K_r + \alpha) / \alpha) + G / ((K_r + \alpha)$$
$$(1 - (V_t + \alpha \cdot \theta) \wedge (-(K_r + \alpha) / \alpha))) \qquad (31)$$

it is important to note that when $K_r = 0$, Eq. (31) reduces to

$$C_o = C_t(V_o / V_t) + (G / V_o) \cdot \theta \qquad (32)$$

where V_o is predialysis V and V_e is V at the end of the dialysis.

The rate of interdialytic expansion is represented by the constant term α in Eq. (29) and is calculated as the total interdialytic weight gain divided by the length of the interval θ. The rate of contraction during dialysis is represented by the constant term Q_f, which is calculated from total weight loss during dialysis divided by the length of dialysis, t. The urea generation and removal terms, Gu and (K_e +

$K_r)C$, are identical with the FVSP model. As noted above, when $K_r = 0$, Eq. (31) reduces to Eq. (32), which is similar to Eq. (19) but with varying volume. It is important to note that Eq. (30) becomes discontinuous when $Q_f = 0$ and Eq. (31) is discontinuous when $\alpha = 0$. The reason for this can be seen from expansion of the accumulation term in Eq. (26), $d/(VC)/dt$, which becomes $V(dC/dt) + C(dV/dt)$. When Q_f or α are zero, $C(dV/dt) = 0$ and Eq. (26) reduces to Eq. (17). On a practical note, this problem can easily be resolved in programming these expressions for clinical use by simply entering a very small value for the interdialytic weight gain or intradialytic weight loss such as 0.0001 kg when either of these is in fact zero.

Solution of Eq. (30) for the end dialysis volume V_t is

$$V_t = (Q_f \cdot t) / (((G - C_t(K_e + K_r - Q_f)) / \\ (G - C_o(K_e + K_r - Q_f))) \,^\wedge \\ \times (Q_f / (K_e + K_r - Q_f)) - 1) \quad (33)$$

and solution of Eq. (31) for G gives

$$G = (K_r + \alpha)(C_o - C_t((V_t + \alpha \cdot \theta) \,^\wedge (-(K_r + \alpha) / \alpha))) / \\ (1 - (V_t + \alpha \cdot \theta) \,^\wedge (-(K_r + \alpha) / \alpha)) \quad (34)$$

Equation (34) is very useful for clinical application of urea kinetics. In order to calculate a prescription, which is quan-

titatively expressed as spKt/V, it is necessary to determine V_t in the individual patient. A second equally important use of the V_t calculation is for monitoring the technical quality of delivered dialysis therapy. If there are technical problems resulting in an error in the Kt delivered, the magnitude of Kt error can be assessed quantitatively from the error in calculated V_t. These relationships will be considered in detail later.

Clinical application of urea kinetics was initially based on measurement of C_{o1}, C_{t1}, and C_{o2} during the first and second dialyses of the week on a thrice weekly schedule and iteration of Eqs. (33) and (34) until unique values for V_t and G are found satisfying both expressions. Although this is a rigorous method for measurement of these parameters, it is not logistically practical because three BUN measurements from two consecutive dialyses are required. This is more costly and also subject to incomplete data collection due to missed samples.

A much more clinically acceptable and equally rigorous approach can be based on measured (m) C_o and C_t samples from a single dialysis (C_{om}, C_{tm}) with iterative solution of the equations using the specified treatment schedule until steady state concentrations are reached matching the values for the measured dialysis. This method is illustrated in Fig. 7–3 and begins with solution of Eq. (33) for V_t using K_e calculated from Q_e, Q_{di} and the in vivo dialyzer K_oA, an esti-

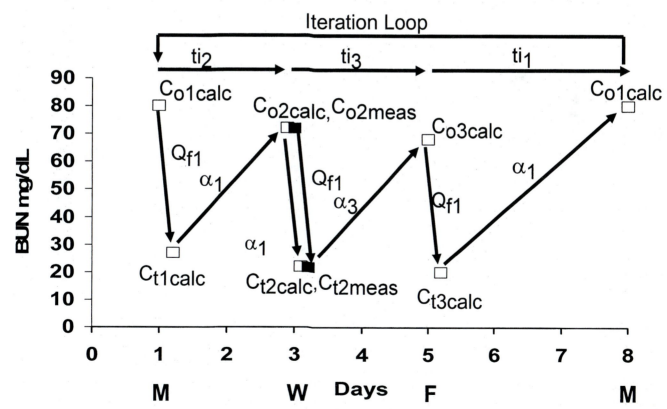

Figure 7–3. Illustration of the iteration loop for calculation of Vt, spG, eG, and hence spKt/V, eKt/V, ePCR, and eNPCR. A thrice-weekly schedule is depicted; C_{o2} and C_{t2} are measured and all other values calculated.

mated Gu and then subsequent sequential iterative solution of Eq. (31) or Eqs. (32), (33), and (34) until the calculated values for C_o and Ct (C_{oc} and C_{tc}) values are constant. Thus each iteration begins with solution of Eq. (33) for V_t from the measured C_o and C_t and other input parameters as discussed above. The analysis proceeds with sequential solution of Eq. (31) or Eqs. (32), (33), and (34) through weekly loops until C_o calculated for the analyzed dialysis, cC_o, is *constant*, i.e., it varies less than 0.1 percent from last value. It may differ substantially from the mC_o for the analyzed dialysis which will reflect error in the assumed spG. After steady state is reached for cC_o, spG is adjusted ($_{aj}$spG) in direct proportion to the deviation of the ratio cC_o/mC_o from unity in accordance with

$$_{aj}spG = [mC_o / cC_o](spG) \quad (35)$$

where spG is value at the end of the current loop. The new value for $_{aj}$spG is used in Eq. (33) to calculate a new V_t and again Eq. (31) or Eqs. (32), (33), and (34) are solved sequentially starting again with the mCt value to find a new steady state cC_o which is again used to calculate a new $_{aj}$spG and V_t. When cC_o/mC_o is constant the iteration is terminated and if it does not match the measured value for mC_o, the G is again adjusted and the iterative process repeated until the C_o and C_t match the measured values. The three BUN method provides an estimate of PCR for the specific time interval between the C_{t1} and C_{o2} while the two BUN method will provide a more average value for PCR over the week. Once V_t has been calculated, the spKt/V is calculated simply as $K_e \cdot t/V_t$. However, as discussed below, this value must be corrected for double pool kinetic effects to obtain the most accurate results.

Approaches to Approximation of Single-Pool Kinetics for Clinical Use. There have been many attempts to find simple solutions of the VVSP urea model.[13-15] However, the only reliable solution has been the "Daugirdas equation."[16] Daugirdas derived an accurate empirical approximation equation to estimate spKt/V from C_t/C_o, treatment time, weight loss, and body weight. He developed empirical coefficients which reliably estimate the effects of t, Q_f, and Gu on the spKt/V calculation in accordance with

$$spKt / V = -\ln(R_t / R_o + .008t)$$
$$+ (4 - 3.5 * (R_t / R_o))(Q_{FT}) / BWt \quad (36)$$

As noted above, this equation correlates closely with formal VVSP calculation of spKt/V over a wide range of dialysis dose. However, with the Daugirdas approximation equation the V is not calculated, only the ratio, spKt/V, is

estimated, so it is not possible to check that the calculated spKt/V makes sense from evaluation of the calculated volume. Further, the PCR cannot be calculated since V is not determined. Daugirdas and Depner have published an algorithm to calculate the normalized NPCR,[17] which appears to correlate well with formal VVSP UKM. The only weakness of this approach is that V is not estimated to calculate actual protein intake, i.e., PCR.

APPLIED DOUBLE-POOL KINETIC MODELING

The Fixed-Volume Double-Pool (FVDP) Urea Model

The actual anatomical distribution of urea is comprised of blood plasma and red cell water (V_{bw}), interstitial (V_i), and intracellular (V_I) water. Transfer between these compartments is diffusive and can, in analogy with the dialyzer, be described by the product of a volumetric mass transfer coefficient and the difference in concentration between the compartments. The whole-body mass transfer coefficient across the capillary bed is extremely high for most low-molecular-weight solutes and so concentration equilibrium is assumed between V_{bw} and V_i and these two compartments can be treated as a single extracellular compartment, V_e.[18] A FVDP model for urea is illustrated in Fig. 7–1B where typical assumed ratios for V_c/V_e and $V_c + V_e \cong$ TBW are depicted. The intercompartmental transfer coefficient for an average patient is indicated to be 500 mL/min or 15 mL/L of ($V_c + V_e$). The generation of urea nitrogen is assumed to be into V_e since it is produced in the liver and promptly diffuses into V_e. In the FVDP models, urea is removed from V_e by the dialyzer resulting in a transcompartmental urea concentration gradient from V_c to V_e down which urea diffuses at a rate equal to the product $K_c(C_cU - C_eU)$. As a consequence of these mechanisms of urea transport, little urea is removed from V_c until a sizable concentration gradient develops over the first half hour of dialysis. Subsequently, the concentration gradient remains constant during the remainder of dialysis. Immediately after dialysis, urea continues to diffuse from V_c to V_e until concentration equilibrium is reached. This results in a rapid rebound increase in C_eU with the magnitude of the rebound proportional to the magnitude of the end-dialysis concentration gradient and the compartment volumes. In the case of a double pool creatinine model, generation of creatinine is due to hydration and release of a small constant fraction of the muscle creatine pool and consequently it would be modeled as generation into the cellular compartment. The rate equations describing mass balance in the general FVDP model are

$$V_c(dCc / dt) = -K_c(C_c - C_e) \quad (37)$$

$$V_e(dCe / dt) = G + K_c(C_c - C_e) - (K_e + K_r)C_e \quad (38)$$

when generation into V_e is assumed while as in the case of creatinine, mass balance would be described as

$$V_c(dCc / dt) = G - K_c(C_c - C_e) \qquad (39)$$

$$V_e(dCe / dt) = K_c(C_c - C_e) - (K_e + K_r)C_e \qquad (40)$$

Analytic solutions of the FVDP model have been derived previously (19). In the case of a solute such as urea with generation into V_e solutions for C_{et} and C_{ct} are

$$
\begin{aligned}
C_{et} = &(C_{eo} \cdot K_c / V_e + C_{eo} \cdot K_e / V_c + G / V_b \\
&- (G \cdot K_c / V_e \cdot V_c)(1 / \beta) - C_{eo}) \\
&\cdot \beta(\exp(-\beta t / (\alpha - \beta))) \\
&- (C_{co} \cdot Kc / V_e + C_{eo} \cdot K_c / V_c \\
&- (G \cdot K_c / V_e \cdot V_c)(1 / \alpha) - C_{eo} \cdot \alpha) \\
&(\exp(-\alpha \cdot t / (\alpha - \beta))) \\
&+ G \cdot K_c / (V_e \cdot V_c \cdot \alpha \cdot \beta)
\end{aligned}
\qquad (41)
$$

$$
\begin{aligned}
C_{ct} = &((C_{eo} K_c / V_c) + (C_{co}(K_c + K_r + K_d) / V_e) \\
&- (GK_c / V_e V_c)(1 / \beta) - C_{co}\beta)(\exp(-\beta t) / \\
&(\alpha - \beta)) - ((C_{eo} K_c / V_c) \\
&+ (C_{co}(K_c + K_r + K_d) / V_e) \\
&- (GK_c / V_e V_c)(1 / \alpha) - C_{co}\alpha)(\exp(-\alpha t)(\alpha - \beta)) \\
&+ GK_c / (V_e V_c \alpha \beta)
\end{aligned}
\qquad (42)
$$

in the case of generation into V_c the solutions are

$$
\begin{aligned}
C_{et} = &(C_{eo} \cdot K_c / V_e + C_{eo} \cdot K_e / V_c + (G \cdot K_c / V_e \cdot V_c) \\
&\times (1 / \beta) - C_{eo}) \cdot \beta(\exp(-\beta t / (\alpha - \beta))) \\
&- (C_{co} \cdot K_c / V_e + C_{eo} \cdot K_c / V_c - (G \cdot K_c / V_e \cdot V_c) \\
&\times (1 / \alpha) - C_{eo} \cdot \alpha)(\exp(-\alpha t / (\alpha - \beta))) \\
&+ G \cdot K_c / (V_e \cdot V_c \cdot \alpha \cdot \beta)
\end{aligned}
\qquad (43)
$$

$$
\begin{aligned}
C_{ct} = &((C_{eo} K_c / V_c) + (C_{co}(K_c + K_r + K_d) / V_e) \\
&+ (G / V_e) - (G(K_c + K_r + K_d) / V_e V_c) \\
&\times (1 / \beta) - C_{co}\beta)(\exp(-\beta t) / (\alpha - \beta)) \\
&- ((C_{eo} K_c / V_c) + (C_{co}(K_c + K_r + K_d) / V_e) \\
&+ (G / V_e) - (G(K_c + K_r + K_d) / V_e V_c) \\
&\times (1 / \alpha) - C_{co}\alpha)(\exp(-\alpha t)(\alpha - \beta)) \\
&- G(K_c + K_r + K_d) / (V_e V_c \alpha \beta)
\end{aligned}
\qquad (44)
$$

where, in both cases,

$$
\begin{aligned}
\alpha = &0.5((K_C / V_c) + (K_c + K_r + K_d) / V_e \\
&+ (((K_c / V_c) + ((K_c + K_r + K_d) / V_e))^2 \\
&- 4((K_c(K_r + K_d) / V_e V_c)))^{0.5})
\end{aligned}
\qquad (45)
$$

$$
\begin{aligned}
\beta = &0.5((K_c / V_c) + (K_c + K_r + K_d) / V_e \\
&- (((K_c / V_c) + ((K_c + K_r + K_d) / V_e))^2 \\
&- 4((K_c(K_r + K_d) / V_e V_c)))^{0.5})
\end{aligned}
\qquad (46)
$$

Equations (41) to (46) provide analytic solutions to the FVDP model in terms of (1) the two compartment volumes, (2) intercompartmental transport coefficient, (3) dialyzer clearance, (4) residual renal clearance, and/or (5) treatment time or interdialytic interval. They can be solved both during dialysis and between dialyses to analyze concentration profiles and will be used below to assess the double pool approximation algorithms.

The Variable-Volume Double-Pool (VVDP) Urea Model. A VVDP model describing urea kinetics is depicted in Fig. 7–2B. This model differs from the FVDP model only in that V_e is modeled to contract during dialysis as a function of Q_f and to expand between dialyses as a function of the rate of fluid accumulation, α. The mass balance rate equations for the compartments are more complex consisting of

$$V_c(dC_c / dt) = -K_c(C_c - C_e) \qquad (47)$$

$$d(V_e \cdot C_e) / dt = G + K_c(C_c - C_e) - (K_e + K_r u)(C_e) \qquad (48)$$

$$dV_e / dt = -Q_f \text{ during dialysis and } \alpha \text{ between} \\ \text{dialyses.} \qquad (49)$$

The VVDP model is a more rigorous description of urea kinetics than the VVSP model. However, the physiological model parameters requiring estimation are expanded from two in the VVSP model (G, V_c) to four in the VVDP model (G, V_c, V_e, K_cU). An analytic solution of the VVDP model is not possible so the rate equations must be solved numerically which is inconvenient for clinical use since many intermediate concentrations are required for optimal solution. Even then, attempting to fit the four-model parameters is very difficult and can often result in unrealistic parameters.

A Variable-Volume Double-Pool Model Describing Beta₂-Microglobulin (B2M) Kinetics. Beta₂-microglobulin is an established major uremic toxin resulting in B2M amyloidosis.[20] There is still considerable uncertainty as to what determines the magnitude of amyloid deposition.[21] The plasma concentration becomes very high in renal failure which is thought to be a major determinant of the amyloid deposition[22] although it has not been possible to show a direct correlation of the plasma level and degree of amyloid disease.[23] The anatomic distribution of B2M and its transport kinetics are illustrated in Fig. 7–4. It is usually assumed that B2M is released from cell membranes at a relatively constant rate of about 0.125 mg/min.[24] The filtered B2M is completely catabolized in the proximal tubule so renal clearance is equal to GFR and the normal C_p can be predicted to be very low since it will be determined in steady state by

$$C_pB2M = GB2M / GFR \qquad (50)$$

and, if G = 0.125 mg/min and GFR = 0.10 L/min, C_pB2M = 0.125/0.10 = 1.25 mg/L.[24] The relationships in Eq. (50) also show that if there is a significant level of residual GFR it will have a powerful influence on the plasma concentration of B2M and changes in GFR over time can confound the interpretation of changes in the effects of dialysis therapy.

After release, this small protein is considered to be uniformly distributed in interstitial fluid (V_{is}) and plasma volume (V_p) with the two compartments linked by a transvascular diffusion coefficient (K_v).[24] The total distribution volume ($V_{is} + V_p$) is relatively small, approximately one third of TBW or about 12 L in the average sized patient with V_{is} = 9 L and V_p = 3 L. The K_v is quite small, of the order of 5 mL/L of V_e or 60 mL/min in the average patient, and is, therefore, a bottle neck with respect to removal of B2M with efficient dialyzers. In addition to removal by GFR, there is a relatively constant rate of extrarenal catabolism (K_m) which has been described as a first order metabolic constant with value about 2.5 mL/min.[25] Thus when GFR = 0 and there is no dialyzer clearance, the steady state C_pB2M can be calculated from Eq. (50) as 0.125/0.0025 = 50 mg/L a 40-fold increase over the normal level.

The VVDP model of B2M in Fig. 7–4 differs substantially from the urea model. The generation of B2M is modeled as occurring into V_{is}. The dialytic removal of volume (Q_f) and interdialytic volume accumulation (α) are depicted in Fig. 7–4 to distribute in both volumes in proportion to their sizes, with distribution determined primarily by changes in the plasma protein concentration and oncotic pressure. Consequently both volumes expand and contract and transport from V_{is} to V_p will have a diffusive and important convective component dependent on ultrafiltration rate and the transvascular sieving coefficient (K_s). The mass balance equations for the VVDP B2M model are

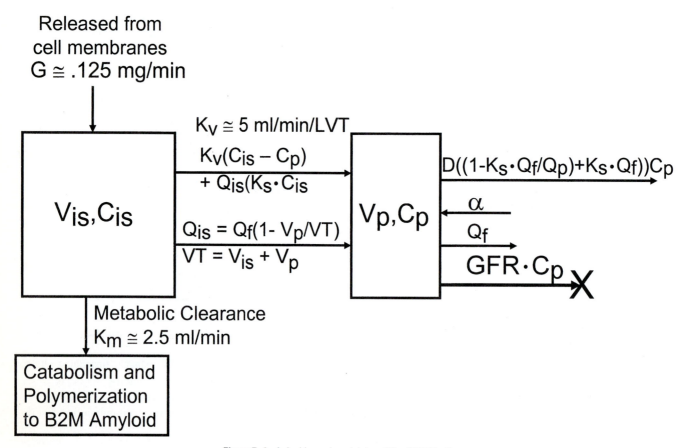

Figure 7–4. A double-pool model describing B2M kinetics.

$$d(V_{is} \cdot C_{is})/dt = G - (K_v + K_m)$$
$$\times (C_{is} - C_p) - Q_f(1 - V_p / V_{is}) \qquad (51)$$

$$d(V_p \cdot C_p)/dt = K_v(C_{is} - C_p) + Q_f(1 - V_p / V_{is})$$
$$-Q_f \cdot C_p - K_e(1 - K_s \cdot Q_f / Q_e) + K_s \cdot Q_f + GFR \cdot C_p \qquad (52)$$

As in the case of the urea VVDP model, analytic solution of the VVDP B2M model is not possible. The solution would similarly require multiple interdialytic and postdialytic B2M concentration measurements and numerical estimation of the parameters resulting in the best fit of the concentration curves. These numerical techniques are not suitable for routine clinical measurement of therapy, which has resulted in the study of techniques to simplify the relationships.

Approaches to Approximations of Double Pool Kinetics for Clinical Use. The physiologic and anatomical bases of double pool kinetics of uremic toxins are not clearly elucidated. The two compartments have been considered to be cellular and extracellular fluid for many years. An alternative model based on the distribution of blood flow to body organs was proposed many years ago.[26] More recent data have been reported which appear to be consistent with such a model.[27] The data

indicate that approximately 80 percent of cardiac output is distributed to visceral organs, which contain only about 30 percent of body water. In contrast, only 20 percent of cardiac output is distributed to muscle, bone, and skin, which contain 70 percent of body water. Isotope dilution kinetics generally indicate tracer uptake in muscle is flow limited and first order, which would suggest that the whole body urea transport coefficient is not a cell membrane constant but is instead a blood flow parameter. The remarkably long time required for Na osmotic distribution equilibrium to occur across cell membranes freely permeable to water[28] is consistent with the flow limitation hypothesis. During passage across the dialyzer, where diffusion distances between red cells and plasma are short, complete Na equilibrium occurs between red cells and plasma.[29] Although the anatomical and physiologic basis of double pool kinetics have not been fully elucidated, considerable progress has been made in understanding and simplification of double-pool kinetics for clinical use in treatment of uremia over the past few years.

The increased complexity of interpretation of pre- and postdialysis solute concentrations due to double pool kinetics is illustrated for urea in Fig. 7–5. The concentration profiles depicted for plasma water, cell water, and mean body water concentration were calculated with Eqs. (41) and (42)

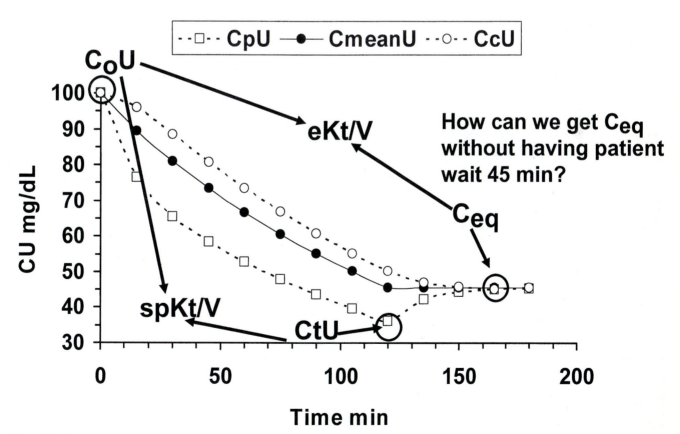

Figure 7–5. Urea concentration profiles for plasma, cell water, and mean body water calculated with double-pool kinetic parameters during and after dialysis. The spKt/V is calculated from the postdialysis C_{tU}, while eKt/V is calculated from the equilibrated value, which does not occur until about 30 min after dialysis.

during dialysis and during postdialysis reequilibration between the two compartments. Note that all three concentrations fall exponentially during dialysis while, during reequilibration, the mean concentration remains stable while C_p and C_c exponentially approach mean concentration of urea in body water (mC) over approximately 30 minutes. As will be discussed in detail below and illustrated in Fig. 7–5, the spKt/V is calculated from C_o and C_t but calculation of the equilibrated Kt/V (eKt/V) requires a value for the C_p after postdialysis equilibration (C_{eq}). It would obviously be much preferable to reliably predict C_{eq} rather than require the patient to remain for blood sampling after equilibration. Several algorithms to predict C_{eq} have been derived and reported.[30–33]

The basis of all C_{eq} prediction algorithms is the observation by Smye[30] that the mathematics of the double pool model dictates that after an initial transient, during which a concentration gradient is established between C_p and C_c, both C_p and mC decrease with equal, log linear slopes as depicted in Fig 7–6. Note that at t = 0 the body water is in concentration equilibrium, $C_p = mC$; mC decreases linearly and after the initial transient is complete at 60 to 90 min both C_p and mC decrease with virtually identical log linear slopes. From the simple slope-intercept linear functions depicted in Fig. 7–6, Smye recognized that from measurement of C_o (predialysis BUN) and intradialytic C_p values at 90 minutes and the end of dialysis, the slope and intercept for $ln(C_p)$ could be readily determined and from this an equation to predict C_{eq} derived (see Fig. 7–7) of the form

$$C_{eq} = C_o (C_s / C_t)^{\wedge}(t / (t - t_s)) \qquad (53)$$

The Smye algorithm is the most rigorous double pool approximation conceptually but it suffers from the effects of small BUN measurement errors, which can result in substantial slope errors based on only 2 numbers. It is the most generalized approximation model because the actual slope and intercept for $ln(C_p) = f(t)$ are measured.

Tattersall[33] derived and reported an algorithm which is also based on the log linear equal slopes shown in Fig. 7–6, but based on the difference in intercept of the two linear curves which he described as a generalizable solute specific time constant (the patient equilibration time, t_p) as depicted in Fig. 7–8,

$$eKt / V = spKt / V(t / (t + t_p)) \qquad (54)$$

This expression is derived from the simplified relationships

$$eKt / V = ln(C_o / C_{eq}) \qquad (55)$$

and

$$spKt / V = ln(C_o / C_t) \qquad (56)$$

thus from Eqs. (54), (55), and (56), we can see that

$$t_p = t(ln(C_o / C_t) - ln(C_o / C_{eq})) / ln(C_o / C_{eq}) \qquad (57)$$

The basis for Eq. (57) is, again, equal log-linear slopes for C_p and mC demonstrated mathematically by Smye. How-

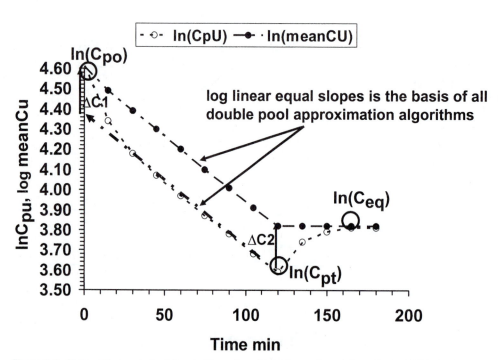

Figure 7–6. Mathematical analysis of the double-pool model by Smye showed that, after an initial transient, the ln(CpU) falls linearly with the same slope as ln(mCu), the mean concentration in total body water.

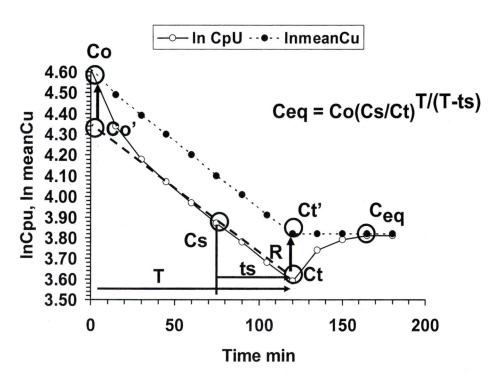

Figure 7–7. The Smye algorithm computed C_{eq} from C_o, C_s at 65 min, and C_t at the end of dialysis. This technique eliminated the need to wait for rebound sampling. The method was subject to error in estimating the log-linear curve from two points.

ever, the Tattersall expression is not as truly generalized as Eq. (53) since t_p is strongly dependent on the ratio K_c/VT and the ratio V_e/V_c as well as K_c, which is dependent on the solute diffusion coefficient which, in turn, is largely molecular size dependent. Since C_o and the actual slope of C_p is measured with the Smye method, these problems are avoided but the problem of error amplification due to small variances in BUNs appears to result in better reproducibility of the Tattersall algorithm. Tattersall reported solute specific t_p values for urea and creatinine of 35 and 65 min, respectively. Subsequent analysis of HEMO data showed similar coefficients.[34]

Daugirdas and Schneditz[31] also reported an algorithm to predict rebound based on similar considerations and in accordance with

$$eKt / V = spKt / V(1 - 36 / t) + 0.03 \quad (58)$$

Rearrangement of Eq. (58) and solution for a Daugirdas "patient constant" (dt_p) results in

$$dt_p = t(\ln(C_o / C_t) - \ln(C_o / C_{eq}) + .03) / \ln(C_o / C_t) \quad (59)$$

Equation (59) differs from Eq. (57) only in that in Eq. (59) the denominator is $\ln(C_o/C_t)$ rather than $\ln(C_o/C_{eq})$ as in Eq. (57). However, inspection of Eq. (58) shows that this difference will result in a discontinuity when t = 36 min and it is gradually approached as t decreases into the range of short

daily dialysis. The ratios of $eKt/V_{Daug}/eKt/V_{Tatt}$ calculated from Eqs. (55) and (58) respectively are plotted in Fig. 7–9 where the anomalous behavior of Eq. (58) as treatment time shortens can be seen. The Tattersall algorithm provides a more reliable estimate of rebound.

Determinants of Patient Rebound Time (t_p), Rebound Rate (k_p), and Total Rebound (R_T). The t_p as defined by Tattersall is the time required to achieve complete postdialysis equilibration between the two modeled compartments. The k_p, discussed below, defines the rate at which this rebound occurs. The mechanisms determining these values can be seen in the FVDP mass balance Eqs. (37) and (38) during the rebound interval which can be written, neglecting the generation term, as

$$dC_c / dt = -(K_c / V_c)(C_c - C_e) \quad (60)$$

$$dC_e dt = (K_c / V_e)(C_c - C_e) \quad (61)$$

Equations (60) and (61) show that the rate of equilibration or rebound will be strongly dependent on the ratio K_c/V_c and K_c/V_e. Since $V_e + V_c = V_T$ (V total), we can write V_e and V_c in terms of V_T by defining a ratio $R_V = V_e/V_T$ and substitution into Eqs. (60) and (61) to give

$$dC_c dt = -(K_c / (1 - R_V) \cdot V_T)(C_c - C_e) \quad (62)$$

$$dC_e / dt = (K_c / (R_v \cdot V_T))(C_c - C_e) \quad (63)$$

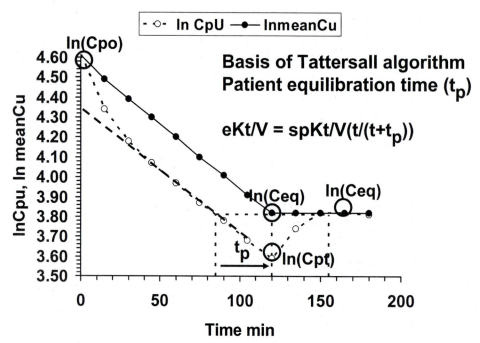

Figure 7–8. Tattersall showed that the separation of the two curves demonstrated by Smye was a generalizable and predictable time constant t_p, 35 min for urea and 65 min for creatinine. This time constant was then used to derive the C_{eq} and eKt/V from spKt/V, as shown here.

Equations (60) to (63) show that the rate of rebound (and hence t_p and k_p) will be strongly dependent on the ratio K_c/V_T and to some extent on R_V. The total rebound will be determined by the magnitude of the end dialysis gradient, $C_c - C_e$, which in turn is primarily dependent on the ratio K_e/K_c or how rapidly the patient is dialyzed relative to the intercompartmental transfer coefficient (K_c). The total rebound will also be somewhat dependent on the site of solute generation, i.e., into V_c or V_e. Removal will be more efficient with generation into V_e, which is the compartment from which solute is directly removed by dialysis and increase the end dialysis gradient somewhat compared to generation into V_c.

These relationships were simulated with the FVDP model and results compared to the Tattersall approximation calculations. The relationships of t_p to K_c/V_T with $R_V = 0.33$ are shown in Fig. 7–10. The FVDP model Eqs. (41) and (42) were solved for C_o, C_t, and C_{eq} over a wide range of K_c/V_T with $R_V = 0.33$ and the results plotted in Fig. 7–10, along with the t_p calculated from the Tattersall algorithm, in the following way. The FVDP equations were used to calculate values for C_o, C_t, and C_{eq}. The Tattersall expression for C_{eq},

$$C_{eq} = C_o(C_t/C_o)^{\wedge}(t/(t+t_p)) \qquad (64)$$

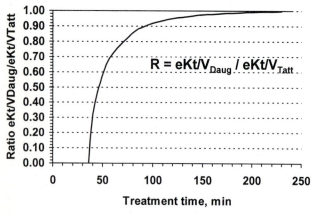

Figure 7–9. The Daugirdas/Schneditz approximation equation to estimate eKt/V becomes a discontinuous treatment time of 36 minutes.

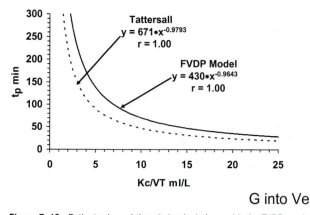

G into Ve

Figure 7–10. Patient rebound time (tp) calculations with the FVDP model and the Tattersall algorithm over a wide range of Kc/VT, with RV = 0.33.

was rearranged to calculate t_p from the C_o, C_t, and C_{eq} values calculated with the FVDP model. In Fig. 7–10 it can be seen that there is a very tight power function dependence of t_p on K_c/V_T but that the Tattersall equation systematically results in somewhat shorter t_p values at all levels of K_c/V_T. The difference is trivial in the case of urea and increases as K_c/V_T decreases. Although the difference reflects divergence of the approximation from true FVDP kinetics, the approximations may be more characteristic for clinical use where the blunting effect of ultrafiltration on the concentration changes during and after dialysis is included in the empiric data reported by Tattersall. The C_{eq} predicted by Eq. (64) agrees perfectly with the C_{eq} values calculated with the FVDP model, which is not unexpected, since t_p was calculated from C_{eq}. In Fig. 7–11 the calculations shown in Fig. 7–10 are repeated with $R_V = 0.25$ (representative of a solute such as B2M) where similar relationships of the FVDP model to the Tattersall equation are again seen.

Inspection of Eqs. (62) and (63) suggest the fractional rate of rebound (k_p) might be expected to conform to a single exponential function over the interval t to t_p and be of the form

$$(C_{t'} - C_t) / (C_{eq} - C_t) = 1 - \exp(-k_p \cdot t') \quad (65)$$

where $C_{t'}$ represents rebound values C_t during the interval (t') from t to t_p as illustrated in Fig. 7–12. The curve labeled FVDP Model was constructed from solutions of the model and, indeed, shows the rebound function to exponentially approach a limiting value defined by t_p. The curve labeled "Tattersall" was calculated from Eq. (64) modified to define the rate of rebound as in Eq. (65) resulting in

$$Ct' = C_o(C_t / C_o) ^ (t / (t + t_p(1 - \exp(-k_p t')))) \quad (66)$$

Equation (66) is a description of the complete rebound curve expected with the Tattersall approximation algorithm. Although it has two unknowns, t_p and k_p, from Eqs. (64)

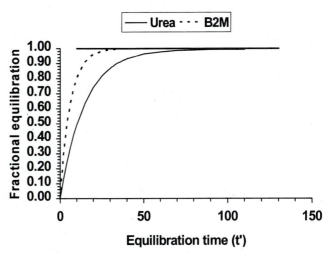

Figure 7–12. Comparison of urea and B2M rebound curves calculated with FVDP model. The model solutions show single exponential rebound curves related to tp. Rebound with the Tattersall algorithm can be modeled as:

$$Ct' = Co((Ct / Co) ^ (t / (t + tp(1 - \exp(-kp \cdot t'e)))))$$

and (65), it can be surmised that k_p will be closely related to K_c/V_T and hence to t_p. This postulate was evaluated by simulations with the FVDP model over a wide range of K_e/V_T with two levels of R_V .33 and .25. The results can be seen in Fig. 7–13 where k_p is shown to be highly correlated to t_p as a power function. The effect of R_V (simulations not shown) was negligible so a single relationship can be defined. From the relationship in Fig. 7–13 we can write

$$C_t' = C_o((C_t / C_o) ^ (t /(t + t_p(1 - \exp(-1.030* (t_p) ^ (-0.659) \cdot t'))))) \quad (67)$$

Equation (67) can be solved iteratively for t_p from measured values for C_o, C_t, t, and three $C_{t'}$ values measured

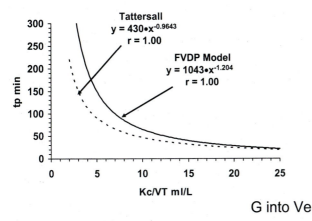

Figure 7–11. Patient rebound time (tp) calculations with FVDP model and the Tattersall algorithm over a wide range of Kc/VT, with RV = 0.25.

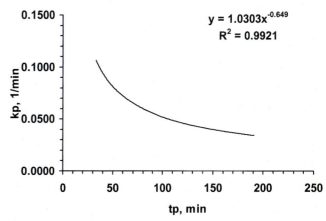

Figure 7–13. Relationship of kp to tp, RV 0.25 and 0.33, where these are defined as:

$$Ct' = Co((Ct / Co) ^ (t / (t + tp(1 - \exp(-kp \cdot te)))))$$
$$Ct' = Co((Ct / Co) ^ (t / (t + tp(1 - 1.030(tp - 0.649) \cdot te)))))$$

randomly over 20 to 30 minutes post dialysis without the need to determine C_{eq}. As part of a study of urea and creatinine generation[9] we obtained C_o, C_t, and $C_{t'}$ values at 15, 30, and 45 minutes postdialysis and used Eq. (67) to determine the t_p value by finding the best fit between the three measured and calculated $C_{t'}$ values. The best-fit t_p values were: urea $t_p = 35 \pm 15$ minutes and creatinine $t_p = 60 \pm 23$ minutes (M ± SD, N = 21). These results compare quite favorably with the values reported by Tattersall who obtained 4 postdialysis samples including C_{eq}.[33] Each of the calculated and observed rebound values are depicted in Figs. 7–14 and 7–15. In Fig. 7–14 a high degree of correlation can be seen with a slope not quite equal to unity. In Fig. 7–15 a Bland Altman plot shows there was a small bias with slight overestimation of early rebound with Eq. (67) but the bias is minimal and overall agreement is excellent. This would appear to provide a simplified method of establishing rebound kinetics for a wide range of solutes.

The total rebound, C_{eq}/C_t, can be expected to be primarily dependent on the rate of dialysis, K_e/K_c, which is the major determinant of the total end dialysis gradient between C_e and C_c. This was evaluated by solving the FVDP model over a wide range of K_e/K_c and K_c/V_T to determine total percent rebound, $100*((C_{eq}/C_t) - 1)$. The results plotted in Fig. 7–16 demonstrate a stepwise increase in rebound as K_e/K_c increases and with relatively little effect of K_c/V_T.

Approximation of the Double-Pool Effect on Kinetic Single-Pool Volume Calculation (Vsp) and spKt/V.

It has long been known that there are systematic errors in volume calculated with the FVSP and VVSP models.[19] Early in dialysis while the transcompartmental gradient is being established and solute removal is primarily from V_e, the V_{sp} is severely underestimated while with a long duration, high Kt/V dialysis it becomes overestimated. The geometric relationships between $\ln(C_e)$ and $\ln(C_m)$ dictated by the double pool effect enabled

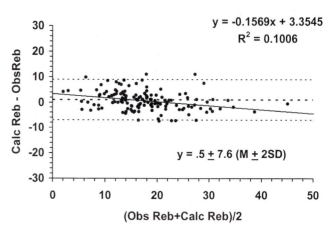

Figure 7–15. Bland Altman plot of the data in Fig. 7–14 shows there is a significant slope with a small positive bias at low levels of rebound and negative bias at high levels of rebound.

Tattersall to derive a simple algorithm to estimate this effect in accordance with

$$cV_{sp} = V_{sp}(t + t_p) / (t + t_p \cdot (Kt/V) \cdot (t/(t + t_p))) \quad (68)$$

In clinical use of UKM the VVSP model should be used to calculate V_{sp} and Kt/V which will minimize systematic errors related to ultrafiltration as described. This value for V can then be corrected with Eq. (68). and the corrected V_{sp}, cV_{sp}, is used to calculate a corrected spKt/V.

Calculation of Double-Pool Effects on PCR and NPCR.

Estimation of the equilibrated eKt/V was described above using Eq. (54). The NPCR is primarily determined by the total decrease in BUN and the reciprocal rise prior to the next dialysis. The postdialysis BUN is artificially low and will rebound as discussed above. This rebound must be accounted for in calculation of equilibrated Gu, PCR, and NPCR (eGu, ePCR, and eNPCR). The rebound increase in BUN must not be included in the generation calculations. The rebound effect on eGu can be calculated by adjusting the K_e (adK_e) to

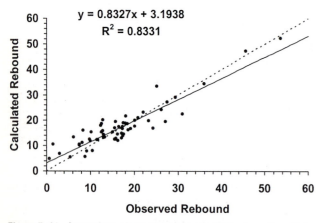

Figure 7–14. Comparison of measured and calculated urea and creatinine percent rebound.

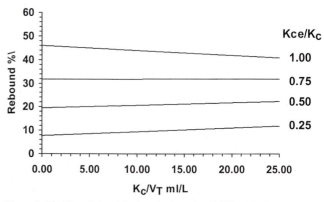

Figure 7–16. The relationship of total rebound to K_c/VT and K_e/K_c.

reflect the value which corresponds to Vsp and eKt/V in accordance with

$$adK_e = V_{sp}(eKt / V) / t \qquad (69)$$

The VVSP equations again must be iterated as described above to calculate an eGu. The iteration routine differs in that the V_{sp} remains constant as the value obtained after correction for double-pool effects. Iteration with the new, lower adK_e will result in a concentration profile resulting in higher post dialysis BUN. The process continues and eGu adjusted until the calculated C_o is equal to the measured C_o and ePCR and eNPCR are then calculated as above from eGu.

Magnitude of Error in V_{sp}. The error in V_{sp} was calculated over a wide range of treatment time and rate of dialysis (the observed Kt/V_{sp}) and error calculated in both L and percent with results shown in Figs. 7–17 and 7–18. The reference simulation V_{sp} was 36 L and the kinetic domains of short daily hemodialysis (SDHD), conventional hemodialysis (CHD), and long nocturnal hemodialysis (LNHD) are indicated in Figs. 7–17 and 7–18. In SDHD the V_{sp} will be consistently underestimated by 3 to 5 L and Kt/V_{sp} by 8 to 12 percent. In the domain of CHD, the error is smaller, ± 2 L and percent error will range about ± 5 percent. In LNHD, the V_{sp} will be consistently overestimated and delivered Kt/V_{sp} underestimated by 5 to 10 percent. The systematic overestimation of dose in SDHD and underestimation in LNHD will result in combined dose error between the two approaches of about 20 percent, i.e., the actual dose in LNHD is about 20 percent higher than the actual dose in SDHD unless these systematic single-pool errors are corrected. The Tattersall algorithm very successfully reduced these errors to near zero.

Magnitude of Error in NPCR and PCR. The error in these parameters was also calculated over a wide range of treatment

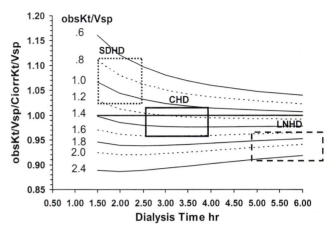

Figure 7–18. The error in observed Kt/Vsp (obsKt/Vsp) calculated as function of t and the obsKt/Vsp.

time and rate of dialysis with results shown in Figs. 7–19 and 7–20. It is interesting to note than the NPCR and PCR are overestimated in all domains of therapy. In SDHD and CHD the underestimation of V_{sp} combined with overestimation of Gu result in maximum overestimation of NPCR since NPCR is proportional to $\Delta BUN/V_{sp}$. The overestimation of PCR is less since PCR is proportional to $\Delta BUN \cdot V_{sp}$. In LNHD the overestimation of V_{sp} leads to greater overestimation of PCR. Thus the nutritional parameters, NPCR and PCR are overestimated substantially in all domains of therapy without correction for double pool effects. Again, correction with the Tattersall algorithm successfully eliminated these errors.

eKt/V, eNPCR, C_0U, and Adequacy of Thrice-Weekly Dialysis. The first rigorous attempt to define an adequate dose of dialysis was the prospectively randomized study, the National Cooperative Dialysis Study (NCDS).[35] The overall study design is illustrated in Fig. 7–21. The intervention

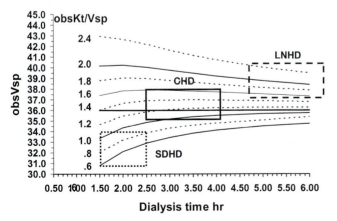

Figure 7–17. The error in observed Vsp (obsVsp) calculated as function of t and the obsKt/Vsp, K_e/K_c.

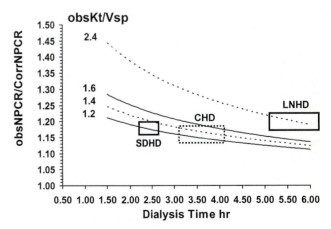

Figure 7–19. The error in observed NPCR (obsNPCR) calculated as function of t and the obsKt/Vsp, model simulation V = 36.0 L.

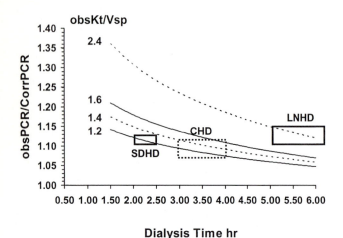

Figure 7–20. The error in observed PCR (obsPCR) calculated as function of t and the obsKt/Vsp.

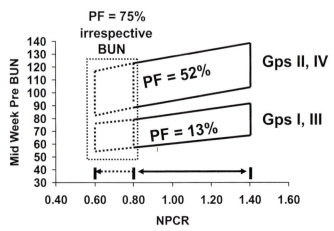

Figure 7–22. The clinical outcome in the NCDS.

was to reduce the amount of thrice weekly dialysis sufficiently to increase the predialysis midweek predialysis BUN (C_o) from about 70 to 110, with both short and long treatment times as shown. The VVSP model was used to prescribe the amount of dialysis from V, K_oA, Q_b, Q_d, and t and to monitor NPCR which was to be held in the region 0.80 to 1.40.

The clinical results were initially quite puzzling as depicted in Fig. 7–22. The probability of clinical outcome failure (PF) was very high in the high BUN groups compared to the low BUN groups when NPCR ≤ 0.80 which fit with the hypothesis as shown in Fig. 7–22. However, the PF was extremely high in both groups irrespective of BUN when NPCR ≤ 0.80. This suggested the possibility of two mechanisms of failure: nutritionally mediated failure in the low NPCR patients and uremic toxicity-mediated failure in the normal range NPCR patients.

The relationships between C_o, NPCR, and spKt/V were not understood when the NCDS was designed. Further development of the VVSP model after the study started

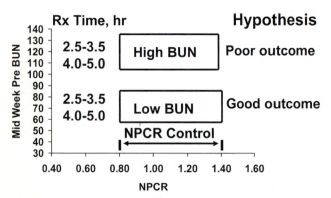

Figure 7–21. The NCDS design called for use of UKM to prescribe two BUN levels with long and short treatment times and the control of NPCR in the range 0.8 to 1.4.

showed that C_o was linearly related to NPCR as a function of spKt/V as depicted in Fig. 7–23. Although it was not recognized at the time of the study design, the relationships in Fig. 7–23 show that there were 3 experimental variables: C_o, NPCR, and spKt/V. The spKt/V was less completely tied to urea per se since it also served as a surrogate for the dialysis dose with respect to removal of other putative low-molecular-weight uremic toxins and, in this sense, might be considered a mechanistic definition of the dialysis dose. Analysis of the NCDS with all three parameters is depicted in Fig. 7–24. Superimposition of the C_o, NPCR, and spKt/V parameters on the clinical outcome data provided a unified explanation for the puzzling domains of high PF. It is apparent in Fig. 7–24 that the two high PF regions were separated from low PF by a spKt/V = 1.00. The analysis depicted in Fig. 7–24 led to the recommendation an adequate dose of dialysis was spKt/V = 1.00. A conclusion that has been been strongly debated over the past 20 years.

In Fig. 7–25 the PF data in Fig. 7–24 are normalized to PF at spKt/V = 1.00, expressed now as relative probability of failure (RPF), and plotted as a function of spKt/V.[2] We recognized that three functions could fit the data equally well—a discontinuous function, a linear function, and an exponential function. We reported all three but concluded that the data conformed best to the discontinuous function which implied an adequate dose of dialysis was defined by spKt/V = 1.0. It was subsequently argued that the exponential function best fit the data[36] which implied improving clinical outcome at much higher doses. Subsequent observational studies suggested that outcome was improved with higher doses[37–39] and resulted in the National Kidney Foundation-Dialysis Outcomes Quality Initiative (NKF-DOQI, subsequently K/DOQI, recommendation of spKt/V at least 1.20 for adequate dialysis.[40] Particularly impressive was the extremely low mortality with very high spKt/V 1.6 reported by Charra.[39] These observations combined with the higher mortality in the U.S. compared to Europe played an impor-

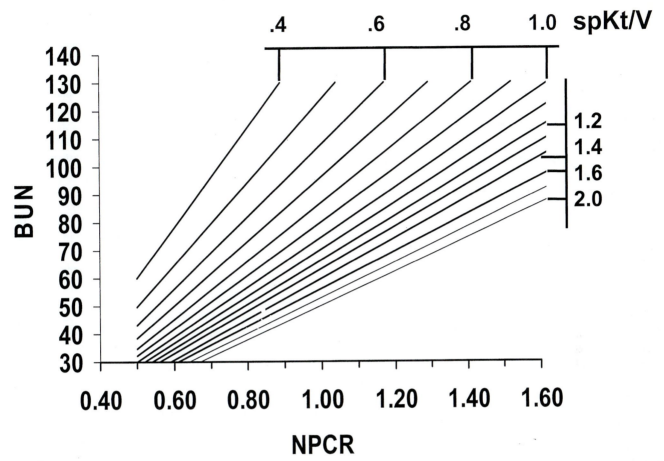

Figure 7–23. Solution of the single-pool urea kinetic model for predialysis midweek BUN as a function of NPCR and spKt/V shows a family of spKt/V curves relating BUN to NPCR.

tant role in stimulating the initiation of the multicenter Hemodialysis (HEMO) study, the second prospectively randomized study of dialysis therapy. This recently completed study had many more patients and a longer follow up of 6 years duration compared to the NCDS.

The original HEMO study design called for a standard therapy arm with spKt/V = 1.2 (eKt/V 1.05) and high dose intervention arm 1.45 (eKt/V 1.20). However, by the time the study got under way, the nephrology community in the United States was already convinced that minimum adequate therapy required a spKt/V in the range of 1.3 to 1.4 so it was considered necessary, because of ethical considerations, to increase the standard dose and intervention arms to recruit patients. The NCDS and NKF-DOQI modeling lines for adequate dialysis are shown in Fig. 7–26 where the domain of the revised HEMO study is also shown. Many were surprised when the results of the HEMO study were published showing no decrease in mortality nor improvement in other outcome measures in the high dose arm compared to the standard arm.[41] This result is depicted in Fig. 7–27 and compared to the NCDS domain. As shown in Fig. 7–27, because of the increase in dosage targets, the HEMO study

does not shed any light on dose response in the region $1.00 \leq spKt/V \leq 1.35$ but it clearly showed that spKt/V > 1.35 was not beneficial. As will be considered further below in the context of the ADEMEX study, there is still uncertainly about adequacy in the dosing range $1.00 \leq spKt/V \leq 1.40$.

The role of urea in renal failure has been recognized (and debated) for over 180 years. The uremic syndrome has long been conceptualized as resulting in part from accumulation in body water of solutes which are normally eliminated by the kidney and have concentration dependent toxicity. The first evidence of this concept was reported in 1821 by Prevot and Dumas[42] who found an elevated blood urea and symptoms mimicking chronic nephritis in nephrectomized animals. In 1826 Bostock[43] and in 1829 Christison[44] reported elevated blood urea concentrations in patients with degeneration of the kidneys. These findings were interpreted to implicate urea as the major toxin of uremia.

However, the urea theory of uremic toxicity was challenged very early on.[45] Of particular interest to the notion of adequate hemodialysis was the report by Richard Bright in 1836 of patients with considerably elevated blood urea concentrations who did not have uremic symptoms.[46] During

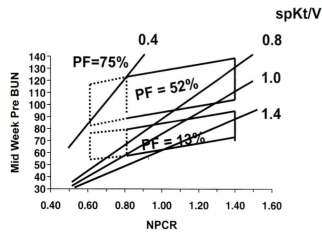

Figure 7–24. The NCDS dilemma: Was uremia BUN-dependent with NPCR ≥ 0.8 and nutrition-dependent with NPCR < 0.8?

the latter part of the nineteenth century, creatinine,[47] potassium,[48] and acidosis due to H^+ retention[49] were suggested to be major toxins in the uremic state. In light of the observations that numerous solutes were accumulating in blood with renal disease, the symptom complex was termed uremia by Piorry[50] to indicate "urine in the blood."

Over the subsequent 160 years many solutes have been shown to accumulate in renal failure and a recent tabulation by Vanholder et al.[51] of the major retained organic substances lists more than 40 compounds ranging in molecular weight from 60 (urea) to greater than 10^6 Da. Unfortunately for almost all of these retained solutes organ-specific toxicities have not been established in the uremic syndrome. Creatinine concentration in the dialysis patient is now known to be inversely related to mortality and appears to be primarily useful as an index of nutrition and skeletal muscle mass.[52] B2M is the only organic compound accumulating in uremia which has been established to be a major long term uremic toxin due to its polymerization into B2M amyloid, which is widely deposited in bone and soft tissues resulting in severe multiple organ system malfunctions.

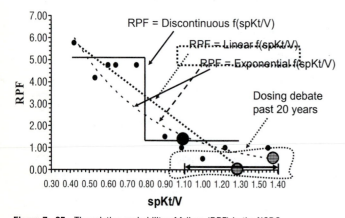

Figure 7– 25. The relative probability of failure (RPF) in the NCDS.

The abnormalities of body fluid and electrolyte composition and acid base balance in renal failure have unquestioned adverse clinical consequences and must be controlled as well as possible for adequate dialysis therapy. Hyperkalemia and hypokalemia, water, and Na retention, acidosis due to H^+ retention and inorganic phosphate retention can result in severe morbidity and fatal consequences.

The initial publication of the NCDS results in 1983 coincided with implementation of the sharply reduced composite rate for reimbursement of dialysis treatment in the United States by the Health Care Financing Administration (HCFA). Analysis of HCFA mortality data presented at the Morbidity, Mortality and Prescription of Dialysis Symposium in 1990[53] showed the gross mortality rate in the United States began to increase quite sharply in 1983 despite no change in the rate of increase in major risk factors.[54] Data presented at that meeting by National Medical Care (which provided dialysis for about 25 percent of all patients in the United States) indicated only predialysis BUN was used to routinely monitor therapy.[52] An analysis of visiting patients in SF indicated that in 98 percent of patients only predialysis BUN was measured and that low treatment time correlated with low BUN and low Kt/V[55] in these patients. Thus is appears that both the academic and clinical nephrology communities in the United States interpreted the NCDS to show that clinical uremia was proportional to BUN and that treatment time could be reduced if BUN was low. The results of reported USRDS data for 1986, 1990, and 1991[56] showed that that median eKt/V ranged from 0.75 to 0.85 in 1986 to 1991 USRDS samples. The median eKt/V finally reached 1.0 in the 1996 Core indicator data[57] but still 50 percent of patients had levels less than 1.0. These data indicate quite severe underdialysis in the United States for many years after initial publication of the NCDS results and the subsequent mechanistic analysis.

In the light of these data three different historical perceptions of the role of urea in uremia can be described as shown in Fig. 7–28. In 1820 high BUN and chronic nephritis were initially observed to correlate with clinical uremia. If we consider Kt/V an analogue of residual renal function normalized to patient size, the patients described in 1820 would be mapped in the domain of low Kt/V, low NPCR, and high BUN as depicted in Fig. 7–28; i.e., patients with far advanced renal failure, anorexia, and reduced protein intake. In contrast, Bright's patients with elevated BUN and minimal clinical abnormalities can be predicted to have had a higher level of residual renal function with less impairment of appetite and higher protein intake and would thus likely fall in the domain of higher Kt/V, higher protein intake and elevated BUN as depicted in Fig. 7–28. A dialysis therapy analogue of this description of Bright's patients has in fact been reported[58,59] and underscores the lack of correlation between BUN per se and clinical uremic toxicity. A third perception of the role of urea in uremia, the low

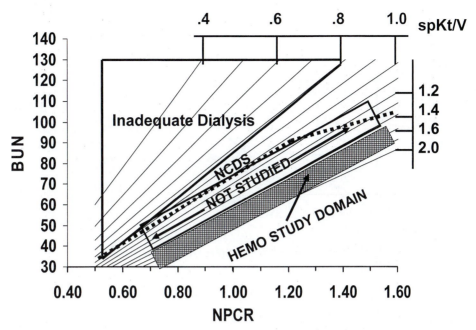

Figure 7–26. The domains of inadequate and adequate dialysis as defined by the NCDS compared to the HEMO domain of study.

NPCR, low BUN, and low Kt/V syndrome of the 1980s depicted in Fig. 7–28 was a likely consequence of interpreting the NCDS to show that the adequacy of dialysis therapy could be monitored from measurement of BUN and that treatment time was not an important determinant of outcome. The ever increasing economic pressures combined with this interpretation of the NCDS resulted in reduction of treatment time, the single most costly component of the prescription, in patients with low BUN due to low NPCR and led to the syndrome depicted in the lower left corner of Fig. 7–28 which likely contributed to the increased mortality in the United States in the 1980s.

The Dilemma Due to the Dual Role of V as Dose Modeling Parameter and a Predictor of Outcome. An unpublished observation made during analysis of the NCDS data was that V_{sp}

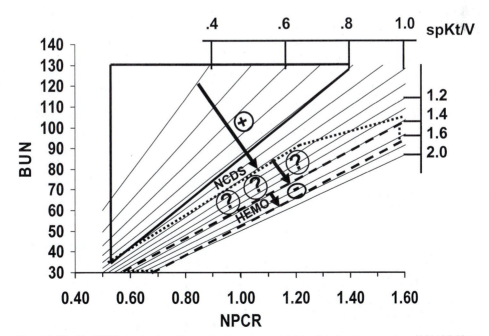

Figure 7–27. The NCDS clearly showed a marked improvement (+) in clinical outcome up to spKt/V of 0.80 to 1.00. The dose range $1.35 \leq spKt/V \leq 1.65$ was studied in HEMO and showed no benefit over this range (–).

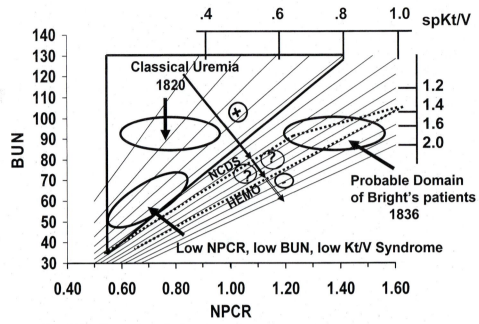

Figure 7–28. The perceived role of urea in renal failure over the past 180 years. See text for details.

was the strongest predictor of clinical outcome. The NCDS data base was probably more suitable than subsequent observational data bases to examine this relationship since the dose, spKt/V, was uniformly distributed across volume in the high and low spKt/V groups so the effect of Vsp was clearly separated from spKt/V. The relationship we observed in this very small data base is reproduced in Fig. 7–29 and is quite striking. A strong inverse relationship of probability of success to V was first formally reported by Lowrie et al.[60] A similar inverse relationship has been observed in the USRDS data base and DOPPS studies.[61,62]

The mechanism(s) underlying the inverse relationship of relative risk (RR) to V are quite obscure. It is suggested

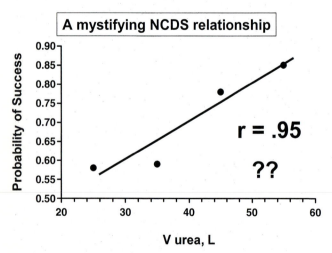

Figure 7–29. Urea distribution volume (V_{urea}) was the best predictor of successful outcome in the NCDS (1981).

that V is a surrogate for nutrition and that poor nutritional status is associated with smaller patients.[63,64] However there is no direct evidence of that, i.e., albumin does not correlate with V.[65] The general relationship of increased RR with small V would dictate that small healthy female patients beginning dialysis are doomed from the start to a higher mortality rate even though they enter with good nutritional status. In our experience small patients tend to have interdialytic weight gains similar to those of large patients, which means that repetitive volume overload relative to size is substantially greater in small patients (unpublished data). We have also noted that NPCR tends to be significantly higher in small compared to large patients. One might also postulate that generation of the unidentified low molecular weight toxins is proportional to some visceral volume index rather than total body water which is heavily influenced by skeletal muscle mass. At present we can only conclude that there appears to be a strong inverse correlation between mortality risk and V but the mechanism underlying the inverse relationship of mortality risk to V is unknown.

Lowrie has recently argued that Kt/V is a flawed parameter of dialysis dose.[66] The qualitative argument he advances is that, since RR decreases as V increases and Kt/V decreases as V increases, expressing the dose as Kt/V "is dividing a 'good' parameter (Kt) by a 'bad' parameter (V)," therefore increasing Kt/V must be associated with decreasing V and increased risk of mortality. To avoid this entanglement of V with Kt he suggests that since Kt is the "good" parameter it should be used to measure dose. This issue, which has been debated thoroughly elsewhere,[67] is important, since dosing is now more complicated since V is an independent predictor of outcome. Wolfe et al. have pointed out that the most rigorous way to study these interactions is to examine relative risk of mortality (RRM) as a function of Kt/V with V held constant at different levels.[68] They have pursued this approach with USRDS and DOPPS data and shown a family of parallel curves with higher RRM at all levels of Kt/V and low V. We recently used that approach with Fresenius Medical Care (FMC) data (unpublished observations) with results shown in Fig. 7–30 where RRM is shown as a function of eKt/V for three tertiles of V. Note there is maximal benefit at eKt/V about 1.2 at all levels of V which corresponds well with the results of HEMO. It should also be noted that there was an effect of volume seen in the HEMO database but was eliminated when gender was included,[69] which showed higher RRM for female patients.

Dialysis Studies of Middle-Molecule Toxicity. Although the NCDS was the only prospective, randomized study of clinical outcome over a wide range of precisely controlled levels of therapy until recently with the completion of the NIH-sponsored HEMO trial,[41] clinical outcomes have been reported from a number of experimental treatment prescriptions over the past 30 years. The concept of toxic middle molecules derived from a comment by Belding Scribner in 1965:

> My impression is that peritoneal dialysis seems to be more effective than hemodialysis to increase well-being for a given amount of urea clearance—because of the leaky peritoneal membrane we may be removing higher molecular weight substances more efficiently than in hemodialysis—we need a more leaky membrane for the hemodialyzer.[70]

This observation spawned an enormous interest in studies with increased clearance of larger molecules. These studies were generally guided by the in vitro dialyzer clearance of vitamin B_{12} and expressed as a vitamin B_{12} dialysis index

(DIB_{12}).[71] The results of many of these studies are plotted in Fig. 7–31 as a function of spKt/V and DI_{B12}. The vertical bar depicts the adequate zone for DI_{B12} (0.9 to 1.0) in accordance with this model.[71] The horizontal bar depicts Kt/V_t 1.0, the transition from inadequate to adequate dialysis in the NCDS.[2] All prescription coordinates above the horizontal bar provided $Kt/V_t > 1.00$, whereas those below provided $Kt/V_t < 1.00$. Prescriptions to the left of the vertical bar provided $DI_{B12} < 1.0$, and those to the right of the bar $DI_{B12} > 1.0$. Figure 7–31 displays the levels of small and middle molecule removal and clinical outcome for a wide spectrum of experimental dialysis, hemofiltration, and hemodiafiltration therapies.

The first four dialysis patients reported in 1960 were dialyzed once weekly[72] and, if the calculated Kt/V_t, DI_{B12} levels for this prescription are divided by 3, very low values of 0.45 and 0.25, respectively, are seen. Clinical outcome was poor, with crippling neuropathy and widespread soft tissue calcification. Clearly failure in these sentinel patients was associated with grossly inadequate clearances of urea and middle molecules. Over the next 10 years, the levels of Kt/V_t and DI_{B12} were empirically increased to eventuate in the 6-hour multiple point support Kiil "gold standard" for therapy with Kt/V_t, DI_{B12} levels 1.1, 1.0 as shown. The four groups of patients in the NCDS (I, II,, III, and IV) are depicted. Groups I and II had successful outcome and had Kt/V_t, DI_{B12} levels of 1.2, 1.0, and 1.0, 0.84, respectively. Groups II and IV from the NCDS failed with prescriptions providing Kt/V_t, DI_{B12} levels of 0.57, 0.88, and 0.54, 0.68, respectively. Teschan et al. compared clinical outcome with Kt/V_t, DI_{B12} levels of 1.0, 1.0 to that with levels of 0.72, 0.82.[73] He found deterioration of central nervous system function that correlated highly with Kt/V_t but not DI_{B12}. Keshaviah et al compared clinical outcome of dialysis therapy with Kt/V_t, DI_{B12} levels of 1.0, 0.75 with outcome using hemofiltration providing Kt/V_t, DI_{B12} 1.0, 3.0.[74,75] Both therapies were successful with no major differences in outcome with Kt/V constant at 1.0, but DI_{B12} ranging from 0.75 to

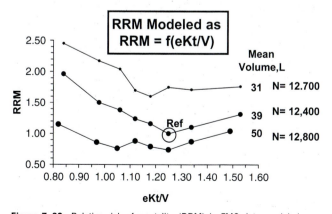

Figure 7–30. Relative risk of mortality (RRM) in FMC data modeled as a function of eKt/V after stratification for V.

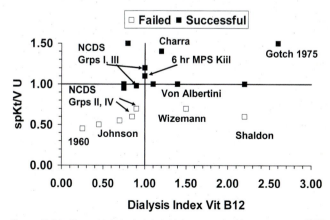

Figure 7–31. Some historical clinical trials mapped with respect to spKt/V and DI vitamin B_{12}.

3.0. Our studies reported in 1975[76] shown in Fig. 7–31 compared clinical outcome with Kt/Vt, DI_{B12} levels of 1.5, 0.75 with outcome with Kt/Vt, DI_{B12} levels of 1.5, 2.6. No differences in clinical outcome were observed regardless of DI_{B12} levels varying from 0.75 to 2.6. High-flux, 2-hour treatments using hemodiafiltration have been reported by von Albertini and Miller.[77,78] The Kt/Vt, DI_{B12} coordinates for this successful therapy are 1.0, 1.35. We also reported similar results.[79] In contrast to these results, Dyck reported a 50 percent failure rate with 1.5- to 2.0-hour treatments.[80] However, as shown in Fig. 7–31, the Kt/Vt, DI_{B12} coordinates for this therapy were 0.56, 0.43, very similar to the coordinates for Group IV patients in the NCDS. Cambi and Laurent presented clinical outcomes with "short"[81] and "long"[82] dialysis. The Kt/Vt, DI_{B12} coordinates for Cambi's prescription were 0.95, 0.72, and for Laurent's prescription the values were 1.4, 1.5. The reports indicated successful outcomes with both approaches although subsequently Charra data from the Tassin center[39] has been widely recognized as providing outstanding results.

Several investigators have studied outcome with renal replacement prescriptions providing Kt/Vt <0.8 and DI_{B12} >1.0 as depicted in the right lower quadrant of Fig. 7–31. The first reported postdilution hemofiltration by Quellhorst.[83] Quellhorst later reported excellent long-term results with similar therapy, but with residual renal function of 5 mL/min after 10 years of therapy.[84] Shaldon reported 2-hour treatments[85] with "mixed hemofiltration" providing Kt/Vt, DI_{B12} levels of 0.65, 2.1. This therapy was abandoned because of poor clinical outcome. Wizemann has reported on 1.75- to 2.0-hour therapy with hemodiafiltration,[86] providing Kt/Vt, DIB12 levels of 0.65, 1.5 which subsequently was abandoned. Inspection of Fig. 7–31 indicates that all therapies with Kt/Vt > 0.90 have been judged successful, whereas all therapies with Kt/Vt < 0.90 have failed. In contrast to the strong correlation between adequacy of therapy and Kt/Vt, DI_{B12} does not appear to be a strong determinant of adequacy of the renal replacement prescription. Successful clinical outcome is reported with DI_{B12} ranging from 0.70 to 3.0 when Kt/Vt is greater than 0.9, although failure is reported from DI_{B12} ranging from .25 to 2.1 when Kt/Vt is <0.80.

The concept of middle molecules was recently resurrected in the form of the Hemodialysis Product (HDP)[87] after publication of the ADEMEX study.[88] The HDP defined therapy exclusively in terms of time in accordance with

$$HDP = N^2 \cdot t \tag{70}$$

where N is number of dialyses per week and t is length of dialysis in hrs. This remarkable proposal eliminated all the fundamental elements of the dialysis procedure—dialyzer clearance, solute concentration, and solute distribution vol-

ume—from consideration in therapy and defined dialysis treatment only in units of time. The basis for this remarkable postulate was the ADEMEX study, which will be considered further below.

As discussed above, there was a growing perception in the clinical literature of the 1990s that levels of spKt/V substantially higher than 1 were required for optimal therapy,[37–39] which contributed heavily to the increase in HEMO target doses. Of particular interest was the low gross mortality rate of 3 percent reported by Charra et al.[39] These data were perceived to indicate that very high mean spKt/V levels of 1.6 with 8-hour treatment times are required to achieve optimal therapy. The patients in this report had a mean age of 47 years and combined incidence of diabetes plus "serious illnesses" of only 9 percent. The patient population was not comparable in age or incidence of diabetes to the large U.S. populations. We reported a gross mortality rate of 14 percent[89,90] with mean age of 62 years, 24 percent incidence of diabetes, mean spKt/Vt 1.4, and mean treatment time of 2.25 hours. We also compared Charra's outcome to our outcome and that of several international data bases normalized for age and diabetes with results shown in Fig. 7–32. It is ironic that the lowest normalized mortality rates were seen with the longest and shortest treatment times.

INORGANIC PHOSPHATE (iP): A SOLUTE THAT DOES NOT FOLLOW FIRST-ORDER KINETICS

Adequacy of the control of inorganic phosphorous (iP) mass balance in current hemodialysis therapy (HD) is usually judged by examination of a single, monthly, predialysis plasma iP concentration (Co_{iP}) so a quantitative approach to management of iP balance has not been possible in clinical practice. The predialysis iP concentration is known to be a major predictor of mortality in dialysis patients.[91] Restric-

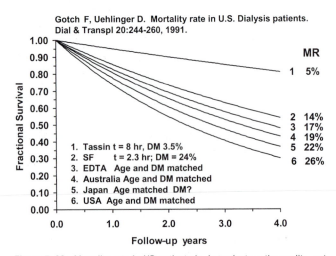

Figure 7–32. Mortality rate in HD patients is dependent on the quality, not necessarily the quantity of treatment time.

tion of iP intake and oral phosphate binders have been the primary methods of controlling iP balance. Compliance with prescribed diet is not regularly quantified and binders may be quite expensive or carry the potential risk of Ca loading. Newer therapies with long overnight dialysis have resulted in iP depletion.[92] The dialysis prescription is not usually written in terms of iP removal and the interacting roles of diet, binders, and dialysis are not quantified. iP intake and removal in HD (iPKM) has been modeled in an attempt to provide more quantitative assessments of the roles of dietary intake, iP binders and highly efficient dialyzers in control of phosphate balance.[93]

Phosphorous mass balance in HD. Since nearly all iP intake is contained in the protein content of foods, the intake or generation of iP (G_{iP}), in milligrams per day, might be predictable from the protein catabolic rate (PCR), in grams per day, unless there is intake of protein with widely varying iP content, assuming there is not excessive intake of dairy products protein. If the iP removed by dialysis (J_{diP}), in milligrams, can be reliably predicted, the amount of iP which must be removed by binders (J_{biP}) can be calculated and, it is hoped, provide a more quantitative approach to control of iP mass balance with different dialysis therapies and binders. Overall iP mass balance can be described in clinical terms by the word equation:

$$
\begin{array}{ccccc}
\text{Accumulation} & & \text{Dietary} & \text{Dialyzer} & \text{Binder} \\
\text{iP} & = & [\text{iP}] & - \ [\text{iP}] & - \ [\text{iP}] \\
\end{array} \quad (71)
$$

$$
\begin{array}{cccc}
\text{in tissues} & \text{Intake} & \text{Removal} & \text{Removal} \\
\Delta T_c P & G_{i_p} & J_{di}P & J_{bi}P \\
\end{array}
$$

This can be expressed more formally as a mass balance equation

$$ d(T_{ciP}) / dt = G_{iP} - J_{diP} - J_{biP} \quad (72) $$

where T_{ci} is tissue content in milligrams.

Over the weekly, asymmetrical treatment cycle, the change in tissue content is given by

$$ \Delta T_{ciP} = G_{iP} - J_{diP} - J_{biP} \quad (73) $$

where all units are expressed as milligrams per day. The therapy goal in dialysis is to maintain $\Delta T_{ciP} = 0$ over complete treatment cycles so in this context, Eq. (73) can be written as

$$ J_{biP} = G_{iP} - J_{diP} \quad (74) $$

Equation (74) could provide a quantitative framework for writing and evaluating the dialysis, binder, and diet prescriptions. If the binding capacity of the prescribed binder

(k_b), in milligrams of iP per tablet is known, the number of binder tablets (N_b) required per day could be calculated as

$$ N_b = J_{biP} / k_b \quad (75) $$

The G_{iP} is derived primarily from catabolized protein. The protein catabolic rate (PCR), in grams per day, can be measured with urea kinetic modeling. An average value of absorbed iP content of protein might be estimated as

$$ G_{iP} = 12(\text{PCR}) \ \text{mg} / \text{day} \quad (76) $$

where the coefficient 12 is estimated from an average iP content of 15 mg/g protein and 80 percent absorption, since most patients are receiving vitamin D analogues.

The magnitude of iP removal by dialysis can be defined as the product dialyzer clearance × average blood concentration × treatment time. In order to estimate J_{diP} it is essential to know the time averaged iP concentration during dialysis (TACiP), the dialyzer plasma water clearance of iP (K_{pwiP}), duration of dialysis (t, or time, in minutes), and number of dialyses per week (N). With this information total iP removal by the dialyzer can be written as

$$ J_{diPT} = K_{pwiP}(t) \ (N) \ (TAC_{iP}) / 7 \quad (77) $$

where J_{diPT} is mg/day.
We can combine Eqs. (75) to (77) to derive

$$ J_{biP} = 12(\text{PCR}) - (K_{pwiP})(TAC_{iP})(t)(N / 7) \quad (78) $$

The information in Eq. (78) could provide quantitative guidance for the dialysis and binder prescriptions as well a tool to evaluate compliance with the dietary and binder prescriptions if the parameters can be reliably measured in the clinical setting, which has not yet been established. A major parameter of concern in Eq. (78) is the feasibility of prediction of K_{pwiP} and TAC_{iP} over a total dialysis.

Calculation of K_{pwiP}. The approach to this problem has been discussed above. It is necessary to develop a K_oA for iP for any specific dialyzer used and then use Eq. (9) to calculate effective blood flow and from the K_oA equation calculate clearance of iP.

An Empiric Mathematical Description of the Normalized, Cumulative Time-Averaged Concentration of iP (nTACiP) during HD

A review of reported serial plasma water iP concentrations at serial time intervals (C_{tiP}) during dialysis indicates that iP must be mobilized (M_{iP}) from other compartment(s) at a sufficiently rapid rate to stabilize plasma concentration during dialysis.[94–97] Although the mechanism(s) operating to cause such rapid mobilization of iP during dialysis are undefined, examination of previously reported concentration profiles suggested that it might be possible to formulate an empiric mathematical description of the net effect of the mobilization process on the plasma concentration profile. We have reported such a mathematical description[93] which can be described as follows:

$$J_{diPT} = C_{oiP}(nTAC_{iP})(K_{pwiP})(t) \qquad (79)$$

where K_{pwiP} is dialyzer blood water clearance, t is treatment time, and C_{oiP} is predialysis plasma iP. Each serial value of C_{tiP} measured during dialysis was normalized to C_{oiP} in each patient studied as

$$C_{niP} = C_{tiP} / C_{oiP} \qquad (80)$$

The mean of C_{niP} (mC_{niP}) for each successive time interval $(1,2,...,n)$ between serial samples (30 to 60 minutes) was calculated as

$$mC_{niP} = [C_{niPn-1} + C_{niPn}] / 2 \qquad (81)$$

The normalized, cumulative time average concentration ($nTAC_{iP}$) for the sequential, cumulative intervals of dialysis time were then computed as

$$nTAC_{iP} = 1/n \cdot ts \sum_{i=ts}^{n} mC_{niP} \cdot ts = 1/t \int_{o}^{t} d(mC_{niP})/dt \qquad (82)$$

where *ts* is length of time interval between samples, *n* is total number of intervals, and mC_{niP} for each interval is defined above. In other words, we computed the sum of the mC_{niP}·ts products and divided by total time for each increasing cumulative time interval during dialysis. We then multiplied the cumulative time axis values by K_{pwiP}/V_{iP} (where V_{iP} is V_e and was estimated as one-third of kinetically measured urea distribution volume) for each patient and examined the relationship

$$nTAC_{iP} = f[K_{pwiP} \cdot t / V_{iP}] \qquad (83)$$

In this way we are able to examine the $nTAC_{iP}$ profile as a generalized function of the total normalized dose of iP dialysis, $K_{pwiP} \cdot t/V_{iP}$.

The serial values observed for $nTAC_{iP}$ vs $K_{pwiP} \cdot t/V_{iP}$ in 23 patients are shown in Fig. 7–33 along with the regression equation fitted to the means at sequential 30 min time intervals. The mean values correspond extremely well to the function

$$nTAC_{iP} = 1 - .44(1 - exp[-1.279(Kt/V_{iP})]) \quad (r = 0.99) \quad (84)$$

It is important to emphasize that Eq. (84) is an empiric, mathematical description of the profound effect on blood iP concentration of undefined physiologic mechanisms operating to rapidly mobilize iP from other sites into the extracellular fluid during its removal by dialysis. Although these

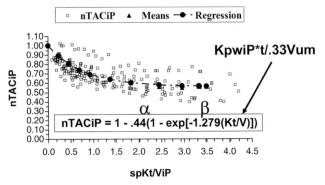

Figure 7–33. The mean values nTACiP plotted as a function of spKt/ViP.

mechanisms are undefined, the relationship in Eq. (84) suggests the feasibility of use of this empirical definition of the iP concentration profile to model and predict dialyzer phosphate removal as

$$J_{diPT} = (1 - \alpha(1 - exp(-\beta(Kt/V_{iP}))))(C_{oiP})$$
$$\times (K_{pwiP})(t)(N)/7 \qquad (85)$$

where N is number of dialyses per week, t is dialysis treatment time, α and β are patient specific constants, and J_{diPT} is total dialyzer removal of iP averaged here as mg/day.

The general function in Eq. (85) was used with blood profiles and dialysate collection[93] to determine patient specific values for α and β in three consecutive dialyses and then over the next 6 months estimate J_{diPT} from K_oA, t, C_o, C_t, and α and β values. A simple method was devised to fit an individualized function to each patient's data set by calculating individualized coefficients α and β in accordance with the relationship

$$nTAC_{iP} = 1 - \alpha(1 - exp[-\beta(K_{pwiP} t/V_{iP})]) \qquad (86)$$

where α was taken as the last measured value for $nTAC_{iP}$ at $K_{pwiP} t/V_{iP}$ in the range 2.5 to 3.5 and β was calculated from

$$\beta = (-ln(1 - [1 - nTAC_{iP}/\alpha]))/K_{pwiP} t/V_{iP} \qquad (87)$$

where $nTAC_{iP}$ and $K_{pwiP} t/V_{iP}$ are the values measured early in dialysis at $K_{pwiP} t/V_{iP} = .50$ to 1.0.

Equation (87) can now be individualized as

$$J_{diPT} = (1 - \alpha(1 - exp[-\beta(Kt/V_{iP})]))C_{oiP}$$
$$\times (K_{pwiP})(t)(N)/7 \qquad (88)$$

where α and β are coefficients established computed for each patient as described above.

The values calculated with Eq. (88) were compared to J_{diPT} measured in total dialysate with results in Figs. 7–34 and 7–35. Inspection of these two figures shows that the correlation between predicted and measured was excellent with no apparent bias.

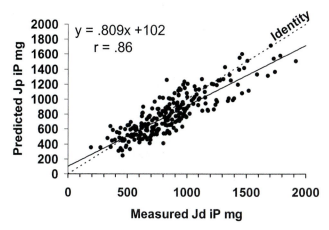

Figure 7–34. The correlation of predicted J_pT_{iP} to measured J_dT_{iP}.

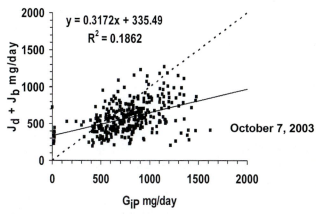

Figure 7–36. Although iP removal by dialysis can be predicted, it is not possible to close a mass balance with the model parameters postulated for phosphorus intake and binder removal. It would appear that generation is overestimated and/or removal by binders is underestimated.

Protein catabolic rate and total binder intake was also measured to evaluate the mass balance expression by comparing $J_{diPT} + J_{biPT}$ to G_{iP} with results shown in Fig. 7–36. The results in Fig. 7–36 clearly show the model parameters for G_{iP} and J_{biPT} must have major errors since mass balance was far from zero. Although the model developed above for mass balance is not suitable for clinical use, the concept should be useful for further refinements in the future.

KINETIC CONTINUOUS AND INTERMITTENT CLEARANCES

There is rapidly growing interest in more frequent dialysis therapy, daily dialysis, and initiation of diaysis therapy at higher levels of continuous renal urea clearance. A National Institutes of Health feasibility study of six times weekly dialysis will soon be underway. Consequently there is a growing need to model the effects of combined continuous and intermittent dialysis and variable frequency and intensity of intermittent dialysis. Daily dialysis therapy has been prescribed empirically, generally comprising five or six dialyses per week and defined primarily by short or long

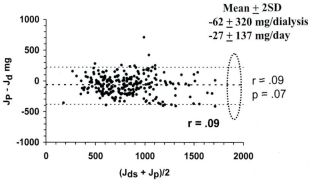

Figure 7–35. A Bland Altman plot shows no bias between J_pT_{iP} and J_dT_{iP} over a wide range of removal. The 95 percent confidence limits are + 137 mg/day.

dialysis time (t). The advocates of long t have reported overnight 7- to 9-hour dialyses (LNHD) while short-time therapy, t ~ 2 hours, has typically been in-center daytime dialysis (SDHD). The dose of dialysis has often been described as a weekly sum of the Kt/Vs (spKt/V) provided by each dialysis and spKt/V has often been estimated with approximation equations (16) which, as shown above, will result in substantial overestimation of dose in SDHD with short treatment times and low eKt/V's and underestimation of dose in LNHD. A theory of dosing parameters suitable for all dialysis schedules with respect to frequency and intensity is developed below.

The eKt/V Is a Quantitative Measure of the Dose of an Individual Dialysis. The most widely used formal definition of the dose of dialysis as developed above is the fractional clearance of body water for urea. The eKt/V required for thrice weekly conventional HD (CHD) is 1.1 to 1.2 and rigidly tied to this fixed thrice weekly dialysis schedule. This target level of eKt/V cannot be logically extrapolated to other frequencies of treatment, continuous therapy, or combinations of continuous and intermittent therapy. A new parameter of dose quantification is required to standardize expression of dose in variable frequency dialysis therapies.

Time-Averaged Clearance (TAK). The dose in more frequent hemodialysis treatment schedules (four to seven times per week) has often been expressed as the weekly sum of Kt/V for each dialysis. The assumption underlying this approach to quantification is that dialysis doses with variable dialysis frequency (N, dialyses per week) can be quantitatively expressed simply as the time averaged total weekly clearance provided or TAK.[94] This calculation implies that the total intermittent clearances provided with any treatment schedule are therapeutically equivalent to the same total amount of continuous clearance over the week. Thus we define TAK as

$$TAK = N \cdot K \cdot t / 10080 \qquad (89)$$

where N is number of dialyses per week, K·t is total clearance for each dialysis, and the constant 10080 is simply number of minutes in a week.

Examination of the mechanism of solute removal by dialysis reveals a major potential flaw in this assumption. The primary pathway through which dialysis therapy ameliorates uremia is believed to be solute removal (or solute restoration as in the case of HCO_3) and correction of abnormal solute concentrations. This is a first-order process driven by the product of clearance and concentration, $K \cdot C$. Since C falls, the ratio (C_t/C_o) falls during each intermittent dialysis, efficiency of solute removal markedly diminishes as eKt/V increases for any individual treatment as illustrated in Fig. 7–37. Note in Fig. 7–37 that the dialyzer clearance (K_d) remains constant but the rate of solute removal decreases at eKt/V = 2.0 to a level of only 15 percent relative to the rate at the start of the dialysis. In any single dialysis the efficiency of solute removal always decreases exponentially in proportion to the dose or intensity of the dialysis, eKt/V. With an eKt/V = 1.0, 63 percent of the body content of urea will be removed while with eKt/v = 2.0, 86 percent of urea will be removed. Thus the amount of solute removal increases by only 39 percent but the eKt/V has increased 100 percent.

The Concept of Equivalent Steady-State Clearance. A rational approach to quantify variable frequency HD and combinations of intermittent HD with continuous dialysis is to express all doses as effective continuous steady state clearances (K_s) which are therapeutically equivalent to the total doses of intermittent clearance. In steady state, the solute generation rate is balanced by (equal to) solute removal rate so concentration (C_s) remains constant in accordance with

$$G = (K_s)(C_s) \qquad (90)$$

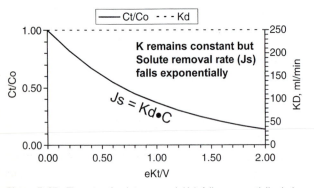

Figure 7–37. The rate of solute removal (Js) falls exponentially during each intermittent dialysis ≈ to C_t/C_o.

The K_s is defined from rearrangement of Eq. (90) to

$$K_s = G / C_s \qquad (91)$$

The continuous K_s is defined as the ratio G/C_s so we can, in theory, calculate a continuous K_s which is equivalent (K_{seq}) to the amount of dialysis provided by any specific intermittent dialysis schedule as follows: (1) define G; (2) calculate the concentration profile for a specified eKt/V, G, V and number of treatments per week (N); (3) define a concentration point on the profile to serve as the equivalent steady state concentration (C_{seq}); and (4) calculate the continuous clearance, which is therapeutically equivalent to the total weekly intermittent clearance in accordance with

$$K_{seq} = G / C_{seq} \qquad (92)$$

This approach has been reported using three different values to represent the concentration profile for definition of C_{seq} as depicted graphically in Fig. 7–38. The BUN concentration profiles in Fig. 7–38 were calculated for HD three and six times weekly, providing eKt/V 1.0 for each dialysis with NPCR 1.0 and V = 35 L. The peak concentration hypothesis[99] defines C_{seq} as the maximum or peak predialysis BUN (C_{pk}) after the longest interdialytic interval to be used to calculate an equivalent continuous clearance (K_{pk})

$$K_{pk} = G / C_{pk} \qquad (93)$$

The mean predialysis BUN (C_{om}) is used[100,101] to define a standard K (stdK) in accordance with

$$stdK = G / C_{om}. \qquad (94)$$

Note that in the case of CHD in Fig. 7–38 the C_{pk} and C_{om} differ only minimally but the difference becomes much greater in more frequent HD schedules. In both cases the time average concentration (TAC) is substantially lower than C_{pk} and C_{om}.

The TAC is used to define the "equivalent renal clearance" (EKR).[95] In this case we write

$$EKR = G / TAC \qquad (95)$$

The EKR is based on the TAC calculated from the total area under the urea concentration curve during a week including the log mean profiles during the short dialysis intervals and the long linear interdialytic profile segments. The clinical validity of these three definitions of K_{seq} can, at present, only be evaluated from analysis of clinical equivalence between CAPD and CHD, two well established continuous and intermittent dialysis therapies which can serve as benchmarks to evaluate the three definitions C_{seq} and will be considered further below.

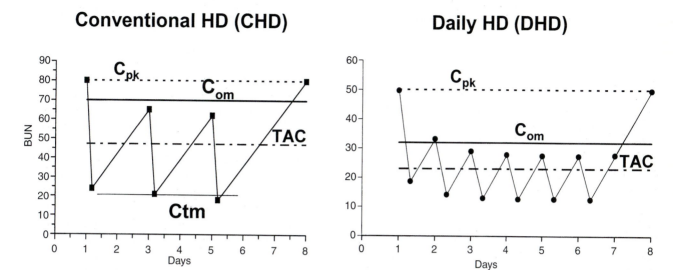

Figure 7–38. Three different definitions of equivalent points on the concentration profile to calculate continuous clearance equivalent to intermittent clearance.

Conceptual Differences between EKR and stdK. As shown in Fig. 7–37 and further in Fig. 7–39, panel A, an exponential decrease in efficiency of solute removal occurs during each intermittent dialysis relative to efficiency at the start of the dialysis. The instantaneous and cumulative log mean ratios of C_t/C_o are depicted as a function of eKt/V in Fig. 7–39A,B. The C_t/C_o ratios in Fig. 7–39A were calculated from Eq(16) and the log mean (C_t/C_o) was calculated from

$$\log \text{mean} \, (C_t / C_o) = (C_o - C_t)/ \ln(C_o / C_t) \quad (96)$$

The geometric description of instantaneous stdK (stdK_t) is shown in Fig. 7–39A as a function of the instantaneous curve for C_t/C_o values. The therapeutic assumption which underlies the definition of stdK is

$$K(C_t) = \text{stdK}_t(C_o) \quad (97)$$

where K is dialyzer urea clearance, stdK_t are instantaneous values for the theoretical continuous equivalent clearance, C_o is the initial urea concentration at time zero of dialysis, C_t is instantaneous urea nitrogen concentration at any time t

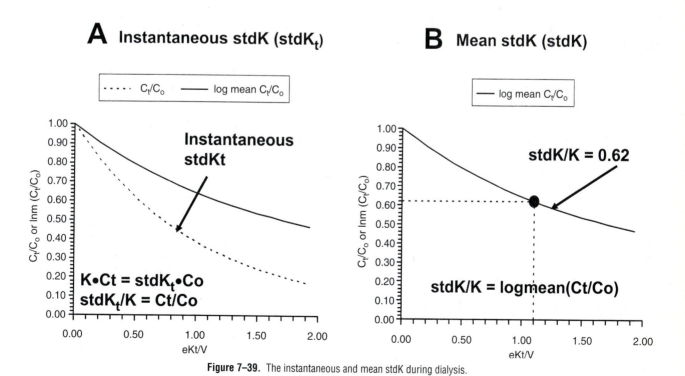

Figure 7–39. The instantaneous and mean stdK during dialysis.

during dialysis, and the equality represents both equivalent rates of solute removal and therapeutic equivalence. It thus follows that

$$stdK_t / K = C_t / C_o \qquad (98)$$

The ratio $stdK_t/K$ in Eq (98) and Fig. 7–39A depict the exponential decline in $stdK_t$ which is required for therapeutic equivalence to the dialyzer clearance. The mean value for the ratio $stdK/K$ for the total dialysis can be similarly computed from the log-mean values for C_t/C_o as shown in Fig. 7–39B and expressed as

$$stdK / K = \log \text{ mean}(C_t / C_o) \qquad (99)$$

Equation (99) defines the level of continuous $stdK$ which is equivalent to the actual dialyzer K over the entire dialysis. It is of interest to note that when eKt/V reaches 1.1 in Fig. 7–39B the value for $stdK/K$ is 0.62, which, as will be discussed further below, is the ratio of adequate continuous weekly CAPD clearance to total weekly clearance provided by eKt/V 1.1 thrice weekly.

The concept of EKR is the inverse of that for $stdK$. We can describe instantaneous values for EKR_t as a function of eKt/V in accordance with

$$EKR_t(C_t) = K(C_o) \qquad (100)$$

$$EKR_t / K = C_o / C_t \qquad (101)$$

and

$$EKR / K = \log\text{–mean}(C_o / C_t) \qquad (102)$$

The EKR would appear to be counterintuitive in that the EKR is maximal at the end of dialysis when the highest value for log mean(C_o/C_t) occurs which is when the rate of solute removal is lowest as shown in Fig. 7–40. The EKR

may have more relevance to describe the continuous equivalent clearance with larger molecular weight solutes such as B2M. Clark has reported detailed solutions with double pool kinetics for higher-molecular-weight solutes[96] and, if evidence accumulates showing the TAC of such solutes are controlling on adequacy of the dialysis prescription, the EKR modeled for B2M may be more relevant for such solutes.

The conceptual notion underlying $stdK$ is that with adequate intermittent dialysis therapy each successive dialysis occurs before there is sufficient interdialytic solute accumulation to result in symptomatology relative to the therapeutic benefit conferred with that schedule and eKt/V. This is the empirical basis for normalizing K_{eq} to C_{om}. In the context of $stdK$ the exponential drop in concentration during the short intradialytic time interval confers no therapeutic benefit. Its only effect is to decrease the efficiency of solute removal and result in a requirement for high clearances. This is the price paid for providing intermittent "catch-up" dialysis as opposed to delivering continuous dialysis. Improvement in outcome compared to CHD may be expected to occur if the frequency of dialysis is increased, which may ameliorate symptoms now clinically accepted with thrice weekly dialysis.

In contrast, the basic concept behind the EKR model is that there is increasing clinical benefit during each dialysis which is proportional to the drop in BUN since equivalent continuous therapy is normalized to the TAC achieved with any treatment schedule. In the author's view, the term "equivalent renal clearance" is highly misleading. The term implies that a continuous renal clearance of urea (Kru) equal to the dialyzer EKR will provide clinical benefits equivalent to the intermittent dialysis treatment. It would seem more precise to identify our goal as definition of a continuous dialyzer clearance which provides clinical benefit equivalent to intermittent dialyzer clearance with specified frequency and intensity. Equivalent continuous dialyzer clearances should not be considered equivalent to the same level of renal urea clearance, a fact recently established for CAPD where it has been shown that dialyzer and renal clearances cannot be simply added.[97]

Generalized Solution of the stdK model. The kinetic descriptions of intermittent and continuous dialysis which follow contain the assumptions of equally spaced dialyses and constant V. Since our goal is to define a steady state continuous clearance, we solve for C_{om} without the dilution of interdialytic fluid gain, which will be erroneously interpreted is higher $stdK$. However, the VVSP model would be required for analysis of *delivered* intermittent dialysis doses in order to accurately estimate the urea distribution volume, V. The assumption of equal spacing simply provides an estimate of the average peak concentration. Although the inputs include single pool Kt/V (spKt/V), correction to equilibrated Kt/V

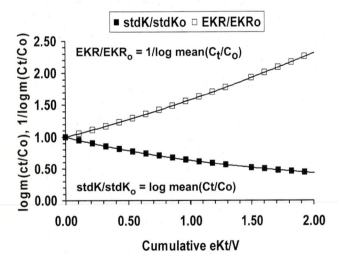

Figure 7–40. Comparison of the mean stdK and mean EKR over the course of a typical dialysis.

(eKt/V) is made in all instances as a function of the rate of dialysis relative to V.[34] Further, in the case of daily HD and combined therapies, the spKt/V prescribed for each HD may be relatively low, i.e., less than 1.1, which may result in spuriously low calculated V,[98,99] which requires the appropriate volume correction algorithm discussed above.

Equation (14) can now be written in general form applicable to both intermittent and continuous therapies in accordance with

$$V(dC / dt) = G - (K_d + K_p + K_r)C \qquad (103)$$

Intermittent therapies consist of either intermittent hemodialysis (IHD) or automated peritoneal dialysis (APD). We can now restate some of the FVSP model solutions derived above for use in development of stdK. The decrease in BUN over each intermittent therapy session is

$$C_t = C_o \exp(-(K_d \text{ or } K_p + K_r)t / V)$$
$$+ (G / (K_d \text{ or } K_p + K_r))$$
$$\times (1 - \exp(-(K_d \text{ or } K_p + K_r)t / V)) \qquad (104)$$

where C_o is predialysis BUN, C_t is postdialysis BUN, K_d, K_p, K_r are dialyzer, peritoneal, and renal urea clearances respectively, t is treatment time, V is urea distribution volume, and all units must be consistent.

FVSP model solution for BUN build up over the intervals between HD or APD results in

$$C_o = C_t \exp(-(K_p + K_r)t_i / V) + (G / (K_p + K_r))$$
$$\times (1 - \exp(-(K_p + K_r)t_i / V)) \qquad (105)$$

or

$$C_o = C_t + G * t_i / V \qquad (106)$$

where C_t is postdialysis BUN as in Eq. (104), C_o is predialysis BUN prior to next IHD or APD treatment, t_i is the interdialytic time interval, and all units must be consistent. Note that Eq. (105) applies if either K_p or K_r are greater than zero while Eq. (106) applies when both are zero between the IHD or APD treatments.

In order to generalize the model and calculate the average predialysis BUN or mC_o it is necessary to combine Eqs. (104) to (106) and to express G as a function of the NPCR as developed in Eqs. (21) and (22), The generalized expression to compute C_o with any combination of frequency of IHD, APD and continuous dialysis (CD) between IHD or APD, sessions is

$$C_{om} = (0.184(PCRn - 0.17) \cdot V / (spKt / V) \cdot V / t))(1 - \exp(-eKt / V)$$
$$\cdot \exp(-(Kp + K_r)(1440 \cdot (7 / N) - t) / V) + (0.184(PCRn - 0.17)$$
$$\cdot V / (Kp + Kr))(1 - \exp(-(Kp + K_r)(1440(7 / N) - t) / V))$$
$$/(1 - \exp(-eKt / V) \cdot \exp(-(Kp + K_r)((7 / N)1440 - t / V)) \qquad (107)$$

where spKt/V is single pool Kdt/V or KptV (for APD); t is duration of intermittent treatment sessions min; N is frequency of IHD or APD per week; eKt/V is the equilibrated Kt/V calculated from spKt/V in accordance with Eq. (54); Kp is any CD between IHD or APD sessions; K_r is included in spKt/V and in CD intervals and all units must be consistent.

In the case when CD is zero during the intervals between IHD or APD sessions, the expression for C_o becomes

$$C_{om} = (0.184(PCRn - .017) \cdot V) / (spKt / V)(V / t))(1 - \exp(-eKt / V)$$
$$+ (0.184(PCRn - 0.17) \cdot V(1440 \cdot (7 / N) - t) / V) / V)$$
$$/(1 - \exp(-eKt / V)) \qquad (108)$$

In the case of continuous clearance only as in normal renal function, chronic renal failure without dialysis and CAPD, Eqs. (107) and (108) reduce to

$$Css = (.184(NPCR - .17)V) / (K_p + K_r) \qquad (109)$$

where C_{ss} is the steady state BUN with continuous clearance.

We can now substitute C_o, found from solution of Eq. (107) or (108) with a specified set of modality input parameters—intermittent dialysis ± continuous dialysis—into Eq. (109), and solve for the standard clearance (stdK) which results in C_{ss} equal to C_{om} at identical NPCR. The appropriate rearrangement of Eq. (109) to find stdK, where stdK= $(K_p + K_r)$ in Eq. (109), is

$$stdK = 0.184(NPCR - 0.17)V / C_{om} \qquad (110)$$

Division of Eq. (110) by V and incoporation of appropriate time constants results in

$$std(Kt / V) = 1440[0.184(NPCR - 0.17)] / C_{om} \qquad (111)$$

daily

$$std(Kt / V) = 7 * 1440[0.184(PCR_n - .17) / C_{om} \qquad (112)$$

weekly

The level of therapy defined by std(Kt/V) can also be expressed as a percent of the normal renal reference standard in accordance with

$$\%ref(Krt / V) = 100[std(Kt / V) / ref(Krt / V)] \qquad (113)$$

The model is now complete. The dose of dialysis can be expressed as an equivalent, normalized continuous clearance for all combinations of intermittent and continuous treatment modalities. Equation (113) permits expression of the std(Kt/V) dose as a percent of the normal renal reference standard but it is probably not appropriate to equate dialyzer clearance to renal clearance.

Comparative Solutions of the EKR and stdK Models. The two models were solved over wide ranges of both frequency (N dialyses per week) and intensity (eKt/V each dialysis) to examine how stdKt/V relates to dialysis frequency and intensity. It is important to specify zero interdialytic fluid accumulation in simulation of these models. As noted above, since we define EKR and stdK as G/C_{seq}, dilution of the BUN profiles by positive fluid balance can result in significant errors in the steady state clearance calculation. Furthermore, we are attempting to conceptualize theoretical steady states with these models and do not consider volume overload a clinical benefit. Values for EKRm and stdKm were determined from BUN profiles calculated with a fixed volume single pool kinetic model for specified levels of eKt/V and PCR = 1.0 with N varied 2 to 7 and eKt/V varied 0.2 to 2.9 for each N which were equally spaced over the week. The TAC was computed from [t·log mean(C_t/Co) + θ· (C_o+C_t)/2]/[t + θ] where t is dialysis time and θ is interdialytic time interval. These calculations will slightly overestimate TAC and underestimate EKRm since a single exponential profile was assumed during dialysis rather than double exponential. The results are shown in Fig. 7–41 where in both panels the values for EKRm and stdKm are plotted as a function of TAK which is also shown on the ordinate scale as the identity line. In Fig. 7–42 the curves in

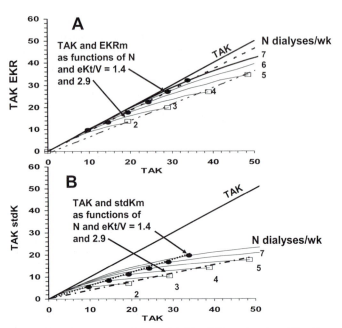

Figure 7–42. Comparisons of EKR and StdK to TAK as a function of N and two levels of eKt/V.

Fig. 7–41 are again shown and in addition discrete values for EKRm and stdKm are plotted at eKt/V = 1.4 and 2.9 for each N. In the case of EKRm it can be observed that for all eKt/V ≤ 1.4, the EKRm is virtually identical to TAK (and would be even a little closer to identity with a double exponential decay of concentration during dialysis). Thus, over the typical range of dialysis intensity with N varied from 2 to 7, the EKRm is nearly identical to TAK calculated by simply averaging the total intermittent clearance over a week. At the very high level of eKt/V = 2.9, which would be typical only of LNHD, the EKRm deviates more from TAK but is still about 80 percent of TAK at eKt/V = 2.9 and N = 6.

In Fig. 7–42 the relationships of stdKm to TAK are also shown as functions of TAK and N with eKt/V varied from .2 to 2.9 and discrete values for eKt/V = 1.4 and 2.9 are shown. The stdKm deviates much more from TAK because it reflects the greatly decreased efficiency at high eKt/V. At eKt/V = 2.9 and N = 6, extrapolation of the curves shows stdKm/TAK is only 0.33.

Generalized Solution of the stdK Model for stdK·t/V. Solution of Eqs. (107) to (112) over wide ranges of eKt/V and N, an average V = 35 and NPCR = 1.00 is shown in Fig. 7–43. Inspection of the points in Fig. 7–43 reveals that stdKt/V appears to increase quite steeply and linearly as N increases but the increase is shallow and logarithmic as eKt/V increases at all fixed levels of N. This reflects the decreasing efficiency of solute removal, which is recognized by the stdKt/V model, as each individual dose increases and blood concentration falls and therefore the driving force for solute

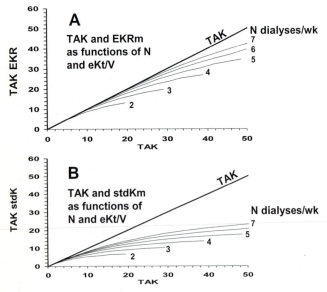

Figure 7–41. Comparisons of EKR and StdK to TAK as a function of N.

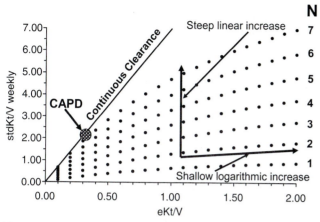

Figure 7–43. Results of solution of stdKt/V model over wide ranges of eKt/V and N.

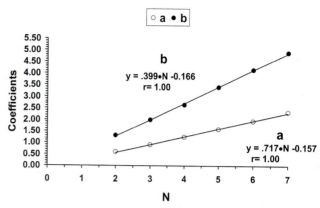

Figure 7–44. Results of fitting the regression coefficients for the functions stdKt/V = a + b·ln(eKt/V) to N.

$$stdKt / V = (0.717 * N - 0.157) + (0.399N - 0.166) * \ln(eKt / V)$$

removal. The line labeled continuous clearance in Fig. 7–43 is calculated as seven times the abscissa values with the understanding (for this calculation) that the eKt/V values on the abscissa are given continuously 7 days per week. Note that the locus of CAPD is indicated on the continuous clearance line. The plot in Fig. 7–43 provides a uniform expression of dialysis dose combining intensity, eKt/V, and frequency, N, in a generalized dosing parameter, stdKt/V. The orderly behavior of the stdKt/V model solutions exhibited in Fig. 7–43 suggests that it might be possible to devise a generalized logarithmic or parabolic regression equation which incorporates both N and eKt/V. Both of these conjectures are true as will be shown below.

An Optimized Regression Equation to Calculate stdKt/V. The conjecture that a logarithmic regression might be fitted to model solutions is schematically depicted in Fig. 7–43. The logarithmic function suggested would be of the form

$$stdKt / V = \alpha \cdot f(N) + \beta \cdot f(N) \cdot \ln(eKt / V) \qquad (114)$$

Further, it is likely that the two coefficients may be linear functions of N. This was evaluated by fitting the model solution points for $0.10 \leq eKt/V \leq 2.00$ at each N varied from 1 to 7 and the values for α and β at each N fit to a linear regression as f(N). The results of this analysis are shown in Fig. 7–44 where virtually perfect linear correlations of the coefficients to f(N) are seen and result in the logarithmic regression algorithm

$$stdKt / V = (0.717 * N - 0.157)$$
$$+ (0.399N - 0.166) * \ln(eKt / V) \qquad (115)$$

The results in Fig. 7–44 strongly suggested that Eq. (115) would be suitable to calculate stdKt/V from N and measurement of eKt/V and would be much simpler than formal solution of the modeling equations. The suitability

of Eq. (115) can be evaluated in Fig. 7–45 where it is apparent the regression fits the modeled values very well for all N with eKt/V ≥ 0.40 but, for eKt/V ≤ 0.40, the equation substantially underestimates the true value of modeled stdKt/V. Although eKt/V <0.40 is not seen in CHD, values in this range may be seen with the advent of short daily hemodialysis and in APD and Eq. (115) would not be suitable to estimate the dose of dialysis in this range.

As noted above it could also be conjectured that a second order regression would fit the model over a wide range. We used the technique described above to fit all modeled values calculated for each level of N and $0.10 \leq eKt/V \leq 2.00$ to a function of the form

$$stdKt / V = a \cdot eKt / V^2 + b \cdot eKt / V + c \qquad (116)$$

the coefficients a , b, and c were then fit as linear functions of N in accordance with

$$stdKt / V = a \cdot f(N) \cdot eKt / V^2$$
$$+ b \cdot f(N) \cdot eKt / V + c \cdot f(N) \qquad (117)$$

with results depicted in Fig. 7–46 where again tight linear correlations are seen and the algorithm derived is shown to be

$$stdKt / V = (- 0.1516 \cdot N + 0.011) \cdot (eKt / V)^2$$
$$+ b \cdot f (0.7884 \cdot N - 0.1606) \cdot eKt / V$$
$$+ (0.0406 \cdot N + 0.0621) \qquad (118)$$

The second-order expression in Eq. (118) was evaluated over the total range of N and eKt/V; the results shown in Fig. 7–47 show that this function fits the model almost perfectly over the entire domains of frequency and eKt/V. The superior performance of Eq. (118) over Eq. (115) is shown graphically in Fig. 7–48 where the error with each

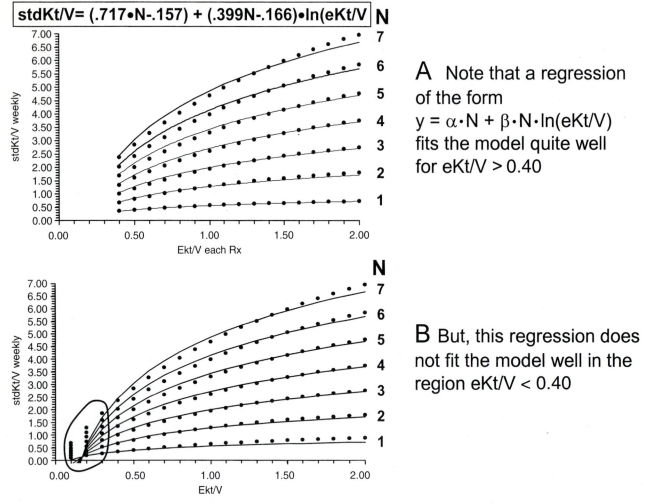

$$\boxed{stdKt/V = (.717 \bullet N - .157) + (.399N - .166) \bullet \ln(eKt/V)}$$

A Note that a regression of the form $y = \alpha \cdot N + \beta \cdot N \cdot \ln(eKt/V)$ fits the model quite well for eKt/V > 0.40

B But, this regression does not fit the model well in the region eKt/V < 0.40

Figure 7–45. A slope intercept logarithmic regression fits model solutions quite well for eKt / V > 0.40 but does not fit the model well for eKt / V < 0.40.

expression is plotted as a function of eKt/V. The large systematic error at low eKt/V for Eq. (115) is readily apparent while there is virtually no systematic error with Eq. (118) which can be used to calculate stdKt/V for any dialysis schedule (N) and eKt/V. It is also useful to note that Eq. (118) can be solved for eKt/V using the quadratic formula in accordance with

$$eKt / V = (-b \pm ((b \wedge 2) - 4 \cdot a \cdot c) \wedge (0.50)) / 2 \cdot a$$

where a=$(-0.152 \cdot N + 0.011)$

b=$(0.788 \cdot N - 0.1606)$ (119)

c=$(0.041 \cdot N + 0.062 - stdKt/V)$

Equation (119) is suitable to calculate the eKt/V required to achieve any desired stdKt/V with any specified frequency of dialysis.

Quantification of the Dose of Intermittent HD Combined with Residual Renal Urea Clearance (K_{ru}). There is a growing be-

lief that starting patients on dialysis at a higher level of residual renal function may have long term benefits on outcome with dialysis therapy.[100] A quantitative method of incorporating residual renal urea clearance (K_{ru}) in the special cases of twice and thrice-weekly dialysis prescription has been derived previously.[8] There is increasing support for initiation of both HD and CAPD at higher levels of residual renal function[101] and the concept of stdKt/V as embodied in Eqs. (107) to (112) is well suited to calculation of the dose of intermittent HD with residual renal function. However the model mathematics are not suitable for derivation of a generalized algorithm such as in Eqs (118) and (119) to cover the entire domains of N, eKt/V and K_{ru}. Instead a family of solutions for each N must be derived to quantify the dose of combined intermittent and continuous clearance. The techniques described above were used to derive N-specific logarithmic and parabolic expressions for stdKt/V = f(N, eKt/V, nK_{ru}) where nK_{ru} is the residual renal urea clearance divided by the patient's urea distribution vol-

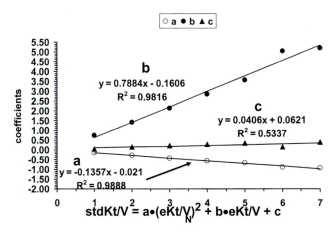

Figure 7–46. Results of fitting regression coefficients for the functions stdKt/V = a · f(N) · eKt/V2 + b · f(N) · eKt/V + c · f(N). The three coefficients show almost perfect linear correlation to N except for c, with slope near 0, and result in the regression equation

$$stdKt / V = (-0.516 \bullet N + 0.011) \bullet (eKt / V)2 + (0.7884 \bullet N - 0.1606)$$

$$\bullet eKt / V + (.0406 \bullet N + 0.621)$$

ume and expressed as ml/L The parabolic regression is depicted in Fig. 7–49 for N 1, 2, 3, and 4. This clearly does not provide a satisfactory general algorithm. It fits the model data perfectly for N = 2 but deviates significantly at high levels of eKt/V for N = 1, 3, and 4 and could not serve as a generalized algorithm.

A logarithmic algorithm relating stdKt/V to N and eKt/V was formulated as

$$stdKt / V = a \cdot f(N) + b \cdot f(N) \cdot \ln(eKt / V) \qquad (120)$$

and specific for each individual N. The logarithmic algorithm derived is illustrated in Fig. 7–50 for N 1, 2, 3, and 4,

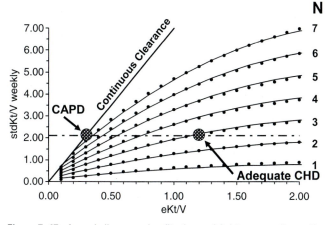

Figure 7–47. A parabolic regression fits the model data very well over the ranges 0.1 ≤ eKt/V ≤ 2.00, 1 ≤ N ≤ 7 and will be the most reliable regression to estimate stdKt/V over this entire range from knowledge of N and eKt/V.

$$stdKt / V = (-0.1516 \bullet N + 0.011) \bullet (eKt / V)2 + (0.7884 \bullet N - 0.1606)$$

$$\bullet eKt / V + (0.0406 \bullet N + 0.0621)$$

where it can be seen to fit the model data very well over the entire domains of N and eKt/V and thus can serve as a reliable algorithm to quantify combined intermittent HD and nK$_r$. In order to make the K$_{ru}$ units more familiar, the plots in Fig. 7–50 are normalized to an average V = 35 L and thus expressed as K$_{ru}$, mL/min rather than nK$_{ru}$. This algorithm should be useful for calculating dialysis dose for patients starting dialysis earlier with higher K$_{ru}$. In each of the plots a reference line for adequate stdKt/V = 2.15 is plotted and a patterned circle marks the point of minimum adequate eKt/V as a function of K$_{ru}$ and N. In panel A it can be seen that if it is elected to initiate HD once a week, the minimum eKt/V required will be 2.0 in a patient with K$_{ru}$ = 6.0 mL/min. The regression lines are almost flat in Fig. 7–50 A so that the minimum K$_{ru}$ for once-weekly dialysis is K$_{ru}$ = 6.0 and might be considered to be a kinetic definition of absolute minimum K$_{ru}$ to initiate hemodialysis once weekly with eKt/V = 2.00. In panels B, C, and D the stdKt/V 2.15 line crosses the K$_{ru}$ regression lines and the levels of minimum eKt/V required as f(N and eKt/V) are depicted as open circles. If higher levels of eKt/V and N are chosen the plots can also provide a quantification of the dose actually selected and prescribed. For example, in panel C the stdKt/V that would result if CHD dialysis were initiated with N = 3 and stdKt/V = 1.2 with K$_{ru}$ 6.0 in the average-sized patient will result in stdKt/V = 3.2. This may be much better therapy than 2.15 but there are no data available at present to make that decision. However, this points up the potential value of using the relationships depicted in Fig. 7–50 to quantify the dose as stdKt/V with earlier initiation of HD and more frequent dialysis. In this way a uniform dosing parameter can be used to examine outcome with the widening range of doses with regard to K$_{ru}$ and N.

Tables of Parabolic and Logarithmic Solutions for the Relationships between stdKt/v, N eKtV, and K$_{ru}$. A summary of the algorithms is shown in Tables 7–1 and 7–2. Table 7–1 provides the individual logarithmic regressions for stdKt/V = f(N, eKt/V and nK$_{ru}$) for each N over the range 1 to 7. The last row in the table lists the general parabolic equation for stdKt/V as f(N and eKt/V) when nK$_{ru}$ = 0. Table 7–2 provides the logarithmic equations for required eKt/V = f(N, stdKt/V and nK$_{ru}$) for each N over the range 1 to 7. The last row in the table shows the quadratic equation to determine eKt/V as f(N, stdKt/V) when nK$_{ru}$ = 0. In this way these two tables summarize all of the algorithms relating stdKt/V, eKt/V, nK$_{ru}$ and N for use in evaluating these relationships in clinical data.

Clinical Evaluation of EKR·t/V and stdK·t/V

As noted above, there are no prospective studies evaluating these two definitions of equivalent continuous clearance over wide ranges but there is a very large body of clinical experience and consensus regarding equivalency between

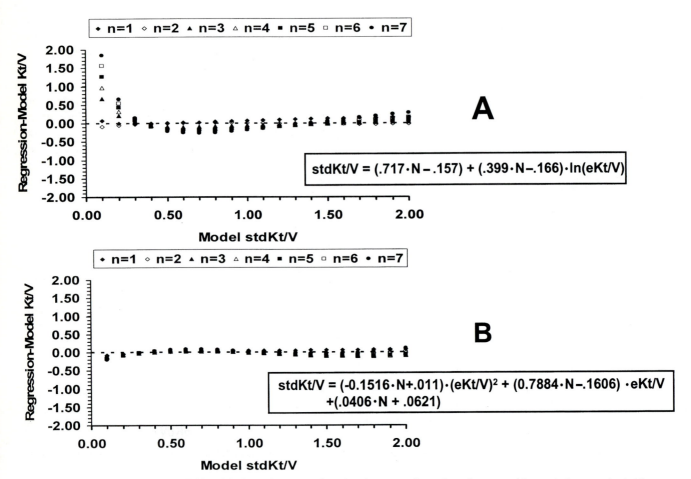

Figure 7–48. The error, difference in stdKt/V model values minus regression values is very small over the entire range of the parabolic regression but becomes very large at eKt/V < 0.40 with the logarithmic regression.

the dose of CAPD and thrice-weekly HD. The DOQI consensus recommendation is a weekly CAPD Kt/V of 2.1 for adequate therapy and adequate thrice weekly HD requires an eKt/V of about 1.1 for each dialysis.[102] Since in CAPD the peritoneal clearance (K_p) is virtually continuous, the total weekly CAPD clearance ($K_p \cdot t/V$) is by definition a steady state clearance and the level of adequate $K_p \cdot t/V$ in CAPD can be used to evaluate the three definitions of K_{seq} described above (K_{pk}, stdK, and EKR). Evaluation of these three definitions of C_{seq} has previously been reported[98] through calculation of a family of weekly concentration profiles EKRt/V, stdKt/V, and pkKt/V with specified V, NPCR = 1, N = 3 and eKt/V varied over a wide a wide range ($0.2 \leq eKt/V \leq 2.2$). These analyses indicated the stdKt/V predicted an adequate $K_p \cdot t/V$ of 2.0 while the EKR·t/V predicted is 3.0 and pkK·t/V predicted about 1.8.

These relationships for EKR and stdKt/V are illustrated in Fig. 7–51 where they are shown in the context of the generalized solutions of the two models. In panel A the EKR model shows that adequate $K_p \cdot t/V$ of 2.1 L/L/wk in CAPD predicts that an adequate eKt/V for CHD would be only 0.70. The model predicts that the adequate dose of eKt/V of 1.1 in HEMO would require a continuous Kpt/V of 3.0 for equivalent CAPD. The EKR model predicts the high dose arm of HEMO with eKt/V 1.45 would require a CAPD dose of nearly 4 L/wk/L for equivalent therapeutic benefit. Clearly, the EKR model does not correctly predict equivalent doses in CAPD and CHD.

The relationships among these therapies as defined by the stdKt/V model are shown in Fig. 7–51B. It can be observed that the adequate CAPD dose agrees quite well with both the standard and high dose arms of HEMO. It also predicts there would be little if any improvement in outcome with very low doses of SDHD with eKt/V 0.5 as described by Kooistra et al.[103] The model, because of the shallow logarithmic increase in stdKt/V as eKt/V increases, indicates there are very small differences in the level of stdKt/V despite wide differences in weekly Kt/V for CAPD, the two arms of HEMO and very low dose SDHD.

The recently reported ADEMEX[88] study is also plotted in Fig. 7–51B. This study showed no improvement in clinical outcome when weekly stdKt/V was increased from 1.75

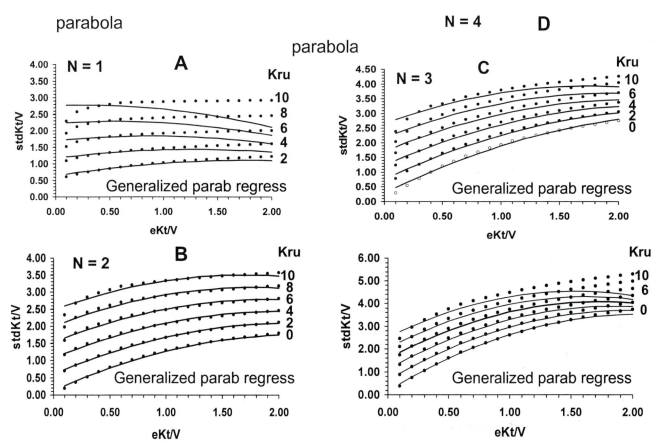

Figure 7–49. The effect of residual Kru on stdKt/V as a function of N and eKt/V. The reference line for adequate thrice weekly stdKt/V = 2.15 is shown on each plot with the coordinates of Kru, eKt/V required for $1 \leq N \leq 4$.

to 2.00. It is of interest to note that the stdKt/V 1.75 indicates therapeutic equivalence with CHD spKt/V of 1.0, which was the dose concluded to be adequate from kinetic analysis of the NCDS 20 years ago.[2] The lower bound of spKt/V studied in HEMO was 1.35 and did not address the dosing domain $1.00 \leq$ spKt/V ≤ 1.35 as depicted in Figs. 7–27 and 7–28. The stdKt/V model indicates there were relatively small differences in dose in all of the studies depicted in Fig. 7–51B and would support a conclusion that the ADEMEX and NCDS studies had similar dose response curves. In sharp contrast to this interpretation, the recently reported HDP concept[87] interpreted the ADEMEX results to show the strong influence of middle molecule removal on clinical outcome and recommended time as the only treatment parameter of importance.

However, there appeared to be a design flaw in the ADEMEX study design which casts some doubt on the generalizability of the study. The baseline therapy was four 2-L exchanges per day irrespective of body size for all patients. Patients were selected for the intervention and stdKt/V increased to 2.0 only if they had inadequate stdKt/V on the current therapy. By definition this criterion must bias patient selection toward recruitment of larger patients with larger anthropometric V who are known to have better outcomes than smaller patients (see Fig. 7–30).

Consideration of the Potential Role of the stdK·t/V Model to Guide Design of Studies of More Frequent Dialysis Therapies. It is of interest to examine dose quantification by the stdKt/V model over a range of potential experimental dialysis therapies. Ideally it would seem logical that such studies should be designed to evaluate N and stdKt/V independently since there is no a priori way to distinguish between the effects of frequency and intensity. A design that would fulfill these requirements is shown in Fig. 7–52 where interventions are distributed nearly independently of N and eKt/V over wide ranges of these parameters. The two most important interventions would seem to be SDHD and LNHD. These both have N = 6 and stdKt/V 3.5 and 5.5 respectively as depicted in Fig. 7–52. Comparison of these two dosages should provide critical outcome information helpful to distinguish between the importance of frequency and intensity on the dose response. The region of low-dose SDHD outlined in Fig. 7–52 should probably not be included in prospective studies of more frequent dialysis since the increase in dose would not appear to be sufficient in the light of previous

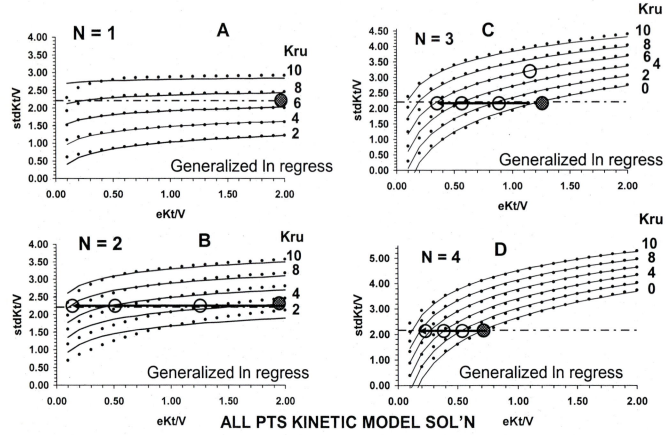

Figure 7–50. The effect of residual Kru on stdKt/V as a function of N and eKt/V. the reference line for adequate thrice weekly stdKt/V = 2.15 is shown on each plot with the coordinates of Kru, eKt/V required for $1 \leq N \leq 4$.

studies and as defined by the stdKt/V model to result in major changes in outcome.[98]

Modeling stdKt/V with Combined CAPD and HD. This combination will be identical to the relationships between N, eKt/V, and K_{ru} so the relationships in Fig. 7–50 would apply directly to this clinical question and the equations in Tables 7–1 and 7–2 can be used to evaluate therapy or calculate prescription combinations. This subject will be considered more fully in Chap. 15.

The Monthly stdKt/V: A Proposed New QA Standard. Although conventional dialysis is administered 13 times per month, technical QA of this therapy is typically based on process-

TABLE 7–1. APPROXIMATION EQUATIONS TO CALCULATE stdKt/V[a]

N	stdKt/V = f(N, eKt/V, nKru)
1	stdKt/V = (7.938·nKru + 0.5816) + (-0.987·nKru + 0.330·ln(eKt/V)
2	stdKt/V = (7.077·nKru + 1.2683) + (-1.173·nKru + 0.676)·ln(eKt/V)
3	stdKt/V = (6.472·nKru + 1.9849) + (-1.400·nKru + 1.075)·ln(eKt/V)
4	stdKt/V = (6.479·nKru + 2.6651) + (-1.393·nKru + 1.488)·ln(eKt/V)
5	stdKt/V = (6.276·nKru + 3.3838) + (-1.480·nKru + 1.938)·ln(eKt/V)
6	stdKt/V = (6.090·nKru + 4.1295) + (-1.512·nKru + 2.429)·ln(eKt/V)
7	stdKt/V = (6.787·nKru + 1.9539) + (-1.5575nKru + 1.111)·ln((eKt/V)
1<N<7, Kr=0	stdKt/V = (-0.152·N + .011)·eKt/V² + (0.788·N − 0.161)·eKt/V + (0.041·N + 0.062)

[a]Approximation equations to calculate stdKt/V urea as a function of eKt/V number of dialyses per week (N) and level of normalized renal urea clearance (nKru). Note that when Kru = 0, a single quadratic equation can be used to calculate stdKt/V for all N and $0.1 \leq eKt/V \leq 2.00$.

TABLE 7–2. APPROXIMATION EQUATIONS TO CALCULATE eKt/V[a]

N	eKt/V = f(stdKt/V, N Kru)
1	eKt/V = exp(((stdKt/V)-(7.938·nKru + 0.582))/(−0.987·nKru + 0.330))
2	eKt/V = exp(((stdKt/V)-(7.077·nKru + 1.268))/(−1.173·nKru + 0.676))
3	eKt/V = exp(((stdKt/V)-(6.472·nKru + 1.985))/(−1.400·nKru + 1.075))
4	eKt/V = exp(((stdKt/V)-(6.479·nKru + 2.665))/(−1.393·nKru + 1.488))
5	eKt/V = exp(((stdKt/V)-(6.276·nKru + 3.384))/(−1.481·nKru + 1.938))
6	eKt/V = exp(((stdKt/V)-(6.090·Kru + 4.130))/(−1.512·Kru + 2.429))
7	eKt/V = exp(((stdKt/V)-(6.787·nKru + 1.954))/(−1.556·nKru + 1.111))
2 ≤ N ≤ 6, Kr=0	eKt/V = −**b** ± ((b^2) - 4·**a**·**c**)^(0.50))/2·a where **a** = (-0.152·N + 0.011) **b** = (0.788·N − 0.1606) **c** = (0.041·N + 0.062)

[a]Approximation equations to calculate eKt/V as a function of stdKt/V, number of dialyses per week (N) and level of normalized renal urea clearance (nKru). Note that when Kru = 0, a single quadratic equation can be used to calculate eKt/V for all N and stdKt/V.

Clinical Correlates of the two models

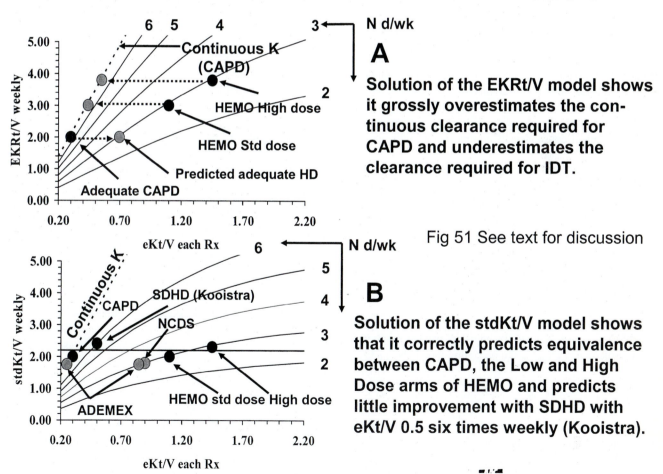

A

Solution of the EKRt/V model shows it grossly overestimates the continuous clearance required for CAPD and underestimates the clearance required for IDT.

Fig 51 See text for discussion

B

Solution of the stdKt/V model shows that it correctly predicts equivalence between CAPD, the Low and High Dose arms of HEMO and predicts little improvement with SDHD with eKt/V 0.5 six times weekly (Kooistra).

Figure 7–51. See text for details.

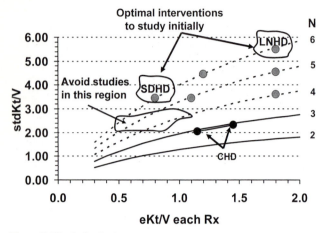

Figure 7–52. A distribution of interventions of more frequent dialysis as defined by the stdKt/V model with frequency (N) and dose stdKt/V (eKt/V) independently distributed.

ing a single set of pre/post BUNs during the month. It has been suggested that there is a strong need to quantitatively communicate to physicians and patients the effects of missed dialyses on the overall dialysis dose (personal communication, Dr J.M. Lazarus, Chief Medical Officer, Fresenius North America). To that end, he believes there is need for development of a monthly stdKt/V (stdKt/V_M) which, in addition to reflecting the eKt/V measured on one analyzed dialysis that month, is also adjusted to reflect the number of dialyses missed during the month. Missed dialyses have a profound effect on the dose of treatment expressed as stdKt/V and there is some evidence to suggest there are associated clinical consequences commensurate with the kinetically defined effect.

The monthly stdKt/V_M must be derived from the weekly stdKt/V reference level. This requires determination of the number of dialysis days (N_d) in the previous month, i.e., the number of days that fall on a scheduled day of dialysis for the patient. From N_d the number of dialysis weeks (N_{dw}) in the month can be calculated as

$$N_{dw} = N_d / 3 \qquad (121)$$

Next add up the actual number of dialyses received that month (N_{dRx}) and calculate the adjusted average number of dialyses per week (N_{adj}) in the preceding month as

$$N_{adj} = N_{dRx} / N_{dw} \qquad (122)$$

Since we are discussing conventional HD with prescribed N = 3 and eKt/V in the range of 1.0, a logarithmic regression will be rigorous (see Fig. 7–45) for calculating the adjusted stdKt/V (stdKt/V_{adj}) from measured eKt/V and N_{adj} in accordance with

$$stdKt / V_{adj} = (0.717 \cdot N_{adj} - 0.157)$$
$$+ (0.399 \cdot N_{adj} - 0.166) \cdot \ln(eKt / V) \qquad (123)$$

Next consider how to convert the adjusted weekly stdKt/V_{adj} to a monthly adjusted stdKt/V_M. The month would probably be represented most realistically as a 13-dialysis-day month for which Ndw = 4.33 in which case the monthly stdKt/V_M is simply calculated as

$$stdKt / V_M = 4.33 \, (stdKt / V_{adj}) \qquad (124)$$

It is very informative to solve Eq. (124) for the adjusted eKt/V (eKt/V_{adj}) corresponding to the stdKt/V_{adj} from rearrangement of Eq. (124),

$$eKt / V_{adj} = \exp(((stdKt / V_{adj})$$
$$- (0.717 \cdot N - 0.157))$$
$$(0.399 \cdot N - 0.166)) \qquad (125)$$

The effect of two missed dialyses is illustrated in Fig. 7–53. In this example the patient is receiving eKt/V 1.20 during each dialysis he attends but by missing two treatments in the month he drops down to an average of 2.54 dialyses per week which reduces stdKt/V_M from 9.44 to 7.87 and reduces the eKt/V_{adj} from 1.20 to 0.84. This could also be expressed as an adjusted treatment time: If t = 3.5 hour for eKt/V = 1.2 the equivalent t for eKt//V.84 is .84/1.2(2.5) = 2.45 hours or reduction of t by about 1 hour for each treatment with no missed dialyses. The reason for this huge effect is not intuitively obvious because of the enduring concern about the danger of any shortening of treatment time. The reason for the large calculated effect is that the last hour of diaysis is far less efficient for solute removal than the first 2.5 hours (see discussion of Fig. 7–40). However, it should also be noted that if large fluid gains are a problem, they would clearly mitigate against the calculated time equivalency.

There is some clinical support for the rather impressive calculations illustrated in Fig. 7–53. USRDS data were analyzed for the effect of skipped treatments compared to shortening dose on relative risk of mortality (RRM).[103,104] The number of skipped treatments was not precisely quantified but reporting a missing treatment was associated with much greater proportional increase in mortality compared to reduction in eKt/V. The findings are illustrated in Fig. 7–54, where it can be seen that a decrease of eKt/V by 7 percent was associated with a 7 percent increase in RRM. Skipping one dialysis decreased stdKt/V by 6 percent but increased RRM by 13 percent, which would define a decrease in eKt/V_{adj} by 13 percent from 1.13 to 0.99. These data are very comparable to the kinetic calculations in Fig. 7–53 and

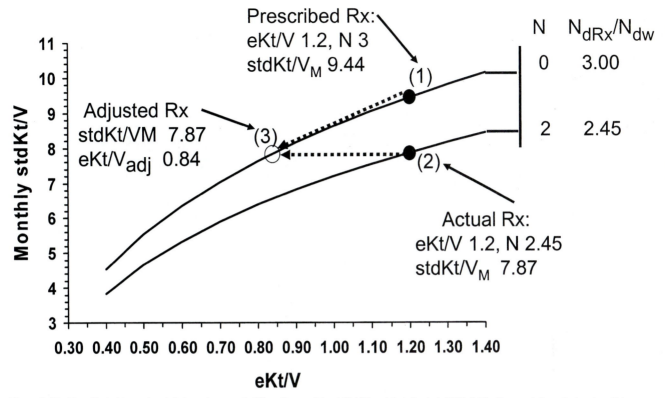

Figure 7–53. The effect of two missed dialyses in a month (N) on the monthly stdKt/VM and the adjusted eKt/Vadj. The therapy delivered when two dialyses are missed in a month is equivalent to reducing eKt/V from 1.2 to 0.84 with no missed dialyses in the month.

provide some clinical support for the calculated effect of missed treatment on dose. This would appear to be a fruitful area for study.

THE PHARMACODYNAMICS OF ERYTHROPOIETIN THERAPY

Anemia in chronic renal failure is often considered due to decreased red cell production, which in turn is caused by inadequate renal production of erythropoietin.[105,106] However, red cell survival is also reduced, not due to random destruction of red cells as is the case in acquired hemolytic anemia, but because of a shortening of the normal red cell life span.[107,108] With the kinetics of dialysis and drug therapy, the removal (clearance) of solutes and drugs is continuous and directly proportional to their concentrations (first order). In contrast, the modeled substance in therapy with recombinant human erythropoietin (rHuEpo) is the red cell, which has a reduced but finite survival or life span. This means that all red cells produced on a specific day survive until their life span is reached, and then all cells in that day's production die and are cleared from the circulation. Consequently, it is necessary to use a finite survival population model to describe the red cell system,[109] and it is inappropriate to refer to a red cell half-life, which applies only

in the case of random destruction observed in hemolytic anemia.

These kinetics dictate that when rHuEpo therapy is begun, it results in an abrupt and constant increase in red cell production (P), in milliliters of red cells per day, and all new cells produced under the influence of rHuEpo will survive and accumulate in the circulating blood volume resulting in a linear rise in hematocrit (H) which will continue until the red cell survival time (τ, days) is reached. When treatment duration equals or exceeds τ, all the cells produced on the first day of rHuEpo therapy will die off, and each day thereafter the cells produced τ days earlier will die. In this way the death rate abruptly increases to equal the rHuEPo-induced increment in production rate and the H will stabilize at a new steady state.

The population kinetics of the red cell system can be described mathematically. In order to better conceptualize this, assume there are no red cells in the system at time zero (t = 0), at which point a constant red cell production, P, is abruptly initiated. Assuming total blood volume (V, mL) remains constant, the mass balance of red cells over the interval τ (where τ is red cell survival time, days) can be described as

Circulating RCM at t days = where RCM is red cell mass daily production rate times t days of production

(126)

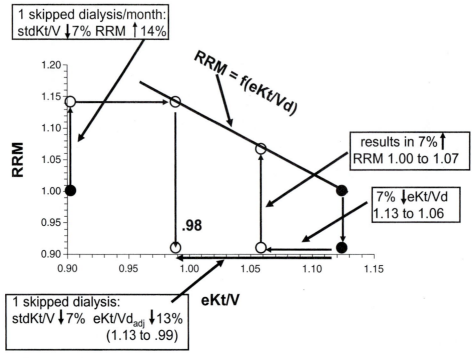

Figure 7–54. Comparison of effect of skipped dialysis to effect of decreased eKt/V on RRM in USRDS data.

or

$$Ht(V) = (P) \cdot t \tag{127}$$

which can be rearranged to give

$$Ht = (P / V) \cdot t \tag{128}$$

Note in Eq. (128) that the H will increase linearly with a slope equal to P/V, which precisely defines the volume of cells which are produced daily and added to the circulating blood volume. As discussed above, when t reaches τ, accumulation will abruptly stop because the death rate of cells will suddenly increase from zero to equal the daily production rate. The steady-state H which is reached is

$$Hss = (P / V)\tau \tag{129}$$

Equation (129) shows that the total increase in H is the product of the slope or daily increase and τ which is the length of time all new red cells accumulate. The relationships in Eq. (129) can be used to quantitatively show the relative effects of P and τ in the anemia of chronic renal failure. Solution of Eq. (129) for P results in

$$P = H \cdot V / \tau \tag{130}$$

If the normal values H = 40 and τ = 120 are substituted into Eq. (123)

$$nP = 0.33V \tag{131}$$

where nP = normal production rate. In the renal patient we can write

$$uP = H \cdot V / \tau \tag{132}$$

where uP = production rate in the uremic patient. We can divide Eq. (132) by Eq. (131), define uP/nP as Rp, the ratio of red cell production in uremia to the average normal rate, and solve for H we find is

$$H = 0.33 \cdot \tau \cdot Rp \tag{133}$$

Note that in Eq. (133) the steady-state H in renal anemia will be equally dependent on Rp and τ, and the degree of anemia is directly proportional to the product of Rp and

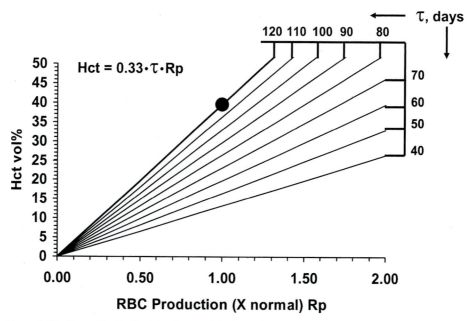

Figure 7–55. The erythrokinetic determinants of the Hct with finite RBC lifetime. The RBC production is expressed relative to normal (Rp). Hct is plotted as a function of Rp constant levels of τ ranging from 40 to 120 days. Note there is a family of straight lines.

τ. Equation (133) is depicted graphically in Fig. 7–55, where it has been solved over an Rp range of 0 to 2.0 at constant τ levels ranging from 120 to 40. Normal erythrokinetics are shown with the large filled circle with coordinates Hct = 40, Rp = 1.00, and τ = 120 days. Figure 7–56 depicts with heavy arrows three pathways for development of uremic anemia with Hct fall from 40 to 20: (1) Isolated de-

crease in Rp; (2) Isolated decrease in red cell survival or τ; and (3) Combined decrease in production and survival of red cells.

Uremic anemia is often considered to be due only to a pure decrease in Rp due to erythropoietin deficiency. Cotes et al.[110] reported very complete studies of the clinical response to rHuEpo therapy, including measurement of τ be-

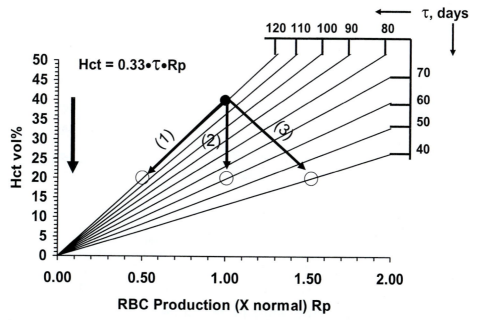

Figure 7–56. The erythrokinetic determinants of anemia in renal failure. Note that the Hct can fall from 40 to 20 by (1) isolated decrease in Rp, (2) isolated decrease in τ, or (3) decrease in τ combined with inadequate compensatory increase in Rp.

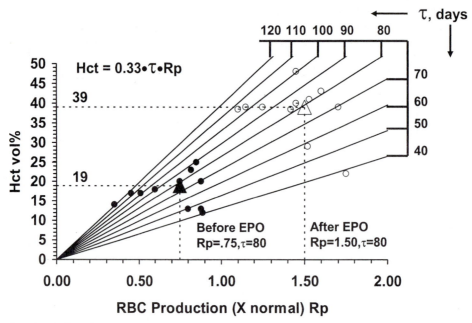

Figure 7–57. The erythrokinetic determinants of the increase in Hct calculated from Cotes data.

fore and after treatment. Values for Rp and finite survival time were calculated from this data and are depicted in Fig. 7–57. Prior to therapy the mean H was 20, τ was 80 days, and Rp was 0.75, indicating both decreased P and τ were contributing to the anemia. After a new steady state was reached with rHuEpo the mean H was 40, the mean Rp was 1.5, and τ was unchanged at 80 days. Thus, the red cell pro-

duction rate had to be increased to 150 percent of normal with rHuEpo therapy to compensate for the substantially shortened survival time in these patients.

We have reported similar data[109] from San Francisco with the mean values observed depicted in Fig. 7–58 and compared to the Cotes data. In our data Rp was initially normal and anemia was due to failure to increase produc-

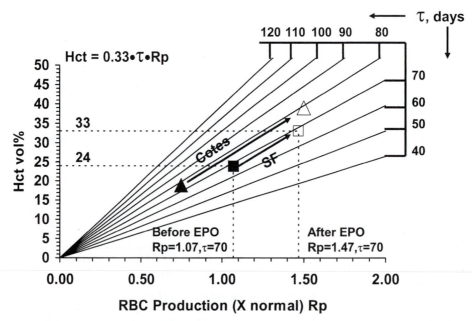

Figure 7–58. Change in mean erythrokinetic parameters observed in 50 San Francisco (SF) patients compared to Cotes data.

tion to compensate for shortened red cell survival. Recovery from anemia resulted in Rp 147 percent of normal, nearly identical to the Cotes data. Clearly, both P and τ must be included in a pharmacodynamic model for clinical guidance of rHuEpo therapy.

We can now develop the model further and attempt to derive a formulation useful for quantitative guidance of rHuEpo therapy. Prior to rHuEpo therapy the typical patient has a steady-state anemia which can be described in accordance with

$$HO = (PO / V) \cdot \tau \qquad (134)$$

where H0 and P0 are baseline levels of H and P immediately prior to rHuEpo therapy. Regular administration of rHuEpo results in an abrupt and constant increase in production, Pe, with accumulation of red cells and linear rise in H over the interval t τ in accordance with

$$Ht = (PO / V) \cdot \tau + (Pe / V) \cdot t \qquad (135)$$

when t = τ, the new steady state with rHuEpo therapy is reached and defined as

$$Hss = (PO / V) \cdot \tau + (Pe / V) \cdot \tau \qquad (136)$$

The correction of anemia achieved with rHuEpo is defined by the increase in H achieved which is exactly equal to the second right-hand term, $(Pe/V)(\tau$, in Eq. (136). Next it is necessary to show how the targeted total rise in H, ΔH, relates to the rHuEpo dose (D). The patient response or sensitivity (S) to rHuEpo can be defined as the induced rate of H increase relative to D or

$$S = (Pe / V) / D \qquad (137)$$

The desired correction of anemia is

$$\Delta H = (Pe / V) \cdot \tau \qquad (138)$$

Combination of Eqs. (137) and (138), and solution for D results in

$$D = (\Delta H / S) \cdot \tau e \qquad (139)$$

We have reported[109] mean values for S = 0.0168 units of H increase per day per 1000 units of total rHuEpo dose per week (administered in three equal iv doses after each dialysis) and τ = 64 days. Incorporation of these mean population values into Eq. (139) results in

$$D = 930 \ (\Delta H) \qquad (140)$$

where D is total units/week.

Equation (140) can be used to estimate the initial rHuEpo dose in a new patient. The H should be measured at least weekly and after 4 or 5 weeks the slope can usually be calculated and used to determine an individualized value for S (Si) for the patient in accordance with

$$Si = (Pe / V)_{observed} / D_{weekly \ dose \ given} \qquad (141)$$

If Si differs substantially from S, a new individualized dose (Di) can be calculated during the accumulation phase (H still rising) from

$$Di = \Delta H / Si \cdot \tau \qquad (142)$$

Frequent H measurements must be continued after dose adjustment. The individual red cell survival time, τi, can be determined when the new slope decreases (second dose was higher than first dose), becomes zero (second dose was equal to first dose), or becomes negative (second dose was less than first dose). A final maintenance dose (Dm) can now be calculated by incorporation of Si and τi into Eq. (142) and solution in accordance with

$$Dm = \Delta H / Si \cdot \tau i \qquad (143)$$

The model is now fully developed and provides a rational approach to individualizing and optimizing the dose of rHuEpo. However, it is difficult to fully utilize such a model without computerized surveillance and analysis of the data base in each patient. Manually calculating slopes during the red cell accumulation phase and identifying the slope changes which signal the onset of the new steady state are very labor intensive. However, even with sophisticated computer assistance, it will be almost impossible to rationally calculate dose changes in some patients because of the arbitrary and irrational HCFA reimbursement policy that requires rHuEpo to be discontinued whenever the H reaches an arbitrary level of 36 percent. This policy results in a broad spectrum of cell cohort ages and death rates which are virtually impossible to track with a model.

Finally, it should be pointed out that a recommended practice of prescribing a high dose of rHuEpo initially to increase the H and a smaller maintenance dose after the target

H is reached is not rational in the light of the pharmacodynamics of the red cell system. The H will rise more rapidly when a large initial dose is given, but when τ is reached the red cells will die off at a high rate, equal to the high production rate, and the H must fall until it reaches a steady state of the production rate achieved with the smaller dose. The pharmacodynamics of the system show that the optimal dose is identical during both the accumulation phase and subsequent new steady state and is a function of both P and τ.

GLOSSARY

An Important Note: all units of mass and volume must be compatible such as mg/mL, mL, or mg/L, L.

A		
α		minimal level of nTACiP reached during dialysis
β		exponent determining the rate at which α is reached
BWt		body weight, kg
C		concentration
	C_c	intracellular concentration
	C_{co}	predialysis intracellular concentration
	C_{ct}	postdialysis intracellular concentration
	C_{cU}	intracellular urea concentration
	C_{do}	dialysate outlet concentration
	C_e	extracellular concentration
	C_{eo}	predialysis extracellular concentration
	C_{eq}	equilibrium concentration
	C_{et}	postdialysis extracellular concentration
	C_{eU}	extracellular urea concentration
	C_{is}	interstitial fluid concentration
	C_o	predialysis concentration
	C_{o1}	C_o before first dialysis of week
	C_{o2}	C_o before second dialysis of week
	C_{oiP}	predialysis inorganic phosphorus
	C_{om}	osmotic concentration of Na
	C_{niP}	postdialysis inorganic phosphorus
	C_p	plasma concentration
	C_{pk}	peak concentration
	C_{pwi}	dialyzer inlet plasma water C
	C_{pwo}	dialyzer outlet plasma water C
	C_s	equivalent steady state concentrations
	C_t	postdialysis concentration
	C_{t1}	postdialysis C after first dialysis of week
	C_{t2}	postdialysis C after second dialysis of week
	C_{ss}	steady state concentration
	C_{tiP}	postdialysis C inorganic phosphorus
CAPD		continuous ambulatory peritoneal dialysis

CHD		chronic hemodialysis
D		dialysance
	Di	dialysate inlet
	Dm	dialysate outlet
DI_{B12}		dialysis index vitamin B_{12}
dtp		change in patient equilibration time
EKR		equivalent renal clearance
EKR_m		mean EKR
EKR_t		mean EKR
G		generation rate
	G_{iP}	generation rate iP
	G_u	generation rate urea
	spG	generation calculated from single pool model
	ajspG	adjusted spG
	eG_u	generation calculated from equilibrated double pool kinetics
H		hemoatocrit
	H0	hematocrit at time zero of EPO administration
	ΔH	change in hematocrit
	Hss	steady state hematocrit on EPO therapy
	Ht	hematocrit after one cell survival time
iP		inorganic phosphorus
J		flux rate, mass/min or mass/hr
	J_b	flux into or out of blood stream
	J_{biP}	Jb inorganic phosphorus
	J_d	flux out of or into dialysate stream
	J_{diP}	flux of Ip into dialysate stream
	J_{diPT}	total flux over a dialysis into dialysate stream
K		
	K_c	transfer coefficient from intracellular compartment
	K_d	dialyzer clearance
	K_e	effective dialyzer clearance
	adK_e	adjusted Ke
	K_m	mean clearance
	K_o	over all permeability of membrane
	K_p	peritoneal clearance
	K_{pk}	peak concentration hypothesis clearance
	K_{pwiP}	plasma water clearance of iP
	K_r	renal clearance
	K_s	sieving coefficient
	K_{rU}	renal clearance of urea
	nKr_U	renal urea clearance normalized to Vu
	K_{seq}	equivalent steady state clearance
	K_v	vascular transfer coefficient
kb		iP binder constant mg/binder tablet
KoA		overall permeability membrane area product
Kt		product of clearance and dialysis time

Kt/V		Kt divided by solute distribution volume
	eKt/V	equilibrated Kt/V
	eKt/V$_{adj}$	adjusted eKt/V
	Kdt/V	dialyzer Kt/V
	Kpt/V	peritoneal Kt/V
	KrtV	renal Kt/V
	pkKt/V	peak concentration hypothesis Kt/V
	spKt/V	single pool Kt/V
	obsKt/V$_{sp}$	observed Kt/V single pool
LNHD		long nocturnal hemodialysis
	mC	mean concentration
	mC$_{niP}$	mean normalized C iP
	mC$_o$	mean predialysis concentration
	M$_{iP}$	mean CiP
Nb		number of binders per day
N$_d$		number of dialyses
	N$_{dadj}$	adjusted number of dialyses per week
	N$_{dRx}$	number of dialyses prescribed per week
	N$_{dw}$	number of dialyses per week
P		production of red cells
	nP	normalized production of red cells
	Up	red cell production in the uremic state
	P$_0$	red cell production prior to initiation of EPO
PCR		protein catabolic rate, gm/day calculated from spKt/V model
	ePCR	protein catabolic rate calculated from eKt/V model
	obsPCR	observed PCR
	NPCR	normalized PCR as defined in text
	obsNPCR	observed NPCR
	spNPCR	NPCR calculated with sp model
	eNPCR	NPCR calculated with eKt/V model
Q		
	Q$_b$	blood flow rate
	Q$_{bi}$	dialyzer inlet blood flow rate
	Q$_d$	dialysate flow rate
	Q$_{di}$	Qd at inlet of dialyzer
	Q$_e$	effective flow rate
	Qecr	effective flow rate for creatinine
	QeiP	effective flow rate for iP
	Qeu	effective flow rate for urea
	Qf	ultrafiltration rate
	QFT	total ultrafiltrate
	Qwbi	whole blood flow rate at blood inlet
R		
	R$_p$	ratio red cell production in uremia to normal
RR		relative risk
SDHD		short daily hemodialysis
stdK		standard clearance for continuous and intermittent therapy

	stdK$_m$	the mean standard clearance during dialysis
	stdK$_t$	standard K at the end of dialysis
	stdKt/V$_{adj}$	adjusted stdKt/V
	stdKt/V$_M$	mean stdKt/V over a week
t		treatment time
	t$_p$	patient time constant for equilibration
τ		red cell survival time
TAC		time average concentration
	nTACiP	normalized TACiP
	TACiP	time average concentration iP
TAK		time average clearance
Tc		collection time
	T$_{ciP}$	collection time for iP
θ		interdialytic time interval
TBW		total body water
V		volume
	V$_b$	blood volume
	V$_{bw}$	blood water volume
	V$_c$	cell volume
	V$_e$	extracellular volume
	V$_{is}$	interstitial fluid volume
	V$_o$	volume predialysis
	V$_p$	plasma volume
	V$_{sp}$	volume calculated with sp kinetics
	V$_t$	end dialysis volume
	VT	total volume

REFERENCES

1. Keane WF, Collins AJ. Influence of co-morbidity on mortality and morbidity in patients treated with hemodialysis. *Am J Kidney Dis* 1994;24:1010.
2. Gotch F, Sargent JA. A mechanistic analysis of the National Cooperative Dialysis Study (NCDS). *Kidney Int* 1985;28:526.
3. Gupta S. A victim of truth. *Nature* 2000;407:677.
4. DeGoulet P, Legrain M, Reach I, et al. Mortality risk factors in patients treated by chronic hemodialysis. *Nephron* 1982;31:103.
5. Kaysen GA, Stevenson FT, Depner T. Determinants of albumin concentration in hemodialysis patients. *Am J Kidney Dis* 1997;29:658.
6. Acchiardo SR, Moore LW, Burk L. Malnutrition as the main factor in morbidity and mortality of hemodialysis patients. *Kidney Int Suppl* 1983;16:S199.
7. Sargent JA, Lowrie E. Which mathematical model to study uremic toxicity? *Clin Nephrol* 1982;17:303.
8. Gotch F. Kinetic modeling in hemodialysis. In: Nissenson AR, Fine RN, Gentile DE, eds. *Clinical Dialysis*, 3d ed. East Norwalk CT: Appleton & Lange, 1995:156.
9. Gotch FA, Panlilio F, Sergeyeva O, et al. Effective diffusion volume flow rates (Qe) for urea, creatinine and inorganic phosphorus (Qeu, Qecr, QeiP) during hemodialysis. *Semin Dial* 2003;16:474.

10. Michaels AS. Operating parameters and performance criteria for hemodialyzers and other membrane-separation devices. *Trans Am Soc Artif Intern Organs* 1967;13:200.

11. Sargent JA, Gotch FA. Principles and biophysics of dialysis Drukker W, Parsons F, Maher J, eds. *Replacement of Renal Function by Dialysis*, 2d ed. Dordrecht/Boston/London: Kluwer, 1983:53.

12. Borah M, Schoenfeld P, Gotch F. Nitrogen balance during intermittent dialysis therapy for uremia. *Kidney Int* 1978; 14:491.

13. Jindal KK, Manuel A, Goldstein MB. Percent reduction in blood urea concentration during hemodialysis (PRU). A simple and accurate method to estimate Kt/V urea. *ASAIO Trans* 1987;33:286.

14. Barth RH. Urea modeling and Kt/V: a critical appraisal. *Kidney Int Suppl* 1993;41:S252.

15. Kovacic V, Roguljich L, Judle I: Comparison of methods for hemodialysis dose calculations. *Dial Transplant* 2003; 32:170.

16. Daugirdas JT. Second generation logarithmic estimates of single pool variable volume Kt/V: and analysis of error. *J Am Soc Nephrol* 4:1205.

17. Depner TA, Daugirdas JT. Equations for normalized protein catabolic rate based on two-point modeling of hemodialysis urea kinetics. *J Am Soc Nephrol* 1996;7:780.

18. Schindhelm K, Farrell P. Patient-hemodialyzer interactions. *ASAIO Trans* 1978;24:357.

19. Sargent JA, Gotch FA. Principles and biophysics of dialysis. In: Jacobs C, Kjellstrand C, Koch K, Winchester J, Eds. *Replacement of Renal Function by Dialysis*, 4th ed. Dordrecht/Boston/London: Kluwer, 1996:114.

20. Jadoul M, Garbar C, Vanholder R, et al. Prevalence of histologic beta$_2$-microglobulin amyloidosis in CAPD patients compared with hemodialysis patients. *Kidney Int* 1998; 54:956.

21. Vincent C, Chanard J, Caudwell V, et al. Lometocs pf 125I-beta$_2$-microglobulin turnover in dialyzed patients. *Kidney Int* 1992;42:1434.

22. Chanard J, Vincent C, Candwell V, et al. Beta$_2$-microglobulin metabolism in uremic patients who are undergoing dialysis. *Kidney Int Suppl* 1993;41:S83.

23. Gorevic PD, Munoz PC, Casey TT, et al. Polymerization of intact beta 2-microglobulin in tissues causes amyloidosis: identification of the glycated sites. *Biochemistry* 1984;33: 12215.

24. Gotch FA, Levin N, Zasuwa G, et al. Kinetics of beta-2-microglobulin in hemodialysis. In: Berlyne GM, Giovanetti S, eds. *Contributions to Nephrology*. Basel: Karger, 1989:132.

25. Floege J, Bartsch A, Schulze M, et al. Clearance and synthesis rates of beta$_2$-microglobulin in patients undergoing hemodialysis and in normal subjects. *J Lab Clin Med* 1991; 118:153.

26. Dedrick R, Gabelnick H, Bischoff B. Kinetics of urea distribution. *N Eng J Med* 1968;10:36.

27. Schneditz D, Van Stone JC, Daugirdas JT. A regional blood circulation alternative to in-series two compartment urea kinetic modeling. *ASAIO J* 1993;39:M573.

28. Heineken FA, Evans MC, Keen ML, et al. Intercompartmental fluid shifts in hemodialysis patients. *Biotechnology Prog* 1988;3:69.

29. Gotch FA, Panlilio FM, Buyaki RA, et al. Mechanisms determining the rate of conductivity clearance to urea clearance. *Kidney Int Suppl* 2004;89:S3.

30. Smye S, Evans J, Will E, et al. Pediatric haemodialysis: estimation of treatment efficiency in the presence of urea rebound. *Clin Phys Physiol Meas* 1992;13:51.

31. Daugirdas JT, Schneditz D. Overestimation of hemodialsis dose depends on dialysis efficiency by regional blood flow but not by conventional two pool urea kinetic analysis. *ASAIO J* 1995;41:M719.

32. Daugirdas JT, Depner TA, Gotch FA, et al. Comparison of methods to predict equilibrated Kt/V in the HEMO Pilot Study. *Kidney Int* 1997;52:1395.

33. Tattersall JE, De Takats D, Chamney P, et al. The post-hemodialysis rebound: predicting and quantifying its effect on Kt/V. *Kidney Int* 1996;50:2094.

34. Daugirdas JT, Greene T, Depner TA, et al. Factors that affect post-dialysis rebound in serum urea concentration, including the rate of dialysis: results from the HEMO study. *J Am Soc Nephrol* 2004;15:194.

35. Lowrie E, Laird N, Parker T, et al. Effect of the hemodialysis prescription on patient morbidity. *N Eng J Med* 1981; 305:1176.

36. Keshaviah P. Urea kinetic and middle molecule approaches to assessing the adequacy of hemodialysis and CAPD. *Kidney Int* 1993;43(suppl):S28.

37. Parker T, Husni L, Huang W, et al. Survival of hemodialysis patients in the United States is improved with a greater quantity of dialysis. *Am J Kidney Dis* 1994;23:670.

38. Hakim R, Breyer J, Ismail N, et al. Effects of dose of dialysis on morbidity and mortality. *Am J Kidney Dis* 1994;23: 661.

39. Charra B, Calemard E, Chazot, et al. Survival as an index of adequacy of dialysis. *Kidney Int* 1992;41:1286.

40. NKF-K/DOQI Clinical Practice Guidelines for Hemodialysis Adequacy: update 2000. *Am J Kidney Dis* 2001;1(suppl 1):S7.

41. Eknoyan G, Beck G, Cheung A, et al. Effects of dialysis dose and membrane flux in hemodialysis patients. *N Engl J Med* 2002;347:2010.

42. Prevot A, Dumas J. Examen du sang et de son action dans les divers phenomenes de la vie. *Ann Chimie Physique* 1821;23:90.

43. Quinan J. The uremic theory. *Maryland Med J* 1880;7:193.

44. Christison R. Observations on the variety of dropsy which depends on diseased kidneys. *Edinburgh Med Surg J* 1829;32:261.

45. Richet G. Early history of uremia. *Kidney Int* 1988;33:1013.

46. Bright R. Cases and observations illustrative of renal disease accompanied by the secretion of albuminous urine. *Guy Hosp Rep* 1836;1:338.

47. Lansois L. Uber die erregung typischer Krampfanfalle nach Behandlung des centralen Nervensystems mit chemischen Substantzen unter besonder Beruchsichtigung der Uramie. *Wien Med Presse* 1887;28:233.

48. Herringham W. An account of some experiments upon the toxicity of normal urine. *J Pathol Bacteriol* 1900;6:158.

49. Von Jaksh R: Uber die aldalescenz des blutes bei krankheiten. *Z Klin Med* 1887;13:350.

50. Fishberg A. *Hypertension and Nephritis*, 2d ed. Philadelphia: Lea & Febiger, 1931:619.

51. Vanholder R, De Smet R, Bogeleere P, et al. The uremic syndrome. In: Jacobs C, Kjellstrand C, Koch K, Winchester J, eds. *Replacement of Renal Function by Dialysis*, 4th ed. Dordrecht: Kluwer, 1996:1.

52. Lowrie E, Lew N. Death risk in hemodialysis patients: the predictive value of commonly measured variables and an evaluation of death rate differences between facilities. *Am J Kidney Dis* 1990;15:458.

53. Eggers P. Mortality rates among dialysis patients in Medicare's end-stage renal disease program. *Am J Kidney Dis* 1990;15:414.

54. Held PJ, Brunner F, Odaka M, et al. Five-year survival for end-stage renal disease patients in the United States, Europe, and Japan. *Am J Kidney Dis* 1990;15:451.

55. Gotch F, Yarian S, Keen M. A kinetic survey of U.S. dialysis prescriptions. *Am J Kidney Dis* 1990;15:511.

56. Held P, Caitlin E, Carroll B, et al. Hemodialysis therapy in the United States: what is the dose and does it matter? *Am J Kidney Dis* 1994;25:974.

57. ESRD Core Indicators Project. *Annual Report, Health Care Financing Administration.* HCFA, Office of Clinical Standards and Quality, 1997.

58. Shapiro J, Argy W, Rakowski A, et al. The unsuitability of BUN as a criterion for prescription dialysis. *ASAIO Trans* 1983;29:129.

59. Gotch F, Sargent J. Discussion of manuscript 22. *ASAIO Trans* 1983;29:133.

60. Lowrie E, Zhu X, Kew B. Primary associates of mortality among dialysis patients: trends and reassessment of Kt/V and URR as outcome based measures of dialysis dose. *Am J Kidney Dis* 1998;32(suppl4):516.

61. Wolfe R, Ashby V, Agodoa L, et al. Dose of hemodialysis, body size and mortality: results from the USRDS special studies. *J Am Soc Nephrol* 2000;35:1.

62. Port FK, Wolfe RA, Hulbert-Shearon TE, et al. High dialysis dose is associated with lower mortality among women but not among men. *Am J Kidney Dis* 2004;43:1014.

63. Wolfe R, Port F. Separating the effects of hemodialysis dose and nutrition: in search of the optimal dialysis dose. *Semin Dial* 1999;12(suppl 1):S99.

64. Lowrie E, Zhu X, Lew N. Primary associates of mortality among dialysis patients: trends and reassessment of Kt/V and URR as outcome based measures of dialysis dose. *Am J Kidney Dis* 1998;32(suppl 4):516.

65. Leavey SF, Strawderman RL, Young EW, et al. Cross-sectional and longitudinal predictors of serum albumin in hemodialysis patients. *Kidney Int* 2000;58:2119.

66. Lowrie E. The normalized treatment ratio (Kt/V) is not the best dialysis dose parameters. *Blood Purif* 2000;18:286.

67. Gotch F. Kt/V is the best dose parameters. *Blood Purif* 2000;18:276.

68. Wolfe R, Ashby V, Daugirdas J, et al. Body size, dose of hemodialysis and morbidity. *Am J Kidney Dis* 2000;35:80.

69. Depner T, Daugirdas J, Greene T, et al. dialysis dose and the effect of gender and body size on outcome in the HEMO Study. *Kidney Int* 2004;65:1386.

70. Scribner B. Discussion, *ASAIO Trans* 11:29, 1965.

71. Babb A, Farrell P, Uvelli D, et al. Hemodialyzer evaluation by examination of solute molecular spectra. *ASAIO Trans* 1972;18:98.

72. Scribner B, Buri R, Caner J, et al. The treatment of chronic uremia by means of intermittent hemodialysis: a preliminary report. *ASAIO Trans* 1960;6:114.

73. Teschan P, Ginn H, Bourne K, et al. A prospective study of reduced dialysis. *ASAIO Trans* 1983;29:108.

74. Keshaviah P, Collins A, Berkseth R, et al. Adequacy, benefit, complications, dose and efficiency of filtration—the Minneapolis experience. *Blood Purif* 1984;2:149.

75. Keshaviah P, Collins A. Rapid high-efficiency bicarbonate hemodialysis. *ASAIO Trans* 1986;32:17.

76. Gotch F, Sargent J, Peters J. Studies on the molecular etiology of uremia. *Kidney Int* 1975;7(suppl 3):276.

77. von Albertini B, Miller J, Gardiner P, et al. High flux hemodiafiltration: under 6 hours/week treatment. *ASAIO Trans* 1984;30:227.

78. Miller J, von Albertini B, Gardner P, et al. Technical aspects of high flux hemodiafiltration for adequate (under 2 hours) treatment. *ASAIO Trans* 1984;30:327.

79. Keen M, Evans M, Gotch F. comparison of morbidity in high flux dialysis (HFD) and conventional dialysis (CD). *Kidney Int* 1987;31:A235.

80. Dyck P, Johnson W, Lamber E, et al. Comparison of symptoms, chemistry and nerve function to assess adequacy of hemodialysis. *Neurology* 1979;29:1361.

81. Cambi V, Garini G, Sovazzi G, et al. Short dialysis. *Proc Eur Dial Transplant Assoc* 1983;20:111.

82. Laurent G, Calemard E, Charra B. Long dialysis: a review of fifteen years experience 1968–1983. *Proc Eur Dial Transplant Assoc* 1983;20:122.

83. Quelhorst E, Schuenemann B, Doth B. A new method for the purification of blood. *Artif Organs* 1978;2:83.

84. Quelhorst E, Schuenemann B, Mietzch G. Long term hemofiltration in "poor risk" patients. *ASAIO Trans* 1987;33: 758.

85. Shaldon S, Beau M, Deschodt G, et al. Mixed hemofiltration (MHF): 18 months experience with ultrashort treatment times. *ASAIO Trans* 1981;27:610.

86. Wizemann V, Kramer W, Knopp G, et al. Ultrashort hemodiafiltration: efficiency and hemodynamic tolerance. *Clin Nephrol* 1983;19:24.

87. Scribner B, Oreopoulos D. The hemodialysis product (HDP): a better index of dialysis adequacy than Kt/V. *Dial Transplant* 2002;31:13.

88. Paniagua R, Amato D, Vonesh E, et al. Effects of increased peritoneal clearances on mortality rates in peritoneal dialysis: ADEMEX, a prospective, randomized, controlled trial. *J Am Soc Nephrol* 2002;13:1307.

89. Gotch F, Uehlinger D. Mortality rate in U.S. dialysis patients. *Dial Transplant* 1991;20:255.

90. Uehlinger D, Keen M, Gotch F. Patient surivival with short-time high flux dialysis therapy. *J Am Soc Nephrol* 1993;4:392.

91. Gotch FA, Sargent JA, Keen ML. Whither goest Kt/V? *Kidney Int* 2002;58(suppl 76):S3.

92. Pierratos A, Ouwendyk M, Farncoeur R, et al. Nocturnal hemodialysis: three years experience. *J Am Soc Nephrol* 1998;9:859.

93. Gotch F, Panlilio F, Sergeyeva O, et al. A kinetic model of inorganic phosphorus mass balance in hemodialysis therapy. *Blood Purif* 2003;21:51.

94. Depner T. Benefits of more frequent dialysis: lower TAC at the same Kt/V. *Nephrol Dial Transplant* 2001;12:2158.

95. Casino F, Lopez. The equivalent renal urea clearance: a new parameter to assess dialysis dose. *Nephrol Dial Transplant* 1996;11:1574.

96. Clark WR, Henderson LW: Renal versus continuous versus intermittent therapies for the removal of uremic toxins. *Kidney Int* 2001;59(suppl 78):S298.

97. Bargman J, Thorpe K, Churchill D, et al. Relative contribution of residual renal function and peritoneal clearance to adequacy of dialysis: a reanalysis of the CANUSA study. *J Am Soc Nephrol* 2001;12:2158.

98. Gotch F. Modeling the dose of home hemodialysis. *Home Hemodial Int* 1999;3:37.

99. Gotch F. Definitions of dialysis dose suitable for comparison of daily hemodialysis and continuous ambulatory peritoneal dialysis to conventional thrice weekly dialysis therapy. *Hemodial Int* 2004;8:172.

100. Bonomini V, Feletti C, Scolari MP, et al. Benefits of early initiation of dialysis. *Kidney Int* 1985;28:S57.

101. Mehrolra R, Saran R, Moore H, et al. Towards targets for initiation of chronic dialysis. *Perit Dial Int* 1997;17:497.

102. NKF-KDOQI Clinical Practice Guidelines for Peritoneal Dialysis Adequacy: update 2000. *Am J Kidney Dis* 2001;1:S65.

103. Kooistra M, Vos J, Koomans A, et al. Daily home haemodialysis in the Netherlands: effects on metabolic control, haemodynamics and quality of life. *Nephrol Dial Transplant* 1998;13:2853.

104. Held P, Port F, Wolfe R, et al. The dose of hemodialysis and patient mortality. *Kidney Int* 1996;50:550.

105. Eschbach J, Egrie J, Downing M, et al. Correction of the anemia of end-stage renal disease with recombinant human erythropoietin: results of a combined phase I and phase II clinical trial. *N Engl J Med* 1987;316:28.

106. Desforges J, Dawson J. The anemia of renal failure. *Arch Intern Med* 1958;101:326.

107. Ragen P, Hagedorn A, Owne C. Radioisotope study of anemia in chronic renal disease. *Arch Intern Med* 1960;105:518.

108. Jandl J, Greenberg M, Honemoto R, et al. Clinical determination of the sites of red cell sequestration in hemolytic anemia. *J Clin Invest* 1956;35:842.

109. Uehlinger D, Gotch F, Sheiner L. A pharmacodynamic model of erythropoietin therapy for uremic anemia. *Clin Trial Ther* 1992;51:56.

110. Cotes P, Pippard M, Reid C, et al. Characterization of the anaemia of chronic renal failure and the mode of its correction by a preparation of human erythropoietin (r-HuEPO): an investigation of the pharmacokinetics of intravenous erythropoietin and its effects on erythrokinetics. *Q J Med* 1989;70:113.

Optimizing Dialysis in Pediatric Patients

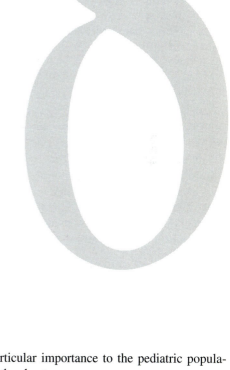

Bradley A. Warady

Optimizing dialysis in the pediatric patient is likely an unrealistic goal. As discussed by Twardowski, *optimal dialysis,* in the truest sense of the term, is the amount of dialysis that yields clinical results that cannot be improved—a target that most clinicians would agree is beyond our scope because of time and cost.[1] On the other hand, *adequate dialysis* is thought of as the quantity of dialysis associated with clinical and biochemical well-being and continues to be the focus of both enthusiastic investigation and controversy.[2–10]

The major portion of this chapter reviews the current information available on the "optimal" approach to the prescription and quantification of peritoneal dialysis (PD) in children, the predominant mode of dialysis therapy from the pediatric period through early adolescence.[11,12] Data on the kinetics of PD, the basis for the peritoneal equilibration test (PET), and the role of this information in dialysis prescription are presented. Finally, a discussion pertaining to the prescription of hemodialysis (HD), with specific emphasis

on issues of particular importance to the pediatric population, concludes the chapter.

It would be negligent not to acknowledge the fact that the provision of the most effective dialysis is dependent on many technical factors (e.g., vascular or peritoneal access) and personal factors (e.g., patient compliance) in addition to the topics raised here. These issues and others pertaining to pediatric PD (Chap. 19) and pediatric HD (Chap. 12) are included in other portions of this text, which should be consulted for a global understanding of the characteristics inherent to the goal of optimal dialysis.

BACKGROUND

PD continues to be the primary dialytic modality for children with end-stage renal disease (ESRD) worldwide.[11,13,14] For example, the North American Pediatric Renal Transplant Cooperative Study (NAPRTCS) found that during the 10-year period from January 1, 1992, to January 1, 2002, 65 percent of more than 4000 index dialysis patients underwent PD.[14] Of patients receiving PD, 69 percent chose automated PD (APD), while the remainder received continuous ambulatory PD (CAPD). Initially, the popularity of PD over HD for children was a result of the properties inherent to CAPD, namely (1) continuous biochemical and fluid control in association with a minimum of four exchanges, (2) patient mobility and freedom from a machine, (3) greatly reduced dietary restrictions, (4) simplicity of operation, and (5) elimination of the need for routine blood access. However, and as noted above, the advent of the automated cycling machine, its positive impact on lifestyle, and its applicability with infants, children, and adolescents has been followed by the establishment of various modifications of APD, including continuous cycling PD (CCPD), nightly intermittent PD (NIPD), and tidal PD (TPD) as common modality selections.[4,7,14]

In recent years, great efforts have been made to optimize PD in the adult patient. Years ago, the experience of the National Cooperative Dialysis Study (NCDS) suggested that the use of urea kinetics as a measure of low-molecular-weight solute clearance may be the best tool for monitoring the efficacy of HD and that clinical outcome failure was least likely to occur in association with an adequate protein intake and intensive dialysis.[15] Extrapolation of this philosophy led to multiple attempts to use urea kinetics and associated clinical manifestations to define adequate—if not optimal—approaches to PD, an issue that continues to evolve to the present day.[8,9,16-20] Residual renal function and ultrafiltration capacity are additional crucial considerations.[18,21] Irrespective of the criteria used to define adequacy, the goal is to prescribe a dialysis regimen that meets the needs of the individual patient, as opposed to a generic prescription that may have to be modified repeatedly, in a reactive manner, as a response to a poor clinical outcome.

In children, practitioners could be said to have the advantage of possessing the growing child as a patient and a "natural laboratory," whose development may ideally reflect either the adequacy of dialysis or the need to modify the dialysis prescription. An indirect estimate of the adequacy might well be achieved by assessing the dialysis and nutritional prescription of a large group of infants or children who receive PD and are growing well, demonstrate normal cognitive development, and have had a minimal number of hospitalizations. Unfortunately, limited data of this type exist at present, although earnest efforts toward this end are being made.[13,22-25] The feasibility of determining clear correlates between solute clearance on dialysis and patient outcome in children is also compromised because of the rapid progression to transplant in most cases.[13,26] Nevertheless, information on the kinetics of PD in children is available, which facilitates a thorough understanding of PD and is necessary if determining the most efficacious approach to

PD prescription (see below) for the individual pediatric patient is the desired goal.

PERITONEAL MEMBRANE FUNCTION IN CHILDREN

A number of years ago, Gruskin et al. provided evidence that apparent variations in peritoneal solute transport characteristics between individuals or populations are often the result of kinetic studies in which the following factors are not incorporated[27]:

1. Constant inflow, dwell, and outflow times for all study exchanges
2. Identical dialysate composition in all study subjects
3. Exchange volume scaled per unit body size in an identical manner
4. Results adjusted according to the body size scaling factor used to determine the exchange volume

Despite the recognition of the Gruskin "principles," attempts to accurately define the solute transport characteristics of the pediatric peritoneal membrane have historically been hampered by the long-standing lack of agreement on what should be considered the appropriate scaling factor, body surface area (BSA), or body weight, for standardizing the test procedure and for proper analysis of test results.

SCALING FACTOR FOR KINETIC STUDIES

Recommendations for the use of BSA as the most appropriate scaling factor were initially derived from evaluations performed more than 100 years ago. Putiloff conducted direct measurements of the peritoneal membrane in a 2.9-kg infant and found the infant's peritoneal surface area (0.15 m^2) to be almost twice that of a 70-kg adult when scaled for body weight (522 cm^2/kg vs. 284 cm^2/kg).[28] The studies were repeated on six adults and six children by Esperanca and Collins in 1966, with similar results.[29] The mean surface area in the infants was 383 cm^2/kg and in the adults, 177 cm^2/kg. In contrast, the ratio between BSA and peritoneal membrane area appears to be age-independent.[30] Accordingly, because the rapidity of solute equilibration between plasma and dialysate is in part dependent on the volume of dialysate into which the dialyzed solute must diffuse—the so-called principle of geometry of diffusion—the use of a weight-based peritoneal exchange volume for studies of solute kinetics, such as the PET (see below), can be expected to result in the provision of a relatively low exchange volume to the youngest patients and the apparent but inaccurate perception of a relatively rapid solute transport capacity in these same children.[31] In contrast, because of the constant relationship between the peritoneal surface area and BSA, scaling of the dialysate volume by BSA will maintain the ratio of dialysate volume to peritoneal surface area constant across populations with any detectable differences in solute mass transfer a result of variations in peritoneal permeability. The importance of scaling the fill volume to BSA has been verified by Kohaut et al., Schaefer et al., deBoer et al., and Warady et al. in association with the Pediatric Peritoneal Dialysis Study Consortium (PPDSC).[32–35]

It is noteworthy that few actual measures of the peritoneum have been published. Although it was originally estimated to equal BSA,[30] it is clear that the size of the membrane that actually participates in an exchange is significantly smaller than that.[36,37] In addition, the total membrane size is likely less relevant than the total membrane pore area or, more precisely, the membrane pore area of that part of the peritoneum which is engaged in exchanges. Of interest, the three-pore model, described below, has been applied to PD studies in infants and children and has verified a linear correlation between peritoneal capillary pore area and BSA.[38]

Finally, the determination of BSA is commonly derived using the method of Dubois and DuBois,[39] and most of the currently available data (PET; see below) are based on this method. However, in an independent comparison, the Gehan and George method[40] was preferred, as more than 400 subjects, including many children, were used to define this formula; in contrast, only 9 subjects were used to define the formula of DuBois and DuBois. The respective formulas are as follows.

DuBois and DuBois method:

$$BSA\ (m^2) = 71.84 \times Wt^{0.425} \times Ht^{0.725}/10{,}000$$

Gehan and George method:

$$BSA\ (m^2) = 0.0235 \times Wt^{0.51456} \times Ht^{0.42246}$$

PERITONEUM AS A DIALYZING MEMBRANE

The peritoneal exchange process is the sum of two simultaneous and interrelated transport mechanisms: diffusion and convection. *Diffusion* refers to the movement of solute down a concentration gradient, whereas *convection* refers to movement of solutes that are "transported" in a fluid flux, the magnitude of which is determined by the ultrafiltration rate.[41]

Several theories have been developed to model the movement of water and solute across the peritoneal membrane, each progressively more complex but each, in turn, more accurate. The development of CAPD in the mid-1970s was accompanied by the development of a distributed pore model. Recently, a more comprehensive model, known as the three-pore model, has been developed. As one would expect from the name, the model postulates three types of pores:

1. Ultrasmall transcellular water pores or channels, which make up perhaps 1 to 2 percent of the total pore area yet account for 40 percent of water flow and are driven by osmotic forces.
2. Small pores 4 to 6 nm in diameter, making up 90 percent of total pore area. These pores are subject to both concentration gradients (diffusive forces) and osmotic gradients (convective forces).
3. Large pores greater than 40 nm in diameter, making up the remaining 5 to 7 percent of total pore area. These pores allow larger molecules, such as albumin, to leave capillaries, probably driven by hydrostatic forces within the capillary bed.

Although water moves through all three pores, only the small and large pores allow convective solute transfer.[38,42,43]

MASS TRANSFER AREA COEFFICIENT

The mass transfer area coefficient (MTAC) characterizes the diffusive permeability of the peritoneal membrane and is for the most part independent of dialysis mechanics.[41,44] The MTAC has been variably defined as the area available for solute transport divided by the sum of resistances to peritoneal diffusion and represents the clearance rate (expressed in milliliters per minute) that would be obtained in the absence of ultrafiltration or solute accumulation in the dialysate.[45] The MTAC, as applied to the current three-pore model of transperitoneal solute and water flux, is equal to the product of the free-diffusion coefficient for the solute, the fractional area available for diffusion (which is a percent of the area of the unrestricted pores), and A_0/Δ_X, which characterizes the diffusion distance across the peritoneum.[46] While there are no simple methods for determining the MTAC and precise estimates require rigorously performed PD exchanges and computer solutions of complex equations, some formulas allow for reasonable estimates of the MTAC. In turn, the use of MTAC data in kinetic modeling of pediatric PD may allow for accurate predictions of fluid removal as well as urea and creatinine clearance for various treatment regimens, thereby assisting in the prescription process.[38,47,48]

To date, very few studies have measured MTACs in pediatric patients. Popovich et al. and later Morgenstern and Baluarte studied a total of only 12 patients and found little difference between children and adults for the MTAC of glucose, creatinine, and urea nitrogen.[49,50] However, test mechanics were not standardized and the reliability of the adult reference data used as a comparison is suspect when viewed in the context of more recent information.[51] Morgenstern and Baluarte did find the MTAC for protein to be significantly greater in children than in adults, corresponding to the greater losses of protein often noted in the pediatric population in clinical practice.[52,53]

Geary et al. determined the MTACs for creatinine and glucose in 28 pediatric patients and provided evidence to suggest that solute transport in children is directly related to age and that more rapid transport per unit of body weight is observed in children than in adult patients.[54] However, the validity of these data has been questioned by some. While determination of the MTAC is usually immune to alterations in dialysis mechanics, Brandes et al. have shown that the use of exceptionally low exchange volumes will decrease the accuracy of the MTAC determination.[55] In turn, the test exchange volume used in Geary's study (32 ± 5 mL/kg) was decidedly low and not standardized in the patients evaluated.

Warady et al. determined the MTACs for urea, creatinine, glucose, and potassium in 95 patients, ranging in age from less than 1 to 20 years, who were evaluated in a standardized manner with a test exchange volume scaled to BSA (i.e., 1100mL/m²).[56] When the MTAC was scaled for BSA and using analysis of variance, there were differences by age only for the MTAC of glucose and potassium (the younger children having a higher value), with the mean MTAC values for creatinine, urea and glucose scaled to 1.73m² BSA being 10.6 ± 4.8, 15.5 ± 5.0, and 13.3 ± 6.4 mL/min, respectively. However, when analyzed using quadratic regression analysis, there was greater transport capacity in the youngest patients (those below 3 years of age) for glucose, potassium, and creatinine. The determination of MTACs in the study of Warady et al. was based on the two-pool model of Pyle-Popovich and was calculated in the following manner[57-59]:

$$\frac{-V_D}{t} \times In\left[\frac{1 - \dfrac{D_E}{P}}{1 - \dfrac{V_0 D_0}{V_D P}}\right]$$

where t = time

D_0 = dialysate concentration at time 0

D_E = dialysate concentration at time 240

P = average plasma concentration

V_0 = volume infused + residual volume

V_D = volume drained + residual volume

The enhanced transport demonstrated in the young patients is likely the result of differences in either permeability, effective surface area, or possibly maturational changes of the peritoneum.[38]

A comparison of the pediatric MTAC data to the adult data of Waniewski et al. reveals a trend of only slightly decreased transport characteristics from the pediatric to adult age groups (Table 8–1).[51] MTAC data have also been determined in children undergoing PD studies, based on the three-pore model; the values for children were found to be similar to those of adults when the former data were scaled to BSA.[60] The fact that the BSA-scaled pediatric MTAC

TABLE 8–1. MASS TRANSFER AREA COEFFICIENT (MTAC) IN CHILDREN AND COMPARED WITH ADULTS[51]

Solute	MTAC		
	mL/min/1.73m²	mL/min/70 kg	Adult Ref.
Creatinine	10.6 ± 4.8[a]	16.1 ± 8.6	8.6 ± 3.2
Urea	15.5 ± 5.0	23.3 ± 9.0	16.7 ± 2.3
Glucose	13.3 ± 6.4	19.9 ± 10.3	10.8 ± 2.0

[a]Data presented as mean + SD.

data are clearly more like the adult data than the body weight-scaled values provides additional indirect support for the use of BSA as the most appropriate scaling factor for pediatric kinetic studies.

ULTRAFILTRATION AND CONVECTION

The amount of body water that must be ultrafiltered depends on the child's daily fluid intake and residual urine output. This aspect of dialysis care is important because the establishment and achievement of the patient's dry weight are major factors influencing blood pressure control.[21] Failure to manage these aspects effectively can have profound ramifications.[61,62] In designing the dialysis prescription in terms of ultrafiltration, children receiving CAPD with 1.5 or 4.25% dextrose should expect the drainage volume to exceed the infused volume of dialysate by 15 to 25 percent and 30 to 40 percent, respectively.[63] On the other hand, children receiving APD with shorter dwell times (e.g., 30 minutes) with 1.5 and 4.25% dextrose dialysis solutions should expect drain volumes that exceed infused volumes by >4 to 8 percent and 12 to 18 percent, respectively.[63] The personal dialysis capacity (PDC) test, a means of modeling PD efficacy based on the three-pore model of peritoneal mass transport, can assist in this process, since it has been shown to model water transport in children accurately.[33,38]

Convective mass transfer, which is dependent on fluid removal, contributes little to the movement of small solutes, yet it is responsible for most large solute removal. Studies by Pyle have demonstrated that the contribution of convection to urea transport in a 4-hour CAPD exchange with 4.25% glucose is 12 percent; it is 45 percent for inulin and 86 percent for total protein.[58]

Early studies and much clinical experience suggest that adequate ultrafiltration can be difficult to achieve in infants and young children. Investigations conducted by Kohaut and Alexander, using a weight-scaled test exchange volume, revealed a more rapid decline in dialysate dextrose concentration and osmolality in the youngest patients, suggestive of enhanced peritoneal transport capacity in the pediatric population.[64] Presumably this was the reason behind the suboptimal ultrafiltration. However, subsequent studies failed to confirm these findings and provided evidence that the apparent age-related differences in ultrafiltration capacity tended to disappear when the exchange volume was scaled to BSA rather than body weight, as discussed above. On the other hand, and as mentioned previously, data generated by Warady et al. revealed slightly higher MTACs for glucose in children <1 year of age in a study suggesting that maturational processes of peritoneal transport may still be present in the first year of life.[56] Schaefer et al., on the other hand, have suggested that the reduced ultrafiltration rate sometimes observed in infancy may actually be related to a greater total fluid "reuptake" or reabsorption rate from the peritoneal cavity.[38] It appears that this reuptake may be secondary to either a higher lymphatic reabsorption rate (see below) or a greater intraperitoneal pressure in the infants, which generates a reversed transcapillary flux of fluid along hydrostatic and oncotic pressure gradients.[38,65]

PERITONEAL FLUID AND LYMPHATIC ABSORPTION

During PD, fluid is continuously lost from the peritoneal cavity, both directly into the tissues surrounding the peritoneal cavity and via lymphatic vessels. Fluid absorption out of the peritoneal cavity remains poorly understood.[66] Initially, flow through lymphatic vessels was felt to be the dominant pathway.[67] More recently, fluid absorption is felt to move primarily directly into the tissues surrounding the peritoneal cavity.[68] Lymphatic absorption is thought to account for only 20 percent of fluid reabsorption.[69] The limited data on lymphatic absorption in children are conflicting.[70,71]

Fluid absorption rates can be determined when a PD exchange is modeled using the three-pore model. It is felt to be driven by intraperitoneal hydraulic pressure[68] and may be explained by the movement of dialysate into interstices within the peritoneal cavity. This allows for water absorption at the same time that ultrafiltration is occurring in the portion of the peritoneum where the bulk of the fluid remains.[66] Data on fluid absorption using the three-pore model in children are limited. In one study, the absorption rate increased with body size in absolute terms but decreased when normalized to body size. The decrease was slight when scaled to BSA but marked when scaled to body weight.[38]

PRINCIPLES OF THE PERITONEAL EQUILIBRATION TEST

The peritoneal equilibration test (PET) was originally popularized by Twardowski et al. as a means of characterizing peritoneal membrane transport characteristics in comparison with population norms in adults.[72] The information obtained was then used to assist the clinician in defining an initial individualized PD prescription or in evaluating the reasons behind inadequate dialysis. The solute transport reference curves developed by Twardowski et al. arose from 103 equilibration tests performed in 18 diabetic and 68 nondiabetic adult patients. The reference curves are based on the kinetics of solute equilibration between dialysate and plasma (D/P ratio), so that the higher the D/P ratio for solutes, such as urea and creatinine, after a specific dwell period, the higher the transport rate. In contrast, since glucose transport is in the opposite direction when compared with other solutes, the higher the ratio of dialysate glucose at a particular time in relation to dialysate glucose at time 0 (D/D_0), the lower the transport rate. These data have made possible the categorization of adult patients into those with high, high-average, low-average, and low peritoneal membrane solute transport capacity and serve as the basis for dialysis prescription (see below).

The results of Twardowski's studies have not enjoyed widespread application in the pediatric dialysis population for two reasons. First, there has been a well-acknowledged but, as noted previously, unproven perception (except possibly in small infants less than 1 year of age) that the solute transport function of the pediatric peritoneal membrane differs from that of the adult.[38,56] The second "flaw" in the evaluation, especially as it pertains to children, is the fact that a test exchange volume of 2000 mL was used in all study patients regardless of size. Obviously this approach does not allow for modification of the exchange volume to reflect differences in body size (e.g., pediatric patient, small adult, large adult) and has contributed to the limited usefulness of this approach in children.

PEDIATRIC PET PROCEDURE

Application of a standardized PET procedure for children has resulted from an appreciation of the previously mentioned age-independent relationship between BSA and peritoneal membrane surface area and the recommended use of an exchange volume scaled to BSA whenever one conducts studies of peritoneal transport kinetics.[32,34,56,73,74] In the largest pediatric study to date, the PPDSC evaluated 95 children using a test exchange volume of 1100 mL/m^2 BSA to develop reference kinetic data (e.g., D/P and D/D_0 ratios), which can be used to categorize an individual pediatric patient's peritoneal membrane solute transport capacity (Figs. 8–1 and 8–2).[56] Similar reference data have been generated from pediatric studies in Europe with a test exchange volume of 1000 mL/m^2 BSA.[74] The procedure is as follows:

1. Dialysate volume for test is scaled to body surface area, the latter value being determined by the Du Bois and Du Bois BSA formula.[39]
2. During the evening prior to the PET study, the patient receives an exchange of 40 mL/kg (range 35 to 45 mL/kg) of 2.5% dextrose dialysis solution.

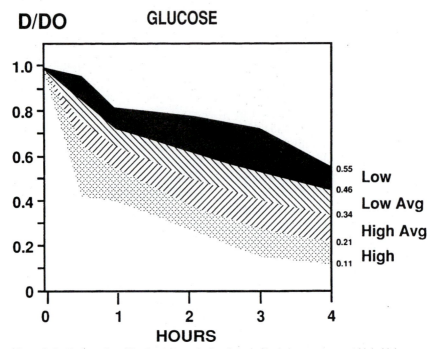

Figure 8–1. Peritoneal equilibration test results for glucose. Shaded areas represent high, high-average, and low transport rates. The white band represents the low-average transport rate. The four categories are bordered by the maximal, mean +1 SD, mean, mean –1 SD, and minimal values for the population. D/D_0, dialysate glucose:initial dialysate glucose concentration ratio. *(Reprinted with permission from Warady BA, Alexander SR, Hossli S, et al. Peritoneal membrane transport function in children receiving long-term dialysis. J Am Soc Nephrol 1996;7:2385–2391.)*

The overnight exchange should dwell for 8 to 12 hours.

3. The overnight dwell is drained over 20 minutes with the patient in the sitting position. The length of the dwell and the volume drained should be recorded.

4. The test exchange infusion is conducted next and consists of a dialysate volume of 1100 mL/m² comprising 2.5% dextrose dialysate (North America, Japan) or 2.3 to 2.4% anhydrous glucose dialysate (Europe) infused over 10 minutes with the patient remaining supine. In early infancy, the volume may not be tolerable. If this occurs, the PET is conducted with the regular daily exchange volume. Note the infusion time.

5. Immediately after completing the infusion, <10 percent of the dialysate is drained into the drip chamber on the drainage line and a 5-mL sample is obtained from the sample port on the administration set at the catheter connection. The effluent volume in the administration set is reinfused from the drip chamber to the point before the sample port back into the peritoneum. The sample is labeled with patient data and time and all dialysate samples are evaluated for glucose and creatinine concentration. The sampling procedure is repeated at 120- and 240-minute dwell times.

6. The test volume is drained with the patient in the upright position 240 minutes after 0 dwell time. The patient should be drained completely with a maximum drain time of 20 minutes. The drain bag is mixed by inverting it three times and a 5-mL sample is obtained.

7. A blood sample is obtained at the midpoint of the PET (120 minutes). The blood is evaluated for glucose and creatinine, with all of the data used to determine the values of dialysate to plasma (*D/P*) creatinine and dialysate glucose to baseline dialysate glucose *(D/D₀)* in the following manner:

$$D/P \text{ ratio} = \frac{\text{dialysate concentration of creatinine}}{\text{plasma concentration of creatinine}}$$

$$D/D_0 \text{ ratio} = \frac{\text{dialysate glucose concentration}}{\text{dialysate glucose concentration at time 0}}$$

An experience with a 2-hour "Fast PET" in children has recently been reported and also appears to provide an accurate assessment of peritoneal membrane transport kinetics in a manner similar to that reported in adults.[75–77]

Proper evaluation of the data obtained during the PET requires that dialysate creatinine values be corrected for glucose interference, since falsely elevated creatinine values may result when creatinine is measured by the Jaffe

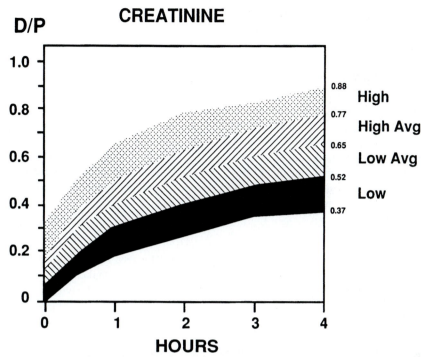

Figure 8–2. Peritoneal equilibration test results for creatinine. Shaded areas represent high, high-average, and low transport rates. The white band represents the low-average transport rate. The four categories are bordered by the maximal, mean +1 SD, mean, mean -1 SD, and minimal values for the population. D/P, dialysate:plasma ratio. *(Reprinted with permission from Warady BA, Alexander SR, Hossli S, et al. Peritoneal membrane transport function in children receiving long–term dialysis. J Am Soc Nephrol 1996;7:2385–2391.)*

method.[72] In addition, the measured plasma solute concentrations must be divided by 0.9 to account for their presence in plasma water only and not in whole plasma. Failure to do so has resulted in solute D/P ratios greater than unity.[51]

Because the transport capacity of the peritoneal membrane is such an important factor to consider in determining the dialysis prescription (see below), the PET evaluation should be conducted soon after the initiation of dialysis.[78,79] However, there is evidence that a PET performed within the first week of PD may yield higher transport results than a PET performed several weeks later.[80] Accordingly, whereas it may be most convenient to perform the initial PET at the conclusion of PD training, the results after 1 month of PD may more accurately reflect peritoneal transport properties.[20,80] While the peritoneal membrane transport capacity is stable early in the course of PD in children and does not mandate routine reevaluation, the PET evaluation should be repeated when knowledge of the patient's current membrane transport capacity is necessary in order to determine the patient's PD prescription, especially when clinical events have occurred (e.g., repeated peritonitis) that may have altered transport characteristics, as previously demonstrated.[81–83] In addition, knowledge of a patient's transport capacity may have a profound impact on his or her overall care because of the important relationships that exist between transport status and patient outcome in children and adults.[24,84–86]

SOLUTE EQUILIBRATION IN CHILDREN

The data accumulated by the PPDSC has allowed for categorization of the solute transport capacity of the individual pediatric patient in a manner identical to that practiced in adults (Figs. 8–1 and 8–2).[56] As popularized by Twardowski et al., values that define the transport categories represent the maximal, mean + 1 SD, mean, mean − 1 SD, and minimum values for the population studied. Low transport is defined as a D/P ratio < mean − 1 SD or D/D_0> mean + 1 SD. Low-average transport is represented by a D/P value between the mean and the mean − 1 SD or a D/D_0 between the mean and the mean + 1 SD. High-average transport is defined by a D/P between the mean and the mean + 1 SD or a D/D_0 between the mean and the mean − 1 SD. Finally, high transport is defined by a D/P > mean + 1 SD or a D/D_0 < mean − 1 SD. It is particularly noteworthy that a comparison of the pediatric equilibration data for creatinine with the data obtained from adults by Twardowski et al. and corrected for the presence of solute in plasma water reveals no significant differences and supports the prior suggestion of

Gruskin et al. that, in large part, the previously perceived differences in solute transport between individuals of different ages can be attributed to the lack of standardized test mechanics.[27,56] However, and as mentioned previously, the evaluation of glucose transport in terms of D/D_0 ratios (as well as the MTAC data shown previously) does reveal findings consistent with more rapid transport in children ≤3 years of age when compared with older children and adults.[56] These findings, at least in part, support prior data from Kohaut and Alexander describing more rapid glucose absorption and poor ultrafiltration in infants vs. older children, which were presumed to be solely artifactual in nature and the result of the relatively small exchange volume used during their studies.[64]

PRESCRIBING PERITONEAL DIALYSIS

In general, the PD prescription for children has evolved empirically from guidelines that adapted adult CAPD for pediatric patients. A CAPD regimen of four to five exchanges per day with an exchange volume of 900 to 1100 mL/m^2 BSA (35 to 45 mL/kg) of 2.5% dextrose dialysis solution has routinely yielded net ultrafiltration volumes of up to 1100 mL/m^2 per day. Using similar exchange volumes, the greatest percentage of children receiving PD receive cycler dialysis with a regimen consisting of 6 to 10 exchanges over 8 to 10 hours per night.

The current goal of achieving dialysis adequacy in the most cost-effective manner has highlighted the need to be cognizant of a patient's BSA, peritoneal membrane solute transport capacity, and residual renal function in designing the dialysis prescription.[56,79,87,88] In most patients (except for rapid transporters), the most effective way to increase solute clearance is to initially increase the exchange volume, followed by an increase in dialysis duration by prolonging the dwell time. In the case of the rapid transporter, an increase in the number of exchanges and a reduction of the dwell time per cycle can result in improved solute clearance. Ideally, the prescription for all children should include an exchange volume of 1100 to 1400 mL/m^2 BSA, as tolerated by the patient. Measurement of the intraperitoneal pressure generated by escalating exchange volumes can be useful in determining the optimal dialysis prescription.[89–93] Calculation of the mean IPP, for which pediatric standards exist (Table 8–2), occurs as follows:

- Patient is at rest, lying in a supine position.
- Connection with the peritoneal system is made (as usual), and the patient's peritoneal cavity is filled with dialysis fluid.
- The PD line is fixed vertically on a bracket, and there is no counterpressure in the distal part of the measurement tubing.
- The level of the column of dialysis fluid in the PD line is read with a scale graduated in centimeters after the height of the column stabilizes, first after deep inspiration (IPP insp) and second after expiration (IPP exp). Mean IPP is calculated as follows:

$$\frac{\text{IPP insp} + \text{IPP exp}}{2}$$

- The zero level of the column is set at the center of the abdominal cavity, on the midaxillary line.
- The peritoneal cavity is emptied after taking the IPP reading, and the volume of the drained dialysis fluid is measured and correlated to the measured mean IPP.
- The IPP is measured at atmospheric pressure without any counterpressure in the distal part of the measurement tubing. The technique used depends on the geometry of the PD system. In disconnect systems, there is no counterpressure in the line or in the empty drainage bag after the line has been connected. In nondisconnect systems, there is almost always a moderate counterpressure, so an air inlet is needed. This is accomplished before the readings are made by introducing a trocar at the injection site of the bag.

As mentioned previously, categorization of a patient's peritoneal membrane transport capacity can best be determined by the performance of a PET and comparison of the individual patient data to reference values.[56] This information makes it possible to optimize the dialysis prescription in terms of dwell time. However, recognizing that it is often impractical to consider the provision of a dialysis prescription based solely on kinetic data without reference to social constraints (e.g., school attendance, working parent), the use of the results of a PET evaluation can also be particularly helpful in determining the most cost- and time-effective approach to PD modality selection (e.g., high transporter-cycling PD, high-average to low-average transporter-CAPD or cycling PD +/– additional daytime exchange) by using one of several computer modeling programs that have been validated in pediatric patients and that can provide accurate estimates of solute clearance.[38,48,94] It must be emphasized that in pediatric patients as well as in adults, predicted values are only estimates and do not substitute for actual measurements of solute clearance (see below). It is, in turn, recommended that measurement of

TABLE 8–2. NORMAL IPP LEVELS FOR CHILDREN GREATER THAN 2 YEARS OF AGE[89]

	IPV mL/m^2	
	990 ± 160	1400 ± 50
IPP cm of water	8.2 ± 3.8	14.1 ± 3.6

solute clearance routinely take place every 4 months in children receiving PD.

The residual renal function, a characteristic that appears to be better preserved by PD vs. HD, is calculated as the average of urea and creatinine clearance and assumes greatest importance in the patient who does not attain target clearances with dialysis alone.[18,20,95–97] There is also evidence to suggest that native renal and dialysis solute clearance are not equivalent, with the former being qualitatively better than the latter.[23] Unfortunately, whereas the contribution of residual renal function toward a target goal may be significant early in the course of dialysis, a progressive loss of residual renal function usually occurs and mandates an associated modification of the dialysis prescription, with enhancement of the dialysis-related solute removal if target clearances are to be maintained.[95,98,99]

ADEQUACY OF PERITONEAL DIALYSIS

Until recently, most studies with adult PD patients in which clinical outcome parameters (e.g., frequency of hospitalization, patient mortality) have been monitored have characterized dialysis adequacy in terms of small solute clearance as a total (residual renal + PD) weekly Kt/V_{urea} greater than or equal to 2.0 and a total weekly creatinine clearance greater than or equal to 60 L/1.73 m^2 for the patient receiving CAPD.[20] Minor differences in the recommendations exist for the cycler dialysis patient. The calculation of the total weekly creatinine clearance is performed in the following manner:

$$CCR\left[L/1.73m^2/week\right] = \left\{\frac{D_{cr} \cdot V_D}{Pcr} + \left[\left(\frac{U_{cr} \cdot V_u}{Pcr} + \frac{U_{ur} \cdot V_u}{Pur}\right) \middle/ 2\right]\right\}$$
$$\cdot \frac{1.73}{BSA} \cdot 7$$

where Dcr, Pcr, and Ucr are the dialysate, plasma, and urinary concentrations of creatinine; U_{ur} and P_{ur} the urinary and plasma concentrations of urea; V_D and V_U the 24-hour dialysate and urine volumes; and BSA the body surface area.

The total weekly Kt/V_{urea} is calculated as follows:

$$\text{Weekly } Kt/V_{urea} = \frac{(D_{ur} \cdot V_D)(U_{ur} \cdot V_u)}{Pur \cdot V} \cdot 7$$

where D_{ur}, U_{ur}, and P_{ur} are the dialysate, urinary, and plasma concentrations of urea; V_D and V_U the 24-hour dialysate and urine volumes; and V the urea distribution volume. In the calculation of Kt/V, it is most important to use an accurate estimate of V, which is considered to be equivalent to the total body water volume (see below).

Despite our increasing ability to measure solute removal accurately, there are few data to support the preference of one solute clearance measure (Kt/V$_{urea}$ vs. creatinine clearance) over another, and discrepancies in the results may occur in as many as 20 percent of patients. This has prompted the recommendation that the evaluation of adequacy be based on the results of both clearance measures and, most importantly, an ongoing assessment of the patient's clinical condition.[100,101] If there is discordance in achieving these targets, it has been suggested that the Kt/V$_{urea}$ be the immediate determinant of adequacy because it directly reflects protein metabolism and is less affected by extreme variations in residual renal function.[20,101]

Implicit in the approach to achieve and maintain dialysis adequacy is the need to repeatedly measure total solute clearance. Ideally, and as mentioned previously, 24-hour collections of urine and dialysate fluid should be obtained three times per year or when there have been significant changes in the patient's clinical status that may influence dialysis performance (e.g., severe or repeated peritonitis).

Over the past several years, two publications have provided data that challenge current PD adequacy recommendations and require consideration. An analysis of data generated in the CANUSA study by Churchill et al. has revealed superior patient and technique survival in the adult CAPD population with low/low average transport capacity and lower total creatinine clearance values compared to those patients who are high transporters.[85] This has resulted in a change of the target creatinine clearance recommendation to 50L/1.73m^2/week for the former subset of patients in the guidelines of the National Kidney Foundation-Kidney Disease Outcomes Quality Initiative (NKF-K/DOQI) and the Canadian Society of Nephrology.[20,102] In the second set of data, derived from the ADEMEX (ADEquacy of PD in Mexico) study, adult CAPD patients were prospectively randomized to their routine PD prescription vs. a prescription targeted to a creatinine clearance of 60L/1.73m^2/week. This study found no improvement in patient survival when the peritoneal clearance of small solutes was increased to the adequacy targets recommended by NKF-K/DOQI.[8,20] However, deaths attributable to uremia and inadequate fluid removal were higher in the control population. Not unexpectedly, this experience has prompted a further reassessment of PD adequacy criteria in adults receiving CAPD, with some experts recommending target weekly Kt/V$_{urea}$ values ≥ 1.7. Additional emphasis has also been placed on close monitoring of the patient's fluid status and overall clinical condition.[4]

Current clinical experience supports the use of similar (or greater) target clearances for children and the need to closely monitor all aspects of the patient's clinical condition. Reports by Höltta et al., McCauley et al., and Chadha et al. have all presented data suggestive of a correlation between patient outcome and solute clearance.[22,23,103,104] The experience of Chadha et al. was also significant for demonstrating the influence that residual renal function has on patient outcome and for providing evidence that contradicts the presumed equivalence of PD and native solute clearance.[23] The contribution of residual renal function is most apparent with respect to total creatinine clearance as well as middle molecule clearance.[105]

Can the solute clearance targets be achieved by children on PD without introducing a prescription that has a significant negative impact on their quality of life? Whereas data by Van der Voort et al. suggest otherwise, the clinical experiences of Höltta et al. and Chadha and Warady provide good evidence that if the dialysis exchange volume is maximized and the frequency of the exchanges is individualized

and adjusted according to the peritoneal membrane transport characteristics, it should be possible to achieve the current NFK-K/DOQI clearance targets, at least for Kt/V_{urea}, in most children receiving CPD.[22,25,106] Algorithms designed to assist clinicians in this process have recently been published (Figs. 8–3 to 8–7).[89,107]

As mentioned above, the ability to accurately estimate a patient's total body water [TBW or (V)] is integral to the determination of Kt/V_{urea} as an adequacy measure. The NKF-K/DOQI guidelines have recommended the use of the gender-specific formulas of Mellits-Cheek for TBW assess-

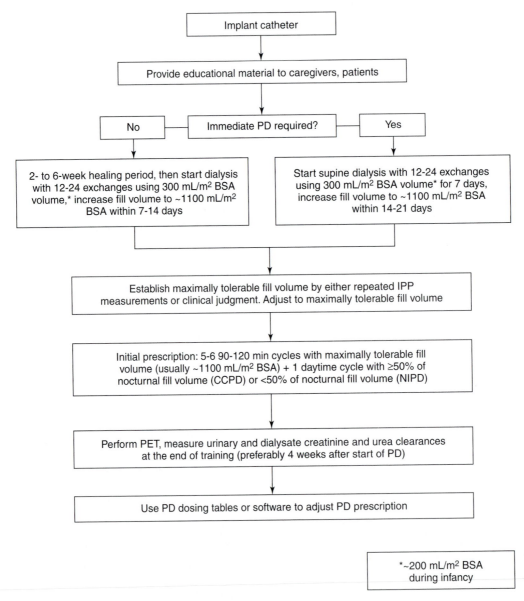

Figure 8–3. Algorithm for initiation of APD.

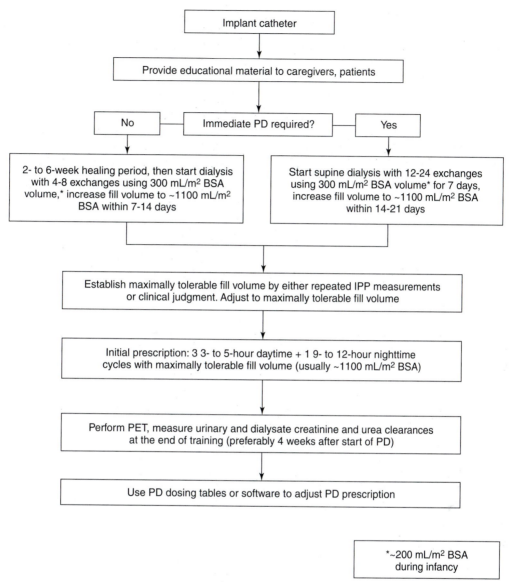

Figure 8–4. Algorithm for initiation of CAPD.

ment despite the fact that the formulas were derived from studies of healthy children.[108] Recently, more accurate estimates of V have at last become feasible, following the analysis of additional body-water data in the literature and after study of pediatric dialysis patients by bioelectrical impedance analysis as well with the use of D_2O or H_2O[18,109–112] The most recent report is that of Morgenstern et al., who studied 47 children between the ages of 4 months and 19 years receiving chronic PD with either D_2O or H_2O[18,112] The equation derived from these studies for estimation of TBW is as follows:

$$TBW = 0.098(Ht \times Wt)^{0.63}$$

The TBW estimates using this formula correlate linearly with BSA estimates, leading to the following formula (using the Gehan and George formula for BSA):

$$TBW = 20.36 \times BSA - 3.68$$

Gender did not affect TBW in these children, in contrast to studies in healthy children. It is also noteworthy that the measured TBW data were significantly different than the estimated results generated by using the Mellits-Cheek equations.[111]

In summary, current knowledge supports the clinical use of a target total weekly Kt/V$_{urea}$ of greater than or equal to 2.0 and a total weekly creatinine clearance of greater than or equal to 60 L/1.73 m^2 to achieve dialysis adequacy in

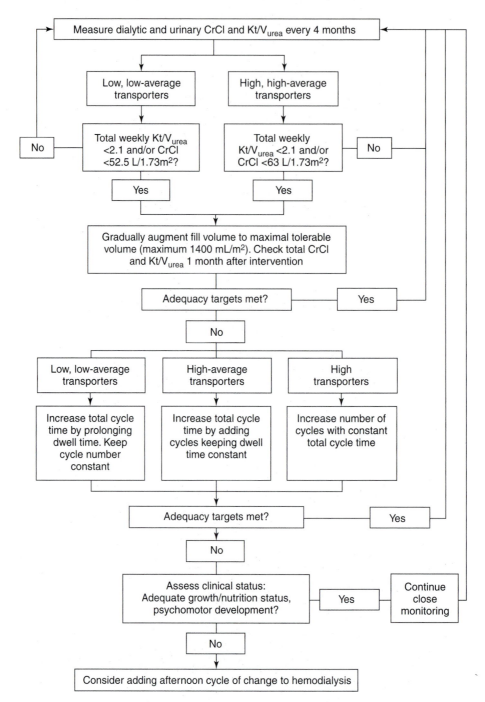

Figure 8–5. Algorithm for maintenance management of CCPD.

most children receiving CAPD.[20] Patients receiving cycling PD likely require slightly greater clearances, and low transporters may do well with lower clearances if the pediatric experience is comparable to that of the adults. Close monitoring of the patient's overall clinical condition is imperative and is an additional means by which adequacy should be assessed. The continued accumulation of patient outcome data is critical to the ongoing evaluation and credibility of these criteria.

DIALYSIS SOLUTION

While a topic not typically associated with a discussion of dialysis adequacy, recognition of the negative impact that standard dialysis solutions can have on peritoneal membrane viability as a result of their inherent bioincompatibility makes brief mention of this topic apropos.[113] In addition, the topic of fluid biocompatibility is particularly relevant to children with ESRD because of their potential long-term

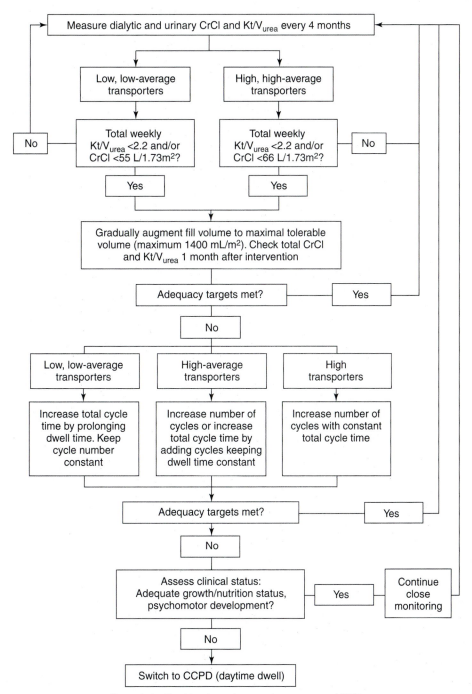

Figure 8–6. Algorithm for maintenance management of NIPD.

dependence on a functioning peritoneal membrane and the preferential use of APD as a PD modality, with its characteristic repeated exposure to fresh fluid.

Icodextrin is a mixture of high-molecular-weight glucose polymer fractions of hydrolyzed cornstarch.[114,115] Icodextrin-based solutions are clearly more biocompatible than their glucose-based counterparts and, theoretically, could be used as an alternative to glucose from the outset of PD. More commonly, and as has been described in children,

icodextrin has been used as "salvage therapy" for patients with ultrafiltration failure. Icodextrin-based solutions have recently been introduced into the United States.

Biocompatible PD fluids buffered with lactate, bicarbonate, or a lactate/bicarbonate mixture have also recently become commercially available in many countries.[116] In a multicenter European study of a bicarbonate-based dialysis solution in children receiving APD, the use of the solution was associated with a more effective correction of meta-

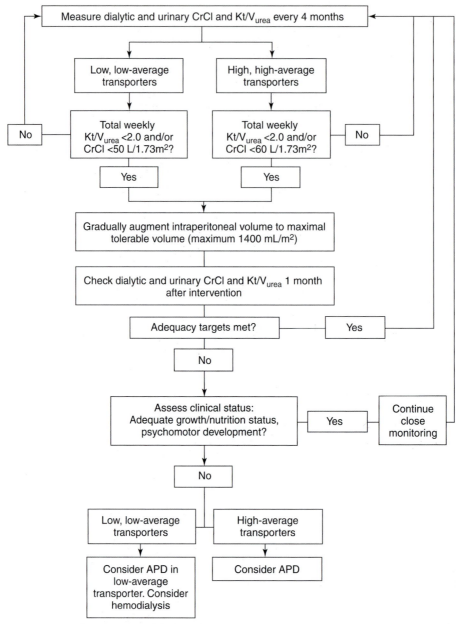

Figure 8–7. Algorithm for maintenance management CAPD.

bolic acidosis and better preservation of the peritoneal cell membrane than a conventional lactate-based solution.[117] Additional studies with these and other solutions are necessary to optimally tailor the various combinations of buffers and osmotic agents to the prescription needs of the individual patient, all with the goal of achieving dialysis adequacy while minimizing the risk of toxicity.[118]

CONCLUSION

Clearly, many of the decisions that have been made to date concerning dialysis prescription in the pediatric PD patient have been based on empiricism rather than data. Lifestyle demands have been a major influence on the popularity of APD. Whether or not the principles presented here will now be routinely incorporated into the planning process for an initial and maintenance dialysis prescription awaits the pediatric nephrology community's assessment of their clinical applicability.

OPTIMIZING HEMODIALYSIS

While PD remains the dialytic modality of choice for children worldwide, an increasing number of children now use HD as a primary alternative. The registry of the North American Pediatric Renal Transplant Cooperative Study

(NAPRTCS) reveals that 35 percent of incident dialysis patients received HD during the years 1992–2003, while the 2003 report of the USRDS has provided data that of the 1050 dialysis patients <19 years of age who initiated dialysis in 2001, 63 percent were on HD.[13] The development of more sophisticated equipment—such as ultrafiltration control devices—has been critical to the safe provision of HD to the smallest infants, while the basic principles and procedures associated with HD remain relatively constant across age groups.[119,120]

Like with PD, many factors contribute to optimizing the HD procedure in children. The choice and maintenance of the vascular access, the incorporation of dialysis machines with capabilities of extremely low blood flow rates and volumetric control of ultrafiltration, noninvasive intravascular monitoring to minimize dialysis-associated morbidity, and the use of biocompatible dialyzers characterized by minimal blood volume and predictable solute clearance and ultrafiltration coefficients are all necessary components and are discussed in Chap. 12.[121–123] This brief discussion is intended to focus on optimizing HD in terms of prescribing and quantifying dialysis. In doing so, we begin by providing an overview of the basic principles that influence solute and fluid removal in pediatric HD, as was discussed with regard to PD. The remainder of the discussion focuses on the use of kinetic modeling as a means of assessing dialysis adequacy and guiding the management of children receiving HD. A more in-depth review of kinetic modeling as it applies to HD can be found in Chap. 7.

PRINCIPLES OF HEMODIALYSIS

Solute removal during HD occurs as a result of diffusion and convection. Diffusion is defined as the movement of solute across a semipermeable membrane. Three major factors influence the diffusive solute clearance inherent to HD; these can be modified if an alteration of solute clearance is desired.[124] The permeability-surface area product (KoA) of the dialyzer characterizes the ability of that dialyzer to transfer a solute and is inversely proportional to the molecular weight of the solute.[125] The clearance (K_D) of a solute is a measure of the capacity of a specific dialyzer to transfer a solute from a patient as a function of the blood-flow rate and dialysate-flow rate. The formula for clearance is:

$$CL(mL/min) = F \times (C_A - C_v)/C_v$$

where F equals the blood-flow rate through the dialyzer in mL/min, C_A is the arterial solute concentration, and C_V is the venous solute concentration.

The third factor is the mass transfer, which is the total quantity of solute removed as a function of K_D, the length of the treatment, the transmembrane concentration or diffusion gradient, and the volume of distribution of the solute in question. The volume of distribution, or the amount of fluid into which a solute is distributed, plays an important role in determining the efficacy of solute removal. Solutes such as urea, which are distributed throughout total body water [e.g., intracellular (ICF) and extracellular (ECF) fluid], have ready access to the ECF and the extracorporeal circuit and are easily removed. In contrast, solutes more confined to the ICF space that do not rapidly equilibrate between the ICF and ECF will be removed in a less efficient manner.[124]

As in the case of PD, a second and less important route of solute removal is convective transport. Convection refers to the movement of solute across the dialyzer membrane as a manifestation of the quantity of ultrafiltrate formed and the sieving property of the dialyzer; it is independent of the concentration gradient.

DIALYSIS PRESCRIPTION

In many cases, the initiation of HD is associated with the potential for large osmolar shifts and the inherent risks for the development of cerebral edema, disequilibrium syndrome, and seizures. In this setting, the first few dialysis treatments should be designed to minimize the osmolar shifts by maintaining a relatively high extravascular osmolality with the use of an infusion of mannitol (0.5 g/kg over 1 hour starting 30 minutes after dialysis initiation) or by limiting the solute clearance that occurs [and thus decreasing the fall in blood urea nitrogen (BUN)].[126] It has been suggested that, to prevent disequilibrium, one should consider targeting a urea clearance of 30 percent for the initial one or two treatments, 50 percent for the next treatment, and >70 percent for all subsequent treatments. If the initial BUN is <100 mg/dL or mannitol is used, a urea clearance of 50 percent can be targeted for the initial session.

Once an initial maintenance dialysis prescription has been designed, monitoring of the efficacy of the individual prescription in terms of its ability to meet adequacy targets can best be conducted with the use of kinetic modeling.

KINETIC MODELING

All methods of HD adequacy measurement base the assessment of dialysis dose on a variation of the fractional urea reduction that occurs as a manifestation of the HD procedure. It is critical to recognize that during the HD procedure, urea is preferentially removed from the intravascular space with rapid subsequent equilibration of urea between the extravascular and intravascular compartments. In contrast, movement of urea from the intracellular to extracellular space is prolonged, and this disequilibrium must be taken into account in calculating the urea removal that actually occurs during a HD session.[127,128] Failure to do so has the potential of calculating an artifactually elevated urea clearance.

The rate of removal of urea is depicted by the term Kt/V [dialyzer urea clearance at a particular blood flow rate (K, mL/min), HD treatment duration (t, min) and the patients pre- and posttreatment weight (kg)]. The interdialytic accumulation of urea reflects the amount of protein catabolized during the time between dialysis treatments and, in a steady state, reflects the ingested dietary protein.

In 1985, The National Cooperative Dialysis Study concluded that adult patients with low levels of urea removal and poor nutrition fared poorly.[129] Based on these data, it was recommended that small solute removal in terms of urea clearance (Kt/V_{urea}) should serve as the guiding principle of HD adequacy and should be the main driving force behind the manipulations that occur in designing the HD prescription. In turn, NKF-K/DOQI has recommended the practice of monthly assessments of urea kinetics with a minimum target delivered Kt/V_{urea} of 1.2 for children and adults, indicative of the provision of "adequate" dialysis.[130]

Formal urea kinetic modeling is a valuable means by which a patient's urea clearance and nutritional status can be evaluated. However, the calculations have been difficult to incorporate into clinical practice and have led to the development of several equations that provide very valid estimates of urea clearance.

The Daugirdas natural logarithm formula (Daugirdas II) provides an excellent approximation of the single pool Kt/V (not accounting for the disequilibrium of the intracellular and extracellular urea that occurs during HD).[131] The formula is as follows:

$$Kt/V = -\ln(C1/C0 - 0.0008 * t) + (4 - 3.5 * C1/C0) * UF/W$$

where C0 = predialysis BUN (mg/dL)
C1 = postdialysis BUN (mg/dL)
t = session duration (hours)
UF = ultrafiltration volume (kg)
W = postdialysis weight (kg)

More recently, Goldstein et al. have provided data that have facilitated the estimation of urea removal, taking into consideration the post-HD rise in BUN that occurs as a manifestation of the reequilibration of urea between the ICF and the ECF.[132] Since urea rebound is primarily characterized by a first-order logarithmic, concentration dependent ICF to ECF urea movement, the equilibrated BUN can be estimated by extrapolating the rise in BUN from 30 seconds to 15 minutes posttreatment. With recognition of the fact that the urea rebound is 69 percent complete at the 15 minute mark, the estimated equilibrated BUN can be determined as follows:

$$estBUN = ((\Delta BUN)/0.69) + BUN_{30sec}$$

This value is then incorporated into the Daugirdas II equation to determine the equilibrated double-pool Kt/V_{urea}.

Finally, the urea reduction ratio (URR) is a means by which the fractional reduction of urea during dialysis can be calculated. It is determined as follows[133]:

$$URR = (preBUN - postBUN)/preBUN * 100\%$$

While easy to calculate, its inability to account for convective solute loss or to provide information related to dietary protein intake makes it an inferior method to assess dialysis efficacy.

ADEQUACY OF HEMODIALYSIS

Despite the recommendation of the NKF-K/DOQI work group regarding the target Kt/V of 1.2 for adults and children receiving HD and the fact that nearly 90 percent of adolescents on HD meet or exceed that target, clear evidence in support of this recommendation is lacking.[134] In addition, even if the 1.2 target has been deemed most appropriate for adults based on prior studies, a reappraisal of the target may well be indicated because of data accumulated in both adult and pediatric patients.

Most recently, the HEMO study evaluated the impact of different levels of equilibrated Kt/V_{urea} and beta$_2$ microglobulin clearance on adult patient outcome (e.g., mortality).[135] In this excellent prospective study of 1846 patients, neither urea clearance (eKt/V of 1.05 vs. 1.45) or beta$_2$ microglobulin clearance (10 mL/min vs. 20 mL/min) had a significant impact on patient deaths and emphasized that something other than solute clearance (e.g., nutrition, inflammation)—or in the manner/quantity HD is currently provided in clinical practice—has a major influence on patient outcome.

In contrast and specific to pediatrics, Tom et al. have previously reported on the occurrence of normal growth, catch-up growth, and normal puberty in children receiving intensive nutritional support and solute clearances that markedly exceed current recommendations.[136] With approximately 15 hours per week of dialysis and a single-pool Kt/V of 2.0 for each session, the mean annual change in height standard deviation score was + 0.3 without the use of growth hormone. What specific role the combination of enhanced nutritional regimen, good blood pressure control and excellent calcium-phosphorus metabolism played in comparison to the solute clearance is unknown.

CONCLUSION

Optimization of HD, like PD, in children can be achieved only if the dialysis prescription is individualized and based on the patient's clinical status and some measure of dialysis delivery. While the adult experience suggests that target values determined with urea kinetic modeling can serve as a starting point, further studies in children are necessary to define the kinetics of urea in the entire pediatric age range and evaluate the validity of measures such as Kt/V before these tools can be applied universally. In addition, while data from a variety of sources ranging from the NCDS to the HEMO study emphasize the fact that solute removal most certainly has a role in the outcome of patients receiving HD, additional observational/interventional efforts are necessary to better define those other important factors that likely contribute to the adequacy of care.[137,138]

REFERENCES

1. Twardowski ZJ. PET—a simpler approach for determining prescriptions for adequate dialysis. *Adv Perit Dial* 1990;6: 186–191.
2. Goldstein SL. Adequacy of dialysis in children: does small solute clearance really matter? *Pediatr Nephrol* 2004;19: 1–5.
3. Chadha V, Warady BA. Adequacy of peritoneal dialysis in pediatric patients. In: Nissenson AR, Fine RN, eds. *Dialysis Therapy*, 3d ed. Philadelphia: Hanley & Belfus, 2002: 493–497.
4. Blake PG. Adequacy of dialysis revisited. *Kidney Int* 2003: 63:1587–1599.
5. Blake PG, Sombolos K, Abraham G, et al. Lack of correlation between urea kinetic indices and clinical outcomes in CAPD patients. *Kidney Int* 1991;39:700–706.
6. Keshaviah PR, Nolph K, Prowant B, et al. Defining adequacy of CAPD with urea kinetics. *Adv Perit Dial* 1990;6: 177.
7. Fischbach M, Stefanidis CJ, Watson AR, European Paediatric Peritoneal Dialysis Working Group. Guidelines by an ad hoc European Committee on Adequacy and the Paediatric Peritoneal Dialysis Prescription. *Nephrol Dial Int* 2002;17: 380–385.
8. Paniagua R, Amato D, Vonesch E, et al. Effects of increased peritoneal clearances on mortality rates in peritoneal dialysis: ADEMEX, a prospective, randomized, controlled trial. *J Am Soc Nephrol* 2002;13:1307–1320.
9. Wang T, Lindholm B. Beyond CANUSA, DOQI, ADEMEX: what's next? *Perit Dial Int* 2002;22:555–562.
10. Eknoyan G, Beck GJ, Cheung AK, et al. Effect of dialysis dose and membrane flux in maintenance hemodialysis. *N Engl J Med* 2002;347:2010–2019.
11. Alexander SR, Honda M. Continuous peritoneal dialysis for children: a decade of worldwide growth and development. *Kidney Int* 1993;43:S65–S74.
12. Warady BA, Alexander SR, Watkins SL, et al. Optimal care of the pediatric end-stage renal disease patient on dialysis. *Am J Kidney Dis* 1999;33:567–583.
13. USRDS Coordinating Center. *United States Renal Data System 2003 Annual Data Report: Atlas of End-Stage Renal Disease in the United States.* Bethesda, MD: National Insti-

tutes of Heatlh, National Institute of Diabetes and Digestive and Kidney Diseases, 2003.
14. Fine RN, Ho M, North American Pediatric Renal Transplant Cooperative Study: The role of APD in the management of pediatric patients: a report of the North American Pediatric Renal Transplant Cooperative Study. *Semin Dial* 2002;15: 427–429.
15. Lowrie EG, Laird NM, Parker TF, et al. Effect of the hemodialysis prescription on patient morbidity. Report from the National Cooperative Dialysis Study. *N Engl J Med* 1981;305: 1176–1181.
16. Teehan BP, Schliefer CR, Brown J. Urea kinetic modeling is an appropriate assessment of adequacy. *Semin Dial* 1992;5: 189–192.
17. Churchill DN. The ADEMEX study: make haste slowly. *J Am Soc Nephrol* 2002;13:1415–1418.
18. Bargman JM, Thorpe KE, Churchill DN, for the CANUSA Peritoneal Dialysis Study Group. Relative contribution of residual renal function and peritoneal clearance to adequacy of dialysis: a reanalysis of the CANUSA study. *J Am Soc Nephrol* 2001;12:2158–2162.
19. Heimburger O. The negative results of the ADEMEX study may be positive for peritoneal dialysis. Time for a paradigm shift in the focus of peritoneal dialysis adequacy? *Perit Dial Int* 2002;22:546–548.
20. *NKF–K/DOQI Clinical Practice Guidelines for Peritoneal Dialysis Adequacy.* New York: National Kidney Foundation, 2001.
21. Konings CJ, Kooman JP, Schonck M, et al. Fluid status in CAPD patients is related to peritoneal transport and residual renal function: evidence from a longitudinal study. *Nephrol Dial Transplant* 2003;18:797–803.
22. Höltta T, Rönnholm K, Jalanko H, et al. Clinical outcome of pediatric patients on peritoneal dialysis under adequacy control. *Pediatr Nephrol* 2000;14:889–897.
23. Chadha V, Blowey DL, Warady BA. Is growth a valid outcome measure of dialysis clearance in children undergoing peritoneal dialysis? *Perit Dial Int* 2001;21:S179–S184.
24. Schaefer F, Günter K, Mehls O, The Mid–European Pediatric Peritoneal Dialysis Study Group. Peritoneal transport properties and dialysis dose affect growth and nutritional status in children on chronic peritoneal dialysis. *J Am Soc Nephrol* 1999;10:1786–1792.
25. Chadha V, Warady BA. What are the clinical correlates of adequate peritoneal dialysis? *Semin Nephrol* 2001;21: 480–489.
26. *North American Pediatric Renal Transplant Cooperative Study (NAPRTCS) 2003 Annual Report.* Rockville, MD: EMMES Corporation, 2003.
27. Gruskin AB, Lerner GR, Fleischman LE. Developmental aspects of peritoneal dialysis kinetics. In: Fine RN, ed. *Chronic Ambulatory Peritoneal Dialysis (CAPD) and Chronic Cycling Peritoneal Dialysis (CCPD) in Children.* Boston: Martinus Nijhoff, 1987:33–46.
28. Putiloff PV. Materials for the study of the laws of growth of the human body in relation to the surface areas of different systems: the trial on Russian subjects of planigraphic anatomy as a means for exact anthropometry; one of the problems of anthropology. Report of Dr. P.V. Putiloff at the

meeting of the Siberian Branch of the Russian Geographic Society. 1884.

29. Esperanca MJ, Collins DL. Peritoneal dialysis efficiency in relation to body weight. *J Pediatr Surg* 1966;1:162–169.

30. Wegner G. Chirurgische Bemerkungen umlautuber die peritoneal Humlautohle, mit besonder Berucksichtigung der Ovariotomie. *Arch Klin Chir* 1887;20:51.

31. Morgenstern BZ. Equilibration testing: close, but not quite right. *Pediatr Nephrol* 1993;7:290–291.

32. Kohaut EC, Waldo FB, Benfield MR. The effect of changes in dialysate volume on glucose and urea equilibration. *Perit Dial Int* 1994;14:236–239.

33. Schaefer F, Haas S, Mehls O. Analysis of peritoneal transport characteristic by peritoneal dialysis capacity (PDC) test in children. *Perit Dial Int* 1996;16:S11.

34. de Boer AW, van Schaijk TCJG, Willems HL, et al. The necessity of adjusting dialysate volume to body surface area in pediatric peritoneal equilibration tests. *Perit Dial Int* 1997;17:199–202.

35. Warady BA, Alexander S, Hossli S, et al. The relationship between intraperitoneal volume and solute transport in pediatric patients. *J Am Soc Nephrol* 1995;5:1935–1939.

36. Chagnac A, Herskovitz P, Weinstein T, et al. The peritoneal membrane in peritoneal dialysis patients: estimation of its functional surface area by applying stereological methods to computerized tomography scans. *J Am Soc Nephrol* 1999;10:342–346.

37. Flessner MF, Lofthouse J, Zakaria ER. Improving contact area between the peritoneum and intraperitoneal therapeutic solutions. *J Am Soc Nephrol* 2001;12:807–813.

38. Schaefer F, Haraldsson B, Haas S, et al. Estimation of peritoneal mass transport by three–pore model in children. *Kidney Int* 1998;54:1372–1379.

39. DuBois D, DuBois EF. A formula to estimate the approximate surface area if height and weight be known. *Arch Intern Med* 1916;17:863–971.

40. Gehan EA, George SL. Estimation of human body surface area from height and weight. *Cancer Chemother Rep* 1970;54:225–235.

41. Rippe B, Stelin G. Simulations of peritoneal transport during CAPD. Application of two-pore formalism. *Kidney Int* 1989;35:1234–1244.

42. Fischbach M, Haraldsson B. Dynamic changes of the total pore area available for peritoneal exchange in children. *J Am Soc Nephrol* 2001;12:1524–1529.

43. Flessner MF. The peritoneal dialysis system: importance of each component. *Perit Dial Int* 1997;17:S91–S97.

44. Popovich RP, Moncrief JW, Okutan M, et al. A model of the peritoneal dialysis system. *Proc 25th Ann Conf Eng Med Biol* 1972;14:172.

45. Morgenstern BZ, Pyle WK, Gruskin AB, et al. Transport characteristics of the pediatric peritoneal membrane. *Kidney Int* 1984;25:259–264.

46. Haraldsson B. Assessing the peritoneal dialysis capacities of individual patients. *Kidney Int* 1995;47:1187–1198.

47. Vonesch EF, Burkart J, McMurray SD, et al. Peritoneal dialysis kinetic modeling: validation in a multicenter clinical study. *Perit Dial Int* 1996;16:471–481.

48. Warady BA, Watkins SL, Fivush BA, et al. Validation of PD Adequest 2.0 for pediatric dialysis patients. *Pediatr Nephrol* 2001;16:205–211.

49. Morgenstern BZ, Baluarte HJ. Peritoneal dialysis kinetics in children. In: Fine RN, ed. *Chronic Ambulatory Peritoneal Dialysis (CAPD) and Chronic Cycling Peritoneal Dialysis in Children (CCPD).* Boston: Martinus Nijhoff, 1987:41–61.

50. Popovich RP, Pyle WK, Rosenthal DA, et al. Kinetics of peritoneal dialysis in children, In: Moncrief JW, Popovich RP, eds. *CAPD Update.* New York: Masson, 1981:227–241.

51. Waniewski J, Heimburger D, Werynski A, et al. Aqueous solute concentrations and evaluation of mass transport coefficients in peritoneal dialysis. *Nephrol Dial Transplant* 1992;7:50–56.

52. Balfe JW, Vigneaux A, Williamson J, et al. The use of CAPD in the treatment of children with end–stage renal disease. *Perit Dial Bull* 1981;1:35–38.

53. Quan A, Baum M. Protein losses in children on continuous cycler peritoneal dialysis. *Pediatr Nephrol* 1996;10:728–731.

54. Geary DF, Harvey EA, Balfe JW. Mass transfer area coefficients in children. *Perit Dial Int* 1994;14:30–33.

55. Brandes J, Emerson P, Campbell D, et al. The relationship between body size, fill volume and mass transfer area coefficient (MTAC) in PD. (abstract) *J Am Soc Nephrol* 1992;9P.

56. Warady BA, Alexander SR, Hossli S, et al. Peritoneal membrane transport function in children receiving long–term dialysis. *J Am Soc Nephrol* 1996;7:2385–2391.

57. Popovich RP, Pyle WK, Moncrief JW. Kinetics of peritoneal transport: *In Peritoneal Dialysis,* Boston, Martinus Nijhoff, 1981.

58. Pyle WK. Mass transfer in peritoneal dialysis (PhD dissertation). 47–62. 1987. Austin: University of Texas.

59. Vonesh EF, Lysaght MJ, Moran J, et al. Kinetic modeling as a prescription aid in peritoneal dialysis. *Blood Purif* 1991;9:246–270.

60. Bouts AH, Davin JC, Groothoff JW, et al. Standard peritoneal permeability analysis in children. *J Am Soc Nephrol* 2000;11:943–950.

61. Mitsnefes MM, Daniels SR, Schwartz SM, et al. Changes in left ventricular mass in children and adolescents during chronic dialysis. *Pediatr Nephrol* 2001;16:318–323.

62. Ates K, Nergizoglu G, Keven K, et al. Effect of fluid and sodium removal on mortality in peritoneal dialysis patients. *Kidney Int* 2001;60:767–776.

63. Gruskin AB, Rosenblum H, Baluarte HJ, et al. Transperitoneal solute movement in children. *Kidney Int* 1983;24:S95.

64. Kohaut EC, Alexander SR: Ultrafiltration in the young patient on CAPD, in CAPD Update, edited by Moncrief JW, Popovich RP, New York, Masson, 1981, pp 221–226.

65. Schaefer F, Fischbach M, Heckert KH, et al. Hydrostatic intraperitoneal pressure in children on peritoneal dialysis. (abstract) *Perit Dial Int* 1996;16:S79.

66. Leypoldt JK. Solute transport across the peritoneal membrane. *J Am Soc Nephrol* 2002;13:S84–S91.

67. Mactier RA, Khanna R, Twardowski ZJ, et al. Contribution of lymphatic absorption to loss of ultrafiltration and solute

clearances in continuous ambulatory peritoneal dialysis. *J Clin Invest* 1987;80:1311–1316.

68. Flessner MF. Transport kinetics during peritoneal dialysis, In: Leypoldt JK, Austin RG, eds. *The Artificial Kidney: Physiological Modeling and Tissue Engineering.* Landes, 1999:59–89.

69. Rippe G. Is lymphatic absorption important for ultrafiltration? *Perit Dial Int* 1995;15:203–204.

70. Mactier RA, Khanna R, Moore H, et al. Kinetics of peritoneal dialysis in children: role of lymphatics. *Kidney Int* 1988;34:82–88.

71. Schroder CH, Reddingius R, van Dreumel JA, et al. Transcapillary ultrafiltration and lympatic absorption during childhood continuous ambulatory peritoneal dialysis. *Nephrol Dial Transplant* 1991;6:571–573.

72. Twardowski ZJ, Nolph KD, Khanna A, et al. Peritoneal equilibration test. *Perit Dial Bull* 1987;7:378–383.

73. Sliman GA, Klee KM, Gall–Holden B, et al. Peritoneal equilibration test curves and adequacy of dialysis in children on automated peritoneal dialysis. *Am J Kidney Dis* 1994;24: 813–818.

74. Schaefer F, Lagenbeck D, Heckert KH, et al. Evaluation of peritoneal solute transfer by the peritoneal equilibration test in children. *Adv Perit Dial* 1992;8:410–415.

75. Twardowski ZJ. The fast peritoneal equilibration test. *Semin Dial* 1990;3:141–142.

76. Twardowski ZJ, Prowant BF, Moore HL, et al. Short peritoneal equilibration test: impact of preceding dwell time. *Adv Perit Dial* 2003;19:53–58.

77. Jennings J, Warady BA. The fast PET in pediatrics (abstr). *Perit Dial Int* 2004;24:S49.

78. Warady BA. The peritoneal equilibration test (PET) in pediatrics. *Contemp Dial Nephrol* 1994;March:21–41.

79. Blake P, Burkart JM, Churchill DN, et al. Recommended clinical practices for maximizing peritoneal dialysis clearances. *Perit Dial Int* 1996;16:448–456.

80. Rocco MV, Jordan JR, Burkart JM. Changes in peritoneal transport during the first month of peritoneal dialysis. *Perit Dial Int* 1995;15:12–17.

81. Warady BA, Fivush BA, Andreoli SP, et al. Longitudinal evaluation of transport kinetics in children receiving peritoneal dialysis. *Pediatr Nephrol* 1999;13:571–576.

82. Yoshino A, Honda M, Fukuda M, et al. Changes in peritoneal equilibration test values during long-term peritoneal dialysis in peritonitis-free children. *Perit Dial Int* 2001;21: 180–185.

83. de Boer AW, van Schaijk TCJG, Willems HL, et al. Follow–up study of peritoneal fluid kinetics in infants and children on peritoneal dialysis. *Perit Dial Int* 1999;19:5 72–577.

84. Fried L. Higher membrane permeability predicts poorer patient survival. *Perit Dial Int* 1997;17:387–388.

85. Churchill DN, Thorpe KE, Nolph KD, et al. Increased peritoneal membrane transport is associated with decreased patient and technique survival for continuous peritoneal dialysis patients. The Canada-USA (CANUSA) Peritoneal Dialysis Study Group. *J Am Soc Nephrol* 1998;9: 1285–1292.

86. Kagan A, Bar-Khayim Y. Role of peritoneal loss of albumin in the hypoalbuminemia of continuous ambulatory peritoneal dialysis patients: relationship to peritoneal transport of solutes. *Nephron* 1995;71:314–320.

87. Burkart JM, Schreiber M, Korbet SM, et al. Solute clearance approach to adequacy of peritoneal dialysis. *Perit Dial Int* 1996;16:457–470.

88. Rocco MV. Body surface area limitations in achieving adequate therapy in peritoneal dialysis patients. *Perit Dial Int* 1996;16:617–622.

89. Fischbach M, Terzic J, Laugel V, et al. Measurement of hydrostatic intraperitoneal pressure: a useful tool for the improvement of dialysis dose prescription. *Pediatr Nephrol* 2003;18:976–980.

90. Fischbach M, Terzic J, Becmeur F, et al. Relationship between intraperitoneal hydrostatic pressure and dialysate volume in children on PD. *Adv Perit Dial* 1996;12:330–334.

91. Fischbach M, Terzic J, Menouer S, et al. Impact of fill volume changes on peritoneal dialysis tolerance and effectiveness in children. *Adv Perit Dial* 2000;16:321–323.

92. Fischbach M, Terzic J, Menouer S, et al. Optimal volume prescription for children on peritoneal dialysis. *Perit Dial Int* 2000;20:603–606.

93. Aranda RA, Romao JE, Kakehashi E, et al. Intraperitoneal pressure and hernias in children on peritoneal dialysis. *Pediatr Nephrol* 2000;14:22–24.

94. Verrina E, Amici G, Perfumo F, et al. The use of the PD Adequest mathematical model in pediatric patients on chronic peritoneal dialysis. *Perit Dial Int* 1998;18:322–328.

95. Feber J, Scharer K, Schaefer F, et al. Residual renal function in children on haemodialysis and peritoneal dialysis therapy. *Pediatr Nephrol* 1994;8:579–583.

96. Rocco MV, Frankenfield DL, Prowant B, et al for the Centers for Medicare & Medicaid Services Peritoneal Dialysis Core Indicators Study Group. Risk factors for early mortality in U.S. peritoneal dialysis patients: impact of residual renal function. *Perit Dial Int* 2002;22:371–379.

97. Fischbach M, Terzic J, Menouer S, et al. Effects of automated peritoneal dialysis on residual daily urinary volume in children. *Adv Perit Dial* 2001;17:269–273.

98. Canada-USA (CANUSA) Peritoneal Dialysis Study Group. Adequacy of dialysis and nutrition in continuous peritoneal dialysis: association with clinical outcomes. *J Am Soc Nephrol* 1996;7:198–207.

99. Lutes R, Perlmutter J, Holley JL, et al. Loss of residual renal function in patients on peritoneal dialysis. *Adv Perit Dial* 1993;9:165–168.

100. Chen HH, Shetty A, Afthentopoulos IE, et al. Discrepancy between weekly Kt/V and weekly creatinine clearance in patients on CAPD. *Adv Perit Dial* 1995;1:83–87.

101. Twardowski ZJ. Relationship between creatinine clearance and Kt/V in peritoneal dialysis: a response to the defense of the DOQI document. *Perit Dial Int* 1999;19:199–203.

102. Churchill DN, Blake PG, Jindal KK, et al. Clinical practice guideline for initiation of dialysis. *J Am Soc Nephrol* 1999; 10:S289–S291.

103. McCauley L, Champoux S, Parvex P, et al. Enhanced growth in children on peritoneal dialysis (PD): dialysis dose, nutri-

tion, and metabolic control (abstr). *Perit Dial Int* 2000;20: S89.

104. Champoux S, McCauley L, Sharma A, et al. Enhanced response to growth hormone in children on peritoneal dialysis (abstr). *Perit Dial Int* 2001;21:S86.

105. Montini G, Amici G, Milan S, et al. Middle molecule and small protein removal in children on peritoneal dialysis. *Kidney Int* 2002;61:1153–1159.

106. van der Voort JH, Harvey EA, Braj B, et al. Can the DOQI guidelines be met by peritoneal dialysis alone in pediatric patients? *Pediatr Nephrol* 2000;14:717–719.

107. Warady BA, Schaefer F, Alexander SR, et al. *Care of the Pediatric Patient on Peritoneal Dialysis.* Baxter Healthcare Corporation, 2004:1–89.

108. Mellits ED, Cheek DB. The assessment of body water and fatness from infancy to adulthood. *Monogr Soc Res Child Dev* 1970;35:12–26.

109. Morgenstern B, Sreekumaran NK, Lerner G, et al. Impact of total body water errors on Kt/V estimates in children on peritoneal dialysis. *Adv Perit Dial* 2001;17:260–263.

110. Wühl E, Fusch CH, Schäarer K, et al. Assessment of total body water error in paediatric patients on dialysis. *Nephrol Dial Transplant* 1996;11:75–80.

111. Morgenstern B, Warady BA. Estimating total body water in children based upon height and weight: a reevaluation of the formulas of Mellits and Cheek. *J Am Soc Nephrol* 2002;13: 1884–1888.

112. Morgenstern BZ, Mahoney DW, Wuehl E, et al. Total body water (TBW) in children on peritoneal dialysis (abstr). *J Am Soc Nephrol* 2002;13:2A.

113. Holmes CJ, Faict D. Peritoneal dialysis solution biocompatibility: definitions and evaluation strategies. *Kidney Int* 2003;64:S50–S56.

114. de Boer AW, Schroder CH, van Vliet R, et al. Clinical experience with icodextrin in children: ultrafiltration profiles and metabolism. *Pediatr Nephrol* 2000;15:21–24.

115. Schroder CH. New peritoneal dialysis fluids: practical use for children. *Pediatr Nephrol* 2003;18:1085–1088.

116. Dratwa M, Wilkie M, Ryckelynck JP, et al. Clinical experience with two physiologic bicarbonate/lactate peritoneal dialysis solutions in automated peritoneal dialysis. *Kidney Int* 2003;64:S105–S113.

117. Haas S, Schmitt CP, Arbeiter K, et al for the Mid European Pediatric Peritoneal Dialysis Study Group. Improved acidosis correction and recovery of mesothelial cell mass with neutral-pH bicarbonate dialysis solution among children undergoing automated peritoneal dialysis. *J Am Soc Nephrol* 2003;14:2632–2638.

118. Vardhan A, Zseers MM, Gokal R, et al. A solutions portfolio approach in peritoneal dialysis. *Kidney Int* 2003;64: S114–S123.

119. Goldstein SL. Hemodialysis in the pediatric patient: state of the art. *Adv Renal Replace Ther* 2001;8:173–179.

120. Donckerwolke RA, Bunchman TE. Hemodialysis in infants and small children. *Pediatr Nephrol* 1994;8:103–107.

121. Sheth RD, Brandt ML, Brewer ED, et al. Permanent hemodialysis vascular access survival in children and adolescents with ESRD. *Kidney Int* 2002;62:1864–1869.

122. Jain SR, Smith L, Brewer ED, et al. Non-invasive intravascular monitoring in the pediatric hemodialysis population. *Pediatr Nephrol* 2001;16:15–18.

123. Goldstein SL, Smith CA, Currier H. Noninvasive interventions to decrease hospitalization and associated costs for pediatric patients receiving hemodialysis. *J Am Soc Nephrol* 2003;14:2127–2131.

124. Harmon WE, Jabs K. Hemodialysis. In: Holliday MA, Barratt TM, Avner ED, eds. *Pediatric Nephrology.* Baltimore: Williams & Wilkins, 1994:1354–1372.

125. Gotch FA, Autian J, Colton C, et al. The evaluation of hemodialyzers. DHEW Publ No NIH-73–103. Washington, DC: Department of Health, Education, and Welfare, 1973.

126. Goldstein SL, Jabs K. Hemodialysis. In: Avner ED, Harmon WE, Niaudet P, eds. *Pediatric Nephrology,* 5th ed. Philadelphia: Lippincott Williams & Wilkins, 2004:1375–1394.

127. Pedrini LA, Zereik S, Ramsy S. Causes, kinetics and clinical implications of post-hemodialysis urea rebound. *Kidney Int* 1998;34:817–824.

128. Goldstein SL, Sorof JM, Brewer ED. Evaluation and prediction of urea rebound and equilibrated Kt/V in the pediatric hemodialysis population. *Am J Kidney Dis* 1999;34:49–54.

129. Gotch FA, Sargent JA. A mechanistic analysis of the National Cooperative Dialysis Study (NCDS). *Kidney Int* 1985; 28:526–534.

130. NKF–K/DOQI Clinical practice guidelines for hemodialysis adequacy: update 2000. *Am J Kidney Dis* 2001;37:S7–S64.

131. Daugirdas JT. Second generation logarithmic estimates of single-pool variable volume Kt/V: an analysis of error. *J Am Soc Nephrol* 1993;4:1205–1213.

132. Goldstein SL, Brewer ED. Logarithmic extrapolation of a 15-minute postdialysis BUN to predict equilibrated BUN and caclulate double-pool Kt/V in the pediatric hemodialysis population. *Am J Kidney Dis* 2000;36:98–104.

133. Borah MF, Schoenfeld PY, Gotch FA, et al. Nitrogen balance during intermittent dialysis therapy of uremia. *Kidney Int* 1978;14:491–500.

134. Frankenfield DL, Neu AM, Warady BA, et al. Anemia in pediatric hemodialysis patients: results from the 2001 ESRD CPM project. *Kidney Int* 2003;64:1120–1124.

135. Cheung AK, Levin NW, Greene T, et al for the HEMO Study Group: Effects of high-flux hemodialysis on clinical outcomes: results of the HEMO study. *J Am Soc Nephrol* 2003;14:3251–3263.

136. Tom A, McCauley L, Bell L, et al. Growth during maintenance hemodialysis: impact of enhanced nutrition and clearance. *J Pediatr* 1999;134:464–471.

137. Goldstein SL. Adequacy of dialysis in children: does small solute clearance really matter? *Pediatr Nephrol* 2004;19: 1–5.

138. Sharma AK. Reassessing hemodialysis adequacy in children: the case for more. *Pediatr Nephrol* 2001;16:383–390.

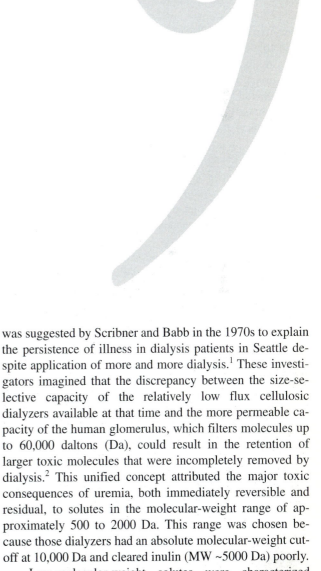

Clinical Implications of Larger Molecules

Victoria A. Kumar
Thomas A. Depner

THE RESIDUAL SYNDROME

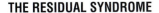

The immediate life-threatening aspects of the uremic syndrome result mostly from the accumulation of a variety of toxins—including electrolytes, organic acids, inorganic salts, and metabolic end products such as urea and creatinine—that diffuse easily across cellulosic membranes. While dialysis corrects many of the derangements associated with uremia, some clinical symptoms usually persist despite adequate removal of low-molecular-weight solutes. This "residual syndrome," experienced by most dialysis patients, includes anorexia, muscle wasting, neuropathy, pruritus, increased susceptibility to infection, prolonged recovery from infection, and poor wound healing. Today, mortality rates remain high in dialysis-dependent patients, even in those who are well dialyzed by currently accepted standards. The so-called middle molecule (MM) hypothesis

was suggested by Scribner and Babb in the 1970s to explain the persistence of illness in dialysis patients in Seattle despite application of more and more dialysis.[1] These investigators imagined that the discrepancy between the size-selective capacity of the relatively low flux cellulosic dialyzers available at that time and the more permeable capacity of the human glomerulus, which filters molecules up to 60,000 daltons (Da), could result in the retention of larger toxic molecules that were incompletely removed by dialysis.[2] This unified concept attributed the major toxic consequences of uremia, both immediately reversible and residual, to solutes in the molecular-weight range of approximately 500 to 2000 Da. This range was chosen because those dialyzers had an absolute molecular-weight cutoff at 10,000 Da and cleared inulin (MW ~5000 Da) poorly.

Low-molecular-weight solutes were characterized much earlier than MMs and can be defined as compounds that diffuse easily across a cellulosic dialysis membrane. Most authors have distinguished small solutes arbitrarily as those with a molecular weight of less than 500 Da, although this cutoff point has increased in recent years with the advent of high-flux (more permeable) membranes. Solutes in the mid-molecular-weight range diffuse poorly and require more time to equilibrate across cellulosic membranes. These theoretical compounds have a molecular weight greater than 500 Da, but the upper range is poorly defined, usually in the range of 2000 to 15,000 Da, although some authors would include all molecules with a molecular weight lower than that of albumin (approximately 65,000 Da) or even higher. The definition has become blurred during the last decades for two reasons: (1) failure to identify specific toxic compounds in the previously described molecular-weight range of 500 to 2000 Da and (2) persistence of the residual syndrome in patients treated with high-flux dialyzers that significantly clear solutes up to 10,000 Da. Some small solutes can behave like MMs due to protein binding, sequestration in remote body compartments, or interaction with tissue membranes. Larger molecules are removed more efficiently by convection than diffusion.

Although retention of toxic solutes explains the life-saving effects of dialysis, the uremic state is complex, probably caused by a myriad of accumulated solutes, including commonly measured urea and creatinine, and involving several indirect mechanisms. A review of uremic toxins by the European Uremic Toxin Work Group (EUTox) identified 90 organic compounds that are retained in the uremic state[3]; 68 of which had a molecular weight lower than 500 Da. Of these, 45 were classified as water-soluble (Table 9–1). Of the remaining 22 molecules, 12 exceeded 12,000 Da (Table 9–2). Of the retained uremic solutes, 25 were bound to serum proteins, and most of these were small molecules (Table 9–3). Since uremic retention products comprise a spectrum of compounds with a continuous array of molecular weights, any classification according to size is artificial. However, it is important to distinguish water-soluble compounds, protein-bound compounds, and higher-molecular-weight compounds because the latter two classes are not efficiently removed by conventional hemodialysis.

Several criteria have been proposed to rationally classify a uremic retention product as a true uremic toxin.[3] First, the compound must be identified and quantified in biological fluids, such as serum, urine, or ultrafiltrate. The solute levels in uremic subjects must be higher than in nonuremic subjects, and the concentration should correlate with specific symptoms or biological dysfunction. When the solute level is reduced by dialysis, transplantation, or other technology, specific symptoms should improve. The biological activity of a uremic toxin should be proven in vitro or in vivo and toxicity should be exhibited for the specific range of concentrations found in uremic subjects. Thus

TABLE 9–1. NON-PROTEIN-BOUND LOW-MOLECULAR-WEIGHT SOLUTES THAT ACCUMULATE IN UREMIA

Solute	Molecular Weight (Da)	Compound Classification
1-methyladenosine	281	Ribonucleoside
1-methylguanosine	297	Ribonucleoside
1-methylinosine	282	Ribonucleoside
Asymmetrical dimethylarginine	202	Guanidine
α-keto-δ-guanidinovaleric acid	151	Guanidine
α-N-acetylarginine	216	Guanidine
Arab(in)itol	152	Polyol
Arginic acid	175	Guanidine
Benzylalcohol	108	
β-guanidinopropionic acid	131	Guanidine
β-lipotropin	461	Peptide
Creatine	131	Guanidine
Creatinine	113	Guanidine
Cytidine	234	Purine
Dimethylglycine	103	
Erythritol	122	Polyol
γ-guanidinobutyric acid	145	Guanidine
Guanidine	59	Guanidine
Guanidinoacetic acid	117	Guanidine
Guanidinosuccinic acid	175	Guanidine
Hypoxanthine	136	Purine
Malondialdehyde	71	
Mannitol	182	Polyol
Methylguanidine	73	Guanidine
Myoinositol	180	Polyol
N^2,N^2-dimethylguanosine	311	Ribonucleoside
N^4-acetylcytidine	285	Ribonucleoside
N^6-methyladenosine	281	Ribonucleoside
N^6-threonylcarbamoyladenosine	378	Ribonucleoside
Orotic acid	174	Pyrimidine
Orotidine	288	Pyrimidine
Oxalate	90	
Phenylacetylglutamine	264	
Pseudouridine	244	Ribonucleoside
Symmetrical dimethylarginine	202	Guanidine
Sorbitol	182	Polyol
Taurocyamine	174	Guanidine
Threitol	122	Polyol
Thymine	126	Pyrimidine
Uracil	112	Purine
Urea	60	
Uric acid	168	Purine
Uridine	244	Pyrimidine
Xanthine	152	Purine
Xanthosine	284	Ribonucleoside

TABLE 9–2. HIGHER-MOLECULAR-WEIGHT SOLUTES THAT ACCUMULATE IN UREMIA

Solute	Molecular Weight (Da)	Compound Classification
Adrenomedullin	5,729	Peptide
Atrial natriuretic peptide	3,080	Peptide
β_2-microglobulin	11,818	Peptide
β-endorphin	3,465	Peptide
Cholecystokinin	3,866	Peptide
Clara cell protein	15,800	Peptide
Complement factor D	23,750	
Cystatin C	13,300	Peptide
Degranulation inhibiting protein I[c]	14,100	Peptide
Delta sleep–inducing peptide	848	Peptide
Endothelin	4,283	Peptide
Hyaluronic acid	25,000	Peptide
Interleukin-1β	32,000	Cytokine
Interleukin-6	24,500	Cytokine
κ-Ig light chain	25,000	Peptide
λ-Ig light chain	25,000	Peptide
Leptin	16,000	Peptide
Methionine-enkephalin	555	Peptide
Neuropeptide Y	4,272	Peptide
Parathyroid hormone	9,225	Peptide
Retinol-binding protein	21,200	Peptide
Tumor necrosis factor-α	26,000	Cytokine

TABLE 9–3. PROTEIN-BOUND SOLUTES THAT ACCUMULATE IN UREMIA

Solute	Molecular Weight (Da)	Compound Classification
2-methoxyresorcinol	140	Phenol
3-deoxyglucosone	162	AGE[a]
3-carboxy-4-methyl-5-propyl-2-furanpropionic acid	240	
Fructoselysine	308	AGE
Glyoxal	58	AGE
Hippuric acid	179	Hippurate
Homocysteine	135	
Hydroquinone	110	Phenol
Indole-3-acetic acid	175	Indole
Indoxyl sulfate	251	Indole
Kinurenine	208	Indole
Kynurenic acid	189	Indole
Leptin	16,000	Peptide
Melatonin	126	Indole
Methylglyoxal	72	AGE
N^ϵ-(carboxymethly)lysine	204	AGE
p-Cresol	108	Phenol
Pentosidine	342	AGE
Phenol	94	Phenol
P-OH hippuric acid	195	Hippurate
Putrescine	88	Polyamine
Quinolinic acid	167	Indole
Retinol-binding protein	21,200	Peptide
Spermidine	145	Polyamine
Spermidine	202	Polyamine

[a]Advanced glycation end product.

very few of the identified uremic retention products can be classified as bona fide uremic toxins.

Conventional hemodialysis alleviates many uremic symptoms, but the morbidity and mortality associated with end-stage renal disease (ESRD) remains high. Some complications, such as dialysis related amyloidosis (DRA), develop in long-term survivors of ESRD and are clearly the result of inadequate treatment. Adequacy of hemodialysis is currently based on small solute clearance, yet larger molecules may also contribute to the complications of ESRD and thus represent uremic toxins. While it is evident that larger solutes accumulate in patients with renal failure and may exert toxic effects, most data indicate that uremic toxicity as a whole correlates better with clearance of small solutes.

Because the originally proposed MMs were theoretical, attempts were subsequently made to prove their existence and to demonstrate their toxicity in the uremic state. Simultaneously, developers of dialysis membranes sought to improve the removal of MMs by developing membranes with increased porosity (flux). Increases in membrane flux have paralleled improvements in dialysis technology, including membrane composition and biocompatibility, confounding attempts to evaluate the clinical impact of increased larger molecule clearance.

MORBIDITY, MORTALITY AND LARGER RETAINED SOLUTES

In the late 1970s, the U.S. National Institutes of Health (NIH) sponsored the National Cooperative Dialysis Study (NCDS) in an attempt to define adequacy of hemodialysis and assess the impact of both small and larger solute clearance on morbidity. Patients were randomly assigned to one of four different treatment schedules, with either a short or long treatment time and either a low or high time-averaged urea concentration (TAC_{urea}). During this 6-month study, the highest morbidity was found in patients in the high TAC_{urea} group given a short treatment time, but all patients with a high TAC_{urea} had higher morbidity than patients with a low TAC_{urea}.[4] However, patients with a higher urea generation rate, resulting in a higher TAC_{urea}, fared better than those with a lower generation rate. A later analysis of NCDS data in terms of fractional urea clearance, expressed as Kt/V_{urea}, found that morbidity increased dramatically as Kt/V_{urea} fell below 0.8 volumes per dialysis.[5] Although the longer dialysis treatment time produced a borderline significant improvement in morbidity, two-compartment modeling was not used to examine urea kinetics, so TAC_{urea} was likely higher in the short-time arm than was reported (rebound was not assessed).[4] The absence of an independent impact of dialysis treatment time on morbidity suggested that removal of larger molecules was less important as a determinant of short-term morbidity.

While the NCDS clearly demonstrated the impact of small solute clearance on survival, the impact of MM clearance on survival remained untested in a rigorous fashion until the NIH-sponsored HEMO Study. The HEMO Study was a prospective randomized multicenter clinical trial designed to examine the impact of hemodialysis dose and membrane flux on survival.[6] Patients were randomized to one of four treatment groups: (1) standard Kt/V_{urea} and high-flux membrane; (2) standard Kt/V_{urea} and low-flux membrane; (3) high Kt/V_{urea} and high-flux membrane; (4) high Kt/V_{urea} and low-flux membrane. The standard-Kt/V_{urea} treatment groups targeted an equilibrated Kt/V_{urea} (eKt/V) of 1.05, while the high-Kt/V_{urea} treatment groups targeted an eKt/V_{urea} of 1.45. A low-flux dialyzer was defined as one that had a mean beta$_2$-microglobulin (β_2M) clearance < 10 mL/min during the first use, while a high-flux dialyzer was defined as one that had a mean β_2M clearance > 20 mL/min and an ultrafiltration coefficient > 14 mL/h/mmHg. Dialyzer reprocessing was permitted in the HEMO Study, and various reprocessing techniques were utilized. The study found no significant impact of the dialysis dose or of membrane flux on patient survival. In the subgroup analysis, however, there was a nonsignificant trend toward improved survival in patients on dialysis > 3.7 years who were treated with high-flux membranes, suggesting that patients with different durations (vintage) of dialysis may benefit from high-flux dialysis.[7]

Leypoldt et al. retrospectively examined the impact of dialysis membranes with respect to pore size and chose vitamin B_{12} (1355 Da) as the large solute marker.[8] Using data from the 1991 Case Mix Adequacy Study of the U.S. Renal Data System (USRDS), these investigators found that patients treated with membranes that provided a 10 percent higher calculated vitamin B_{12} clearance had an approximately 5 percent lower mortality risk if Kt/V_{urea} remained constant. If B_{12} clearance remained constant, patients treated with a 0.1-unit higher single-pool Kt/V urea had a 7.5 percent lower mortality risk. While this report demonstrated a role for larger molecules in determining survival, the results could be explained by other variables, such as membrane biocompatibility, nutritional status, or reprocessing technique. Another retrospective analysis of 715 patients treated exclusively with more biocompatible polysulfone membranes found a lower mortality in patients treated with high-flux vs. low-flux hemodialysis.[9] In contrast,

Charra et al. report the highest survival rate in the world for their patients treated with long, slow dialysis (8 hours) thrice weekly using standard cuprophane membranes.[10,11] Since cuprophane membranes do not provide an appreciable clearance of β_2M, survival in this particular population may be related to other factors, such as improvements in extracellular volume and blood pressure control or, alternatively, to improved clearance of solutes in the range of 500 to 2000 Da.[12]

IDENTIFICATION, CHARACTERIZATION, AND BIOACTIVITY OF LARGER UREMIC TOXINS

The identification of the toxins responsible for the uremic state has frustrated scientists for several decades. After the MM hypothesis was proposed, numerous attempts were made to isolate compounds in the molecular-weight range of 500 to 2000 Da from body fluids of uremic patients. The combination of gas chromatography and mass spectrometry was used to identify low-molecular-weight compounds in uremic blood, but this technique was not suitable for analysis of higher-molecular-weight or nonvolatile compounds.[13] Early studies of larger retained solutes relied on ion-exchange chromatography followed by gel filtration for separation and purification of a compound.[14] This was combined with gas chromatography and derivatization for volatile compound formation. Identification and determination of structure was then carried out with mass spectrometry, which demonstrated peaks corresponding to the molecular weight of a compound and characteristic peaks from other ion fragments. Progress in the identification of these larger solutes was slow, however, due to the diversity of methods used for their separation and characterization. Comparison of fractions obtained by different methods was difficult since isolation techniques were so variable. While many suspected fractions were identified in various uremic fluids, chemical composition and bioactivity remained unknown for several years.

Early studies of uremic MMs suggested that they were peptides[14–18] or amino acid conjugates.[19,20] In 1979, Abiko et al. purified and characterized three components from uremic ultrafiltrate, including a heptapeptide (752 Da), a pentapeptide (688 Da), and a tripeptide (340 Da). These efforts were considered major advancements in the research to identify MMs.[16–18] In vitro studies of the biological activity of MMs subsequently demonstrated an inhibition of E-rosette formation,[21] leukocyte migration [22] and proliferation,[23] glucose utilization,[24] phagocytosis[25,26] and platelet aggregation.[27,28] These studies were limited by their small size and lack of control samples from nonuremic patients, but they were the first reports to include the structure and biological activity of mid-molecular-weight peptides.

Analytic techniques continued to advance with the development of size exclusion, ion exchange, affinity, and reversed-phase chromatography.[29–32] The development of high-performance liquid chromatography (HPLC) allowed faster separation and better resolution than conventional liquid chromatography and demonstrated that MM fractions identified by earlier techniques were contaminated by numerous small molecules.[33] Liquid chromatography/mass spectrometry using newer ionization methods is currently the preferred method for analysis of higher-molecular-weight compounds. Other major technologic advances in the analysis of higher-molecular-weight compounds include fast atom bombardment, liquid secondary ion mass spectrometry, and matrix-assisted laser desorption ionization/time-of-flight-mass spectrometry (MALDI-TOFMS).[13] This last technique utilizes a soft-ionization source (MALDI) that vaporizes and ionizes molecules in the range of 500 to 300,000 Da, which are then mass analyzed by TOFMS to determine molecular weight.

Chu et al. have identified six MM compounds in the range of 800 to 2015 Da.[34] These investigators used gel chromatography followed by anion-exchange chromatography, desalting on a Sephadex G column, and characterization by IR, UV, and MALDI-TOFMS. Further separation of a subfraction using HPLC yielded the six compounds that were identified in uremic sera and normal urine but not in uremic urine. The bioactivity of these compounds remains unknown, however.

Kaplan et al. utilized SDS electrophoresis and HPLC to isolate peptides (MW = 520 to 1500 Da) from uremic sera.[35] Amino acid sequencing followed by tandem mass spectrometry revealed that the majority of these peptides were derived from the alpha and beta chains of fibrinogen. The investigators hypothesized that such fibrinogen fragments accumulate in uremic blood and occupy the glycoprotein GPIIb-IIIa receptor on platelet membranes, leading to reduced platelet aggregation and a bleeding diathesis.

Increased concentrations of numerous peptides have now been identified in uremic sera, including parathyroid hormone, β_2M, granulocyte inhibitory proteins, degranulation-inhibiting proteins, and chemotaxis-inhibiting proteins.[13,29–31,36–39] The clinical significance of these molecules is discussed below.

BETA$_2$ MICROGLOBULIN AND DIALYSIS-RELATED AMYLOIDOSIS

Dialysis-related amyloidosis (DRA), a major cause of morbidity in a minority of dialysis patients, is characterized by amyloid deposits primarily in joints and periarticular structures. β_2M was identified as the major constituent of DRA, although a number of other proteins were later discovered in amyloid deposits.[40,41] Accumulation of β_2M in dialysis patients, due to poor or absent elimination by the native kidneys, is most likely the major factor predisposing to the formation of amyloid deposits. β_2M is an 11,800-Da polypeptide that is freely filtered by the glomerulus and then reabsorbed and metabolized by the proximal tubule.[42] Normal β_2M production is 20 to 30 mg/kg/week and serum concentrations are usually less than 2 mg/L. Serum β_2M levels in dialysis patients vary but may be as high as 15 to 30 times normal. β_2M concentrations in the dialysis population depend on residual renal function, properties of the dialysis membrane including flux and adsorption, generation rate, and the modality of renal replacement (convection vs. diffusion).

Clinical manifestations of DRA include carpal tunnel syndrome (CTS), spondyloarthropathies, joint pain and immobility, and, rarely, cardiac and gastrointestinal involvement.[43–46] Arthralgias are usually bilateral and often involve the shoulders, although other joints such as knees, wrists, and small joints of the hand may be involved. DRA is generally reported in long-term survivors of hemodialysis, but it has also been reported prior to the initiation of renal replacement therapy and in CAPD patients.[47,48] To date, β_2M deposits have not been observed in nonuremic subjects. In general, DRA is observed after more than 6 years of dialysis, and the incidence appears to increase with time on dialysis.[49] Symptoms are more common in patients over 40 years of age at the time hemodialysis is initiated and appear to occur earlier in older patients.[50]

Since most amyloid deposits do not appear to cause clinical symptoms[37] and β_2M levels do not correlate with the extent or severity of amyloid deposition,[51] other modifying factors are thought to be involved in the development and pathogenesis of DRA, such as posttranslational modification of proteins via the Maillard reaction. In the initial part of the Maillard reaction, glucose reacts nonenzymatically with protein amino groups to initiate glycation via a Schiff base and subsequent Amadori products. Amadori products can undergo rearrangement to produce highly reactive carbonyl compounds, such as 3-deoxyglucosone. The latter reacts with the free amino groups on proteins to form advanced glycation end products (AGEs). AGEs are characterized by browning, fluorescence, cross-linking, and activation of AGE-specific receptors. Serum levels of 3-deoxyglucosone are elevated in both diabetic and uremic patients. Reaction of 3-deoxyglucosone with β_2M may promote polymerization of the latter and promote DRA.

The observation that β_2M is modified by AGEs such as pentosidine[52] and N^ε (carboxymethyl) lysine[53] led to the proposal that these modifications are necessary for the development of DRA. β_2M that is modified by AGEs can bind to biologically active specific receptors. Such binding has been invoked as an explanation for enhanced chemotaxis of human monocytes in vitro[54] and secretion of bone-resorbing cytokines such as interleukin-1 (IL-1), IL-6, and tumor necrosis factor (TNF). Sakata et al. examined serum pentosidine levels in 127 dialysis patients in a cross-sectional study.[55] Pentosidine levels, but not intact parathyroid hormone levels (iPTH) or β_2M levels, were significantly elevated in patients with DRA defined by spondyloarthropathy and CTS. A greater concentration of pentosidine has been demonstrated in the carpal tunnel ligaments of hemodialysis patients compared to patients with idiopathic CTS.[56] Since diabetic dialysis patients have markedly higher circulating AGE levels than nondiabetic dialysis patients but no higher prevalence of DRA,[57] the clinical significance of AGE-modified proteins in DRA remains uncertain.

Clinical symptoms of DRA are nonspecific, making diagnosis difficult. The "gold standard" for diagnosis remains a biopsy demonstrating Congo-red staining and immunohistochemistry staining of β_2M. The sternoclavicular joint is considered by many to be the best site for biopsy,[46] although one group recommended biopsy of the knee.[37] Alternatives to biopsy include computed tomography, magnetic resonance imaging, and ultrasonography, but the specificity and sensitivity of these diagnostic techniques remain unknown. Scintigraphy using radiolabeled isotopes reveals increased uptake in involved joints. Procedures that utilized radiolabeled serum amyloid P component of β_2M (SAP) or radiolabeled β_2M are most specific.[58,59] Routine screening for DRA is not recommended by the National Kidney Foundation–Kidney Disease Outcomes Quality Initiative (NKF-K/DOQI), since therapies other than renal transplantation remain clinically unproven.

GRANULOCYTE–INHIBITING PROTEINS

Several granulocyte-inhibiting proteins (GIPs) have been isolated and purified from uremic ultrafiltrate and peritoneal effluent. GIP-1 in nanomolar concentrations has been shown to inhibit polymorphonuclear leukocyte glucose uptake, chemotaxis, oxidative metabolism, and intracellular killing of bacteria in vitro.[29] GIP-I has a molecular mass of 28,000 Da and shows 80 percent homology with kappa light chains. GIP-II has an amino acid sequence identical to β_2M and inhibits leukocyte glucose uptake and oxidative metabolism[38] but β_2M does not impair leukocyte function. It is possible that modification of β_2M with AGEs leads to GIP-II formation.

Two degranulation-inhibiting proteins (DIPs) have been isolated from uremic ultrafiltrate obtained from patients undergoing high-flux hemodialysis. DIP-I has a molecular mass of 14,400 Da and is identical to the protein angiogenin.[30] It appears to be involved in lactoferrin release from leukocytes in vitro.[60] DIP-II has been identified as complement factor D.[39] Another GIP has been identified that inhibits leukocyte chemotaxis and shows complete homology to the protein ubiquitin.[31] Since intact ubiquitin does not impair leukocyte chemotaxis, it may also undergo posttranslational modification, possible by AGEs, to form a chemotaxis-inhibiting protein.

PARATHYROID HORMONE

Parathyroid hormone (PTH) is a small polypeptide (84 amino acids) that accumulates in uremia and contributes significantly to co-morbid pathology, most notably osteitis fibrosa. Normal serum levels are between 10 and 65 pg and rise as GFR falls below 50 to 70 mL/min.[61] The major determinant of PTH secretion is the ionized serum calcium concentration, but low serum calcitriol levels and elevated phosphorus levels also stimulate PTH secretion and accelerate the development of secondary hyperparathyroidism. The "trade-off" hypothesis proposed by Bricker in 1972 is based on the effects of uremia on the balance between serum calcium, phosphorus, and PTH levels.[61] The elevations in PTH that occur early in chronic kidney disease help to restore serum calcium and phosphorus levels to normal but subsequently lead to hyperplasia of the parathyroid gland and secondary hyperparathyroidism (trade-off). The response of normal target tissues to PTH is also impaired, at least partially due to decreased expression of PTH receptors but also to decreased numbers of vitamin D– and calcium-sensing receptors.[62]

The most significant consequence of hyperparathyroidism in uremia is the development of osteitis fibrosis, but elevations in serum PTH also promote soft tissue calcifications and contribute to metabolic abnormalities and electroencephalographic changes seen in uremic patients.[63] PTH excess contributes to muscle dysfunction, cardiomyopathy, leukocyte and T-cell dysfunction, and insulin resistance.[64] Bone biopsy remains the gold standard for the diagnosis of osteitis fibrosa. Treatment of secondary hyperparathyroidism includes aggressive control of serum phosphate levels, supplementation with synthetic vitamin D, and parathyroidectomy for refractory cases.

PROTEIN-BOUND UREMIC TOXINS

Several protein-bound compounds have been identified that accumulate in renal failure and exhibit bioactive behavior. Most of these are small solutes and only 2 (leptin and retinal binding protein) of the 25 known protein-bound solutes are above 500 Da in size. The best-known substances in this group include p-cresol, indoxyl sulfate, hippuric acid, 3-carboxy-4-methyl-5-propyl-2-furan-propionic acid (CMPF), and homocysteine. The prototypic protein bound toxin is p-cresol, a small solute that is generated as an end product of protein metabolism and normally is nearly 100 percent bound to plasma protein. Levels of free p-cresol are increased in patients with renal failure, and toxicity appears to be enhanced by increases in the free fraction.[65] High levels of free p-cresol have a negative impact on leukocyte functional capacity, including leukocyte adhesion to endothelium[66] and in vitro chemiluminescence production. Both hypoalbuminemia and increased levels of total p-cresol can increase the free fraction of p-cresol.[67] Displacement by other retained solutes may also contribute to toxicity of albumin or tissue-bound toxins.[68] Hypoalbuminemia is a strong predictor of survival in dialysis patients and is associated with malnutrition and/or inflammation,[69] but it could potentially contribute to uremic toxicity by increasing the free concentration of albumin-bound toxic solutes. Extracorporeal removal of p-cresol using existing technology is low in comparison with that of other small solutes; however low-protein diets and supplementation with *Lactobacillus acidophilus* may lower total levels of p-cresol. Oral sorbents also appear to lower intestinal levels of p-cresol.

Other protein-bound solutes include indoxyl sulfate, a product of gut bacterial metabolism, and indoxyl-β-D-glucuronide, both of which have been measured in uremic sera using HPLC with fluorescence detection. Indoxyl sulfate is 90 percent bound to serum albumin. It accumulates in renal failure and is available for removal during hemodialysis only in the free form (10 percent). Indoxyl sulfate inhibits drug binding to serum albumin in uremic patients and inhibits hepatic transport of tetraiodothyronine, leading to low triiodothyronine (T_3) levels in uremic patients.[70] It also stimulates the progression of renal failure in rats[71] via the synthesis of transforming growth factor beta$_1$ (TGF-β_1).[72,73] Both p-cresol and indoxyl sulfate decrease endothelial proliferation and inhibit wound repair.[66] Levels of indoxyl-β-D-glucuronide in serum are markedly increased in undialyzed uremic patients but are also increased in hemodialysis and CAPD patients. Despite a protein-bound ratio of about 50 percent, indoxyl-β-D-glucuronide is efficiently removed by hemodialysis. Administration of the oral sorbent AST-120 markedly reduces serum and urine levels of both indoxyl sulfate and indoxyl-β-D-glucuronide in undialyzed uremic patients.

Mass spectrometry and nuclear magnetic resonance has been identified 3-carboxy-4-methyl-5-propyl-2-furanpropionic acid (CMPF) and, more recently, by HPLC with UV detection.[74,75] It is nearly 100 percent bound to albumin and has been found to inhibit albumin binding of drugs in uremic sera.[75-77] It also inhibits erythroid colony formation and may contribute to the anemia of renal disease.[78] Along with indoxyl sulfate, it may account for low T_3 levels in uremic patients.[70] While CMPF is not removed by hemodialysis, the loss of albumin that occurs in CAPD may lead to lower levels in CAPD patients.[78]

ANEMIA AND LARGER RETAINED SOLUTES

Anemia is a major and nearly universal finding in patients with advanced chronic kidney disease, largely due to erythropoietin deficiency. While the use of recombinant human erythropoietin has drastically improved the anemia associated with kidney disease, some patients remain resistant to this agent for a variety of reasons, including iron deficiency, infection and inflammation,[36] hyperparathyroidism, aluminum toxicity, and vitamin deficiencies. Adequate dialysis, including removal of small and medium-sized molecules, is necessary for the correction of anemia. A prospective randomized study of 135 dialysis patients found that increasing dialysis dose led to an improvement in response to erythropoietin in patients who were inadequately dialyzed.[79] This study utilized high-flux biocompatible dialysis membranes, so it is possible that removal of higher-molecular-weight solutes played a role in correcting the anemia. Other investigators have reported improvements in anemia in patients treated with high-flux membranes, but the studies were nonrandomized, lacking in a control group, or lacking in strict exclusion criteria.[80,81] A more recent prospective randomized clinical trial examined the impact of high-flux biocompatible membranes in selected patients and found no improvement in hemoglobin levels after 3 months of treatment.[82] The study protocol appropriately excluded patients who were underdialyzed, malnourished, iron- or vitamin-deficient, or had evidence of either aluminum bone disease or hyperparathyroidism.

ELIMINATION OF BETA$_2$ MICROGLOBULIN BY DIALYSIS, HEMOFILTRATION, AND ADSORPTION

High-flux hemodialysis and ultrapure bicarbonate dialysate may postpone the appearance of DRA, but the role of the dialysis membrane and type of renal replacement remains unclear.[83-85] Several controlled trials have found that polysulfone membranes remove more β_2M from serum than cuprophane membranes, but total removal remains a fraction of daily production.[86-88] Other mechanisms of removal appear to be active. Lower β_2M levels correlate with a lower incidence of DRA, as evidenced by CTS, bone cysts, and decreased synovial thickness by shoulder ultrasound.[86] Patients treated solely with polyacrylonitrile membranes (AN69) also have fewer signs and symptoms of DRA than those treated with cellulosic membranes.[50] Newer synthetic membranes are more biocompatible, however, and may stimulate less β_2M formation and release during dialysis.[89,90]

In a retrospective study of DRA, Schiffl et al. found the lowest prevalence in patients treated with high-flux biocompatible membranes and in patients treated with less contaminated dialysate.[91] Other investigators found that membrane flux is a more important determinant of serum β_2M levels than membrane biocompatibility.[83] Potential disadvantages of high-flux membranes include loss of albumin when bleach is used for reprocessing and backflow of nonsterile dialysate.[92,93] Dialysate purity may be a more important factor than biocompatibility, since CAPD patients also develop DRA and have no exposure to foreign membranes. The incidence of CTS after 10 years of dialysis using ultrapure dialysate was 7 percent in another retrospective analysis,[94] much lower than the incidence reported by other investigators.[50,95]

Hemofiltration was initially introduced as a renal replacement modality with the advantages of convective removal of higher-molecular-weight solutes and improved cardiovascular stability. Convective removal of solutes using biocompatible membranes also offers potential survival advantages and reduced morbidity due to DRA.[95,96] However, adequate removal of small solutes has been difficult, especially during early applications of hemofiltration, and urea clearances have been generally lower than afforded by hemodialysis. The additional diffusive clearance provided by predilutional infusion of replacement fluids has improved small solute clearance in more recent applications.

Predilutional hemofiltration reduces the serum concentration of β_2M more than low-flux hemodialysis and is associated with greater postdialysis rebound, but the ultimate effect is a lower predialysis serum concentration at subsequent dialysis sessions.[82,97] The net β_2M reduction provided by hemofiltration performed daily using the AN69 membrane was 36 percent per session in one study.[98] Unfortunately, daily treatments were necessary to remove a significant mass of β_2M, and they were unable to normalize serum levels. To enhance β_2M removal, Lornoy et al. examined the impact of convection and diffusion combined with a high-flux biocompatible membrane. The investigators studied high-dose predilutional hemodiafiltration (6 L/h) and conventional hemodialysis, both performed in 4-hour treatments with high-flux membranes.[99] The clearance of β_2M by hemodiafiltration was nearly twice that of hemodialysis (116.8 vs. 63.8 mL/min).

Sorbents remove solutes from solution by specific or nonspecific adsorption. Specific adsorbents utilize highly selective ligands or antibodies, but their clinical use is limited by cost and a low capacity for toxin removal. Nonspecific adsorbents rely on hydrophobic interactions, ionic attraction, and van der Waals forces and have a high capacity for toxin removal. Charcoal and resins are inexpensive, nonspecific sorbents, but they may have poor hemocompatibility.[100] Sorbents are considered an adjunct to hemodialysis, since they adsorb water, urea, and acids poorly. Commercially available devices provide nonspecific β_2M removal that may also deplete other small proteins and peptides. Abe et al. used high-flux dialysis to treat patients with

dialysis-related amyloidosis for 1 year and found no change in β_2M levels.[101] These patients were subsequently treated with a commercially available adsorption column in series with a high-flux dialyzer and were found to have significantly lower serum β_2M levels, increased pinch strength, and reduced median motor latency after 1 year of treatment.

The recent addition of a hemocompatible coating to nonspecific sorbents may allow more widespread use.[102] Combined hemodialysis and hemoperfusion using biocompatible resin beads reduced plasma β_2M levels by approximately 70 percent in a preliminary study and produced no changes in albumin concentration, platelet counts, or leukocyte counts.[103] The investigators also observed reductions in other MMs, including leptin and angiogenin. The vortexflow plasmapheretic reactor is another specific adsorption device based on high-affinity immunoadsorption of β_2M.[104] In a preliminary study, this device cleared β_2M from human whole blood below detectable limits after 2 hours of hemoperfusion and resulted in no hemocompatibility complications. While newer technologies have improved β_2M clearance, they are costly and still not widely available.

PERITONEAL DIALYSIS

Plasma β_2M levels are lower in CAPD patients than in hemodialysis patients—a finding that could be explained by better preservation of residual renal function or by higher permeability of the peritoneal membrane.[41,105,106] Plasma β_2M levels correlate inversely with residual renal function for both hemodialysis and CAPD patients.[107–109] Several studies have demonstrated that plasma β_2M levels remain lower in CAPD patients than in hemodialysis patients matched for residual renal function and duration of dialysis therapy.[107,110] However, Tan et al. performed SAP scintigraphy in peritoneal dialysis patients and found that the prevalence of DRA based on positive scan results was similar for hemodialysis and CAPD patients.[111] A recent autopsy study also failed to find a statistically significant difference in the incidence of amyloid deposition in CAPD and hemodialysis patients.[112] Daily removal of β_2M averages 38 mg in CAPD patients and directly correlates with plasma levels of β_2M. CAPD may provide lower serum β_2M levels than hemodialysis with cuprophane membranes, but the reported incidence of CTS is not lower in patients treated with CAPD.[48,113] Although plasma β_2M levels may be lower in CAPD, this may only serve to delay the onset of DRA.

DAILY AND NOCTURNAL HEMODIALYSIS

While the HEMO Study showed no significant difference in the survival of patients randomized to different conventional hemodialysis schedules, more frequent hemodialysis schedules show greater potential for improvements in morbidity and mortality. The recent literature documents better control of blood pressure, dry weight, and, in some cases, decreases in erythropoietin doses in patients receiving short daily (1.5 to 2.5 h/day) hemodialysis.[114,115]

Nocturnal hemodialysis (performed nightly for 6 to 10 hours) increases removal of both low- and higher-molecular-weight solutes—including urea, phosphorus, and β_2M—and reduces or eliminates the requirement for phosphate binders for most patients.[116] Raj et al. studied β_2M kinetics in 10 anuric patients in a crossover trial of conventional hemodialysis performed thrice weekly and six nocturnal sessions per week using slower blood and dialysate flow rates.[117] While weekly removal of urea and creatinine were comparable for the two modalities at the flow rates studied, the mass of β_2M removed was significantly higher for nocturnal hemodialysis (585 vs. 127 mg), with a reduction in serum levels of 38.8 vs. 20.5 percent. No correlation was made between clinical symptoms and serum β_2M levels in this study. A study in patients treated with short daily hemodialysis for 6 months revealed lower levels of pentosidine-like AGE compounds measured by total fluorescence compared to corresponding levels in patients treated with either conventional hemodialysis or CAPD.[118] Predialysis levels of protein-linked pentosidine were also significantly lower in patients treated with daily hemodialysis. The same investigators also found that serum levels of the protein-bound solutes indole-3-acetic acid, indoxyl sulfate, and p-cresol were lower for patients treated with daily hemodialysis.

TREATMENT AND PREVENTION OF DRA

Renal transplantation rapidly reduces serum β_2M levels[119] and may improve signs and symptoms of DRA, but radiographic evidence of DRA remains unchanged by transplantation even after many months of follow-up.[120–122] Indeed, β_2M amyloid deposits have been identified in joint structures 10 years after successful renal transplantation.[123,124] The mechanism of joint pain relief may be related more to the anti-inflammatory effect of steroids and less to the regression of amyloid. Disease progression does appear to be arrested radiographically, as evidenced by the absence of changes in bone cyst size after transplantation. Transplant recipients have other bone disorders largely due to the adverse effects of steroids, including epiphyseal necrosis, tendon rupture, and septic arthritis.

More conservative therapy includes use of nonsteroidal anti-inflammatory drugs (NSAIDs), topical steroid ointments, and surgical interventions such as carpal tunnel decompression and resection of amyloid deposits. One group reported improvement in symptoms of DRA after change from cuprophane membranes to biocompatible

membranes, but placebo effects could also explain the results.[125]

CONCLUSIONS

A wide variety of compounds—including small- and larger-molecular-weight solutes as well as protein-bound toxins—accumulate in uremic patients. Despite advances in renal replacement therapies, many of these compounds are not effectively removed by currently available technology and may have an adverse clinical impact. β_2M is the best-studied larger molecule, and numerous studies show that it can cause significant morbidity in long-vintage patients. Other larger solutes contribute to specific clinical derangements, including impaired immune response, endocrine abnormalities. and neurologic dysfunction. While the balance of current data indicates that the immediate life-threatening risks associated with the uremic state are caused by small solutes, the obvious complexity of the residual uremic milieu and limited findings to date from clinical research suggest a potential role for larger solutes.

REFERENCES

1. Scribner BH, Farrell PC, Milutinovic J, Babb AL. Evolution of the middle molecule hypothesis. In: Villareal H, ed. *Proceedings of the Fifth International Congress of Nephrology.* Basel: Karger, 1974:190–199.
2. Babb AL, Popovich RP, Christopher TG, Scribner BH. The genesis of the square meter-hour hypothesis. *Trans Am Soc Artif Intern Organs* 1971;17:81–91.
3. Vanholder R, De Smet R, Glorieux G, et al. Review on uremic toxins: classification, concentration, and interindividual variability. *Kidney Int* 2003;63:1934–1943.
4. Lowrie EG, Laird NM, Parker TF, Sargent JA. Effect of the hemodialysis prescription of patient morbidity: report from the National Cooperative Dialysis Study. *N Engl J Med* 1981;305:1176–1181.
5. Gotch FA, Sargent JA. A mechanistic analysis of the National Cooperative Dialysis Study (NCDS). *Kidney Int* 1985;28:526–534.
6. Eknoyan G, Beck GJ, Cheung AK, et al. Effect of dialysis dose and membrane flux in maintenance hemodialysis. *N Engl J Med* 2002;347:2010–2019.
7. Cheung AK, Levin NW, Greene T, et al. Effects of high-flux hemodialysis on clinical outcomes: results of the HEMO study. *J Am Soc Nephrol* 2003;14:3251–3263.
8. Leypoldt JK, Cheung AK, Carroll CE, et al. Effect of dialysis membranes and middle molecule removal on chronic hemodialysis patient survival. *Am J Kidney Dis 1999;33:* 349–355.
9. Woods HF, Nandakumar M. Improved outcome for haemodialysis patients treated with high-flux membranes. *Nephrol Dial Transplant* 2000;15(suppl 1):36–42.

10. Charra B, Calemard M, Laurent G. Importance of treatment time and blood pressure control in achieving long–term survival on dialysis. *Am J Nephrol* 1996;16:35–44.

11. Charra B, Calemard E, Ruffet M, et al. Survival as an index of adequacy of dialysis. *Kidney Int* 1992;41:1286–1291.

12. Charra B, Chazot C, Jean G, et al. Long 3 × 8 hr dialysis: a three-decade summary. *J Nephrol* 2003;16(suppl 7): S64–S69.

13. Niwa T. Mass spectrometry in the search for uremic toxins. *Mass Spectrom Rev* 1997;16:307–332.

14. Furst P, Zimmerman L, Bergstrom J. Determination of endogenous middle molecules in normal and uremic body fluids. *Clin Nephrol* 1976;3:178–188.

15. Klein A, Sarnecka–Keller M, Hanicki Z. Middle-sized ninhydrin-positive molecules in uraemic patients treated by repeated haemodialysis. II. Chief peptide constituents of the faction. *Clin Chim Acta* 1978;90:7–11.

16. Abiko T, Onodera I, Sekino H. Isolation, structure and biological activity of the Trp-containing pentapeptide from uremic fluid. *Biochem Biophys Res Commun* 1979;89: 813–821.

17. Abiko T, Kumikawa M, Higuchi H, Sekino H. Identification and synthesis of a heptapeptide in uremic fluid. *Biochem Biophys Res Commun* 1978;84:184–194.

18. Abiko T, Kumikawa M, Ishizaki M, et al. Identification and synthesis of a tripeptide in ECUM fluid of an uremic patient. *Biochem Biophys Res Commun* 1978;83:357–364.

19. Zimmerman L, Jornvall H, Bergstrom J, et al. Characterization of a double conjugate in uremic body fluids. *FEBS Lett* 129:237–240, 1981.

20. Bergstrom J, Furst P, Zimmerman L. Separation, isolation, and identification of middle molecules. *Artif Organs* 1981;4(suppl):5–7.

21. Abiko T, Kumikawa M, Sekino H. Inhibition effect of rosette formation between human lymphocytes and sheep erythrocytes by specific heptapeptide isolated from uremic fluid and its analogs. *Biochem Biophys Res Commun* 1979; 86:945–952.

22. Cichocki T, Hanicki Z, Klein A, et al. Influence of middle-molecular-weight solutes from dialysate on the migration rate of leukocytes. *Kidney Int* 1980;17:231–236.

23. Navarro J, Contreras P, Touraine JL, et al. Effect of middle molecules on immunological functions. *Artif Organs* 1981;4(suppl):76–81.

24. Dzurik R, Hupkova V, Cernacek P, et al. The isolation of an inhibitor of glucose utilization from the serum of uraemic subjects. *Clin Chim Acta* 1973;46:77–83.

25. Vanholder R, Ringoir S, Dhondt A, Hakim R. Phagocytosis in uremic and hemodialysis patients: a prospective and cross sectional study. *Kidney Int* 1991;39:320–327.

26. Ringoir SM, van Landschoot N, De Smet R. Inhibition of phagocytosis by a middle molecular fraction from ultrafiltrate. *Clin Nephrol* 1980;13:109–112.

27. Gallice P, Fournier N, Crevat A, et al. "In vitro" inhibition of platelet aggregation by uremic middle molecules. *Biomedicine* 1980;33:185–188.

28. Maejima M, Takahashi S, Hatano M. Platelet aggregation in chronic renal failure—whole blood aggregation and effect of guanidino compounds. *Nippon Jinzo Gakkai Shi* 1991;33: 201–212.

29. Horl WH, Haag-Weber M, Georgopoulos A, Block LH. Physicochemical characterization of a polypeptide present in uremic serum that inhibits the biological activity of polymorphonuclear cells. *Proc Natl Acad Sci USA* 1990;87: 6353–6357.

30. Tschesche H, Kopp C, Horl WH, Hempelmann U. Inhibition of degranulation of polymorphonuclear leukocytes by angiogenin and its tryptic fragment. *J Biol Chem* 1994;269: 30274–30280.

31. Cohen G, Rudnicki M, Horl WH. Isolation of modified ubiquitin as a neutrophil chemotaxis inhibitor from uremic patients. *J Am Soc Nephrol* 1998;9:451–456.

32. Nyberg G, Sanderson K, Andren P, et al. Isolation of haemorphin-related peptides from filter membranes collected in connection with haemofiltration of human subjects. *J Chromatogr A* 1996;723:43–49.

33. Schoots AC, Mikkers FE, Claessens HA, et al. Characterization of uremic "middle molecular" fractions by gas chromatography, mass spectrometry, isotachyphoresis, and liquid chromatography. *Clin Chem* 1982;28:45–49.

34. Chu J, Yuan Z, Liu X, et al. Separation of six uremic middle molecular compounds by high performance liquid chromatography and analysis by matrix-assisted laser desorption/ionization time-of-flight mass spectrometry. *Clin Chim Acta* 2001;311:95–107.

35. Kaplan B, Cojocaru M, Unsworth E, et al. Search for peptidic "middle molecules" in uremic sera: isolation and chemical identification of fibrinogen fragments. *J Chromatogr B Analyt Technol Biomed Life Sci* 2003;796: 141–153.

36. Horl WH. Are new toxins appearing on the horizon? *Contrib Nephrol* 2001;28[AU6]–41.

37. Jadoul M, Garbar C, Noel H, et al. Histological prevalence of beta 2-microglobulin amyloidosis in hemodialysis: a prospective post-mortem study. *Kidney Int* 1997;51: 1928–1932.

38. Haag-Weber M, Mai B, Cohen G, Horl WH. GIP and DIP: a new view of uraemic toxicity. *Nephrol Dial Transplant* 1994;9:346–347.

39. Balke N, Holtkamp U, Horl WH, Tschesche H. Inhibition of degranulation of human polymorphonuclear leukocytes by complement factor D. *FEBS Lett* 1995;371:300–302.

40. Gejyo F, Yamada T, Odani S, et al. A new form of amyloid protein associated with chronic hemodialysis was identified as beta 2-microglobulin. *Biochem Biophys Res Commun* 1985;129:701–706.

41. Gorevic PD, Casey TT, Stone WJ, et al. Beta 2-microglobulin is an amyloidogenic protein in man. *J Clin Invest* 1985;76:2425–2429.

42. Karlsson FA, Wibell L, Evrin PE. Beta 2-microglobulin in clinical medicine. *Scand J Clin Lab Invest Suppl* 1980;154: 27–37.

43. Dzido G, Sprague SM. Dialysis-related amyloidosis. *Minerva Urol Nefrol* 2003;55:121–129.

44. Campistol JM, Sole M, Munoz-Gomez J, et al. Systemic involvement of dialysis-amyloidosis. *Am J Nephrol* 1990;10: 389–396.

45. Campistol JM, Cases A, Torras A, et al. Visceral involvement of dialysis amyloidosis. *Am J Nephrol* 1987;7: 390–393.

46. Zingraff JJ, Noel LH, Bardin T et al: Beta 2-microglobulin amyloidosis in chronic renal failure. *N Engl J Med* 1990;323:1070–1071.

47. Moriniere P, Marie A, el Esper N, et al. Destructive spondyloarthropathy with beta 2-microglobulin amyloid deposits in a uremic patient before chronic hemodialysis. *Nephron* 1991;59:654–657.

48. Benz RL, Siegfried JW, Teehan BP. Carpal tunnel syndrome in dialysis patients: comparison between continuous ambulatory peritoneal dialysis and hemodialysis populations. *Am J Kidney Dis* 1988;11:473–476.

49. Onishi S, Andress DL, Maloney NA, et al. Beta 2-microglobulin deposition in bone in chronic renal failure. *Kidney Int* 1991;39:990–995.

50. van Ypersele dS, Jadoul M, Malghem J, et al. Effect of dialysis membrane and patient's age on signs of dialysis-related amyloidosis. The Working Party on Dialysis Amyloidosis. *Kidney Int* 1991;39:1012–1019.

51. Gejyo F, Homma N, Suzuki Y, Arakawa M. Serum levels of beta 2-microglobulin as a new form of amyloid protein in patients undergoing long-term hemodialysis. *N Engl J Med* 1986;314:585–586.

52. Miyata T, Taneda S, Kawai R, et al. Identification of pentosidine as a native structure for advanced glycation end products in beta 2-microglobulin-containing amyloid fibrils in patients with dialysis-related amyloidosis. *Proc Natl Acad Sci USA* 1996;93:2353–2358.

53. Niwa T, Sato M, Katsuzaki T, et al. Amyloid beta 2-microglobulin is modified with N epsilon-(carboxymethyl) lysine in dialysis-related amyloidosis. *Kidney Int* 1996;50: 1303–1309.

54. Miyata T, Hori O, Zhang J, et al. The receptor for advanced glycation end products (RAGE) is a central mediator of the interaction of AGE-beta2-microglobulin with human mononuclear phagocytes via an oxidant-sensitive pathway. Implications for the pathogenesis of dialysis-related amyloidosis. *J Clin Invest* 1996;98:1088–1094.

55. Sakata S, Takahashi M, Kushida K, et al. The relationship between pentosidine and hemodialysis-related connective tissue disorders. *Nephron* 1998;78:260–265.

56. Takahashi M, Hoshino H, Kushida K, et al. The advanced glycation endproduct, pentosidine, in the carpal ligament in patients with carpal tunnel syndrome undergoing hemodialysis: comparison with idiopathic carpal tunnel syndrome. *Nephron* 1998;80:444–449.

57. Lehnert H, Jacob C, Marzoll I, et al. Prevalence of dialysis-related amyloidosis in diabetic patients. Diabetes Amyloid Study Group. *Nephrol Dial Transplant* 1996;11:2004–2007.

58. Nelson SR, Hawkins PN, Richardson S, et al. Imaging of haemodialysis-associated amyloidosis with 123I-serum amyloid P component. *Lancet* 1991;338:335–339.

59. Floege J, Burchert W, Brandis A, et al. Imaging of dialysis-related amyloid (AB-amyloid) deposits with 131I-beta 2-microglobulin. *Kidney Int* 1990;38:1169–1176.

60. Schmaldienst S, Oberpichler A, Tschesche H, Horl WH. Angiogenin: a novel inhibitor of neutrophil lactoferrin release during extracorporeal circulation. *Kidney Blood Press Res* 2003;26:107–112.

61. Slatopolsky E, Rutherford WE, Hoffsten PE, et al. Non-suppressible secondary hyperparathyroidism in chronic progressive renal disease. *Kidney Int* 1972;1:38–46.

62. Martin-Salvago M, Villar-Rodriguez JL, Palma-Alvarez A, et al. Decreased expression of calcium receptor in parathyroid tissue in patients with hyperparathyroidism secondary to chronic renal failure. *Endocr Pathol* 2003;14:61–70.

63. Klahr S, Slatopolsky E. Toxicity of parathyroid hormone in uremia. *Annu Rev Med* 1986;37:7171–7178.

64. Slatopolsky E, Martin K, Hruska K. Parathyroid hormone metabolism and its potential as a uremic toxin. *Am J Physiol* 1980;239:F1–12.

65. De Smet R, Van Kaer J, Van Vlem B, et al. Toxicity of free p-cresol: a prospective and cross-sectional analysis. *Clin Chem* 2003;49:470–478.

66. Dou L, Cerini C, Brunet P, et al. P-cresol, a uremic toxin, decreases endothelial cell response to inflammatory cytokines. *Kidney Int* 2002;62:1999–2009.

67. De Smet R, Van Kaer J, Van Vlem B, et al. Toxicity of free p-cresol: a prospective and cross-sectional analysis. *Clin Chem* 2003;49:470–478.

68. Gulyassy PF, Bottini AT, Stanfel LA, et al. Isolation and chemical identification of inhibitors of plasma ligand binding. *Kidney Int* 1986;30:391–398.

69. Kaysen GA. Biological basis of hypoalbuminemia in ESRD. *J Am Soc Nephrol* 1998;9:2368–2376.

70. Lim CF, Bernard BF, de Jong M, et al. A furan fatty acid and indoxyl sulfate are the putative inhibitors of thyroxine hepatocyte transport in uremia. *J Clin Endocrinol Metab* 1993;76:318–324.

71. Niwa T, Ise M, Miyazaki T. Progression of glomerular sclerosis in experimental uremic rats by administration of indole, a precursor of indoxyl sulfate. *Am J Nephrol* 1994;14:207–212.

72. Miyazaki T, Ise M, Hirata M, et al. Indoxyl sulfate stimulates renal synthesis of transforming growth factor-beta 1 and progression of renal failure. *Kidney Int Suppl* 1997;63:S211–S214.

73. Miyazaki T, Ise M, Seo H, Niwa T. Indoxyl sulfate increases the gene expressions of TGF-beta 1, TIMP-1 and pro-alpha 1(I) collagen in uremic rat kidneys. *Kidney Int Suppl* 1997;62:S15–S22.

74. Spiteller M, Spiteller G. Occurrence of alpha-alkyl-substituted malic acids, and beta-hydroxy-beta-alkyl-substituted dicarboxylic and tricarboxylic acid derivatives in normal urine (author's transl). *J Chromatogr* 1979;164:319–329.

75. Niwa T, Kawagishi I, Ohya N. Rapid assay for furancarboxylic acid accumulated in uremic serum using high-performance liquid chromatography and on-line mass spectrometry. *Clin Chim Acta* 1994;226:89–94.

76. Mabuchi H, Nakahashi H. Isolation and characterization of an endogenous drug-binding inhibitor present in uremic serum. Nephron 1986;44:277–281.

77. Mabuchi H, Nakahashi H. Profiling of endogenous ligand solutes that bind to serum proteins in sera of patients with uremia. *Nephron* 1986;43:110–116.

78. Niwa T, Yazawa T, Kodama T, et al. Efficient removal of albumin-bound furancarboxylic acid, an inhibitor of erythropoiesis, by continuous ambulatory peritoneal dialysis. *Nephron* 1990;56:241–245.

79. Ifudu O, Feldman J, Friedman EA. The intensity of hemodialysis and the response to erythropoietin in patients with end-stage renal disease. *N Engl J Med* 1996;334: 420–425.

80. Yamada S, Kataoka H, Kobayashi H, et al. Identification of an erythropoietic inhibitor from the dialysate collected in the hemodialysis with PMMA membrane (BK-F). *Contrib Nephrol* 1999;125:159–172.

81. Depner TA, Rizwan S, James LA. Effectiveness of low dose erythropoietin: a possible advantage of high flux hemodialysis. *ASAIO Trans* 1990;36:M223–M225.

82. Locatelli F, Andrulli S, Pecchini F, et al. Effect of high-flux dialysis on the anaemia of haemodialysis patients. *Nephrol Dial Transplant* 2000;15:1399–1409.

83. Pickett TM, Cruickshank A, Greenwood RN, et al. Membrane flux not biocompatibility determines beta-2-microglobulin levels in hemodialysis patients. *Blood Purif* 2002;20:161–166.

84. Baz M, Durand C, Ragon A, et al. Using ultrapure water in hemodialysis delays carpal tunnel syndrome. *Int J Artif Organs* 1991;14:681–685.

85. Lonnemann G, Koch KM. Beta(2)-microglobulin amyloidosis: effects of ultrapure dialysate and type of dialyzer membrane. *J Am Soc Nephrol* 2002;13(suppl 1):S72–S77.

86. Kuchle C, Fricke H, Held E, Schiffl H. High-flux hemodialysis postpones clinical manifestation of dialysis-related amyloidosis. *Am J Nephrol* 1996;16:484–488.

87. Mayer G, Thum J, Woloszczuk W, Graf H. Beta-2-microglobulin in hemodialysis patients. Effects of different dialyzers and different dialysis procedures. *Am J Nephrol* 1988;8:280–284.

88. Ward RA, Schaefer RM, Falkenhagen D, et al. Biocompatibility of a new high-permeability modified cellulose membrane for haemodialysis. *Nephrol Dial Transplant* 1993;8:47–53.

89. Zaoui PM, Stone WJ, Hakim RM. Effects of dialysis membranes on beta 2-microglobulin production and cellular expression. *Kidney Int* 1990;38:962–968.

90. Hakim RM, Wingard RL, Husni L, et al. The effect of membrane biocompatibility on plasma beta 2-microglobulin levels in chronic hemodialysis patients. *J Am Soc Nephrol* 1996;7:472–478.

91. Schiffl H, Fischer R, Lang SM, Mangel E. Clinical manifestations of AB-amyloidosis: effects of biocompatibility and flux. *Nephrol Dial Transplant* 2000;15:840–845.

92. Ikizler TA, Flakoll PJ, Parker RA, Hakim RM. Amino acid and albumin losses during hemodialysis. *Kidney Int* 1994;46:830–837.

93. Kaplan AA, Halley SE, Lapkin RA, Graeber CW. Dialysate protein losses with bleach processed polysulphone dialyzers. *Kidney Int* 1995;47:573–578.

94. Kleophas W, Haastert B, Backus G, et al. Long–term experience with an ultrapure individual dialysis fluid with a batch type machine. *Nephrol Dial Transplant* 1998;13:3118–3125.

95. Locatelli F, Marcelli D, Conte F, et al. Comparison of mortality in ESRD patients on convective and diffusive extracorporeal treatments. The Registro Lombardo Dialisi e Trapianto. *Kidney Int* 1999;55:286–293.

96. Koda Y, Nishi S, Miyazaki S, et al. Switch from conventional to high-flux membrane reduces the risk of carpal tunnel syndrome and mortality of hemodialysis patients. *Kidney Int* 1997;52:1096–1101.

97. Ward RA, Schmidt B, Hullin J, et al. A comparison of online hemodiafiltration and high-flux hemodialysis: a prospective clinical study. *J Am Soc Nephrol* 2000;11: 2344–2350.

98. Canaud B, Assounga A, Flavier JL, et al. Beta-2 microglobulin serum levels in maintenance dialysis. What does it mean? *ASAIO Trans* 1998;34:923–929.

99. Lornoy W, Becaus I, Billiouw JM, et al. On-line haemodiafiltration. Remarkable removal of beta2 microglobulin. Long-term clinical observations. *Nephrol Dial Transplant* 2000;15(suppl 1):49–54.

100. Pond SM. Extracorporeal techniques in the treatment of poisoned patients. *Med J Aust* 1991;154:617–622.

101. Abe T, Uchita K, Orita H, et al. Effect of beta(2)-microglobulin adsorption column on dialysis-related amyloidosis. *Kidney Int* 2003;64:1522–1528.

102. Ronco C, Brendolan A, Winchester JF, et al. First clinical experience with an adjunctive hemoperfusion device designed specifically to remove beta(2)-microglobulin in hemodialysis. *Blood Purif* 2001;19:260–263.

103. Winchester JF, Ronco C, Brady JA, et al. The next step from high-flux dialysis: application of sorbent technology. *Blood Purif* 2002;20:81–86.

104. Ameer GA, Grovender EA, Ploegh H, et al. A novel immunoadsorption device for removing beta2-microglobulin from whole blood. *Kidney Int* 2001;59:1544–1550.

105. Catizone L, Cocchi R, Fusaroli M, Zucchelli P. Relationship between plasma beta 2-microglobulin and residual diuresis in continuous ambulatory peritoneal dialysis and hemodialysis patients. *Perit Dial Int* 1993;13(suppl 2):S523–S526.

106. Scalamogna A, Imbasciati E, De Vecchi A, et al. Beta-2 microglobulin in patients on peritoneal dialysis and hemodialysis. *Perit Dial Int* 1989;9:37–40.

107. Tielemans C, Dratwa M, Bergmann P, et al. Continuous ambulatory peritoneal dialysis vs haemodialysis: a lesser risk of amyloidosis? *Nephrol Dial Transplant* 1988;3:291–294.

108. Duranti E, Sasdelli M. Serum B2 microglobulin (B2M) in CAPD. *Adv Perit Dial* 1989;5:195–199.

109. Vincent C, Revillard JP, Galland M, Traeger J. Serum beta2-microglobulin in hemodialyzed patients. *Nephron* 1978;21: 260–268.

110. Kabanda A, Goffin E, Bernard A, et al. Factors influencing serum levels and peritoneal clearances of low molecular weight proteins in continuous ambulatory peritoneal dialysis. *Kidney Int* 1995;48:1946–1952.

111. Tan SY, Baillod R, Brown E, et al. Clinical, radiological and serum amyloid P component scintigraphic features of beta2-microglobulin amyloidosis associated with continuous ambulatory peritoneal dialysis. *Nephrol Dial Transplant* 1999;14:1467–1471.

112. Jadoul M, Garbar C, Vanholder R, et al. Prevalence of histological beta2-microglobulin amyloidosis in CAPD patients compared with hemodialysis patients. *Kidney Int* 1998;54:956–959.

113. Gonzalez T, Cruz A, Balsa A, et al. Erosive azotemic osteoarthropathy of the hands in chronic ambulatory peritoneal dialysis and hemodialysis. *Clin Exp Rheumatol* 1997;15:367–371.

114. Lindsay RM, Kortas C. Hemeral (daily) hemodialysis. *Adv Renal Replace Ther* 2001;8:236–249.

115. Klarenbach S, Heidenheim AP, Leitch R, Lindsay RM. Reduced requirement for erythropoietin with quotidian hemodialysis therapy. *ASAIO J* 2002;48:57–61.

116. Pierratos A, Ouwendyk M, Francoeur R, et al. Nocturnal hemodialysis: three-year experience. *J Am Soc Nephrol* 1998;9:859–868.

117. Raj DS, Ouwendyk M, Francoeur R, Pierratos A. beta(2)-microglobulin kinetics in nocturnal haemodialysis. *Nephrol Dial Transplant* 2000;15:58–64.

118. Fagugli RM, Vanholder R, De Smet R, et al. Advanced glycation end products: specific fluorescence changes of pentosidine-like compounds during short daily hemodialysis. *Int J Artif Organs* 2001;24:256–262.

119. Edwards LC, Helderman JH, Hamm LL, et al. Noninvasive monitoring of renal transplant function by analysis of beta 2-microglobulin. *Kidney Int* 1983;23:767–770.

120. Jadoul M, Malghem J, Pirson Y, et al. Effect of renal transplantation on the radiological signs of dialysis amyloid osteoarthropathy. *Clin Nephrol* 1989;32:194–197.

121. Campistol JM, Ponz E, Munoz-Gomez J, et al. Renal transplantation for dialysis amyloidosis. *Transplant Proc* 1992;24:118–119.

122. Bardin T, Lebail-Darne JL, Zingraff J, et al. Dialysis arthropathy: outcome after renal transplantation. *Am J Med* 1995;99:243–248.

123. Sethi D, Brown EA, Cary NR, et al. Persistence of dialysis amyloid after renal transplantation. A case report. *Am J Nephrol* 1989;9:173–174.

124. Kessler M, Aymard B, Pourel J. Persistence of beta 2-microglobulin amyloid 10 years after renal transplantation. *Nephrol Dial Transplant* 1994;9:333–334.

125. Hardouin P, Flipo RM, Foissac–Gegoux P, et al. Dialysis-related beta 2 microglobulin-amyloid arthropathy. Improvement of clinical symptoms after a switch of dialysis membranes. *Clin Rheumatol* 1988;7:41–45.

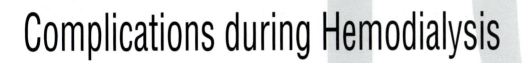

Complications during Hemodialysis

Shubho R. Sarkar
Charoen Kaitwatcharachai
Nathan W. Levin

Over the past three decades, hemodialysis (HD) has evolved into a safe and less stressful procedure for both patients and caregivers. Enormous improvements in every aspect of dialysis technology have resulted in major reductions in intradialytic complications. Although modern technology has improved the safety and efficacy of the treatment, there is still much to be done. Because of the acute, intermittent nature of dialysis, the short duration of treatments, the use of an artificial membrane, and the requirements of extracorporeal circulation, intradialytic complications are to be expected.

Intradialytic complications still cause considerable patient morbidity and, rarely, mortality. The monetary costs of intradialytic complications are enormous. Measures to assess and prevent complications are expensive but clearly cost-effective when a formal cost-benefit analysis is performed.

According to the recent U.S. Renal Data System (USRDS) *Annual Data Report*, 51 percent of incident HD patients are aged 65 or older, and, diabetes continues to be the primary cause of end-stage renal disease (ESRD) across racial and ethnic groups (44.8 percent in incident patients). The proportion of patients beginning ESRD treatment with three or more comorbid conditions has increased since 1995, while the percent with no reported comorbidity has fallen over the same period. HD continues to be the major form of renal replacement therapy, with 64.5 percent of prevalent patients on in-center HD. Therefore increasing number of patients with multiple risk factors for cardiovascular events are on HD treatment.[1] Thus it is easy to understand why intradialytic complications continue to be a major problem in the older, complex patient population.

Intradialytic complications should be routinely assessed as part of an ongoing quality improvement program. The emergence of computerized data systems, which help the dialysis staff record each treatment's intradialytic complications, is itself a major development of the past few years. An analysis of 22,514 dialysis treatments performed on 531 patients in five outpatient units helps provide an understanding of the incidence and significance of many intradialytic events (Tables 10–1 and 10–2).[2]

TABLE 10–1. INTRADIALYTIC COMPLICATIONS BY PATIENT AGE: PERCENTAGE OF TREATMENTS WITH SPECIFIC SYMPTOMS

	Age (years)			
	<30	30–50	51–70	>70
Number of treatments	1314	5355	11,085	4800
Percentage of treatments with:				
Hypotension	18.1	19.7	25.2	34
Nausea	8.0	6.8	8.1	8.8
Vomiting	3.4	2.3	3.7	6.2
Cramps	11.4	13.3	10.2	6.7
Chest pain	0.9	1.2	1.5	1.3
Fever	0.6	0.2	0.2	0.1

TABLE 10–3. INTRADIALYTIC COMPLICATIONS BY PATIENT AGE: CUMULATIVE PERCENTAGE OF PATIENTS WITH SYMPTOMS OVER A 5-MONTH PERIOD

	Age (years)			
	<30	30–50	51–70	>70
Number of treatments	26	109	212	95
Percentage of treatments with:				
Hypotension	80.8	88.9	90.6	96.8
Nausea	69.2	62.4	74.5	72.6
Vomiting	42.3	31.2	51.8	57.9
Cramps	57.7	81.6	67.9	56.8
Chest pain	38.5	30.3	35.4	33.7
Fever	19.2	11.0	6.6	0.4

CARDIOVASCULAR COMPLICATIONS

Intradialytic Hypotension

Hypotension is a frequent complication of dialysis. Decreases in blood pressure (BP) range in severity from relatively asymptomatic episodes to marked declines resulting in myocardial ischemia; cardiac arrhythmias; cerebral, splanchnic, and peripheral vascular thromboses; loss of consciousness; seizures; or death. Associated vomiting may be accompanied by aspiration.

Table 10–1 and Table 10–3 show the frequency of hypotensive episodes in different age groups and the cumulative percentage of patients with this symptom over a 5-month period.

A functional definition of hypotension is that level of BP low enough to require nursing or medical intervention. However, when hypotension is defined as that level of BP requiring saline or a change in patient position, the frequency is lower.[2]

A decline in BP is observed regularly during chronic HD treatments. BP fall is commonly observed during the first 10 to 20 percent of the treatment, followed by a more gradual decrease and a sharp rebound immediately after dialysis.[2] In most patient BP falls during the course of dialysis because of ultrafiltration, the decrease being within the normal range and with minimal symptoms. The incidence

TABLE 10–2. NUMBER OF TREATMENTS ASSOCIATED WITH HYPOTENSION BY PATIENT AGE

	Age (years)			
	<30	30–50	51–70	>70
Number of treatments	1314	5355	11,085	4800
Percentage of treatments with:				
Hypotension	18.1	19.7	25.2	34
Hypotension requiring intervention	11.2	12.5	17.3	21.7

of hypotension is variously reported in between 20 and 50 percent of HD sessions, depending on the population of patients studied.[3]

Patients with frequent symptomatic hypotension were found to be older (64.4 vs. 56.9 years) and to develop hypotension during the early part of the dialysis session.[4] Other factors correlated with the incidence of hypotension were female gender, diabetes, left ventricular hypertrophy, and coronary artery disease (CAD).

Hypotension in HD patients can develop during the course of HD (intradialytic period) or may be present at the beginning of the treatment (interdialytic period) session.

A recent analysis of 1846 patients participating in the HEMO Study provides further insight into dialysis-related hypotension. It was found that intradialytic hypotensive episodes (IDHE) occurred in 17.8 percent of treatments. IDHE was defined as an episode where a drop in BP required administration of intravenous saline, lowering of the ultrafiltrtion (UF) rate, or use of a head-low (Trendelenburg) position. There were only slight differences in UF rate and percent of cramping between sessions vs. those without IDHE. Baseline patient predictors of IDHE included advanced age, diabetes, high comorbidity status, and female gender. The mean maximum intradialytic decrease in systolic BP was 33 percent in sessions with IDHE and 19 percent in sessions without IDHE. Those with maximum percent intradialytic decline in systolic BP had the maximum incidence of IDHE. IDHE was strongly, continuously, and inversely associated with both predialytic systolic and diastolic BP.[5]

Etiology. Dialytic hypotension has a multifactorial etiology that can be divided into patient- and procedure-related factors (Table 10–4). It is also important to rule out other uncommon causes of hypotension (such as pericardial tamponade, myocardial infarction, arrhythmias, internal bleeding, septicemia, dialyzer reactions, hemolysis, and air embolism). A careful analysis of patients' dialysis records,

TABLE 10–4. ETIOLOGY OF DIALYSIS-INDUCED HYPOTENSION

Patient-Related Factors	Procedure-Related Factors	Uncommon Causes
• Impaired plasma refilling (? decreased UF coefficient of vascular wall)	• Decreased plasma osmolality (relatively large surface area membrane, high starting BUN)	• Pericardial tamponade
• Decreased cardiac reserve (diastolic or systolic dysfunction)	• Excess absolute volume and rate of fluid removal (large interdialytic weight gain)	• Myocardial infarction
• Impaired venous compliance	• Change in serum electrolyte (hypocalcemia, hypokalemia)	• Aortic dissection
• Autonomic dysfunction (diabetic, uremic)	• Dialysate-acetate, too warm dialysate	• Internal hemorrhage
• Arrhythmias	• Membrane blood interaction	• Septicemia
• Anemia	• Hypoxia	• Air embolism
• Drug therapy (vasodilators, β blockers, calcium channel blockers)		• Pneumothorax
• Alteration of vasoactive substances in the blood		• Hemolysis
• Eating during treatment (increased splanchnic blood flow)		
• Low dry-weight estimation		

careful physical examination, and bedside chest x-ray and echocardiography can rule out most of these causes.

Pathogenesis. The pathogenesis of dialytic hypotension is complex. Many of its causes have been described, including cardiac, endocrine, autocrine, mechanical, physical, and nervous system factors. The effects of hypotension are usually adverse (Table 10–5). Consequently, the development of effective preventive and therapeutic interventions is extremely important and challenging.

Ultrafiltration. Intradialytic hypotension (IDH) is rare in the absence of an UF-induced reduction in blood volume. The frequency of IDH increases with an increasing UF rate.[6]

Vascular refilling and physiologic compensation is limited and an ultrafiltration rate of >0.35 mL/min/kg produces a decrease in BP in most patients.[7] At slower UF rates in patients who are not prone to hypotension and depending on the extent of hypervolemia, an absolute decrease in plasma volume of up to 20 percent can generally be tolerated without significant hypotension.

The basic dialytic processes of diffusion and UF determine the rate of fluid shifts between body compartments. Net fluid transfer between the intra- and extracellular compartments is influenced by the urea gradient between cells and interstitial water created as urea is rapidly removed from the plasma and interstitial compartments through the

TABLE 10–5. EFFECTS OF HYPOTENSION IN REDUCING DIALYSIS EFFICIENCY (REDUCED DELIVERED KT/V)

• Increased cardiopulmonary recirculation
• Vasoconstriction leading to reduced perfusion of large-volume areas with sequestration of solutes
• Alarms reducing useful dialysis time

dialyzer. A small, usually clinically insignificant reduction in BP may occur at the beginning of dialysis as water enters the intracellular compartment. Water transfer between the plasma and interstitial compartment, far more important clinically, is driven by the combined transvascular (capillary) oncotic and hydraulic pressure gradients. The rate is determined by the whole-body vascular UF coefficient, which is an average representing all of the body capillary beds.

As emphasized by Gotch, it is the gradient between intracellular and extracellular osmolality rather than the concentration gradient between plasma and dialysate that is primarily responsible for the decrease in BP noted early in dialysis.[8] Intracellular fluid shift resulting in an initial reduction in BP is usually clinically insignificant unless the patient is volume-depleted at the beginning of dialysis treatment. The interstitial fluid compartment plays an essential role in determining the rate of plasma refilling. The compliance of the interstitial fluid compartment is very high.[9] Its high compliance and the marked interindividual variability of fluid flux makes it difficult to recognize when the patient is euvolemic. Tissue compliance decreases, and interstitial pressure may become negative as the interstitial volume falls below normal. This can cause a decrease in the rate of water transfer into the vascular compartment. Patients with low extracellular fluid volumes have substantial decreases in blood volume and BP with UF during dialysis.[10] On the other hand, overhydration results in high tissue compliance with rapid intravascular volume repletion during UF. The predialysis state of hydration is therefore an important predictor of patient response to UF. Predialysis mean arterial BP, age, the use of antihypertensive drugs, or duration on dialysis did not correlate with refilling of the plasma compartment.[9] Gotch has suggested that there is an optimal interstitial volume for each patient that will be controlled by targeting both the blood sodium at the end of dialysis and the dry body weight.[11]

Underestimation of dry weight with low tissue compliance will result in slower filling of the intravascular space. The dry body weight, defined as the state where there is no excess extracellular fluid volume, is not only difficult to define but also a difficult state to achieve. This is primarily because of the complex physiologic actions controlling the interstitial compartment volume. Intense research has focused on the ways to determine the dry weight (blood volume monitoring, cyclic guanosine monophosphate (c-GMP), inferior vena cava (IVC) diameter estimation, bioimpedance, and others). The lack of correlation between the change in intravascular volume and the UF rate makes it difficult to define the fluid fluxes in various segments (arm, trunk, and leg) of the body, which might have some bearing on various complications seen during dialysis treatment such as hypotension and cramps. We have used a segmental bioimpedance approach for defining these fluid fluxes in the various segments of the body during the course of HD treatment. Our results show that the leg is the last segment to become dry (by bioimpedance criteria) and that makes it the ideal place to test the achievement of dry weight (Fig. 10–1).[12] This approach might be an objective way to determine dry weight—namely, the state where the interstitial space in the leg contains no excess extracellular fluid.

Factors Affecting the Response to Ultrafiltration. In a patient undergoing thrice-weekly dialysis and gaining approximately 1.5 kg/day, the therapeutic requirement of fluid removal equals absolute plasma volume.[13] If not for the plethora of compensatory mechanisms, all patients would

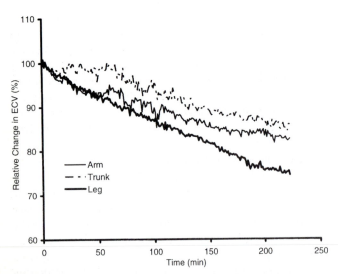

Figure 10–1. Relative change in segmental volume (arm, trunk, and leg) as estimated by segmental bioimpedance analysis. The leg is the segment showing maximum change in extracellular volume compared to other segments. *(Reproduced with permission from Zhu et al.[12])*

develop profound hypovolemic shock. The various compensatory mechanisms, which are activated with the fall of BP, prevent this from happening, and patients are able to maintain normal BP until the end of the treatment. The usual response to a reduction in circulating plasma volume is an increase in cardiac output, peripheral vascular resistance, and venoconstriction. The primary mechanism is the acute stimulation of the sympathetic nervous system with an increase in stroke volume and heart rate and vasoconstriction. Arteriolar vasoconstriction results in decreased mean intracapillary hydraulic pressure, which favors refilling of the plasma volume in the capillary bed. Venous pooling is prevented by venoconstriction, which results in better cardiac filling (preload), which then improves cardiac output (Starling's law) and prevents BP from falling (except when patients have systolic cardiac dysfunction). These changes slow the rate of reduction in plasma volume during UF. Hypotension can occur when one or more responses are defective. Impaired sympathetic activity, cardiac dysfunction, and arteriolar and venous dysfunction can, in various combination, act to break the coordinated feedback protective mechanism.

Plasma Refilling. Plasma refilling is essential for the prevention of cardiac underfilling, which would otherwise occur in the presence of continuous UF and decreases in blood volume. Because of refilling, despite the removal of one entire plasma volume during the course of HD, the blood volume typically drops by 5 to 20 percent. The source of refilling fluid is primarily the interstitial space. The larger the interstitial space volume (i.e., the more fluid overloaded a patient is), the more rapid the plasma refilling rate and the smaller the decrease in blood volume during UF. Thus, patients who are hypervolemic (e.g., edematous) are less prone to IDH than euvolemic patients are, while those who are hypovolemic are at increased risk.[14] Excess refilling in the face of inadequate venoconstriction can itself predispose to hypotension, as was shown by a study finding that excess plasma refilling, due to a decrease in intracapillary hydraulic pressure, can itself predispose to hypotension.[15] Plasma refilling at the capillary level also affects measurement of the hematocrit and interferes with the determination of relative change in blood volume. Blood volume shifts from the micro- to the macrocirculation can change the systemic hematocrit due to differing hematocrit levels in the two compartments.[16] For this reason, relative blood volume calculated from hematocrit during hypovolemia may not be accurate.

Blood Volume Regulation. Maintenance of blood volume is central to all the compensatory mechanisms and an assessment of changes in blood volume provides a direct measure of their efficacy. It is known from the detailed hemodynamic analysis of IDH episodes that in some patients there is a sudden decrease in plasma volume just before a hypotensive episode, likely caused by a decrease in cardiac output engendered by reduced cardiac filling. The pathophysiologic problem in hypovolemic hypotension is in getting blood into the heart, not getting it out (in those with no systolic dysfunction). Reduced atrial filling (because of increased heart rate or reduced atrial pressure) triggers the Bezold-Jarish reflex, which produces paradoxical vasodilatation, bradycardia, and hypotension. This happens because of stimulation of cardiac mechanoreceptors as the heart contracts vigorously in a virtually empty ventricular cavity. The result is a strong inhibitory signal to the brain and withdrawal of the central sympathetic outflow, resulting in a decrease of peripheral resistance and hypotension. This phenomenon is similar to what is seen in idiopathic postural hypotension and neurocardiogenic syncope.[17]

Relative blood volume change during dialysis can be measured by monitoring the change in hematocrit by ultrasound (or other) sensors. As fluid is removed during dialysis, the hematocrit increases, because plasma water is removed but the volume of cellular elements remains constant. Although a number of studies have reported continuous intradialytic changes in blood volume measured simultaneously with arterial pressure, a precise relationship between the blood volume changes and the BP response has yet to be defined. Some have defined blood volume or hematocrit values below which a BP drop appears ("crash crit"), whereas others have failed to demonstrate any relationship between the degree of hypovolemia, hypotension, and the hematocrit. In fact, blood volume is one of the many factors that come into play to determine pressure levels during HD with simultaneous UF. Central blood volume is preferentially preserved rather than the peripheral circulation. In a study of 20 patients, it was shown that UF causes the blood volume to fall but is associated with an increase in peripheral vascular resistance, which maintains BP, preferentially conserving central blood volume. Failure of a peripheral vascular response was found to lead to intradialytic hypotension.[18]

A recent study used a computer model-based approach of cardiovascular response to hypotension. Three categories of patients were identified. The first group consisted of hypotension prone patients in whom the hypotensive response was due to a lack of efficacy of both capacity (venous) and resistance (arteriolar) regulation. In this group of patients, BP was highly sensitive to blood volume changes, as both arteriolar and venous regulation were impaired. This represented the group of hypotensive patients who had a predialysis systolic BP of <100 mmHg. The second group consisted of patients with an unstable response to UF with delayed hypotension, in which the control of venous capacity was not effective and resistance control alone kept the BP stable only when relative blood volume reduction (5 percent) was minimal. This is the group in which there was likely a failure of sympathetic nervous system activity during the course of dialysis. The third group of patients had a

hypotension resistance response to UF—an efficient compensation of capacitance vessels was seen. This group of patients tolerated UF and had an efficient cardiovascular response to blood volume reduction.[15]

Venous Capacity. Most of an individual's blood volume is normally contained in the venous bed. With hypovolemia, arteriolar resistance increases, which in turn increases systemic BP not only by increasing total peripheral resistance but also by decreasing pressure in the highly compliant venous bed. This decrease in venous bed pressure favors passive venous recoil, resulting in translocation of blood in the central vessels and maintenance of cardiac filling (DeJager-Krogh phenomenon). Splanchnic venous capacity decreases by 10 percent with UF, indicating the likely importance of this phenomenon in dialysis patients.[19] The effectiveness of this protective mechanism may vary substantially among dialysis patients.[20, 21] Higher levels of compliance (and thus more recoil and venous return with a given decrease in pressure) correlate with a smaller decrease in central venous pressure with UF, again suggesting the importance of this mechanism in IDH. Failure of this phenomenon could predispose to IDH, as was suggested by one study[22] in which investigators found that increases in venous distensibility with increased peripheral pooling of blood occured in patients who were prone to dialysis hypotension. This shift of volume was found to aggravate the effects of UF.

Cardiac Function. Diastolic dysfunction,[23] decreased cardiac contractility (systolic dysfunction), and susceptibility to arrhythmias are all major cardiac factors that can lead to hypotension.

Diastolic cardiac dysfunction is common in dialysis patients; however, it is difficult to identify clinically. Normal cardiac output (and BP) is maintained in these patients by high left ventricular filling pressure. Rapid UF can cause a sudden fall in filling pressure and profound hypotension. A recent study in non-renal-failure patients tried to determine the relative significance of various clinical findings in differentiating between systolic and diastolic cardiac dysfunction. Systolic dysfunction was characterized by a history of previous myocardial infarction, presence of dyspnea, jugular venous distention, tachycardia, hypotension, edema, physical evidence of cardiomegaly (displaced and diffuse cardiac apex), S3 gallop, left bundle branch block, anterior q-wave on electrocardiography (ECG), and reduced ejection fraction on two-dimensional echocardiography (2D-ECHO). Isolated diastolic dysfunction, on the other hand, was characterized by older age, obesity, hypertension, no history of smoking or CAD, and no physical evidence of cardiac enlargement.[24,25] These findings are likely relevant to HD patients as well.

Patients with left ventricular hypertrophy (LVH) on echocardiography were almost tenfold more likely to develop IDH than those with normal echocardiograms.[26] LVH (leading to diastolic dysfunction) results in decreased cardiac filling in diastole, with resultant decreased cardiac output. A hypertrophied left ventricle requires higher filling pressure to maintain cardiac output during dialysis than a compliant, nonhypertrophied ventricle. One study showed that patients with the shortest left ventricular filling times were the most hemodynamically unstable during dialysis.[27] Late, atrial-assisted filling does not increase in a compensatory fashion. The ratio of early to late ventricular filling is far lower in patients with frequent IDH than in those with stable intradialytic BP, indicating the general importance of left atrial contraction in maintaining cardiac output during dialysis and its particular importance in those with LVH. Thus, theoretically, atrial fibrillation is likely to be a major risk factor for the development of IDH. Cardiac contractility reserve as assessed by dobutamine stress echocardiography is impaired in IDH-prone patients.[28] In part, this could be due to electrolyte changes that occur during dialysis (decrease in serum potassium, increase in serum HCO_3^-, and change in serum calcium) or may be due to intrinsic myocardial dysfunction (cardiomyopathy).

Arteriolar Tone. As mentioned previously, the integrity of the autonomic nervous system is important for maintaining arteriolar tone and normal cardiac compensation. Arteriolar tone modulates filling of the venous system. Sudden arteriolar dilatation can cause pooling of blood in the venous bed with cardiac underfilling and resultant hypotension. Normal arteriolar tone and vasoconstrictor response can maintain the BP and interrupt a vicious cycle of vasodilatation, cardiac underfilling, and hypotension. Several factors affect vasoconstriction during dialysis, and vasodilatation can result from the following: autonomic dysfunction, inadequate vasoactive response, generation of neurohormones and cytokines, particularly interleukin-1 (IL-1), thermal stress (i.e., heat accumulation), acetate in dialysate, increased adenosine level, food intake.

Autonomic Nervous System and Vasoactive Response. Sympathetic activity is increased in uremia. Plasma catecholamine levels are higher in hypotension-prone patients; however, the pressor response to exogenous norepinephrine is blunted. This suggests that despite the sympathetic overactivity, the cardiovascular response to adrenergic stimuli in hypotensive dialysis patients is reduced. There is a reduced cardiovascular response to vasopressor agents (such as norepinephrine and angiotensin II), associated with a downregulation of their receptors. Thus, the apparent sympathetic dysfunction is attributable to a reduced cardiovascular responsiveness to sympathetic stimulation rather than to a primary autonomic defect. Zucchelli and Santoro have explored this phenomenon and categorized hypotensive dialysis patients into two pathogenetic groups[29]: tachy-

cardic and bradycardic. The first group describes patients in whom the normal compensatory mechanisms are inadequate despite increases in cardiac output and vasoconstriction. These patients most often have impaired left ventricular systolic function. In the bradycardic type, which these authors believe accounts for more than 50 percent of hypotensive episodes during dialysis, sudden severe reductions in BP may occur ("crashes"). In this syndrome, there is sudden loss of sympathetic vasoconstrictor tone when left ventricular chamber volume is small and ventricular filling is slow. This compromises venous return to an adrenergically stimulated heart, which contracts forcefully on an almost empty chamber, stimulating ventricular mechanoreceptors. Paradoxically, general sympathetic tone is then markedly reduced, since the information delivered centrally from cardiac efferents is similar to that which occurs in situations of *hyper*volemia. This phenomenon has been demonstrated in experimental animals.[30] In this situation, a small bolus of fluid infused intravenously will raise the BP immediately.

Autonomic dysfunction is more marked in hypotension-prone dialysis patients. The response to Valsalva maneuver, considered an indirect measure of the entire baroreflex arc, is impaired in hypotensive more than in normotensive patients. The efferent sympathetic pathway is impaired and there is a reduction of baroreceptor sensitivity with relative preservation of the parasympathetic pathway responses. Sympathetic dysfunction is manifest by the following important clinical observations: (1) Patients with dialysis-induced hypotension (DIH) have a decreased heart-rate-variability response to head tilting [31] and (2) hypotension seen in the later part of a dialysis session is preceded by sudden failure of sympathetic nervous system compensation,[17] as described previously.

Neurohormonal Agents. The cardiac index, heart rate, or stroke volume is very similar in hypotensive and normotensive HD patients, whereas total peripheral resistance is lower in the former (except for those with preexisting systolic dysfunction, who will have a reduced cardiac index and stroke volume). The blood concentration of vasodilator substances such as nitric oxide (NO), adrenomedullin, and adenosine are raised in hypotensive patients, which might be related to the inflammatory state of uremia. Acetate in the dialysis fluid can activate human monocytes to produce IL-1 and tumor necrosis factor (TNF).[32] It has been proposed that cytokines (IL-1 and TNF-α) released during HD can induce production of NO in vascular smooth muscle cells and endothelial cells.[33,34] Nitric oxide could be an important mediator of the hypotensive response.[34-36] Some investigators have found raised concentrations of adenosine metabolites before the onset of the hypotensive episode. Adenosine inhibits the release of norepinephrine. The concept of a vicious cycle was postulated in some patients with sudden hypotension-inducing ischemia, which results in increased levels of adenosine and consequent inhibition of norepinephrine release, vasodilatation, and deepening hypotension.[37]

Acetate. While acetate is used currently in only a small number of dialysis units, it is a powerful vasodilator.[38] The maximum rate of acetate metabolism is approximately 300 mM/h.[39] During HD with high-efficiency dialyzers (see below), acetate diffuses from dialysate to plasma at rates greater than this. In addition to hypotension, the patient may develop nausea, vomiting, disorientation, and fatigue. Acetate-free biofiltration is a technique by which most acetate is replaced by bicarbonate, resulting in better cardiac stability, better control of predialysis mean arterial BP,[40] and fewer hypotensive episodes.[41]

Thermal Stress and Dialysate Temperature. UF is thought to raise body temperature in part by the compensatory vasoconstriction it induces, leading to the retention of body heat. Body temperature change during HD can be modulated by varying the dialysate temperature. Much of the recent focus has been on the regulation of dialysate temperature, as such regulation is relatively easy to carry out with modern dialysis equipment and has a direct effect on arteriolar resistance. The first report documenting the influence of dialysate temperature on dialysis-induced hypotension was published over 20 years ago.[42] This was substantiated by the theoretical model proposed by Gotch et al. in 1989. They showed that the UF process, with the accompanying reduction in circulating blood volume, evokes peripheral vasoconstriction, which tends to impair the dissipation of heat through the skin.[43] It is well known that standard HD (using a dialysate temperature of 36.9 to 37.5°C) induces an increase in core temperature averaging 0.67°C. This small increase in core temperature can cause substantial hemodynamic changes, with an increase in cardiac output and a decrease in peripheral resistance. In addition to heat stress, HD treatment causes hypovolemic stress due to fluid removal through the UF process. This stress causes a hemodynamic response of the peripheral circulation, which is the opposite of that caused by heat—namely, vasoconstriction instead of vasodilatation. However, studies in patients have shown that the response to heat stress takes precedence over the response to hypovolemic stress.

Since the first report, many studies have confirmed that if dialysate temperature is adjusted to the range of 34 to 35.5°C, cardiovascular tolerance to HD is better than if dialysate temperature is set to 37°C or higher. Low dialysate temperature may itself inflict an empiric cold stress.[44] Therefore the dialysate temperature should be modulated according to the needs of the individual patient, because pre-HD temperature varies widely.[45] Blood temperature monitors (BTMs) on some dialysis machine are able to modulate the blood temperature and keep the patient in thermal balance when the reference goal is set. By keeping the UF constant, changes in the dialysate temperature alter the core body temperature. Recent work has shown that when UF is increased, more heat must be removed through the extracorporeal circuit to keep the body temperature unchanged (isothermal dialysis).[46] We studied 51 dialysis treatments in 27 patients during isothermic dialysis (body temperature variation of +/- 0.1°C) and found that approximately 6 percent of the energy expenditure must be removed through the extracorporeal circulation for each percent UF induced body-weight change. The use of isothermic dialysis was found to be better tolerated by patients, as overall heat transfer was reduced. This study showed that rather than using fixed low-temperature dialysate in all patients at risk of hypotension, a maneuver that is not well tolerated by most patients,[47] one should remove only the surplus heat accumulated in the body as a result of the dialysis process (blood flow and UF) by automatic changes in the dialysate temperature during the treatment. The benefit of this approach was also confirmed by a large multicenter, randomized crossover trial in which isothermic dialysis was compared with thermoneutral dialysis (in which any thermal energy transfer in the extracorporeal circuit was prevented).[48] Hypotension-prone patients were carefully selected and randomized to both arms of the study. Other than the changes in the dialysate temperature, all the treatment parameters were unchanged. Isothermic dialysis was found to halve the frequency of sessions complicated by symptomatic hypotensive episodes without significantly impairing treatment efficacy.

Treatment Prevention of Intradialytic Hypotension. The immediate treatment of intradialytic hypotension is the restoration of the circulating blood volume with isotonic saline or by various hypertonic agents (which enhance the mobilization of interstitial fluid). Intravenous boluses of 100 to 250 mL of 0.9 percent saline are often used for therapy (albumin has little added value but great expense). Hypotensive dialysis patients should be placed in the Trendelenburg position, with precautions to avoid aspiration if vomiting should occur. The UF rate should be reduced. In rare instances (often septic patients with acute or chronic renal failure), continuous infusion of pressor agents (e.g., metaraminol, norepinephrine, levarterenol) during HD has been employed. This can maintain BP during the dialysis procedure and allow for some fluid removal. However, once the procedure has concluded, many patients will become profoundly hypotensive because they lack the intrinsic mechanisms to maintain BP. The major defense against hypovolemia developing during dialysis and UF is movement of fluid from the interstitial compartment to the intravascular space. Since this movement can be hindered by osmotic disequilibrium induced by rapid solute removal from plasma, an appropriate dialysate sodium concentration can partially compensate by causing movement of fluid back into the plasma compartment.[49]

Prevention (Table 10–6).

Low-Sodium Dialysate. The dialysate sodium concentration has a significant impact on the changes in blood volume accompanying any given amount of fluid removal. Routinely, no specific attempt is made to ensure accurate removal of sodium gained in the interdialytic interval. Sometimes the patient has more than the required sodium removal during the dialysis session, which can lead to IDH. It is well established that increasing the dialysate sodium level results in better preservation of plasma volume (due to mobilization of fluid from the intracellular compartment ICW) and helps to prevent IDH. The level to which the dialysate sodium can be increased, however, is limited by the development of postdialysis hypernatremia (relative to the patient's usual

plasma sodium concentration), which is associated with thirst, hypertension, and increased interdialytic weight gain, thus making UF more difficult during subsequent dialyses.

Variations in dialysate sodium during treatment, termed sodium profiling, have been widely advocated and used to obtain the hemodynamic benefits of high dialysate sodium without its complications. High dialysate sodium is used early in the treatment, with levels declining often abruptly in the latter phase of the treatment. However, there is no evidence that using a relatively low dialysate sodium during the terminal phase of dialysis (commonly done to avoid postdialysis hypernatremia) is of any benefit if the time-averaged concentration of dialysate sodium remains high. In other words, a linear decline in dialysate sodium from 150 to 140 meq/L over the course of a treatment will produce approximately the same serum sodium after dialysis as when a dialysate sodium of 145 meq/L is used throughout the treatment. Thus, high dialysate sodium can be used when it is thought that plasma volume support is needed, and this can be accomplished by using a biofeedback system incorporated into the dialysis machine.[50]

In prescribing dialysis using a sodium gradient, it is important to monitor the patient for evidence of a progressive increase in total body sodium. A sodium gradient protocol can be utilized in such a way that the amount of sodium exchanged is the same as with a fixed sodium dialysate while better preserving blood volume during UF. A recent study found that the use of a sodium-gradient protocol was associated with better preservation of stroke volume (and hence cardiac output) without a significant decrease in blood volume.[51] A profiled dialysis regimen based on a mathematical model in which baseline patient characteristics are used to construct a patient-specific sodium-profile dialysate before each treatment, showed improved clinical tolerance.[52] Thus, sodium-balanced sodium-profiled HD is the best way of providing hemodynamic stability without increasing the overall sodium load. However, this approach is not currently available for clinical use.

The same principle is used for blood volume-controlled HD. This is a relatively new concept. A number of biosensors are fitted onto the dialysis circuit to feed patient-related information back to a special biofeedback unit integrated into the dialysis machine that automatically transmits specific on-line patient status information to permit real-time adjustment of the dialysis fluid composition and machine technical parameters. This can successfully prevent sudden excessive fall in blood volume and the consequent side effects.[53,54]

TABLE 10–6. PRESCRIPTION CHOICES INFLUENCING INTRADIALYTIC BLOOD PRESSURE

Choice	Result	Mechanism
High Kuf (without ultrafiltration control)	Hypovolemia	Inadequate plasma refilling from interstitial fluid
High small molecule clearance, especially with high predialysis BUN	Hypovolemia	Large gradient between intracellular and extracellular compartments attenuating plasma refilling
Low dry weight	Decreased plasma volume	Inadequate plasma refilling
Low dialysate sodium	Hypovolemia	Decreased plasma osmolality with slow refilling from cells
Acetate dialysate	Decreased compensatory vasoconstriction	Direct vascular and cardiac effects with acidosis, hypoxia, IL-1 generation, and metabolic consequences of catabolism of acetate
Low calcium dialysate	Decreased compensatory vasoconstriction and myocardial inotropic response	Less than usual increase in ionized calcium
Dialysate temperature ~37°C	Vasodilatation	Increased skin blood flow
Bioincompatible membranes	? Decreased compensatory vasoconstriction	?Release of cytokines ?Effect of hypoxia

Cool Dialysate. Cooler dialysate has been clearly demonstrated to reduce the incidence of hypotension. Isothermic dialysis (which can be performed only by using a BTM module in the dialysis machine) at this point seems to be the best approach for reducing the core temperature without any discomfort to the patient. The guidelines of the Association for the Advancement of Medical Instrumentation (AAMI) for dialysate temperature state that, under normal operating conditions, the system shall maintain the temperature of the dialysate between 33 and 40°C and within ± 1°C of its set point value.[55] This is well within the range of the temperature variation needed for the cool dialysate required for isothermic dialysis.

UF Rate. The relationship between UF and decrease in plasma volume is determined by the excess fluid in the interstitial space and the rate of UF and plasma refilling. When the UF rate is less rapid, the plasma volume is maintained better by plasma refilling. Thus, a major therapeutic consideration in patients with frequent IDH is slowing the UF rate by prolonging the treatment time. This, however, is not practicable in day-to-day clinical practice in most dialysis units. A nonlinear UF rate can be useful in some patients, even though its application is largely dependent on guesswork. Another common practice is use of UF without dialysis for a short period (often 1 hour, with two-thirds of fluid removal) preceding dialysis. This, however, has no benefit if the total treatment time is unchanged. If the treatment time is prolonged, the benefits are not better than with continuous slow UF during the same extended treatment time. The value of pulsed UF over continuous slow UF has not been fully documented, although its ability to predict hemodynamic stability has been shown in a small group of patients.[56]

Dry Weight. Often patients are below their true dry (or euvolemic) weight. The most immediate step that can prevent IDH in such patients is revision of the prescribed dry weight to a higher value. This will increase the size of the interstitial space and minimize the decline in plasma volume associated with large amounts of UF.

Dialysate Calcium. Variations of the concentration of dialysate calcium can affect hemodynamic stability during dialysis. Routine practice is to keep the dialysate calcium low (1.25 mmol/L) because of problems of calcium deposition and its associated complications. However, high dialysate calcium might be beneficial to avoid IDH.

In a crossover trial, a high dialysate calcium concentration (3.75 meq/L) was associated with significantly less decrease in both systolic and mean arterial BP than a low calcium dialysate (2.75 mEq/L). In patients with ejection fraction < 40 percent a dialysate calcium of 3.5 mmol/L offered clear hemodynamic benefits over a 2.5 mmol/L dialysate. An increase in blood calcium concentration (produced by increased dialysate calcium) was found to affect BP primarily through changes in left ventricular output rather than by peripheral vascular resistance.

Thus, it would seem that in patients who are prone to intradialytic hypotension, avoidance of a low dialysate calcium concentration might be of benefit. A trial of high dialysate calcium levels can be used in patients with IDH who are incompletely responsive to other therapies (midodrine, cool dialysate, etc). However, high levels should not be used in the presence of hypercalcemia, hyperphosphatemia, or an elevated calcium phosphorus product.[57,58]

Other Electrolytes. Both potassium and magnesium can increase the BP; however, there is no direct evidence of their benefit to minimize IDH in any long-term clinical trials. A lower dialysate bicarbonate level is associated with higher intradialytic BP. This is probably due to higher ionized calcium levels in the former.

Blood Pressure Medications. The benefits in reducing IDH of withholding BP medications prior to dialysis are undocumented. Although this seems rational clinically, the benefits of such an approach are unclear. Table 10–7 shows the removal of antihypertensive drugs during dialysis, which should be reviewed before making changes in BP medications.

Dialyzer Choice. For a long time it was believed that IDH was more likely when bioincompatible dialysis membranes

TABLE 10–7. REMOVAL OF CARDIAC DRUGS BY HEMODIALYSIS

Drug Group	Removed with HD	Not Extensively Removed with HD
Antihypertensives		
Sympatholytics	Methyldopa	Clonidine, guanabenz
Alpha/beta blockers		Prazosin, labetalol
Beta blockers	Atenolol, metoprolol, nadolol	Propanolol, esmolol, bisoprolol
ACE inhibitors	Captopril, enalapril, lisinopril	Fosinopril
Calcium channel blockers	None	All
Vasodilators	Minoxidil, diazoxide, nitroprusside	Hydralazine
Antiarrhythmic		
Class 1	Procainamide, flecainide, propafenone	Disopyramide, lidocaine, mexiletine, phenytoin, quinidine
Class 2	Atenolol	Propranolol
Class 3		Bretylium, amiodarone
Class 4		Diltiazem, verapamil
Unclassified		Digitoxin, digoxin

SOURCE: Adapted with permission from Nicholls AJ. Heart and circulation, Chap. 3 in Ing TS, *Handbook of Dialysis*, 3d ed. Philadelphia: Lippincott Williams & Wilkins, 2001;595, 597, 598.[94a]

were used. None of the studies published to date, however, have supported this concept, although there may be numerous other reasons to choose biocompatible high-flux dialyzers for chronic dialysis therapy.

Drugs.[59] Various drugs that act by modulating the sympathetic nervous system have been tried for the treatment of IDH. These include ephedrine, fludrocortisone, vasopressin, L-carnitine, midodrine,[60] sertraline[61,] and L-threo-3,4-dihydroxyphenylserine[62] (which counters sympathetic nervous system dysfunction), caffeine[63] (which counters the rise of adenosine), and methylene blue (which counters action of NO).[64] It appears that only a few of these drugs are efficacious, well tolerated, safe, and easy to administer. They include carnitine, sertraline, and midodrine.

Midodrine is an alpha agonist that has been used for orthostatic hypotension in patients with autonomic dysfunction. Recently it has been used to prevent and treat IDH. Midodrine administered approximately 30 minutes before dialysis (dose range, 2.5 to 30 mg) has been shown to blunt the decrease in BP both during and at the completion of HD. In prospective studies, this benefit has been demonstrated in patients with severe IDH resistant to most other interventions. In addition, both hypotensive symptoms as well as interventions required to treat IDH were reduced. Midodrine also remained effective chronically (it has now been employed effectively for several years) and, most importantly, it has been well tolerated and found to be safe in high-risk patients (patients who are elderly and those who have diabetes mellitus, CAD, cardiomyopathy, or peripheral vascular disease). The only major contraindication in ESRD patients is the presence of active myocardial ischemia. Table 10–8 shows the current recommendations for the use of midodrine to prevent dialysis-induced hypotension. Carnitine (20 to 30 mg/kg per treatment) has been reported to have several benefits, including an improvement in the stability of intradialytic BP and a reduction in hypotensive symptoms. It has been used in dialysis patients with increased episodes of hypotension. Carnitine supplementation has been approved by the U.S. Food and Drug Administration not only for treatment but also for the prevention of carnitine depletion in dialysis patients.

Sertraline in a dose of 50 to 100 mg per day reduced bouts of IDH in approximately 50 percent of patients studied. This selective serotonin reuptake inhibitor (SSRI) also decreased the number of interventions required to treat hypotension.

Hemodialysis-Associated Hypertension

A rise in BP during or immediately after dialysis, though a less frequent occurrence than hypotension, is a significant intradialytic complication. Hypertension in HD patients is mainly systolic, with only 3 percent having isolated diastolic hypertension.[65,66] Systolic hypertension in HD patients is mainly caused by vascular stiffening, which may be due to various factors including hyperparathyroidism with increased calcium phosphorus product, increased circulating endothelin and angiotensin II levels, and sympathetic activation.[65] At any mean arterial pressure level, HD patients have higher systolic BP, lower diastolic BP, and higher pulse pressure values than control subjects with normal renal function who are matched for age, sex, diabetes mellitus, and body mass index.[67] These factors were also found to be associated with increased mortality.[68,69]

Pathophysiology. Many explanations for the phenomenon of intradialytic hypertension have been proposed (Table 10–9). Extracellular fluid volume expansion is the most consistent finding in hypertensive HD patients. This is because of the presence of arteriovenous (AV) fistula/graft, anemia, and fluid and salt retention. Mechanisms involve inappropriately increased angiotensin II, increased vascular sensitivity

---

TABLE 10–8. DIRECTIONS FOR MIDODRINE THERAPY IN ESRD PATIENTS WITH IDH

- Initiate midodrine therapy 30 minutes before HD.
- Start with 2.5 mg if patient weight < 70 kg or with 5 mg if weight >70 kg.
- Titrate dose to correct blood pressure and symptoms; maximum dose approximately 30 mg predialysis.
- If blood pressure is still low during the last half of dialysis or postdialysis despite maximizing predialysis dose:
    Administer second dose of midodrine at midway point of dialysis.
    Start with 2.5 mg and titrate up to correct blood pressure.
    Maximum dose approximately 10 mg.
- Avoid midodrine in patients with active myocardial ischemia.

SOURCE: Perazella,[59] with permission.

TABLE 10–9. FACTORS CONTRIBUTING TO INTRADIALYTIC HYPERTENSION

- Genetic predisposition
- Preexisting hypertension
- Extracellular volume excess
- ↑ Renin-angiotensin system activity
- ↑ Sympathetic activity
- ↑ Ratio of endothelin 1 to nitric oxide
- Uremic toxins (homocysteine, ADMA)
- EPO use (↑ blood viscosity)
- Correction of hypoxia-induced vasoconstriction
- Secondary hyperparathyroidism
- ↑Dialysate sodium
- Hemodialysis regimen

ABBREVIATIONS: ADMA = asymmetrical dimethyl arginine; EPO = erythropuietin.

to endogenous pressors, increased cardiac output in the presence of high peripheral vascular resistance, and failure to fully suppress the vasoconstrictor system.[71] Lowering of BP and improved survival occurs with improved control of extracellular fluid volume.[72,73]

Rapid plasma volume contraction and negative sodium balance during dialysis therapy may induce an increase in plasma catecholamine levels. Maintenance HD may thus be associated with chronically increased sympathetic nerve discharge, which may not correlate with nonadrenalin levels or plasma renin activity.[74,75] Bilateral nephrectomy might lower BP by interfering with this mechanism.[74] As discussed previously, HD is associated with low levels of nitric oxide (NO) due to the accumulation of asymmetrical dimethyl arginine (ADMA), hyperparathyroidism and uremia per se) and this may contribute to hypertension by the unopposed action of endothelin 1 and other vasoconstrictor agents.

In 20 to 30 percent of ESRD patients, regular administration of recombinant human erythropoietin (rHuEpo) is accompanied by de novo hypertension or aggravation of preexisting hypertension.[70] The increase in BP occurs within a few weeks to months after initiation of rHuEpo therapy.[76,77] The dose of rHuEpo has largely been found to have no effect on the degree of hypertension[78]; however, there are some conflicting reports.[76] Factors responsible for an EPO-induced increase in BP include an increase in hematocrit with an attendant increase in peripheral resistance[79] and cardiac afterload[80]; activation of various neurohormonal systems[81]; correction of hypoxia-mediated vasodilatation[82]; upregulation of genes implicated in the regulation of vascular functions[83]; elevated cytosolic free calcium in the vascular smooth muscle cells, which increases vascular smooth muscle tone[84]; inhibition of NO synthesis[85]; low baseline hematocrit levels[86]; and rapid correction of anemia.[87] The use of calcium channel blockers can normalize intracellular calcium, abrogate rHuEpo-induced hypertension, and reverse downregulation of NO production.[88]

Secondary hyperparathyroidism facilitates entry of calcium into smooth muscle cells of the vessel wall, which favors vasoconstriction and an increase in peripheral vascular resistance.[89]

Treatment

According to the JNC 7 report, lifestyle modifications such as weight reduction, dietary modification, sodium restriction, physical activity, and moderation of alcohol consumption can reduce systolic BP from 2 to 14 mmHg. In addition, most patients with chronic kidney disease require aggressive BP management to reach target values of less than 130/80 mmHg. This might require the use of three or more antihypertensive drugs,[90] usually including angiotensin-converting enzyme (ACE) inhibitors or angiotensin receptor blockers (ARBs) .

Aerobic exercise can improve BP control in dialysis patients. In a controlled trial of 40 stable chronic HD patients, stationary cycling during each HD treatment for 6 months resulted in 13 (54 percent) of patients in the exercise group having a reduction of antihypertensive medication, as opposed to 4 (12.5 percent) in the control group ($p = 0.008$). The average relative benefit of exercise was a 36 percent reduction in antihypertensive medications.[91]

Sodium restriction is the next step in the treatment of hypertension in dialysis patients. This will limit interdialytic weight gain and make it easier to reach dry weight. Studies have shown that those having a interdialytic weight gain of 4.8 percent or more had a 12 percent higher mortality than those gaining less than 2.3 percent.[65] Adjustment of dry weight on a regular basis is important to prevent both hyper- and hypotension during HD.[92] Poorly controlled hypertension is often attributed to chronic volume overload. Gradual reduction of postdialysis weight over a few weeks along with salt restriction, longer dialysis, or extra dialysis sessions may yield a significant benefit.[93]

Withholding antihypertensive agents on days of dialysis and use of submaximal antihypertensive therapy are significant barriers to BP control. Current evidence suggests that ACE inhibitors and beta blockers should be used in preference to calcium channel blockers.[94] ACE inhibitors improve left ventricular dilatation in addition to reducing aortic stiffness. With all three groups of drugs, there is more reduction of systolic than of diastolic BP, which effectively reduces the pulse pressure. In prescribing antihypertensive agents (and other cardiac drugs), one should be aware of their renal clearances and prescribe accordingly (Table 10–10).

Low compliance with the dialysis regimen is associated with hypertension. Patients skipping or shortening one or more dialysis treatments have higher BPs than compliant patients.[95] Short or prolonged daily dialysis has been shown to improve fluid removal and is associated with excellent BP control and improved mortality rates. Nocturnal HD performed 8 to 10 hours during sleep at home for 6 to 7 days per week allows BP control with fewer medications and fewer episodes of sleep apnea.[96] Longer and/or more frequent dialysis regimens, in addition to removing excess fluid, might act by removing pressor substances and mitigating autonomic activation.[97] Despite good control of extracellular volume, the normal nocturnal dipping of BP is not fully restored.[98]

Thus, a combination of exercise, diet, regular dialysis therapy, and drugs is needed in most HD patients in order to get BP under control. In refractory cases, consideration should be given to reducing the EPO dose and to prolonging weekly dialysis time by increasing either the time or frequency of treatment sessions. The pathophysiology and treatment of hypertension in dialysis patients is reviewed in detail in Chap. 27B.

TABLE 10–10. DOSAGE ADJUSTMENT OF SELECTED CARDIAC DRUGS IN HEMODIALYSIS PATIENTS

Drug	Dose Method	GFR > 50 (mL/min)	GFR 10–50 (mL/min)	GFR < 10 (mL/min)	Supplemental Dose after Hemodialysis	CAPD	CRRT
Acebutolol	D	100%	50%	30–50%	None	None	Dose for GFR 10–50
Adenosine	D	100%	100%	100%	None	None	Dose for GFR 10–50
Amiloride	D	100%	50%	Avoid	NA	NA	NA
Amiodarone	D	100%	100%	100%	None	None	Dose for GFR 10–50
Amlodipine	D	100%	100%	100%	None	None	Dose for GFR 10–50
Amrinone	D	100%	100%	50–75%	No data	No data	Dose for GFR 10–50
Atenolol	D, I	100% q24h	50% q48h	30–50% q96h	25–50 mg	None	Dose for GFR 10–50
Benazepril	D	100%	50–75%	25–50%	None	None	Dose for GFR 10–50
Bepridil		Unknown	Unknown	Unknown	None	None	No data
Bisoprolol	D	100%	75%	50%	Unknown	Unknown	Dose for GFR 10–50
Bleomycin	D	100%	75%	50%	None	Unknown	Dose for GFR 10–50
Bretylium	D	100%	25–50%	25%	None	None	Dose for GFR 10–50
Captopril	D, I	100% q8–12 h	75% q12–18 h	50% q24h	25–30%	None	Dose for GFR 10–50
Carvedilol	D	100%	100%	100%	None	None	Dose for GFR 10–50
Cilazapril	D, I	75% q24h	50% q24–48h	10–25% q72h	None	None	Dose for GFR 10–50
Clonidine	D	100%	100%	100%	None	None	Dose for GFR 10–50
Diazoxide	D	100%	100%	100%	None	None	Dose for GFR 10–50
Digitoxin	D	100%	100%	50–75%	None	None	Dose for GFR 10–50
Digoxin	D, I	100% q24h	25–75% q36h	10–25% q48h	None	None	Dose for GFR 10–50
Dilevalol	D	100%	100%	100%	None	None	Unknown
Diltiazem	D	100%	100%	100%	None	None	Dose for GFR 10–50
Disopyramide	I	q8h	q12–24h	q24–40h	None	None	Dose for GFR 10–50
Dobutamine	D	100%	100%	100%	No data	No data	Dose for GFR 10–50
Doxazosin	D	100%	100%	100%	None	None	Dose for GFR 10–50
Enalapril	D	100%	75–100%	50%	20–25%	None	Dose for GFR 10–50
Felodipine	D	100%	100%	100%	None	None	Dose for GFR 10–50
Flurazepam	D	100%	100%	100%	None	Unknown	NA
Fosinopril	D	100%	100%	75–100%	None	None	Dose for GFR 10–50
Furosemide	D	100%	100%	100%	None	None	NA
Guanabenz	D	100%	100%	100%	Unknown	Unknown	Dose for GFR 10–50
Guanadrel	I	q12h	q12–24h	q24–48h	Unknown	Unknown	Dose for GFR 10–50
Guanethidine	I	q24h	q24h	q24–36h	Unknown	Unknown	Avoid
Guanfacine	D	100%	100%	100%	None	None	Dose for GFR 10–50
Hydralazine	I	q8h	q8h	q8–16h	None	None	Dose for GFR 10–50
Isosorbide	D	100%	100%	100%	10–20 mg	None	Dose for GFR 10–50
Isradipine	D	100%	100%	100%	None	None	Dose for GFR 10–50
Labetalol	D	100%	100%	100%	None	None	Dose for GFR 10–50
Lidocaine	D	100%	100%	100%	None	None	Dose for GFR 10–50
Lisinopril	D	100%	50–75%	25 to 50%	20%	None	Dose for GFR 10–50
Losartan	D	100%	100%	100%	Unknown	Unknown	Dose for GFR 10–50
Metaproterenol	D	100%	100%	100%	Unknown	Unknown	Dose for GFR 10–50
Methyldopa	I	q8h	q8–12h	q12–24h	250 mg	None	Dose for GFR 10–50
Metolazone	D	100%	100%	100%	None	None	NA
Metoprolol	D	100%	100%	100%	50 mg	None	Dose for GFR 10–50
Mexiletine	D	100%	100%	50–75%	None	None	None
Midodrine		5–10 mg q8h	5–10 mg q8h	Unknown	5 mg q8h	No data	Dose for GFR 10–50
Milrinone	D	100%	100%	50 to 75%	No data	No data	Dose for GFR 10–50
Minoxidil	D	100%	100%	100%	None	None	Dose for GFR 10–50
Nadolol	D	100%	50%	25%	40 mg	None	Dose for GFR 10–50

(continued)

TABLE 10–10. DOSAGE ADJUSTMENT OF SELECTED CARDIAC DRUGS IN HEMODIALYSIS PATIENTS (*Continued*)

Drug	Dose Method	GFR > 50 (mL/min)	GFR 10–50 (mL/min)	GFR < 10 (mL/min)	Supplemental Dose after Hemodialysis	CAPD	CRRT
Nicardipine	D	100%	100%	100%	None	None	Dose for GFR 10–50
Nifedipine	D	100%	100%	100%	None	None	Dose for GFR 10–50
Nimodipine	D	100%	100%	100%	None	None	Dose for GFR 10–50
Nisoldipine	D	100%	100%	100%	None	None	Dose for GFR 10–50
Nitroglycerin	D	100%	100%	100%	No data	No data	Dose for GFR 10–50
Nitroprusside	D	100%	100%	100%	None	None	Dose for GFR 10–50
Penbutolol	D	100%	100%	100%	None	None	Dose for GFR 10–50
Perindopril	D	100%	75%	50%	25–50%	Unknown	Dose for GFR 10–50
Phenytoin	D	100%	100%	100%	None	None	None
Pindolol	D	100%	100%	100%	None	None	Dose for GFR 10–50
Prazosin	D	100%	100%	100%	None	None	Dose for GFR 10–50
Procainamide	I	q4h	q6–12h	q8–24h	200 mg	None	Dose for GFR 10–50
Propafenone	D	100%	100%	100%	None	None	Dose for GFR 10–50
Propranolol	D	100%	100%	100%	None	None	Dose for GFR 10–50
Quinapril	D	100%	75–100%	75%	25%	None	Dose for GFR 10–50
Quinidine	D	100%	100%	75%	100–200 mg	None	Dose for GFR 10–50
Quinine	I	q8h	q8–12h	q24h	Dose after dialysis	Dose for GFR < 10	Dose for GFR 10–50
Ramipril	D	100%	50–75%	25–50%	20%	None	Dose for GFR 10–50
Reserpine	D	100%	100%	Avoid	None	None	Dose for GFR 10–50
Sotalol	D	100%	30%	15–30%	80 mg	None	Dose for GFR 10–50
Spironolactone	I	q6–12h	q12–24h	Avoid	NA	NA	Avoid
Terazosin	D	100%	100%	100%	Unknown	Unknown	Dose for GFR 10–50
Thiazides	D	100%	100%	Avoid	NA	NA	NA
Ticlopidine	D	100%	100%	100%	Unknown	Unknown	Dose for GFR 10–50
Tocainide	D	100%	100%	50%	200 mg	None	Dose for GFR 10–50
Urokinase	D	Unknown	Unknown	Unknown	Unknown	Unknown	Dose for GFR 10–50
Verapamil	D	100%	100%	100%	None	None	Dose for GFR 10–50
Warfarin	D	100%	100%	100%	None	None	None

ABBREVIATIONS: CAPD = chronic ambulatory peritoneal dialysis; CRRT = continuous renal replacement therapies; D = decreasing individual doses; GFR = glomerular filtration rate; HD = hemodialysis; I = increasing individual doses; NA = not applicable.

SOURCE: Adapted with permission from Aronoff GR, Brier ME. Prescribing drugs in renal disease. In: Brenner BM, ed. *Brenner & Rector's The Kidney,* 7th ed. Philadelphia: Saunders; 2004:2857–2865.

Cramps

Approximately 20 percent of dialysis treatments are accompanied by muscle cramps.[99] These are painful, sustained contractions of skeletal muscles, mainly of the lower extremities, that may occur progressively toward the end of a dialysis session. While the majority are associated with the dialysis treatment, the differential diagnosis is extensive and includes the following conditions: idiopathic cramps, contractures (occurring in conditions such as metabolic myopathies and thyroid disease), tetany (due to hypocalcemia), and dystonias (occupational cramps, antipsychotic medications). Other leg problems, such as restless leg syndromes and periodic leg movements, must be distinguished from cramps.[100]

Cramps are more pronounced in patients who require high UF rates and are dialyzed below their dry weight. Such cramps are presumably related to the reduction in muscle perfusion that occurs in response to hypovolemia. In addition to the effects of reduction in intravascular volume on limb perfusion, compensatory vasoconstrictive responses may shunt blood centrally during dialysis and could play a role in promoting muscle cramps. Electrolyte and acid-base changes may also contribute to these symptoms, especially when intra- vs. extracellular gradients are altered. Under such circumstances, potassium intra-/extracellular balance and changes in the concentration of ionized calcium may also produce alterations of neuromuscular transmission with involuntary contraction of muscles or group of muscle fibers.

A recent study found that peripheral vascular disease, although common in dialysis patients, is not associated with an increased prevalence of intradialytic cramps,[101] which confirms that processes related to the dialytic treatment are likely responsible for the cramps.

Treatment. Many of the treatment strategies are similar to those used to treat intradialytic hypotension. Physical maneuvers that might help include massage of the calf muscles and dorsiflexion of the foot. This approach can relieve pain within a few minutes in a nondialysis setting[100] but is often ineffective in HD patients.

The immediate treatment is to increase intravascular volume by interrupting or slowing UF and administering saline, mannitol, or glucose. In addition to effecting an intravascular shift of water, hypertonic solutions may directly improve blood flow to the muscles. Use of dialysate sodium, potassium, or calcium modeling may help to prevent this complication, using the previously described principle of preserving the intravascular volume during the early part of the treatment. The individualization of dialysate composition seems to be a good preventive approach. Equally important are the careful reassessment of the dry weight, counseling the patient to reduce intradialytic weight gain, and using bicarbonate dialysis.

Drugs that have been tested to treat muscle cramps in dialysis patients include carnitine,[102] quinine,[103] prazosin,[104] vitamins E and C,[105] and Japanese herbal medicine.[106]

L-Carnitine is an essential cofactor in fatty acid and energy metabolism, and some HD patients have been found to have low levels of free L-carnitine and decreased skeletal muscle stores. Administration of L-carnitine has been found to improve symptoms of cramps and of intradialytic hypotension, cardiac function, and anemia in dialysis patients. In addition to reduced muscle cramps, it has been claimed to improve exercise performance and increase muscle strength and mass.[107] L-carnitine doses that have been tried vary from 5 to 100 mg/kg administered intravenously, orally, or via the dialysate. The majority of studies used intravenous administration after each dialysis session.[102]

Quinine appears to decrease the excitability of the motor endplate, thereby reducing muscle contractility. A dosage of 200 to 300 mg of quinine every night has not been shown to cause significant side effects. Nevertheless, quinine should be used in low doses and cautiously, especially in the elderly, and should be avoided in patients with liver disease.[103]

One study used low dose prazosin to treat muscle cramps based on the premise that sympathetic nervous system response to volume stress is more marked in patients with frequent HD-associated skeletal muscle cramps than in patients who cramp infrequently.[104] One study found vitamin E alone to be as useful as quinine in the setting of muscle cramps without any of quinine's side effects.[108] This might make vitamin E an attractive treatment option. In another study, vitamin C (250 mg) and vitamin E (400 mg) given together were found to be effective and safe in reducing HD cramps over a short period.[105]

If these treatments are to be accepted for routine practice, they all need validation in larger groups of patients in controlled trials.

Arrhythmias

The mortality rates of patients on dialysis are high and increasing. ESRD patients on chronic HD have a variable yearly mortality rate ranging from 6 to 20 percent, depending on country and region, which is attributable primarily to cardiovascular disease (CVD). Congestive heart failure, ventricular arrhythmias, sudden cardiac death, and acute myocardial infarction are responsible for 40 percent of deaths.[109] Cardiac arrest or arrhythmias are responsible for more than 20 percent of cardiac deaths.[110]

Arrhythmias occur frequently in HD patients. The prevalence of both atrial and ventricular arrhythmias has been reported to range from 17 to 76 percent of the total HD population.[111] They are frequent in patients with myocardial hypertrophy, heart failure, or IHD. Both patient- and treatment-related factors are involved in their occurrence. Patient-related factors include age, heart and/or lung failure, rapid reduction of extracellular fluid volume, electrolyte and acid base derangements, cardiac and major vascular surgery, digoxin therapy, sympathetic dysfunction, and possibly increased phosphate and PTH levels. Treatment-related factors include changes in serum potassium, calcium, and acid base status; hypovolemia; and sympathetic stimulation produced by dialysis per se. Patients with reduced heart rate variability and increased QT dispersion are at particular risk for arrhythmias.[112]

A lower incidence of arrhythmias has been noted using bicarbonate dialysis instead of acetate; this reduction may be explained by the more regular correction of acidosis with the use of bicarbonate.

Atrial Arrhythmias. About 50 percent of HD patients have (asymptomatic) atrial extrasystoles when they are evaluated by Holter monitoring.[113] However, most of these are of no clinical consequence. A 1-year follow-up study reported an incidence of atrial fibrillation in HD patients at 13.6 percent; 9.4 percent of these were of the permanent type. Approximately 1 in 3 HD patients with atrial fibrillation had thromboembolic complications within 1 year of follow-up. These findings suggest that the consensus contraindication of prophylactic anticoagulation therapy for this group of patients may need to be reconsidered.[114]

Ventricular Arrhythmias. There is evidence of interstitial myocardial fibrosis in experimental uremia and in patients on chronic HD; this can predispose to ventricular arrhythmias due to electrical instability and reentry.[110,115] The incidence of ventricular premature beats (VPBs) is significantly higher during HD and for the following 4 hours than before HD.[116] Complex VPBs and nonsustained ventricular tachycardia (VT) frequently appear during HD. Q-T, Q-Tc (corrected QT), Q-Td (QT dispersing defined as the difference between the maximal and minimal QT interval on a standard ECG), and Q-Tcd (corrected Q-Td) are all longer in chronic HD patients than in those not on dialysis and rise after HD to levels seen in nonuremic patients after myocardial infarction.[109] Q-Td originally was proposed as a direct measure of the regional heterogeneity of myocardial repolarization. It was thought that increased repolarization heterogeneity, or Q-Td, predisposed to reentrant pathways and ventricular arrhythmias. However, it has more recently been proposed that QT-d should be viewed more as an approximation for repolarization abnormalities rather than a true measure of regional heterogeneity of myocardial refractoriness. In one study, QTcd of >74 ms was found to be an independent marker of overall and cardiovascular-related mortality, with a trend toward prediction of arrhythmias and sudden death.[113] Other investigators, however, have not shown any clinical significance of Q-Td and its attendant arrythmogenic potential in HD patients.[117,118] In these studies, Q-T does not reflect the full range of ventricular repolarization in homogeneity, and the prognostic value of Q-Td as an independent marker to predict electrical instability is limited. This may be related to the technical difficulties in measuring Q-T. Indeed, Q-Td is a poorly reproducible ECG parameter, with 30 to 40 percent interobserver relative error.[119,120]

Parathyroid hormone (PTH) may be responsible for uremic cardiomyopathy and for the generation of VPBs. Other factors implicated in ventricular arrhythmias are a decrease in the extracellular volume, rapid correction of metabolic acidosis, increase in levels of free fatty acid, differences between serum and intracellular potassium concentrations, and impaired magnesium metabolism. The changes in potassium fluxes induced by HD may influence cardiac cell electrophysiology and may predispose to cardiac arrythmias.[121] Marked intracellular potassium depletion can exist despite a normal potassium concentration in the blood. In one study, it was found that 89 percent of the HD patients on digoxin had serious VT.[122] This occurred most prominently in those who were dialyzed against a low-potassium bath (2 meq/L). When the potassium concentration in the bath was increased to 3.5 meq/L, there was a significant reduction in VPBs. Signal-averaged ECG (SAECG), still in the development stage, can be used to analyze ventricular late potential (LP), which can detect patients prone to reentry and sustained VT as well as cardiac arrest.[123,124]

Management

Many of the arrhythmias are transient and do not require treatment if the patient is asymptomatic and hemodynamically stable. Maintenance of hemoglobin level, prevention of hypoxia during dialysis, evaluation for any cause of hypotension (if present), and investigation for a possible underlying cardiac condition suffice in most patients. Patients with suspected silent ischemic heart disease might benefit from ambulatory ECG monitoring. Patients on digitalis might need an increase of the dialysate potassium to 3 to 3.5 meq/L to prevent hypokalemia. Intracellular shift of potassium can be minimized by reducing dialysis solution glucose (from 200 to 100 mg/dL) and, when acid base status permits, bicarbonate level.[125]

In patients with arrhythmias during dialysis, blood samples should be immediately drawn for measurement of sodium, potassium, calcium, magnesium, bicarbonate, and glucose levels. An ECG should be obtained and evaluated for supraventricular or ventricular arrhythmia. Treatment is based on the same principles as for nondialysis patients. User-friendly automated external defibrillators (AEDs) should be available in every dialysis unit and can have significant impact on rates of mortality due to arrhythmias.

Amiodarone can be used for the treatment of chronic arrhythmias and does not need any adjustment in dosing for HD patients. It is not dialyzable and no unique problems in dialysis patients have been found with its use. It is safe and effective in chronic kidney disease (CKD) patients and in those with concurrent low cardiac ejection fraction. There may be a small risk of development of torsades de pointes, which could theoretically be increased by hypokalemia during HD. Its various side effects and drug interactions (especially with digoxin and coumadin), however, may result in low patient compliance. The digoxin dose must be reduced by 25 percent compared to the nondialysis dose regimen.[125]

In patients with symptoms or hemodynamic instability dialysis may have to be discontinued before considering defibrillator use or loading with any antiarrythmic drug.

Hypoxemia

During HD, PaO_2 falls by about 10 to 20 mmHg. This decrease has no clinical consequences in patients with normal oxygen tension. In seriously ill patients, however, with predialysis hypoxemia, the drop in PaO_2 can be catastrophic. The cause of hypoxemia is multifactorial, but it is principally related to the use of acetate dialysate (which is now rarely used) and bioincompatible membranes. Acetate causes hypoxemia by at least two mechanisms: increased oxygen consumption in the metabolism of acetate to bicarbonate and intradialytic loss of CO_2. In addition, hypocapnia may be an initial adaptation to chronic metabolic acidosis in CKD patients. This condition has a key role in the pathogenesis of periodic breathing, which is also augmented by increased chemoreceptor sensitivity, as seen in patients with ESRD.[126] A high prevalence of sleep apnea syndrome (SAS) of 54 to 80 percent has been reported in patients with ESRD. SAS in such patients is characterized by both obstructive (due to upper airway occlusion) and central (central destabilization of ventilatory control) apnea. This can also lead to arterial hypoxemia in HD patients. The known complications of sleep apnea include arrhythmias, pulmonary hypertension, and systemic hypertension. In addition, sleep apnea has been implicated in CAD and strokes.[127,128] SAS is also postulated to result in altered autonomic control, which might be a potential mechanism whereby hypoxemia triggers cardiovascular events as well as hypotension in dialysis patients.[129] Improvement in sleep apnea was found with daily HD, possibly by improving oxygenation, because the HD membrane acted as an artificial lung. Patients have increased respiration associated with improved neuroregulation of respiration.[126,130]

Dialysis-induced hypoxemia can be attenuated by interventions that increase the CO_2 content of the dialysate, either by direct administration or by using bicarbonate-buffered dialysate.

The interaction between blood and cellulose membranes activates the alternate complement pathway, which leads to activation of neutrophils. Neutrophil activation results in increased expression of receptors specific for phagocytosis and adhesion as well as of other receptors, which cause adhesion of neutrophils to endothelium with possible sequestration in pulmonary circulation. Neutropenia occurs maximally at 15 minutes with new cuprophane membranes and is followed by a rebound leukocytosis at 120 minutes. Resultant pulmonary microemboli of leukocytes may lead to an impairment of pulmonary gas diffusion and consequent hypoxia.

In critically ill patients, who may already have some degree of predialytic hypoxia, it is necessary to increase the ventilated volumes and/or the percentage of FiO_2 during dialysis. The use of bioincompatible membranes and acetate dialysis should be avoided.

Sudden Death and Cardiac Arrest

HD patients may die suddenly and unexpectedly from a number of causes. Such events may be divided into those due directly to and occurring during HD, those occurring while the patient is not undergoing dialysis, and death that can occur at any time (Table 10–11).[131]

Hypokalemia as a cause of sudden death should be suspected in patients with preexisting conduction system abnormalities, CAD, left ventricular hypertrophy, treatment with digitalis and diuretics, and use of low dialysate potassium. Low blood potassium after death strongly suggests antemortem hypokalemia, as blood potassium rises after death.

TABLE 10–11. CAUSES OF DEATH IN HEMODIALYSIS PATIENTS

Death during Dialysis	Death off Dialysis	Death during or off Dialysis
Hypokalemia	Cardiac tamponade	Cardiovascular disease
Anaphylactoid reactions	Suicide	
Brain herniation	External hemorrhage	Arteriosclerosis
Overheated dialysate		Hyperkalemia
Hemopericardium caused by catheters		Internal hemorrhage
Electrocution		
Third-degree heart block caused by triglyceride emulsion		
Contaminated dialysate		
Acute hemorrhage		
Air embolism		

SOURCE: Reprinted, with permission, from Cohle SD, Graham MA. *J Forensic Sci* 1985;30(1):158–166, copyright ASTM International, 100 Barr Harbor Drive, West Conshohockem, PA 19428.

Anaphylactic reactions to cuprophane membranes are now an uncommon cause of sudden death but should be kept in mind. In addition, anaphylaxis can occur because of allergic reactions to ethylene oxide, with which dialyzers may be sterilized, and/or due to improper priming of the dialyzers before a dialysis session, with inadequate rinse-out of ethylene oxide. One recent study reported cases of sudden death related to the use of a particular brand of diacetate cellulose dialyzer.[132]

Fatal brain herniation results from brain edema and can cause sudden death on dialysis. Brain edema is caused by rapid dialysis leading to a decrease in the pH of the cerebrospinal fluid (CSF) and thus retention of hydrogen ions. In addition, rapid lowering of blood urea can produce an osmotic gradient favoring water movement from the extracellular fluid into the central nervous system. Overheated dialysate can cause disseminated intravascular coagulation (DIC) or hyperkalemia. This can result from a faulty heater alarm system but is extremely rare with modern dialysis machines.

The introduction of a subclavian line in an emergency setting can result in perforation of the superior vena cava and resultant hemopericardium. This can lead to cardiac tamponade over a very short of period of time, even with a blood collection of as little as 300 mL.

Electrocution, triglyceride emulsion, and dialysate contamination with aluminum, calcium, or fluoride are other rare causes of sudden death during dialysis.

Acute hemorrhage can result from line separation in the dialysis machine or needle dislodgment. Air embolism can result from a low level of blood in the venous drip chamber or leakage of air in blood connections on the negative pressure side of the line. Air detectors usually prevent this from happening.

Cardiac tamponade can occur in the interdialytic period as well as during dialysis. The underlying causes include uremic pericarditis and bleeding following heparin used for the dialysis treatment.

Suicide accounts for approximately 1 percent of deaths among HD patients. Their rate of suicide is about 10 to 100 times higher than that of the general population. Methods of suicide peculiar to dialysis patients include exsanguination by disconnecting or otherwise interrupting the vascular access and excessive intake of salt, potassium, or fluid.

Death at anytime can occur following hemorrhage at various locations (subdural, retroperitoneal, gastrointestinal, mediastinal, etc). Cardiovascular causes, however, top the list of causes of death per the latest USRDS data (42 percent of total deaths in dialysis patients, of which 22.4 percent are related to cardiac arrest or arrhythmia.[133]

The incidence of sudden death and cardiac death is greater on Monday (for Monday, Wednesday, and Friday shift patients) and on Tuesday (for Tuesday, Thursday, and Saturday patients).[133] These increased deaths on particular days are postulated to be due to the increased volume and potassium accumulation over the longer weekend interval as well as the development of postdialysis hypotension from the removal of large amounts of fluid.[133] Another study reported similar findings for Monday but not for Tuesday.[134] This study focused on patients having in-facility cardiac arrest, who were found to be older, to have diabetes, and more likely to be using a catheter for vascular access.

Dialysis Dysequilibrium Syndrome

Dialysis dysequilibrium syndrome (DDS) was initially described as the worsening of a preexisting mental confusion, headache, and sometimes muscle twitching and was thought to be due to delayed urea clearance from the cerebrospinal fluid.[135] It is a neurologic disorder, more common in patients just starting on dialysis, especially if they had a high predialysis blood urea nitrogen (BUN). It was also common in elderly and pediatric patients, in patients with preexisting brain lesions (such as recent stroke, head trauma, subdural hematoma, brain tumor) or conditions characterized by cerebral edema (such as malignant hypertension, hyponatremia, hepatic encephalopathy), and in those with severe metabolic acidosis.

Minor symptoms include headache, nausea/vomiting, drowsiness, restlessness, and muscle cramps; moderate symptoms are asterixis, myoclonus, disorientation, and somnolence, while in more severe forms, hypertension, confusion, disorientation, blurred vision, seizures, coma, and possibly death are observed. Symptoms usually occur toward the end of a dialysis session but may be delayed for up to 24 hours.[136] The syndrome is typically self-limited, although full recovery can take several days. DDS must be diagnosed clinically, since laboratory tests, including elec-troencephalography (EEG), are nonspecific.[137] Full-blown disequilibrium syndrome has become rare in recent years. Most of the seizures, coma, and deaths were reported before 1970, and symptoms reported after the 1980s have generally been mild.[135] Improvements in dialysis delivery technology, including bicarbonate dialysate,[138] high dialysate sodium concentration,[139] and controlled UF[140] are responsible for the decreasing frequency and severity of DDS. In addition, the number of patients initiating dialysis with severe azotemia has declined over the years.

Pathophysiology. Consistent findings in patients with DDS are elevation of CSF pressure and urea levels compared to those in blood. Very early, it was realized that the clinical features of DDS are in fact largely due to brain swelling, which occurs because of the dialysis process. The presence of higher CSF urea levels led to the "reverse urea hypothesis." This assumes that urea concentrations are similar in plasma, CSF, and brain tissue water. With rapid HD, it was assumed that clearance of urea would be more rapid from plasma than from the brain tissue. This would lead to the relative increase of brain tissue osmolality compared to that of plasma. This, in turn, would cause net movement of water from plasma into the brain with, resultant cerebral edema.

In experimental studies with uremic animals, however, no significant difference was found between urea levels in brain tissue and plasma. Elevated levels of CSF urea can be explained by the small surface area available for exchange of CSF with blood and the "sink action" of the CSF, which is intact in uremia. The osmolality of brain and CSF has been found to be essentially equal, while plasma and brain differ by about 5 mOsm/Kg H_2O. Determination of brain pH by the radioactive dimethadione (DMO) method and magnetic resonance spectroscopy (MRS) suggests paradoxical acidemia of CSF and brain tissue in both patients and experimental animals treated with rapid HD.[141] Most of the decrement in CSF pH was due to a decrease in CSF bicarbonate rather than any increase of CSF PCO_2. There is no increase of CSF lactate (which can occur in presence of hypoxia and ischemia). The decrement in CSF pH could be due to the presence of organic acid anions (idiogenic osmoles), whose identity is still elusive.[142] These strong organic acid(s) could increase brain tissue osmolality by two mechanisms—(1) displacement of intracellularly bound Na^+ and K^+ ions from protein anions by H^+ ions, which can then become osmotically active, and (2) organic acids per se could raise brain osmolality.[143]

The differential diagnosis of DDS should include the following: intracerebral vascular lesions/cerebral infarction; subdural, subarachnoid, and intracerebral hemorrhage; metabolic disorders such as hyperosmolar states, hypercalcemia, hypoglycemia, and hyponatremia; hypotension, and aluminum intoxication.[144] Serum electrolytes (sodium, potassium, calcium), blood glucose, serum osmolality,

ECG, and computed tomography (CT) scan of the head can rule out many of these conditions. DDS in the modern era should always be a diagnosis of exclusion.

Intervention. DDS is generally a self-limited condition; however, for severe symptoms, dialysis should be discontinued. If seizures are present, glucose should be given after blood samples have been withdrawn. If seizures persist, diazepam 5 to 10 mg IV can be slowly infused. This can be repeated at 5-minute intervals to a maximum total dosage of 30 mg. Diazepam therapy can be followed by loading and maintenance doses of phenytoin (one should be aware of altered phenytoin pharmacodynamics in HD patients). In several studies, DDS has been treated by addition of osmotically (or oncotically) active solutes (albumin, glycerol, glucose, fructose, NaCl, mannitol) to the dialysate.[143]

Prevention. As noted previously, severe symptoms associated with DDS have become rare with improved dialysis delivery. Since brain edema appears to underlie the symptomatology, identification of high-risk patients is of major importance. The recommended prevention method is to limit urea reduction to 30 percent. One small study however found that urea reduction ratios of 60 to 85 percent could be safely achieved with minimal symptoms by increasing dialysate osmolality to equal the extraosmotic contribution of urea in patients requiring acute dialysis with BUN values up to 250 mg/dL.[145]

The simplest strategy for the prevention of DDS is to reduce dialysis efficiency by using small dialyzers, decreasing blood flow, using sequential dialysis, or increasing dialysis time. Therapy can be initiated with 2 hours of dialysis at a relatively low blood flow rate of 150 to 250 mL/min with a small-surface-area dialyzer. If the patient shows no signs of DDS, the blood flow rate can be increased by 50 mL/min per treatment (up to 300 to 400 mL/min) and the duration of dialysis increased in 30-minute increments. Patients who also have marked fluid overload can be treated with UF, followed by a short period of HD (sequential dialysis). Additional strategies include prophylactic administration of osmotic agents—such as mannitol, glucose, fructose, glycerol, urea, and sodium chloride—either intravenously or via the dialysate, with the aim of minimizing the decline in serum osmolality. Intravenous mannitol, 20% at a rate of 50 mL/h, together with intravenous diazepam is the simplest way to prevent DDS in high-risk patients. Because modern dialysis machines can easily change the dialysate sodium levels, the use of high-sodium dialysate may be the most convenient approach. Initiation of dialysis in a timely manner, before severe azotemia occurs, should prevent symptoms of disequilibrium.

Air Embolism

Air embolism, or the entry of air into the vascular system, can result in serious morbidity and even death. With the de-

velopment of the modern HD machine, the incidence of life-threatening air embolism has markedly diminished due to the use of air-bubble detectors, which can stop the blood pump if air is in the circuit. However, cases of air embolism are still occasionally reported.[146,147]

Types and Mechanism. There are two broad categories of air embolism—venous and arterial—which are distinguished by the mechanism of air entry and the site where the embolism ultimately lodges. The inadvertent entry of air through the HD circuit is a potential source of embolism in HD patients due to the combination of the blood pump and a long extracorporeal circuit. There are three main vulnerable areas for air entry: First, between the patient and the blood pump, where a high negative pressure of up to 250 mmHg routinely develops, making it possible for air to get sucked into the circuit. Leaks in this segment, including loose connectors, or a crack in the Silastic tubing of the blood pump may result in air embolism.[148] Second, air in the dialysate fluid diffuses across the dialysis membrane into the blood and forms bubbles in the venous air trap (however, no major episodes of air embolism have yet resulted from this mechanism).[148] Third, central venous catheters, a more important source of air entry today, are frequently used for vascular access for HD. Air embolization has been reported during catheter insertion or removal and also when the catheter gets disconnected from the line.[146,147,149] Significant contributing factors include the patient's body position and hydration status. An upright position will accentuate the normal decrease in intravenous pressure that occurs within the central veins during inspiration. Hypovolemia can cause a low intravenous or intracardiac pressure and facilitate the entry of air into the central venous system.

Clinical Manifestations. The clinical manifestations of air embolism are nonspecific. The absolute quantity and rapidity of air entry, the cardiovascular status of the patient, the patient's body position, and the areas affected determine the clinical presentation. In arterial air embolism, the symptoms are caused by end-artery obstruction. Although obstruction is possible in any artery, occlusion of either the coronary arteries or the nutritive arteries of the brain are especially serious complications, as even small amounts of air often produce severe clinical manifestations.

The basic disturbance in venous air embolism is obstruction to right ventricular blood ejection; this disturbance may be at the pulmonary outflow tract or at the level of the pulmonary arterioles.[150,151] Symptoms are nonspecific and may be transient; they include dyspnea, chest pain, and cough. Significant emboli result in tachypnea and frequently hypotension. In humans, the volume of air that can be tolerated is unknown, but accidental injection of 100 to 300 mL of air has been reported to be fatal.[151,152] Air that has entered the venous circulation can manage to enter the systemic arterial circulation and cause symptoms of end-artery obstruction. This can happen by "paradoxical embolism" via a patent foramen ovale (which is present in 30 percent of the general population), passage through physiologic pulmonary AV shunts, or due to incomplete filtering of a large air embolus by the pulmonary capillaries.[146,151,153,154] Elevated pulmonary arterial pressure due to venous air embolism may result in elevated right atrial pressure, making it possible for a bubble to be transported through a patent foramen ovale. The decrease in left atrial pressure caused by controlled ventilation, the use of positive end-expiratory pressure, and systemic hypotension may also create a pressure gradient across the patent foramen ovale. Because the majority of patients present with nonspecific symptoms, air embolism may be difficult to diagnose in the absence of a high level of suspicion. The most important diagnostic criterion is the patient's history. Air embolism should be suspected in patients during HD or following insertion/manipulation/removal of a central venous catheter who have the sudden onset of cardiopulmonary or neurologic decompensation with either encephalopathic features (i.e., acute confusional state, akinetic mutism, coma, or generalized seizure) or focal neurologic signs (i.e., hemiparesis, homonymous hemianopia, aphasia).[155] Foam in the venous blood line should make one suspect that air is entering the dialysis system. Air embolization may be documented by audible air aspiration ("sucking sound").[149] The "millwheel" murmur, a splashing auscultatory sound due to the presence of air in the cardiac chambers and great vessels, is often present only after cardiovascular deterioration and can be auscultated by a precordial or esophageal stethoscope. Air bubbles in the vessels of the retina can occasionally be demonstrated.

Typically, gas exchange demonstrates initial hypercarbia with hypoxemia. Increased right-sided pressures are evident with central venous and pulmonary artery pressure monitors. ECG abnormalities may demonstrate dysrhythmias and a right ventricular strain pattern. Doppler ultrasonography is a sensitive and practical means of detecting intracardiac air. A more sensitive and definitive method for detecting intracardiac air is transesophageal echocardiography.[156] Cerebral air embolism due to either arterial or paradoxical air embolism can sometimes be demonstrated on CT scan in the early stages. However, this method is not reliable and may fail to detect embolism if the symptoms are mild. This is also true of MRI.

Treatment and Prevention. The primary goal of treatment is the protection and maintenance of vital functions. Whenever air embolism is suspected, further entry of air must be prevented. Clamping and disconnecting the circuit, correct positioning of the patient, infusion of fluid to replace blood loss in the dialyzer and blood tubing, and administration of oxygen are the only measures readily available in the dialysis unit. Flat, supine positioning over the traditionally advocated left lateral (Duran's position) and the Trendelenburg position are now recommended for both venous and arterial air embolism.[149,151] This new recommendation is based on the echocardiographic observation that in the lateral position, air persists longer in the right ventricle, thus worsening and prolonging right ventricular dilatation. The buoyancy of air bubbles is not sufficient to counteract blood flow propelling such bubbles toward the head, even when the patient is placed in a head-down position. In addition, the head-down position may aggravate the cerebral edema that develops in these patients. However, Duran's position is an advantageous one for aspiration of air via the catheter if the air emboli are within the right atrium or pulmonary outflow tract.[149] Adequate oxygenation is often possible only with an increase in the oxygen concentration of the inspired gas up to 100%. Supplemental oxygen also reduces the size of the air embolus by increasing the gradient for the egress of nitrogen from the bubble. Evacuation of air embolism has been described in patients with a preexisting central venous catheter. It has a variable success rate. Cardiopulmonary resuscitation (CPR) may be necessary.

With hyperbaric-oxygen therapy, the patient breathes 100% oxygen at pressure above that of the atmosphere at sea level. The therapeutic effects result from two features of the treatment: the mechanical effects of increased pressure and the physiologic effects of hyperoxia. This therapy may help prevent cerebral edema by reducing the permeability of blood vessels while supporting the integrity of the blood-brain barrier. Further, hyperbaric oxygen diminishes the adherence of leukocytes to the damaged endothelium, which contributes to the cerebral injury. Baskin et al.[157] has reported that eight of nine HD patients with severe cardiorespiratory and neurologic decompensation made full recoveries within minutes of hyperbaric therapy. Thus, as soon as cardiopulmonary stabilization has been achieved, the patient with arterial air embolism and/or venous embolism with evidence of neurologic changes should be transferred to a hyperbaric chamber, particularly patients not responding to conventional measures. It should be noted, however, that controlled trials comparing this therapy with standard measures have not been conducted. Prevention of air embolism has centered mainly on the development of dialysis machines with air-bubble traps and foam detectors distal to the dialyzer at the venous end. Tripping a detector simultaneously activates an alarm, stops the blood pump, and clamps the venous return tubing to prevent air entry into the circulation. Dialysis should never be performed with the air-detection alarm system inoperative (some machines make this impossible). The patient undergoing catheter insertion or removal should be positioned so that the insertion site is at least 5 cm below the right atrium. Patients can assist by performing a Valsalva maneuver, breath-holding, or humming—maneuvers that increase central venous pressure. Whenever possible, the patient should be euvolemic. The dialysis catheter should not be used for routine blood drawing except by dialysis staff or in an emergency. If such a catheter needs to be used for this purpose, the patient should be placed supine and the lines clamped firmly before opening the caps. Luer-lock-type syringes should be used for the blood drawing.

Dialysis-Related Reactions

During the dialysis procedure, reactions may occur due to exposure of large blood volumes to many foreign materials in the dialyzer, blood tubing, sterilant agents, and dialysate. These are responsible for adverse clinical consequences ranging from clinically insignificant to potentially fatal events[158,159] and may contribute directly to increased mortality among patients on long-term HD.[160]

Dialysis-related reactions are usually categorized into type A or anaphylactoid reactions (AR) and type B or mild reactions.[159,161] In general, type A reactions are more severe and more rapid in onset compared to type B reactions, but the incidence of type A is lower. In the early years of dialysis, both types of reactions were found primarily in patients dialyzed with new dialyzers (the "first-use syndrome"). More recently, these reactions were reported in reused dialyzers as well.

Type A or Anaphylactoid Reactions (AR).

AR are anaphylactic in character and can be severe, resulting in respiratory arrest and death. They result from the direct release of mediators by the host cells. The incidence is rare. A preliminary survey from 20,228 patients found that the prevalence rate of AR during HD is 7.0 per 1000 patients per year.[162] The onset of these reactions is usually immediate or within the first 5 minutes; however, the onset may be delayed up to 30 minutes into treatment. Diagnostic criteria for AR have been defined by Daugirdas and Ing.[163] Major criteria include (1) onset within 20 minutes of starting dialysis, (2) dyspnea, (3) burning/heat sensation at the access site or throughout the body, and (4) angioedema. The minor criteria are (1) reproducibility of symptoms during subsequent dialysis when using the same type or band of dialyzer, (2) urticaria, (3) rhinorrhea or lacrimation, (4) abdominal cramping, and (5) itching. AR is diagnosed by three major criteria or two major and one minor criterion. Other symptoms include chest tightness, laryngeal edema, swelling or fullness in the mouth or throat, numbness or tingling of the fingers, toes, lips, or tongue, and flushing of the skin.

Several etiologies have been documented to explain these reactions. Among these, ethylene oxide (ETO) and the polyacrilonitrile (PAN) membrane, especially AN69, in patients treated with ACE inhibitors are well-defined causes of AR. ETO was the most common cause of AR, particularly in patients using new cuprammonium cellulose dialyzers, between 1982 and 1988. The incidence declined in the late 1980s with more thorough rinsing of dialyzers before use and switching from ETO to other sterilization methods. ETO hypersensitivity occurred despite switching to a more biocompatible membrane such as PAN.[164] Patients with a history of atopy, high IgE levels, eosinophilia, or allergic reactions during dialysis have an increased risk of type A reactions.[164,165] Since 1990, a number of clinical studies have shown a strong association of PAN with induced AR.[166–172] Recently, AR has been reported in a patient using a surface-treated AN69 membrane (Nephral ST, 500).[173]

Treatment and Prevention of Dialysis-Related Reactions

If AR is suspected, HD should be discontinued immediately and the blood not returned to the patient. Management is symptomatic and supportive. It depends on the severity and the cause of the reaction. Oxygen administration, antihistamines, adrenaline, and corticosteroids may be required. After the patient has been stabilized, HD can be resumed with a more biocompatible dialyzer membrane, preferably not sterilized with ETO.

As mentioned, reactions usually occur with the first use of a new dialyzer. Reuse of the membrane, particularly with formadehyde, may prevent these reactions. This finding can be explained by changes of the surface charge of PAN membrane, washing out of ethylene oxide, or fixing of the plasma-absorbed protein to the membrane.[171,174,175] Membrane reprocessing with hypochlorite (bleach) removes the adsorbed plasma proteins, restoring the original properties to the membrane. Use of ETO should be avoided. It is mandatory to avoid the combination of PAN with ACE-inhibitor therapy. Use of angiotensin II–receptor antagonists instead of ACE inhibitors and use of dialysate with a calcium concentration of 3.5 meq/L may lower the risk of AR.[176]

Type B or Mild Reactions

The primary symptoms are chest and back pain. Type B reactions often occur 20 to 40 minutes into the dialysis treatment and disappear or lessen dramatically during the subsequent hours of dialysis.[159,161] The pathogenesis of type B reactions is not clear. It is generally believed that they might be related to complement activation. At first, reactions were reported with new bioincompatible membranes, particularly cuprammonium cellulose capillary dialyzers. However, current data do not support the role of membrane biocompatibility in the development of type B reactions.[177] Treatment with oxygen and analgesics is usually sufficient.

Electrolyte and Acid-Base Disturbances

Technical or human errors induce intradialytic electrolyte and acid-base imbalances. Modern dialysis machines improve accurate proportioning of treated water and salts.

Therefore severe electrolyte and acid-base abnormalities during HD are rare. Fortunately, these errors are avoidable as well. Early recognition and proper treatment result in favorable outcomes.

Metabolic Acidosis

Most hemodialyzed patients have mild acidosis due to their inability to excrete protons. The predialysis serum HCO_3^- generally averages approximately 20 meq/L.[178,179] Transient, mild metabolic acidosis is commonly observed during the first 30 to 60 minutes of dialysis with acetate buffer, particularly in patients with low acetate metabolic conversion (such as women, patients who are small in size, elderly and/or cachetic patients, etc.) and in high-efficiency HD, as the rate of bicarbonate loss across the dialyzer membranes exceeds the metabolic conversion rate of acetate. The serum bicarbonate concentration increases rapidly in the first 2 hours of the dialysis treatment and then changes very little during the remainder of the treatment.

An acute, severe intradialytic metabolic acidosis is rare. It can be due to dialysate fluid that contains improper ratios of acid and base concentrates in the form of acetate or bicarbonate.[180–183] Acidosis can also develop as a result of the accidental use of an acidic concentrate instead of acetate, in error, and due to computer software malfunction of the machine. Since the proportioning unit is able to dilute acid concentrate to the proper conductivity, these patients suffer from severe metabolic acidosis without setting off the alarm of the conductivity cell device (which is designed for controlling osmolar and sodium balance). A severe metabolic acidosis was also reported in bicarbonate-buffered HD using sorbent regenerative dialysis, particularly in the first hour into treatment. This is because of the capacity of the regenerating cartridge to release protons.[184,185] At the same time, CO_2 is produced that is dissolved in the dialysate, resulting in increased Pa_{CO_2}, which leads to combined metabolic and respiratory acidosis.[185]

Metabolic acidosis causes nonspecific symptoms including malaise, nausea, headache, general discomfort, and hypotension; it also predisposes to ventricular arrhythmias. These symptoms may continue during the following 24 hours. The diagnosis is usually suggested by the acute onset of hyperventilation during dialysis and then confirmed by blood chemistry/blood gas analysis and biochemical analysis of the dialysate. Blood obtained from the arteriovenous fistula is equivalent to arterial blood for the measurement of pH and Pa_{CO_2}.[186] Blood analysis discloses hyperchloremic acidosis in such cases. Intravenous administration of bicarbonate and dialysis with bicarbonate dialysate of a correct concentration is the appropriate treatment. All HD machines should be fitted with a pH meter and alarms that will prevent the extreme acid load caused by an inappropriately prepared bicarbonate dialysate. Conductivity checks are vital.

Metabolic Alkalosis

Metabolic alkalosis (MA) is an uncommon occurrence in maintenance HD. Despite dialysis using bicarbonate dialysate concentrate up to 39 to 40 meq/L, the highest postdialysis serum HCO_3^- values are typically only 31 to 33 meq/L, and the value rapidly drops into the high 20s.[179] The most common cause of metabolic alkalosis in dialysis patients is loss of hydrogen and chloride ions as a result of vomiting or nasogastric suction.[187] Other less common causes of MA are technical errors during HD and malfunction of the dialysis machine's pH monitor and proportioning system, such as the reversed connection of bicarbonate and acid concentrate containers to the entry ports.[188]

Metabolic alkalosis can result in intradialytic symptoms such as headache, fatigue, and a feeling of ill health. This appears to be at least partially related to hypoxia and a decrease in cerebral blood flow. Acute, severe metabolic alkalosis with pH values greater than 7.55 or an HCO_3^- concentration greater than 55 meq/L may result in tissue hypoxia, arrhythmia, seizure, delirium, or stupor. The diagnosis of metabolic alkalosis is signaled by a 4- to 5-meq/L increase in bicarbonate concentration from its usual value.[187]

Dialysis with standard bicarbonate dialysis solution (a bicarbonate level of 35 to 40 meq/L) in patients with metabolic alkalosis can aggravate or perpetuate this complication. Several reports have shown that applying HD therapy with specially formulated low-bicarbonate, low-acetate, or acid dialyses is a safe and effective intervention for severe metabolic alkalosis.[189,190] A recent report showed that severe metabolic alkalosis could be corrected rapidly and safely with bicarbonate concentrates dialysate between 25 and 28 meq/L.[191]

Hyperkalemia

Serious hyperkalemia is common in HD patients; it is seen in about 10 percent and contributes to 3 to 5 percent of deaths.[192] Several causes and factors render these patients susceptible to hyperkalemia, including excessive dietary K intake, metabolic acidosis, acute infection with marked catabolism, rhabdomyolysis, mineralocorticoid deficiency, and medications. Dialysis-induced hyperkalemia is rare. It has been reported in HD patients from dialysis against a dialysate potassium concentration of 10 mmol/L,[193] from hemolysis, or from accidental acute 20-mmol potassium infusion.[194]

Hyperkalemia should be suspected in any dialysis patient with weakness, dysrhythmia, or hypotension. Patients with accidental, acute potassium infusion may complain of burning in the injected vessel.[194] The effects of hyperkalemia on cardiac electrophysiology are of greatest concern in the clinical setting. Hyperkalemia is associated with reduced myocardial conduction velocity and accelerated repolarization. Although serum potassium concentrations in excess of 6.5 meq/L are usually associated with ECG changes, patients with extreme hyperkalemia (more than 9 meq/L) have been reported to show a normal ECG.[195] A recent study demonstrated that HD patients with hyperkalemia might not exhibit the usual ECG sequel of hyperkalemia, possibly due in part to fluctuations in serum calcium concentration.[196] Therefore the ECG is less reliable in detecting the severity of potential lethal hyperkalemia in HD patients.

Because hyperkalemia is unpredictable and lethal, Ahmed et al.[192] have suggested that patients with serum potassium levels greater than 6.5 meq/L with or without ECG changes or ECG changes consistent with hyperkalemia regardless of the serum potassium level should undergo emergency therapy. Intravenous calcium and insulin administration for acute hyperkalemia is usually acceptable. Albuterol, a selective beta$_2$-adrenoceptor agonist, and bicarbonate should never be used as single agents for the treatment of such cases. HD is the most effective and rapid way to remove potassium and reverse hyperkalemia. Some studies have shown that a rapid decrease in serum potassium concentration induces ventricular ectopy and that the removal of potassium is largely determined by the potassium concentration gradient between the plasma and the dialysate. Therefore continuous cardiac monitoring is needed for all patients dialyzed for hyperkalemia against a 0 to 1 meq/L bath. High-risk patients with underlying CHD, left ventricular hypertrophy, and digoxin use may benefit from gradually decreasing concentrations of potassium and by extending the treatment time to allow for the secondary egress of potassium from the intracellular compartment. Because of the inequality in the rates of potassium flux across the dialyzer and the cell membranes, a rebound in serum potassium is always seen. This rebound correlates with the predialysis potassium. Thus, potassium measurement should be done 2 to 3 hours after HD and HD for hyperkalemia may have to be repeated if hyperkalemia persists.

Hypokalemia

The majority of HD patients will have their pre- and postdialysis plasma potassium concentration within the range of 6 and 3 meq/L, respectively, with a 2-meq/L dialysate potassium concentration. Most patients tolerate this well and do not suffer from complications of hypokalemia if postdialysis serum potassium is kept at 2 to 3 meq/L. However, it is clear that life-threatening hypokalemia can occur during HD. Severe intradialytic hypokalemia has been reported to occur even when the dialysate contained a higher potassium concentration than the predialysis serum potassium concentration.[197] Patients with a history suggesting prolonged potassium loss, marked acidosis, and moderate hypokalemia are prone to these complications. The cause of the hypokalemia is a rapid shift of potassium from the extracellular to the intracellular space secondary to correction of acidosis. Thus, the dialysate potassium concentration should be higher than normal (between 4 and 5 meq/L), and frequent determinations of the serum potassium level should be performed in these patients.[198]

Another major problem associated with low serum potassium concentrations is an increased risk of cardiac arrhythmias in patients with underlying heart disease, particularly in the setting of digoxin therapy. In order to prevent hypokalemia during dialysis, the use of dialysate with 3.0 meq/L of potassium is recommended unless there is chronic, severe hyperkalemia.[199] Use of very low dialysate potassium (0 to 1 meq/L) should be discouraged (unless predialysis serum potassium is followed before each treatment). A sudden reduction in the plasma potassium concentration during the initial portion of the dialysis treatment has been shown to unfavorably alter the Q-Tc (a marker of risk of ventricular arrhythmias). Such an increase of the Q-Tc dispersion was totally blunted during HD in absence of plasma potassium decrease.[200] Dialysis with the modeling of the dialysate potassium concentration, which maintained a constant blood-to-dialysate potassium gradient, decreased premature ventricular complexes.[201]

Hyponatremia

Hyponatremia can occur at the start of dialysis if an error is made in connecting concentrate containers or during dialysis if containers run dry and conductivity monitors fail.[202,203] Acute hyponatremia increases intracellular volume, producing cerebral edema and symptoms that may mimic those of dialysis dysequilibrium syndrome. In addition, it can produce hemolysis and hyperkalemia.[203] Patients may complain of restlessness, anxiety, cramps, dizziness and pain in the vein receiving blood from the dialyzer, chest pain, headache, and nausea. Pallor, vomiting, and seizures may be observed. Treatment of dialysis-induced hyponatremia consists of clamping the blood lines and discarding the hemolyzed blood present in the dialysis tubing. Anticonvulsants are indicated for seizures and blood transfusion may be needed for severe anemia. High-flow oxygen should be administered. Cardiac monitoring is required because of the possibility of hyperkalemia-induced arrhythmias. Use of hypertonic saline in hyponatremia may be life-threatening. Dialysis should be resumed promptly with freshly prepared dialysate.

It is well known that rapid correction of chronic hyponatremia can lead to the development of osmotic demyelination syndrome. Patients with a high BUN from renal failure and hyponatremia may not be as vulnerable as patients with normal renal function to the development of osmotic demyelination syndrome when hyponatremia is rapidly corrected during HD.[204] Experimental studies have revealed that chronically hyponatremic rats with azotemia tolerated large increases in serum sodium without significant brain damage.[205] Rapid reaccumulation of brain organic osmolytes, particularly myoinositol, after correction of chronic hyponatremia partially explain the resistance of azotemic brains to injury resulting from rapid correction of hyponatremia.[206] However, there is a paucity of literature about the safety of HD in patients with dialysis-induced hyponatremia, the risk of demyelinosis being the concern. There is at least one report of a patient with severe hyponatremia developing osmotic demyelination syndrome following HD along with hypertonic saline administration.[207] In addition, there is no need to increase the serum sodium concentration by more than 1 to 2 meq/L/h even in the most acute symptomatic hyponatremia. Therefore serum sodium should be corrected in dialysis patients, using the guidelines currently accepted for correction of hyponatremia in nonuremic patients. Stern and Silver have suggested that the sodium levels of dialysis solution should not be higher than 15 to 20 meq/L above the plasma level.[208]

Hypernatremia

Hypernatremia can occur when the conductivity monitors of the dialysis machine are not functioning or the alarms are not set properly.

Dialysate conductivity can be incorrectly sensed as low by the coated conductivity cells (which become coated by granules from a less soluble batch of sodium bicarbonate powder). The consequence is that an increasing amount of "acid" concentrate, with its accompanying electrolytes, can be delivered to the dialyzer.[209] The clinical expression of hypernatremia is due to the effect of hyperosmolality and intracellular volume depletion as water shifts into the extracellular space. Symptoms include headache, profound thirst, nausea and vomiting, convulsions, and coma or death. High dialysate Na concentration causes hypernatremia and hypertension. A high index of suspicion and aggressive treatment are mandatory. This often requires hospitalization. Some recommend resuming dialysis but changing to a dialysate with a sodium level 2 meq/L lower than the plasma sodium concentration while infusing isotonic saline. Dialyzing against a sodium level 3 to 5 meq/L less than the plasma sodium level increases the risk of disequilibrium syndrome. However, Pazmino and Pazmino describe three patients with severe hypernatremia (sodium levels of 178, 172, 182 meq/L) who were treated successfully with dialysate sodium 110 meq/L without significant side effects.[210]

Febrile Reactions

Febrile reactions, defined as a rise in temperature during HD of at least 0.5°C and a rectal or axillary temperature during dialysis of at least 38.0 or 37.5°C, respectively, are among the major complications in patients undergoing maintenance HD. The majority of febrile reactions are associated with preexisting infections (such as vascular infections, urinary and respiratory tract infections), which account for more than 70 percent of the cases.[211,212] In considering febrile episodes resulting directly from the performance of HD, these complications are usually associated with localized infection of the vascular access site or with exposure to bacterial organisms or products from the apparatus used in HD treatment.[213] Other causes include blood-dialyzer membrane reactions, neoplasm, vasculitis, and unidentified causes in some patients.[212]

Despite significant advances in reducing the risk of infection over the past four decades, HD procedures subject patients to the risk of exposure to bacteremia and/or bacterial products, including those due to contaminated dialysis machines, contaminated water or bicarbonate dialysate, or reprocessing of dialyzers. These exposures result in bloodstream infections, particularly from hydrophilic gram-negative bacteria (i.e., *Pseudomonas, Acinetobacter, Xanthomonas, Alcaligenes,* etc.) and nontuberculous mycobacterium (i.e., *Mycobacterium fortuitum, Mycobacterium chelonae,* etc.), and/or pyrogenic reactions, which are related to exposure of the patient's blood to bacterial endotoxin/liposaccharide (LPS).[214–220] Theoretically, intact hollow-fiber dialysis membranes, cellulose-derived or cellulosic membrane, or synthetic membranes present an excellent barrier to contamination with organisms or with pyrogens such as endotoxin.[221,222] Despite high levels of bacteria and endotoxin in bicarbonate dialysate at the point of use, the passage of endotoxin in dialysate across intact dialyzer membranes during conventional dialysis or across intact polysulfone or polyamide membranes during high-flux HD cannot go undetected. Blockage of endotoxin is seen to a greater extent with polysulfone and polyamide dialyzers compared to cellulosic or modified cellulosic membranes. However, bacteremia can occur in certain circumstances—i.e., if there are defects in membrane integrity, if the level of bacterial contamination in the dialysate is high enough to allow the organism to grow through the membrane, or if extrinsic contamination in the blood compartment occurs during dialyzer reprocessing.

Pyrogenic reactions are defined as chills (visible rigors) and/or fever (oral temperature ≥37.8°C) in a patient who was afebrile and who had no signs or symptoms of infection before the dialysis treatment.[221] The fever and chills are often associated with malaise, nausea, and hypotension (in 17 to 20 percent of cases).[221,223] Some of these episodes can be very severe. The symptoms rapidly disappear after cessation of HD. The presence of circulating endotoxin in 42 percent of febrile episodes (using the limulus lysate test) but in none of the samples taken from the same patients when afebrile establishes a close relationship between endotoxin and PR.[223] In in vitro studies, LPS interacts with plasma LPS Binding Protein (LBP) and mediates cytokine production, including pyrogenic cytokines such as IL-1 and TNF, producing a transient febrile reaction. The reactions during HD may be triggered by monocyte activation at the dialyzer surface or from transfer of low-molecular-weight endotoxin to blood, particularly the lipid A moiety and some monosaccharide precursors, that could be small enough to pass through the membrane pores.[222]

The National Surveillance of Dialysis-Associated Diseases in the United States, reported by the Centers for Disease Control and Prevention (CDC), found that PR without bacteremia was reported by about 19 to 22 percent of HD centers, and these reactions were more frequent in centers reusing dialyzers and using high-flux dialyzers for at least some of their patients.[224,225] Unfortunately, the incidence in individual centers was not reported. A prospective study conducted in three HD centers showed no increased risk of PR for patients treated by conventional, high-efficiency, or high-flux HD or with prior reuse. The incidence of PR was low (i.e., 0.7 episodes per 1000 treatments), even with high levels of bacteria and endotoxin in the dialysate.[226]

Vascular access infections remain a leading cause of morbidity and mortality. These infections account for one-third of the bacterial infections and more than one-half of the bacteremias. Recent data show that the rate of vascular access infection and bacteremia is dependent on the type of access used: 0.9 for 0.2 of 1000 dialysis treatments for arteriovenous fistulas, 2.0 for 0.4 of 1000 dialysis treatments for arteriovenous grafts, 12.2 for 5.5 of 1000 dialysis treatments for tunneled catheters, and 29.2 for 10.5 of 1000 dialysis treatments for temporary catheters.[227] Generally, vascular access infections, whether related to temporary central venous catheters or to permanent fistulas or grafts, are easily diagnosed. However, signs and symptoms of inflammation—such as tenderness, warmth, redness, swelling, or local drainage—at the infected site can be subtle both in polytetrafluoroethylene and catheter-associated infections.[228–230] Singh and Depner[230] have described four patients using an indwelling venous catheter for dialysis access who had no symptoms or fever before HD; then, all of them developed symptoms of chills, rigors, nausea, or a combination of these during the dialysis treatment. Fever resolved after removal of the catheter. The investigators proposed that the fever was probably induced by blood flow through the catheter, termed "flow-induced catheter sepsis." Table 10–12 shows various causes of pyrogenic reactions in HD patients.

In general, the differential diagnosis of fever in dialysis patients is developed by a careful history, clinical exami-

nation, and simple laboratory studies including complete blood count, urine, blood cultures, and chest x-ray. The diagnosis of clinically silent vascular access infections requires a high index of suspicion and may be made only after repeated or prolonged episodes of bacteremia or when the patient is cured by access removal. The probability of catheter-related sepsis is increased in patients who have fever temporally related to dialysis, but the development of fever during HD does not always implicate catheter sepsis, and catheter sepsis may account for fever before dialysis as well. Therefore other types of bacterial infection should be diligently sought before it is assumed that symptoms and signs of sepsis/bacteremia are due to subclinical vascular access infection. Patients with clotted grafts who present with fever of unknown origin should be investigated with an indium scan. PR is a diagnosis of exclusion and septicemia should first be ruled out, because the clinical consequences of sepsis are potentially much more serious. The mortality rate of bacteremia in HD patients is 50 times higher than that in the general population.[236] Many of these patients develop metastatic infections such as osteomyelitis, septic arthritis, and infective endocarditis; the incidence of these is 21 to 54 times higher in HD patients than in the general population.[237] The diagnosis of infective endocarditis is often delayed in dialysis patients because of the lack of characteristic features; moreover, the presentation may be obscured by other HD-related problems.

Even if febrile HD patients have no obvious source of infection, aggressive management is prudent because of the high frequency and high risk of complications, including access loss and metastatic infection. Blood cultures must be obtained and antibiotics started immediately until the culture results are negative or another etiology is established. Management of PR is largely supportive and empiric. A cluster of similar cases should prompt a review of the water used for reprocessing and the dialysate, the processing procedure, and the bicarbonate system. Most outbreaks in HD units have resulted from inadequate disinfection of water-treatment and distribution systems, reprocessed dialyzers, or other reused equipment.

There are several steps to the prevention of infection. One of the most important ways to prevent vascular access infection is to reduce the use of catheters for HD. In order to reduce the susceptibility to infections, optimal adequacy of HD should be attained, malnutrition should be prevented and/or treated, optimal hemoglobin concentration should be maintained, iron overload should be avoided, and high-biocompatibility dialysis membranes should be used.[238] To reduce *Staphylococcus aureus* infections, nasal carriage screening should be performed and carriers should be treated. Many of the PR/bacteremia outbreaks could have been prevented by adequate water treatment, proper disinfection of the water system and dialysis machines, adherence to recommended reprocessing protocols in reusing dia-

TABLE 10–12. SOURCES OF ENDOTOXIN/BACTERIAL CONTAMINATION IN PYROGENIC REACTIONS (PR)/BLOODSTREAM INFECTION (BSI) RELATED TO HEMODIALYSIS PROCEDURES

Source of PR/BSI	(Possible) Related Organism	Manifestations/Comment
Related to dialyzer reprocessing		
O-ring in Hemoflow F-80 dialyzers [231]	*Pseudomonas cepacia, Xanthomonas maltophilia, Citrobacter freundii, Acinetobacter calcoaceticus* var. *anitratus,* and *Enterobacter cloacae*	BSI, procedures should include measure to ensure adequate disinfection of O-ring.
Inadequate disinfectant concentration [218,232]	*Mycobacterium chelonei*	BSI, soft tissue infection, access-graft infection and disseminated infection, may be difficult to diagnosis unless specific cultures for mycobacteria are obtained.
Inadequate mixture of disinfectant [214]	*Pseudomonas cepacia, Xanthomonas maltophilia, Alcaligenes denitrificans* spp.	PR and BSI, failure to mix Renalin resulted in low germicide level, elevated bacterial and endotoxin levels in the blood compartments of dialyzers.
Contaminated tap water and product water [217]	*Pseudomonas* spp, *Enterobacter* spp, unidentified gram-negative cocci	PR/endotoxin/bacteria can contaminate every step of reprocessing; i.e.. rinsing (tap water), cleaning and disinfectant/sterilization (product water) in this report
Cross-contamination by technician's glove during reprocessing [233]	*Klebsiella pneumoniae*	BSI, glove-changing and adequate dialyzer disinfection procedures are required
Related to water treatment		
Inadequate disinfection of water distribution system and machine[218]	*Mycobacterium chelonei*	BSI, soft tissue infection, access-graft infection and disseminated infection, relatively resistant to chemical germicides.
Related to dialysate		
Bicarbonate concentrate [221]	*Pseudomonas* spp, *Xanthomonas maltophilia, Alcaligenes denitrificans*	PR; despite high levels of bacteria and endotoxin in bicarbonate dialysate, the incidence of PR is low.
Related to dialysis machines		
Incompetent valve allowing backflow from contaminated dialysis machine waste-handling option into patient blood tubings [216]	*Enterobacter cloacae*	PR and BSI, highlights the importance of following special manufacturer's recommendations for specific equipment items.
Improper disinfection of HD machine [234]	*Enterobacter cloacae, Klebsiella oxytoca, Pseudomonas cepacia, Xanthomonas maltophilia*	PR and BSI, illustrates need for the use of proper procedures when performed microbial assays
Related to central venous catheter		
Contaminated chlorhexidine-cetrimide solution [235]	*Burkholderia cepacia*	BSI, improper aseptic technique was the source of an outbreak.

lyzers, and more stringent quality-control monitoring. Use of pyrogen filters in the dialysis machines provides further protection against endotoxemia.

Intradialysis Hemolysis

Hemolysis in HD patients is rarely reported today but is a potentially fatal event. The CDC reported 30 patients developing hemolysis while on HD from three U.S. states, 2 of 30 of these patients died and 10 of 30 were admitted to intensive care units.[239] Hemolysis even to a minor degree is highly undesirable; it potentially aggravates the anemia of renal disease and increases the overall cost of the therapy (due to need for higher doses of recombinant erythropoietin).

Accelerated red blood cell (RBC) destruction arises from renal failure itself or its therapy. Most available reports support at least a moderate reduction in RBC survival.[240] RBC half-life in renal failure is one-half to one-third normal, which is related to an intrinsic increase in RBC membrane fragility. In addition, blood that is passed through an extracorporeal system passes through a hostile environment that causes blood cell damage. There are numerous reported causes of acute hemolysis during HD, including oxidant damage (from chloramines, copper, zinc, or nitrate contamination of the dialysate), reduction injury (from formaldehyde used to disinfect reprocessed dialyzers or water-treatment systems), osmolar injury (from hypo/hypertonic dialysate), thermal injury (from overheated dialysate exceeding 108°F), and mechanical injury. Most of these risks have disappeared today through the introduction of appropriate safety systems in dialysis machines and the water-treatment system. The main cause of hemolysis today is mechanical injury to RBCs.[239,241,242] High shear stress is known to rupture the cell membrane. This effect has been demonstrated clearly in the case of tube kinking,[242,243] narrowed aperture of the blood tubing sets,[239] pump malocclusion, inappropriate single-needle dialysis[244] and the presence of a blood clot at the tip of a subclavian catheter,[245] where the blood is pushed through a narrow passage. High-pressure gradients and high velocities in narrow segments increase shear force, which can hemolyze RBCs.

Clinical manifestations of hemolysis vary; they include hypertension, abdominal pain, nausea, vomiting, chest/back pain, shortness of breath, cyanosis, and diarrhea.[239] Pancreatitis, as indicated by a serum lipase higher than 500 U/L or double the baseline value, frequently develops after a hemolytic episode.[241,242] Most reported cases of traumatic hemolysis were described as acute hemolysis occurring during the dialysis treatment. The onset of symptoms is approximately 2.5 hours (range, 20 to 275 minutes) into the dialysis treatment. Symptoms may develop after HD as well.[246] By contrast, chronic mild hemolysis may be clinically inapparent and may be recognized only in the course of an investigation for erythropoietin resistance. The diagnosis of acute major hemolysis during ongoing treatment, particularly in outbreaks, is comparatively easy. In the HD circuit, some sites are more prone to generate high-shear hemolysis and are easily missed. The most important of these is a kink in the tubing segment between the roller blood pump and the inlet to the dialyzer, since it usually precludes the detection of venous and arterial pressure.[242,243]

Causes of hemolytic anemia, which might be first noticed or become symptomatic during dialysis, include autoimmune hemolytic anemia, paroxysmal hemoglobinuria, hemoglobinopathy, and hemolytic uremic syndromes. These must be ruled out by appropriate tests whenever indicated.

Treatment. As soon as acute hemolysis is suspected or diagnosed, the blood pump should be stopped, the venous blood lines clamped, and the blood discarded. Oxygen should be administered and steps taken to obtain cross-matched or type-specific blood. Dialysis should be resumed as soon as the patient is stable, because hyperkalemia is a potential complication of hemolysis in dialysis patients.

The cornerstone of prevention of hemolysis in dialysis patients is recognizing that the dialysis procedure is a dynamic one and that it requires careful and frequent monitoring to meet recommended standards. Care should be taken to screen blood lines and avoid using small needles. Shear stress problems can be prevented by keeping blood flow in the dialyzer circuit within acceptable limits and minimizing resistance to blood flow by the use of large needles/cannulas with the application of an optimal relationship between dialyzer blood flow and access diameter. The use of highly negative arterial pressure settings (exceeding 150 mmHg) should be avoided, and the correct positioning of tubing in the roller pumps should be ensured.[247] Table 10–13 shows causes and associated findings of hemolysis in HD patients.

Uremic Pruritus

Pruritus is one of the most common and bothersome symptoms of patients undergoing dialysis. The prevalence of uremic pruritus in HD patients ranges from 25 to 90 percent.[252–254] The prevalence of itching in dialysis patients has steadily declined over the past 30 years. This has occurred coincident with a general trend toward improved dialysis techniques and efficacy.[255] A recent study showed that in 47 percent of pruritic subjects, itching appeared within the first year of HD, 27 percent developed itching 1 year after the start of HD, the remaining 26 percent noted itching before the initiation of HD.[254] In general, the underlying renal disease, patient's gender, and duration of HD do not seem to influence either the appearance or the severity of pruritus.

Although a variety of factors induced by the uremic state and by HD treatment have been considered to be involved in the pathogenesis of uremic pruritus, its definitive cause is still poorly understood. This symptom is purported to be associated with various chemical mediators including histamine, protease, serotonin, leukotrienes, prostaglandins, substance P, and opioids. The common abnormalities in ESRD per se—such as xerosis, peripheral neuropathy, hypercalcemia, hyperphosphatemia, hypermagnesemia, zinc depletion, and hypervitaminosis A—have been suggested to play a role in the pathogenesis as well. However, no correlation is found between standard biochemical tests (blood urea nitrogen, creatinine, calcium, phosphate, parathyroid hormone) and uremic pruritus.[256] Theoretically, contact be-

TABLE 10–13. CAUSES AND FINDINGS OF DIALYSIS-ASSOCIATED HEMOLYSIS

Type of Injury and Examples	Associated Findings
Osmolar injury: hypoosmolar[248] and hyperosmolar dialysate[249]	Neurologic manifestations
Thermal injury: overheated dialysate[250]	Sensation of being hot, increased osmotic fragility and spherocyte formation
Oxidant: chloramines, copper, aluminum, zinc, nitrate contamination of dialysate[240]	High level of methemoglobinemia and sulfhemoglobinemia, Heinz body, green dialysate color in copper contamination[251]
Reduction: formaldehyde	
Mechanical: central venous catheter, kinked blood line, narrowed aperture of the blood tubing set	Fragmented red blood cells

tween the patient's blood and the dialysis membrane may induce the release of inflammatory and potentially pruritogenic substances. The data concerning a possible relationship between pruritus and type of dialyzer is not clear. Rollino et al.[257] could not demonstrate the role of sensitization with fragments of tubing sets and fragments of different dialyzer membranes including cuprophane, polymethylmethacrylate, and polysulfone in the occurrence of uremic pruritus.

The severity of pruritus varies from patient to patient and from time to time in the same individual. Pruritus is generalized in 19 to 50 percent of cases.[252,258] The forehead, upper back, and volar part of the forearm are considered typical sites.[259] Pruritus in many patients can occur or be exacerbated during or soon after HD. This might be related to the HD procedure, as in allergic reactions to ethylene oxide or porcine heparin. Formaldehyde and iodine (iodized antiseptics) have been reported as sensitizing agents in uremic patients with eczematous lesions.[260] Alternatively, the effect of forced inactivity and the psychological effect of discomfort during HD cannot be excluded.

Before considering the treatment of uremic pruritus, the clinician should evaluate its cause (whether dermatologic or due to other systemic diseases), which might suggest the most appropriate therapeutic approach. History, physical examination, and blood tests including stool examination for parasites and occult blood and a chest x-ray will detect most skin or systemic diseases that produce itching. Determination and avoidance of potential dialysis-related factors include iodine, ethylene oxide, formaldehyde, and porcine or bovine heparin. Efforts should be made to optimize serum calcium, phosphate, and magnesium, maintain parathyroid hormone, and ensure adequate dialysis. Extrapolation of the data indicates that itching may be greatly reduced once Kt/V is 1.5 or more.[255] Even though the relationship between a type of membrane and uremic pruritus is not clear, highly permeable and biocompatible membranes are preferable.

In general, treatment is mainly empiric and individualized. The results are highly variable from patient to patient, but often no treatment is effective. The only definite treatment is a successful renal transplantation. Fortunately, pruritus often remits spontaneously.[252,259]

Following are the reported effective medications and methods for pruritus in uremic patients[259, 261,262]:

Treatment of xerosis: Reduced use of bathing, skin emollients, etc.

Capsaicin: To deplete and prevent the reaccumulation of substance P from local type C sensory nerve terminals that transmits itching sensation.

H₁-receptor antagonists (such as hydroxyzine, diphenhydramine): These are recommended for 2 to 3 weeks, even though they are often ineffective.

Phototherapy with ultraviolet B (UVB) light: This has been the treatment of choice in patients with uremic pruritus.[262] Treatment with UVB is generally well tolerated, the most common side effect being sunburn. Exposure to UVB light may have carcinogenic potential. Several controlled and uncontrolled studies have clearly shown that phototherapy with UVB light is more effective in reducing pruritus than UVA light. The mechanism of actions remains unclear. Recent studies have revealed that UVB results in a significant decrease in the expression of inducible nitric oxide synthase and hence nitric oxide production. This may in part explain the anti-inflammatory and antipruritic properties of UVB radiation. UVB can be performed three times a week for 3 weeks. Photosensitive drugs should be avoided. Remission time is about 3 months.

Other drugs: Thalidomide, nicergoline, lidocaine, mexiletine, cholestyramine to reduce bile acid absorption, activated charcoal to adsorb an unidentified pruritogen, and opioid antagonists may be considered for patients with severe and intractable pruritus.

Other modalities: Acupuncture, electric needle stimulation, and sauna.

Most of the aforementioned methods are of limited usefulness due to their poor efficacy, poor patient acceptance, unacceptable risk of adverse effects, or drug interactions.

Bleeding

Uremic patients have an increased risk of bleeding, primarily due to platelet dysfunction and ineffective platelet-vessel interaction.[263] Although effective dialysis partially improves platelet abnormality,[264,265] the risk still exists and is amplified with anticoagulation for clotting prevention in the extracorporeal circuit, comorbid diseases such as liver failure, sepsis, and certain medications (particularly antiplatelet drugs). In general, the bleeding risk in stable HD patients, with intermittent heparin dosing, is small (except that due to heparin-induced thrombocytopenia).[267] In chronic HD patients, this risk may be augmented by the presence of inadequate control of hypertension or gastrointestinal diseases.

The incidence of bleeding in HD patients is based on the assessment of risk of bleeding more than the actual dose of heparin used.[268–271] At present, the incidence of bleeding is apparently declining.[271] As a rule, spontaneous organ bleeding is rare.

Common clinical manifestations are ecchymoses and prolonged bleeding from puncture sites.[272] Hemorrhage during HD tends to be largely iatrogenic, such as that due to disconnection of blood tubings or needles or catheter insertion. The more serious spontaneous internal bleeding complications that occur with increased incidence in patients on

HD include hemorrhagic pericarditis, gastrointestinal bleeding, intracranial hemorrhage, hemorrhagic pleural effusion, and bleeding in the anterior eye chamber and retropharyngeal space.[273,274]

Treatment in patients with bleeding is similar to that in non-HD patients, consisting of volume and blood replacement, identification of the bleeding sites, and appropriate definitive therapy, which depends on the severity and site of bleeding. Relatively small amounts of blood loss may be enough to produce symptoms and signs in anemic patients. The underlying etiology of bleeding influences the therapeutic modality. Therefore bleeding and coagulating-time screening are mandatory in patients with repeated bleeding episodes.

If the bleeding time is prolonged, cryoprecipitate (10 unit every 12 to 24 hours; onset is 30 minutes and duration up to 36 hours), deamino-D-arginine vasopressin (DDAVP) (intravenously 0.3 µg/kg or intranasally 3 µg/kg, maximal effect at 6 hours, duration up to 8 hours) or conjugated estrogen (Premarin 25 mg/day for 7 days, initial effect at 6 hours, duration up to 21 days) can be used acutely.

If the PTT is prolonged, protamine may be helpful. Generally, 1 mg for every 100 units of heparin can be used if heparin was given within a few minutes of presentation. If 30 minutes to 1 hour has elapsed, 0.5 mg per 100 units of heparin should be used. If more than 2 hours have elapsed, further reduction to 0.25 mg per 100 units is recommended. Since rapid administration is associated with a higher likelihood of side effects such as hypotension and anaphylactoid-like syndromes, the rate of administration should not exceed 50 mg/10 min. Infusion of fresh frozen plasma may be indicated in such circumstances.

Prevention. HD patients can be categorized for bleeding risk as proposed by Swartz and Port into very high risk, high-risk, moderate-risk, and low-risk groups.[269]

Table 10–14 shows various alternatives to conventional heparin dosing in HD patients. In patients with a low risk for bleeding, low-dose conventional heparin (loading dose 50 IU/kg followed by 800 to 1000 IU/h and maintenance of an activated partial thromboplastin time (PTT) at 150 percent of their predialysis values) or, preferably, low-molecular-weight heparin (LMWH) (due to its convenience of use and fewer side effects) can be used for systemic anticoagulation.[275] Several strategies have evolved specifically to anticoagulate patients at high risk for bleeding. These include regional anticoagulation with heparin and protamine, low-dose heparin, use of LMWH, heparin-free dialysis, regional citrate anticoagulation, and prostacyclin (PGI₂). All these methods, however, have their unique complications, which may be more severe than those of heparin itself: for example, severe life-threatening hypocalcemia and metabolic alkalosis with citrate anticoagulation and hypotension with prostacyclin use.

TABLE 10–14. ALTERNATIVE METHODS TO CONVENTIONAL HEPARIN IN HIGH-RISK PATIENTS

Methods	Problems
Heparin-free dialysis	Requires hemodynamic stability to tolerate the high blood flow and close monitoring of arterial and venous pressure and of clot formation
Regional heparinization with protamine reversal	Rebound anticoagulant effect can be observed; bleeding complication appear to be more frequent than with low-dose heparin
Low-dose heparin	Systemic anticoagulation augments the risk of bleeding
Low-molecular-weight heparin	As low-dose heparin
Prostacyclin	Flushing and hypotension may occur
Regional citrate anticoagulation	Complexity of the technique, severe metabolic alkalosis and hypocalcemia are potentially life-threatening complications

Treatment with regional heparinization, which involves infusion of heparin into the blood entering the dialyzer and neutralization by infusion of protamine into the heparinized blood as it returns to the patients, should be avoided due to its technical difficulty and, more importantly, one prospective study in patients at high risk of bleeding found that regional heparinization induced a significantly higher risk of bleeding complications compared to that seen with low-dose heparin.[275]

Low-dose heparinization aims to increase the clotting time by 20 to 50 percent. It permits a reduction in the heparin dose by 50 to 70 percent without causing clotting in the dialyzer, at the same time reducing bleeding complications.[273] The major disadvantage is the risk of bleeding, since this approach will still result in systemic anticoagulation and errors in technique during heparin administration may occur.[276]

LMWH consists of fragments of unfractionated heparin. In terms of hemorrhagic risk, there is only a minor difference between LMWM and conventional heparin. One study found that LMWH induced significant systemic anticoagulation in comparison to citrate.[277] Thus it is not preferable to citrate for patients with a bleeding risk.

The advantage of citrate anticoagulation is that systemic anticoagulation can be completely avoided because 60 percent of the calcium-citrate complexes are removed from the blood by the dialyzer and the citrate entering the body is rapidly metabolized by the tricarboxylic acid pathway, primarily in the liver and skeletal muscle. A recent study showed that regional citrate anticoagulation with a conventional calcium-containing dialysate is safe and effective.[278] However, the potential complications from the use of citrate—such as volume overload, hypernatremia, metabolic alkalosis, and serum-ionized calcium disturbance—are still a concern.

PGI$_2$ is a vasodilator and inhibitor of platelet aggregation. Several reports have demonstrated that PGI$_2$ can be used safely in HD patients with a high bleeding risk.[279] Infusion of PGI$_2$ is advocated to watch for side effects like facial flushing, headache, and hypotension. The most important drawback of PGI$_2$ is its high cost.

The EBPG Expert Group on Haemodialysis has stated that heparin-free regional citrate or prostacyclin (PGI$_2$) during HD is recommended in patients at high risk for bleeding.[275] If long-term avoidance of anticoagulation is required, such as after subarachnoid hemorrhage, conversion of these patients to peritoneal dialysis should be considered.

REFERENCES

1. USRDS: the United States renal data system. *Am J Kidney Dis* 2003;42(6 Pt 6):1–230.
2. Levin NW, Kupin WL, Zasuwa G, Venkat KK. Complications during hemodialysis. In: *Clinical Dialysis,* 2d ed. Norwalk, CT: Appleton & Lange, 1990:172–201.
3. Santoro A, Mancini E, Basile C, et al. Blood volume controlled hemodialysis in hypotension-prone patients: a randomized, multicenter controlled trial. *Kidney Int* 2002;62(3):1034–1045.
4. Tisler A, Akocsi K, Harshegyi I, et al. Comparison of dialysis and clinical characteristics of patients with frequent and occasional hemodialysis-associated hypotension. *Kidney Blood Press Res* 2002;25(2):97–102.
5. Daugirdas J, Levin N, Bailey J, Cheung A. Occurrence of intradialytic hypotension (IH) as a risk factor for mortality in the HEMO Study. *J Am Soc Nephrol* 14:711A, 2003.
6. Ronco C, Feriani M, Chiaramonte S, et al. Impact of high blood flows on vascular stability in haemodialysis (review). *Nephrol Dial Transplant* 1990;5(suppl 1):109–114.
7. Ronco C, Brendolan A, Bragatini L, et al. Technical and clinical evaluations of different short, highly efficient techniques. *Contrib Nephrol* 1988;61:46–68.
8. Gotch FA. Dialysis of the future. *Kidney Int Suppl* 1988;24:S100—S104.
9. Koomans KA, Geers AB, Dorhout Mees EJ. Plasma volume recovery after ultrafiltration in patients with chronic renal failure. *Kidney Int* 1984;26:848–854.
10. Kouw PM, Olthof CG, TerWee PM, et al. Assessment of post-dialysis dry weight: an application of the conductivity measurement method. *Kidney Int* 1992;41:440–444.
11. Sargent JA, Gotch FA. Mathematic modeling of dialysis therapy. *Kidney Int Suppl* 1980;suppl (Sept) 10:S2–S10.
12. Zhu F, Kaysen G, Morris AT, et al. Estimation of dry weight in hemodialysis patients by continuous segmental bioimpedance analysis (abstr.) *J Am Soc Nephrol* 13:30A.
13. Daugirdas JT. Pathophysiology of dialysis hypotension: an update (review). *Am J Kidney Dis* 2001;38(4 suppl 4):S11—S17. Review.
14. de Vries JP, Kouw PM, van der Meer NJ, et al. Noninvasive monitoring of blood volume during hemodialysis: its relation with post-dialytic dry weight. *Kidney Int* 1993;44(4):851–854.
15. Cavalcanti S, Cavani S, Santoro A. Role of short-term regulatory mechanisms on pressure response to hemodialysis-induced hypovolemia. *Kidney Int* 2002; 61(1):228–328.
16. Lee JS. 1998 Distinguished Lecture: biomechanics of the microcirculation, an integrative and therapeutic perspective (review). *Ann Biomed Eng* 2000;28(1):1–13.
17. Converse RL Jr, Jacobsen TN, Jost CM, et al. Paradoxical withdrawal of reflex vasoconstriction as a cause of hemodialysis-induced hypotension. *J Clin Invest* 1992;90(5):1657–1665.
18. Prakash S, Reddan D, Heidenheim AP, et al. Central, peripheral, and other blood volume changes during hemodialysis. *ASAIO J* 2002;48(4):379–382.
19. Yu AW, Nawab ZM, Barnes WE, et al. Splanchnic erythrocyte content decreases during hemodialysis: a new compensatory mechanism for hypovolemia. *Kidney Int* 1997;51(6):1986–1990.
20. Kooman JP, Gladziwa U, Bocker G, et al. Role of the venous system in hemodynamics during ultrafiltration and bicarbonate dialysis. *Kidney Int* 1992;42(3):718–726.
21. Kooman JP, Wijnen JA, Draaijer P, et al. Compliance and reactivity of the peripheral venous system in chronic intermittent hemodialysis. *Kidney Int* 1992;41(4):1041–1048.
22. Nakamura Y, Ikeda T, Takata S, et al. The role of peripheral capacitance and resistance vessels in hypotension following hemodialysis. *Am Heart J* 1991;121:1170–1177.
23. Furukawa K, Ikeda S, Naito T, et al. Cardiac function in dialysis patients evaluated by Doppler echocardiography and its relation to intradialytic hypotension: a new index combining systolic and diastolic function. *Clin Nephrol* 2000;53(1):18–24.
24. Badgett RG, Lucey CR, Mulrow CD. Can the clinical examination diagnose left-sided heart failure in adults? *JAMA* 1997;277(21):1712–1719.
25. De Santo NG, Cirillo M, Perna A, et al. The heart in uremia: role of hypertension, hypotension, and sleep apnea (review). *Am J Kidney Dis* 200138(4 suppl 1): S38–S46.
26. Sherman RA. Intradialytic hypotension: an overview of recent, unresolved and overlooked issues (review). *Semin Dial* 2002;15(3):141–143.
27. Rozich JD, Smith B, Thomas JD, et al. Dialysis-induced alterations in left ventricular filling: mechanisms and clinical significance. *Am J Kidney Dis* 1991;17(3):277–285.
28. Poldermans D, Man in `t Veld AJ, Rambaldi Ret al. Cardiac evaluation in hypotension-prone and hypotension-resistant hemodialysis patients. *Kidney Int* 1999; 56(5):1905–1911.
29. Zucchelli P, Santoro A. Dialysis induced hypotension. A fresh look at pathophysiology. *Blood Purif* 1993;11:85–98.
30. Oberg B, Thoren P. Increased activity in left ventricular receptors during hemorrhage or occlusion of caval veins in the cat: a possible cause of the vaso-vagal reactions. *Acta Physiol Scand* 1972;85:164–173.
31. Yalcin AU, Kudaiberdieva G, Sahin G, et al. Effect of sertraline hydrochloride on cardiac autonomic dysfunction in pa-

tients with hemodialysis-induced hypotension. *Nephron* 2003;93(1):P21–P28.

32. Noris M, Todeschini M, Casirighi F, et al. Effect of acetate, bicarbonate dialysis, and acetate-free biofiltration on nitric oxide synthesis: implications for dialysis hypotension. *Am J Kidney Dis* 1998;32(1):115–124.

33. Beasley D, Brenner BM. Role of nitric oxide in hemodialysis hypotension. *Kidney Int* 1992;42(suppl 38):S96–S100.

34. Nishimura M, Takahashi H, Maruyama K, et al. Enhanced production of nitric oxide may be involved in acute hypotension during maintenance hemodialysis. *Am J Kidney Dis* 1998;31(5):809–817.

35. Lin SH, Chu P, Yu FC, et al. Increased nitric oxide production in hypotensive hemodialysis patients. *ASAIO J* 1996; 42(5):M895–M899.

36. Raj DS, Vincent B, Simpson K, et al. Hemodynamic changes during hemodialysis: role of nitric oxide and endothelin. *Kidney Int* 2002;61(2):697–704.

37. Shizato T, Miwa M, Nakai S, et al. Role of adenosine in dialysis-induced hypotension. *J Am Soc Nephrol* 1994; 4(12): 1987–1994.

38. Pagel MD, Ahmad S, Vizzo JE, Scribner BH. Acetate and bicarbonate fluctuations and acetate intolerance during dialysis. *Kidney Int* 1982;21:513–518.

39. Lewis EJ, Tolchin N, Roberts J. Estimation of the metabolic conversion of acetate to bicarbonate during hemodialysis. *Kidney Int* 1980;18:551–555.

40. Schrander-yd Meer AM, ter Wee PM, Kan G, et al. Improved cardiovascular variables during acetate free biofiltration. *Clin Nephrol* 1999;51(5):304–309.

41. Hmida J, Balma A, Lebben I, et al. [Clinical evaluation of acetate-free biofiltration at 84 0/00 in patients with chronic renal insufficiency](French.) *Tunis Med* 2002;80(8): 473–484.

42. Maggiore Q, Pizzarelli F, Zoccali C, et al. Effect of extracorporeal blood cooling on dialytic arterial hypotension. *Proc Eur Dial Transplant Assoc* 1981;18:597–602.

43. Gotch FA, Keen ML, Yarian SR. An analysis of thermal regulation in hemodialysis with one and three compartment models. *ASAIO Trans* 1989;35(3):622–624.

44. Schneditz D. Temperature and thermal balance in hemodialysis (review). *Semin Dial* 2001;14(5):357–364.

45. Fine A, Penner B. The protective effect of cool dialysate is dependent on patients' predialysis temperature. *Am J Kidney Dis* 1996;28(2):262–265.

46. Rosales LM, Schneditz D, Morris AT, et al. Isothermic hemodialysis and ultrafiltration. *Am J Kidney Dis* 2000;36(2): 353–361.

47. Orofino L, Marcen R, Quereda C, et al. Epidemiology of symptomatic hypotension in hemodialysis: is cool dialysate beneficial for all patients? *Am J Nephrol* 1990;10(3): 177–180.

48. Maggiore Q, Pizzarelli F, Santoro A, et al. The effects of control of thermal balance on vascular stability in hemodialysis patients: results of the European randomized clinical trial. *Am J Kidney Dis* 2002;40(2):280–290.

49. Van Stone JC, Bauer J, Carey J. The effect of dialysate sodium concentration on body fluid distribution during hemodialysis. *ASAIO Trans* 1980;26:383–386.

50. Ronco C, Brendolan A, Milan M, et al. Impact of biofeedback-induced cardiovascular stability on hemodialysis tolerance and efficiency. *Kidney Int* 2000;58(2):800–808.

51. Straver B, De Vries PM, Donker AJ, ter Wee PM. The effect of profiled hemodialysis on intradialytic hemodynamics when a proper sodium balance is applied. *Blood Purif* 2002;20(4):364–369.

52. Coli L, Ursino M, De Pascalis A, et al. Evaluation of intradialytic solute and fluid kinetics. Setting up a predictive mathematical model. *Blood Purif* 2000;18(1):37–49.

53. Santoro A, Mancini E, Basile C, et al. Blood volume controlled hemodialysis in hypotension-prone patients: a randomized, multicenter controlled trial. *Kidney Int* 2002;62(3): 1034–45.

54. Wolkotte C, Hassell DR, Moret K, et al. Blood volume control by biofeedback and dialysis-induced symptomatology. A short-term clinical study. *Nephron* 2002;92(3):605–609.

55. Association for the Advancement of Medical Instrumentation. *Hemodialysis Systems, ANSI/AAMI.* RD5:2003. Arlington, VA: Association for the Advancement of Medical Instrumentation, 2003.

56. Mitra S, Chamney P, Greenwood R, Farrington. Linear decay of relative blood volume during ultrafiltration predicts hemodynamic instability. *Am J Kidney Dis* 2002;40(3): 556–565.

57. Kyriazis J, Glotsos J, Bilirakis L, et al. Dialysate calcium profiling during hemodialysis: use and clinical implications. *Kidney Int* 2002;61(1):276–287.

58. Alappan R, Cruz D, Abu-Alfa AK, et al. Treatment of severe intradialytic hypotension with the addition of high dialysate calcium concentration to midodrine and/or cool dialysate. *Am J Kidney Dis* 2001;37(2):294–299.

59. Perazella MA. Pharmacologic options available to treat symptomatic intradialytic hypotension (review). *Am J Kidney Dis* 2001;38(4 suppl 4):S26–s36.

60. Lim PS, Yang CC, Li HP, et al. Midodrine for the treatment of intradialytic hypotension. *Nephron* 1997;77(3):279–283.

61. Yalcin AU, Kudaiberdieva G, Sahin G, et al. Effect of sertraline hydrochloride on cardiac autonomic dysfunction in patients with hemodialysis-induced hypotension. *Nephron* 2003;93(1):P21–P28.

62. Iida N, Koshikawa S, Akizawa T, et al. Effects of L-threo-3,4-dihydroxyphenylserine on orthostatic hypotension in hemodialysis patients. *Am J Nephrol* 2002;22(4):338–346.

63. Shizato T, Miwa M, Nakai S, et al. Role of adenosine in dialysis-induced hypotension. *J Am Soc Nephrol* 1994; 4(12):1987–1994.

64. Peer G, Itzhakov E, Wollman Y, et al. Methylene blue, a nitric oxide inhibitor, prevents haemodialysis hypotension. *Nephrol Dial Transplant* 2001;16(7):1436–1441.

65. Agarwal R. Systolic hypertension in hemodialysis patients. *Semin Dial* 2003;16(4):334.

66. Agarwal R, Lewis RR. Prediction of hypertension in chronic hemodialysis patients. *Kidney Int* 2001;60(5):1982–1989.

67. Tozawa M, Iseki K, Iseki C, et al. Evidence for elevated pulse pressure in patients on chronic hemodialysis: a case-control study. *Kidney Int* 2002;62(6):2195–2201.

68. Klassen PS, Lowrie EG, Reddan DN, et al. Association between pulse pressure and mortality in patients undergoing maintenance hemodialysis. *JAMA* 2002;287(12):1548–1555.

69. Foley RN, Herzog CA, Collins AJ, United States Renal Data System. Blood pressure and long-term mortality in United States hemodialysis patients: USRDS Waves 3 and 4 Study. *Kidney Int* 2002;62(5):1784–1790.

70. Horl MP, Horl WH. Hemodialysis-associated hypertension: pathophysiology and therapy (review). *Am J Kidney Dis* 2002;39(2):227–244.

71. Mailloux LU. Hypertension in chronic renal failure and ESRD: prevalence, pathophysiology, and outcomes (review). *Semin Nephrol* 2001;21(2):146–156.

72. Charra B, Calemard E, Ruffet M, et al. Survival as an index of adequacy of dialysis. *Kidney Int* 1992;41(5):1286–1291.

73. Innes A, Charra B, Burden RP, et al. The effect of long, slow haemodialysis on patient survival. *Nephrol Dial Transplant* 1999;14(4):919–922.

74. Converse RL Jr, Jacobsen TN, Toto RD, et al. Sympathetic overactivity in patients with chronic renal failure. *N Engl J Med* 1992;327(27):1912–1918.

75. Grekas D, Kalevrosoglou I, Karamouzis M, et al. Effect of sympathetic and plasma renin activity on hemodialysis hypertension. *Clin Nephrol* 2001;55(2):115–120.

76. Raine AE, Roger SD. Effects of erythropoietin on blood pressure (review). *Am J Kidney Dis* 1991;18(4 suppl 4): 76–83.

77. Canadian Erythropoietin Study Group. Effect of recombinant human erythropoietin therapy on blood pressure in hemodialysis patients. *Am J Nephrol* 1991;11(1):23–26.

78. Mittal SK, Kowalski E, Trenkle J, et al. Prevalence of hypertension in a hemodialysis population. *Clin Nephrol* 1999;51(2):77–82.

79. Lebel M, Kingma I, Grose JH, Langlois S. Hemodynamic and hormonal changes during erythropoietin therapy in hemodialysis patients. *J Am Soc Nephrol* 1998;9(1):97–104.

80. Mayer G, Horl WH. Cardiovascular effects of increasing hemoglobin in chronic renal failure (review). *Am J Nephrol* 1996;16(4):263–267.

81. Campese VM. Neurogenic factors and hypertension in chronic renal failure (review). *J Nephrol* 1997;10(4): 184–187.

82. Roger SD, Grasty MS, Baker LR, Raine AE. Effects of oxygen breathing and erythropoietin on hypoxic vasodilation in uremic anemia. *Kidney Int* 1992;42(4):975–980.

83. Fodinger M, Fritsche-Polanz R, Buchmayer H, et al. Erythropoietin-inducible immediate-early genes in human vascular endothelial cells. *J Invest Med* 2000;48(2):137–149.

84. Neusser M, Tepel M, Zidek W. Erythropoietin increases cytosolic free calcium concentration in vascular smooth muscle cells. *Cardiovasc Res* 1993;27(7):1233–1236.

85. Kusano E, Akimoto T, Inoue M, et al. Human recombinant erythropoietin inhibits interleukin-1beta-stimulated nitric oxide and cyclic guanosine monophosphate production in cultured rat vascular smooth-muscle cells. *Nephrol Dial Transplant* 1999;14(3):597–603.

86. Buckner FS, Eschbach JW, Haley NR, et al. Hypertension following erythropoietin therapy in anemic hemodialysis patients. *Am J Hypertens* 1990;3(12 Pt 1):947–955.

87. Eschbach JW, Egrie JC, Downing MR, et al. Correction of the anemia of end-stage renal disease with recombinant human erythropoietin. Results of a combined phase I and II clinical trial. *N Engl J Med* 1987;316(2):73–78.

88. Ni Z, Wang XQ, Vaziri ND. Nitric oxide metabolism in erythropoietin-induced hypertension: effect of calcium channel blockade. *Hypertension* 1998;32(4):724–729.

89. Massry SG, Iseki K, Campese VM. Serum calcium, parathyroid hormone, and blood pressure (review). *Am J Nephrol* 1986;6(Suppl 1):19–28.

90. Chobanian AV, Bakris GL, Black HR, et al. National Heart, Lung, and Blood Institute Joint National Committee on Prevention, Detection, Evaluation, and Treatment of High Blood Pressure; National High Blood Pressure Education Program Coordinating Committee. Evaluation, and Treatment of High Blood Pressure: the JNC 7 report. *JAMA* 2003;289(19):2560–2572.

91. Miller BW, Cress CL, Johnson ME, et al. Exercise during hemodialysis decreases the use of antihypertensive medications. *Am J Kidney Dis* 2002;39(4):828–833.

92. Charra B. "Dry weight" in dialysis: the history of a concept. *Nephrol Dial Transplant* 199813(7):1882–1885.

93. Katzarski KS, Charra B, Luik AJ, et al. Fluid state and blood pressure control in patients treated with long and short haemodialysis. *Nephrol Dial Transplant* 1999;14(2):369–375.

94. Zazgornik J, Biesenbach G, Forstenlehner M, Stummvoll K. Profile of antihypertensive drugs in hypertensive patients on renal replacement therapy (RRT). *Clin Nephrol* 1997;48(6): 337–340.

94a. Nicholls AJ. Heart and circulation. In: Ing TS, ed. *Handbook of Dialysis,* 3d ed. Philadelphia: Lippincott Williams & Wilkins, 2001:595, 597, 598.

95. Rahman M, Fu P, Sehgal AR, Smith MC. Interdialytic weight gain, compliance with dialysis regimen, and age are independent predictors of blood pressure in hemodialysis patients. *Am J Kidney Dis* 2000;35(2):257–265.

96. Hanly PJ, Pierratos A. Improvement of sleep apnea in patients with chronic renal failure who undergo nocturnal hemodialysis. *N Engl J Med* 200111;344(2):102–107.

97. Kielstein JT, Boger RH, Bode-Boger SM, et al. Asymmetric dimethylarginine plasma concentrations differ in patients with end-stage renal disease: relationship to treatment method and atherosclerotic disease. *J Am Soc Nephrol* 1999;10(3):594–600.

98. Fagugli RM, Reboldi G, Quintaliani G, et al. Short daily hemodialysis: blood pressure control and left ventricular mass reduction in hypertensive hemodialysis patients. *Am J Kidney Dis* 2001;38(2):371–376.

99. Wilkinson R, Barber SG, Robson V. Cramps, thirst and hypertension in hemodialysis patients—the influence of dialyzate sodium concentration. *Clin Nephrol* 1977;7(3):101–105.

100. Riely JD, Antony SJ. Leg cramps: differential diagnosis and management (review). *Am Fam Physician* 1995;52(6): 1794–1798.

101. Brass EP, Adler S, Sietsema K, et al. Peripheral arterial disease is not associated with an increased prevalence of intradialytic cramps in patients on maintenance hemodialysis. *Am J Nephrol* 2002;22(5–6):491–496.

102. Ahmad S. L-carnitine in dialysis patients (review). *Semin Dial* 2001;14(3):209–117.

103. Mandal AK, Abernathy T, Nelluri SN, Stitzel V. Is quinine effective and safe in leg cramps (review)? *J Clin Pharmacol* 1995;35(6):588–593.

104. Sidhom OA, Odeh YK, Krumlovsky F, et al. Low-dose prazosin in patients with muscle cramps during hemodialysis. *Clin Pharmacol Ther* 1994;56(4):445–451.

105. Khajehdehi P, Mojerlou M, Behzadi S, Rais-Jalali GA. A randomized, double-blind, placebo-controlled trial of supplementary vitamins E, C and their combination for treatment of haemodialysis cramps. *Nephrol Dial Transplant* 2001;16(7):1448–1451.

106. Hyodo T, Taira T, Kumakura M, et al. The immediate effect of Shakuyaku-kanzo-to, traditional Japanese herbal medicine, for muscular cramps during maintenance hemodialysis. *Nephron* 2002;90(2):240.

107. Goral S. Levocarnitine and muscle metabolism in patients with end-stage renal disease (review). *Renal Nutr* 1998;8(3):118–121.

108. Roca AO, Jarjoura D, Blend D, et al. Dialysis leg cramps. Efficacy of quinine versus vitamin E. *ASAIO J* 1992;38(3):M481–M485.

109. Meier P, Vogt P, Blanc E. Ventricular arrhythmias and sudden cardiac death in end-stage renal disease patients on chronic hemodialysis (review). *Nephron* 2001;87(3):199–214.

110. Ritz E, Rambausek M, Mall G, et al. Cardiac changes in uremia and their possible relationship to cardiovascular instability on dialysis (review). *Nephrol Dial Transplant* 1990;5(suppl 1):93–97.

111. Erem C, Kulan K, Tuncer C, et al. Cardiac arrhythmias in patients on maintenance hemodialysis. *Acta Cardiol* 1997;52(1):25–36.

112. Kantarchi G, Ozener C, Tokay S, et al. QT dispersion in hemodialysis and CAPD patients. *Nephron* 2002;91(4):739–741.

113. Beaubien ER, Pylypchuk GB, Akhtar J, Biem HJ. Value of corrected QT interval dispersion in identifying patients initiating dialysis at increased risk of total and cardiovascular mortality. *Am J Kidney Dis* 2002;39(4):834–842.

114. Vazquer E, Sanchez-Perales C, Borrego F,et al. Influence of atrial fibrillation on the morbido-mortality of patients on hemodialysis. *Am Heart J* 2000;140(6):886–890.

115. Roithinger FX, Punzengruber C, Rossoll M, et al. Ventricular late potentials in haemodialysis patients and the risk of sudden death. *Nephrol Dial Transplant* 1992;7(10):1013–1018.

116. Kimura K, Tabei K, Asano Y, Hosoda S. Ventricular tachyarrhythmia treated by parathyroidectomy in a chronically hemodialyzed patient. *Nephron* 1989;53(2):176–177.

117. Gussak HM, Gellens ME, Gussak I, Bjerregaard P. Q-T interval dispersion and its arrhythmogenic potential in hemodialyzed patients: methodological aspects. *Nephron* 1999;82(3):278.

118. Coumel P, Maison-Blanche P, Badilini F. Dispersion of ventricular repolarization. Reality? Illusion? Significance? *Circulation* 1998;97(25):2491–2493.

119. de Bruyne MC, Hoes AW, Kors JA, et al. QTc dispersion predicts cardiac mortality in the elderly: the Rotterdam Study. *Circulation* 1998;97(5):467–472.

120. Kautzner J. QT interval measurements (review). *Card Electrophysiol Rev* 2002;6(3):273–277.

121. Redaelli B, Locatelli F, Limido D, et al. Effect of a new model of hemodialysis potassium removal on the control of ventricular arrhythmias. *Kidney Int* 1996;50(2):609–617.

122. Morrison G, Michelson EL, Brown S, Morganroth J. Mechanism and prevention of cardiac arrhythmias in chronic hemodialysis patients. *Kidney Int* 1980;17(6):811–819.

123. Lindsay BD, Ambos HD, Schechtman KB, et al. Noninvasive detection of patients with ischemic and nonischemic heart disease prone to ventricular fibrillation. *J Am Coll Cardiol* 1990;16(7):1656–1664.

124. Morales MA, Gremigni C, Dattolo P, et al. Signal-averaged ECG abnormalities in haemodialysis patients. Role of dialysis. *Nephrol Dial Transplant* 1998;13(3):668–673.

125. Nicholls AJ. Heart and circulation. In: Daugirdas JT, Blake PG, Todd SI, eds. *Handbook of Hemodialysis*, 3d ed. Philadelphia: Lippincott Williams & Wilkins, 2001:594–596.

126. Hanly PJ, Pierratos A. Improvement of sleep apnea in patients with chronic renal failure who undergo nocturnal hemodialysis. *N Engl J Med* 2001;344(2):102–107.

127. Kraus MA, Hamburger RJ. Sleep apnea in renal failure (review). *Adv Perit Dial* 1997; 13:88–92.

128. De Santo NG, Cirillo M, Perna A, et al. The heart in uremia: role of hypertension, hypotension, and sleep apnea (review). *Am J Kidney Dis* 2001;38(4 suppl 1):S38–s46.

129. Zoccali C, Mallamaci F, Tripepi G, Benedetto FA. Autonomic neuropathy is linked to nocturnal hypoxaemia and to concentric hypertrophy and remodelling in dialysis patients. *Nephrol Dial Transplant* 2001;16(1):70–77.

130. Friedman EA. Hemodialysis as an artificial lung in sleep apnea. *N Engl J Med* 2001;344(2):134–135.

131. Cohle SD, Graham MA. Sudden death in hemodialysis patients. *J Forens Sci* 1985;30(1):158–166.

132. Garcia Lopez FJ, Anchuela OT, Lopez-Abente G. Sudden death related to a brand of diacetate cellulose dialyzers. *J Am Soc Nephrol* 2002;17:579A.

133. Bleyer AJ, Russell GB, Satko SG. Sudden and cardiac death rates in hemodialysis patients. *Kidney Int* 1999;55(4):1553–1559.

134. Karnik JA, Young BS, Lew NL, et al. Cardiac arrest and sudden death in dialysis units. *Kidney Int* 2001;60(1):350–357.

135. Harris CP, Townsend JJ. Dialysis dysequilibrium syndrome (clinicopathologic conference). *West J Med* 1989;151:52–55.

136. Burn DJ, Bates D. Neurology and the kidney. *J Neurol Neurosurg Psychiatry* 1998;65:810–821.

137. Kiley JE, Woodruff SE, Pratt KL. Evaluation of encephalopathy by EEG frequency analysis in chronic dialysis patients. *Clin Nephrol.* 1976;5:245–260.

138. Graefe U, Milutinovich J, Follette WC, et al. Less dialysis-induced morbidity and vascular instability with bicarbonate in dialysate. *Ann Intern Med* 1978;88:332–336.

139. Port FK, Johnson WJ, Klass DW. Prevention of dialysis disequilibrium syndrome by use of high sodium concentration in the dialysate. *Kidney Int* 1973;3:327–333.

140. Kishimoto T, Yamagami S, Tanaka H, et al. Superiority of hemofiltration to hemodialysis for treatment of chronic renal failure: comparative studies between hemofiltration and he-

modialysis in dialysis disequilibrium syndrome. *Artif Organs* 1980;4:86–93.

141. Arieff AI, Guisado R, Massry S, et al. Central nervous system pH in uremia and the effect of hemodialysis. *J Clin Invest* 1976;58:306–311.

142. Lien YH, Shapiro JI, Chan L. Study of brain electrolytes and organic osmolytes during correction of chronic hyponatremia: implications for the pathogenesis of central pontine myelinolysis. *J Clin Invest* 1991;88:303–309.

143. Arieff AI. Dialysis disequilibrium syndrome: current concepts on pathogenesis and prevention (editorial). *Kidney Int* 1994;45(3):629–635.

144. Nicholls AJ. Nervous system. In: Daugirdas JT, Blake PG, Todd SI, eds. *Handbook of Hemodialysis*, 3d ed. Philadelphia: Lippincott Williams & Wilkins, 2001: 656–666.

145. Macon EJ. Dialysis disequilibrium after acute dialysis: must the urea reduction ratio be limited to 30%? *J Am Soc Nephrol* 1998;9:259A.

146. Yu ASL, Levy EV. Paradoxical cerebral air embolism from a hemodialysis catheter. *Int J Kidney Dis* 1997;29:453–455.

147. Ely EW, Hite RD, Baker AM, et al. Venous air embolism from central venous catheterization: a need for increased physician awareness. *Crit Care Med* 1999;27:2113–2117.

148. Ward MK, Shadforth M, Hill AVL, Kerr DNS. Air embolism during haemodialysis. *Br J Med* 1971;3:74–78.

149. Vesely TM. Air embolism during insertion of central venous catheters. *J Vasc Intervent Radiol* 2001;12;1291–1295.

150. Orebaugh SL. Venous air embolism: clinical and experimental considerations. *Crit Care Med* 1992;20:1169–1177.

151. Muth CM, Shank ES. Gas embolism. *N Engl J Med* 2000;342;476–482.

152. Toung TJK, Rossberg MI, Hutchins GM. Volume of air in a lethal venous air embolism. *Anesthesiology* 2001;94: 360–361.

153. Black M, Calvin J, Chan KL, Walley VM. Paradoxical air embolism in the absence of an intracardiac defect. *Chest* 1991;99;754–755.

154. Thackray NM, Murphy PM, McLean RF, Delay JL. Venous air embolism accompanied by echocardiographic evidence of transpulmanary air passage. *Crit Care Med* 1996;24: 359–361.

155. Heckmann JG, Lang CJ, et al. Neurologic manifestations of cerebral air embolism as a complication of central venous catheterization. *Crit Care Med* 2000;28:1621–1625.

156. Palmon SC, Moore LE, Lundberg J, Toung T. Venous air embolism: a review. *J Clin Anesth* 1997;9:251–257.

157. Baskin SF, Woznizk RF. Hyperbaric oxygenation in the treatment of hemodialysis-associated air embolism. *N Engl J Med* 1975;293;184–185.

158. Lazarus JM, Owen WF. Role of bioincompatibility in dialysis morbidity and mortality. *Am J Kidney Dis* 1994;24: 1019–1032.

159. Jaber BL, Pereira BJG. Dialysis reactions. *Semin Dial* 1997;10 158–165.

160. Hakim RM, Held PJ, Stannard DC, et al. Effect of the dialysis membrane on mortality of chronic hemodialysis patients. *Kidney Int* 1996;50:566–570.

161. Salem M, Ivanovich PT, Ing TS, Daugirdas JT. Adverse effects of dialyzers manifesting during the dialysis session. *Nephrol Dial Transplant* 1994;9(suppl 2);127–137.

162. Bright RA, Torrence ME, McMlellan WM. Preliminary survey of the occurrence of anaphylactoid reactions during haemodilaysis. *Nephrol Dial Transplant* 1999;14:799–800.

163. Daugirdas JT, Ing TS. First-use reactions during hemodialysis: A definition of subtypes. *Kidney Int* 1988;33(suppl 24);S37–S43.

164. Kraske GK, Shinaberger JH, Klaustermeyer WB. Severe hypersensitivity reaction during hemodialysis. *Ann Allergy Asthma Immunol* 1997;78:217–220.

165. Lemke HD, Heidland A, Schaefer RM. Hypersensitivity reactions during haemodialysis: role of complement fragments and ethylene oxide antibodies. *Nephrol Dial Transplant* 1990;5:264–269.

166. Tielemans C, Madhoun P, Lenaers M, et al. Anaphylactoid reactions during haemodialysis on AN69 membranes in patients receiving ACE inhibitors. *Kidney Int* 1990;38: 982–984.

167. Parnes EL, Shapiro WB. Anaphylactoid reactions in hemodialysis patients treated with AN69 dialyzer. *Kidney Int* 1991;40:1148–1152.

168. Verresen L, Fink E, Lemke HD, Vanrenterghem Y. Bradykinin is a mediator of anaphylactoid reactions during haemodialysis with AN69 membranes. *Kidney Int* 1994;45: 1497–1453.

169. John B, Anijeet HKI, Ahmad R. Anaphylactic reactions during haemodialysis on AN69 membrane in a patient receiving angiotensin II receptor antoagonist. *Nephrol Dial Transplant* 2001;16:1955–1956.

170. Schaefer RM, Schaefer L, Horl WH. Anaphylactoid reactions during hemodialysis. *Clin Nephrol* 1994:42 (suppl 1);S44–S47.

171. Schulman G, Ikizler TA, Hakim R. Angiotensin-converting enzyme inhibitors and hemodialysis membranes. *Semin Dial* 1999;12(suppl 1):S88–S91.

172. Krieter DH, Grude M, Lemke HD, et al. Anaphylactoid reactions during hemodialysis in sheep are ACE inhibitor dose-dependent and mediated by bradykinin. *Kidney Int* 1998;53:1026–1035.

173. Peces R. Anaphylactoid reaction induced by ACEI during haemodialysis with a surface-treated AN69 membrane. *Nephrol Dial Transplant* 2002;17:1859–1860.

174. Dumler F, Zasuwa G, Levin NW. Effect of dialyzer reprocessing methods on complement activation and hemodialyzer-related symptoms. *Artif Organs* 1987;11:128–131.

175. Mahiout A, Meihold H, Kessel M, et al. Dialyzer membranes: effect of surface area and chemical modification of cellulose on complement and platelet activation. *Artif Organs* 1987;11:149–154.

176. Van der Niepen P, Sennesael JS, Verbeelen DL. Prevention of anaphylactoid reactions to high flux membrane dialysis and ACE inhibitors by calcium. *Nephrol Dial Transplant* 1994;9:87–89.

177. Locatelli F, Manzoni C. Biocompatibility in haemodialysis: fact and fiction. *Curr Opin Nephrol Hypertens* 1997;6: 528–532.

178. Messa P, Mioni G, Maio G et al. Derangement of acid-base balance in uremia and under hemodialysis. *J Nephrol* 2001;14(suppl 4);S12–S21.

179. Gennari FJ. Acid-base balance in dialysis patients. *Semin Dial* 2000;13:235–239.

180. Hartmann A, Reisaeter A, Holdaas H,. Accidental metabolic acidosis during hemodialysis. *Artif Organs* 1994;18: 214–217.

181. Gainza FJ, Zarraga S, Minguela I, Lampreabe I. Accidental substitution of acid concentrate for acetate in dialysis fluid concentrate: a cause of severe metabolic acidosis. *Nephron* 1995;69:480–482.

182. Fourtounas C, Kopelias I, Dimitriadis G, et al. Severe metabolic acidosis during haemodialysis: a rare but life threatening complication. *Nephrol Dial Transplant* 2001;16: 2416–2417.

183. Navarro JF, Mora-Fernandez C, Garcia J. Errors in the selection of dialysate concentrates cause severe metabolic acidosis during bicarbonate hemodialysis. *Artif Organs* 1997;2: 966–968.

184. Brezis M, Brown RS. An unsuspected cause for metabolic acidosis in chronic renal failure: sorbent system hemodialysis. *Am J Kidney Dis* 1985;6:425–427.

185. Reyes A, Turchetto E, Bernis C, Cereijo E. Acid-base derangements during sorbent regenerative hemodialysis in mechanically ventilated patients, *Crit Care Med* 1991;19; 554–559.

186. Gennari FJ, Rimmer JM. Acid-base disorders in end-stage renal disease: Part I. *Semin Dial* 1990: 3: 81–85.

187. Gennari FJ, Rimmer JM. Acid-base disorders in end-stage renal disease: Part II. *Semin Dial* 1990;3:161–165.

188. Sethi D, Curtis JR, Topham DL, Gower PE. Acute metabolic alkalosis during haemodialysis. *Nephron* 1989;51:119–120.

189. Gerhardt RE, Koethe JD, Glickman JD, et al. Acid dialysate correction of metabolic alkalosis in renal failure. *Am J Kidney Dis* 1995;25;343–345.

190. Leblanc M, Farah A. Severe metabolic alkalosis corrected by hemodialysis. *Clin Nephrol* 1997;48:65.

191. Hsu SC, Wang MC, Liu HL, et al. Extreme metabolic alkalosis treated with normal bicarbonate hemodialysis. *Am J Kidney Dis* 2001;37:E31.

192. Ahmed J, Weisberg LS. Hyperkalemia in dialysis patients. *Semin Dial* 2001;14:348–356.

193. Brady HR, Goldberg H, Lunski C, Uldall PR. Dialysis-induced hyperkalemia presenting as profound muscle weakness. *Intern J Artif Organs* 1988;11:43–44.

194. Romagnoni M, Beccari M, Sorgato G. Life-threatening hyperkalemia during a haemodialysis session: an avoidable risk. *Nephrol Dial Transplant* 1998;13:2480–2481.

195. Szerlip HM, Weiss J, Singer I. Profound hyperkalemia without electrocardiographic manifestation. *Am J Kideny Dis* 1986;7:461–465.

196. Aslam S, Friedman EA, Ifudu O. Electrocardiography is unreliable in detecting potential lethal hyperkalaemia in haemodialysis patients. *Nephrol Dial Transplant* 2002;17: 1639–1642.

197. Wiegand CF, Davin TD, Raij L, Kjellstrand CM. Severe hypokalemia induced by hemodialysis. *Arch Intern Med* 1981;141:167–170.

198. Van Stone JC. Individualization of the dialysate prescription in chronic hemodialysis. *Dial Transplant* 1994;23: 624–635, 663.

199. Morrison G, Michaelson EL, Brown S, Morganroth J. Mechanisms and prevention of cardiac arrhythmias in chronic hemodialysis patients. *Kidney Int* 1980;17:811–819.

200. Cupsti A, Galetta F, Caprioli R, et al. Potassium increases the QTc interval dispersion during hemodialysis. *Nephron* 1999;82:122–126.

201. Redaelli B, Locatelli F, Limido D, et al. Effect of a new model of hemodialysis potassium removal on the control of ventricular arrhythmias. *Kidney Int* 1966;50:609–617.

202. Olivero JJ, Dichoso C. Severe hyponatremia in a home-dialysis patient. *JAMA* 1978;239:108–109.

203. Said R, Quintanilla A, Levin N, Ivanovich P. Acute hemolysis due to profound hypo-osmolality. A complication of hemodialysis. *J Dial* 1977;1:447–452.

204. Oo TN, Smith CL, Swan SK. Does uremia protect against the demyelination associated with correction of hyponatremia during hemodialysis? A case report and literature review. *Semin Dial* 2003;1:68–71.

205. Soupart A, Penninckx R, Stenuit A, Decaux G. Azotemia (48 h) decreases the risk of brain damage in rats after correction of chronic hyponatremia. *Brain Res* 2000;852:167–172.

206. Soupart A, Silver S, Schroeder B, et al. Rapid (24-hour) reaccumulation of brain organic osmolytes (particularly *myo*-inositol) in azotemic rats after correction of chronic hyponatremia. *J Am Soc Nephrol* 2002;13:1433–1441.

207. Peces R, Ablanedo P, Alvarez J. Central pontine and extrapontine myelinolysis following correction of severe hyponatremia. *Nephron* 1988;49:160–163.

208. Sterns RH, Silver SM. Hemodialysis in hyponatremia: is there a risk? *Semin Dial* 1990;3:3–4.

209. Williams DJ, Jugurnauth J, Harding K, et al. Acute hypernatraemia during bicarbonate-buffered haemodialysis. *Nephrol Dial Transplant* 1994;9:1170–1173.

210. Pazmino PA, Pazmino BP. Treatment of acute hypernatremia with hemodialysis. *Am J Nephrol* 1993;13:260–255.

211. Kolmos HJ, Moller S. The epidemiology of febrile reactions in haemodialysis. *Acta Med Scand* 1978;203:345–349.

212. Evers J. Approach to fever in dialysis patients. *Nephron* 1995;69:110.

213. Gaynes R, Fridman C, Foley MK, Swartz R. Hemodialysis-associated febrile episodes: surveillance before and after major alteration in the water treatment system. *Int J Artif Organs* 1990;13:482–487.

214. Beck-Sague CM, Jarvis WR, Bland LA,. Outbreak of gram-negative bacteremia and pyrogenic reactions in a hemodialysis center. *Am J Nephrol* 1990;10;397–403.

215. CDC. Outbreaks of bacterial gram-negative bacterial blood stream infections traced to probable contamination of hemodialysis machines. *MMWR Morb Mortal Wkly Rep* 1998;47: 55–59.

216. Jochimsen EM, Frenette C, Delorme M, et al. A cluster of bloodstream infections and pyrogenic reactions among hemodialysis patients trace to dialysis machine waste-handling option units. *Am J Nephrol* 1998;18:485–489.

217. Gordon SM, Tipple M, Bland LA, Jarvis WR. Pyrogenic reactions associated with the reuse of disposable hollow-fiber hemodialyzers. *JAMA* 1988;260;2077–2081.

218. Bolan G, Reingold AL, Carson LA, et al. Infections with *Mycobacterium chelonae* in patients receiving dialysis and using processed hemodialyzers. *J Infect Dis* 1985;152; 1013–1019.

219. Rudnick JR, Arduino MJ, Bland LA, et al. An outbreak of pyrogenic reactions in chronic hemodialysis patients associated with hemodialyzer reuse. *Artif Organs* 1995;19; 289–294.

220. Roth VR, Jarvis WR. Outbreaks of infection and/or pyrogenic reactions in dialysis patients. *Semin Dial* 2000;13: 92–96.

221. Gordon SM, Oettinger CW, Bland LA, et al. Pyrogenic reactions in patients receiving conventional, high flux-efficacy, or high-flux hemodialysis treatments with bicarbonate dialysate containing high concentrations of bacteria and endotoxin. *J Am Soc Nephrol* 1992;2:1436–1444.

222. Felice AD, Cappelli G, Facchini F, et al. Ultrafiltration and endotoxin removal from dialysis fluids. *Kidney Int* 1993; 43(suppl 41):S201–S204.

223. Raij L, Shapiro FL, Michael AF. Endotoxemia in febrile reaction during hemodialysis. *Kidney Int* 1973; 4:57–60.

224. Tokars JI, Alter MJ, Favero MS, et al. National surveillance of hemodialysis associated diseases in the United States, 1990. *ASAIO J* 1993;39:71–80.

225. Tokars JI, Miller ER, Alter MJ, Arduino MJ. National surveillance of dialysis-associated disease in the United States, 1997. *Semin Dial* 2000:13;75–85.

226. Pegues DA, Oettinger CW, Bland LA, et al. A prospective study of pyrogenic reactions in hemodialysis patients using bicarbonate dialysis fluid filtered to remove bacteria and endotoxin. *J Am Soc Nephrol* 1992;3:1002–1007.

227. Stevenson KB, Hannah EL, Lowder CA, et al. Epidemiology of hemodialysis vascular access infections from longitudinal infection surveillance data: predicting the impact of NKF-DOQI Clinical Practice Guideline for vascular access. *Am J Kidney Dis* 2002;39;549–555.

228. Ayus JC, Sheikh–Hamad D. Silent infection in clotted hemodialysis access grafts. *J Am Soc Nephrol* 1998;9: 1314–1317.

229. Nassar GM, Ayus JC. Clotted arteriovenous grafts: a silent source of infection. *Semin Dial* 2000;13:1–3.

230. Singh B, Depner TA. Catheter related bacterial infections mimic reactions to exogenous pyrogens during hemodialysis. *ASAIO J* 1994; 40: M674–M677.

231. Flaherty JP, Garcia-Houchins S, Chudy R, Arnow PM. An outbreak of gram-negative bacteremia traced to contaminated O-rings in reprocessed dialyzers. *Ann Intern Med* 1993;119:1072–1078.

232. Lowry PW, Beck-Sague CM, Bland LA, et al. *Mycobactium chelonae* infection among patients receiving high-flux dialysis in a hemodialysis clinic in California. *J Infect Dis* 1990;161:85–90.

233. Welbel SF, Schoendorf K, Bland LA, et al. An outbreak of gram-negative bloodstream infections in chronic hemodialysis patients. *Am J Nephrol* 1995;15:1–4.

234. Jackson BM, Beck-Sague CM, Bland LA, et al. Outbreak of pyrogenic reactions and gram-negative bacteremia in a hemodialysis center. *Am J Nephrol* 1994;14:85–89.

235. Kaitwatcharachai C, Silpapojakul K, Jitsurong S, Kalnauwakul S. An outbreak of *Burkholderia cepacia* bacteremia in hemodialysis patients: an epidemiologic and molecular study. *Am J Kidney Dis* 2000;36:199–204.

236. Sarnak MJ, Jaber BL. Mortality caused be sepsis in patients with end-stage renal disease compared with the general population. *Kidney Int* 2000;58:1758–1764.

237. Brueck M, Rauber K, Wizemann V, Kramer W. Infective tricuspid valve endocarditis with septic pulmonary emboli due to puncture of an endogenous arteriovenous fistula in a chronic hemodialysis patient. *J Infect* 2003; (3):188–191.

238. The EBPG Expert Group on Haemodialysis. Hemodialysis-associated infection. *Nephrol Dial Transplant* 2002;17(suppl l7):72–87.

239. Duffy R, Tomashek K, Spangencerg M, et al. Multistate outbreak of hemolysis in hemodialysis patients traced to faulty blood tubing sets. *Kidney Int* 2000;57:1668–1674.

240. Eaton JW, Leida MN. Hemolysis in chronic renal failure. *Semin Nephrol* 1985:5:133–139.

241. Daul AE, Schafers RF, Wenzel RR, et al. Acute hemolysis with subsequent life-threatening pancreatitis in hemodialysis. A complication which is not preventable with current dialysis equipment. *Dtsch Med Wochenschr* 1994; 119(38): 1263–1269.

242. Sweet SJ, McCarty S, Steingart R, Callaham T. Hemolytic reactions mechanically induced by kinked hemodialysis blood lines. *Am J Kidney Dis* 1996;27:262–266.

243. Gault MH, Duffett S, Purchase L, Murphy J. Hemodialysis intravascular hemolysis and kinked blood lines. *Nephron* 1992;62:267–271.

244. Dhaene M, Gulbis B, Lietaer N, et al. Red blood cell destruction in single-needle dialysis. *Clin Nephrol* 1989;31: 327–331.

245. Nand S, Bansal VK, Kozeny G, et al. Red cell fragmentation syndrome with the use of subclavian hemodialysis catheter. *Arch Intern Med* 1985;145:1421–1423.

246. Roman-Latorre J. Postdialysis hemolysis with acute pigmentation in a chronic hemodialysis patient. *Semin Dial* 1999;12:50–52.

247. Section III. Biocompatibility. *Nephrol Dial Transplant* 2002;17(suppl 7):32–44.

248. Said R, et al. Acute hemolysis due to profound hypo-osmolarity. A complication of hemodialysis. *J Dial* 1977;1: 447–452.

249. Mulligan I, Parfrey P, Phillips ME, et al. Acute haemolysis due to concentrated dialysis fluid. *Br J Med* 1982;284: 1151–1152.

250. Fortner RW, Nowakowski A, Carter CB, et al. Death due to overheated dialysate during dialysis. *Ann Intern Med* 1970; 9:443–444.

251. Manzler AD, Schreiner AW. Copper-induced acute hemolysis anemia: a new complication of hemodialysis. *Ann Intern Med* 1970;73:409–412.

252. Gilchrest BA, Stern RS, Steinman TI, et al. Clinical features of pruritus among patients undergoing maintenance hemodialysis. *Arch Dermatol* 1982;118:154–156.

253. Balaskas EV, Chu M, Uldall RP, et al. Pruritus in continuous ambulatory peritoneal dialysis and hemodialysis patients. *Perit Dial Int* 1993;13(suppl 2):S527–S532.

254. Szepietowski JC, Sikora M, Kusztal M, et al. Uremic pruritus: a clinical study of maintenance hemodialysis patients. *J Dermatol* 2002;29:621–627.

255. Masi CM, Cohen EP. Dialysis efficacy and itching in renal failure. *Nephron* 1992;62:257–261.

256. Virga G, Mastrosimone S, Amici G, et al. Symptoms in hemodialysis patients and their relationship biochemical and demographic parameters. *Int J Artif Organs* 1998;21:788–793.

257. Rollino C, Goitre M, Piccoli G, et al. What is the role of sensitization in uremic pruritus? *Nephron* 1991;57:319–322.

258. Ponticelli C, Bencini PL. Uremic pruritus: a review. *Nephron* 1992;60:1–5.

259. Schwartz IF, Iaina A. Uraemic pruritus. *Nephrol Dial Transplant* 1999;14:834–839.

260. Kessler M, Moneret-Vautrin DA, Cao-Huu T, et al. Dialysis pruritus and sensitization. *Nephron* 1992;60:241–251.

261. Schwartz IF, Iaina A. Management of uremic pruritus. *Semin Dial* 2000;13;177–180.

262. Urbonas A, Schwartz RA, Szepietowski JC. Uremic pruritus—an update. *Am J Nephrol* 2001;21:343–350.

263. Noris M, Remuzzi G. Uremic bleeding: closing the circle after 30 years of controversies? *Blood* 1999;94:2569–2574.

264. Di Minno G, Martinez J, McKean M, et al. Platelet dysfunction in uremia. Multifaceted defect partially corrected by dialysis. *Am J Med* 1985;79:552–559.

265. Malyszko J, Malyszko JS, Mysliwiec M. Comparison of hemostatic disturbances between patients on CAPD and patients on hemodialysis. *Perit Dial* 2001;21:158–165.

266. Biggers JA, Remmers AR, Glassford DM, et al. The risk of anticoagulation in hemodialysis patients. *Nephron* 1977;18:109–113.

267. Reilly BF. The pathophysiology of immune-mediated heparin-induced thrombocytopenia. *Semin Dial* 2003;16:54–60.

268. Swartz RD. Hemorrhage during high-risk hemodialysis using heparinization. *Nephron* 1981;28:65–69.

269. Swartz RD, Port FK. Preventing hemorrhage in high-risk hemodialysis: regional versus low-dose heparin. *Kidney Int* 1979;16:513–518.

270. Flanigan MJ, Brecht JV, Freeman RM, Lim VS. Reducing the hemorrhagic complications of hemodialysis: a controlled comparison of low-dose heparin and citrate anticoagulation. *Am J Kidney Dis* 1987;9:147–153.

271. Locatelli F, Del Vecchio L, Manzoni C. Morbidity and mortality on maintenance hemodialysis. *Nephron* 1998;8;380–400.

272. Weigert AL, Schafer AI. Uremic bleeding: pathogenesis and therapy. *Am J Med Sci* 1998;316;94–104.

273. Lohr JW, Schwab SJ. Minimizing hemorrhagic complications in dialysis patients. *J Am Soc Nephrol* 1991;2:961–975.

274. Janssen MJFM, van der Meulen J. The bleeding risk in chronic haemodialysis: preventive strategies in high-risk patients. *Netherlands J Med* 1996;48:198–207.

275. The EBPG Expert Group on Haemodialysis. Chronic intermittent haemodialysis and prevention of clotting in the extracorporal system. *Nephrol Dial Transplant* 2002;17(suppl 7):63–71.

276. Ouseph R, Ward RA. Anticoagulation for intermittent hemodialysis. *Semin Dial* 2000;13:181–187.

277. Janssen MJFM, Deegens JK, Kapinga TH et al. Citrate compared to low molecular weight heparin anticoagulation in chronic hemodialysis patients. *Kidney Int* 1996;49:806–813.

278. Evenepoel P, Maes B, Vanwalleghem J, et al. Regional citrate anticoagulation for hemodialysis using a conventional calcium-containing dialysate. *Am J Kidney Dis* 2002;39;315–323.

279. Caruana RJ, Smith MC, Clyne D, et al. Controlled study of heparin versus epoprostenol sodium (prostacyclin) as the sole anticoagulant for chronic hemodialysis. *Blood Purif* 1991;9;296–304.

11

Dialyzer Reuse

Bruce M. Robinson
Harold I. Feldman
Sidney M. Kobrin

Reuse of flat-plate (Kiil) hemodialyzers dates back to the earliest days of dialysis.[1,2] In the 1960s, because flat-plate dialyzers were assembled from their component parts by the user and required sterilization prior to each use, little additional hazard was thought to arise from dialyzer reprocessing and reuse. Subsequently, disposable coil and hollow-fiber dialyzers did not require sterilization prior to use, and they were designed and labeled principally for single use. However, dialyzer reuse remained commonplace in the United States, chiefly as a means of reducing costs, although claims were also made in the 1970s and 1980s of clinical benefits related to improved biocompatibility.[3–7] Since the mid-1980s, a substantial majority of American dialysis units have practiced dialyzer reuse.

The practice of dialyzer reuse remains controversial. It is much less common in countries other than the United States and is prohibited in some, such as France and Japan.[8] Some authors have suggested that the high prevalence of dialyzer reuse in the United States may contribute to the relatively high mortality reported among dialysis patients in this country.[9] Recent literature, although inconclusive, has consistently raised concerns about possible adverse effects of dialyzer reuse, including decline in solute clearance with some reprocessing techniques, loss of protein into the dialysate with other techniques, increased risk of infection if proper reprocessing techniques are not observed, and the possibility of decreased patient survival. Furthermore, the 2002 publication of the hemodialysis (HEMO) trial, a major multicenter clinical trial sponsored by the National Institutes of Health (NIH) showing no statistically significant overall improvement in clinical outcomes with the use of high- rather than low-flux dialyzers,[10] also raises questions about the economic justification for reuse programs, many of which have been perpetuated in an effort to deliver dialysis with relatively expensive high-flux dialyzers.

This chapter reviews patterns of dialyzer reuse, methods of dialyzer reprocessing, and the effects of hemodialyzer reprocessing on biocompatibility, solute clearance, and clinical outcomes. Evaluation of economic factors that influence decisions to practice dialyzer reuse is beyond the scope of this chapter and is addressed in several recent publications.[11-15]

EVOLUTION OF DIALYZER REUSE IN THE UNITED STATES

Data on the number of times a single dialyzer is used as well as the sterilizing agents employed by dialysis units have been collected by the Centers for Disease Control (CDC) in most years since 1976. These surveys, summarized in Table 11–1, represent greater than 90 percent of Medicare-certified dialysis units.[16,17] In the 1980s, the proportion of dialysis units reprocessing hemodialyzers rose rapidly, from 19 percent in 1980 to above 70 percent by 1990. During this decade, it became recognized that dialysis with reprocessed unsubstituted (e.g., regenerated or cuprammonium) cellulosic dialyzers reduced intradialytic symptoms.[3] The increase in dialyzer reuse has also been attributed to the 1983 Health Care Financing Administration's (HCFA; now, Centers for Medicare and Medicaid Services, or CMS) imposition of a cost-control measure known as the "composite rate" as reimbursement to facilities for dialysis treatments, which has led to a progressive decrease in payment adjusted for inflation. The proportion of dialysis units practicing reuse peaked at 82 percent in 1997 and was 80 percent in 2000. The proportion of hemodialysis patients reusing dialyzers in the United States is believed to closely mirror the proportion of reprocessing centers.[16] Between 1986 and 1997, the mean and median number of uses per patient rose from 10 to 17 and 9 to 15, respectively.

Certain aspects of dialyzer reprocessing technology have changed substantially since the practice was first introduced. In the early 1980s, multiple-use dialyzers were reprocessed manually. By contrast, the CDC reported that 61 percent of centers practicing dialyzer reuse in 1994 used automated reprocessing systems exclusively, while 14 percent of centers used a combination of automated and manual systems.[16] Subsequent to 1994, the CDC has not collected information from dialysis facilities about whether they use automated or manual reprocessing systems. Automation of dialyzer reprocessing is believed to have lessened the risk of infection with dialyzer reuse,[18] although empiric support for

TABLE 11–1. USE OF DIALYZER REPROCESSING IN THE UNITED STATES

Year	Number of Dialysis Facilities	Number (%) of Dialysis Facilities Reprocessing	Frequency of Dialyzer Reuse (mean number of dialysis sessions)	Chemical Germicide Used (%) among Facilities Reprocessing Dialyzers			
				Formaldehyde	Peracetic Acid	Glutaraldehyde	Heat
1976	750	135 (18)	NA	NA	NA	NA	NA
1980	956	179 (19)	NA	NA	NA	NA	NA
1982	1015	435 (43)	NA	NA	NA	NA	NA
1983	1120	579 (52)	NA	94	5	<1	—
1984	1201	693 (58)	NA	86	12	3	—
1985	1250	764 (61)	NA	80	17	3	—
1986	1350	855 (63)	10	69	28	3	—
1987	1486	948 (64)	11	62	34	4	—
1988	1586	1058 (67)	11	54	40	6	—
1989	1726	1172 (68)	12	47	46	7	—
1990	1882	1310 (70)	13	43	49	8	—
1991	2046	1453 (71)	14	42	50	9	—
1992	2170	1569 (72)	14	40	52	8	<1
1993	2304	1688 (73)	15	40	51	8	1
1994	2449	1835 (75)	15	40	52	7	1
1995	2647	2048 (77)	15	38	54	7	1
1996	2808	2261 (81)	15	36	54	7	3
1997	3077	2523 (82)	17	34	56	7	3
1999	3478	2788 (80)	NA[a]	33	58	6	3
2000	3669	2935 (80)	NA	31	59	5	4

[a]Not available.
SOURCE: Data from Tokars JI, Miller ER, Alter MJ, Arduino MJ. National surveillance of dialysis-associated diseases in the United States, 1997. Semin Dial 2000;13:75–85, and Tokars JI, Frank M, Alter MJ, Arduino MJ. National surveillance of dialysis-associated diseases in the United States, 2000. Semin Dial 2002;15:162–171, with permission.

this hypothesis is lacking and no association of automated reprocessing with improved survival has been found.[19,20]

Because of concerns about long-term health effects of occupational formaldehyde exposure, the percentage of dialysis units using formaldehyde as the reprocessing germicide has decreased from 94 percent in 1983 to 31 percent in 2000.[17] Over this time, a combination of hydrogen peroxide and acetic acid (referred to in this chapter as *peracetic acid*) has emerged as the most commonly used germicide, with its use increasing from 5 to 59 percent of reprocessing dialysis centers. Glutaraldehyde, used by a small minority of dialysis facilities since 1983, is currently used by approximately 5 percent of reprocessing dialysis centers. Recently, heated citric acid has been used for disinfecting dialyzers.[21,22] As of 2000, some 4 percent of dialysis facilities in the United States utilize this method.

In addition to dialyzers, other components of the extracorporeal dialysis circuit are also reprocessed and reused. In 1994, a total of 64 percent of dialysis facilities disinfected and reused dialyzer caps.[16] Reuse of blood tubing, relatively common in the early days of dialyzer reuse, was practiced by only 8 to 14 percent of facilities in 1994.[16] Blood tubing reprocessing has become unattractive to dialysis providers because (1) it is cumbersome and not readily automated and (2) CMS regulations limit blood tubing reuse to those situations where the manufacturer has developed a specific reuse protocol that has been accepted by the U.S. Food and Drug Administration (FDA) through premarket notification [section 510(k) of the provisions of the Food, Drug and Cosmetic Act].[23] As of the late 1990s, the FDA had accepted only one such protocol. Reuse of transducer filters, practiced by 25 percent of facilities in 1986, is now specifically prohibited by CMS regulations.[23]

REGULATION OF DIALYZER REUSE IN THE UNITED STATES

The federal government regulates dialyzer reuse in the United States through CMS and the FDA.[18] The FDA influences reuse practices by regulation of the sale of medical devices including dialyzers, blood tubing, automated reprocessing equipment, and germicides used to disinfect reprocessed dialyzers. Until the mid-1990s, dialyzers were typically labeled for single use only; reprocessing and reuse were carried out as an "off-label" practice. Recently, however, the FDA has determined that manufacturers' labeling must reflect the actual commercial marketing and intended clinical use of hemodialyzers. The 1995 FDA publication *Guidance for Hemodialyzer Reuse Labeling* stipulates that each dialyzer manufacturer is required to label its reusable dialyzers for multiple use, to recommend appropriate reprocessing methods, and to demonstrate that the in vitro and in vivo performances are sustained over 15 reuses when these

methods are used.[24] Dialyzer manufacturers retain the option to label their dialyzers for single use only, with the expectation that such products will not be sold to facilities that reuse dialyzers. Documentation to demonstrate that dialyzers labeled for single use are not being reused may be required from manufacturers selling these dialyzers to facilities that practice some reuse.

CMS imposes reuse and reprocessing practice requirements directly on ESRD facilities as a condition of reimbursement. These *Conditions for Coverage of Suppliers of End-Stage Renal Disease Services* are part of the Code of Federal Regulations (CFR).[23] The regulations require that ESRD facilities practicing reuse comply in full with the *Reuse of Hemodialyzers* guidelines developed by the Association for Advancement of Medical Instrumentation (AAMI).[18] These guidelines were last updated in 2002. CMS also imposes other requirements on facilities that reuse dialyzers:

1. Reprocessed dialyzers may not be exposed to more than one chemical germicide. For the purposes of these regulations, bleach is considered a cleaning agent rather than a germicide.
2. ESRD facilities must have in place a surveillance program to identify and act on unexplained incidents of bacteremia or pyrogenic reactions.
3. Reuse of transducer protectors is prohibited and reuse of blood tubing is strictly limited (as described above).

REPROCESSING TECHNIQUES

Most of the technology in the dialyzer reprocessing field has been developed for hollow-fiber dialyzers. Accordingly, this chapter focuses on the reprocessing techniques used for these devices. Coil and parallel plate dialyzers are not reprocessed or reused, since their compliant blood compartment makes it impossible to measure residual surface area simply and inexpensively as a proxy for solute clearance after each use. This may have contributed to the decline in the use of these types of dialyzers in the United States.[25]

A brief summary of a typical reprocessing procedure follows. Both manual and automated reprocessing systems utilize these same general steps. The reader is referred to *Reuse of Hemodialyzers: AAMI Recommended Practice,* which represents a consensus of expert opinion, for a detailed consideration of dialyzer reprocessing and reuse procedures and quality assurance.[18] This publication was last updated in 2003. As noted previously, CMS regulations[23] require that ESRD facilities practicing reuse comply in full with these guidelines. Additionally, the *NKF-K/DOQI Clinical Practice Guidelines for Hemodialysis Adequacy, 2000* recommend that reused dialyzers be reprocessed according to AAMI standards, with the exception of the AAMI guideline regarding baseline measurement of residual fiber bundle volume (FBV) detailed below.[26]

Labeling

Dialyzer labels should clearly record patient name, the number of prior reprocessings, and the date of the last reprocessing. Performance test results may also be included. Dialysis units should use multiple checks by the staff and patients to ensure that once a dialyzer is reprocessed, it is used exclusively by the same patient until it is discarded.

Rinsing/Cleaning

After a dialyzer has been used, residual blood must be rinsed from the device to preserve the patency of the individual fibers as well as reduce the organic matter that could potentiate bacterial growth. The rinsing process is initiated when the patient's blood is returned with a saline rinseback. It is continued by flushing both the blood and dialysate compartments of the dialyzer with water. Water used for this purpose, as for other steps of the reprocessing procedure, is expected to meet requirements set in the AAMI publication *Water Treatment Equipment for Hemodialysis Applications: AAMI Recommended Practice.*[27]

Many facilities combine an initial manual rinse with an automated rinsing and cleaning process, which follows. For manual techniques, the water pressure and flow must be specified, so that rinsing is performed consistently and effectively. Automated reprocessing equipment is programmed by the manufacturer to accomplish effective rinsing.

Proteinaceous deposits adsorb to both sides of the reused dialysis membrane with reuse, leading to occlusion of membrane fibers and the potential for decreased solute (especially middle-molecule) clearance. Chemical cleaning agents may be used to remove remaining blood and dissolve adsorbed deposits.[28–30] Dilute solutions of sodium hypochlorite (bleach), hydrogen peroxide, or peracetic acid are used most frequently for this purpose. Certain automated systems use peracetic acid for both cleaning and disinfection. Special care is necessary in using bleach because high concentrations (>2%), elevated temperature, or prolonged exposure (>10 minutes) may weaken hemodialysis membranes, lessen biocompatibility, and increase the risk of albumin loss into the dialysate.[31,32] Even using recommended techniques, bleach may cause structural damage to reprocessed dialysis membranes[30,33,34] (see "Effects on Dialysis Delivery," below).

When combinations of chemicals are used for reprocessing, each chemical must be removed before the next is added unless mixing is known to be safe and effective for reprocessing. The combination of bleach with formalde-

hyde or peracetic acid may produce noxious fumes and degrade the germicide.

Performance Measurements

After the dialyzer has been rinsed and cleaned, its functional and structural integrity should be tested to ensure that it will effectively transport solute and ultrafilter fluid and remain intact during its next use. Ideally, the in vitro clearance of a small molecule such as urea should be used as the actual clearance criterion for rejection. By AAMI mandate, up to a 10 percent decrease in clearance when compared with a new dialyzer is acceptable.[18,35]

Direct measurement of clearance during follow-up dialyses with a reused dialyzer is impractical and expensive in most clinical settings. A surrogate measure in common practice involves determination of the residual volume within the hollow fibers (residual fiber bundle volume, or FBV).[18,36–38] The residual FBV can be determined manually by measuring the volume of fluid displaced by a nitrogen flush, but it is now typically measured electronically by automated reprocessing equipment. When the residual FBV drops to ≤ 80 percent of the initial measured volume or manufacturer's stated volume, the dialyzer should be discarded, as this cutoff is believed to approximate a decrease in small molecule clearance to ≤ 90 percent of the reference value. In a given patient, repeated failure to reach a target number of reuses because of FBV test failure suggests excessive clot formation during dialysis and should prompt a review of the heparin prescription.[39,40]

AAMI standards permit new-dialyzer FBV to be determined by batch testing and/or the use of a manufacturer's stated volume. However, the *NKF-K/DOQI Clinical Practice Guidelines for Hemodialysis Adequacy, 2000,* recommend that FBV be measured directly prior to first use for any new hemodialyzer that is intended for reuse, due to concerns about considerable dialyzer-to-dialyzer FBV variability within a single lot.[26,41,42]

In 1989, severely decreased urea clearance within certain lots of reprocessed unsubstituted cellulosic (cuprophane) dialyzers was demonstrated despite preservation of FBV.[43] In these instances, alterations in the geometry of the dialyzer capillary fibers may have led to maldistribution of flow between blood and dialysate. Because of notable FBV test failures such as this, periodic urea kinetic modeling and in vitro clearances to corroborate the results of FBV testing are warranted by dialysis facilities to provide assurance about adequate dialysis delivery in the setting of dialyzer reuse.[18,35] Concerns that have recently been raised about the validity of the FBV performance test as a meaningful measure of decrease in received dialysis dose with reuse are addressed later in this chapter (see "Quantification of Changes in Delivered Dialysis Dose with Reuse").

The measurement of the in vitro ultrafiltration coefficient (K_{uf}) is not recommended as a measure of in vivo ultrafiltration performance of a dialyzer because the former overestimates the latter in hollow fiber dialyzers.[18] Instead, failure to achieve expected weight loss during treatment, uncommon in recent times with the advent of volumetric control machines, should result in evaluation of the reprocessing method if no alternative clinical explanation is evident.

A membrane integrity test, such as the air-pressure leak test, checks the ability of a reprocessed dialyzer to resist membrane rupture. Failure to withstand a pressure 20 percent above the highest operating pressure necessitates that the dialyzer be discarded. Leak tests also screen for defects in the dialyzer O-rings, potting compound, and end caps.

Disinfection

The blood and dialysate compartments of a functionally and structurally intact dialyzer must then be subjected to high-level disinfection (not sterilization).[18] The hemodialyzer is filled with germicide until the concentration in the dialyzer is $\geq 90\%$ of the prescribed concentration. The presence of the germicide in adequate concentrations should be confirmed either in all dialyzers or in a random sample. The ports of the hemodialyzer filled with germicide should be disinfected and then capped with new or disinfected caps. The apparatus must then remain in contact with germicide for a mandated number of hours before subsequent reuse.

Formaldehyde, peracetic acid, and glutaraldehyde are the most common chemical germicides used. To ensure adequate disinfection and avoid the possibility of structural damage, regulator and manufacturer instructions should be followed closely. For formaldehyde, the CDC recommends that a 4% solution be used for both the blood and dialysate compartments, with a minimum contact time of 24 hours at a temperature of at least 20°C (68.0°F). Low-level disinfection is sufficient for the exterior of the device. Soaking or wiping with 0.05% bleach is usually suitable for this purpose.

Heat has emerged as an alternative to chemical germicides for disinfection of reprocessed dialyzers. Reprocessing with water heated to 100°C (212.0°F) for 20 hours destroys all infective agents but may also result in structural damage to the dialyzer.[21] For polysulfone dialyzers, equivalent microbiological effects are produced by an automated reprocessing system using 1.5 percent citric acid heated to 95°C (203.0°F) for 20 hours. This method has appeal because it avoids the use of chemical germicides. In vitro testing has shown that mechanical properties of the polysulfone membrane are not affected by heated citric acid.[44] As with other reprocessing systems that do not include bleach, protein adsorption on both sides of the membrane, which occurs with reuse, is incompletely cleared by heated citric acid reprocessing.

Germicide Removal and Preparation for Dialysis

To rinse germicide from the dialyzer, saline is typically circulated in the blood compartment and dialysate is run in single-pass fashion through the dialysate compartment. Rinse to below established toxic levels of germicide must be accomplished within a rinse-out period established for the particular germicide, usually from 10 to 45 minutes. Residual germicide concentrations measured by reagent strips must be < 5 parts per million (ppm) for formaldehyde and < 1 ppm for peracetic acid.[18]

Final Inspection

Finally, a visual inspection of the dialyzer for cracks, chips, or defects in the plastic housing, as well as for esthetic appearance, should be performed after reprocessing. Dialyzers that are not structurally intact or display a large quantity of discolored fibers should be discarded.

Monitoring of Clinical Parameters

The clinical course of each patient should be monitored during each dialysis to identify possible complications due to reprocessed dialyzers. Unexplained fever and/or chills, pain in the blood access arm at the onset of dialysis, deviation from the expected ultrafiltration volume, or deterioration of a patient's condition not explained on other clinical grounds should prompt attention to the possibility of complications consequent to the reprocessing procedure.[18]

EFFECTS ON DIALYSIS DELIVERY

Recently published clinical studies illustrate that, in centers practicing reuse, precise knowledge of the membrane material, reprocessing technique, and their interaction is important to understand the effects of dialyzer reprocessing and reuse on hemodialysis delivery.

Urea Clearance

Several small single-center clinical studies published in recent years have used crossover design (reuse with one dialysis membrane followed by reuse with another membrane) to evaluate the effects on urea clearance of the reuse of high- and low-flux dialyzers reprocessed by a variety of germicides with or without bleach.[28,45,46] In three patients using low-flux cellulosic and high-flux polysulfone dialyzers reprocessed with glutaraldehyde and bleach, Sridhar et al. found no significant decline in Kt/V urea at repeated measures between reuses one and eight.[45] In six patients using low-flux cellulosic and high-flux cellulosic or polysulfone dialyzers reprocessed with peracetic acid without bleach, Leypoldt et al. found no significant decline in urea, creatinine, or phosphate clearance at repeated measures between reuses 1 and 15.[28] In six patients using high-flux polysulfone and high-efficiency cellulosic membranes processed with formaldehyde and bleach, Murthy et al. reported that urea clearance from new to 20th reuse did have a modest but statistically significant decrease for the polysulfone membrane (241 to 221 mL/min) but not the cellulosic membrane.[46]

The finding of these single-center studies, that urea clearance is minimally altered by dialyzer reuse, was confirmed in the epidemiologic setting by Cheung et al. in 1999. These investigators published a report of the effects of dialyzer reuse on urea clearance in 1189 patients who used reprocessed dialyzers in the HEMO study, a clinical trial to examine the effects of different Kt/V urea and types of dialysis membranes on clinical outcomes in chronic hemodialysis patients.[30] Reprocessing techniques included automated systems of peracetic acid alone, heated citric acid alone, bleach followed by formaldehyde, bleach followed by glutaraldehyde, and a manual system of bleach followed by peracetic acid. The dialyzers included high- and low-flux cellulosic and polysulfone membranes. Dialysis units used their usual criteria for discarding reprocessed dialyzers, although the maximum number of dialyzer reuses was limited to 20 and later decreased to 6 for units using peracetic acid without bleach. Among the key findings regarding reuse, Kt/V urea decreased linearly but modestly (approximately 1 to 2 percent total decline) over the first 10 reuses, regardless of membrane flux or reprocessing method.

These encouraging findings regarding the preservation of urea clearance with reuse in a variety of experimental settings are tempered by a 1994 observational study, by Sherman et al., which found a somewhat larger impact of dialyzer reprocessing on urea clearance in 436 patients chosen randomly from 34 American dialysis units.[47] Patients received their typical care, and dialyzers were reprocessed and reused in each unit's usual manner. By formal urea kinetic modeling monthly for 3 months, Kt/V urea for the treatment using the dialyzer with the most reuses for each patient (mean number reuses 13.8; mean Kt/V 1.05) was significantly lower than that for the fewest reuses (mean number reuses 3.8; mean Kt/V 1.10; *p* for mean Kt/V <0.01). Prescribed Kt/V by most and fewest reuses was identical. Substantial variability by center was observed. Although the reprocessing germicide could not be shown to influence the extent to which reuse impaired dialysis delivery, peracetic acid and glutaraldehyde were used in only five and six centers, respectively. Because FBV was not reported, it is unknown whether the decreased Kt/V with increasing number of reuses occurred due to nonadherence with AAMI guidelines or despite guideline adherence. Nonetheless, this study raises concern that reuse procedures as practiced may yield suboptimal dialysis delivery.

This possibility is addressed by the *NKF-K/DOQI Clinical Practice Guidelines for Hemodialysis Adequacy, 2000,* which recommends that to prevent the delivered hemodialysis dose from falling below the recommended Kt/V 1.2, the prescribed hemodialysis dose should be Kt/V 1.3.[26] Inadequate dialyzer reprocessing related to inadequate quality control of reuse is listed as one of several factors that may compromise delivered urea clearance.

Beta$_2$-Microglobulin (β_2-MG) Clearance

Because β_2-MG clearance is modest with low-flux membranes, it is not altered appreciably by reuse or choice of reprocessing system.[28,30,40,46] However, reuse of high-flux dialyzers has been repeatedly found by recent single-center experimental studies[28,29,33,40,46,48] to have substantially more impact on middle- to large-solute clearance than on the clearance of small molecules. Whether β_2-MG clearance increases or decreases with reuse of high-flux dialyzers depends principally on whether or not bleach is included in the reprocessing cycle.

Reprocessing of high-flux cellulosic or polysulfone dialyzers with peracetic acid alone has been shown to significantly decrease middle-molecule clearance,[28,29] consistent with the hypothesis that adsorption of plasma protein onto the dialyzer membrane surface diminishes the effective size of large pores and that peracetic acid alone is relatively ineffective in removing these proteinaceous deposits.[30] On the other hand, reprocessing of high-flux polysulfone dialyzers with bleach in addition to formaldehyde has been shown consistently to increase clearance of β_2-MG and other larger solutes at 15 to 20 reuses in vitro[34] and in the clinical setting.[33,46] For high-flux cellulosic dialyzers, bleach/formaldehyde reprocessing increased larger solute permeability in one[34] but not another clinical study.[46] It is likely that bleach increases membrane porosity by (1) removing the protein layer that accumulates with repeated dialyses and (2) altering the structure of the residual membrane.[30] Using x-ray spectroscopy, Krautzig et al. found that exposure to bleach markedly reduced the polyvinylpyrrolidone (PVP) content of the polysulfone-PVP polymer of which polysulfone membranes are made.[32]

The HEMO study investigators confirmed that changes in β_2-MG clearance with reuse of high-flux dialyzers vary chiefly with whether or not bleach is used, but that the effect is modulated by choice of dialyzer and germicide.[30] For high-flux cellulosic dialyzers treated with peracetic acid without bleach, β_2-MG clearance declined rapidly in the first 4 reuses and then more slowly up to the 14th reuse.

Mean decrease from the first to the 10th to 14th reuses was 13.4 mL/min. A modest β_2-MG clearance decline was observed with reuse of high-flux polysulfone dialyzers treated with peracetic acid but no bleach. The use of bleach increased β_2-MG clearance most rapidly for high-flux polysulfone dialyzers when used with formaldehyde in the first 7 reuses (mean increase 3.3 mL/min per reuse), though some increase persisted through the 20th reuse. The increase in β_2-MG clearance with reuse was smaller for reprocessing with bleach and peracetic acid and smallest, though still statistically significant, for bleach and glutaraldehyde. Reuse of high-flux cellulosic dialyzers yielded modest (mean 0.3 mL/min per reuse) increases in β_2-MG clearance when processed with bleach combined with formaldehyde or glutaraldehyde. For high-flux polysulfone dialyzers processed with heated citric acid alone, β_2-MG clearance increased linearly at 2.3 mL/min per reuse for up to 7 reuses. Other than the HEMO study, in vivo data regarding the effect of reuse with heated citric acid on dialyzer clearance are very limited.

Quantification of Changes in Delivered Dialysis Dose with Reuse

Urea kinetic modeling repeated sequentially after dialysis with reprocessed dialyzers is used extensively in experimental settings to study the effects of dialyzer reuse on delivered dialysis dose, but it is impractical in the clinical setting. The criterion for FBV ≥ 80 percent (see "Performance Measurements" above) after each dialyzer reuse as a cutoff for urea clearance ≥ 90 percent of its value prior to first use was developed in the early 1980s for dialyzers using low-permeability cellulosic membranes reprocessed with formaldehyde.[36,37] In its 1997 position paper, the National Kidney Foundation-Kidney Disease Outcomes Quality Initiative (NKF-K/DOQI) Task Force on Reuse of Dialyzers voiced caution because this relationship had not been demonstrated extensively in high-flux, synthetic membranes or with use of germicides such as peracetic acid, now in common use.[35] In addition, the Task Force questioned the use of FBV ≥ 80 percent as the "universal yardstick" for dialyzer acceptability because of the unclear understanding of its relationship to clearance of middle and large molecules, such as β_2-MG.

Several authors have shown FBV to be preserved with current reuse techniques. Garred et al., in 1990, were unable to detect a negative impact of automated polysulfone dialyzer reprocessing with peracetic acid on FBV and the dialyzer mass transfer coefficient.[41] Losses for each of these two parameters were negligible—1 percent and 3 percent, respectively—for 102 dialyzers used a mean of 14.4 times and tested on average on the seventh use. Direct measures of solute clearance were not reported. In 1997, Ouseph et

al. found that FBV remained ≥ 80 percent and Kt/V urea remained ≥ 90 percent over at least 10 peracetic acid–reprocessed dialyzer reuses for 9 patients using high-flux polysulfone membranes and 8 patients using high-flux cellulosic membranes.[29] Because FBV was ≥ 80 percent at all measured occasions, this study does not definitively validate FBV ≥ 80 percent as a cutoff for urea clearance ≥ 90 percent of its initial value in the modern dialysis setting.

The same study by Ouseph et al. did demonstrate that FBV ≥ 80 percent may not be a valid cutoff for adequacy of β_2-MG clearance. Despite FBV in nine subjects remaining ≥ 80 percent from the first to tenth dialyzer reuses, β_2-MG clearance dropped from 30 to 12 percent for users of polysulfone membranes ($p = 0.04$) and from 18 to 12 percent for users of cellulosic membranes ($p = 0.28$).[29] This finding suggests that if middle- or large-molecule clearance is to become an important component of prescribed dialysis dose, change in FBV is not a sensitive test to identify reused dialyzers that no longer clear these solutes effectively. At this time, practical methods to reliably evaluate the clearances of larger solutes by reused dialyzers on a routine clinical basis are not available.[35]

Albumin Loss

Concern has been raised that reprocessing of high-flux dialyzers with bleach, while favorably increasing β_2-MG clearance, can also lead to the deleterious loss of larger proteins such as albumin. Ikizler et al. found that losses of albumin into dialysate using formaldehyde-reprocessed high-flux polysulfone membranes averaged in excess of 12g per treatment by the 23rd to 25th reuse, with only modest increase in β_2-MG removal.[49] Kaplan et al. also showed that formaldehyde-reprocessed high-flux polysulfone membranes became increasingly permeable to albumin following successive reprocessing cycles with bleach.[33] When bleach was removed from the reprocessing cycle for these 11 patients, albumin loss into the dialysate ceased and serum albumin concentrations increased. No such changes were observed when the membranes were exposed to either formaldehyde or peracetic acid without bleach.

On the other hand, Kaysen et al. reported much lower levels of albumin loss (less than 1 g during the 15th use) for dialyzers containing polysulfone membranes processed for reuse with bleach and formaldehyde.[50] These conflicting observations regarding the magnitude of protein loss may be related to the conditions of bleach exposure in addition to the composition of the starting membrane material. It is not known to what extent similar phenomena may occur with other synthetic polymer membranes.

While most work has focused on the impact of dialyzer reprocessing techniques on protein loss into dialysate, particle movement from dialysate to blood can also be affected. For example, transfer of bacterial products from dialysate to blood is facilitated by the change in polysulfone membranes induced by bleach exposure.[51]

EFFECTS ON HOSPITALIZATION AND SURVIVAL

The effect of dialyzer reuse on patient outcomes has been in dispute since the practice was introduced more than three decades ago.[20] Because no longitudinal studies of clinical outcomes have randomly assigned patients to reuse or non-reuse practice, inference about possible causal associations between dialyzer reuse and adverse patient events has been derived from a series of observational epidemiologic studies.

Early work indicated that clinical outcomes might be better at reuse facilities than at noreuse facilities.[52–55] Wing et al., in 1978, found that 1-year mortality in five countries reporting statistics to the European Dialysis and Transplant Association was similar or lower than in facilites not reprocessing dialyzers.[52] However, it is quite possible that this apparent benefit of reuse was confounded by the treatment of less stable patients in hospital facilities, where reprocessed dialyzers were rarely used, while healthier patients were treated in freestanding outpatient dialysis units. Pollak et al., in 1986, compared 2-year mortality rates of 1318 American dialysis patients in two units that reprocessed dialyzers with the regional rates reported by the local end-stage renal disease (ESRD) networks to which these dialysis units belonged.[54] The reported mortality rates in these facilities were 70 and 96 percent of the corresponding ESRD networks' rates, but were unadjusted for numerous facility- and patient-level confounding variables. The use of network rates for comparisons may have masked greater differences in survival, because many dialysis units in these networks also reprocessed dialyzers during the study period. In 1987, Held et al. reported findings from CDC and Medicare data for 4661 patients who began dialysis in 1977 and survived until at least 1982. Among these patients, mortality in dialysis facilities practicing dialyzer reuse was 12 percent lower than in facilities not reusing dialyzers.[55] The implications of this finding were limited because only long-term survivors were studied and the analyses did not account for clustering among patients treated by the same dialysis provider, which would tend to incorrectly increase the statistical significance of the findings. For each of these earlier studies, generalizability to current practice is limited because the germicide formaldehyde, used in most reuse dialysis units during the 1970s and 1980s, is now used in only approximately one-third of units reprocessing dialyzers.

In 1994, Held et al. published an analysis of Medicare and CDC data from 845 freestanding dialysis units that included approximately 33,000 patients at the start of 1989 or 1990 who had survived dialysis for at least 90 days.[19] Compared to patients in nonreuse units, patients treated in dialysis units that disinfected dialyzers with peracetic acid, glutaraldehyde, and formaldehyde had 1-year relative risks for mortality, adjusted for facility-level and demographic factors, of 1.17 (95 percent CI 1.06 to 1.21, $p = 0.01$), 1.13 (95 percent CI 1.04 to 1.31, $p < 0.001$), and 1.06 (95 percent CI 0.99 to 1.14, $p = 0.09$), respectively. For each germicide, no statistically significant differences in mortality were found between manual and automated reprocessing techniques. The restriction of this analysis to units using predominantly conventional (low-flux) dialyzers limits its generalizability to current practice, in which the use of reprocessed high-flux dialyzers is common. Further, the exclusion of patients incident to ESRD precludes the application of the study's results to the early period of dialysis, when mortality rates are especially high.

In 1996, Feldman et al. reported the relationship of dialyzer reuse to mortality over 4.5 years of follow-up among 27,938 patients identified by Medicare who began hemodialysis in 1986 or 1987.[56] Dialysis in freestanding facilities reprocessing dialyzers with peracetic acid was associated with greater mortality (RR 1.10; 95 percent CI 1.02 to 1.18, $p = 0.02$) than treatment in facilities not reprocessing dialyzers. However, there were no significant differences in survival between freestanding facilities not reprocessing dialyzers and freestanding facilities reprocessing dialyzers with formaldehyde (RR 1.03; 95 percent CI 0.96 to 1.10, $p = 0.45$) or glutaraldehyde (RR 1.13; 95 percent CI 0.95 to 1.35, $p = 0.18$). There were also no statistical differences in survival between hospital-based facilities not reprocessing dialyzers and hospital-based facilities reprocessing dialyzers by peracetic acid, formaldehyde, or glutaraldehyde. Sensitivity analyses demonstrated that possible misclassification of exposure to dialyzer reuse (by using facility reuse characteristics to assign individual-level reuse exposure) would not have caused important distortions of the reported relationships between dialyzer reuse and survival. Within the same cohort, rates of hospitalization of patients in freestanding reuse facilities using peracetic acid (RR 1.11; 95 percent CI 1.04 to 1.18, $p < 0.01$) and formaldehyde (RR 1.07; 95 percent CI 1.00 to 1.14, $p = 0.04$) were higher than in patients in freestanding facilities practicing dialyzer nonreuse.[57] Reprocessing with glutaraldehyde in freestanding facilites was not associated with an increased rate of hospitalization (RR 1.00; 95 percent CI 0.89 to 1.13, $p = 0.97$). There were no differences among hospitalization rates in hospital-based facilities reprocessing dialyzers and those not practicing reuse.

The finding by Feldman et al., that dialysis in freestanding facilities reprocessing dialyzers with peracetic acid was associated with greater mortality than treatment in facilities not reprocessing dialyzers, was consistent with the 1994 results of Held et al., despite differences in the source population studied and analytical techniques. However, confounding due to comorbidity, quality of delivered care at the dialysis facility, or other parameters not fully captured by the Medicare and CDC databases used for both analyses remained possible alternative explanations for the studies' findings. To specifically investigate the possibility that the apparent relationships between dialyzer reuse and survival might be attenuated after further adjustment for comorbidity, Feldman et al. examined survival among 1491 hemodialysis patients in freestanding facilities who had extensive comorbidity and laboratory data available as part of the USRDS Study of Case Mix, a 1989 sample of approximately 7.5 percent of the U.S. dialysis patients who had begun dialysis in 1986 or 1987.[57] Reuse of dialyzers, obtained from facility-level CDC data, was associated with a higher rate of death than dialyzer nonreuse both before (RR 1.25; 95 percent CI 0.97 to 1.61, $p = 0.08$) and after comorbidity adjustment (RR 1.25; 95 percent CI 1.03 to 1.52, $p = 0.02$). Dialyzer reuse was similarly associated with increased hospitalization risk. These findings suggested that the relationships of dialyzer reuse in freestanding dialysis facilities to elevated rates of death and hospitalization demonstrated by earlier studies did not result from confounding due to different comorbidity levels among patients treated in facilities that reuse compared with patients treated in facilities that do not reuse. However, because they were unable to control for aspects of hemodialysis care other than reuse, Feldman et al. could not directly address the possibility that differences in outcome according to facility reuse practice were due to dialyzer reuse per se or to other associated aspects of dialysis care provided in facilities that reuse dialyzers. This study was also not powered to detect differences in outcomes among the different reprocessing germicides.

In 1998, Collins et al. reported analyses of Medicare and CDC data from approximately 34,000 patients, representing a 10 percent random sample from the HCFA ESRD database between 1989 and 1993.[58] Patients prevalent to ESRD at the beginning of each study year or who had received at least 90 days of hemodialysis at any time during that year were then followed until death, loss to follow-up, or year's end. In an effort to derive a study population similar to those in prior studies, this study was restricted to patients in facilities that reported to the CDC the use of high-flux dialysis in no more than 25 percent of patients. Advantages claimed over prior publications included the inclusion of more recent data and the adjustment for unit characteristics including unit age, size, and profit status.

From a series of survival-time analyses comparing reuse to nonreuse that were stratified according to four combinations of freestanding or hospital-based facility status and years 1989–1990 or 1991–1993, Collins et al. reported that greater survival was associated with formaldehyde reprocessing (RR 0.82; 95 percent CI 0.72 to 0.93) and peracetic acid reprocessing (RR 0.83; 95 percent CI 0.72 to 0.96) among patients dialyzed in freestanding facili-

ties than among patients dialyzed in nonreuse facilities in 1991–1993.[58] Additionally, survival in 1989–1990 or 1991–1993 was compared across 21 levels of a composite variable representing combinations of facility-level profit status, freestanding vs. hospital-based status, automated vs. manual reprocessing technique, and germicide used, with patients in nonreuse, not-for-profit, hospital-based units serving as baseline. By this approach, the authors reported that manual reprocessing with peracetic acid was associated with increased mortality in for-profit, freestanding facilities in 1989–1990 (RR 1.36; 95 percent CI 1.17 to 1.59). While this finding corroborated prior associations over roughly the same time period reported by both Held et al. and Feldman et al.,[19,56] Collins et al. did not observe this association in 1991–1993. Elevated mortality associated with reuse in 1991–1993 was limited to (1) glutaraldehyde reuse in freestanding, for-profit units and (2) automated formaldehyde reuse in not-for-profit, hospital-based units, accounting together for reuse practices in fewer than 3 percent of all dialysis units. However, inconsistencies such as the reported association of manual peracetic acid reprocessing with improved survival in not-for-profit, freestanding facilities in 1989–1990 raise concern about the stability of this analysis and the possibility that some reported statistically significant findings were due to chance alone.

In the same publication, Collins et al. also reported increased adjusted mortality in for-profit compared to not-for-profit freestanding dialysis units during both 1989–1990 and 1991–1993,[58] lending further credence to the possibility raised by other authors that the associations of reuse with mortality found in prior studies may have been confounded by an unbalanced distribution of facility-level factors.[19,56,57] For this reason and because they found no consistent adjusted associations of any reprocessing germicide with mortality, Collins et al. concluded that a meaningful causal link between dialyzer reuse and mortality was unlikely.

As follow-up to their 1998 publication, Ebben and Collins et al., in 2000, published an analysis intended to address the possibility that other factors associated with survival might have a greater influence on survival than did hemodialyzer reuse.[59] Using five cohorts of all Medicare patients prevalent to hemodialysis in the first 6 months of each year from 1991 to 1995, mortality over the following year as a function of dialysis unit reprocessing germicide was examined in a series of progressively more complex multivariable models incorporating Medicare and CDC data. In the base model—adjusted for patient age, prior ESRD time, dialysis unit age and size, water treatment method, dialysate, and germicide—greater survival or nonsignificant trend toward greater survival was reported for most years within units reprocessing with formaldehyde, peracetic acid, or glutaraldehyde compared to units not practicing reuse. No temporal trend in survival by reprocessing germicide was found. The base model associations of reuse with greater survival were no longer present after more extensive adjustment for facility-level factors including dialyzer type (> or ≤ 25 percent use of high flux dialyzers, representing 41 percent of units in 1991 and 77 percent in 1995), dialysis unit profit status, ICD-9 comorbidity, a Medicare database-derived index of disease severity, and hematocrit level. Further, the authors reported that because they found comorbidity, disease severity, and hematocrit level to not be randomly distributed across type of reuse germicide, they again postulated that factors such as these were likely, in part, to explain prior associations found between germicide and mortality.

In 2001, Port et al. described mortality risk during 1994–1995 among 12,791 patients prevalent to hemodialysis in the Dialysis Morbidity and Mortality Study (DMMS), a random sample of US chronic hemodialysis patients stratified by ESRD network.[20] By dialysis facility chart abstraction, the DMMS collected detailed data on patient demographics, comorbidity, delivered dialysis dose, and facility- and patient-level characteristics including dialyzer specifications and reuse practices. Notably, the Port et al. study is the only study published to date reporting associations between reuse practices and outcomes that has adjusted for delivered dialysis dose.

The principal finding of this study was that no significant difference was detected in the adjusted death rates for patients at facilities reporting a predominant practice of dialyzer reuse compared with patients at facilities not reusing dialyzers (RR 0.96; 95 percent CI, 0.86 to 1.08; p > 0.51).[20] Pooled relative risks for mortality according to reprocessing germicide compared to dialyzer nonreuse were not reported, but several findings in a series of subgroup analyses incorporating patient-level dialyzer reuse data are consistent with prior published findings. Among these, patients using peracetic acid-reprocessed dialyzers had a 10 percent greater adjusted mortality than patients using formaldehyde-reprocessed dialyzers, although this association was not statistically significant (RR 1.10; 95 percent CI, 0.98 to 1.23; p = 0.13). Comparing subgroups with the two most common reprocessing agent by bleach practices, patients using dialyzers reprocessed by peracetic acid without bleach (96 percent of peracetic acid-reprocessed dialyzers) had a 15 percent greater adjusted mortality (RR 1.15; 95 percent CI 0.99 to 1.30; p = 0.07) than users of formaldehyde with bleach (73 percent of formaldehyde-reprocessed dialyzers). Among subgroups classified further by membrane type and flux, patients using dialyzers reprocessed with peracetic acid without bleach had higher mortality than patients using dialyzers reprocessed with formaldehyde and bleach in all five subgroups, with four of five achieving statistical significance. These patient-level associations between peracetic acid reprocessing and mortality corroborate prior facility-level findings by Held et al.[19] and Feldman et al.[56, 57] but contrast with the results of Collins et

al.[58] and Ebben et al.[59] In their DMMS analysis, Port et al.[20] also reported somewhat greater mortality with glutaraldehyde than with formaldehyde reprocessing, again consistent with earlier reports by Held et al.[19] and Feldman et al.,[56] although the small sample sizes in the glutaraldehyde subgroups limits interpretation and generalizability of these data. Within the same membrane by flux subgroups, the authors also reported that patients in nonreuse units had increased mortality (statistically significant in two of four subgroups) compared to patients using dialyzers reprocessed with formaldehyde and bleach.

The Port et al. study[20] of DMMS data was the first to publish analyses examining the possible association of bleach reprocessing with improved survival, and the authors raise the possibility that bleach may explain, in part, the disparate accumulated findings regarding associations of reuse with outcome. In addition to the subgroup analyses summarized above, Port et al. reported that the pooled death rate—adjusted for reprocessing germicide, membrane type, and patient characteristics—for patients using membranes reprocessed without bleach was 24 percent higher (RR 1.24; 95 percent CI, 1.01 to 1.48; p = 0.04) for all types of synthetic membranes and 23 percent higher for high-flux synthetic membranes alone (p = 0.11) than for patients using dialyzers reprocessed with bleach.[20] Among users of high and/or low flux cellulosic membranes, survival was not associated with bleach use. The authors postulated that the overall associations of bleach with improved outcomes might reflect the increased middle- and large-molecule clearance with bleach reprocessing compared to reprocessing without bleach.[30] However, this hypothesis is now difficult to reconcile with the results of the HEMO Study published in 2002,[10] which found no overall survival benefit to subjects randomized to high- rather than low-flux dialysis.

In summary, associations between dialyzer reuse and elevated mortality were reported in a variety of observational studies using individual-level Medicare and facility-level CDC data from the late 1980s.[19,57] By contrast, hemodialyzer reuse did not appear to measurably modify overall mortality risk compared with nonreuse in subsequent observational studies examining Medicare and CDC data predominantly from the early to mid 1990s.[20,58,59] Because these later studies incorporated more detailed characterization of dialytic care into their adjusted analyses, it is possible that the prior reported associations of reuse with mortality were confounded by factors such as quality of care. While it does not appear at this time that dialyzer reuse as a whole carries substantial mortality risk, caution is still warranted for several reasons:

1. Recent studies showing no association of survival with reuse[20,58,59] comprised primarily patients prevalent to hemodialysis. Pathophysiologic consequences of reuse, if any, may manifest more clearly

in patients who have recently begun hemodialysis and who tend to be sicker than those patients who survive to enroll in a prevalent hemodialysis cohort.

2. The possibility that peracetic acid reprocessing carries a stronger link with mortality than formaldehyde reprocessing has been raised by some[19,20,56] but not all[58,59] studies. Analyses of the associations of glutaraldehyde with mortality have been hampered by small sample sizes, and no epidemiologic data have been published that examine the relationship of heated citric acid reprocessing to clinical outcomes.

3. The possibility that bleach influences mortality, reported by Port et al. in 2001,[20] deserves further investigation.

Because reuse practices, patient case-mix severity, and other aspects of dialytic therapy continue to change over time, the need is clear for further studies to continue monitoring for potential risks and benefits associated with dialyzer reprocessing techniques.

INFECTION RISK

Bacteria

The practice of reuse is considered safe by the CDC if performed according to recognized protocols.[17] However, outbreaks of infection in reuse dialysis centers that have resulted in increased patient morbidity and mortality have been well documented. Most of these outbreaks have been linked to inadequate sterilization or cross-contamination, and the risk of infection due to failure to observe proper reprocessing techniques remains one of the greatest potential hazards facing any reprocessing program.

Nontuberculous mycobacterial (NTM) infection represents a particular risk to dialysis patients because of NTM's predilection to colonize water used in hemodialyzer reprocessing. A 1988 CDC survey of NTM recovery from water used by 115 dialysis centers found NTM at 83 percent of centers and in 50 percent of all water samples from those centers.[60] These data demonstrate the importance of using disinfecting agents that are effective in eradicating NTM, such as 4% formaldehyde, and of achieving a final adequate germicide concentration in the dialyzer, estimated to be equal to 90 percent of the stock concentration.[35,61] In a 1985 outbreak in Louisiana, attributed to inadequate preparation of formaldehyde by the staff of the dialysis unit, 27 patients became infected with a rapidly growing NTM, *Mycobacterium chelonei*.[62] Over a 1-year period, 14 of these patients died due to multiple medical problems. Another outbreak of *M. chelonei* was reported in 1990 from a dialysis center in California.[63]

Outbreaks of gram-negative bloodstream infections in reuse centers also have been described on several occasions over the past two decades.[64–68] The CDC reported in 1986 on nine patients in several dialysis units who developed gram-negative bacteremia due to bacterial contamination of reprocessed dialyzers.[64] In an infection outbreak described in 1983, nine pyrogenic reactions and five gram-negative bacteremias occurred over an 18-day period in 11 patients for whom reprocessed dialyzers were used, whereas no pyrogenic reactions or bacteremias were observed during this same period among patients in the same diaysis unit who used only new dialyzers.[66] Germicide (peracetic acid) concentrations were found to vary markedly in manually reprocessed dialyzers during the epidemic period, suggesting that failure to mix germicide properly during dilution may have accounted for its inadequate concentrations in some dialyzers. More recently, a 1995 report describing a dialysis unit outbreak of *Klebsiella pneumoniae* bacteremia implicated cross-contamination of other dialyzers by failure to observe proper aseptic technique during reprocessing of a dialyzer used by a patient with a *K. pneumoniae* arteriovenous fistula infection.[67]

A series of articles in the early 1990s described outbreaks of gram-negative bacteremia due to contamination of the dialyzer header, including the O-ring component, by nonsterile product water when the header was removed for cleaning. An outbreak of bacteremia in 11 patients treated with reprocessed high-flux dialyzers was attributed to inadequately sterilized dialyzer O-rings;[69] the CDC reported the failure of reprocessing to remove bacteria from high-flux dialyzer header spaces and O-rings,[70] and a "header sepsis syndrome" due to *Xanthomonas* has been described.[71] Some centers now avoid the problem of header area infection by dipping the header and O-ring in germicide before reassembling the dialyzer.[35]

In summary, exposure to dialyzer reprocessing leads to the potential for enhanced vulnerability to bloodborne bacterial infection and breakdowns in reprocessing technique were implicated in all case series (described above) reporting infection outbreaks with dialyzer reuse in the 1980s and early 1990s. While the number of reports of outbreaks of invasive infection in reprocessing dialysis units has subsequently decreased, no reliable estimates exist of current infection risk attributable to dialyzer reuse, and controlled studies examining the potential association of dialyzer reuse with infectious morbidity are not likely to be undertaken. Nonetheless, it is now hoped that improvements in dialyzer reprocessing techniques, including standardization and automation, have resulted in an acceptably low risk of bacterial infection with modern dialyzer reuse.

Pyrogenic Reactions

As part of their annual survey of dialysis practices, the CDC reported from 1986 to 1994 on the risk of pyrogenic reactions associated with dialyzer reuse.[16,72,73] Later CDC surveys[17,74,75] have not collected these data. In the 1994 report (1992 data), 24 percent of reprocessing facilities and 14 percent percent of nonreprocessing facilities reported one or more pyrogenic reactions, and 2.9 percent of reprocessing facilities and 1 percent of nonreprocessing facilities reported clusters of pyrogenic reactions. In adjusted models, dialyzer reuse (RR 1.4 compared to nonreuse) was an independent predictor of pyrogenic reactions, as was high-flux dialysis (RR 1.2 compared to low-flux dialysis).[76] Although centers reporting pyrogenic reactions were three times more likely than nonreprocessing centers to report patients with dialysis-related sepsis, reported episodes of septicemia were not statistically related to dialyzer reuse.

While many pyrogenic reactions are assumed to represent a systemic response to circulating bacteria, it is conceivable that others may be a manifestation of poor compatability with the dialyzer membrane. Associations of reuse with blood-membrane interactions and acute allergic reactions are discussed under "Effects on Biocompatibility," below.

Viral Pathogens

Dialyzer reuse has not been associated with transmission of bloodborne viruses.[77] However, the CDC advises that dialyzers should not be reused on Hepatitis B surface antigen (HBsAg)-positive patients. Because Hepatitis B (HBV) is efficiently transmitted through occupational exposure to blood, the practice of reprocessing dialyzers from HBsAG-positive patients might place HBV-susceptible staff members at increased risk for infection. By contrast, reprocessing of dialyzers from Hepatitis C (HCV)-positive or HIV-positive patients should not place staff members or other patients at increased risk for infection. Consequently, the CDC recommends that "universal" infection control precautions recommended for all hemodialysis patients are sufficient to prevent HIV and HCV transmission in dialysis units, and that both HCV-positive and HIV-positive patients can participate in dialyzer reuse programs. Nonetheless, the reuse of dialyzers from HIV-positive patients remains an emotionally charged issue, and it is believed that many dialysis units exclude HIV-infected patients from their dialyzer reprocessing programs.[77]

The CDC has published descriptive data from the year 2000 about the incidence and prevalence of HCV infection by dialysis center reuse status.[17] A total of 1239 of 1519 (82 percent) reuse facilities practiced dialyzer reuse for HCV-positive patients. Anti-HCV antibody prevalence in centers that reused dialyzers on anti-HCV antibody patients (8.7 percent) was similar to the prevalence in reuse centers that did not reuse on anti-HCV antibody-positive patients (7.6 percent) and in centers that did not reuse dialyzers on any patients (8.9 percent). Among centers that reused dialyzers, anti-HCV antibody incidence rate in 2000 was slightly higher at centers that reused on anti-HCV antibody-positive patients (0.16 vs. 0.27 percent).[17] Although this finding could result from environmental contamination due to improper handling of reused dialyzer products (i.e., a true infection risk associated with dialyzer reuse among anti-HCV antibody-positive patients), the reported incidence rates are so small that bias or confounding could easily influence their ratio substantially. Data describing HIV infection by dialysis center reuse status have, to our knowledge, not been collected.

EFFECTS ON BIOCOMPATIBILITY

Dialysis with reused dialyzers was long believed to be associated with a lower incidence of intradialytic symptoms than dialysis with new but otherwise similar diayzers,[53,78–82] but the relationship between first-use and intradialytic complications is now less apparent. The term *first-use syndrome* has referred to a broad group of clinical events—ranging in intensity from symptoms such as mild chest and back pain to bronchospasm to, rarely, anaphalactic reactions and shock—that occurred typically with dialyzers used for the first time.[83,84] However, the argument for reusing dialyzers to improve blood-membrane biocompatibility has now become substantially less persuasive because (1) the incidence of the "first-use syndrome" has diminished,[73,85] (2) allergic reactions occurring with the use of reprocessed dialyzers are now recognized,[86–88] and (3) concern has been raised that chronic inflammatory responses linked to dialyzer reuse may be deleterious, although data regarding this possibility are preliminary.[85]

Exposure to Manufacturing Residuals

The decline in the incidence of the first-use syndrome has been attributed in large part to efforts to lessen patient exposure to ethylene oxide and other manufacturing residuals in new dialyzers. Ethylene oxide was used in the 1980s by most manufacturers to sterilize new hollow-fiber dialyzers, and it tended to accumulate in the dialyzer potting compound. A high proportion of type A (anaphylactic) dialyzer reactions in the late 1980s was associated with elevated serum titers of IgE antibody to ethylene oxide.[89–91] These reactions were observed exclusively during first use of dialyzers, often after less than adequate rinsing.[80] However, ethylene oxide reactions to new dialyzers are now uncommon because of steps taken by manufacturers to remove most ethylene oxide and other residuals from dialyzers prior to shipment.[35] Additionally, it is now common for centers, whether practicing dialyzer reuse or not, to "preprocess" dialyzers before their first clinical use to minimize the content of undesirable manufacturing residuals.

Blood-Membrane Interactions

Other cases of first-use syndrome have occurred in the absence of an anti-ethylene oxide immune response. In the case of unsubstituted cellulosic membranes, it is believed that many of these cases were mediated by alternative pathway complement activation precipitated by the contact of blood with membrane during first use of the dialyzer. This process appears to be initiated by the deposition of C3b, an activated form of C3, on the first-use dialyzer membrane, and is modulated by the binding of serum complement regulatory proteins to the membrane.[35,92] Deposition of C3b may be facilitated by the presence on the membrane surface of nucleophilic groups such as the hydroxyl groups present on the surface of unsubstituted cellulose.[93] Activation of the complement cascade leads to the release of small complement fragments that are biologically active and act as anaphylatoxins, causing vasodilatation, bronchospasm, and increased vascular permeability.[5-7,94-96] Stimulation of interleukin-1 (IL-1) and kinin contributes further to the adverse effects mediated by complement activation.[3] Another effect is neutropenia, caused by aggregation of white blood cells and their subsequent trapping in the pulmonary circulation.[4,6,94,95,97] Pulmonary leukostasis partially accounts for the hypoxemia that may complicate dialysis treatments.

Adequate reprocessing of unsubstituted cellulosic membranes was shown in the 1970s and 1980s to ameliorate the adverse biochemical and hematologic effects that can occur with the first use of these dialyzers. Significantly less complement activation occurs with reprocessed than first-use dialyzers,[4-6] and the neutrophil count drops by between 40 and 50 percent compared with 90 percent for first-use dialyzers.[4,5] Hypoxemia and other measures of respiratory dysfunction early during dialysis also improve with reprocessing of unsubstituted cellulosic dialyzers.[82,98]

The mechanism by which reprocessing an unsubstituted cellulosic dialyzer with formaldehyde or peracetic acid[81] results in a more biocompatible dialyzer than an unused dialyzer involves exposure of the membrane to both plasma and a germicide.[4,6,7,81,97,99] A protein layer forms on the membrane surface when the dialyzer is first exposed to plasma. Subsequent rinsing with formaldehyde cross-links these proteins, binding C3b firmly to the membrane and rendering the dialyzer much less capable of activating complement further.[100] Thus, exposure of the unsubstituted cellulosic dialyzer to blood during dialysis with subsequent fixation of certain moieties to the membrane by germicide during reprocessing seems to limit additional blood-membrane interaction.

Variation by Dialyzer Type. The robust literature and mechanistic insights just described that support the improved biocompatibility of unsubstituted cellulosic membranes with reuse may have limited applicability to the dialysis membranes more commonly used at this time in the United States. In 1991, Cheung et al. were unable to detect any reduction in symptoms with reprocessed substituted cellulosic (e.g., cellulose acetate) hollow-fiber dialyzers,[101] although this finding may have resulted in part from the improved removal over the years of residual noxious substances from new dialyzers. Heierli et al. in 1988 demonstrated that formaldehyde reprocessing had a positive effect on leukopenia observed with cuprammonium cellulosic membranes but not cellulose acetate or synthetic membranes.[102] Numerous other studies have shown that synthetic membranes—including polysulfone, polymethyl-methacrylate, and polyacrylonitrile—do not activate the complement cascade and demonstrate enhanced biocompatibility prior to first use that is similar to reprocessed membranes.[103-105]

Acute Allergic Reactions

In 1992, Pegues et al. described a cluster of 12 anaphylactoid reactions in 10 patients that occurred within 10 minutes of starting dialysis with cuprammonium cellulosic, cellulose acetate, or polysulfone membranes reprocessed with peracetic acid at a single dialysis center over 4 months.[86] The events occurred at a minimum of 4 and maximum of 19 reuses. The event rate among these 10 patients was greater in sessions with a reused dialyzer (12 of 70) than sessions with a first-use dialyzer (0 of 31; $p = 0.016$). This report was the first to describe an outbreak of anaphylactoid reactions associated exclusively with reused dialyzers.[86] Although its characteristics suggest contamination as a cause, CDC investigators found no specific reprocessing deficiencies that explained the event cluster.

Pegues et al. observed that patients experiencing an event during this outbreak were significantly more likely than those who did not receive an angiotensin-converting-enzyme (ACE) inhibitor (7/10 vs. 3/34; RR 7.9, 95 percent CI 2.5 to 25.2).[86] None of the ACE inhibitor users had just started using the drug at the time of the clinical event. The association of anaphylactoid reactions with ACE inhibitor use is reminiscent of similar reactions developing when certain new polyacrylonitrile membranes are used in conjunction with ACE inhibitor therapy. These have been attributed to bradykinin generation facilitated by the interaction between blood constituents and the dialyzer membrane.[35,106] Although none of the patients who experienced an anaphylactoid reaction in the Pegues report were using a polyacrylonitrile membrane, it has been proposed that a similar process may plausibly occur due to effects of reuse that diminish membrane biocompatibility among patients who are taking ACE inhibitors. Vienken et al. have hypothesized that reprocessing causes partial denaturation and oxidation of proteins on the dialyzer membrane, leading to the formation of negative charges which support contact activation and bradykinin formation with subsequent dialyzer reuse.[105]

This hypothesis is supported by the demonstration of oxidized proteins on the surface of polysulfone membranes reprocessed with peracetic acid.[107]

A 1989 questionnaire of 1290 dialysis centers by the CDC did not demonstrate convincing epidemiologic evidence linking reuse with acute dialyzer reactions. Some 3 percent of all centers reported acute allergic reactions with new dialyzers, and 4 percent of centers reprocessing dialyzers reported acute allergic reactions with reused dialyzers.[87,88] The report did, however, implicate reprocessing with bleach as a possible risk factor for acute dialyzer reactions.[87,88,108] Because bleach denatures proteins, this epidemiologic association lends further support to the hypotheses described above that invoke breakdown and oxidation of membrane proteins as a mechanism by which reuse may lessen membrane biocompatibility.

Taken as a whole, the evidence to date that dialyzer reuse may impair biocompatibility remains inconclusive. To our knowledge, no case series subsequent to the Pegues publication[86] have been published, and the CDC no longer collects epidemiologic data regarding this topic.

Chronic Inflammatory Responses

It has been proposed that chronic inflammatory responses to reused dialyzers contribute to the higher mortality associated with hemodialysis in the United States than in other countries.[9] As mechanistic rationale, the hypothesis has been advanced that endotoxin and adsorbed protein fragments trapped in the dialyzer during reprocessing may serve as inflammatory stimuli during subsequent dialyzer use. However, the few papers published to date that address this hypothesis have yielded inconclusive results. After in vitro reprocessing with formaldehyde, cytokine-inducing substances in one study were retained and remained biologically active on polyamide membranes and the protein layer covering the membranes.[109] On the other hand, several in vitro studies have found greater decrease in the release of IL-1β,[109,110] as well as TNF-α and IL-6,[110] after the start of dialysis with a variety of reused membranes than with new membranes. Clinical studies have found no difference in cytokine release[111] and decreased levels of oxidative stress markers[112] before and after several weeks of dialyzer reuse, although these publications lack comparative data for single use dialyzers. In 1996, Pereira et al. found no significant difference in plasma levels of IL-1 receptor antagonist-alpha, C3a, or lipopolysaccharide binding protein among 37 patients after random assignment to 12 weeks of dialysis using either cellulosic dialyzers without reuse or with reuse by glutaraldehyde and bleach processing.[113] Further studies are needed before the effect of reuse on cytokine generation, oxidative stress, and their clinical sequelae can be clarified.[112,114]

TOXICITY OF GERMICIDE EXPOSURE

Controversy exists regarding the effects of long-term patient exposure to small amounts of residual germicide not removed by rinsing. Formaldehyde was the only reprocessing germicide available for many years. Due in large part to concerns about long-term occupational exposure, its prevalence has decreased substantially, but it was still used in 2000 by 31 percent of reprocessing dialysis units.[17] While only a single case of a life-threatening anaphylactoid reaction to formaldehyde has been described,[115] considerable attention has been paid to immune-mediated and oncologic complications of exposure to residual formaldehyde.

During the early experience with dialyzer reuse in the mid-1970s, it was reported that dialysis patients exposed to formaldehyde-packed or reprocessed dialyzers had an unusually high incidence of a cold agglutinin identified as an antibody to blood group N (anti-N-like antibody).[116,117] This undesired immunologic response results in structural changes in the red cell membrane and has been linked to the development of hemolytic anemia and to destruction of kidney grafts when they were not warmed prior to insertion in recipients with these antibodies. It has been hypothesized that formaldehyde may alter the M antigen, found on red cell fragments adherent to reprocessed dialyzer membranes, to an N antigen,[118] and that these modified fragments may reenter the systemic circulation and instigate immune hemolysis.[119] The mandated reduction of the residual formaldehyde concentration in reprocessed dialyzers to <5 ppm[18,23] has been associated with decreased reported frequency of this problem.[120] However, anti-N-like antibody formation and immune hemolysis have developed in patients chronically exposed to formaldehyde concentrations as low as 2 ppm.[121,122]

Formaldehyde is carcinogenic in animal species, and the Occupational Safety and Health Administration (OSHA) has established limits for employee exposure to this chemical.[123] However, these limits apply to fumes, not to intravenous exposure. Ideally, all of the formaldehyde should be rinsed from a dialyzer before use. In practice this is not possible, however, because of the long and expensive rinsing procedures that would be necessary. Most facilities rinse dialyzers until a sensitive test, such as that using Schiff's reagent, demonstrates residual formaldehyde level <5 ppm. It is nonetheless likely that small amounts of the germicide are delivered to the patient with each use. While the long-term consequences of this systemic exposure are unknown, the latency period for most cancers may be sufficiently long that an increased cancer rate due to dialyzer reprocessing is unlikely to be manifest among dialysis patients due to their shortened life spans.

Staff in the dialysis unit and reprocessing area are also potentially at risk from occupational exposure to chemical toxins and infectious agents. Measures to minimize these risks should include ensuring adequate ventilation of the reprocessing area to reduce levels of potentially toxic fumes to OSHA-mandated levels.[123] Other measures to reduce the risk of injury include observing universal infection control measures.[85] Agents of known or suspected toxicity should be handled with durable gloves, eye protection, and protective clothing in areas with adequate ventilation, washing facilities, eyewash stations, and spill control materials.

Peracetic acid has been the most widely used germicidal agent since 1990.[5] Because it was adopted for use more recently than formaldehyde, considerably fewer data are available about the long-term effects of peracetic acid exposure.

INFORMED CONSENT

The question of whether informed consent should be required for the use of reprocessed hemodialyzers has been contentious.[18] Some opponents of mandated informed consent for dialyzer reuse argue that reuse is customary medical practice. As such, consent for dialyzer reuse does not require specific consent procedures because it can be properly inferred from consent for hemodialysis therapy, just as are many other aspects of dialytic care. Proponents of consent procedures for dialyzer reuse have cautioned that reuse programs can be motivated by, or perceived to be motivated by, financial incentives rather than by overt improvement in quality of care. As such, it is possible that reuse programs may be viewed skeptically by some patients, and obtaining informed consent is believed by some to be one means to address this mistrust.

The AAMI and CMS and the NKF-K/DOQI Task Force on Dialyzer Reuse do not provide specific recommendations or requirements regarding the need to obtain informed consent prior to dialyzer reuse, but they stress the importance of keeping the patient informed regarding the risks and benefits of and rationale for dialyzer reuse.[18,35,124] The 1996 CMS *Conditions for Coverage of Suppliers of End-Stage Renal Disease Services* stated that all patients in a dialysis facility will be fully informed regarding reuse of dialyzers.[124] In the 1997 position paper by the NKF-K/DOQI Task Force on Dialyzer Reuse, it was argued that "it is an ethical and regulatory requirement that each patient participating in reuse programs understands, to the degree he or she desires, the risks and benefits of reuse."[85] The committee responsible for the 2002 AAMI publication on technical aspects of dialyzer reuse wrote as part of their rationale that in any facility practicing dialyzer reuse and regardless of informed consent practice, "sharing information with patients, responding to questions, and eliminating any impression of secrecy are encouraged."[18]

SUMMARY AND FUTURE DIRECTIONS

Dialyzer reuse is a highly prevalent practice in the United States today, with 80 percent of all U.S. dialysis units reprocessing hemodialyzers in 2000.[17] In the past, reuse programs were motivated in part by the belief that dialyzer reuse might benefit the health of ESRD patients by moderating complement activation and cytokine release. However, the decreased incidence of "first-use syndrome," attributed to the now widespread use of synthetic and newer cellulosic membranes and to alterations in dialyzer manufacturing techniques, has rendered this justification for dialyzer reuse obsolete. At this time, economic motivations remain the major reason for widespread dialyzer reuse, but the economic benefits of reuse deserve ongoing reevaluation as the price of newer membranes decreases and as other aspects of dialysis care and the market forces that influence dialysis providers continue to evolve.

As for the safety and efficacy of dialyzer reuse as it is currently practiced, certain issues have become more clearly understood while many other questions remain unanswered. Although epidemiologic studies have failed to clearly implicate dialyzer reuse as a whole as a cause of higher morbidity or mortality in the U.S. ESRD population, it remains unclear whether certain reprocessing techniques are independently associated with worse outcomes than others. Numerous case reports have demonstrated potential infectious dangers of dialyzer reuse when reprocessing procedures fail to achieve well-established technical standards recommended by the AAMI and endorsed by the CMS, but reported outbreaks of invasive infection in reprocessing dialysis units have become less common in recent years and the CDC now asserts that modern dialyzer reuse performed according to established guidelines carries an acceptably low infection risk. Regarding adequacy of delivered dialysis, urea clearance appears to be substantially preserved after multiple uses with reprocessed membranes. Clearance of larger solutes, decreased after multiple uses with membranes reprocessed without bleach, may actually increase after bleach reprocessing. Nonetheless, bleach reprocessing may cause excessive protein losses into the dialysate. The hypothesis has also been advanced in recent years that a chronic inflammatory response to reused dialyzers may adversely influence patient outcomes, but clinical data supporting this possibility are as yet very limited. Finally, the possible risks associated with chronic exposure of patients and health care workers to germicides in the modern reuse setting have yet to be fully characterized. As hemodialysis care in the United States continues to evolve, it seems prudent to continue critical evaluation of the net health benefits of dialyzer reuse from the perspective of individual dialysis patients and the U.S. ESRD population as a whole.

REFERENCES

1. Scribner B, Buri R, Caner J, et al. The treatment of chronic uremia by means of intermittent dialysis: a preliminary report. *ASAIO Trans* 1960;6:114.

2. Pollard T, Barnett B, Eschbach J, Scribner B. A technique for storage and multiple reuse of the Kiil dialyzer and blood tubing. *ASAIO Trans* 1967;13:24.

3. Lowrie EG, Hakim RM. The effect on patient health of using reprocessed artificial kidneys. *Proc Clin Dial Transplant Forum* 1980;10:86–91.

4. Hakim RM, Lowrie EG. Effect of dialyzer reuse on leukopenia, hypoxemia and total hemolytic complement system. *Trans Am Soc Artif Intern Organs* 1980;26:159–164.

5. Chenoweth DE, Cheung AK, Ward RA, Henderson LW. Anaphylatoxin formation during hemodialysis: comparison of new and reused dialyzers. *Kidney Int* 1983;24:770–774.

6. Stroncek DF, Keshaviah P, Craddock PR, Hammerschmidt DE. Effect of dialyzer reuse on complement activation and neutropenia in hemodialysis. *J Lab Clin Med* 1984;104:304–311.

7. Hakim R, Breillott J, Lazarus M, Port F. Complement activation and hypersensitivity reactions to dialysis membranes. *N Engl J Med* 1984;311:878–882.

8. Stragier A. Dialyzer reuse in Europe: current status and perspectives. *Nephrol News Issues* 1998;12:44.

9. Shaldon S. The influence of dialysis time and dialyser reuse on survival. *Nephrol Dial Transplant* 1995;10(suppl)3:57–62.

10. Eknoyan G, Beck GJ, Cheung AK, et al. Effect of dialysis dose and membrane flux in maintenance hemodialysis. *N Engl J Med* 2002;347:2010–2019.

11. Baris E, McGregor M. The reuse of hemodialyzers: an assessment of safety and potential savings. *CMAJ* 1993;148:175–183.

12. Manns BJ, Taub K, Richardson RM, Donaldson C. To reuse or not to reuse? An economic evaluation of hemodialyzer reuse versus conventional single-use hemodialysis for chronic hemodialysis patients. *Int J Technol Assess Health Care* 2002;18:81–93.

13. Ozgen H, Ozcan YA. A national study of efficiency for dialysis centers: an examination of market competition and facility characteristics for production of multiple dialysis outputs. *Health Serv Res* 2002;37:711–732.

14. Powe NR, Thamer M, Hwang W, et al. Cost-quality tradeoffs in dialysis care: a national survey of dialysis facility administrators. *Am J Kidney Dis* 2002;39:116–126.

15. Sullivan JD. The economics of dialyzer reuse in ESRD. *Nephrol News Issues* 2002;16:32–34,36,38.

16. Tokars JI, Alter MJ, Miller E, et al. National surveillance of dialysis associated diseases in the United States—1994. *ASAIO J* 1997;43:108–119.

17. Tokars JI, Frank M, Alter MJ, Arduino MJ. National surveillance of dialysis-associated diseases in the United States, 2000. *Semin Dial* 2002;15:162–171.

18. *Reuse of Hemodialyzers: AAMI Recommended Practice, ANSI/AAMI RD47:2002 & RD47:2002/A1:2003.* Arlington, VA: Association for the Advancement of Medical Instrumentation, 2003.

19. Held PJ, Wolfe RA, Gaylin DS, et al. Analysis of the association of dialyzer reuse practices and patient outcomes. *Am J Kidney Dis* 1994;23:692–708.

20. Port FK, Wolfe RA, Hulbert-Shearon TE, et al. Mortality risk by hemodialyzer reuse practice and dialyzer membrane characteristics: results from the USRDS dialysis morbidity and mortality study. *Am J Kidney Dis* 2001;37:276–286.

21. Levin NW, Parnell SL, Prince HN, et al. The use of heated citric acid for dialyzer reprocessing. *J Am Soc Nephrol* 1995;6:1578–1585.

22. Schoenfeld P, McLaughlin M, Mendelson M. Heat disinfection of polysulfone hemodialyzers. *Kidney Int* 1995;47:638–642.

23. Department of Health and Human Services, Health Care Financing Administration. *Conditions for Coverage of Suppliers of End-Stage Renal Disease (ESRD) Services. Condition: Reuse of Hemodialyzers and Other Dialysis Supplies.* Code of Federal Regulations 42 CFR Part 405 Sec 2150. Washington, DC: DHHS/HCFA, October 1, 1997.

24. Food and Drug Administration, Center for Devices and Radiological Health, Office of Device Evaluation. *Guidance for Hemodialyzer Reuse Labeling.* Washington, DC: FDA, October 6, 1995.

25. Center for Infectious Diseases. *National Surveillance of Dialysis-Associated Diseases in U.S. 1989.* Atlanta, GA: Centers for Disease Control, Public Health Service, Department of Health and Human Service, 1992.

26. National Kidney Foundation. KDOQI Clinical Practice Guidelines for Hemodialysis Adequacy, 2000. *Am J Kidney Dis* 2001;37(suppl 1):S7–S64.

27. *Water Treatment Equipment for Hemodialysis Applications: AAMI Recommended Practice.* ANSI/AAMI RD62:2001. Arlington, VA: Association for the Advancement of Medical Instrumentation, 2001.

28. Leypoldt JK, Cheung AK, Deeter RB. Effect of hemodialyzer reuse: dissociation between clearances of small and large solutes. *Am J Kidney Dis* 1998;32:295–301.

29. Ouseph R, Smith BP, Ward RA. Maintaining blood compartment volume in dialyzers reprocessed with peracetic acid maintains Kt/V but not beta2-microglobulin removal. *Am J Kidney Dis* 1997;30:501–506.

30. Cheung AK, Agodoa LY, Daugirdas JT, et al. Effects of hemodialyzer reuse on clearances of urea and beta2-microglobulin. The Hemodialysis (HEMO) Study Group. *J Am Soc Nephrol* 1999;10:117–127.

31. Deane N, Bermis J. *Multiple Use of Hemodialyzers.* New York: Manhattan Kidney Center: National Institute of Arthritis, Diabetes, Digestive, and Kidney Diseases, 1981:64–90.

32. Krautzig S, Mahiout A, Koch KM, Lemke H. Reuse with oxidizing agents leads to a loss of polyvinylpyrrolidone from polysulfone membranes. *Blood Purif* 1994;12:176.

33. Kaplan AA, Halley SE, Lapkin RA, Graeber CW. Dialysate protein losses with bleach processed polysulphone dialyzers. *Kidney Int* 1995;47:573–578.

34. Scott MK, Mueller BA, Sowinski KM, Clark WR. Dialyzer-dependent changes in solute and water permeability with bleach reprocessing. *Am J Kidney Dis* 1999;33:87–96.

35. National Kidney Foundation. Report on Dialyzer Reuse. Task Force on Reuse of Dialyzers, Council on Dialysis, National Kidney Foundation. *Am J Kidney Dis* 1997;30: 859–871.

36. Gotch F. Mass transport in reused dialyzers. *Proc Clin Dial Transplant Forum* 1980;10:81–85.

37. Gotch FA. Correlation of transport properties with total cell volume of new and reused hollow fiber dialyzers. In: Deane N, Beamis JA, eds. *Multiple Use of Hemodialyzers.* National Institutes of Arthritis, Diabetes, Digestive, and Kidney Diseases contract NO1–AM–9–2214. New York: Manhattan Kidney Center, 1981.

38. Krivitski NM, Kislukhin VV, Snyder JW, et al. In vivo measurement of hemodialyzer fiber bundle volume: theory and validation. *Kidney Int* 1998;54:1751–1758.

39. Ouseph R, Brier ME, Ward RA. Improved dialyzer reuse after use of a population pharmacodynamic model to determine heparin doses. *Am J Kidney Dis* 2000;35:89–94.

40. Matos JP, Andre MB, Rembold SM, et al. Effects of dialyzer reuse on the permeability of low–flux membranes. *Am J Kidney Dis* 2000;35:839–844.

41. Garred LJ, Canaud B, Flavier JL, et al. Effect of reuse on dialyzer efficacy. *Artif Organs* 1990;14:80–84.

42. Saha L, Van Stone J. Differences between Kt/V measured during dialysis and Kt/V predicted from manufacturer clearance data. *Int J Artif Organs* 1992;15:465–469.

43. Delmez JA, Weerts CA, Hasamear PD, Windus DW. Severe dialyzer dysfunction undetectable by standard reprocessing validation tests. *Kidney Int* 1989;36:478–484.

44. Cornelius RM, McClung WG, Richardson RM, et al. Effects of heat/citric acid reprocessing on high-flux polysulfone dialyzers. *ASAIO J* 2002;48:45–56.

45. Sridhar NR, Ferrand K, Reger D, et al. Urea kinetics with dialyzer reuse—a prospective study. *Am J Nephrol* 1999;19: 668–673.

46. Murthy BV, Sundaram S, Jaber BL, et al. Effect of formaldehyde/bleach reprocessing on in vivo performances of high-efficiency cellulose and high-flux polysulfone dialyzers. *J Am Soc Nephrol* 1998;9:464–472.

47. Sherman RA, Cody RP, Rogers ME, Solanchick JC. The effect of dialyzer reuse on dialysis delivery. *Am J Kidney Dis* 1994;24:924–926.

48. Diaz RJ, Washburn S, Cauble L, et al. The effect of dialyzer reprocessing on performance and beta 2-microglobulin removal using polysulfone membranes. *Am J Kidney Dis* 1993;21:405–410.

49. Ikizler TA, Flakoll PJ, Parker RJ, Hakim RM. Amino acid and albumin losses during hemodialysis. *Kidney Int* 1994; 46:830–837.

50. Kaysen GA, Rathore V, Shearer GC, Depner TA. Mechanisms of hypoalbuminemia in hemodialysis patients. *Kidney Int* 1995;48:510–516.

51. Sundaram S, Barrett TW, Meyer KB, et al. Transmembrane passage of cytokine-inducing bacterial products across new and reprocessed polysulfone dialyzers. *J Am Soc Nephrol* 1996;7:2183–2191.

52. Wing AJ, Brunner F, Brynger H, et al. Mortality and morbidity of reusing dialyzers. *Br Med J* 1978;2:853–855.

53. Kant KS, Pollak VE, Cathey M, et al. Multiple use of dialyzers: safety and efficacy. *Kidney Int* 1981;19:728–738.

54. Pollak VE, Kant KS, Parnell SL, Levin NW. Repeated use of dialyzers is safe: long-term observations on morbidity and mortality in patients with end-stage renal disease. *Nephron* 1986;42:217–223.

55. Held PJ, Pauly M, Diamond L. Survival analysis of patients undergoing dialysis. *JAMA* 1987;257:645–650.

56. Feldman HI, Kinosian M, Bilker WB, et al. Effect of dialyzer reuse on survival of patients treated with hemodialysis. *JAMA* 1996;276:620–625.

57. Feldman HI, Bilker WB, Hackett MH, et al. Association of dialyzer reuse with hospitalization and survival rates among U.S. hemodialysis patients: do comorbidities matter? *J Clin Epidemiol* 1999;52:209–217.

58. Collins AJ, Ma JZ, Constantini EG, Everson SE. Dialysis unit and patient characteristics associated with reuse practices and mortality: 1989–1993. *J Am Soc Nephrol* 1998;9: 2108–2117.

59. Ebben JP, Dalleska F, Ma JZ, et al. Impact of disease severity and hematocrit level on reuse-associated mortality. *Am J Kidney Dis* 2000;35:244–249.

60. Carson L, Bland L, Cusic L, et al. Prevalence of nontuberculous mycobacteria in water supplies of hemodialysis centers. *Appl Environ Microbiol* 1988;54:3122–3125.

61. Arduino M, McAllister S, Bland L. Assuring proper germicide concentrations in reprocessed hemodialyzers. *Dial Transplant* 1993;22.

62. Bolan G, Reingold AL, Carson LA, et al. Infections with *Mycobacterium chelonei* in patients receiving dialysis and using processed hemodialyzers. *J Infect Dis* 1985;152: 1013–1019.

63. Lowry PW, Beck-Sague CM, Bland LA, et al. *Mycobacterium chelonae* infection among patients receiving high-flux dialysis in a hemodialysis clinic in California. *J Infect Dis* 1990;161:85–90.

64. Centers for Disease Control. Bacteremia associated with reuse of disposable hollow-fiber hemodialyzers. *MMWR Morb Mortal Wkly Rep* 1986;35:417–418.

65. Vanholder R, Vanhaecke E, Ringoir S. *Pseudomonas* septicemia due to deficient disinfectant mixing during reuse. *Int J Artif Organs* 1992;15:19–24.

66. Beck–Sague C, Jarvis W, Bland L, et al. Outbreak of gram-negative bacteremia and pyrogenic reactions in a hemodialysis center. *Am J Nephrol* 1990;10:397–403.

67. Welbel SF, Schoendorf K, Bland LA, et al. An outbreak of gram-negative bloodstream infections in chronic hemodialysis patients. *Am J Nephrol* 1995;15:1–4.

68. Vanholder R, Vanhaecke E, Ringoir S. Waterborne *Pseudomonas* septicea. *ASAIO Trans* 1990;36:M215–M216.

69. Flaherty JP, Garcia-Houchins S, Chudy RE, Arnow PM. An outbreak of gram-negative bacteremia traced to contaminated O-rings in reprocessed dialyzers. *Ann Intern Med* 1993;119:1072–1078.

70. Bland L, Arduino M, Aguero S, Favero M. Recovery of bacteria from reprocessed high flux dialyzers after bacterial contamination of the header spaces and o-rings. *ASAIO Trans* 1989;35:315–316.

71. Roberts B, Alvarado N, Garcia W, et al. "Header sepsis" syndrome: waterborne *Xanthomonas*-induced fevers. *Dial Transplant* 1994;23:464–472.

72. Alter M, Favero M, Miller J, et al. Reuse of hemodialyzers: results of nationwide surveillance for adverse effects. *JAMA* 1988;260:2073–2076.

73. Tokars JI, Alter MJ, Favero MS, et al. National surveillance of dialysis associated diseases in the United States, 1991. *ASAIO J* 1993;39:966–975.

74. Tokars JI, Miller ER, Alter MJ, Arduino MJ. National surveillance of dialysis associated diseases in the United States, 1995. *ASAIO J* 1998;44:98–107.

75. Tokars JI, Miller ER, Alter MJ, Arduino MJ. National surveillance of dialysis-associated diseases in the United States, 1997. *Semin Dial* 2000;13:75–85.

76. Tokars JI, Alter MJ, Favero MS, et al. National surveillance of dialysis associated diseases in the United States, 1992. *ASAIO J* 1994;40:1020–1031.

77. Recommendations for preventing transmission of infections among chronic hemodialysis patients. www.cdc.gov/mmwr/PDF/RR/RR5005.pdf.

78. Bok DV, Pascual L, Herberger C, et al. Effect of multiple use of dialyzers on intradialytic symptoms. *Proc Clin Dial Transplant Forum* 1980;10:92–99.

79. Robson MD, Charoenpanich R, Kant KS, et al. Effect of first and subsequent use of hemodialyzers on patient well-being. Analysis of the incidence of symptoms and events and description of a syndrome associated with new dialyzer use. *Am J Nephrol* 1986;6:101–106.

80. Charoenpanich R, Pollak VE, Kant KS, et al. Effect of first and subsequent use of hemodialyzers on patient well-being: the rise and fall of a syndrome associated with new dialyzer use. *Artif Organs* 1987;11:123–127.

81. Dumler F, Zasuwa G, Levin NW. Effect of dialyzer reprocessing methods on complement activation and hemodialyzer-related symptoms. *Artif Organs* 1987;11:128–131.

82. Vanholder R, Ringoir S. Influence of reuse and of reuse sterilants on the first-use syndrome. *Artif Organs* 1987;11:137–139.

83. Ogden DA. New dialyzer syndrome. *N Engl J Med* 1980;302:1262.

84. Agar JW, Holl JD, Kaplan M, et al. Acute cardiopulmonary decompensation and complement activation during hemodialysis. *Ann Intern Med* 1979;90:792–793.

85. National Kidney Foundation report on dialyzer reuse. *Am J Kidney Dis* 1988;11:1–6.

86. Pegues DA, Beck-Sague CM, Woollen SW, et al. Anaphylactoid reactions associated with reuse of hollow-fiber hemodialyzers and ACE inhibitors. *Kidney Int* 1992;42:1232–1237.

87. Centers for Disease Control. Acute allergic reactions associated with reprocessed hemodialyzers: United States, 1989–1990. *MMWR* 1991;40:153–154.

88. Centers for Disease Control: Update: acute allergic reactions associated with reprocessed hemodialyzers—United States, 1989–1990. *MMWR* 1991;40:147.

89. Marshall CP, Shimizu A, Smith E, et al. Ethylene oxide allergy in a dialysis center: prevalence in hemodialysis and peritoneal dialysis population. *Clin Nephrol* 1984;21:346–349.

90. Dolovich J, Marshall CP, Smith EKM, et al. Allergy to ethylene oxide in chronic hemodialysis patients. *Artif Organs* 1984;8:334–337.

91. Grammer LC, Paterson BF, Roxe D, et al. IgE against ethylene oxide-altered human serum albumin in patients with anaphylactic reactions to dialysis. *J Allergy Clin Immunol* 1985;76:511–514.

92. Cheung AK, Parker CJ, Wilcox L, Janatova J. Activation of the alternative pathway of complement by cellulosic hemodialysis membranes. *Kidney Int* 1989;36:257–265.

93. Chenoweth D, Henderson L. Complement activation during hemodialysis: laboratory evaluation of hemodialyzers. *Artif Organs* 1987;11:155–162.

94. Craddock P, Fehr J, Brigham K, et al. Complement and leukocyte-mediated pulmonary dysfunction in hemodialysis. *N Engl J Med* 1977;296:769–774.

95. Amadori A, Candi P, Sasdelli M, et al. Hemodialysis leukopenia and complement function with different dialyzers. *Kidney Int* 1983;24:775–781.

96. Ivanovitch P, Chenoweth D, Schmidt R, et al. Symptoms and activation of granulocytes and complement with two dialysis membranes. *Kidney Int* 1983;24:758–763.

97. Hakim RM, Fearon DT, Lazarus JM. Biocompatibility of dialysis membranes: effects of chronic complement activation. *Kidney Int* 1984;26:194–200.

98. Davenport A, Williams AJ. The effect of dialyzer reuse on peak expiratory flow rate. *Respir Med* 1990;84:17–21.

99. Bauer H, Brunner H, Franz HE. Experience with the disinfectant peroxyacetic acid (PES) for hemodialyzer reuse. *Trans Am Soc Artif Intern Organs* 1983;29:662–665.

100. Chenoweth D, Cheung A, Henderson L. Anaphylatoxin formation during hemodialysis: effects of different dialyzer membranes. *Kidney Int* 1983;24:764–769.

101. Cheung AK, Dalpias D, Emmerson R, Leypoldt JK. A prospective study on intradialytic symptoms associated with reuse of hemodialyzers. *Am J Nephrol* 1991;11:397–401.

102. Heierli C, Markert M, Lambert PH, et al. On the mechanism of haemodialysis-induced neutropenia: a study with five new and reused membranes. *Nephrol Dial Transplant* 1988;3:773–783.

103. Dumler F, Zawusa G, Levin NW. Effect of dialyzer reprocessing methods on complement activation and hemodialyzer-related symptoms. *Artif Organs* 1987;11:128–131.

104. Kuwahara T, Markert M, Wauters JP. Biocompatibility aspects of dialyzer reprocessing: a comparison of 3 reuse methods and 3 membranes. *Clin Nephrol* 1989;32:139–143.

105. Klinkmann H, Grassmann A, Vienken J. Dilemma of membrane biocompatibility and reuse. *Artif Organs* 1996;20:426–432.

106. Verresen L, Fink E, Lemke H, Vanrenterghem Y. Bradykinin is a mediator of anaphylactoid reactions during hemodialysis with AN69 membranes. *Kidney Int* 1994;45:1497–1503.

107. Sodemann K, Lubrich-Birkner I, Berger O, Mahiout A. Identification of oxidized protein and bradykinin generation in dialyzer reuse with polysulfone membranes. *Nephrology* 1997;3:S438.

108. Schmitter L, Sweet S. Anaphylactic reactions with the addition of hypochlorite to reuse in patients maintained on reprocessed polysulfone hemodialyzers and ACE inhibitors. *Am Soc Artif Int Organs* 1993:A75.

109. Lufft V, Mahiout A, Shaldon S, et al. Retention of cytokine-inducing substances inside high-flux dialyzers. *Blood Purif* 1996;14:26–34.

110. Qian J, Yu Z, Dai H, et al. The study of IL-1 beta, TNF-alpha, IL-6 gene expression and plasma levels on hemodialysis before and after dialyzer reuse. *Chin Med J (Engl)* 1997;110:508–511.

111. Pereira BJ, King AJ, Poutsiaka DD, et al. Comparison of first use and reuse of cuprophane membranes on interleukin-1 receptor antagonist and interleukin-1 beta production by blood mononuclear cells. *Am J Kidney Dis* 1993;22:288–295.

112. Kose K, Dogan P, Gunduz Z, et al. Oxidative stress in hemodialyzed patients and the long-term effects of dialyzer reuse practice. *Clin Biochem* 1997;30:601–606.

113. Pereira BJ, Natov SN, Sundaram S, et al. Impact of single use versus reuse of cellulose dialyzers on clinical parameters and indices of biocompatibility. *J Am Soc Nephrol* 1996;7:861–870.

114. Trznadel K, Luciak M, Pawlicki L, et al. Superoxide anion generation and lipid peroxidation processes during hemodialysis with reused cuprophane dialyzers. *Free Radic Biol Med* 1990;8:429–432.

115. Bousquet J, Maurice F, Rivory J, et al. Allergy in long-term hemodialysis. II. Allergic and atopic patterns of a population of patients undergoing long-term hemodialysis. *J Allergy Clin Immunol* 1988;81:605–610.

116. Shaldon S, Chevallet M, Marqovi M, Mion C. Dialysis associated auto-antibodies. *Proc EDTA* 1976;13:339–347.

117. Koch K, Frei U, Fassbinder W. Hemolysis and anemia in anti-N-like antibody positive hemodialysis patients. *Trans Am Soc Artif Int Organs* 1978;24:709–712.

118. White W, Miller G, Kaehny W. Formaldehyde in the pathogenesis of hemodialysis-related anti-N antibodies. *Transfusion* 1977;17:443–447.

119. Ng YY, Yang AH, Wong KC, et al. Dialyzer reuse: interaction between dialyzer membrane, disinfectant (formalin), and blood during dialyzer reprocessing. *Artif Organs* 1996;20:53–55.

120. Lewis K, Dewar P, Ward M, Kerr D. Formation of anti-N-like antibodies in dialysis patients: effects of different methods of dialyzer rinsing to remove formaldehyde. *Clin Nephrol* 1981;15:39–43.

121. Vanholder R, Noens L, De Smet R, Ringoir S. Development of anti-N-like antibodies during formaldehyde reuse in spite of adequate predialysis rinsing. *Am J Kidney Dis* 1988;11:477–480.

122. Ng YY, Chow MP, Wu SC, et al. Anti-N form antibody in hemodialysis patients. *Am J Nephrol* 1995;15:374–378.

123. Occupational Safety and Health Administration, Department of Labor. *Part 1910—Occupational Safety And Health Standards*. Washington, DC: OSHA, July 1, 1998.

124. Department of Health and Human Services, Health Care Financing Administration. *Conditions for Coverage of Suppliers of End-Stage Renal Disease (ESRD) Services. Conditions: Patients' Rights and Responsibilities*. U.S. Code of Federal Regulations, 42 CFR chap IV Sec 405.2138 (a–4), p. 112. Washington, DC: DHHS/HCFA, October 1, 1996.

Hemodialysis in Children

Stefan G. Kiessling
Michael J. G. Somers

THE CHANGING FACE OF PEDIATRIC HEMODIALYSIS

The widespread use of hemodialysis in adults with both acute and chronic renal failure has, over the course of the last four decades, led to its introduction and more widespread application in children of all ages and sizes in need of some period of renal replacement therapy.[1,2] According to data from the most recent report of the U.S. Renal Data System (USRDS), over 1200 children and adolescents develop end-stage renal disease (ESRD) in the United States each year.[3] Although the majority of these pediatric patients with chronic kidney failure will eventually be treated by renal transplantation, nearly half come to be placed on hemodialysis while awaiting grafts.

In addition to this cadre of children with chronic dialysis needs, advancements in pediatric intensive care and pediatric surgery, most notably cardiothoracic surgery, have led to an ever-increasing population of children with acute renal insufficiency who may require a period of hemodialysis during acute illness and recuperation. For instance, it is estimated that up to 5 percent of children develop renal failure after cardiac surgery.[4] Especially as a result of the grow-

ing number of hospitalized pediatric patients at risk for acute renal insufficiency, it is increasingly likely that pediatric clinicians will be caring for children in need of dialysis therapy.

Concurrent discoveries and refinements in biotechnology have also led to the introduction of equipment that makes the application of hemodialysis in pediatric patients more likely to be clinically tolerated and successful.[5] In fact, the development of smaller long-term vascular catheters, the introduction of a broader array of dialyzers and dialysis tubing of smaller caliber and length, and the ongoing development of hemodialysis machines with increasingly precise pumps and accurate ultrafiltration controls has made it possible to provide hemodialysis even to small infants.[6,7]

Pediatric Concerns

Beyond the technical challenges posed by pediatric hemodialysis, there are ongoing clinical concerns unique to children receiving dialysis that, in many ways, make the application of this therapy even more problematic. As with adult patients, the primary objective in providing hemodialysis to children is to remove metabolic waste products, toxic solutes, and extra fluid volume in as efficient, effective, and safe a manner as possible. With chronic dialysis therapy requiring repeated treatments over significant periods of time every week, a long-term challenge faced by the clinician is to strike a balance between delivering optimal medical care to the patient while minimizing the treatment's impact on the patient's life outside the dialysis unit. With acute hemodialysis, the same primary goal exists for the dialysis therapy, but with the focus of therapy aimed at optimizing the child's recovery from the acute insult that has caused renal failure.

With children, the whole task of providing care becomes even more daunting as the physical and psychosocial effects of hemodialysis and especially chronic hemodialysis therapy may adversely affect important aspects of normal growth and development. Moreover, since pediatric patients are usually dependent on parents, family members, or other adult caregivers for their direct physical and emotional well-being, the effect of the child's illness and dialysis therapy on the child's immediate and extended family and their subsequent ability to care and support this child cannot be either underestimated or overlooked.[8]

As a result, the availability of nonphysician staff—such as dialysis nurses, renal dieticians, and renal social workers, all trained, comfortable, and familiar with aspects of pediatric hemodialysis and working to provide information and professional support to both the pediatric patient and his or her family—is invaluable in providing long-term successful dialysis care to the pediatric patient and underscores the importance of a multidisciplinary team approach to the child with ESRD. Because of the small number of children who develop ESRD, there are much more limited data to direct the clinical care of the child requiring hemodialysis than exists for the adult population. With adults with ESRD, the development of guidelines over the last decade to optimize outcome and high-quality care has helped to build a better consensus as to standards of dialysis adequacy, management of vascular access, and management of anemia. These guidelines, though primarily derived from the experiences of adult dialysis patients, often provide at least minimal standards of care for children on hemodialysis as well.[9]

EPIDEMIOLOGY

Patient Characteristics and Demographics

USRDS registry data suggest that the incidence of ESRD in the pediatric population has remained stable over the last 30 years, with only 11 to 14 children per million individuals below 20 years of age being diagnosed annually.[3] Recent data from the North American Pediatric Renal Transplant Cooperative Study (NAPRTCS) registry suggest that, on average, 300 to 500 children initiate chronic dialysis each year, with about 30 percent of those starting on hemodialysis.[10] USRDS data suggest that there is a more even distribution of dialysis modalities in children. With both NAPRTCS and USRDS data, the proportion of children receiving hemodialysis rather than peritoneal dialysis has been slowly increasing in recent years.

Across all pediatric age groups, about 60 percent of new dialysis patients are boys.[3] This male predominance has been seen for some time and most likely represents long-term sequelae of obstructive uropathy in male infants.

About half of children who start dialysis each year are white, between 20 and 25 percent are black, and about 20 percent are Hispanic, demonstrating a disproportionate representation of blacks and Hispanics in the pediatric dialysis population in comparison to the general pediatric population.[3,11] According to the NAPRTCS registry, about 60 percent of white children on hemodialysis are at least 12 years old, compared to almost 70 percent of blacks.[10] For over a decade, the peak age range for initiation of chronic dialysis in the pediatric population has been between 13 and 17 years.[10]

Renal dysplasia, focal segmental glomerulosclerosis (FSGS), and obstructive uropathy remain the most common underlying etiologies of ESRD in children, each occurring in about 15 percent of children requiring renal replacement therapy.[10] Looking at etiology by race, FSGS is the cause of renal failure in one-quarter of all black dialysis patients, followed by renal dysplasia in about 10 percent.[10] In comparison, renal dysplasia and obstructive uropathy remain equally prevalent for white dialysis patients (between 15 and 20 percent of new dialysis cases), followed by FSGS in just over 10 percent.[10]

Availability of Pediatric-Specific Care

Over one-third of children and adolescents undergoing ESRD care are actually managed by health care providers trained in internal medicine and other adult-focused specialties.[12] Due to the relatively small number of pediatric nephrologists and their concentration at academic medical centers, barriers to access will most likely continue to exist, preventing a larger segment of pediatric hemodialysis patients from receiving care at pediatric facilities.

There is evidence to suggest that pediatric ESRD patients who receive their care from adult nephrologists are more likely to receive hemodialysis than peritoneal dialysis. A recent survey found that 65 percent of American pediatric nephrologists preferentially placed patients on peritoneal dialysis, despite the fact that less than half of all pediatric dialysis patients in the United States are actually receiving peritoneal dialysis.[13] This study also found that pediatric nephrologists were more likely to forego placing children on hemodialysis regardless of their prior training in hemodialysis, their prior exposure to children on hemodialysis, their years in practice, their practice setting, their geographic location, or pertinent patient characteristics.

These data underscore that perceptions about appropriate patient care and practice patterns may vary substantially between physicians trained to provide pediatric care and other clinicians. It is often assumed that, as a group, pediatric nephrologists are most likely to take into account important developmental issues, such as growth, pubertal changes, and regular school attendance that are more germane to pediatric practice and pediatric training in general.

To complicate care further, even highly experienced and trained dialysis staff accustomed to adult patients may feel uncomfortable with their skills or competence when dealing with a child. This discomfiture is often accentuated in adolescent patients, where more rigid and inflexible routines may conflict with the adolescent's burgeoning independence, and in families where the child has always previously been healthy and no coping skills for illness have developed.[8] Family-centered care must not only establish clear goals and expectations for the pediatric patient and the adult caregivers but also allow the child and family to have as much control as possible over schedule, diet, and medications. The importance of these principles cannot be underestimated, and hemodialysis will succeed best where the dialysis staff is familiar with the needs of pediatric patients and their families.

PHYSIOLOGY OF HEMODIALYSIS IN CHILDREN

Since the pediatric clinician may be prescribing dialysis to children of a wide array of ages, sizes, and body weights, the exact physiologic principles involved in the process of hemodialysis and the factors that influence solute clearance and ultrafiltration from an extracorporeal circuit must be well understood, so that therapy can be individualized to each child's needs. Certainly, the hemodialysis prescription for an 80-kg hemodynamically stable adolescent on chronic dialysis will differ dramatically from the orders developed for a 4-kg hypotensive infant in an intensive care unit (ICU). Since pediatric hemodialysis patients are more likely to have clinically relevant variations in body size and total blood volume than adults undergoing dialysis, the quantity of dialysis that a pediatric patient is to undergo is much more likely to be precisely calculated and readjusted than it is in adult patients. Nonetheless, the basic physical and physiologic principles underlying hemodialysis are identical in both populations.

Solute Clearance

In hemodialysis, the patient's blood is pumped through the hollow fibers of a dialyzer. At the same time, the fibers in the dialyzer are bathed by a physiologic dialysate solution being pumped countercurrent to the blood flow in the circuit. The dialyzer fibers act as a bundle of multiple, semipermeable membranes that allow the passage of solutes down concentration gradients between the blood and dialysate spaces and the movement of water based on osmotic or hydrostatic forces.

For easier understanding, the blood and dialysate compartments may be pictured as being separated by a sheet perforated by multiple small holes.[14] The holes allow free passage of water from one side to another but restrict the passage of solutes, depending on their size or other physical or electrochemical factors relative to the size, physical, or electrochemical characteristics of the holes in the sheet.

There are two mechanisms by which solutes can come to pass through the holes of this sheet or the pores of a dialysis membrane. Diffusion is the result of relatively random movement of smaller molecules from one side of a membrane to the other. Factors directly related to the likelihood that a solute will cross from one side to the other include the concentration gradient of the molecule between the two sides, the size of the molecule, and the membrane itself. The higher the concentration of a solute on one side of the membrane and the smaller the physical size of the solute in comparison to the pore size of the membrane, the more likely is it that the solute will move to the contralateral side. In addition to size, any charge on the solute may interact with any charge present on the membrane pore. Thus, if a membrane is negatively charged, small, negatively charged particles will pass across the membrane less readily than neutrally charged solutes of similar size that may themselves pass less readily than positively charged solutes.

The second mechanism of solute transport is related to convection or solute drag. With semipermeable membranes, water can move from one side to the other based on osmotic or hydrostatic pressure gradients. For instance, if there is a relative surfeit of solute on one side of the semipermeable membrane, water will tend to move by osmosis to equilibrate the relative solute concentration on both sides. If a hydrostatic force is applied to the system, water will move independent of osmotic forces in the direction it is being propelled. As the water passes from one side of the membrane to the other, either by osmotic or hydrostatic mechanisms, any solute dissolved in the water will be "dragged" along as the water moves. Thus, any solute that is physically and electrochemically predisposed to traverse the pores of the semipermeable membrane will move along with the water in this process, called *convection*.

Determinants of Solute Clearance

During the process of hemodialysis, only a small fraction of the total body water—the plasma water—is exposed to the dialyzer. Any solute that needs to be cleared from the patient during dialysis must, therefore, be distributed well in the plasma water and must, in addition, meet the physical and electrochemical requirements to allow ready movement across the pores of the dialyzer from the blood space into the dialysate space. Substances that are sequestered in large concentration outside of the plasma water or that are, for instance, bound to large plasma proteins will be less effectively cleared.

For the diffusional component of solute clearance, the major factors affecting the final solute concentration (C_{final}) in a hemodialysis treatment include the initial solute concentration in the plasma water ($C_{initial}$), the duration of the treatment (t), how intrinsically permeable the dialyzer is to solute that needs to be cleared based on physical and electrochemical properties of the dialyzer as well as the blood and dialysate flows through the circuit (K), and the volume of the total body water that needs to be cleared of the solute (V). This diffusional solute clearance during hemodialysis can be mathematically modeled by the equation

$$C_{final}/C_{initial} = e^{-Kt/V}$$

The component of solute clearance achieved by convection is directly related to the amount of ultrafiltration achieved during the dialysis treatment. Consequently, during a treatment in which there is extensive ultrafiltration, more convective solute losses will occur than in a hemodialysis treatment of similar duration with little ultrafiltration. Ultrafiltration is limited by hemodynamic considerations in that only a fraction of the plasma water can be removed over any period of time without causing significant perturbation in the patient's effective circulating volume. As a result, in the typical hemodialysis treatment, although some solute will be cleared by convection in the process of ultrafiltration, diffusional solute losses comprise the vast majority of solute clearance. Thus, the desired amount of clearance of a solute during a hemodialysis treatment can be prescribed by the clinician, specifying the use of a certain sized dialyzer, specific blood and dialysate flow rates, and a set duration of dialysis therapy according to the equation

$$C_{final}/C_{initial} = e^{-Kt/V}$$

(See Case 12–1.)

DIALYSIS PRESCRIPTION–PEDIATRIC ISSUES

Individualization of Prescription

As noted above, with the pediatric patient, individualization of the dialysis prescription is more important than with the adult patient because of the relative diversity in size and blood volume of any population of children. Using "standard" or "protocol" hemodialysis routines with relatively little variation in circuit blood flows, dialysate flows, and duration of treatment across a whole patient population may result in little clinically relevant variation in a 70- or 80-kg

---

Case 12–1. Calculation of Dialysis Prescription in the Child

Urea reduction can be accurately prescribed by using the following equation:

$$-\ln (C_t / C_0) = Kt/V$$

Case: A 12-year-old boy will undergo his first hemodialysis treatment. He weighs 40 kg and his current BUN is 100 mg/dL. His volume of distribution is estimated at (0.6 × body weight in kilograms) or 24,000 mL. A circuit blood-flow (Q_B) rate of 250 mL/min has been chosen (5 to 7 mL/kg/min). A dialyzer with a surface area of 1.4 m^2 and a K_{Urea} of 240 mL/min will be used. Duration of dialysis needed for a urea reduction rate of 30 percent can be calculated as follows:

$$-\ln (70/100) = 240 \text{ mL/min} \times t/24,000$$

or

$$0.35 = 240 \text{ mL/min} \times t/24,000 \text{ mL}$$

$$t = 0.35 \times 24,000 \text{ mL}/240 \text{ mL/min}$$

or

$$t = 35 \text{ min}$$

t = time on dialysis or duration of treatment

Pre- and postdialysis BUN levels should be checked with every acute dialysis treatment and actual urea reduction compared to calculated goals.

---

adult and may also work well in the average-sized older adolescent, but it could result in potentially catastrophic fluid and electrolyte shifts in a 10- or 20-kg preschool child. Hence, a much more important aspect of hemodialysis therapy in children is actually calculating the parameters of dialysis dependent on the desired reduction in concentration of a solute and what is thought to be physiologically tolerable in terms of blood flow or ultrafiltration volume or change in serum osmolality.

Most children will tolerate acute decreases in blood urea nitrogen (BUN) of 30 to 40 mg/dL over a relatively short period of time without the development of any dialysis disequilibrium.[15] To that extent, most clinicians experienced in pediatric hemodialysis aim for a slow but steady increase in effective solute reduction over the course of the first four or five hemodialysis sessions, aiming for an eventual urea reduction rate near 70 percent for a dialysis session or a calculated Kt/V for a chronic dialysis patient exceeding 1.2.

Although the use of mannitol infusions to decrease fluxes in serum osmolality as urea is cleared by dialysis was once very much in vogue as a way to decrease adverse central nervous system effects in pediatric hemodialysis, its clinical effectiveness was never studied, and it is probably safer and just as effective to do more frequent sequential dialysis sessions aiming for a gradual stepwise reduction in serum BUN to target levels rather than to try to maintain high osmolality by replacing mannitol for urea. In situations such as increased intracranial pressure, where it would be useful not to shift the serum osmolality, mannitol infusion may indeed be beneficial.

Ramifications of Circuit Volumes in Children

An issue infrequently encountered in adult nephrology is the need to keep extracorporeal circuit volumes to less than 10 percent of the patient's estimated blood volume. Although some patients may tolerate larger extracorporeal volumes, it is the general approach to follow this guideline so as to minimize potential cardiodynamic compromise, especially in children requiring acute dialysis.

The total blood volume for a child may be estimated at 75 mL/kg of body weight. The blood volume of the circuit tubing and dialyzer are specified by the manufacturers. Thus, in a 10-kg child, the estimated blood volume is 750 mL, and there would be concern using a dialysis circuit that exceeded 75 mL (10 percent of 750 mL) without priming that circuit. Most often, the prime would consist of packed red blood cells diluted with 5% albumin to a hematocrit of 40 percent. At the conclusion of dialysis, the lines would be clamped and the blood left in the dialyzer and tubing would not be reinfused into the patient. As a result, there would be no substantive net loss or gain of blood from the patient due to the dialysis treatment.

In some circumstances, there may be concern that hemodynamically unstable patients may not tolerate extracorporeal blood volumes less that 10 percent of estimated blood volume. In those cases, lines may be primed with a blood/albumin solution or, alternatively, 5% albumin or a 0.9% NaCl saline solution. In instances where saline or albumin is used as a prime, at the conclusion of dialysis, all blood in the tubing and dialyzer would be reinfused into the child. The prime volume, if desired, could be included in the ultrafiltration goal of the treatment so that the child does not receive any extra volume.

Ultrafiltration

With acute hemodialysis in children, there is often no clear sense of the patient's dry weight or actual volume of distribution and the initial dialysis treatment is prescribed based on a "best guess" estimate. In that case, assaying pre- and post-BUN levels and solving the equation $C_{final}/C_{initial} = e^{-Kt/V}$ for V will allow for more precise calculation of subse-quent treatments, as a better sense of the patient's volume status and actual estimated dry weight evolves (see Case 12–2). Ill children who are small will have less of a reserve in terms of ability to tolerate ultrafiltration of any absolute volume from their vascular space than if this same absolute volume is removed from an equally ill adult. Thus, again, it is vital to make assessment of ultrafiltration goals on each pediatric patient dependent on individual clinical circumstance rather than some standard targeted ultrafiltration volume.

Given that most pediatric hemodialysis treatments will be shorter in duration than the 4-hour treatment commonly encountered in adults, difficulty in achieving adequate ultrafiltration during the prescribed period of hemodialysis may arise. This situation is most often encountered in the pediatric patient with acute renal failure who is quite volume overloaded and initiating hemodialysis. In those cases, the time necessary to achieve the targeted reduction in urea may be too brief to allow for the desired volume of ultrafiltration. In that case, doing ultrafiltration without dialysis for a period of time, when the child is first placed on the extracorporeal circuit, can allow for achieving the ultrafiltration goal without risking too rapid clearance and disequilibrium. Generally, the period of extended ultrafiltration should precede the dialysis, since ultrafiltration from the intravascular space in the setting of higher serum osmolality will result in more movement of water from the extravascular spaces to the intravascular space to maintain effective circulating volume than if this ultrafiltration is done with reduction in effective serum osmolality.

With chronic hemodialysis, the use of in-line circuit monitoring of hematocrit may allow more precise control of ultrafiltration. In a study of 200 pediatric dialysis treatments, children who underwent hemodialysis with concomitant noninvasive monitoring of their hematocrits had fewer dialysis-associated difficulties such as hypotension, cramping, or the need for repetitive nursing interventions.[16] The benefits of such monitoring was most apparent in children weighing less than 35 kg and suggested that children best tolerated ultrafiltration rates that did not exceed 8 percent of estimated blood volume in the first hour and 4 percent with each subsequent hour.

VASCULAR ACCESS

As with most decisions involving hemodialysis in children, the choice of vascular access should be based on each patient's individual needs, with special emphasis on the acuity of dialysis and the estimated duration of therapy. In addition, a recent review of North American children receiving hemodialysis found that access is highly age-dependent: children less than 6 years of age receive hemodialysis almost exclusively via percutaneous catheters, while older

Case 12–2. Readjustment of Estimated Volume of Distribution

In a significant number of patients, especially in the setting of acute hemodialysis, the child's exact dry weight is unknown. The initial calculation of dialysis time will therefore be based on an estimated dry weight and should be adjusted according to the actual urea reduction rate achieved by the treatment.

Case: The 12-year-old boy in Case 12–1 underwent his first hemodialysis treatment. His estimated dry weight was 40 kg, leading to an estimated volume of distribution (0.6 × body weight in kilograms) of 24,000 mL. A circuit blood flow (Q_B) rate of 250 mL/min was used with a dialyzer with a surface area of 1.4 m^2 and a K_{Urea} of 240 mL/min. the goal was a urea reduction of 30 percent. At the end of the treatment, although all specifications of the dialysis prescription were met, the urea reduction rate was only 20 percent instead of the calculated 30 percent goal.

Returning to the formula:

$$-\ln(C_t / C_0) = Kt/V$$

$-\ln$ = the negative natural log

it is important to make a correction to discern the actual volume of distribution:

$$-\ln(80/100) = (240 \text{ mL/min})$$
$$\times (35 \text{ min}/X)$$

or

$$0.22 = (240 \text{ mL/min}) \times (35 \text{ min}/X)$$

or

$$X = (240 \text{ mL/min}) \times (35 \text{ min}/0.22)$$

$$X = 38,180 \text{ mL}$$

or some 14 L higher than estimated.

Given the fact the actual volume of distribution in the patient was higher, the dialysis time to reduce the urea by 30 percent should have been 55 minutes instead of 35 minutes:

$$-\ln(70/100) = (240 \text{ mL/min}) \times (t/38,180 \text{ mL})$$

$$0.35 = (240 \text{ mL/min}) \times (t/38,180 \text{ mL})$$

$$t = 56 \text{ min}$$

Calculations for the next hemodialysis treatment should be based on the actual volume of distribution.

children are more likely to have arteriovenous fistulas (AVFs) or arteriovenous grafts (AVGs) created, likely reflecting the technical challenge of surgically creating a vascular access that can mature in young children with small-caliber blood vessels.[1]

It is important to establish a hemodialysis access that allows sufficient blood flow and is not unduly predisposed to clotting or infection, allows for the provision of adequate solute clearance and ultrafiltration, and minimizes the need for repetitive medical procedures or hospitalizations to deal with access malfunctions or complications. Currently, the most common reason for hospitalization in a hemodialysis patient is an access-related issue.[17]

Access Modalities

Access modalities can be separated into four categories—temporary intravascular catheters, longer-term or "permanent" intravascular catheters, AVFs formed from native vasculature, and AVGs formed from a combination of native vasculature and synthetic material. Besides technical feasibility in any specific child, the choice of catheter versus fistula or graft is often driven by the relative urgency to initiate dialysis and the forecast length of therapy. Children who require immediate dialysis cannot wait the several weeks to several months necessary for a fistula or graft to heal after its surgical creation.[18,19] Moreover, even if a vascular access can be surgically created with success, it makes little sense to contemplate more permanent access if the child's predicted need for dialysis is brief.

In the vast majority of children below elementary school age, an intravascular catheter will be placed for either temporary or longer-term access. For temporary access, catheters are often uncuffed and not tunneled, whereas catheters for more permanent access are cuffed and tunneled in an attempt to reduce both infection and access displacement over time.

The size of the hemodialysis catheter should correspond to the size of the patient's vasculature. Over the last decade, an increased number of dialysis catheters have become commercially available, allowing vascular access even in babies. Besides standard dual-lumen hemodialysis lines, triple-lumen catheters sized for children are also now manufactured. A guide to appropriately sized pediatric hemodialysis catheters based on patient weight can be found in Table 12–1.

As with adult hemodialysis patients, most hemodialysis lines in children are placed in the subclavian, jugular, or femoral veins.[10] The actual site of catheter placement is dependent on several factors, including the expertise of the clinician placing the vascular line, the predicted chronicity of dialysis, and individual patient factors. Thus, in the child with an acute exposure to a dialyzable toxin, the pediatric intensivist may wish to place a femoral dialysis line, since

TABLE 12–1. OPTIONS FOR DIALYSIS CATHETERS IN CHILDREN

Age	Weight	Catheter Size (available lengths)
Small infant	< 3 kg	5F UAC and 8F UVC
		Dual-lumen 7F (10, 15, 20 cm)
Large infant	3–10 kg	Dual- or triple-lumen 7F (10, 15, 20 cm)
Older baby		Dual-lumen 8F (12, 15, 18, 24 cm)
Small toddler		Dual-lumen 9F (12, 15, 20 cm)
Large toddler	11–30 kg	Dual-lumen 9F (12, 15, 20 cm)
Preschool child		Dual-lumen 10F (15, 19.5 cm)
Young elementary		
Older school-age	> 30 kg	Dual-lumen 11.5F (12, 13.5, 15, 16, 19.5, 20 cm)
adolescent		Dual- or triple-lumen 12.5F (12, 15, 17, 19, 23, 28 cm)

this can be accomplished quickly in the ICU and the presumed duration and chronicity of dialysis is brief, making some of the usual concerns regarding femoral line placement—such as limited patient mobility and increased infection risk—less concerning. On the other hand, in a child with dense acute tubular necrosis from sepsis and ongoing hemodynamic compromise and nephrotoxin exposure, an acute hemodialysis catheter placed in the internal jugular vein may be preferred.

Access Placement in the Child

In any child with presumed chronic renal insufficiency or actual ESRD, vascular access will be of lifelong importance. To that extent, a multidisciplinary team approach to vascular access planning—involving transplant or vascular surgeons, interventional radiologists, and nephrologists, all familiar with the needs of patients with ESRD—is of paramount importance, especially since vascular disease and issues of long-term vascular integrity are occasionally encountered in the usual pediatric patient.[20] Moreover, the child may benefit from avoiding the placement of percutaneously inserted central catheters or other long vascular lines, which are increasingly being utilized in children to afford more durable intravenous access for the provision of intravenous medications or fluids during hospitalization. Such lines may compromise the suitability of a vessel for later vascular access creation. Therefore, if a patient requires longer-term access for a reason other than dialysis and typical peripheral intravenous lines are thought inappropriate, it is again prudent to consult a transplant or vascular surgeon regarding the placement of a central vascular line.

Since children as a group are far less likely to require dialysis than adults, many skilled pediatric clinicians are unfamiliar with vascular access requirements for hemodialysis and assume that standard long-term pediatric catheters, such as Broviac or Hickman right atrial catheters, can be utilized. Such catheters should not be utilized for hemodialysis, since their length and relative flexibility limit effective blood flow and increase resistance in an extracorporeal circuit.

Occasionally, in a newborn infant who needs acute hemodialysis, umbilical lines can be considered, with a 5F umbilical arterial line drawing blood from the baby into the circuit and an 8F umbilical venous line returning blood. The umbilical line may be placed either above or below the liver. Even in babies, however, careful consideration should be made to the placement of a 7F dual-lumen formal hemodialysis line, which can afford better access in terms of consistent blood flows and lower circuit resistance.

Although the availability of pediatric-sized acute and chronic hemodialysis catheters has allowed more choices in terms of dialysis vascular access, long-term complication-free catheter performance remains rare. One study showed that half of uncuffed acute dialysis lines were lost within 2 months, generally because of infection or kinking of the line.[21] In this same study, cuffed and tunneled lines did tend to perform more reliably for longer periods, but 1-year line survival rates were only 25 percent, and line infection was again a frequent problem, often leading to the replacement or removal of vascular lines. Catheters with diameters 9F or lower were significantly more likely to malfunction due to kinking, again frequently requiring replacement or repositioning of the line.

Fistulas and Grafts in Children

In children with AVFs or AVGs, vascular access tends to be longer-lived.[22] In one large pediatric hemodialysis center, 5-year patency rates near 50 percent in fistulae or grafts have been demonstrated, approximating the long-term patency rates seen in adults with AVFs or AVGs.[23] Because children have smaller blood vessels that may not mature after creation of a native vascular access to allow reliable needle placement, primary access failure with an AVF is seen more often than primary failure of an AVG. On the other hand, once an AVF has matured and is functioning well, rates of thrombosis, stenosis, and infection are generally lower than with an AVG.

In children with an AVF or an AVG, vascular stenosis may become problematic, adversely affecting dialysis access and adequacy and requiring the services of vascular surgeons or interventional radiologists skilled in addressing access thrombosis in children. Pediatric patients with AVFs or AVGs may benefit from the routine use of ultrasound dilution technology to assess vascular flow through an access. By studying venous outflow patterns in individual patients on a regular basis, for instance monthly, the detection of decreased access flow from baseline can be used as a reliable predictor of outflow stenosis, and angioplasty can be performed in the access prior to the formation of critical stenotic lesions predisposing to access thrombosis. One study suggested a nearly threefold decline in access thrombosis when angioplasty was performed within 48 hours after flow rates had fallen below 650 mL/min/1.73 m^2.[24] As is the case with many pediatric measurements, the correction of raw data for surface area makes individual measurements more comparable, since the range of absolute flow rates will vary dramatically in any cohort of children, depending on their age and size. There is some evidence to suggest that a venous outflow rate >700 mL/min/1.73 m^2 indicates a pediatric vascular access with robust enough flow to make thrombosis unlikely.[25]

As would be expected, AVFs and AVGs are more commonly used in adolescents than younger children, due both to technical feasibility and the likelihood that an older child will remain on hemodialysis for a longer period of time than a small child, in whom more rapid transplantation may be optimal. The Brescia-Cimino fistula, a surgically placed side-to-side anastomosis between the radial artery and the cephalic vein, is frequently the AVF of choice in adolescents, allowing relatively easy access for venipuncture, generally providing a good blood flow rate, and likely to have an acceptable complication rate. In a study of 112 children with Brescia-Cimino AVFs, thrombosis was the main complication, although two-thirds of fistulas were still patent 4 years after surgical creation.[22]

ACUTE HEMODIALYSIS AND ACUTE RENAL FAILURE IN CHILDREN

Etiologies of Pediatric Acute Renal Failure

As in adults, causes of acute renal failure requiring hemodialysis in children can be divided into three categories: prerenal states due to decreased renal perfusion or decreased effective circulating volume, intrinsic renal failure due to renal parenchymal injury, and postrenal states related to urinary tract outflow obstruction.

Prerenal acute renal failure as a consequence of hypovolemia, hypoperfusion, and shock with secondary acute tubular necrosis is the leading cause of acute renal failure in children. The prognosis in these children is largely dependent on the severity of the underlying acute disease process and is guarded in children with multiorgan system failure. Acute tubular necrosis itself is likely to resolve over time, but diligent fluid and electrolyte management as well as judicious exposure to nephrotoxins and the avoidance of further renal insults may optimize outcome. Occasionally, children may have so severe an ischemic injury that there is widespread cortical necrosis and irreversible renal injury. Most children with acute tubular necrosis, however, will regain renal function and no longer need dialytic support within a few weeks of clinical recovery, although in some

cases dialytic support may have to continue for several months.[26]

The second category includes children with intrinsic renal disease, either as a primary process or as part of a more systemic disease process. The majority of young children with intrinsic renal disease requiring acute hemodialysis carry the diagnosis of hemolytic uremic syndrome, whereas older children are likely to have a fulminant acute nephritis as the underlying cause of the renal failure. Again, the general prognosis for recovery of eventual renal function is excellent as long as the child survives the acute illness.

The third category of acute renal failure, postrenal etiologies, is rare in children and involves acute obstruction of the lower urinary tract from stones, tumor, or blood clot. Most often, dialysis can be avoided if the obstruction is relieved prior to prolonged oligoanuria. Congenital obstruction of the urinary tract predisposes to chronic renal insufficiency and these children will rarely present outside of the neonatal period with acute failure.

As opposed to ESRD, which is more commonly seen in adolescents than in younger children, acute renal failure requiring hemodialysis presents across all pediatric age groups. In one series of 280 cases of acute renal failure in children, 22 percent were in neonates, 15 percent were in babies from 1 to 12 months of age, 13 percent were in children 1 to 5 years of age, 34 percent were in children 6 to 14 years of age, and 16 percent were in adolescents above 15 years of age.[27] In another single-center series spanning 20 years and 228 children with acute renal failure, 39 percent of the patients were less than 2 years of age, 21 percent were 2 to 4 years of age, and 40 percent were above 5 years of age.[28]

Dialytic modalities used to treat children with acute renal failure include continuous hemofiltration or hemodiafiltration in addition to intermittent hemodialysis and peritoneal dialysis. For the pediatric nephrologist, the choice of a specific modality is patient-dependent and reflects specific clinical factors, dialytic goals, and clinician and institutional expertise.[29] With the advent of continuous modalities, more pediatric nephrologists appear to be utilizing extracorporeal circuits to treat acute renal failure than was the case prior to 1995, and the potential now exists for multimodal therapy, with children transitioning to intermittent hemodialysis after undergoing a period of continuous dialysis during initial hemodynamic instability.[28,30]

Indications for Hemodialysis in Pediatric Acute Renal Failure

Indications to initiate hemodialysis for acute renal failure must be individualized to the child's current clinical condition and renal function in the foreseeable future. For instance, the 6-year-old with early fulminant hemolytic uremic syndrome, symptomatic anemia, and oliguria may require dialysis when creatinine and BUN levels are only moderately elevated, whereas another 6-year-old who is status postrepair of a congenital cardiac lesion with a complicated postoperative course may have much worse laboratory values, but if he is maintaining adequate urine output and beginning to exhibit more stable cardiodynamics, he is likely to show spontaneous recovery of renal function without hemodialysis therapy. Clinicians inexperienced with renal failure or dialysis in children often become anxious as renal function laboratory values deteriorate; by themselves, however, these values are rarely the proximate reason for initiating acute therapy; more often, they represent one of several important factors.

In the child with acute renal failure, hypervolemia is often the primary indication for acute hemodialysis. Proper assessment of a child's fluid status and careful management of further fluid and electrolyte therapy are of extreme importance. In the hospitalized child, accurate daily weights and an accurate tally of input and output is invaluable to prevent inadvertent fluid overload or provide a more objective assessment of the degree of hypervolemia. Careful assessment of blood pressures and signs of volume overload on physical examination are also useful adjuncts. In children with an indwelling central line, measurement of the central venous pressure can also be helpful in assessing the fluid status correctly, but it is still far less common for critically ill children to have their central venous pressures or pulmonary wedge pressures assessed than for critically ill adults. There is a growing body of clinical data to suggest that the degree of volume overload at initiation of dialysis may be a critical prognostic factor in children in ICU settings.[31,32] As such, early recognition of evolving hypervolemia and prevention of its exacerbation are crucial maneuvers. Conservative management—including fluid and salt restriction as well as parenteral diuretic therapy—should be attempted if the child's hemodynamic state allows, but early hemodialysis or ultrafiltration may have to be considered in the case of a suboptimal response.

In addition to uremia and hypervolemia, other indications for acute hemodialysis in children include life-threatening electrolyte perturbations or intractable acidosis unresponsive to medical management and the presence of a dialyzable toxin. These toxins may be exogenous, such as inadvertent or purposeful drug overdoses, or endogenous, as seen in infants and children with certain inherited metabolic anomalies such as urea cycle defects.

Inborn Errors of Metabolism and Pediatric Hemodialysis

In children with some of the inborn errors of metabolism, hemodialysis is an especially useful modality, since it generally allows the very rapid clearance of toxin from the patient's blood space.[33] This advantage of hemodialysis in these situations should not be underestimated since, in some conditions, long-term neurologic prognosis may be affected

by the degree and duration of early metabolic derangement.[34] In certain conditions, special metabolic "cocktails" may have to be infused to blunt production of the toxin. It is vital that this adjunctive therapy be initiated as quickly as possible, as otherwise toxin levels will rebound dangerously following intermittent hemodialysis. In certain instances, following an intermittent hemodialysis treatment it may be useful to place the child on a continuous regimen with hemofiltration or hemodiafiltration if ongoing significant production of a toxin is predicted.

If one of these metabolic cocktails is being infused, its composition must be considered carefully with the initiation of hemodialysis. Certain of these mixes will themselves contain drugs that may be readily cleared by hemodialysis, because they are small solutes that are not protein-bound. Thus, to allow the child to maintain therapeutic drug levels, the rate of infusion of these drugs must be adjusted upward during dialysis to compensate for any drug removed. Otherwise, if there is no adjustment, the child will rapidly be cleared of the therapeutic agents during dialysis and there will be no ongoing intervention to prevent the production of toxin.

Many of these therapeutic mixes may present an acid load to the child, and there may be concern, in clinicians unfamiliar with hemodialysis, that rapid infusion rates of these solutions may predispose to the development of a dangerous acidosis. Since larger volume infusion would be ongoing only during the hemodialysis treatment itself, any evolving acidosis would actually be counterbalanced by the bicarbonate-rich dialysate solution. An example of the approach to hemodialysis in an infant with an inborn error of metabolism is summarized in Case 12–3.

HEMODIALYSIS IN CHRONIC RENAL FAILURE

Even though the general consensus among pediatric nephrologists is that renal transplantation is the best treatment for children with ESRD, only one-fourth of children will receive a preemptive transplant.[10] That means that most children with ESRD will require dialysis for some period of time. During this time, children must be followed closely for a variety of problems that accompany ESRD.

Anemia

The majority of children with ESRD, including the population on hemodialysis, develop a normocytic normochromic anemia requiring medical treatment.[35] This anemia stems primarily from reduced erythropoietin (EPO) production by the diseased kidneys and is usually present once the glomerular filtration rate (GFR) declines to less than 40 mL/min/1.73 m^2. Other important factors contributing to

Case 12–3. Dialysis in a Newborn with Hyperammonemia

A 3.5-kg term newborn with feeding difficulties since birth is found to be floppy and somnolent on the fourth day of life. During the initial emergency department evaluation, he has a brief convulsion; blood work is remarkable for an acidosis and an ammonia level of 1080 μmol/L (normal <50 μmol/L). A urea cycle defect is suspected and, because of his degree of hyperammonemia, hemodialysis is initiated with a 0.4-m^2 dialyzer, a circuit blood flow (Q_B) of 35 mL/min, and a dialysate rate of 500 mL/min. With this size dialyzer and this blood flow, the K_{Urea} will be 49 mL/min.

An intravenous infusion of a metabolic cocktail containing sodium benzoate, sodium phenylacetate, and arginine is started to provide substrate for alternative pathways of waste nitrogen synthesis and excretion. Once hemodialysis is initiated, these therapeutic agents will also be cleared. To maintain a steady blood level of those agents during hemodialysis, the removal rate by hemodialysis must be equal to the infusion rate, or

$$\text{Infusion rate} = K_{Urea} \times C$$

where K is the dialyzer urea clearance (50 mL/min) and C is the desired steady-state concentration of the substance in milligrams per milliliter.

As an example, the desired steady-state concentration for sodium benzoate is 2 mmol/L and its molecular weight is 144 mg/mmol.

$$C = (2 \text{ mmol/L}) \times (144 \text{ mg/mmol}) = 288 \text{ mg/L} = 0.288 \text{ mg/mL}$$

This means that the required infusion rate for sodium benzoate is:

$$(49 \text{ mL/min}) \times (0.288 \text{ mg/mL}) = 14 \text{ mg/min}$$

anemia in the child on hemodialysis include inadequate iron stores and other nutritional deficiencies, frequent blood loss from phlebotomy, and additional blood loss from entrapment in dialyzers or tubing.

Intravenous replacement of recombinant human EPO is the treatment of choice for children on chronic hemodialysis. Because intravenous administration of EPO during chronic hemodialysis therapy is easy to coordinate and ensures some measure of compliance, this route is commonly preferred over subcutaneous injection. Although bioavailability is higher with intravenous EPO, EPO dosing requirements are higher with intravenous dosing due to a reduced duration of effect.[36] Assessment of iron parameters (serum iron, total iron binding capacity, transferrin saturation, and ferritin) and initiation of oral or intravenous iron supplementation should be considered in every patient. According to the National Kidney Foundation–Dialysis Outcomes Quality Initiative (NKF-DOQI) guidelines, pediatric dialysis patients should be maintained at a hematocrit above 33 percent or a hemoglobin greater than 11 g/dL.[35]

In children, there may be a significant dose-response variation to EPO from patient to patient, and frequent reassessment is crucial. Infants and younger children tend to require higher doses of EPO than children 12 years of age and above.[10] For instance, in infants, EPO doses up to 300 U/kg per week are not uncommon.[36] Race and gender do not seem to affect the required dose. After initiation or dose change of EPO, blood work should be repeated every 1 to 2 weeks until stabilization is achieved. After that, a monthly review is recommended, according to the DOQI Guidelines, with prompt readjustment of EPO dosing if indicated. Children on hemodialysis receiving intravenous EPO require up to three times more EPO supplementation than children on peritoneal dialysis receiving subcutaneous EPO.[37,38]

The importance of maintaining adequate iron stores in children should not be underestimated. Many pediatric hemodialysis patients require intravenous iron infusions; overall, children tolerate this therapy with minimal side effects.[39,40]

Osteodystrophy

In children receiving chronic hemodialysis, bone disease is heterogeneous and bone biopsy is needed to determine the exact histologic changes. In one study, patterns of bone disease were described in 21 adolescents who had been on chronic hemodialysis for a mean of 35 months and all of whom underwent periodic bone biopsy.[41] Although a small number of patients had normal histology, three major aberrant histologic groups were identified: osteitis fibrosa, mild hyperparathyroidism, and aplastic or adynamic bone disease. Levels of serum parathyroid hormone (PTH) tended to correlate with the histology results. Children with chronically unsuppressed secondary hyperparathyroidism tended to have osteitis fibrosa, whereas those whose PTH was controlled down to normal levels actually seemed to have bone turnover and remodeling interrupted and had adynamic disease. As a result, aiming for intact PTH values at two to three times normal is the goal in children on hemodialysis so as to optimize bone homeostasis.

By helping to suppress secondary hyperparathyroidism, the provision of vitamin D in oral or intravenous forms plays a critical role in the prevention and treatment of renal bone disease.[42] ESRD leads to impaired hydroxylation of vitamin D to bioactive 1,25-dihydroxyvitamin D_3 (calcitriol). As discussed above, timely initiation of vitamin D therapy is necessary to avoid long-term orthopedic complications in children, most importantly alterations in skeletal integrity and growth potential.

In children, dietary phosphate restriction and calcium-based phosphate binders are generally used to treat the hyperphosphatemia that accompanies a decreased GFR and also contributes to alterations in normal calcium, phosphorus, and bone balance. Since, as a group, children are more likely to ingest larger quantities of dairy products, dietary phosphate restrictions may prove problematic. In addition, since children are often dependent on adult caregivers to provide them with medication at the appropriate time, inconsistencies often arise with the use of repetitive daily doses of oral phosphate binders with meals and snacks. Since many children are unable to swallow pills or capsules, the types of phosphate binders that can be used may also be limited, and this explains why some of the non-calcium-based binders, such as sevelamer, are less popular with children.

Growth

Children on chronic hemodialysis are at significant risk for severe growth failure. Most children begin hemodialysis with a significant preexisting growth delay that has accrued during a period of chronic renal insufficiency.[43] According to the *NAPRTCS 2003 Annual Report,* the mean height standard deviation score for all children 1 month after initiation of hemodialysis is −1.55, and this growth lag actually increases to −1.94 standard deviations 24 months after hemodialysis initiation.[10] Height deficits are worse for boys and for younger children at hemodialysis initiation and at any subsequent time point.

This growth failure is most likely multifactorial in etiology. Children with GFRs less than 40 mL/min/1.73 m^2 often have high levels of IGF binding proteins due to decreased renal clearance and thus are unable to utilize endogenous growth hormone efficaciously. In addition, children with renal failure often also suffer from poor nutrition, acidosis, anemia, and chronic bone disease.[44] Despite the recognition of growth failure during the evolution of chronic renal insufficiency into ESRD, most children exhibit little or no catch-up growth with medical management of their renal insufficiency.[45] There is also some concern that growth failure is associated with more clinical complications and an increased risk of death in children with kidney failure.[46]

Children are most vulnerable to factors adversely affecting growth potential during two phases of rapid growth—infancy and puberty. It is important to remember that hemodialysis does not correct any underlying endocrine abnormalities that may contribute to poor growth and that even children with excellent measures of dialysis adequacy will be at great risk for further growth delay. Moreover, efficacy of recombinant human growth hormone therapy is better in preadolescent children than adolescents, further underscoring the importance of initiating early therapy when appropriate.[47]

Unfortunately, despite the increased availability of recombinant human growth hormone, most children with ESRD in North America do not receive growth hormone therapy. In the chronic pediatric hemodialysis population, only about 10 percent of children receive supplemental growth hormone, even after 2 or 3 years of chronic dialysis therapy.[10] Although there is hope that, following renal transplant and the return of effective renal function, the child will begin to exhibit more normal growth parameters, there is little likelihood of any child regaining all the growth that is needed to make up for any sustained period of lost growth potential. To that extent, a more substantial number of children with growth potential on chronic dialysis would likely benefit from growth hormone use, and some practitioners have used these data to support the development of practice guidelines designed to decrease variability in the treatment of growth retardation in pediatric hemodialysis patients as well as to suggest that aggressive nutritional support and early nephrology referral may optimize growth.[48,49]

Cognitive Effects

There is evidence that children on chronic hemodialysis may exhibit a number of abnormalities on neurologic or cognitive screens.[50] This has led to speculation regarding the effect of hemodialysis on developmental progress and academic achievement.

The etiology of these deficits is unclear. There has been concern that the relatively acute changes in serum osmolality that accompany dialysis lead to injury in cells in the central nervous system as fluid fluxes into and out of cells in response to changes in osmotic gradients.[51] For children on chronic dialysis, this repetitive insult over time can contribute to neurocognitive deficits.

In children who have been chronically hyperosmolar, an additional concern is the role of intracellular idiogenic osmoles such as inositol or taurine.[52] These organic solutes are generated by the cell in response to extracellular hyperosmolality to maintain cell volume by reducing the transcellular osmotic gradient. With dialysis, the extracellular osmolality drops, but the presence of these previously generated intracellular osmoles contributes to fluid flux into the cell and the cell swells.

In addition to these potential physiologic effects, children on hemodialysis are less likely to attend school than children on peritoneal dialysis. Data from the NAPRTCS registry have shown consistently that only about 40 percent of children on hemodialysis are regular in their school attendance.[10] The proportion of children attending school does not seem to vary across all pediatric age groups. This decreased exposure to classroom instruction is problematic not only in terms of academic achievement but also of socialization skills and opportunities to interact with peers.

Although tutoring can ameliorate some of the potential academic challenges, there are often logistic and motivational barriers to its provision, either on dialysis or at regular intervals at home. Some pediatric dialysis centers have attempted to augment opportunities for peer interaction by establishing patient groups that meet at regular intervals, so that the children can engage in discussion and projects together. With preschool children, community-based early intervention programs may serve the same purpose.

COMPLICATIONS OF HEMODIALYSIS

Acute Problems

The acute complications seen with hemodialysis in children are largely related to volume shifts and electrolyte adjustments that occur over a relatively short period of time. The more chronic complications stem from the inherent inability of current intermittent dialysis technology and practice to replace all aspects of normal renal homeostasis on a long-term basis.

Hypotension occurs in up to 30 percent of hemodialysis treatments, most often arising from the need to remove large volumes of fluid with rapid ultrafiltration.[14] Efforts to minimize intradialytic weight gains and the extension treatment times will likely reduce the appearance of symptoms during hemodialysis. As previously discussed, noninvasive hematocrit monitoring in the dialysis circuit may also play a role in preventing too rapid ultrafiltration and symptoms related to effective volume depletion.[53] Children treated with vasodilators for hypertension may have exaggerated sensitivity to volume depletion, and readjustment of the timing of these medications on dialysis days may be worthwhile. Treatment of acute hypotension during dialysis includes stopping any ongoing ultrafiltration, placing the child in the Trendelenburg position, and infusing aliquots of saline.

Muscle cramps also occur in up to 20 percent of hemodialysis patients and, although their etiology is unclear, there are three factors that seem to play a role in the evolution of cramps during dialysis: excessive ultrafiltration goals, frank hypotension leading to ineffective perfusion, and low-sodium dialysate.[14] There is evidence to suggest that children on dialysis can benefit from the use of the sodium modeling capacities of many modern dialysis machines, whereby the sodium dialysate concentration can be varied during dialysis to minimize potential excessive shift of fluid between body compartments.[54]

Up to 10 percent of hemodialysis patients experience episodes of nausea and emesis during or just following the treatment.[14] The etiology of this distress is also thought to be multifactorial, with both hypotension and early disequilibrium implicated. Disequilibrium syndrome consists of a constellation of neurologic symptoms including nausea, vomiting, headache, and restlessness as well as more serious compromise such as seizures and coma.[55,56] Disequilibrium is thought to occur when a rapid clearance of solute from the blood space causes a relatively hypertonic cerebral environment in relation to the plasma osmolality, with consequent inflow of water into the brain cells. Disequilibrium tends to occur more often during initiation of dialysis than with established patients undergoing maintenance treatments. The treatment for disequilibrium is mainly symptomatic, but the infusion of hypertonic sodium or glucose solutions to decrease the osmotic gradient has been beneficial in some cases. The chances of disequilibrium occurring can be reduced by limiting the extent by which serum osmolality is decreased in any patient who has been in a hyperosmolar state chronically. Current custom in children requiring acute hemodialysis is to increase the intensity and duration of dialysis in a stepwise fashion, reaching a full treatment time in four to five sessions.

Dialysis Mortality

Available data on patient survival in pediatric ESRD indicate the superiority of transplantation over hemodialysis as a mode of renal replacement therapy.[3,10,57] Currently in the United States, 1-year patient survival on dialysis is above 90 percent in all children above 1 year of age and, in children older than 12 years, as high as 98 percent. On the other hand, children who initiate dialysis before their first birthday have only an 84 percent survival rate after a year of dialysis. With protracted courses of chronic dialysis, patient survival across all pediatric age groups falls significantly. Most recent NAPRTCS data show that, after 36 months of chronic dialysis, the survival rates for children who initiated dialysis at less than 2 years of age approximates only 70 percent; for children who initiated between 2 and 5 years of age, 3-year survival is 85 percent; and for children older than 6 years at initiation, 3-year survival is near 90 percent.[10] In comparison, 5-year patient survival following an initial renal transplant is more than 95 percent in all pediatric age groups.

What underlies the morbidity and mortality in long-term pediatric dialysis is unclear. Since most of these children will achieve more than adequate dialysis by current assessments of dialysis adequacy, factors beyond urea clearance must be implicated.[38,58] Across all pediatric age groups, cardiopulmonary complications appear as the most common cause of death, exceeding by nearly a factor of two the deaths due to infection.[10] Asymptomatic children on chronic hemodialysis do indeed tend to have frequent abnormal measures of cardiodynamics when assessed by echocardiography, again unrelated to adequacy of dialysis.[59] Other risk factors investigated as contributing to cardiac disease in children on hemodialysis include anemia, hypertension, hyperlipidemia, left ventricular hypertrophy, calcium phosphate imbalance, and hyperhomocysteinemia.[60]

Others have contended that anemia and hypoalbuminemia may serve as surrogate markers for inadequate dialysis and may portend poor outcome in pediatric dialysis patients.[61] Despite the availability of synthetic erythropoietin, anemia remains a problem for children on chronic hemodialysis. In fact, if anemia exists when hemodialysis is initiated, there is a high likelihood that it will still be present months later, despite the close contact these children experience with the health care system.[61] To date, there is no evidence that anemia in children influences long-term patient outcome and there are very limited data implicating hypoalbuminemia and poor nutrition.

There is evidence that children on dialysis do have higher measurable markers of inflammation. One recent study showed that levels of various cytokines such as tumor necrosis factor-alpha and interleukin-1β as well as C-reactive protein levels were chronically altered in pediatric hemodialysis patients.[62] This state of chronic inflammation seemed to be related to the adequacy of hemodialysis and may suggest that intensified hemodialysis regimens could be useful to counteract the effect of this inflammation. Whether this inflammatory state is a direct mediator of pediatric dialysis morbidity and mortality remains unclear, however, since there is evidence that exceeding current suggested dialysis adequacy in children does not decrease patient morbidity.[63]

ADEQUACY OF HEMODIALYSIS

The relationship between the delivered dose of hemodialysis and long-term patient outcome has been clearly documented in a number of studies in adults and underlies current recommendations for the adequacy of hemodialysis in adults.[64] Unfortunately, to date little is known about hemodialysis adequacy and patient survival in the pediatric hemodialysis population. As discussed above, ESRD is uncommon in children, and most, in comparison to adults, spend a relatively brief time on hemodialysis. The paucity of data has lead to the adoption of adult guidelines for assessing adequate pediatric hemodialysis. Given the wide range of metabolic needs and patient size in pediatrics, the appropriateness of this approach remains controversial.[63,65]

Both "single-pool" and "double-pool" approaches to kinetic modeling are being used to assess the adequacy of dialysis. Underlying these calculations is the net change in BUN level before initiation to postcompletion of a dialysis treatment. Single-pool kinetics are based on a blood sample drawn immediately after the treatment ends (usually within 30 seconds) and do not, unlike double-pool calculations, take the logarithmic equilibration phase of urea nitrogen, which happens 30 to 60 minutes thereafter, into account. There are concerns that by discounting the reequilibration, single-pool sampling may overestimate Kt/V by more than 15 percent. On the other hand, the logistics of keeping children at the dialysis facility for an extra hour to do the delayed postdialysis blood work necessary to calculate double-pool kinetics has been a stumbling block to its more widespread adoption.

Urea kinetic modeling integrates pre- and posttreatment BUN levels, dialyzer urea clearance rates for a known blood flow rate Q_B, dialysis time, and the patient's pre- and posttreatment weight into an equation, allowing calculation of the urea distribution volume V_D and urea generation rate G. Consequently, urea clearance by means of the Kt/V equation and nutritional status by the normalized protein catabolic rate equation, PCR = $(6.5 \times G) + (0.17 \times weight)$, can readily be assessed.

According to the NKF-DOQI guidelines for adults and also currently applied in children, the recommended Kt/V$_D$ in hemodialysis based on single-pool analysis is >1.2, equaling, in most cases, a urea reduction rate of greater than 65 percent.[64] Recent studies including only pediatric dialysis patients have shown that most children on hemodialysis now attain Kt/V exceeding 1.2.[37,63] Not surprisingly, the delivered Kt/V is inversely correlated with the age of the patients, since younger children generally have a smaller V_D to clear due to their smaller body size.[63]

There is preliminary evidence that optimizing caloric intake and diet and intensifying dialysis to achieve higher than normally targeted measures of adequacy, improves growth and pubertal development in children.[66] At this point, however, additional data will be necessary to determine whether exceeding the currently recommended amount of dialysis does have an impact on the overall long-term prognosis and outcome in children.

REFERENCES

1. Leonard MB, Donaldson LA, Ho M, et al. A prospective cohort study of incident maintenance dialysis in children: a NAPRTC study. *Kidney Int* 2003;63:744.
2. Goldstein SL. Hemodialysis in the pediatric patient: state of the art. *Adv Renal Replace Ther* 2001;8:173.
3. U.S. Renal Data System. *USRDS 2002 Annual Data Report: Atlas of End-Stage Renal Disease in the United States.* Bethesda, MD: National Institutes of Health, National Institute of Diabetes and Digestive and Kidney Diseases, 2002.

4. Ramage IJ, Beattie TJ. Acute renal failure following cardiac surgery. *Nephrol Dial Transplant* 1999;14:2777.

5. Fischbach M, Terzic J, Menouer S, et al. Hemodialysis in children: principles and practice. *Semin Nephrol* 2001;21:470.

6. Shroff R, Wright E, Ledermann S, et al. Chronic hemodialysis in infants and children under 2 years of age. *Pediatr Nephrol* 2003;18:378.

7. Sadowski RH, Harmon WE, Jabs K. Acute hemodialysis of children weighing less than five kilograms. *Kidney Int* 1994;45:903.

8. Corsini E, Hoffman R, Knight F. Adolescent issues in renal treatment. *Adv Renal Replace Ther* 1998;5:120.

9. Jabs K, Warady BA. The impact of the Dialysis Outcome Quality Initiative guidelines on the care of the pediatric end-stage renal disease patient. *Adv Renal Replace Ther* 1999; 6:97.

10. North American Pediatric Renal Transplant Cooperative Study (NAPRTCS). *NAPRTCS 2003 Annual Data Report*, 2003.

11. Balinsky W: Pediatric end-stage renal disease: incidence, management, and prevention. *J Pediatr Health Care* 2000;14: 304.

12. Furth SL, Powe NR, Hwang W, et al. Does pediatric specialization influence treatment choice in chronic disease management? Dialysis choice for children with ESRD. *Arch Pediatr Adolesc Med* 1997;151:545.

13. Furth SL, Hwang W, Yang C, et al. Relation between pediatric experience and treatment recommendations for children and adolescents with kidney failure. *JAMA* 2001;258:1027.

14. Daugirdas JT, Ing TS. Complications in dialysis. In: Daugirdas JT, Blake PG, Ing TS, eds. *Handbook of dialysis*, 3d ed. Philadelphia: Lippincott Williams & Wilkins, 2000:148.

15. Harmon WE, Jabs KL. Hemodialysis. In: Barratt TM, Avner ED, Harmon WH, eds. *Pediatric Nephrology,* 4th ed. Baltimore: Williams & Wilkins, 1999:1267.

16. Jain SR, Smith L, Brewer ED, et al. Noninvasive intravascular monitoring in the pediatric hemodialysis population. *Pediatr Nephrol* 2001;16:15.

17. Morduchowicz G, Boner G. Hospitalizations in dialysis end-stage renal failure patients. *Nephron* 1996;73:413.

18. NKF-K/DOQI. Clinical Practice Guidelines for Vascular Access: Update 2000. *Am J Kidney Dis* 2001;37(S1):S137.

19. Bourquelot P, Cussenor O, Corbi P, et al. Microsurgical creation and follow-up of arteriovenous fistulae for chronic haemodialysis in children. *Pediatr Nephrol* 1990;4:156.

20. Patel NH, Ravenur VK, Khanna A, et al. Vascular access for hemodialysis: an in depth review. *J Nephrol* 2001;14:146.

21. Goldstein SL, Macierowski CT, Jabs K. Hemodialysis catheter survival and complications in children and adolescents. *Pediatr Nephrol* 1997;11:74.

22. Bagolan P, Spagnoli A, Ciprandi G, et al. A ten-year experience of Brescia-Cimino arteriovenous fistula in children: technical evolution and refinements. *J Vasc Surg* 1998;27: 640.

23. Sheth RD, Brandt ML, Brewer ED, et al. Permanent hemodialysis vascular access survival in children and adolescents with end-stage renal disease. *Kidney Int* 2002;62:1864.

24. Goldstein SL, Allstead A, Smith CM, et al. Proactive monitoring of pediatric hemodialysis vascular access: effects of ultrasound dilution on thrombosis rates. *Kidney Int* 2002;62: 272.

25. Goldstein SL, Allsteadt A. Ultrasound dilution evaluation of pediatric hemodialysis vascular access. *Kidney Int* 2001;59: 2357.

26. Somers MJG. Acute renal failure. In: Burg FD, Ingelfinger JR, Polin RA, Gershon A, eds. *Current Pediatric Therapy,* 17th ed. Philadelphia: Saunders, 2002:809.

27. Stickle SH, Brewer ED, Goldstein SL. Pediatric acute renal failure update: epidemiology and outcome from a three and one-half year experience. *J Am Soc Nephrol* 2002;13:642A.

28. Flynn JT. Choice of dialysis modality for management of pediatric acute renal failure. *Pediatr Nephrol* 2002;17:61.

29. Williams DM, Sreedhar SS, Mickell JJ, et al. Acute kidney failure: a pediatric experience over 20 years. *Arch Pediatr Adolesc Med* 2002;156:893.

30. Warady BA, Bunchman T. Dialysis therapy for children with acute renal failure: survey results. *Pediatr Nephrol* 2000;15: 11.

31. Goldstein SL, Currier H, Graf CD, et al. Outcome in children receiving continuous hemofiltration. *Pediatrics* 2001;107: 1309.

32. Michael M, Kuehnle I, Goldstein SL. Fluid overload and acute renal failure in pediatric stem cell transplant patients. *Pediatr Nephrol* 2004;19:91.

33. Schaefer F, Straube E, Oh J, et al. Dialysis in neonates with inborn errors of metabolism. *Nephrol Dial Transplant* 1999; 14:910.

34. Puliyanda DP, Harmon WE, Peterschmitt MJ, et al. Utility of hemodialysis in maple sugar urine disease. *Pediatr Nephrol* 2002;17:239.

35. *NKF-DOQI Clinical Practice Guidelines for the Treatment of Anemia of Chronic Renal Failure*. New York: National Kidney Foundation, 1997.

36. Van Damme-Lombaerts R, Herman J. Erythropoietin treatment in children with renal failure. *Pediatr Nephrol* 1999;13: 148.

37. Brem AS, Lambert C, Hill C, et al. Outcome data on pediatric dialysis patients from the end-stage renal disease clinical indicators project. *Am J Kidney Dis* 2000;36:310.

38. Frankenfield DL, Neu AM, Warady BA, et al. Adolescent hemodialysis: results of the 2000 ESRD clinical performance measures project. *Pediatr Nephrol* 2002;17:10.

39. Chavers BM, Roberts TL, Herzog A, et al. Prevalence of anemia in erythropoietin-treated pediatric as compared to adult chronic dialysis patients. *Kidney Int* 2004;65:266.

40. Morgan HEG, Gautam M, Geary DF. Maintenance intravenous iron therapy in pediatric hemodialysis patients. *Pediatr Nephrol* 2001;16:779.

41. Mathias R, Salusky I, Harmon W, et al. Renal bone disease in pediatric and young adult patients on hemodialysis in a children's hospital. *J Am Soc Nephrol* 1993;3:1938.

42. Malluche HH, Monier-Faugere MC, Koszewski NJ. Use and indication of vitamin D and vitamin D analogues in patients with renal bone disease. *Nephrol Dial Transplant* 2002; 17:6.

43. Neu AM, Ho PL, McDonald RA, et al. Chronic dialysis in children and adolescents. The 2001 NAPRTCS annual report. *Pediatr Nephrol* 2002;17:656.

44. Warady BA, Alexander SR, Watkins S, et al. Optimal care of the pediatric end-stage renal disease patient on dialysis. *Am J Kidney Dis* 1999;33:567.

45. Furth SL, Hwang W, Yang C, et al. Growth failure, risk of hospitalization and death for children with end-stage renal disease. *Pediatr Nephrol* 2002;17:450.

46. Seikaly MG, Ho PL, Emmett L, et al. Chronic renal insufficiency in children: the 2001 annual report of the NAPRTCS. *Pediatr Nephrol* 2003;18:796.

47. Haffner D, Schaefer F. Does recombinant growth hormone improve adult height in children with chronic renal failure? *Semin Nephrol* 2001;21:490.

48. Furth SL, Alexander DC, Neu AM, et al. Does growth retardation indicate suboptimal clinical care in children with chronic renal disease and those undergoing dialysis? *Semin Nephrol* 2001;21:463.

49. Furth SL, Stabelin D, Fine RN, et al. Adverse clinical outcomes associated with short stature at dialysis initiation: a report of the North American Pediatric Renal Transplant Cooperative Study. *Pediatrics* 2002;109: 909.

50. Polinsky MS, Kaiser BA, Stover JA, et al. Neurologic development of children with severe chronic renal failure from infancy. *Pediatr Nephrol* 1987;1:157.

51. Brownbridge G, Fielding DM. Psychosocial adjustment to end-stage renal failure: comparing haemodialysis, continuous ambulatory peritoneal dialysis and transplantation. *Pediatr Nephrol* 1992;5:612.

52. Arieff AI, Massry SG, Barrientos A, et al. Brain water and electrolyte metabolism in uremia: effects of slow and rapid hemodialysis. *Kidney Int* 1973;4:177.

53. Goldstein SL, Smith CM, Currier H. Noninvasive interventions to decrease hospitalizations and associated costs for pediatric patients receiving hemodialysis. *J Am Soc Nephrol* 2003;14:2127.

54. Sadowski RH, Allred EN, Jabs K. Sodium modeling ameliorates intradialytic and interdialytic symptoms in young hemodialysis patients. *J Am Soc Nephrol* 1993;4:1192.

55. Kleeman CR: Metabolic coma. *Kidney Int* 1989;36:1142.

56. Fraser CL, Arieff AI. Nervous system complications in uremia. *Ann Intern Med* 1988;109:143.

57. Wolfe RA, Ashby VB, Milford EL, et al. Comparison of mortality in all patients on dialysis, patients on dialysis awaiting transplantation, and recipients of a first cadaveric transplant. *N Engl J Med* 1999;341:1725.

58. Sharma AK. Reassessing hemodialysis adequacy in children: the case for more. *Pediatr Nephrol* 2001;16:383.

59. Lipshultz SE, Somers MJG, Lipsitz S, et al. Serum cardiac troponin and subclinical status in pediatric chronic renal failure. *Pediatrics* 2003;112:79.

60. Chavers B, Schnaper HW. Risk factors for cardiovascular disease in children on maintenance hemodialysis. *Adv Renal Replace Ther* 2001;8:180.

61. Wong CS, Gipson DS, Gillen DL, et al. Anthropometric measures and risk of death in children with end-stage renal disease. *Am J Kidney Dis* 2000;36:811.

62. Goldstein SL, Currier H, Watters L, et al. Acute and chronic inflammation in pediatric patients receiving hemodialysis. *J Pediatr* 2003;143:653.

63. Brem AS, Lambert C, Hill C, et al. Clinical morbidity in pediatric dialysis patients: data from the network 1 clinical indicators project. *Pediatr Nephrol* 2001;16:854.

64. *NKF-DOQI Clinical Practice Guidelines for Hemodialysis Adequacy.* New York: National Kidney Foundation, 1997.

65. Harmon WE. Urea kinetic modeling to describe hemodialysis for children. In: Nissenson AR, Fine RN, eds. *Dialysis Therapy.* Philadelphia: Hanley & Belfus, 1986:240.

66. Tom A, McCauley L, Bell L, et al. Growth during maintenance hemodialysis: impact of enhanced nutrition and clearance. *J Pediatr* 1999;134:464.

13

Peritoneal Access Devices: Design, Function, and Placement Techniques

Stephen R. Ash
David J. Carr
Jose A. Diaz-Buxo
John H. Crabtree

To transform the peritoneum from a lubricating system to an excretory system, only two items are required: an access device and a sterile, balanced salt solution. A successful peritoneal access device must transfer large volumes of dialysate into and out of the peritoneal cavity in a minimal amount of time while maintaining normal anatomy, histology, bacteriology, and physiology of the surrounding tissues.

Filling the peritoneal cavity is easily accomplished with any peritoneal catheter. Drainage of the abdomen is, however, less than consistent with all access devices. Outflow time usually exceeds inflow time, even if the volumes of dialysate and pressure gradients are similar. From 5 to 25 percent of Tenckhoff-type catheters are removed because of outflow obstruction, which sometimes occurs shortly after placement and sometimes much later, especially after peritoneal infection. Avoiding this one-way obstruction has been the principal goal of design of the intraperitoneal portion of the catheter.

FLUID FLOW IN PERITONEAL CATHETERS—THEORY AND OBSERVATIONS

Flow through a peritoneal catheter is theoretically simple. The rate of flow depends on the pressure gradient, the hydraulic resistance of the fluid pathway, and the viscosity of the dialysis solution. For Newtonian fluids such as peritoneal dialysate, the flow rate (Q) through a certain pathway is described by

$$Q = \Delta P/R$$

where Q =   flow rate in mL/min

ΔP =   pressure gradient in cmH2O or mmHg
between the endpoints of the
fluid pathway

R =   hydraulic resistance of the system, as
cmH$_2$O/mL/min or mmHg/mL/min,
which depends on the
shape of the fluid channels
and fluid viscosity

In most peritoneal dialysis (PD) systems, pressure gradients are created by gravity. A bag is lifted above the patient to infuse fluid and lowered below the patient to drain fluid. The pressure gradient is calculated by measuring the difference in height between the air-fluid interface in the bag and the umbilicus, taking into account the intraperitoneal pressure. Intraperitoneal pressure may be conveniently measured by allowing the sterile air in peritoneal dialysate bags to enter the patient's tubing line, waiting for flow to cease, and then measuring the distance between the umbilicus and the air-fluid interface. Fluid flow rate and extraperitoneal volume are easily measured by hanging the drain bag on a commercially available spring scale.

Intraperitoneal pressure depends on a number of factors, including compliance of the abdomen (change in volume/change in pressure), the size and build of the patient, muscle tone, position, activity, and volume of infused fluid.[1] The patient's tolerance of intraperitoneal volumes is dependent more on the pressure than the volume in the peritoneum. A pressure greater than 7 cmH$_2$O (referenced to the umbilicus) diminishes respiratory tidal volume,[2] and a 15-cm intraperitoneal pressure diminishes cardiac output.[3] Patients with chronic lung or heart disease may tolerate even less of an increase in intraabdominal pressure. Figure 13–1

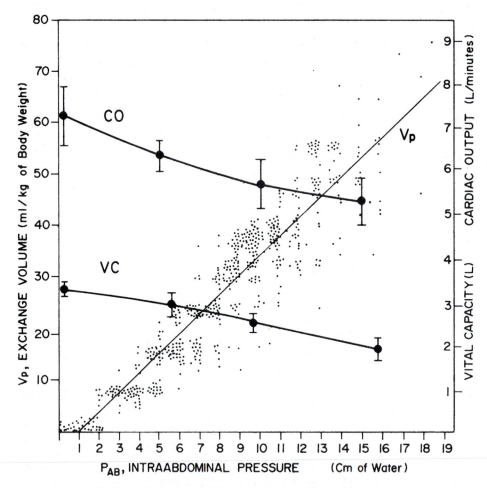

Figure 13–1. Relationship between intraabdominal pressure (P_{AB}) (measured at umbilicus level, intraperitoneal volume (Vp/kg), cardiac output (L/min), and vital capacity (L) in adult patients on peritoneal dialysis. P_{AB}, Vp, and cardiac output determined in supine patients. Vital capacity–P_{AB} relationship determined in patients at 45 degrees of elevation of head. (From Gotloib et al.,[2,3] with permission.)

indicates the relationship of intraperitoneal pressure to volume and the effect of this pressure on both vital capacity and cardiac output with the patient in the supine position. Standard fluid volume in an average-size patient results in intraperitoneal pressures below 10 cmH$_2$O. For a 70-kg patient in the supine position, $P_{AB} = 1 + (0.0038$ cmH$_2$O/ΔmL fill volume).[2]

Once the intraperitoneal pressure is known, it is easy to predict the rate of fluid flow into and out of the peritoneal cavity. Figure 13–2 demonstrates the measurement points for calculating the pressure gradient during the inflow and outflow of peritoneal fluid. During inflow, the air-fluid interface in the hanging 2-L bag diminishes by a distance D, which is related to the cross-sectional area of the hanging bag. During outflow, the air-fluid interface in the drainage bag increases by D, related to the large cross-sectional area of the horizontally supported bag. Because the intraperitoneal pressure is always positive, it would be expected to slow the rate of inflow and increase the rate of outflow. If, from this simplistic model, the hydraulic resistance of the peritoneal catheter is constant, the rate of outflow would be higher than the rate of inflow (Fig. 13–3).

This hydraulic analysis indicates that a peritoneal catheter could drain the abdomen as well from the top of the abdomen as from the bottom. Fluid can easily flow uphill initially if the rest of the course is downhill, as long as the fluid pathway is filled with liquid rather than air. In fact, coiled Tenckhoff catheters have migrated to the upper part of the abdomen[4] or have been placed there purposefully without outflow obstruction. When catheters spontaneously migrate to the upper abdomen, they usually do so because of attachment of the omentum. It is the omental attachment

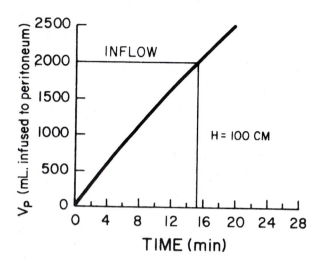

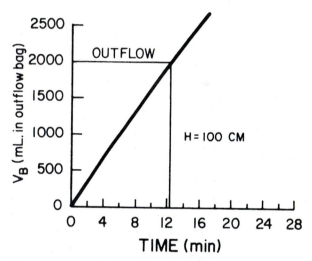

Figure 13–3. Theoretical prediction of inflow and outflow rate during gravity-flow peritoneal dialysis, assuming constant hydraulic resistance. (See text for explanation.)

rather than the catheter position that results in outflow obstruction. The column-disk (Lifecath) catheter had a disk affixed to the parietal peritoneum of the anterior abdominal wall.[5–7] This catheter drained the peritoneum well even though the intraperitoneal disk is located considerably above the lowest part of the abdomen; fluid flows along the parietal peritoneal surface to enter the disk and then flows down and out through the catheter and external tubing (see below). There is pooling of peritoneal fluid in the lower abdomen when a PD patient is standing and there is generally less omental surface in the pelvis, so the optimal location for the tip of a Tenckhoff catheter is in the lower abdominal quadrants; however, if placed peritoneoscopically to an area free of adhesions in the mid abdomen, Tenckhoff catheters can still function well. When the patient is lying down, as during nighttime cycler therapy, a catheter in the midabdomen will work just as well as one in a lower quadrant.

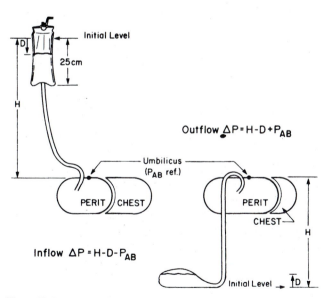

Figure 13–2. Measurements necessary for determination of pressure gradients during gravity-flow peritoneal dialysis. H and P_{AB} measured in reference to the umbilicus, not the tip of the catheter.

It is more difficult to drain the peritoneal cavity than to fill it. Flow at the start of outflow is fast, but it decelerates later in outflow. Figure 13–4 demonstrates outflow after infusion of 2 L of dialysate through a standard straight Tenckhoff catheter. The first 1500 mL drains at a constant rapid rate, but the last 500 mL exits more slowly and irregularly. The overall flow rate is best described by two straight lines: 200 mL/min up to 8 minutes and 35 mL/min after 8 minutes ($r^2 = 0.953$). The diminution in flow rate for the last quarter of intraperitoneal volume can be explained only by an increased hydraulic resistance within the peritoneal cavity.

A peritoneal catheter contacts a variety of parietal and visceral tissues. As intraperitoneal dialysate volume decreases, these structures come closer to the catheter. Negative pressure exerted by fluid flowing into the catheter accelerates movement of the abdominal contents toward the catheter. The pressure of fluid next to a flowing stream is decreased according to the linear velocity of the stream ($\Delta P = \frac{1}{2} pV^2$, the Bernoulli effect).[8] The cross-sectional area of the hole at the tip of a straight Tenckhoff catheter is 0.07 cm^2, and the cross-sectional area of the thirty-two 1-mm-diameter side holes is 0.25 cm^2, creating a total hole area of 0.32 cm^2. At an outflow rate of 200 mL/min, there is a linear velocity of 10 cm/s through the holes. This results in a pressure diminution of 50 cmH$_2$O on tissues adjacent to the flow routes into the holes of the catheter.

Tissues near the tip of the Tenckhoff straight catheter are subjected to the greatest negative pressure, as the tip is larger and has a higher initial flow rate than any side hole. As tissues approach the tip of the catheter, they diminish the flow pathway further. Velocity of fluid then increases, negative pressure increases, and the tip occludes early in outflow, as shown in Fig. 13–5A. After the tip occludes, outflow proceeds entirely through the side holes. This results in a small increase in flow resistance, because the total cross-sectional area of the side holes is much larger than that of the tip (0.25 vs. 0.07 cm^2).

The increase in hydraulic resistance at the end of outflow is due to apposition of abdominal contents around the side holes of the catheter. As shown in Fig. 13–5, this can occur in one of two ways. Bowel loops can align themselves along the length of the catheter, as shown in Fig. 13–5B, or omentum can approach the catheter to form plate-like channels between omentum and abdominal wall, as in Fig. 13–5C. For bowel loops to increase hydraulic resistance enough to cause the diminished flow rate at the end of outflow, three triangular channels must form with an average radius of 0.03 cm around the catheter. For approaching omentum to cause the same increase in hydraulic resistance, the distance between omentum and abdominal wall must be 0.004 cm over a width of 10 cm.

To determine the actual fluid pathways for flow into and out of a Tenckhoff catheter, we performed x-ray studies on a straight Tenckhoff catheter which had been placed immediately prior to the x-ray procedure. The radiolucent catheter was implanted under peritoneoscopy to ensure that it was placed in a clear space between visceral and parietal peritoneum, in an area free of adhesions. After one exchange of peritoneal dialysate which left 400 mL residual, a 250-mL bag of Renografin-60 was placed 1 m above the umbilicus and infused into the abdomen. Figure 13–6A indicates the passage of radiopaque dye through the catheter after 1 second of inflow. Flow into the abdomen is entirely through the tip; the Bernoulli principle predicts that fluid flowing through the inside of a straight Tenckhoff catheter would create a negative pressure at each perpendicular side hole, drawing fluid in through the holes rather than exiting from them.

Figure 13–6B indicates the flow of dye 3 seconds after the start of inflow. The dye flows in two general directions: out of the tip to move inferolateral to the catheter and back-

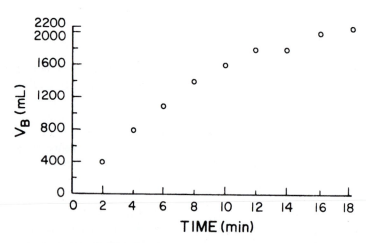

Figure 13–4. Outflow volume (*VB*) vs. time of drainage for a straight Tenckhoff catheter. Obtained using a 60-cmH$_2$O hydrostatic pressure head after infusion of 2 L of fluid.

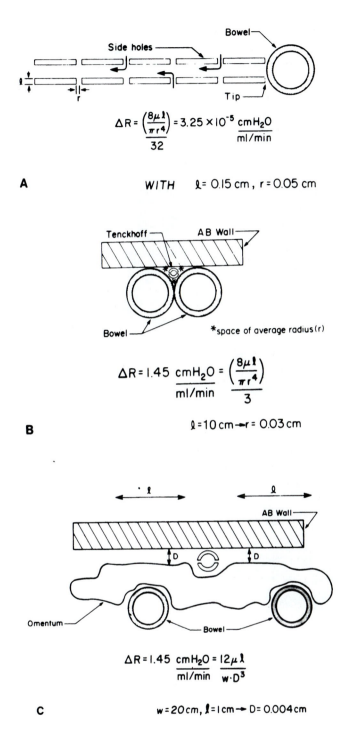

A   WITH $\ell = 0.15$ cm, $r = 0.05$ cm

$$\Delta R = \dfrac{\left(\dfrac{8\mu\ell}{\pi r^4}\right)}{32} = 3.25 \times 10^{-5} \dfrac{cmH_2O}{ml/min}$$

B

$$\Delta R = 1.45 \dfrac{cmH_2O}{ml/min} = \dfrac{\left(\dfrac{8\mu\ell}{\pi r^4}\right)}{3}$$

$\ell = 10$ cm $\rightarrow r = 0.03$ cm

C

$$\Delta R = 1.45 \dfrac{cmH_2O}{ml/min} = \dfrac{12\mu\ell}{w\cdot D^3}$$

$w = 20$ cm, $\ell = 1$ cm $\rightarrow$ D = 0.004 cm

Figure 13–5. Three theoretical mechanisms for increasing hydraulic resistance during late outflow of a straight Tenckhoff catheter. A. Attraction of bowel loops over the tip of catheter. Minimal increase in resistance occurs, since side holes are numerous. B. Attraction of bowel loops toward the catheter and abdominal wall, forming triangular channels for fluid flow along the outside of the catheter. The measured increase in resistance during late outflow could be explained if these channels were 10-cm long and had a 0.03-cm average cross-sectional radius. C. Approach of omentum toward the catheter and abdominal wall, forming plate-like channels for fluid flow on either side of the catheter. The width of the channel is assumed to be the same as the side-hole region of the catheter (10 cm); therefore the total width of the channel is 20 cm. The measured increase in resistance during late outflow could be realized if these channels were 20 cm wide, 1 cm long, and 0.004 cm in height.

wards along the catheter in two linear tracks. The change of fluid-flow direction near the catheter tip indicates that peritoneal surfaces in this area have absorbed some of the kinetic energy of the inflowing fluid. The maximum pressure that is exerted at this point could nearly equal the hydrostatic pressure head (100 cmH$_2$O). This would occur only if flow were diverted 180 degrees, as when the catheter is placed into the pelvic cul-de-sac. This amount of pressure will result in visceral pain. The small channels forming parallel to the catheter during early inflow are essentially the same as those that develop at the end of outflow and create the increase in outflow resistance. Because these tracts are created in spaces that are in turn created by the contacting surfaces of the catheter and neighboring bowel loops, the tracts are generally triangular in shape.

Figure 13–6C is taken after 3 seconds of outflow. The absence of radiopaque dye in the radiolucent catheter shows and persistence of radiopaque dye surrounding the catheter tip indicates that the most recently infused fluid did not leave the abdomen first. The irregular dye-filled space in the peritoneum below the catheter remains unchanged during the first 10 seconds of outflow. From this study and others, it is apparent that fluid pathways change during inflow and outflow. The "last-in, first-out" phenomenon of the lungs does not pertain to peritoneal fluid flow through dialysis catheters. In the peritoneum, the first infused fluid is not the first to leave during outflow, due to diversion of the fluid by bowel loops during inflow, obstruction of the catheter tip during outflow, and irregular channels for fluid flow within the peritoneum.

When Tenckhoff catheters migrate to the upper part of the abdomen, they often drain less than the infused volume of peritoneal fluid. The simple hydraulic model demonstrated in Fig. 13–2 would predict the same outflow rate whether the catheter is in the lower or upper part of the abdomen, and, in fact, peritoneal catheters placed in the upper abdomen next to the parietal peritoneum (such as the Lifecath) can function quite well. Peritoneoscopic inspection of Tenckhoff catheters that have migrated and developed outflow failure almost invariably indicates that these catheters are firmly entangled in omentum; they are difficult to free and relocate with the peritoneoscope or with obturators.[9] When these catheters are removed, omentum must often be stripped from the side holes. This omental attachment brings omental and bowel tissue next to the catheter, and it is this proximity of visceral surfaces that promotes the outflow obstruction. This obstruction is similar to outflow obstruction found with intravenous catheters when the tip is near the vein wall.[10]

In coiled Tenckhoff catheters, the tip is somewhat protected from tissue contact since it sits within the center of the terminal spiral of the catheter. There are more side holes, and the ones facing adjacent catheter loops are also somewhat protected from the approach of adjacent visceral peritoneal surfaces. However, the time and degree of decelera-

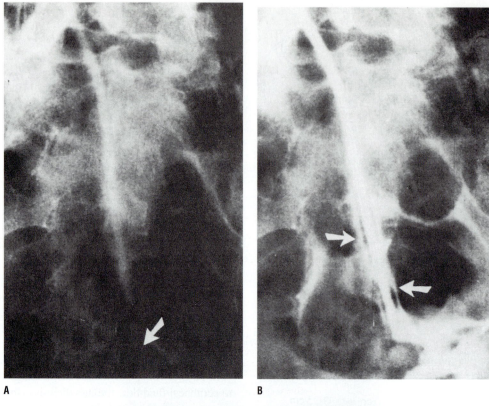

A   B

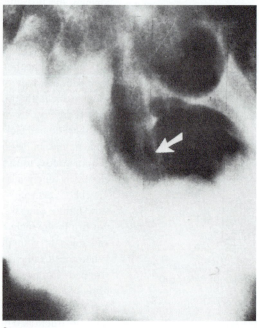

C

Figure 13–6. Radiographs taken during infusion and drainage of Renografin-60 through a radiolucent straight Tenckhoff catheter in a supine patient. The catheter was placed by peritoneoscopy between bowel loops and the anterior abdominal wall, in the left lower quadrant. The abdomen was drained of dialysate to a residual of 400 mL, and 50 mL of Renografin-60 was infused from a bag 1 m above the umbilicus through a standard CAPD patient line. *A.* Radiograph taken after 1 second of inflow, as dye reached the tip of the catheter. The arrow indicates dye in the catheter. Note the lack of flow through the side holes during inflow. *B.* Radiograph taken after 3 seconds of inflow. Arrows indicate dye flowing backward along the catheter, through narrow channels, and dye diverting laterally after exiting from the tip. *C.* Radiograph taken after 3 seconds of outflow of dye (bag 1 m below the umbilicus). The arrow indicates the catheter, now radiolucent. Note that the last fluid in, the dye, is not the first fluid to leave. (X-rays performed by Dr. Paul Webster, Radiology Department, and photographs prepared by Audio Visual Department, St. Elizabeth Hospital, Lafayette, IN.)

tion of flow occurring with the curled Tenckhoff catheter is similar to that of straight catheters, in part because the longer intraperitoneal portion of the curled Tenckhoff catheter creates greater hydraulic resistance and in part because the catheter lies within the same visceral tissues as the straight Tenckhoff catheter. Catheters that place drainage ports next to the parietal peritoneum, such as the column-disk (Lifecath), pail-handle (Cruz), and T-shaped Advantage (Ash) catheters, have outflow that continues at a rapid rate until most of the intraperitoneal volume is drained; subsequent flow is about 25 mL/min. The parietal peritoneum is a smooth, relatively flat surface, which does not collapse around the catheter and is continuous with distant portions of the abdomen.

DESIGNS OF CATHETERS FOR CHRONIC PERITONEAL DIALYSIS—HYDRAULIC FUNCTION AND BIOCOMPATIBILITY

Perfect hydraulic function of a peritoneal catheter would mean that the catheter allows fluid to flow out of the peritoneal cavity with the same ease as with inflow and that all the peritoneal fluid is drained completely. Biocompatibility of an implanted device means that it operates without altering the physiology, anatomy, bacteriology, biochemistry, or reparative function of neighboring tissues.[11] The evolution of chronic PD catheters reflects the goals of attaining adequate hydraulic function and perfect biocompatibility which includes the following features:

1. Peritoneal membrane without sclerosis or adhesions
2. Abdominal wall without leaks or hernias
3. Subcutaneous tract without infection
4. Skin exit site without infection
5. Peritoneum without infection and without adhesions between viscera or to the catheter
6. Resolution of peritonitis as well as if the catheter were not present (catheter or biofilm not harboring bacteria)

HISTORY AND CHRONOLOGY OF PERITONEAL DIALYSIS CATHETERS

Today's PD catheters are the most successful of all transcutaneous access devices, with longevity and successful function measured in years rather than days to months. They are made of soft materials like silicone rubber or polyurethane. The intraperitoneal portion usually contains 1-mm side holes but one version has linear grooves or slots rather than side holes. All chronic PD catheters have one or two extraperitoneal Dacron cuffs, which promote a local inflammatory response. In a unique example of beneficial bioincompatibility the sclerotic process produces a fibrous plug to fix the catheter in position, prevent fluid leaks, and prevent bacterial migration around the catheter. In spite of general success, peritoneal access failure is still a continued source of frustration for all PD programs, and catheter failure is the reason for "dropout" from such programs in about 25 percent of patients. Increasing the success of a PD program requires optimizing the function of peritoneal catheters. Currently, the method of placement of the catheter has more effect on the outcome of the catheter than the choice of catheter type.[12,13]

Since the first attempts to perform PD, there have been many different peritoneal catheter designs (Fig. 13–7). The conspicuous feature of all chronic peritoneal catheters is that they contain numerous holes or pathways by which fluid can enter the peritoneal cavity. It was learned very early that catheters with only one hole at the tip resulted in outflow obstruction. Early peritoneal catheters (1923–1950) were created from a variety of materials, but all had multiple side holes for peritoneal drainage (Fig. 13–7A).[14–17]

The stainless steel coiled-spring design of Rosenak and Oppenheimer provided excellent outflow of fluid (Fig. 13–7A, part 2) for up to 1 month of acute PD.[18] The small slits between the coils of stainless steel wire avoided omental attachment to the catheter, as did the small side holes in later silicone rubber catheters. Grollman used a short-beveled, 17-gauge needle, intermittently inserted to support dogs with acute renal failure by PD, and a 17F catheter with side holes to support patients with acute renal failure (Fig. 13–7A, parts 3 and 4).[19] Similar 17F semirigid catheters were used by Legrain and Merrill[20] and Maxwell and Rockney[21] in treating uremic patients. As reviewed by Odel and Ferris, there were "numerous" episodes of infection, bowel perforation, outflow failure, and subcutaneous leaks with these catheters.[17]

The problems in placement and use of these early catheters led to the design of permanently placed guides in the abdominal wall to intermittently replace plastic catheters. Boen and Mulinari used an indwelling rubber button for repeated introduction of a semirigid catheter.[22,23] Barry used a PVC tube with a balloon on the anterior abdominal wall.[24] The high protein loss during dialysis with this device was possibly due to peritoneal reaction to its vinyl material.[25] Henderson and Merrill[26] used a Teflon guide to direct plastic catheters through the abdominal wall; Dean[27] used knitted fabric; Gotloib[28] used a nylon funnel with the open end under the skin. These transabdominal devices did not diminish the problems of bowel perforation, subcutaneous infection, or outflow obstruction that occurred with intermittently placed catheters.[27]

In 1961, Boen described a latex rubber "permanent" indwelling catheter for chronic PD. This rubber catheter had no cuffs and had side holes one half the diameter of the catheter.[29] The catheter drained poorly and also had a high

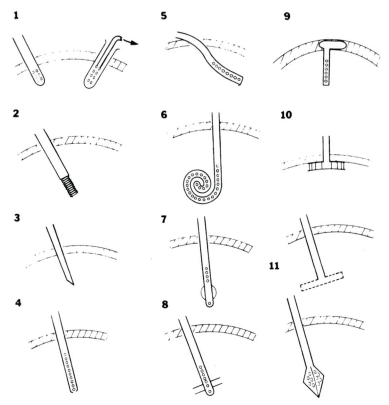

Figure 13–7A. *A.* A variety of intraperitoneal catheter designs utilized from 1923 to the present. (For explanation, see text.)

infection rate, causing Boen to develop a rubber button through which nylon catheters could be introduced.[23]

In 1964, Palmer and Quinton described a rubber peritoneal catheter with a curled intraperitoneal portion, a 90-degree bend at the parietal peritoneal surface, a flange within the abdominal musculature, and a long subcutaneous portion (without cuffs).[30–32] Silicone rubber as a peritoneal catheter was first proposed by Gutch[25] and clinically tested by Gutch and Stevens.[33] They also defined the proper size of the catheter side holes (1-mm diameter) that would allow adequate fluid flow without omental attachment (Fig. 13–7A, part 5). Subcutaneous infection and outflow obstruction were fairly common, although protein loss was less than that produced by the polyvinyl chloride (PVC) catheter guide of Barry.[24]

In 1965, Weston and Roberts[34,35] described a new placement technique for a straight nylon catheter, now known as the "acute" dialysis catheter. A metal stylet inside the catheter punctures the abdominal wall and peritoneum, creating a hole that is then dilated by the catheter. Outflow problems with this catheter are routine, requiring frequent repositioning. Infections of the catheter and peritoneum limit its use to 3 days or less. From the current perspective, any patient needing acute dialysis should have a chronic peritoneal catheter placed for safer and more effective peritoneal access.[36,37]

In 1968, Tenckhoff described two types of silicone catheters, one straight like the Gutch catheter and one coiled like the Palmer catheter (Fig. 13–7A, parts 5 and 6). Tenckhoff's contribution was to place two Dacron cuffs around the catheter, one to lie within or just outside the abdominal musculature and one just below the skin surface[38] (Fig. 13–8). Tenckhoff's studies (with himself as a subject) showed that Dacron felt induces a classic inflammatory reaction in neighboring tissues: a fibrin clot, ingrowth of granulocytes and fibroblasts, and finally a granuloma with giant cells.[39] The resulting fibrous plug represents a curious case of beneficial bioincompatibility; it prevents bacteria from entering the subcutaneous space from the skin surface or from the peritoneum during peritonitis. At the skin exit site, stratified squamous epithelium grows along the surface of the catheter, ending in granulation tissue near the preperitoneal cuff.[39] At the peritoneal surface, simple squamous epithelium grows around the catheter, penetrating the abdominal wall and ending at the deep cuff (Fig. 13–9). Grossly, this results in a smooth, glistening surface surrounding the catheter, leading to the deep Dacron cuff.

Single-cuff catheters were originally described by Tenckhoff as acute catheters; they avoided the need for subcutaneous tunneling, but these have also been used as chronic catheters, with the single cuff sewn into muscle tissue or placed in the subcutaneous tissue.[40,41]

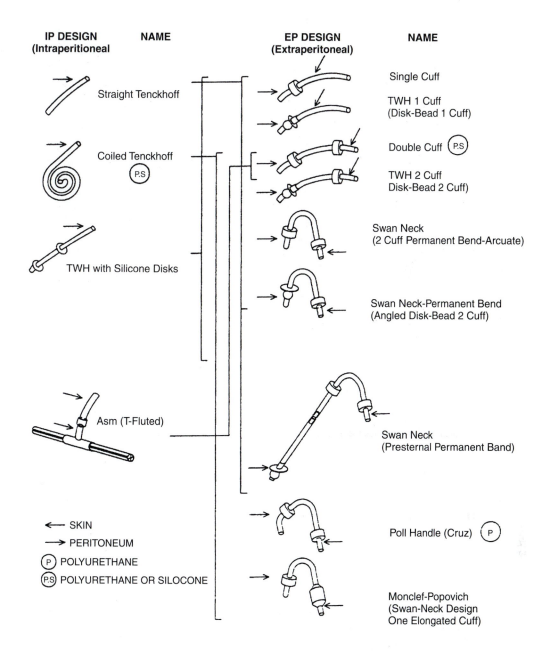

Figure 13–7B. *B.* Currently available chronic peritoneal catheters; combinations of IP and EP designs.

Several modifications of the Tenckhoff catheter have been made in the past 25 years. Each has been designed to avoid specific hydraulic or biocompatibility problems of the original catheter (Fig. 13–7A). The "swan-neck" catheter includes a preformed 150-degree bend in the catheter between the two cuffs, which ensures that the exit site is directed downward in the same general direction as the intraperitoneal portion, following Tenckhoff's original description of the desired course of the subcutaneous segment. As Tenckhoff recommended, this brings the skin exit site below the belt line, allows flexibility between the deep and superficial cuffs, and places the deep and superficial

cuffs in proper positions without the strain that results from bending a straight subcutaneous segment. The downward-directed exit site prevents debris from entering the tract during showering or bathing.[42] Although there are no comparative studies to prove that the swan-neck bend in the subcutaneous tract results in fewer exit complications than the dual-cuff Tenckhoff catheter, the overall success of the catheter in studies within single centers and the popularity of the design indicate that it is generally successful.

The Toronto Western Hospital (TWH) catheter has two silicone disks perpendicular to the catheter to hold bowel and omentum away from the catheter (Fig. 13–7A, part 8).[43]

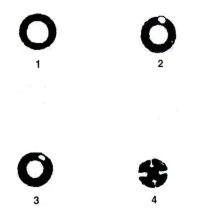

Figure 13–7C. *C.* Comparison of cross-sectional dimensions of the intraperitoneal portion of several peritoneal catheters: (1) Flexneck Tenckhoff catheter (silicone), (2) Cruz Tenckhoff catheter (polyurethane), (3) standard Tenckhoff (silicone), (4) one intraperitoneal limb of the T-fluted catheter (Ash Advantage, silicone).

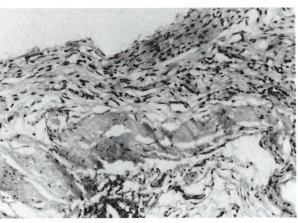

Figure 13–9. Section through tissue surrounding a Tenckhoff catheter between the deep cuff and the parietal peritoneum. Simple squamous epithelium is seen at the top.

These disks are not totally effective; outflow obstruction occurs in 10 percent or more of these catheters.[40,43–46] The Model 2 TWH catheter has a Dacron disk and a silicone bead, between which the peritoneum is sewn. The bead and disk immobilize the catheter and diminish pericatheter leaks. One-year survival of this catheter is similar to, but not greater than, that of the straight Tenckhoff catheter,[43] and removal of the catheter is more difficult.

The "Missouri" catheter combines some features of the swan-neck and TWH catheters. The catheter portion between the two cuffs has a 150-degree arc, like the swan-neck catheter. The deep cuff is contiguous with a Dacron disk and an adjacent silicone bead, between which the peritoneum is sewn during surgical placement. The disk is fixed at a 45-degree angle to the catheter to help direct the in-

traperitoneal portion of the catheter toward the pelvis. This catheter is associated with a low incidence of exit-site infection and pericatheter leak, due principally to the fixed position of the deep and superficial cuffs relative to the parietal peritoneum.

The Lifecath catheter (no longer available) had a 2-inch-diameter disk that rests against the parietal peritoneum (Fig. 13–10). The large size of the peripheral port created a low-velocity fluid flow into the peritoneum, and the location on the parietal peritoneum provided contact with a smooth surface communicating with the entire peritoneum, resulting in a high rate of outflow throughout the majority of outflow.[47] The rapid-outflow portion was prolonged for 1 to 2 minutes further than for standard Tenckhoff catheters, resulting in a shorter total outflow time. The adequate hy-

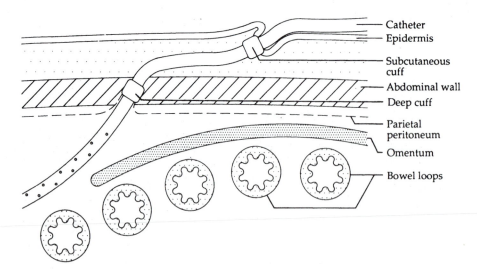

Figure 13–8. Proper location of a dual-cuff Tenckhoff catheter and relation to various tissues. (From Ash et al.,[37] with permission.)

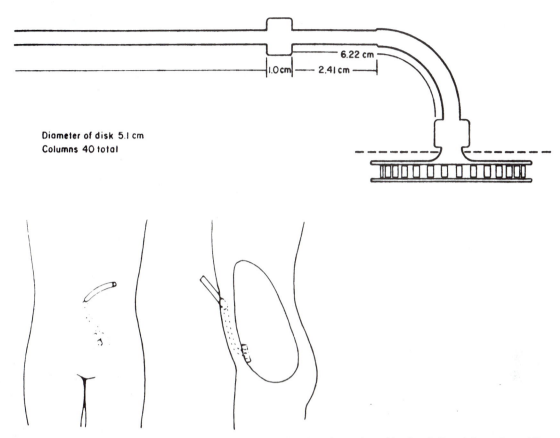

Diameter of disk 5.1 cm
Columns 40 total

Figure 13–10. The column-disk peritoneal catheter (Lifecath) (top) and one intraperitoneal location (halfway between the umbilicus and symphysis pubis). The dotted line indicates the peritoneal membrane, closed between the preperitoneal cuff and disk (bottom).

draulic function of this catheter proved that a catheter does not have to be placed in the lowest part of the abdomen as long as the parietal peritoneal surface is available for fluid flow up to the catheter and there are no adhesions to the catheter (see above). The fixed position of the disk and deep cuff relative to the parietal peritoneum largely avoided pericatheter hernias, exit-site erosion, and exit-site infections.[48–50] Inflow pain did not occur due to the low velocity of fluid flowing through the larger peripheral port of the disk. The overall half-life of the catheters was over 36 months, due mostly to a diminished incidence of the late complications often seen with Tenckhoff catheters.[48] Some centers have found an increased incidence of early leakage with the Lifecath, due probably to the need for a larger peritoneal incision during placement.[51] Approximately 6 percent of Lifecaths developed outflow obstruction within the first 6 months, due to omental attachment to the disk.[47,48] This omental attachment has been demonstrated during peritoneoscopy or laparoscopy and by cross-table x-rays after pneumoperitoneum with 400 mL filtered air. Surprisingly, this outflow obstruction could occur even if the omentum attaches to only one half of the peripheral port. This brings the omental sheet close enough to the disk to create a one-way obstruction during outflow. Partial omen-

tectomy at the time of Lifecath placement was found to diminish outflow obstruction to nearly zero, but this would have represented a fairly major surgical procedure in most patients.

CURRENT DESIGNS OF PERITONEAL DIALYSIS CATHETERS

As shown in Fig. 13–7B, there appears at first to be a bewildering variety of chronic peritoneal catheters available today. However, each portion of the catheter has only a few basic design options.[52]

There are four designs of the intraperitoneal portion:

Straight Tenckhoff, with a 8-cm portion containing 1-mm side holes
Curled Tenckhoff, with a coiled 16-cm portion containing 1-mm side holes
Straight Tenckhoff, with perpendicular disks (TWH, rarely used)
T-fluted catheter (Ash Advantage), with grooved limbs positioned against the parietal peritoneum

There are three basic shapes of the subcutaneous portion between the muscle wall and the skin exit site:

Straight, or gently curved

A 150-degree bend or arc (swan neck)

A 90-degree bend, with another 90-degree bend at the peritoneal surface (Cruz pail-handle catheter)

There are three positions and designs for Dacron cuffs:

Single cuff around the catheter, usually placed in the rectus muscle but sometimes on the outer surface of the rectus

Dual cuffs around the catheter, one in the rectus muscle and the other in subcutaneous tissue

Disk-ball deep cuff, with parietal peritoneum sewn between the Dacron disk and silicone ball (TWH and Missouri catheters)

There are three internal diameters of PD catheters, each having outer diameter of approximately 5 mm (see Fig. 13–7C):

2.6 mm, standard Tenckhoff catheter size

3.1 mm, Cruz catheter

3.5 mm, Flexneck catheter

There are two materials of construction:

Silicone rubber (nearly all catheters)

Polyurethane (Cruz catheter)

The various intraperitoneal designs were all created to diminish outflow obstruction due to the normal diminution in flow which occurs as peritoneal surfaces approach the catheter, or due to omental attachment to the catheter. The shape of the curled Tenckhoff catheter and the disks of the TWH catheter hold visceral peritoneal surfaces away from the side holes of the catheter to some degree (as described above). The grooves of the Advantage catheter distribute flow over the surface of the limbs that contact the parietal peritoneum, providing a much larger surface area for drainage than side holes provide. An irritated omentum attaches firmly to side holes of a catheter but only weakly to grooves on a catheter (as demonstrated by the Blake surgical drain, with grooves on the catheter surface).

By virtue of their shape, the subcutaneous components of all PD catheters provide an exit site in the lateral or downward direction. This minimizes the risk of exit-site infection. An upwardly directed exit site collects debris and fluid, thus increasing the risk of exit-site infection.

The optimal location for the standard deep cuff is within the rectus muscle (described below). The subcutaneous cuff provides additional protection from bacterial contamination of the subcutaneous tunnel. The disk-ball deep cuff provides security of position of the catheter, since with the peritoneum sewn between the Dacron disk and intraperitoneal ball the catheter is fixed in position and cannot migrate outward. Similarly, the T-shape of the Advantage catheter places the intraperitoneal limbs against the parietal peritoneum, preventing outward migration of the catheter.

Double-Lumen Catheters for Continuous-Flow Peritoneal Dialysis

A series of novel catheters have been designed for potential use with continuous-flow peritoneal dialysis (CFPD) (see Chap. 16 for a detailed description of CFPD). The ideal catheter for CFPD should allow continuous inflow and drainage in the range of 150 to 250 mL/min and good mixing of the peritoneal solution with minimal streaming and recirculation. In addition, it should have the other attributes previously mentioned, such as being cosmetically acceptable (small diameter and minimal bulk), ease of implantation, biocompatibility, reliability of function, and safety. These demands have stimulated the design of several novel catheters, all of which are either experimental or have seen only limited clinical use.

The representative prototypes are presented in Fig. 13–11. The simplest of these devices are double-lumen catheters with barrels of different lengths.[53,54] The internal configuration of the lumen is either circular or double "D." The infusion barrel is generally shorter than the drain barrel. The difference in barrel lengths is meant to achieve separation of the flow streams and to improve mixing. The longer barrel can be straight or coiled. In addition, disks similar to those used in the TWH catheter have been added to the longer segment of the catheter to reduce omental wrapping. The main problem with these catheters has been the high degree of streaming and mixing observed. Preliminary clinical experiences suggest that recirculation can be as high as 50 percent with certain catheters and can be significantly reduced with good separation of the catheter limbs or with the use of two separate catheters.[55,56] In response to the poor mixing observed with the double-lumen catheters, a novel catheter was recently designed incorporating several old and new features.[57] It is a double-lumen catheter, with maximum internal separation of the two tubes, that can be implanted peritoneoscopically or laparoscopically. The two distinct lumens use a novel cross-sectional configuration whereby one tube, slightly oval-shaped, nests within the other, a crescent-shaped tube. This geometric arrangement allows maximal internal diameters (cross sections) and a minimal external diameter. The tubes are bonded where they pass through the abdominal wall and subcutaneous tissue. Externally, they are separate, for convenience and ease of use. Internally, they are also separate, each tube terminating with an appropriately sized fluted section similar to the fluted-T Ash Advantage design.[58] The internal tubes take a double J configuration which fits near the parietal peritoneum. This double-J shape causes the cranial and caudal limbs to separate by 180 degrees. This configuration, combined with the functional separation provided by the flutes, translates into a minimal physical flow separation of 13 cm and a probable functional separation of around 20 cm. This unique design permits passive flow

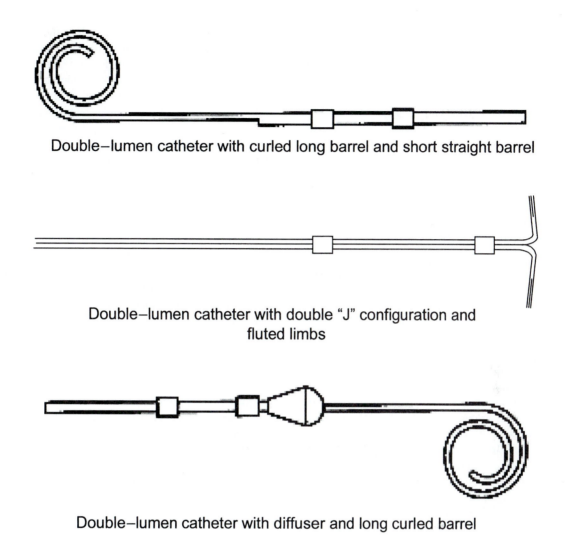

Double–lumen catheter with curled long barrel and short straight barrel

Double–lumen catheter with double "J" configuration and fluted limbs

Double–lumen catheter with diffuser and long curled barrel

Figure 13–11. Double-lumen catheters with barrels of different lengths.

rates well within the required CFPD parameters. In vitro studies indicate that inflow and outflow rates are within acceptable margins. However, clinical validation is not yet available.

The latest novel design is the dual catheter with diffuser.[59] This catheter incorporates a thin-walled silicone diffuser within the intraperitoneal segment closest to the abdominal wall. This lumen is used for infusion and designed to gently diffuse the infusate. The holes on the diffuser are positioned to allow dialysate to exit perpendicularly 360 degrees from the diffuser in order to improve mixing of the fluid. The longer segment has a coiled configuration and is used for drainage. The potential theoretical advantages of this design also await clinical validation.

A final dual-lumen catheter option can be created by using two separate peritoneal catheters (any type). The catheters can be inserted through the abdominal musculature at two separate points of entry to the peritoneum, each

then being connected to a dual-lumen catheter segment that includes the subcutaneous cuff and passes outward through the skin. Historically, almost all clinical experience with flow-through PD has involved two separate catheters placed into the peritoneum. This approach has the advantage of limiting the shunting of peritoneal fluid along the catheter from one end to the other, since the inflow and outflow catheters are completely separate. For optimal drainage of the peritoneum at rates of fluid flow of up to 200 mL/min, the drainage catheter can be of a design to allow maximum drainage (such as the two-limbed Advantage catheter), and the infusion limb can be much smaller (a catheter similar to the Tesio IJ catheter would work). Each catheter limb can be placed in locations to allow optimal function and with tips in different quadrants of the abdomen (preferable). The obvious disadvantage is that two punctures of the peritoneum must be made; but if the catheter is being placed laparoscopically or peritoneoscopically, it is not difficult to make a second puncture safely under vision in an airspace. For example, the peritoneoscopic cannula insertion could be made at the lateral border of the rectus, the infusion catheter limb placed through the midline with a direction toward the contralateral lower quadrant (under vision), and the drainage catheter then placed through the Quill guide at the site of the peritoneoscopic cannula. This approach of using two catheters for flow through dialysis access has been validated clinically in early studies but not proven with more modern catheter types.

COMPLICATIONS RELATED TO THE DESIGN OF PERITONEAL DIALYSIS CATHETERS

Randomized, prospectively controlled studies have generally shown little effect of catheter design on the success of peritoneal catheters (see Table 13–1,[60]). One study by Nielson demonstrated a longer 3-year survival of coiled vs. straight Tenckhoff catheters.[13] If properly placed, dual-cuff Tenckhoff catheters have a lower incidence of exit-site infection and longer lifespan than single-cuff catheters,[12,13,61,62] though properly placed single-cuff catheters can work as well.[63] Curled Tenckhoff catheters have been shown in some studies to be associated with a lower incidence of outflow failure than straight catheters.[13,63] However, only one in three randomized studies has indicated a difference in the incidence of flow or infectious complications of straight versus coiled Tenckhoff catheters. In some studies, a lower incidence of exit-site infection has been seen with swan-neck catheters than those with straight subcutaneous segments.[64] However, none of three randomized studies showed an advantage of the swan-neck subcutaneous bend versus straight (gently bent) subcutaneous segments. This means that in randomized, controlled studies in experienced centers with uniform placement and training procedures, the advantages of curled tips or sharply arcuate subcutaneous segments have not been proven. In general practice, swan-neck catheters may have an educational function, ensuring that the physician places the catheter with a downward exit-site direction.

Some Tenckhoff catheters, such as the silicone rubber Flexneck, have a larger internal diameter and thinner walls than standard catheters (Fig. 13–7C). Flexneck catheters are more pliable and create less tension between deep and superficial cuffs during normal patient activities. This decreased tension may result in a lower incidence of pericatheter leaks and hernias and fewer exit-site and tunnel erosions over time, but this benefit has not been proven. These catheters, like the Cruz catheter, create a higher rate of inflow and initial outflow vs. the standard Tenckhoff catheters, with smaller internal diameters. Rapidity of flow at the end of outflow for the Cruz catheter is also aided by the 90-degree angle of the catheter at the parietal surface, which positions the coiled portion next to the parietal peritoneal surface (like the Palmer catheter).[12,50] Catheters made of polyurethane (such as the Cruz) have excellent strength and biocompatibility. The glue bonding of the Dacron cuffs to the catheters, however, may fail over 1 to 2 years of use, resulting in leaks and infections.[52] A problem with Flexneck catheters is that they are also prone to crimping in the subcutaneous tunnel if they are angled sharply. If the physician follows a template to create the subcutaneous tunnel with a gentle downward curve, crimps in the subcutaneous tract are eliminated.

The Advantage catheter contains a straight portion that is adjacent to the parietal peritoneum, ensuring a stable position and fluid flow along the parietal peritoneal surface; this avoids the possibility of extrusion of the deep cuff and subsequent exit-site erosion (like the disk-ball catheters and the older Lifecath catheter).[65] Further, the grooves of the catheter allow fluid inflow from every direction over every part of the intraperitoneal portion. Advantage catheters placed in patients beginning PD and those with previous Tenckhoff failures demonstrate a 1-year survival of 85 percent, higher than the 50 to 80 percent survival of Tenckhoff catheters in numerous other studies (Fig. 13–12). During follow-up of 70 patients with Advantage catheters in place for up to 4 years, only a few patients developed a pericatheter leak early or late (resolved usually by delaying continuous ambulatory peritoneal dialysis (CAPD) or im-

TABLE 13–1. RANDOMIZED, PROSPECTIVELY CONTROLLED TRIALS OF TENCKHOFF VARIATION CATHETERS

Study	Catheter		Outcome	Significance
Akyol, 1990[165]	Tenckhoff straight vs. coiled, 20 patients	1-year survival	90% straight; 70% coiled	NS
Nielson, 1995[166]	Tenckhoff straight vs. coiled, 72 patients	3-year survivial	78% coiled; 40% straight	$p<0.01$
Scott, 1994[167]	Straight vs. coiled vs. Toronto-Western, 90 patients		No difference in complications	NS
Eklund, 1994[168]	Straight vs. swan neck, 40 patients	2-year survival	78%	NS
Eklund, 1995[64]	Straight vs. swan neck, 40 patients	3-year survival	90% swan neck; 80% Tenckhoff	NS
Lye, 1996[131]	Straight vs. swan neck coiled, 40 patients	1-year survival Swan neck	95% swan neck; 90% straight Less exit-site infection	NS

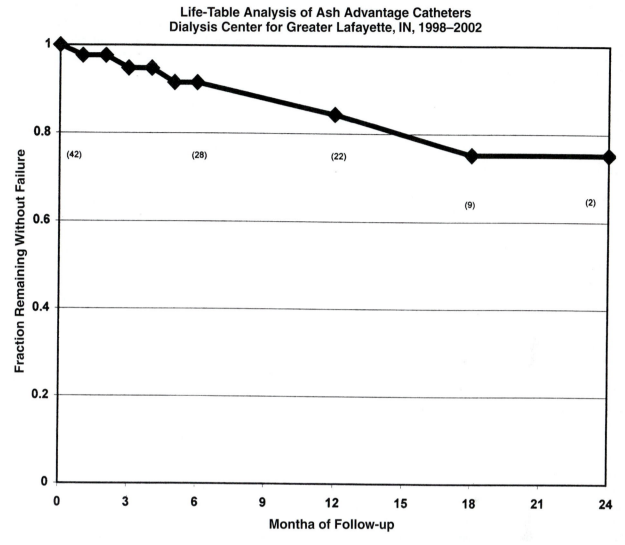

Figure 13–12. Life-table analysis of survival of the Ash Advantage peritoneal dialysis catheter placed in patients with previous Tenckhoff catheter failures and those new to peritoneal dialysis. (From Ash.[12])

plementing dry days and cycler therapy at night). No patient developed a pericatheter hernia, and late exit-site infection was rare (less than 10 percent in 2 years). Pericatheter leak with the Advantage catheter has occurred in only a few patients, with evidence of deep cuff infection and subsequent lack of ingrowth to the catheter cuffs (though this infection was not always evident before operation and cuff culture). The outflow rate of PD fluid is on average equal to that of the best-functioning Tenckhoff catheters (including the large-internal-diameter Flexneck catheters). Outflow volume is more consistent with the Advantage catheter. In CAPD exchanges with the same glucose concentration and dwell time, the Advantage catheter has a standard deviation of 2 percent, vs. 10 percent for Tenckhoff catheters. The consistent peritoneal outflow is probably due to more complete drainage of the peritoneum, with a diminished residual

volume. Diminished residual volume is important, since if residual volume is decreased by 300 to 500 mL, the inflow volume can be increased by the same amount, thus increasing the peritoneal clearance by 10 to 20 percent without increasing patient discomfort by overfilling the abdomen.

Advantage peritoneal catheters diminish the risk of outflow failure but do not eliminate this risk. The mechanism of outflow failure is different from that of Tenckhoff catheters. Omentum does not directly attach to the intraperitoneal portion of the catheter but rather surrounds the long, slotted catheter's intraperitoneal limbs and traps them against the parietal peritoneum. Infusion of iodine dye during fluoroscopy demonstrates that the dye does not pass freely in many directions out of the grooves of the catheter but rather stays near the catheter and exits from the ends of the intraperitoneal limbs. Laparoscopic removal of adhesions from around the catheter can often result in a perfectly functioning PD catheter. In clinical trials, this device maintains a fixed position, provides high outflow rates, and generally avoids outflow failure even in patients with prior complications of Tenckhoff catheters.[66,67] Direct attachment to a groove or slot is more difficult for the omentum than to a cylindrical side hole, and no direct attachment has been found in animal or clinical studies of the Advantage catheter.)

There are advantages and also disadvantages of other current catheter designs. The larger internal diameter of the Cruz and Flexneck catheters provides lower hydraulic resistance and more rapid dialysate flow during the early phase of outflow. In the latter part of outflow, the resistance to flow is determined mostly by the spaces formed by peritoneal surfaces as they approach the catheter. The Advantage catheter provides much larger area of entry ports for drainage of peritoneal fluid; limited clinical studies have demonstrated faster drainage of the peritoneum in early and late phases of outflow and a decrease in residual peritoneal volume at the end of outflow.

Changes in the construction material of peritoneal catheters has not changed the incidence of most complications. Polyurethane catheters are not associated with a lower incidence of peritonitis or omental attachment leading to outflow failure than are silicone catheters. Polyurethane PD catheters have generally had a weaker bond to the Dacron cuff, and loosening of this bond has led to a high incidence of pericatheter leaks. These leaks can be quite slow, resulting in little palpable local edema yet still creating overall outflow failure. Using ultrasound, however, fluid can usually be seen around the deep cuff and in the subcutaneous area. Surprisingly, most chronic central venous catheters for dialysis are also made of polyurethane and have Dacron cuffs, but they rarely show separation of the catheter from the cuff even when used for some years.

Nonrandomized studies of specific catheters have indicated various advantages; for example, it has been found that catheters with the best fixation of the deep cuff (such as the Missouri and Advantage catheters) have a very low incidence of exit-site infection.[68] Catheters with devices to affix them to the parietal peritoneal surface or perpendicular disks within the peritoneum (the Missouri, Missouri Pre-Sternal, and TWH catheters) must be placed surgically. Catheters with arcuate subcutaneous segments (such as the swan neck) require more skill and judgment in placement than straight catheters so as to ensure that the subcutaneous course of the catheter fits the catheter design; an extra skin incision at the apex of the catheter is sometimes used for placement (though in most cases an arcuate tunnel can be created).[42]

Dacron cuffs are not totally effective in preventing infection of the subcutaneous catheter tract (the tunnel). Clinical studies have demonstrated subcutaneous catheter infec-

tion in up to 35 percent of Tenckhoff catheters in 1 year (Table 13–2). Infection of the deep cuff is usually a prelude to peritonitis, and chronic exit-site infection often leads, eventually, to peritonitis. If the subcutaneous cuff begins to erode through the skin, a local infection usually follows. Removal of this cuff from the catheter sometimes resolves the infection. The infection may persist, however, resulting in persisting peritonitis or tunnel infection. In these cases, the peritoneal catheter must be removed. Catheters with a fixed position of the deep cuff have a diminished incidence of exit-site infection (Missouri, Missouri Pre-Sternal, and TWH ball-disk).

There is some evidence that bacterial contamination of the catheter and cuffs during or after catheter placement can result in subsequent peritonitis, even without signs of deep or superficial cuff infection. Moncrief and Popovich developed a catheter placement technique that can be applied to all two-cuff Tenckhoff catheters but which they first tested with a dual-cuff, coiled, and arcuate catheter with a 3-cm superficial cuff (rather than the usual 1-cm length).[69] The catheters are placed in the usual manner and the external portion is then shortened, occluded, and buried under the skin. Both the primary and secondary incisions are then closed. When the catheter is needed for dialysis (weeks to months later), the secondary incision is opened, the tunnel is incised, and the outer portion is exteriorized (see discussion below).

Subcutaneous leak of peritoneal fluid occurs if there is insufficient tissue ingrowth around the deep cuff of the catheter or if the deep cuff is outside the abdominal musculature and the preperitoneal tunnel becomes weakened. Early fluid leak impairs tissue ingrowth to both cuffs; fibroblasts are poor swimmers and move through a fibrous clot much more easily than through water. Fluid leaks are more likely if intraperitoneal fluid has increased pressure in the first 2 weeks after catheter placement. To avoid catheter leaks, a number of break-in procedures have been developed to ensure patency of the catheter without risking peritoneal catheter leaks. The common denominator of these procedures is that the abdomen is left dry during part of each day, or at least every few days, and fluid is infused through the catheter daily or at least weekly. Catheter leakage is also affected by the number of cuffs used (one or

TABLE 13–2. INCIDENCE COMPLICATIONS LEADING TO REMOVAL OF CHRONIC PERITONEAL DIALYSIS CATHETERS DURING LIFETIME OF CATHETER, ARRANGED ACCORDING TO METHOD OF PLACEMENT[a]

Insertion Method	Infections	Outflow Failure	Leaks
Blind: trocar or guidewire	0.24	0.16	0.17
Surgical: dissection	0.35	0.07	0.06
Peritoneoscopic	0.13	0.06	0.06

[a]Summary of 70 published studies on all types of catheters.
Source: Adapted from Nolph,[1] with permission.

two) and the method of catheter placement. A break-in technique can usually be chosen that is also therapeutic for uremia, without causing leaks. However, the fewest leaks occur if the catheter is not used for several weeks or if the catheter is "buried," as in the Moncrief-Popovich technique.[69]

Pericatheter hernias are a late complication of Tenckhoff catheters. The incidence of this problem depends on the location of the deep cuff of the catheter. If it is outside the abdominal musculature, the peritoneal membrane surrounding the catheter creates a potential hernial sac surrounding it. If the abdominal wall is weak, then a golfball-size hernia can develop around the cuff. With surgical and peritoneoscopic placement, the deep cuff is placed within the abdominal musculature. Nevertheless, the abdominal incision and the catheter exit site itself weaken the wall and thus may eventually allow pericatheter hernias to develop. Catheters with devices to fix their position relative to the parietal peritoneum have a decreased incidence of pericatheter leaks (Lifecath, Missouri, Missouri Pre-Sternal, TWH ball-disk, and T-fluted catheters).

The silicone rubber of Tenckhoff catheters is not completely compatible with the peritoneum. Inadequate drainage occurs in up to 16 percent of catheters (Table 13–2). Omental attachment is one reflection of bioincompatibility. Outflow failure due to omental attachment occurs spontaneously in the first few days of use in some patients, especially in young, thin males with active omentum, and is frequent after severe peritonitis (outflow failure may also be due to malposition of the catheter or constipation). In most catheters removed for outflow failure, the omentum is so firmly attached to all of the side holes that omentum is pulled through the exit site with the catheter.[40,45,70–74]

Omental attachment is not totally the fault of the material; it is also related to the design of the catheter and factors that irritate the peritoneum (bioincompatibility of the dialysate and infection). Omental adhesion to Tenckhoff catheters is almost immediate when these catheters are used for dialysis of animals.[11,33,66] Irritation of the peritoneum by lactate-based PD solution contributes to the adhesion, since Tenckhoff catheters that are left in place in dogs with the external portion "buried" work well hydraulically when brought through the skin months later and used for PD exchanges, but then only for a day or so.[69] The Lifecath and T-fluted catheters (described above) are generally successful in PD of animals, apparently because of the port design; omentum grasps a slot or groove less readily than it does cylindrical side holes.[40,66] Omental attachment to side holes increases dramatically if the side holes are larger than 1 mm in diameter.[33] The phenomenon of outflow failure is related more to the design than the material of PD catheters. Outflow failure of coiled Tenckhoff two-cuff polyurethane catheters has not proved to be less frequent than with silicone catheters, and the T-fluted catheter is made of the same silicone material as standard Tenckhoff catheters.

A major disadvantage of all current peritoneal catheters is that they can serve as a nidus for infection. Omental attachment and persistent infection after peritonitis illustrate that Tenckhoff catheters are less biocompatible with regenerating peritoneal surfaces than with the normal peritoneum. Different catheter materials may help diminish the risk of catheter infection. Polyurethane has been used to create coiled peritoneal catheters by VasCath and Corpak (the Cruz catheter). The surface of polyurethane is smoother than that of silicone, so insertion through catheter guides and cannulas is easier. Its strength is greater, so the wall thickness can be smaller, resulting in either a smaller outer diameter or large internal diameter. The tunnel that forms around the subcutaneous portion is thinner than that around silicone catheters. So far, however, general experience and a few studies have failed to show a decreased tendency to bacterial seeding of polyurethane than of silicone. There appears to be hydrolysis of the polyurethane surface and cracking of the material after exposure to polyethylene glycol or alcohol.[60,75] Mupirocin ointment (Bactroban) can cause ballooning and cracking of the catheter due to its base—polyethylene glycol.[76] Polyurethane catheters are susceptible to alcohol and other organic solvents that are frequently encountered in the clinical environment.[77]

Antibacterial catheter surfaces should prevent bacterial growth and thus minimize biofilm formation. Experiments with miniaturized column-disk catheters have indicated that sterling silver is compatible with the peritoneum, in spite of the metallic, inflexible shape.[78] Silver has known bacteriostatic/bacteriocidal activity. Catheter surface treatment with ion beam–assisted deposition of silver has been investigated with flexible catheters in animal studies.[79,80] Evaporated silver is allowed to condense as a thin coating on the catheter surface. Adhesion of this film to the catheter surface is facilitated by high-energy ion-beam bombardment. While preliminary laboratory studies have shown antibacterial activity, no clinical trials utilizing this coating process with PD catheters have been performed. Treatment of PD catheters by surface imbedding (no coating) of silver ions with high-energy beam bombardment did not reduce dialysis-related infections in a randomized controlled clinical trial.[81] Failure to demonstrate a clinical effect in reducing infectious complications may have been due to the low surface availability of silver. In addition, current ion-beam technologies do not permit treatment of the internal surface of the catheter. Silver catheter impregnation can also cause local irritation of the exit site and simulate peritonitis. Peritoneal catheters with a long-term and effective antibacterial surface are still an elusive goal.

A silicone or polyurethane catheter is not completely inert in the peritoneum. Although in most patients the anatomy remains normal,[82] in some there is thickening of the peritoneum, with loss of ultrafiltration capacity,[70] and inclusions of aluminum and silica have been found in the membrane.[83] A peripheral eosinophilia occurs in some patients in the first 3 days after catheter placement, and eosinophilic (noninfectious) peritonitis occurs in some during the first week after placement.[51] This eosinophilia may occur in the absence of general anesthesia, infection, or infusion of peritoneal fluid. Daugirdas and colleagues demonstrated that intraperitoneal air injection could cause eosinophilia in peritoneal fluid, raising the possibility that air entering the peritoneal cavity during catheter placement could cause dialysate eosinophilia.[84] Nonetheless, air is used for insufflation of the peritoneum during peritoneoscopic placement of catheters, and fewer than 1 in 100 patients develop peritoneal fluid eosinophilia.[85] Other possible causes of peritoneal eosinophilia include talc contamination of catheters during placement, antibiotics used in peritoneal fluid or adhering to the catheter,[86] and an intrinsic allergy to silica or barium (the component that makes a white stripe) or to the silicone polymer. During the first weeks of residence in the peritoneum, silicone catheters become more biocompatible, as native glycoproteins form a biofilm on the surfaces. Bacteria introduced during placement of the catheter may become a part of this biofilm, creating peritoneal infections much later.[11,87] The development of a stable biofilm is probably why outflow failure is less common after the first month of catheter use and why catheters that are placed and "buried" for some months work well when brought through the skin.[69]

PLACEMENT OF CATHETERS FOR CHRONIC PERITONEAL DIALYSIS

Overview

There is general agreement on the proper location of the components of chronic peritoneal catheters (see Fig. 13–8):

The intraperitoneal portion should be between the parietal and visceral peritoneum and directed toward the pelvis to the right or left of the bladder.
The deep cuff should be within the medial or lateral border of the rectus sheath.
The subcutaneous cuff should be approximately 2 cm from the skin exit site.

Placement of the deep cuff within the rectus muscle promotes tissue ingrowth and therefore avoids pericatheter hernias, leaks, catheter extrusion, and exit-site erosion.[13,52,88] At the parietal peritoneal surface, the squamous epthelium reflects along the surface of the catheter to reach the deep cuff. If the deep cuff is outside the muscle wall, the peritoneal extension creates a potential or actual pericatheter hernia. At the skin surface, the stratified squamous epthe-

lium follows the surface of the catheter until it reaches the superficial cuff. If the tunnel from subcutaneous cuff to exit site is longer than 2 cm, the squamous epithelium disappears before reaching the cuff and granulation tissue is left, leading to an exit site with continued "weeping" of serous fluid; thus the potential for exit-site infection is increased. If the subcutaneous cuff is too close to the exit site, the cuff will irritate the dermis and the exit site will be continually reddened and inflamed.

Some peritoneal catheters have components that provide greater fixation of the deep cuff within the musculature. When the Missouri and TWH catheters are placed, the parietal peritoneum is closed between the ball (inside the peritoneum) and disk (outside the peritoneum). When the T-fluted (Ash Advantage) catheter is placed, the wings open in position adjacent to the parietal peritoneum and perpendicular to the penetrating tube. With these two catheters, outward migration of the catheter is impossible.

In placing peritoneal catheters, especially by blind or peritoneoscopic approaches, it is best to choose a deep cuff location that is free of major blood vessels (Fig. 13–13). The superficial epigastric arteries course from the femoral artery and ligament toward the umbilicus, anterior to the rectus sheath. The inferior epigastric arteries lie behind the rectus muscles, roughly in the middle of the rectus sheath. Considering the position of these arteries, the safest locations for inserting a needle or cannula to place the catheter are in the medial or lateral borders of the rectus muscle. By physical examination, the lateral border of the rectus can be determined by asking the patient to tense the abdomen and palpating the lateral border; for all patients, this border is located halfway between the anterosuperior iliac spine and the midline. The medial border is located approximately

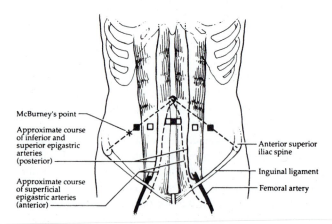

Figure 13–13. Primary placement sites for the deep cuff of a chronic peritoneal dialysis catheter. The solid squares are the safest penetration sites for blind and peritoneoscopic insertion. The open squares are locations of the primary incision during dissective (surgical) placement, to safely place the deep cuff within the rectus muscle. (From Ash and Daugirdas,[217] with permission.)

1 cm from midline, below the umbilicus. The exact location of the medial and lateral border of the rectus muscle can be determined more precisely using ultrasound (as with the Site-Rite) by moving the probe laterally from midline to flank. Positioning the probe over potential sites for catheter placement in an orientation to detect vertical movement of the viscera also allows a qualitative assessment of motion and a determination of which sites are most freely mobile and therefore less likely to contain dense adhesions.

There are three methods for the placement of chronic peritoneal catheters: dissective (surgical), blind, and peritoneoscopic.[89] All of these methods are used by surgeons and nephrologists, in a variety of locations within the hospital, so defining placement techniques as merely "medical" or "surgical" is imprecise. Dissective placement means separating tissues by sharp and blunt instruments to the level of the peritoneum, creating a small hole in the peritoneum, lifting the abdominal wall, advancing the catheter through the small hole into the pelvis by "feel" to avoid entanglement in omentum or bowel loops, and closing the abdominal musculature around the deep cuff. Blind placement is performed using the Tenckhoff trocar[90] or a needle/guidewire/split-sheath technique, both of which involve advancing the catheter into the abdomen without any visualization, and both of which usually place the deep cuff just outside the abdominal musculature.[91] The peritoneoscopic technique uses a small-diameter, long scope to direct a cannula and surrounding spiral-wound Quill guide to the desired location of the catheter; the Quill guide is left in place to direct the catheter to the chosen location. Expansion of the guide allows the cuff to enter the musculature. Acute PD catheters (without Dacron cuffs) are almost always placed blindly. The risks associated with their insertion are higher than the risks of inserting chronic catheters, and because of their rigidity and lack of cuffs, acute catheters can be used safely for only a few days. Each reinsertion poses a higher risk of bowel perforation. For treatment of acute renal failure by PD, it is best to insert a chronic PD catheter right at the start.[92]

Figure 13–13 indicates the safest locations for the deep cuff of a chronic PD catheter, placed by any technique. Since the inferior and superficial epigastric arteries generally pass under and over the middle of the rectus muscle, the deep cuff of the catheter should be placed at the medial or lateral border of the rectus muscle. Dissective placement can penetrate the rectus more toward the middle, since any artery that may be encountered can be avoided. However, it is still best not to place the cuff of the catheter against an inferior epigastric artery. Blind and peritoneoscopic placements are safest if directed at the outer and inner borders of the rectus, so as to avoid major vessels. This will allow the deep cuff to be placed in musculature even if the tract is lateral to the rectus muscle, or to be placed halfway into the linea alba if the tract is medial to the rectus. For all catheter placement techniques, the entry site can be made higher or lower on the border of the rectus than shown in Fig. 13–13, to avoid having the exit site of the catheter at the level of the belt line (if a belt is worn). A higher (cephalad) deep cuff location is advisable in obese patients, to avoid dissection through the panniculus. However, the paramedian approach to the right rectus should not be attempted above the umbilicus because of the risk of entering the falciform ligament.

The internal portion of the Tenckhoff catheter should be directed toward the left or right lower quadrant, behind the femoral ligament, since the lower abdomen has less omentum than the upper portion. In Tenckhoff's manual, he suggests placing the catheter into the cul-de-sac between rectum and bladder.[90] This location is not reached in most placements with the standard Tenckhoff catheter, which measures only 15 cm from the deep cuff to the tip or coil of the catheter. If the catheter actually does enter the cul-de-sac, inflow of fluid will almost always produce pain (due to pressure on the peritoneum as flow is deflected 180 degrees). In large patients, the left-lower-quadrant position is best reached by inserting the catheter in the left midquadrant. In small patients, the right-midquadrant approach can place the catheter behind the left inguinal ligament. During peritoneoscopic placement, catheters are placed into the largest clear area between viscera and peritoneum, regardless of direction.

Preoperative Planning

Planning for the correct implantation of a PD catheter begins in the clinic in advance of the procedure. This provides an opportunity to examine the patient dressed and in the sitting position to determine belt-line location and other body habitus features that will influence selection of catheter type, insertion site, and exit-site location. The choice of catheter type and insertion site represents a balance between what location will produce a deep pelvic position of the catheter tip and an exit site that is not under a belt line, within a skin crease, or on the blind side of a skin fold. Postimplantation, patients quickly appreciate the value of an exit site that is easy to visualize during daily care and that is not prone to trauma or infection. Physicians who perform implantation procedures should not be fixated on attempts to hide the catheter below the belt line. Educating patients about the importance of a good exit-site location and their observation of the care taken to determine the most optimal catheter exit-site eliminates any concerns about whether the tubing comes out above or below the belt.

The incision through which the catheter will be inserted corresponds to the final location of the deep catheter cuff. For each style and size of catheter, the insertion site is determined by noting the position of the deep catheter cuff when the upper border of the catheter coil (first side hole of straight-tip catheters) is aligned with the upper border of the symphysis pubis (Fig. 13–14). This ensures that the coil is located deep in the true pelvis but not so deep that redundant tubing produces pressure discomfort or buckles out of the pelvis. A paramedian location of the insertion point is planned so that the catheter will traverse the rectus muscle toward the medial aspect of the rectus sheath to avoid the epigastric vessels. Typically, a point 3 cm lateral of midline is selected.

Once the insertion site and deep cuff location are determined, planning the tunnel tract configuration and exit-site location for a catheter with a preformed swan-neck bend is simple. The course of the subcutaneous tunnel tract of an appliance with a preformed bend must precisely follow the shape of the catheter. One or two exit-site options at distances 2 and 3 cm beyond the superficial cuff are indicated on the skin in line with the external catheter limb.

Catheters with straight intramural segments require special consideration. An algorithm is used to plan the tunnel tract of a Tenckhoff-style catheter to reduce the tendency for superficial cuff extrusion through the exit site that results from the shape memory of a straight tube bent into an arcuate configuration (Fig. 13–15). With the deep cuff

maintained at the position as previously determined, a point 2 cm cephalad of the superficial cuff is marked on the skin in the same paramedian line. Using the catheter as a compass, a 90-degree arc is inscribed from the point 2 cm above the superficial cuff to the lateral transverse plane of the abdomen. The circumference of the 90-degree arc is divided into thirds. The planned exit site is the junction of the medial two-thirds and the lateral third on the arc. With the deep cuff maintained in the fixed position, a point 4 cm cephalad to the superficial cuff on the tubing is arched over with the convexity oriented upward until the 4-cm point intersects with the planned exit site. The shape of the arc and the position of the superficial cuff are traced on the skin. This will correspond to the planned tunnel tract and superficial cuff location. The shape of the arch will give the catheter a lateral and slightly downward direction as it exits the skin. At the time of implantation, the superficial cuff will be 4 cm from the skin exit site. The amount of tube straightening that occurs over time is a balance between the resilience forces of the tubing and the resistive forces of the tissues and will be different from patient to patient. In the worst-case scenario, in which the tube straightens, the cuff will come no closer than 2 cm of the exit wound. The algorithm is meant to serve as a guide. Exit-site selection can be shifted on the arc as

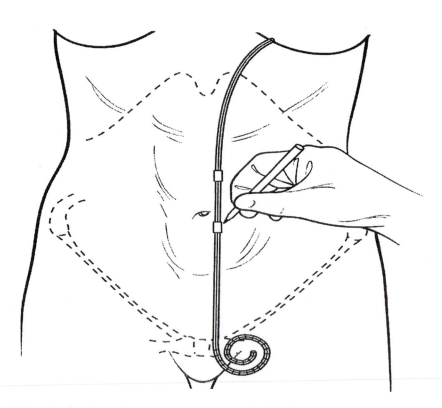

Figure 13–14. Schematic drawing showing the manner in which the proper catheter insertion site and deep cuff location are selected in order to achieve proper pelvic positioning of the coiled-tip catheter.

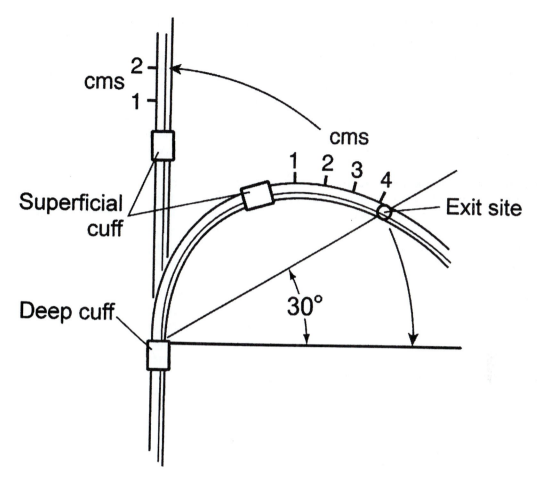

Figure 13–15. Diagram representing the algorithm used to plan the tunnel tract and exit-site location for Tenckhoff-style peritoneal dialysis catheters. (From Crabtree,[81] with permission.)

long as it is remembered that upwardly directed exit sites collect debris and that increasingly downward configurations add to tubing stress.

Because patients come in all sizes and shapes, it should be apparent that several catheter styles and sizes should be available. Insertion and exit-site locations for several catheter types are mapped out while the patient is in the recumbent operative position. The patient is examined in the sitting position to determine which catheter appliance would result in an exit-site free of the belt line, skin creases, or folds. The catheter style that results in the best exit-site location without compromising correct pelvic position is the device that should be used. The proposed incision, tunnel tract, and exit site are marked with indelible ink or measurements are recorded in relation to suitable anatomic landmarks—e.g., umbilicus—to permit remapping in the operating room. The use of plastic stencils that incorporate the above geometric considerations for multiple catheter styles and sizes greatly simplifies tunnel tract and exit-site planning.[93] A sterilized version of the selected stencil can be used to retrace the incision site, tunnel-tract configuration, and exit-site location at the time of the implantation procedure.

Preparation of the Patient and the Procedure

Preoperatively, patients are fasted for 8 hours; however, essential medications are permitted with a sip of water. Preparation includes a shower on the day of surgery with a chlorhexidine soap abdominal wash. Preoperative bowel preparation is not performed unless there is a previous history of constipation. Removal of body hair is performed in the preoperative holding area, preferably with electric clippers. Hair removal should be limited to that necessary to facilitate performance of the procedure. Patients are instructed to empty the bladder prior to the implantation procedure; otherwise, a Foley catheter should be placed. A single dose of a prophylactic antibiotic to provide anti-staphylococcal coverage is administered prior to the procedure. A first-generation cephalosporin is most commonly used. Vancomycin is substituted in the event of cephalosporin allergy.

The operating room provides the best environment for PD catheter implantation. A procedure room may serve as an alternate site provided that it is suitably designed and equipped to perform catheter implantation and conforms to all applicable government regulations. Everyone in the room should wear a cap and mask (including the patient), and the physician and assistant must wear gowns and gloves. Sterile instrument packs, drapes, and disposable kits should be opened shortly before the procedure. The selected PD catheter is prepared by soaking the tubing and flushing the lumen with saline to remove any particulate residues from the manufacturing process. No antibiotics should be added to the soak solution. The air bubbles are squeezed from the Dacron cuffs before insertion to promote better tissue ingrowth.

Surgical skin preparation is performed with povidone-iodine (scrub solution or gel) or chlorhexidine gluconate scrub. Sterile surgical towels are placed around the operative field, exposing only that portion of the abdominal skin required to perform the procedure. A laparotomy sheet or other suitable drape is used to cover the rest of the patient.

Surgical Implantation by Open Dissection

Implantation of the dialysis catheter by an open dissection technique currently remains the most common method of providing peritoneal access.[94] Some catheter devices equipped with a silicone bead and Dacron flange that are positioned at the level of the peritoneum and posterior rectus sheath can be implanted only by this approach. Implantation by open dissection is generally performed under local or general anesthesia in the operating room by surgeons.

A 5- to 8-cm paramedian incision through the skin and subcutaneous tissues is made to expose the rectus sheath at a level on the abdominal wall that corresponds to the planned deep catheter cuff location. The anterior rectus sheath is incised and the muscle is split parallel with its fibers to expose the posterior rectus sheath. After the posterior rectus sheath and peritoneum have been lifted up with forceps, a 0.5-cm incision is made with Metzenbaum scissors or a scalpel to enter the peritoneal cavity. A purse-string suture of absorbable material is placed around the peritoneal opening under direct vision, with care to avoid puncturing the bowel or accidentally including the omentum in the stitch. The peritoneum and fascia are elevated to create an air space between the parietal and underlying viscera. The catheter, usually straightened over an internal stylet, is advanced through the peritoneal incision toward the pelvis. The stylet is partially withdrawn as the catheter is advanced until the deep cuff abuts the posterior fascia. If resistance is encountered during insertion, the catheter is

withdrawn and redirected until it advances easily. After satisfactory placement has been achieved, the stylet is completely withdrawn and the purse-string suture tied.

The catheter tip can be encouraged to remain oriented toward the pelvis by oblique passage of the catheter through the rectus sheath in a craniocaudal direction.[95] The catheter tubing and superficial cuff are passed through the anterior rectus sheath at least 2.5 cm cephalad to the level of the purse-string suture and deep cuff. If the anterior rectus sheath was opened with a transverse incision, the oblique tunneling is performed using a clamp to pull the catheter through a small hole in the anterior fascia above the level of the fascial incision.[95] If the rectus sheath was opened vertically, the catheter is passed between two fascial sutures at the cephalad end of the incision.[96]

Although not commonly practiced, prophylactic resection of the omentum at the time of the implantation procedure has been used in an attempt to prevent catheter obstruction. Reported case series include omentectomy performed in all patients or in selected cases according to the surgeon's preference, the latter without clear criteria for its use.[97–99] Utilizing a selective policy, partial omentectomy should be performed only if the omentum spontaneously exited through the wound, was noted to be large, and/or was situated in the pelvis; this approach has been shown to improve catheter survival free of obstruction.[100] Assessing omental characteristics through a limited peritoneotomy can be unreliable, however. Omentectomy is performed by teasing the omentum out of the peritoneal incision and resecting as much as possible. Despite the use of prophylactic partial omentectomy, the incidence of flow obstruction still complicates 2 to 10 percent of cases.[97–99,101]

Subcutaneous tunneling of the catheter to the selected exit site is discussed further on. After the establishment of careful wound hemostasis, the fascia, subcutaneous tissue, and skin are sutured in separate layers.

Blind Percutaneous Placement

Placement of catheters by blind percutaneous puncture is performed using a modification of the Seldinger technique.[102–105] The advantage of this approach is that it can be performed at the bedside under local anesthesia using prepackaged self-contained kits that include the dialysis catheter. The abdomen is usually prefilled with dialysis solution instilled with a needle inserted through a 2-cm incision in the midline 3 cm below the umbilicus. Alternatively, a lateral abdominal site may be used at a point just lateral of the rectus sheath, on a line between the umbilicus and anterior superior iliac spine. Having the patient push out and tense the abdominal wall facilitates needle placement. By gravity, 1 to 4 L of dialysis solution is infused through the needle until the abdomen becomes moderately tense. A guidewire is passed through the same needle into the peritoneal cavity. The needle is withdrawn. A dilator with overlying peel-away sheath is advanced through the fascia over the guidewire. The guidewire and dilator are removed. Stiffened over a stylet, the dialysis catheter is directed through the sheath toward the pelvis. As the deep catheter cuff advances, the sheath is peeled away. When the deep cuff stops at the level of the fascia, the remainder of the sheath is removed from around the catheter. Subcutaneous tunneling of the catheter to the selected exit site is discussed in a separate section to follow. After the establishment of careful wound hemostasis, the subcutaneous tissue and skin are sutured in separate layers.

Radiologically Guided Percutaneous Placement

Interventional nephrologists and radiologists have used fluoroscopy to guide insertion of PD catheters.[106–108] The procedure is similar to that described for blind percutaneous placement except that the abdomen is not prefilled with dialysate. Needle entry into the peritoneal cavity is confirmed with fluoroscopy by observing the flow of injected contrast solution around loops of bowel. The guidewire is advanced into the pelvis under fluoroscopic control. The remainder of the procedure proceeds as described for blind placement. Although the radiopaque tubing stripe permits the radiologist to observe the final intraperitoneal configuration of the catheter, the proximity of adhesions or omentum cannot be assessed. As with blind placement, the deep catheter cuff is located just outside of the fascia.

Peritoneoscopic Implantation with Y-Tec and Quill Catheter Guide

Peritoneoscopic placement of chronic peritoneal catheters is increasingly popular and is now more frequently performed than blind placement. The basic components for peritoneoscopic implantation of Tenckhoff catheters are fairly simple (Fig. 13–16). The trocar and surrounding spiral Quill catheter guide are just over 2 mm in diameter and 150 mm in length. The tapered and coiled Quill guide is made of very thin plastic attached to the end of the cannula by a tab. The tab is secured in place by the internal trocar.[37] A small peritoneoscope can be advanced through the cannula after the trocar is removed. Peritoneoscopic placement differs from both blind and dissective techniques in several ways.

To begin placement, a 2-cm incision is made in the skin, and subcutaneous tissue is anchored to the abdominal musculature with hemostats. The trocar with stylet and surrounding Quill catheter guide is advanced to the abdominal wall (Fig. 13–17), and then with a rotating motion is advanced into the peritoneum. The trocar is removed, and the peritoneoscope is advanced into the trocar. The patient is asked to take several deep breaths; the passage of smooth,

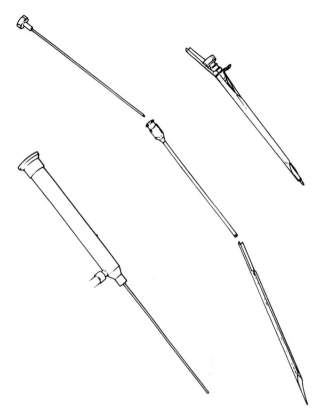

Figure 13–16. The basic components of the Y-Tec system for peritoneoscopic implantation of a chronic peritoneal dialysis catheter, showing the stylet, cannula, Quill catheter guide, and peritoneoscope. (From Ash and Daugirdas,[217] with permission.)

glistening surfaces with blood vessels past the tip of the peritoneoscope confirms the intraperitoneal location of the cannula. The peritoneoscope is then removed, and 600 mL of air is injected using a disposable bulb and two one-way valves.

The peritoneoscope is reinserted into the cannula, and the cannula is retracted under vision until a clear airspace appears between the bowel and the anterior abdominal wall. The cannula is advanced under vision into the longest and clearest space between the visceral and parietal peritoneum until the hub of the cannula reaches the skin level, or the tip reaches tissues at the end of the airspace. The peritoneoscope and cannula are removed from the Quill guide and dilators are advanced to spread the guide and surrounding abdominal musculature to a diameter of 6 mm. The peritoneal catheter with this internal stylet is then advanced through the guide. The deep cuff proceeds through the guide, stopping at the anterior fascia of the musculature. The deep cuff is advanced into the musculature with a cuff-positioner tool that stops automatically when the cuff is in the proper location. While the catheter is held in place, the spiral guide is retracted around the catheter; at this point, 50

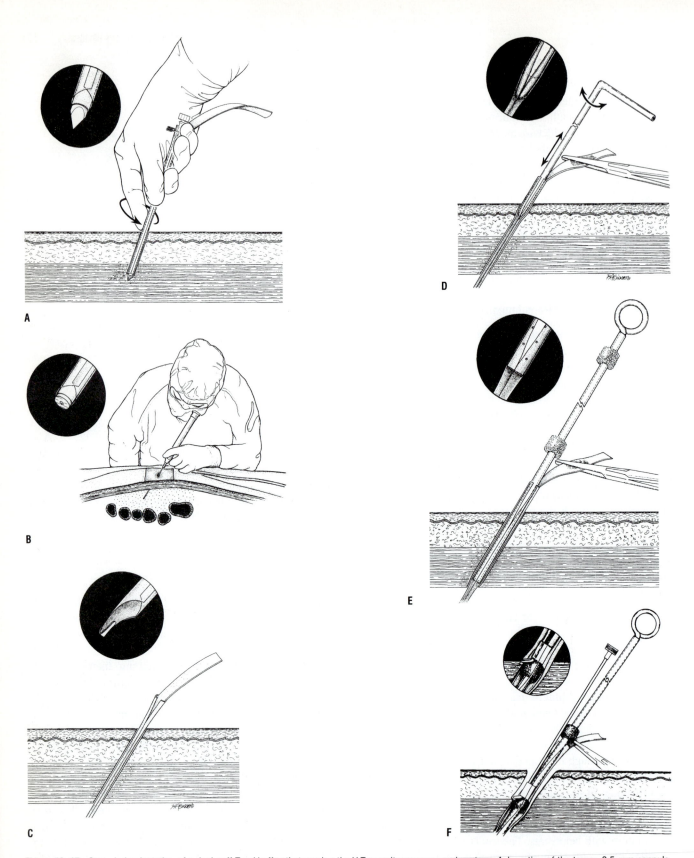

Figure 13–17. Steps in implantation of a dual-cuff Tenckhoff catheter using the Y-Tec peritoneoscope and system. *A.* Insertion of the trocar, 2.5-mm cannula, and coiled Quill guide through the abdominal wall. *B.* After removal of the trocar, visual inspection confirms the intraperitoneal location of the cannula; subsequent air insufflation creates a space through which the cannula and Quill guide are advanced, adjacent to the parietal peritoneum. *C.* The Quill guide in the desired catheter location. *D.* Radial dilation of the coiled Quill guide to 6-mm diameter. *E.* Insertion of the Tenckhoff catheter (with internal stylet) through the dilated Quill guide; the deep cuff stops at the outer fascia. *F.* The cuff-positioner tool is used to advance the deep cuff through the Quill guide into the abdominal musculature. The Quill guide is removed while the catheter is held stationary, and the stylet is removed. The free end of the catheter is then tunneled subcutaneously to place the superficial cuff 2 cm from the exit site. (From Ash and Daugirdas,[217] with permission.)

mL of saline is injected into the catheter. The easy return of some of this fluid, and changes in the level of an air-fluid interface in the catheter during respiration, confirms that the catheter is located in the peritoneum and has no kinks.

The desired skin exit site is chosen after laying the catheter over the skin and incising the skin with a #11 blade. The gently curved Tunnelor tool is advanced from the skin exit site through the subcutaneous tissue, through the primary incision. For arcuate (swan-neck) catheters, the tip of the Tunnelor is directed under the course of the catheter as it lies on the skin surface. The catheter is attached to this tool and pulled through the exit site. Hemostats are compressed around the catheter and advanced with the catheter until they reach the desired location of the subcutaneous cuff. The hemostats are then opened and removed through the primary incision. While a hemostat secures the catheter near the deep cuff, the catheter is drawn through the subcutaneous tunnel, bringing the subcutaneous cuff into the desired location. Sutures are not used at the skin exit site. The primary incision is closed with nylon or other skin sutures.

Surgical Laparoscopic Implantation

With the revolutionary introduction of laparoscopic cholecystectomy into surgical practice, surgeons have endeavored to apply the laparoscope to virtually every abdominal procedure. However, laparoscopic techniques used by surgeons to establish PD access are still evolving. Currently, there is no standardized methodology for laparoscopic PD catheter implantation. The process is partially impeded by the attempted use of ordinary laparoscopic equipment that is familiar to surgeons but is not suitably adapted to catheter insertion. As a consequence, reported outcomes have been extremely variable and frequently demonstrate no clear advantage to implantation of catheters by standard open dissection.

The strength of laparoscopy is that it allows an opportunity to visibly address problems that adversely affect catheter outcome, namely, catheter tip migration, omental entrapment, and peritoneal adhesions.[109–111] The identification and preemptive correction of these problems at the time of the implantation procedure are potential advantages of surgical laparoscopy over other catheter insertion techniques.

One of the impediments for accepting laparoscopy as a means of implanting PD catheters has been the necessity for general anesthesia. Insufflation of CO_2 gas to create the pneumoperitoneum produces pain and requires general anesthesia. In addition, insufflation of carbon dioxide can produce metabolic acidosis and cardiac arrhythmias. Recently, the use of an alternative insufflation gas (nitrous oxide, helium), which is painless and metabolically inert, has permitted safe laparoscopy under local anesthesia.[111,112]

The implantation of a laparoscopic dialysis catheter is accomplished using a two-port technique. The peritoneal catheter is inserted through a port at the previously designated paramedian site while the implant procedure is continuously monitored with a laparoscope from a second port location. Any patient who is a candidate for catheter insertion by open dissection is a candidate for laparoscopic implantation. A history of previous abdominal surgery and the location of surgical scars only dictate the manner in which the gas insufflation needle (Veress needle) and the initial camera port are inserted. Under local anesthesia, with the patient protruding and tensing the abdominal wall to create a rigid platform, the Veress needle is safely inserted using the closed method through a pararectus incision on the side opposite of the planned catheter insertion site. Under general anesthesia, closed insertion of the Veress needle can be achieved at the lateral border of the rectus sheath below the costal margin in either of the upper abdominal quadrants. Alternatively, and in the event of midline scars or multiple previous abdominal surgeries, the initial port is placed by opening the peritoneum under direct vision.

After insertion of the camera port and creation of a satisfactory pneumoperitoneum, laparoscopic exploration of the peritoneal cavity is performed. The laparoscope permits evaluation for undiagnosed abdominal wall hernias, redundant omentum, and adhesions that create compartmentalization or obscure the planned catheter insertion site. Adjunctive procedures to address redundant omentum and adhesions are discussed further on. Abdominal wall hernias are covered in a separate section.

Under laparoscopic control, the port cannula through which the catheter will be placed is inserted at the predetermined paramedian site and tunneled through the rectus sheath in a craniocaudal direction for 4 to 6 cm before entry into the peritoneal cavity. An example of an atraumatic port device that permits safe tunneling through the rectus sheath by a process of radial expansion (instead of cutting with trocar blades) is shown in Fig. 13–18. Rectus sheath tunneling is important for maintaining pelvic orientation of the catheter to prevent migration of the catheter tip.[101,111,113,114] In addition, the tangential passage of the catheter through the abdominal wall reduces the risk of pericannular leak or hernia.

The PD catheter, straightened over a stylet, is advanced through the port under laparoscopic control. The stylet is partially withdrawn as the catheter is advanced. The catheter tip is positioned in the retrovesical space. To make sure that the deep cuff has passed through the anterior rectus sheath, the catheter is advanced until the cuff is visible in the peritoneal cavity. Once the port and stylet are removed, the catheter is gently withdrawn until the deep cuff is just below the anterior rectus sheath. Subcutaneous tunneling of the catheter to the selected exit site is discussed further on. After the establishment of careful wound hemo-

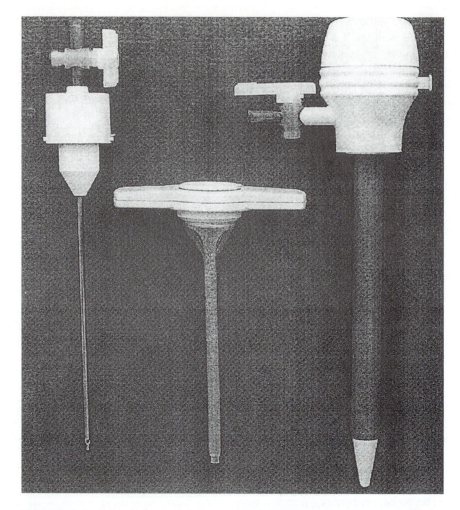

Figure 13–18. Laparoscopic atraumatic port system includes, from left to right, Veress-type needle for pneumoperitoneum, radially expandable plastic sleeve, and 7/8-mm dilator-cannula assembly. Needle with overlying sleeve is tunneled through rectus sheath. Needle is withdrawn and sleeve serves as conduit for introduction of dilator-cannula assembly. Dilator is withdrawn and cannula serves as port for insertion of dialysis catheter.

stasis, the subcutaneous tissue and skin are sutured in separate layers.

Redundant, thin, filmy omentum that extends into the pelvis and lies in juxtaposition to the catheter tip increases the risk of omental entrapment. The performance of an omental tacking-up procedure (omentopexy) eliminates this complication.[115,116] The procedure is performed only when the omentum is found to extend into the pelvis. The employment of selective criteria for omentopexy eliminates the performance of unnecessary procedures and minimizes cost. Omentopexy requires insertion of an additional port through which grasping forceps are used to pull the omentum into the upper abdomen (Fig. 13–18). Here it is fixed to the abdominal wall or falciform ligament with a suture or tacking device. Laparoscopic resection of the omentum has been performed but requires more instrumentation and procedure time without increasing the benefit provided by omentopexy. Alternatively, the omentum may be teased out through one of the port incision sites; this has permitted partial omental resection. Although the procedure is shorter than laparoscopic resection and requires no extra instrumentation, partial omentectomy is still followed with an incidence of flow obstruction as high as 10 percent.[97–99,101]

Adhesions from previous abdominal surgery may involve the parietal peritoneum at the planned site for catheter insertion or form intraperitoneal compartments that potentially contribute to poor drainage function. When these lesions are detected laparoscopically, additional ports may be inserted to permit adhesiolysis with laparoscopic scissors, cautery, or an ultrasonic shears device (ultrasonic scalpel). However, it is neither necessary nor desirable to mobilize every adhesion. Omental adhesions to the abdominal wall above the level of the pelvis that will not interfere with drainage of dialysate from the upper abdomen may even protect from omental entrapment of the catheter. Extensive adhesiolysis to create a dialyzable space has met with variable success.[109,110] Damage to the parietal peritoneum may result in insufficient dialyzable surface area. Immediate use of the created space by standard volumes of dialysate is necessary to prevent obliteration of the peritoneal cavity from acute adhesions between raw surface areas. Dialysate fluid leaks through laparoscopic port sites and around the catheter may still occur despite attempts to obtain watertight closure. In addition, prolonged anesthesia time and conversion to an open laparotomy to control bleeding or repair accidental enterotomies can potentially complicate such heroic attempts to create a space suitable for PD.

Presternal Implantation

The presternal PD catheter is utilized when an abdominal catheter exit site is not suitable.[117] The device consists of an abdominal catheter component that is joined to an extension tube capable of reaching the upper chest wall. The catheter is ideally suited for patients who are obese, those with abdominal ostomies, incontinent children and adults with diapers, and those individuals who wish to take deep tub baths without risking exit-site contamination.

The abdominal catheter currently provided with the presternal catheter system has a 12-mm Silastic bead and a 20-mm Dacron flange just distal to a single deep catheter cuff (Missouri catheter). The large bead and flange can be implanted only by the open dissection technique. A single-cuff Tenckhoff-style catheter is substituted for the bead-and-flange device to enable laparoscopic implantation of the abdominal segment.[118] Laparoscopic implantation of the abdominal component is accomplished as described above. Fig. 13–19 shows the general configuration and position of the components of the presternal catheter.

The location of the presternal catheter's exit site should be planned preoperatively. The exit site should avoid the open collar area, bra line, and fleshy part of the breast. The subcutaneous tract should be parasternal in location and not cross the midline in the event that the patient should subsequently require a midline sternotomy for cardiovascular surgery. The alignment of the swan-neck presternal segment is such that the exit limb is oriented medially with the exit site at least 2.5 to 3 cm off the midline.

After the abdominal segment is implanted, a 3- to 4-cm transverse or vertical incision is made 4 to 5 cm lateral to the midline at the level of the second or third intercostal space. An 8-mm vascular tunneler (vascular tunneler, sheath, and tip, Scanlan International, St. Paul, MN) is passed from the abdominal wound to the chest incision. The tunneler is advanced in a plane as close to the fascia as possible. The presternal segment of the catheter is pulled through the tunneler, taking care to keep the radiopaque guide stripe straight. The tunneling sheath is then carefully withdrawn, leaving the catheter in the subcutaneous tract. When the catheter is appropriately positioned, the desired lengths of the tubes are measured and the redundant portions are trimmed. A length of the presternal segment is temporarily pulled into the abdominal wound to enable this process. It is important to preserve at least a 5-cm segment of the abdominal catheter above the fascia in order to facilitate insertion of the connector. The titanium connector is inserted into the catheter ends and secured with 2–0-Prolene sutures tied over the respective connector grooves of the abdominal and presternal segments and then to each other. The connector is placed in the subcutaneous tract and the presternal segment is pulled back into its proper position. A subcutaneous pocket is created under the upper portion of the chest incision to accommodate the swan-neck bend of the intercuff catheter segment. Subcutaneous tunneling of the catheter to the selected exit site is discussed further on. After establishing careful wound hemostasis, subcutaneous tissue and skin are sutured in separate layers.

On occasion, patients may be encountered in whom the lower abdomen is not suitable for a catheter exit site owing to obesity or from having sustained massive weight loss with a resultant large panniculus or floppy skin folds. The upper abdomen is frequently an acceptable site in these individuals, but standard catheters will not reach far enough without significantly compromising the deep pelvic location of the catheter tip and predisposing the device to omental entrapment. Although they may be ideal candidates, some patients refuse a presternal catheter because of body image concerns. An alternative application of the presternal catheter system is to use the extension tube to reach the upper abdominal region. This provides an environmentally friendly exit site that is easily visible to the patient without sacrificing proper pelvic location of the catheter tip. Insertion and connection techniques are exactly the same as described for presternal catheter placement, the only difference being that the extension tube is tailored to reach the upper abdomen instead of the chest. The exit limb alignment of the swan-neck extension segment can be oriented medially or laterally in the upper abdomen, depending on which configuration produces the best exit-site location.

Testing Catheter Patency and Hydraulic Function

It is important to test catheter patency and flow function before accepting intraperitoneal placement of the catheter and ending the procedure. If the catheter has poor flow function at the outset, it is unreasonable to presume that somehow it will improve by the time the patient reaches the postoperative recovery area. Catheter position should be revised until

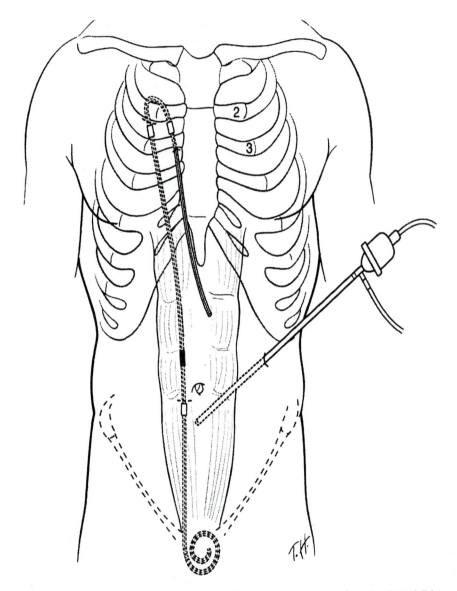

Figure 13–19. Schematic view of the laparoscopically implanted swan-neck presternal peritoneal dialysis catheter, showing the relative positions of incisions, exit wound, catheter cuffs, titanium connector, subcutaneous catheter tunnel tract, and laparoscopic port site. (From Crabtree,[118] with permission.

satisfactory flow function is achieved before quitting the operation.

Checking patency can be as simple as injecting 50 mL of saline into the catheter. The easy return of some of this fluid, and changes in the level of an air-fluid interface in the catheter during respiration, confirms that the catheter is located in the peritoneum and has no kinks. Alternatively, trial irrigation can be performed to identify potential problems with flow function. With the patient in reverse Trendelenburg position, a standard 1-L bag of normal saline for intravenous administration with heparin (1000 U/L) is observed for unimpeded inflow and drainage by gravity. A residual of

250 to 300 mL is left in the abdomen to reduce the likelihood of intraperitoneal structures sucking up against the catheter toward the end of the drainage process.

It is advisable to check for catheter patency and flow function prior to exteriorizing the catheter through the exit site. This will prevent unnecessary tunnel tract and exit-site trauma in the event that catheter repositioning is required. If poor flow function occurs during laparoscopic implantation, visual evaluation for the usual causes (omental wrap, epiploic appendices, uterine tubes) can be performed and problems resolved without disturbing the catheter. Therefore, to save operative time during laparoscopic implantation, testing for flow function is conducted after tunnel tract and exit-site construction. The primary surgical wound is closed and dressings are applied during the trial irrigation procedure.

Primary Exteriorization of the Catheter: Construction of Subcutaneous Tunnel and Exit Site

The same principles apply to subcutaneous tunnel tract and exit-site construction irrespective of the technique utilized to implant the catheter. The catheter should exit the skin facing in a lateral or downward direction to discourage pooling of cutaneous detritus, water, and bacteria in the skin exit sinus. The configuration of the subcutaneous tunnel tract and exit-site location should be determined prior to the implantation procedure and is discussed under "Preoperative Planning," above.

The catheter is tunneled from the insertion site to the designated exit site with a tunneling tool that does not exceed the diameter of the catheter. The exit site should be the smallest hole possible that permits passage of the catheter tubing. There are a number of commercially available devices specifically designed for this purpose. The use of hemostat clamps, laparoscope ports, and other oversized instruments to tunnel catheters result in large, patulous pericannular wounds that increase the risk for exit-site and tunnel tract infection, catheter infection-related peritonitis, and catheter loss.[119]

Tunneling stylets are available that feature recessed, ribbed stems over which the catheter end is attached with a friction grip. The other ends of these devices possess varying degrees of curvature and sharp trocar tips to facilitate arcuate passage through the subcutaneous tissues and penetration of the skin. Tunneling stylets of this design are passed from the primary incision toward the exit site. Another tunneling tool design is passed from a small incision made at the designated exit site toward the primary incision. The tip of the catheter is attached to the tool and the catheter pulled through the subcutaneous tissue and out the exit site. Once the end of the catheter has emerged through the exit site, sharp-tipped tunneling tools should be removed and set aside. Insertion of the catheter adapter into the end of the tubing at this point will prevent inadvertent retraction of the catheter tip through the exit wound. The remainder of the catheter and superficial cuff is pulled through the subcutaneous tract with care not to kink the tubing or displace the deep catheter cuff. Applying a hemostat lightly to the catheter tubing outside of the superficial cuff facilitates the process of seating the cuff in the subcutaneous tract. As the catheter is pulled through the tract, the tips of the hemostats are drawn into the tunnel. When the tips of the hemostats reach the desired position of the subcutaneous cuff, the tips are spread and the hemostat removed. The catheter is pulled through the exit wound and the superficial cuff is drawn into the tunnel until it rests at the designated location within 2 to 4 cm of the exit site.

To reduce the risk of infection, no sutures are used to anchor the catheter at the exit site. The tubing is stabilized near the exit wound with tincture of benzoin and sterile adhesive strips. The exit site and other operative incisions are covered with a sterile nonocclusive gauze dressing held in place with tape or an air-permeable adhesive sheet. The catheter adapter and transfer set should be assembled to the catheter at the time of the implantation procedure to eliminate performing these necessary plumbing connections in a less sterile environment. The entire catheter assembly is flushed with 20 mL of heparin (100 U/mL) to prevent fibrin plugging of the catheter.

Catheter-Burying Procedure with Secondary Exteriorization

Traditional surgical implantation of Tenckhoff catheters involves immediate exteriorization of the external segment through the skin, so that the catheter can be used for supportive PD or for intermittent infusions during the break-in period. In order to prevent blockage and confirm function, the catheter is flushed weekly with saline or dialysate; each exchange carries the same risk of peritonitis as does CAPD therapy. The catheter must also be bandaged and the skin exit site must be kept clean in the weeks after placement to avoid bacterial contamination of the exit site. The patient must therefore be trained in some techniques of catheter care. It has always been difficult to decide when to place a PD catheter in a patient with chronic kidney disease. If the catheter is placed too early, the patient may spend weeks to months caring for a catheter that is not used for dialysis. If the catheter is placed after the patient becomes uremic, it is often used for PD therapy without a break-in period.

Moncrief and Popovich devised a placement technique in which the entire peritoneal catheter can be buried under the skin some weeks or months before it is used.[120] The catheter burying technique was first described for placement of a modified Tenckhoff catheter with a 2.5-cm superficial cuff, but the technique has been adapted for standard dual-cuff Tenckhoff catheters.[121–123] In the original technique, the external portion of the catheter was brought through a 2- to 3-cm skin exit site (much larger than the usual 0.5-cm incision). The catheter was then tied off with silk suture, coiled, and placed into a "pouch" created under the skin. The skin exit site was then closed. Weeks to months later, the original skin exit site was opened and the free end of the catheter brought through the original large skin exit site.[120,121]

Burying the entire external limb of the catheter under the skin in a subcutaneous tunnel eliminates an exit wound.[121] Healing and tissue ingrowth into the cuffs occurs while the catheter is buried in this sterile environment. At a later date, 3 to 5 weeks after insertion, a small incision is made 2 to 4 cm distal to the subcutaneous cuff and the external limb of the catheter is brought out through the skin. The catheter may be left in place under the skin for many months. During this time, the patient is not faced with exit-site maintenance issues or risks of infection. Full-volume PD may be initiated immediately following exteriorization without concerns of pericannular leak. The goal of burying the PD catheter was to allow ingrowth of tissue into the catheter cuffs without any chance of bacterial colonization and to allow a transcutaneous exit site to be created after tissue had fully grown into the deep and subcutaneous cuffs. Burying the catheter effectively eliminated early peri-catheter leaks and decreased the incidence of peritonitis. In 66 months of follow-up, patients with the buried Tenckhoff catheter had peritonitis infection rates of 0.017 to 0.37 infections per year, vs. 1.3 to 1.9 infections per year in control patients.[120] In a study of 26 buried Tenckhoff catheters, the incidence of infectious complications during PD was 0.8 infections per year, and catheter-related peritonitis was only 0.036 per patient-year.[121] A retrospective study confirmed a significantly lower catheter infection and peritonitis rate in patients having had buried catheters and a significantly longer catheter life,[124] although the procedure was not effective when used for single-cuff catheters.[125] Exit-site infections were not decreased in catheters that were buried, but this is understandable, since a large exit site was created when the catheter was buried, and a similarly large site was recreated when the catheter was exteriorized. Creating the pouch under the skin requires a considerable amount of dissection and trauma near the exit site. The size of the pocket limits the length of catheter that can be coiled and buried under the skin, thus also limiting the external length of the catheter after exteriorization. The exit site must be opened widely to remove the catheter, because the coil rests in a position distant from the skin exit site. Subcutaneous adhesions to the silk suture around the catheter further restrict removal. Increased trauma near the exit site during placement and removal of the catheter have caused an increased incidence of early exit-site infection with this technique.[12,13,52,88] In one study of "embedded" catheters in 26 adult patients (with mean subcutaneous residence of 79.5 days), 2 patients developed local seromas and 12 developed subcutaneous hematomas (5 of which were revised surgically).[68] At catheter "activation," there were a number of flow problems: 9 patients developed fibrin thrombi (2 requiring operative clearance) and 4 patients had omental catheter obstruction (4 requiring omentectomy).

When the Tenckhoff catheter was buried by standard techniques, there were a total of 27 complications in 26 catheter placements, with 13 requiring corrective surgery. Despite initial reports by the authors of reduction in the rate of peritonitis and colonization of bacterial biofilms in the catheter segments between the two cuffs, a controlled randomized study has failed to confirm these claims.[69,126,127] A possible reason for the failure to reduce the incidence of infectious complications may be the inability of the body to provide an effective "seal" around the external cuff while the catheter is buried, partly because the external cuff and coiled external tubing are buried in a pouch under the skin, according to the initially described procedure. Therefore, upon exteriorization of the catheter, the process of healing starts all over again. Prischl et al. have also reported a high incidence of seromas, subcutaneous hematomas and fibrin thrombi postoperatively with this technique.[128] Other methods of placement—such as tunneling the catheter straight toward the skin, making a bend in the catheter, and then tunneling toward a temporary exit site under the umbilicus—may diminish general trauma near the external cuff, allow better bonding of the cuff to surrounding subcutaneous tissues, and diminish the size of exit site created in exteriorizing the catheter, all leading to a decreased incidence of early exit-site infection after exteriorization.

Burying of the external limb of the catheter can be performed as a component of any of the implantation techniques. The particular implantation procedure employed is conducted as previously described up to the point of preparation for subcutaneous tunneling of the catheter. At this juncture, a 1- to 1.5-cm secondary incision is made at the designated exit site; the catheter is tunneled and exteriorized through this secondary incision. Downward from the secondary incision, a linear subcutaneous tunnel is dissected by sharp and blunt dissection for a distance of 5 to 6 cm. The external segment of the catheter is trimmed to fit the length of the created tunnel. The catheter is flushed with heparinized saline and the end of the tubing is plugged. With care not to bend or curl the tubing, the external limb is introduced into the subcutaneous tunnel with a hemostat or other suitable instrument. The primary and secondary incisions are closed and sterile dressings are applied.

For best results, the catheter is allowed to reside in the subcutaneous tissues for a period of at least 3 to 5 weeks. This allows for adequate tissue ingrowth into the catheter cuffs. Secondary exteriorization of the external catheter limb can be performed under local anesthesia. The patient is prepped and draped in the manner as described for implantation. Caution must be exercised during infiltration of the local anesthetic to prevent accidental puncture of the catheter tubing. A 0.5-cm incision is made through or near the previous secondary incision scar. A hemostat is used to dissect down to the catheter and lift it up and out of the wound. The length of the external end of the catheter is pulled from the subcutaneous tunnel. Since tissue ingrowth into the superficial cuff has already occurred, application of gentle traction when exteriorizing the external limb can be performed without concern for displacement of the deeper transabdominal portion. The tubing is unplugged, an adapter and transfer set attached, and catheter patency checked with a saline flush. Although the exit site may appear patulous, no sutures should be used to repair it. Since movement of the catheter at the exit site may slow wound healing, the catheter should be immobilized with tincture of benzoin and sterile adhesive strips. A nonocclusive dressing is applied as described for primary exteriorization.

When catheters are placed by the Y-Tec procedure, the Quill and cannula of the system can be reassembled and used to bury the external portion of dual-cuff Tenckhoff and Advantage catheters in a linear direction under the umbilicus through only one exit site (Fig 13–20). The catheter exit site is made slightly larger than the standard exit site. The Quill and cannula are inserted through this exit site to create a long, straight tunnel for the external end of the catheter. The catheter is blocked with an internal plug rather than an external silk suture. We have used this technique to bury and then remove over 40 Tenckhoff and Advantage catheters. There have been few early complications of hematoma, seroma, exit-site infection, or outflow failure, and all catheters have functioned after exteriorization.

The first portion of the Y-Tec placement procedure is exactly as usual for a dual-cuff Tenckhoff catheter.[61,62,129,130] The only difference is that the skin exit site is chosen slightly more distal from the subcutaneous cuff than usual, and the exit-site incision is made slightly larger (1 cm, or two widths of the No. 11 scalpel blade, rather than the usual 0.5-cm stab wound). After the catheter is tunneled and exteriorized through the exit site, the steps for burying the catheter are as follows:

1. The Quill guide is reattached to the cannula, first inserting the trocar to lock the tab into place and then clicking the body of the Quill over the cannula.
2. The Quill guide and cannula are laid over the skin, in a direction just below the umbilicus (for laterally placed catheters). The catheter is then cut so that the free end of the catheter reaches the end of the Quill guide.
3. An injection of 10 mL of sterile saline with 1000 units of heparin is made into the catheter; then the "bullet" end of the Tunnelor tool is inserted and the tip is broken off by rotating the tool backward and forward. The outer end of the bullet is advanced into the catheter a few millimeters, using hemostats.
4. The Quill/trocar assembly is inserted into skin just next to the catheter, at an angle to reach the middle of the subcutaneous space.
5. The Quill is advanced in a direction parallel to the skin surface, directing it into the subcutaneous space just below umbilicus. The tip of the Quill is kept in the middle of the subcutaneous tissue, be-

tween the musculature and the skin. If pain develops, the Quill is redirected to avoid the muscle layer, dermis, or fibrous adhesions.
6. The trocar and cannula are removed from the Quill, and the tab of the Quill is grasped with a hemostat. The Quill is dilated with the small dilator and then the larger 6-mm dilator.
7. The catheter is gently grasped with nontoothed forceps or hemostat and the free end of the catheter is advanced into the Quill guide.
8. The catheter is continued to be advanced into the Quill guide until the bend of the catheter reaches the skin level. The bend of the catheter is held under the skin with forceps and the Quill guide is withdrawn from around the catheter.
9. The skin exit site is closed with an absorbable suture; the needle tip is pointed upward, away from the catheter, when it is being advanced through the subcutaneous tissue.

To exteriorize the catheter some weeks or months later, our current technique is as follows:

1. The original skin exit site is anesthetized, being careful to not inject too deeply (if necessary, the edges of the incision may be raised with toothed forceps).
2. The original exit-site skin incision is opened using mosquito hemostats (if less than 2 months have passed since placement) or scalpel (if more than 2 months of healing). Using larger hemostats, the exit site and subcutaneous tissue are opened to the original 1-cm width.
3. The wound is probed with a hemostat until the catheter is found in its tunnel.
4. Tissue is spread parallel to the tunnel, freeing the tunnel from subcutaneous tissue along its medial and lateral borders.
5. The tip of the hemostat is advanced under the tunnel, and the tunnel and catheter are lifted until they are at skin level.
6. If the tunnel is very thin and wispy, it is broken open by being grabbed with toothed forceps; portions are then pulled off the catheter. If the tunnel is thick and substantial, it is grasped with small-toothed forceps, and the grasped portion is cut just below the forceps with Metzenbaum scissors.
7. One jaw of a smooth-tipped forceps is advanced under the catheter, grasping and lifting the catheter and pulling it through the skin exit site. The outside portion is held with the fingers while the tunneled portion is grabbed and pulled out. This is repeated until the tunneled portion is completely removed.
8. The plug is expressed outward and removed by pressing on the sides of the catheter.

1.   Reattach the Quill guide to cannula, first inserting the trocar to "lock" the tab into place and then "clicking" the body of the Quill over the cannula

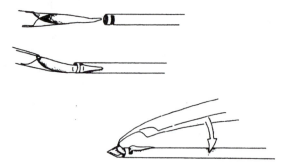

2.   Lay the Quill guide and cannula over the skin, in direction just below the umbilicus (for laterally placed catheters). Then cut the catheter so that free end of catheter reaches the end of the Quill guide.

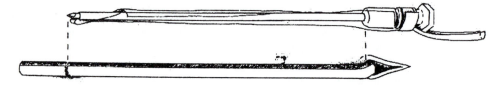

3.   Inject 10 cc sterile saline with 1000 units of heparin into the catheter, then insert the "bullet" end of the Tunnelor tool, and break off the tip by rotating the tool backward and forward. Advance the outer end of the bullet into the catheter a few millimeters, using hemostats.

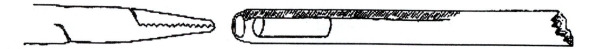

4.   Insert the Quill/trocar assembly into skin just next to the catheter, at an angle to reach the middle of the subcutaneous space.

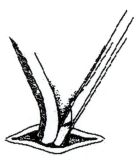

5.   Advance the Quill in a direction parallel to the skin surface, directing it into the subcutaneous space just below umbilicus. Keep the tip of the Quill in the middle of the subcutaneous tissue, between the musculature and the skin. If pain develops, redirect the Quill to avoid the muscle layer, the dermis, of fibrous adhesions.

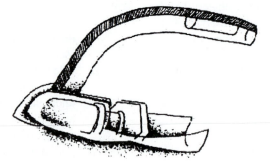

Figure 13–20. Steps for "burying" the external portion of a peritoneal dialysis catheter after bringing the external portion through the skin exit site, using the Cannula and Quill components of the Y-Tec system for placement of peritoneal dialysis catheters.

6. Remove the trocar and cannula from the Quill, and grasp the tab of the Quill with a hemostat. Dilate the Quill with the small dilator then a larger 6-mm dilator.

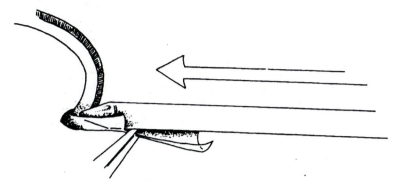

7. Gently grasp the catheter with nontoothed forceps or hemostat and advance the free end of the catheter into the Quill guide.

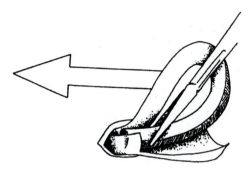

8. Continue to advance the catheter into the Quill guide until the bend of the catheter reaches the skin level. Then hold the bend of the catheter under the skin with forceps, and withdraw the Quill guide from around the catheter.

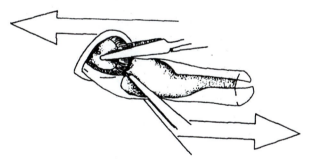

9. Close the skin exist site with an absorbable suture; point the needle tip upward away from the catheter when advancing it through the subcutaneous tissue.

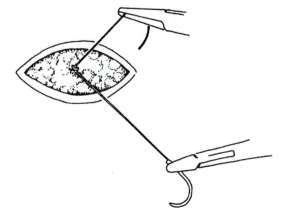

Figure 13–20. (*cont.*)

9. A suitable long-term connector is attached to the end of the catheter, injected with 50 mL of sterile saline, and checked for free outflow of fluid and change in air-fluid level with respiration, indicating that it is completely open.

10. The exit site should not be closed with suture. A bandage and nonocclusive dressing should be applied over the catheter exit site, as is done for chronic catheter care in CAPD.

Our technique for exteriorization of the first 20 catheters included a method for creating a tighter exit site near the original exit site. The catheter was exteriorized through the original exit site just as above. Using a scalpel, a stab wound (0.5 cm) was made through the skin just 1 cm lateral to the original exit site. Hemostats were advanced through the new exit site, under the skin, and through the original exit site. The tip of the external portion of the catheter was grasped with the hemostats and brought back under the skin and through the new exit site. The original skin exit site was closed with subcutaneous sutures.

At Dr. Ash's center, dual-cuff Tenckhoff and Advantage catheters have been buried after placement since 1993. Patients selected for this type of placement were those with a trend of kidney function indicating a need for PD within 1 to 6 months. That is, peritoneal catheters were placed when PD therapy was anticipated rather than when it was immediately necessary. The first 30 catheters placed by this technique were studied, with time from placement to exteriorization being 1 week to 1 year. On exteriorization, all of the buried catheters were immediately used for PD, and no patient required hemodialysis while awaiting tissue ingrowth to the catheter cuffs or resolution of problems with the PD catheter. Follow-up analysis of these catheters ranged from 3 to 12 months.

Previous publications regarding the burying of PD catheters have indicated a number of minor complications following the procedure. Complications seen with these 30 catheters in our practice have included bruising or hematoma formation over the buried portion of the catheter (3 patients), outflow failure on first use (1 patient), exit-site redness (10 patients when using a second exit site, 3 patients using the original site), exit-site infection within 4 weeks of use (1 patient), and peritonitis within 4 weeks of use (1 patient). Long-term rates of peritonitis for these patients have been compared to those of patients with catheters exteriorized immediately on implantation. Peritonitis rates are lower for patients with buried catheters though not statistically different from those in patients with immediately exteriorized catheters.

In planning for hemodialysis of patients with end-stage renal disease (ESRD), it is common practice to place a fistula or graft several months before the need for initiation of dialysis, so that they can mature before use. PD catheters also mature after placement, with fibrous tissue ingrowth into the cuffs and development of a fibrous tunnel. The fully ingrown catheter is more resistant to infection of cuffs and the surface of the catheter. The technique of burying PD catheters after placement allows this maturation to occur before the catheter is used, much as with fistulas and grafts. It also permits the time of catheter insertion to be separated from the time of use, without requiring the patient to learn how to care for the catheter site or observe the catheter site for potential complications. At the time of initiation of dialysis, the patient and physician can focus attention on the proper performance of the technique and patient response rather than on function of the catheter. The patient can be trained in full-volume CAPD techniques rather than in the break-in or cycler techniques used for immediately exteriorized catheters.

A curious aspect of the burying technique is that it seems contrary to "the rules" of catheter break-in. In immediately exteriorized catheters, it is necessary to infuse and drain dialysate or saline (with or without heparin) at least weekly, to prevent outflow failure or obstruction of the catheter. However, with the completely buried catheter, there is no infusion of any fluid for periods up to a year. Why is this possible? It may be that in the exteriorized catheter, stress and strain on the catheter and its compliance allows some fluid to enter and exit the side holes during patient movement. The buried catheter has less motion and with a secure blockage there is very little fluid inflow/outflow through the holes during normal activity. Further, the infusion of saline or dialysate during break-in techniques adds a bioincompatible fluid to the abdomen at a time before the catheter is "biolized" or protein/lipid coated. The catheter becomes biolized in the absence of dialysate or saline in the peritoneum. When PD is begun, the catheter is already biolized and less likely to develop omental attachment, even in patients with active omentum. Studies of catheters buried after surgical placement have still shown some early loss of catheters due to outflow failure, but the rates are not higher than in immediately exteriorized catheters.[68,131] In our study, the peritoneoscopic technique was used for placement of the intraperitoneal portion of the catheter. This method places the catheter against the parietal peritoneum in an area free of adhesions or bowel loops, and this method for placement has already shown a very low incidence of outflow failure on immediately exteriorized catheters. Outflow failure is not increased in incidence by burying the catheter for weeks to months.

POSTOPERATIVE CATHETER CARE

Postoperative management for catheters that are exteriorized primarily includes catheter irrigation with 1 L of heparinized saline performed as an in-and-out flush within 72 hours following surgery and weekly thereafter until PD is initiated. PD is generally delayed for a minimum of 2 weeks to permit complete wound healing. Unless excessive drainage is present, dressings are changed weekly for 2 weeks, at which time the patient begins a routine of daily exit-site cleansing with antibacterial soap. The patient is permitted to resume showering after 1 month if wound healing has been uncomplicated. Sterile gauze dressing over the exit site is encouraged. Tub bathing and swimming with immersion of the exit-site is discouraged. Catheters that are exteriorized secondarily can be used immediately for full volume PD. Exit-site management for secondarily exteriorized catheters is the same as described for primary exteriorization.

EFFECTS OF PLACEMENT TECHNIQUES ON THE SUCCESS OF CATHETERS FOR CHRONIC PERITONEAL DIALYSIS

The success of peritoneal catheters depends more on placement technique than on the catheter's design.[12,52,68,131] Peritoneoscopic placement results in the lowest incidence of catheter complications and a catheter half-life of over 3 years.[88] Randomized, controlled studies have confirmed that catheter survival is approximately twice as long for those placed by peritoneoscopy vs. catheters placed by dissective techniques.[129,130] In these studies, nephrologists placed the catheters peritoneoscopically and surgeons placed the catheters by dissection. Table 13-2 summarizes the results of over 70 studies on the incidence of serious catheter complications (infection, outflow failure, and pericatheter leak) during an average follow-up of 13 months after catheter placement. Catheters included all types of Tenckhoff-type catheters and TWH catheters. Infectious complications are defined as any peritoneal or catheter infection except randomly occurring peritonitis with differing organisms. Results are organized according to the type of catheter and method of placement.[12,52,68] The table does not differentiate catheters of silicone or polyurethane construction.

Among methods of placement, the peritoneoscopic method (generally performed by nephrologists) has the lowest incidence of infectious complications over the life of the catheters. This may relate to the decreased amount of tissue trauma and smaller incision size of the peritoneoscopic placement vs. dissective placement, and better assurance that the cuff is placed within the muscle vs. blind placement. Outflow failure and leaks are comparable between peritoneoscopic placement and surgical dissection, but they are higher with blind placement. This relates to the lack of peritoneal visualization during positioning of the catheter with blind techniques and the positioning of the cuff outside the rectus sheath rather than within the rectus muscle (in general).

There are also differences in the use of catheters according to the method of placement. Peritoneoscopically-placed catheters may be used for PD treatments immediately to support the patient without need for hemodialysis in almost any schedule that does not include full volume of the peritoneum during times of activity. This includes nighttime cycler therapy or overnight exchanges but excludes full-volume CAPD.[52] Surgically placed catheters can also be used immediately if the deep cuff is secured by sutures within the rectus muscle.

Successful creation of reliable long-term PD access is as dependent on operator skill as it is on the method used to insert the catheter. Attention to detail, commitment to excellence, and adherence to demonstrated best practices are essential attributes of physicians who perform implantation procedures. The recognized best practices for implantation as listed in should be incorporated into the procedure regardless of the implantation approach used.[13] Although surgeons continue to perform the majority of PD access procedures, surgical training programs often lack adequate instruction in catheter implantation. Perceptions that PD access is less challenging and glamorous than hemodialysis vascular access and the persistent view that PD is a "second-class treatment"[132] frequently leads to delegation of catheter insertion procedures to lower-level surgical trainees with little or no supervision. The scarcity of surgical champions in peritoneal access has impeded the advancement of implantation science and the development of standardized catheter placement methodologies. These deficiencies have served as an ongoing impetus for nephrologists to develop and practice implantation techniques that can be performed independently of the surgeon and the operating room. However, it is recognized that not all nephrologists wish to develop an interventional role in establishing PD access, and it is probable that surgeons will continue to perform the majority of catheter placement procedures. Therefore, to overcome current deficiencies, efforts should focus on developing processes through which interested surgeons are identified and mentored. Possible venues for educational activities to improve PD access include developing or expanding professional societies and symposia that jointly include nephrologists and surgeons.

Each catheter implantation approach is associated with its own inherent strengths and weaknesses. Although clinical success with PD access may be influenced by operator skill, certain of the catheter placement methods tend to produce more predictable outcomes (see Table 13–2).

While catheter implantation by blind puncture can be conveniently performed at the bedside under local anesthesia, this procedure has innate disadvantages. Contrary to recognized best practices, catheter insertion by blind puncture with or without fluoroscopic guidance usually places the deep catheter cuff outside of the muscle. This accounts for a high incidence of reported pericannular leaks (Table 13–2). Moreover, due to poor deep cuff fixation, the catheter may shift outward toward the skin, leading to superficial cuff extrusion through the exit site. The formation of pericannular hernias and the occurrence of late leaks are associated with deep cuff positions outside of the rectus muscle.[133] Previous abdominal surgery with the possibility of adhesions and associated risk of intestinal perforation (1 to 2 percent incidence) constitutes a relative contraindication for blind or fluoroscopically guided percutaneous puncture methods. Lack of peritoneal visualization during the implantation procedure is associated with a 16 percent average incidence of outflow failure but ranges up to 36 percent of cases.

Catheter placement by open dissection permits visual confirmation of entry into the peritoneal cavity. However, exploration of the abdominal cavity is still limited to what can be seen or felt through a small hole in the peritoneum. Despite the openness of this procedure, the catheter is advanced mostly by feel, therefore, blindly, into the peritoneal cavity. The incidence rate of catheter flow dysfunction following placement by open dissection averages 7 percent but ranges up to that reported for blind and fluoroscopically guided puncture approaches. Catheter infection rates associated with open dissective placement are higher compared to percutaneous puncture methods, possibly due to larger incision size and greater tissue trauma (Table 13–2). When open dissection placement is performed through a paramedian approach with the deep cuff positioned in the rectus sheath, the incidences of pericannular leak and hernia are low. Certain catheters (Missouri or TWH catheters) can be implanted only by an open dissection approach.

Laparoscopy (peritoneoscopy) offers patients the advantage of a minimally invasive approach while providing greater visibility of the peritoneal cavity during the catheter implantation procedure. The laparoscopic approach is associated with the lowest incidence of infectious complications, outflow dysfunction, and pericatheter leaks (Table 13–2). Laparoscopic implantation using the Y-Tec system provides accurate placement with reproducible results because the technique involves equipment specifically designed for implantation and utilizes standardized methodology that embodies demonstrated best practices. The wide variety of laparoscopic methods and equipment employed by surgeons to implant catheters and the inconsistent use of recognized best practices accounts for a broader range of outcomes. As a result, the reported outcomes of laparoscopic implantation procedures performed by surgeons often demonstrate no advantage over traditional open dissection approaches. One difference between the Y-Tec (peritoneoscopic) approach and surgical laparoscopy is that the former is practiced as a one-puncture technique whereas the latter utilizes two or more puncture sites in the abdominal wall. Another difference is that the Y-Tec procedure is performed under local anesthesia and the laparoscopic approach is under general anesthesia. Although multiple punctures are involved in laparoscopy, the extra port sites allow an opportunity to visibly address problems that adversely affect catheter outcome, namely, catheter tip migration, omental entrapment, and peritoneal adhesions. Identifying and preemptively correcting these problems at the time of the implantation procedure are potential advantages of surgical laparoscopy over other catheter insertion techniques.

Secondary exteriorization of buried dialysis catheters following 3 to 5 weeks of subcutaneous rest reportedly reduces the incidence of subsequent pericatheter infection and peritonitis. In addition, patients are not bothered with interim catheter care until dialysis is needed and there is no catheter break-in period following exteriorization. To optimally utilize this technique, the need for dialysis must be anticipated at least 3 weeks in advance. Patients who require urgent initiation of dialysis are not candidates for this approach. Concern for the extra cost of performing a second procedure to exteriorize the buried catheter may be offset by the cost benefits of a lower infection rate and longer catheter survival.[124]

NEW PLACEMENT TECHNIQUES

Several publications have recently described the use of laparoscopic techniques for the placement of peritoneal catheters. These techniques use 5- to 10-mm diameter trocars generally used for laparoscopic surgery. These are much larger than the 2.2-mm peritoneoscope used in the Y-Tec system and provide much better visualization of the peritoneal space. However, there are several disadvantages to laparoscopic placement: the procedure usually requires general anesthesia, the carbon dioxide used to inflate the abdomen is more irritating to the peritoneum than air, the procedure usually requires two punctures to the peritoneum (one for the scope and one for the catheter), and placement of the deep cuff is not automatically assured to be within the rectus. If the catheter is advanced through a 5-mm split sheath, the deep cuff will be outside the external rectus sheath. If the catheter is advanced through a 10-mm cannula, the deep cuff will end up within the intraperitoneal space or outside the rectus muscle. Some adjustment of cuff position is almost always necessary after the catheter is first placed. As opposed to catheters placed with specially designed equipment, those placed by the laparoscopic technique have no advantage in longevity over those placed by dissection.

MANAGEMENT OF CATHETER COMPLICATIONS

Exit-Site Infection, Cuff Extrusion, and Tunnel Tract Infection

The characteristics of a well-healed catheter exit site include a natural, dark, or pale pink skin color, mature epidermis in the visible skin sinus, and a dry tract or minute, nonpurulent wetness in the deepest portion of the visible skin sinus.[134] Specks of crust may normally be observed on the covering dressing.

An acute exit-site infection is diagnosed if signs of redness (>13-mm border to border including diameter of catheter) and purulent and/or bloody discharge are present. The epidermis within the exit sinus may be partially replaced with granulation tissue. A scab may be present but crusting alone is not indicative of an infection. Pain may accompany physical findings. Chronic exit-site infection is arbitrarily defined as inflammation persisting for more than 4 weeks. Pain and skin erythema may be absent at this stage. External cuff infection is usually accompanied with chronic purulent, bloody, or gluey discharge. Exuberant granulation tissue may be present deep in the visible sinus. The tissue around the cuff may be indurated or tender on palpation. Pressure over the cuff may produce drainage through the exit site.[134] Signs of tunnel tract infection include induration or redness over the subcutaneous course of the catheter associated with tenderness and pain, with or without abscess formation. Advanced tunnel tract infections may spread to the deep cuff and peritoneal cavity and result in concurrent peritonitis.[135]

If signs of infection are present, specimens of exit-site drainage should be collected for culture and Gram's stain. Exit-site, cuff, and tunnel tract infections require antibiotic therapy. The initial antibiotic therapy for gram-positive organisms is oral administration of either a first-generation cephalosporin or penicillinase-resistant penicillin.[13,136] Quinolones are commonly used as initial therapy for gram-negative organisms.[137,138] When the results of the Gram's stain are not immediately available, ciprofloxacin is a suitable empiric choice for first line treatment of exit-site infections.[134] Ciprofloxacin provides antistaphylococcal coverage equal to that of cephalosporins and is the first-line antibiotic for gram-negative organisms. Therapy is modified according to the results of antibiotic susceptibility testing and continued for 14 days. Local exit-site care should be increased to 2 to 3 times daily. Hypertonic saline compresses to the exit-site have been of value.[139] Exuberant granulation tissue can be treated with silver nitrate sticks. Failure of the exit-site infection to resolve after two courses of appropriate antibiotic therapy and intensified exit-wound care usually indicates cuff and tunnel tract infection even in the absence of other findings.

Surgical treatment can successfully resolve chronic exit-site, superficial cuff, and tunnel tract infection provided that intervention is performed before the infectious process extends to the deep cuff. Catheter implantation techniques that place the deep cuff within the rectus muscle increase the resistance to deep cuff infection and improve the likelihood of a successful surgical outcome. Surgically unroofing the skin and subcutaneous tissue overlying the infected portion of the catheter tract permits drainage of pus, debridement of granulation tissue, and shaving of the superficial

cuff.[95,140–144] However, if, during the course of the procedure, the infectious process is found to extend to the deep cuff, the catheter should be removed. Patients with concurrent peritonitis are not candidates for this procedure. The primary advantage of the unroofing/cuff-shaving procedure is that PD is not interrupted. When the technique is applied for the appropriate indications, it is effective in resolving chronic exit-site and tunnel infection in 80 to 100 percent of cases.[142–144]

The unroofing/cuff-shaving procedure is performed under local anesthesia in the operating room or other suitable procedure room. The peritoneal cavity should be drained before the operation in case it is discovered during the procedure that catheter removal is required. Skin preparation, draping, and use of sterile technique are performed as described for implantation procedures. Exercise caution during infiltration of the local anesthetic to prevent accidental puncture of the catheter tubing.

An elliptical incision is made around the exit site and is extended through the skin and subcutaneous tissues along the course of the catheter until the superficial cuff is identified. The cuff is mobilized from the tissues. The exit-site skin and all inflammatory tissue are completely excised to healthy tissue. A #15 scalpel blade, applied parallel to the cuff surface, is used to excise the cuff in repetitive slices until all of the cuff material is removed. The scalpel blade is changed frequently to ensure ease in performing the shave without applying undue pressure on the tubing. The wound is irrigated with saline.

The catheter should be immobilized in its new position. Tubing motion will impair wound healing. The catheter and the shaved tubing segment are directed out of the medial aspect of the incision and stabilized in this position by securing it to the adjacent skin surface with tincture of benzoin and sterile adhesive strips. In selected cases, in the absence of abscess or cellulitis, the redundant lateral portion of the wound is loosely approximated with absorbable sutures. The rest of the wound is packed open with saline soaked gauze as a wet to dry dressing.

Postoperatively, patients are permitted to resume PD immediately. Oral antibiotic therapy is continued for 2 to 4 weeks after the unroofing procedure until healthy granulation tissue appears. Patients are permitted to resume showering once the wound is covered with granulation tissue. Saline wet-to-dry dressings are changed daily until the wound is completely healed, after which, the patient resumes the routine exit-site protocol of daily antibacterial soap wash and a sterile gauze covering dressing. Wound healing is usually complete within 4 to 6 weeks.

Extrusion of the subcutaneous cuff through the skin exit site can occur if the cuff was placed too close to the skin or when the deep cuff is not seated properly within the muscle and subsequently permits the catheter to shift outward from the abdominal wall. Cuff extrusion or impending extrusion through the exit site with or without infection can be managed by cuff shaving. A hemostat is used to gently separate and stretch the skin at the exit site to complete the exteriorization of the cuff. Minimal division and debridement of overlying skin may be required. The cuff is completely shaved off as previously detailed. Local wound care is performed as described for exit-site infection or the unroofing procedure depending on the magnitude of skin disruption.

An alternative surgical treatment approach for chronic exit-site and cuff infection is replacement of the infected external tubing segment by catheter splicing.[145–148] After skin preparation, the infected exit site is isolated from the primary surgical field during draping and managed in the final step to prevent contamination of the new catheter and wound. An incision is made through the previous insertion-site scar to expose the uninvolved intercuff segment of the catheter. If the infectious process is discovered to extend to the intercuff segment but does not involve the deep cuff, the procedure should be converted to unroofing of the subcutaneous tract and shaving of the superficial cuff. If infection has extended to the deep cuff, the peritoneal catheter should be removed. Otherwise, the catheter is divided in the intercuff segment to preserve a 1- to 1.5-cm stump on the deep cuff side. A new catheter is divided in the intercuff segment and the external half is joined to the stump of the deep cuff end of the former catheter with a titanium connector. The catheter ends are secured with 2–0 Prolene sutures tied over the respective grooves of the titanium connector. The external segment of the spliced catheter is tunneled to a suitable exit location remote from the infected exit site. The wound is closed and dressings are applied. In the final step, the external part of the old catheter is removed and the wound is debrided and packed open with saline wet-to-dry dressings. Antibiotics are continued for 2 to 4 weeks until the wound is healed. PD is continued uninterrupted.

The disadvantages of catheter splicing include the expense of additional catheter materials, the potential for intraluminal contamination when the tubing is opened, and the new catheter segment may be seeded with bacteria from the old tunnel tract. Infectious complications and catheter loss following splicing techniques have been reported as high as 35 percent.[146] Catheter splicing appears to work only in chronic exit-site infections when the superficial cuff is close to the skin. There appears to be no clear advantage of catheter splicing over unroofing/cuff-shaving procedures. Perhaps, the best use of catheter splicing is in the case of mechanical damage of the catheter where the tubing is too short to perform an external repair.

Patients with the incidental finding of an infected deep cuff at the time of a catheter salvage procedure should have their catheters removed. The clinical picture will dictate whether simultaneous insertion of a new catheter can be accomplished after a repeat surgical prep and use of new drapes and instruments, or staged implantation performed at a later date. Patients with recognized deep tunnel-tract infections with or without associated peritonitis could be considered for planned simultaneous insertion of a new catheter and removal of the infected catheter at the same procedure.[149,150] In a summary of multiple studies, the overall success rate for this approach is 93 percent for exit-site/tunnel-tract infections and 86 percent when the infection is associated with peritonitis.[151] Peritonitis associated with tunnel-tract infection should be under control at the time of simultaneous catheter replacement/removal procedures (see following section). The placement of the new catheter (clean step) should precede the removal of the infected catheter (dirty step) to reduce the risk of infectious complications. The subcutaneous tissue and skin layers of an infected tunnel tract should be left open, packed daily with a saline wet-to-dry gauze dressing, and allowed to heal by secondary intention.

Relapsing Peritonitis from Catheter Infection

Relapsing peritonitis is arbitrarily defined as a repeat episode of peritonitis caused by the same organism that produced the previous infection and occurs within 4 weeks of completing appropriate antibiotic therapy.[152] Relapsing peritonitis related to the peritoneal catheter is due to bacteria harbored in the biofilm covering the intraperitoneal portion of the tubing or from seeding of the peritoneum by direct extension of a deep cuff and tunnel infection.[153] Although antibiotics may temporarily control the clinical signs of infection, the residual bacterial nidus will eventually proliferate and lead to a recrudescence of overt infection. Relapsing episodes of peritonitis related to catheter infection must be differentiated from other intraperitoneal causes, such as diverticulitis or abscess.

Catheter removal should be considered at the time of the third episode of peritonitis caused by the same organism. Although the optimal time of implantation of a new catheter is not known, a period of at least 3 weeks has been recommended.[152] Simultaneous catheter replacement and removal at the same procedure can be considered if antibiotic treatment resolves clinical signs of infection, the dialysate leukocyte count is <100/mm^3, and the infecting organisms are not mycobacteria, fungi, or enteric in origin.[149,150,153] Antibiotic therapy should be continued for 2 weeks following the catheter replacement-removal procedure and for as long as 3 to 4 weeks for *Pseudomonas* infections. Insertion of the new catheter should precede removal of the infected catheter. The success rate of this approach has been reported between 83 to 98 percent.[149–151,153] Lower success rates (70 percent) have been associated with *Pseudomonas* infections; therefore these patients should be carefully selected for simultaneous catheter replacement/removal.[151,153]

Mechanical Flow Dysfunction

Catheter flow dysfunction is usually manifest as outflow failure; therefore, the volume of drained dialysate is substantially less than the inflow volume. The most common cause of outflow dysfunction is constipation. Mechanical kinking of the catheter tubing or an intraluminal fibrin clot may be accompanied with two-way obstruction. A KUB (kidney-ureter-bladder) x-ray is often helpful in identifying a kink in the catheter tubing or a fecal-filled rectosigmoid colon. Displacement of the catheter tip into the upper abdomen is presumptive evidence of omental entrapment. If the x-ray excludes tubing kinks or displacement, and flow function is not restored with correction of constipation, then fibrinolytic therapy (heparin, urokinase, tissue plasminogen activator, streptokinase) may be attempted. If these measures are not successful in restoring drainage function, the catheter is presumed to be obstructed by omentum or other adherent intraperitoneal structures. Fluoroscopic guidewire manipulation,[154,155] endoluminal brushes,[156] and Fogarty balloons[157] have been used to redirect displaced and obstructed catheters. Frequently, multiple manipulations are required, with long-term flow function restored in 70 to 80 percent of cases. Higher failure rates occurred if catheters became obstructed during the first 3 months following catheter implantation.

Laparoscopy has become an invaluable method of evaluating and resolving catheter flow obstruction. Because laparoscopy can reliably identify the source of flow dysfunction and provide a means for definitive treatment, it is often considered as the next step in the management sequence after the diagnoses of constipation and fibrin plug have been excluded.[109,158] Laparoscopic rescue of peritoneal catheters from mechanical dysfunction is performed in the operating room under local or general anesthesia. The rescue procedure can be performed under local anesthesia provided that painless insufflation gases are used) e.g., nitrous oxide or helium), as discussed in connection with laparoscopic implantation.[111,112,150] The dialysis catheter can frequently be used to perform the initial gas insufflation of the abdomen, since most catheter obstructions represent outflow problems. Alternatively, a Veress needle is used for insufflation as described for implantation.

Surgical skin preparation is performed, including the exit site and the catheter tubing out to the level of the adapter-transfer set junction. Since there is no practical way to adequately clean the external catheter assembly, it should not be exposed or handled by the surgical team during the course of the procedure. Surgical drapes are applied to the abdomen and exclude the exit site and catheter tubing from the field. After satisfactory creation of a pneumoperitoneum, access to the peritoneal cavity for the laparoscope and instruments is provided by insertion of 5-mm port devices along a line lateral to the rectus sheath on the side opposite of the peritoneal catheter. Preliminary exploration with a 5-mm laparoscope is performed to determine the source of the flow dysfunction. One or more 5-mm ports are inserted as needed depending on the instrumentation required to resolve the problem. Omental entrapment is relieved by using grasping forceps to strip the omentum from the catheter (Fig 13–21). The catheter tip is temporarily exteriorized through one of the port sites to facilitate removal of residual intraluminal tissue debris. An omentopexy is performed to prevent recurrent obstruction. Failure to treat the omentum at the time of the laparoscopic rescue procedure results in recurrent entrapment in nearly 30 percent of cases.[119] Omentopexy is preferred to laparoscopic omental resection because it can be performed in a fraction of the time at a fraction of the cost with an outcome that is equal or better.

The practice of laparoscopic suturing of the catheter tip in the pelvis to prevent migration should be abandoned. The tacking-up procedure demonstrates a lack of understanding that the majority of catheter migrations are caused by omental wraps. Not recognizing that redundant omentum is the underlying cause is frequently rewarded with recurrent catheter obstruction produced by omentum adherent to the tack-up site. Another concern is that the opening, bordered by the catheter, the abdominal wall, the point of peritoneal entry of the tubing, and the tack-up site, creates a potential space for internal herniation of intestine. Incorporating rectus sheath tunneling as a component of the implantation procedure can prevent catheter tip migration not related to omental entrapment and eliminates the need for catheter tacking-up maneuvers.

On occasion, the obstruction may be due to the catheter tip being walled-off against the parietal peritoneum by adherent epiploic appendices of the sigmoid colon. The catheter is gently pulled free without disturbing the adhesions. Leaving the epiploic appendices adherent to the peritoneum will prevent recurrent obstruction. Rarely, the fimbria of the uterine tubes may produce flow dysfunction. Laparoscopic resection of the uterine tube prevents recurrent obstruction. Adhesiolysis for poor drainage function, especially after peritonitis, is associated with a high failure rate (30 percent) secondary to reforming of adhesions.[119]

Laparoscopic rescue procedures can be accomplished on an outpatient basis. Frequently, the need for temporary hemodialysis is avoided. Using small port sizes and meticulous watertight wound closures enable many patients to immediately resume a modified PD schedule following surgical interventions. During the first postoperative week, patients are managed with low volume automated PD using 10 exchanges over 10 hours with 1-L volumes while recumbent and a dry abdomen while ambulatory. In the absence of leaks, the volume is increased to 1.5 L during the second week. Patients are permitted to resume their normal preoperative dialysis schedule by the third week.

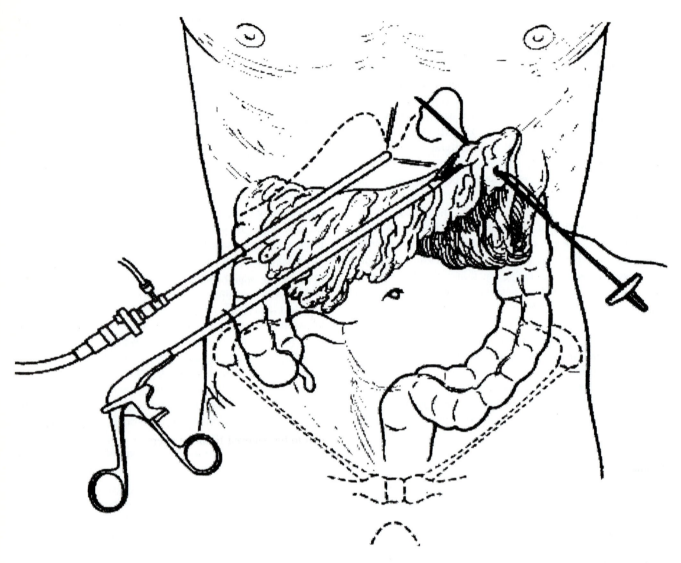

Figure 13–21. Schematic drawing demonstrating the manner in which the omentopexy is performed under laparoscopic vision with the use of a grasping forceps and tacking needle. (From Crabtree,[115] with permission).

Abdominal Wall Hernias and Leaks

Preoperatively identified hernias should be repaired in conjunction with the implantation procedure. Once dialysis is initiated, previously undiagnosed umbilical, inguinal, and incisional hernias may present as obvious bulges, genital swelling, abdominal wall edema, weight gain, or apparent ultrafiltration failure. When an occult hernia is suspected, computed tomography with dialysis fluid containing radiocontrast[159] or scintigraphy with radionucleotide-containing dialysate[160] can confirm the location. After mobilization from surrounding soft tissues, hernia sacs may be inverted to avoid entry into the peritoneal cavity. If the hernia sac is excised, an attempt should be made to obtain a watertight closure of the peritoneum. The abdominal wall defect is preferably closed with native fascial tissues buttressed with an overlying prosthetic patch. If only a prosthetic patch bridges the abdominal wall defect and is exposed to the peritoneal cavity, fluid leak will occur through or around the material until the interstices become reperitonealized a number of weeks later. Under these circumstances, temporary hemodialysis will be required. In addition, a prosthetic material exposed to the peritoneal surface may be predisposed to infection in the event of a subsequent occurrence of dialysis-related peritonitis. Removal of the prosthetic material may be required to resolve the infection. After uncomplicated hernia repair, patients are allowed to resume a modified PD schedule with low-volume automated exchanges as described for laparoscopic rescue procedures.

Pericatheter leaks may occur as a consequence of early institution of PD or technical problems associated with catheter placement, e.g., purse-string suture failure, poor wound repair, or midline catheter insertion. Delaying initiation of dialysis usually results in spontaneous cessation of the leak. Persistent leaks are susceptible to tunnel infection and peritonitis and warrant repair or catheter replacement. Late pericatheter leaks are caused by pericannular hernia or occult tunnel-tract infections with separation of the cuffs from the surrounding tissues. The occurrence of pericannular hernia is largely influenced by the location of the deep cuff. At the parietal peritoneal surface, the mesothelium reflects along the surface of the catheter to reach the deep cuff. If the deep cuff is outside of the muscle wall, the extension of the peritoneal lining above the muscle layer creates a potential or actual pericannular hernia. If the abdominal wall is weak, a "golf-ball" size hernia can develop around the cuff. Pericannular hernias require repair, frequently employing prosthetic mesh to reinforce the abdominal wall. Larger hernias may require catheter replacement through a different abdominal wall location in addition to the hernia repair. The best strategy is to avoid the problem altogether by adopting an implantation technique that places the deep cuff within the rectus muscle to assure firm tissue ingrowth.

Hydrothorax from dialysate leak through a pleuroperitoneal connection occurs in 1 to 2 percent of PD patients. Dyspnea is the first clinical clue to the diagnosis of pleural leak. Hydrothorax is usually unilateral, most commonly on the right side, and occurs during the first year on dialysis. Diagnosis is confirmed by recovery of fluid on thoracentesis containing low protein content and high glucose concentration relative to measured blood levels. Conservative management in the form of peritoneal rest and intermittent low-volume dialysis is rarely successful. Thoracoscopic pleurodesis with talc poudrage or mechanical rub produces nearly a 100 percent success rate in resolving pleural leaks and should be the first choice of therapeutic methods for pleuroperitoneal communication.[161–163]

REMOVING PERITONEAL CATHETERS

Peritoneal catheters are removed under local anesthesia in the operating room or a suitable procedure room. When possible, the abdomen should be drained of dialysate before the procedure. Skin preparation, draping, and sterile technique are practiced as described for implantation. Although the catheter exit site is prepped, draping should exclude this area from the remainder of the operative field.

The previous surgical implantation scar is incised. Extending the incision a little further laterally than the original scar facilitates exposure of the superficial cuff. Blunt spreading dissection through the subcutaneous tissues is performed with a hemostat and finger until the catheter within its fibrous capsule is palpated. Army-navy retractors, or ribbon retractors facilitate exposure in a narrow wound of this sort. A clamp may be inserted deep to the catheter and fibrous capsule in the intercuff segment and used to elevate the tubing toward the skin. Metzenbaum scissors, scalpel, or a cautery device is used to enter the fibrous capsule and expose the catheter tubing. If excessive heating of the tissues is avoided, the cautery can be applied directly to the capsule surrounding the catheter without damage to the rubber tubing. Using upward traction with a hemostat applied to the catheter, the cautery is used to unroof the fibrous tissue capsule overlying the tubing toward the fascia until the deep cuff is encountered. The cuff can be freed from the attached muscle by blunt and sharp dissection but cautery dissection is easier and associated with less bleeding. The cautery is kept close to the surface of the cuff with care to remove all of the cuff material. When the deep border of the cuff is recognized, the edge of the fibrous capsule is undercut to expose the tubing. At this point, intraperitoneal structures such as bowel may become visible and care should be taken not to cause injury with a sharp instrument or cautery tip. The capsule is divided circumferentially to completely free the peritoneal end of the catheter. A hand is used to shield the catheter as the coiled tip is withdrawn from the peritoneal cavity to prevent splattering of fluid as the catheter tip flips out of the wound. The catheter is conveniently divided with scissors in the intercuff segment to allow the peritoneal portion to be removed from the operative field. A clamp is applied to the tubing of the superficial segment and used as a handle for traction. In like manner, the cautery is used to divide the surrounding tissue capsule until the superficial cuff is identified. The catheter is divided with scissors on the skin side of the superficial cuff to permit this segment to be removed. Upon lifting the edge of the drapes, a clamp is used to withdraw the remainder of the catheter from the exit wound. The external portion of the catheter is left under the drapes and the clamp is set aside. Careful hemostasis is established and the wound is irrigated with saline. The fascial defect in the rectus sheath is repaired with absorbable 0-polygalactic suture. The subcutaneous tissues and skin are closed as separate layers. If the catheter is being removed for tunnel tract infection, debridement of infected granulation tissue is performed and the wound is managed open with saline wet-to-dry gauze dressings changed daily. The exit site is left open and covered with gauze.

REMAINING CHALLENGES IN PERITONEAL CATHETER DESIGN

There are two major remaining challenges for all transcutaneous catheters: to diminish infection of the catheter and the surrounding biofilm and to avoid outflow failure due to adhesions. A variety of antibacterial coatings have been developed for central venous catheters but these coatings have not demonstrated a lower infection rate for coated catheters. To prevent exit-site infection and catheter seeding, which results in persistent peritonitis, antibacterial materials must be applied to the inside and outside of the peritoneal catheter. In long-term use, silver and sulfa compounds tend to disappear from the surface of the catheter, diminishing effectiveness, but several new approaches to bacterial inactivation of biofilm are now being evaluated.

A final challenge is to limit the growth of adventitial tissue around and onto catheters, as in fibrous sheathing of central venous catheters and omental attachment to peritoneal catheters. Some new materials are being evaluated that are both bactericidal and mildly cytocidal to determine whether these can prevent fibrous attachment and sterilize catheter surfaces and biofilm. These materials must be applied to the catheter body and not the cuffs, so that tissue ingrowth can occur normally to the cuffs while the catheter body avoids such ingrowth.

Other features related to PD catheters are the method of making sterile connections between the catheter and the dialysate fluid ("connectology"), and the access of the catheter at or above the skin surface. Obviously it would be ideal if there were an access device that worked at skin level, or were even buried below skin surface, to eliminate the need for bandages and the "bulk" of all the external tubing and connectors now worn by our patients. One approach that has been tried is a subcutaneous port or graft segment into which needles can be placed, passing through the skin. This works reasonably well but requires that the PD set be attached to a fistula-type needle. This general approach has not proven to diminish incidence of infection when tested as the "Mouse" access by Utah in the 1970s or as the Vasca port in Europe more recently. Other methods are available that will eventually allow low-level access at the skin level.

REFERENCES

1. Nolph KD. Presentation at 2d Annual National Conference on Pediatric and Adult CAPD. Kansas City, MO, 1982.
2. Gotloib L, Garmizo L, Varak I, Mines J. Reduction of vital capacity due to increased intra-abdominal pressure during peritoneal dialysis. *Perit Dial Bull* 1981;1:63–64.
3. Gotloib L, Mines M, Garmizo L, Varak I. Hemodynamic effects of increasing intra-abdominal pressure in peritoneal dialysis. *Perit Dial Bull* 1981;1:41–43.
4. Rottembourg J, Dominque J, VonLanthen M, et al. Straight or curled Tenckhoff peritoneal catheter for continuous ambulatory peritoneal dialysis (CAPD). *Perit Dial Bull* 1981;1: 123–124.
5. Ash SR, Johnson H, Hartman J, et al. The column disc peritoneal catheter: a peritoneal access device with improved drainage. *ASAIO Trans* 1980;3:109–113.
6. Thornhill JA, Ash SR, Dhein CR, et al. Peritoneal dialysis with the Purdue column disc catheter. *Minn Vet* 1980; 20:27–33.
7. Ash SR, Struewing JD. Clinical trials of the column disc peritoneal catheter (Lifecath). *Perit Dial Bull* 1983;3:77–80.
8. Keller KH. Fluid mechanics and mass transfer in artificial organs. *ASAIO Trans* (special publication) 1973;20:28–30.
9. Ash SR, Wolf GC, Bloch R. Placement of the Tenckhoff peritoneal dialysis catheter under peritoneoscopic visualization. *Dial Transplant* 1981;10:383–386.
10. Roberts RK. Microprocessor Control of Blood Flow in a Reciprocating Dialyzer. Thesis. West Lafayette, IN: School of Mechanical Engineering, Purdue University, 1980.
11. Ash SR. Chronic peritoneal dialysis catheters: effects of catheter design, materials, and location. *Semin Dial* 1990;3: 39–46.
12. Ash SR. Chronic peritoneal dialysis catheters: effects of catheter design, materials and location. *Semin Dial* 1990; 3(1):39–46.
13. Gokal R, Alexander S, Ash S, et al. Peritoneal catheters and exit site practice: toward optimum peritoneal access: 1998 update. *Perit Dial Int* 1998;18(1):11–33.
14. Ganter G. Uber die Beseitigung giftiger Stoffe aus dem Blute durch Dialyse. *Munch Med Wochenschr* 1923;70: 1478–1480.
15. Frank HA, Seligman AM, Fine J. Treatment of uremia after acute renal failure by peritoneal irrigation. *JAMA* 1946; 703–705.
16. Frank HA, Seligman AM, Fine J. Further experiences with peritoneal irrigation for acute renal failure. *Ann Surg* 1948;128(3):561–608.
17. Odel HM, Ferris DO, Power MH. Peritoneal lavage as an effective means of extrarenal excretion. *Am J Med* 1950;9: 63–77.
18. Rosenak SS, Openheimer GD. An implanted drain for peritoneal lavage. *Surgery* 1948;23:832.
19. Grollman A, Turner LB, McLean JA. Intermittent peritoneal lavage in nephrectomized dogs and its application to the human being. *Arch Intern Med* 1951;87:379–380.
20. Legrain M, Merrill JP. Short-term continuous transperitoneal dialysis. *N Engl J Med* 1953;248:126–129.
21. Maxwell MH, Rockney RE, Kleeman CR, Twiss MR. Peritoneal dialysis I, techniques and applications. *JAMA* 1959; 170:917–924.
22. Boen ST, Mulinari AS, Dillard DH, et al. Periodic peritoneal dialysis in the treatment of chronic uremia. *ASAIO Trans* 1962;8:256–262.
23. McBride P, Fred TS, Boen MD: The man who brought science to the art of peritoneal dialysis. *Perit Dial Bull* 1982; 2:50–53.
24. Barry KG, Shambaugh GE, Goler D, Matthews FE. A new flexible cannula and seal to provide prolonged access to the peritoneal cavity for dialysis. *ASAIO Trans* 1963;9:105–107.
25. Gutch CF. Peritoneal dialysis. *ASAIO Trans* 1964;10: 406–408.
26. Henderson LW, Merrill JP, Crane C. Further experience with the inlying plastic conduit for chronic peritoneal dialysis. *ASAIO Trans* 1963;9:108–120.
27. Jacob GB, Deane N. Repeated peritoneal dialysis by the catheter replacement method; description of technique and a replaceable prosthesis for chronic access to the peritoneal cavity. *Proc Eur Dial Transplant Assoc* 1967;4:136.

28. Gotloib L, Nisencorn I, Garmizo AL, et al. Subcutaneous intraperitoneal prosthesis for maintenance of peritoneal dialysis. *Lancet* 1975;1:1318–1320.

29. Boen ST. Kinetics of peritoneal dialysis: a comparison with the artificial kidney. *Medicine* 1961;40:243–287.

30. Palmer RA, Quinton W, Gray JE. Prolonged peritoneal dialysis for chronic renal failure. *Lancet* 1964;1:700–702.

31. Palmer RA, Newel JE, Gray EJ, Quinton WE. Treatment of chronic renal failure by prolonged peritoneal dialysis. *N Engl J Med* 1966;274:248–253.

32. Palmer RA. Peritoneal dialysis by indwelling catheter for chronic renal failure, 1963–68. *Can Med Assoc J* 1971; 105(4):376–386.

33. Gutch CF, Stevens, SC. Silastic catheter for peritoneal dialysis. *ASAIO Trans* 1966;12:106–107.

34. Weston RE, Roberts M. Clinical use of stylet-catheter for peritoneal dialysis. *Arch Intern Med* 1965;115:659–662.

35. Roberts M. Paracentesis stylet catheter. US Patent 3459188, August 5, 1969.

36. Weber J, Mettang T, Hubel E, et al. Survival of 138 surgically placed straight double-cuff Tenckhoff catheters in patients on continuous ambulatory peritoneal dialysis. *Perit Dial Int* 1993;13:224–227.

37. Ash SR, Handt AE, Bloch R. Peritoneoscopic placement of the Tenckhoff catheter: further clinical experience. *Perit Dial Bull* 1983;3:8–12.

38. Tenckhoff H, Schechter H. A bacteriologically safe peritoneal access device. *ASAIO Trans* 1968;14:181–186.

39. Striker GE, Tenckhoff HAM. A transcutaneous prosthesis for prolonged access to the peritoneal cavity. *Surgery* 1971; 69:70–74.

40. Flanigan MJ, Ngheim DD, Schulak JA, et al. The use and complications of three peritoneal dialysis catheter designs—a retrospective analysis. *ASAIO Trans* 1987;33:33–38.

41. Diaz-Buxo JA, Geissinger G. Single cuff versus double cuff Tenckhoff catheter. *Perit Dial Bull* 1984;5(suppl 3): S100–S102.

42. Twardowski ZJ, Nolph KD, Khanna R, et al. The need for a "swan neck" permanently bent, arcuate peritoneal dialysis catheter. *Perit Dial Bull* 1985;5:219–223.

43. Ponce SP, Pierratos A, Izatt S, et al. Comparison of the survival and complications of three permanent peritoneal dialysis catheters. *Perit Dial Bull* 1982;2:82–85.

44. Kim D, Burke D, Izatt S, et al. Single- or double-cuff peritoneal catheters? A prospective comparison. *ASAIO Trans* 1984;30:232–235.

45. Schmidt RW, Blumenkrantz M. Peritoneal sclerosis: a "sword of Damocles" for peritoneal dialysis. *Arch Intern Med* 1981;141:1265–1266.

46. Grefberg N, Danielson BG, Nilsson P, Wahlberg J. Comparison of two catheters for patients undergoing CAPD. *Scand J Urol Nephrol* 1983;17:343–346.

47. Thornhill JA, Dhein CR, Johnson H, Ash SR. Drainage characteristics of the column disc catheter: a new chronic peritoneal access catheter. *Proc Clin Dial Transplant Forum* 1980;3:119–125.

48. Ash SR, Slingeneyer A, Schardin KE. Further clinical experience with the Lifecath peritoneal implant. *Perspect Perit Dial* 1983;1:9–11.

49. Steinberg SM, Culter SJ, Novak JW, Nolph KD. *Report of the National CAPD Registry, Division of NIADDK.* Washington, DC: National Institutes of Health, 1986:41.

50. US Renal Data Systems (USRDS). USRDS 1992 Annual Data Report. Chapter VI: catheter-related factors and peritoneal risk in CAPD patients. *Am J Kidney Dis* 1992; 20(2):48–54.

51. Digenis GE, Khanna R, Pantalony D. Eosinophilia after implantation of the peritoneal catheter. *Perit Dial Bull* 1982;2: 98–99.

52. Ash SR, Carr DJ, Diaz-Buxo JA. Peritoneal access devices: hydraulic function and biocompatibility. In: Nissenson AR, Fine RN, Gentile DE, eds. *Clinical Dialysis.* Norwalk, CT: Appleton & Lange, 1995:295–321.

53. Mineshima M, Watanuki M, Yamagata K, et al. Development of continuous recirculating peritoneal dialysis using a double lumen catheter. *ASAIO J* 1992;38:M377–M381.

54. Diaz-Buxo JA. Renal Care 2000—Peritoneal Dialysis. Prospects for PD in the future. *Nephrol News Issues* 1999;3: 12–16.

55. Diaz-Buxo JA: Continuous flow peritoneal dialysis: clinical applications. *Blood Purif* 2002;20:36–39.

56. Amerling R, DeSimone L, Inciong-Reyes R, et al. Clinical experience with continuous flow and flow-through peritoneal dialysis. Semin Dial 2001;14:388–390.

57. Diaz-Buxo JA. Streaming, mixing and recirculation: Role of the peritoneal access in continuous flow peritoneal dialysis (clinical considerations). *Adv Perit Dial* 2002;18:87–90.

58. Ash SR, Janle EM. Continuous flow-through peritoneal dialysis: comparison of efficiency to IPD, TPD and CAPD in an animal model. *Perit Dial Int* 1997;17:365–372.

59. Ronco C, Gloukhoff A, Dell'Aquila R, Levin NW. Catheter design for continuous flow peritoneal dialysis. *Blood Purif* 2002;20:40–44.

60. Gokal R, Alexander S, Ash S, et al. Peritoneal Catheters and Exit-Site Practices Toward Optimum Peritoneal Access: 1998 Update (Official Report from the International Society for Peritoneal Dialysis). *Perit Dial Int* 1998;18:11–33.

61. Kim D, Burke D, Izatt S, et al. Single- or double-cuff peritoneal catheters? A prospective comparison. *Trans Am Soc Artif Intern Organs* 1984;30:232–235.

62. Eklund B, Honkanen E, Kyllonen L, et al. Peritoneal dialysis access: prospective randomized comparison of single-cuff and double-cuff straight Tenckhoff catheters. *Nephrol Dial Transplant* 1997;12(12):2664–2666.

63. Nielsen PK, Hemmingsen C, Friis SU, et al. Comparison of straight and curled Tenckhoff peritoneal dialysis catheters implanted by percutaneous technique: a prospective randomized study. *Perit Dial Int* 1995;15(1):18–21.

64. Eklund BH, Honkanen EO, Kala A-R, Kyllonen LE. Peritoneal dialysis access: prospective randomized comparison of the Swan Neck and Tenckhoff catheters. *Perit Dial Int* 1995;15(18):353–356.

65. Ash SR, Janle EM. T-fluted peritoneal dialysis catheter. *Adv Perit Dial* 1993;9:223–226.

66. Ash SR, Janle EJ. T-fluted peritoneal dialysis catheter. *Adv Perit Dial* 1993;9:223–226.

67. Piraino B, Bernardini J, Peitzman A, Sorkin M. Failure of peritoneal catheter cuff shaving to eradicate infection. *Perit Dial Bull* 1987;7(3):179–182.

68. Ash SR. Bedside peritoneoscopic peritoneal catheter placement of Tenckhoff and newer peritoneal catheters. *Adv Perit Dial* 1998;14:75–79.

69. Moncrief JW, Popovich RP, Broadrick LJ, et al. The Moncrief-Popovich catheter: a new peritoneal access technique for patients on peritoneal dialysis. *ASAIO Trans* 1993;39:62–65.

70. Khanna R, Nolph KD. Ultrafiltration failure and sclerosing peritonitis in peritoneal dialysis patients. In: Nissenson AR, Fine RN, eds. *Dialysis Therapy.* Philadelphia: Hanley & Belfus, 1986:122–125.

71. Oreopoulos DG, Zellerman G, Izatt S, Gotloib L. Catheters and connectors for chronic peritoneal dialysis: present and future. In: Atkins RC, Thomson NM, Farrell PC, eds. *Peritoneal Dialysis.* New York: Churchill Livingstone, 1981: 313–319.

72. Tucker CT, Cunningham JT, Nichols AM, et al. Cannulography with peritoneal air contrast study. *Contemp Dial* 1982; 3:9–16.

73. Tank ES. Catheter placement in children for continuous ambulatory peritoneal dialysis. In: *Proceedings of the 2d Annual National Conference on Pediatric & Adult CAPD.* Columbia, MO: University of Missouri Press, 1982:388–392.

74. Scott DF, Marshall VC. Insertion and complications of Tenckhoff catheters—surgical aspects. In: Atkins RC, Thomson NM, Farrell PC, eds. *Peritoneal Dialysis.* New York: Churchill Livingstone, 1981:61–72.

75. Cruz C. Clinical experience with a new peritoneal access device, in Ota K, Maher JF, Winchester JF, Hirszel P, eds. *Current Concepts in Peritoneal Dialysis.* Amsterdam, 1992: 164–169.

76. Rao SP, Oreopoulos DG. Unusual complications of a polyurethane PD catheter. *Perit Dial Int* 1997;17:410–412.

77. Crabtree JH. Clinical biodurability of aliphatic polyether based polyurethanes as peritoneal dialysis catheters. *ASAIO J* 2003;49:290–294.

78. Bauer BA. Diabetic/renal time-line. *Perit Dial Int* 1988;8: 65.

79. Dasgupta MK. Silver peritoneal catheters reduce bacterial colonization. *Adv Perit Dial* 1994;10:196–198.

80. Kathuria P, Moore HL, Mehrotra R, et al. Evaluation of healing and external tunnel histology of silver-coated peritoneal catheters in rats. *Adv Perit Dial* 1996;12:203–208.

81. Crabtree JH, Burchette RJ, Siddiqi RA, et al. The efficacy of silver-ion implanted catheters in reducing peritoneal dialysis-related infections. *Perit Dial Int* 2003;23:368–374.

82. Sorkin MI, Luger AM, Rowant B, et al. Histology and functional characteristics of the peritoneal membrane of a diabetic patient after 34 months of CAPD. *Perit Dial Bull* 1982;2:24–27.

83. Verger C, Berry JP, Galle P, et al. Foreign material inclusions in the peritoneum of CAPD patients: a study with x-ray microanalysis. *Perit Dial Bull* 1982;2:138–139.

84. Daugirdas JT, Leehey DJ, Popli S, et al. Induction of peritoneal-fluid eosinophilia by intraperitoneal air in patients on continuous ambulatory peritoneal dialysis. *N Engl J Med* 1985;313(23):1481.

85. Handt AE, Ash SR. Longevity of Tenckhoff catheters placed by the Vitec peritoneoscopic technique. *Perspect Perit Dial* 1984;2(2)30–33.

86. Helfrich GB, Winchester JF. What is the best technique for implantation of a peritoneal catheter? *Perit Dial Bull* 1982; 2:132–133.

87. Reed WP, Light PD, Newman KA. Biofilm on Tenckhoff catheters: a possible source for peritonitis. In: Maher JF, Winchester JF, eds. *Frontiers in Peritoneal Dialysis.* New York: Field, Rich, 1986:176–180.

88. Eklund BH. Surgical implantation of CAPD catheters: presentation of midline incision-lateral placement method and review of 100 procedures. *Nephrol Dial Transplant* 1995;10: 386–390.

89. Copley JB, Smith BJ, Koger DM, et al. Prevention of postoperative peritoneal catheter-related infections. *Perit Dial Int* 1988;8:195–197.

90. Tenckhoff H. *Chronic Peritoneal Dialysis Manual.* Seattle, WA: University of Washington School of Medicine, 1974.

91. Gupta A, Vas S, Simons M, Oreopoulos DG. Usefulness of catheter tunnel ultrasound in CAPD patients (abstr). *Perit Dial Int* 1992;12(suppl 2):S51.

92. Ash SR. Peritoneal dialysis for acute renal failure: the safe, effective, and low cost modality. *14th Annual Conference on Peritoneal Dialysis 1994; Proceedings.* Columbia, MO: University of Missouri School of Medicine; 1994: 339–345.

93. Crabtree JH: Construction and use of stencils in planning for peritoneal dialysis catheter implantation. *Perit Dial Int* 2003;23:395–398.

94. Twardowski ZJ, Nolph KD, Khanna R, et al. Computer interaction: catheters. *Adv Perit Dial* 1994;10:11–18.

95. Helfrich GB, Pechan BW, Alijani MR, et al. Reduction of catheter complications with lateral placement. *Perit Dial Bull* 1983;3:S2–S4.

96. Favazza A, Petri R, Montanaro D, et al. Insertion of a straight peritoneal catheter in an arcuate subcutaneous tunnel by a tunneler: long-term experience. *Perit Dial Int* 1995; 15:357–362.

97. Stone MM, Fonkalsrud EW, Salusky IB, et al. Surgical management of peritoneal dialysis catheters in children: five-year experience with 1,800 patient-month follow-up. *J Pediatr Surg* 1986;21:1177–1181.

98. Rinaldi S, Sera F, Verrina E, et al. The Italian registry of pediatric chronic peritoneal dialysis: a ten-year experience with chronic peritoneal dialysis catheters. *Perit Dial Int* 1998;18:71–74.

99. Reissman P, Lyass S, Shiloni E, et al. Placement of a peritoneal dialysis catheter with routine omentectomy—does it prevent obstruction of the catheter? *Eur J Surg* 1998;164: 703–707.

100. Nicholson ML, Donnelly PK, Burton PR, et al. Factors influencing peritoneal catheter survival in continuous ambulatory peritoneal dialysis. *Ann R Coll Surg Engl* 1990;72: 368–372.

101. Draganic B, James A, Booth M, et al. Comparative experience of a simple technique for laparoscopic chronic ambulatory peritoneal dialysis catheter placement. *Aust NZ J Surg* 1998;68:735–739.

102. Allon M, Soucie JM, Macon EJ. Complications with permanent peritoneal dialysis catheters: experience with 154 percutaneous placed catheters. *Nephron* 1988;48:8–11.

103. Zappacosta AR, Perras ST, Closkey GM. Seldinger technique for Tenckhoff catheter placement. *Am Soc for Artif Organs Trans* 1991;37:13–15.

104. Mellotte GJ, Ho CA, Morgan SH, et al. Peritoneal dialysis catheters: a comparison between percutaneous and conventional surgical placement techniques. *Nephrol Dial Transplant* 1993;8:626–630.

105. Ozener C, Bihorac A, Akoglu E. Technical survival of CAPD catheters: comparison between percutaneous and conventional surgical placement techniques. *Nephrol Dial Transplant* 2001;16:1893–1899.

106. Jacobs IG, Gray RR, Elliott DS, Grossman H. Radiologic placement of peritoneal dialysis catheters: preliminary experience. *Radiology* 1992;182:251–255.

107. Savader SJ, Geschwind JF, Lund GB, Scheel PJ. Percutaneous radiologic placement of peritoneal dialysis catheters: long-term results. *J Vasc Radiol* 2000;11:965–970.

108. Georgiades CS, Geschwind JF. Percutaneous peritoneal dialysis catheter placement for the management of end-stage renal disease: technique and comparison with the surgical approach. *Tech Vasc Interv Radiol* 2002;5:103–107.

109. Kimmelstiel FM, Miller RE, Molinelli BM, Lorch JA. Laparoscopic management of peritoneal dialysis catheters. *Surg Gynecol Obstet* 1993;176:565–570.

110. Brandt CP, Franceschi D. Laparoscopic placement of peritoneal dialysis catheters in patients who have undergone prior abdominal operations. *J Am Coll Surg* 1994;178: 515–516.

111. Crabtree JH, Fishman A. A laparoscopic approach under local anesthesia for peritoneal dialysis access. *Perit Dial Int* 2000;20:757–765.

112. Crabtree JH, Fishman A, Huen IT. Videolaparoscopic peritoneal dialysis catheter implant and rescue procedures under local anesthesia with nitrous oxide pneumoperitoneum. *Adv Perit Dial* 1998;14:83–86.

113. Gerhart CD. Needleoscopic placement of Tenckhoff catheters. *J Soc Laparoendosc Surg* 1999;3:155–158.

114. Poole GH, Tervit P. Laparoscopic Tenckhoff catheter insertion: a prospective study of a new technique. *Aust NZ J Surg* 2000;70:371–373.

115. Crabtree JH, Fishman A. Selective performance of prophylactic omentopexy during laparoscopic implantation of peritoneal dialysis catheters. *Surg Laparosc Endosc Percutan Tech* 2003;13:180–184.

116. Ogunc G. Videolaparoscopy with omentopexy: a new technique to allow placement of a catheter for continuous ambulatory peritoneal dialysis. *Surg Today* 2001;31:942–944.

117. Twardowski ZJ, Nichols WK, Nolph KD, Khanna R. Swan neck presternal ("bathtub") catheter for peritoneal dialysis. *Adv Perit Dial* 1992;8:316–324.

118. Crabtree JH, Fishman A. Laparoscopic implantation of swan neck presternal peritoneal dialysis catheters. *J Laparoendosc Adv Surg Tech* 2003;13:131–137.

119. Crabtree JH, Fishman A, Siddiqi RA, et al. The risk of infection and peritoneal catheter loss from implant procedure exit-site trauma. *Perit Dial Int* 1999;19:366–371.

120. Moncrief JW, Popovich RP, Simmons EE, et al. The Moncrief-Popovich catheter: a new peritoneal access technique for patients on peritoneal dialysis. *Trans Am Soc Artif Intern Organs* 1994;39(1):62–65.

121. Moncrief JW, Popovich, Simmons EE, et al. Peritoneal access technology. *Perit Dial Int* 1993:13(2):S112–S123.

122. Moncrief JW, Popovich RP, Oreopoulos DG, et al. Continuous ambulatory peritoneal dialysis. In: Gokal R, Nolph KD, eds. *Textbook of Peritoneal Dialysis.* Dordrecht, The Netherlands: Kluwer, 1994:357–398.

123. Moncrief JW, Popovich RP, Seare W, et al. Peritoneal dialysis access technology: the Austin Diagnostic Clinic experience. *Perit Dial Int* 1996;16:S327–S329.

124. Caruso DM, Gray DL, Kohr JM, et al. Reduction of infectious complications and costs using temporary subcutaneous implantation of PD catheters. *Adv Perit Dial* 1997;13:183–189.

125. Stegmayr BG, Wikdahl AM, Arnerlov C, Petersen E. A modified lateral technique for the insertion of peritoneal dialysis catheters enabling immediate start of dialysis. *Perit Dial Int* 1998;18(3):329–331.

126. Moncrief JW, Popovich RP, Dasgupta M, et al. Reduction in peritonitis incidence in continuous ambulatory peritoneal dialysis with a new catheter and implantation technique. *Perit Dial Int* 1993;13:S329–S331.

127. Danielsson A, Blohme L, Tranaeus A, Hylander B. A prospective randomized study of the effect of a subcutaneously "buried" peritoneal dialysis catheter technique versus standard technique on the incidence of peritonitis and exit-site infection. *Perit Dial Int* 2002;22:211–219.

128. Prischl FC, Wallner M, Kalchmair H, et al. Initial subcutaneous embedding of the peritoneal dialysis catheter—a critical appraisal of this new implantation technique. *Nephrol Dial Transplant* 1997;12:1661–1667.

129. Gadallah MF, Pervez A, el-Shahawy MA, et al. Peritoneoscopic versus surgical placement of peritoneal dialysis catheters: a prospective randomized study on outcome. *Am J Kidney Dis* 1999;33(1):118–122.

130. Pastan S, Gassensmith C, Manatunga AK, et al. Prospective comparison of peritoneoscopic and surgical implantation of CAPD catheters. *Trans Am Soc Artif Intern Organs* 1991;37: M154–M156.

131. Lye WC, Kour NW, van der Straaten JC, et al. A Prospective randomized comparison of the Swan Neck, coiled, and straight Tenckhoff catheters in patients on CAPD. *Perit Dial Int* 1996;16(suppl 1):S333–S335.

132. Shaldon S, Koch KM, Quellhorst E, et al. CAPD is a second-class treatment. *Contrib Nephrol* 1985;44:163–172.

133. Diaz-Buxo JA, Geissinger G. Single cuff versus double cuff Tenckhoff catheter. *Perit Dial Bull* 1984;4:100–102.

134. Khanna R, Twardowski ZJ. Recommendations for treatment of exit-site pathology. *Perit Dial Int* 1996;16:S100–S104.

135. Piraino B, Bernardini J, Sorkin M. The influence of peritoneal catheter exit-site infections on peritonitis, tunnel infections, and catheter loss in patients on continuous ambulatory peritoneal dialysis. *Am J Kidney Dis* 1986;8: 436–440.

136. Flanigan MJ, Hochstetter LA, Langholdt D, Lim VS. CAPD catheter infections: diagnosis and management. *Perit Dial Int* 1994;14:248–254.

137. Taber TE, Hegeman TF, York SM, et al. Treatment of *Pseudomonas* infections in peritoneal dialysis patients. *Perit Dial Int* 1991;11:213–216.

138. Kazmi HR, Raffone FD, Kliger AS, Fenkelstein FO. *Pseudomonas* exit-site infections in CAPD patients. *J Am Soc Nephrol* 1992;2:1498–1501.

139. Strauss FG, Holmes DL, Nortman DF, Friedman S. Hypertonic saline compresses: therapy for complicated exit-site infections. *Adv Perit Dial* 1993;9:248–250.

140. Nichols WK, Nolph KD. A technique for managing exit site and cuff infection in Tenckhoff catheters. *Perit Dial Bull* 1983;3:S4–S5.

141. Scalamogna A, De Vecchi A, Maccario M, et al. Cuff-shaving procedure. A rescue treatment for exit-site infection unresponsive to medical therapy. *Nephrol Dial Transplant* 1995;10:2325–2327.

142. Glickman JD, Rafanello T, Gerhardt RE, et al. Surgical treatment of persistent exit-site infections. *Adv Perit Dial* 1996;12:209–210.

143. Suh H, Wadhwa NK, Cabralda T, et al. Persistent exit-site/tunnel infection and subcutaneous cuff removal in PD patients. *Adv Perit Dial* 1997;13:233–236.

144. St. Laurent M, Surendranath C, Saad T, et al. A new salvage procedure for peritoneal dialysis catheters with exit site infections. *Am Surg* 1998;12:1215–1217.

145. Roman J. Tenckhoff catheter repair by the splicing technique. *Perit Dial Bull* 1984;4:89–91.

146. Cheung AHS, Wheeler MS, Limm WML, et al. A salvage technique for continuous ambulatory peritoneal dialysis catheters with exit-site infections. *Am J Surg* 1995;170:60–61.

147. Wu YM, Tsai MK, Chao SH, et al. Surgical management of refractory exit-site/tunnel infection of Tenckhoff catheter: technical innovations of partial replantation. *Perit Dial Int* 1999;19:451–454.

148. Fukasawa M, Matsushita K, Tanabe N, et al. A novel salvage technique that does not require catheter removal for exit-site infection. *Perit Dial Int* 2002;22:618–621.

149. Cancarini GC, Manili L, Brunori G, et al. Simultaneous catheter replacement-removal during infectious complications in peritoneal dialysis. *Adv Perit Dial* 1994;10:210–213.

150. Posthuma N, Borgstein PJ, Eijsbouts Q, ter Wee PM. Simultaneous peritoneal dialysis catheter insertion and removal in catheter-related infections without interruption of peritoneal dialysis. *Nephrol Dial Transplant* 1998;13:700–703.

151. Mitra A, Teitelbaum I. Is it safe to simultaneously remove and replace infected peritoneal dialysis catheters? Review of the literature and suggested guidelines. *Adv Perit Dial* 2003;19:255–259.

152. Keane WF, Bailie GR, Boeschoten E, et al. Adult peritoneal dialysis-related peritonitis treatment recommendations: 2000 update. *Perit Dial Int* 2000;20:396–411.

153. Swartz R, Messana J, Reynolds J, Ranjit U. Simultaneous catheter replacement and removal in refractory peritoneal dialysis infections. *Kidney Int* 1991;40:1160–1165.

154. Honkanen E, Eklund B, Laasonen L, et al. Reposition of a displaced peritoneal catheter: the Helsinki whiplash method. *Adv Perit Dial* 1990;6:159–164.

155. Hevia C, Bajo MA, Aguilera A, et al. Alpha replacement method for displaced peritoneal catheter: a simple and effective maneuver. *Adv Perit Dial* 2001;17:138–141.

156. Kumwenda MJ, Wright FK. The use of a channel-cleaning brush for malfunctioning Tenckhoff catheters. *Nephrol Dial Transplant* 1999;14:1254–1257.

157. Gadallah MF, Arora N, Arumugam R, Moles K. Role of Fogarty catheter manipulation in management of migrated, nonfunctional peritoneal dialysis catheters. *Am J Kidney Dis* 2000;35:301–305.

158. Crabtree JH, Fishman A. Laparoscopic epiplopexy of the greater omentum and epiploic appendices in the salvaging of dysfunctional peritoneal dialysis catheters. *Surg Laparosc Endosc* 1996;6:176–180.

159. Leblanc M, Ouimet D, Pichette V. Dialysate leaks in peritoneal dialysis. *Semin Dial* 2001;14:50–54.

160. Canivet E, Lavaud S, Wampach H, et al. Detection of subclinical abdominal hernia by peritoneal scintigraphy. *Adv Perit Dial* 2000;16:104–107.

161. Jagasia MH, Cole FH, Stegman MH, et al. Video-assisted talc pleurodesis in the management of pleural effusion secondary to continuous ambulatory peritoneal dialysis report of three cases. *Am J Kidney Dis* 1996;28:772–774.

162. Okaka H, Ryuzaki M, Kotaki S, et al. Thoracoscopic surgery and pleurodesis for pleuroperitoneal communication in patients on continuous ambulatory peritoneal dialysis. *Am J Kidney Dis* 1999;34:170–172.

163. Tang S, Chui WH, Tang AW, et al. Video-assisted thoracoscopic talc pleurodesis is effective for maintenance of peritoneal dialysis in acute hydrothorax complicating peritoneal dialysis. *Nephrol Dial Transplant* 2003;18:804–808.

164. Cruz C, Faber M, Melendez A. Peritoneoscopic implantation of Tenckhoff catheters for CAPD: effect on catheter function, survival and tunnel infection (abstr). *Perit Dial Int* 1989;9:S1.

165. Akyol AM, Porteous C, Brown MW. A comparison of two types of catheters for continuous ambulatory peritoneal dialysis (CAPD). *Perit Dial Int* 1990;10:63–66.

166. Nielson PK, Hemmingsen C, et al. Comparison of straight and curled Tenckhoff peritoneal dialysis catheters implanted by the subcutaneous technique: a prospective randomized study. *Perit Dial Int* 1995;15:18–21.

167. Scott PD, Bakran A, et al. Peritoneal dialysis access. Prospective randomized trial of three different peritoneal catheters. Preliminary report. *Perit Dial Int* 1994;14:289–290.

168. Eklund BH, Honkanen EO, et al. Peritoneal dialysis access. Prospective randomized comparison of the Swan neck and Tenckhoff catheters. *Perit Dial Int* 1995;15:353–356.

169. Cruz C, Faber M, Melendez A. A peritoneoscopic implanation of Tenckhoff catheters for CAPD: effect on catheter function, survival and tunnel infection (abstr). *Perit Dial Int* 1989;9:51.

170. Dasgupta MK, McKay S, Olsen M, Costerton JW. Silver-coated peritoneal catheter reduces colonization by *Staphylococcus aureus* in a rabbit model of peritoneal dialysis (abstr). *Perit Dial Int* 1994;14(suppl 1):S86.

171. Tenckhoff H, Schechter H. A bacteriologically safe peritoneal access device. *ASAIO Trans* 1968;14:181–185.

172. Bierman M, Kasperbauer J, Kisek A, et al. Peritoneal catheter survival and complications in end stage renal disease. *Perit Dial Bull* 1985;5:229–233.

173. Valenti G, Cresseri D, Bianchi ML, et al. Surgical complications during continuous ambulatory peritoneal dialysis. *Perit Dial Bull* 1985;5:39–42.

174. Slingeneyer A, Mion C. Peritoneal catheters: update 1985. In: LaGreca G, Chiabamontes S, Fabris A, et al, eds. *Peritoneal Dialysis.* Milan: Wichtig Editore, 1986:171–173.

175. Nebel M, Marczewski K, Finke K. Three years of experience with the Swan-Neck Tenckhoff catheter. *Adv Perit Dial* 1991;7:208–213.

176. Scalamogna A, De Vecchi A, Castelnovo C, Ponticelli C. Peritoneal catheter outcome effect of mode of placement. *Perit Dial Int* 1994;14(suppl 1):S81.

177. Brewer TE, Caldwell FT, Patterson RM, Flanigan WJ. Indwelling peritoneal (Tenckhoff) dialysis catheter: experience with 24 patients. *JAMA* 1972;219:1011–1015.

178. Thomas C, Mahoney JF, Darlison P, et al. Peritoneal dialysis using a semi-permanent intra-abdominal catheter. *Med J Aust* 1973;2:1037–1039.

179. Giordano C, Desanto NG, Papa A, et al. Short daily peritoneal dialysis. *Kidney Int* 1975;7:425–430.

180. Karanicolas S, Oreopoulos DG, Pylychuk G, et al. Home peritoneal dialysis: three years experience in Toronto. *Can Med Assoc J* 1977;116:266–269.

181. Khanna R, Oreopoulos DB, Dombros N, et al. CAPD after three years: still promising treatment. *Perit Dial Bull* 1981; 1:24–34.

182. Rottembourg J, Dominque J, Von Lantehen M, et al. Straight or curled Tenckhoff peritoneal catheter for continuous ambulatory peritoneal dialysis (CAPD). *Perit Dial Bull* 1981;1:123–124.

183. Odor A, Alessio-Robles L, Leuchter J, et al. Experience with 150 consecutive peritoneal catheters in patients on CAPD. *Perit Dial Bull* 1985;5:226–229.

184. Flanigan MJ, Hgheim DD, Schulak JA, et al. The use and complications of three peritoneal dialysis catheter designs—a retrospective analysis. *ASAIO Trans* 1987;33:33–38.

185. Gibel LJ, Quintana BJ, Tzamaloukas AH. Soft tissue complications of Tenckhoff catheters (abstr). *Perit Dial Int* 1989; 9:S1.

186. Baker WB, Pratt J, Stone K, et al. Peritonitis and exit site infection rates using single-cuff Tenckhoff Missouri swan-neck peritoneal catheters (abstr). *Perit Dial Int* 1989;9:51.

187. Davis DS, McMorrow RG. The importance of surgical expertise in preventing peritoneal catheter complications (abstr). *Perit Dial Int* 1989;9:S1.

188. Stegmayr V, Hedberg B, Sandzen B, Wikdahl AM. Absence of leakage by insertion of peritoneal dialysis catheter through the rectus muscle. *Perit Dial Int* 1990;10: 53–55.

189. Piraino B, Bernardini J, Centa PK, et al. The effect of body weight on CAPD related infections and catheter loss. *Perit Dial Int* 1991;11:64–68.

190. Shah GM, Sabo A, Nguyen T, Juler GL. Peritoneal catheters: a comparative study of column disc and Tenckhoff catheters. *Int J Artif Organs* 1990;13:267–272.

191. Rubin J, Didlake R, Raju S, Hsu H. A prospective randomized evaluation of chronic peritoneal catheters. *ASAIO Trans* 1990;36:M497–M500.

192. Buijsen JGM, Kox C, Boeschoten EW, Strujik DG. Randomised trial to compare single cuff (Sc) with double cuff (Dc) straight Tenckhoff catheter (Tc) in CAPD patients (pt)(abstr). *Artif Organs* 1993;17:466.

193. Alvaro F, Romero JR, Selgas R, et al. Moncrief's technique for peritoneal catheter placement—a three years experience. *Perit Dial Int* 1994;14(suppl 1):S10.

194. Handt AE, Ash SR. Longevity of Tenckhoff catheters placed by the Vitec peritoneoscopic technique. *Perspect Perit Dial* 1984;2:30–33.

195. Cruz C, Melendez A, Faber M, et al. Can the incidence of peritoneal catheter tunnel infections be reduced (abstr)? *Perit Dial Int* 1988;8:72.

196. Adamson AS, Kelleher JP, Snell ME, Hulme B. Endoscopic placement of CAPD catheters: a review of one hundred procedures. *Nephrol Dial Transplant* 1992;7:855–857.

197. Donate T, Rousaud F, Oliva JA, et al. Peritoneal catheter (PC) implantation through Y-Tec system (abstr). *Perit Dial Int* 1993;13(suppl 1):S39.

198. Swartz DA, Sandroni SE, Moles KA. Laparoscopic Tenckhoff catheter placement: a single center's experience (abstr). *Perit Dial Int* 1993;13:S31.

199. Lindblad AS, Novak JS, Nolph KD, et al. Final report of the national CAPD Registry. *National Institute of Diabetes and Digestive and Kidney Diseases.* July 1988:7–67.

200. Bozhurt F, Keller E, Schollmeyer P. Swan neck peritoneal dialysis catheter can reduce catheter complications in CAPD patients. *Perit Dial Bull* 1987;7:S9.

201. Ishizaki M, Suzuki K, Kurosawa K, et al. Swan neck Sendai catheter: a modification of the swan neck Tenckhoff catheter. *Perit Dial Int* 1988;8:221–222.

202. Multicentric Group of study of Continuous Ambulatory Peritoneal Dialysis (Spain). Multicentric prospective study of swan neck peritoneal catheters with intraperitoneal (IP) segment straight or coiled (abstr). *Perit Dial Int* 1991; 11(suppl 1):203.

203. Twardowski ZJ, Khanna R, Nichols WK, et al. Low complication rates with swan neck short tunnel peritoneal catheter. *Perit Dial Bull* 1987;7(suppl 1):80.

204. Twardowski ZJ, Prowant BF, Khanna R, et al. Long-term experience with Swan Neck Missouri catheters. *ASAIO Trans* 1991;36:M154–M156.

205. Twardowski ZJ, Prowant BF, Nichols WK, et al. Six-year experience with swan neck catheters. *Perit Dial Int* 1992;12: 384–389.

206. Swartz R, Rocher L, Messana J, et al. The curled catheter: optimal access choice for chronic peritoneal dialysis (CPD). *ASAIO Abstr* 1989;18:77.

207. Swartz R, Messana J, Rocher L, et al. The curled catheter: dependable device for percutaneous peritoneal access. *Perit Dial Int* 1990;10:231–235.

208. Pastan S, Gassensmith C, Manatunga AK, et al. Prospective comparison of peritoneoscopic and surgical implantation of CAPD catheters. *ASAIO Trans* 1991;37:M154–M156.

209. Scalamogna A, Castelnovo C, De Vechhi A, Ponticelli C. Exit-site and tunnel infections in continuous ambulatory peritoneal dialysis patients. *Am J Kidney Dis* 1991;6: 674–677.

210. Dryden MS, Ludlam HA, Wing AJ, Phillips I. Active intervention dramatically reduces CAPD-associated infection. *Adv Perit Dial* 1991;7:125–128.

211. Scabardi M, Ronco C, Chiaramonte S, et al. Dynamic catheterography in the early diagnosis of peritoneal catheter malfunction. *Int J Artif Organs* 1992;15:358–364.

212. Chadha I, Mulgaonkar S, Jacobs M, et al. Outcome of laparoscopic Tenckhoff catheter insertion (LTCI) versus surgical Tenckhoff catheter insertion (STCI): a prospective randomized comparison. *Perit Dial Int* 1994;14(suppl 1):S89.

213. Han DC, Cha HK, So IN, et al. Subcutaneously implanted catheters reduce the incidence of peritonitis during CAPD by eliminating infection by periluminal route. *Adv Perit Dial* 1992;8:298–300.

214. Wadhwa NK, Cabralda T, Suh H, et al. Exit-site/tunnel infection and catheter outcome in peritoneal dialysis patients. *Adv Perit Dial* 1992;8:325–327.

215. Gokal R, Ash SR, Helfrich GB, et al. Peritoneal catheters and exit-site practices: toward optimum peritoneal access. *Perit Dial Int* 1993;13:29–39.

216. Brandt CP, Franceschi D. Laparoscopic placement of peritoneal dialysis catheters in patients who have undergone prior abdominal operations. *J Am Coll Surg* 1994;178: 515–516.

217. Ash SR, Daugirdas JT. Peritoneal access devices. In: Ing TS, Daugirdas JT, eds. *Handbook of Dialysis*. Boston, MA: Little, Brown, 1994:274–300.

218. Oreopoulous DG, Baird-Helfrich G, Khanna R, et al. Peritoneal catheters and exit-site practices: current recommendations. *Perit Dial Bull* 1987;7(3):130–138.

219. Diaz-Buxo JA, Turner MW, Nelms M. Fluoroscopic manipulation of Tenckhoff catheters: outcome analysis. *Clin Nephrol* 1997;47:384–388.

220. Hwang SJ, Chang JM, Chen HC, et al. Smaller insertion angle of Tenckhoff catheter increases the chance of catheter migration in CAPD patients. *Perit Dial Int* 1998;18: 433–443.

221. Kappel JE, Ferguson GMC, Kudel RM, et al. Stiff wire manipulation of peritoneal dialysis catheters. *Adv Perit Dial* 1995;11:202–207.

222. Kim JH, Lee TW, Ihm CG, Kim MJ. Use of fluoroscopy-guided wire manipulation and/or laparoscopic surgery in the repair of malfunctioning peritoneal dialysis catheters. *Am J Nephrol* 2002;22:532–538.

223. Twardowski ZJ. Peritoneal dialysis catheter exit site infections: prevention, diagnosis, treatment, and future directions. *Semin Dial* 1992;5:305–315.

224. Ash SR, Sutton JM, Mankus RA, et al. Clinical trials of the T-fluted (Ash Advantage) peritoneal dialysis catheter. *Adv Renal Replace Ther* 2002;(9):133–143.

225. Verger C, Chesneau A-M, Thibault M, Bataille N. Biofilm on Tenckhoff catheters: a negligible source of contamination. *Perit Dial Bull* 1987;7(3):174–178.

226. Rubin J, Raju S, Teal N, et al. Abdominal hernia in patients undergoing continuous ambulatory peritoneal dialysis. *Arch Intern Med* 1982;142:1453–1455.

227. O'Connor J, Rutland M. Demonstration of pleuro-peritoneal communication with radionuclide imaging in a CAPD patient. *Perit Dial Bull* 1981;1:153.

228. Cancarini GC, Manili L, Brunori G, et al. Simultaneous catheter replacement-removal during infectious complications in peritoneal dialysis. *Adv Perit Dial* 1994;10: 210–213.

229. Canivet E, Lavaud S, Wampach H, et al. Detection of subclinical abdominal hernia by peritoneal scintigraphy. *Adv Perit Dial* 2000;16:104–107.

Physiology of Peritoneal Dialysis

Zbylut J. Twardowski

ANATOMY OF THE PERITONEUM

The Peritoneum and the Peritoneal Cavity

The peritoneum is a living membrane consisting of two principal parts: (1) the parietal peritoneum lining the inner surface of the abdominal and pelvic walls, including the diaphragm, and (2) the visceral peritoneum, which covers visceral organs and forms the omentum and the visceral mesentery, connecting loops of bowel.[1–3] The peritoneum forms a closed sac in the male and is continuous with the mucous membrane of the uterine tubes in the female. The uterine tubes are ordinarily collapsed; thus there is normally no free communication between the peritoneal sac and the exterior. The peritoneum contains only small amounts of fluid (probably less than 100 mL) and is ordinarily nearly collapsed. In an adult of normal size, the space can be enlarged by instillation of fluid; 2 or more L of fluid can be accommodated without causing discomfort. The surface of the membrane is a shiny layer of mesothelial cells, beneath which lies supporting interstitium containing extracellular fluid, connective tissue fibers, blood vessels, and lymphatics. The mesentery, as well as the omentum, consists of two sheets of mesothelium that enclose a layer of connective tissue. The total surface area of the peritoneal mesothelium (parietal and visceral) is believed to approximate the surface area of skin. As a result of very careful measurements, Wegner found a total peritoneal surface area averaging 1.782 m^2 in cadavers with an average body surface area of 1.750 m^2.[4] Hertzler obtained somewhat higher values in 20 cadavers, but again the mean total peritoneal surface area of 2.199 m^2 and the mean total body surface area of 2.217 m^2 were very similar.[5] Children have a proportionally larger peritoneal area than adults.[6]

The Parietal Peritoneum. The parietal peritoneum is attached to the fascia endoabdominalis, which lines the structures of the abdominal wall.[5] This is composed of the transversalis fascia, quadratus fascia, the fascia of the pelvis, the diaphragm, etc. The peritoneum is so closely attached to it in certain regions (e.g., transversalis fascia) that, for practical purposes, surgeons consider it a single structure.

The endoabdominal fascia of the anterior abdominal wall is covered by the peritoneum almost without interruption with the exception of the attachment of the round ligament of the liver to the umbilicus and the attachment of the falciform ligament of the liver to the transversalis fascia and the posterior rectus sheath. Fascia of the pelvis in the male is covered uninterruptedly by the peritoneum. In the female, the peritoneum is interrupted by the interface with the mucous membranes of the uterine tubes. The passage of the peritoneum over the posterior abdominal wall is interrupted by the mesoappendix, the mesentery, the transverse mesocolon, and the sigmoid mesocolon. The diaphragmatic area of the peritoneum is interrupted by the coronary ligament of the liver, the falciform ligament of the liver, and the gastrophrenic ligament. The coronary ligament of the liver borders the bare area of the liver where the liver is in direct contact with the diaphragm.

The Visceral Peritoneum. The visceral peritoneum begins in the posterior abdominal wall as a two-layer structure with the roots of mesentery, mesocolon, mesoappendix, and sigmoid mesocolon; it covers corresponding organs as a single layer structure. The ascending and descending colon lie retroperitoneally. In the diaphragmatic area, the visceral peritoneum begins with the coronary ligament of the liver, falciform ligament of the liver, and gastrophrenic ligament attaching to the greater stomach curvature. Except for the bare area, the liver lies intraperitoneally, covered by a single peritoneal layer. At the porta hepatis, the peritoneum reduplicates, covering the hepatoduodenal ligament and hepatogastric ligament attaching to the lesser stomach curvature. This part of the peritoneum forms the lesser omentum.

The stomach is covered with a single layer of the peritoneum. The peritoneum again reduplicates at the greater curvature, covering the gastrophrenic, gastrosplenic, and gastrocolic ligaments. The gastrosplenic ligament ensheathes the splenic vessels entering the hilum of the spleen. Along the greater-stomach curvature, from the spleen to the duodenum, extends the greater omentum.[7] The gastrocolic ligament constitutes the upper part of the greater omentum. The liver, spleen, stomach, small intestine, transverse and sigmoid colon, appendix, ligaments attached to these organs, mesentery, both transverse and sigmoid mesocolon, and mesoappendix are covered with the visceral peritoneum. The peritoneum of the gastrocolic ligament attaches to the transverse colon and descends as a free part of the greater omentum over the abdominal viscera.

The omental bursa (the lesser sac) is situated behind the gastrocolic ligament, stomach, lesser omentum, and liver, and in front of the transverse mesocolon, parietal peritoneum covering the pancreas, the inferior vena cava, the aorta, and the diaphragm.

The remainder of the space between the parietal and visceral peritoneum forms the greater sac. The greater sac communicates with the omental bursa through the epiploic foramen of Winslow. It is bound superiorly by the caudate lobe of the liver, inferiorly by the superior part of the duodenum, posteriorly by the inferior vena cava, and anteriorly by the lesser omentum. The foramen readily admits two fingers. Figure 14–1 portrays schematically the greater and lesser sac of the peritoneum. Note that the second and third layers of the omentum are fused at the transverse colon. Thus, the omental bursa does not descend below the transverse colon into the greater sac.

Blood Supply. The parietal peritoneum receives its blood supply from the vasculature of the adjacent structures covered by the peritoneum: phrenic, abdominal wall muscle, retroperitoneal, and pelvic vessels. The arterial blood sup-

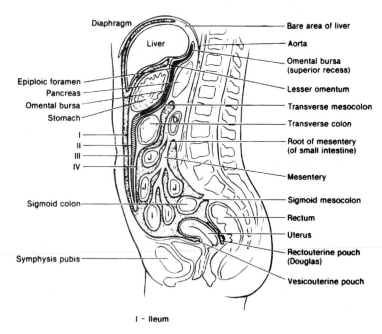

Figure 14–1. Sagittal section of the female abdomen showing the greater and lesser sacs. In adults, the omental bursa does not descend below the transverse colon because layers II and III of the greater omentum are completely fused at this level.

I - Ileum

ply to the visceral peritoneum comes from the celiac, superior, and inferior mesenteric arteries and their branches:

1. Left gastric to the stomach and lesser omentum
2. Common hepatic to the liver, through the right gastric artery to the stomach and lesser omentum, through the right gastroepiploic artery to the stomach and greater omentum
3. Splenic to the spleen and through the gastroepiploic artery to the stomach and greater omentum
4. Superior mesenteric to the mesentery, mesoappendix, and transverse mesocolon
5. Inferior mesenteric to the mesosigmoid colon

Almost all venous blood from the visceral peritoneum and a majority of that from the parietal peritoneum covering the retroperitoneal space is drained through the inferior and superior mesenteric, splenic, and left gastric veins that ultimately drain to the portal vein of the liver.

The exact ratio of parietal to visceral peritoneal surface area is unknown, but the many folds of visceral mesentery obviously represent a larger fraction of the total peritoneal surface area; therefore parietal peritoneum participation in solute transport during peritoneal dialysis is usually considered to be less than the participation of visceral peritoneum. Portions of the parietal peritoneum, however, may be more vascular than some of the avascular sections of mesentery, and the true fractional contributions of the parietal and visceral peritoneum to solute transport during peritoneal dialysis have not yet been determined. There is, however, little doubt that most blood from the peritoneum is drained through the portal vein.

The absolute peritoneal capillary blood flow that participates in peritoneal dialysis exchange is not known. Total splanchnic blood flow in adult humans at rest ranges between 1000 to 2400 mL/min.[8] Most of this blood is, however, on its way to visceral organs, not to the small vessels of the peritoneum. In fact, observations of the rat peritoneum suggest that the mesentery itself is not particularly vascular and that most of the small vessels capable of participating in exchange may be located at sites where the peritoneum reflects over loops of bowel.[9] Blood flow through the peritoneal capillaries probably does not exceed 200 mL/min (see "Solute Transfer by Diffusion," below).

Lymph Drainage. The lymphatics from both the small and large intestines drain through chains of mesenteric lymph nodes following the branches of the superior mesenteric vessels, eventually interconnect with preaortic chains of nodes, and ultimately drain through the cisterna chyli to the thoracic duct.[3] This route, however, drains lymph mainly from the gastrointestinal (GI) tract and does not seem to participate in lymphatic drainage from the peritoneal cavity.

Lymphatic drainage from the peritoneal cavity follows two major pathways: diaphragmatic and omental. The di-

aphragmatic pathway seems to be the most important one for transporting fluid from the peritoneal cavity. After leaving the diaphragm, lymph primarily enters the large collecting ducts associated with the internal mammary vessels to reach the anterior mediastinal lymph nodes, and ultimately drains into the right lymphatic duct. In addition to this major lymphatic pathway, vessels from the diaphragm also travel up in the mediastinum to the bronchial lymph nodes and then to the thoracic duct. The substernal pathway is the principal one in many experimental animals and in humans.[10,11] Courtice and Steinbeck found that only 20 percent of labeled plasma protein introduced into the peritoneal cavity passed into the thoracic duct in cats.[11]

There are two primary routes of lymphatic drainage from the omentum: to the right toward the subpyloric nodes and to the left toward the splenic nodes.[7] Both routes are interconnected with celiac nodes that ultimately drain lymph to the thoracic duct above the cisterna chyli.[12] The lymphatic vessels in the omentum seem to play a minor role in the removal of fluid from the peritoneal cavity, because omentectomy does not significantly influence the peritoneum's absorptive capacity.[13,14]

In rabbits, Courtice and Steinbeck showed that the lymphatic absorption of proteins is slower in the pelvis-down posture, because less fluid reaches the diaphragm, the site of predominant protein absorption.[15] Lymphatic drainage from the parietal peritoneum, including pelvic but excluding diaphragmatic peritoneum, is of minor importance in animals and probably in humans. This route may be more important after the infusion of dialysis solution into the peritoneal cavity (see the "Lymphatic Absorption," below).

Mesothelium. The mesothelium as a continuous monolayer formed by flattened cells was described in rabbits by Henle,[16] and an underlying homogeneous basement membrane was described in 1845 by Todd and Bowman.[16] The free surface area of the mesothelium shows many cytoplasmic prolongations or microvilli that were first described by Kolossow.[17] It is not known whether mesothelial microvilli influence transport. In mice, these are usually 1.5 to 3.0 μm long and 40 to 90 nm wide.[18] Microvilli markedly increase gross surface area. Surface charges may trap water between microvilli and prevent friction of adjacent surfaces.[19] The open ends of surface vesicles can be seen at the base of microvilli.[20]

The mesothelial layer is approximately 0.5 μm thick. Nuclei, oval or reniform, are generally located in the central region of the cell and occupy 12 percent of the mesothelial surface area.[20] Nucleoli are absent or rare.[21,22] Most cells bear single cilium.[23] The cytoplasm contains mitochondria, endoplasmic reticulum, and Golgi apparatus, suggesting high-energy consumption and protein synthesis.

The ultrastructure of mesothelial cells has been found to be similar to that of type II pneumocytes. Both mesothelial cells and type II pneumocytes contain lamellar bodies known to be storage vesicles for surfactant, the essential constituent of which is phosphatidylcholine.[23] Both cells secrete lamellar bodies to decrease surface tension in the lungs and the peritoneal cavity, respectively, as well as for easier alveolar expansion in the lungs and better lubrication in the peritoneal cavity.

Round and oval pinocytotic vacuoles are common in all observed mesothelial cells.[24,25] According to Gotloib and colleagues,[21] the vesicles have a mean diameter of 71.7 nm with a fairly normal frequency distribution curve, which suggests that there is in fact only one size of vesicle, with smaller values representing vesicles cut at a distance from their maximal diameter. Vesicles are concentrated at both the basal and the luminal cell borders and are able to transport large molecules, such as iron dextran.[25]

Mesothelial cells contain cancer antigen 125 (CA 125), which was originally detected in ovarian tumor tissue (OC 125).[26] This antigen was found in various fetal tissues, amniotic fluid, and, in adults on the epithelium of the female genital tract and on mesothelial cells of the pleura, pericardium, and peritoneum.[27] CA 125 is a glycoprotein with a molecular weight exceeding 700 kDa.[28] High concentrations of CA 125 in ascitic fluid, markedly exceeding those in plasma, indicate that the peritoneal mesothelial cells are the source of the antigen in peritoneal fluid.[29] In vitro studies of mesothelial cells in monolayers, as well as studies of drained dialysate, concluded that CA 125 is locally produced in the peritoneal cavity during continuous ambulatory peritoneal dialysis (CAPD) and that the mesothelial cells are the major source of this CA 125.[30] This finding led to studies demonstrating that dialysate CA 125 concentration may serve as a marker of mesothelial cell mass in peritoneal dialysis patients.[31]

Mesothelial cells contain aquaporins, or water-selective pores. These are morphologic equivalents of "transcellular" pores in the "three-pore" model of peritoneal transport (see below). The presence of aquaporin-1 (AQP-1) in mesothelial cells was first demonstrated by Lai et al. in 2001.[32] The presence of aquaporin-3 (AQP-3), which is selective for the passage of not only water but also of other small molecules like glycerol and urea, has recently been established in human peritoneal mesothelial cells.[33]

Mesothelial cells have tortuous boundaries, thus increasing the area of contact between cells. Adjacent cells are connected with tight junctions at the luminal surface.[34] Adherent junctions are present subjacent to the tight junctions. Desmosomes are observed deeper than the adherent junctions with microfilaments anchored on the inner aspect of the plasma membrane of two adjoining cells.[35] The abluminal portions of cell interfaces show open intercellular channels approximately 50 nm wide. Intercellular tight junctions are absent in some portions of the mesothelium, resulting in stomata, more prominent on the diaphragmatic peritoneum.[36–38]

A homogenous basement membrane underlying the mesothelial cells is 38.6 nm thick in rabbits[21] and 25 to 40 nm thick in mice.[39] There are some openings in the basement membrane, particularly in the diaphragmatic peritoneum subjacent to the mesothelial stomata, allowing direct contact between the peritoneal cavity and the lymphatics. Some studies indicate that the basement membrane is absent under the omental mesothelium.[39]

Interstitium. The interstitium is filled with isolated fibers or bundles of collagen, a few fibroblasts, occasional macrophages, and blood and lymphatic vessels submerged in a mucopolysaccharide matrix. Hyaluronan (hyaluronic acid, or HA) is the major constituent of the matrix. HA is polysaccharide of varying length made up by repeating disaccharide units of N-acetylglucosamine and glucuronic acid. It is produced by fibroblasts and its molecular weight ranges from 10^6 to 10^7 Da. In the interstitium, it keeps water bound in a gel-sol fashion, hindering water flow.[40] Lubrication is its major role in synovial fluid.[40]

A low concentration of HA is present in noninfected peritoneal dialysate, but it increases tenfold during peritonitis.[41] Mesothelial cells are also likely to produce HA.[41] Lubricating properties of the peritoneal membrane may be augmented by the presence of HA.

In the rabbit mesentery and the diaphragmatic and parietal peritoneum, bundles of collagen arranged in rows parallel to the mesothelial surface form a latticed layer immediately beneath the basement membrane.[35] Parietal peritoneum may have up to six layers of collagen bundles. In the peritoneal interstitium of the small intestine, the superficial collagen fibers are arranged along the longitudinal axis of the intestine and placed between the basement membrane and an underlying elastic network. These two layers, with an approximate thickness of 35 μm, are free of blood and lymphatic capillaries.[42]

Blood and lymphatic vessels are located in the deep-latticed collagenous layer, which is 60 μm thick.[42] In other regions of the peritoneum, the distance between the capillaries and the peritoneal lumen seems to be shorter.

Blood Vessels. Information about the density of the peritoneal microcirculatory net is incomplete. In the rabbit mesentery, only 2.6 percent of the mesothelial surface area covers subjacent capillaries.[21] In rat omentum and mesentery, six to ten capillaries emerge from an arteriole and end in a venule.[43] True capillaries constitute the main population of mesenteric microvessels. They have a single layer of endothelium lying on a continuous basement membrane and occasional perithelial cells. The luminal diameter of true capillaries is up to 7.2 μm and the mean wall thickness is

0.4 μm. Most capillaries have a continuous layer of endothelium. Fenestrated capillaries are found in rabbit diaphragmatic and human parietal peritoneum.[44] Whereas only 1.7 percent of capillaries in humans are fenestrated, the incidence of fenestrated capillaries in the rabbit diaphragmatic peritoneum is 29 percent.[44] An electronegatively charged network (the fibrous glycocalyx) covering the luminal surface of fenestrated capillaries and anionic fixed charges distributed along the subendothelial basement membranes suggest that there is little or no transfenestral passage of macromolecular anionic proteins. It has been hypothesized that fenestrations may explain the high permeability of some peritoneal capillaries to noncharged larger molecules such as vitamin B_{12} and inulin. It has also been proposed that fenestrae could contain a high density of small pores. Better understanding of the role of fenestrated capillaries in peritoneal transport may depend on studies in single perfused microvessels.[45]

The luminal diameter of vessels transitional between true capillaries and postcapillary venules is up to 9.2 μm, and the mean wall thickness is 0.8 μm.[35] The diameter of postcapillary venules ranges between 9.4 and 20.6 μm, with a mean of 12.6 μm and a mean wall thickness of 1.7 μm.[35] With increasing diameter, there is a disproportionately higher increase in wall thickness due to increasing numbers of perithelial cells.

Endothelial cells have oval, elongated, and occasionally kidney-shaped nuclei. The cell cytoplasm contains mitochondria, a rudimentary Golgi apparatus, and rough endoplasmic reticulum.[35] Plasmalemmal or cytoplasmic vesicles with a mean outer diameter of 61.6 nm occupy up to 7 percent of the endothelial cell volume.[35,43] These vesicles open on either aspect of the endothelial cells through a neck with a mean diameter of 16.1 nm.[21] Two-thirds of the vesicles on the surface of the endothelial cells are open at any given time.[46,47] Chains of two or more vesicles form channels open on both sides of the endothelial cells. Such channels are more frequent in the venular segment of the capillary.[48] Adjacent endothelial cells are connected by a labyrinth of irregular adhesion lines in the interendothelial clefts.[49] The slit width appears to be about 20 nm except for a few constricted portions with a slit width of 6 to 7 nm.[50] Capillary and venule endothelia contain AQP-1. The presence of AQP-1 or aquaporin-CHIP in the peritoneal vasculature was first described in 1996[51] before it was found in the mesothelial cells.[32] Aquaporin-2 (AQP-2), regulated by vasopressin, has not been demonstrated in the endothelium of peritoneal capillaries.[52]

Lymphatics. Diaphragmatic lymphatics are the major route of particulate matter absorption from the peritoneal cavity. They begin as terminal channels or lacunae, which anastomose freely with each other and are located beneath the mesothelial covering of the peritoneal surface of the diaphragm.[53] Lacunae are covered with a roof consisting of three layers: (1) a sheet of mesothelial cells, (2) a layer of connective tissue forming a lattice of fibers, and (3) an inner endothelial layer.[54]

The mesothelial cells overlying the lacunae are smaller than those covering the rest of the peritoneal membrane, and gaps between the cells are seen in light and electron microscopy.[54] These gaps correspond to peritoneal stomata, first observed by Von Recklinghausen on silver stain preparations as openings capable of accommodating frog erythrocytes, which are 23 μm in diameter.[36] This observation has been confirmed by others.[37,38] These stomata are located at the junction of several mesothelial cells. Along the margin of the stomata, mesothelial and endothelial cells are joined creating a channel that leads from the peritoneal cavity into the lumen of the lacuna. The submesothelial connective tissue is interrupted and its structure is modified to accommodate the channel.[55,56] During expiration, the stomata are open and the lacunae dilated; the pressure gradient favors peritoneal fluid flow into the lacunae. During inspiration, the lacunae are constricted, the overlapping flaps of endothelium and mesothelium close the stomata, and the fluid is forced into the deeper lymphatics rather than returning to the peritoneal cavity.[57,58]

In the omentum, the lymphatics form an irregular interconnecting system of flattened tubes.[12] The saccular terminal lymphatics are located within the vascular system of the milky spot and are in direct contact with the abdominal cavity because of the gaps in the mesothelial lining.[59–61]

Milky spots were first observed by Ranvier, who believed them to be lymph nodes[62]; however, they differ from lymph nodes by the absence of sinus architecture, germ center, and capsule.[63] Carr proposed calling the spots "lymphoreticular organs," because they contain numerous phagocytic elements.[64] Milky spots are not preformed structures but rather extremely dynamic structures that form in response to specific immune reactions.[65]

Uremic Peritoneum

The morphology of the peritoneum in uremia and after exposure to the dialysis solution has been extensively studied and reported by the International Peritoneal Biopsy Registry.[66] The most prominent difference between the normal and uremic peritoneum is in the structure of the mesothelial cells. About one-third of specimens taken from the parietal peritoneum at the time of a first catheter implantation show distinctive inclusion bodies. They are formed in the cistern of the rough endoplasmic reticulum and burst out to lie free in the cytosol. Cells containing a large number of these inclusions become detached from the basement membrane. As a consequence, localized areas of peritoneal membrane with defoliated mesothelium are formed. The etiology of these inclusions is not known, but they seem to be associated with the uremic state, because they are not observed after initiation of peritoneal dialysis.

Peritoneum in Peritoneal Dialysis

Constant exposure to the dialysis solution causes reactive proliferation of mesothelium, giving rise to an increased number of cells per unit area. Scanning electron microscopy shows a decrease in density of microvilli leading to a decrease in cell membrane reserve.[66] The number of micropinocytotic vesicles is also reduced. The most characteristic feature of cell cytoplasm is the hyperplasia of the rough endoplasmic reticulum, indicating an adaptive response to constant removal of secretory products in dialysate.

In nondiabetic patients, the basement membrane of mesothelium and stromal blood vessels may undergo diabetiform transformation. The membrane becomes thickened and reduplicated; pericyte debris is present in the walls of blood vessels, implicating increased cell death and turnover. These changes are particularly pronounced after episodes of peritonitis. Dobbie et al.[66] speculated that the exposure to high glucose concentration causes nonenzymatic glycosylation of proteins, resulting in diabetiform alterations of the basement membrane. The loss of mesothelium during and for some time after peritonitis exposes stroma to glucose concentrations 10 to 40 times greater than those found in normal serum. This concept of pathogenesis is further supported by observations that nondiabetic patients without a history of peritonitis may have no basement membrane alterations.

Any agent that causes irritation of the mesothelial layer and induces serositis or single severe or multiple episodes of peritonitis resulting in mesothelial loss predisposes the peritoneum to fibroneogenesis.[67] Fibrin deposition and fibrinolysis, hyalinization of the superficial stromal collagen—possibly tanned through nonenzymatic glycosylation by dialysate glucose, and the proliferative potential of mesothelial stem cells play important and possibly interdependent roles in the excessive fibroneogenesis in certain patients on CAPD.

These observations led Dobbie et al.[66] to challenge the wisdom of using glucose-based dialysis solution during peritonitis episodes. Recent report of the Peritoneal Biopsy Registry,[68] based on studies of the parietal peritoneal membranes of 130 patients undergoing peritoneal dialysis, confirmed and extended previous studies on smaller number of samples. Samples from peritoneal dialysis patients were compared with the peritoneal membranes of normal individuals, uremic predialysis patients, and patients undergoing hemodialysis. The median thickness of the submesothelial compact collagenous zone was 50 μm for normal subjects, 140 μm for uremic patients, 150 μm for patients undergoing hemodialysis, and 270 μm for patients undergoing peritoneal dialysis (PD). Compact-zone thickness in-

creased progressively with the duration of PD therapy from 180 μm in first two years of therapy, to 240 μm at 2 to 4 years, 300 μm at 5 to 6 years, and 750 μm at 7 to 8 years. Vascular changes, which included progressive subendothelial hyalinization with luminal narrowing or obliteration, were seen in 56 percent of biopsies from patients undergoing PD. The prevalence of vasculopathy progressed with therapy duration. These vascular changes are associated with and may be related to increased activity of nitric oxide synthase (NOS), which increases local nitric oxide activity in long-term peritoneal dialysis patients. NOS activity is increased fivefold in long-term PD patients compared with control subjects and is positively correlated with the duration of PD. These changes are associated with upregulation of vascular endothelial growth factor (VEGF) mostly along the endothelium lining peritoneal blood vessels co-localized with the advanced glycation end-product deposits.[69] It is widely believed that conventional acidic, lactate-buffered glucose-containing dialysis solutions contribute to both the structural and functional changes in the dialyzing peritoneal membrane.[70]

PHYSIOLOGY OF THE PERITONEUM

Primary Functions of the Peritoneum

The primary function of the peritoneum is to provide a smooth surface of contact between intraabdominal organs and the abdominal wall. Microvilli, with their glycocalyx charges, may trap water, lubricate the surface, and prevent friction.[19] Healthy humans have minimal amounts of fluid in the peritoneal cavity. Fluid is constantly filtered into the peritoneal cavity from the capillaries and absorbed at the same rate. It seems that the fluid turnover in the normal human is approximately 1 L per day.[71] The rate of absorption of electrolyte solutions infused into the peritoneal cavity depends on crystalloid osmotic pressure; it is most rapid when serum osmolality greatly exceeds that of the peritoneal fluid.[72–74] Isosmotic fluids are absorbed at the same rate as whole plasma.[10,75] The principal route of fluid absorption from the peritoneal cavity is convective transport through diaphragmatic lymphatics.[76]

Whole blood is also removed from the peritoneal cavity; however, the red blood cells are absorbed more slowly than is the plasma. Blood transfusions have been given via the intraperitoneal route, particularly in children and in the fetus in utero.[77–79] Red blood cells are absorbed mostly through diaphragmatic lymphatics. Thus, particles up to 23 μm in size are cleared through the diaphragmatic lymphatic system.

The omentum has been called an "abdominal policeman" because of its role in combating and localizing intraperitoneal infection.[80] Living bacteria introduced into the peritoneal cavity induce antibody production in the cells comprising the milky spots.[81] Omental milky spots probably act as the first line of defense in the peritoneal cavity and contain macrophages and lymphocytes. Macrophages form clusters near the peritoneal surface of the milky spots and are oriented toward the peritoneal cavity for migration. Clusters of B and T lymphocytes are typically found in the periarteriolar locations within the milky spots. The spots are analogous to regional lymph nodes.[82] Omentectomy lowers the resistance to abdominal infections.[7] Various foreign bodies, including bacteria and tissue particles, are absorbed by the omentum.[83,84] This omental absorption has been most impressively shown after intraperitoneal administration of suspended charcoal.[85] When the omentum is intact, most charcoal is taken up by the omentum; however, after omentectomy, the particles are scattered around the abdominal cavity. If particle size exceeds the omental absorption capacity, particles are encapsulated by tissue pouches.[86] Omental adhesions also develop after intraperitoneal trauma, ischemia, and/or infection. Suction of the omentum into the ports of peritoneal dialysis catheters causes entanglement.

The Peritoneum as a Dialysis System

After intraperitoneal infusion of 2000 mL of peritoneal dialysis solution in patients without intraabdominal organomegaly and/or any clinical suspicion of fluid maldistribution and as evaluated in the supine position, approximate fluid contents in the intraperitoneal spaces are: pelvis, 30 to 55 percent; paracolic gutter, 15 to 30 percent; perisplenic and perihepatic, 10 to 20 percent each; and lesser sac, 1 to 3 percent (Figs. 14–2 and 14–3). A small amount of fluid is retained in the peritoneal cavity after drainage in the supine position, but usually no fluid is seen after drainage in the upright position.[87] Although the peritoneum was not designed for dialysis, it serves this purpose amazingly well. Peritoneal dialysis does not infringe on the "lubricating" function of the peritoneum, but its ability to combat and localize infection is compromised. Absorptive functions of the peritoneum may be altered depending on the composition of the solution instilled into the peritoneal cavity and on increased intraabdominal pressure.

Resistance to Solute and Water Transport. Solutes moving from peritoneal capillaries into the peritoneal cavity encounter at least six sites of resistance[88]: R_1, fluid films within peritoneal capillaries; R_2, the capillary endothelium; R_3, the capillary basement membrane; R_4, the interstitium; R_5, the mesothelium; and R_6, stagnant fluid films within the peritoneal cavity. These sites and their hypothesized dimensions are diagrammatically shown in Fig. 14–4.

The exact route taken by solutes traversing the peritoneal cellular layers has not been established. Fluid films within peritoneal capillaries present little resistance because

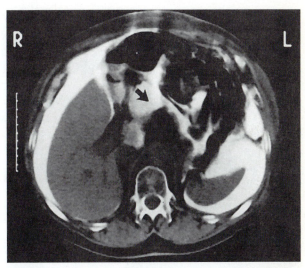

Figure 14–2. Computed tomography of the upper abdomen after filling the peritoneal cavity with 2 L of dialysis solution containing 100 mL of 60% diatrizoate meglumine. Most of the fluid is distributed in the perihepatic and perisplenic areas in the supine position. The lesser sac (arrow) is usually filled with the peritoneal fluid.

of the very short distance the molecules have to pass. The capillary endothelium constitutes a very selective barrier for solute diffusion. Since the original suggestion by Grotte,[89] a "two-pore model" has been supported by a large number of investigators.[90–92] It is generally accepted that small pores are located within the interendothelial clefts (see "Blood Vessels," above). The morphologic equivalent of the large pores is uncertain. The large pores are represented either by channels of fused vesicles or a few interendothelial gaps, which occur particularly in the venular part of the capillary, similar to those produced by mediators of inflammation[52] (see above). Molecules larger than 4.2 nm in radius are excluded by the small pores and transported through the large pores that constitute only 1/30,000 of the total number of pores.[89] It has not been determined whether fenestrated capillaries play a role in the transport of large molecules. In the early 1990s, Rippe et al.[93] developed a "three-pore" model which better conforms to experimental data. The model assumed the existence of small "paracellular" pores (radius 47 Å), "large" pores (radius 250 Å), and ultrasmall, "transcellular" pores (radius 4 to 5 Å). The ultrasmall pores are permeable to water but impermeable to almost all solutes and it is clear now that they are aquaporins localized in peritoneal capillaries[51,52] and mesothelial cells[32,33] (see above for discussion of aquaporins).

Based on this model, computer-simulated curves for intraperitoneal dialysate volume versus time made a good fit with those obtained experimentally in adult patients using solutions of various dextrose concentrations.[93] The model predicts the fall in dialysate sodium concentration as a function of the rate of ultrafiltration (a phenomenon re-

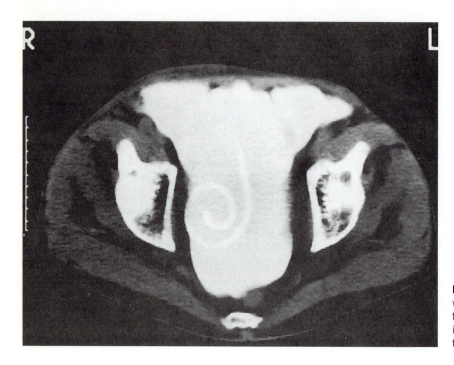

Figure 14–3. Computed tomography of the pelvis with the same technique as in Fig. 14–2. The conditions for fluid drainage are best if the catheter tip is in the rectovesical pouch, which is usually filled with the dialysate.

lated to the well-known sodium sieving characteristics of the peritoneal membrane) and agrees with the peritoneal equilibration test data (see below).

Wayland[94] suggests that the endothelium is a low-resistance barrier to small solute movement from peritoneal capillary blood into the peritoneal cavity. When rats are injected with a fluorescein-tagged small solute, extensive migration of the solute into the interstitium is observed. This contrasts with observations after injection of fluorescein-tagged albumin, where movement of albumin across vascular walls is not obvious over many minutes unless agents that increase vascular permeability are administered in solutions bathing the peritoneum.[94]

The basement membrane seems to offer little resistance to solute diffusion when molecular mass is less than 30,000 Da.[90,95] Patients on chronic peritoneal dialysis may develop a multilayered basal lamina in postcapillary venules and mesothelium of the parietal peritoneum.[96] It is not known whether these reduplications of the peritoneal basement membranes affect transport.

The interstitial solute path probably represents a relatively long distance[88] and, as shown in Fig. 14–4, may range

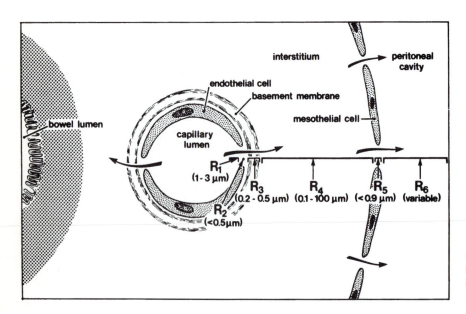

Figure 14–4. Schematic representation of six hypothetical resistance sites to solute movement in peritoneal dialysis and their dimensions. *(From Nolph et al.,[88] with permission.)*

from 0.1 to 100 μm. A distributed model of peritoneal-plasma transport assumes capillaries to be uniformly distributed in the interstitium with some capillaries so distant from the mesothelium that the concentration gradient between plasma and interstitium approaches zero.[97] The situation may be even more complex. Wayland and Silberberg[98] suggest that the interstitium may represent a network of aqueous channels through mucopolysaccharide and collagenous gels. Hypertonic peritoneal dialysis solutions may dehydrate the interstitium, and although the total distance for a solute to traverse before it reaches the peritoneal cavity may be shortened, the aqueous network of channels could become more tortuous and the resistance to solute movement could actually increase.

The mesothelium appears to be more permeable than the endothelium, possibly because of the larger intercellular gaps between mesothelial cells.[99] The permeability of the peritoneal mesothelium apparently is not uniform; it has been suggested that the visceral peritoneum is more permeable than the parietal peritoneum.[100]

Studies in rabbits have noted very tight intercellular mesothelial cell junctions and numerous intravital plasmic vesicles.[101,102] Following intravenous injection of iron dextran, an electron dense tracer, the iron dextran is found primarily in vesicles in the peritoneum of the rabbit. Additional work is needed to determine the relative role of intracellular gaps and vesicles in passive solute transport across the peritoneum. This may vary from species to species in different areas of the peritoneum and for solutes of different molecular weight. In addition, it is not clear how peritoneal morphology and solute transport in animals relates to humans. In addition, it is not clear how tissue processing may artificially misrepresent the number of vesicles and/or the dimensions of the intracellular gaps in vivo. Finally, in vivo inflammation, such as peritonitis, may widen intercellular gaps resulting in a misrepresentation of the normal morphology.[103]

Peritoneal clearances, glucose absorption, and protein losses increase during peritonitis.[103,104] In addition to widening of intercellular gaps, there is a loss of mesothelial microvilli; there may also be interstitial edema, vasodilatation, and interstitial cellular infiltration. Thus, it is impossible to determine whether transport changes are primarily the result of mesothelial, interstitial, or vascular alterations. In the rat, heat injury, which morphologically appears to be confined to the mesothelium, also induces enhancement of transport.[103] Morphologic changes are similar to those seen during peritonitis, supporting the contention that mesothelial integrity may influence peritoneal transport. It is not known whether mesothelial microvilli influence transport.

Dialysate within the many folds of the mesentery always remains relatively stagnant, even with rapid cycling.[105–107] External massage of the abdomen has been shown to increase clearances in rats.[108] Dialysate channels are relatively wide and stagnant pools of fluid in the peritoneal cavity constitute substantial fluid film resistances.[107]

Solute Transfer by Diffusion. The diffusive mass transfer (M) may be presented by the equation

$$M = I\frac{A}{R}(C_{PB} - C_D) \quad (1)$$

where I = coefficient of proportionality
A = effective peritoneal surface area
R = sum of all resistances to diffusion
C_{PB} = peritoneal capillary blood solute concentration
C_D = peritoneal dialysate solute concentration

Dividing both sides of the equation by peripheral blood solute concentration (C_B), the instantaneous clearance (K_i) may be calculated as follows:

$$\frac{M}{C_B} = K_i = I\frac{A}{R}\left(\frac{C_{PB}}{C_B} - \frac{C_D}{C_B}\right) \quad (2)$$

At infinite peritoneal blood flow $C_{PB} = C_B$, and

$$K_i = I\frac{A}{R}\left(1 - \frac{C_D}{C_B}\right) \quad (3)$$

If dialysate flow is also infinite, then $C_D = 0$ and the maximal clearance (K_{max}) that may be achieved is

$$K_{max} = I\frac{A}{R} \quad (4)$$

Thus, with infinite peritoneal capillary blood and dialysate flows, the clearance is directly proportional to the effective peritoneal surface area and inversely proportional to the overall resistance. It is impossible to achieve infinite blood and dialysate flows; therefore, the maximal clearance cannot be measured. The closest measurable value, the mass-transfer-area coefficient (MTAC), was introduced to separate the influences of dialysate flow rate and convective transport on solute transfer. Based on kinetic models of the solute mass-transfer process, this coefficient is the inverse of peritoneal diffusion resistance and represents the clearance rate that would be realized in the absence of both ultrafiltration and solute accumulation in the dialysate. This approach has been explored by several investigators.[109–114]

To determine MTAC, a test exchange is performed with at least two measurements of dialysate and plasma solute concentrations at different dwell times. The more data points, the more precise the measurement. Popovich and Moncrief[115] reported a mean MTAC of 33.5 mL/min for urea and 23.5 mL/min for creatinine. The bigger the molecule the lower the MTAC (Fig. 14–5). The MTAC measurement is seldom utilized in routine clinical practice.

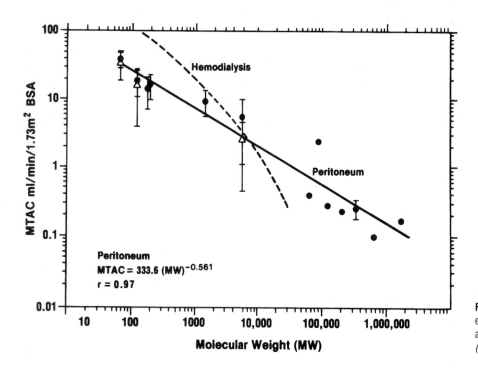

Figure 14–5. Peritoneal mass transfer area coefficients normalized to 1.73 m² body surface area versus molecular weight of the solutes. *(From Popovich et al.[115] with permission.)*

The efficiency index most commonly used by clinicians is the clearance rate of a solute from the plasma. This is calculated by dividing the amount of solute removed per unit time, the mass transfer rate, by the concentration of solute in plasma. This calculation expresses the volume of plasma cleared of that solute per unit time (usually expressed in milliliters per minute, liters per day, or liters per week). The clearance term is independent of the blood solute concentration and expresses the efficiency of removal. Thus

$$K = \frac{C_D V_t}{C_B t} \qquad (5)$$

where K = average clearance per exchange
C_D = dialysate solute concentration
V_t = dialysate volume at time t
C_B = peripheral blood solute concentration
t = total exchange time

So calculated, clearance represents the mean clearance rate per exchange. The instantaneous clearance is highest and is close to MTAC at the beginning of an exchange when the dialysis solution solute concentration is near zero and the diffusion gradient is maximal. The instantaneous clearance approaches zero exponentially as the dialysate solute concentration approaches equilibrium with blood.

Peritoneal dialysis clearance is a function of three parameters: the peritoneal capillary flow rate, the dialysate flow rate, and the MTAC.[115] The clearance can never exceed the lowest value of these three parameters. At infinite blood

and dialysate flow rates, the clearance will be equal to the MTAC and would be mass-transfer-limited. High molecular weight solutes are mass-transfer-limited; thus their clearances do not increase significantly with high dialysate flow. The clearance of a solute is considered as dialysate flow rate limited if the value of dialysate flow rate is markedly lower than the other two parameters. Such a situation is typical for CAPD, where urea clearance is close to the dialysate flow rate. Figure 14–6 illustrates these concepts. It must be realized that this analysis assumes an ideal system

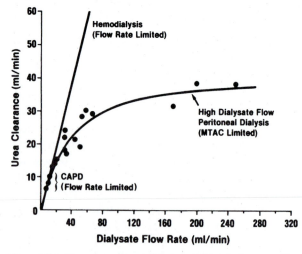

Figure 14–6. Urea clearance as a function of dialysate flow rate. *(From Popovich et al.[115] with permission.)*

with dialysate and blood flows in the immediate vicinity of endothelium and mesothelium, as well as complete contact of the peritoneal membrane area with dialysate.

In clinical practice, the effective dialysate turnover rate is influenced by the intraperitoneal volume of dialysate and mixing of dialysate present in the peritoneal cavity with fresh dialysis solution. The MTAC may be influenced both by the physical characteristics of the dialysis solution and by pharmacologic agents.

During manual intermittent peritoneal dialysis in adults where dialysis solution is instilled and drained by gravity, it is customary to use 2.0 L exchanges with inflow duration of 10 minutes, a dwell time of 30 minutes, and a drainage period of 20 to 30 minutes. Thus, dialysate flow rate potentially limits peritoneal dialysis clearances of small, highly diffusible solutes. With 1.5% dextrose dialysis solution (which is usually slightly hypertonic to azotemic plasma), a typical drainage volume is 2100 to 2200 mL per exchange. With a 70-minute exchange, this represents an average dialysate turnover rate near 30 mL/min. If a solute equilibrated completely between plasma and dialysate during such an exchange (and even urea does not), the maximum clearance possible would be 30 mL/min. Urea clearance is usually 18 to 20 mL/min with this type of exchange.[116]

Clearances of small solutes can be increased by more rapid exchanges. As dwell time is shortened, however, the portion of exchange time occupied by inflow and drainage increases. During inflow and drainage, there is less volume in the peritoneal cavity, which reduces clearances during those times and so reduces the final average clearance per exchange. Thus, although clearances can be increased by increasing dialysate flow, a point of diminishing returns is eventually reached. Boen[117] has shown that urea clearance decreases at flow rates above 3.5 L/h. Other studies support this finding.[118,119] Tenckhoff et al.,[120] using automated cycling equipment, later showed that urea clearance might increase to over 40 mL/min with dialysate flow rates of 12 L/h.

The discrepancy between studies showing a point of diminishing returns[117] and constant increase in efficiency with increased solution dose[120] may be dependent on the techniques used. Efficiency of dialysis in a particular individual, at the same dialysis solution dose, is enhanced by increased contact time between dialysate and the peritoneal dialysis membrane.[121] For this purpose a drain time should be shortened as much as possible because solute transport is reduced when little fluid is present in the peritoneal cavity. The principle of full contact dialysis is relevant only in peritoneal dialysis regimens with short exchange times.

It is possible to achieve higher dialysis solution turnover rates without increasing inflow and drainage times by continuous flow through two catheters or a double-lumen catheter.[106,107,122,123] Clearances of urea may approach 40 mL/min using an 18 L/h solution flow.[123] Dialy-

sis solution may be utilized single pass[105] or be recycled after passage through an extracorporeal dialysis system.[106] A shortcoming limiting this approach is channeling, whereby the dialysis solution streams from lumen to lumen, mixing poorly with the remaining volume of dialysate.[122] Abdominal pain and catheter obstruction due to suction of tissue into catheter holes were common at flow rates above 12 L/h.[106]

Reciprocating peritoneal dialysis involves rapid in-and-out cycling of dialysate (100 to 300 mL, in 1 minute and out the next), with an intraperitoneal dialysate reservoir of approximately 2 L.[123,124] Dialysate regeneration was often used to decrease the cost of dialysis. In studies of semicontinuous peritoneal dialysis Di Paolo[125] used a single catheter, assisted inflow and outflow with pumps, and used a high dialysis solution dose up to 50 L/8 h. After an initial fill with 1000 to 1500 mL of solution, a 100 to 110 mL portion of fluid was drained and replaced with 100 mL of fresh solution during frequent cycles. No regeneration system was used. These techniques can accommodate net flow rates of 6 L/h or more with better patient tolerance and without the manipulations of patient position often required for complete drainage. Urea clearances of 30 to 40 mL/min may be achieved. Studies in rats also show that maintaining a fluid reservoir in the peritoneal cavity and exchanging only a portion of the fluid yields urea clearances more than 30 percent higher at the same dialysis solution doses when compared to the complete drainage technique.[126]

Still another technique to enhance peritoneal clearances is called tidal peritoneal dialysis (TPD).[127–130] The technique is similar to semicontinuous peritoneal dialysis. In TPD, a bolus of fluid is infused into the peritoneal cavity at the beginning of the treatment, but unlike a typical complete volume drainage technique, only part of the fluid is drained leaving a reserve volume (RV), on top of which a tidal volume (TV) of fresh solution is cycled. TPD efficiency depends on the maintenance of a sufficient reserve volume to ensure adequate contact of dialysate with the peritoneal membrane, a suitable tidal volume to assure adequate mixing of dialysate with fresh dialysis solution, and a high dose of dialysis solution to provide a high concentration gradient between plasma and dialysate. In our studies, we found the highest efficiency with tidal and reserve volumes constituting 50 percent of the total intraperitoneal volumes of 2 to 3 L in adults. The gain in dialysis efficiency depends on the dose of dialysis solution. The higher the dose, the greater the gain. At low doses of dialysis solution (< 2 L/h) the gain is negligible; at higher doses (3 to 3.5 L/h), the gain is significant. In our studies using 27 L/8 h (3.4 L/h), we found gains in creatinine and urea clearances of about 20 percent compared to intermittent-flow peritoneal dialysis (IPD) at a similar dose of peritoneal dialysis solution (26 L/8 h or 3.3 L/h). It must be realized that to achieve a very high dose of dialysis solution with IPD, the dwell time must be eliminated and drain time must be maximally shortened. Consequently, the drainage is incomplete, the residual volume is increased and this technique is no longer IPD but rather TPD. Thus, the comparison of IPD with TPD at very high doses of dialysis solutions (>3.7 L/h) is difficult, if not impossible, as both techniques become the same i.e., TPD. This may explain why in some studies the increase in small molecule clearances with TPD is not significantly different compared to IPD.[131]

In CAPD, dialysis solution dose may be increased by more frequent exchanges or by augmented volume per exchange. Some normal-sized adults tolerate up to 4 L of intraperitoneal volume without discomfort and such patients have been maintained on continuous ambulatory peritoneal dialysis with 2.5- or 3-L exchanges.[132,133] Clearance increases with 3-L volumes as compared to 2-L volumes at fixed cycle times are primarily a function of the increased dose of dialysis solution rather than increased fluid membrane contact.[134]

Maximum dialysate contact with the peritoneal membrane ensures maximum clearances if other parameters are constant. Studies with intraperitoneal volumes of 2 vs. 3 L did not show differences in fluid-membrane contact[134,135]; however, Spencer and Farrell[136] found higher mass transfer area coefficients with 2-L volumes than with 1-L intraperitoneal volumes, indicating that 1 L of intraperitoneal fluid is not in full contact with the entire peritoneal surface area. Thus, for optimal efficiency, the minimal volume of fluid in the peritoneal cavity should be higher than 1 L but need not be higher than 2 L in adults.

Dialysis solution temperature influences solute movement into the peritoneal cavity, and higher temperatures enhance solute diffusion and presumably cause vasodilation.[137] Theoretically, very cold solutions should reduce clearances. Nevertheless, no significant differences in peritoneal clearances at room temperature as compared to body temperature have been found.[138] Perhaps this reflects rapid heat exchange between dialysis solutions and body fluids, so that temperature differences are not sustained. Thus, the temperature of the instilled solution may be of little clinical importance relative to its impact on peritoneal transport. This should be particularly true for long dwell exchanges, when any differences in temperature would exist for only a small portion of the exchange time. With rapid cycling techniques, cold dialysis solution may decrease body temperature.[139]

A high dialysate pH may increase net clearances of anions of weak acids such as urate and barbiturate. As these acids diffuse into more alkaline dialysate, fractions are converted to the charged, less diffusible anionic salts. This helps keep the diffusible acid concentration low on the dialysate side and tends to "trap" the solute in a less diffusible form.[140,141]

For solutes bound to protein, the addition of protein to the dialysis solution may enhance clearances. The diffusible free solute binds to protein in the dialysate, maintaining a very low dialysate water concentration of the free, diffusible form.[142]

Peritoneal dialysis solutions made hypertonic with dextrose increase clearances.[143] This is partly accounted for by the convective transport effects of osmotically induced ultrafiltration during such exchanges. Clearances often, however, remain elevated when less hypertonic exchanges are resumed, which may be due to vasodilatory effects of the hyperosmolar solutions.

Maximum urea clearances in adult humans usually do not exceed 40 mL/min, even with the most rapid cycling.[105,106,117–119,122–125] A possible explanation may be that maximum urea clearances are approaching effective peritoneal capillary blood flow and that this blood flow does not exceed 40 mL/min. Abundant indirect evidence suggests, however, that peritoneal capillary blood flow is at least two to three times higher than the maximum urea clearance.[88,116] Measurement of blood flow in animals using radioactive microspheres gave results exceeding 100 mL/min.[144] The strongest support for this notion is provided by peritoneal clearances of CO_2 gas in humans and hydrogen gas in rabbits, which are two to three times the maximum respective urea clearances.[116,145] Gas clearances should also be limited by effective peritoneal capillary flow and should not exceed urea clearances to any great extent if capillary flow was the main determinant of urea clearance. The fact that they are higher indicates that the blood flow markedly exceeds urea clearances. The blood flow through the peritoneal capillaries in humans, as measured by carbon dioxide diffusion, was estimated to range from 100 to 200 mL/min.[146] Carbon dioxide seems to be particularly suitable for these measurements because of low tissue resistance to its diffusion.

Many drugs have been given systemically or intraperitoneally with the expectation of increasing dialysis efficiency. An extensive review of pharmacologic agents influencing peritoneal transport has recently been published.[147] Unfortunately, most agents augmenting transport of uremic toxins also increase protein losses.

Peritoneal clearances are primarily MTAC limited. Moreover, there is a wide variation of MTAC among patients. Garred and associates reported a mean creatinine MTAC of 10 with a range from 2.6 to 21.4 mL/min.[114] Popovich and Moncrief reported an average value of 23.5 mL/min and a minimum of 5.1 mL/min.[115]

For practical clinical purposes, we prefer to perform the peritoneal equilibration test (PET) and present the peritoneal transport characteristics as simple dialysate-to-plasma ratios of solutes during and after 4-hour dwell time. Glucose transport is presented as dialysate concentration during and after 4-hour dwell time divided by its concentration at zero dwell time.[148,149] In an "abridged" test, only D/D0 glucose and D/P creatinine ratios and drain volumes are measured.[150] Although an abridged PET is useful in daily practice,[150,151] a full, "unabridged" test is needed for complete characterization of the peritoneal membrane function (see "Measurements of Peritoneal Functions, below").

Figure 14–7 portrays creatinine dialysate-to-plasma ratios, dialysate volume, and creatinine clearance versus dwell time in patients with extremely low and high transport rates using dialysis solution with a 2.5 percent glucose

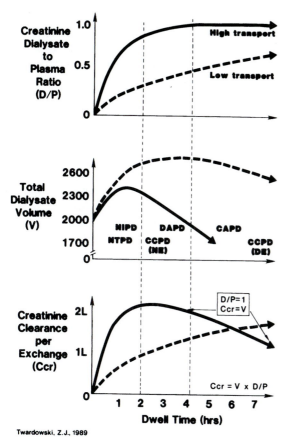

Twardowski, Z.J., 1989

Figure 14–7. Idealized curves of creatinine and water transport during exchange with 2 L of 2.5% glucose dialysis solution in patients with extremely low and high peritoneal transport characteristics. Upper panel shows dialysate to plasma ratio (D/P); middle panel shows total dialysate volume (V), which is the sum of infusion volume and ultrafiltration; and lower panel shows creatinine clearance per exchange (Ccr). The curves in the lower panel are derived from those of the upper and middle panels. Nightly intermittent peritoneal dialysis (NIPD) and nightly tidal peritoneal dialysis (NTPD) utilize short-dwell exchanges and are more suitable for patients with high peritoneal transport. Continuous ambulatory peritoneal dialysis (CAPD) and diurnal exchanges of continuous cyclic peritoneal dialysis [CCPD (DE)] utilize long-dwell exchanges and are more suitable for patients with low peritoneal transport. Daytime ambulatory peritoneal dialysis (DAPD) and nocturnal exchanges (NE) of continuous cyclic peritoneal dialysis (CCPD) usually operate within an intermediate range of dwell times (2 to 4 hours) and are also suitable for patients with high rates of peritoneal solute transport. Diurnal exchanges (DE) of CCPD are not suitable for patients with high transport rates. *(From Twardowski,[151] with permission.)*

concentration. In patients with low transport rates, peak ultrafiltration occurs late during dwell time and net ultrafiltration is still obtained after a long dwell time. In addition, D/P ratios increase almost linearly during the dwell, consequently clearances per exchange increase also almost linearly throughout the long-dwell exchange. In these patients, time of dialysis is crucial for adequate clearances and they benefit from continuous regimens such as CAPD or continuous cyclic peritoneal dialysis (CCPD) with diurnal exchanges. Because of a well-maintained dialysate/plasma concentration gradient for an extended period during dwell, clearances per unit time are augmented relatively little by rapid exchange techniques such as IPD or TPD. Consequently, intermittent regimens require long treatment times for adequate clearances. On the contrary, patients with high peritoneal transport rates have poor ultrafiltration on standard CAPD with dwell times exceeding 4 hours. In these patients, peak ultrafiltration occurs early during the dwell time and is followed by dialysate absorption. If dialysate is drained after a 4-hour dwell, there is minimal or no net ultrafiltration. In addition, the mass transfer of small molecular weight solutes in long-dwell exchanges decreases proportionately with the reduction in drain volume. After several hours of dwell, the clearance per exchange is less than in patients with low peritoneal transport rates (crossing point in Fig. 14–7). Reducing the dwell time in patients with high transport rates captures maximum ultrafiltration while maintaining near complete equilibration of small molecular weight solutes and so increases net solute removal. These patients are not good candidates for long-dwell exchanges.[151,152] They benefit from techniques utilizing rapid exchanges and may achieve adequate clearances with intermittent peritoneal dialysis regimens of relatively short duration. Patients with transport rates between these two extremes have intermediate patterns.

There is a renewed interest in continuous flow peritoneal dialysis (CFPD), as it is believed that an improved peritoneal access may make this modality successful. One of these accesses, a fluted double-lumen catheter, has recently been described by Diaz-Buxo.[153] Internally the tubes are separated, with each tube terminating with a fluted section. Another catheter, a double-lumen catheter with diffuser, has been recently developed by Ronco et al.[154] The intraperitoneal segment of the outflow tubing has a coiled design. The intraperitoneal segment of the inflow tubing is a short, thin-walled, silicone rubber, round tapered diffuser with multiple side holes, which allow the inflowing dialysis solution to be dispersed just below the parietal peritoneum, far away from the outflow tubing tip. Clinical trials with these new catheters are needed to determine whether CFPD can be revived.

A recent comparison of IPD, TPD with CFPD in 5 patients, using glucose-based, low pH solution (Dianeal PD1 1.36%; Baxter Healthcare, Castlebar, Ireland) at a rate of

100 mL/min, and two catheters (a permanent for outflow and an acute for inflow) showed increased clearances, due not only to increased diffusive gradient but also to more than doubling of MTAC creatinine in all 5 patients.[155] Fresh dialysis solution has vasodilatory properties.[156] Therefore this MTAC augmentation may be related to long-lasting vasodilatation with constant delivery of fresh dialysis solution and upregulation of NOS; it may be dangerous in the long term.

Ultrafiltration. Ultrafiltration (Q_f), that is, solvent (water) movement across the peritoneal membrane, is proportional to the transmembrane pressure (TP), the membrane area (A), and its hydraulic permeability (L_p):

$$Q_f = TP \cdot A \cdot L_p \qquad (6)$$

Transmembrane pressure is the result of differences in hydrostatic and osmotic pressure between the peritoneal capillaries and the peritoneal cavity. If the peritoneum were ideally impermeable to solutes but permeable to water, the osmotic pressure difference could be easily computed from the "blood and bath" osmolalities and the results converted into millimeters of mercury by van't Hoff's equation (1 mOsm = 19.3 mmHg at body temperature). Furthermore, if peritoneal membrane area and hydraulic permeability were known, it would be possible to compute the ultrafiltration rate in any clinical setting. Unfortunately, none of these parameters is known. The peritoneal membrane is permeable for even very large molecules and a correction factor, Staverman's reflection coefficients (σ),[157] is required to calculate the "effective" transmembrane pressure difference.[158]

$$TP = \Delta H + \delta\pi\sigma_1 + \delta\pi\sigma_2 + \cdots + \delta\pi\sigma_n \qquad (7)$$

where ΔH = transmembrane hydrostatic pressure gradient
  $\Delta\pi\sigma_1$ = the osmotic driving gradient for solute 1
  $\Delta\pi\sigma_2$ = the osmotic driving gradient for solute 2
  $\Delta\pi\sigma_n$ = the osmotic driving gradient for each of n solutes present on each side of the membrane

Each gradient favoring ultrafiltration has a positive value and each gradient opposing ultrafiltration has a negative value.

The situation is even more complicated due to transmembrane diffusion of solutes that dissipates the osmotic driving force. The reflection coefficient for these solutes ranges between 0.0 and 1.0. High-molecular-weight solutes such as albumin, hemoglobin, and dextran sulfate have reflection coefficients close to unity, whereas the reflection coefficient of glucose (MW = 180 Da) is 0.02.[159] Most commercially available peritoneal dialysis solutions contain glucose as an osmotic agent; however, glucose is not an ideal osmotic agent, and many substances have been proposed as its replacement.[160] Regardless of the lower osmolality of high- compared to low-molecular-weight solutes at the same percentage concentration, the high reflection coefficient of the former leads to a high osmotic driving force. Moreover, due to the slower absorption of larger molecules, ultrafiltration is sustained longer when such solutes are present.[160] We have evaluated several high-molecular-weight solutes as potentially useful osmotic agents for peritoneal dialysis.[161–163] As predicted, these agents induce more sustained ultrafiltration than does glucose; however, synthetic cations and anions are toxic,[162] and cross-linked gelatins at the concentration required for adequate ultrafiltration are absorbed through the lymphatics at a rate markedly exceeding a permissible metabolic load.[164] Low-molecular-weight solutes like glycerol and amino acids, because of their low reflection coefficients and rapid absorption, provide lower ultrafiltration than glucose at the same percentage concentrations, in spite of higher osmolality.[160,164]

Mistry and Gokal[165] have been working for many years on polyglucose, a nonionic, high-molecular-weight osmotic agent, which generates sustained ultrafiltration and is slowly absorbed from the peritoneal cavity. After absorption, polyglucose is metabolized into glucose, maltose, and maltotriose. Since human blood does not contain maltase, the circulating maltose is slowly metabolized in the tissues and partly excreted into the urine and dialysate. Several studies have shown that icodextrin (polyglucose) is safe and efficacious, particularly in patients with poor ultrafiltration in long dwell exchanges.[166–168]

Solute Transfer by Convection. Solutes accompany the bulk flow of water from the peritoneal capillary blood into the peritoneal cavity by convection. At equilibrium, greater amounts of low-molecular-weight solutes are removed with hypertonic exchanges because of increased drainage volumes.[169,170] In addition, high-molecular-weight solutes are removed in greater amounts with ultrafiltration because convective transport is more effective than diffusive. Convective transport is similar in its nature to mixing in a sense that the movement of solute molecules is caused by movement of solvent molecules (solvent drag). Very large protein molecules are probably transported almost exclusively by convection. Protein losses are usually higher with more hypertonic exchanges, which are associated with higher ultrafiltration.[169]

Solute Sieving. Most solutes do not accompany the bulk flow of water in proportion to their concentration in extracellular water.[171] The peritoneum offers greater resistance to accompanying solutes than to water, so that the concentration of solutes in the ultrafiltrate is less than in plasma water (solute sieving). Hence, convective solute transport (J_s) is the product of water flux (J_w), the sieving coefficient (S), which equals (1 − σ), and the mean solute concentration in the peritoneal capillaries (C_{pc}). That is,

$$J_s = J_w \cdot S \cdot C_{pc} \qquad (8)$$

Consequently, the contribution of convective mass transfer to overall solute transport diminishes during the dwell time as water flux decreases. The concentration gradient for net diffusion of a solute from blood to dialysis solution is enhanced by ultrafiltration. With longer dwell times, the sieving effects of disproportionate water removal are obliterated by greater net diffusion into the peritoneal dialysis solution.

Although the sieving effect influences each solute, the most important clinical consequences of sieving are related to sodium. Convective net removal of sodium per liter of ultrafiltrate is usually well below extracellular fluid concentration. Thus, dialysate sodium concentration is initially reduced due to solute sieving with ultrafiltration and tends to increase later in the dwell time due to diffusion and diminished ultrafiltration rate.[148,169,171,172] Dialysate sodium concentration decreases more in patients with low peritoneal transport characteristics.[148] Although the sieving effect creates a concentration gradient for some diffusion, during short dwell exchanges, net electrolyte removal per liter of ultrafiltrate remains far below the extracellular fluid concentration and severe hypernatremia may develop.[173,174]

The sieving of sodium through artificial membranes impermeable to proteins is close to unity.[175] In the early days of peritoneal dialysis, it was surprising that the "leaky" peritoneal membrane, permeable to high-molecular-weight protein, can deter convective movement of low molecular weight sodium during ultrafiltration. Nolph and colleagues presented a hypothesis to explain this phenomenon.[176] The primary assumption is that most ultrafiltration takes place across the proximal capillaries where the effective pore width is small when compared to that in the distal capillaries. There is substantial evidence that the width of intercellular gaps progressively increases from proximal to distal portions of the capillaries, with the most permeable portions in the small venules,[94] whereas artificial membranes are more homogenous. Hydrostatic pressure is higher at the proximal end of the capillaries, and glucose should be more osmotically effective across this tighter portion of the capillary than at the distal portion, where it may be readily absorbed and exert little osmotic pressure.[177] Thus, combined hydrostatic and osmotic pressure could induce maximum ultrafiltration rates across portions of the capillary that are least permeable. Several other possible mechanisms have been also postulated.[178] Ultimately the mystery was solved in the early 1990s with the formulation of the "three-pore" model by Rippe et al.[93] and discovery of aquaporins (see above).

The most important consequences of sodium sieving during dialysis are hypernatremia, thirst, and hypertension, which are frequently observed in patients treated with short-dwell peritoneal dialysis. This problem may be overcome by lowering the sodium concentration in the dialysis solution to increase the diffusion gradient. The sodium concentration in dialysis solutions has been progressively lowered. In the 1920s and 1930s, the solutions contained more than 150 meq/L of sodium.[179–181] Rhoads used a solution containing a sodium concentration of 276 meq/L.[182] In the 1940s and 1950s, sodium concentrations between 140 and 145 meq/L were generally used,[183–185] and only a few authors recommended sodium concentrations of 130 to 131 meq/L.[186,187] Boen used 140 meq/L of sodium when he worked in Amsterdam[188] and later used 135 meq/L when working in Seattle.[189] The use of solutions with sodium concentrations close to 140 resulted in severe thirst and poor blood pressure control.[190] Hypernatremia over 160 meq/L has been reported.[173,174,191] Many patients did not develop hypernatremia because of high water intake during dialysis due to severe thirst.[190] In the late 1960s and early 1970s, when hypernatremia was explained by molecular sieving,[171] the concentration of sodium in the dialysis solutions was decreased. Ahearn and Nolph[192] recommended a sodium concentration of 110 meq/L for 7% glucose solution. Tenckhoff recommended 130 meq/L for solutions with a lower glucose content.[193] In 1973, a special workshop recommended a sodium concentration of 132 meq/L and a maximum glucose concentration of 4.5%.[194] Since that time, most commercial solutions contain such a concentration of sodium. Notwithstanding this lower sodium concentration, many patients continue to have thirst, hypernatremia, and poor blood pressure control on IPD. In 1978, Shen and coworkers[195] proposed a sodium concentration of 118 for 2.5% glucose solution and 109 meq/L for 4.5% glucose solution. At that time, CAPD was introduced and the disappearance of problems of thirst and poor blood pressure control was noted within a few days after conversion from IPD to CAPD.[196] A dialysis solution sodium concentration of 132 meq/L seems appropriate for most patients treated with CAPD.

Treatment with nightly intermittent peritoneal dialysis (NIPD) may be associated with thirst and more difficult blood pressure control in some patients with low serum sodium concentration and/or low peritoneal permeability times area using a dialysis solution containing 132 meq/L of sodium.[149,197] Since the number of patients treated with NIPD has increased, it would be desirable to have dialysis solutions with lower sodium concentration, e.g., 120 meq/L. Mixing this solution in various proportions with a solution containing sodium concentration of 132 meq/L, it would be possible to obtain final solutions with sodium concentrations between these two values.

Sodium sieving is an excellent indicator of ultrafiltrate generation. Figure 14–8 shows two curves of dialysate to plasma ratio versus time, superimposed on the population study, in a patient with excellent ultrafiltration (first study) and ultrafiltration failure (second study) after an episode of severe *Staphylococcus aureus* peritonitis. Whereas in the first study there was a significant drop of dialysate sodium

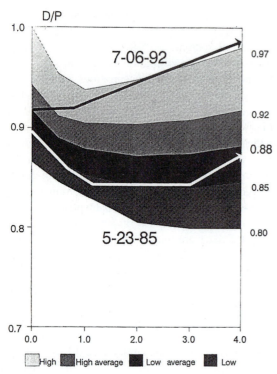

Figure 14–8. Ratios of dialysate to plasma sodium concentration vs. time (hours) in a patient with high ultrafiltration (first study 05–23–85) and poor ultrafiltration (second study 07–06–92). The curves are superimposed on the population study. Whereas sodium dialysate concentration markedly decreased in the first study, due to high generation of ultrafiltrate with sodium sieving, the dialysate sodium concentration immediately started to rise in the second study because of poor generation of ultrafiltrate. *(From Dobbie et al.,[198] with permission.)*

concentration due to high generation of ultrafiltrate, in the second study no decrease of dialysate sodium was observed. Another significant observation in this patient was extremely high protein concentration (381 mg/dL) in the overnight exchange prior to an unabridged PET (normal 8 to 168 mg/dL). Almost complete denudation of the mesothelium and significant peritoneal sclerosis were observed in this patient.[198] Such observations support the hypothesis of a significant role of mesothelial cells in restriction of protein loss into dialysate and the importance of mesothelial "transcellular" pores (aquaporins) in the generation of solute-free ultrafiltrate. A modification of the original PET to improve characterization of the peritoneal membrane was proposed by Krediet.[199] Instead of a 2.27% test solution, Krediet proposes a 3.86% glucose solution, which exaggerates the sodium dip at one hour of equilibration. This sodium dip is a rough measure of the aquaporin-mediated water transport. To determine the mesothelial cell mass, he proposed measuring CA125 at 4-hour equilibration.

Lymphatic Absorption. "The older investigators regarded the peritoneal cavity as a huge lymph sac" (Ref. 5, page 1) and

much of the work done in experimental animals indicates that the lymphatic system draining the peritoneal cavity is very active. However, most of the research into peritoneal dialysis physiology focused on solute and fluid movement between peritoneal capillary blood and the dialysis solution; the role of peritoneal lymphatics was neglected. The observation that 60 percent of cross-linked gelatin (mean MW 25,000 Da) was absorbed from the peritoneal cavity of rats within 8 hours[164] stimulated our interest in the role of lymphatics in peritoneal dialysis.[76,200,201] Because solutes of more than 19,400 Da are absorbed almost exclusively by lymphatics,[202] and lymphatic absorption is by convection, our data indicated that most of the fluid is absorbed from the peritoneal cavity through lymphatics.

The lymphatics probably having the greatest impact on peritoneal transport kinetics are those immediately beneath the mesothelial layer on the caudal surface of the diaphragm. Diaphragmatic contractions actively pump fluid from the peritoneal cavity into and through the diaphragmatic lymphatics and lymph drains mainly via the right lymphatic duct into the venous circulation (see "Lymph Drainage," above).

Lymphatic absorption (LA) in CAPD can be calculated from the rate of disappearance of albumin (MW 68,000 Da) from the peritoneal cavity, as charged molecules above 10,000 Da are absorbed by convection.[203] Thus,

$$LA = \frac{C_0}{C_G}\left(IPV_0\right) - \frac{C_t}{C_G}\left(IPV_t\right) \qquad (9)$$

where C_0 = dialysate albumin concentration at 0 dwell time
C_t = dialysate albumin concentration at t dwell time
C_G = geometric mean dialysate albumin concentration
IPV_0 = intraperitoneal volume at 0 dwell time
IPV_t = intraperitoneal volume at t dwell time

One study of 10 CAPD patients using albumin as a marker showed that the cumulative lymphatic drainage from the peritoneal cavity during a 4-hour exchange averaged 358 ± 47 mL and reduced cumulative net transcapillary ultrafiltration by 58 ± 7.2 percent.[204] Extrapolated to four 2-L, 2.5 percent, 6-hour exchanges per day, lymphatic drainage may reduce potential daily net ultrafiltration by 83.2 ±10.2 percent. Reduction of lymphatic drainage, therefore, would be beneficial for augmentation of ultrafiltration.

In 16 CAPD patients, studies with albumin were done with 4-hour dwell exchanges on two separate days.[205] During day 1, patients received intraperitoneal administration of 10 g/L of human albumin. Some patients received albumin from one batch and other patients from another batch of human albumin. The transport of all measured solutes was found increased during the administration of batch A compared to control experiments (urea + 78%, creatinine

+96%, inulin +27%, and IgG +126%). The use of batch A was also associated with increased white cell counts in the drainage. With batch B, there were no changes in solute transport and white cell count. The authors suggest that the effects on solute transport and white cell count with batch A were caused by a relatively higher concentration of prekallikrein activator (30.1 U/L compared to 0 in batch A and B, respectively). They warn about possible artifacts when human albumin is used for simultaneous measurement of peritoneal fluid and solute kinetics. This is a very important observation since albumin is used to assess absorption kinetics from the peritoneal cavity.

Lymphatic absorption rate was measured in CAPD patients using intraperitoneal dextran 70 and a rapid, highly accurate high-performance liquid chromatography (HPLC) method that was not influenced by glucose.[206] Lymphatic absorption rate ranged from 0.1 to 3.5 mL/min with a median value of 1 mL/min (60 mL/h).

Transcapillary ultrafiltration, lymphatic absorption rate, and intraperitoneal volume were measured utilizing intraperitoneally administered polydispersed dextran 70 in CAPD patients during a 4-hour dwell exchange with 1.36% glucose solutions.[207] The recovery of dextran was 88 percent. Lymphatic absorption rate calculated from the amount of dextran loss and dialysate dextran concentration averaged 1.3 mL/min. Dextran 70 had no measurable effect on solute transport. Changes in intraperitoneal volume (due to net ultrafiltration) were highly dependent on lymphatic absorption rate and effective peritoneal surface area as represented by mass transfer area coefficients of low molecular weight solutes. The authors conclude that dextran 70 is a useful marker for the measurement of peritoneal cavity fluid kinetics, even with glucose present in the solutions.

Measurements of lymphatic flow from the peritoneal cavity by measuring plasma appearance of a tracer after its infusion into the peritoneal cavity yield markedly lower values than those measured by tracer disappearance.[208]

Direct measurements of lymph flow provide lower values than those obtained by the disappearance of macromolecules from the peritoneal cavity. In sheep undergoing peritoneal dialysis, lymph was collected from the caudal mediastinal lymph node and the thoracic duct, both of which are involved in lymphatic drainage of the peritoneal cavity.[209] Based on the appearance of tracer in lymph, drainage of peritoneal fluid into the caudal lymphatics was calculated to be 3.1 and 14.1 mL per hour in anesthetized and conscious sheep, respectively. Drainage into the thoracic duct was 1.32 and 14.7 mL/h in anesthetized and conscious sheep, respectively. Johnston,[210] in an overview of the work of the same group, notes that under the conditions of their studies in sheep, lymph flows derived from tracer movement into the cannulated lymph compartments and from the appearance of tracer in the bloodstream were very similar. Calculations of lymph flow based on the disappear-

ance of tracer from the peritoneal cavity appeared to overestimate lymphatic drainage.

Another group also studied lymphatic absorption during peritoneal dialysis in sheep with lymphatic flow rate measured through cannulated lymphatic vessels, draining subdiaphragmatic lymphatics.[211] They agree with the above workers that studies in anesthetized animals may yield underestimates of diaphragmatic lymph flow. These investigators noted increased lymph flow with the infusion of endotoxin into awake sheep and with the infusion of Ringer's solution into the abdominal cavity. This last observation indicates that the infusion of a solution into the peritoneal cavity increases lymphatic flow due to increased intraabdominal pressure or through some other mechanism.

Flessner feels that 5 to 25 percent of total fluid loss from the peritoneal cavity is via lymphatics and that the remaining absorption is directly into tissue surrounding the peritoneal cavity.[212] He feels that the driving force for convection into tissue is the hydrostatic pressure gradient between the peritoneal cavity and the tissue. He argues that more data on the mechanical properties of the peritoneal tissue space and its response to hydrostatic pressure in the cavity are required to fully understand fluid transport kinetics at the tissue level.

Rippe and colleagues postulate that fluid loss from the peritoneal cavity is dominated by capillary fluid absorption and that lymphatic absorption accounts for a smaller fraction of peritoneal-to-blood absorption of fluid in peritoneal dialysis.[213] Nagy has observed interstitial fluid uptake of intraperitoneally injected soluble macromolecules by fluorescent microscopy into the parietal peritoneal wall in animals with increased peritoneal pressure.[214] Additional nonlymphatic pathways for peritoneal absorption therefore appear to exist in mice, in accord with the opinions of Flessner and Rippe mentioned above. In the studies by Nagy, the uptake of tagged red cells estimated peritoneal lymphatic absorption at 1.6 L/min in normal awake mice.

Khanna and Mactier focused on the conflicting results with two indirect methods of lymph flow, namely plasma appearance and peritoneal disappearance of tracer colloids.[215] They emphasize that direct measurements of lymph flow rates through cannulation of mediastinal lymph vessels suggest a significant flow through lymph channels in response to intraperitoneal fluid instillation; but lymph-flow modifications at the lymph-node level may prevent use of this technique to assess the precise role played by lymphatics in fluid kinetics. They cite numerous animal and clinical studies suggesting that reabsorption is predominantly through subdiaphragmatic lymphatics and in CAPD patients may be at least 1 L/day.

Thus, the debate continues; it remains to be established whether more fluid is absorbed from the peritoneal cavity through diaphragmatic lymphatics or through the capillaries in the tissues surrounding the peritoneal cavity.

Neostigmine reduces lymphatic drainage in rats,[216] presumably by constricting diaphragmatic stomata. Diaphragmatic stomata contain actin filaments,[57,217] and thus may react to muscle constrictors. Attempts to enhance ultrafiltration by reducing lymphatic absorption have not been successful so far.

Measurements of Peritoneal Functions

Mass Transfer Area Coefficient (MTAC). The first peritoneal function test, MTAC, as described above (see section: Solute transfer by diffusion) is rarely used at present because new, less complex tests have been developed.

Accelerated Peritoneal Examination (APEX). APEX was developed by Verger.[218] The test summarizes in a single number the peritoneal permeability both to glucose and urea; it represents the time at which glucose and urea equilibration curves (using percentages as units) cross; the shorter the APEX time, the higher the peritoneal permeability and, conversely, the longer this time is, the lower the peritoneal permeability is.

Peritoneal Dialysis Capacity (PDC). The PDC test was developed by Haraldsson in 1995.[219] It is designed to mimic ordinary CAPD and is performed by the patient with minimal requirements of nursing time. The three-pore model of Rippe et al. (see above) is used to describe the PDC using three physiologic parameters:

1. The "area" parameter ($A_0/\Delta x$), which determines the unrestricted pore area (A_0) available over the diffusion distance (Δx) (Fig. 14–9).

2. The final reabsorption rate of fluid from the abdominal cavity to blood (Jv_{AR}), after the glucose gradient disappears (Fig. 14–10).
3. The large pore flux of plasma (Jv_L), which determines the loss of protein to the dialysate.

To facilitate the calculations of these parameters, a computer program has been developed (PDC, Gambro Lundia AB, Lund, Sweden). A recent multicenter study evaluated this program and showed its usefulness in describing peritoneal membrane transport characteristics. The test was renamed personal dialysis capacity (PDC) but retained the same acronym.[220]

Peritoneal Equilibration Test (PET). PET is the most widely used peritoneal function test, because of its standardization, simplicity, and usefulness for diagnostic and prognostic purposes. An abridged test[150] looking only at D/D0 glucose and D/P creatinine ratios, and drain volumes, is commonly used.

Based on PET, a computer model (PD ADEQUEST, Baxter Healthcare Corporation, Round Lake, Illinois) has been developed that permits prediction of small solute clearances and ultrafiltration for various alternative prescriptions of peritoneal dialysis. An excellent agreement between predicted and measured values has been validated in 111 patients.[221]

In the original PET, which established standard values for membrane categorization in 1987, a glucose solution was used for the preceding exchange.[148,149] Recently many patients, particularly those with ultrafiltration problems, use polyglucose solution for nightly exchanges. Lilaj et al.[222] found that polyglucose containing solutions used for the preceding exchange increase D/P ratios of creatinine, phos-

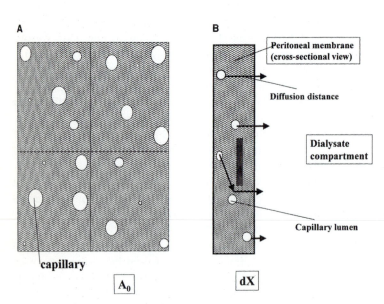

Figure 14–9. Interpretation of $A_0/\Delta x$. The area parameter, $A_0/\Delta x$, is composed of two components that cannot be separated because they both determine the diffusive properties of the membranes in an interrelated way. A. A_0 reflects the total pore area available for transport. This is determined by the total surface of the peritoneal membrane (shaded square) and the number of perfused capillaries per surface area (open circles). B. Δx is the "diffusion path distance" (i.e., the distance that molecules have to travel from the capillary space before they reach the dialysate compartment). It should be noted that also the "resistance" of the interstitium plays a role in this "distance." If the interstitium contains parts where no diffusion is possible (e.g., because of fibrosis, in the picture schematically represented by shaded area), the diffusion path distance will be longer than the actual distance between the capillary and the dialysate compartment. *(From Van Biesen et al.,[220] with permission.)*

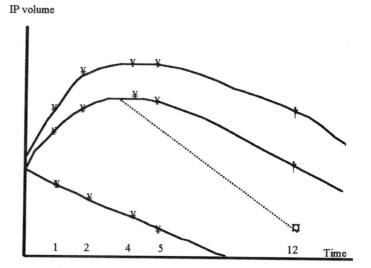

Figure 14–10. Determination of Jv_{AR}. Jv_{AR} is the rate of reabsorption of fluid after osmotic equilibrium has been reached. It is calculated as the slope of the final part of the intraperitoneal volume over time curve. It is of note that in the PDC test, the initial part of the curve is based on four data points of drained volume (the short dwells during the day, represented by ¥) whereas the final part is only based on one data point, the drained volume after the long night dwell (in the figure represented by †). Therefore small mistakes in the drain volume after the night dwell will have a big impact on Jv_{AR}. As the most common mistake is incomplete drainage (represented in figure by ϶), resulting in an underestimation of the intraperitoneal volume, and thus an overestimation of Jv_{AR} (dotted line). Different full-line curves represent different osmotic agents and different osmotic concentrations. Note that the slope of the final part (and thus Jv_{AR}) is independent of the osmotic agent used. *(From Van Biesen et al.,[220] with permission.)*

phate, and sodium, as well as glucose absorption, measured during the test. Therefore, they recommend that patients using icodextrin solution during the nighttime should perform their nighttime exchange with conventional glucose solution before a scheduled PET.[222]

The preceding exchange dwell time was 8 hours in the original PET. This was convenient when almost all patients were on continuous ambulatory peritoneal dialysis; however, now that many patients are on some form of automated peritoneal dialysis (APD), an 8-hour exchange prior to the PET requires changes in the dialysis schedule. Our recent study[223] evaluated the differences in 2-hour equilibration curves with standard, ~8-hour, and 3-hour preceding exchange. The values for D/P creatinine and urea, as well as D/D0 glucose, were almost identical throughout the 2-hour PET dwell after long and short exchanges. D/P protein values tended to be higher in the PET after the long exchange. We concluded that for creatinine and glucose equilibration, any dwell time between 3 and 12 hours was acceptable for the preceding exchange, and the equilibration test might be performed with a 2- or 4-hour dwell. The protein values obtained with a 3-hour prior dwell are different than with a long prior exchange.[223]

However, for a full characterization of peritoneal membrane function, an unabridged test as described in 1987,[148,149] which include D/P urea, protein, creatinine, and D/D0 glucose (Fig. 14–11), as well as D/P potassium, sodium, and corrected creatinine, drain volume and residual volumes (Fig. 14–12) should be used. Exact values presented in Figs. 14–11 and 14–12 are shown in Tables 14–1, 14–2, and 14–3. Although this test is extremely reliable and valuable in the characterization of peritoneal membrane function, it is rarely used because of its complexity and considerable nursing time requirement; nonetheless, it should

be used in cases where full characterization of peritoneal function is necessary. An unabridged test should be performed shortly after the break-in period of peritoneal dialysis as a baseline for future comparisons.

Peritoneal Function after Long-Term Exposure to Peritoneal Dialysis Solutions

Long-term peritoneal dialysis is associated with progressive loss of ultrafiltration capability. There are two possible mechanisms leading to this phenomenon. First, effective peritoneal surface area progressively increases in long-term PD patients. This is related to an increased number and surface area of peritoneal capillaries as a response to increased NOS activity and upregulation of VEGF. Second, the peritoneal membrane is gradually denuded of mesothelial cells, leading to a loss of mesothelial aquaporins, which are ultra-small pores responsible for free water transport. A gradual decline of CA 125 concentration in dialysate, a marker of mesothelial cell mass, has been found in long-term peritoneal dialysis patients,[224] and loss of mesothelial cells in patients with ultrafiltration failure has been determined by peritoneal biopsy.[198]

The structural and functional alterations in the membrane in long-term peritoneal dialysis are thought to be the consequence of the toxicity of glucose through the formation of glucose degradation products (GDPs) or the formation of advanced glycation end products generated during the sterilization process.[225] Replacing glucose by other osmotic agents, such as icodextrin,[166,226] changing the sterilization process, replacing the lactate buffer by bicarbonate, and blocking the formation of GDPs may be a significant step forward to improved membrane preservation during long-term peritoneal dialysis treatment.[227]

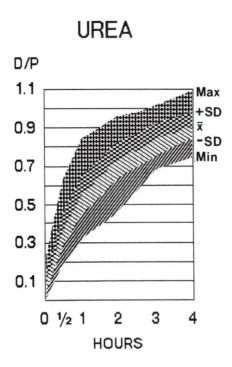

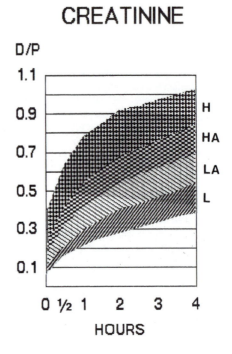

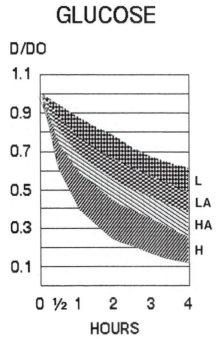

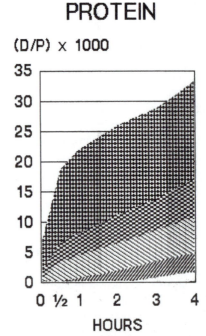

Figure 14–11. The results of the equilibration test in the study population. Areas shaded in different patterns portray results representing high (H), high-average (HA), low-average (LA), and low (L) peritoneal transport rates. For urea, creatinine, and protein, the higher dialysate-to-plasma ratio (D/P), the higher the transfer rate. Because glucose transport direction is opposite to that of other solutes, the higher the concentration ratio of dialysate glucose at particular dwell time to dialysate glucose at 0 dwell time (D/D0), the lower the transfer rate. Areas of H, HA, LA, and L transfer rate categories have the same shade pattern. Maximal, mean + 1SD, mean, mean - 1SD, and minimal values border the four categories. *(From Twardowski et al.,*[148] *with permission.)* Urea D/P ratios at 2-hour dwell are most dispersed and best for discrimination among transport categories. A very high protein concentration in dialysate, exceeding maximal values shown in this figure, is characteristic for denudation of mesothelium in patients with ultrafiltration failure.[198]

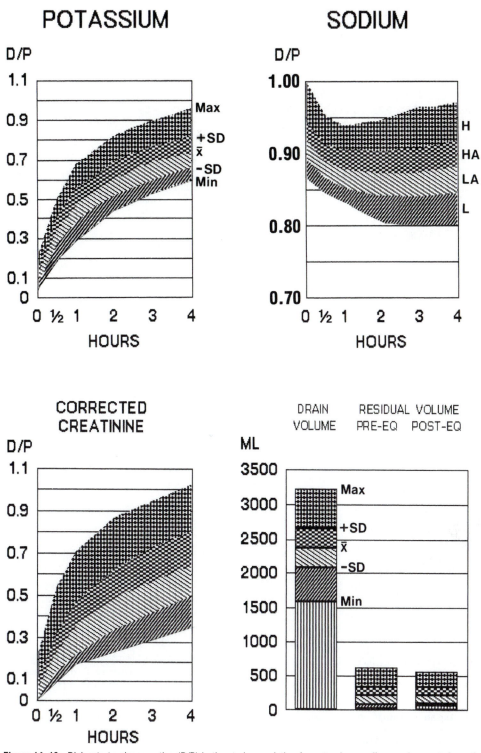

Figure 14–12. Dialysate-to-plasma ratios (D/P) in the study population for potassium, sodium, and corrected creatinine, as well as drain and residual volumes. Dialysate creatinine concentrations were corrected for glucose interference with the Jaffe reagent. Areas shaded in the same pattern represent the same category of transfer rate. See Fig. 14–11 for further explanations. *(From Twardowski et al.,[148] with permission.)*

TABLE 14–1. DIALYSATE-TO-PLASMA RATIOS (D/P)

	Urea						Creatinine					
Dwell time (h)	0	0.5	1	2	3	4	0	0.5	1	2	3	4
Minimal value	0.00	0.19	0.32	0.46	0.68	0.75	0.08	0.22	0.22	0.28	0.33	0.38
Mean – 1 SD	0.05	0.29	0.45	0.64	0.75	0.84	0.12	0.22	0.30	0.40	0.47	0.54
Mean	0.10	0.38	0.55	0.73	0.84	0.91	0.18	0.32	0.42	0.54	0.62	0.69
Mean + 1 SD	0.16	0.47	0.65	0.83	0.92	0.98	0.24	0.42	0.54	0.68	0.76	0.84
Maximal value	0.24	0.64	0.84	0.96	1.01	1.08	0.40	0.64	0.78	0.92	0.97	1.03

	Protein [(D/P) × 1000]						Corrected Creatinine					
Dwell time (h)	0	0.5	1	2	3	4	0	0.5	1	2	3	4
Minimal value	0.00	0.00	0.00	0.00	0.95	1.71	-0.01	0.08	0.17	0.23	0.29	0.34
Mean – 1 SD	0.00	0.08	0.81	1.98	3.43	4.8	0.02	0.14	0.22	0.34	0.42	0.50
Mean	0.92	3.37	4.55	6.59	8.60	10.96	0.07	0.23	0.35	0.48	0.57	0.65
Mean + 1 SD	1.84	6.67	8.29	11.20	13.76	17.13	0.12	0.32	0.47	0.62	0.73	0.81
Maximal value	7.13	18.61	21.91	25.91	28.87	33.22	0.24	0.54	0.71	0.87	0.95	1.03

	Potassium						Sodium					
Dwell time (h)	0	0.5	1	2	3	4	0	0.5	1	2	3	4
Minimal value	0.04	0.19	0.29	0.44	0.53	0.60	0.866	0.846	0.832	0.805	0.799	0.799
Mean – 1 SD	0.08	0.27	0.39	0.52	0.60	0.66	0.892	0.868	0.853	0.841	0.840	0.846
Mean	0.13	0.34	0.47	0.60	0.69	0.74	0.918	0.890	0.879	0.872	0.874	0.882
Mean + 1 SD	0.17	0.41	0.56	0.69	0.77	0.82	0.943	0.912	0.905	0.904	0.908	0.918
Maximal value	0.23	0.50	0.68	0.82	0.90	0.96	1.000	0.954	0.938	0.948	0.963	0.970

Source: Modified from Twardowski et al.,[149] with permission.

TABLE 14–2. DIALYSATE GLUCOSE–TO-DIALYSATE AT 0 DWELL TIME (D/D0)

Dwell time (h)	0	0.5	1	2	3	4
Minimal value	1.00	0.61	0.40	0.24	0.17	0.12
Mean – 1 SD	1.00	0.74	0.60	0.44	0.35	0.26
Mean	1.00	0.81	0.69	0.55	0.46	0.38
Mean + 1 SD	1.00	0.88	0.78	0.66	0.57	0.49
Maximal value	1.00	0.94	0.88	0.78	0.67	0.61

Source: Modified from Twardowski et al.,[149] with permission.

TABLE 14–3. DRAIN VOLUMES AND RESIDUAL VOLUMES (ML)

	Drain Volume after 4-h dwell	Preequilibration Residual Volume	Postequilibration Residual Volume
Minimal value	1580	17	63
Mean – 1 SD	2085	95	102
Mean	2368	218	222
Mean + 1 SD	2650	341	342
Maximal value	3226	624	569

Source: Modified from Twardowski et al,.[149] with permission.

REFERENCES

1. Cunningham RS. The physiology of the serous membranes. *Physiol Rev* 1926;6 (April):242–280.
2. Putnam TJ. The living peritoneum as a dialyzing membrane. *Am J Physiol* 1923;63(Feb):548–565.
3. Clemente CD. *Anatomy. A Regional Atlas of the Human Body,* 3d ed. Baltimore and Munich: Urban & Schwarzenberg, 1987.
4. Wegner G. Chirurgische Bemerkungen über die Peritonealhöhle, mit besonderer Berücksichtigung der Ovariotomie. *Arch Klin Chir* 1877;20:51–145.
5. Hertzler AE. *The Peritoneum.* St. Louis: Mosby, 1919.
6. Esperanca MJ, Collins DL. Peritoneal dialysis efficiency in relation to body weight. *J Pediatr Surg* 1966;1(2):162–169.
7. Liebermann Meffert D, White H. *The Greater Omentum.* Berlin: Springer-Verlag, 1983.
8. Bradley SW, Childs AW, Combes B, et al. The effect of exercise on the splanchnic blood flow and splanchnic blood volume in normal man. *Clin Sci (Lond)* 1956;15(3):457–463.
9. Miller FN, Nolph KD, Johsua IG. The osmolality component of peritoneal dialysis solutions. In: Legrain M, ed. *Continuous Ambulatory Peritoneal Dialysis.* Amsterdam:. Excerpta Medica, 1980;12–17.

10. Brown KP. Peritoneal lymphatic absorption: an experimental investigation to determine the value of lymphaticostomy. *Br J Surg* 1928;15:538–544.

11. Courtice FC, Steinbeck AW. Absorption of protein from the peritoneal cavity. *J Physiol (London)* 1951;114:336–355.

12. Nylander G, Tjernberg B. The lymphatics of the greater omentum. An experimental study in the dog. *Lymphology* 1967;2(1):3–7.

13. Simer PH. The drainage of particulate matter from the peritoneal cavity by lymphatics. *Anat Rec* 1944;88(Feb): 175–192.

14. Higgins GM, Bain CG. The absorption and transference of particulate material by the great omentum. *Surg Gynecol Obstet* 1930;50(May):851–860.

15. Courtice FC, Steinbeck AW. Effects of lymphatic obstruction and of posture on the absorption of protein from peritoneal cavity. *Aust J Exp Biol Med Sci* 1951;29:451–458.

16. Todd RB, Bowman W. *The Physiological Anatomy and Physiology of Man*. London: Parker, 1857:129–130.

17. Kolossow A. Ueber die Struktur des Endothels der Pleuroperitonealhöhle der Blut- und Lymphgefässe. *Biol Centralbl Erlang* 1892;12:87–94.

18. Baradi AF, Rao SN. A scanning electron microscope study of mouse peritoneal mesothelium. *Tissue Cell* 1976;8(1): 159–162.

19. Andrews PM, Porter KR. The ultratructural morphology and possible functional significance of mesothelial microvilli. *Anat Rec* 1973;177(3):409–426.

20. Baradi AF, Rayns DG. Mesothelial intercellular junctions and pathways. *Cell Tissue Res* 1976;173(1):133–138.

21. Gotloib L, Rabinovich S, Rodella H, et al. Ultrastructure of the rabbit mesentery. In: Gahl GM, Kessel M, Nolph KD, eds. *Advances in Peritoneal Dialysis: Proceedings of the Second International Symposium on Peritoneal Dialysis*. West Berlin, June 16–19, 1981. Amsterdam: Excerpta Medica, 1981:27–31.

22. Odor DL. Observations of the rat mesothelium with the electron and phase microscopes. *Am J Anat* 1954;95(3):433–465.

23. Dobbie JW. New concepts in molecular biology and ultrastructural pathology of the peritoneum: their significance for peritoneal dialysis. *Am J Kidney Dis* 1990; 15(2):215–219.

24. Casley-Smith JR. The dimensions and numbers of small vesicles in cells, endothelial and mesothelial and the significance of these for endothelial permeability. *J Microsc* 1969;90(3): 251–268.

25. Fukata H. Electron microscopic study on normal rat peritoneal mesothelium and its changes in absorption of particulate iron dextran complex. *Acta Pathol Jpn* 1963;13(Oct): 309–325.

26. Bast RC Jr, Feeney M, Lazarus H, et al. Reactivity of a monoclonal antibody with human ovarian carcinoma. *J Clin Invest* 1981;68(5):1331–1337.

27. Kabawat SE, Bast RC Jr, Bhan AK, et al. Tissue distribution of a coelomic-epithelium-related antigen recognized by the monoclonal antibody OC125.*Int J Gynecol Pathol* 1983;2(3): 275–285.

28. O'Brien TJ, Hardin JW, Bannon GA, et al. CA 125 antigen in human amniotic fluid and fetal membranes. *Am J Obstet Gynecol* 1986;155(1):50–55.

29. Molina R, Filella X, Bruix J, et al. Cancer antigen 125 in serum and ascitic fluid of patients with liver diseases. *Clin Chem* 1991;37(8):1379–1383.

30. Koomen GC, Betjes MG, Zemel D, et al. Cancer antigen 125 is locally produced in the peritoneal cavity during continuous ambulatory peritoneal dialysis. *Perit Dial Int* 1994;14(2): 132–136.

31. Krediet RT. Dialysate cancer antigen 125 concentration as marker of peritoneal membrane status in patients treated with chronic peritoneal dialysis. *Perit Dial Int* 2001;21(6): 560–567.

32. Lai KN, Li FK, Lan HY, et al. Expression of aquaporin-1 in human peritoneal mesothelial cells and its upregulation by glucose in vitro. *J Am Soc Nephrol* 2001;12(5):1036–1345.

33. Lai KN, Leung JC, Chan LY, et al. Expression of aquaporin-3 in human peritoneal mesothelial cells and its up-regulation by glucose in vitro. *Kidney Int* 2002;62(4):1431–1439.

34. Baradi AF, Hope J. Observations on ultrastructure of rabbit mesothelium. *Exp Cell Res* 1964;34(March):33–44.

35. Gotloib L. Anatomy of the peritoneal membrane. In: La Greca G, Biasoli S, Ronco C, eds. *Peritoneal Dialysis*. Milan: Wichtig Editore, 1982:19–30.

36. von Recklinhausen FT. Zur Fettresorption. *Arch Pathol Anat Physiol (Berl)* 1863;26:172–208.

37. Allen L. The peritoneal stomata. *Anat Rec* 1936;67(Dec): 89–103.

38. Simer PH: The passage of particulate matter from the peritoneal cavity into the lymph vessels of the diaphragm. *Anat Rec* 1948;101(July):333–351.

39. Dalton AJ, Felix MD. A comparison of mesothelial cells and macrophages in mice after the intraperitoneal inoculation of melanin granules. *J Biophys Biochem Cytol* 1956;2(4, suppl): 109–114.

40. Laurent TC, Laurent UB, Fraser JR. The structure and function of hyaluronan: an overview. *Immunol Cell Biol* 1996;74(2):A1–A7.

41. Yung S, Coles GA, Williams JD, Davies M. The source and possible significance of hyaluronan in the peritoneal cavity. *Kidney Int* 1994;46(2):527–533.

42. Baron MA. Structure of the intestinal peritoneum in man. *Am J Anat* 1941;69(Nov):439–497.

43. Simionescu M, Simionescu N, Palade G. Segmental differentiation of cell junctions in the vascular endothelium. The microvasculature. *J Cell Biol* 1975; 67(3):863–885.

44. Gotloib L, Shustak A, Bar-Sella P, Eliali V. Fenestrated capillaries in human parietal and rabbit diaphragmatic peritoneum. *Nephron* 1985;41(2):200–202.

45. Gotloib L, Shostak A. In search of a role for submesothelial fenestrated capillaries. *Perit Dial Int* 1993;13(2):98–102.

46. Palade GE, Simionescu M, Simionescu N. Structural aspects of the permeability of the microvascular endothelium. *Acta Physiol Scand Suppl* 1979;463:11–32.

47. Renkin EM. Relation of capillary morphology to transport of fluid and large molecules: a review. *Acta Physiol Scand Suppl* 1979;463:81–91.

48. Simionescu N, Simionescu M, Palade G. Structural basis of permeability in sequential segments of the microvasculature of the diaphragm. II. Pathways followed by microperoxidase across the endothelium. Microvasc Res 1978;15(1):17–36.

49. Bundgaard M. The three-dimensional organization of tight junctions in a capillary endothelium revealed by serial-section electron microscopy. *J Ultrastruct Res* 1984;88(1):1–17.

50. Rippe B, Haraldsson B. Capillary permeability in rat hindquarters as determined by estimations of capillary reflection coefficients. *Acta Physiol Scand* 1986;127(3):289–303.

51. Pannekeet MM, Mulder JB, Weening JJ, et al. Demonstration of aquaporin-CHIP in peritoneal tissue of uremic and CAPD patients. *Perit Dial Int* 1996;16(suppl 1):S54–S57.

52. Devuyst O, Nielsen S, Cosyns JP, et al. Aquaporin-1 and endothelial nitric oxide synthase expression in capillary endothelia of human peritoneum. *Am J Physiol* 1998;275 (1 Pt 2):H234–H242.

53. McCallum WG. On the mechanism of absorption of granular materials from the peritoneum. *Johns Hopkins Hosp Bull* 1903;14:105–115.

54. French JE, Florey HW, Morris B. The absorption of particles by the lymphatics of the diaphragm. *Q J Exp Physiol Cogn Med Sci* 1960;45(Jan):88–103.

55. Leak LV, Rahil K. Permeability of the diaphragmatic mesothelium: the structural basis for "stomata." *Am J Anat* 1978;157(4):557–594.

56. Tsilibary EC, Wissig SL. Lymphatic absorption from the peritoneal cavity: regulation of patency of mesothelial stomata. *Microvasc Res* 1983;25(1):22–39.

57. Allen L, Vogt E. A mechanism of lymphatic absorption from serous cavities. *Am J Physiol* 1937; 119(Aug):776–782.

58. Casley-Smith JR. Endothelial permeability. The passage of particles into and out of diaphragmatic lymphatics. *Q J Exp Physiol* 1964;49(Oct):365–383.

59. Borisov AV. Lymphatic capillaries and blood vessels of milky spots in the human greater omentum. *Fed Proc Trans Suppl* 1964;23(Jan-Feb):150–154.

60. Mironov VA, Gusev SA, Baradi AF. Mesothelial stomata overlying omental milky spots: scanning electron microscopic study. *Cell Tissue Res* 1979;201(2):327–330.

61. Beelen RHJ, Fluitsma DM, Hoefsmit ECM. The cellular composition of omentum milky spots and the ultrastructure of milky spot macrophages and reticulum cells. *J Reticuloendothel Soc* 1980;28(6):585–599.

62. Ranvier L. I. Recherches sur la formation des mailles du grand épiploon. II. Du developpement et de l'accroissment des vaisseaux sanguines. III. Note sur les vaisseaux sanguines et la circulation dans les muscles rouges. *Arch Physiol Normale Pathol Par* 1874; 2ᵉ serie,1:421–428,429–445,446–450, et planche XVIII, XIX.

63. Seifert E. Studien am Omentum majus des Menschen. *Langenbecks Arch Klin Chir Berl* 1923;123:608–683.

64. Carr I. The fine structure of the cells of the mouse peritoneum. *Z Zellforsch Mikrosk Anat* 1967;80(4):534–555.

65. Beelen RHJ, Fluitsma DM, Hoefsmit ECM. Peroxidatic activity of mononuclear phagocytes developing in omentum milky spots. *J Reticuloendothel Soc* 1980;28(6):601–609.

66. Dobbie JW, Lloyd JK, Gall CA. Categorization of ultrastructural changes in peritoneal mesothelium, stroma and blood vessels in uremia and CAPD patients. In: Khanna R, Nolph KD, Prowant BF, et al, eds. *Advances in Peritoneal Dialysis, Selected Papers from the Tenth Annual Conference on Peritoneal Dialysis*. Dallas, TX, February 1990. Toronto: Peritoneal Dialysis Bulletin, 1990;6:3–12.

67. Dobbie JW. Pathogenesis of peritoneal fibrosing syndromes (sclerosing peritonitis) in peritoneal dialysis. *Perit Dial Int* 1992;12(1):14–27.

68. Williams JD, Craig KJ, Topley N, et al. Peritoneal Biopsy Study Group. Morphologic changes in the peritoneal membrane of patients with renal disease. *J Am Soc Nephrol* 2002; 13(2):470–479.

69. Combet S, Miyata T, Moulin P, et al. Vascular proliferation and enhanced expression of endothelial nitric oxide synthase in human peritoneum exposed to long-term peritoneal dialysis. *J Am Soc Nephrol* 2000;11(4):717–728.

70. Devuyst O, Topley N, Williams JD. Morphological and functional changes in the dialysed peritoneal cavity: impact of more biocompatible solutions. *Nephrol Dial Transplant* 2002; 17(suppl 3):12–15.

71. Courtice FC, Simmonds WJ. Physiological significance of lymph drainage of the serous cavities and lungs. *Physiol Rev* 1954;34(3):419–448.

72. Orlow WN. Einige Versuche über die Resorption in der Bauchhöhle. *Arch Ges Physiol Bonn* 1894;59:170–200.

73. Bolton C. Absorption from the peritoneal cavity. *J Pathol Bacteriol Cambr* 1921;14:429–445.

74. Clark AJ. Absorption from the peritoneal cavity. *J Pharmacol Exper Ther Balt* 1920–1921;16:415–433.

75. Courtice FC, Steinbeck AW. Rate of absorption of heparinized plasma and of 0.9 per cent NaCl from the peritoneal cavity of the rabbit and guinea-pig. *Austr J Exp Biol Med Sci* 1950;28:171–182.

76. Khanna R, Mactier R, Twardowski ZJ, Nolph KD. Peritoneal cavity lymphatics. *Perit Dial Bull* 1986;6(3):113–121.

77. Siperstein DM. Intraperitoneal transfusion with citrated blood. *Am J Dis Child* 1923;25(Mar):202–221.

78. Cole WCC, Montogomery JC. Intraperitoneal blood transfusion. Report of two hundred and thirty-seven transfusions on one hundred and seventeen patients in private practice. *Am J Dis Child* 1929; 37(Mar):497–510.

79. Liley AW. Intrauterine transfusion of the fetus in haemolytic disease. *Br Med J* 1963; 2(5365):1107–1109.

80. Morison R. Remarks on some functions of the omentum. *Br Med J Lond* 1906;1:76–78.

81. Portis B. Role of omentum of rabbits, dogs, and guinea pigs in antibody production. *J Infect Dis* 1924; 34(Feb): 159–185.

82. Shimotsuma M, Shields JW, Simpson-Morgan MW, et al. Morpho-physiological function and role of omental milky spots as omentum-associated lymphoid tissue (OALT) in the peritoneal cavity. *Lymphology* 1993;26(2):90–101.

83. Muscatello G. Ueber den Bau und das Aufsaugungsvermögen des Peritonäum. Anatomische und experimentalle Unterschungen. *Virchows Arch Pathol Anat* 1895;142:327–359.

84. Durham HE. The mechanism of reaction to peritoneal infection. *J Pathol Bact Edinb Lond* 1896–7;4:338–383.

85. Wilkie DPD. Some functions and surgical uses of omentum. *Br Med Lond* 1911;2:1103–1106.

86. de Renzi E, Boeri G. Das Netz als Shutzorgan. *Berl Klin Wochnschr* 1903;40:773–775.

87. Twardowski ZJ, Tully RJ, Ersoy FF, Dedhia NM. Computerized tomography with and without intraperitoneal contrast for

determination of intraabdominal fluid distribution and diagnosis of complications in peritoneal dialysis patients. *ASAIO Trans* 1990;36(2):95–103.

88. Nolph KD, Miller F, Rubin J, Popovich RP. New directions in peritoneal dialysis concepts and applications. *Kidney Int* 1980;18(suppl 10):111–116.

89. Grotte G. Passage of dextran molecules across the blood-lymph barrier. *Acta Chir Scand* 1956;(suppl 211):1–84.

90. Karnovsky MJ. The ultrastructural basis of capillary permeability studied with peroxidase as a tracer. *J Cell Biol* 1967;35(1):213–236.

91. Wissig SL. Identification of small pore in muscle capillaries. *Acta Physiol Scand Suppl* 1979;463:33–44.

92. Rippe B, Kamiya A, Folkow B. Transcapillary passage of albumin, effects of tissue cooling and of increases in filtration and plasma colloid osmotic pressure. *Acta Physiol Scand* 1979;105(2):171–187.

93. Rippe B, Stelin G, Haraldsson B. Computer simulations of peritoneal fluid transport in CAPD. *Kidney Int* 1991;40(2):315–325.

94. Wayland H. Transmural and interstitial molecular transport. In: Legrain M, ed. *Continuous Ambulatory Peritoneal Dialysis: Proceedings of an International Symposium*. Paris, November 2, 3, 1979. Amsterdam: Excerpta Medica, 1980:18–27.

95. Cotran RS. The fine structure of the microvasculature in relation to normal and altered permeability. In: Reeve EB, Guyton AC, eds. *Physical Basis of Circulatory Transport: Regulation and Exchange*. Philadelphia: Saunders, 1967.

96. Gotloib L, Bar-Sella P, Shostak A. Reduplicated basal lamina of small venules and mesothelium of human parietal peritoneum: ultrastructural changes of reduplicated peritoneal basement membrane. *Perit Dial Bull* 1985;5(4):212–215.

97. Flessner MF, Dedrick RL, Schultz JS. A distributed model of peritoneal plasma transport: theoretical considerations. *Am J Physiol* 1984;246(4 Pt 2):R597–R607.

98. Wayland H, Silberberg A. Blood to lymph transport. *Microvasc Res* 1978;15(3):367–374.

99. Tsilibary EC, Wissig SL. Absorption from the peritoneal cavity: SEM study of the mesothelium covering the peritoneal surface of the muscular portion of the diaphragm. *Am J Anat* 1977;149(1):127–133.

100. Cascarano J, Rubin AD, Chick WL, Zweifach BW. Metabolically induced permeability changes across mesothelium and endothelium. *Am J Physiol* 1964;206(Feb):373–382.

101. Gotloib L, Digenis GE, Rabinovich S, et al. Ultrastructure of normal rabbit mesentery. *Nephron* 1983;34(4):248–255.

102. Digenis GE, Rabinovich S, Medline A. Electron microscopic study of the peritoneal kinetics of iron dextran during peritoneal dialysis in the rabbit. *Nephron* 1984;37(2):108–112.

103. Verger C, Luger A, Moore HL, Nolph KD. Acute changes in peritoneal morphology and transport properties with infectious peritonitis and mechanical injury. *Kidney Int* 1983;23(6):823–831.

104. Rubin J, McFarland S, Hellems EW, Bower JD. Peritoneal dialysis during peritonitis. *Kidney Int* 1981;19(3):460–464.

105. Lange K, Treser G, Mangalat J. Automatic continuous high flow rate peritoneal dialysis. *Arch Klin Med* 1968;214(3):201–206.

106. Stephen RL, Atkin-Thor E, Kolff WJ. Recirculating peritoneal dialysis with subcutaneous catheter. *Trans Am Soc Artif Intern Organs* 1976;22:575–584.

107. Goldschmidt ZH, Pote HH, Katz MA, Shear L. Effect of dialysate volume on peritoneal dialysis kinetics. *Kidney Int* 1974;5(3):240–245.

108. Rubin J, Kirchner K, Bower J. Evaluation of stagnant fluid films during simulated peritoneal dialysis: in vitro and in vivo studies. *Clin Exp Dial Apheresis* 1981;5(3):285–292.

109. Randerson DH. Continuous ambulatory peritoneal dialysis—a critical appraisal. Thesis. Sydney, Australia: University of New South Wales, 1980.

110. Pyle WK. Mass transfer in peritoneal dialysis. Thesis. Austin, TX: University of Texas, 1981.

111. Farrell PC, Randerson DH. Mass transfer kinetics in continuous ambulatory peritoneal dialysis. In: Legrain M, ed. *Proceedings of the First International Symposium on Continuous Ambulatory Peritoneal Dialysis*. Amsterdam: Excerpta Medica, 1980:34–41.

112. Pyle WK, Moncrief JW, Popovich RP. Peritoneal transport evaluation in CAPD. In: Moncrief JW, Popovich RP, eds. *CAPD Update*. New York: Masson, 1981:35–52.

113. Pyle WK, Popovich RP, Moncrief JW. Mass transfer in peritoneal dialysis. In: Gahl GM, Kessel M, Nolph KD, eds. *Advances in Peritoneal Dialysis*. Amsterdam: Excerpta Medica, 1981:41–46.

114. Garred LJ, Canaud B, Farrell PC. A simple kinetic model for assessing peritoneal mass transfer in continuous ambulatory peritoneal dialysis. *ASAIO J* 1983;6:131–137.

115. Popovich RP, Moncrief JW. Kinetic modeling of peritoneal transport. In: Trevino-Bacerra A, Boen FST, eds. Today's Art of Peritoneal Dialysis. Contributions to Nephrology. Vol 17. Basel: Karger, 1979:59–72.

116. Nolph KD, Popovich RP, Ghods AJ, Twardowski Z. Determinants of low clearances of small solutes during peritoneal dialysis. *Kidney Int* 1978;13(2):117–123.

117. Boen ST. Kinetics of peritoneal dialysis: A comparison with the artificial kidney. *Medicine (Baltimore)* 1961;40(Sept): 243–287.

118. Penzotti SC, Mattocks AM. Effects of dwell time, volume of dialysis fluid, and added accelerators on peritoneal dialysis of urea. *J Pharm Sci* 1971;60(10):1520–1522.

119. Pirpasopoulos M, Lindsay RM, Rahman M, Kennedy AC. A cost-effectiveness study of dwell times in peritoneal dialysis. *Lancet* 1972;2(7787):1135–1136.

120. Tenckhoff H, Ward G, Boen ST. The influence of dialysate volume and flow rate on peritoneal clearance. *Proc Eur Dial Transpl Assoc* 1965;2:113–117.

121. Trivedi HS, Twardowski ZJ. Long-term successful nocturnal intermittent peritoneal dialysis: a ten-year case study. In: Khanna R, ed. *Advances in Peritoneal Dialysis. Selected Papers from the Fourteenth Annual Conference on Peritoneal Dialysis*. Orlando, Florida, January 24–26, 1994. Toronto: Dialysis Publications, 1994;10:81–84.

122. Miller JH, Gipstein R, Margules R, et al. Automated peritoneal dialysis: analysis of several methods of peritoneal dialysis. *Trans Am Soc Artif Intern Organs* 1966;12:98–105.

123. Kablitz C, Stephen RL, Duffy DP, et al. Technological augmentation of peritoneal urea clearance: past, present, and future. *Dial Transplant* 1980;9(8):741–778.

124. Warden GD, Maxwell JG, Stephen RL. The use of reciprocating peritoneal dialysis with a subcutaneous peritoneal catheter in end-stage renal failure in diabetes mellitus. *J Surg Res* 1978;24(6):495–500.

125. Di Paolo N. Semicontinuous peritoneal dialysis. *Dial Transplant* 1978;7:839,842.

126. Finkelstein FO, Kliger AS. Enhanced efficiency of peritoneal dialysis using rapid, small-volume exchanges. *ASAIO J* 1979;2(3):103–106.

127. Twardowski ZJ, Nolph KD, Khanna R, et al. Tidal peritoneal dialysis. In: Avram MM, Giordano C, eds. *Ambulatory Peritoneal Dialysis; Proceedings of the IVth Congress of the International Society for Peritoneal Dialysis.* Venice, Italy, June 29–July 2, 1987. New York: Plenum, 1990:145–149.

128. Twardowski ZJ, Prowant BF, Nolph KD, et al. Chronic nightly tidal peritoneal dialysis (NTPD). *ASAIO Trans* 1990; 36(3):M584–588.

129. Twardowski ZJ. Tidal peritoneal dialysis—acute and chronic studies. *EDTNA/ERCA J* 1990;15 (Sept):4–9.

130. Twardowski ZJ. Tidal peritoneal dialysis. In: Nissenson AR, Fine RN, eds. *Dialysis Therapy.* Philadelphia: Hanley & Belfus, 1993:153–156.

131. Piraino B, Bender F, Bernardini J. A comparison of clearances on tidal peritoneal dialysis and intermittent peritoneal dialysis. *Perit Dial Int* 1994;14(2):145–148.

132. Twardowski Z, Janicka L. Three exchanges with a 2.5 liter volume for continuous ambulatory peritoneal dialysis. *Kidney Int* 1981;20(2):281–284.

133. Twardowski ZJ, Prowant BF, Nolph KD, et al. High volume, low frequency continuous ambulatory peritoneal dialysis. *Kidney Int* 1983;23(1):64–70.

134. Twardowski ZJ, Nolph KD, Prowant BF, Moore HL. Efficiency of high volume low frequency continuous ambulatory peritoneal dialysis (CAPD). *Trans Am Soc Artif Intern Organs* 1983;29:53–57.

135. Krediet RT, Boeschoten EW, Zuyderhoudt FMJ, Arisz L. Differences in the peritoneal transport of water, solutes and proteins between dialysis with two- and with three-litre exchanges. In: Krediet RT, ed. Peritoneal permeability in continuous ambulatory peritoneal dialysis patients. Thesis. Amsterdam: University of Amsterdam, 1986;129–146.

136. Spencer PC, Farrell PC. Applications of kinetic monitoring in CAPD. In: Weimar W, Fieren MWJA, Diderich PPNN, op de Hoek, CT, eds. *Continuous Ambulatory Peritoneal Dialysis: Proceedings of the Fourth Benelux Symposium.* Rotterdam; November 24, 1984. Amsterdam: Excerpta Medica, 1985, pp. 9–23.

137. Gross M, McDonald HP Jr. Effects of dialysate temperature and flow rate on peritoneal clearance. *JAMA* 1967;202(4):363–365.

138. Indraprasit S, Namwongprom A, Sooksriwongse C, Buri PS. Effect of dialysate temperature on peritoneal clearance. *Nephron* 1983;34(1):45–47.

139. Gjessing J, Barsa J, Tomlin PJ. A possible means of rapid cooling in the emergency treatment of malignant hyperpyrexia. *Br J Anaesth* 1976;48(5):469–473.

140. Knochel JP, Mason AD. Effect of alkalinization on peritoneal diffusion of uric acid. *Am J Physiol* 1966;210(5):1160–1164.

141. Deger GE, Wagoner RD. peritoneal dialysis in acute uric acid nephropathy. *Mayo Clin Proc* 1972;47(3):189–192.

142. Campion DS, North JDK. Effect of protein binding of barbiturates on their rate of removal during peritoneal dialysis. *J Lab Clin Med* 1965;66(4):549–563.

143. Henderson LW, Nolph KD. Altered permeability of the peritoneal membrane after using hypertonic peritoneal dialysis fluid. *J Clin Invest* 1969;48(6):992–1101.

144. Granger DN, Ulrich M, Perry MA, Kvietys PR. Peritoneal dialysis solutions and feline splanchnic blood flow. *Clin Exp Pharmacol Physiol* 1984;11(5):473–481.

145. Aune S. Transperitoneal exchange. II. Peritoneal blood flow estimated by hydrogen gas clearance. *Scand J Gastroenterol* 1970;5(2):99–104.

146. Grzegorzewska AE, Antoniewicz K. An indirect estimation of effective peritoneal capillary blood flow in peritoneally dialyzed uremic patients. *Perit Dial Int* 1993;13(suppl 2):S39–S40.

147. Hirszel P, Lameire N, Bogaert M. Pharmacologic alteration of peritoneal transport rates and pharmacokinetics of the peritoneum. In: Gokal R, Nolph KD, eds. *The Textbook of Peritoneal Dialysis.* Amsterdam: Kluwer, 1994:69–113.

148. Twardowski ZJ, Nolph KD, Khanna R, et al. Peritoneal equilibration test. *Perit Dial Bull* 1987;7(3):138–147.

149. Twardowski ZJ, Khanna R, Nolph KD. Peritoneal dialysis modifications to avoid CAPD dropouts. In: Khanna R, Nolph KD, Prowant BF, et al, eds. *Advances in Continuous Ambulatory Peritoneal Dialysis: Proceedings of the Seventh Annual CAPD Conference.* Kansas City, MO, February 1987. Toronto: Peritoneal Dialysis Bulletin, 1987:171–178.

150. Twardowski ZJ. Clinical value of standardized equilibration tests in CAPD patients. *Blood Purif* 1989;7(2–3):95–108.

151. Twardowski ZJ. Nightly peritoneal dialysis (why? who? how? and when?). *ASAIO Trans* 1990;36(1):8–16.

152. Nolph KD, Moore HL, Prowant BF, et al. Continuous ambulatory peritoneal dialysis with a high flux membrane. *ASAIO J* 1993;39(3):M566–M568.

153. Diaz-Buxo JA. Streaming, mixing, and recirculation: role of the peritoneal access in continuous flow peritoneal dialysis (clinical considerations). *Adv Perit Dial* 2002;18:87–90.

154. Ronco C, Gloukhoff A, Dell'Aquila R, Levin NW. Catheter design for continuous flow peritoneal dialysis. *Blood Purif* 2002;20(1):40–44.

155. Freida P, Issad B. Continuous flow peritoneal dialysis: assessment of fluid and solute removal in a high-flow model of "fresh dialysate single pass." *Perit Dial Int* 2003;23(4):348–355.

156. Miller FN, Nolph KD, Harris PD, et al. Microvascular and clinical effects of altered peritoneal dialysis solutions. *Kidney Int* 1979;15(6):630–639.

157. Staverman AJ. The theory of measurement of osmotic pressure. *Rec Trav Chim Pays-Bas Belg* 1951;70:344–352.

158. Henderson L. Ultrafiltration with peritoneal dialysis. In: Nolph KD, ed. *Peritoneal Dialysis*, 2d ed. Boston: Martinus Nijhoff, 1985:159–177.

159. Rippe B, Perry MA, Granger DN. Permselectivity of the peritoneal membrane. *Microvasc Res* 1985;29(1):89–102.

160. Twardowski ZJ, Khanna R, Nolph KD. Osmotic agents and ultrafiltration in peritoneal dialysis. *Nephron* 1986;42(2):93–101.

161. Twardowski ZJ, Nolph KD, McGary TJ, Moore HL. Polyanions and glucose as osmotic agents in simulated peritoneal dialysis. *Artif Organs* 1983;7(4):420–427.

162. Twardowski ZJ, Moore HL, McGary TJ, et al. Polymers as osmotic agents for peritoneal dialysis. *Perit Dial Bull* 1984;4(suppl 3):125–131.

163. Twardowski ZJ, Hain H, McGary TJ, et al. Sustained UF with gelatin dialysis solution during long dwell peritoneal dialysis exchanges in rats. In: Maher TF, Wincheser TF, eds. *Frontiers in Peritoneal Dialysis: Proceedings of the Third International Symposium on Peritoneal Dialysis.* Washington, DC, 1984. New York: Field, Rich, 1986:249–254.

164. Twardowski ZJ, Nolph KD, Khanna R, et al. Charged polymers as osmotic agents for peritoneal dialysis. *Mater Res Soc Sym Proc* 1986;55:319–326.

165. Mistry CD, Gokal R. Glucose polymer as an osmotic agent in CAPD. *Adv Exp Med Biol* 1989;260:149–156.

166. Wolfson M, Piraino B, Hamburger RJ, Morton AR. Icodextrin Study Group. A randomized controlled trial to evaluate the efficacy and safety of icodextrin in peritoneal dialysis. *Am J Kidney Dis* 2002;40(5):1055–1065.

167. Krediet R, Mujais S. Use of icodextrin in high transport ultrafiltration failure. *Kidney Int Suppl* 2002; (81):S53–S61.

168. Plum J, Gentile S, Verger C, et al. Efficacy and safety of a 7.5% icodextrin peritoneal dialysis solution in patients treated with automated peritoneal dialysis. *Am J Kidney Dis* 2002;39(4):862–871.

169. Twardowski Z, Książek A, Majdan M, et al. Kinetics of continuous ambulatory peritoneal dialysis (CAPD) with four exchanges per day. *Clin Nephrol* 1981;15(3):119–131.

170. Nolph KD, Twardowski ZJ, Popovich RP, Rubin J. Equilibration of peritoneal dialysis solutions during long dwell exchanges. *J Lab Clin Med* 1979;93(2):246–256.

171. Nolph KD, Hano JE, Teschan PE. Peritoneal sodium transport during hypertonic peritoneal dialysis: physiologic mechanisms and clinical implications. *Ann Intern Med* 1969;70(5):931–941.

172. Nolph KD, Sorkin MI, Moore H. Autoregulation of sodium and potassium removal during continuous ambulatory peritoneal dialysis. *Trans Am Soc Artif Intern Organs* 1980;6: 334–337.

173. Boyer J, Gill GN, Epstein FH. Hyperglycemia and hyperosmolality complicating peritoneal dialysis. *Ann Intern Med* 1967;67(3):568–572.

174. Miller RB, Tassistro CR. Peritoneal dialysis. *N Engl J Med* 1969;281(17):945–949.

175. Nolph KD, New DL. Effects of ultrafiltration on solute clearances in hollow fiber artificial kidneys. *J Lab Clin Med* 1976;88(4):593–600.

176. Nolph KD, Miller FN, Pyle WK, et al. A hypothesis to explain the characteristics of peritoneal ultrafiltration. *Kidney Int* 1981;20(5):543–548.

177. Starling EH. On the absorption of fluids from the connective tissue spaces. *J Physiol Cambridge* 1896; 19:312–326.

178. Nolph KD, Twardowski ZJ. The peritoneal dialysis system. In: Nolph KD, ed. *Peritoneal Dialysis,* 3d ed. Dordrecht/Boston/London: Kluwer, 1989:13–27.

179. Ganter G. Ueber die Beseitigung giftiger Stoffe aus dem Blute durch Dialyse. *Münch Med Wochnschr* 1923(Dec);70:1478–1480.

180. Balázs J, Rosenak S. Zur Behandlung der Sublimaturie durch peritoneale Dialyse. *Wien Klin Wochnschr* 1934; 47(July):851–854.

181. Wear JB, Sisk IR, Trinkle AJ. Peritoneal lavage in treatment of uremia: Experimental and clinical study. *J Urol* 1938; 39(Jan):53–62.

182. Rhoads JE. Peritoneal lavage in the treatment of renal insufficiency. *Am J Med Sci* 1938;196(Nov):642–647.

183. Frank HA, Seligman AM, Fine J. Further experiences with peritoneal irrigation for acute renal failure including modifications and methods. *Ann Surg* 1948;128(Sept):561–608.

184. Odel HM, Ferris DO, Power MH. Peritoneal lavage as an effective means of extrarenal excretion. A clinical appraisal. *Am J Med* 1950;9(July):63–77.

185. Maxwell MH, Rockney RE, Kleeman CR, Twiss RM. Peritoneal dialysis. I. Technique and applications. *JAMA* 1959;170(8):917–924.

186. Abbott WE, Shea P. The treatment of temporary renal insufficiency by peritoneal lavage. *Am J Med Sci* 1946;21(March):312–319.

187. Legrain M, Merrill JP. Short-term continuous transperitoneal dialysis: A simplified technique. *N Engl J Med* 1953;248(4):125–129.

188. Boen ST. Peritoneal dialysis (thesis). Amsterdam: University of Amsterdam, 1959.

189. Boen ST, Mulinari AS, Dillard DH, Scribner BH. Periodic peritoneal dialysis in the management of chronic uremia. *Trans Am Soc Artif Intern Organs* 1962;8:256–262.

190. Twardowski Z, Lebek R, Hakuba A, et al. Treatment of chronic irreversible renal insufficiency by means of repeated peritoneal dialysis. *Acta Med Pol* 1970;11(4):343–362.

191. Gault MH, Ferguson EL, Sidhu JS, Corbin RP. Fluid and electrolyte complications of peritoneal dialysis. Choice of dialysis solutions. *Ann Intern Med* 1971;75(2):253–262.

192. Ahearn DJ, Nolph KD. Controlled sodium removal with peritoneal dialysis. *Trans Am Soc Artif Intern Organs* 1972;17:423–428.

193. Tenckhoff H. Choice of peritoneal dialysis solutions. *Ann Intern Med* 1971;75(2):313–314.

194. Vidt DG. Recommendations on choice of peritoneal dialysis solutions. *Ann Intern Med* 1973;78(1):144–146.

195. Shen FH, Sherrard DJ, Scollard D, et al. Thirst, relative hypernatremia and excessive weight gain in maintenance peritoneal dialysis. *Trans Am Soc Artif Intern Organs* 1978;24:142–145.

196. Oreopoulos DG, Khanna R, McCready W, et al. Continuous ambulatory peritoneal dialysis in Canada. *Dial Transpl* 1980;9(3):224–226.

197. Twardowski ZJ, Nolph KD, Khanna R, et al. Daily clearances with continuous ambulatory peritoneal dialysis and nightly peritoneal dialysis. *ASAIO Trans* 1986;32(1):575–580.

198. Dobbie JW, Krediet RT, Twardowski ZJ, Nichols WK. A 39-year-old man with loss of ultrafiltration. *Perit Dial Int* 1994;14(4):384–394.

199. Krediet RT. Evaluation of peritoneal membrane integrity. *J Nephrol* 1997;10(5):238–244.

200. Mactier RA, Khanna R, Twardowski ZJ, Nolph KD. Role of peritoneal cavity lymphatic absorption in peritoneal dialysis. *Kidney Int* 1987;32(2):165–172.

201. Nolph KD, Mactier R, Khanna R, et al. The kinetics of ultra-filtration during peritoneal dialysis: the role of lymphatics. *Kidney Int* 1987;32(2):219–226.

202. Flessner MF, Dedrick RL, Schultz JS. Exchange of macro-molecules between peritoneal cavity and plasma. *Am J Physiol (Heart Circ Physiol 17)* 1985;248(1 Pt 2):H15–H25.

203. Cheek TR, Twardowski ZJ, Moore HL, Nolph KD. Absorp-tion of inulin and high molecular weight gelatin isocyanate solutions from the peritoneal cavity of rats. In: Avram MM, Giordano C, eds. *Ambulatory Peritoneal Dialysis—Proceed-ings of the IVth Congress of the International Society for Peritoneal Dialysis.* Venice, Italy, June 29–July 2, 1987. New York: Plenum, 1990:149–152.

204. Mactier RA, Khanna R, Twardowski Z, et al. Contribution of lymphatic absorption to loss of ultrafiltration and solute clearances in continuous ambulatory peritoneal dialysis. *J Clin Invest* 1987;80(5):1311–1316.

205. Struijk DG, Bakker JC, Krediet RT, et al. Effect of intraperi-toneal administration of two different batches of albumin so-lutions on peritoneal solute transport in CAPD patients. *Nephrol Dial Transplant* 1991;6(3):198–202.

206. Koomen GC, Krediet RT, Leegwater AC, et al. A fast reliable method for the measurement of intraperitoneal dextran 70, used to calculate lymphatic absorption. *Adv Perit Dial* 1991;7:10–14.

207. Krediet RT, Struijk DG, Koomen GCM, Arisz L. Peritoneal fluid kinetics during CAPD measured with intraperitoneal dextran 70. *ASAIO Trans* 1991;37(4):662–667.

208. Flessner MF. Peritoneal transport physiology: insights from basic research. *J Am Soc Nephrol* 1991;2(2):122–135.

209. Tran L, Rodela H, Abernethy NJ, et al. Lymphatic drainage of hypertonic solution from peritoneal cavity of anesthetized and conscious sheep. *J Appl Physiol* 1993;74(2):859–867.

210. Johnston MG. Studies on lymphatic drainage of the peri-toneal cavity in sheep. *Blood Purif* 1992;10(3–4):122–131.

211. Drake RE, Gabel JC. Diaphragmatic lymph vessel drainage of the peritoneal cavity. *Blood Purif* 1992;10(3–4):132–135.

212. Flessner MF. Net ultrafiltration in peritoneal dialysis: Role of direct fluid absorption into peritoneal tissue. *Blood Purif* 1992;10(3–4):136–147.

213. Rippe B, Zakaria ER. Lymphatic versus nonlymphatic fluid absorption from the peritoneal cavity as related to the peri-toneal ultrafiltration capacity and sieving properties. *Blood Purif* 1992;10(3–4):189–202.

214. Nagy JA. Lymphatic and nonlymphatic pathways of peri-toneal absorption in mice: Physiology versus pathology. *Blood Purif* 1992;10(3–4):148–162.

215. Khanna R, Mactier R. Role of lymphatics in peritoneal dialy-sis. *Blood Purif* 1992;10(3–4):163–172.

216. Mactier RA, Khanna R, Twardowski Z, Nolph KD. Lym-phatic absorption in CAPD. In: Avram MM, Giordano C, eds. *Ambulatory Peritoneal Dialysis—Proceedings of the IVth Congress of the International Society for Peritoneal Dialysis.* Venice, Italy, June 29–July 2, 1987. New York: Plenum, 1990:71–75.

217. Leak LV. The structure of lymphatic capillaries in lymph for-mation. *Fed Proc* 1976;35(8):1863–1871.

218. Verger C. How to use the peritoneum as a dialysis membrane. Methods of surveillance, criteria of efficacy and longevity as a dialysis membrane, consequences with respect to tech-niques of peritoneal dialysis (in French). *Nephrologie* 1995;16(1):19–31.

219. Haraldsson B. Assessing the peritoneal dialysis capacities of individual patients. *Kidney Int* 1995;47(4):1187–1198.

220. Van Biesen W, Carlsson O, Bergia R, et al. Personal dialysis capacity (PDC) test: a multicentre clinical study. *Nephrol Dial Transplant* 2003;18(4):788–796.

221. Vonesh EF, Burkart J, McMurray SD, Williams PF. Peritoneal dialysis kinetic modeling: validation in a multicenter clinical study. *Perit Dial Int* 1996;16(5):471–481.

222. Lilaj T, Dittrich E, Puttinger H, et al. A preceding exchange with polyglucose versus glucose solution modifies peritoneal equilibration test results. *Am J Kidney Dis* 2001;38(1):118–126.

223. Twardowski ZJ, Prowant BF, Moore HL, et al. Short peri-toneal equilibration test: impact of preceding dwell time. *Adv Perit Dial* 2003;19:53–58.

224. Sanusi AA, Zweers MM, Weening JJ, et al. Expression of cancer antigen 125 by peritoneal mesothelial cells is not in-fluenced by duration of peritoneal dialysis. *Perit Dial Int* 2001;21(5):495–500.

225. Mortier S, De Vriese AS, Lameire N. Recent concepts in the molecular biology of the peritoneal membrane—implications for more biocompatible dialysis solutions. *Blood Purif* 2003;21(1):14–23.

226. Frampton J, Plosker G. Icodextrin: a review of its use in peri-toneal dialysis. *Drugs* 2003;63(19):2079–2105.

227. Passlick-Deetjen J, Schaub TP, Schilling H. Solutions for APD: special considerations. *Semin Dial* 2002;15(6):407–413.

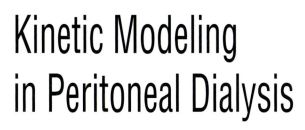

Kinetic Modeling in Peritoneal Dialysis

Frank A. Gotch
Marcia L. Keen

The clinical purpose of kinetic modeling in peritoneal dialysis (PD) broadly considered is the development of mathematical models to (1) reliably predict water and solute removal with various PD regimens, (2) quantify the dose of delivered dialysis, and (3) guide prescription of adequate dialysis.

All forms of peritoneal dialysis in clinical use are fundamentally batch dialysis systems with intraperitoneal dialysate infusion followed by variable dwell time and subsequent drainage. Modern single-pass hemodialysis systems provide constant rates of ultrafiltration and solute clearance during each dialysis,[1] while with the batch or exchange system of peritoneal dialysis, quantitative descriptions of the rates of ultrafiltration and clearance are more complex. These rates are maximal at the beginning of each exchange and decrease continuously to near zero as exchange or dwell time increases. In order to prescribe specified levels of fluid and solute removal for individual patients, the time course of ultrafiltration and clearance with varying infusion volumes and exchange times must be reliably predicted.

ULTRAFILTRATION IN PERITONEAL DIALYSIS

Ultrafiltration can be described as the bulk flow rate of water from blood to dialysate across an artificial membrane in hemodialysis (HD) and across the peritoneal membrane in PD. The rate of ultrafiltration (Q_f, mL/h) is controlled by the product of the membrane hydraulic permeability-area product (K_f, mL/h/mmHg) and the hydraulic driving force (mmHg) across the membrane in accordance with

$$Q_f = (K_f) \cdot (\text{Hydraulic Driving Force}) \qquad (1)$$

The two components of the driving force in all dialysis systems are transmembrane hydraulic pressure (*TMHP*) and transmembrane osmotic pressure (*TMOP*). Thus,

$$Qf = Kf \, (TMHP + TMOP) \qquad (2)$$

In hemodialysis, Kf is a well-defined property for any individual dialyzer (Kfd) and TMHP is determined by the mean blood compartment minus mean dialysate compartment pressure. The TMOP is small compared with TMHP and negative since it is approximately equal to plasma protein oncotic pressure opposing ultrafiltration from blood to aqueous dialysate. The TMHP can be precisely controlled with modern hemodialysis delivery systems so that accurate levels of Qf can be prescribed and achieved throughout each HD treatment in accordance with

$$Qf = Kfd(TMHP) \qquad (3)$$

In peritoneal dialysis, the forces controlling ultrafiltration are more complex and less amenable to precise control. The primary driving force is osmotic and the TMHP is relatively insignificant. A variable TMOP is achieved by adjusting the dextrose concentration of dialysate which can be varied from 1.5 to 4.25 of hydrated dextrose, equivalent to 1.36 and 3.86 g/dL of dextrose. The osmolalities due to glucose in these solutions range from 76 to 214 mOsm/L. These osmolalities, if separated from pure water by a semipermeable membrane impermeable to glucose but permeable to water, would require a hydraulic pressure in the range of 1450 to 4050 mmHg to prevent water flow into the glucose solution. The effective osmotic pressures in the peritoneal dialysate are far less than this since the membrane is permeable to glucose, which is absorbed during the exchange, with a $t_{1/2}$ of about 2.5 hours. Many investigators have reported Kfp values.[2–8] The average Kfp is approximately 2 mL/h/mmHg[8] and the total Qf over 2 hours is approximately 400 and 1200 mL, respectively, with 1.5 and 4.25% dextrose, indicating mean effective glucose osmotic pressures of only 100 and 300 mmHg. The hydraulic permeability of high-flux hemodialysis membranes is much higher and in the range of 50 to 100 mL/h/mmHg.

Maximal ultrafiltration occurs at the beginning of each exchange and exponentially falls to near zero over about 2 hours reflecting the exponential decrease in glucose concentration due to first order transport into blood from dialysate. There also is continuous lymphatic absorption of dialysate and the combined effects of glucose transfer and lymphatic flow result in a complex ultrafiltration profile originally described in a study by Mactier and colleagues.[9] They measured both the accumulation of fluid and lymphatic reabsorption and clearly distinguished between total and net ultrafiltrate as illustrated in Fig. 15–1. Note that the total ultrafiltrate (upper curve) exponentially approaches a limiting value while the net ultrafiltrate peaks in about 2

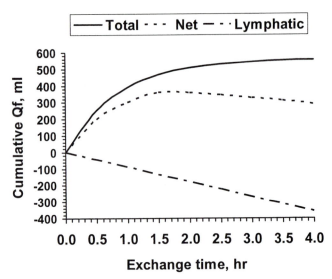

Figure 15–1. Typical cumulative total ultrafiltrate, net ultrafiltrate, and lymphatic reabsorption. Note that net ultrafiltrate reaches a maximum at about 1.5 to 2.0 hours and then falls reflecting lymphatic absorption.

hours and then falls due to continuous lymphatic absorption after the rate of ultrafiltration falls to zero. Analysis of the curve of total Qf in Fig. 15–1 is helpful for modeling Qf in PD. The M ± 2 SD values for the total ultrafiltrate profile in Fig. 15–1 are plotted in Fig 15–2. The M, +2SD and –2SD reported (Fig. 15–1) are each fit to a function of the form

$$QFt = QFT[1 - \exp(-k)] \qquad (4)$$

where QFt is the amount of Qf accumulated at any dwell time; QFT is the total amount of Qf which will accumulate during an infinite dwell; and k is a fitted time constant with

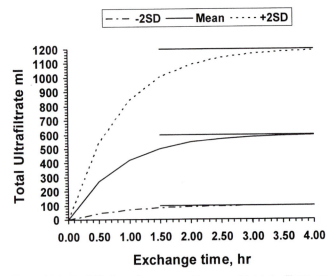

Figure 15–2. Total Qf at any time over a wide range of total ultrafiltrate can be described generally as Qft = QFT [1 – exp(–0.0200(t)] and specifically as Qft = QFT [1 – exp(-0.0200(t)] where QFT is total ultrafiltrate formed in an exchange and t is exchange time in minutes.

units of 1/min. Note that the three data sets can be fit with a single k = 0.02, although QFT varies from 100 to 1200 mL, with a mean value of 600 mL. The time constant of 0.02 indicates that over a wide range of QFT, the time course of Qf accumulation is similar and about 90 complete in 2.0 hours. This agrees well with a similar formulation previously used by Randerson.[10]

Equation (4) provides a generalized description of the time course of ultrafiltration during an exchange. It is also useful to develop relationships between the total ultrafiltrate (QFT) and the osmotic driving force expressed as the initial percent dextrose concentration. In clinical usage, the primary interest is to predict the net ultrafiltrate volume (QFnt) which will be present at time t when the exchange is drained. As shown in Fig. 15–1, the rate of lymphatic absorption (Ql) is constant and continuous so that

$$QFnt = QFT[1 - \exp(-.0200 \cdot t)] - Q1 \cdot t \quad (5)$$

Note in Eq. (5) that during the first 2 hours of dwell the QFnt is dependent on QFT, the time constant, k, and Ql·t, while after 2 hours, it is dependent on QFT and Ql·t. In order to model and predict QFnt, we need to know QFT and Ql. We can solve Eq. (5) for QFT, resulting in

$$QFT = (QFnt + Q1 \cdot t)/[1 - \sim\exp(-\sim0.02t)] \quad (6)$$

The net ultrafiltrate (QFnt) can be directly measured from the drain volume at any exchange time. Therefore, QFT can be calculated from Eq. (6) using an estimated value for Ql. Drain volumes with 1.5 and 4.5% dextrose for 4956 ambulatory exchanges on 15 patients have been reported.[11] These authors found the rate of decrease in drain volume from 2.5 to 12 hours to be linear with a slope ~0.7 mL/min, which is considered equal to Ql in these ambulatory data. QFT was calculated using Eq. (6) from these data and is shown in Fig. 15–3 plotted as a function of percent dextrose (%D). We have obtained similar data in San Francisco with 2.5% dextrose, which are also shown in Fig. 15–3. These data

(mean, ±1 SD and ±2 SD) were fitted to a logarithmic function with an intercept fixed at 0.7%D, corresponding to approximately 39 mOsm/L, in accordance with

$$QFT = a + b \ln(\%D) \quad (7)$$

It can be noted that the mean QFT reported for 2.5% dextrose (610 mL) in supine studies[9] is almost identical to the mean for our ambulatory observations (650 mL). The measured Ql was 1.5 mL/min for the supine studies[9] and 0.7 mL/min for the ambulatory studies.[11] However, it is of considerable interest to note that QFT values for 2.5% dextrose were almost identical, 650 mL ambulatory and 610 mL supine. Thus, the mean logarithmic regression in Fig. 15–3 can be used to estimate QFT for either CAPD or supine automated peritoneal dialysis (APD) as a function of percent dextrose. However, the predicted net ultrafiltrate (QFnt) would be predicted to be different in CAPD and APD due to the variance in Ql. For CAPD, from the data in Fig. 15–3:

$$QFnt = [184 + 512 \ln(\%D)][1\sim\exp(\sim0.02t)] -\sim0.7t \quad (8)$$

and for APD:

$$QFnt = [184 + 512 \ln(percentD)] \\ \times [1\sim\exp(\sim0.02t)] -\sim1.5t \quad (9)$$

Equations (8) and (9) can serve as modeling equations to predict QFnt as a function of the exchange time or they can be solved for percent dextrose and used to calculate the percent dextrose required to achieve a desired level of QFnt for the average patient with specified exchange time. Solution of Eq. (8) for percent dextrose as a function of desired Qfnt and exchange time, t, gives

$$\%D = \exp((Qfnt - 184 \langle(1 - \exp(-0.02t)) + 0.7t))/ \\ (512(1 - \exp(-.02t))) \quad (10)$$

and solution of Eq. (9) for percent dextrose gives

$$\%D = \exp((Qfnt - 184 \langle(1 - \exp(-0.02t)) + 1.5t))/ \\ (512(1 - \exp(-0.02t))) \quad (11)$$

These expressions provide a general description of ultrafiltration but are not always reliable, particularly in APD with high volume exchanges. In practice the percent dextrose must often be prescribed from empiric data correlating Qfnt with the percent dextrose used in an individual patient.

Solute Transport in Peritoneal Dialysis. The operational definition of the dose of peritoneal dialysis is the total clearance provided by the sum of peritoneal and residual renal clearance (KprT) normalized to body water volume as KprT/V. The term KprT/V represents the fractional clearance of body water and is an analogue of Kt/V in hemodialysis. The total

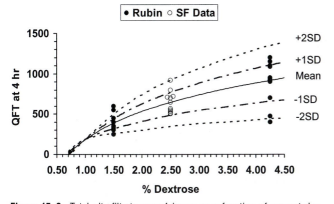

Figure 15–3. Total ultrafiltrate over 4 hours as a function of percent dextrose in the exchange.

daily peritoneal clearance is the sum of clearances provided by each exchange. As will be described quantitatively below, clearance (Kp) is not constant during an exchange; it is maximal at the beginning and decreases exponentially during the exchange. Although the clearance profile is somewhat complex, the total clearance provided by an exchange is very easily calculated from

$$Kpt = RtVt \qquad (12)$$

where Kpt is the clearance at exchange time t, Rt is the ratio of dialysate to plasma solute concentration at t (commonly termed the D/P ratio), and Vt is the volume of drained dialysate. The total clearance during each 24 hours is the sum of Kpts for each exchange:

$$KpT = RtVt1 + Rt2Vt2+ \ldots +RtNVtN \qquad (13)$$

The total clearance, KpT, can be calculated from the sum of RtVts measured on each individual exchange or from RtVt of the batched total drained dialysate for a day.

In contrast to Kp, which oscillates exponentially during each exchange, the renal clearance, Kr, is constant throughout the 24-hour period. It is calculated from a timed urine collection in accordance with

$$Kr = Cur(Vur) / Cp(t) \qquad (14)$$

where Cur is urine solute concentration; Vur is volume of urine collected; Cp is plasma solute concentration; and t is the collection time with all units compatible. The total daily renal clearance, KrT, is simply the product of Kr (usually expressed as mL/min or L/min) times 1440. As mentioned above, the KprT is normalized to V, and the dose is expressed as KprT/V. In hemodialysis, the V term is calculated from urea kinetics (see Chap. 8), but in PD this is not possible. Consequently, V must be estimated from gender and body surface area.[16]

As with ultrafiltration, solute clearance in PD varies greatly during each exchange, while in contrast, it is constant throughout dialysis in modern single-pass hemodialyzers. In PD, solute clearance is maximal at the beginning and falls exponentially during each exchange. The peritoneal dialysis system can be schematically depicted as in Fig. 15–4 where well-mixed body (Vb) and dialysate compartments (Vd) are linked by a peritoneal membrane mass transfer coefficient (MTC) and combined first order diffusive, MTC (Cb – Cd), and convective, Qf·Cb, transport are shown. In addition, lymphatic convection of solute from Vd to Vb, Ql·Cd, is also depicted. The term MTC is a constant that is exactly analogous to the term "dialysance" used for hemodialyszers and has units of L/min or ml/min. It can be thought of as the diffusive peritoneal clearance at the exact moment an exchange starts when Cd is approximately zero. As Cd rises, clearance falls but MTC remains constant. Figure 15–4 shows three rate equations, which are the differential equations underlying several kinetic models of the system. Both analytic and numerical solutions of this system of varying complexity[12–27] have been reported and have been recently reviewed.[8]

Fixed-Volume Model. Equation (15) in Fig. 15–4

$$Vd(dCd / dt) = MTC(Cb – Cd) \qquad (15)$$

attributes all solute flux to diffusion, neglects convective transport, and was the first quantitative description of solute equilibration in peritoneal dialysis.[17] Assuming constant Cb and Vd, integration of Eq. (15) results in

$$Cdt = Cb – (Cb – Cdo) \cdot \exp(–MTC \cdot t / Vt) \qquad (16)$$

where Cdo is dialysate concentration at t = 0; Vt is the drained volume at the end of the exchange; and MTC is the diffusive transport constant as discussed above.

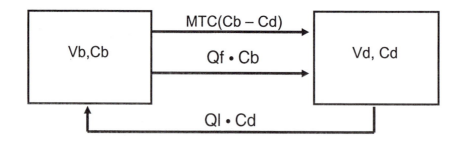

$$\text{Eq} \cdot (15)\text{: } Vd(dCd)/dt = MTC(Cb – Cd)$$

$$\text{Eq} \cdot (23)\text{: } d(Vd \cdot Cd)/dt = MTC(Cb – Cd) + QF \cdot Cb – Ql \cdot Cd$$

$$\text{Eq} \cdot (24)\text{: } d(Vd \cdot Cd)/dt = MTC(Cb – Cd) + (QF – Ql) \cdot Cb$$

Figure 15–4. A schematic illustration of the peritoneal dialysis system. The equation numbers are found in the text descriptions.

Since the primary clinical interest is the total clearance provided by the exchange, it is helpful to divide Eq. (16) by Cb, which gives

$$Rt = 1 - (1 - Ro) \cdot \exp(-MTC \cdot t / Vt) \qquad (17)$$

where R represents Cd/Cb or the commonly referred to dialysate/plasma or D/P ratio. The D/P ratio should always be expressed as the dialysate solute concentration divided by the concentration in plasma water, which is calculated as Cb/0.94. Since total clearance (Kpt, L) is by definition

$$Kpt = [Solute\ Removed)/Cb] = [Cdt(Vt)/Cb] = RtVt \qquad (18)$$

we can predict the total peritoneal clearance provided by an individual exchange by combining Eqs. (17) and (18) to give

$$Kpt = Rt(Vt) = (1 - (1 - Ro \cdot \exp(-MTC \cdot t / Vt)))Vt \qquad (19)$$

In order to predict Rt, and hence the total clearance which will be achieved with a prescribed exchange, we need to know the patient specific transport parameter, MTC. This can be determined from clinical data using Eq. (17) solved for MTC:

$$MTC = In((1 - Ro) / (1 - Rt))(Vt / t) \qquad (20)$$

Clinical calculation of the MTC from Eq. (20) theoretically requires measurement of the Ro or D/P ratio immediately after infusion, and in the drained dialysate at the end of the exchange (Rt), the volume of dialysate drained (Vt) and the exchange time. Measurement of Ro requires mixing of dialysate by rolling the patient from side to side immediately after infusion and then withdrawing a small sample. The R is never zero because there is always some equilibrated dialysate remaining from the previous exchange. In clinical practice, Ro can usually be reliably estimated as approximately 0.10 for CAPD therapy.

There is always some ambiguity about estimation of the effective exchange time during the inflow and outflow intervals of the exchange. If flow is constant during these intervals, it is reasonable to estimate the effective time for the exchange as one half of the inflow and outflow time segments. The inflow and outflow intervals are of little consequence in analyzing long CAPD exchanges, but they become significant in APD, where they occupy an increasing fraction of exchange time as dwell time decreases, as is discussed below quantitatively.

Variable-Volume Model. Although the fixed-volume model (FVM) of peritoneal transport provides a reliable method to determine MTC during the isovolumic exchange phase,[18] it will overestimate MTC during the early part of an exchange when there is substantial ultrafiltration since it does not account for the convective component of transport. The rate of

ultrafiltration can be quite high during the first hour, depending on the dextrose concentration. The ultrafiltration rate (Qf), in milliliters per minute, expected can be calculated directly from differentiation of Eq. (5) to give

$$Qf = 0.02QFT \cdot \exp(-.02 \cdot t) \qquad (21)$$

The Qf with variable percent dextrose can be computed by estimation of QFT from Eq. (9) and incorporation into Eq. (21) to give

$$Qf = 0.02(184 + 512In(\%D)) \cdot \exp(-.02 \cdot t) - Q1 \quad (22)$$

The Qf profiles expected for CAPD with 1.5, 2.5, and 4.25% dextrose were calculated with Eq. (22) and plotted in Fig. 15–5, where they can be seen to range up to nearly 20 mL/min during the first 1/2 hour of the exchange. Since MTC values for urea range from 10 to 20 mL/min, it is apparent that Qf of 10 to 20 mL could account for a substantial amount of transport early in an exchange if there is negligible solute rejection of low molecular weight solutes during ultrafiltration.[20] However, this is not strictly correct and is considered more fully below with continuous flow peritoneal dialysis (CFPD).

The variable volume model (VVKM) was first described by Babb et al.[19]:

$$d(Vd \cdot Cd)/dt = MTC(Cb - Cd) + QF \cdot Cb - QI \cdot Cd \qquad (23)$$

where QF is total ultrafiltrate and QI is lymphatic reabsorption. This model has been simplified by Garred[20] and Qf defined as the measurable net ultrafiltration rate in accordance with

$$d(Vd \cdot Cd)/dt = MTC(Cb - Cd) + (Qf - Qf) \cdot Cb \quad (24)$$

where (Qf – QI) is considered to operate only on Cb. Analytic solution of Eq. (24) by Garred results in

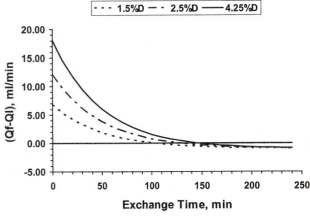

Figure 15–5. Instantaneous values for net ultrafiltration rate (Qf – QI) calculated as a function of exchange time and percent dextrose with typical hydraulic permeability of the peritoneum.

$$Rt = 1 - Vo/VT(1-Ro) \cdot \exp(-MTC \cdot t/MV) \qquad (25)$$

where Vo is the initial volume of the exchange, Vt is the volume at the end of the exchange, and MV is the mean intraperitoneal volume during the exchange. The MV can be calculated from integration of Eq. (5), to give

$$MV = Vo + QFT(1-(50/tc)(1-\exp(-0.02tc))) \\ -0.00075 \cdot tc \qquad (26)$$

where tc is the length of each exchange cycle and Q1 is taken to be 1.5 mL/min.

Solution of Eq. (25) for MTC is

$$MTC = (MV/t) \cdot \ln(VO(1-Ro)/(Vt(1-Rt))) \qquad (27)$$

It is important to also note that Eq. 27 can be rearranged to give:

$$\ln[Vt(Cb - \tilde{}\, Cdt)] = \ln[VO(Cb - \tilde{}\, Cdo)] \\ -(MTC \cdot t / MV) \qquad (28)$$

The development of the VVM by Garred,[20] as described in Eqs. (23) through (28) includes the assumptions that there is no solute rejection with ultrafiltration (sieving coefficient, S = 1) and that KoA is proportional to MV as intraperitoneal volume increases with Qf. This proportionality has recently been confirmed.[28,29] The increase in intraperitoneal volume over time is calculated using Eq. (5) and the measured drained volume and MV with Eq. (24). It should be noted that this is actually the net ultrafiltrate and implicit in this model is the concept that convective transport can be described as (Qf – Q1)Cb as in Eq. (24), Fig. 15–4. The MTC parameter can be calculated from either Eq. (27) with only two D/P ratios or graphically with Eq. (28) using a series of Cdt values since a plot of lnVt(Cb – Cdt) as a function of time will be linear and the slope will equal KoA/MV. The VVM [Eqs. (27) and (28)] can be used to compute KoA at any elapsed exchange time for solutes where S = 1, while the FVM will give valid results only if used for analysis of Rt after ultrafiltration is complete. Since dialysate equilibration with plasma is exponential [Eqs. (17) and (23)] the rate of equilibration can also be expressed as the time required for 50 percent equilibration (PT50), in hours. This is a useful clinical expression of the rate of equilibration for individual patients. The average PT50 for urea is 1.2 hours. If there is low transport, the PT50 may increase to 3 hours, which immediately informs the physician that to achieve 95 percent equilibration, 4 half-times or 12 hours are required and the patient is not a candidate for PD therapy.

Automated Peritoneal Dialysis

Automated peritoneal dialysis (APD) is a method developed to increase the throughput of dialysate batches using automated control with shortened exchange time to achieve increased clearance.[31-41] Although the relationship between clearance and exchange time in APD is complex and depends on several interacting parameters, the general relationship between efficiency and rate of dialysate throughput can be stated very simply as

$$Kph = Rt \cdot (DFR + QFnh) \qquad (29)$$

where Kph is the hourly clearance (L/h); Rt is the D/P ratio of each drained exchange; DFR is the dialysate flow rate (L/h); and Qfnh is the hourly net rate of ultrafiltration (hourly ultrafiltrate minus hourly lymphatic reabsorption).

Dialysate flow is intermittent during APD and occurs in the form of discrete exchange volumes. The number of cycler exchanges per hour (Nch) can be expressed as

$$Nch = 1 / tc \qquad (30)$$

where tc is the total time in hours required for each exchange cycle.

The DFR can now be expressed as

$$DFR = Nch(Vf) = Vf / tc \qquad (31)$$

where Vf is the fill or total volume infused for each exchange. We can solve Eq. (31) for tc to show

$$tc = Vf / DFR \qquad (32)$$

Equation (32) shows that tc is exactly determined by the ratio Vf/DFR and must always decrease as DFR increases. The tc is comprised of dwell time (td), inflow time (ti), and outflow or drain time (to). The concept of effective exchange time (te) was discussed briefly above in the context of CAPD where tc is very long—4 to 8 hours—and ti and to are very short relative to tc. We can now define te more precisely for cycler therapy where inflow and outflow occupy a larger fraction of tc. Actually, the MTC is increasing from near zero to some value normalized to Vf during ti and again decreasing to near zero during to. It would add considerable complexity to compute Rt with a variable MTC during ti and to. It is much simpler technically and rigorous (since transport is directly related to the MTC·t product) to adjust ti and to in proportion to the expected change in MTC. Since MTC appears to be proportional to intraperitoneal volume,[28,29] we can define te as the product of the ratio (mean intraperitoneal volume during ti or to)/(Vf) and the inflow or outflow time. Thus,

$$tei = (MVi / Vf)(ti) \qquad (33)$$

and

$$teo = (MVo / Vf)(to) \tag{34}$$

where tei and teo are effective dialysis times during ti and to; MVi and MVo are mean intraperitoneal volumes during inflow and outflow; and Vf is the filled intraperitoneal volume as described above.

We can describe the effective dialysis time during fill and drain (te) for each exchange as

$$te = tei + teo = \beta i(ti) + \beta o(to) \tag{35}$$

where βi and βo refer to MVi/Vf and MVo/Vf, respectively. Current cycler technology generally does not permit analysis of flow profiles during ti and to, which must be known to precisely define βi and βo. If the flow curves were complex (such as an exponential outflow curve with rapid early flow which progressively decreases) determination of mean V would require double integration of the flow rate profile. In the absence of a flow rate monitor during ti and to, we must simply assume constant flow during these intervals in which case,

$$\beta i = \beta o = \beta = 0.5 \tag{36}$$

and Eq. (35) educes to

$$te = \beta(ti + to) = 0.5(ti + to) \tag{37}$$

The total effective dialysis time during each exchange cycle can now be defined as

$$
\begin{aligned}
tec &= tc - \sim (ti + to) + te \\
tec &= tc \sim - (ti + to) + \beta(ti + to) \\
tec &= tc - (1 - \beta)(ti + to)
\end{aligned}
\tag{38}
$$

Describing ti and to as functions of exchange volume is also very useful. We can write $ti = \alpha i(Vf)$ and $to = \alpha o(Vf)$, and thus

$$ti + to = (\alpha i + \alpha o)Vf \tag{39}$$

where αi and αo are the estimated or measured minutes per liter required to fill and drain the exchange, respectively. We can combine Eqs. (30), (38), and (39) to write

$$tec = (Vf / DFR) \sim - (1 - \sim \beta)(\alpha i + \alpha o)Vf \tag{40}$$

If we set $\beta = 0.5$ and express DFR as L/h in Eq. (40), we can write the more generalized relationship

$$tec = Vf[(60 / DFR) \sim - 0.5(\alpha i + \alpha o)] \tag{41}$$

Equation (41) provides a generalized definition of effective dialysis time for each exchange cycle as a function of Vf, DFR, and the specific fill and drain time constants αi and αo. As shown below, this development is essential to analyzing and predicting the efficiency of APD over a wide range of DFR.

In the case of tidal peritoneal dialysis (TPD), where the dialysate is not completely drained at the end of each exchange, the relationships between MVi/Vf and MVo/Vf in Eqs. (33) and (34) must be modified to reflect the effect of residual volume. The two volume moieties of the exchange in TPD are the tidal volume (VTi) and residual volume (Vr), which can be related in accordance with

$$r = VTi / (VTi + Vr) \tag{42}$$

The total intraperitoneal volume at the end of inflow (corresponding to Vf above) and the start of outflow is (VTi + Vr). The ratio MV/(VTi + Vr) during inflow and outflow is

$$MV / (VTi + Vr) = (Vr + \beta \cdot VTi) / (VTi + Vr) \tag{43}$$

For Eq. (41), recall that Vr remains in the abdomen throughout ti and to, and βVTi is identical to the definition in Eqs. (35) and (36). Combination of Eqs. (42) and (43), and simplification results in

$$MV / VTi + Vr) = (1 - r) + \beta \cdot r \tag{44}$$

and the analogue for TPD of the relationship in Eq. (38) can be seen to be

$$te = ((1 - r) + \beta \cdot r)(ti + to) \tag{45}$$

and the total effective dialysis time during each exchange cycle in TPD is

$$
\begin{aligned}
tec &= tc - (ti + to) + te \\
&= te - (ti + to) + ((1 - r) + \beta \cdot r)(ti + to) \\
tec &= tc - r(1 - \beta)(ti + to)
\end{aligned}
\tag{46}
$$

Letting $\beta = 0.5$, we derive for TPD

$$tec = tc - 0.5r(ti + to) \tag{47}$$

we can now write the TPD analogue of Eq. (41),

$$tec = VTI((60 / DFR) - 0.5r(\alpha i + \alpha o)) \tag{48}$$

Equation (48) is suitable for both regular cycler therapy and TPD which differ only with respect to r. In Cycler therapy r is often considered 1, but is actually never quite 1 because of the small residual volume of about 200 mL after "complete" drainage. Thus, r is approximately 0.1 in regular cycler therapy. In TPD, r usually varies from 0.25 to 0.75. Equation (48) will be used to calculate tec in the further development of cycler analysis, which follows.

One further step is required to develop a completely generalized model of APD. We can define Ro in cycler dialysis from simple solute mass balance as

$$Ro = (Rt \cdot Vr) / (VTi + Vr) \tag{49}$$

We can combine Eqs. (48) and (49) and Eq. (29) and solve for Rt,

$$
\begin{aligned}
Rt = Qfn + (VTi + Vr)(1 - \exp(-MTC/MV) \\
\times (VTi(60/DFR - (1 - \beta)r(\alpha i + \alpha o)))) / \\
Qfn + VTi + Vr \cdot (1 - \exp(-MTC/MV) \\
\times (VTi(60/DFR - (1 - \beta)r(\alpha i + \alpha o))))
\end{aligned}
\tag{50}
$$

where QFn is net ultrafiltration per exchange and MV is calculated using Eq. (26).

The efficiency of any defined cycler dialysis regimen can now be predicted by combining Eqs. (50) and (29), which results in

$$
\begin{aligned}
Kph = (Qfn + (VTi + Vr)(1 - \exp(-MTC/MV) \\
\times (VTi((60/DFR) - 0.5r(\alpha i + \alpha o)))) / \\
(Qfn + VTi + Vr \cdot (1 - \exp(-MTC/MV) \\
\times (VTi(60/DFR - 0.5r(\alpha i + \alpha o)))))) \\
\times (DFR + Qfh)
\end{aligned}
\tag{51}
$$

Although the VVM was derived with the assumption of S = 1.00, this would result in substantial overestimation of clearance in Eqs. (29) and (51) because there is significant sieving of urea, creatinine, uric acid, and glucose. Therefore a further approximation is needed to include a more realistic estimate of the contribution of Qfn. The effective net ultrafiltrate (Qfen) corrected for estimated mean concentration for coupled diffusion and convection, Eqs. (43) and, (44), as reported previously [Eq. (42)], can be defined as

$$QfenU = 0.50 \,\backslash\! Qfn \quad \text{for urea} \tag{52}$$

$$QfenCr = 0.44 \,\backslash\! Qfn \quad \text{for creatinine} \tag{53}$$

$$QfenUA = 0.42 \,\backslash\! Qfn \quad \text{for uric acid} \tag{54}$$

$$QfenGluc = 0.26 \,\backslash\! Qfn \quad \text{for glucose} \tag{54}$$

At the start of an APD treatment session, if r is substantially less than 0.9, Eq. (48) is not rigorous for the first few exchanges because Rt will be increasing until a steady state is reached. During the first few exchanges Eq. (51) will overestimate Kph because Rt has not reached steady state (recall Kph = Rt·(DFR + Qfnh). However, with typical transport parameters the underestimation with respect to the entire treatment will be quite small.

Effect of drain profile and MTC on efficiency of CPD, TPD

Examination of Eq. (51) shows that the hourly clearance achieved with APD will be determined by the DFR, MTC, drain profile constants (β, αI, and αo), Qf and the ratio of VTi/MV. The primary technical problems encountered with APD are inefficient drain cycles. Four theoretical drain profiles are shown in Fig. 15–6 where a typical 2-L fill volume is depicted. Profiles (1) and (2) are optimal with linear and quite brisk drainage times of 5 and 10 min for 2 L.

Equation (51) was used to calculate hourly clearances of urea and creatinine with profiles (1) and (2) as a function of DFR, 2-L fill volume, Qfen 0 and r varied from 1.0 to 0.25 with results shown in Fig. 15–7 panels A, B, C, and D. Note that when r = 1.00 Keu is maximal in the DFR region of 2.0 to 2.5 L/h with both profiles (Fig 15–7A,C). As r decreases from 1.00 to 0.25 (and VTi decreases from 2.0 to 0.50) the efficiency steadily decreases. With very efficient drain rates, efficiency is improved by the longer dwell time and continued clearance. The creatinine clearance profiles in Fig. 15–7B,D are much flatter because of the lower MTC and very little is gained for DFR greater than 1.5 to 2.0 L/h and R = 1.00 still provides the most efficient therapy.

Drain profiles (3) and (4) in Fig. 15–6 are much less efficient than profiles (1) and (2). Profile (3) is linear but

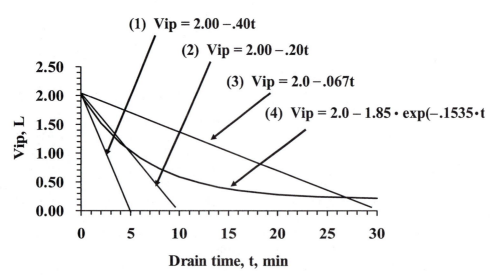

Figure 15–6. Four drain profiles that would have profoundly differing effects on efficiency of APD and TPD.

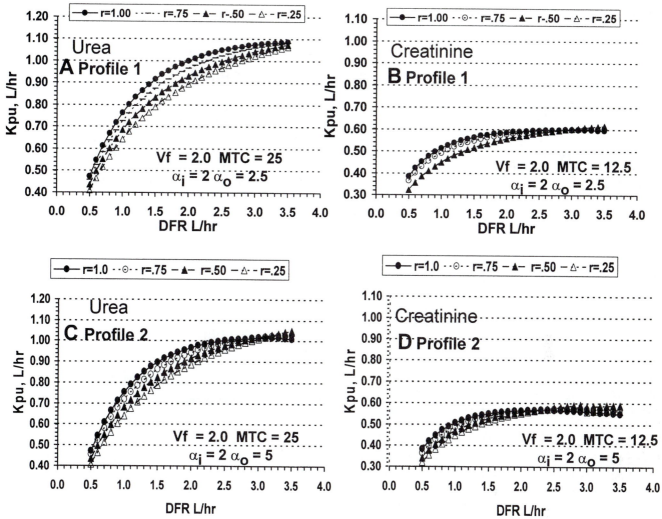

Figure 15–7. The effects of drain profiles on APD clearance.

quite slow with 30 minutes required to drain 2.0 L. The effects of this profile on efficiency is depicted in Fig. 15–8A,B for urea and creatinine. Note in Fig. 15–8A that in the case of urea, regular exchanges with r = 1.00 are the most efficient at DFR over the range 0.5 to about 1.7, but the maximum Kpu achieved is 0.80 L/h. At higher flow rates efficiency falls off very rapidly with r = 1.00 but continues to increase in inverse proportion to r with maximal Kpu of 1.00 L/h with r = .25 at maximal DFR 3.5 L/h. Thus even with this poor drainage profile quite high clearances can theoretically be achieved by optimizing the tidal volume but there would be increased cost associated with higher dialysate requirement. In Fig. 15–8B the creatinine clearances are computed. Again these are much flatter profiles but they tend to mirror the urea clearances and the most efficient therapy is achieved with r = .25 and high DFR.

The effects on clearance of the exponential drain profile (4) in Fig. 15–6 are depicted in Fig. 15–8C,D. Note that

these profile effects are even more striking than the long linear profile (3) which reflects the exponential nature of the curve with quite rapid drain early in the cycle which then exponentially decays to a minimum residual volume of about 0.2 L. By taking advantage of the drain profile with r = .25, clearances equal to profile (1) can be achieved for both urea and creatinine.

The profiles calculated in Figs. 15–7 and 15–8 are done with Qf = 0. In Fig. 15–9 a total Qf of 1.5 is calculated with each profile. Note that the curves disperse and are higher but still have very much the same shape.

There has been very little work done on optimization of APD as a function of defined drain profiles. The variability and shape of drain profiles are usually not defined in clinical management of APD. Instead, a generous drain time is usually programmed to minimize alarms but little effort is made to optimize efficiency. This approach would require software to analyze the drain profile and calculate the optimal r with respect to achievable clearance. The curves

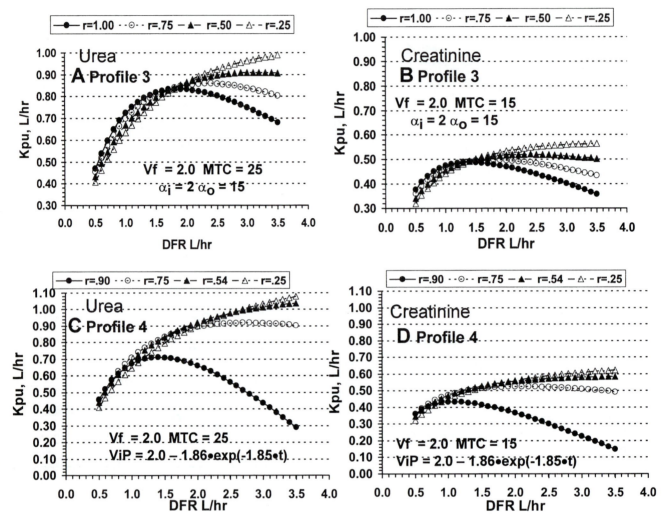

Figure 15–8. Drain profile effects on APD clearances.

in Figs.15–7 and 15–8 must be considered a great extent theoretical but do point up an area for needed research. It is important to recall that one important assumption in generation of these profiles is that the intraperitoneal dialysate is well mixed dialysate. Another variable that could affect the drain profile is the fill volume.

Creatinine-to-Urea Clearance Ratios in APD

It is apparent in Figs. 15–7 and 15–8 that the ratio Kpcr/Kpu will vary in CAPC and APD. This can be explicitly examined from a plot of Kpcr/Kpu ratios calculated from the clearance profiles in Figs. 15–7 and 15–8. Note that r = 1.00 and DFR = 0.5 define typical CAPD exchanges so the profiles provide a continuum from CAPD to the most efficient APD. The ratios are plotted in Fig. 15–10 for all profiles. The ratio falls exponentially from 0.8 in CAPD to 0.5 in maximally efficient APD. There is no known clinical signif-

icance related to this since clinical outcome is considered similar in APD and CAPD.

Continuous Flow Peritoneal Dialysis (CFPD). This is a very different form of automated peritoneal dialysis which was first described by Shinaberger[45] many years ago and more recently by several authors.[42,46–48] The process requires two peritoneal access catheters and a system which can deliver and monitor continuous single pass or recirculating peritoneal dialysate at high flow rates.

The process first reported by Shinaberger is depicted schematically in Fig. 15–11B where the abdominal cavity filled with well mixed peritoneal dialysate (Vp, Cp) is joined to well mixed body solute (Vb, Cb) by a first order transport coefficient (MTC) as described above. Note in Fig. 15–11B that dialysate is recirculating in series between Vp, Cp and the "blood compartment" of an external dialyzer which has single pass countercurrent dialysate flow

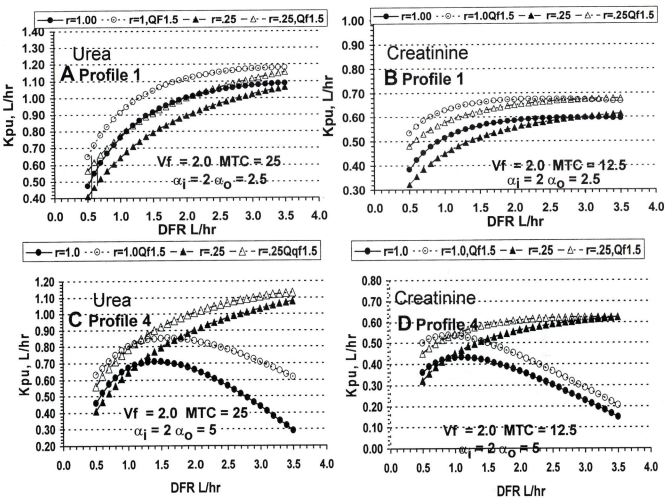

Figure 15–9. Effects of drain profile on APD clearance with ultrafiltration.

(Q_d, C_d). Thus this a recirculating/single pass (RSP) CFPD system as labeled in Fig. 15–11B. The transport of solute into the system from Vb, Cb is depicted as MASS IN and removal of solute across the dialyzer in QdCd is depicted as MASS OUT. The kinetics defining this system[48] will be derived below.

The CFPD system shown in Fig. 15–11A is a single-pass (SP) system with continuous flow of fresh dialysate through the peritoneal cavity. This system would require very large amounts of dialysate of quality suitable for direct infusion into the peritoneal cavity and would thus almost certainly be prohibitively expensive. However, experimental results with such a system have been recently reported.[42]

Rationale for CFPD. There are two theoretical mechanisms by which CFPD may greatly increase the efficiency of PD relative to APD. The first mechanism, as depicted in Fig. 15–12, could be greatly improved dialysate flow distribution with high, continuous DFR. Panel A in Fig. 15–12 is a schematic illustration of poor dialysate flow distribution

which is theorized to be the case in APD. The most sensitive index of flow distribution is the MTC which can be predicted to be strongly dependent on the amount of peritoneal membrane area which is exposed to dialysate as well as the thickness of the dialysate film. If the dialysate is flowing through stagnant pools, as in panel A, severe reduction of MTC would be expected. If uniform flow distribution could be achieved, as depicted in panel B, a substantial improvement in the MTC would be predicted.

The second mechanism is the inherent kinetic superiority of continuous dialysis systems compared to batch systems as illustrated in Fig. 15–13. Average peritoneal clearance is plotted as a function of exchange time for a family of MTC values and methods of PD. Note that in all batch modalities (APD and CAPD) clearance decays steadily as a function of exchange time due to dissipation of the concentration gradient from blood to dialysate as the batch equilibrates. In contrast, continuous average clearance nearly equal to the MTC would be predicted in CFPD where dialysate concentration build up is prevented.

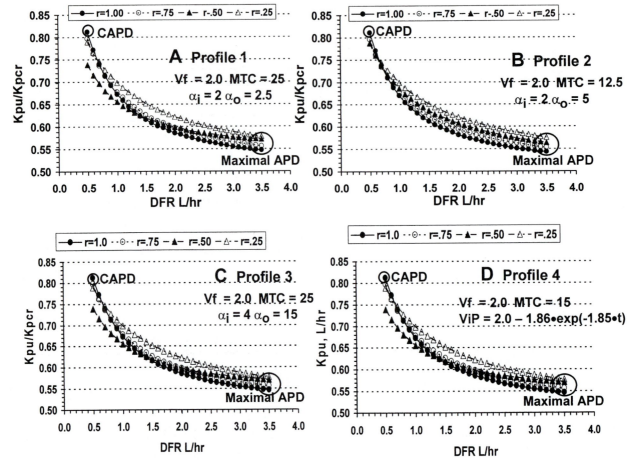

Figure 15–10. Effect DFR and drain profile on ratio Kpu/Kpcr.

Kinetic Model of Single Pass CFPD. This system is depicted in Fig. 15–11A. After an initial transient during buildup of a low level of dialysate solute concentration, it is characterized by virtual steady state over short intervals but with a slow fall in Cb and Cp over the course of a dialysis. The mass removed from the peritoneal dialysate (Mass Out) is given by the product of solute concentration and flow rate of outflow peritoneal dialysate stream, Qpo·Cp. Solute is transferred across the peritoneal membrane into the dialysate primarily by diffusion, MTC (Cb–Cp) but also by convection where convection is defined as the product of the ultrafiltration rate, a sieving coefficient and the mean concentration in the membrane. Convective transport is thus defined as Qf·S·(0.67Cb + 0.33Cp) where S is the sieving coefficient and the concentration term, (0.67Cb + 0.33Cp), is an approximation of mean concentration for coupled diffusion and convection suggested by Villaroel.[43] Mean values of S reported by Lysaght[44] are urea 0.74, creatinine 0.65, uric acid 0.63, and glucose 0.40.

After steady state is reached, we can write mass balance in peritoneal dialysate as

$$d(V_pC_p) / dt = 0 = MTC(C_b - C_p) \tag{55}$$
$$+ Q_f \cdot S(0.67C_b + 0.33C_p) - (Q_p + Q_f)(C_p)$$

which can be rearranged to

$$MTC(C_b - C_p) + Q_f \cdot S(0.67C_b + 0.3C_p)) \tag{56}$$
$$= (Q_p + Q_f)(C_p)$$

divide Eq(56) by Cb which results in

$$MTC(1 - C_p / C_b) + Q_f \cdot S(0.67 + 0.33C_p / C_b) \tag{57}$$
$$= (Q_p + Q_f)(C_p / C_b)$$

Solve Eq. (58) for Cp/Cb,

$$C_p / C_b = (MTC + 0.67Q_f \cdot S) / \tag{58}$$
$$(MTC + Q_p + Q_f(1 + .33S)$$

Note that effective peritoneal clearance (Kpe) is

$$Kpe = (Q_p + Q_f)(C_p / C_b) \tag{59}$$

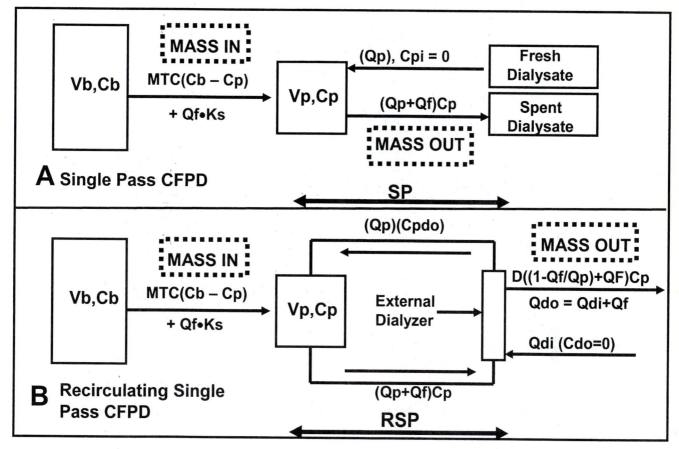

Figure 15–11. Single-pass (SP) and recirculating/single-pass (RSP) continuous flow peritoneal dialysis (CFPD) systems.

Combine Eqs. (58) and (59) and solve for Kpe,

$$Pke = ((MTC + 0.67Qf \cdot S)(Qp + Qf)) / \qquad (60)$$
$$(MTC + Qp + Qf(1 + .33S))$$

Eq. (60) when solved for MTC results in

$$MTC = (Kpe(Qf(1 + 0.33S) + Qp) - 0.67Qf \cdot S \qquad (61)$$
$$(Qp + Qf)) / (Qp + Qf - Kpe)$$

Kinetic Model of Recirculating/Single Pass CFPD

This system is shown in Fig. 15–11B, where it can be seen that the dialyzer operates directly on the peritoneal dialysate leaving the peritoneal cavity to flow through the dialyzer. The dialyzer will reduce concentration in the external peritoneal dialysate stream in direct proportion to the dialyzer clearance relative to peritoneal dialysate flow rate. Thus this system is represented by two first order transport sites arranged in series and comprised of the peritoneal membrane and the external dialyzer. The solute concentration in the peritoneal dialysate will be zero at the start of therapy and rise fairly rapidly to reach near steady state since the

blood concentration will fall quite slowly due to the large distribution volume compared to the external circuit. The mass into Vp will equal mass out of Vp as depicted in Fig. 15–11B. When quasi–steady state is reached we can write

$$d(VpCp) / dt = 0 \qquad (62)$$

and thereforen as shown in Fig. 15–11B,

$$0 = MTC(Cb - Cp) + Qf \cdot S(.67Cb + .33Cp) \qquad (63)$$
$$- (Qp + Qf)Cp + Qp(Cpdo)$$

The rate of solute transfer into the dialysate (Jd) as

$$Jd = (D(1 - Qf / (Qp + Qf)) + Qf)Cp \qquad (64)$$

We can also describe Jd from mass balance across the "blood compartment" of the dialyzer,

$$Jd = (Qp + Qf)Cp - Qp(Cpdo) \qquad (65)$$

Combine Eqs. (64) and (65), and substitute into Eq. (63) and simplify to show

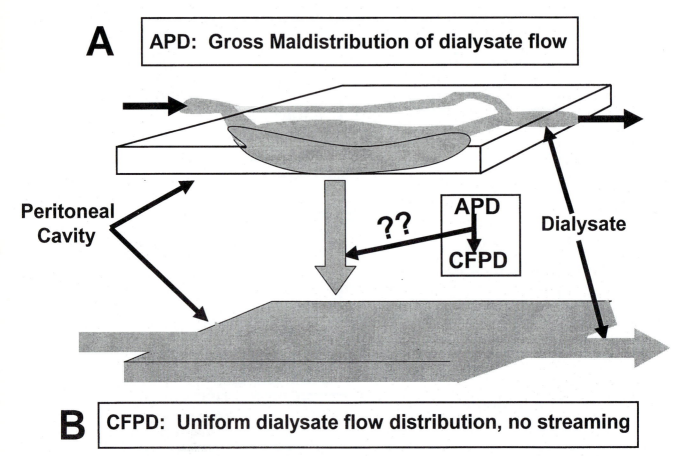

Figure 15–12. Schematic illustration of peritoneal dialysate streaming in stagnant batch exchanges (APD) vs. (it is hoped) uniform distribution in high-flow CFPD.

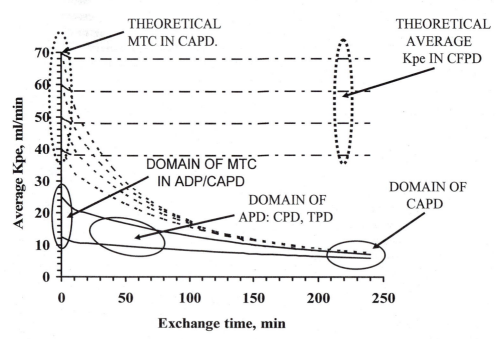

Figure 15–13. The spectrum of mass-transfer coefficients (MTC) and peritoneal clearances (Kp) in CAPD and APD batch modalities (CPD, TPD) compared to continuous-flow PD (CFPD). Both higher MTC and the elimination of the concentration gradient decay are postulated for CFPD.

$$MTC(Cb - Cp) + Qf \cdot S(0.67Cb + 0.33Cp) \quad (66)$$
$$= (D(1 - Qf / (Qp + Qf)) + Qf)Cp$$

Divide Eq. (66) by Cb and solve for Cp/Cb:

$$Cp / Cb = (MTC + 0.67Qf \cdot S) /$$
$$(MTC + D(1 - Qf / \quad (67)$$
$$(Qp + Qf)) + Qf(1 - 0.33S))$$

Recalling that Kpe is solute removal from Vp (which equals the rate of solute transport across the dialyzer) divided by Cb we can combine Eqs. (64) and (67),

$$Kpe = ((MTC + .67Qf \cdot S)(D(1 - Qf /$$
$$(Qp + Qf)) + Qf)) / (MTC$$
$$+ D(1 - Qf / (Qp + Qf)) + Qf \quad (68)$$
$$(1 - 0.33S))$$

Equation (68) when solved for MTC gives

$$MTC = (Kpe(Qf(1 + 0.33S + Qp) - 0.67Qf \quad (69)$$
$$\cdot S(Qp + Qf)) / (Qp + Qf - Kpe)$$

Note that Kpe and MTC are defined in Eqs. (68) and (69) only in terms of each other, Qp, Qf, and D, so the generalized relationships between them can be explored. In clinical work Kpe can be readily measured from concentration measurements,

$$Kpe = (D(1 - Qf / (Qp + Qf)) + Qf)(Cp / Cb) \_ \quad (70)$$

after a sufficiently long interval to assure a quasi–steady state has been reached. Note that when Qf is zero, Eqs. (68) and (69) reduce to

$$Kp = MTC / (1 + MTC / D) \quad (71)$$

and

$$MTC = Kpe / (1 - MTC / D)) \quad (72)$$

Relationships between Kpe, MTC, and D. It is instructive to solve Eq. (71) over a wide range of MTC and D to examine the dependence of Kpe on these two parameters of CFPD therapy as illustrated in Fig. 15–14. A family of curves with MTC varied from zero to 150 mL/min and constant levels of D ranging from 25 to 300 mL/min. Note that in the left lower corner Kpe is permeability or is MTC limited and is virtually independent of D. Over the right edge of the plot at high MTC levels, Kpe is dependent on D or is dialysance limited demonstrating that both high dialysance and high MTC are required to achieve high Kpe.

The results of Shinaberger's RSP studies[45] are depicted in Fig. 15–15, where they can be seen to disperse very widely over the domain of MTC and D. The three SP studies reported by Cruz[42] appear quite reproducible. The Shinaberger data are also shown in Fig. 15–16 where MTC is plotted in Fig. 15–16 A as a function of Qp and in. Fig. 15–16B as a function of Qp expressed as DFR for comparison to APD therapy. The plots show an impressive increase in MTC to a mean level of 52 mL/min but with considerable scatter and SD 27 mL/min. In comparison, the mean MTC for urea in

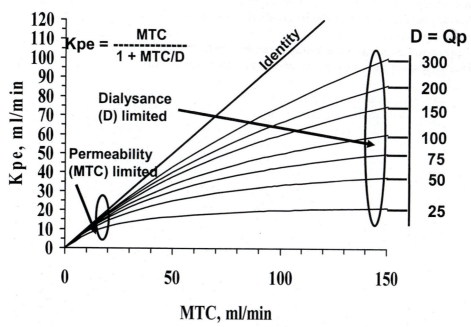

Figure 15–14. Solution of the CFPD models for effective peritoneal clearance (Kpe) as a function of MTC and either single pass dialysate flow rate (Qp) or dialysance (D) with D = Qp. Note that there are permeability limited (MTC) and dialysance/flow limited regions.

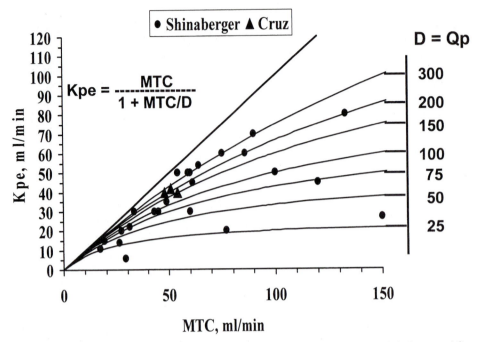

Figure 15–15. Continuous flow peritoneal dialysis clinical data (Kpe, Qp, Qd) reported by Shinaberger and Cruz with calculated MTC values.

APD is 25 mL/min so the mean has increased by a little more than 100 percent in CFPD.

The clearance results to date with CFPD are summarized in Fig. 15–17 and compared to APD in region A. It would appear that substantial improvement as in region B should be possible to attain based on data to date. Performance in region B would result in hourly clearance levels (KpH) of 2 to 3 L/h compared to maximum of about 1 L/h with APD and TPD. It remains to be seen if greatly improved and reliable performance in region C can be achieved with Kph of 3 to 4 L/h in clinical use.

Modeled Glucose Absorption in CFPD compared to CAPD. Batch dialysate systems are inefficient with respect to the amount of ultrafiltrate achieved relative to the amount of glucose absorbed. Equation (22) was used to calculate the intstantaneous ultrafiltration profile with variable D concentrations and is depicted as a function of exchange time in Fig. 15–18A. In batch exchanges it is necessary to use a high concentration of glucose to get adequate total Qf because the glucose is reabsorbed quite rapidly diminishing the gradient and also there is continuing lymphatic reabsorption of fluid. In CFPD high initial glucose concentrations might not be necessary because there is not a long dwell period with unopposed reabsorption. As shown in Fig. 15–18B, it would be predicted that ultrafiltration will be constant at the rate reflecting the initial concentration which can be held nearly constant with high fresh dialysate flow rate. As shown in Fig. 15–19, it can be calculated from the transport parame-

ters that typical glucose caloric absorption in CFPD is predicted to be 35 to 40 percent lower than in CAPD.

Optimization of PD Catheters for CFPD. Catheter design will almost certainly be critical to achieve further improvement of CFPD. Realistic study of catheter design in vitro is virtually impossible since it is not possible to realistically simulate the peritoneal cavity. The most rational approach to catheter studies would be the use of temporary study catheters so that a long-term commitment to any experimental catheter is not required. It intuitively would seem likely that the inflow catheter should be in the upper abdomen and outflow in pelvic area. Since it is anticipated that the MTC will be a function of Qp, studies with any catheter should be conducted over a wide range of Qp. The data in Fig. 15–16 are widely dispersed but best fit empirically to a power function as shown. In order to compare catheter designs it will be necessary to develop profiles of MTC as a function of Qp to compare catheter efficiency. The set of theoretical profiles shown in Fig. 15–20 is highly idealized but they serve to crudely illustrate the study data required to evaluate catheters for CFPD.

Urea Kinetic Modeling in CAPD. Since the patient is considered to be at steady state with virtually continual dialsis in CAPD. urea nitrogen mass balance can be decribed as

$$V(dC / dt) = G- \sim KprC \tag{73}$$

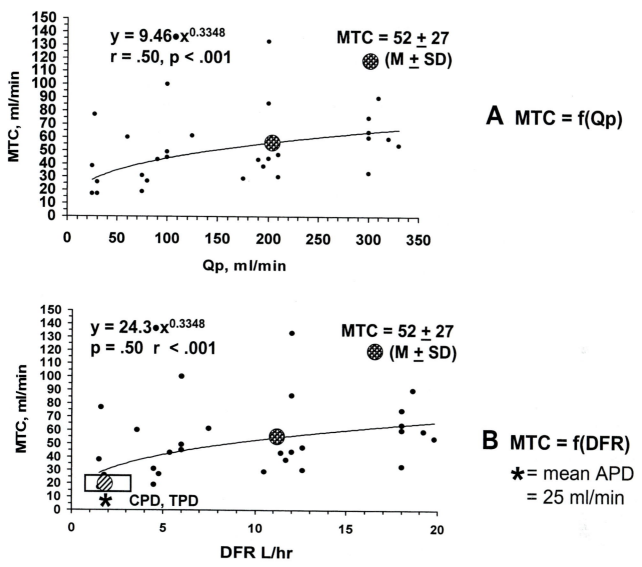

Figure 15–16. MTC values calculated from Shinaberger and plotted as f(Qp) and f(DFR).

where V is urea distribution volume, C is BUN, and Kpr is the sum of continuous peritoneal and renal urea clearances. Since Kpr is continuous and body urea content is at steady state, V(dc/dt) = 0, and Eq. (73) reduces to

$$G = Kpr \langle C \qquad (74)$$

the net protein catabolic rate (PCR) is a function of G,

$$PCR = 9.35G + 0.29V \text{ (see chapter HD)} \qquad (75)$$

Equation (75) also describes the relationship of PCR to G in PD but in PD there are additional amino acid and dialysate protein losses[49]; each of these is approximately 0.1 g/kg/day, so that the normalized dietary protein requirement (NDPR) to maintain zero nitrogen balance is approximately

$$NDPR = NPCR + 0.2g / kg / day \qquad (76)$$

Although the NDPR is an essential nutritional parameter, the NPCR is presumably more relevant to the dose of dialysis since uremia is related to protein catabolic products such as H^+, K^+, PO_4, and urea, among others. Note that there is no volume term in Eq. (74), which has units of mg/min of urea nitrogen. In order to express G in terms of NPCR, which is PCR normalized to volume, both G and Kpr must be normalized to volume by first dividing Eq. (74) by V:

$$G / V = (Kpr / V)(C) \qquad (77)$$

Substitution of Eq. (77) into Eq. (76), expression of Kpr as KprT, total liters per day per liter of body water of urea clearance, and reconciliation of units results in

$$BUN = [26.5 / (KprT / V)](NPCR \sim 0.17) \qquad (78)$$

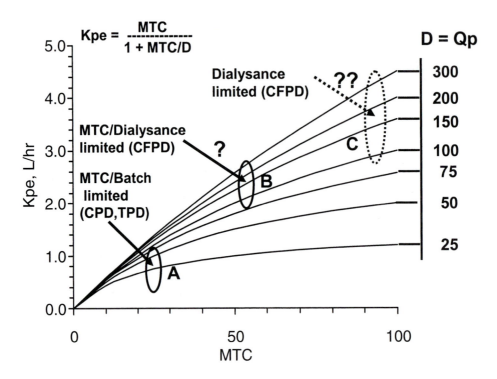

Figure 15–17. Comparison of Kpe expressed as L/h achieved with CPD/TDP to that with CFPD to date. The Cruz data were quite reproducible and suggest MTC 50 and Kpe 2 to 2.5 L/h are possible with CFPD.

In Eq. (78), BUN is expressed as the aqueous concentration in body water, while the plasma BUN is only 94 percent of this level due to the void volume of plasma protein. So we can write

$$BUNpd = [(25 / KprT / V)](NPCR \sim 0.17) \qquad (79)$$

Equation (79) describes the linear dependence of BUN on NPCR with slope inversely related to KprT/V. Solution of Eq. (79) over a wide range of KprT/V (expressed as L/week/L body water) and NPCR provides a urea kinetic map for CAPD therapy relating BUNpd, NPCR, and KprT/V as shown in Fig. 15–21. It can be seen in Eq. (79) and Fig. 15–21 that BUN increases linearly with NPCR with slope inversely proportional to KprT/V. The regions of inadequate and adequate CAPD as defined by DOQI are shown. As in the case for HD, it is important to note that BUN alone is not helpful to define adequate CAPD and that BUN can only be properly interpreted with knowledge of both NPCR and KprT/V, as illustrated by points A and B in Fig. 15–21. Point A depicts a low BUN with inadequate Kprt/V and very low NPCR while point B is a high BUN with adequate Kprt/V and high protein intake.

Equivalent Doses of Dialysis in PD and HD— The Standard Kt/V (stdKt/V)

A very detailed discussion of this issue and derivation of the equivalency equations in contained in Chap. 7 and should be reviewed in conjunction with the following material.

There is some redundancy in the following material because of the considerable importance of this concept to both HD and PD. It currently is an area of particular importance because of the renewed interest in more frequent dialysis and in earlier initiation of CAPD and CHD at higher levels of residual renal urea clearance (Kru). The concept of stdKt/V addresses the need for uniform quantification of dialysis with respect to intensity of each dialysis (eKt/V, Kprt/V), the number of dialyses per week (N), and the presence or absence of associated continuous clearance such as Kru and/or CAPD. A rational approach to quantify variable frequency HD and combinations of intermittent HD with continuous dialysis is an expression of all doses as equivalent continuous steady state clearances (Ks) which are therapeutically equal to the summed doses of intermittent clearance. In steady state the solute generation rate is balanced by (equal to) solute removal rate so concentration (Cs) remains constant in accordance with

$$G = (Ks)(Cs) \qquad (80)$$

The Ks is defined from rearrangement of Eq. (80) to give

$$Ks = G / Cs \qquad (81)$$

It can be seen in Eq. (81) that continuous Ks is defined as the ratio G/Cs so we can in theory calculate a continuous Ks which is equivalent (Ks_{eq}) to the amount of dialysis provided by any specific intermittent dialysis schedule as fol-

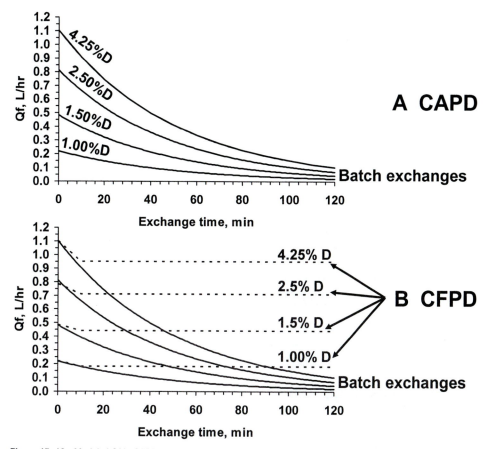

Figure 15–18. Modeled Qf in CAPD and CFPD. The elimination of long dwell times should increase the efficiency of Qf per gram of glucose absorbed.

lows: (1) define G; (2) calculate the concentration profile for a specified eKt/V, G, V, and number of treatments per week (N); (3) define a concentration point on the profile to serve as the equivalent steady state concentration (Cs_{eq}); (4) calculate the continuous clearance which is therapeutically equivalent to the total weekly intermittent clearance in accordance with

$$Ks_{eq} = G / Cs_{eq} \qquad (82)$$

This approach has been reported using three different values to represent the concentration profile for definition of C_{seq} as depicted graphically in Fig. 15–22. The peak concentration hypothesis[50] defines Cs_{eq} as the maximum or peak predialysis BUN (C_{pk}) after the longest interdialytic interval to be used to calculate an equivalent continuous clearance (Ks_{pk})

$$Ks_{pk} = G / Cs_{pk} \qquad (83)$$

The mean predialysis BUN (Co_m) is used[51,52] to define the standard K (stdK) in accordance with

$$stdK = G / C_{om}. \qquad (84)$$

Note that in the case of thrice weekly CHD (see Fig. 17–38) the Cs_{pk} and C_{om} differ only minimally but the difference becomes much greater in more frequent HD schedules. In all cases the time average concentration (C_{TAC}) is substantially lower than C_{pk} and C_{om}.

The C_{TAC} is used to define the "equivalent renal clearance" (K_{EKR}).[53,54] In this case we write

$$K_{EKR} = G / C_{TAC} \qquad (85)$$

The K_{EKR} is based on the C_{TAC} calculated from the total area under the urea concentration curve during a week including the log mean profiles during the short dialysis intervals and the long linear interdialytic profile segments. The clinical validity of these three definitions of Ks_{eq} can at present only be evaluated from analysis of clinical equivalence between CAPD and CHD, two well-established continuous and intermittent dialysis therapies which can serve as benchmarks to evaluate the three definitions C_{seq} and will be considered further below.

Mathematical Development of the stdK Model. The kinetic descriptions of intermittent and continuous dialysis which follow contain the assumptions of equally spaced dialyses and constant V. Since our goal is to define a steady

Modeled Glucose Absorption in CAPD
[1] MTC Dextrose = 10 ml/min
[2] Four 6 hr, 2L, 2.5%D exchanges
[3] Blood glucose 150 mg/dL
$Rt=1-(Vo/VT)(1-Ro\bullet exp(-MTC\bullet t/MV)$
$Rt=1-(2/2.5)(1-11.8\bullet exp(-.01\bullet 360/2.25)$
$Rt = 2.0$
$Abs=((11.8\bullet 2)-(2.5\bullet 2))(4) =149$ gm/day
$Abs = 520$ kcal/day

Modeled Glucose Absorption in CFPD
[1] MTC Dextrose = 20 ml/min
[2] 8 hr CFPD D = 170 ml/min
[3] 1.25%D, Blood glucose 150 mg/dL
$$\frac{\text{Dextrose flux}}{\text{into blood}} = \frac{\text{Dextrose flux}}{\text{out of dialysate}}$$
$(MTC(Cdo-Cb) = D(Cdi-Cdo)$
$Cdo = (.17(11.9)+.02(2))/(.17+.02)$
$\qquad = 10.8$ gm/L
$G = MTC(Cdo-Cb)=.02(10.8-2.0)=.21$ gm/min
$G = .212(60)(8)=1.2$ gm/day = 355 kcal/day

Summary Modeled Dextrose Absorption in CAPD and CFPD

CAPD

Estimated average Abs = 149 g/day, 540 kcal/day

CFPD

Estimated average Abs = 102 g/day, 355 kcal/day

Figure 15–19. The predicted improved efficiency of Qf/absorbed glucose is expected to reduce calorie uptake from dialysate.

state continuous clearance, we solve for C_{om} without the dilution of interdialytic fluid gain which will be erroneously interpreted as higher stdK. However, the VVSP model would be required for analysis of *delivered* intermittent dialysis doses in (eKt/V) order to accurately estimate the urea distribution volume, V. The assumption of equal spac-

ing simply provides an estimate of the average peak concentration. Although the inputs include single pool Kt/V (spKt/V), correction to equilibrated Kt/V (eKt/V) is made in all instances as a function of the rate of dialysis relative to V.[7] Further, in the case of daily HD and combined therapies, the spKt/V prescribed for each HD may be relatively

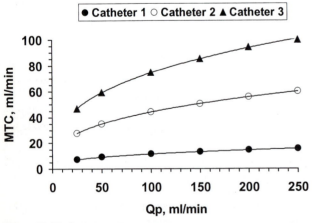

Figure 15–20. Four theoretical catheter dependent profiles for catheter function expressed as MTC = ƒ(Qp). Catheter 3 would obviously be much superior to catheter 1. How can we obtain this kind of experimental data?

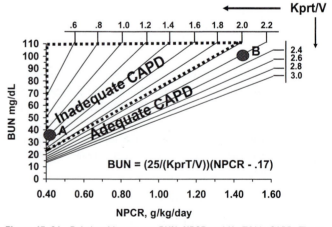

Figure 15–21. Relationships among BUN, NPCR and KprT/V in CAPD. The regions of inadequate and adequate CAPD are depicted as defined by DOQI guidelines. Note that BUN alone provides little knowledge about therapy. Point A shows BUN 35 with NPCR 0.40 and KprT/V 1.2 while point B show NPCR 1.5 and Kpr/T/V 2.2.

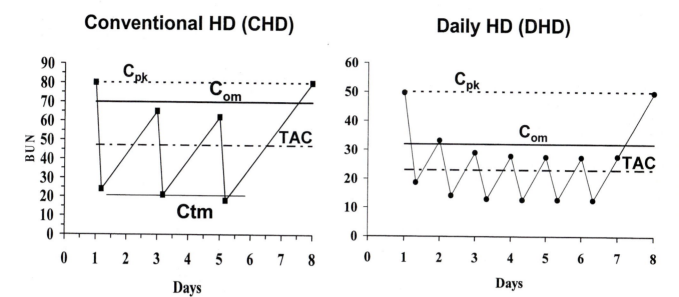

Figure 15–22. Three different definitions of equivalent points on the concentration profile to calculate continuous clearance equivalent to intermittent clearance.

low, i.e., less than 1.1, which may result in spuriously low calculated $V^{55,56}$ which requires the appropriate volume correction algorithm discussed above.

Equation (73) can now be written in general form applicable to both intermittent and continuous therapies in accordance with

$$V(dC/dt) = G - (Kd + Kp + Kr)C \qquad (86)$$

Intermittent therapies consist of either intermittent hemodialysis (IHD) or automated peritoneal dialysis (APD). We can now restate some of the FVSP model solutions derived in Chap. 7 for use in development of stdK. The decrease in BUN over each intermittent therapy session is

$$
\begin{aligned}
C_{tm} = C_{om} Co \exp[-Kd \text{ or } Kp+Kr)t/V] \\
+ [G/(Kd \text{ or } kp+Kr)][1 \\
-\exp[-Kd \text{ or } kp+Kr)t/V]]
\end{aligned} \qquad (87)
$$

where C_{om} is mean predialysis BUN, C_{tm} is mean post dialysis BUN, Kd, Kp, and Kr are dialyzer, peritoneal, and renal urea clearances respectively, t is treatment time, V is urea distribution volume, and all units must be consistent.

Solution of Eq. (86) for BUN buildup over the intervals between HD or APD results in

$$
\begin{aligned}
C_{om} = C_{tm} \langle\exp[-(Kp + Kr)ti / V] \\
+ [G / (Kp + Kr)][1 - \exp[-Kp + Kr)ti / V]]
\end{aligned} \qquad (88)
$$

or

$$C_{om} = C_{tm} + G * ti / V \qquad (89)$$

where C_{tm} is mean postdialysis BUN as in Eq. (82), C_{om} is mean predialysis BUN prior to next IHD or APD treatment, ti is the interdialytic time interval, and all units must be consistent. Note that Eq. (88) applies if either Kp or Kr are greater than zero while Eq. (89) applies when both are zero between the IHD or APD treatments.

In order to generalize the model and calculate the mean predialysis BUN or C_{om} it is necessary to combine Eqs (86)–(89) and to express G as a function of the normalized protein catabolic rate (NPCR) as developed in Eq. (75). The generalized expression to compute C_{om} with any combination of frequency of IHD, APD, or CFPD and CAPD between IHD, APD, or CFPD sessions is

$$
\begin{aligned}
C_{om} &= (0.184 \text{ PCRn} - 0.17) \cdot V / (spKt / V) \cdot V/t))(1 - \exp(-eKt/V) \\
&\cdot \exp(-(Kp + K_r)(1440 \cdot (7/N) - t) / V)) + (0.184(\text{PCRn} - 0.17) \\
&\cdot V / (Kp + Kr))(1 - \exp(-(Kp + K_r)(1440(7/N) - t) / V)) \\
&/(1 - \exp(-eKt / V) \cdot \exp(-(Kp + K_r)((7 / N)1440 - t / V))
\end{aligned} \qquad (90)
$$

where spKt/V is single pool Kdt/V for HD or KptV (for APD); t is duration of intermittent treatment sessions in minutes; N is frequency of IHD or APD per week; eKt/V is the *equilibrated* Kt/V calculated from spKt/V in accordance with Eq (91) below[56]; Kp is any CD between IHD or APD sessions; Kr is included in spKt/V and in CD intervals; and all units must be consistent.

$$eKt / V = spKt / V[t / (t + 35)] \qquad (91)$$

In the case when CAPD and Kr zero, during the intervals between IHD or APD sessions, the expression for C_{om} becomes

$$C_{om} = (0.184(PCRn - .017) \cdot V) / (spKt / V)V / t))(1 - exp(-eKt / V)$$
$$+ (0.184(PCRn - 0.17) \cdot V \cdot (1440(7/N) - t) / V) / V \ (1 - exp(-eKt / V) \quad (92)$$

In the case of continuous clearance only as in normal renal function, chronic renal failure and CAPD with neither IHD nor APD,

$$Css = (0.184(NPCR - 0.17)\langle V) / (Kp + Kr) \quad (93)$$

where Css is the steady state BUN with continuous clearance and an exact analogue of Eq. (79) for CAPD.

We can now substitute C_{om}, found from solution of Eq. (90) or (92) with a specified set of modality input parameters—intermittent dialysis ± continuous dialysis—into Eq. (84), and solve for the *standard* urea clearance (stdK) which results in Cs_{eq} equal to C_{om} at identical NPCR as given by

$$stdK = .184(NPCR - .17) \cdot V / Com \quad (94)$$

Division of Eq. (94) by V and incorporation of appropriate time constants results in

$$std(Kt / V) = 1440[0.184(PCRn - 0.17)] / Com \ daily \quad (95)$$

$$std(Kt / V) = 7 * 1440[0.184(PCRn - 0.17) \\ / Com \ weekly \quad (96)$$

The model is now complete. The dose of dialysis can be expressed as an equivalent, normalized continuous clearance for all combinations of intermittent and continuous treatment modalities and residual Kru.

Generalized Solution of the stdKt/V Model

Solution of Eqs. (90), (92), and (96) over wide ranges of eKt/V, N, an average V = 35 and NPCR = 1.00 is shown in Fig. 15–23. Inspection of the points in Fig. 15–23 reveals that stdKt/V appears to increase quite steeply and linearly as N increases, but the increase is shallow and logarithmic as eKt/V increases at a fixed level of N. This reflects the inefficiency of intermittent dialysis as each individual dose increases and blood concentration, the driving force for solute removal, falls. The line labeled continuous clearance in Fig. 15–23 is calculated as seven times the abscissa values with the understanding that for this calculation the eKt/V is given continuously 7 days per week. Note the locus of CAPD is indicated on the continuous clearance line and illustrates the greatly increased efficiency of continuous therapy compared to intermittent therapy. The plot in Fig. 15–23 provides a uniform expression for dialysis dose combining intensity, eKt/V, and frequency, N, in the generalized dosing parameter, stdKt/V. The orderly behavior of the

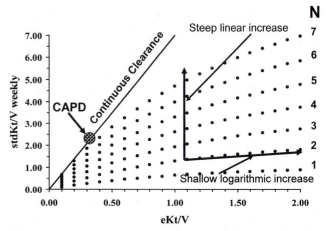

Figure 15–23. Results of solution of stdKt/V model over wide ranges of eKt/V and N. Note that by inspection stdKt/V appears to increase linearly as N increases and logarithmically with eKt/V. Can we fit a generalized regression equation to the entire range of eKt/V and N and thus calculate stdKt/V from only eKt/V and N?

stdKt/V model solutions exhibited in Fig. 15–23 suggests that it might be possible to devise a generalized logarithmic or parabolic regression equation which incorporates N and eKt/V. Both of these conjectures are true, fully derived in Chap. 7 and summarized in the following.

The logarithmic expression derived for stdKt/V = f(N, eKt/V) is

$$stdKt / V = (0.717 \cdot N - 0.157) \\ + (0.399N - 0.166) \cdot \ln(eKt / V) \quad (97)$$

and is illustrated in Fig. 15–24. The regression equation solution is displayed by the solid curves and can be compared to individual points calculated from the stdKt/V model. Note that the logarithmic algorithm agrees with the model very well for eKt/V ≤ 0.40 but underestimates the model values for eKt/V < 0.40.

The second order function derived for stdKt/V = f(N, eKt/V),

$$stdK / V - (-0.1516 \cdot N + 0.11) \cdot (eKt / V)2 \\ + (0.8994 \cdot N - 0.1606) \cdot eKt / V \quad (98) \\ + \ (.0406 \ N + 0.0621)$$

is illustrated in Fig. 15–25. Evaluation of Eq. (98) over the total range of N and eKt/V in Fig. 15–25 shows this function fits the model almost perfectly over the entire domains of frequency and eKt/V. The superior performance of Eq. (98) over Eq. (97) is shown graphically in Fig. 15–26 where the error with each expression is plotted as a function of eKt/V. The large systematic error at low eKt/V for Eq. (97) is readily apparent while there is virtually no systematic

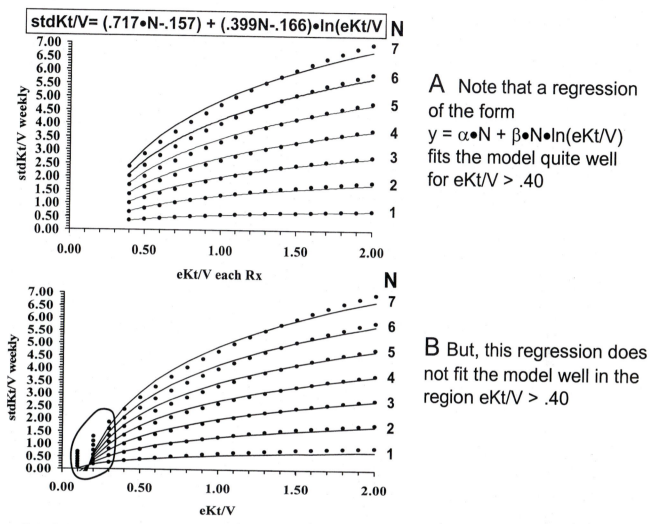

Figure 15–24. A slope intercept logarithmic regression fits model solutions quite well for eKt/V > 0.40 but does not fit the model well for eKt/V < 0.40.

error with Eq (98). Thus Eq (98) can be used to calculate stdKt/V for any dialysis schedule (N) and eKt/V. It is also useful to note that Eq. (98) can be solved for eKt/V using the quadratic formula in accordance with

$$eKt / V = (-b \pm ((b^2) - 4 \cdot a \cdot c)^{(0.50)}) / 2 \cdot a$$

where
$$a = (-0.152 \cdot N + 0.11)$$
$$b = (0.788 \cdot N - 0.1606) \tag{99}$$
$$c = (0.041 \cdot N + 0.062 - stdKt/V)$$

Equation (99) can be used to calculate the eKt/V required to achieve any desired stdKt/V with any specified frequency of dialysis. This regression equation fits the model calculations almost perfectly over the entire range of N and eKt/V and clearly can provide the best method to calculate stdKt/V from N and eKt/V.

Quantification of the Dose of Intermittent HD Combined with Residual Renal Urea Clearance (Kru)

There is a growing belief that starting patients on dialysis at a higher level of residual renal function may have long-term benefits on outcome with dialysis therapy.[57] There is increasing support for initiation of both HD and CAPD at higher levels of residual renal function.[58] A quantitative method of incorporating residual renal urea clearance (Kru) in the special cases of twice and thrice weekly dialysis prescription has been derived previously.[58,59] The concept of stdKt/V as embodied in Eqs. (90) to (96) is well suited to generalize calculation of the dose of intermittent HD with residual renal function. However, it is not possible to derive a generalized algorithm such as in Eqs. (97) and (98) to cover the entire domains of N, eKt/V and Kru. Instead a family of solutions for each N must be used to quantify the dose of combined intermittent and continuous clearance.

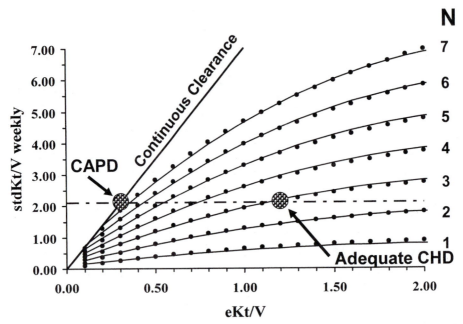

Figure 15–25. A parabolic regression fits the model data very well over the ranges 0.1 ≤ eKt/V ≤ 2.00, 1 ≤ N ≤ 7 and will be the most reliable regression to estimate stdKt/V over this entire range from knowledge of N and eKt/V.

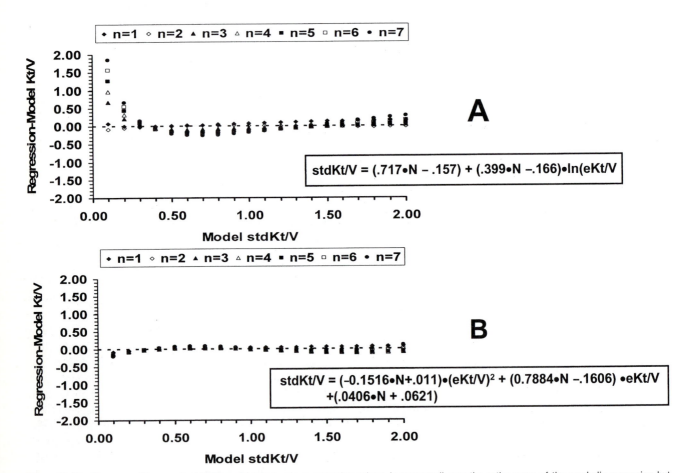

$$stdKt/V = (.717 \cdot N - .157) + (.399 \cdot N - .166) \cdot \ln(eKt/V)$$

$$stdKt/V = (-0.1516 \cdot N + .011) \cdot (eKt/V)^2 + (0.7884 \cdot N - .1606) \cdot eKt/V + (.0406 \cdot N + .0621)$$

Figure 15–26. The error, difference in stdKt/V model values minus regression values, is very small over the entire range of the parabolic regression but becomes very large at eKt/V < 0.40 with the logarithmic regression.

We derived N specific logarithmic and parabolic expressions (see Chap. 7) for stdKt/V = f(N, eKt/V, nKru) where nKru is the residual renal urea clearance divided by the urea distribution volume and expressed as mL/L.

The parabolic regression derived for stdKt/V = f(N, eKt/V, nKu) is depicted in Fig. 15–27 for N 1, 2, 3, and 4. In order to make the Kru units more familiar, for the plots in Fig. 15–27, nKru was further normalized to an average V = 35 L and thus expressed as a more familiar parameter, Kru, mL/min. Examination of the plots in Fig. 15–27 clearly shows the parabolic expression does not provide a satisfactory algorithm. It fits the model data perfectly for N = 2 but deviates significantly from model calculated values at high levels of eKt/V for N = 1, 3, and 4 and could not serve as a generalized algorithm.

The logarithmic algorithm relating stdKt/V to N and eKt/V is of the form

$$stdKt / V = a \cdot f(N) + b \cdot f(N) \cdot \ln(eKt / V) \qquad (100)$$

and is specific for each individual N. The logarithmic algorithm derived is illustrated in Fig. 15–28 for N 1, 2, 3, and 4, where it can be seen to fit the model calculations very well,

over the entire domains of N and eKt/V and thus can serve as a reliable algorithm to quantify combined intermittent HD and Kru normalized to V = 35 L. The logarithmic equations should be very useful to evaluate patients who may be starting dialysis at higher levels of Kru. In each of the plots a reference line for adequate stdKt/V = 2.15 is plotted and a patterned circle marks the point of minimum adequate eKt/V as a function of Kru and N. In panel A it can be seen that if it is elected to initiate HD once a week, minimum eKt/V 2.0 and minimum Kru = 6.0 ml/min will be required for the average sized patient with V = 35 L. The regression lines are almost flat in Fig. 15–28A and show that increasing eKt/V with N = 1 does not significantly increase the dose expressed as stdKt/V. Consequently the minimum Kru for once weekly dialysis with eKt/V 2.00 is Kru = 6.0 and might be considered to be a kinetic definition of absolute minimum Kru to initiate hemodialysis once weekly.

In Fig. 15–28, panels B, C, and D the stdKt/V 2.15 line crosses several Kru regression contour lines and the levels of minimum eKt/V required as f(N and stdKt/V) are depicted as open circles. If higher levels of eKt/V and N are chosen the plots also provide a quantification of how much the dose is increased. For example, in panel C the stdKt/V

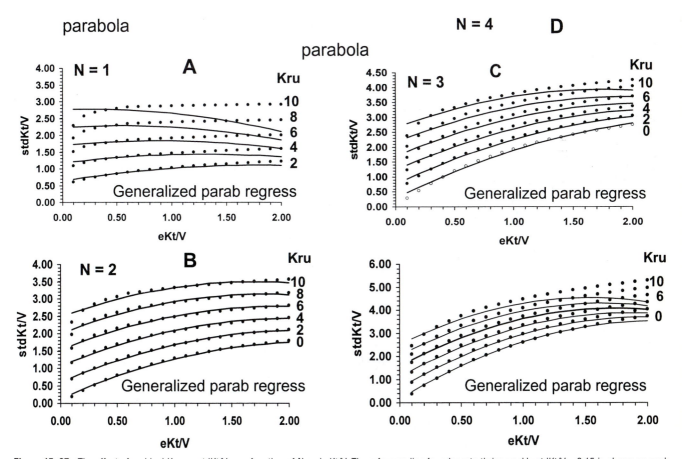

Figure 15–27. The effect of residual Kru on stdKt/V as a function of N and eKt/V. The reference line for adequate thrice-weekly stdKt/V = 2.15 is shown on each plot with the coordinates of Kru, eKt/V required for 1 ≤ N ≤ 4.

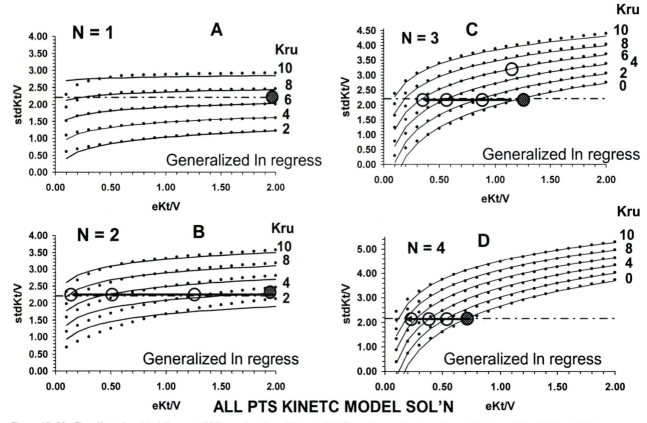

Figure 15–28. The effect of residual Kru on stdKt/V as a function of N and eKt/V. The reference line for adequate thrice-weekly stdKt/V = 2.15 is shown on each plot with the coordinates of Kru, eKt/V required for $1 \leq N \leq 4$.

resulting with initiation of CHD (N = 3, eKt/V = 1.15) with Kru 6.0 in the average sized patient will result in stdKt/V = 3.2. This may be better therapy than 2.15, but there are no data available to make a decision. However, this does point up the potential value of using the relationships depicted in Fig. 15–28 to quantify the dose as stdKt/V with both earlier initiation of HD and more frequent dialysis. In this way a uniform dosing parameter can be used to examine outcome

in a period of rapidly changing frequency and intensity of dialysis.

Tables of Parabolic and Logarithmic Solutions for the Relationships between stdKt/v, N eKtV, and Kru. A summary of the algorithms is shown in Tables 15–1 and 15–2. Table 15–1 gives the individual logarithmic regressions for stdKt/V =

TABLE 15–1. APPROXIMATION EQUATIONS TO CALCULATE stdKT/V UREA AS A FUNCTION OF eKT/V NUMBER OF DIALYSES PER WEEK (N) AND LEVEL OF NORMALIZED RENAL UREA CLEARANCE (nKru)[a]

	stdKt/V = f(N, eKt/V, nKru)
1	stdKt/V = (7.938·nKru + 0.5816) + [(−0.987·nKru + 0.330·ln(eKt/V)]
2	stdKt/V = (7.077·nKru + 1.2683) + [(−1.173·nKru + 0.676)·ln(eKt/V)]
3	stdKt/V = (6.472·nKru + 1.9849) + [(−1.400·nKru + 1.075)·ln(eKt/V)]
4	stdKt/V = (6.479·nKru + 2.6651) + [(−1.393·nKru + 1.488)·ln(eKt/V)]
5	stdKt/V = (6.276·nKru + 3.3838) + [(−1.480·nKru + 1.938)·ln(eKt/V)]
6	stdKt/V = (6.090·nKru + 4.1295) + [(−1.512·nKru + 2.429)·ln(eKt/V)]
7	stdKt/V = (6.787·nKru + 1.9539) + [(−1.5575nKru + 1.111)·ln((eKt/V)]
1<N<7, Kr=0	stdKt/V = (−0.152·N + .011)·eKt/V² + [(0.788·N − 0.161)·eKt/V + (0.041·N + 0.062 −stdKt/V)]

[a]Note that when Kru = 0, a single quadratic equation can be used to calculate stdKt/V for all N and 0.1 < eKt/V < 2.00

TABLE 15–2. APPROXIMATION EQUATIONS TO CALCULATE eKT/V AS A FUNCTION OF stdKT/V, NUMBER OF DIALYSES PER WEEK (N), AND LEVEL OF NORMALIZED RENAL UREA CLEARANCE (nKru)

N	eKt/V = f(stdKt/V, N Kru)[a]
1	eKt/V = exp[(stdKt/V)-(7.938·nKru + 0.582)]/(-0.987·nKru + 0.330)
2	eKt/V = exp[(stdKt/V)-(7.077·nKru + 1.268)]/(-1.173·nKru + 0.676)
3	eKt/V = exp[(stdKt/V)-(6.472·nKru + 1.985)]/(-1.400·nKru + 1.075)
4	eKt/V = exp[(stdKt/V)-(6.479·nKru + 2.665)]/(-1.393·nKru + 1.488)
5	eKt/V = exp[(stdKt/V)-(6.276·nKru + 3.384)]/(-1.481·nKru + 1.938)
6	eKt/V = exp[(stdKt/V)-(6.090·Kru + 4.130)]/(-1.512·Kru + 2.429)
7	eKt/V = exp[(stdKt/V)-(6.787·nKru + 1.954)]/(-1.556·nKru + 1.111)
2<N<6, Kru=0	eKt/V = -b + [(b^2) - 4·a·c)^(0.50)]/2·a where a = (-0.152·N + 0.011) b = (0.788·N − 0.1606) c = (0.041·N + 0.062 − stdKt/V)

[a]Note that when Kru = 0, a single quadratic equation can be used to calculate eKt/V for all N and stdKt/V.

f(N, eKt/V, and nKru) for each N over the range 1 to 7. The last row in Table 15–1 gives the general parabolic equation for stdKt/V as f(N and eKt/V) when nKru = 0. Table 15–2 provides solutions of the logarithmic equations required to calculate eKt/V = f(N, stdKt/V and nKru) for each N over the range 1 to 7. The last row in Table 15–1 shows the quadratic equation to calculate eKt/V as f(N, stdKt/V) when nKru = 0. These two tables summarize all of the algorithms relating stdKt/V, eKt/V, nKru, and N for use in evaluating these relationships in clinical data.

Modeling the Dose of Peritoneal Dialysis

There are a remarkably large number of interacting parameters which can significantly affect the dose of dialysis in both CAPD and APD. Ideally, these should all be optimized to select the regimen that delivers adequate therapy and is most compatible with the patient's life-style. The parameters that can be optimized in CAPD are exchange volume, exchange times, number of exchanges, and distribution of exchanges over the 24-hour period. These can all be individualized according to patient-specific MTC, Kr, and V. Attempting manual mathematical evaluation of the many possible options is completely unrealistic; they can be calculated almost instantaneously and displayed for review with an appropriately designed kinetic program written for the personal computer. Similarly, the options for APD can be quickly surveyed by computer analysis. This is illustrated in Fig. 15–29, which depicts an analysis of APD with respect to dialysis time and total dialysate required in a patient with drain profile[4] in Fig 15–6. The curves in Fig. 15–29 show the relationship of required cycler treatment time to achieve the prescribed stdKt/V of 2.15 (with a specified set of patient parameters) as a function of total

dialysate (QdT) used. It is clear from inspection of Fig. 15–29 that with r = 1.00 a time minimum of 13 h is reached with QdT of 16 L. A minimum time of 11 h is feasible with all r ≤ .75 and QdT about 20 L. Little is gained by further increase in DFR, which would be wasteful of dialysate.

Peritoneal Dialysis Quantification Tests

Peritoneal membrane transport and therapy quantification tests provide useful information on one or more important patient- and peritoneal-specific characteristics. The information may include MTC, the actual level of treatment provided with a given PD prescription, protein nutritional information, and the consistency or reproducibility of

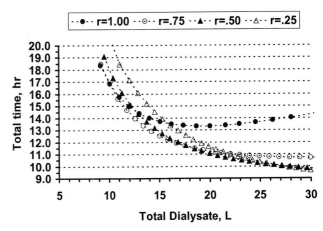

Figure 15–29. Modeled APD treatment time and dialysate required for drain profile[4] depicted in Fig. 15–6. Note that with r = 1.00, t reaches a minimum of 13 hours with total dialysate about 20 L. The most suitable therapy would be r = 0.50 or 0.25 and trade off between t and total dialysate can be seen clearly in the plot.

peritoneal transport and/or delivered peritoneal dialysis treatment over time.

There are a number of issues to be considered when selecting one or more of the peritoneal dialysis or membrane transport quantification techniques in clinical use. These issues include the reliability and validity of the quantification technique, the ease of clinical application for patient and clinic staff, the solute(s) of interest for quantification, and the utility and comprehensiveness of the information generated from the test(s).

Peritoneal Equilibration Test

Twardowski and colleagues described the first specific quantification technique for peritoneal dialysis,[61,62]—the peritoneal equilibration test (PET), which measures the dialysate to plasma ratio (D/P) of creatinine and dialysate dextrose concentration (Dt) over beginning dialysate dextrose concentration (Dt/D0) as a measure of ultrafiltration capability. The classic PET is standardized to a 2-L, 2.5% dextrose exchange and a 4-hour dwell, and there are specific instructions to ensure mixing of the dialysate solution in the peritoneal cavity during inflow and sampling procedures. Dialysate samples are drawn immediately after inflow of dialysate, at 2 hours of dwell duration when a blood sample is drawn, and at the end of the 4-hour dwell, when the exchange is drained for measurement of total volume

and concentrations. A simplification of the PET, which uses only two dialysate samples, has also been described[63]; this test has been reported to provide comparable accuracy to the classic PET.[64,65]

The measured dialysate to plasma ratio values are plotted as a function of dwell duration as shown in Fig. 15–30. The results from the test are compared with mean (M) values ±1 and ±2 SD determined from previous studies to classify peritoneal transport. Thus, the peritoneal transport categories are high (+2SD), high-average (+1SD), average (M), low-average (–1SD), and low (–2SD). Utilizing these categories assists in the evaluation of potential PD modalities. The PET has been widely used to measure peritoneal membrane transport in patients, and published data suggest that the PET is reproducible and stable over repetitive measurements in patients.[66,67] The five transport categories and a set of high quality PET data are shown for creatinine in Fig. 15–30.

Creatinine and glucose are the primary solutes measured with the PET, which allows determination of solute removal and expected ultrafiltration. Creatinine was originally selected by Twardowski as the marker solute because it appeared to correlate better with the clinical status of the patient and was more reproducible and stable than urea nitrogen in repetitive measurements.[61] Recent data suggest that low serum creatinine concentrations rather than high values are more highly correlated with the relative risk of

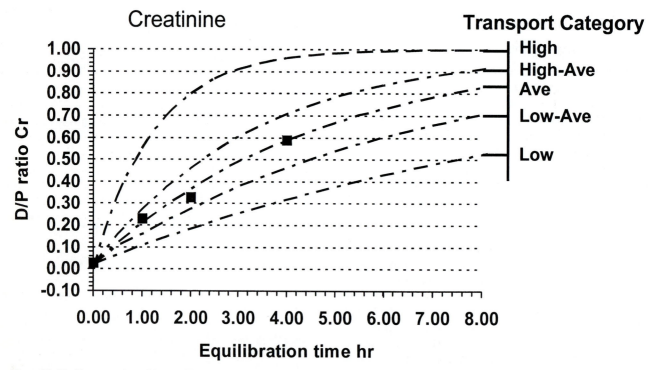

Figure 15–30. The range of creatinine equilibration curves for the PET. A high-quality set of four sequential PET D/P ratios are shown for a patient with average transport.

death in hemodialysis patients,[68] implying a close correlation to skeletal muscle mass and nutritional status.

Using the PET to prescribe and monitor PD therapy has some limitations. In order to determine the total daily or weekly therapy provided with the current prescription, the results obtained with a single, carefully measured exchange must be extrapolated to 24 or 168 hours to assess total daily or weekly peritoneal clearance. Some data suggest that extrapolation of the PET is not a reliable method of estimating the total delivered dose of dialysis, while others indicate that this extrapolation is accurate.[69,70] However, this may be problematic if the prescribed PD regimen uses an alternative exchange volume, dextrose concentration, or dwell duration. Predicting or modeling the effect of any of these modifications, which would be necessary if the clinician wanted to further individualize the PD prescription, is not possible. Other data suggest that the procedural steps in the PET may actually overestimate peritoneal membrane transport and underestimate the variation in peritoneal transport that may occur under actual clinical conditions.[71] In summary, the PET is a standardized and reproducible test, which has been widely used to measure and categorize the peritoneal membrane for creatinine clearance and ultrafiltration characteristics. The results from the PET assist in the evaluation of alternative PD modalities. These objective data are combined with patient preferences or life-style to assist in the selection of the peritoneal dialysis modality most appropriate for the individual patient.

24-Hour Batch Dialysate Test

The 24-hour batch test has been used to monitor the amount of treatment provided with a PD prescription. Individual drained dialysate exchanges over a 24-hour period are collected and brought to the clinic where the drained exchanges are measured, pooled, and well mixed, and an aliquot is obtained and analyzed for urea nitrogen and creatinine. In some centers, a sample is obtained from each drained exchange as a constant volume or as a proportional sample of each exchange, and these samples are combined and analyzed as a single sample. Residual renal function is measured over the period of the dialysate collection. The total peritoneal urea clearance, KpT (L/day), can be calculated from the dialysate collection and normalized to urea distribution volume, KpT/V. Residual renal urea clearance, KrT/V, is added to give KprT/V, the combined fractional urea clearance.

Total liters of peritoneal and renal creatinine clearance can be calculated and normalized to time and body surface area (KprT [L/week/1.73 m^2 body surface area]). In addition to measured total creatinine clearance provided by peritoneal membrane and renal function, creatinine can also be used to assess patient adherence to the dialysis prescription. This is described more fully below.

There are a number of additional parameters that cannot be determined from the PET but can be calculated from the batch collection. Net protein catabolism [PCR (g/day)] can be calculated from dialysate and urine collections. Protein intake is an important nutritional measure in PD patients. It has been recommended that PD patients should ingest 1.2 g/kg/day of protein to maintain zero nitrogen balance,[72] while others have reported that neutral or positive nitrogen balance is achieved in CAPD patients with NPCR values <1.0.[73] If total protein is measured on the collection, dialysate protein losses can also be determined and added to the PCR, to give a more complete picture of net protein balance over the interval of the collection. Protein losses via dialysate are variable but average around 8 to 9 g/day.[74] Once these data have been calculated, they can be displayed on the three-variable therapy map, relating BUN concentration, total fractional urea clearance, KprT/V, and calculated NPCR, as shown in Fig. 15–21.

Some advantages of the batch collection are that the test is completed by the patient in the home, under actual clinical conditions, and the results represent actual delivered treatment for that day. The disadvantages of the batch collection include the need for the patient to transport 8 to 12 L of dialysate and a concern about mixing the entire collection adequately to obtain a true mean dialysate concentration. Sufficient time and effort must be expended in the mixing process to ensure a homogenous collection.

Peritoneal transport characteristics are generally not calculated from the pooled collection. The failure to determine specific peritoneal transport characteristics makes it difficult to predict the effect of changing the number or volume of exchanges on total clearance. While the batch collection gives information about the total clearance for the day, it does not allow review of the consistency of delivered exchanges over the testing interval.

In summary, the 24-hour batch collection is done in the home and measures the total clearance of urea nitrogen and creatinine over the testing period. A number of interesting and useful patient and treatment parameters can be calculated from this collection, which makes the information generated from this test even more useful than that from the PET. However, the lack of calculated peritoneal MTC values limits its usefulness for optimizing the dialysis prescription.

Peritoneal Function Test

The rigid testing conditions of the PET, the need to extrapolate from one well-controlled exchange to 24 hours or 7 days of therapy, and the difficulties inherent in the batch collection led to the development of an alternative quantification technique, the peritoneal function test (PFT). This test was used and validated in a multicenter study[75,76.] In this clinical evaluation, each patient had at least two PFT measurements done at 4- to 6-week intervals, which provided information on reproducibility of the test.

This test consists of (1) a sample of each exchange and a written record of exchange inflow and outflow volume, and duration of dwell for each exchange in the 24 hours before a clinic visit; (2) a urine collection over 20 to 30 hours; and (3) one blood sample at the time of the clinic visit. The dialysate exchange samples are analyzed for urea, creatinine, glucose, and total protein, and the urine sample is analyzed for urea, creatinine, and volume. The blood sample is analyzed for urea, creatinine, glucose, total protein, and albumin. Each exchange is analyzed with the variable-volume kinetic model described above to determine the MTC and data is displayed as a PT50 value, which is the time required for the dialysate concentration to reach 50 percent of corrected plasma concentration of urea nitrogen and creatinine. Total body water or urea volume [V (L)] is calculated from patient height, weight, and gender.[77]

The PFT calculates the actual daily treatment for urea and creatinine achieved with the peritoneal dialysis prescription. The following indices are calculated from the PFT: (1) the daily total peritoneal urea clearance [KpT (L)]; (2) daily total renal urea clearance [KrT (L)]; (3) the combined peritoneal and renal urea clearance [KprT (L)]; (4) KprT normalized to total body water or V (KprT/V); (5) peritoneal and renal creatinine clearance normalized to body surface area [KpT and KrT (L/week/1.73 m² body surface area), respectively]; (6) protein catabolic rate based on urea nitrogen generation [PCR (g/kg/day)] and normalized to body water [NPCR (g/kg/day)]; (7) dialysate protein losses and normalized to body water [DP (g/day) and NDP

(g/kg/day)]; (8) the sum of PCR and DP and amino acid loss expressed as total dietary protein requirements to maintain zero nitrogen balance and normalized to body water [DPR (g/day) and NDPR (g/kg/day)]; (9) residual renal urea and creatinine clearances [KrU and KrCr (mL/min), respectively]; (10) fluid loss by peritoneal and renal mechanisms; (11) Pt50 values for urea, creatinine, and glucose for each exchange; (12) predicted creatinine generation rate as a function of gender, age, and weight [PGCr (mg/kg/day)][78] and measured creatinine generation rate from the exchanges [(MGCr (mg/kg/day)]; (13) estimated resting energy expenditure [EREE (kcal/day and kcal/kg/day)]; (14) glucose calories absorbed from dialysate [GA (kcal/day and kcal/kg/day)]; and (15) ratio of GA/EREE.

The calculation of the individual peritoneal and renal clearance components for urea and creatinine allows the evaluation of the level of treatment with the current prescription when renal function is lost.

The spectrum of PFT urea equilibration curves (expressed as percent equilibration) are shown as a function of exchange time in Fig. 15–31. The transport categories as defined by the PET are noted for the five curves. The relationship between PT50 and transport category is also illustrated. Note each point at which the line of 50 percent equilibration on the ordinate crosses a transport category contour line defines the PT50 on the abscissa. As described above, usually four or five exchanges are examined with the PFT. A high-quality PFT data set for urea are shown in Fig. 15–32. The solid line is the regression line calculated for the data set and defines for this patient a urea MTC 16 ml/min and PT50 1.5 h. In Fig. 15–33 a high quality creati-

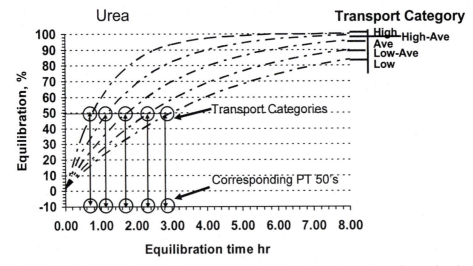

Figure 15–31. The range of urea equilibration curves for the urea PFT with transport categories noted as defined in the PET. It is readily apparent from inspection of the curves that measurements of PFT beyond 4 hours is nearly meaningless because of virtual complete equilibration for all levels of transport capacity. The paired values for transport category and PT 50 are noted.

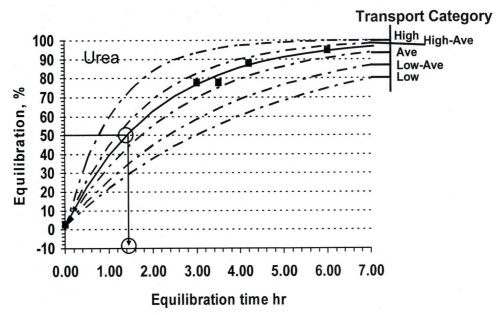

Figure 15–32. The spectrum of urea equilibration profiles for the PFT with transport. categories noted as defined in the PET. A high-quality data set is shown for a patient with PT50 of 1.5 h and MTC for urea of 16 mL/min as defined by the solid regression line calculated from the data set.

nine PFT data set is depicted. The data set shows a high MTC of 12 ml/min and short PT50 1.6 h compared to an average value of 3.2 h. This data reliably demonstrates the patient is a fast transporter.

The PFT allows inspection of the consistency with which the patient performs the individual exchanges. Figure 15–34 shows a set of urea PFT values demonstrating poor quality data. The mean MTC calculated is 10 ml/min but

the scatter in the points indicate a serious technical problem with the exchanges. This data provides a strong indication to discuss therapy technique with the patient and explore common technical errors such as inaccurate reporting of dwell times and/or incomplete inflow or drain of the exchange.

The calculation of peritoneal MTC values for urea, creatinine, and glucose from each exchange provides the

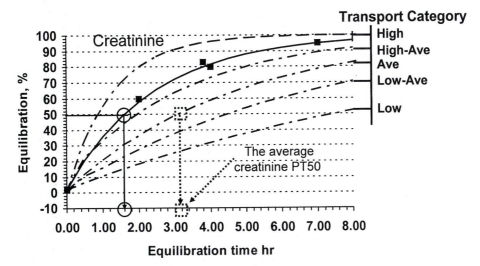

Figure 15–33. A high-quality set of PFT creatinine equilibration values is shown for a patient with a transport profile category between high-average and high. The solid regression line is calculated from the data and defines a creatinine MTC of 12 mL/min and short PT50 of 1.6 h compared to the average PT50 of 3.2 h.

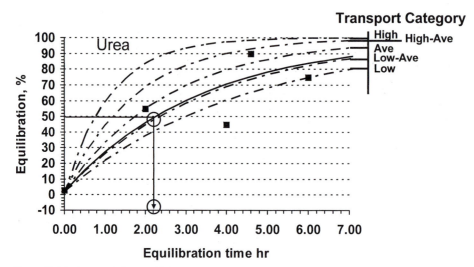

Figure 15–34. A poor-quality urea PFT data set is shown for a patient with PT50 2.2 h, MTC for urea 10 mL/min and transport classification low average. However, it is apparent the data are of poor quality and suggest technical errors in sampling which should be discussed with the patient.

necessary information to model the prescription, if modifications are desired or necessary. As a consequence, individualized prescriptions which consider exchange volume, dextrose concentration, and duration of dwell to optimize the prescription can be calculated.

Several indices of protein/calorie nutrition can be calculated from the PFT, including PCR and NPCR from the dialysate and urine collections. The combination of PCR and NPCR with measured dialysate protein losses [DP (g/day) and NDP (g/kg/day)] and an assumed amino acid loss of 0.1 g/kg/day gives a better approximation of dietary protein intake over the interval of the collection, which is important in assessing dietary protein requirements in PD patients.

The PFT can provide information on glucose calories absorbed from dialysate. Using the creatinine generation information described below, lean body mass can be calculated, but this value may be in error due to poor compliance with the dialysis prescription (skipping dialyses). As a function of the lean body mass, the estimated resting energy expenditure (EREE [kcal/day]) and normalized EREE (NEREE, kcal/kg/day) can be calculated. The measurement of dextrose on each exchange for the PFT allows a quantitative estimate of the fraction of EREE that is being delivered from the dialysate.

The major advantages of the PFT are as follows: (1) The test is done by the patient in the home and reflects the actual treatment delivery on the day of study; (2) it reduces the impact of therapy monitoring on the clinic staff and schedule; (3) a large amount of patient- and peritoneal-specific information is generated; and (iv) modifications in the prescription can be rationally calculated from the data obtained. The analysis of individual samples yields much

more information than a pooled collection, and the ability to calculate MTC allows modeling of the prescription if modifications are desired. The major limitations of the full PFT is the increased work load for the patient at home and the laboratory costs incurred with multiple samples for PD monitoring. Preliminary data indicate that after a complete PFT, routine monitoring may be done with the simplified PFT, which consists of a written record of 24 hours of individual exchanges, a urine collection, a blood sample at the time of the clinic visit, and a single sample from an exchange outflow in the clinic.[75] The PFT was validated by comparison of two values 4 to 6 weeks apart in 60 patients. The KpT/V for the second measurement was calculated only from the written record of the exchanges and a blood sample. This calculated value was then compared with the KpT/V measured from the exchanges and blood sample. The calculated mean error between the predicted and actual KpT/V was ~1.1 ± 14.4 percent (mean ± 2SD).

In summary, the PFT is a quantification test that has been developed and validated to measure a broad spectrum of treatment and patient information. This test allows the clinician to assess total delivered therapy for urea and creatinine, protein and calorie nutrition, fluid balance, and peritoneal transport. The transport information can be used to further individualize or optimize the peritoneal dialysis prescription.

Creatinine can be used as a way of assessing patient adherence with the PD prescription. The elimination pathways (Kr and Kp) can be modeled as first order clearances, KrCr and KpCr, respectively. There is metabolic degradation of creatinine in the gut lumen, which can also be expressed as a first order clearance mechanism, KgCr, and which averages 0.36 L/kg/day.[79] The measured creatinine generation can be expressed as

$$MGCr = (KprCrT)CpCr + KgCrT(CpCr) \quad (101)$$

where KprCrT is total creatinine clearance; CpCr is plasma creatinine concentration (mg/dL); and KgCrT is gut clearance of creatinine.

The rate of creatinine generation can be predicted (PGCr [md/day]) as follows:

$$PGCr \text{ in males} = [28 - \sim 0.20(age, years)] \quad (102)$$
$$(body weight, kg)$$

$$PGCr \text{ in females} = [24 - \sim 0.17(age, years)] \quad (103)$$
$$(body weight, kg)$$

With the assumptions of (1) steady-state conditions and (2) the best estimate of true creatinine generation is PGCr, one can compare the MGCr with PGCr.[80] Therefore, one can assess the ratio of MGCr to PGCr as a measure of patient adherence to the prescription. If the patient has omitted one or more exchanges in the 7 to 10 days preceding the scheduled test and clinic visit, there has been an accumulation of creatinine in the body and serum creatinine increases. On the day of study, when all the exchanges are done, more creatinine is removed than would be predicted. This finding represents a falling body content of creatinine rather than the steady-state conditions usually assumed.

This approach was used to assess compliance in the multicenter study cited above.[80] The ratio of MGCr over PGCr ratio was 1.29 ± 0.31 rather than the expected normal distribution with a mean of 1.00. This indicated that 29 percent more creatinine was removed on the day of study than would be predicted from body composition. If one expresses this as the mean KprT Cr over measured KprT Cr, the average KprT Cr was only 0.78 ± 0.28 of the measured KprT/V on the day of study. This suggested that, on the average, only 78 percent of the PD prescription was delivered in this patient population. This has challenged with the argument that the Cockcroft-Gault underestimates creatinine generation in younger patients.[80] However, these data support the possibility that elective deviation from the PD prescription may be more common than previously assumed. They suggest that therapy must be monitored frequently to assure that the level of treatment prescribed is routinely delivered in order to evaluate its relationship to clinical outcomes. This becomes particularly important for studies which attempt to evaluate causal relationships between the dose in peritoneal dialysis and selected clinical outcome variables. Reported monitoring intervals of several months may not be appropriate to evaluate patient adherence with

sufficient confidence. Close monitoring is required so that the dialysis dose can be adjusted as necessary to maintain a constant level of treatment while the clinical outcome is being observed.

REFERENCES

1. Keen M, Gotch F. Dialyzers and delivery systems. In: Cogan MC, Schoenfeld PY, eds. *Introduction to Dialysis*, 2d ed. New York: Churchill Livingstone, 1991:1–67.
2. Smeby LC, Wideroe TE, Jorstad S. Individual differences in water transport in continuous peritoneal dialysis. *ASAIO J* 1981;4:17–27.
3. Jaffrin MY, Odell RA, Farrell PC. A model of ultrafiltration and glucose mass transfer kinetics in peritoneal dialysis. *Artif Organs* 1987;11:198–207.
4. Flessner MF, Dedrick RL, Schuh JS. A distributed model of peritoneal transport: theoretical considerations. *Am J Physiol* 1984;246:596–637.
5. Popovich RP, Moncrief JW. Kinetic modeling peritoneal transport. *Contrib Nephol* 1979;17:59–72.
6. Ronco C, Borin D, Brendolan A, et al. Studies on peritoneal UF loss: the UF coefficient (K) as an index of the PM filtration efficiency. In: Maher JF, Winchester JF, eds. *Frontiers in Peritoneal Dialysis*. New York: Field, Rich, 1986:100–105.
7. Rippe B, Perry MA, Granger DN. Permselectivity of the peritoneal membrane. *Microvasc Res* 1985;29:89–102.
8. Lysaght MJ, Farrell PC. Membrane phenomena and mass transfer kinetics in peritoneal dialysis. *J Membrane Sci* 1989;44:5–33.
9. Mactier RA, Khanna R, Rwardowski Z, Nolph KD. Contribution of lymphatic absorption to loss of ultrafiltration and solute clearances in continuous ambulatory peritoneal dialysis. *J Clin Invest* 1987;80:1311–1316.
10. Randerson DH, Farrell PC. Mass transfer properties of the human peritoneum. *ASAIO J* 1980;3:140–146.
11. Rubin J, Nolph KD, Popovich RP, et al. Drainage volumes during continuous ambulatory peritoneal dialysis. *ASAIO J* 1979;2:54–60.
12. Hasbargen JA, Smith BJ, Rodgers AJ. Ultrafiltration failure at the initiation of CAPD. *Perit Dial Bull* 1986;6:46–57.
13. Sligeneyer A, Canaud B, Mion C. Permanent loss of ultrafiltration capacity of the peritoneum in long-term peritoneal dialysis: an epidemiological study. *Nephrology* 1983;33:133–138.
14. Gandhi VC, Ing TS, Jablokow VR, et al. Thickened peritoneal dialysis membranes in maintenance peritoneal dialysis patients. *Kidney Int* 1979;14:675.
15. Twardowski ZJ, Nolph KD, Khanna R, et al. Peritoneal equilibration test. *Perit Dial Bull* 1987;7:138–147.
16. Hume R, Weyers E. Relationship between total body water and surface area in normal and obese subjects. *J Clin Pathol* 1971;24:234–238.
17. Henderson LW, Nolph KD. Altered permeability of the peritoneal membrane after using hypertonic peritoneal dialysis fluid. *J Clin Invest* 1969;48:992–1001.

18. Lindholm B, Serynski A, Bergstrom J. Kinetics of peritoneal dialysis with glycerol and glucose as osmotic agents. *ASAIO Trans* 1987;33:19–27.

19. Babb AL, Johansen PJ, Strand MJ, et al. Bi-directional permeability of the human peritoneum to middle molecules. *Proc Eur Dial Transplant Assoc* 1973;10:247–262.

20. Garred LJ, Canaud B, Farrell PC. A simple kinetic model for assessing peritoneal mass transfer in chronic ambulatory peritoneal dialysis. *ASAIO J* 1983;6:131–137.

21. Leypoldt JK, Pust AH, Frigon RP, Henderson LW. Dialysate volume measurements required for determining peritoneal solute transport. *Kidney Int* 1988;34:254–262.

22. Pust AH, Leypoldt JK, Frigon RP, Henderson LW. Peritoneal dialysate volume determined by indicator dilution measurements. *Kidney Int* 1988;33:64–70.

23. Werynski A, Lindholm B. A model of solute transport in CAPD: impact of peritoneal tissue and lymphatic flow (abstr). *Blood Purif* 1987;7:316,317.

24. Villaroel F. Kinetics of intermittent and continuous peritoneal dialysis. *J Dial* 1977;1:333–347.

25. Villaroel F, Popovich RP, Nolph KD. Evaluation of permeance in peritoneal dialysis. *J Dial* 1977;2:361–378.

26. Pyle WK. Mass transfer in peritoneal dialysis. Dissertation. Austin: University of Texas, 1981.

27. Krediet RT, Zemel D, Imholz ALT, Struijk DG. Impact of square area and permeability on solute clearances. *Perit Dial Int* 1994;14(suppl):S70–S78.

28. Schoenfeld PY, Diaz-Buxo J, Keen M, Gotch FA. The effect of body position (P), surface area (BSA) and intraperitoneal exchange volume (Vip) on the peritoneal transport constant (KoA)(abstr). *J Am Soc Nephrol* 1993;4:416.

29. Keshaviah P, Emerson PF, Vonesh EF, Brandes JC. Relationship between body size, fill volume, and mass transfer area coefficient in peritoneal dialysis. *J Am Soc Nephrol* 1994;4:1820–1826.

30. Boen ST. Kinetics of peritoneal dialysis: a comparison with the artificial kidney. *Medicine* 1961;40:243.

31. Diaz-Buxo JA, Farmer CD, Walter PJ, et al. Drainage volumes during CAPD. *ASAIO J* 1979;2:54–60.

32. Diaz-Buxo JA, Walter PJ, Farmer CD, et al. Continuous cyclic peritoneal dialysis (CCPD)(abstr). *Kidney Int* 1981;19:145.

33. Dobbie J, Serkes K, Kenley R, et al. Eight hour tidal peritoneal dialysis matches 24 hour CAPD and surpasses 8 hour nightly intermittent peritoneal dialysis clearances (abstr). *Perit Dial Bull* 1987;7 (suppl):S79.

34. Twardowski ZJ, Nolph KD, Khanna R, et al. Tidal peritoneal dialysis. In: Avram MM, Giordano C, eds. *Ambulatory Peritoneal Dialysis.* New York: Plenum Medical, 1991:145–149.

35. Glanigan M, Pflederer T, Doyle C, et al. Tidal peritoneal dialysis in children: initial experiences. *Dial Transplant* 1993;22:554–563.

36. Flanigan MJ, Lim VS, Pflederer TA. Tidal peritoneal dialysis: kinetics and protein balance. *Am J Kidney Dis* 1993;5:700–707.

37. Balaskas EV, Izatt S, Chu M, Oreopoulos DG. Tidal volume peritoneal dialysis versus intermittent peritoneal dialysis. *Adv Perit Dial* 1993;9:105–110.

38. Steinhauer HB, Keck I, Lubrich-Birkner I, Schollmeyer P. Increased dialysis efficiency in tidal peritoneal dialysis compared to intermittent peritoneal dialysis. *Nephron* 1991;58:500–501.

39. Quellhorst E, Solf A, Hildebrand U. Tidal peritoneal dialysis (TPD) is superior to intermittent peritoneal dialysis (IPD) in long-term treatment of patients with chronic renal insufficiency (CRI)(abstr). *Perit Dial Int* 1991;11(suppl):217.

40. Lubrich-Birkner I, Wichary R, Schollmeyer P, Steinhauer HB. Ultrafiltration and solute clearances in tidal peritoneal dialysis (TPD) compared to intermittent peritoneal dialysis (IPD)(abstr). *Perit Dial Int* 1992;12(suppl):138.

41. Piraino B, Bernardini J, Bender F. Comparison of clearances (CL) on intermittent peritoneal dialysis (IPD) and tidal peritoneal dialysis (TPD)(abstr). *J Am Soc Nephrol* 1991;2:366.

42. Diaz-Buxo JA, Cruz C, Gotch FA, Advances in end-stage renal diseases 2000. Continuous-flow peritoneal dialysis. Preliminary results. *Blood Purif* 2000;18(4):361–365.

43. Villaroel F, Klein E, Holland F. Solute flux in hemodialysis and peritoneal dialysis membranes. *Trans Am Soc Artif Intern Organs* 1977,23:225–233.

44. Lysaght M. The kinetics of continuous peritoneal diaysis. Doctoral thesis. University of New South Wales, Sydney Australia, 1989.

45. Shinaberger JH, Shear L, Barry KG. Increasing efficiency of peritoneal dialysis. Experience with peritoneal-extracorporeal recirculation dialysis. *Trans Am Soc Arfic Intern Organs* 1965;11:76–82.

46. Kraus MA. Ultrafiltration peritoneal dialysis and recirculating peritoneal dialysis with a portable kidney. *Dial Transplant* 1983;12(5):385–388.

47. Tobe SW, Purcell L, Sokaiphoo CS, et al. High efficiency peritoneal dialysis (HEPF): a new method of performing peritoneal dialysis (PD)(abstr). *Perit Dial Int* 1994;14:S24.

48. Gotch F. Kinetic modeling of continuous flow peritoneal dialysis. *Semin Dial* 2001;14:378–384.

49. Sargent J, Gotch F. Principles and biophysics of dialysis. In: Maher J, eds. *Replacement of Renal Function by Dialysis,* 3d ed. Boston: Kluwer, 1989:87–144.

50. Keshaviah PR, Nolph KD, Van Stone JC. The peak concentration hypothesis: a urea kinetic approach to comparing the adequacy of continuous ambulatory peritoneal dialysis (CAPD) and hemodialysis. *Perit Dial Int* 1989;9:257–260.

51. Gotch F. The current place of urea kinetic modeling with respect to different dialysis modalities. *Nephrol Dial Transplant* 1998;13(suppl 1):S109–S115.

52. Gotch F. Definitions of dialysis dose suitable for comparison of daily hemodiaysis and continuous ambulatory peritoneal dialysis to conventional thrice weekly dialysis therapy. *Hemodial Int* 2004; 8:172–183.

53. Casino F, Lopez F. The equivalent renal urea clearance: a new parameter to assess dialysis dose. *Nephrol Dial Transplant* 1996;11:1574–1581.

54. Depner T. Benefits of more frequent dialysis: lower TAC at the same Kt/V. *Nephrol Dial Transplant* 13:(suppl 6):20–24, 1998.

55. Kooistra M, Vos J, Koomans A, Vos P. Daily home hemodialysis in the Netherlands: effects on metabolic control, haemo-

dynamics, and quality of life. *Nephrol Dial Transplant* 1998; 13:148–152.

56. Tattersall J, De Takats D, Chamney P, et al. The post dialysis rebound: predicting its effect on Kt/V. *Kidney Int* 1992;50: 2091–2102.

57. NKF-K/DOQI Clinical Practice Guidelines for Hemodialysis Adequacy: update 2000. *Am J Kidney Dis* 2001;1(suppl 1): S7-S64.

58. NKF-K/DOQI Clinical Practice Guidelines for Peritoneal Dialysis Adequacy: update 2000. *Am J Kidney Dis* 2001; 1(suppl 1):S65–S136.

59. Gotch F. Kinetic modeling in hemodialysis. In: Nissenson A, Fine R, Gentille E, eds. *Clinical Dialysis*, 3d ed. Stamford, CT: Appleton & Lange, 1984:156–189.

60. Twardowski ZJ. Clinical value of standardized equilibration tests in CAPD patients. *Blood Purif* 1989;7:95–108.

61. Twardowski ZJ, Nolph KD, Khanna R, et al. Peritoneal equilibration test. *Perit Dial Bull* 1987;7:138–147.

62. Twardowski ZJ. The fast peritoneal equilibration test. *Semin Dial* 1990;3:141–142.

63. Adcock A, Fox K, Walter P, Raymond K. Clinical experience and comparative analysis of the standard and fast peritoneal equilibration tests (PET). *Adv Perit Dial* 1993;8:59–61.

64. Teixido J, Borras M, Bonet J, et al. Peritoneal function tests: usefulness of simplified methods. *Adv Perit Dial* 1992;8: 177–180.

65. Davies SJ, Brown B, Bryan J, Russel GI. Clinical evaluation of the peritoneal equilibration test: a population based study. *Nephrol Dial Transplant* 1993;8:64–70.

66. Steiner R, Blakely P, Freidman L, Kaiser J. Reproducibility and relationship of PET data to clinical parameters in CAPD patients. *Perit Dial Int* 1993;13(suppl):S86.

67. Lowrie EG, Lew NL. Death risk in hemodialysis patients: the predictive value of commonly measured variables and an evaluation of death rate differences between facilities. *Am J Kidney Dis* 1990;5:458–482.

68. Burkhart JM, Jorden JR, Rocco MV. Assessment of dialysis dose by measured clearance versus extrapolated data. *Perit Dial Int* 1993;13:184–188.

69. Wolf CJ, Polsky J, Ntoso KA, et al. Adequacy of dialysis in CAPD and cycler PD: the PET is enough. *Adv Perit Dial* 1992;8:208–211.

70. Gotch F, Schoenfeld PY, Gentile DE. The peritoneal equilibration test (PET) is not a realistic measure of peritoneal clearance (PC)(abstr). *J Am Soc Nephrol* 1991;2:361.

71. Blumenkrantz MJ, Kopple JD, Moran JK, Coburn JW. Metabolic balance studies and dietary protein requirements in patients undergoing continuous ambulatory peritoneal dialysis. Kidney Int. 1982;21:849–861.

72. Bergstrom J, Alvestrand A, Lindholm B, Tranaeus A. Relationship between Kt/V and protein catabolic rate is different in continuous peritoneal dialysis and hemodialysis patients (abstr). *J Am Soc Nephrol* 1991;2:358.

73. Coronel F, Tornero F, Macia M, et al. Peritoneal clearances, protein losses and ultrafiltration in diabetic patients after four years on CAPD. *Adv Perit Dial* 1991;7:33–38.

74. Keen ML, Gotch FA. Peritoneal function test as a basis for assessment of adequate therapy and for urea kinetic modeling. *Nieren Hochdruckkranh.* In press.

75. Gotch F, Gentile DE, Schoenfeld PY. CAPD prescription in current clinical practice. *Adv Perit Dial* 1993;9:69–72.

76. Hyme R, Weyers E. Relationship between total body water and surface area in normal and obese subjects. *J Clin Pathol* 1971;1:24:234–238.

77. Cockroft DW, Gault MH. Prediction of creatinine clearance from serum creatinine. *Nephon* 1976;16:31–41.

78. Mitch W, Walzer M. A proposed mechanism for reduced creatinine excretion in severe chronic renal failure. *Nephon* 1978; 21:248–254.

79. Keen ML, Lipps BJ, Gotch FA. The measured creatinine generation rate in CAPD suggests only 78% of prescribed dialysis is delivered. *Adv Perit Dial* 1993;9:73–75.

80. Perez R, Blake P, Spanner E, et al. High creatinine excretion ratio predicts a good outcome in peritoneal dialysis patients. *Am J Kidney Dis* 2000;36:362–367.

Clinical Use of Peritoneal Dialysis

Jose A. Diaz-Buxo

PERITONEAL DIALYSIS: HISTORIC MILESTONES, EVOLUTION, AND CURRENT STATUS

Historic Milestones

The term *peritoneum* derives from the Greek *peritonaion*, meaning "to stretch around." The first known recorded reference to the peritoneal cavity appears in the Ebers papyrus in 1550 BC.[1] However, it is evident that, long before then, the Egyptians became familiar with the sac that envelops the internal abdominal organs during their meticulous separation of the viscera from the rest of the corpse prior to embalmment. Galen and many other prominent physicians of antiquity observed the peritoneum in the open abdomens of injured gladiators. The early anatomists and surgeons described the extent of the peritoneal membrane, named its surfaces and attachments, but did not elaborate on its function or fine structure.

It was not until the discovery of cells that the peritoneal membrane became of physiologic interest to anatomists. The first description of the gross and cellular anatomy of the peritoneum was provided by von Recklinghausen in 1862.[2,3] Shortly afterward, Wegner described the effects of changes in body temperature occurring after intraperitoneal (IP) infusion of solutions of different temperatures.[4] He also reported the effects of concentrated dextrose or glycerin solutions on the volume of outflow obtained in the peritoneal effluent, perhaps the first evidence of osmotic ultrafiltration (UF). Starling and Tubby expanded these observations by studying the bidirectional transfer of molecules across the peritoneal and pleural membranes and demonstrated the rapid absorption of isotonic solutions and slow absorption of serum.[5] By 1920, it had been recognized that, regardless of the infusate's osmolality, the fluid was completely absorbed within 20 hours of infusion.[6–8] These observations led to the administration of IP fluids to infants with severe dehydration when use of the oral route was not possible.[9,10] This was perhaps the first therapeutic use of the peritoneal membrane.

The first quarter of the twentieth century established the physiologic milestones for peritoneal dialysis (PD). There was significant activity in the study of the relationship between osmolality of the fluids and peritoneal ultrafiltration and absorption.[7,11] It was shown that, in addition to water, bidirectional flux of small molecules readily occurred between the peritoneal cavity and the intravascular compartment. The contributions of Orlow, Clark, Putnam, and others confirmed the peritoneal membrane's permeability for sodium and other minerals.[12–16] The concept of osmotic equilibrium between peritoneal fluid and plasma was established by Putnam in 1922; he concluded that mass transfer was driven by passive concentration gradients rather than active membrane transport.[13] Furthermore, Klapp showed that heat applied to the anterior abdominal wall could accelerate the exchange of substances between the IP cavity and the blood compartment.[15] This observation was a precursor to the concept of augmentation dialysis. In 1921, Clark confirmed these findings by using IP infusions of warm solutions, suggesting that the accelerated rate of exchange was a consequence of vasodilatation.[16]

Evolution

Ganter first applied the concept of peritoneal lavage to treat renal insufficiency more than 80 years ago.[17] The initial uremic models consisted of rabbits and guinea pigs subjected to ureteral ligation. IP exchanges lasting 2 to 4 hours were utilized. Although there was moderate absorption of the dialysate due to its hypotonicity relative to uremic plasma, definite clinical improvement was noted in the animals after dialysis. Ganter also reported the first experience with PD for the treatment of a woman with obstructive uropathy. This experience was followed by scattered reports with variable outcomes using the continuous perfusion technique.[18,19]

In 1938, Rhoads used intermittent peritoneal dialysis (IPD) to treat two nephrotic patients.[20] Dwell times of 50 minutes and total dialysate volumes of 6 to 11 L were used. In 1951, Grollman et al. reported their classic work on the use of intermittent peritoneal lavage in uremic dogs and its application to humans.[21,22] The next serious contributions to the clinical use of PD were the recognition of the need for frequent intermittent dialysis, the maintenance of a sterile setting, and the concomitant use of a conservative chronic renal failure (CRF) program consisting of dietary restrictions and nutritional supplements. In 1964, Boen published the first textbook on PD for use in clinical medicine, emphasizing its importance in the treatment of acute renal failure (ARF) and further contributing to the basic physiology, indications, and complications of this technique.[23] Due to the success of hemodialysis (HD) as chronic renal replacement therapy, PD remained dormant for several decades. Nonetheless, interest in PD was renewed by the availability of permanent catheters, commercial dialysate, and automated delivery systems in the 1960s. The novel concept of equilibration dialysis, however, transformed PD into a popular, effective, and acceptable form of renal substitution therapy.[24] The interest in continuous peritoneal dialysis (CPD) and the large number of patients undergoing this therapy have stimulated significant technologic advances

for the provision of dialysis as well as systematic studies of peritoneal transport that are defining the role of PD as renal substitution therapy. The quest for the optimal prescription and dose of dialysis remain an important subject of investigation, generating a vast body of literature in recent years.

Current Status

The growth of CPD is the result of patient satisfaction with therapy, the excellent clinical outcomes obtained during the first few years of therapy, and technologic advances. In 1979, there were fewer than 5000 patients undergoing chronic PD worldwide. In contrast, the world prevalence of dialysis patients is now estimated at 1.14 million, of which 126,000 are treated by PD. The dialysis modality distribution for selected countries is shown in Fig. 16–1. The proportion of patients on PD as a percentage of end-stage renal disease (ESRD) patients varies widely in different countries. At the extremes of this distribution are third world countries, with more than 75 percent of patients on continuous ambulatory peritoneal dialysis (CAPD) and highly industrialized countries with lower proportions. The proportion of PD patients treated by continuous cyclic peritoneal dialysis (CCPD) and other forms of automated PD (APD) has increased more rapidly in recent years and has surpassed the proportion treated with CAPD in a few countries (Fig. 16–2). The growth of APD modalities is probably due to the recognition that certain patients benefit from higher flow, shorter dwell times due to increased peritoneal transport rates, to the adoption of CCPD in the treatment of pediatric patients and in response to adequacy guidelines demanding higher doses.[25,26] Many anuric patients with large body mass require APD to achieve the target doses.[27]

MODALITIES OF PERITONEAL DIALYSIS

Continuous Ambulatory Peritoneal Dialysis

In 1976, Popovich and coworkers conceived the theory of a continuous peritoneal system comprising equilibration PD and a low flow rate.[24] The equilibration peritoneal system allows the continuous presence of dialysate in the peritoneal cavity, interrupted only by the brief periods required for drainage and infusion of new dialysate. The process of transperitoneal equilibration between dialysate and plasma is mostly affected by time of exposure of the dialysate to the peritoneum and the molecular size of the solute. Small molecules such as urea (60 Da) will achieve virtual equilibration within 4 hours, whereas larger molecules such as vitamin B_{12} (1355 Da) accomplish a dialysate-to-plasma ratio of approximately 0.4 during the same time interval.[28] Therefore small molecules in the range of 60 to 500 DA will accomplish rapid equilibration during the first 2 hours of dialysate dwell. Consequently, for small solutes, clear-

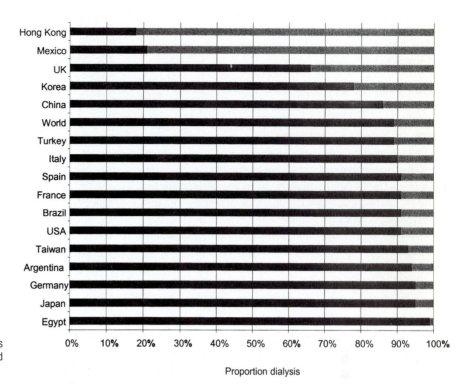

Figure 16–1. Global distribution of dialysis modalities. Black bars denote hemodialysis and gray bars peritoneal dialysis.

ances could be expected to be reduced with dwell times beyond 3 or 4 hours, making continuous equilibration dialysis relatively ineffective. Nevertheless, the continuous nature of the system compensates for this deficiency and allows weekly clearances for small molecules generally superior to those of intermittent peritoneal dialysis (IPD). For large molecules in the range of 500 to 5000 Da, the process of

equilibration continues for long periods of time, favoring continuous equilibration dialysis over IPD. Clearance of these larger solutes will fall proportionately less rapidly with prolonged exchanges of up to 15 hours than will clearances of small solutes.

Protein concentrations in dialysate show a linear increase with time. Net protein removal is essentially depen-

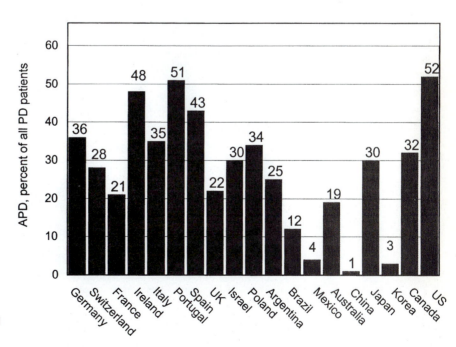

Figure 16–2. Utilization of automated peritoneal dialysis in selected countries.

dent on membrane surface area and permeability.[29] The weekly loss of protein is similar in IPD and continuous long-dwell PD.[28,30,31]

Standard CAPD. The first application of the continuous equilibration dialysis concept was reported by Popovich and Moncrief and referred to as CAPD.[24,32] The technique consists of four or five 2 to 3 L dialysate exchanges, each lasting 4 to 8 hours.[33] Diurnal cycles are shorter, lasting 4 to 6 hours and the nocturnal cycle generally lasting 8 to 10 hours (Fig. 16–3). Approximately 30 to 35 minutes are required for drainage and instillation of the dialysate. The initial technique used 2 L of commercial dialysate in glass bottles delivered via plastic tubing connected to the permanent catheter. Using glass bottles, patients had to disconnect the tubing from the catheter for each dialysate infusion and drainage unless the bottle could be left in place and connected to the tubing until the next instillation. Because of the many connections and disconnections required, the incidence of peritonitis was high (approximately one episode every 8 to 10 patient weeks). Nonetheless, good control of body chemistries and hydration state aroused interest and promoted the development of more convenient and safer techniques.

A major breakthrough occurred with the introduction of dialysate in plastic, disposable, collapsible containers.[34,35] Following the instillation of dialysate into the peritoneal cavity, the plastic bag could be rolled and attached to the body until the end of the prescribed cycle. For drainage, the patient simply unrolled the bag and allowed it to drain by gravity for 15 to 20 minutes. Following complete drainage, the bag was disconnected from the tubing and a

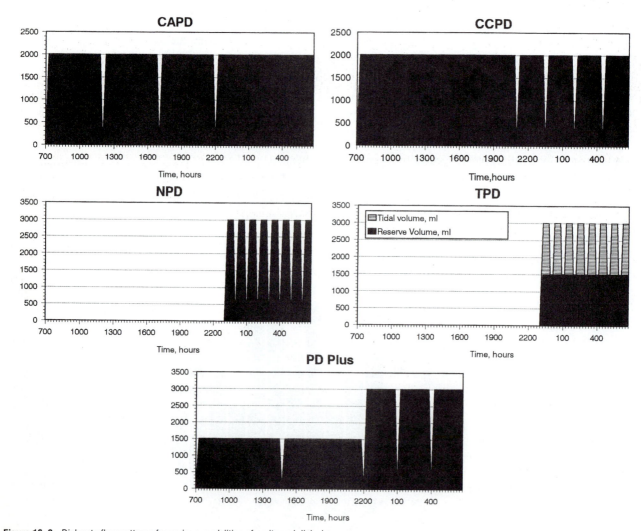

Figure 16–3. Dialysate flow patterns for various modalities of peritoneal dialysis.

new container attached. The new technique allowed convenience and freedom of movement. It also resulted in significant reduction in the number of connections and in incidence of peritonitis. The convenience, efficiency, and competitive costs of CAPD influenced the dramatic growth of this therapy.

The increased number of patients treated with CAPD and the persistent high rate of peritonitis stimulated the development of various connection systems and devices. These devices can be categorized as (1) connectors attached to disposable CAPD bags and transfer sets and (2) devices to sterilize or to connect and disconnect automatically. The first category includes titanium connectors, Luer-locks, friction-fit spikes, and devices with an outer sleeve surrounding the male connector. Sponges impregnated with disinfectant and chambers filled with disinfectant solution for bathing the connecting site have also been incorporated into some of these systems. The second category comprises more complex and sophisticated devices such as in-line filters,[36] sterilizing machines with an ultraviolet light source,[37] heat sterilization, thermic splicing of transfer lines,[38] and mechanical aids for patients with impaired eye-hand coordination. Of these, devices with an ultraviolet source for disinfection and a capability to automatically connect and disconnect proved to be the most popular. Although the impact they made on the rate of peritonitis was marginal, some reports suggested greater influence in lowering peritonitis rates.[33] The training in self-dialysis was also facilitated by most of these systems, and specific patient groups benefited from their availability. The advent of modern disconnect systems removed the need for these devices.

CAPD Y-Set. Notwithstanding the worldwide acceptance of CAPD, several problems persisted that generated significant technical improvements of the standard CAPD system. The high frequency of peritonitis and the inconvenience resulting from wearing an empty bag between exchanges stimulated the design of bagless CAPD systems. A variety of such systems were designed.[39–47] Some were reusable while others were discarded after a single use. Most recently, many systems have eliminated the connection between the bag and the Y-set; these are known as double-bag systems.

The rationale behind Y-sets is twofold: the convenience and freedom from not carrying a bag and a lower rate of peritonitis. From the very beginning, the rates of peritonitis were noted to be particularly low with these types of devices, often dropping below one episode every 2 years. Although most of the clinical experience first took place in Europe,[40–45,48,49] the recent experience in North America has confirmed the superiority of these systems in reducing peritonitis.[33,46,47] Port et al. reported a national study comparing CAPD with standard technique and Y-sets with a large sample of patients from many centers.[33] The standard set had a

peritonitis rate indicator of 9 months per episode, while the Y-set had a rate of 15 months per episode, or an average 67 percent longer interval between episodes of peritonitis.

These in vitro and clinical experiences suggest that the main reason for the lower rate of peritonitis is the direction of flow following a connection.[50,51] The first event to occur when the system is opened is outflow of the used dialysate. It is likely that a potential contamination is flushed by spent dialysis, particularly if the organisms responsible are of low adhesiveness. The experience with CAPD Y-sets has confirmed this hypothesis by showing a significant decrease in peritonitis rates.[40,43,46,47] The in vitro experiences have also confirmed the value of "flush-before-fill" techniques in preventing peritonitis from organisms with low adhesiveness, such as *Staphylococcus epidermidis*.[50,51]

The new double-bag systems incorporate preattached solution and drain bags to the Y-set and retain the flush-before-fill feature. In addition, some systems also use "snap disconnect" and/or disks to dial the direction of dialysate flow.[52] The reported peritonitis rates with these systems have further improved to the range of 0.27 to 0.33 episodes per year.[52]

Automated Peritoneal Dialysis

IPD and Early Developments in APD. In 1962, Boen and associates introduced an automatic PD machine in an attempt to control peritonitis and simplify the provision of chronic PD.[53] This device used a 40-L dialysate container and a closed sterile system that provided 2-L exchanges for 10 hours. This development minimized the time required for clamping and opening the fluid lines and reduced the rate of peritonitis by eliminating the many connections and disconnections necessary for dialysate exchanges with the manual method. In 1966, Lasker designed an automated cycler that provided exchanges with relatively short dwell times of approximately 30 minutes at prescribed time intervals.[54] The peritoneal cycler proved simpler and its smaller size allowed its use at home.

In 1969, automated equipment using reverse osmosis–treated water and a proportioning system to mix the treated water with dialysate concentrate was introduced.[55] It had the advantage of providing large amounts of dialysate at a relatively low cost. Furthermore, treatment could be provided at night while the patient rested, allowing complete freedom of movement during the day. The typical prescription consisted of 10 hours of intermittent dialysis every other night, exchange volumes of 2 L, and dwell times of 15 to 20 minutes for the average adult. Commercial dialysate concentrate with glucose concentrations that ultimately provided 1.5 and 2.5% dialysate glucose was used. Higher glucose concentrations could be attained by adding additional hypertonic glucose to the mixture. Regardless of the complexity of the equipment and the relatively costly and complex maintenance required, for the first time, the reverse osmosis (R/O) system allowed the training of many patients to provide self-PD at home.

Between 1970 and 1976, IPD became widely used, with more than 800 patients treated.[56] Nonetheless, at the peak of interest in IPD, the proportion of patients receiving PD remained low compared with the total population of ESRD patients.[57] The convenience and freedom provided by IPD as well as its relative simplicity permitted many patients to train for home dialysis with or without a partner. The initial enthusiasm and the excellent results obtained by many programs around the world[58–67] led to multiple reports comparing IPD with HD and concluded that it was an effective alternative for HD.[59–63,67]

During the first 2 years of therapy, with a few exceptions, most investigators reported comparable biochemical profiles to those achieved by HD. The early survival rates with IPD proved similar to those obtained in patients treated with HD in the same centers. Tenckhoff reported patients on IPD surviving up to 8 years, many of whom were treated for over 4 years.[65] Diaz-Buxo et al. observed several patients for 4 to 6 years without significant clinical deterioration.[68] These authors reported a patient survival rate of 83 percent after 2 years and a simultaneous technique survival rate of 70 percent.[69] Further analysis of their experience revealed evidence of malnutrition, reductions in hematocrit level, recurrence of metabolic acidosis, and poor control of hydration state after the second year. Most patients transferred to HD due to malnutrition and inadequate dialysis, and the mortality rate escalated between the third and fourth years. Many other centers experienced a significant increase in mortality rate after the second year.[34,35,70–72] The principal cause for the high dropout rate among the adult, nondiabetic population on IPD was inadequate dialysis. The clinical deterioration occurred concomitantly with a reduction in residual renal function (RRF).

In retrospect, it is evident that most of the patients—those with with satisfactory chemistries and good nutritional status—surviving many years while undergoing IPD had several characteristics in common. The majority of patients who did well were females with relatively small body mass who showed compliance with diet and medical therapy and in many instances dialyzed more than 40 h/week. Many of the patients maintained a small but significant RRF. The good results observed during the first year of IPD are most likely due to the additive benefits of residual native renal clearance and peritoneal clearance.

Small molecule clearances in PD are flow-dependent. The peritoneal urea clearance averages 12 mL/min when 1 L/h of dialysate is used and 20 mL/min with 2 L/h. Up to 40 mL/min can be accomplished with dialysate flow rates of 10 to 12 L/h.[73] The typical patient undergoing IPD for 40 h/week can accomplish a total weekly urea clearance of 50 L/week. Therefore small molecule clearances are very limited in IPD when compared with HD and slightly lower than in CAPD or CCPD.

Middle molecule clearances are a function of time of exposure of the solute to the peritoneal membrane and the surface area of the membrane. Because dialysis time is limited to 35 to 40 h/week in a typical IPD program, middle molecule removal is also inferior to that of continuous equilibration dialysis and HD.

IPD should be considered only for the occasional patient with RRF in need of supplemental dialysis; for those awaiting a renal transplant; as temporary therapy while adequate blood access is created for HD; and in chronically debilitated, institutionalized patients requiring in-center PD. Although IPD has been largely replaced by more effective methods of therapy, the early experiences with IPD broadened our knowledge of peritoneal kinetics, prevention and treatment of peritonitis, and general physiology of the peritoneal membrane. Most importantly, IPD established the value of chronic PD as therapy for patients with uremia.

Modern APD. The enthusiasm generated by CAPD in the late 1970s identified problems that stimulated the development of new modalities of APD. Foremost among the problems encountered with CAPD were the inconvenience of performing multiple daily exchanges and the relatively high frequency of peritonitis. These obstacles were particularly limiting in treating pediatric patients. An alternative mode of continuous equilibration dialysis, CCPD, was introduced in 1980.[30,74–76] The anticipated advantages of this new approach were a lower incidence of peritonitis—brought about by a reduction in the number of manual connections required, and the convenience of performing all procedures at home with total freedom during the day while providing continuous equilibration dialysis.

Further experience with chronic PD has identified a significant segment of the population as having high peritoneal transport. These patients enjoy adequate peritoneal clearances but fail to ultrafilter adequately with a continuous equilibration system. Nocturnal intermittent PD (NIPD) has been effectively used in their treatment.[77] The extended use of CAPD and CCPD has also identified patients who require more aggressive therapy due to their body size and loss of RRF. High-flow PD systems—including CCPD with more frequent exchanges, tidal peritoneal dialysis (TPD), hybrids of CAPD and CCPD (PD Plus) and continuous-flow peritoneal dialysis (CFPD)—are being utilized or considered to enhance peritoneal clearances.[78] Figure 16–3 summarizes the dialysate flow patterns of the various APD modalities.

Cyclers. APD is possible only with the use of an automated device capable of delivering a measured volume of dialysate into the peritoneal cavity, providing both a specific dwell of the dialysate in the peritoneal cavity and automated drainage of the spent dialysate. Modern electronics and computerized programs have been used to change the traditional mechanical cyclers into reliable, efficient, versatile devices. Today's cyclers vary from simple, inexpensive, relatively small devices to specialized, highly automated machines with very sophisticated functions (Fig. 16–4).

The early cyclers used gravity for both infusion and drainage of dialysate into and out of the peritoneal cavity. However, it soon became evident that pump assistance for delivery of dialysate from the floor to an overhead bag above the peritoneal cavity both reduced the patient's effort in setting up the equipment and allowed the use of larger bags, which reduced cost. The addition of a pump to deliver dialysate from the ground to a level above the patient can also reduce the size of the cycler.

Active infusion and drainage of dialysate is possible with the use of pumps. This feature also accelerates fluid inflow and outflow and eliminates the cycler stand. Some modern cyclers use cassettes containing two fluid chambers and a series of channels for solution flow. Air pressure is applied to one chamber to generate positive pressure, thus pressing fluid out of the chamber and into the patient or the drain line, depending on the function selected (inflow or prime). Negative pressure draws fluid in from the patient (during drain) or from the heater bag. Similarly, air can be used to open and close the valves that control flow of solution from various sources and destinations. The measurement of fluid volume flowing through the cassette can also be used for volumetric control.[79]

Tubing Sets, Connectors, and Other Disposables. The introduction of disposable, one-step-setup cassettes that include all of the necessary tubing for the cycler has simplified the procedure of setting up the equipment. This has been particularly useful for blind patients and those with impaired coordination due to arthritis or neuropathy. The utilization of an empty solution bag as the next day's drain bag has also resulted in a significant reduction in the cost of disposables and as much as 40 percent less disposable plastic per exchange than with standard cycler sets.

APD has shared the same connectors developed for CAPD to effect connections among dialysis solution bags, the transfer sets, and the peritoneal catheter. The use of external occlusion for the disconnection procedure during APD has markedly simplified the procedure and has probably contributed to a reduced rate of peritonitis.[74,80] The device consists of a simple, disposable plastic clamp to occlude the patient's cycler line distal to its connection with the peritoneal catheter. The line is then cut with sterile scissors. The procedure is simple and safe, prevents accidental contamination (since the system always remains closed), and can be completed in a few seconds by most patients.

Continuous Cyclic Peritoneal Dialysis. Introduced in the late 1970s, CCPD is a virtual reversal of CAPD.[30,76] Multiple exchanges are automatically provided during the night, using variable volume, for a total cycling time of approximately 10 hours. Before disconnection in the morning, a predetermined amount of fluid is left in the peritoneal cavity, which dwells during the day for approximately 14 hours until the next nocturnal session. The typical prescription consists of three to four exchanges during the night, with volumes ranging from 2 to 3 L, and a prolonged dwell time with 1.5 to 2 L of dialysate. Utilization of larger dialysate

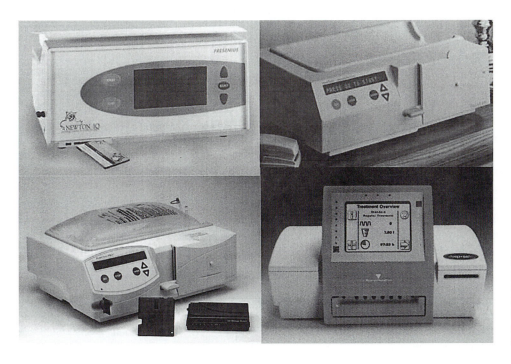

Figure 16–4. Modern peritoneal dialysis cyclers. Top left: Newton IQ (Fresenius Medical Care). Top right: HomeChoice PRO (Baxter Healthcare Corporation). Bottom left: Serena (Gambro). Bottom right: sleep•safe (Fresenius Medical Care).

containers can reduce the number of connections between the bags and the cycler tubing set. The system is opened only once to connect the peritoneal catheter to the cycler line in the evening. Disconnection takes place in the morning, allowing the patient freedom of ambulation without bags.

Ultrafiltration (UF) is achieved by varying the dextrose concentration of the nocturnal bags and/or providing shorter dwell times for the nocturnal exchanges. Because of the prolonged diurnal dwell and significant absorption of dextrose from the peritoneal cavity after 4 to 6 hours of dwell, the use of hypertonic solutions (usually 4.25% dextrose) is recommended. Conversely, the diurnal cycle can be divided by adding an additional exchange and using lower glucose concentrations.[81] This modification of the standard CCPD regimen (PD Plus) not only reduces the use of hypertonic solutions, but significantly enhances small solute removal.[27,82] The diurnal cycle is extremely important in maintaining a steady concentration of nitrogenous waste product concentrations in plasma. The elimination of the diurnal cycle results in a loss of urea clearance in the order of 10 to 18 percent and creatinine clearance of 18 to 25 percent.[83] Large volumes of dialysate during the day may generate significant intraabdominal pressure (IAP) when the patient is sitting and standing. For that reason, it is important to reduce the volume according to patient's tolerance. Most adult patients can tolerate at least 1.5 L during the day without an increase in the frequency of complications such as hernias and gastrointestinal reflux while still providing significant clearance of small and middle size molecules. The elimination of the diurnal cycle results in intermittent therapy and significantly diminishes solute clearance.

The efficiency of CCPD is comparable to that of CAPD. Middle molecule clearances are virtually identical to CAPD, since the clearance is mostly dependent on membrane surface area, time of contact between the peritoneal dialysate and the membrane, and peritoneal permeability. Small molecule clearances can be enhanced by either increasing the dialysate flow rate or the exchange volume.

Nocturnal and Intermittent Peritoneal Dialysis. NPD is IPD performed nightly. The total exchange time is 8 to 10 hours using cycle times of 20 to 60 minutes. Like other schedules of IPD, NPD has the disadvantage of not providing a steady physiologic state. It is also more expensive due to the relatively high dialysate flows and the fact that it requires an automated delivery system capable of infusing large amounts of dialysate during each session. It has, however, several specific indications, which fall into two principal categories: patients with high peritoneal transfer rates (or increased membrane permeability) with poor UF and those suffering complications associated with increased IAP.

Patients suffering from a high peritoneal transport rate achieve glucose and osmotic equilibration within a rela-

tively short period of time. Consequently, UF is impaired due to rapid absorption of glucose. Nevertheless, faster solute equilibration for metabolic waste products also occurs. Therefore the use of short, frequent peritoneal exchanges will result in adequate UF and improved solute removal. Long dwell exchanges result in dialysate absorption and should be avoided. Twardowski et al. have studied the effect of 8-hour NPD using dialysate volumes ranging from 14 to 26 L per session in patients with average, high, and low peritoneal permeability.[84,85] Their results confirm that although the clearances obtained with NPD are inferior to those of CAPD in patients with average peritoneal permeability, clearances of urea and creatinine are superior and generally satisfactory among patients with high peritoneal permeability.

Although the diagnosis of increased peritoneal solute transport rate is a good indication for transferring the patient from CAPD or CCPD to NPD, clinical experience is inconclusive regarding the long-term safety and efficiency of this technique. It has been speculated that patients with progressive increases in peritoneal transport rate may eventually develop peritoneal sclerosis if PD is continued.[86] Therefore it is strongly recommended that patients with very high peritoneal permeability undergoing NPD be closely monitored for changes in transport rates.

Patients suffering from hernias, bladder or uterine prolapse, intractable low back pain, restrictive lung disease, severe cardiovascular instability, gastrointestinal reflux, and/or abdominal discomfort associated with the infusion of dialysate may benefit from NPD, since the abdominal cavity is kept drained during the day and the IAP generated by dialysate at night is significantly lower.[83] Whenever possible however, a diurnal cycle with whatever volume of dialysate is tolerated should be used in order to enhance larger molecule clearance.

Tidal Peritoneal Dialysis. TPD was first introduced in 1978 as reciprocating PD to enhance clearances by improving mixing of the PD fluid and reducing the nondialytic transit time through the creation of a tidal flow.[87] TPD consists of an initial infusion followed by a variable dwell and a partial drain of solution (Fig. 16–5). A reserve volume (RV) is left in the peritoneal cavity until the final cycle. A tide is created by the serial partial infusions and drains. Several reports suggested better small solute clearances when compared to CAPD, CCPD, and IPD.[88–93] However, when exchange volume and dialysate flow rates were controlled, TPD did not show any superiority over intermittent modalities[94–99] TPD could be considered an intermediate phase between the intermittent and the continuous techniques. As the ratio of tidal volume (TV) to total exchange volume (V_{ip}) diminishes, the tides become smaller and the flow eventually becomes continuous (Fig. 16–6). Theoretically, one would expect a lower TV/V_{ip} to be associated with better clearances,

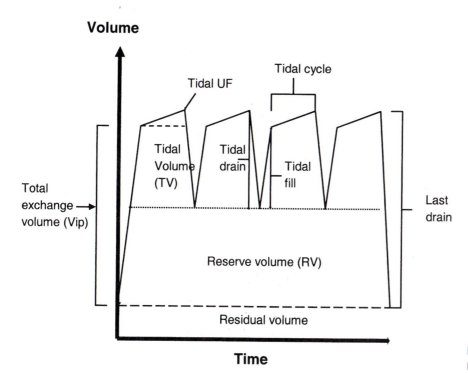

Figure 16-5. Schematic representation of a tidal peritoneal dialysis flow pattern.

since they more closely resemble CFPD, known to enhance small solute clearance.[100] In practice, however, the best clearances are observed with a $TV/V_{ip} = 0.5$.[101] The discrepancies between theory and practice and the apparent limitations of TPD may be due to the poor mixing of dialysate achieved with conventional catheters and lost dialytic time while the solution is in transit. Most investigators are of the opinion that TPD using conventional catheters has little to offer over other forms of automated IPD techniques. Some clinicians have reserved its use for patients with poor catheter outflows; however, it is difficult to justify its higher cost based on solute removal profiles.

Continuous-Flow Peritoneal Dialysis. The continuous-flow technique attracted the attention of the pioneers of PD.[102,103] It employs two catheters or a double-lumen catheter to pro-

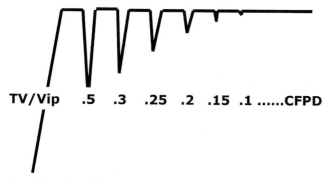

Figure 16-6. Illustration of various tidal volumes (TV) to total exchange volume (V_{ip}) ratio. As the ratio diminishes, the tides become smaller and the flow eventually becomes continuous.

vide continuous inflow of solution via one catheter and simultaneous outflow through the other. The mechanical principles are (1) elimination of the nondialytic transit time, (2) maintenance of a fixed V_{ip} by controlling the inflow and outflow of solution, and (3) use of a high dialysate flow rate (DFR) limited only by the catheter flow. Theoretically, such a system should improve mixing with a properly designed catheter and provide effective peritoneal clearances (Kp) close to the mass transfer coefficient (MTC).

In 1965, Shinaberger et al. designed a simple experiment using two catheters, conventional hemodialysis equipment to regenerate the spent peritoneal dialysate, and peritoneal dialysate flow rates (Qp) between 120 and 300 mL/min.[104] They observed Kp_{urea} of 46 to 125 mL/min and similar improvement in creatinine and phosphorus clearances compared to IPD. This experience stimulated various investigators to perform CFPD using diverse techniques for solution generation and clinical protocols.[105–112] Despite promising results, progress was halted due to limited technology and economic constraints.

The main limitations of CFPD are the need for very large volumes of solution as well as adequate catheters to obtain good mixing of fluid in the peritoneal cavity and minimal recirculation. Various methods for solution generation or regeneration of spent dialysate have been used, including fresh solution in standard bags, large batches of solution, proportioning systems to mix reverse osmosis (RO)-treated water with dialysate concentrate, on-line preparation of dialysate using hemodiafiltration technology, or dialysate regeneration by sorbents or HD technique.[113] The latter method simply uses a standard HD machine and filter, circulating the spent peritoneal dialysate through the "blood circuit."[114] In other words, the spent dialysate is dialyzed against a standard bicarbonate-based hemodialysate. The advantages of this method are that the technology is readily available, the priming PD solution is soon converted into a bicarbonate-based solution, and high flows can be achieved at a modest cost.

Double-lumen peritoneal access has presented a significant challenge. The catheter must be of sufficient diameter to allow dialysate flows in the range of 200 to 300 mL/min but small enough to be cosmetically acceptable. The design must provide adequate mixing with minimal recirculation of dialysate. This has led to various designs and practices: two conventional peritoneal catheters placed in opposite lower abdominal quadrants[100]; a single conventional catheter used with a "single-needle HD device"[115]; double-lumen catheters with internal limbs of different lengths and configurations[116–118] designed to improve mixing; fluted catheters intended to enhance mixing[119]; catheters with diffusers in the proximal IP segment used for infusion; and long tubular segments located in the pelvis used for outflow.[120] The clinical experience is insufficient to determine whether any of these will prove adequate for use with CFPD.

SELECTION OF THERAPY

Selection between HD and PD

Forty years after HD became established as chronic renal substitution therapy and more than 20 years after PD became clinically feasible, we still have no consensus on the definite indications for one or the other. For practical reasons, no controlled, randomized studies have been performed to establish the relative merits of these therapies. The utilization of HD and PD varies widely globally and within specific countries. At the end of 2001, HD remained the more frequent dialysis treatment modality with approximately 89 percent of all dialysis patients worldwide (1,015,000 patients) compared to PD with only 11 percent (126,000 patients).[121] PD growth rates in 2001 were an average of 5 percent below those of HD. The marked variation in patient distribution is shown in Fig. 16–1. Various important determinants of selection between HD and PD have been identified (Table 16–1) and deserve consideration.

Patient Choice. Patient choice should be considered the most important factor in the selection of dialytic therapy. Unfortunately, patient choice is complicated by its dependency on many other factors. Foremost among them is predialytic education on dialysis modality selection. Proper education before the start of dialysis affects dialysis modality selection. Multiple studies have shown that when patients are given proper information on dialytic options, many

TABLE 16–1. DETERMINANTS OF SELECTION BETWEEN HEMODIALYSIS AND PERITONEAL DIALYSIS

Patient choice
Early referral
Physician and nurse bias
Residual renal function
Comorbidity
Survival
Quality of life
Cost and nonmedical factors

more choose PD than when no information is given.[122–129] In all of these series, the proportion of patients selecting PD was significantly higher than the prevalent utilization of PD for that particular country. Patient choice is also influenced by the availability of services, desire for independence, the ability to assume self-care, social and family support, home and environmental conditions conducive to adequate self-care, and economic factors. Various studies have identified several predictors of dialysis modality choice favoring PD: younger age, white race, married status, predialysis counseling, employment status, fewer comorbid conditions, and greater distance to hemodialysis center.[126,129,130]

Early Referral. Early referral to a renal team provides the time necessary to educate the patient on options of therapy and the cause and prevention of uremic complications. The experience from the USRDS Wave 2 study showed that patients selecting PD were exposed to nephrologic care earlier and more often participated in deciding their mode of treatment.[131] When dialysis is urgently required, there is little time for patient education; consequently, most patients are started and maintained on HD.[127]

Physician and Nurse Bias. Physician or nurse bias is an influential factor in selection of dialytic therapy. Previous training and continuous education and experience with PD, the availability of the infrastructure required for patient training, institutional support, and reimbursement for professional care affect the physician's comfort with PD. The reimbursement for professional services according to modality of therapy varies considerably in different countries and could well influence physicians' preferences and the time devoted to predialytic education.[132] Nephrologists in the United States and Canada have been polled regarding their opinions on the optimal utilization of HD and PD.[133,134] Their opinions were mostly influenced by patient preference, quality of life, morbidity, and mortality and not by reimbursement. In Canada, the actual vs. expressed optimal utilization of modality are very close, while in the United States they are markedly different. The results suggest that U.S. nephrologists would support more PD and home HD but have not done so, suggesting a more complex set of factors influencing their actions.

Residual Renal Function. Residual renal function is and should be an important determinant of modality selection. As will be seen later, the degree of RRF is an important determinant of patient survival. If PD can preserve renal function better than HD, it would be reasonable to assume a significant advantage in selecting PD as first therapy upon reaching ESRD. Various studies have shown a strong correlation between total small solute clearances and survival, which is mostly attributable to the renal contribution, but not to the peritoneal contribution to solute removal.[135–139] The apparent lack of correlation between peritoneal clearance (dose of PD) and survival is difficult to explain but may be due to the overwhelming benefits of RRF (regulatory and endocrine renal contributions) that may mask the peritoneal contribution to clearance or to the fact that in order to show a benefit from peritoneal clearance, much larger doses than those used clinically are necessary. Among anuric patients treated with PD in a single study, a statistically significant correlation between dose and survival has been reported.[140] The implications of these observations are evident: patients with RRF should fare better on PD than patients with anuria; less demanding PD prescriptions can be used for very large patients with sufficient RRF; and patients with RRF could save procedural time and funds by initiating PD therapy in a gradual manner to achieve the standards of adequacy while they enjoy sufficient renal function.[141]

PD has been reported to preserve RRF better than HD in several studies.[142–149] The factors potentially responsible for this better preservation of RRF among PD patients are hemodynamic stability, less fluctuations in osmotic load and intravascular volumes, stable glomerular capillary pressure, chronic mild volume overload, lower protein intakes, and reduced nephrotoxicity from blood-membrane interactions. However, not all investigators have observed better preservation of RRF among PD patients.[149,150] Differences in practice, patient selection, and the use of biocompatible HD membranes may be responsible for the discrepant results. Actually, the authors attest to the use of biocompatible membranes and ultrapure water in their HD population. In addition, Lang et al. observed a significantly higher preservation of RRF in HD patients on polysulfone vs. cuprophane membranes, indicating the possible role of biocompatibility—such as less generation of nephrotoxic substances by the membrane.[148]

Another important consideration is the possibility that PD may retard the progression of renal failure. In a small retrospective study, Berlanga et al. tested whether PD influences the natural course of the progression of CRF in humans.[151] Their investigation included 14 patients with predialysis follow-up longer than 12 months, renal creatinine clearance 20 mL/min or more at the start of predialysis follow-up, follow-up while on PD longer than 6 months, and renal creatinine clearance above 0 m/min at the start of PD. The main outcome measure was RRF calculated as renal creatinine clearance. A lower mean rate of decline of RRF was observed during PD than during the predialysis period ($-0.06 + 0.16$ vs. $-0.94 + 0.74$ mL/min/month, $p < 0.0005$). The rate of decline in renal creatinine clearance was faster in every patient during the predialysis period than during his or her time on PD. These preliminary data support the hypothesis that PD may contribute to the slowing of the natural progression of renal disease in humans as it does in rodents. Prospective studies involving a larger number of patients are needed to settle the question.

Aside from dialytic modality, other predictors of loss of RRF among new dialysis patients have been identified in recent years. Female gender, nonwhite race, prior history of diabetes mellitus, prior history of congestive heart failure, and time to follow-up were predictive of RRF loss in a large study using a national random sample of PD and HD patients.[152] Treatment with PD, higher serum calcium, use of angiotensin-converting enzyme inhibitors, and use of calcium channel blockers were independently associated with decreased risk of RRF loss. The observation of demographic groups at risk and potentially modifiable factors and therapies have generated testable hypotheses regarding therapies that may preserve RRF among ESRD patients.

Comorbidity. Comorbidity has a marked influence on patient outcome. Several studies have concluded that the main differences in survival observed between HD and PD, the variable survival rates observed in specific countries, and the differences in survival between nations and series are highly dependent on the frequency and severity of comorbid factors. Valuable data have been obtained from many clinical trials that could be favorably used in the selection of dialytic therapy in order to improve patient outcome. Among the most ominous predictors of death among dialysis patients are hypoalbuminemia and malnutrition.[153] PD patients are often severely hypoalbuminemic and malnourished at the initiation of dialysis due to diabetes and uremia. In addition, PD patients are at higher risk of malnutrition due to constant protein losses in the dialysate effluent, which are significantly higher among high peritoneal transporters and during episodes of peritonitis. It is imperative to screen for malnutrition and to take it into serious consideration during the dialytic selection process.[154] If PD is selected, the patient's nutritional status must be closely monitored and proper nutritional supplements recommended when malnutrition is present.

Other conditions that often make PD difficult or even impossible are extensive previous abdominal surgeries, stomas, and conditions related to and aggravated by increased IAP (gastroesophageal reflux, back pain, hemorrhoids, uterine prolapse, severe obstructive lung disease, and hernias).

Survival. Patient survival is not an important consideration in the initial selection of dialytic therapy. Many registry, multicenter, and single-center reports comparing survival rates between PD and HD have provided similar, lower, or even better outcomes for PD. In order to accurately compare patients on HD and PD, it is necessary to adjust for patient selection (age, sex, race, education, compliance, and body mass), comorbid conditions, quality of care, vintage (time at which dialysis was initiated), period of time on dialysis, and dose of dialysis. In addition, there are factors that are more difficult to quantitate, such as background mortality among certain ethnic groups. One important variable that is possible to measure but seldom considered in this analysis is the delivered dose of dialysis. Keshaviah et al. compared survival between HD and PD patients based on matched doses of delivered therapy; they observed that carefully matching the therapies with delivered Kt/V resulted in little difference in the survival outcome of the patients.[155] Another important variable to be considered in judging the published results comprises the differences in statistical analysis. This is best illustrated by two studies using national mortality rates for PD and HD extracted from the USRDS annual reports from 1987 to 1993.[156] When incident patients and those with prior transplant were used, no difference in relative risk (RR) of death was found. Unlike previous studies restricted to prevalent-only patients,[157] this national study of both prevalent and incident patients found little or no difference in overall mortality between PD and HD.

In an attempt to understand and resolve these discrepancies, an exhaustive literature search and metanalysis was performed to compare survival in HD and PD patients using published data from both registry and nonregistry studies.[158] The study was based on data from 82 published nonregistry studies, 55 published registry studies, and two registry reports, which were censored for modality switches, transplants, and dropouts and unadjusted for case mix. The results were inconclusive because survival and mortality outcomes varied with the data sources and formats for outcomes analyzed. Although limited data suggested that differences in case mix may contribute to differences in survival outcomes, adjustments for case mix (predialysis comorbid conditions, adequacy of dialysis, and other important patient level covariates) were not possible because of the paucity of available data. These findings highlight the limitations inherent in current literature reports.

At present, it is reasonable to conclude that the survival of PD and HD patients during the first few years of therapy are comparable assuming similar patient selection and quality of therapy. After the first 4 years of dialysis and

especially among anuric patients, HD has a survival advantage.

Fewer Viral Infections. The rate of seroconversion of hepatitis C has been reported to be 0.15 per patient-year for HD patients vs. 0.03 for PD patients, resulting in a hazard ratio of 5.7. The risk of seroconversion for hepatitis B after 2 years was 38.9 percent for HD vs. 1.5 percent for PD.[159] These differences could not be explained by the rate of blood transfusion. Studies using serotyping suggest that the major cause is environmental and not related to transfusions.[160–162] Patients on chronic dialysis are at increased risk of acquiring nosocomially transmitted hepatitis. The clinical consequences are particularly devastating among transplanted patients. Compared to HD, PD patients have been reported to have a lower incidence of hepatitis B, C, and G. The total prevalence of hepatitis G has been reported to be slightly higher in HD patients (15.4 percent) as compared to PD patients (10.3 percent).[163] Multiple blood transfusions should be considered the main factor in the transmission of this viral disease. We must consider however, that most or all HD patients included in these series were being treated in center and not at home.

Better Renal Transplant Outcomes. Several studies have shown a lower incidence of delayed graft function, infection,[164] and acute renal failure[165] as well as better immediate recovery of renal function[166,167] among transplanted PD patients when compared to those transplanted while on HD. Graft thrombosis rate seems to be unaffected by the prior mode of dialysis.[168] PD has been recommended for the treatment of delayed graft function. PD can be undertaken with a small risk of peritonitis and other PD-related complications.[168] However, late renal transplant failure is considered an adverse prognostic factor for initiation of PD.[169] Aside from the multiple factors associated with a late transplant failure, including the devastating effects of aggressive immunosuppression therapy, it has been reported that these patients also tend to exhibit high peritoneal transport rates.[170]

Quality of Life. Several reports have addressed the potential advantages of PD on preservation of quality of life (QOL). However, it is impossible to differentiate the actual influence of PD per se against the home factor and other circumstances that affect the decision to embrace self-care. In a large cross-sectional study, Diaz-Buxo et al. showed comparable QOL scores using the SF-36.[171] HD and PD patients scored similarly for scales reflecting physical processes. PD patients scored higher for mental processes, but only after statistical adjustment for laboratory measures. Scores on scales reflecting physical processes were worse, and those reflecting mental processes were better among CCPD than CAPD patients. HD and CAPD scores were similar. CCPD patients perceived themselves as more physically impaired but better adjusted than HD or CAPD patients. These descriptive data show that perception of QOL among PD and HD patients is similar before adjustment, but PD patients score higher for mental processes with adjustment. CCPD patients score worse for physical function and better for mental function than either CAPD or HD patients. We cannot, however, exclude the influence of therapy selection.

Morris and Jones[172] and Merkus et al.[173] reported improved QOL among CAPD patients compared to those on in-center HD. The latter reported lower levels of QOL among HD compared to PD patients on physical functioning, role-functioning, emotional factors, mental health, and pain. However, on the multivariate analysis, they could demonstrate an impact of dialysis modality only on mental health. Gudex et al. evaluated cohorts from the general population, transplanted patients, center HD, home HD, and CAPD patients regarding social, leisure, and sex life.[174] The various groups scored in the following order from best to worst: general population, transplanted patients, home HD, CAPD, and center HD.

Cameron et al. performed a metanalysis to compare emotional distress and psychological well-being across renal replacement therapies and examined whether differences could be explained by treatment modalities, case mix, or methodologic rigor.[175] Successful renal transplantation was associated with lower distress and greater well-being than center HD and lower distress and greater well-being than experienced by CAPD patients. CAPD patients were characterized by greater well-being than center HD patients, and center HD was associated with greater distress than home HD. The analysis suggested that the published findings indicating differential QOL across therapies may be attributable to valid differences in effective renal replacement, reduced medical complications, and lifestyles afforded by these treatment modalities; case-mix differences in the patient samples; or both of these alternative explanations.

Employment status has been shown to be better for PD than for HD patients.[172,173,176,177] Once again, it is impossible to determine whether this is attributable to the physical benefits of therapy, the freedom afforded by PD, or to patient selection. The likely answer is the multifactorial effect of all these circumstances.

Cost of Therapy. The size of the ESRD population has been expanding at a rate of 7 percent per year. Total therapy cost per patient per year in the United States is approximately $66,000. Assuming that this figure is a reasonable global average, the present annual worldwide cost of maintenance ESRD therapy, excluding renal transplantation, exceeds $75 billion U.S. dollars.[178] If current trends in ESRD prevalence continue, the ESRD population will exceed 2 million patients by the year 2010 and the aggregate cost of treating ESRD during the coming decade will exceed $1 trillion.

Such estimates certainly favor the most cost-effective dialytic therapies.

The cost of delivering therapy must be precisely defined in order to compare its impact on the payer, the patient, and society. If only the cost of supplies and provision of dialytic services is considered, PD in general and CAPD specifically must be considered significantly lower in cost in most markets. Some exceptions have been reported in developing Asian countries, where the cost of supplies for PD is sometimes higher than for HD.[179] The major reason for the variation in utilization of PD worldwide does not seem to relate to discrepancies in the incidence of ESRD but to economic factors. There is a strong correlation between incidence of new ESRD and the gross national product (GNP) for most countries.[180] There is also a good correlation between national health care expenditures per capita and incidence/prevalence of ESRD. Lo has analyzed these issues and related them to the utilization of PD, concluding that the less spending on health care, the higher penetration of PD in developed countries, where PD is less expensive; but this is not the case in developing countries, where PD is often more expensive.[179]

There is solid evidence that PD is less expensive than HD in most regions, particularly during the early stages of ESRD, when RRF is still present. Furthermore, the prolongation of RRF may further reduce the cumulative cost.[181] Figure 16–7 provides a cost comparison for HD and PD in the United States from three different series.[182–184] The results show a uniform and significantly higher cost for HD of approximately $15,000, mostly attributable to higher cost of hospitalization and erythropoietin therapy. The bulk of this increase is related to the creation and maintenance of vascular access for HD. Most of these figures have been obtained from center HD and CAPD patients. If APD patients are added to the case mix, the cost of supplies and equipment will increase according to the penetration of APD in that particular market. All factors considered, PD has a cost advantage over HD in most regions.

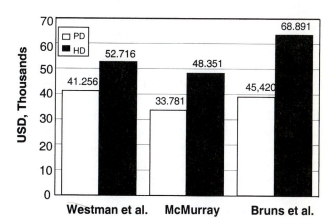

Figure 16–7. Cost comparisons for peritoneal dialysis and hemodialysis in the United States.

Other Nonmedical Factors. Aside from financial considerations, resource availability, and caregiver biases, there are other significant nonmedical factors that affect the selection of PD as renal replacement therapy.[185] Social mores, sociocultural habits, and religious beliefs may have a major influence in the selection of dialytic therapy. It is important to know each patient in depth and consider his or her background and social circumstances before selecting a specific therapy.

PERITONEAL DIALYSIS SOLUTIONS

Evolution

The composition of peritoneal dialysis fluids (PDF) parallels our understanding of physiology, peritoneal transport, biocompatibility, and manufacturing processes. The first infusion into the peritoneal cavity of a substance for therapeutic purposes recorded in the medical literature appears in 1744, when Warrick used red wine as peritoneal lavage fluid for the treatment of ascites.[186] Ganter used plain physiologic saline for his first PD treatment.[17] Heusser improved UF by the addition of dextrose.[18] Rhoads added lactate to peritoneal dialysate as a source of bicarbonate in 1938.[20] By 1969, Boen was mixing solutions containing acetate 35 meq/L, sodium 130 to 140 meq/L, and glucose in concentrations ranging from 1.5 to 5 g/dL—a formulation that remained popular for several decades.[187] The slow rate of change in the composition of PDF was due to three factors: relatively good patient tolerance of the available dialysate, manufacturing limitations, and poor understanding of the effects of the chemical composition and physical characteristics of PDF on peritoneal microcirculation and mass transport mechanisms. The increasing number of patients successfully treated with PD, the high proportion of diabetics, and the possible deleterious effects of the currently used formulations on peritoneal permeability dictated the need for change.

Formulation

PDF is available in containers varying in volume from 250 mL for pediatric use to 6 L for cycler use. Most bags are made of polyvinyl chloride (PVC). Some new solutions are distributed in polyurethane or polyolifine containers. The latter has the advantage of being plasticizer-free; moreover, upon incineration, it releases only water and carbon dioxide, thus improving bio- and ecologic compatibility. The composition of materials used for PDF containers, their potential toxicity, and potential environmental effects have been extensively reviewed by Feriani et al.[188] Table 16–2 summarizes the composition of the various commercial PDFs.

TABLE 16–2. COMPOSITION OF PERITONEAL DIALYSIS SOLUTIONS

Solute	Concentration Range
Glucose (percent)	1.5–4.25
Polyglucose (percent)	7.5
Sodium (meq/L)	132–141
Potassium (meq/L)	0
Calcium (meq/L)	2.5–3.5
Magnesium (meq/L)	0.5–1.5
Lactate (meq/L)^a	35–40
Bicarbonate (meq/L)^a	34–39

^{a}A solution may contain lactate, bicarbonate, or a combination of both.

Osmotic Agents. The ideal osmotic agent should be effective in inducing UF, biocompatible, nonabsorbable or totally inert, easy to manufacture, and inexpensive. Many substances have been used, but none has challenged glucose and its derivatives in terms of cost and relative safety. At present, only glucose- and polyglucose-containing solutions are commercially available.

Glucose. Fluid removal during PD depends on the creation of an osmotic gradient between dialysate and plasma. Glucose has been added to dialysate since the early experimental days and has proven effective as an osmotic agent; it is relatively safely metabolized and inexpensive. However, glucose-containing PDFs have certain disadvantages. The low pH of the dialysate required to prevent the glucose from caramelizing during sterilization may be responsible for inflow pain in some patients. The low pH has also been shown to inhibit polymorphonuclear phagocytosis and to interfere with intracellular killing of bacteria.[189] More recent evidence has shown that the presently used pH (around 5.5) is associated with the generation of glucose degradation products (GDPs) during heat sterilization.[190,191] These GDPs may be ultimately responsible for the deleterious effects of conventional solutions on peritoneal cell function and membrane survival (see "Biocompatibility"). Higher glucose concentrations have also been shown to inhibit the respiratory burst of peritoneal phagocytes, thus reducing effective phagocytosis.[192] Other studies have also suggested that hyperosmolality has a toxic effect on peritoneal cells and negatively affects phagocytic function.[193,194]

The high rate of peritoneal absorption of glucose, as observed when 4.25% dextrose solutions are used, may lead to undesirable nutritional and metabolic consequences, such as hypertriglyceridemia, hyperinsulinemia, obesity, and marked fluctuations in blood glucose levels in diabetic patients. A 2-L peritoneal exchange with a dwell time of 4 to 6 hours with a 1.5 or 4.25% glucose concentration provides approximately 200 to 600 mL of ultrafiltrate volume, respectively.[30,195] The caloric load provided by the absorbed glucose supplies approximately one-third of the patient's daily caloric intake.[35,196] This extra caloric load often results in obesity, hyperinsulinemia, and lipid abnormalities. The carbohydrate load provided by the chronic absorption of glucose may also result in loss of appetite and decreased protein intake.

Diabetic patients undergoing PD may be particularly affected by the continuous absorption of glucose and poorly controlled glycemia. In the presence of hyperglycemia, the metabolism of glucose may shift from the hexose glucose-6-phosphate pathway to the alternate polyol pathway, resulting in intracellular accumulation of fructose, with its potential deleterious effects.[197,198] Because of these concerns, the search for alternatives to dextrose for osmotic UF in PD has been intensified.

Polyglucose. Glucose polymers are derived from cornstarch and used in mixtures of oligopolysaccharides of variable chain length. The molecular weight (MW) varies depending on the number of glucose units, with a typical mean MW of 15,000 to 17,000 Da. The glucose molecules are linked by $\alpha1$–4 alpha glucosidic bonds (more than 90 percent) and $\alpha1$–6 alpha glucosidic bonds (5 to 10 percent). The $\alpha1$–6 links limit the complete enzymatic degradation of glucose polymer in humans.[199] The typical solution contains polyglucose 7.5%, sodium 133 meq/L, calcium 1.75 mmol/L, magnesium 0.25 mmol/L, chloride 96 meq/L, and lactate 40 mmol/L.

Polyglucose is absorbed mainly through lymphatic flow. The absorption of polyglucose has been reported to be 14.4 percent at 6 hours and 28.1 percent at 12 hours.[200] The oligosaccharide fraction with chain length less than G12 are absorbed at rates similar to that of glucose (75 to 80 percent), whereas the remaining fraction greater than G12 are absorbed slowly (20 to 30 percent of the initial load).[201] While the absorption of polyglucose is thought to occur mainly by the lymphatic flow, fractions with small MW undoubtedly diffuse across the peritoneal membrane. The extent to which larger fractions are degraded in the peritoneal cavity into relatively small molecules capable of diffusion across the membrane has not been fully characterized. The degradation of glucose polymers within the peritoneal cavity has been considered negligible in ex vivo studies that may not necessarily reflect the in vivo condition.[202]

Absorbed oligosaccharides are hydrolysed in plasma by α-amylases to maltose (G2), maltotriose (G3), and isomaltose (α l to 6 G2).[203] The presence of larger oligosaccharides (G4 to >G9) in plasma, in addition to di- and trisaccharides, suggests either that some oligosaccharides are not degraded in the plasma of uremic patients or that the metabolic capacity of the plasma α-amylases is exceeded.

Davies incubated plasma samples of CAPD patients treated with glucose containing solutions in vitro with 5 mg/mL of glucose polymer.[204] A decline of high-MW frac-

tions and a rise in G2 to G9 molecules was observed. Although this investigation suggests rapid degradation of polymers in plasma, the steady-state level of larger oligosaccharides in plasma of CAPD patients treated with polyglucose for at least 1 month supports the hypothesis of limited degradation potential in plasma.[203–205]

The MIDAS study revealed that, after 1 month of polyglucose treatment, elevated steady-state levels of oligosaccharides were maintained.[203–205] Maltose (G2) reached levels 30 times higher than before exposure to polyglucose and even higher elevations of the G3 to G9 fraction, reaching values 90 times higher than baseline. This observation lends further support to the possibility of limited degradation of higher-MW oligosaccharides by α-amylases into maltose (G2) in blood, depending on residual renal function. Despite the magnitude of these elevations of oligosaccharides in plasma, the clinical consequences are not clear.

The metabolism of maltose, isomaltose (α l to 6 G2) and maltotriose, is limited by the absence of maltase activity (splitting of G2 into G1) in the human circulation.[206,207] Both maltase[208] and debranching enzyme (responsible for splitting the α l to 6 linkage of isomaltose) activities[209] are relatively high in renal tissue of healthy subjects and contribute to the elimination of intravenously infused disaccharides.[206] However, in renal failure, these enzymes are absent or reduced, causing the accumulation of maltose, isomaltose, and maltotriose in the blood and other tissues. Icodextrin may not be suitable for use in more than one daily exchange due to progressive accumulation.

Isoosmolar polyglucose solutions achieve peritoneal UF by colloid osmosis, allowing net UF during long dwell exchanges due to slow absorption. The UF achieved after 12 hours is superior to that of glucose 4.25%, particularly for patients with high peritoneal transport.[210,211] Isoosmolar glucose polymer solutions have been shown to achieve sustained peritoneal UF for periods of up to 12 hours with minimal insulin response.[212,213] Amici et al., in preliminary studies, report that the chronic use of icodextrin in the long nighttime dwell can reduce serum insulin levels and increase insulin sensitivity in CAPD patients.[214] Although the percentage absorption of total glucose polymer infused from the peritoneal cavity is lower than that of comparable glucose solutions, the total amount of carbohydrate absorbed can be greater, providing a higher caloric load.[215] Table 16–3 compares the caloric load provided by various solutions during an 8-hour dwell.[216]

The use of commercially available polyglucose solutions has been associated with various side effects and manufacturing problems. Hypersensitivity to polyglucose has been reported.[217–221] The reactions include widespread maculopapular rashes, exfoliative dermatitis, vesicular rash, and transient scaly rashes. The prevalence of these skin reactions varies between 0.6 and 15 percent.[217,219,221] The patho-

TABLE 16–3. CALORIC LOAD CONTRIBUTED BY GLUCOSE AND POLYGLUCOSE

	Icodextrin, 7.5%	Dextrose, 2.5%	Dextrose, 4.25%
Grams CHO/2L	150 g	45.4 g	77.2 g
Percent absorbed/ 8-hour dwell	~ 25%	~ 86%	~ 86%
~ Grams CHO absorbed	37.5	39	66
~ Kcal per dwell	150	156	266

SOURCE: Based on Gokal et al.,[216] with permission.

genesis of these reactions is not well characterized. Given the structural similarities between icodextrin and the naturally occurring glucose polymer (dextran), an allergic reaction should be considered. The glucose units in polyglucose are mostly connected by α 1 to 4 links and 5 to 10 percent by α 1 to 6 links, while dextrans are mostly α 1 to 6 links. Dextrans are well known to cause allergic reactions, including anaphylaxis. A similar mechanism for hypersensitivity with polyglucose could be invoked based on the same or similar epitopes and antibodies. Aanen et al. studied patients exposed to polyglucose PDF with no problems and with rashes or peritonitis after exposure to the solution and compared them to a control group of patients on glucose-based PDFs.[222] They measured the concentration of dextran antibodies in the three groups and failed to correlate the concentration with the presence or absence of side effects. This is similar to dextran hypersensitivity, where only severe anaphylactoid reactions are related to hypersensitivity. The authors concluded that dextran antibodies are present in some patients never exposed to polyglucose and that chronic exposure may lead to higher levels in some patients, but no relationship with skin rashes or culture-negative peritonitis could be established.

Recurrent culture-negative peritonitis associated with exposure to polyglucose PDF has been well documented.[223–233] The reactions are characterized by cloudy fluid, a significant increase in peritoneal white blood cell (WBC) count, and abdominal pain, with or without diarrhea and vomiting. The episodes are recurrent with rechallenge in some patients and may occur early in the course of treatment or many months later. The etiology of these episodes has not been fully characterized. However, it is likely that peptidoglycans are responsible for the development of sterile peritonitis as they have been found in increased concentrations in the PDF of some afflicted patients. Peptidoglycans are components of the bacterial wall and have a MW between 1000 and 20,000 daltons. Thus they are difficult to eliminate with the currently used techniques. Other potential causes could be an increased amount of protein byproducts from the corn itself, if the initial isolation step to separate starch from all other constituents is not completely successful, or a hypersensitivity reaction.

An overestimation of blood glucose measured by the glucose dehydrogenase (GDH) method in comparison to the glucose oxidase and the hexokinase methods has been reported.[234] The GDH enzyme probably reacts with the free reducing group of maltose and the other saccharides derived from polyglucose as well as with the reducing group of glucose. This can lead to dangerous overestimation of blood glucose and may mask true hypoglycemia or induced hypoglycemia by overdosing insulin in diabetic patients.[235]

Glucose polymers are promising alternative osmotic agents for the care of diabetics with renal insufficiency and those patients with low UF due to high peritoneal transport rates. Further experience with various types of glucose polymers and advances in manufacturing processes could bring us closer to the ideal osmotic agent.

Alternate Osmotic Agents. Clinical and experimental trials of substances such as gelatin, xylitol, sorbitol, mannitol, fructose, dextrans, glucose polymers, polyanions, glycerol, and amino acids have been reported.[13,102,197,198,212,234–248] Table

TABLE 16–4. ALTERNATE OSMOTIC AGENTS USED IN PERITONEAL DIALYSIS SOLUTIONS

Osmotic Agents	Potential Complications
Gelatin	Prolonged half-life and immunogenicity of some preparations[236]
Xylitol	Peritoneal pain,[237] lactic acidosis, hyperuricemia,[237,249] carcinogenicity,[249] and deterioration of liver function[237,250]
Sorbitol	Metabolized via polyol pathway which may aggravate neuropathy,[197,198,238,239] lactic acidosis, hyperuricemia,[249] and hyperosmolality[240, 251]
Mannitol	Lactic acidosis and hyperuricemia[239,249]
Fructose	Metabolized via polyol pathway which may aggravate neuropathy,[197,198,239] hypernatremia,[252] lactic acidosis, hyperuricemia, and hypertriglyceridemia[236,249,253]
Dextrans	Risk of bleeding[254] and systemic absorption[236]
Polyanions	Damage to peritoneum and cardiovascular instability[236,254]
Amino acids	Increased concentration of nitrogenous products in blood, increased hydrogen ion generation,[244,245] expensive, optimal formulation not yet determined,[236,246] difficult to sterilize in combination with glucose,[239] and nonphysiologic high plasma levels of amino acids
Glycerol	Retention, hypertriglyceridemia, sterile peritonitis, greater ultrafiltration than glucose but of short duration resulting in low net ultrafiltration capacity,[241,242] and hyperosmolality[243]
Glucose polymers	Prolonged half-life, impaired metabolism in uremia, accumulation of maltose,[212,213] and potential for high caloric loads[215,236,255,256]

16–4 summarizes the potential complications reported with these osmotic agents.[197,198,212–215,236–256] Many of these substances are principally of historical importance, but recent clinical research suggests potential clinical application for others.

The use of amino acids as osmotic agents and nutritional supplements was proposed by Gjessing in 1968.[257,258] Oreopoulos and colleagues studied the effects of amino acid–containing solutions in an attempt to reduce amino acid losses from peritoneal effluent and prevent hypertriglyceridemia and obesity.[245,259,260] Early human studies indicated that amino acids may be osmotic agents without significantly interfering with nitrogenous waste product removal. The preliminary experience of Williams and associates and Oren and coworkers showed a mean plasma amino acid concentration increment of approximately two- to threefold following instillation of amino acid–containing dialysate but falling to preinstillation values after 6 hours.[244,245] Total body nitrogen and transferrin levels increased, suggesting an improved nutritional status. Although the peak plasma levels of most amino acids after peritoneal instillation were not greater than those normally observed after ingestion of a large protein meal, it is of concern that the levels of methionine, elevated prior to IP instillation of amino acids, rose threefold in one of these studies.[244] In light of various observations suggesting that induction of nitrogen balance is highly dependent on the maintenance of a normal ratio of essential and nonessential amino acids in plasma, it is apparent that most amino acid–containing solutions for IP infusion have been suboptimal.[236,261,262]

Bonzel and colleagues studied the loss of amino acids during CAPD and the influence of IP amino acid infusions on plasma and intracellular amino acid concentrations.[246] They observed an absence of correlation between intra- and extracellular amino acid levels, indicating that plasma amino acids are not representative of total body amino acid balance in CAPD patients and that the rate of peritoneal transfer was highly variable for individual amino acids. These data once again suggest that in supplementing amino acids in CAPD patients, one should consider intracellular amino acid levels and the rate of peritoneal amino acid transfer. Additional shortcomings to the use of amino acid solutions include the significant and progressive increase in blood urea nitrogen (BUN) concentration and the development of an anion gap, suggesting the eventual development of clinical metabolic acidosis.[245]

Although several authors have recommended the use of continuous or intermittent IP nutrition with hypertonic glucose and amino acid solutions, claiming the advantages of a possible continuous and steady absorption of both nutrients in quantities comparable to total parenteral nutrition, of good UF, and of no significant electrolytic imbalance, others have recommended caution with its use.[263,264]

In a 6-month study, Dombros et al. found amino acids ineffective in improving the nutritional status of five patients, perhaps due to their low caloric intake.[265] An increase in dialysate protein losses secondary to prostaglandin E_2 synthesis has also been reported.[266] Park et al. compared the effects of equimolar glucose and amino acid solutions on solute transport and UF.[267] There was no significant difference between the solutions on peritoneal transport of solutes; however, UF tended to be lower with the amino acid solutions. Also, the hypertonic amino acid solution yielded nonphysiologic high plasma levels of several amino acids. Qamar et al., in a 3-month study in children, concluded that although amino acid solutions were equally effective in UF and creatinine clearance and produced no adverse clinical or biochemical effects, they provided no additional nutritional benefits.[268]

The latest and longest clinical trial with amino acid–containing PDF has been slightly more encouraging.[269] This 3-year, randomized, prospective controlled study of amino acid dialysate in malnourished Chinese patients on CAPD showed that patients maintained on conventional glucose-based PDF experienced a decrease in serum albumin and cholesterol concentrations, while those receiving one daily exchange of the amino acid–containing PDF remained stable or experienced an increase concentration. The two groups had similar mortality, hospitalization duration, and dropout rates.

Peptides have been used in recent years in an attempt to reduce the osmolarity of the PDF and to improve UF and nutritional status. The first use of peptides as osmotic agents was reported by Klein et al.[270] The early experiments showed superior UF to 2.5% glucose PDF, very low absorption, and no toxic effects. More recently, mixtures of peptides and glucose have been used with modest effect on UF, no apparent toxicity, and no differences in plasma amino acid profiles.[271] The results are encouraging enough to justify further research.

Glycerol is a naturally occurring trivalent alcohol with a MW of 92 Da. The theoretical advantages of this compound as an alternative osmotic agent to glucose are as follows: (1) it does not require insulin for metabolism, which could make it most attractive in the treatment of diabetic patients; (2) it has a higher pH than glucose; and (3) glycerol does not react with amino acids and can be sterilized as a mixture of amino acids and glycerol without causing caramelization. Although the caloric load obtained from glycerol may be 30 percent lower than that with corresponding glucose solutions, experience has shown that because of the inferior UF capacity of glycerol solutions, the resulting caloric load when equivalent fluid removal is obtained is similar to that of glucose.[272] Matthys and colleagues reported their long-term experience with glycerol-containing dialysate in diabetic CAPD patients.[243,272] These authors observed good patient tolerance to glycerol-containing PDF, stable biochemical profiles, and maintenance of a stable peritoneal UF capacity. The daily blood glucose profiles were remarkably constant and the IP insulin dose required for good control of glycemia was 50 to 67 U/day, which is probably lower than the dose usually reported for patients using glucose dialysate.[28,273–276] On the other hand, the use of glycerol PDF resulted in high levels of free glycerol in plasma, one case of hyperosmolar syndrome, hypertriglyceridemia, and an unusually high incidence of culture-negative peritonitis. The net UF capacity of the various glycerol solutions tested was considerably lower than that accomplished with comparable glucose dialysates.[241,272]

Sodium. The concentration of sodium in PDF has varied very little throughout the years despite a wealth of interesting experimental data that both emphasize the complexities of sodium balance in PD and the potential advantages of tailoring the sodium concentration to the specific prescription. To better understand the complexities of determining the ideal sodium concentration in PDFs, it is important to consider that sodium balance is a function of diffusive and convective transport and is influenced by UF rate, dialysate and plasma concentrations of sodium, and intravascular volume.[276,277] This has clear implications in designing solutions for CAPD or for high-flow APD.

Dialysate sodium concentrations have historically varied from 118 to 141 meq/L. The lower concentrations have been recommended for IPD, where short dwell times and hypertonic glucose solutions often result in a disproportionately greater removal of extracellular water than sodium (sodium sieving) and consequently lead to hypernatremia.[276–282]

To better illustrate the importance of considering UF rate, dialysate flow, and the combined effect of all the factors influencing sodium balance in PD, let us consider the case of CFPD using very high peritoneal dialysate flow (200 mL/min) and achieving UF rates of 6 to 7 mL/min.[100] Significant increases in serum sodium will result due to excessive water removal relative to sodium through the ultrasmall pores. Solutions with lower sodium concentrations should be recommended to avoid hypernatremia.

Very low PDF sodium concentrations have been used in CAPD to increase sodium and water removal.[278,280,283] Using PDF sodium concentrations in the range of 98 to 102 meq/L, these investigators achieved significant sodium removal; thus they increased transcapillary UF and achieved marked reductions in body weight and arterial blood pressure among fluid-overloaded CAPD patients.

At present, most PDFs used for conventional continuous PD provide sodium concentrations of 132 to 141 meq/L. Proper manipulation of the dialysate glucose concentration can provide a daily UF of 0.5 to 3 L with four 2-L exchanges. Nomograms and kinetic models have been developed that predict the net sodium and potassium removal adjusted for glucose concentration of the solution.[276,284]

Potassium. Potassium balance in PD is the result of serum and dialysate potassium concentrations, acid-base balance, Na-K cellular pump activity, and insulin availabity. Diffusion is the primary mechanism for potassium removal.[285] Most PD solutions do not contain potassium. Some patients on PD require potassium in concentrations of 2 to 3 meq/L in PDF in order to maintain a normal blood concentration. Maintenance of normokalemia is particularly important in digitalized patients. The addition of potassium chloride to dialysate is simple and relatively safe, but caution must be exercised due to the increased risk of contaminating the solution. Hypokalemia is usually prevented by liberalizing the dietary potassium content or by oral supplementation. It is apparent that the total potassium removed in the dialysate is less than the total potassium intake, yet significant hyperkalemia is uncommon. Balance studies suggest that the difference can be accounted for by fecal potassium excretion.

Calcium. Calcium concentrations range from 2.4 to 3.5 meq/L in most PDFs. Peritoneal calcium transit is mostly determined by the diffusive gradient of ionized calcium between plasma and dialysate.[286] The normal range of serum ionized calcium is 2.3 to 2.6 meq/L. A significant amount of PDF calcium (~30 percent) is chelated, mostly by lactate, leaving 70 percent as ionized.[287] Ionized calcium crosses the peritoneum faster than chelated calcium and thus is more important in the determination of calcium balance. The rapid increase in pH that occurs after infusion of conventional solutions or the higher pH of newer biocompatible solutions also decreases the ionized calcium fraction.[287]

The use of 3.5 meEq/L resulted in positive calcium balance in most patients undergoing CAPD prior to the generalized use of vitamin D supplements and calcium salts as phosphate binders.[288,289] The use of hypertonic solutions and high UF can result in negative calcium balance in the absence of calcium supplementation.[289,290] However, the introduction of calcium salts as phosphate binders and the common use of active forms of vitamin D in the treatment of renal osteodystrophy can markedly increase calcium loads in dialysis patients and require a reduction in the calcium concentration of the solutions.[291–296]

Transperitoneal calcium balance depends not only on the serum ionized calcium but also on UF.[294,295] Therefore the dialysate calcium concentration for a specific patient should be determined according to the patient's UF needs, serum ionized calcium, and need for calcium salts as phosphate binders and vitamin D supplementation for suppression of PTH secretion. For PDFs in general, the old standard calcium concentration (3.5 meq/L) is considered to be too high to permit adequate doses of calcium-based phosphate binders. When the calcium concentration is reduced to 2.0 to 2.5 meq/L, sufficient phosphate control and administration of active vitamin D compounds are made possible without the risk of hypercalcemia. Weinreich et al. demonstrated that dialysate calcium levels of 2.0 meq/L resulted in a loss of calcium into the dialysate even at low ultrafiltration volumes and serum calcium levels.[297] Reduction in dialysate calcium (2.5 vs. 3.5 meq/L) revealed that reduced calcium concentrations resulted in less hypercalcemia.[294] Furthermore, application of the 2.5-meq/L calcium dialysate resulted in negative mass transfer when serum ionized calcium was lower than conventional dialysate calcium with a low glucose concentration. Calcium mass transfer was always found to be negative when the highest glucose concentrations were used, due to ultrafiltration and solute drag.

Calcium-free solutions have been used in patients with severe extraosseous calcifications and to treat hypercalcemia with some success.[293,298] Calcium-free dialysate is not commercially available but can be easily prepared in the hospital pharmacy. Since the solution is calcium- and magnesium-free, a 1.5 to 5% dextrose solution containing 30 meq bicarbonate, 135 meq sodium, and 105 meq chloride can be prepared using standard intravenous solutions.

The influence of calcium concentration in PD solutions on host defenses remains somewhat controversial. The use of low-calcium dialysate (2 and 2.5 meq/L) has been reported to reduce proliferation of peritoneal fibroblasts and production of interleukin-1 and interferon, thus preventing peritoneal fibrosis.[299,300] However, the same authors have shown that low calcium concentrations reduce the effectiveness of macrophage killing of *S. epidermidis* and that improved killing was accomplished by increasing the calcium level of the solution.[301] The use of higher calcium concentrations (3.5 meq/L) increases macrophage cytosolic calcium levels, superoxide generation, and bacterial killing power.[302] Piraino and coworkers have also shown that there is an increased risk of *S. epidermidis* peritonitis in patients undergoing PD with low dialysate calcium concentrations.[303]

Magnesium. Magnesium is generally present in concentrations of 0.5 to 1.5 meq/L in PDF. Dialysate glucose concentrations of 1.5% result in net magnesium absorption, and 4.25% solutions promote magnesium removal.[287,289] The average patient on continuous equilibration dialysis maintains serum magnesium concentrations in the normal range.

Limited interest has been expressed in using magnesium hydroxide antacids as phosphate binders. Magnesium-containing antacids are nonconstipating, palatable, and possibly effective phosphate binders. Their use is limited by the availability of effective and safe modern binders; however, because of their low cost, magnesium-containing binders may be attractive in certain areas. In order to adopt magnesium phosphate binders, the dialysate magnesium must be

eliminated or its concentration markedly reduced to prevent hypermagnesemia.[304]

Buffer Bases. Lactate and acetate were traditionally used as a source of bicarbonate in PDFs. Both of these anions have similar effects on the maintenance of acid-base balance. Lactate is provided as a racemic mixture of dextro (D) and levo (L) isomers. L-lactate is metabolized faster by humans than the D-isomer; however, the accumulation is minimal in an equilibration system. Levoacetate is converted to pyruvate, which, in turn, can be converted to acetyl-CoA. The metabolism of the dextro form appears to be through a different enzyme, D-2-hydroxy acid dehydrogenase. While levolactate is metabolized at a rate of 54 to 61 meq/h, dextrolactate is only metabolized at 28 meq/h. Therefore the tolerance is totally dependent on the rate of introduction of lactate into the system. In the typical CAPD or CCPD patient, this does not pose a problem. However, during prolonged periods of high-flow PD, the use of D-isomer could represent a problem.[305–307]

La Greca et al. have shown that the use of acetate results in a stable blood pH but also a high and potentially bothersome serum acetate level, whereas lactate is safer and provides a more stable blood pH and bicarbonate concentration.[307] Because of the potential differences in metabolism between lactate and acetate, many others have recommended the use of acetate or bicarbonate solutions in the treatment of acutely ill patients or those with lactic acidosis.[308–311]

Acetate has been proposed as a causative factor in development of loss of UF and peritoneal sclerosis among patients undergoing chronic PD. The bulk of the evidence rests on North American experience with IPD using acetate-buffered concentrate[312–314] and that of several European investigators with CAPD patients.[315] Acetate is an active vasodilator and diffuses easily into the cells, where it is metabolized.[316] Lactate penetrates into cells with difficulty and is metabolized in the liver.[317] These differences may help explain the increased glucose transfer rates observed in some patients using acetate-containing dialysate.

Extensive studies by Miller and coworkers have shown that commercial dialysate causes an initial and transient vasoconstriction in the rat parietal peritoneum, followed by significant vasodilatation.[318,319] The visceral peritoneum responds with immediate vasodilatation. Analysis of their data suggests that the observed vasodilatation is due to acetate or lactate and the hypertonicity of the solution, rather than glucose concentration per se or the low pH.[320] Clinical studies with physiologic pH solutions have failed to improve clearance.[321] Furthermore, Nielsen et al. carried out chronic PD in rats and found that acetate was associated with protracted peritoneal infection and more profound functional and morphologic membrane alterations than was lactate.[322] Nonetheless, there is no conclusive evidence that acetate is the sole or even the primary factor responsible for reduced UF and peritoneal sclerosis.[323] An international study including 29 centers failed to explain rapid glucose absorption and low UF on the sole basis of acetate used as a buffer anion, since some of the cases observed used lactate-containing solutions.[324] Other investigators have also observed these complications in patients using lactate dialysate exclusively.[325]

Although, in theory, sodium salts of lactate, acetate, citrate, α-ketoglutarate, pyruvate, succinate, malate, and others could be utilized as PD buffers, it is commonly known that these organic anions are poorly metabolized in patients with lactic acidosis, diabetes, Addison's disease, or alcoholic cirrhosis.[326] Thus the use of these buffers could result in aggravation of the preexisting acidosis. Feriani and colleagues have measured some Krebs cycle intermediate metabolites (citrate, α-ketoglutarate, malate, and oxalacetate) in the peritoneal effluent of patients undergoing CAPD.[327] They observed increased malate values, reflecting the fact that the Krebs cycle is deranged in patients on CAPD. The derangement can be explained by a shift of acetate compounds (CoA) to malate production. Because acetate and lactate are metabolized to acetyl CoA, their use in dialytic solutions could overload the Krebs cycle and influence the metabolic status of CAPD patients.

Bicarbonate-containing dialysate could be considered ideal for the correction of metabolic acidosis and the maintenance of acid-base balance during PD. Bicarbonate is the natural physiologic buffer, it does not require metabolism, and its use in dialysate minimizes its loss in the peritoneal effluent. Bicarbonate-buffered solutions are also considered more biocompatible by maintaining adequate concentration of cytoplasmic calcium in peritoneal macrophages and mesothelial cells.[299] There are, however, two major limitations related to dialysate manufacturing of bicarbonate-based solutions. The solutions must be formulated at an acid pH to prevent glucose from caramelizing. Furthermore, calcium precipitates in the presence of bicarbonate and an alkaline pH.

Ing and coworkers devised a method of preparing peritoneal dialysate containing bicarbonate, calcium, magnesium, and glucose by using an automated dialysate delivery system that mixes treated water, acid concentrate, and basic concentrate.[328] This system has potential utility for patients on IPD or CCPD, but it would require the use of a complex proportioning system.

The development of a peritoneal dialysate containing bicarbonate was limited by three major problems.[329] First is the problem of calcium carbonate precipitating during sterilization:

$$NaHCO_3 + CaCl_2 \rightarrow CaCO_3 + NaCl + HCl$$

Second is the loss of CO_2 from plastic containers. It is necessary to maintain a relatively high Pco_2 inside the dialysate container in order to drive the following reaction to the left and thus keep soluble calcium bicarbonate in the solution:

$$Ca(HCO_3)_2 \leftrightarrow CaCO_3 + H_2O + CO_2$$

Third is the hazard of infusing an acid or alkaline dialysate into the patient before proper mixing, potentially causing chemical peritonitis.

Recognizing these problems, Feriani et al. developed a system using a double-lined plastic bag, divided by a partition with the upper compartment filled with acid solution and the lower with basic solution.[329] The acid solution contains calcium and acetic or lactic acid, which reacts with sodium bicarbonate and generates the Pco_2 needed to maintain calcium in the solution:

$$NaHCO_3 + CH_3COOH \rightarrow CH_3COONa + H_2O + CO_2$$

Prior to use, the septum is broken and the two solutions are mixed, resulting in a solution with physiologic pH (Fig. 16–8). Clinical trials have shown the system to be effective in correcting uremic acidosis, safe, and well tolerated in adults and children.[330–332] Inflow pain has also been reported to be reduced with the use of bicarbonate-containing solutions.[331]

An alternate solution to the problem of calcium precipitation has been offered by Yatzidis with the use of glycylglycine.[333,334] Glycylglycine added to bicarbonate forms a buffer with an optimum pH of 7.35. The solutions can be sterilized by filtration and remain stable at room temperature for prolonged periods of time. Studies in animals have suggested that these solutions are safe and that net UF is superior to that achieved with lactate-based solutions.[334–336] Although the precise mechanism for the enhanced UF is not known, the maintenance of a higher transperitoneal osmotic gradient and the reduction in lymphatic absorption through an increase in phosphatidylcholine concentration in the peritoneal cavity have been proposed. The main limitation to the use of glycylglycine is the need for sterilizing by filtration, which may not prove adequate for commercial dialysate manufacturing.

Other Additives. Heparin is often added to the peritoneal dialysate to prevent fibrin strand formation and obstruction of the peritoneal catheter. Its use is particularly important during episodes of peritonitis, when there is increased debris and fibrin deposition and the catheter is not being used for prolonged periods of time, as is the case with IPD and NPD. Heparin has also been recommended to prevent IP adhesions.[337] The use of IP heparin in recommended doses does not result in systemic heparinization.[338,339] It can, however, interfere with the activity of other additives simultaneously added to the dialysate.[340]

Insulin is commonly added to dialysis solutions in the treatment of diabetic patients. This practice is common in many centers, and the experience with glycemic control has

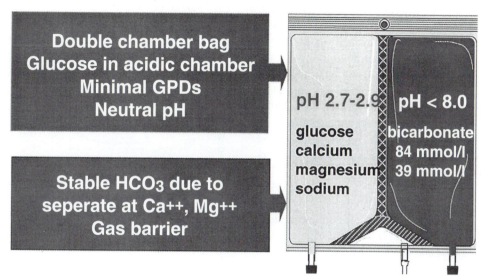

Figure 16–8. Schematic representation of a double chamber bicarbonate dialysate bag. Glucose and electrolytes are kept in the acidic compartment and bicarbonate in the alkaline compartment. After the septum is broken, the two solutions are mixed and the resulting solution has a physiologic pH. *(Courtesy of Fresenius Medical Care, AG, Bad Homburg, Germany.)*

been reported to be similar to that observed with subcutaneous (SC) administration and with insulin pumps (see below).

The addition of vasodilators, such as nitroprusside, has been suggested for use in patients with reduced small molecule clearances; however, protein losses increase with vasodilatation, limiting this approach.[341] Vasodilators may also be considered for situations in which increased protein losses are desirable, as in the treatment of multiple myeloma or amyloidosis.[341,342]

Peritoneal lymphatic absorption has been shown to have significant influence on peritoneal UF.[343,344] Studies in rats have demonstrated that neostigmine can reduce peritoneal lymphatic absorption and thus effect a significant increase in net UF and solute clearance without altering peritoneal transport.[344]

Atrial natriuretic peptide (ANP) is a hormone with well-known diuretic and vasodilating properties. Wang et al. have recently reported that ANP may decrease peritoneal fluid absorption (by 51 percent), partially because of decreasing the direct lymphatic absorption, resulting in a significant increase in peritoneal fluid removal and small solute clearances.[345] While the basic diffusive permeability of the peritoneal membrane did not change, the peritoneal glucose absorption was retarded by adding ANP to peritoneal dialysate, perhaps through the interaction of ANP with glucose metabolism.

In yet another report, Kuriyama et al. observed increased peritoneal ultrafiltration volume after administration of tranexamic acid in patients on CAPD.[346] It is possible that pharmacologic manipulation of peritoneal UF may eventually find its place in the treatment of PD patients. However, at present no clinical application has been found for these practices.

The use of small amounts of sodium hydroxide to neutralize the acid pH of solutions has been practiced with some success in patients extremely sensitive to the infusion of commercial dialysate.[58] Also a 1 or 2% xylocaine solution added to the dialysate (5 mL/L) may relieve the pain.

Antibiotics are commonly added to peritoneal dialysate in the treatment of peritonitis. The recommended loading and maintenance doses are provided in Chap. 17.

Biocompatibility

PD has been considered a physiologic therapy using unphysiologic solutions; however, recent progress in our understanding of the unphysiologic aspects of PDF—identification of the more toxic factors in PDF affecting the peritoneal membrane and how to overcome these deficiencies—have markedly improved the biocompatibility of solutions. The peritoneal cavity is exposed to huge cumulative volumes of PDF. In order to illustrate the importance of biocompatibility of these fluids, consider the fact that the typical annual exposure for CAPD patient is 3000 L, that of an APD patient is approximately 7000 L, and that of a CFPD patient more than 35,000 L! A relationship between time on PD and functional and morphologic changes of the peritoneal membrane has been observed.[347–350] The functional manifestations are an increase in transperitoneal solute transport and decreased net ultrafiltration. The predominant morphologic changes consist of reduplication of the basal lamina, interstitial fibrosis, hyalinization of blood vessels, and neoangiogenesis. The pathophysiology of membrane failure is thought to follow an inflammatory process that in turn causes functional vascular changes and ultimately results in morphologic vascular, mesothelial, and interstitial changes. The possible triggering factors include peritonitis, glucose, pH of the solution, osmolality, glucose degradation products (GDPs), advanced glycation end-products (AGEs), plasticizers, lactate, and other toxic products associated with PDFs. While the presence of several of these factors has been correlated with the development of membrane failure, it has been more difficult to characterize the specific role and importance of each of these factors in causing functional and morphologic changes of the peritoneal membrane. For example, a correlation between AGE content of the peritoneal membrane and number of peritonitis episodes has been reported.[351] However, this observation alone does not implicate peritonitis per se as the responsible factor for AGE deposition, since peritonitis is associated with peritoneal vasodilatation and reduced ultrafiltration (requiring higher concentrations of glucose), which in turn may be associated with the generation of more GDPs and thus may promote the formation of AGEs. Another confounding factor is the effect that uremia per se may have on significant peritoneal membrane deterioration, independent of the influence of PDFs.[352–354]

Conventional PDFs are manufactured with a relatively low pH (5.5) in order to prevent caramelization during heat sterilization. This pH is still too high to prevent formation of toxic GDPs. Experimental data have shown that conventional solutions contain significant concentrations of GPDs (aldehydes and carbonyls), whose concentrations increase with time and exposure to heat.[191,355,356] The heat applied during sterilization leads to the degradation of glucose. The extent of this degradation depends on a number of factors, such as heating time, temperature, pH, glucose concentration, and catalyzing substances. The ideal pH to minimize the development of GPDs during heat sterilization is around 3.2 (Fig. 16–9).[191] Based on these principles, novel biocompatible solutions with minimal GDP concentrations have been introduced. The basic design consists of a double-chamber bag (Fig. 16–8) containing the electrolytes and glucose at a very low pH (2.8 to 3.2) in one compartment and another solution consisting of lactate or other buffer base at a high pH (8.0 to 8.6) in the second compartment. Maintaining the glucose at a low pH during heat sterilization markedly reduces the formation of GDPs. Mixing the fluids of both chambers, by breaking the septum dividing them prior to use, results in the delivery of a ready-to-use fluid with physiologic pH (6.8 to 7.4) and a low concentration of GDPs.

Glucose vs. GDP Toxicity. The precise toxicity of glucose as an osmotic agent has become a controversial subject. Glu-

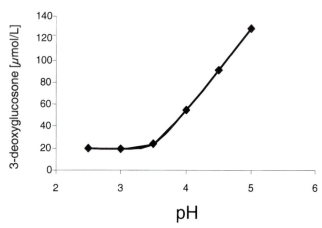

Figure 16–9. Reduction in GDP formation by lowering pH during sterilization. *(Courtesy of Prof. Jutta Passlick-Deetjen, Bad Homburg, Germany.)*

cose per se is a physiologic substance present in all humans in substantial concentrations. However, hyperglycemia is well known to be deleterious, and chronically elevated glucose levels in the presence of tissue proteins promote the formation of AGEs. On the other hand, GPD cytotoxicity is dose-dependent; the reduction or elimination of GDPs reduces cytoxicity and improves cellular function and survival, regardless of glucose concentration, and GDPs accelerate AGE formation more than glucose per se.[357] This raises the following question: Is the culprit glucose or GDP concentration in the PDF?

Several in vitro studies with either fibroblasts or with isolated human peritoneal mesothelial cells (HPMC) have demonstrated that GDPs impair cellular growth, reduce cell viability, and significantly decrease the cellular release from cells of interleukin-6 and other cytokines or chemokines into the incubation medium.[349,358–364] Furthermore, Igaki et al. showed that when serum albumin was incubated with 3-deoxyglucosone (3-DG), a potent GDP, or with glucose alone, 3-DG accelerated the formation of AGEs significantly more than glucose.[357]

Mortier et al. reported another interesting series of experiments designed to differentiate the role of glucose, GDPs, pH, and lactate in peritoneal hemodynamics.[363] The authors studied the effect of conventional and new PD solutions on the hemodynamics of peritoneal membrane of Wistar rats. Conventional PDF with high GDP concentrations that were lactate-based resulted in maximal vasodilatation. PDF containing lactate but minimal GDP concentrations caused only transient vasodilatation. Bicarbonate-based PDF with minimal concentrations of GDPs did not cause any hemodynamic changes.

There are abundant data, mostly generated from in vitro experiments, that support the deleterious effects of unphysiologic pH, GDPs, lactate, and high osmolality on peritoneal cell function, survival and host defenses, mesothelial cell viability, and inflow pain during PDF infusion.[349,358–362,364–367] Most data on standard and new dialysis solutions presently available are based on in vitro and ex vivo experiments showing cytotoxic effects of single fluid components (e.g., acidic pH, lactate buffer, glucose, and GDPs). However, hardly any data are available presenting significant evidence that the in vitro and ex vivo results of these models are clinically relevant to long-term PD. According to the available clinical data, only CA 125 seems to be useful as an IP marker for mesothelial cell mass and mesothelial cell regeneration during PD treatment.[358,359,368–371] Indeed, the preliminary data with new solutions characterized by physiologic pH and low GDP, containing either lactate or bicarbonate, have shown significantly higher levels of CA 125, reflective of better mesothelial cell preservation or regeneration.[369,371–373]

TECHNIQUES TO ASSESS PERITONEAL FUNCTION

The success of PD depends to a large extent on our ability to evaluate membrane function. Characterization of solute transport rate and ultrafiltration upon initiation of PD is of considerable value to formulate an adequate prescription and to establish a baseline to monitor future performance of the peritoneum as a dialyzing membrane. The concepts of diffusive mass transfer, convection, dialysance, clearance, and Kt/V have been discussed in previous chapters. Our discussion here is limited to clinical issues and the tests most commonly used for assessment of peritoneal function.

The selection of urea or creatinine kinetics for the assessment of peritoneal adequacy has been a most controversial topic.[374,375] The discriminating power of creatinine as a predictor of clinical outcomes has been cited by some as a reason for its preference.[376] Others have found that creatinine kinetics do not show sufficient discriminative capacity

in terms of adequacy of dialysis.[377] In the absence of controlled studies to determine the superiority of one parameter over the other, the clinician should evaluate both measures in addition to the general clinical picture.

While there are no definite data on the superiority of small or larger solutes as the best indices of adequacy in dialysis, it is evident that when patients develop uremic signs and symptoms, we generally respond with maneuvers intended to increase small solute clearance and that have minimal if any effects on middle molecule clearance. This approach usually succeeds in ameliorating or eliminating the symptoms.[378] Another reason for the popularity of small solutes, and specifically urea kinetics and modeling, in the evaluation and monitoring of PD function is the wealth of information accumulated with HD using urea as a marker, the utility of urea as a surrogate for protein metabolism, and the widespread use of the peritoneal equilibration test (PET) worldwide.

Peritoneal Equilibration Test

The PET was first described by Twardowski et al. to evaluate peritoneal solute transport.[379,380] It requires the collection of peritoneal effluent samples at timed intervals over 4 hours, using a standard protocol and a midpoint blood sample. The samples are analyzed for urea, creatinine, glucose, and sodium. The results are expressed as dialysate to plasma ratios (D/P) for the specific times for urea, creatinine, and sodium or as dialysate dextrose concentration (Dt) at a certain time over dialysate dextrose concentration at time 0 (D0). The results are plotted as D/P or Dt/D0 versus time in hours (Fig. 16–10). The results are compared to the mean of a large population +1 and 2 SD. The values are categorized as high-average, high, low-average, and low, accordingly. The PET has been serially repeated and found to be stable and reproducible over time.[381–383]

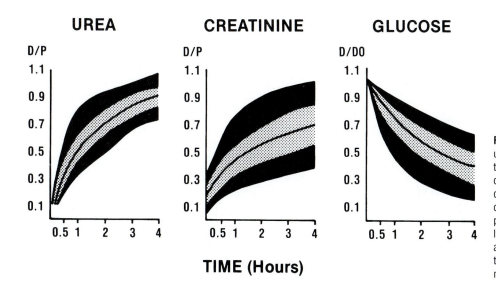

Figure 16–10. Equilibration test curves for urea, creatinine and glucose. D/P refers to the dialysate-to-plasma ratio of urea and creatinine. D/D_0 denotes the ratio of dialysate glucose concentration at time t to dialysate glucose concentration immediately postinfusion (sample 0). The continuous line represents the mean; the lightly shaded area comprises ± 1 SD from the mean, and the heavily shaded area minimal and maximal values.

The PET has been useful in categorizing patients according to peritoneal transport rates, in developing appropriate PD prescriptions, and in monitoring membrane function. The periodic testing of the patient with the PET can alert the physician to significant changes in peritoneal transport and the need for transfer to a more efficient therapy for that particular patient to maintain adequate dialysis. There is evidence that some patients develop a high-permeability syndrome after some time on CPD. The serial application of the PET will characterize this phenomenon and allow appropriate modifications in individual prescriptions for the provision of adequate dialysis.

While the PET has been shown to be a practical and very valuable diagnostic and prognostic tool, it also has certain limitations. The test must be performed using strict standardized methodology. The results can be compared to a reference population or the individual patient if previous tests are available. However, the results of a single PET should never be extrapolated to predict daily clearances. In other words, the sum of four PETs is not equivalent to a day of CAPD. While the PET is performed in a standardized manner, the actual patient's therapy varies significantly throughout the day. The use of alternate peritoneal exchange volumes, glucose concentrations, position, and activity of the patient will influence the D/P ratios of solutes. Gotch et al. have suggested that the procedural steps in the PET may overestimate peritoneal membrane transport and underestimate the variation in peritoneal transport that may occur under actual clinical conditions.[384]

Modified or Fast PET

The fast PET was designed to simplify the procedure, reduce cost, and improve compliance with testing.[385,386] It requires only one dialysate sample; eliminates the supervised inflow procedure, the baseline, and 2 hour measurements; and substitutes dialysate glucose at 4 hours for the ratio of the 4-hour value to baseline glucose dialysate value (D_4/D_0). The results of the dialysate sample are interpreted using a standard table that classifies the results by transport categories.[386] The main limitations of this test are the lack of internal controls and its reproducibility.

Accelerated Peritoneal Equilibration Examination (APEX Time)

Verger et al. designed the APEX time using the same protocol as their initial equilibration test with 3.86% glucose solution.[387] The time at which the D/P_{urea} and Dt/D0 curves intersect is called the APEX time (Fig. 16–11). The higher the permeability, the shorter the time, and vice versa. The typical range of time recorded is between 39 and 89 minutes.[388] The main advantages of the test are that it combines both transport rates for urea and glucose into a single number

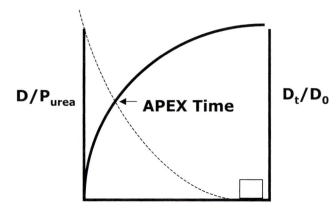

Figure 16–11. Accelerated peritoneal equilibration examination. The intersection between the two curves is referred to as APEX time.

and it is generally shorter than a PET, since most patients exhibit a crossing of the curves before 2 hours.

Batch Peritoneal Dialysate Test

The 24-hour batch test is used to monitor the actual amount of treatment provided. All individual dialysis exchanges are brought to the clinic to be measured, pooled, and mixed. An aliquot is obtained and analyzed for urea and creatinine, from which peritoneal Kt/V and creatinine clearance are determined. The addition of a 24-hour urine collection makes it possible to calculate the net protein catabolic rate (PCR), and obtaining a blood sample provides a good measure of delivered dialysis dose, regardless of the type of prescription.[389,390] The main disadvantage is the required collection of individual drains and their measurement. Unless the patient is well trained and reliable, it is best to perform the measurements and sampling at the clinic. According to one study, the 24-hour D/Pcr correlates well with the PET transport information.[390]

Peritoneal Function Test (PFT)

The Peritoneal Function Test (PFT) was developed by Gotch et al. and has been extensively used and validated in multicenter studies.[391–394] The test allows the clinician to assess total delivered therapy for urea and creatinine, protein and calorie nutrition, fluid balance, and peritoneal transport. The transport information can be used to further individualize or optimize the peritoneal dialysis prescription. The results are expressed as Pt50 or the time required for a solute to achieve 50 percent equilibration between dialysate and plasma. The PFT has been extensively used as part of a kinetic modeling program. The accumulated data can be displayed for individual patients, clinics, or regional groups of dialysis centers. This feature makes it practical for continuous quality improvement.

Dialysis Adequacy and Transport Test (DATT)

The DATT was developed to more conveniently assess peritoneal transport and dialysis adequacy with a single 24-hour dialysate collection and one blood sample.[395] Good correlation between the 4- and the 24-hour D/Pcr was reported in a cross-sectional study of CAPD patient.[395] It has also been found useful to monitor for changes in peritoneal transport over time.[396] The test is validated only for patients undergoing CAPD with four 2-L exchanges per day. The accuracy among patients undergoing alternate CAPD prescriptions is diminished.[397] The test is not recommended for assessment of patients on cyclers. Other studies have shown correlation but not agreement between the PET and DATT results.[398]

Standard Peritoneal Permeability Analysis (SPA)

The SPA is a modification of the PET.[399] Glucose 1.5% and Dextran 70, 1 g/L, is used for the calculation of fluid kinetics with a volume consistent with the patient's usual prescription. The study is performed in the clinic over a period of 4 hours. It requires two blood samples and many timed effluent samples. The SPA is useful in assessing mass-transfer area coefficient (MTAC) of low-MW solutes, clearances of proteins, and change in IP volume.

Personal Dialysis Capacity (PDC)

The PDC was designed in response to a need for a noninvasive test to measure transperitoneal passage of fluid and solutes under normal PD conditions.[400] The patients collect the data themselves during an almost normal CAPD day, using a carefully designed protocol. Nursing time is kept to a minimum. The three-pore model is used to describe the PDC[401] with three physiologic parameters: (1) the "area" parameter (A_o/x), which determines the diffusion of small solutes and the hydraulic conductance of the membrane (L_pS); (2) the final reabsorption rate of fluid from the abdominal cavity to blood ($J_{v_{AR}}$) when the glucose gradient has dissipated; and (3) the large-pore fluid flux of plasma, (J_vL), which determines the loss of protein to the PDF. In the adult PD population the normal area parameter has been determined to be 23,600 cm/1.73 m^2, with an SEM of 650.[400] The $J_{v_{AR}}$ was 1.49 mL/min/1.73 m^2 and J_vL was 0.078 mL/min/1.73 m^2. The PDC parameters were reproducible and could adequately predict the concentrations of the test solutes as well as that of beta$_2$-microglobulin. The results in terms of clearance, "UF volume," and nutritional consequences were presented on easily understandable graphs, whereby patient compliance was improved. These physiologic parameters are highly dynamic, as evidenced by the marked increases observed during peritonitis. The PDC can be a useful tool to achieve adequate dialysis and enhance the understanding of PD exchanges.

Calculation of Estimated Glomerular Filtration Rate (GFR)

In calculating glomerular filtration rate from the traditional determinations of small solute clearances from 24-hour urine collections, it is important to consider the basic physiologic processes involved in the excretion of these solutes. Much of the creatinine appearing in the urine in advanced renal failure is secreted by the proximal tubule, thus overestimating the magnitude of GFR.[378] Conversely, urea is reabsorbed by the renal tubules and underestimates GFR. A practical compromise is to use the average of both urea and creatinine clearances in the estimation of GFR. This amount, in liters per day, can then be added to the peritoneal creatinine clearance to obtain the total daily clearance in the evaluation of adequacy.

TECHNIQUES TO ASSESS PERITONEAL ANATOMY

Peritoneoscopy

PD efficiency can be severely limited by the compartmentalization of the peritoneal cavity and restriction of fluid distribution due to fibrous adhesions or entrapment of the peritoneal catheter. Rigid or flexible peritoneoscopy is possible and sometimes useful in the anatomic evaluation of the peritoneal cavity (Fig. 16–12). It requires however, a 1-cm incision, which may lead to postoperative dialysate leakage and prevent PD for days or weeks after the proce-

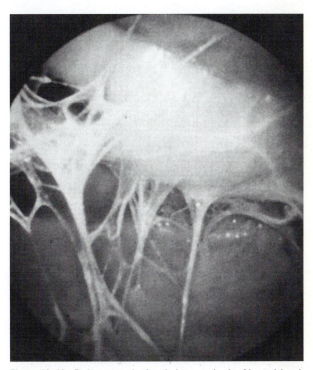

Figure 16–12. Peritoneoscopic view during an episode of bacterial peritonitis. *(Courtesy of Dr. C. Thomas Tucker.)*

dure. The use of the needlescope for initial implantation of the catheter can provide adequate evaluation of the peritoneal cavity at the time of initiation of dialysis and assure proper placement of the intraabdominal portion of the catheter.[402,403]

Cannulography with Peritoneal Air-Contrast Studies

The insufflation of nitrous oxide into the peritoneal catheter combined with infusion of radiographic contrast material can provide an air-contrast image with high resolution capable of identifying the presence of adhesions, fibrous bands, and catheter migration into blind pouches of the peritoneum.[404-406] Figure 16–13 shows a normal peritoneal cavity air-contrast study with a free space in the anterior peritoneal compartment. By contrast, Fig. 16–14 demonstrates the presence of adhesions to the anterior abdominal wall and above the catheter. This information may prove valuable in assessing the causes of poor dialysate flow and reduced peritoneal clearances.

For those patients with adhesions to the anterior abdominal wall who require either catheter replacement or diagnostic peritoneoscopy, blind penetration of the peritoneum may result in bowel perforation. Prior identification of these patients can be facilitated by air-contrast studies and simple x-rays. This technique may also help in selecting patients who would benefit from surgical placement of

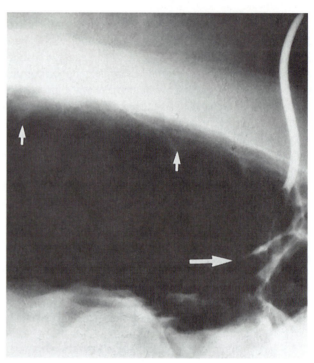

Figure 16–14. Adhesions to the anterior abdominal wall (small arrows) and around the catheter (large arrow) are demonstrated with air-contrast study. *(Courtesy of Dr. C. Thomas Tucker).*

catheters. Air-contrast studies may prove invaluable in diagnosing the presence of potential spaces or abscesses in the subcutaneous catheter tunnel. These abscesses may be responsible for episodes of recurrent peritonitis or indolent catheter infections. Figure 16–15 demonstrates a subcutaneous air collection following nitrous oxide insufflation in a patient who had developed a pseudohernia around the peritoneal catheter. After injection of contrast material, the patient was placed in the elbow-knee position, allowing the contrast media to gravitate around the catheter and into the pseudohernial sac. The contrast media clearly delineated the intramural cavity. This technique is relatively safe, and although strict aseptic surveillance is mandatory, it can be most helpful in the anatomic evaluation of the peritoneal cavity.

Peritoneal Scintigraphy

Scanning of the peritoneal cavity following infusion of a small dose of radionuclide can provide valuable anatomic information in patients undergoing PD.[407-413] The most commonly used technique consists of injecting technetium-99m sulfur colloid (1 mCi) into a fresh bag of dialysate. The labeled dialysate is infused into the peritoneal cavity via the PD catheter after thorough mixing. Imaging can be performed in the supine and upright positions with a large gamma camera from the anterior, lateral, right, and left anterior oblique projections.

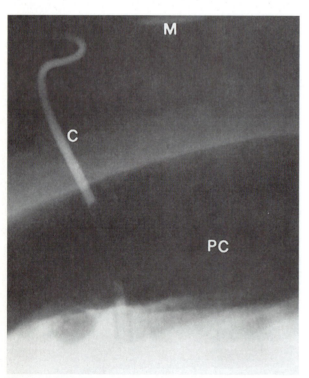

Figure 16–13. Normal air-contrast study. M denotes marker at the umbilicus; C is the Tenckhoff catheter; and PC is the peritoneal cavity. *(Courtesy of Dr. C. Thomas Tucker.)*

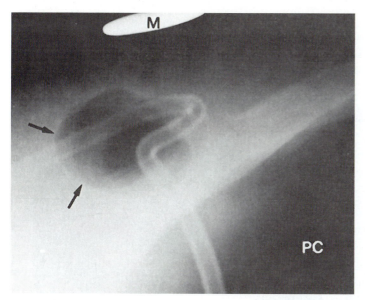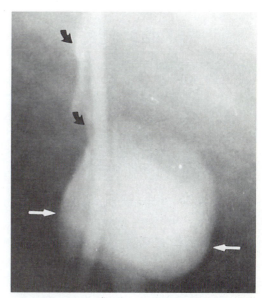

Figure 16–15. Left: Subcutaneous air collection (arrows) following nitrous oxide insufflation. M denotes the marker at the umbilicus and PC is the peritoneal cavity. Right: Contrast medium (dark arrows) draining from the peritoneal cavity, along the catheter, and into a large cavity (white arrows). The crosstable roentegenogram was taken with the patient in the elbow-knee position. *(Courtesy of Dr. C. Thomas Tucker.)*

Radioisotopic scanning has proven of value in the diagnosis of pleuroperitoneal communications, hernias, pericatheter leaks (leading to abdominal and genital edema), and labial or scrotal swelling from the presence of a patent processus vaginalis. Repeat scintigram after drainage of the labeled dialysate is helpful in showing the persistent activity of the isotope in soft tissues and hernial cavities. The disappearance of the radioisotopic activity from the pleura after drainage also establishes the presence of a pleuroperitoneal communication.

Figure 16–16 demonstrates a patent processus vaginalis in a patient with severe scrotal edema after the insertion of a peritoneal catheter and initiation of PD. After surgical correction of the patent processus vaginalis, PD was restarted. Two weeks later, he developed a large right pleural effusion, which was confirmed by peritoneal scintigraphy (Fig. 16–17). Upon termination of PD and transfer to HD, the pleural effusion completely resolved.

Computed Tomography Scanning

Computed tomography (CT) scanning can be useful in the diagnosis of certain complications of PD for which high resolution is needed.[414,415] Enhancement with radiographic contrast material can be achieved in a manner similar to that described for cannulography. This technique has been useful in the diagnosis of small subcutaneous leaks responsible for genital and abdominal wall edema, where other techniques have failed.

Ultrasonography

Although abdominal ultrasound is of limited value in the diagnosis of small dialysate leaks or intraabdominal adhe-

sions, it is a useful, safe, and noninvasive technique for the diagnosis of intraabdominal and anterior abdominal wall abscesses and fluid collections. Simple ultrasonographic studies can differentiate a fluid collection (abscess, liquified hematoma) from fibrous or calcific tissue. Figure 16–18 illustrates the use of ultrasound in the diagnosis of a large peritoneal catheter tunnel abscess in an obese patient with mild abdominal tenderness but no overt inflammation or peritonitis. Surgical removal of the peritoneal catheter confirmed a deep-seated abscess contained between the two dacron cuffs of the catheter.[416,417]

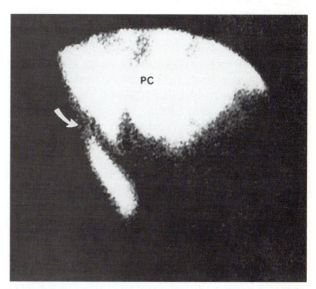

Figure 16–16. Peritoneal scintigraphy with technetium-99 m sulfur colloid in the anterior upright position demonstrating a patent processus vaginalis (arrow). (PC) Peritoneal cavity.

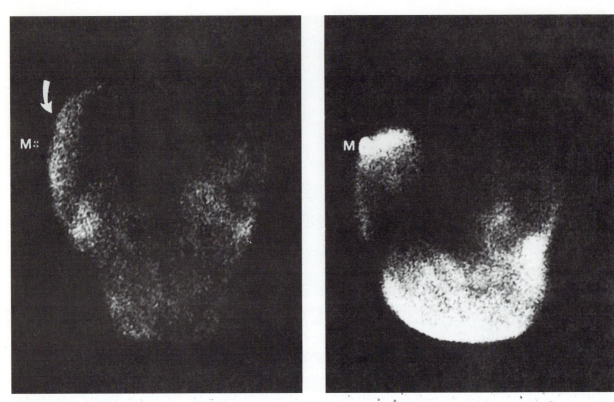

Figure 16–17. Peritoneal scintigraphy in a patient with pleuroperitoneal communication and right hydrothorax. Left: Right hydrothorax (arrow) above the level of the marker (M) is seen with the patient in the supine position. Right: Drainage of the right hydrothorax into the peritoneal cavity with patient in the upright position.

ADEQUACY OF PERITONEAL DIALYSIS

Adequate PD implies sufficient removal of toxins and excessive fluid from the blood to provide good clinical outcomes. Of course, we should aim for optimal PD or the amount and quality of PD that will provide the best clinical outcomes using the most biocompatible and physiologic processes. Adequacy has become a very important topic of discussion for good reasons. The mortality of patients on PD varies tremendously in different countries but remains high compared with most other diseases. This high mortality has been considered by many to be the result of inadequate dialysis. It has also become clear that as RRF is lost, the survival of PD patients diminishes. These observations have raised many questions: Should we compensate loss of RRF with higher doses of PD? What is the equivalency of PD dose and RRF? What parameters best define adequacy?

When we compare the clearances provided by our natural kidneys to those provided by PD or HD (Table 16–5), it becomes evident that the kidneys are significantly more efficient than either dialytic therapy and that the degree of renal solute removal is similar for low- and middle-molecular-weight solutes. There is abundant evidence in the literature demonstrating a direct correlation between the dose of PD, defined as small solute clearance, and clinical outcomes. These data are particularly impressive when we focus on mortality risk below a certain dose of dialysis. One decade ago, Teehan et al. showed significantly better survival among CAPD patients with $Kt/V_{urea} > 1.89$.[418–419] Similarly, in a longitudinal 5-year survey of urea kinetic parameters in CAPD patients, Lameire et al. showed significantly better survival among those with a $Kt/V_{urea} > 1.89$.[420] Several other investigators confirmed these findings, and a minimum dose range of 1.7 to 2.0 Kt/V_{urea} was established.[421–423] Also significant was the finding that when equivalent doses of PD and HD were provided to patients in the same age groups, based on the peak concentration hypothesis, the survival was almost identical.[424] This relationship held true for both diabetic and nondiabetic patients.

In 1996, the CANUSA study further cemented the importance of dose.[425] The CANUSA study reported a decrease of 0.1 U of Kt/V_{urea} per week to be associated with a 5 percent increase in the RR of death and a decrease of 5 L/1.73 m^2 creatinine clearance (Ccr) per week to be associated with a 7 percent increase in the RR of death. The average baseline GFR for this population was 3.8 mL/min. This analysis was unfortunately based on total weekly clearances without consideration of the specific contributions of peritoneal and RRF. In other words, it assumed that the peritoneal and renal contributions were equivalent, which they are not.

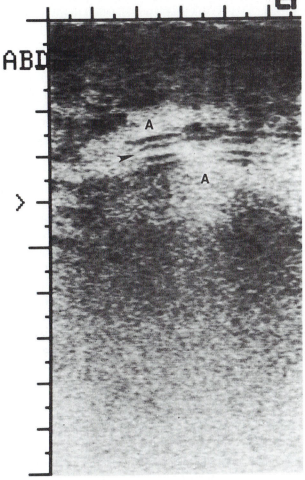

Figure 16–18. Ultrasound of the anterior abdominal wall demonstrating a large peritoneal catheter tunnel abscess. The arrow points at the catheter and the "A" denotes the abscess.

Several recent studies have shown a significant correlation between RRF and survival among PD patients but no correlation between peritoneal clearances and survival.[135–139] The reduction in the RR of death associated with RRF was considerable. In view of these findings we should raise the following question: Is the contribution of peritoneal clearance important? It obviously is, since anuric patients die within a very short time without dialysis and survive for many years on PD.

TABLE 16–5. COMPARATIVE CLEARANCES FROM NATIVE KIDNEYS, HEMODIALYSIS AND CAPD

	Kidneys	HD	CAPD
Urea (L/wk)	750	130	70
Vitamin B_{12} (L/wk)	1200	30–60	40
Insulin (L/wk)	1200	10–40	20
B_2 microglobulin (mg/wk)	1000	0–300	250

Szeto et al. studied 140 anuric patients and found that even in the absence of RRF, higher dialysis doses were associated with better actuarial survival.[140] The significant protection associated with a higher dose remains valid for both the Kt/V_{urea} and C_{cr} models. In another study, Bhaskaran and coworkers observed a RR of death of only 0.54 when the Kt/V_{urea} was >1.85 in their regression model among 122 functionally anuric PD patients.[426] However, this lower RR failed to achieve statistical significance, perhaps related to the cohort size and variability of results.

This brings us to the latest major study addressing the importance of dose among patients undergoing PD. The ADEMEX study is the first randomized trial designed to evaluate the effects of small solute clearance on clinical outcomes.[427] A total of 965 patients from 24 Mexican centers were randomly assigned to control and intervention groups in a 1:1 ratio. All patients between ages 18 and 70 years were eligible if they were undergoing CAPD with a prescription of four daily 2-L exchanges and exhibited a measured peritoneal C_{cr} <60 L/1.73 m^2/week, irrespective of RRF. The control group continued their standard CAPD prescription. The prescription for the intervention group was modified in order to achieve the minimal C_{cr} by increasing the volume of exchange and/or the number of exchanges. Death was the primary endpoint for the study. The secondary endpoints were hospitalizations, therapy-related complications, correction of anemia, and nutritional status.

A clear average separation of clearances across the study was achieved and maintained. The mean difference for C_{cr} was 10.87 L/1.73 m^2/week (control group 46.1 + 0.45, intervention group 56.9 + 0.48, p < 0.001). The survival rates for both groups in intent-to-treat and as-treated analyses were essentially the same (1- and 2-year control 85.5 and 68.3 percent, intervention 83.9 and 69.3 percent). The mortality remained the same for both groups despite adjustments. Should we then assume that peritoneal dose is irrelevant to survival? Probably not. A closer look at ADEMEX opens the doors to more interesting interpretations.

Consistent with previous studies, the ADEMEX results may be simply explained by the fact that peritoneal and renal contributions are not equivalent and that the effects of RRF overwhelm the benefits associated with peritoneal dose.[135–139] By extension, we may propose that the dose range achieved by the study is insufficient to detect the influence of peritoneal dose on outcome.

Although there was no difference in patient survival between the groups, there was a statistically significant increase in the proportion of deaths due to uremia and fluid overload in the control group. The death rate due to congestive heart failure and uremia in the control group was 25.6 percent, compared with 10.8 percent in the intervention group. Also, 5 percent of the patients in the control group withdrew from the study because of uremia, while none in the intervention group did so (p < 0.0001).

We cannot discount the possibility that patients were inadvertently selected for the trial due to higher V (total body water), a known protective factor among HD patients.[428] Since the prestudy (Kt) dose in Mexico was fixed at four 2-L exchanges per day and the selection criterion was the inability to attain a peritoneal C_{cr} >60 L/1.73 m^2/week, we must assume that those selected for the study either had low peritoneal solute transport or a high V. In HD patients at least, the sensitivity to dose among patients with high V is less and mortality is lower. Among PD patients, a low peritoneal transport rate is also a protective factor.[429–432] Thus, the inclusion criteria per se could have introduced a selection bias.

Churchill has noted that the subjects comprised a mixture of incident and prevalent dialysis patients.[433] The prevalent patients (58 percent) were equally distributed between the control and intervention groups. The prevalent patients represent a survivor cohort with a probable over-representation of low transporters, once again a known protective factor. The higher transporters are more likely to transfer to HD or die. A PET would have been ideal to clarify the distribution of peritoneal transport in this population of patients. Unfortunately a DATT was done instead. The PET and DATT have shown correlation but not agreement.[398]

Several other considerations to explain the results of the ADEMEX are the relatively young age of the patients compared to other large series, the very low prevalence of cardiovascular disease (cardiac failure was an exclusion criterion), and uncertain compliance monitoring rigor. ADEMEX has reiterated the difficulties in designing the perfect study and the complexities of clinical trials and statistical analysis.

More recently, Lo et al. examined the effect of Kt/V on patient outcome in a randomized, prospective study of 320 incident patients from Hong Kong.[434] Patients with a total weekly Kt/V < 1.7 had significantly more clinical problems and severe anemia, but there was no difference in outcome when compared to those receiving doses between 1.7 and 2.0. Once again, it is possible that the limited follow-up, the excellent background survival of the population studied, the effect of RRF, and other factors related to the medical care received by the patients may have influenced the results. Nonetheless, it is important to note that while doses below a certain level are associated with inferior clinical outcomes, no correlation between dose of PD and survival has been established.

Intuitively and biologically we can maintain that peritoneal dose is indeed important. It has been clearly established that adequacy is much more than dialytic dose, but dose remains an important component of adequacy. It is fortunate that the therapeutic armamentarium allows us to individualize care of patients according to their metabolic needs and personal preferences. CAPD remains an excellent therapy for some at a certain stage of the spectrum of renal insufficiency; APD, HD, and transplantation fulfill the needs of many others. It is imperative to approach each patient with an open mind and provide the most adequate dose based on a well-balanced interpretation of the literature. However, the bulk of the extensive clinical experience with PD strongly suggests that the average patient can be adequately dialyzed with PD as long as a reasonable dose (weekly Kt/V > 1.75) is provided together with adequate and constant volume and blood pressure control and good nutrition.

Based on a thorough review of the literature, the National Kidney Foundation Dialysis Outcomes Quality Initiative (NKF-DOQI) published PD guidelines recommending weekly Kt/V doses above 2.0 and weekly C_{Cr} above 60 L/1.73 m^2 for CAPD patients and slightly higher for patients on APD.[25,435] Other national organizations in North America, Europe, and Australia have followed with modifications of the original NKF-DOQI guidelines. The recently published Canadian Society of Nephrology (CSN) Guidelines for Peritoneal Dialysis Adequacy[26] differ in a number of ways from the NKF-DOQI guidelines on the same topic. The three main differences are that (1) the CSN targets are the same for CAPD and APD, whereas the DOQI targets are higher for APD; (2) the CSN guidelines have a lower creatinine clearance (CCr) target of 50 L/week for low and low-average transporters compared to 60 L/week for high and high-average transporters, but no such distinction is made by DOQI; and (3) the CSN has set lower limit targets as well as preferred targets for Kt/V and C_{Cr}.[436] Other differences are that the CSN recommendations do not give Kt/V the same primacy over C_{Cr} that DOQI does. Also, the CSN recommendations give greater emphasis to the risks associated with high transport status.

THE PERITONEAL DIALYSIS PRESCRIPTION

Inadequate dialysis has been implicated as a causal factor in the transfer of patients from CAPD to other therapies in up to 29 percent of cases.[437,438] The long-term survival of CAPD patients has, however, improved; consequently the number of patients without RRF has also increased. Although the ideal marker for adequacy of dialysis has not been identified and the role of middle molecules as uremic toxins has not been totally ruled out, urea kinetic modeling (UKM) has been used by many as a predictor of nutritional and dialysis adequacy in CPD.[378,391,419,439–447] Despite the positive relationship between dialysis dose in terms of normalized urea clearance and normalized protein catabolic rate (NPCR), the ability of UKM to predict clinical outcome and nutrition has not been confirmed by all investigators.[448] The main argument in favor of UKM for the prescription of PD is the fact that in the presence of uremic symptoms, significant improvement is usually obtained by enhancing urea clearance.

In order to optimize the PD prescription, it is essential to understand the determinants of peritoneal clearance and the practical ways to increase it. Table 16–6 summarizes the factors determining dose among PD patients. The total clearance is determined by both prescription and factors not related to prescription, including RRF, body size, and the peritoneal transport characteristics.

By far the most common way to improve small solute clearance is to increase the dialysate flow rate. This can be done by either increasing the frequency and number of dialysate exchanges or the volume of the exchange. An increase in exchange volume not only improves clearance by increasing the dialysate flow rate, but also has an independent effect.[449–452] A strong relationship between MTAC and dialysate exchange volume has been described.[449–451] Additionally, the MTAC further increases when the patient assumes the supine position.[450] The latter is probably the consequence of increased effective peritoneal surface area. Since larger volumes are better tolerated in the supine position, these data indicate that cycler dialysis therapy with larger volumes may be significantly more efficient than CAPD and should be considered in patients who require a higher Kt/V_{urea}.

Finally, it is important to avoid the very short or very long dwell times. Very short dwells can markedly increase small solute removal and increase UF, but they are very costly due to high dialysate flow rates. Conversely, dwell times in excess of 7 hours are associated with significant glucose absorption and low UF; they become inefficient once equilibration is reached. In order to improve clearances while containing cost, the use of larger exchange volumes for CAPD and addition of daytime exchanges for APD have been used very succesfully.[81,82,453]

The importance of peritoneal transport rate cannot be overstated. Peritoneal transport has been shown to be an important factor in determining clinical outcomes and is an essential factor in the formulation of an appropriate PD prescription. The simplest way of defining peritoneal transport

rate is with a PET. Most patients fall into the low-average to high-average range and can generally undergo CPD (CAPD, CCPD, PD Plus). High transporters have excellent small solute clearances but poor UF with the usual dwell times of CPD due to rapid absorption of glucose and loss of the osmotic gradient. If the UF is insufficient despite moderate use of hypertonic solutions, IPD or NIPD often provide adequate clearances and UF. Due to the limited dialytic time and intermittent nature of IPD, it should be reserved for this condition only.

The integration of all these concepts in the formulation of optimal PD prescriptions has been shown to provide adequate clearances for most patients in the absence of renal function as long as optimal prescriptions are used and patients are compliant with the therapy. A model to assess the possibility of providing a weekly Kt/V_{urea} of 2.0 or more and a CCr of 60 L/1.73 m^2 or more to anuric patients undergoing CAPD and APD (PD Plus) has been reported.[27] The body surface area (BSA) and peritoneal transport rate distributions were obtained from a large population of patients in a cross-sectional study and modeled to calculate the weekly peritoneal Kt/V_{urea} (Kpt/V) and C_{Cr} for the various transport groups and the range of BSA with four PD prescriptions—CAPD, 8 L; CAPD, 10 L; PD Plus, 12 L; and PD Plus, 15 L—using a validated kinetic program. Most patients were able to attain the current standards of adequacy with APD, but few (less than 25 percent) could do so with standard CAPD in the absence of RRF. This and other models clearly demonstrate that while the suggested adequacy guidelines may not be easy to achieve in some patients, application of well established principles may satisfy the metabolic needs of most patients.[454] It also illustrates the importance of preserving membrane function.

CLINICAL OUTCOMES

The clinical outcomes obtained with PD continue to vary greatly among countries and even between centers close to one another. Much attention has been given to this issue; the answer is not clearly found in any particular study but in the global analysis of the accumulated data. The main categories of factors affecting clinical outcome are patient selection, resources available, and quality of care. The quality of the data presented and the variations in the methodology and statistical analysis applied to the data are also important in interpreting the clinical outcomes and in the comparison between renal replacement therapies.

Patient selection is a complex issue with many unquantifiable variables. Patient selection is more than determination of demographic characteristics and comorbid conditions.[129,455] Selection is affected by patient motivation, family and societal support, and general QOL, all of which are very difficult parameters to measure. Early referral to a

TABLE 16–6. FACTORS DETERMINING DOSE AND CLEARANCE AMONG PATIENTS UNDERGOING PERITONEAL DIALYSIS

Nonprescription factors:
  Residual renal function
  Body size
  Peritoneal transport rate
Prescription factors:
  Number/frequency of exchanges
  Exchange volume
  Patient position
  Tonicity of dialysis solution

nephrologist not only increases the proportion of patients selecting self-dialysis[123–126,128,129,456–458] but also allows the time required to provide adequate education and physical preparation of the patient for future dialysis and to ameliorate anxiety. All of these influence the ultimate outcome of therapy. Little attention has been given to background mortality of the general population, social mores, and ethnic differences among PD patient cohorts.[185] The combination of all these factors may well affect compliance and satisfaction with therapy, rate of development of complications, QOL, hospitalization rates, and survival.

The availability of resources is critical in the selection of therapy. Adequate funding is required for the implementation of specific therapies. The distribution of funds also influences the offering of particular forms of treatment. Certain systems promote the use PD due to its low cost, while others interfere with its use due to limited payment to the physician if PD is used.[179] Economic factors also affect the quality of training for physicians and medical personnel and the availability of adequate equipment and training centers. A definite relationship between gross domestic product per capita and dialysis treatment rate has been established; however, the selection of specific dialytic modalities is determined by many other factors.[185,459]

The quality of general care received by the patient is a major factor of clinical outcome for any therapy. Economic factors have some bearing on the quality of care but are not the most important determinant. The time spent by the nephrologist with the patient and in training the nurses caring for the patient must be considered in judging the variations in outcome. The knowledge, experience, integrity, and enthusiasm of the medical professionals involved in patient care may be considered the most important determinant of good outcome.

The typical training time for CAPD and APD has varied from 5 to 14 sessions in most centers, with most patients requiring 5 to 7 sessions.[30,69,289,460–470] Although the majority of patients become proficient in the mechanics of PD in a few sessions, most of the time is used to familiarize the patient with the rationale for medications, diet, and variations in the prescription.

The clinical and laboratory results observed with CAPD and APD seem comparable to those obtained with HD. The mean body weight has been reported to increase, particularly during the first year of CAPD, and to remain stable thereafter.[460,471–475] Excellent blood pressure control has been reported in the majority of patients and, indeed, a significant number who previously required complex antihypertensive therapy can be maintained on CAPD or APD without chemical intervention.[289,476] In fact, a small percentage of patients have experienced episodes of hypotension that can be easily corrected by liberalizing sodium and fluid intake.

Hemoglobin concentrations generally increase during the first few months of therapy on CAPD and remain stable thereafter. The early improvement in hemoglobin is probably due to the dual effect of hemoconcentration and improved erythropoiesis.[477–482] Hemoglobin concentrations may rapidly fall during episodes of peritonitis. Patients undergoing PD usually have less severe anemia than those receiving HD.[483,484] Some of the reasons proposed for the less severe anemia include the possibility of lower blood losses, less immune stimulation, longer erythrocyte life due to less trauma, extrarenal erythropoietin production by peritoneal macrophages, higher use of subcutaneous erythropoietin, and the better removal of uremic inhibitors of erythropoietin production.[479,485–501] Higher erythropoietin levels have indeed been reported among PD patients compared with HD patients.[502] The use of erythropoietin for the treatment of anemia among PD patients has become common.[484] The usual route of administration is subcutaneous, since peritoneal absorption is limited, particularly when erythropoietin administered with dialysate in the peritoneal cavity.[503,504] Subcutaneous erythropoietin injections have been shown to be effective in raising hemoglobin concentrations in patients on PD. The use of single weekly subcutaneous injections has been reported satisfactory, with no advantage to more frequent administration.[505–507]

In nondiabetic patients, blood glucose concentrations have not significantly changed over time on CAPD.[508] A few patients have developed diabetes while on PD, which may be the result of the increased glucose load. Although the early CAPD literature stressed the problem of hyperlipoproteinemia, cholesterol and triglyceride levels have usually increased to the point of requiring dietary and chemical intervention only in patients with lipid abnormalities prior to initiation of CAPD. During the first year of therapy, it is not uncommon to see a transient and mild increase in cholesterol and triglycerides, which usually stabilizes or normalizes after 1 year of such therapy.[474,509,510] Significant concern has been expressed about the effect of chronic dyslipidemia on the clinical outcome of PD patients. Recent publications have reviewed this topic in depth and offered conservative and pharmacologic intervention.[511–517]

Serum sodium levels have remained stable and normal in most patients undergoing CAPD. A small number of patients have developed hypokalemia, requiring dietary potassium supplementation. Very few patients will need the addition of potassium chloride to the dialysate in order to maintain normokalemia. Acid-base balance has been adequately maintained in the majority of patients on CAPD.

Serum albumin concentrations tend to decrease during the first few months of therapy and usually stabilize in the low-normal or slightly low range. Some patients develop progressive hypoalbuminemia requiring nutritional supplementation. A definite relationship between serum albumin concentration and survival has been shown for patients on PD as well as for those on HD.[418,518] It is thus imperative to monitor serum albumin levels and to determine the possible causes of any significant drop. Nutritional supplementation and/or increments in dialysis dose are recommended. Much progress has been made in correlating adequacy of dialysis, nutrition, and inflammatory stress.[519–529] This important subject is covered in Chap. 21.

Peritonitis rates have markedly dropped for CAPD during the last decade with the use of disconnect systems, while that of APD has remained relatively stable. Nonetheless, lower peritonitis rates for APD when compared to CAPD are still being reported by the vast majority of investigators. Table 16–7 summarizes the incidence of peritonitis for CAPD and APD from the recent literature.[80,530–537] There are only two randomized studies comparing the peritonitis rates of CAPD and APD.[538,539] De Fijter et al. reported a median time to a first episode of peritonitis of 11 months in the patients using CAPD with a Y connector compared with 18 months in those using CCPD ($p = 0.06$).[538] Bro et al. reported 0.31 and 0.17 episodes per year for CAPD and APD, respectively, but the difference was not significant due to the small population studied.[539]

The number of hospitalization days among chronic PD patients also varies greatly between series, with an average range of 15 to 20 days per year. This rate of hospitalization has been found to be heavily dependent on the analytic starting point and on whether intention-to-treat or treatment-received analyses are used.[540] A significant proportion of hospitalizations are due to peritonitis. A correlation between dialysis dose and frequency of hospitalization has also been reported for PD as well as HD, emphasizing the importance of dialysis adequacy in the development of complications.[420,541] Several series have reported significantly lower annual cost for hospitalization for PD compared to HD patients.[183,184] The difference is likely due to the higher cost of maintaining a vascular access for hemodialysis.

Patient dropout has been generally reported to be higher with PD than with HD.[542–547] Technique survival is strongly influenced by patient selection, patient age, proportion of high-risk patients included in the series, and the

methodology used for reporting. The most common indications for discontinuation of PD are inadequate dialysis, peritonitis, noncompliance with therapy, and malnutrition.[548–552] Port et al. reported a significantly better technique survival among patients using Y sets compared with patients using standard connectology[33] In the 1980s peritonitis was reported as the most frequent cause of transfer from PD to HD; but more recently, inadequate dialysis leads as the most common cause for transfer. The potential reasons for this reversal in the etiology of PD technique failure are the significant progress in reducing peritonitis and the greater emphasis on adequacy, particularly after RRF is lost.

The determinants of mortality in PD and HD are patient selection (age, sex, education, compliance, etc.), dose, background mortality, rate of transplantation, comorbid conditions, quality of general care, vintage (time period of the study), and sequence of therapeutic modalities.[553,554] The mortality rates of CAPD/CCPD patients compared to HD patients have been variously reported in the literature as significantly higher, lower, or not significantly different (Table 16–8).[157,545,546,555–562] The most likely source of discrepancy among the series is the statistical analysis used. Schaubel et al. reported significantly decreased adjusted mortality rates for CAPD/CCPD relative to HD based on an "as treated" analysis.[563] Most of the protective effect of CAPD/CCPD was concentrated in the first 2 years. Based on an "intent-to-treat" analysis, the estimated CAPD/CCPD effect was greatly reduced. There are other examples of the effect of statistical analysis on reported mortality rates. Using the same national mortality data extracted from the USRDS annual reports from 1987 to 1993, Bloembergen et al. and Vonesh and Moran reached totally different conclusions.[157,564] Bloembergen et al. restricted their analyses to prevalent-only patients and concluded that the PD cohort was at significantly higher risk of death than HD patients.[157] Conversely, Vonesh and Moran, using both prevalent and incident patients, found little or no difference in overall mortality between PD and HD.[564]

Selection bias can also materially influence the comparative mortality of PD and HD. Murphy et al. concluded that the apparent survival advantage of PD patients in Canada is due to lower comorbidity and lower burden of acute onset of ESRD at the inception of dialysis and that HD and PD, as practiced in Canada, are associated with similar overall survival rates.[540] PD seems to confer a survival advantage during the first few years of therapy and HD has a late survival advantage over PD.[164,562,565–567] The most likely reason for these observations is better preservation of RRF with PD. Foley et al. have also suggested that preexistent low albumin is a major marker of increased late mortality, once again underscoring the importance of comorbidity and selection bias.[565]

Van Biesen et al. observed that the survival of patients remaining more than 48 months on their initial modality

TABLE 16–7. INCIDENCE OF PERITONITIS FOR CAPD AND APD FROM THE RECENT LITERATURE

Reference	Disconnect CAPD	APD
de Fijter et al.,[531] 1991	1.20	0.60
Gahrmani et al.,[532] 1995	0.52	0.83
Viglino et al.,[533] 1995	0.32	0.30
Diaz-Buxo et al.,[80] 1998	0.60	0.46
Troidle et al.,[534] 1998	1.15	1.20
Locatelli et al.,[530] 1999	1.44	0.63
Rodriguez et al.,[535] 1999	0.64	0.31
Perez-Fontan et al.,[536] 1999	0.75	0.34
Huang et al.,[537] 2001	0.28	0.15

TABLE 16–8. COMPARISON OF MORTALITY BETWEEN CAPD/CCPD AND HD

Country	Reference	Year	Sampling	RR	Remarks
U.K.	Burton and Walls[555]	1987	Single center	0.77	
Italy	Maiorca et al.[556]	1988	Single center	1.34	PD better in elderly
U.S.	Serkes et al.[545]	1990	Multicenter	0.62	$p=0.08$ non-DM
					0.90 DM
U.S.	Wolfe et al.[557]	1990	Statewide	0.98	
Italy	Maiorca et al.[546]	1991	Multicenter	1.24	NS
Spain	Gentil et al.[558]	1992	Multicenter	1.22	$p=0.33$
U.S.	Held et al.[559]	1994	National	0.84	$p=0.25$ non-DM
					1.26 $p=0.03$ DM
U.S.	Bloembergen et al.[157]	1995	National	1.19	$p<0.001$
Aust-N.Z.	Disney[560]	1995	National	1.31	
Italy	Locatelli et al.[561]	1995	Regional	1.42	
Canada	Fenton et al.[562]	1997	National	0.73	NS

SOURCE: Modified from Schaubel et al.,[563] with permission.

was lower for PD patients.[554] However, patients started on PD and transferred to HD had better survival than those maintained on HD—a very strong argument to use an integrated approach to dialytic therapy and using PD as a first line of treatment. Finally, a metanalysis to compare survival of HD and PD—including 82 independent studies, 55 registry studies, and 2 registry reports—proved inconclusive.[158] The main reasons for the inability to establish comparative survivals were attributed to the wide variability between studies, the many formats, and the paucity of data available for case-mix adjustments. Despite all these limitations, it is fair to say that the survival rates of patients undergoing PD are comparable to those of HD patients, particularly during the first few years of therapy.

COMPLICATIONS

Infectious complications are discussed in Chaps. 17 and 18; those associated with the peritoneal catheter in Chap. 13; nutritional complications in Chaps. 21 and 22; acid-base factors in Chap. 20; and gastrointestinal, cardiovascular, endocrine, and other metabolic complications in their respective chapters.

Complications Associated with Increased Intraabdominal Pressure

A positive correlation between IP volume (V_{ip}) and IAP has been established.[568] Although a linear correlation between IAP and V_{ip} is maintained, a change in position further affects IAP.[465,569] The highest IAP for the same volume is observed with the patient in the sitting position, followed by the standing and supine positions. This phenomenon probably explains the higher incidence of certain complications in patients undergoing CAPD, those on CCPD using high diurnal volumes, and patients using more than 2 L of

dialysate per exchange compared with patients undergoing IPD or NPD. Most adult patients can tolerate infusion volumes of 3 L without discomfort and even higher volumes in the supine position.[570]

Aside from the dialysate volume, there are other factors that may influence the rate of development of these complications, such as intraabdominal masses, large polycystic kidneys, previous abdominal surgery, and weak abdominal walls. Furthermore, certain activities—such as coughing, Valsalva maneuvers, bending, and squatting—further increase IAP.[571] Dialysate leaks are often the result of these circumstances. Table 16–9 outlines the complications of PD resulting from increased IAP.

Hernias. Hernia formation is not related to infusion volume but rather to the IAP resulting from the interaction of volume with patient size, abdominal wall muscle tone, patient position, and activities. Other risk factors include older age, female gender, multiparity, time on PD, previous hernia repair, previous abdominal surgeries, polycystic kidney dis-

TABLE 16–9. COMPLICATIONS DUE TO INCREASED INTRAABDOMINAL PRESSURE

Hernias
Dialysate leaks
Low back pain
Gastrointestinal reflux
Hemorrhoids
Uterine prolapse
Vaginal leaks
Cardiac compromise
Vasovagal syncope
Pulmonary compromise
Sleep disturbances

ease, obesity, and malnutrition.[572,573] Hernias have been described with higher frequency among patients undergoing CAPD than those on IPD, NPD, or CCPD with reduced diurnal volumes.[574] The cumulative incidence of hernias among PD patients has ranged between 2 and 15 percent.[573–575] The mean time for developing hernias is 1 year, with the risk increasing 20 percent for each year on CAPD.[572] The most frequent types of hernias are inguinal, umbilical, catheter incision site (with linea alba placement predominating), processus vaginalis, epigastric, cystocele, and diaphragmatic.[409,573,575–586] Dissection of the anterior abdominal wall from a pericatheter dialysate leak (pseudohernia) has also been described.[574]

Most hernias present as painless swelling.[587] When pain appears, a complication must be considered. Incarceration and strangulation of bowel may occur with any kind of hernia but is more frequent with smaller ones. Although large hernias carry little measurable risk of bowel incarceration, they are unsightly and prone to enlarge. A hernia may present as a tender lump, recurrent peritonitis (particularly with gram-negative organisms), or bowel obstruction. In any patient with an abdominal hernia and peritonitis, an intestinal perforation must be considered. Bowel herniation through the diaphragm at the foramen of Morgagni can present as a retrosternal air-fluid level. Another area of potential weakness for herniation is the processus vaginalis. In fetal life, after testes migration, the processus vaginalis may or may not undergo obliteration. In the latter case, the increased abdominal pressure generated by the peritoneal fluid may push bowel into it, resulting in an indirect inguinal hernia, or dialysis fluid forced through the processus vaginalis may result in genital edema.

Pericatheter hernias may develop during the creation of the subcutaneous tunnel. Their frequency is related to the incision size, abdominal pressure, and the distance between peritoneum and inner cuff (more frequent with larger incisions, higher pressure, and greater distance). The pericatheter hernia may cause peritoneal fluid leaks and subcutaneous edema. The frequency of such hernias is lower with fixed catheter cuffs.

Hernias should be repaired before or during catheter placement. Pericatheter hernias must be treated if dialysis fluid leakage is present or if the hernial diameter is equal to or more than 3 cm. Midline incision should be avoided, since this is an anatomically weak area; a paramedian incision through the rectus muscle results in fewer perioperative leaks and less frequent hernia formation.[588–590]

If a hernia recurs, the patient may benefit from a transfer to APD with lower diurnal volumes and normal nocturnal volumes to lower IAP. Repair may be done with traditional surgical procedures. In some cases, reinforcement of the abdominal wall with polypropylene mesh may be necessary.[591,592] The repair may prove inadequate in some patients with severe malnutrition.

Lower Back Pain. Lower back pain can be caused by the infusion of large volumes into the peritoneum, particularly in patients suffering from chronic lumbosacral strain. High IAP increases the lordotic curvature of the spine, which is associated with lumbosacral strain and pain.[593] The use of exercises to strengthen the paravertebral and anterior abdominal wall muscles may ameliorate these symptoms. In some patients, however, reduction in exchange volume or even discontinuation of PD may become necessary.

Other Complications of Increased IAP. Increased IAP may result in several gastrointestinal side effects, such as gastroesophageal reflux (GERD), hemorrhoids, and early satiety after a meal. These symptoms may result in decreased calorie or protein intake and malnutrition. GERD can be caused or aggravated by increased IAP. The collection of dialysis fluid in the lesser sac can push on the stomach and aggravate the symptoms.[594,595] There are conflicting data concerning the effects of increased IAP on reflux. In one study, esophageal sphincter pressures, as determined by esophageal manometric studies, did not show systematic changes with the infusion of 1.5 to 2.5 L, although some of these patients had chronic complaints.[596] Similar results were found in another study, but symptomatic patients experienced more frequent reflux episodes, as determined by 24-hour esophageal pH monitoring[597] The recommended treatment of GERD among PD patients is to avoid large meals and adopt more frequent small meals, avoid foods known to reduce sphincter pressure (chocolate and alcohol), reduce infusion volume, and to use H_2 blockers, prokinetic agents (cisapride or domperidone), and erythromycin. Prokinetic agents are often not effective in the treatment of reflux. However, erythromycin has been shown to mimic the effect of the gastrointestinal polypeptide motilin on gastrointestinal motility. Erythromycin and other members of the macrolide class of antibiotics inhibit the binding of motilin to its receptor on the smooth muscle membranes while acting as motilin agonists. Erythromycin has been successfully used as an alternative drug to stimulate gastrointestinal motility.[598]

Vaginal leaks without evidence of pelvic wall perforation have also been attributed to increased IAP and leakage of dialysate through the fallopian tubes.[599] Uterine prolapse, a relatively common condition among postmenopausal women, can become more frequent with increased IAP.[600] Similarly, hemorrhoids may become worse or appear de novo as a consequence of high IAP.

Significant decreases in cardiac output and stroke volume, regardless of a higher heart rate, have been described following IP infusion of dialysate.[568,601,602] These changes have occurred even with small exchange volumes ranging between 15 to 26 mL/kg of body weight.[568] These hemodynamic changes are probably the result of preload reduction from increased IAP and compression of the inferior vena cava. Although the effects of IAP on hemodynamics have been well documented, the presence of up to 2 L of IP dialysate in the normal adult does not seem to adversely affect the hemodynamics of most patients on PD or their ability to cope with postural changes.[603,604] In patients with pre-existing cardiac compromise—such as those with left ventricular hypertrophy, cardiomyopathy, or valvular disease—cautious monitoring of cardiac hemodynamics is recommended following initiation of PD.[604,605]

Vasovagal syncope related to PD infusion has been observed by several investigators.[606,607] The precise pathophysiologic mechanism for this complication is uncertain; the possibilities include peritoneal irritation from unphysiologic solutions, hyperosmolality, and acute abdominal distention. Despite this controversy, a hemodynamic disturbance caused by increased IAP and resulting in decreased cardiac output, possibly secondary to a reduction in venous return from the inferior vena cava to the heart, seems most likely. When venous return is reduced, the activity of cardiac baroreceptors diminishes, which, in turn, promotes sympathetic stimulation. The use of atropine and scopolamine has been advocated to minimize vasovagal reflex during the implantation of a peritoneal catheter.[606]

Pulmonary function is also affected by increased IAP. A significant negative correlation between IAP and vital capacity has been observed by Gotloib and colleagues.[608] A 62 percent reduction in vital capacity was observed with IAPs above 7 cmH$_2$O. Twardowski and coworkers have also reported a significant decrease in forced vital capacity and forced expiratory volume with V_{ip}s greater than 3 to 4 L.[569] Interestingly, the values did not decrease significantly in the upright position. Several other investigators have reported reduction of most lung volumes as a consequence of dialysate infusion.[609–614] Regardless of these relationships, clinical experience has shown that only a few patients with severe chronic obstructive lung disease have been intolerant to continuous PD.[615] Actually, the changes in lung volumes have not been found to be any more severe in patients with preexisting obstructive lung disease; thus, lung disease should not be regarded as a contraindication to the use of PD.[611,616] The exchange volume of these patients should, however, be individualized, taking into consideration their pulmonary function capacity.

One reason why the clinical observations have been somewhat inconsistent and the effect of PDF on pulmonary volumes has been transient could be the beneficial effect of increased V_{ip} on respiratory function. The presence of PDF in the peritoneal cavity increases the upward curvature of the diaphragm, which, in turn, may improve diaphragmatic contractility by changing the force-length ratio and improving pulmonary function.[613,617,618]

Wadhwa and coworkers have studied the subjective and objective effects of PD on sleep parameters in a prospective randomized study.[619] The patients were assigned to PD using 2 L of PDF and without PDF in the peritoneal cavity during the night. A significant relationship between PD patients with chronic sleep disturbance and sleep apnea syndrome was reported. The data suggested that apneic patients may be susceptible to oxygen desaturation due to the increased IAP caused by the presence of dialysate in the peritoneal cavity.

Complications Due to Congenital and Anatomic Abnormalities

Acute hydrothorax is a well-recognized complication of PD.[620–631] The incidence is estimated to be less than 5 percent, although it has been reported to be as high as 10 percent.[621,629,632–636] The diagnosis is usually made shortly after initiation of dialysis. The rapid accumulation of pleural fluid in a patient undergoing PD should alert the physician to a potential pleuroperitoneal communication. Most hydrothoraces occur on the right side. The most common types of pleuroperitoneal communications are congenital diaphragmatic weaknesses or open foramina in the posterior lateral region (Bochdalek hernia) or the more rare hernia in the anterior and parasternal region (Morgagni hernia). These communications may not become apparent except by the stress imposed by increased IAP in patients undergoing PD.

The diagnosis can be easily established using radiographic or scintigraphic techniques, as previously described. The presence of a pleuroperitoneal communication has been generally regarded as a contraindication to PD.[625] If, however, PD is the preferred or only available option of treatment, surgical closure of the communication[630] or pleurodesis by insufflation of talc into the pleural cavity,[626,629] intrapleural injection of oxytetracycline,[635–638] autologous blood,[639, 640] or the use other irritants has been recommended.[635, 641]

Severe genital edema can result from leakage of dialysate around the peritoneum into the preperitoneal space or from a patent processus vaginalis.[415] When genital edema is due to the latter, it can present shortly after initiation of dialysis or as a late complication. In some instances, the hernial opening is very small and the flow of dialysate will occur only under stress due to increased intraabdominal dialysate volumes, cough, or other causes of increased IAP. The diagnosis can be made through scintigraphy, cannulography, or CT scanning. Surgical correction can easily be accomplished.

Respiratory Complications

PD may affect respiration in two different ways: by the physical presence of dialysate in the abdominal cavity, with its indirect effects on the mechanics of breathing, or from the glucose load provided by the dialysis fluid, which can affect intermediary metabolism and respiration. The effect of IP fluid on respiration is somewhat unclear and the clinical data are often difficult to interpret. Early studies reported compromised respiratory function in acutely ill patients.[642] Subsequent studies showed that although the presence of 2 L of PDF in the abdominal cavity causes a reduction in lung volume[610–614] and functional residual capacity, these changes pretty much normalize within 2 weeks.[611] Furthermore, not all investigators have been able to observe arterial hypoxymia as a result of PDF infusion.[611,643]

Substrate-induced changes in respiration have also been described.[644] Carbohydrate and to a certain extent lactate loads lead to increased ventilation, minute volume, oxygen consumption, and CO_2 excretion[645,646] (Fig. 16–19). The glucose and lactate content of the dialysis fluid is absorbed through the peritoneal membrane and incorporated into the Krebs cycle. Minute ventilation and oxygen consumption increase. Some of the glucose is metabolized without oxygen requirement, but the process does produce carbon dioxide. The increased carbon dioxide production is removed by hyperventilation.[646] If the patient cannot hyperventilate, respiratory acidosis results. A lower concentration of glucose in the dialysate and eventual use of bicarbonate-based PDF may prove beneficial.

PDF in the peritoneal cavity per se only aggravates sleep disturbances among patients with obstructive sleep apnea. The frequency of sleep apnea among PD patients is unknown, since the few studies available describe only preselected patients with sleep disturbances. Sleep disturbances and obstructive sleep apnea are well-known complications of uremic patients and those undergoing both PD and HD.[647–650] Actually the ESRD population has a high incidence of sleep disorders, including sleep apnea and periodic limb movements during sleep (PLMS). Sleep disorders result in sleep deprivation, which can negatively affect immune function and cardiovascular-related outcomes, common causes of death in patients with ESRD. Benz et al. found that the indices based on PLMS and total arousals per hour from sleep were strongly associated with mortality in patients with ESRD with sleep disorders independent of other factors and may be novel predictors of near-term mortality.[651] Other pulmonary complications—such as basal atelectasis, pneumonia presumably resulting from increased IAP, and aspiration of gastric contents—have been reported.[642]

Gastrointestinal Complications

Aside from the gastrointestinal complications related to increased IAP, mentioned above, a few other should be considered. Delayed gastric emptying is relatively common among PD patients, both diabetics and nondiabetics. Delayed gastric emptying of solids and liquids has been detected in symptomatic and asymptomatic CAPD patients.[652] Gastrointestinal motor function is a complex series of events coordinated by the sympathetic and parasympathetic nervous systems. Among patients with abnormal gastric emptying, a return to normal has been noted when the peritoneal cavity is drained, suggesting a mechanical or neurogenic mechanism triggered by the presence of intraabdominal fluid.[653] The treatment of delayed gastric emptying consists of oral or IP metoclopramide. Cisapride can successfully treat this condition, but its use in dialysis patients is restricted due to the risk of cardiac arrhythmias. Erythromycin has been successfully used as an alternative drug to stimulate gastrointestinal motility.[598]

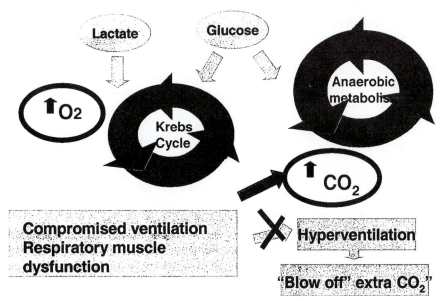

Figure 16–19. Substrate-induced changes in respiration. See text for details.

Acute pancreatitis is an infrequent but serious complication of CPD. Pannekeet et al. have reported an incidence of acute pancreatitis of 0.46 per 100 treatment-years.[654] The risk factors identified included hypercalcemia, hyperparathyroidism, and hyperlipidemia. Although acute pancreatitis has been observed by many clinicians among patients undergoing chronic PD, it is difficult to attribute a definite correlation to the procedure itself, since pancreatic abnormalities are not uncommon among uremic patients.[655,656] Gupta et al. were not able to find a connection between pancreatitis and PD therapy among Canadian patients.[657]

Persistent ascites has been commonly reported after discontinuing PD and transferring to HD or after renal transplantation. In most cases, this complication is self-limited; however, it may occasionally be progressive and accompanied by significant abdominal pain and disfigurement. In the absence of valvular heart disease, hepatic dysfunction, or congestive heart failure, complete drainage followed by IP infusion of nonabsorbable steroids has been used with some success.[658]

Many other infrequent or less important gastrointestinal complications include bowel or visceral perforations from pressure necrosis from the peritoneal catheter; ischemic colitis and necrotizing enteritis, related to hypoperfusion of the bowel after a hypotensive episode; gastrointestinal bleeding from dilated submucosal vessels or arteriovenous malformations in the bowel; pneumoperitoneum from air infused during the procedure or from perforated bowel; and portal vein thrombosis.[659–663] In addition, fibroblastic proliferation and a condition known as subcapsular liver steatosis have been observed in patients receiving IP insulin.[664–666] However, the clinical significance of these findings remains uncertain. Nevalainen et al. reported a high incidence of hepatic subcapsular steatosis among patients receiving IP insulin, but they failed to observe this anomaly among patients on subcutaneous (Sc) insulin.[667] Maximal thickness of the lesion correlated directly with transport rate and inversely with PCR. This complication may be related to protein malnutrition, high glucose and insulin loads, and a condition resembling kwashiorkor that is associated with hepatic steatosis. A rare instance of malignant omentum syndrome with trapping of insulin has also been described with the use of IP insulin.[668]

Inflammatory Peritoneal Processes

The long-term success of PD depends on the maintenance of adequate peritoneal membrane function. Although many patients are able to remain on chronic PD for several years without evidence of clinical deterioration, there is undeniable evidence for the development of peritoneal dysfunction among a significant segment of the population undergoing PD.[307,339,669–672] Two distinct clinical pathologic pictures have been described—UF failure and peritoneal fibrosis and sclerosis.

Ultrafiltration Failure. The syndrome of UF failure is characterized by a progressive increase in peritoneal solute transport rates that results in rapid absorption of dialysate glucose with prompt blunting of the osmotic gradient between dialysate and plasma. Various studies using the PET have demonstrated the presence of peritoneal hyperpermeability from the onset of PD, suggesting that, in certain individuals, UF failure is not the consequence of chronic exposure to dialysate but a preexisting condition.[671,672] In many cases, however, it is a progressive condition that manifests itself after prolonged PD therapy.[673] The reported incidence of ultrafiltration failure varies from 14 percent to as high as 51 percent.[674] Most reports demonstrate an increasing prevalence with time of dialysis. For patients on PD for as long as 6 years, the reported prevalence is in the range of 20 to 35 percent.[674,675] The precise etiology remains unclear and may very well prove to be multifactorial, but—as noted in the section on biocompatibility—several likely factors have been identified as responsible for the increase in peritoneal solute transfer.

Due to the high peritoneal solute transport rate, UF is impaired but adequate solute removal can be accomplished. Proper evaluation of peritoneal permeability is mandatory in any patient who fails to achieve adequate UF with CAPD or CCPD and those who progressively require a higher proportion of hypertonic exchanges in order to achieve adequate UF. In mild or moderately severe cases, a transfer to NPD, with its higher flow rates, using shorter dwell times and elimination of all prolonged dwells, may prove satisfactory.

Periodic monitoring of peritoneal permeability is necessary in order to diagnose further deterioration in peritoneal function and the possible need for discontinuation of PD and transfer to HD. A temporary transfer to HD or the use of IPD or NPD may restore normal permeability in some patients.[670] Resting the membrane in order to restore ultrafiltration capacity has been described, with good success.[676–678] A retrospective study of patients undergoing periodic PETs showed a change in transport toward average, whereby many patients with low UF due to rapid transport improved with time and those with slow transperitoneal transport also normalized.[679] No correlation was found between the change in transport and peritonitis rates.

Peritoneal Sclerosis. The most serious complication of PD is peritoneal sclerosis. This condition is characterized by progressive thickening of the peritoneal membrane, culminating in the formation of a leathery "cocoon" that envelops all intraabdominal organs and results in strangulation of the bowel and patient death (sclerosing encapsulating peritonitis).[312,680] The condition has been sporadically reported in patients undergoing IPD and CAPD. Peritoneal sclerosis results in impairment of solute and water movement across the peritoneal membrane due to loss of peritoneal permeability and surface area. It may present as simple solute and fluid transport failure, nausea, vomiting, bloody effluent, or bowel obstruction.[681–683] The macroscopic and microscopic findings are thickening and sclerotic changes of the peritoneal membrane with or without adhesions, encasement of the bowel by a new membrane (cocoon), and dense and fibrous tissue permeated with chronic inflammatory infiltrate and loss of mesothelial cells.[662,681,684–688] In its most severe clinical form, the diffuse sclerosing process extends transmurally, incorporating the inner circular muscular layer and myenteric plexus of the small bowel in the fibrosing process. Laboratory findings may include blood in the peritoneal effluent, evidence of loculated ascites, adherent bowel loops with narrowed lumina and thickening of the peritoneum with calcifications on CT scan, and low concentrations of CA 125 in the peritoneal effluent. The incidence varies from 1.5 to 4.6 per 1000 patients per year[687] and the prevalence from 2.6 to 4.2 per 1000 patients per year.[681,689–691] Peritoneal sclerosis often occurs after prolonged periods on PD, but it can present shortly after initiation of therapy.[682] The possible pathogenesis includes loss of the normal cellular structure, loss of plasminogen activation from damaged mesothelial cells, impaired fibrinolysis, fibrosis, and elevated levels of type I and III procollagen propeptides. The postulated etiologies include recurrent peritonitis,[304] acetate-containing dialysate,[307,692] hyperosmolar dialysate,[693] chlorhexidine,[694,695] plasticizers, formaldehyde, pyrogen, particulate matter,[696] multiple abdominal surgeries, and beta blockers[697]; many other agents have also been implicated.[698–701] No single factor can be incriminated and the etiology is likely to be multifactorial.

Inasmuch as many patients with peritoneal sclerosis first present with UF failure and the use of acetate-containing dialysate has been proposed as an etiologic agent for both conditions, there is the possibility that they are manifestations of the same spectrum of complications. While some patients progress from a state of high peritoneal transport to the adynamic state of peritoneal sclerosis, the frequency of this phenomenon remains unclear.[702,703]

The prevention of peritoneal sclerosis probably rests on avoiding the postulated agents and conditions responsible for its cause. Based on the literature, the best therapeutic advice is to avoid surgical intervention and try conservative measures, reserve surgical procedures for obstruction and necrosis of the bowel, transfer to HD when the diagnosis is established (although a dry peritoneum may accelerate the encapsulating process), and, as a last resort, try the use of prednisone, azathioprine, or tamoxifen.[86,704–707] The prognosis has been reported to be poor in most series, with a mortality of 37 to 93 percent.[681]

Peritoneal calcification has been observed in a small number of patients.[685,708–714] Presenting symptoms have been abdominal pain, incomplete bowel obstruction, and/or recurrent ileus or hemoperitoneum. X-rays or CT scan of the abdomen show either patches of peritoneal calcification or a generalized eggshell pattern. Histologically, there has been fibrosis of the parietal peritoneum and progressive calcification of the visceral peritoneum. The precise etiology of this condition is not known, but many of the reported cases included hyperparathyroidism, recurrent peritonitis, or hemoperitoneum. With the scanty data available, it is impossible to suggest therapy other than correction of hyperparathyroidism and a high calcium-phosphorus product. The outcome of some of the cases has been benign compared to that of sclerosing encapsulating peritonitis; however, some patients have progressed to require laparotomy and eventually die.

Hemoperitoneum

A bloody peritoneal effluent is a common sign of intraabdominal injury and one that allows a prompt diagnosis. Hemoperitoneum as a complication of catheter placement is discussed in Chap. 13; other causes are discussed below.

Hemoperitoneum Unrelated to the Dialytic Procedure. A bloody effluent is often not associated to the PD procedure and may reflect both pathologic or physiologic processes. Perhaps the most common cause of hemoperitoneum is "retrograde menstruation," with an incidence varying between 6 and 57 percent among premenopausal women.[715–717] The likely route for uterine tissue and blood to reach the peritoneal cavity is through the retrograde course via the fallopian tubes, although the possibility of direct bleeding from peritoneal endometriosis must also be considered.[718] Periodic bleeding in females has also been described at the time of ovulation or from ruptured ovarian cysts.[715,716,719,720] An association between hemoperitoneum resulting from periodic bleeding and peritonitis has been suggested but not established.[715,721,722]

Other causes of hemoperitoneum are coagulopathies and excessive anticoagulation,[715,723] neoplasia,[724–728] polycystic kidneys,[729,730] amyloidosis,[731] pancreatitis,[715] cholecystitis,[732] radiation,[733] diagnostic interventions,[715,732,734,735] splenic infarct,[736] IgA nephritis,[737] connective tissue diseases, and miscellaneous sources of spontaneous bleeding.[738–742]

Hemoperitoneum Related to Peritoneal Dialysis. Hemoperitoneum is a common manifestation of sclerosing peritonitis[715,743] and calcific peritonitis.[719] Irritation from the catheter tip can cause a bloody effluent or erosion into a viscera or the abdominal wall.[744,745]

Chyloperitoneum

This complication manifests itself as a milky effluent—the consequence of lymph in the peritoneal fluid. The milky effluent can be persistent or intermittent. It is usually seen in the absence of pain or increased cell counts in the PDF. The cause of chyloperitoneum is a disruption in the abdominal lymphatic system due to trauma, surgery, tumor, or inflammatory processes (pancreatitis, tuberculosis, cirrhosis, or cardiac congestion).[746–752] It is treated by correcting the causative factor.

Water, Electrolyte, and Acid-Base Derangements

Many of these problems are discussed under "Peritoneal Dialysis Solutions," above.

Hypernatremia. The occurrence of hypernatremia has not been uncommon among patients undergoing IPD. Occasionally, a malfunction of the conductivity meter, which is responsible for the adequate dilution of the concentrate to provide a physiologic dialysate sodium concentration, can result in significant hypernatremia. More frequently hypernatremia is the consequence of inappropriate selection of sodium concentrations in the commercial peritoneal concentrate. The amount of sodium in relation to water in the peritoneal ultrafiltrate bears a close relationship to the length of the dwell time, being lower with short exchanges.[268,269] Therefore it is more likely that hypernatremia will result during IPD than during CAPD with the same level of dialysate sodium concentration. Postdialysis hypernatremia, thirst, and excessive interdialytic weight gain are not uncommon with IPD when a concentrate that provides a dialysate sodium concentration of 132 meq/L is used. The adoption of a reduced dialysate sodium concentration of 118 to 120 meq/L can correct this problem in the majority of patients.

Hypokalemia/Hyperkalemia. Hypokalemia has occasionally been seen in patients undergoing IPD. The addition of potassium in concentrations of 2 to 4 meq/L of dialysate ordinarily restores serum potassium levels to normal. Although hypokalemia has been reported as a frequent complication of PD, it is easily correctable in most instances by increasing dietary potassium intake.

Hyperkalemia has been less frequent with the use of CPD. It usually results from the excessive ingestion of dietary potassium or highly catabolic states. Dietary potassium restriction and an increase in dialysate flow can correct this complication. Geographic and seasonal variations in the incidence of hyperkalemia among patients undergoing CAPD or CCPD are observed and are probably related to the availability and increased consumption of fresh vegetables and fruits. It is important to recognize the potential sources of potassium and to educate the patient and dialysis personnel in order to correct the problem.

Hypovolemia/Hypervolemia. Marked fluctuations in intravascular volume result from inadequate fluid intake, excessive losses of fluid from the gastrointestinal tract, or inappropriate selection of dialysate. It is imperative to devote enough time during the training of the PD patient to assessment of the hydration state and to teach the necessary maneuvers to correct dehydration and overhydration. Specific therapy should be given to treat states of excessive gastrointestinal fluid losses from emesis or diarrhea.

Acid-Base Abnormalities. These abnormalities in dialysis patients are discussed in Chap. 20. Metabolic alkalosis during PD is rare but can result from the use of inappropriately high dialysate buffer concentrations or high UF, leading to contraction alkalosis.[753,754] It can be corrected by the intravenous infusion of saline. Metabolic acidosis has been reported in patients with liver insufficiency dialyzing with lactate-containing dialysate.[754] This can be corrected by the intravenous infusion of bicarbonate and the use of bicarbonate dialysate.

Miscellaneous Medical Complications

Cardiac arrhythmias may result from electrolyte abnormalities or hypothermia. Hypotension is a frequent occurrence among hypovolemic patients undergoing chronic PD. It can be readily corrected by reducing dialysate osmolality or increasing dietary sodium. Conversely, uncontrolled hypertension is often due to hypervolemia. The first step in the management of hypertensive patients undergoing PD is to evaluate their hydration status. If edema, increased venous pressure, or evidence of pulmonary congestion is noted, increased UF should be attempted prior to initiation of antihypertensive therapy.

Beta$_2$-microglobulin has been recognized as a precursor of a type of amyloidosis in renal patients. The clinical manifestations are carpal tunnel syndrome, bone cysts, and bone fractures. The molecular weight of the beta$_2$-microglobulin molecule is 11,815 Da; thus it should be partially dialyzed via the peritoneal route.[755] Elevated beta$_2$-microglobulin levels have been found in patients undergoing CAPD. Although the claim has been made that patients on CAPD may have a lower level of beta$_2$-microglobulin than patients undergoing HD,[756] it is important to recognize that plasma levels are primarily a reflection of RRF and length of uremia.[755] The role of PD in the prevention of beta$_2$-microglobulin amyloidosis remains controversial.[757–768] A postmortem study of patients on chronic CAPD reported a relatively high prevalence of amyloid deposition. Long-term studies on the frequency of this complication among PD patients are necessary.

Hypermyoglobinemia has been reported among CAPD patients.[769,770] This phenomenon has been reported among HD patients as well and is not thought to be influenced by the type of dialysis.[770] Some patients have been reported to respond to carnitine supplementation.[769] Hypermyoglobinemia is probably due to metabolic changes in muscle.

An increased incidence of nephrolithiasis has been reported among patients undergoing CAPD. Many of these patients have calcium oxalate monohydrate stones. The mean urine ionic calcium concentration of CAPD patients has been found to be lower than that of normal subjects, whereas the mean urine ionic oxalate concentration has been significantly higher than that of normal subjects.[771] Although the urine ionic calcium concentration is lower in CAPD patients than in normal subjects, there is a relative increase in its concentration, which appears to be associated with an increased risk of kidney stone formation. The relative hypercalciuria may be a consequence of vitamin D supplementation. Secondary oxalosis is also known to occur among patients with CRF.[772] The increased dietary protein intake in certain patients undergoing CAPD and the poor clearance of oxalate with PD have been proposed as possible risk factors for secondary oxalosis. Measurements of plasma oxalate and ascorbate concentrations in CAPD and HD patients have failed to show a significant difference.

PERITONEAL DIALYSIS IN THE TREATMENT OF SPECIFIC MEDICAL CONDITIONS

Acute Renal Failure

For many years, PD was reserved for the treatment of ARF or for those patients awaiting transplantation or the availability of HD. Although PD is nowadays mostly used as chronic renal replacement therapy, it remains a valuable tool in the management of ARF. There are many reasons to consider the use of PD in the treatment of ARF, most of which relate to its simplicity and widespread availability. PD can be provided in any hospital with the use of the manual technique of dialysis exchanges or with the added convenience of a dialysate cycler. Peritoneal access can easily be achieved by inserting a semirigid acute catheter or a single-cuff Tenckhoff catheter (see Chap. 13). PD avoids the need for systemic anticoagulation, making it most desirable in treating patients in the immediate postoperative period and those with severe trauma, intracerebral hemorrhage, and hypocoagulable states. In the postoperative period after major surgery, acute tubular necrosis may develop, requiring dialysis. These patients are often septic and hypercatabolic. Consequently they may require central hyperalimentation as well as parenteral antibiotics, both of which require a constant infusion of fluid as well as continuous fluid removal. Whenever possible, it is recommended that

PD be initiated early in the course of ARF so that adequate removal of nitrogenous waste products and fluid can be accomplished. The use of hypertonic glucose solutions results in removal of large amounts of fluid in these patients while simultaneously allowing administration of a proportionate volume of parenteral nutrition and a significant glucose load through peritoneal glucose absorption (150 to 200 g/day).[196] Because of the gradual correction of the electrolytic imbalance and removal of nitrogenous waste products, PD seldom results in the dysequilibrium syndrome. Similarly, PD may be most suitable for the treatment of patients with an unstable cardiovascular system, which is a frequent characteristic of the patient with ARF in the postoperative setting.

Finally, PD has provided convenient and satisfactory therapy for children with ARF.[773,774] One of the major impediments to adequate dialysis in small patients is the creation of adequate blood access for extracorporeal circulation. Peritoneal access can be obtained without great difficulty with a technique similar to that used in adults. The selection of a hemodialyzer of appropriate size is also a limiting factor in the treatment of children. With PD, it is easy to calculate the exchange volume of dialysate necessary for adequate therapy. Most infants will tolerate 50 mL/kg of body weight of dialysate. Children 3 to 8 years old tolerate 40 mL/kg. Older children weighing 25 kg or more do best with dialysate volumes of 28 to 35 mL/kg. There are very few contraindications for acute PD. PD may, however, prove difficult or impossible in postsurgical patients with multiple abdominal drains, patients with intraabdominal adhesions, those with hernias, and those with severe gastroesophageal reflux. Fluid dynamics may be inadequate and insertion of catheters difficult in patients with intestinal ileus due to the increase in IAP and the absence of a potential IP space. Peritoneal clearances may be reduced in the presence of vasculitis or disseminated intravascular coagulation.[775] PD is not indicated in patients with pleuroperitoneal communications, since large pleural effusions may result from dialysate infusion into the abdomen.

Although PD is frequently used for the treatment of ARF, there is a scarcity of data in the recent literature regarding the clinical experience and its comparison with HD. Interpretation of the available data is further complicated by the comorbid factors present in patients in each particular series. Orofino and associates reported their experience with 82 ARF patients, 52 percent of whom were treated with PD.[776] The mortality rate was 52 percent for those treated with PD and 61 percent for those treated with HD. The highest mortality was found in cases of sepsis and trauma. Once again, the most important determinants of mortality were sepsis and age. Firmat and Zucchini compiled 1101 cases from the medical literature and from their own series of ARF treated with PD.[777] They concluded that similar results can be obtained with PD and HD. Notwithstanding a significant number of deaths from sepsis, none of this mortality was directly related to the dialytic procedure.

The incidence of peritonitis ranges between 1.2 and 2.5 percent of all procedures.[777] Although peritonitis represents an added risk whenever PD is used in the treatment of patients with ARF, it has seldom been responsible for the patient's death, most cases being promptly treated with IP antibiotics. Whenever semirigid catheters are used, they should be removed within 72 hours of insertion in order to prevent this complication. The use of closed systems and automated delivery systems has reduced the frequency of peritonitis considerably.

Although very few series have compared morbidity or mortality between HD and PD for the treatment of ARF, no evident difference has been found.[778,779] The enthusiasm for PD in managing ARF has varied considerably among clinicians.[780] The choice of therapy for ARF is not an easy one, and although there may be a few definite indications for one therapy over the other, in the majority of cases the physician will be faced with making a decision with no evidence to substantiate the choice. Thus, the final selection should be made based on the availability of equipment, the experience with the particular mode of therapy, and the patient's individual circumstances.

Diabetes Mellitus

The treatment of the diabetic patient is discussed in detail in Chap. 32. Due to the importance of PD in the treatment of this segment of the uremic population and the special considerations necessary for proper treatment, a few additional remarks are included here.

Diabetes is the fastest-growing cause of ESRD and comprises a very large and growing segment of the PD population. In recent years the estimated proportion of diabetics on PD is 45 percent in the United States, 30 percent in Canada, 35 percent in Japan, and 25 percent in Europe.[781,782]

The reasons for the preferential selection of PD in the treatment of diabetic patients with renal failure in many industrialized countries are listed in Table 16–10. Vascular access deserves particular attention, since so many diabetics have vascular calcifications, thrombosis, and generalized atherosclerosis, which limit the use of arteriovenous fistulas and vascular grafts. Diabetic patients are at increased risk of infection and death from neck lines and grafts.[783]

Volume and blood pressure control among diabetics undergoing PD is a more complex subject. While it is well accepted that the steady state provided by continuous therapy is beneficial, it is also thought that PD patients are often overhydrated as compared to those on HD. However, much technologic progress has been made in HD during recent years, resulting in better control of volume and hypertension. Many reports supporting the role of PD as efficient volume-control therapy are from single-center obser-

TABLE 16–10. POTENTIAL ADVANTAGES AND DISADVANTAGES OF PD IN THE TREATMENT OF THE DIABETIC PATIENT

ADVANTAGES
No need for vascular access
Continuous therapy
Gradual ultrafiltration
Fewer episodes of hypotension
Better preservation of renal function
Steady blood pressure control
Better control of anemia
Systemic coagulation not required
More liberal diet
Intraperitoneal administration of insulin
Lifestyle advantages
DISADVANTAGES
Higher incidence of high transporters among diabetic patients starting PD (UF failure)
Nutritional problems
Autonomic neuropathy
Metabolic
    Hyperosmolar states
    Dyslipidemia

vations.[784–787] In a recent analysis of incident data on more than 100,000 new ESRD patients from the Center for Medicare and Medicaid Services in the United States, Stack et al. concluded that new ESRD patients with a clinical history of congestive heart failure experienced poorer survival when treated with PD than with HD.[788] We cannot extrapolate this study to volume control in diabetics but should pay particular attention to the optimal control of volume among diabetic patients on PD and seriously consider better volume control in the selection of specific modalities of dialysis.

Preservation of vision is an important consideration in the selection of dialytic modality for diabetic patients. Prospective studies designed to evaluate the changes in visual function among type I and II diabetic patients undergoing PD and HD have shown a strong correlation between control of arterial hypertension and preservation of vision in both types of diabetes, regardless of dialysis modality.[789–791] Thus, a dialytic therapy capable of better regulation of blood pressure should be favored for the treatment of the progressively blind diabetic.

The potential disadvantages of PD in the treatment of the diabetic patient are the higher incidence of fast peritoneal solute transporters among diabetics as compared to nondiabetics, nutritional problems, autonomic neuropathy, and the metabolic problems inherent to diabetes (Table 16–10).

Serlie et al. reported lower transcapillary ultrafiltration among diabetic patients compared with nondiabetics—

matched for age, gender, and duration of CAPD—shortly after initiation of PD.[792] However, no significant difference was observed 1 year later. These results suggest that long-term exposure to high glucose concentrations in diabetics prior to CAPD may cause changes in the capillary wall aquaporins, similar to those observed after prolonged exposure to high glucose concentration. These findings may explain the published discrepancies on the presence or absence of increased peritoneal permeability among diabetic patients. It is possible that differences were observed when diabetics were compared to nondiabetics early in the course of the disease but not after many years of therapy, when both groups could have had abnormally high permeability.

High leakage of albumin across capillary walls is characteristic of diabetic microvascular disease. This increase in capillary permeability is not confined to the renal or retinal capillaries and has been documented in the peritoneal capillaries as well.[793] Shostak and Gotloib demonstrated increased permeability in the peritoneal capillaries of diabetic rats, and Krediet et al. made similar observations in humans.[792–794] This decreased permselectivity may be due to a reduction in the fixed negative charges of the capillary basement membrane.[793,795]

The potential clinical consequences of high peritoneal permeability are obvious in view of the well-recognized correlation between high peritoneal transport and morbidity and mortality.[377,432,795] High peritoneal transport inversely correlates with serum albumin concentration (SAC), and SAC is a powerful marker of mortality.[153]

Nakamoto et al. have recently confirmed that high peritoneal membrane transport and protein permeability are higher among diabetic patients undergoing PD.[796] The authors attributed the hypoproteinemia observed among their diabetic patients to the higher permeability of the membrane to protein. Cueto-Manzano et al. have further characterized high peritoneal permeability as an independent risk factor among diabetics on PD.[433] No difference in peritoneal transport has been observed between type I and type II patients.[797]

Diabetic patients often develop fluid overload for reasons other than poor UF. A significant number of diabetic patients are nephrotic at the time of initiation of dialysis. Even if their peritoneal UF is satisfactory, they have difficulty mobilizing fluid from the interstitial compartment due to low oncotic pressure.

Another factor that may contribute to malnutrition in the diabetic patient on PD is diabetic gastroparesis. Gastroparesis can be a complication of diabetes and can be aggravated by the infusion of dialysate. Kim et al. observed that gastric emptying is delayed by dialysate infusion and returns to normal after drainage of PDF.[798] This effect is observed among both diabetics and nondiabetics.

Regardless of the substantial improvement in survival rates obtained with PD in the treatment of diabetics, long-term survival remains lower than among nondiabetic patients.[799] Figure 16–20 shows the adjusted survival for incident patients treated with PD from 1987 to 1996. Although the survival rates for diabetic patients on PD and HD have improved over this time, the survival of diabetic patients is definitely worse that for those with other leading diagnoses. PD offers equal or better survival than hemodialysis for younger diabetic patients during the early years of dialysis.[800] PD technique survival does not appear different between diabetic and nondiabetic patients but is inferior to HD technique survival.

Glycemic control of the diabetic patient is critical in assuring the best clinical outcomes. A metanalysis of the effects of intensive blood glucose control on the development of late complications of insulin-dependent diabetics concluded that "long-term intensive blood glucose control significantly reduces the risk of diabetic retinopathy and nephropathy progression."[801] Other studies support the beneficial effects of strict glycemic control before ESRD and during dialysis on survival.[802]

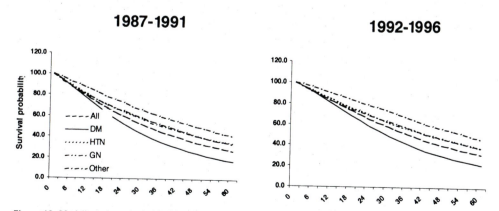

Figure 16–20 Adjusted survival of incident PD patients by diagnosis. Left panel: 1987 to 1991. Right panel: 1992 to 1996. (*Data from USRDS Annual Data Report, 2003.*[799])

Satisfactory glycemic control is possible in diabetic patients undergoing PD with the use of divided doses of insulin administered subcutaneously, with insulin pumps, or intraperitoneally. The available clinical data have not provided proof of superiority for one method over the other.

Intraperitoneal Insulin Administration. Glycemic control in diabetic patients undergoing PD can be facilitated by the constant infusion of glucose and insulin into the peritoneal cavity.[789,803–809] Maintenance of a balanced glucose-insulin administration via the IP route can theoretically result in better glucose utilization, more physiologic insulin administration, and avoidance of wide fluctuations in the plasma concentration of both substances. Consequently, improvement in glycemic control and nutrition, reduction of hyperinsulinemia, and elimination of multiple daily injections would be expected. The effects on lipid metabolism and their ultimate influence on clinical outcomes are more difficult to assess.

Insulin injected into the peritoneal cavity is absorbed into the portal circulation, mimicking endogenously secreted insulin.[810] The portal circulation transports insulin to the liver where 50 percent is bound to receptors in a single pass and the remainder reaches the systemic circulation. The intrahepatic concentration is regulated by the glucose and amino acid concentrations in blood. Insulin inhibits hepatic glycogenolysis, gluconeogenesis, and ketogenesis and enhances glycogen and fatty acid synthesis. Insulin clearance during the first pass through the liver regulates its plasma concentration and reduces hyperinsulinemia. IP insulin use is associated with lower basal insulin levels and faster insulin release in response to acute glucose loads. Insulin absorption is faster when administered into an empty peritoneal cavity than when diluted with PD solution. Insulin kinetics have demonstrated better and more predictable absorption of IP insulin whereas SC administration is affected by tissue degradation of insulin and regional variations in absorption due to fluctuations in tissue perfusion or sequestration.

Hyperinsulinemia has been associated with a high risk of atherosclerosis. Therefore, reducing the circulating levels of insulin should reduce atherogenic risk. However, the literature offers conflicting results. The effects of IP insulin on serum lipids have been reported to be beneficial by some and detrimental by others.[811–813] The confusing interpretation of the available data may be related to methodologic differences among the studies, poor understanding of the ultimate effects of specific lipid profiles on clinical outcome, lack of adjustment for comorbid conditions, and incomplete databases.

Determinants of Insulin Dose. The total dose of IP insulin required for glycemic control is significantly higher than that which the patient was receiving SC prior to initiation of PD.

The reasons for this increment in insulin dose are several.[814–817] Insulin doses increase by approximately 15 percent after initiation of PD, probably due to the increased glucose load resulting from absorption of glucose from PD solutions (90 to 150 g/day). The total caloric load varies with the patient's specific transport rate, ultrafiltration requirements, and the use of hypertonic exchanges. In addition, the total IP insulin dose increases by 100 to 200 percent over the total previous SC dose due to hepatic binding, adsorption to the solution bags and tubing, and unabsorbed insulin discarded in the peritoneal effluent. It is estimated that 50 to 60 percent of the insulin is discarded in the peritoneal effluent. Another 15 percent is bound to the plastic bag and administration tubing.

The PD prescription also influences the insulin dose. The uniform time intervals of CAPD throughout the day provide the opportunity to adjust the insulin dose according to the caloric load and glucose monitoring. However, simple and reliable methods for IP insulin administration in CCPD and in NIPD have also been used with remarkably good results.

Regimens for Intraperitoneal Insulin Administration. There are a few practical considerations worth mentioning before administering IP insulin. The goal is to maintain the fasting blood glucose levels near 100 mg/dL, with postprandial sugars of < 200 mg/dL. Only regular insulin should be administered intraperitoneally. NPH insulin cannot be used intraperitoneally because it precipitates and is poorly absorbed across the peritoneal membrane. The insulin should be mixed with the dialysis solution before infusion by inverting the bags several times. The diluted insulin solution will result in slow and continuous diffusion. Frequent blood sugar monitoring is necessary for tight glycemic control. The insulin dose should never be adjusted without consultation with the physician. Additional monitoring is required during episodes of peritonitis.

The following are general guidelines for IP insulin administration with various PD modalities. It is imperative to understand, however, that these are only general principles and that each patient may respond differently. Thus, close monitoring of blood sugar concentrations is critical.

Daily Insulin Dose Determination. Add the total daily insulin dose administered predialysis and multiply that total by 2 for the initial daily dose of insulin in the well-controlled diabetic. Gradually adjust the dose according to glycemic control. The final dose is usually three times the prior total NPH plus regular dose. A sliding scale can be used based on blood glucose monitoring: Increase insulin by 2 U for blood glucose >200, 4 U for blood glucose >400, and 6 U for blood glucose >600 mg/dL. Insulin should be decreased by 2 U for blood glucose <100 mg/dL.

For patients on CAPD, 85 percent of the total insulin dose should be divided among the diurnal exchanges and 15 percent in the nocturnal exchange. The dose for individual exchanges should be adjusted according to glycemic control. For patients undergoing CCPD, 50 percent of the total daily dose should be administered in the nocturnal exchanges and 50 percent in the diurnal exchange. The diurnal and nocturnal doses are adjusted according to glycemic control. PD Plus patients usually require 40 percent of the total daily dose to be administered in the nocturnal exchanges and 60 percent in the diurnal exchange. Again, the diurnal and nocturnal doses are adjusted according to glycemic control.

Advantages and Disadvantages of IP Insulin Administration.

Table 16–11 summarizes the potential advantages and disadvantages of IP insulin administration in PD patients. Aside from the improved glycemic control, a more physiologic route of absorption through the portal circulation, reduced hyperinsulinemia, and avoidance of insulin injections, some interesting observations have been made related to other metabolic processes. Hepatic functions, not related to carbohydrate or lipid metabolism, have been reported to improve with IP insulin administration.[818] Likewise, higher levels of plasma hydroxy-vitamin D have been observed with IP insulin as compared to SC administration in patients with comparable glycemic control.[819]

There are also a few disadvantages to the use of IP insulin in PD. The need for higher total insulin doses adds to the cost of therapy. Subcapsular liver steatosis and focal necrosis have been reported as necropsy findings.[667] At Toronto Western Hospital, 11 of 12 diabetics who received IP insulin showed varying degrees of steatosis involving the subcapsular area of the liver.[665,666] The steatosis appeared to be more severe in patients with severe obesity and higher serum triglycerides. The clinical implications of these observations remain unclear. In vitro studies suggest that IP insulin may have long-term adverse effects on peritoneal

structure including proliferation of fibroblasts in mice.[664] A rare instance of malignant omentum syndrome has also been reported, whereby insulin is trapped in the omentum in response to foreign protein.[668]

Based on the available literature, the incidence of peritonitis in diabetic patients is not significantly different than in nondiabetics, and the use of IP or SC insulin does not seem to influence peritonitis rates, particularly among APD patients.[820] Protein losses are not affected by the addition of insulin to the dialysate. As previously discussed, the effect of IP insulin on lipid profiles and their clinical consequences remains controversial.

Some concern has been expressed regarding the possibility of promoting insulin antibody production when the IP route is used. Groop and associates have shown that free insulin levels in serum are higher for patients using IP insulin than in those undergoing HD and that the ratio of total insulin to free insulin does increase, suggesting that there is no increase in insulin antibody production.[821]

Edema

PD has proven successful in the treatment of intractable edema states, as in congestive heart failure or severe and refractory nephrotic syndrome.[822,833] Adequate and gradual UF can be achieved by modifying the concentration of the osmotic agent in the dialysate and also the dwell time. Temporary therapy with PD has been beneficial in the treatment of patients with cardiomyopathy or life-threatening CHF in the absence of renal insufficiency. It may also benefit nephrotic patients with cardiopulmonary compromise while awaiting a response to specific therapy for parenchymal renal disease.

Hyperkalemia

PD can successfully correct hyperkalemia with a minimum of effort or equipment. It has proven to be a lifesaving procedure in many instances for treatment of acute hyperkalemia when HD facilities were not available. During PD, equilibrium between extracellular potassium and dialysate is achieved relatively fast.[23,752] Although the clearances for potassium are similar to those of urea, Nolph has pointed out that PD is not very efficient in effecting a rapid potassium removal from the body.[834] In fact, a 30-g ion exchange resin may be more efficient in removing potassium from extracellular fluids. Nonetheless, PD improves hyperkalemia by several means. In addition to slow removal of potassium, it also provides improvement of the acid-base status by generating bicarbonate that raises the pH of the body fluids and results in a shift of potassium into cells. It also provides a glucose load that may favor a shift of potassium into the intracellular compartment.

TABLE 16–11. ADVANTAGES AND DISADVANTAGES OF IP INSULIN OVER SQ INSULIN IN PD

Advantages	Disadvantages	No difference
Better glycemic control	Higher total insulin doses	Peritonitis rates
More physiologic absorption	Subcapsular steatosis and focal necrosis	Protein losses
Avoidance of injections	Malignant omentum syndrome	Lipid profiles (?)
Less hyperinsulinemia		
Higher vitamin D levels		

Hypercalcemia

Acute PD can correct hypercalcemia, but the slow rate of calcium removal warrants the use of HD with a low calcium bath whenever possible. PD is justified only in the treatment of hypercalcemia when renal function is compromised and HD is either unavailable or contraindicated. Calcium-free solutions have been useful in treating severe extraosseous calcifications and hypercalcemia.[292,298]

Metabolic Acidosis

PD is effective in the correction of metabolic acidosis. Conventional dialysate containing lactate as buffer can be utilized or bicarbonate-containing dialysate may be readily prepared for immediate use. The relative efficiency of PD varies according to the plasma bicarbonate concentration, as the rate of transperitoneal bicarbonate movement is influenced by bicarbonate plasma concentrations. Aside from the correction of uremic acidosis, PD can be used for the correction of acutely induced exogenous metabolic acidosis from intoxications. The use of pure bicarbonate solutions can markedly enhance resolution of metabolic acidosis, particularly among patients with liver insufficiency and in neonates.[331,332,835]

Pancreatitis

Since the first reports of treatment of acute pancreatitis with PD in 1960, a significant number of patients have been treated with this modality.[836–840] Severe pancreatitis carries an extremely poor prognosis, with an estimated mortality of 19 percent.[841] The preferred type of treatment remains a controversial issue.

The clinical picture observed in acute pancreatitis—including its multiple complications, which are largely responsible for the associated morbidity and mortality—is due to the release of pancreatic enzymes into the abdominal cavity and subsequent absorption into the circulation. The rationale for using PD in the treatment of acute pancreatitis is based on the belief that removal of these enzymes may prevent or control the inflammatory and necrotic process.[839,842,843] Not only is significant plasma clearance of lipase and amylase possible through PD but actual removal of the free enzymes from the peritoneal cavity is possible through peritoneal drainage.

However logical the approach that PD offers in the treatment of this catastrophic disease, some problems preclude its universal use.[842] The high concentrations of glucose used as osmotic agents in dialysis and the glucose intolerance often seen with acute destruction of the pancreas may present difficulties in controlling hyperglycemia. Patients with hyperglycemia often develop intestinal ileus, which may interfere with proper dialysate flow and make it diffi-

cult to maintain a patent peritoneal catheter. Respiratory compromise is a consequence of abdominal distention and can be aggravated by the addition of dialysate into the peritoneal cavity. The possibilities of peritonitis and peripancreatic abscess, which may complicate and further injure the already debilitated patient suffering from acute pancreatitis, must also be considered. Interestingly, acute pancreatitis has developed in a small but significant number of patients undergoing CAPD (see "Complications," above).

Hypothermia

Hypothermia may be the consequence of accidental exposure or cold water immersion, central nervous system disorders, intoxication, sepsis, or burns.[844] A core temperature below 34°C is considered hazardous chiefly due to the high incidence of ventricular arrhythmias at that level.[845] Core temperatures below 24°C add the danger of respiratory arrest and possible rhabdomyolysis secondary to uncontrolled shivering, which may lead to ARF. PD with solutions warmed to between 40 and 45°C can gradually and effectively achieve a body core temperature of 34°C within a few hours.[844–847] Core temperatures above 34°C are seldom associated with cardiac rhythm disturbances. An additional advantage of PD in cases of drug-induced hypothermia is the possible clearance of the toxic substance responsible for hypothermia.

Drug Overdose

PD plays a minor role in the treatment of drug overdose.[848] Although it is capable of removing toxic drugs—such as barbiturates, methanol, amphetamines, glutethimide, boric acid, salicylates, meprobamate, lithium salts, and other substances that are responsible for a relatively high percentage of overdoses—the removal rate efficiency index is in most cases quite low.[834,849] For some of these substances, forced diuresis is often superior. Furthermore, the availability of HD and charcoal hemoperfusion and their efficient removal of most common toxins make PD a poor alternative under normal circumstances.

The efficiency of PD in the treatment of certain intoxications can be enhanced by adding specific substances to the dialysate. In the treatment of salicylate and barbiturate overdose, addition of albumin to the dialysate increases protein binding and prevents reabsorption of the drug.[850,851] Dialysate pH can be altered to enhance anion diffusion.[852] The IP administration of vasoactive agents to augment peritoneal clearances has also been used.[849]

PD as a detoxifying tool should be reserved for drugs known to be removed with a certain degree of efficiency when HD or charcoal hemoperfusion is unavailable and for the very occasional patient in whom other techniques are contraindicated. Winchester and colleagues have reviewed the subject of dialysis and hemoperfusion of poisons and drugs and offer excellent guidelines for the treatment of acute intoxication.[853]

Miscellaneous

Acute PD has been used in the treatment of patients with hypoglycemia associated with the use of oral hypoglycemic agents,[854] hepatic coma,[855] psoriasis,[856] and in severe hyperuricemia associated with gouty nephropathy.[857,858] IP deferoxamine has been used for chelation of aluminum.[859] The IP use of deferoxamine in CAPD patients has been shown to be an efficacious and potentially safer practice than IV administration.[859,860]

Peritoneal Dialysis in Children

For a full discussion of this subject, see Chap. 19.

REFERENCES

1. Cunningham RS. The physiology of the serous membranes. *Physiol Rev* 1926;6:242.
2. von Recklinghausen FT. *Die Lymphgefässe und ihre Beziehung zum Bindegewebe.* Berlin: Hirshwald, 1862.
3. von Recklinghausen FT: Zur Fettresorption. *Virchows Arch* 1863;26:172.
4. Wegner G. Chirurgische Bermekungen über die Peritonealhöle, mit besonderer Berucksichtigung der Ovariotomie. *Arch Klin Chir* 1877;20:51.
5. Starling EH, Tubby AH. The influence of mechanical factors on lymph production. *J Physiol (London)* 1894;16:140.
6. Cunningham RS. Studies on absorption from serous cavities, III. *Am J Physiol* 1920;53:488.
7. Schechter AJ, Cary MK, Carpentieri AL, et al. Changes in composition of fluids injected into the peritoneal cavity. *Am J Dis Child* 1933;46:1015.
8. Hamburger HJ. Ueber die Regelung der osmotischen Spannkraft von Flüssigkeiten in Bauch-und Pericardialhöhle. *Archiv Phys Bois-Reymond* 1895;281.
9. Blackfan KD, Maxcy KF. The intraperitoneal injection of saline solution. *Am J Dis Child* 1918;15:19.
10. Weinberg M. Die Anwendung der intraperitonealen Infusion beim wasserverarmten Saügling. *Z Kinderheilk* 1921;29:15.
11. Leathes JB, Starling EH. On the absorption of salt solutions from the pleural cavities. *J Physiol* 1895;18:106.
12. Orlow WN. Einige Versuche über die Resorption in der Bauchhöle. *Arch Phys Pflüger* 1895;59:170.
13. Putnam TJ. The living peritoneum as a dialyzing membrane. *Am J Physiol* 1922;63:548.
14. Abbott WE, Shea P. The treatment of temporary renal insufficiency by peritoneal lavage. *Am J Med Sci* 1946;211:312.
15. Klapp R. Ueber Bauchfelresorption. *Mitt Grenzgeb Med Chir* 1902;10:254.
16. Clark AJ. Absorption from the peritoneal cavity. *J Pharmacol* 1921;16:415.
17. Ganter G. Ueber die Beseitigung giftiger Stoffe aus dem Blute durch Dialyse. *Munch Med Wochschr* 1923;70:1478.
18. Heusser H, Werder H. Untersuchungen über Peritonealdialyse. *Bruns Beiträge Klin Chir* 1927;141:38.
19. Balázs J, Rosenak S. Zur Behandlung der Sublimatanurie durch peritoneale Dialyse. *Wien Med Wochnschr* 1934;47:851.
20. Rhoads JE. Peritoneal lavage in the treatment of renal insufficiency. *Am J Med Sci* 1938;196:642.
21. Grollman A, Turner LB, Levitch M, et al. Hemodynamics of bilaterally nephrectomized dogs subjected to intermittent peritoneal lavage. *Am J Physiol* 1951;165:167.
22. Grollman A, Turner LB, McLean JA. Intermittent peritoneal lavage in nephrectomized dogs and its application to the human being. *Arch Intern Med* 1951;87:379.
23. Boen ST. *Peritoneal Dialysis in Clinical Medicine.* Springfield, IL: Charles C Thomas, 1964.
24. Popovich RP, Moncrief JW, Decherd JF, et al. The definition of a novel portable/wearable equilibrium peritoneal dialysis technique (abstr). *Trans Am Soc Artif Intern Organs* 1976;5:64.
25. National Kidney Foundation–Kidney Disease Outcomes Quality Initiative. NKF-K/DOQI Clinical Practice Guidelines For Peritoneal Dialysis Adequacy: Update 2000. *Am J Kidney Dis* 2002;37:S65.
26. Churchill DN. Clinical Practice Guidelines of the Canadian Society of Nephrology for Treatment of Patients with Chronic Renal Failure: Introduction. *J Am Soc Nephrol* 1999;10(suppl 13):287.
27. Diaz-Buxo JA, Gotch FA, Folden TI, et al. Peritoneal dialysis adequacy: a model to assess feasibility with various modalities. *Kidney Int* 1999;55:2493.
28. Nolph KD, Twardowski ZJ, Popovich RP. Equilibration of peritoneal dialysis solutions during long-dwell exchanges. *J Lab Clin Med* 1979;93:246.
29. Rubin J, Nolph KD, Arfania D, et al. Protein losses in continuous ambulatory peritoneal dialysis. *Nephron* 1981;28:218.
30. Diaz-Buxo JA, Farmer CD, Walker PJ, et al. Continuous cyclic peritoneal dialysis: A preliminary report. *Artif Organs* 1981;5:157.
31. Blumenkrantz MJ, Gahl GM, Kopple JD, et al. Protein losses during peritoneal dialysis. *Kidney Int* 1981;19:593.
32. Popovich RP, Moncrief JW, Nolph KD, et al. Continuous ambulatory peritoneal dialysis. *Ann Intern Med* 1978;88:449.
33. Port FK, Held PJ, Nolph KD, et al. Risk of peritonitis and technique failure by CAPD connection technique: a national study. *Kidney Int* 1992;42:967.
34. Oreopoulos DG. Peritoneal dialysis is reinstated. *J Dial* 1978;3:295.
35. Oreopoulos DG, Robson M, Izatt S, et al. A simple and safe technique for continuous ambulatory peritoneal dialysis. *Trans Am Soc Artif Intern Organs* 1978;24:484.
36. Mion C, Slingeneyer A, Liendo-Liendo C, et al. Reduction in incidence of peritonitis associated with CAPD. *Proc Clin Dial Transplant Forum* 1979;9:63.

37. Nolph KD, Prowant B, Serkes KD, et al. A randomized multicenter clinical trial to evaluate the effects of an ultraviolet germicidal system on peritonitis rate in continuous ambulatory peritoneal dialysis. *Perit Dial Bull* 19855:19.

38. Hamilton R, Charytan C, Kurtz S, et al. Reduction in peritonitis frequency by the Dupont sterile connector device. *Trans Am Soc Artif Intern Organs* 1985;31:651.

39. Buoncristiani U, Quintaliani G, Cozzari M, et al. Current status of the Y set, in Gahl GM, Kessel M, Nolph KD, eds. *Proceedings of the Second International Symposium on Peritoneal Dialysis. Advances in Peritoneal Dialysis.* Berlin, Germany: Excerpta Medica, 1981:165.

40. Bazzato G, Landini S, Coli U, et al. A new technique of continuous ambulatory peritoneal dialysis (CAPD): double-bag system for freedom to the patient and significant reduction of peritonitis. *Clin Nephrol* 1980;13:251.

41. Bazzato G, Coli U, Landini S, et al. Connection devices: experience of Umberto I Hospital, Venice-Mestre. In: La Greca G, Chiaramonte S, Fabris A, eds. *Peritoneal Dialysis.* Milan: Wichtig Editore, 1986:183.

42. Buoncristiani U, Carobi C, Cozzari M, et al. Clinical application of a miniaturized variant of the Perugia CAPD connection system. In: Maher JF, Winchester JF, eds. *Frontiers in Peritoneal Dialysis.* New York: Field, Rich, 1986:193.

43. Maiorca R, Cancarini GC, Broccoli R, et al. Prospective controlled trial of a Y-connector and disinfectant to prevent peritonitis in continuous ambulatory peritoneal dialysis. *Lancet* 1983;2:642.

44. Maiorca R, Cancarini GC, Colombrita D, et al. Further experience with Y-system in continuous ambulatory peritoneal dialysis. *Adv Perit Dial* 1986;2:172.

45. Cantaluppi A, Scalamogna A, Castelnovo C, et al. Peritonitis prevention in continuous ambulatory peritoneal dialysis: long-term efficacy of a Y-connector and disinfectant. *Perit Dial Bull* 1986;6:58.

46. Suki WN, Walshe JJ, Ashebrook DW, et al. Multicenter evaluation of a bagless CAPD system. *ASAIO Trans* 1986;32:572.

47. Diaz-Buxo JA, Walshe JJ, Flanigan M. Multicenter experience with Y-set CAPD system (Freedom Set)(abstr). *Perit Dial Bull* 1987;7(suppl):S23.

48. Maiorca R, Vonesh EF, Cavalli PL, et al. A multicenter, selection-adjusted comparison of patient and technique survivals on CAPD and hemodialysis. *Perit Dial Int* 1991;11:118.

49. Maiorca R, Cancarini GC, Manili L, et al. Peritonitis rate and CAPD results. In: La Greca G, Ronco C, Feriani M, et al, eds. *Peritoneal Dialysis: Proceedings of the Fourth International Course on Peritoneal Dialysis.* Milan: Wichtig Editore, 1991:223.

50. Verger C, Luzar MA. In vitro study of CAPD Y-line system. *Adv Perit Dial* 1986;2:160.

51. Verger C, Faller B, Ryckelynck JPH, et al. Comparison between the efficacy of CAPD Y-lines without "in-line" disinfectant and standard systems: A multicenter prospective controlled trial. *Perit Dial Bull* 1987;7(suppl):S82.

52. Li PKT, Law MC, Chow KM, et al. Comparison of clinical outcome and ease of handling in two double-bag systems in continuous ambulatory peritoneal dialysis: a prospective, randomized, controlled, multicentre study. *Am J Kidney Dis* 2002;40:373.

53. Boen ST, Mulinari AS, Dillard DH, et al. Periodic peritoneal dialysis in the management of chronic uremia. *Trans Am Soc Artif Intern Organs* 1962;8:256..

54. Lasker N, McCauley EP, Passarotti CT. Chronic peritoneal dialysis. *Trans Am Soc Artif Intern Organs* 1966;12:94.

55. Tenckhoff H, Shilipetar G, van Paasschen WH, et al. A home peritoneal dialysate delivery system. *Trans Am Soc Artif Intern Organs* 1969;15:103.

56. Boen ST. Overview and history of peritoneal dialysis. *Dial Transplant* 1977;6:12.

57. *Annual Report to Congress—End Stage Renal Disease Program.* Baltimore, MD: Health Care Financing Administration; Department of Health, Education and Welfare, 1979.

58. Gutman RA. Automated peritoneal dialysis for home use. *Q J Med* 1978;47:261.

59. von Hartitzsch B, Medlock TR. Chronic peritoneal dialysis—a regime comparable to conventional hemodialysis. *Trans Am Soc Artif Intern Organs* 1976;22:595.

60. Diaz-Buxo JA, Farmer CD, Chandler JT. Chronic peritoneal dialysis at home—an alternative for the patient with renal failure. *Dial Transplant* 1977;6:64.

61. Diaz-Buxo JA, Walker PJ, Chandler JT, et al. Impact of peritoneal dialysis on renal replacement therapy. *Dial Transplant* 1979;8:1061.

62. Fenton SSA, Cattran DC, Barnes NM, et al. Home peritoneal dialysis—a major advance in promoting home dialysis. *Trans Am Soc Artif Intern Organs* 1977;23:194.

63. Karanicolas S, Oreopoulos DG, Pylypchuk G, et al. Home peritoneal dialysis: three years' experience in Toronto. *Can Med Assoc J* 1977;116:266.

64. Tenckhoff H, Blagg CR, Curtis KF, et al. Chronic peritoneal dialysis. *Proc Eur Dial Transplant Assoc* 1973;10:363.

65. Tenckhoff H. Advantages and shortcomings of peritoneal dialysis in the management of chronic renal failure. *Semin Uronephrol* 1977;1:107.

66. Diaz-Buxo JA, Haas VF. The influence of automated peritoneal dialysis in an established dialysis program. *Dial Transplant* 1979;8:531.

67. Roxe DM, del Greco F, Krumlovsky F, et al. A comparison of maintenance hemodialysis to maintenance peritoneal dialysis in the maintenance of end-stage renal disease. *Trans Am Soc Artif Intern Organs* 1979;25:81.

68. Diaz-Buxo JA, Chandler JT, Farmer CD, et al. Long-term observation of peritoneal clearances in patients undergoing peritoneal dialysis. *Trans Am Soc Artif Intern Organs* 1983;6:21.

69. Diaz-Buxo JA, Walker PJ, Chandler JT, et al. Experience with intermittent peritoneal dialysis and continuous cyclic peritoneal dialysis. *Am J Kidney Dis* 1984;4:242.

70. Ahmad S, Gallagher N, Shen F. Intermittent peritoneal dialysis: status reassessed. *Trans Am Soc Artif Intern Organs* 1979;25:86.

71. Schmidt RW, Blumenkrantz MJ. IPD, CAPD, CCPD, CRPD—peritoneal dialysis: past, present and future. *Int J Artif Organs* 1981;4:124.

72. Ghantous WN, Salkin MS, Adelson BN, et al. Limitations of peritoneal dialysis in the treatment of ESRD patients. *Trans Am Soc Artif Intern Organs* 1979;25:100.

73. Tenckhoff H, Ward G, Boen ST. The influence of dialysate volume and flow rate on peritoneal clearance. *Proc Eur Dial Transplant Assoc* 1965;2:113.

74. Diaz-Buxo JA, Walker PJ, Farmer CD, et al. Continuous cyclic peritoneal dialysis (CCPD) (abstr). *Kidney Int* 1981; 19:145.

75. Nakagawa D, Price C, Stinebaugh B, et al. Continuous cyclic peritoneal dialysis: A viable option in the treatment of chronic renal failure. *Trans Am Soc Artif Intern Organs* 1981;27:55.

76. Price C, Suki W. New modifications of peritoneal dialysis: Options in the treatment of patients with renal failure. *Am J Nephrol* 1981;1:97.

77. Graham W. Nightly intermittent peritoneal dialysis prescription and power. In: Ronco C, Feriani AG, Virga G, eds. *Contributions to Nephrology.* Basel: Karger, 1999:109.

78. Diaz-Buxo JA. Automated peritoneal dialysis: a therapy in evolution. In: Ronco C, Feriani AG, Virga G, eds. *Contributions To Nephrology.* Basel: Karger, 1999:1.

79. Diaz-Buxo JA. Peritoneal dialysis cyclers and other mechanical devices. In: Nissenson A, Fine R, eds. *Dialysis Therapy,* 3d ed. Philadelphia: Hanley & Belfus, 2001:89.

80. Diaz-Buxo JA. Continuous ambulatory and continuous cycling peritoneal dialysis. In: LaGreca G, Chiaramonte S, Fabris A, et al, eds. *Peritoneal Dialysis.* Milan: Wichtig Editore, 1986:257.

81. Diaz-Buxo JA. Enhancement of peritoneal dialysis: The PD Plus concept. *Am J Kidney Dis* 1996;27:92.

82. Diaz-Buxo JA, Youngblood B, Torres A. Delivered dialysis dose with PD Plus therapy: a mulitcenter study. *Am Soc Nephrol* 1998;18:520.

83. Diaz-Buxo JA, Farmer CD, Chandler JT, et al. CCPD: wet is better than dry. In: Avram MM, Giordano C, eds. *Ambulatory Peritoneal Dialysis.* New York: Plenum Medical, 1990: 259.

84. Twardowski ZJ, Nolph KD, Khanna R, et al. Daily clearances with continuous ambulatory peritoneal dialysis and nightly peritoneal dialysis. *ASAIO Trans* 1986;32:575.

85. Twardowski ZJ, Nolph KD, Khanna R, et al. Choice of peritoneal dialysis regimen based on peritoneal transfer rates. *Perit Dial Bull* 1987;7(suppl):S79.

86. Diaz-Buxo JA. Peritoneal sclerosis in a woman on continuous cyclic peritoneal dialysis. *Semin Dial* 1992;5:317.

87. Stephen RL. Reciprocating peritoneal dialysis with a subcutaneous peritoneal catheter. *Dial Transplant* 1978;7:834.

88. Flanigan MJ, Lim VS, Pflederer TA. Tidal peritoneal dialysis: kinetics and protein balance. *Am J Kidney Dis* 21993;2: 700.

89. Twardowski ZJ, Nolph K, Khanna R, et al. Eight hr tidal peritoneal dialysis (TPD) matches 24 hr CAPD and surpasses 8 hr nightly intermittent peritoneal dialysis (NIPD) clearances (C) (abstr). *Perit Dial Bull* 1987;7(suppl):S79.

90. Twardowski ZJ, Prowant BF, Nolph KD, et al. Chronic nightly tidal peritoneal dialysis. *Trans Am Soc Artif Intern Organs* 1990;36:M584.

91. Steinhauer HB, Keck I, Lubrich-Birkner I, Schollmeyer P. Increased dialysis efficiency in tidal peritoneal dialysis compared to intermittent peritoneal dialysis. *Nephron* 1991;58: 500.

92. Rodríguez AMF, Díaz NV, Cubillo LP, et al. Adequacy of dialysis in automated peritoneal dialysis: a clinical experience. *Perit Dial Int* 1997;7:442.

93. Quellhorst E, Solf A, Hildebrand U. Tidal peritoneal dialysis (TPD) is superior to intermittent peritoneal dialysis (IPD) in long-term treatment of patients with chronic renal insufficiency (CRI)(abstr). *Perit Dial Int* 1991;11(suppl 1):217.

94. Piraino B, Bender F, Bernardini J. A comparison of clearances on tidal peritoneal dialysis and intermittent peritoneal dialysis. *Perit Dial Int* 1994;14:145.

95. Rodríguez AMF, Diaz NV, Cubillo LP, et al. Automated peritoneal dialysis: a Spanish multicentre study. *Nephrol Dial Transplant* 1998;13:2335.

96. Vychytil A, Lilaj T, Schneider B, et al. Tidal peritoneal dialysis for home-treated patients: should it be preferred. *Am J Kidney Dis* 1999;33:334.

97. Shah J, Lane D, Shrivastava D, et al. Isovolemic tidal technique does not increase clearances in intermittent peritoneal dialysis (IPD)(abstr). *J Am Soc Nephrol* 1992;3:419.

98. Aasarod K, Wideroe TE, Flakne SC. A comparison of solute cleaerance and ultrafiltration volume in peritoneal dialysis with total or fractional (50%) intraperitoneal volume exchange with the same dialysate flow rate. *Neprhol Dial Transplant* 1997;12:2128.

99. Juergensen PH, Murphy AL, Pherson KA, et al. Tidal peritoneal dialysis: comparison of different tidal regimens and automated peritoneal dialysis. *Kidney Int* 2000;57:2603.

100. Cruz C, Melendez A, Gotch FA, et al. Single-pass continuous flow peritoneal dialysis using two catheters. *Semin Dial* 2001;14:391.

101. Twardowski ZJ. New approaches to intermittent peritoneal dialysis therapies. In: Nolph KD, ed. *Peritoneal Dialysis.* Dordrecht: Kluwer, 1989:133.

102. Frank HA, Seligman AM, Fine J. Further experiences with peritoneal irrigation for acute renal failure. *Ann Surg* 1948;128:561.

103. Legrain M, Merrill JP: Short-term continuous transperitoneal dialysis: A simplified technique. *N Engl J Med* 1953; 248:125.

104. Shinaberger JH, Shear L, Barry KG. Increasing efficiency of peritoneal dialysis. Experience with peritoneal extracorporeal recirculation dialysis. *Trans Am Soc Artif Intern Organs* 1965;11:76.

105. Lange K, Treser G. Automatic continuous high flow rate peritoneal dialysis. *Trans Am Soc Artif Intern Organs* 1967; 13:164.

106. Stephen RL, Atkin-Thor E, Kolff WJ. Recirculating peritoneal dialysis with subcutaneous catheter. *Trans Am Soc Artif Intern Organs* 1976;22:575.

107. Gordon A, Lewin AJ, Maxwell MH, Morales ND Augmentation of efficiency by continuous flow sorbent regeneration peritoneal dialysis. *Trans Am Soc Artif Intern Organs* 1976; 22:599.

108. Kramer MS, Rosenbaum JL. Recirculation peritoneal dialysis with sorbent REDY cartridge. *Trans Am Soc Artif Intern Organs* 1967;12:134.

109. Kablitz C, Kessler T, Dew P, et al: Subcutaneous peritoneal catheter: 2 1/2 years experience. *Artif Organs* 1979;3:210.

110. Tobe SW, Purcell L, Saiphoo CS, et al. High efficiency peritoneal dialysis (HEPD): a new method of performing peritoneal dialysis (PD)(abstr). *Perit Dial Int* 1994;14(suppl 1):S24.

111. Kraus MA. Ultrafiltration peritoneal dialysis and recirculating peritoneal dialysis with a portable kidney. *Dial Transplant* 1983;12:385.

112. Uechi M, Iida E, Watanabe T, et al. Peritoneal dialysis using a recycling system in dogs. *J Vet Med Sci* 1993;55:723.

113. Diaz-Buxo JA. Evolution of continuous flow peritoneal dialysis and the current state of the art. *Semin Dial* 2001;14:373.

114. Diaz-Buxo JA. Continuous flow peritoneal dialysis: Clinical applications. *Blood Purif* 2002;20:36.

115. Raj DS, Self M, Work J. Hybrid dialysis: recirculation peritoneal dialysis revisited. *Am J Kidney Dis* 2000;36:58.

116. Mineshima M, Watanuki M, Yamagata K, et al. Development of continuous recirculating peritoneal dialysis using a double lumen catheter. *ASAIO J* 1992;38:M377.

117. Diaz-Buxo JA. Renal care 2000—peritoneal dialysis. Prospects for PD in the future. *Nephrol News Issues* 1999; 3:12.

118. Passlick-Deetjen J, Quellhorst E. Continuous flow peritoneal dialysis (CFPD): a glimpse into the future. *Nephrol Dial Transplant* 2001;16:2296.

119. Diaz-Buxo JA. Streaming, mixing and recirculation: role of the peritoneal access in continuous flow peritoneal dialysis (clinical considerations). *Adv Perit Dial* 2002;18:87.

120. Ronco C, Gloukhoff A, Dell'Aquila R, Levin NW. Catheter design for continuous flow peritoneal dialysis. *Blood Purif* 2002;20:40.

121. Moeller S, Gioberge S, Brown G. ESRD patients in 2001: global overviews of patients, treatment modalities and development trends. *Dial Transplant* 2002;17:2071.

122. Ahlmen J, Carlsson L, Schonborg C. Well-informed patients with end-stage renal disease prefer peritoneal dialysis to hemodialysis. *Perit Dial Int* 1993;13(suppl 2):S196.

123. Prichard S. Treatment modality selection in 150 consecutive patients starting ESRD therapy. *Perit Dial Int* 1996;16:69.

124. Levin A, Lewis M, Mortiboy P, et al. Multidisciplinary predialysis programs: quantification and limitations of their impact on patient outcomes in two Canadian settings. *Am J Kidney Dis* 1997;29:533.

125. Lameire N, Van Biesen W, Dombros N, et al. The referral pattern of patients with ESRD is a determinant in the choice of dialysis modality. *Perit Dial Int* 1997;17(suppl 2):S161.

126. Little J, Irwin A, Marshall T, et al. Predicting a patient's choice of dialysis modality: experience in a United Kingdom renal department. *Am J Kidney Dis* 2001;37:981.

127. Gil Gomez C, Valido P, Celadilla O, et al. Validity of a standard information protocol provided to ESRD patients and its effect on treatment selection. *Perit Dial Int* 1999;19:471.

128. Wuerth DA, Finkelstein SH, Schwetz O, et al. Patient's descriptions of specific factors leading to selection of chronic

129. Stack AG. Determinants of modality selection among incident US dialysis patients: results from a national study. *J Am Soc Nephrol* 2002;13:1279.

130. Miskulin DC, Meyer KB, Athienites NV, et al. Comorbidity and other factors associated with modality selection in incident dialysis patients: the CHOICE study. *Am J Kidney Dis* 2002;39:324.

131. The USRD Dialysis Morbidity and Mortality Study: Wave 2. *Am J Kidney Dis* 1997;30(suppl 1):S67.

132. Lozano J: Issues and controversies in U.S. dialysis mortality. *Dial Transplant* 1994;23:42.

133. Mendelssohn DC, Mullaney SR, Jung B, et al. What do American nephrologists think about dialysis modality selection? *Am J Kidney Dis* 2001;37:22.

134. Jung B, Blake PG, Mehta RL, Mendelssohn DC. Attitudes of Canadian nephrologists toward dialysis modality selection. *Perit Dial Int* 1999;19:263.

135. Diaz-Buxo JA, Lowrie EG, Lew NL, et al. Associates of mortality among peritoneal dialysis patients with special reference to peritoneal transport rates and solute clearance. *Am J Kidney Dis* 1999;33:523.

136. Szeto CC, Wong TYH, Leung CB, et al. Importance of dialysis adequacy in mortality and morbidity of Chinese CAPD patients. *Kidney Int* 2000;58:400.

137. Rocco M, Soucie JM, Pastan S, McClellan WM. Peritoneal dialysis adequacy and risk of death. *Kidney Int* 2000;58:446.

138. Bargman JM, Thorpe KE, Churchill DN, for the Canada-USA (CANUSA) Peritoneal Dialysis Group. The relative contribution of residual renal function and peritoneal clearance to adequacy of dialysis: a re-analysis of the Canada-USA (CANUSA) study. *J Am Soc Nephrol* 2001;12:2158.

139. Termorshuizen F, Korevaar JC, Dekker FW, et al. The relative importance of residual renal function compared with peritoneal clearance for patient survival and quality of life: An analysis of the Netherlands cooperative study on the adequacy of dialysis (NECOSAD)-2. *Am J Kidney Dis* 2003; 41:1293.

140. Szeto CC, Wong TYH, Chow KM, et al. Impact of dialysis adequacy on the mortality and morbidity of anuric Chinese patients receiving continuous ambulatory peritoneal dialysis. *J Am Soc Nephrol* 2001;12:355.

141. Burkart JM, Satko SG. Incremental initiation of dialysis: one center's experience over a two-year period. *Perit Dial Bull* 2000;20:418.

142. Lysaght MJ, Vonesh EF, Gotch F, et al. The influence of dialysis treatment modality on the decline of remaining renal function. *Trans Am Soc Artif Intern Organs* 1991;37: 598.

143. Rottembourg J. Residual renal function and recovery of renal function in patients treated by CAPD. *Kidney Int* 1993; 43(suppl 40):S106.

144. Cancarini GC, Brunori G, Camerini C, et al. Renal function recovery and maintenance of residual diuresis in CAPD and hemodialysis. *Perit Dial Bull* 1986;6:77.

145. Kim DJ, Park JA, Huh W, et al. The effect of hemodialysis during break-in period on residual renal function in CAPD patients. *Perit Dial Int* 2000;20:784.

146. Lameire N, Biesen WV. The impact of residual renal function on the adequacy of peritoneal dialysis. *Perit Dial Int* 1997;17(suppl 2):S102.

147. Misra M, Vonesh E, Van Stone JC, et al. Effect of cause and time of dropout on the residual GFR: a comparative analysis of the decline of GFR on dialysis. *Kidney Int* 2001;59:754.

148. Lang SM, Bergner A, Topfer M, Schiffl H. Preservation of residual renal function in dialysis patients: effects of dialysis-technique-related factors. *Perit Dial Int* 2001;21:52.

149. Tattersall JE. Is continuous ambulatory peritoneal dialysis an adequate long-term therapy for end-stage renal disease? *Semin Dial* 1995;8:72.

150. McKane W, Chandna SM, Tattersall JE, et al. Identical decline of residual renal function in high-flux biocompatible hemodialysis and CAPD. *Kidney Int* 2002;61:256.

151. Berlanga JR, Marron B, Reyero A, et al. Peritoneal dialysis retardation of progression of advanced renal failure. *Perit Dial Int* 2002;22:239.

152. Moist LM, Port FK, Orzol SM, et al. Predictors of loss of residual renal function among new dialysis patients. *J Am Soc Nephrol* 2000;11:556.

153. Lowrie EG, Huang WH, Lew NL. Death risk predictors among peritoneal dialysis and hemodialysis patients: a preliminary comparison. *Am J Kidney Dis* 1995;26:220.

154. Chung SH, Lindholm B, Lee HB. Influence of initial nutritional status on continuous ambulatory peritoneal dialysis patient survival. *Perit Dial Int* 2000;20:19.

155. Keshaviah P, Collins AJ, Ma JZ, et al. Survival comparison between hemodialysis and peritoneal dialysis based on matched doses of delivered therapy. *J Am Soc Nephrol* 2002; 13(suppl 1):S48.

156. Vonesh EF, Moran J. Mortality in end-stage renal disease: a reassessment of differences between patients treated with hemodialysis and peritoneal dialysis. *J Am Soc Nephrol* 1999;10:354.

157. Bloembergen WE, Port FK, Mauger EA, Wolfe RA. A comparison of mortality between patients treated with hemodialysis and peritoneal dialysis. *J Am Soc Nephrol* 1995; 6:177.

158. Ross S, Dong E, Gordon M, et al. Meta-analysis of outcome studies in end-stage renal disease. *Kidney Int* 2000;57(suppl 74):S28.

159. Cendoroglo NM, Draibe SA, Silva AE, et al. Incidence of and risk factors for hepatitis B virus and hepatitis C virus infection among haemodialysis and CAPD patients: evidence for environmental transmission. *Nephrol Dial Transplant* 1995;10:240.

160. Pascual J, Teruel JL, Mateos H, et al. Nosocomial transmission of hepatitis C virus infection in the hemodialysis unit during two years of prospective follow-up (abstr). *J Am Soc Nephrol* 1992;3:386.

161. Jadoul M, Cornu C, van Ypersele De Strihou C. Incidence and risk factors for hepatitis C seroconversion in hemodialysis: a prospective study. The UCL Collaborative Group. *Kidney Int* 1993;44:1322.

162. Izopet J, Pasquier C, Sandres K, et al. Molecular evidence for nosocomial transmission of hepatitis C virus in a French hemodialysis unit. *J Med Virol* 1999;58:139.

163. Campo N, Sinelli N, Brizzolara R, et al. Hepatitis G virus infection in haemodialysis and in peritoneal dialysis patients. *Nephron* 1999;82:17.

164. Van Biesen W, Vanholder R, Lameire N. The role of peritoneal dialysis as the first-line renal replacement modality. *Perit Dial Int* 2000;20:375.

165. Van Biesen W, Vanholder R, Van Loo A, et al. Peritoneal dialysis favorably influences early graft function after renal transplantation compared to hemodialysis. *Transplantation* 2000;69:508.

166. Fontán MP, Rodriguez-Carmona A, Bouza P, et al. Delayed graft function after renal transplantation in patients undergoing peritoneal dialysis and hemodialysis. *Adv Perit Dial* 1996;12:10.

167. Bleyer AJ, Burkart JM, Russell GB, Adams PL. Dialysis modality and delayed graft function after cadaveric renal transplantation. *J Am Soc Nephrol* 1999;10:154.

168. Gokal R, Kost S. Peritoneal dialysis immediately post transplantation. *Adv Perit Dial* 1999;15:112.

169. Sasal J, Naimark D, Klassen J, et al. Late renal transplant failure: an adverse prognostic factor at initiation of peritoneal dialysis. *Perit Dial Int* 2001;21:405.

170. Wilmer WA, Pesavento TE, Bay WH, et al. Peritoneal dialysis following failed kidney transplantation is associated with high peritoneal transport rates. *Perit Dial Int* 2001;21:411.

171. Diaz-Buxo JA, Lowrie EG, Lew NL, et al. Quality-of-life evaluation using short form 36: comparison in hemodialysis and peritoneal dialysis patients. *Am J Kidney Dis* 2000; 35:293.

172. Morris PL, Jones B. Transplantation versus dialysis: a study of quality of life. *Transplant Proc* 1988;20:23.

173. Merkus MP, Jager KJ, Dekker FW, et al. Quality of life in patients on chronic dialysis: self-assessment 3 months after the start of treatment. *Am J Kidney Dis* 1997;29:584.

174. Gudex CM. Health–related quality of life in endstage renal failure. *Qual Life Res* 1995;4:359.

175. Cameron JI, Whiteside C, Katz J, Devins GM. Differences in quality of life across renal replacement therapies: a meta-analytic comparison. *Am J Kidney Dis* 2000;35:629.

176. Julius M, Kneisley JD, Carpentier-Alting P, et al. A comparison of employment rates of patients treated with continuous ambulatory peritoneal dialysis vs in-center hemodialysis. *Arch Intern Med* 1989;149:839.

177. Wolcott DL, Nissenson AR. Quality of life in chronic dialysis patients: a critical comparison of continuous ambulatory peritoneal dialysis (CAPD) and hemodialysis. *Am J Kidney Dis* 1988;11:402.

178. Lysaght MJ. Maintenance dialysis population dynamics: current trends and long-term implications. *J Am Soc Nephrol* 2002;13(suppl 1):S37.

179. Lo WK. What factors contribute to differences in the practice of peritoneal dialysis between Asian countries and the West? *Perit Dial Int* 2002;22:249.

180. Blake PG. Peritoneal dialysis in Asia: an external perspective. *Perit Dial Int* 2002;22:258.

181. Trivedi HS, Pang MM, Campbell A, Saab P. Slowing the progression of chronic renal failure: economic benefits and patients' perspectives. *Am J Kidney Dis* 2002;39:721.

182. Westman J, George S, Scheel PJ Jr, et al. Options for dialysis providers in a global capitated environment. *Nephrol News Issues* 1996;10:26.

183. McMurray SD, Miller JH. Impact of capitation on free-standing dialysis facilities. Can you survive? *Am J Kidney Dis* 1997;30:542.

184. Bruns F, Seddon P, Saul M, Zeidel ML. The cost of caring for end-stage kidney disease patients: an analysis based on hospital financial transaction records. *J Am Soc Nephrol* 1998;9:884.

185. Nissenson AR, Prichard SS, Cheng IKP, et al. Non-medical factors that impact on ESRD modality selection. *Kidney Int* 1993;43(suppl 40):S120.

186. Warrick C. An improvement on the practice of tapping by which that application instead of a relief of symptoms, becomes an absolute cure for the ascites. *Philos Trans R Soc Lond* 438:1744–1745.

187. Boen ST: Peritoneal dialysis. Thesis. Amsterdam, The Netherlands: University of Amsterdam, 1959.

188. Feriani M, Catizone L, Fracasso A. Peritoneal dialysis solutions and systems. In: Gokal R, Khanna R, Krediet R, Nolph K, eds. *Textbook of Peritoneal Dialysis,* 2nd ed. Dordrecht: Kluwer, 2000:253.

189. Vas SI, Suwe A, Weatherhead J. Natural defense mechanisms of the peritoneum. The effect of peritoneal dialysis fluid on polymorphonuclear cells. In: Atkins RC, Thomson NM, Farrell PC, eds. *Peritoneal Dialysis.* Edinburg; Churchill Livingstone, 1981:41.

190. Wieslander A, Forsbäck G, Svensson E, Lindén T. Cytotoxicity, pH, and glucose degradation products in four different brands of PD fluid. *Adv Perit Dial* 1996;12:57.

191. Kjellstrand P, Martinson E, Wieslander A, et al. Degradation in peritoneal dialysis fluids may be avoided by using low pH and high glucose concentration. *Perit Dial Int* 2001;21:338.

192. de Fijter CW, Verbrugh HA, Peters ED, et al. Another reason to restrict the use of a hypertonic glucose-based peritoneal dialysis fluid: its impact on peritoneal macrophage function in vivo. *Adv Perit Dial* 1991;17:150.

193. de Fijter CWH, Verbrugh HA, Oe LP, et al. Biocompatibility of a glucose-polymer-containing peritoneal dialysis fluid. *Am J Kidney Dis* 1993;21:411.

194. Liberek T, Topley N, Jörres A, et al. Peritoneal dialysis fluid inhibition of phagocyte function: effects of osmolality and glucose concentration. *J Am Soc Nephrol* 1993;3:1508.

195. Rubin J, Nolph KD, Popovich RP, et al. Drainage volumes during CAPD. *Trans Am Soc Artif Intern Organs* 1979;2:54.

196. Grodstein GP, Blumenkrantz MJ, Kopple JD, et al. Glucose absorption during continuous ambulatory peritoneal dialysis. *Kidney Int* 1981;19:564.

197. Ward JD, Barnes CG, Fisher DJ, et al.: Improvement in nerve conduction following treatment in newly diagnosed diabetics. *Lancet* 1971;1:428.

198. Winegrad AI, Simmons DA, Martin DB: Has one diabetic complication been explained? *N Engl J Med* 1983;308:152.

199. Alsop RM: History, chemical, and pharmaceutical development of icodextrin. *Perit Dial Int* 1994;14(suppl 2):S5.

200. Mistry C, Gokal R, Mallick N. Ultrafiltration with an iso-osmotic solution during long peritoneal dialysis exchanges. *Lancet* 1987;2:178.

201. Mistry CD, Gokal R. Icodextrin in peritoneal dialysis: early development and clinical use. *Perit Dial Int* 1994;14(suppl 2):S13.

202. Diaz-Buxo JA, Passlick-Deetjen J, Gotloib L. Potential hazards of polyglucose. *ASAIO J* 2002;47:602.

203. Mistry CD, Gokal R, Peers E, MIDAS Study Group. A randomized multicenter clinical trial comparing isosmolar icodextrin with hyperosmolar glucose solutions in CAPD. *Kidney Int* 1994;46:496.

204. Davies DS: Kinetics of icodextrin. *Perit Dial Int* 1994; 14(suppl 2):S45.

205. Gokal R, Mistry CD, Peers E, MIDAS Study Group. A United Kingdom multicenter study of icodextrin in continuous ambulatory peritoneal dialysis. *Perit Dial Int* 1994; 14(suppl 2):S22.

206. Weser E, Sleisenger MH. Metabolism of circulating disaccharides in man and the rat. *Clin Invest* 1967;46:499.

207. Van Handel E. Trehalase and maltase in the serum of vertebrates. *Comp Biochem Physiol* 1968;26:561.

208. Ohneda A, Yamagata S, Tsutsumi K, Fujiwara H. Distribution of maltose intravenously administered to rabbits and its metabolism in the kidney. *Tohoku J Exp Med* 1974;112:141.

209. Silverman M. Brush border disaccharidases in dog kidney and their spatial relationship to glucose transport receptors. *Clin Invest* 1973;52:2486.

210. Ho-Dac-Pannekeet MM, Schouten N, Langendijk MJ, et al. Peritoneal transport characteristics with glucose polymer based dialysate. *Kidney Int* 1996;50:979.

211. Douma CE, Hiralall JK, De Waart DR, et al. Icodextrin with nitroprusside increases ultrafiltration and peritoneal transport during long CAPD dwells. *Kidney Int* 1998;53:1014.

212. Gokal R. Osmotic agents in peritoneal dialysis. In: Coles GA, Davies M, Williams JD, eds. *Contributions to Nephrology.* Basel: Karger, 1990:126.

213. Mistry CD, Gokal R. Single daily overnight (12-h dwell) use of 7.5% glucose polymer (Mw 18 700; Mn 7300) + 0.35% glucose solution: a 3-month study. *Nephrol Dial Transplant* 1993;8:443.

214. Amici G, Orrasch M, Da Rin G, Bocci C. Hyperinsulinism reduction associated with icodextrin treatment in continuous ambulatory peritoneal dialysis patients. *Adv Perit Dial* 2001; 17:80.

215. Mistry CD, Gokal R, Mallick NP. Glucose polymer as an osmotic agent in CAPD. In: Maher JF, Winchester JF, eds. *Frontiers in Peritoneal Dialysis.* New York: Field, Rich, 1986:241.

216. Gokal R, Moberly J, Mujais S. Metabolic and laboratory effects of icodextrin. *Kidney Int* 2002;62(suppl 81):S62.

217. Lam Po Tang MK, Bending MR, Kwan JTC. Icodextrin hypersensitivity in a CAPD patient. *Perit Dial Int* 1997;17:82.

218. Wilkie ME, Plant MJ, Edwards L, Brown CB. Icodextrin 7.5% dialysate solution (glucose polymer) in patients with ultrafiltration failure: extension of CAPD technique survival. *Perit Dial Int* 1997;17:84.

219. Wilkie ME, Brown CB. Polyglucose solutions in CAPD. *Perit Dial Int* 1997;17(suppl l2):S47.

220. Queffeulou G, Michel C, Vrtovsnik F, et al. Toxidermie severe a l'Icodextrine chez une patiente en dialyse peritoneale. *Bull DP* 1999;9:44.

221. Goldsmith D, Jayawardene S, Sabharwal N, Cooney K. Allergic reactions to polymeric glucose-based peritoneal dialysis fluid icodextrin in patients with renal failure. *Lancet* 2000;355:897.

222. Aanen MC, De Waart DR, Williams PF, et al. Dextran antibodies in peritoneal dialysis patients treated with icodextrin. *Perit Dial Int* 2002;22:513.

223. Pinerolo M, Porri M, D'Amico G. Recurrent sterile peritonitis at onset of treatment with icodextrin solution. *Perit Dial Int* 1999;19:491.

224. Goffin E, Scheiff JM. Transient sterile chemical peritonitis in a CAPD patient using icodextrin. *Perit Dial Int* 2002;22:90.

225. Williams PF, Foggensteiner L. Sterile/allergic peritonitis with icodextrin in CAPD patients. *Perit Dial Int* 2002;22:89.

226. Reichel W, Schulze B, Dietze J, Mende W. A case of sterile peritonitis associated with icodextrin solution. *Perit Dial Int* 2001;21:414.

227. Jenkins SB, Leng BL, Shortland JR, et al. Sclerosing encapsulating peritonitis: a case series from a single U.K. center during a 10-year period. *Adv Perit Dial* 2001;17:191.

228. Montagnac R, Slingeneyer A, Schillinger F. Aseptic peritonitis: role of icodextrin. *Nephrol Dial Transplant* 2001;16:435.

229. Del Rosso G, Di Liberato L, Perilli A, et al. A new form of acute adverse reaction to icodextrin in a peritoneal dialysis patient. *Nephrol Dial Transplant* 2000;15:927.

230. Heering P, Brause M, Plum J, Grabensee B. Peritoneal reaction in a female patient. *Perit Dial Int* 2001;21:321.

231. Bassi S, Dagostino F. Recurrent sterile peritonitis associated with icodextrin solution in a patient of automated peritoneal dialysis. *Perit Dial Int* 2002;22:17.

232. Boer WH, Vos PF, Fieren MW. Culture-negative peritonitis associated with the use of icodextrin-containing dialysate in twelve patients treated with peritoneal dialysis. *Perit Dial Int* 2003;23:33.

233. Basile C, Padova F, Montanaro A et al. The impact of relapsing sterile icodextrin-associated peritonitis on peritoneal dialysis outcome. *J Nephrol* 2003;16:384.

234. Wens R, Collart F, Mestrez F, et al. Overestimation of blood glucose measurements by auto-analyser method in CAPD patients (pts) treated with icodextrin (abstr). *J Am Soc Nephrol* 1997;8:275.

235. Dratwa M, Wens R, Tammine M, Tranaeus A. Interference in blood glucose determination for PD patients (pts) on icodextrin (ICO). *Perit Dial Int* 1998;18:121.

236. Winchester JF. Alternative osmotic agents to dextrose for peritoneal dialysis. In: La Greca G, Chiaramonte S, Fabris A, eds. *Peritoneal Dialysis*. Milan: Wichtig Editore, 1985:135.

237. Bazzato G, Coli U, Landini S, et al. Xylitol and low doses of insulin: new perspectives for diabetic uremic patients on CAPD. *Perit Dial Bull* 1982;2:161.

238. Yotuc W, Ward G, Shilipeter G, et al. Substitution of sorbitol for dextrose in peritoneal irrigation fluid: a preliminary report. *Trans Am Soc Artif Intern Organs* 1967;13:168.

239. Dolkart RE, Lameire N. Alternative osmotic agents to glucose for CAPD. *Perit Dial Bull* 1987;7:4.

240. Bischel MD, Barbour BH. Peritoneal dialysis with sorbitol versus dextrose dialysate. *Nephron* 1974;12:449.

241. Heaton A, Ward MK, Johnston DG, et al. Short-term studies on the use of glycerol as an osmotic agent in continuous ambulatory peritoneal dialysis (CAPD). *Clin Sci* 1984;69:121.

242. Daniels FH, Leonard EF, Cortell S. Glucose and glycerol compared as osmotic agents for peritoneal dialysis. *Kidney Int* 1984;25:20.

243. Matthys E, Dolkart R, Lameire N. Potential hazards of glycerol dialysate in diabetic CAPD patients. *Perit Dial Bull* 1987;7:16.

244. Williams PF, Marliss EB, Anderson GH, et al. Amino acid absorption following intraperitoneal administration in CAPD patients. *Perit Dial Bull* 1982;2:124.

245. Oren A, Wu G, Anderson GH, et al. Effective use of amino acid dialysate over four weeks in CAPD patients. *Perit Dial Bull* 1983;3:66.

246. Bonzel KE, Distler G, Bonatz K, et al. Plasma and granulocyte amino acids and peritoneal transfer of amino acids in children on CAPD. *Perit Dial Bull* 1987;7(suppl):S8.

247. Jirka J, Kotkova E. Peritoneal dialysis in iso-oncotic dextran solution in anesthetized dogs. Intraperitoneal fluid volume and protein concentration in the irrigation fluid. *Proc Eur Dial Transplant Assoc* 1967;4:141.

248. Twardowski ZJ, Nolph KD, McGary TJ, et al. Polyanions and glucose as osmotic agents in simulated peritoneal dialysis. *Artif Organs* 1983;7:420.

249. Wang YM, van Eys J. Nutritional significance of fructose and sugar alcohols. *Ann Rev Nutr* 1981;1:437.

250. Buoncristiani U, Carobi C, Cozzari M. Xylitol as osmotic agent in CAPD: a reappraisal. *Perit Dial Bull* 1987;7(suppl):S11.

251. Raja RM, Moros JG, Kramer MS, Rosenbaum JL. Hyperosmotic coma complicating peritoneal dialysis with sorbitol dialysate. *Ann Intern Med* 1970;73:993.

252. Robson MD, Levi J, Rosenfeld JB. Hyperglycaemia and hyperosmolarity in peritoneal dialysis: its prevention by the use of fructose. *Proc Eur Dial Transplant Assoc* 1969;6:300.

253. Woods HF, Alberti KG. Dangers of intravenous fructose therapy. *Lancet* 1972;2:1354.

254. Twardowski ZJ, Moore HL, McGary TJ. Polymers as osmotic agents for peritoneal dialysis. *Perit Dial Bull* 1984;4(suppl 2):S125.

255. Winchester JF, Stegink LD, Ahmad S. Comparison of glucose polymers in dextrose as osmotic agents in continuous ambulatory peritoneal dialysis. In; Maher JF, Winchester JF. eds. *Frontiers in Peritoneal Dialysis.*, New York: Field, Rich, 1985:231.

256. Mistry CD, Gokal R. The use of glucose polymers (GP) in CAPD: a seven day study. *Perit Dial Bull* 1987;7(suppl):S54.

257. Gjessing J. Addition of amino acids to peritoneal dialysis fluid. *Lancet* 1968;2:812.

258. Gjessing J. Absorption of amino acids and fat from the peritoneum. *Opusc Med* 1968;13:251.

259. Oreopoulos DG, Crassweller P, Katirtzoglou A, et al. Amino acids as an osmotic agent (instead of dextrose). In: Legrain M, ed. *CAPD: Proceedings of an International Symposium*. Amsterdam: Excerpta Medica, 1980.

260. Oreopoulos DG, Balfe JW, Khanna R, et al. Further experience with the use of amino acid containing dialysate (Amino-Dianeal) in peritoneal dialysis. In: Moncrief JW, Popovich RW, eds. *CAPD Update—Continuous Ambulatory Peritoneal Dialysis.* New York: Masson, 1980:109.

261. Alvestrand A, Ahlberg M, Furst P, et al. Clinical results of long-term treatment with a low protein diet and a new amino acid preparation in patients with chronic uremia. *Clin Nephrol* 1982;19:67.

262. Mitch WE, Walser M, Steinman TI, et al. The effect of a keto-amino acid supplement to a restricted diet on the progression of chronic renal failure. *N Engl J Med* 1984; 311:623.

263. Alvaro de F, Jimeno A, Perez-Diaz V, et al. Continuous parenteral nutrition by peritoneum with highly hypertonic glucose and amino acid solutions. *Perit Dial Bull* 1987; 7(suppl):S21.

264. Perez-Diaz V, Alvaro de F, Jimeno A. Continuous peritoneal nutrition versus parenteral central venous nutrition. *Perit Dial Bull* 1987;7(suppl):S58.

265. Dombros N, Prantis K, Tong M, et al. Six-month overnight intraperitoneal amino acid in CAPD patients: no effects on nutritional status. *Nephrol Dial Transplant* 1988;3:55.

266. Steinhauer HB, Lubrich-Birker I, Kluthe R, et al. Amino acid dialysate stimulates peritoneal prostaglandin E2 generation in humans. *Adv Perit Dial* 1988;4:21.

267. Park MS, Heimbürger O, Bergström J, et al. Peritoneal transport during dialysis with amino acid-based solutions. *Perit Dial Int* 1993;13:280.

268. Qamar IU, Levin L, Balfe JW, et al. Effects of 3-month amino acid dialysis compared to dextrose dialysis in children on continuous ambulatory peritoneal dialysis. *Perit Dial Int* 1994;14:34.

269. Li FK, Chan YYC, Ho SKN, et al. A 3-year, prospective, randomized, controlled study on amino acid dialysate in patients on CAPD. *Am J Kidney Dis* 2003;42:173.

270. Klein E, Ward RA, Williams TE, Feldhoff PW. Peptides as substitute osmotic agnet for glucose in peritoneal dialysis. *ASAIO Trans* 1986;32:550.

271. Imholz ALT, Lameire N, Faict D, et al. Evaluation of short-chain polypeptides as an osmotic agent in continuous ambulatory peritoneal dialysis patients. *Perit Dial Int* 1994;14: 215.

272. Matthys E, Dolkart RE, Lameire N. Extended use of glycerol-containing dialysate in diabetic CAPD patients. *Perit Dial Bull* 1987;7:10.

273. Amair P, Khanna R, Liebel B, et al. Continuous ambulatory peritoneal dialysis in diabetics with end-stage renal disease. *N Engl J Med* 1982;306:62.

274. Grefberg N, Danielson BG, Nilsson P. Continuous ambulatory peritoneal dialysis in the treatment of end-stage diabetic nephropathy. *Acta Med Scand* 1984;215:427.

275. Madden MA, Zimmerman SW, Simpson DP. Continuous ambulatory peritoneal dialysis in diabetes mellitus. The risks and benefits of intraperitoneal insulin. *Am J Nephrol* 1982;2:133.

276. Nolph KD, Sorkin ML, Moore H. Autoregulation of sodium and potassium removed during continuous ambulatory peritoneal dialysis. *Trans Am Soc Artif Intern Organs* 1980;26: 334.

277. Shen FH, Sherrard DJ, Scollard D, et al. Thirst, relative hypernatremia, and excessive weight gain in maintenance peritoneal dialysis. *Trans Am Soc Artif Intern Organs* 1978;24: 142.

278. Imholz ALT, Koomen GCM, Struijk DG, et al. Fluid and solute transport in CAPD patients using ultralow sodium dialysate. *Kidney Int* 1994;46:333.

279. Leypoldt JK, Charney DI, Cheung AK, et al. Ultrafiltration and solute kinetics using low sodium peritoneal dialysate. *Kidney Int* 1996;48:1959.

280. Nakayama N, Kawaguchi Y, Yokoyama K, et al. Anti-hypertensive effect of a low sodium concentration (120 mmol/L) solution for CAPD patients. *Clin Nephrol* 1996;41:188.

281. Vande Walle J, Raes A, Castillo D, et al. Advantages of HCO₃ solution with low sodium concentration over standard lactate solutions for acute peritoneal dialysis. *Adv Perit Dial* 1997;13:179.

282. Ortega O, Gallar P, Carreno A, et al. Peritoneal sodium mass removal in continuous ambulatory peritoneal dialysis and automated peritoneal dialysis: influence on blood pressure control. *Am J Nephrol* 2001;21:189.

283. Nakayama N, Yokoyama K, Kawaguchi Y, Sakai O. Effect of ultra low sodium concentration dialysate (ULNaD) in patients with UF loss (abstr). *Perit Dial Int* 1991;11(suppl 1):187.

284. Walker PJ, Juhasz NM, Taber TE, et al. Initial clinical experience with a new model of mass transfer for peritoneal dialysis. *Adv Perit Dial* 1993;9:65.

285. Nolph KD. Kinetics of ultrafiltration and electrolyte transport during peritoneal dialysis. In: La Greca G, Chiaramonte S, Fabris A, et al, eds. *Peritoneal Dialysis.* Milan: Wichtig Editore, 1985:47.

286. Parker A, Nolph KD. Magnesium and calcium net mass transfers during CAPD. *Trans Am Soc Artif Intern Organs* 1980;26:194.

287. Kwong MBL, Lee JSK, Chan MK. Transperitoneal calcium and magnesium transfer during an 8-hour dialysis. *Perit Dial Bull* 1987;7:85.

288. Nolph KD, Parker A. The composition of dialysis solutions for continuous ambulatory peritoneal dialysis. In: *Proceedings of the First International Symposium on CAPD.* Amsterdam: Excerpta Medica, 1980:341.

289. Oreopoulos DG, Robson M, Faller B. Continuous ambulatory peritoneal dialysis: a new era in the treatment of chronic renal failure. *Clin Nephrol* 1979;11:125.

290. Delmez JA. Bone and mineral metabolism in continuous ambulatory peritoneal dialysis. In: Twardowski ZJ, Nolph KD, Khanna R, eds. *Contemporary Issues in Nephrology.* Edinburgh: Churchill Livingstone, 1990:191.

291. Martis L, Serkes KD, Nolph KD. Calcium carbonate as a phosphate binder: is there a need to adjust peritoneal dialysate calcium concentrations for patients using CaCO₃? *Perit Dial Int* 1989;9:325.

292. Cruz C, Schmidt R, Dumler F, et al. Successful treatment of hypercalcemia and tumoral calcifications with calcium-free peritoneal dialysis. *Perit Dial Int* 1992;12:109.

293. Hutchison AJ, Merchant M, Boulton HF, et al. Calcium and magnesium mass transfer in peritoneal dialysis patients using 1.25 mmol/L calcium, 0.25 mmol/L magnesium dialysis fluid. *Perit Dial Int* 1993;13:219.

294. Montenegro J, Saracho R, Aguirre R, et al. Calcium mass transfer in CAPD: the role of convective transport. *Nephrol Dial Transplant* 1993;8:1234.

295. Banalagay EE, Bernardini J, Piraino B. Calcium mass transfer with 10-hour dwell time using 1.25 versus 1.75 mmol/L calcium dialysate. *Adv Perit Dial* 1993;9:271.

296. Malberti F, Corradi B, Imbasciati E. Calcium mass transfer and kinetics in CAPD using calcium-free solutions. *Adv Perit Dial* 1993;9:274.

297. Weinreich T, Colombi A, Echterhoff HH, et al. Transperitoneal calcium mass transfer using dialysate with a low calcium concentration (1.0 mM). *Perit Dial Int* 1993;13(suppl 2):S467.

298. Mars RL. Successful use of zero calcium dialysate to treat hypercalcemia in a postsurgical peritoneal dialysis patient. *Adv Perit Dial* 1993;9:284.

299. Carozzi S, Caviglia PM, Nasini MG, et al. Peritoneal dialysis solution pH and Ca^{++} concentration regulate peritoneal macrophage and mesothelial cell activation. *ASAIO J* 1994;40:20.

300. Carozzi S, Nasini MG, Cantaluppi A, et al. Peritoneal dialysis solution calcium concentration regulates peritoneal fibroblast proliferation in CAPD. *ASAIO J* 1992;38:M585.

301. Carozzi S, Nasini MG, Schelotto C, et al. Ca^{++} and 1,25(OH)2D3 enhanced peritoneal macrophage antimicrobial functions in CAPD. *Adv Perit Dial* 1989;5:103.

302. Carozzi S, Nasini MG, Schelotto C, et al. Peritoneal dialysis fluid Ca^{++} and 1,25(OH)2D3 modulated peritoneal macrophage antimicrobial activity in CAPD patients. *Adv Perit Dial* 1990;6:110.

303. Piraino B, Bernardini J, Holley JL, et al. Increased risk of staphylococcus epidermidis peritonitis in patients on dialysate containing 1.25 mmol/L calcium. *Am J Kidney Dis* 1992;19:371.

304. Hutchison AJ, Gokal R. Improved solutions for peritoneal dialysis: physiological calcium solutions, osmotic agents and buffers. *Kidney Int* 1992;42(suppl 38):S153.

305. Burgess WP, Diaz-Buxo JA, Walker PJ, et al. Observations on inadequate buffer concentration in peritoneal dialysis solutions for CCPD. *Trans Am Soc Artif Intern Organs* 1983;29:58.

306. Robson M, Pinto T, Kao E, et al. The metabolism of lactate and bicarbonate in CAPD.In: Atkins RC, Thompson NM, Farrell PC, eds. *Peritoneal Dialysis*. Edinburgh: Churchill Livingstone, 1981:211.

307. La Greca G, Biasioli S, Chiaramonte S, et al. Acetate, lactate and bicarbonate kinetics in peritoneal dialysis. In: Atkins RC, Thomson NM, Farrell PC, eds. *Peritoneal Dialysis*. Edinburgh: Churchill Livingstone, 1981:217.

308. Jurgessen JC. Dialysis for lactic acidosis. *N Engl J Med* 1968;278:1350.

309. Hayat JC. The treatment of lactic acidosis in the diabetic patient by peritoneal dialysis using sodium acetate. A report of two cases. *Diabetologia* 1974;10:485.

310. Vaziri ND, Ness R, Wellikson L, et al. Bicarbonate buffered peritoneal dialysis—an effective adjunct in the treatment of lactic acidosis. *Am J Med* 1979;67:392.

311. Vaziri ND, Warner AS. Peritoneal dialysis clearance of endogenous lactate. *J Dial* 1979;3:107.

312. Gandhi VC, Ing TS, Jablokow JT, et al. Thickened peritoneal membrane in maintenance peritoneal dialysis patients. *Kidney Int* 1978;14:675.

313. Gandhi VC, Humayun HM, Ing TS, et al. Sclerotic thickening of the peritoneal membrane in maintenance peritoneal dialysis patients. *Arch Intern Med* 1980;140:1201.

314. Ing TS, Daugirdas JT, Gandhi VC. Peritoneal sclerosis in peritoneal dialysis patients. *Am J Nephrol* 1984;4:173.

315. Faller B, Marichal JF. Loss of ultrafiltration in continuous ambulatory peritoneal dialysis: a role for acetate. *Perit Dial Bull* 1984;4:10.

316. Rubin J, Nolph KD, Arfania D, et al. Clinical studies with nonvasoactive peritoneal dialysis solution. *J Lab Clin Med* 1979;93:910.

317. Drukker W: Sclerosing peritonitis. *Dial Transplant* 1984;13:768A.

318. Miller FN. Effects of peritoneal dialysis on rat microcirculation and peritoneal clearances in man. *Dial Transplant* 1978;7:818.

319. Miller FN, Wiegman DL, Joshua IG, et al. Effects of vasodilators and peritoneal dialysis solution on the microcirculation of the rate cecum. *Proc Soc Exp Biol Med* 1979;161:605.

320. Miller FN, Nolph KD, Joshua IG. The osmotic component of peritoneal dialysis solutions. In: *Proceedings of the First International Symposium on CAPD*. Amsterdam: Excerpta Medica, 1980:12.

321. Nolph KD, Rubin J, Wiegman DL, et al. Peritoneal clearances with three types of commercially available peritoneal dialysis solutions: effects of pH adjustment and intraperitoneal nitroprusside. *Nephron* 1979;24:35.

322. Nielsen LH, Nolph KD, Khanna R, et al. Sclerosing peritonitis on CAPD; the acetate-lactate controversy. *Kidney Int* 1985;27:183.

323. Katirtzoglou A, Digenis GE, Kontensis P, et al. Is peritoneal ultrafiltration influenced by acetate or lactate buffers? In: Maher JF, Winchester JF, eds. *Frontiers in Peritoneal Dialysis*. New York: Field, Rich, 1986:270.

324. Nolph KD, Ryan L, Moore H, et al. A survey of ultrafiltration in continuous ambulatory peritoneal dialysis. An international cooperative study—second report. *Perit Dial Bull* 1984;4:137.

325. Rottembourg J, Gahl GM, Poignet JL, et al. Severe abdominal complication in patients undergoing continuous ambulatory peritoneal dialysis. *Proc Eur Dial Transplant Assoc* 1983;20:236.

326. Biasioli S, Fabris A, Feriani M, et al. Sodium lactate and other buffers for peritoneal dialysis. *Contemp Dial* 1982;3:46.

327. Feriani M, Biasioli S, Fabris A, et al. The Krebs cycle derangements in CAPD patients. *Perit Dial Bull* 1987;7(suppl):S30.

328. Ing TS, Gandhi VC, Daugirdas JT, et al. Peritoneal dialysis using bicarbonate-containing dialysate produced by automated dialysate delivery machine. *Artif Organs* 1982;6:67.

329. Feriani M, Biasioli S, Borin D, et al. Bicarbonate buffer for peritoneal dialysis: dream or reality? In: La Greca G, Chiaramonte S, Fabris A, eds. *Peritoneal Dialysis*. Milan: Wichtig Editore, 1985:143.

330. Feriani M, Dissegna D, La Greca G, et al. Short-term clinical study with bicarbonate-containing peritoneal dialysis solution. *Perit Dial Int* 1993:13:296.

331. Feriani M, Kirchgessner J, La Greca G, Passlick-Deetjen J. Randomized long-term evaluation of bicarbonate-buffered CAPD solution. *Kidney Int* 1998;54:1731.

332. Schmitt CP, Haraldsson B, Doetschmann R, et al. Effects of pH-neutral, bicarbonate-buffered dialysis fluid on peritoneal transport kinetics in children. *Kidney Int* 2002;61:1527.

333. Yatzidis H. A new stable bicarbonate dialysis solution for peritoneal dialysis: preliminary report. *Perit Dial Int* 1991; 11:224.

334. Yatzidis H. A new single bicarbonate CAPD solution In: La Greca G, Ronco C, Feriani M, et al, eds. *Peritoneal Dialysis.* Milan: Wichtig Editore, 1991:151.

335. Slingeneyer A, Faller B, Michel C, et al. Increased ultrafiltration capacity using a new bicarbonate CAPD solution (abstr). *Perit Dial Int* 1993;13(suppl 1):S57.

336. Yatzidis H. Enhanced ultrafiltration in rabbits with bicarbonate glycylglycine peritoneal dialysis solution. *Perit Dial Int* 1993;13:302.

337. Mion CM, Boen ST. Analysis of factors responsible for formation of adhesion during chronic peritoneal dialysis. *Am J Med Sci* 1965;250:675.

338. Furman KL, Gomperts ED, Hockley J. Activity of intraperitoneal heparin during peritoneal dialysis. *Clin Nephrol* 1978;9:15.

339. Thayssen P, Pindborg T. Peritoneal dialysis and heparin. *Scand J Urol Nephrol* 1978;12:73.

340. Regamey C, Schabery D, Kirby WMM. Inhibitory effect of heparin on gentamicin concentration in blood. *Antimicrob Agents Chemother* 1972;4:329.

341. Nolph KD, Sorkin MI, Gloor HJ. Considerations for dialysis solution modifications. In: Atkins RC, Thomson NM, Farrell PC, eds. *Peritoneal Dialysis.* Edinburgh: Churchill Livingstone, 1981:236.

342. Russell JA, Ritzharris BM, Corringham R. Plasma exchange versus peritoneal dialysis for removing Bence-Jones protein. *Br Med J* 1978;2:1397.

343. Mactier RA, Khanna R, Twardowski ZJ, et al. The role of peritoneal cavity lymphatic absorption in peritoneal dialysis. *Kidney Int* 1987;32:165.

344. Mactier RA, Khanna R, Nolph KD, et al. Neostigmine increases ultrafiltration and solute clearances in peritoneal dialysis by reducing lymphatic drainage. *Perit Dial Bull* 1987;7(suppl):S50.

345. Wang T, Cheng HH, Heimbürger O, et al. Intraperitoneal atrial natriuretic peptide increases peritoneal fluid and solute removal. *Kidney Int* 2001;60:513.

346. Kuriyama S, Nakayama M, Tomonari H, et al. Tranexamic acid increases peritoneal ultrafiltration volume in patients on CAPD. *Perit Dial Int* 1999;19:38.

347. Davies SJ, Bryan J, Phillips L, Russell GI. Longitudinal changes in peritoneal kinetics: The effects of peritoneal dialysis and peritonitis. *Nephrol Dial Transplant* 1996;11: 498.

348. Nakayama M, Kawaguchi Y, Yamada K, et al. Immunohistochemical detection of advanced glycosylation end-products in the peritoneum and its possible pathophysiological role in CAPD. *Kidney Int* 1997;51:182.

349. Witowski J, Wisniewska J, Korybalska K, et al. Prolonged exposure to glucose degradation products impairs viability and function of human peritoneal mesothelial cells. *J Am Soc Nephrol* 2001;12:2434.

350. Honda K, Nitta K, Horita S, et al. Accumulation of advanced glycation end products in the peritoneal vasculature of continuous ambulatory peritoneal dialysis patients with low ultrafiltration. *Nephrol Dial Transplant* 1999;14:1541.

351. Park MS, Lee HA, Chu WS, et al. Peritoneal accumulation of age and peritoneal membrane permeability. *Perit Dial Int* 2000;20:452.

352. Williams JD, Craig KJ, Topley N, et al. Morphologic changes in the peritoneal membrane of patients with renal disease. *J Am Soc Nephrol* 2002;13:470.

353. Craig KJ, Topley N, Williams GT, Williams JD. Morphological changes in the peritoneal membrane of patients on peritoneal dialysis correlate with total glucose exposure and with peritonitis rates (abstr). *Perit Dial Int* 2002;22(suppl 2):S24.

354. Devuyst O, Topley N, Williams JD. Morphological and functional changes in the dialysed peritoneal cavity: impact of more biocompatible solutions. *Nephrol Dial Transplant* 2002;17:12.

355. Millar DJ, Dawnay AB: Heat sterilization of PD fluid promotes advanced glycation end products (AGE) formation (abstr). *J Am Soc Nephrol* 1995;6:551.

356. Tauer A, Schmitt R, Knerr T, et al. Formation of the glucose degradation product (GDP) 3-deoxyglucosone and other carbonyl compounds in single and double chamber bag PD fluids (abstr). *Perit Dial Int* 2000;20:142.

357. Igaki N, Sakai M, Hata H, et al. Effects of 3-deoxyglucosone on the Maillard reaction. *Clin Chem* 1990;36:631.

358. Jörres A, Gahl GM, Frei U. Peritoneal dialysis biocompatibility: does it really matter? *Kidney Int* 1994;46(suppl 48): S79.

359. Topley N. Membrane longevity in peritoneal dialysis: impact of infection and bio-compatible solutions. *Adv Renal Repl Ther* 1998;5:179.

360. Struik DG, Douma CE. Future research in peritoneal dialysis fluids. *Semin Dial* 1998;11:207.

361. Wieslander AP, Nordin MK, Kjellstrand PT, Boberg UC. Toxicity of peritoneal dialysis fluids on cultured fibroblasts, L-929. *Kidney Int* 1991;40:77.

362. Witowski J, Korybalska K, Wisniewska J, et al. Effect of glucose degradation products on human peritoneal mesothelial cell function. *J Am Soc Nephrol* 2000;11:729.

363. Mortier S, De Vriese A, Passlick-Deetjen J, Lameire N. Hemodynamic effects of conventional and new peritoneal dialysis (PD) solutions on the microcirculation of the rat peritoneal membrane (PM). *Perit Dial Int* 2001;21(suppl 2):S18.

364. Duwe AK, Vas SI, Weatherhead JW. Effects of the composition of peritoneal dialysis fluid on chemoluminescence, phagocytosis, and bactericidal activity in vitro. *Infect Immun* 1981;33:130.

365. Liberek T, Topley N, Jörres A, et al. Peritoneal dialysis fluid inhibition of polymorphonuclear leucocyte resiratory burst activation is related to the lowering of intracellular pH. *Nephron* 1993;65:260.

366. Douvdevani A, Rappoport J, Konforty A, et al. Intracellular acidification mediates the inhibitory effect of peritoneal dialysate on peritoneal macrophages. *J Am Soc Nehprol* 1995;6:207.

367. Arbeiter K, Bidmon B, Endemann M, et al. Peritoneal dialysate fluid composition determines heat shock protein expression patterns in human mesothelial cells. *Kidney Int* 2001;60:1930.

368. Passlick-Deetjen J, Pischetsrieder M, Witowski J, et al. In vitro superiority of dual-chambered peritoneal dialysis solution with possible clinical benefits. *Perit Dial Int* 2001; 21(suppl 3):S96.

369. Lage C, Pischetsrieder M, Aufricht C, et al. First in vitro and in vivo experiences with stay-safe balance, a pH-neutral solution in a dual-chambered bag. *Perit Dial Int* 2000;20(suppl 5):S28.

370. Mackenzie RM, Lage C, Craig KJ, et al. Continuous treatment with low GDP solution (CAPD Balance) is associated with an increase in effluent CA125 and a decrease in HA content: Data from the multicentrer European Balance Trial. *Perit Dial Int* 2002;22:101.

371. Passlick-Deetjen J, Schaub TP, Schilling H. Solutions for APD: special considerations. *Semin Dial* 2002;15:407.

372. Haas S, Schmitt CP, Schaub T, Schaefer F. Use of pH-neutral, bicarbonate buffered PD fluids in children on APD: results of a randomized cross-over trial (abstr). *Perit Dial Int* 2002;22(suppl 1):S71.

373. Schmitt CP, Haas S, Passlick-Deetjen J, Schaefer F. Randomized crossover administration of pH-neutral, bicarbonate-buffered verses conventional peritoneal dialysis fluid in children on APD. *Perit Dial Int* 2002;22:32.

374. Gotch FA. Relationships between creatinine clearance and Kt/V in peritoneal dialysis: a defense of the DOQI document. *Perit Dial Int* 1999;19:107.

375. Mehrotra R, Saran R, Nolph KD, et al. Evidence that urea is a better surrogate marker of uremic toxicity than creatinine. *ASAIO J* 1997;43:M858.

376. Brandes JC, Piering WF, Beres JA, Blumenthal SS. Clinical outcome of CAPD predicted by urea and creatinine kinetics (abstr). *J Am Soc Nephrol* 1990;1:384.

377. Selgas R, Bajo MA, Fernandez-Reyes MJ, et al. An analysis of adequacy of dialysis in a selected population on CAPD for over 3 years: the influence of urea and creatinine kinetics. *Nephrol Dial Transplant* 1993;8:1244.

378. Keshaviah P. Adequacy of CAPD: a quantitative approach. *Kidney Int* 1992;42(suppl 38):S160.

379. Twardowski ZJ, Nolph KD, Khanna R, et al. Peritoneal equilibration test. *Perit Dial Bull* 1987;7:138.

380. Twardowski ZJ. Clinical value of standardized equilibration tests in CAPD patients. *Blood Purif* 1989;7:95.

381. Davies SJ, Brown B, Bryan J, Russel GI. Clinical evaluation of the peritoneal equilibration test: a population based study. *Nephrol Dial Transplant* 1993;8:64.

382. Steiner R, Blakely P, Freidman L, Kaiser J. Reproducibility and relationship of PET data to clinical parameters in CAPD patients. *Perit Dial Int* 1993;13(suppl):S86.

383. Trivedi H, Khanna R, Lo WK, et al. Reproducibility of the peritoneal equilibration test in CAPD patients. *ASAIO J* 1994;40:M892.

384. Gotch F, Schoenfeld PY, Gentile DE. The peritoneal equilibration test (PET) is not a realistic measure of peritoneal clearance (PC) (abstr). *J Am Soc Nephrol* 1991;2:361.

385. Twardowski ZJ. Nightly peritoneal dialysis (why? who? and when?). 1990;*ASAIO Trans* 36:8.

386. Twardowski ZJ. The fast peritoneal equilibration test. *Semin Dial* 1990;3:141.

387. Verger C, Larpent L, Veniez G, et al. L'APEX....description et utilization. *Bull Dial Perit* 1991;1:36.

388. Fischbach M, Mengus L, Birmelé B, et al. Solute equilibration curves, crossing time for urea and glucose during peritoneal dialysis: a function of age in children. *Adv Perit Dial* 1991;7:262.

389. Mooraki A , Kliger A, Gorban-Brennan NL, et al. Weekly Kt/V urea and selected outcome criteria in 56 randomly selected CAPD patients. *Adv Perit Dial* 1993;9:92.

390. Busch S, Schreiber M, Bodnar D, et al. The 24-hour D/P ratio is a convenient screen for identifying altered peritoneal transport rates. *Adv Perit Dial* 1993;9:119.

391. Gotch F, Gentile DE, Schoenfeld PY. CAPD prescription in current clinical practice. *Adv Perit Dial* 1993;9:69.

392. Smith L, Folden T, Youngblood B, et al. Clinical evaluation of a peritoneal dialysis kinetic modeling set. *Adv Perit Dial* 1996;12:46.

393. Gotch FA, Lipps BJ, Keen ML, Panlilio F. Computerized urea kinetic modeling to prescribe and monitor delivered Kt/V (pKt/V, dKt/V) in peritoneal dialysis. *Adv Perit Dial* 1996;12:43.

394. Gotch FA, Lipps BJ, Pack PD. A urea kinetic modeling computer program for peritoneal dialysis. *Perit Dial Int* 1997;17(suppl 2):S126.

395. Rocco MV, Jordan JR, Burkart JM. Determination of peritoneal transport characteristics with 24-hour dialysate collections: dialysis adequacy and transport test. *J Am Soc Nephrol* 1994;5:13.

396. Rocco MV, Jordan JR, Burkart JM. 24-hour dialysate collection for determination of peritoneal membrane transport characteristics: longitudinal follow-up data for the dialysis adequacy and transport test (DATT). *Perit Dial Int* 1996; 16:590.

397. Szeto CC, Wong TY, Chow KM, et al. Dialysis adequacy and transport test for characterization of peritoneal transport type in Chinese peritoneal dialysis patients receiving three daily exchanges. *Am J Kidney Dis* 2002;39:1287.

398. Paniagua R, Amato D, Correa-Rotter R, et al. Correlation between peritoneal equilabration test and dialysis adequacy and transport test, for peritoneal transport type characterization. *Perit Dial Int* 2000;20:53.

399. Panneekeet MM, Imholz ALT, Koomen GCM et al. The standard peritoneal permeability analysis: a tool for the assessment of peritoneal permeability characteristics in CAPD patients. *Kidney Int* 1995;48:866.

400. Haraldsson B. Assessing the peritoneal dialysis capacities of individual patients. *Kidney Int* 1995;47:1187.

401. Rippe B, Stelin G, Haraldsson B: Computer simulations of peritoneal fluid transport in CAPD. *Kidney Int* 1991;40:315.

402. Ash SR, Wolf GC, Bloch R. Placement of the Tenckhoff peritoneal dialysis catheter under peritoneoscopic visualization. *Dial Transplant* 1981;10:383.

403. Ash SR, Handt AE, Bloch R. Peritoneoscopic placement of the Tenckhoff catheter: further clinical experience. *Perit Dial Bull* 1983;3:8.

404. Tucker CT, Cunningham JT, Nichols AM, et al. Cannulography with peritoneal air contrast study. *Contemp Dial* 1982;3:9.

405. Diaz-Buxo JA. Assessing the adequacy of peritoneal access. *Contemp Dial* 1982;9:5.

406. Scanziani R, Dozio B, Caimi F, et al. Peritoneography and peritoneal computerized tomography: a new approach to non-infectious complications of CAPD. *Nephrol Dial Transplant* 1992;7:1035.

407. O'Connor J, Rutland M. Demonstration of pleuroperitoneal communication with radionuclide magnification in a CAPD patient. *Perit Dial Bull* 1981;1:153.

408. Schrugers MLC, Boelaert JRO, Danells RFS, et al. Open processus vaginalis. *Perit Dial Bull* 1983;1:30.

409. Orfei R, Seybold K, Blumberg A. Genital edema in patients undergoing continuous ambulatory peritoneal dialysis. *Perit Dial Bull* 1984;4:251.

410. Ducassou D, Vuillemin L, Wone C, et al. Intraperitoneal injection of technetium—99m sulfur colloid in visualization of peritoneo-vaginalis connection. *J Nucl Med* 1984;25:68.

411. Kennedy JM. Procedures used to demonstrate a pleuroperitoneal communication: a review. *Perit Dial Bull* 1985;5:168.

412. Kopecky RT, Frymoyer PA, Witanowski LS, et al: Complications of continuous ambulatory peritoneal dialysis: diagnostic value of peritoneal scintigraphy. *Am J Kidney Dis* 1987;10:123.

413. Kopecky RT, Frymoyer PA, Witanowski LS, et al. Prospective peritoneal scintography in patients beginning continuous ambulatory peritoneal dialysis. *Am J Kidney Dis* 1990;25:228.

414. Twardowski ZJ, Tully RJ, Nichols WK, et al. Computerized tomography CT in the diagnosis of subcutaneous leaks during continuous ambulatory peritoneal dialysis. *Perit Dial Bull* 1984;4:163.

415. Singal K, Segel DP, Bruns FJ, et al. Genital edema in patients on continuous ambulatory peritoneal dialysis. *Am J Nephrol* 1986;6:471.

416. Diaz-Buxo JA, Black EB, Tyroler J. Ultrasonography in the diagnosis of peritoneal dialysis catheter tunnel abscess. *Perit Dial Int* 1988;8:218.

417. Plum J, Sudkamp S, Grabensee B. Results of ultrasound-assisted diagnosis of tunnel infections in continuous ambulatory peritoneal dialysis. *Am J Kidney Dis* 1994;23:99.

418. Teehan BP, Schleifer CR, Brown J. Urea kinetic modeling is an appropriate assessment of adequacy. *Semin Dial* 1992;5:189.

419. Teehan BP, Schleifer CR, Brown JM, et al. Urea kinetic analysis and clinical outcome in CAPD: a five-year longitudinal study. *Adv Perit Dial* 1990;6:181.

420. Lameire NH, Vanholder R, Veyt D, et al. A longitudinal, five year survey of urea kinetic parameters in CAPD patients. *Kidney Int* 1992;42:426.

421. de Alvaro F, Bajo MA, Alvarez-Ude F, et al. Adequacy of peritoneal dialysis: does Kt/V have the same predictive value as in HD? A multicenter study. *Adv Perit Dial* 1992;8:93.

422. Maiorca R, Brunori G, Zubani R, et al. Predictive value of dialysis adequacy and nutritional indices for mortality and morbidity in CAPD and HD patients. A longitudinal study. *Nephrol Dial Transplant* 1995;10:2295.

423. Genestier S, Hedelin G, Schaffer P, et al. Prognostic factors in CAPD patients: a retrospective study of a 10-year period. *Nephrol Dial Transplant* 1995;10:1905.

424. Keshaviah P, Ma J, Thorpe K, et al. Comparison of 2 year survival on hemodialysis (HD) and peritoneal dialysis (PD) with dose of dialysis matched using the Peak Concentration Hypothesis. *J Am Soc Nephrol* 1995;6:540.

425. Churchill DN, Taylor DW, Keshaviah PR, CANUSA Peritoneal Dialysis Study Group. Adequacy of dialysis and nutrition in continuous peritoneal dialysis: Association with clinical outcomes. *J Am Soc Nephrol* 1996;7:198.

426. Bhaskaran S, Schaubel DE, Jassal SV, et al. The effect of small solute clearances on survival of anuric peritoneal dialysis patients. *Perit Dial Int* 2000;20:181.

427. Paniagua R, Amato D, Vonesh EF, et al. for the Mexican Nephrology Collaborative Study Group. Effects of increased peritoneal clearances on mortality rates in peritoneal dialysis: ADEMEX, a prospective randomized, controlled trial. *J Am Soc Nephrol* 2002;13:1307.

428. Lowrie EG, Chertow GM, Lew NL, et al. The urea [clearance × dialysis time] product (*Kt*) as an outcome-based measure of hemodialysis dose. *Kidney Int* 1999;56:729.

429. Chung SH, Chu WS, Lee HA, et al. Peritoneal transport characteristics, comorbid diseases and survival in CAPD patients. *Perit Dial Int* 2000;20:541.

430. Cueto-Manzano AM, Correa-Rotter R. Is high peritoneal transport rate an independent risk factor for CAPD mortality? *Kidney Int* 2000;57:314.

431. Hung KY, Lin TJ, Tsai TJ, et al. Impact of peritoneal membrane transport on technique failure and patient survival in a population on automated peritoneal dialysis. *ASAIO J* 1999;45:568.

432. Churchill DN, Thorpe KE, Nolph KD, et al. Increased peritoneal membrane transport is associated with decreased patient and technique survival for continuous peritoneal dialysis patients. *J Am Soc Nephrol* 1998;9:1285.

433. Churchill, DN. The ADEMEX study: make haste slowly. *J Am Soc Nephrol* 2002;13:1415.

434. Lo WK, Ho YW, Li CS, et al. Effect of Kt/V on survival and clinical outcome in CAPD patients in a randomized prospective study. *Kidney Int* 2003;64:649.

435. NKF DOQI: Clinical practice guidelines for peritoneal dialysis adequacy. *Am J Kidney Dis* 1997;30(suppl 2):S67.

436. Blake PG: Comparison between DOQI and Canadian guidelines for peritoneal dialysis. *Perit Dial Int* 2000;20:487.

437. Diaz-Buxo JA. Inadequacy of dialysis—a preventable cause of drop out. In: La Greca G, Chiaramonte S, Fabris A, et al, eds. *Peritoneal Dialysis*. Milan: Wichtig Editore, 1988:177.

438. Banks JE, Langenohl KM, Brandes JC. Inadequate dialysis is a major reason for transfer from CAPD to hemodialysis. *Perit Dial Int* 1992;12:97.

439. Vanholder R. Middle molecules as uremic toxins: still a viable hypothesis? *Semin Dial* 1994;7:65.

440. Gotch F. The application of urea kinetic modeling to CAPD. In: LaGreca G, Ronco C, Ferrini M, et al, eds. *Peritoneal Dialysis.* Milan: Wichtig Editore, 1991:47.

441. Keshaviah P. Quantitative approaches to prescribing peritoneal dialysis. In: LaGreca G, Ronco C, Feriani M, et al, eds. *Peritoneal Dialysis.* Milan: Wichtig Editore, 1991:53.

442. Keshaviah PR, Nolph KD, Prowant B, et al. Defining adequacy of CAPD with urea kinetics. *Adv Perit Dial* 1990; 6:173.

443. Keshaviah PR, Nolph KD, Van Stone JC. The peak concentration hypothesis: a urea kinetic approach to comparing the adequacy of continuous ambulatory peritoneal dialysis (CAPD) and hemodialysis. *Perit Dial Int* 1989;9:257.

444. Nolph KD, Moore HL, Twardowski ZJ, et al. Cross-sectional assessment of weekly urea and creatinine clearances in patients on continuous ambulatory peritoneal dialysis. *ASAIO J* 1992;38:M139.

445. Nolph KD, Keshaviah P, Popovich R. Problems in comparisons of clearances prescriptions in hemodialysis and continuous ambulatory peritoneal dialysis. *Perit Dial Int* 1991;11: 298.

446. Teehan BP, Schleifer CR, Sigler MH, et al. A quantitative approach to the CAPD prescription. *Perit Dial Bull* 1985;5: 152.

447. Teehan BP, Brown JM, Schleifer CR. Kinetic modeling in peritoneal dialysis. In: Nissenson AR, Fine R, Gentile D, eds. *Clinical Dialysis.* Norwalk, CT: Appleton & Lange, 1990:319.

448. Harty J, Boulton H, Heelis N, et al. Limitations of kinetic models as predictors of nutritional and dialysis adequacy in continuous ambulatory peritoneal dialysis patients. *Am J Nephrol* 1993;13:454.

449. Keshaviah P, Emerson PF, Vonesh EF, Brandes JC. Relationship between body size, fill volume, and mass transfer area coefficient in peritoneal dialysis. *J Am Soc Nephrol* 1994;4: 1820.

450. Schoenfeld P, Diaz-Buxo JA, Keen M, Gotch FA. The effect of body position (P), surface area (BSA), and intraperitoneal exchange volume (Vip) on the peritoneal transport constant (K_oA). *J Am Soc Nephrol* 1993;4:416.

451. Harty J, Boulton H, Venning M, Gokal R. Impact of increasing dialysis volume on adequacy targets: a prospective study. *J Am Soc Nephrol* 1997;8:1304.

452. Chagnac A, Herskovitz P, Ori Y, et al. Effect of increased dialysate volume on peritoneal surface area among peritoneal dialysis patients. *J Am Soc Nephrol* 2000;13:2554.

453. Cruz C, Dumler F, Schmidt R, Gotch F. Enhanced peritoneal dialysis delivery with PD-PLUS. Adv Perit Dial 1992;8:288.

454. Blake P, Burkart JM, Churchill DN, et al. Recommended clinical practices for maximizing peritoneal dialysis clearances. *Perit Dial Int* 1996;16:448.

455. McLaughlin K, Manns B, Mortis G, et al. Why patients with ESRD do not select self-care dialysis as a treatment option. *Am J Kidney Dis* 2003;41:380.

456. Ahlmen J, Carlsson L, Schonborg C. Well-informed patients with end-stage renal disease prefer peritoneal dialysis to hemodialysis. *Perit Dial Int* 1993;13(suppl 2):S196.

457. Stack AG. Impact of timing of nephrology referral and pre-ESRD care on mortality risk among new ESRD patients in the United States. *Am J Kidney Dis* 2003;41:310.

458. Winkelmayer WC, Owen WF Jr, Levin R, Avorn J. A propensity analysis of late versus early nephrologist referral and mortality on dialysis. *J Am Soc Nephrol* 2003;14: 486.

459. Blake PG. Peritoneal dialysis in Asia: An external perspective. *Perit Dial Int* 2002;22:258.

460. Kurtz SB, Johnson WJ. A four-year comparison of continuous ambulatory peritoneal dialysis and home hemodialysis: a preliminary report. *Mayo Clin Proc* 12984;59:659.

461. Weinman EJ, Lacke C, Kozak SM, et al. Continuous ambulatory peritoneal dialysis: initial experience as a hometraining and an in-hospital procedure. *Dial Transplant* 1980;9: 749.

462. Diaz-Buxo JA, Walker PJ, Farmer CD, et al. Continuous cyclic peritoneal dialysis—a practical form of equilibration dialysis, in Schreiner GE, Mendelson BF, eds. *Controversies in Nephrology.* Washington, DC: Georgetown University, 1983:225.

463. Diaz-Buxo JA, Walker PJ, Burgess WP, et al. Current status of CCPD in the prevention of peritonitis. *Adv Perit Dial* 1986;2:145.

464. Walls J, Smith BA, Feehally J, et al. CCPD—an improvement on CAPD. *Adv Perit Dial* 1981;2:141.

465. Diaz-Buxo JA: CCPD is even better than CAPD. *Kidney Int* 1985;28(suppl 17):S26.

466. Brem AS, Toscano AM. Continuous cycling peritoneal dialysis for children: an alternative to hemodialysis treatment. *Pediatrics* 1984;74:254.

467. Southwest Pediatric Nephrology Study Group. Continuous ambulatory and continuous cyclic peritoneal dialysis in children. *Kidney Int* 1985;27:558.

468. Fine RN, Salusky IB. CAPD/CCPD in children: four years' experience. *Kidney Int* 1986;30(suppl 18):S7.

469. Spinelli C, d'Adamo G, Balducci A, et al. Indications of inadequacy of automated peritoneal dialysis in 74 patients. *Adv Perit Dial* 1991;7:51.

470. King LK, Kingswood JC, Sharpstone P. Comparison of the efficacy cost and complication rate of APD and CAPD as long-term outpatient treatments for renal failure. *Adv Perit Dial* 1992;8:123.

471. Nolph KD, Sorkin M, Rubin J. Continuous ambulatory peritoneal dialysis: three year experience at one center. *Ann Intern Med* 1980;92:609.

472. Ramos JM, Gokal R, Siamopolous K, et al. Continuous ambulatory peritoneal dialysis: three years experience. *Q J Med* 1983;206:165.

473. Bouma SF, Dweyer JT. Glucose absorption and weight change in 18 months of continuous ambulatory peritoneal dialysis. *J Am Diet Assoc* 1984;84:194.

474. Lindholm B, Bergström J. Nutritional aspects of CAPD, in Gokal R, ed. *Continuous Ambulatory Peritoneal Dialysis.* London: Churchill Livingstone, 1986:228.

475. Diaz-Buxo JA, Burgess WP. Is weight gain inevitable in most chronic peritoneal dialysis patients? *Adv Perit Dial* 1992;8:334.

476. Khanna R, Wu G, Vas S, et al. Mortality and morbidity on continuous ambulatory peritoneal dialysis. *Trans Am Soc Artif Intern Organs* 1983;6:197.

477. Moncrief JW, Popovich RP, Nolph KD, et al. Clinical experience with continuous ambulatory peritoneal dialysis. *Trans Am Soc Artif Intern Organs* 1979;2:114.

478. Lamperi S, Icardi A, Carozzi S, et al. Effect of CAPD on renal anemia. *Int J Nephrol Urol Androl* 1981;1:43.

479. Lamperi S, Corozzi S, Icardi A. In vitro and in vivo studies of erythropoiesis during continuous ambulatory peritoneal dialysis. *Perit Dial Bull* 1983;3:94.

480. Summerfield GP, Gyde OHB, Forbes AMW, et al. Haemoglobin concentration and serum erythropoietin in renal dialysis and transplant patients. *Scand J Haematol* 1983;30:389.

481. De Paepe MBJ, Schelstraete KHG, Ringoir SG, et al. Influence of continuous ambulatory peritoneal dialysis on the anemia of end-stage renal disease. *Kidney Int* 1983;23:744.

482. Zappacosta AR, Caro J, Erslev A. Normalization of hematocrit in patients with end-stage renal disease on continuous ambulatory peritoneal dialysis. The role of erythropoietin. *Am J Med* 1982;72:53.

483. Zimmerman S, Johnson CA. *Peritoneal Dialysis and Epoietin Therapy*. New York: Global Medical Communications, 1992.

484. Korbet SM. Anemia and erythropoietin in hemodialysis and continuous ambulatory peritoneal dialysis. *Kidney Int* 1993; 43(suppl 40):S111.

485. Nissenson AR, Strobos J. Iron deficiency in patients with renal failure. *Kidney Int* 1999;69(suppl 69):S18.

486. Shaver MJ, Golper TA. Clinical applications of iron management in peritoneal dialysis patients. *Semin Dial* 1999; 12:257.

487. Hocken AG, Marwah PK. Iatrogenic contribution to anaemia of chronic renal failure. *Lancet* 1971;1:164.

488. Schaefer RM, Schaefer L. Iron monitoring and supplementation: how do we achieve the best results? *Nephrol Dial Transplant* 1998;13:9.

489. Kooistra MP, Marx JJ. The absorption of iron is disturbed in recombinant human erythropoietin-treated peritoneal dialysis patients. *Nephrol Dial Transplant* 1998;13:2578.

490. Milman N. Iron absorption measured by whole body counting and the relation to marrow iron stores in chronic uremia. *Clin Nephrol* 1982;17:77.

491. Roccatello D, Formica M, Cavalli G, et al. Serum and intracellular detection of cytokines in patients undergoing chronic hemodialysis. *Artif Organs* 1992;16:131.

492. Ismail N, Becker BN, Hakim RM. Water treatment for hemodialysis. *Am J Nephrol* 1996;16:60.

493. Lufft V, Mahiout A, Shaldon S, et al. Retention of cytokine-inducing substances inside high-flux dialyzers. *Blood Purif* 1996;14:26.

494. Gault MH, Duffett AL, Murphy JF, Purchase LH. In search of sterile, endotoxin-free dialysate. *ASAIO J* 1992;38: M431.

495. Lonnemann G, Haubitz M, Schindler R. Hemodialysis-associated induction of cytokines. *Blood Purif* 1990;8:214.

496. Casadevall N. Cellular mechanism of resistance to erythropoietin. *Nephrol Dial Transplant* 1995;10:27.

497. Gunnell J, Yeun JY, Depner TA, Kaysen GA. Acute-phase response predicts erythropoietin resistance in hemodialysis and peritoneal dialysis patients. *Am J Kidney Dis* 1999;33: 63.

498. Salahudeen AK, Keavey PM, Hawkins T, Wilkinson R. Is anaemia during continuous ambulatory peritoneal dialysis really better than during haemodialysis? *Lancet* 1983;2: 1046.

499. Raja R, Bloom E, Johnson R, Goldstein M. Improved response to erythropoietin in peritoneal dialysis patients as compared to hemodialysis patients: role of iron deficiency. *Adv Perit Dial* 1994;10:135.

500. Macdougall IC, Roberts DE, Coles GA, Williams JD. Clinical pharmacokinetics of epoietin (recombinant human erythropoietin). *Clin Pharmacokinet* 1991;20:99.

501. Opatrna S, Opatrny K Jr, Cejkova P, et al. Relationship between anemia and adequacy of continuous ambulatory peritoneal dialysis (letter). *Nephron* 1997;77:359.

502. Chandra M, Clemons GK, McVicar M, et al. Serum erythropoietin levels and hematocrit in end-stage renal disease: influence of the mode of dialysis. *Am J Kidney Dis* 1988; 12:208.

503. MacDougall IC, Roberts DE, Neubert P, et al. Pharmacokinetics of recombinant human erythropoietin in patients on continuous ambulatory peritoneal dialysis. *Lancet* 1989;1: 425.

504. Lui SF, Chung WW, Leung CB, et al. Pharmacokinetics and pharmacodynamics of subcutaneous and intraperitoneal administration of recombinant human erythropoietin in patients on continuous ambulatory peritoneal dialysis. *Clin Nephrol* 1990;33:47.

505. Lui SF, Law CB, Ting SM, et al. Once weekly versus twice weekly subcutaneous administration of recombinant human erythropoietin. *Clin Nephrol* 1991;36:246.

506. Bunke M, Bartlett DK, Brier ME, et al. Infrequent dosing of subcutaneous erythropoietin for the treatment of anemia in patients on CAPD. *Adv Perit Dial* 1993;9:331.

507. Kaufman JS, Reda DJ, Fye CL, et al. Subcutaneous versus intravenous administration of erythropoietin in hemodialysis patients. *N Engl J Med* 1998;339:578.

508. Lindholm B, Karlander SG. Glucose tolerance in patients undergoing continuous ambulatory peritoneal dialysis. *Acta Med Scand* 1986;220:477.

509. Lindholm B, Norbeck HE. Serum lipids and lipoproteins during continuous ambulatory peritoneal dialysis. *Acta Med Scand* 1986;220:143.

510. Khanna R, Breckenridge C, Roncari D, et al. Lipid abnormalities in patients undergoing continuous ambulatory peritoneal dialysis. *Perit Dial Bull* 1983;3(suppl 1):S13.

511. Iliescu EA, Marcovina SM, Morton AR, et al. Apolipoprotein(a) phenotype and lipoprotein(a) level predict peritoneal dialysis patient mortality. *Perit Dial Int* 2002;22:492.

512. Moberly JB, Attman PO, Samuelsson O, et al. Alterations in lipoprotein composition in peritoneal dialysis patients. *Perit Dial Int* 2002;22:220.

513. Cheng SC, Chu TS, Huang KY, et al. Association of hypertriglyceridemia and insulin resistance in uremic patients undergoing CAPD. *Perit Dial Int* 2001;21:282.

514. Ozdemir FN, Guz G, Sezer S, et al. Atherosclerosis risk is higher in continuous ambulatory peritoneal dialysis patients than in hemodialysis patients. *Artif Organs* 200125:448.

515. Johansson AC, Samuelsson O, Attman PO, et al. Dyslipidemia in peritoneal dialysis—relation to dialytic variables. *Perit Dial Int* 2000;20:306.

516. Fontan M, Rodriguez-Carmona A, Cordido F, Garcia-Buela J. Hyperleptinemia in uremic patients undergoing conservative management, peritoneal dialysis, and hemodialysis: a comparative analysis. *Am J Kidney Dis* 1999;34:824.

517. Fried L, Hutchison A, Stegmayr B, et al. Recommendations for the treatment of lipid disorders in patients on peritoneal dialysis. *Perit Dial Int* 1999;19:7.

518. Lowrie EG, Lew NL. Death risk in hemodialysis patients: the predictive value of commonly measured variables and an evaluation of death rate differences between facilities. *Am J Kidney Dis* 1990;15:458.

519. National Kidney Foundation-DOQI Clinical Practical Guidelines for Nutrition in Chronic Renal Failure. *Am J Kidney Dis* 2000;35(suppl 2):S1.

520. Brunori G, Guerini S. Can the vicious inflammation-malnutrition circle be corrected? In: Ronco C, Dell'Aquila R, Rodighiero MP, eds. *Peritoneal Dialysis Today.* New York: Karger, 2003:122.

521. Chung SH, Heimburger O, Stenvinkel P, et al. Influence of peritoneal transport rate, inflammation, and fluid removal on nutritional status and clinical outcome in prevalent peritoneal dialysis patients. *Perit Dial Int* 2003;23:174.

522. Garibotto G, Saffioti S, Russo R, et al. Malnutrition in peritoneal dialysis patients: causes and diagnosis. In: Ronco C, Dell'Aquila R, Rodighiero MP, eds. *Peritoneal Dialysis Today.* New York: Karger, 2003:112.

523. Heaf J. High transport and malnutrition-inflammation-atherosclerosis (MIA) syndrome. *Perit Dial Int* 2003;23:109.

524. Wang Q, Bernardini J, Piraino B, Fried L. Albumin at the start of peritoneal dialysis predicts the development of peritonitis. *Am J Kidney Dis* 2003;41:664.

525. Tzamaloukas AH, Servilla KS, Murata GH, Hoffman RM. Nutrition indices in obese continuous peritoneal dialysis patients with inadequate and adequate urea clearance. *Perit Dial Int* 2002;22:506.

526. Flanigan MJ, Frankenfield DL, Prowant BF, et al. Nutritional markers during peritoneal dialysis: data from the 1998 Peritoneal Dialysis Core Indicators Study. *Perit Dial Int* 2001;21:345.

527. Jager KJ, Merkus MP, Huisman RM, et al. Nutritional status over time in hemodialysis and peritoneal dialysis. *J Am Soc Nephrol* 2001;12:1272.

528. Lo WK, Tong KL, Li CS, et al. Relationship between adequacy of dialysis and nutritional status and their impact on patient survival on CAPD in Hong Kong. *Perit Dial Int* 2001;21:441.

529. Thodis E, Passadakis P, Vargemezis V, Oreopoulos DG. Peritoneal dialysis: better than, equal to, or worse than hemodialysis? Data worth knowing before choosing a dialysis modality. *Perit Dial Int* 2001;21:25.

530. Locatelli A, Marcos G, Gomez M, et al. Comparing peritonitis in continuous ambulatory peritoneal dialysis patients versus automated peritoneal dialysis patients. *Adv Perit Dial* 1999;15:193.

531. de Fijter CWH, Oe PL, Nauta JJP, et al. A prospective, randomized study comparing the peritonitis incidence of CAPD and Y-connector (CAPD-Y) with continuous cyclic peritoneal dialysis (CCPD). *Adv Perit Dial* 1991;7:186.

532. Gahrmani N, Gorban-Brennan N, Kliger AS, Finkelstein FO. Infection rates in end-stage renal disease patients treated with CCPD and CAPD using the UltraBag system. *Adv Perit Dial* 1995;11:164.

533. Viglino G, Gandolfo C, Virga G, Cavalli PL. Role of automated peritoneal dialysis within a peritoneal dialysis program. *Adv Perit Dial* 1995;11:134.

534. Troidle L, Gorban-Brennan N, Kliger AS, Finkelstein FO. Continuous cycler therapy, manual peritoneal dialysis therapy, and peritonitis. *Adv Perit Dial* 1998;14:137.

535. Rodríguez-Carmona A, Fontán MP, Falcón TG, et al. A comparative analysis on the incidence of peritonitis and exit-site infection in CAPD and automated peritoneal dialysis. *Perit Dial Int* 1999;19:253.

536. Perez-Fontan M, Rodríguez-Carmona A, García-Falcón T, et al. Incidence of peritonitis (P) and exit site infection (ESI) in CAPD and automated PD (APD). A comparative study. *Perit Dial Int* 1999;19(suppl 1):S35.

537. Huang JW, Hung K-Y, Yen CJ, et al. Comparison of infectious complications in peritoneal dialysis patients using either a twin-bag system or automated peritoneal dialysis. *Nephrol Dial Transplant* 2001;16:604.

538. de Fijter CWH, Oe LP, Nauta JJ, et al. Clinical efficacy and morbidity associated with continuous cyclic compared with continuous ambulatory peritoneal dialysis. *Ann Intern Med* 1994;120:264,.

539. Bro S, Bjorner J, Tofte-Jensen P, et al. A prospective, randomized multicenter study comparing APD and CAPD treatment. *Perit Dial Int* 1999;19:526.

540. Murphy SW, Foley RN, Barrett BJ, et al. Comparative hospitalization of hemodialysis and peritoneal dialysis patients in Canada. *Kidney Int* 2000;57:2557.

541. Sehgal AR, Dor A, Tsai AC. Morbidity and cost implications of inadequate hemodialysis. *Am J Kidney Dis* 2001;37:1223.

542. Charytnan C, Spinovitz BS, Galler M. A comparative study of CAPD and in centre HD. *Arch Intern Med* 1986;146:1138.

543. Gokal R, Jakubowski C,King C, et al. Outcome in patients on CAPD and hemodialysis: a four year analysis of a prospective multicentre study. *Lancet* 1987;2:1105.

544. Cavalli P, Viglino G, Goa F, et al. CAPD versus hemodialysis: 7 years experience. *Adv Perit Dial* 1989;5:52.

545. Serkes KD, Blagg CR, Nolph KD, et al. Comparison of patient and technique survival in continuous ambulatory peritoneal dialysis (CAPD) and hemodialysis: a multicenter study. *Perit Dial Int* 1990;10:15.

546. Maiorca R, Vonesh EF, Cavilli P, et al. A Multicenter, selection-adjusted comparison of patient and technique survival on CAPD and hemodialysis. *Perit Dial Int* 1991;11:118.

547. Maiorca R, Cancarini GC, Zubani R et al. CAPD viability: a long-term comparison with hemodialysis. *Perit Dial Int* 1996;16:276.

548. Nolph KD, Cutler SJ, Steinberg SM, et al. Continuous ambulatory peritoneal dialysis in the United States: a three-year study. *Kidney Int* 1985;28:198.

549. Cantaluppi A, Segoloni GP, Cancarini GC, et al. 1980–1984: CAPD Italian multicenter study, *Adv Perit Dial* 1986;2:23.

550. *National CAPD Registry of the National Institute of Health. Bethesda, MD.* National Institute of Health; 1987.

551. Gokal R. Worldwide experience, cost effectiveness and future of CAPD—its role in renal replacement therapy. In: Gokal R, ed. *Continuous Ambulatory Peritoneal Dialysis.* Edinburgh: Churchill Livingstone, 1986:349.

552. Woodrow G, Turney JH, Brownjohn AM. Technique failure in peritoneal dialysis and its impact on patient survival. *Perit Dial Int* 1997;17:360.

553. Loccatelli F, Marcelli D, Conte F. Dialysis patient outcomes in Europe vs the USA. *Nephrol Dial Transplant* 1997;12:1816.

554. Van Biesen W, Vanholder RC, Veys N, et al. An evaluation of an integrative care approach for end-stage renal disease patients. *J Am Soc Nephrol* 2000;11:116.

555. Burton PR, Walls J: Selection-adjusted comparison of life expectancy of patients on continuous ambulatory peritoneal dialysis, haemodialysis and renal transplantation. *Lancet* 1987;1:1115.

556. Maiorca R, Vonesh E, Cancarini CG, et al. A six year comparison of patients in CAPD and HD. *Kidney Int* 1988;34: 518.

557. Wolfe RA, Strawderman RL. Logical and statistical fallacies in the use of Cox regression models. *Am J Kidney Dis* 1996;27:124.

558. Gentil MA, Carriazo A, Pavon MI, et al. Comparison of survival in continuous ambulatory peritoneal dialysis and hospital hemodialysis: a multicenter study. *Nephrol Dial Tranplant* 1991;6:444.

559. Held PJ, Port FK, Turenne MN, et al. Continuous ambulatory peritoneal dialysis and hemodialysis: comparison of patient mortality with adjustment for co-morbid conditions. *Kidney Int* 1994;45:1163.

560. Disney AP. Demography and survival of patients receiving treatment for chronic renal failure in Australia and New Zealand: report on dialysis and renal transplantation treatment from the Australia and New Zealand Transplant Registry. *Am J Kidney Dis* 1995;25:165.

561. Locatelli F, Marcelli D, Conte F, et al. Report on regular dialysis and transplantation in Lombardy. *Am J Kidney Dis* 1995;25:196.

562. Fenton SSA, Schaubel DE, Desmeules M, et al. Hemodialysis versus peritoneal dialysis: a comparison of adjusted mortality rates. *Am J Kidney Dis* 1997;30:334.

563. Schaubel DE, Morrison HI, Fenton SSA. Comparing mortality rates on CAPD/CCPD and hemodialysis. The Canadian experience: fact or fiction? *Perit Dial Int* 1998;18:478.

564. Vonesh EF, Moran J. Mortality in end-stage renal disease: A reassessment of differences between patients treated with hemodialysis and peritoneal dialysis. *J Am Soc Nephrol* 1999;10:354.

565. Foley RN, Parfrey PS, Harnett JD, et al. Mode of dialysis therapy and mortality in end-stage renal disease. *J Am Soc Nephrol* 1998;9:267.

566. Diaz-Buxo JA. Modality selection. *J Am Soc Nephrol* 1998;9(suppl 10):112.

567. Burkart JM. Peritoneal dialysis should be considered as the first line of renal replacement therapy for most ESRD patients. *Blood Purif* 2001;19:179.

568. Gotloib LA, Mines M, Garmizo L, et al. Hemodynamic effects of increasing intra-abdominal pressure in peritoneal dialysis. *Perit Dial Bull* 1981;1:41.

569. Twardowski ZJ, Prowant BF, Nolph KD, et al. High volume, low frequency continuous ambulatory peritoneal dialysis. *Kidney Int* 1983;23:64.

570. Sarkar S, Bernardini J, Fried L, et al. Tolerance of large exchange volumes by peritoneal dialysis patients. *Am J Kidney Dis* 1999;33:1136.

571. Twardowski ZJ, Khanna R, Nolph KD, et al. Intraabdominal pressure during natural activities in patients treated with continuous ambulatory peritoneal dialysis. *Nephron* 1986;44:129.

572. O'Connor JP, Rigby RJ, Hardie IR. Abdominal hernias complicating continuous ambulatory peritoneal dialysis. *Am J Nephrol* 1986;6:271.

573. Digenis GE, Khanna R, Oreopoulos DG. Abdominal hernias in patients undergoing continuous ambulatory peritoneal dialysis. *Perit Dial Bull* 1982;2:115.

574. Diaz-Buxo JA, Geissinger WT. Single cuff versus double cuff Tenckhoff catheter. *Perit Dial Bull* 1984;4(suppl 2): S100.

575. Rocco MV, Stone WJ. Abdominal hernias in chronic peritoneal dialysis patients: a review. *Perit Dial Bull* 1985;5: 171.

576. Suh H, Wadhwa NK, Cabralda T, et al. Abdominal wall hernias in ESRD patients receiving peritoneal dialysis. *Adv Perit Dial* 1994;10:85.

577. Chan MK, Baillod RA, Tanner A, et al. Abdominal hernias in patients receiving continuous ambulatory peritoneal dialysis. *Br Med J* 1981;283:826.

578. Jorkasky D, Goldfarb S. Abdominal wall hernia complicating chronic ambulatory peritoneal dialysis. *Am J Nephrol* 1982;2:323.

579. Rubin J, Raju S, Teal N, et al. Abdominal hernia in patients undergoing continuous ambulatory peritoneal dialysis. *Arch Intern Med* 1982;142:1453.

580. Nelson H, Lindner M, Schuman ES, et al. Abdominal wall hernias as a complication of peritoneal dialysis. *Surg Gynecol Obstet* 1983;157:541.

581. Wetherington GM, Leapman SB, Robison RJ, et al. Abdominal wall and inguinal hernias in continuous ambulatory peritoneal dialysis patients. *Am J Surg* 1985;150:357.

582. Schleifer CR, Morfesis FA, Cupit M, et al. Management of hernias and Tenckhoff catheter complications in CAPD. *Perit Dial Bull* 1984;4:146.

583. Modi KB, Grant AC, Garret A, Rodger RS. Indirect inguinal hernia in CAPD patients with polycystic kidney disease. *Adv Perit Dial* 1989;5:84.

584. Spence PA, Mathews RE, Khanna R, Oreopoulos DG. Improved results with a paramedian technique for the insertion of peritoneal dialysis catheters. *Surg Gynecol Obstet* 1985;161:585.

585. Morris-Stiff G, Coles G, Moore R, et al. Abdominal wall hernia in autosomal dominant PKD. *Br J Surg* 1997;84:615.

586. Del Peso G, Bajo MA, Costero O, et al. Risk factors for abdominal wall complications in peritoneal dialysis patients. *Perit Dial Int* 2003;23:249.

587. Engeset J, Youngson GG. Ambulatory peritoneal dialysis and hernial complications. *Surg Clin North Am* 1984;64: 385.

588. Helfrich BG, Pechan WB, Alijani MR, et al. Reduction of catheter complications with lateral placement. *Perit Dial Bull* 1983;3(suppl 4):S2.

589. Stegmayr BG, Wikdahl AM, Arnerlöv C, Petersen E. A modified lateral technique for the insertion of peritoneal dialysis catheters enabling immediate start of dialysis. *Perit Dial Int* 1998;18:329.

590. Wikdahl AM, Granbom L, Stegmayr BG. Lower catheter-related peritonitis rates with catheter insertion through the rectus muscle, and the internal cuff between the peritoneum and the inner fascia. *Perit Dial Int* 1998;18:331.

591. Abraham G, Nallathambi MN, Bhaskaran S, Srinivasan L. Recurrence of abdominal wall hernias due to failure of mesh repair in a peritoneal dialysis patient. *Perit Dial Int* 1997; 17:89.

592. Imvrios G, Tsakiris D, Gakis D, et al. Prosthetic mesh repair of multiple recurrent and large abdominal hernias in CAPD. *Perit Dial Int* 1994;14:338.

593. Goodman CD, Husserl FE. Etiology, prevention and treatment of back pain in patients undergoing continuous ambulatory peritoneal dialysis. *Perit Dial Bull* 1981;1:119.

594. Bird NJ, Streather CP, O'Doherty MJ, et al. Gastric emptying in patients with chronic renal failure on CAPD. *Nephrol Dial Transplant* 1990;9:287.

595. Redwood NF, Wilkinson R, Jones NA. Vomiting caused by dialysis fluid "pseudocyst." *Br J Surg* 1993;80:224.

596. Hylander BI, Dalton CB, Castell DO, et al. Effect of intraperitoneal fluid volume changes on esophageal pressures. *Am J Kidney Dis* 1991;17:307.

597. Kim MJ, Kwon KH, Lee SW. Gastroesophageal reflux disease in CAPD patients. *Adv Perit Dial* 1998;14:98.

598. de Graaf-Strukowska L, van Hees CA, Ferwerda J, et al.: Two non-diabetic patients with delayed gastric emptying during CAPD effectively treated with erythromycin. *Nephrol Dial Transplant* 1995;10:2349.

599. Caporale N, Perez D, Alegre S. Vaginal leak of peritoneal dialysis liquid. *Perit Dial Int* 1991;11:284.

600. Liberek T, Lichodziejewska-Niemierko M, Kowalewska J, et al. Uterine prolapse—a rare or rarely reported complication of CAPD? *Perit Dial Int* 2002;22:95.

601. Swartz C, Onesti G, Mailloux L. The acute hemodynamic and pulmonary perfusion effects of peritoneal dialysis. *Trans Am Soc Artif Intern Organs* 1969;15:367.

602. Acquatella H, Perez-Rojas M, Burger B, Guinand-Baldo A. Left ventricular function in terminal uremia: a hemodynamic and echocardiographic study. *Nephron* 1978;22:160.

603. Kong CH, Raval U, Thompson FD. Effect of 2 liters of intraperitoneal dialysate on the cardiovascular system. *Clin Nephrol* 1986;26:134.

604. Franklin JO, Alpert MA, Twardowski ZJ. Effect of increasing intraabdominal pressure and volume on left ventricular function in continuous ambulatory peritoneal dialysis (CAPD). *Am J Kidney Dis* 1988;12:291.

605. Alpert MA, Franklin JO, Twardowski ZJ, et al. Impact of increasing intraperitoneal volume on left ventricular function in CAPD patients. *Perit Dial Bull* 1987;7(suppl 1):S2.

606. Caravaca F, Dominguez C, Machado V, et al. Vasovagal syncope related to peritoneal dialysate infusion. *Perit Dial Int* 1993;13:63.

607. Handa SP. Vasovagal syncopy related to peritoneal dialysate infusion. *Perit Dial Int* 1993;13:240.

608. Gotloib LA, Garmizo L, Varak T, et al. Reduction of vital capacity due to increased intra-abdominal pressure during peritoneal dialysis. *Perit Dial Bull* 1981;1:63.

609. Ahluwalia M, Ishikawa S, Gellman M, et al. Pulmonary functions during peritoneal dialysis. *Clin Nephrol* 1982;18: 251.

610. Gomez-Fernandez P, Sanchez Agudo L, Calatravo J, et al. Respiratory muscle weakness in uremic patients under continuous ambulatory peritoneal dialysis. *Nephron* 1984;36: 219.

611. Singh S, Dale A, Morgan B, Sahebjami H. Serial studies of pulmonary function in continuous ambulatory peritoneal dialysis. *Chest* 1984;86:874.

612. Taveira da Silva A, Davis W, Winchester J, et al: Peritonitis, dialysate infusion and lung function in continuous ambulatory peritoneal dialysis (CAPD). *Clin Nephrol* 1985;24:79.

613. O'Brien AA, Power J, O'Brien L, et al. The effect of peritoneal dialysate on pulmonary function and blood gases in CAPD patients. *Irish J Med Sci* 1990;159:215.

614. Gokbel H, Yeksan M, Dogan E, et al. Effect of CAPD applications on pulmonary function (letter). *Perit Dial Int* 1998; 18:344.

615. O'Brien AAJ, Power J, O'Brien L, et al. The effect of 2 L dialysate on respiratory function. *Perit Dial Bull* 1987; 7(suppl 1):S57.

616. Oreopoulos D, Rebuck A. Risks and benefits of peritoneal dialysis. *Chest* 1985;88:6742.

617. Rebuck A. Peritoneal dialysis and the mechanics of diaphragm. *Perit Dial Bull* 1982;2:209.

618. Wanke T, Auinger M: Diaphrogmatic function in patients on CAPD. *Lung* 1994;172:231.

619. Wadhwa NK, Seliger M, Greenberg HE, et al. Sleep related respiratory disorders in end-stage renal disease patients on peritoneal dialysis. *Perit Dial Int* 1992;12:51.

620. Aye AM, Kulatilake AK, Schackman R. Peritoneal dialysis in surgery. *Proc Eur Dial Transplant Assoc* 1965;2:49.

621. Edwards SR, Unger AM. Acute hydrothorax: a new complication of peritoneal dialysis. *JAMA* 1967;199:853.

622. Finn R, Jowett EW. Acute hydrothorax complicating peritoneal dialysis. *Br Med J* 1970;2:94.

623. Holm J, Lieden B, Lindqvist B: Unilateral pleural effusion: a rare complication of peritoneal dialysis. *Scand J Urol Nephrol* 1971;5:84.

624. Haberli R, Stucki P. Akuter hydrothorax als Komplikation bei peritoneal Dialyse. *Praxis* 1971;1:13.

625. Rudnick MR, Coyle JF, Beck LH, et al. Acute massive hydrothorax complicating peritoneal dialysis, report of two cases and a review of the literature. *Clin Nephrol* 1979;12: 38.

626. Posen GA, Sachs HJ. Treatment of recurrent pleural effusions in dialysis patients by talc insufflation (abstr). *Trans Am Soc Artif Intern Organs* 1979;8:75.

627. Milutinevich J, Shyong W, Lindholm DD, et al. Acute massive unilateral hydrothorax: a rare complication of peritoneal dialysis. *South Med J* 1980;73:827.

628. Lorentz WB. Acute hydrothorax during peritoneal dialysis. *J Pediatr* 1979;94:417.

629. Scheldewaert R, Bogaerts Y, Pauwels R, et al. Management of a massive hydrothorax in a CAPD patient: a case report and a review of the literature. *Perit Dial Bull* 1982;2:69.

630. Pattison CW, Rodger RSC, Adu D, et al. Surgical treatment of hydrothorax complicating continuous ambulatory peritoneal dialysis. *Clin Nephrol* 1984;21:191.

631. Garcia Ramon R, Carrasco AM. Hydrothorax in peritoneal dialysis (editorial). *Perit Dial Int* 1998;18:5.

632. Maher J, Schreiner G. Hazards and complications of dialysis. *N Engl J Med* 1965;273:370.

633. Bunchman T, Wood E, Lynch R. Hydrothorax as a complication of peritoneal dialysis. *Perit Dial Int* 1987;7:237.

634. Abraham G, Schoker A, Blake P, Oreopoulos D. Massive hydrothorax in patients on peritoneal dialysis: a literature review. *Adv Perit Dial* 1988;4:121.

635. Nomoto Y, Suga T, Nakajima K, et al. Acute hydrothorax in continuous ambulatory peritoneal dialysis—a collaborative study of 161 centers. *Am J Nephrol* 1989;9:363.

636. Chow CC, Sung JY, Cheung CK, et al. Massive hydrothorax in continuous ambulatory peritoneal dialysis: diagnosis, management and review of the literature. *N Z Med J* 1988; 101:475.

637. Benz R, Schleifer CR. Hydrothorax in CAPD. Successful treatment with intrapleural tetracycline and a review of the literature. *Am J Kidney Dis* 1985;2:136.

638. Green A, Logan M, Medawar W, et al. The management of hydrothorax in continuous ambulatory peritoneal dialysis (CAPD). *Perit Dial Int* 1990;10:271.

639. Hidai H, Takatsu S, Chiba T. Intrathoracic installation of autologous blood in treating massive hydrothorax following CAPD (letter). *Perit Dial Int* 1989;9:221.

640. Okada K, Takahashi S, Kinoshita Y. Effect of pleurodesis with autoblood on hydrothorax due to continuous ambulatory peritoneal dialysis—induced diaphragmatic communication (letter). *Nephron* 1993;65:153.

641. Vlachojannis J, Bloettcher I, Brandt L, Schoeppe W. A new treatment for unilateral recurrent hydrothorax during CAPD. *Perit Dial Int* 1985;5:180.

642. Berlyne GM, Lee HA, Ralston AJ, Woodlock JA. Pulmonary complications of peritoneal dialysis. *Lancet* 1966;2: 75.

643. Blumberg A, Keller R, Marti H. Oxygen affinity of erythrocytes and pulmonary gas exchange in patients on continuous ambulatory peritoneal dialysis. *Neprhon* 1984;38:248.

644. Eiser A. Pulmonary gas exchange during hemodialysis and peritoneal dialysis: interaction between respiration and metabolism. *Am J Kidney Dis* 1985;6:131.

645. Fabris A, Biasioli S, Chiaramonte C, et al. Buffer metabolism in continuous ambulatory peritoneal dialysis (CAPD): relationship with respiratory dynamics. *Trans Am Soc Artif Intern Organs* 1985;28:270.

646. Cohn J, Balk RA, Bone RC. Dialysis-induced respiratory acidosis. *Chest* 1990;98:1285.

647. Hallet M, Burden S, Stewart D, et al. Sleep apnea in ESRD patients on HD and CAPD. *Perit Dial Int* 1996;16(suppl 1):S429.

648. Kraus MA, Hamburger J. Sleep apnea in renal failure. *Adv Perit Dial* 1997;13:88.

649. Williams SW, Tell GS, Zheng B, et al. Correlates of sleep behavior among hemodialysis patients. The kidney outcomes prediction and evaluation (KOPE) study. *Am J Nephrol* 2002;22:18.

650. Zoccali C, Mallamaci F, Tripepi G. Sleep apnea in renal patients. *J Am Soc Nephrol* 2001;12:2854.

651. Benz RL, Pressman MR, Hovick ET, Peterson DD. Potential novel predictors of mortality in end-stage renal disease patients with sleep disorders. *Am J Kidney Dis* 2000;35:1052.

652. Fernstrom A, Hylander B, Gryback P, et al. Gastric emptying and electrogastrography in patients on CAPD. *Perit Dial Int* 1999;19:429.

653. Brown-Cartwright D, Smith HJ, Feldman M. Gastric emptying of an indigestible solid in patients with end-stage renal disease on continuous ambulatory peritoneal dialysis. *Gastroenterology* 1988;95:49.

654. Pannekeet MM, Krediet RT, Boeschoten EW, et al. Acute pancreatitis during CAPD in the Netherlands. *Nephrol Dial Transplant* 1993;8:1376.

655. Avram RM, Iancu M. Pancreatic disease in uremia and parathyroid hormone excess. *Nephron* 1982;32:60.

656. Padilla B, Pollak VE, Pesce A, et al. Pancreatitis in patients with end-stage renal disease. *Medicine* 1994;73:8.

657. Gupta A, Yuan ZY, Balaskas EV, et al. CAPD and pancreatitis: no connection. *Perit Dial Int* 1992;12:309.

658. Diaz-Buxo JA, Chandler JT, Farmer CD, et al. Intraperitoneal infusion of non-absorbable steroids in the treatment of ascites and sterile peritonitis. *J Dial* 1980;4:43.

659. Korzets Z, Golan E, Ben-Dahan J, et al. Decubitus small bowel perforation in ongoing CAPD. *Nephrol Dial Transplant* 1992;7:79.

660. Steiner RW, Halasz NA. Abdominal catastrophes and other unusual events in continuous ambulatory peritoneal dialysis patients. *Am J Kidney Dis* 1990;15:1.

661. Tomson C, Morgan A: Bleeding from small intestinal telangiectases complicating CAPD. *Perit Dial Bull* 1985;5: 258.

662. Rottembourg J, Gahl GM, Poignet JL, et al. Severe abdominal complications in patients undergoing continuous ambulatory peritoneal dialysis. *Proc Eur Dial Transplant Assoc* 1983;20:236.

663. Lambrecht GLY, Malbrain MLNG, Zachée P, et al. Portal vein thrombosis complicating peritonitis in a patient on chronic ambulatory peritoneal dialysis. *Perit Dial Int* 1994; 14:282.

664. Selgas R, Lopez-Rivas A, Alvaro F, et al. Insulin influence on the mitogenic-induced effect of the peritoneal effluent in CAPD patients. *Adv Perit Dial* 1989;5:161.

665. Wanless IR, Bargman JM, Oreopoulos DG, et al. Subcapsular steatosis in response to peritoneal insulin delivery: A clue to the pathogenesis of steatonecrosis in obesity. *Mod Pathol* 1989;2:69.

666. Tzamaloukas AH, Oreopoulos DG. Subcutaneous versus intraperitoneal insulin in the management of diabetics on CAPD: a review. *Adv Perit Dial* 1991;7:81.

667. Nevalainen, PI, Kallio T, Lahtela JT, et al. High peritoneal permeability predisposes to hepatic steatosis in diabetic continuous ambulatory peritoneal dialysis patients receiving intraperitoneal insulin. *Perit Dial Int* 2000;20:637.

668. Harrison NA, Rainford DJ. Intraperitoneal insulin and the malignant omentum syndrome (abstr). *Nephrol Dial Transplant* 1988;3:103.

669. An international cooperative study—second report. A survey of ultrafiltration in continuous ambulatory peritoneal dialysis. *Perit Dial Bull* 1984;4:137.

670. Manuel MA. Failure of ultrafiltration in patients on CAPD. *Perit Dial Bull* 1983;3(suppl 3):S38.

671. Hasbargen JA, Smith BJ, Rodgers DJ. Ultrafiltration failure at the initiation of CAPD. *Perit Dial Bull* 1986;6:46.

672. Diaz-Buxo JA: Natural history of abnormal peritoneal permeability states. In: La Greca G, Chiaramonte S, Fabris A, et al, eds. *Peritoneal Dialysis*. Milan: Wichtig Editore, 1988:181.

673. Slingeneyer A, Canaud B, Mion C. Permanent loss of ultrafiltration capacity of the peritoneum in long-term peritoneal dialysis: an epidemiological study. *Nephron* 1983;33:133.

674. De Vriese AS, Mortier S, Lamiere NH. What happens to the membrane in long-term peritoneal dialysis? *Perit Dial Int* 2001;21(suppl 3):SS9.

675. Selgas R, Bajo MA, Castro MJ, et al. Risk factors responsible for ultrafiltration failure in early stages of peritoneal dialysis. *Perit Dial Int* 2000;20:631.

676. De Alvaro F, Castro MJ, Dapena F, et al. Peritoneal resting is beneficial in peritoneal hyperpermeability and ultrafiltration failure. *Adv Perit Dial* 1993;9:56.

677. Selgas R, Bajo MA, Castro MJ, et al. Managing ultrafiltration failure by peritoneal resting. *Perit Dial Int* 2000;20:595.

678. Rodrigues A, Cabrita A, Maia P, Grimaraes S. Peritoneal rest may successfully recover ultrafiltration in patients who develop peritoneal hyperpermeability with time on continuous ambulatory peritoneal dialysis. *Adv Perit Dial* 2002;18: 78.

679. Lo WK, Brendolan A, Prowant BF, et al. Changes in the peritoneal equilibration test in selected chronic peritoneal dialysis patients. *J Am Soc Nephrol* 1994;4:1466.

680. Gandhi VC, Ing TS, Daugirdas JT, et al. Failure of peritoneal dialysis due to peritoneal sclerosis. *Int J Artif Organs* 1983;6:97.

681. Hendriks PM, Ho-dac-Pannekeet MM, van Gulik TM, et al. Peritoneal sclerosis in chronic peritoneal dialysis patients: analysis of clinical presentation, risk factors, and peritoneal transport kinetics. *Perit Dial Int* 1997;17:136.

682. Mutoh S, Machida J, Ueda S, et al. Sclerosing encapsulating peritonitis occurring after very short term intermittent peritoneal dialysis. *Nephron* 1992;62:119.

683. Krediet RT. The peritoneal membrane in chronic peritoneal dialysis. Nephrology forum. *Kidney Int* 1999;55:341.

684. Dobbie JW. Pathogenesis of peritoneal fibrosing syndromes (sclerosing peritonitis) in peritoneal dialysis. *Perit Dial Int* 1992;12:14.

685. Marichal JF, Faller B, Brignon P, et al. Progressive calcifying peritonitis: a new complication of CAPD? Report of two cases. *Nephron* 1987;45:229.

686. Korzets A, Korzets Z, Peer G, et al. Sclerosing peritonitis. Possible early diagnosis by computerized tomography of the abdomen. *Am J Nephrol* 1988;8:143.

687. Hauglustaine D, van Meerbeek J, Monballyu J, et al. Sclerosing peritonitis with mural bowel fibrosis in a patient on long-term CAPD. *Clin Nephrol* 1984;22:158.

688. Slingeneyer A, Mion C, Mourad G, et al. Progressive sclerosing peritonitis: a late and severe complication of maintenance peritoneal dialysis. *Trans Am Soc Artif Organs* 1983; 29:633.

689. Yokota S, Kumano K, Sakai T. Prognosis for patients with sclerosing encapsulating peritonitis following CAPD. *Adv Perit Dial* 1997;13:221.

690. Rigby RJ, Hawley CM. Sclerosing peritonitis: the experience in Australia. *Nephrol Dial Transplant* 1998;13:154.

691. Nomoto Y, Kawaguchi Y, Kubo H, et al. Sclerosis encapsulated peritonitis in patients undergoing CAPD: a report of the Japanese Sclerosing Encapsulated Peritonitis Study Group. *Am J Kidney Dis* 1996;28:420.

692. Nielsen LH, Nolph KD, Khanna R, et al. Sclerosing peritonitis on CAPD: the acetate-lactate controversy (abstr). *Am J Nephrol* 1984;17:82.

693. Pauli HG, Buttikofer E, Vorburger CH. Clinical experience with peritoneal dialysis. *Helv Med Acta* 1966;33:51.

694. Junor BJR, Briggs JD, Forwell MA, et al. Sclerosing peritonitis—the contribution of chlorhexidine in alcohol. *Perit Dial Bull* 1985;5:101.

695. Lo WK, Chan KT, Leung AC, et al. Sclerosing peritonitis complicating continuous ambulatory peritoneal dialysis with the use of chlorhexidine in alcohol. *Adv Perit Dial* 1990; 6:79.

696. Diaz-Buxo JA. The durability of the peritoneal membrane—clearances. *Perit Dial Bull* 1984;4(suppl 2):S85.

697. Brown P, Baddeley H, Read A, et al. Sclerosing peritonitis. An unusual reaction to a beta-adrenergic blocking drug (Practolol). *Lancet* 1974;2:1477.

698. Bradley JA, McWhinnie DL, Hamilton DN, et al. Sclerosing obstructive peritonitis after CAPD. *Lancet* 1983;2:113.

699. Daugirdas JT, Gandhi VC, McShane AP, et al. Peritoneal sclerosis in continuous ambulatory peritoneal dialysis patients dialyzed exclusively with lactate-buffered dialysate. *J Artif Organ* 1986;9:413.

700. Lasker N, Burke JF Jr, Patchefsky A, Haughey E. Peritoneal reactions to particulate matter in peritoneal dialysis solutions. *Trans Am Soc Artif Intern Organs* 1975;21:342.

701. Ing TS, Daugirdas JT, Gandhi VC. Sclerosing peritonitis after peritoneal dialysis. *Lancet* 1983;2:1080.

702. Verger C, Celicout B. Peritoneal permeability and encapsulating peritonitis. *Lancet* 1985;1:986.

703. Diaz-Buxo JA. Differences between CAPD and CCPD: implications for therapy. *Semin Dial* 1993;6:312.

704. Assalia A, Schein M, Hashmonai M. Problems in the surgical management of sclerosing encapsulating peritonitis. *Isr J Med Sci* 1993;29:686.

705. Slingeneyer A. Preliminary report on a cooperative international study on sclerosing encapsulating peritonitis. *Contrib Nephrol* 1987;57:239.

706. Junor BJ, Mc Millan MA. Immunosupression in sclerosing peritonitis. *Perit Dial Int* 13(suppl 2):S64.

707. Mori Y, Matsuo S, Sutoh H, et al. A case of a dialysis patient with sclerosing peritonitis successfully treated with corticosteroid therapy alone. *Am J Kidney Dis* 1997;30:275.

708. Klemm G. Peritoneal calcification and calciphylaxis. *Nephron* 1989;51:124.

709. Francis DMA, Busmanis I, Becker G. Peritoneal calcification in a peritoneal dialysis patient: a case report. *Perit Dial Int* 199010:237.

710. Fletcher S, Gibson J, Brownjohn AM. Peritoneal calcification secondary to severe hyperparathyroidism. *Nephrol Dial Transplant* 1995;10:277.

711. Warady BA, Bohl V, Alon U, Hellerstein S. Symptomatic peritoneal calcification in a child: treatment with tidal peritoneal dialysis. *Perit Dial Int* 1994;14:26.

712. Farmer CKT, Goldsmith DJA, Sharpstone P, Kingswood JC. Maintenance of adequate dialysis in a patient with peritoneal calcification using tidal peritoneal dialysis. *Clin Nephrol* 1998;49:55.

713. Cox SV, Lai J, Suranyi M, Walker N. Sclerosing peritonitis with gross peritoneal calcification: a case report. *Am J Kidney Dis* 1992;20:637.

714. Wakabayashi Y, Kawaguchi Y, Shigematsu T, et al. Three cases of extensive peritoneal calcification (ECP) in patients with long-term CAPD. *Perit Dial Int* 1993;13(suppl 2):S99.

715. Greenberg A, Bernardini J, Piraino BM, et al. Hemoperitoneum complicating chronic peritoneal dialysis: single-center experience and literature review. *Am J Kidney Dis* 1992;19:252.

716. Harett JD, Gill D, Corbett L, et al. Recurrent hemoperitoneum in women receiving CAPD. *Ann Intern Med* 1987;107:341.

717. Holley JL, Schiff M, Schmidt RJ, et al. Hemoperitoneum occurs in over half of menstruating women on peritoneal dialysis. *Perit Dial Int* 1996;16:650.

718. Blumenkrantz MJ, Gallagher N, Bashore RA, Tenckhoff H. Retrograde menstruation in women undergoing chronic peritoneal dialysis. *Obstet Gynecol* 1981;57:667.

719. Fraley DS, Johnston JR, Bruns FJ, et al. Rupture of ovarian cyst: massive hemoperitoneum in continuous ambulatory peritoneal dialysis patients: diagnosis and treatment. *Am J Kidney Dis* 1988;12:69.

720. Fenton S. Recurrent hemoperitoneum in a middle-aged woman on CAPD. *Perit Dial Int* 1998;18:88.

721. Coward RA, Gokal R, Wise M, et al. Peritonitis associated with vaginal leakage of dialysis fluid in continuous ambulatory peritoneal dialysis. *Br Med J* 1982;284:1529.

722. Coronel F, Marenjo P, Torrente J, Pratts D. The risk of retrograde menstruation in CAPD patients. *Perit Dial Bull* 1984;4:190.

723. Williams PF, Beer S.: Hemoperitoneum in a patient with idiopathic thrombocytopenic purpura (ITP) and renal failure (letter). *Perit Dial Bull* 1985;5:258.

724. Twardowski ZJ, Schreiber MJ. Peritoneal dialysis case forum: a 55 year old man with hematuria and blood-tinged dialysate. *Perit Dial Int* 1992;12:61.

725. Fine A, Novak C. Hemoperitoneum due to carcinomatosis in the liver of a CAPD patient. *Perit Dial Int* 1996;16:181.

726. Peng SJ, Yang CS. Hemoperitoneum in CAPD patients with hepatic tumors. *Perit Dial Int* 1996;16:84.

727. Posthuma N, van Eps RS, ter Wee PM. Hemoperitoneum due to (hapatocellular) adenoma. *Perit Dial Int* 1998;18:446.

728. Wang JY, Lin YF, Lin SH, Tsao TY. Hemoperitoneum due to splenic rupture in a CAPD patient with chronic myelogenous leukemia. *Perit Dial Int* 1998;18:334.

729. Blake P, Abraham G. Bloody effluent during CAPD in a patient with polycystic kieneys (letter). *Perit Dial Int* 1988;8:167.

730. Rutecki GW, Asfoura JY, Whittier FC. Autosomal dominant polycystic liver disease as an etiologiy of hemoperitoneum during CCPD. *Perit Dial Int* 1995;15:367.

731. Min CH, Park JH, Ahn JH, et al. Dialysis-related amyloidosis (DRA) in a patient on CAPD presenting as haemoperitoneum with colon perforation. *Nephrol Dial Transplant* 1997;12:2761.

732. Nace G, George A Jr, Stone W. Hemoperitoneum: a red flag in CAPD. *Perit Dial Bull* 1985;5:42–44.

733. Hassell L, Moore J Jr, Conklin J. Hemoperitoneum during continuous ambulatory peritoneal dialysis: a possible complication of radiation induced peritoneal injury. *Clin Nephrol* 1984;21:241.

734. Bender F. Hemoperitoneum after pericardiocentesis in a CAPD patient. *Perit Dial Int* 1996;16:330.

735. Huserl F, Tapia N. Peritoneal bleeding in a CAPD patient after extracorporial lithotripsy (letter). *Perit Dial Bull* 1987;7:262.

736. Karlagasudaram NS, Macdougall IC, Turney JH. Massive haemoperitoneum due to rupture of splenic infarct during CAPD. *Nephrol Dial Transplant* 1998;13:2380.

737. Rambausek M, Walherr R, Ritz E. Recurrent episodes of bloody dialysate in mesangial IgA-glomerulonephritis during upper respiratory tract infections. *Perit Dial Bull* 1987;7(suppl 1):S62.

738. Campisi S, Cavatorta F, DeLucia E. Iliopsoas spontaneous hematoma: an unusual cause of hemoperitoneum in CAPD patients (letter). *Perit Dial Int* 1992;12:78.

739. Giron FF, Sanchez FH, Alcalde MP, Martinez JG. Hemoperitoneum in peritoneal dialysis secondary to retroperitoneal hematoma. *Perit Dial Int* 1996;16:644.

740. Ramon G, Miguel A, Caridad A, Colomer B. Bloody peritoneal fluid in a patient with tuberous sclerosis in a CAPD program (letter). *Perit Dial Int* 1989;9:353.

741. Shohat J, Shapira Z, Yussim A, Boner G. An unusual cause of massive intraperitoneal bleeding in CAPD. *Perit Dial Bull* 1984;4:257.

742. Goldstein AM, Gorlick N, Gibbs D, Fernandez-del Castillo C. Hemoperitoneum due to spontaneous rupture of the umbilical vein. *Am J Gastroenterol* 1995;90:315.

743. Modi K, Henderson I. Fatal, massive hemoperitoneum after cessation of CAPD (letter). *Clin Nephrol* 1987;27:47.

744. de los Santos CA, von Eye O, d'Avila D, Mottin CC. Rupture of the spleen: A complication of continuous ambulatory peritoneal dialysis. *Perit Dial Bull* 1986;6:203.

745. Van der Niepen P, Sennesael JJ, Verbeelen DL. Massive hemoperitoneum due to spleen injury by a dislocated Tenckhoff catheter. *Perit Dial Int* 1994;14:90.

746. Le Meur Y, Poux JM, Benevent D, Leroux-Robert C. Ascite chyleuse chez quatre patientes traitees par dialyse peri-

toneale continue ambulatoire et revue de la litterature. *Bull Dial Perit* 1991;23:27.

747. Humayun HM, Daugirdas JT, Ing TS, et al. Chylous ascites in a patient treated with intermittent peritoneal dialysis. *Artif Organs* 1984;8:358.

748. Pomeranz A, Reichenberg Y, Schuzz D, Drukker A. Chyloperitoneum: a rare complication of peritoneal dialysis. *Perit Dial Bull* 1984;4:35.

749. Press OW, Press NO, Kaufman SD. Evaluation and management of chylous ascites. *Ann Intern Med* 1982;96:358.

750. Vasko J, Tapper R. The surgical significance of chylous ascites. *Arch Surg* 1967;95:355.

751. Kelley M Jr, Butt H. Chylous ascites: An analysis of etiology. *Gastroenterology* 1960;39:161.

752. Burns RO, Henderson LW, Hager EB, et al. Peritoneal dialysis—clinical experience. *N Engl J Med* 1962;267:1060.

753. Gault MH, Fergusson EL, Sidhu JS, et al. Fluid and electrolyte complications of peritoneal dialysis. Choice of dialysis solutions. *Ann Intern Med* 1971;75:253.

754. Rottembourg J, Allouache M, Musset L, et al. Beta 2-microglobulin kinetics in patients treated by CAPD. *Perit Dial Bull* 1987;7(suppl 1):S64.

755. Dratwa M, Bergmann P, Tielemans C, et al. Less beta 2 microglobulin in CAPD than in hemodialysis patients. *Perit Dial Bull* 1987;7(suppl 1):S26.

756. Maiorca R, Cancarini GC, Brunori G, et al. Morbidity and mortality of CAPD and hemodialysis. *Kidney Int* 1993;43(suppl 40): S4.

757. Maiorca R, Cancarini GC, Camerini C, et al. Is CAPD competitive with haemodialysis for long-term treatment of uraemic patients? *Nephrol Dial Transplant* 1989;4:244.

758. Gagnon RF, Somerville P, Kaye M: Beta-2-microglobulin serum levels in patients on long-term dialysis. *Perit Dial Bull* 1987;7:29.

759. Gokal R: Continuous ambulatory peritoneal dialysis, In: Maher JF, ed. *Replacement of Renal Function by Dialysis.* Dordrecht, The Netherlands: Kluwer, 1989:590.

760. Miguel Alonso JL, Cruz A, Lopex Revuelta K, et al. Continuous ambulatory peritoneal dialysis does not prevent the development of dialysis-associated amyloidosis. *Nephron* 1989;53:389.

761. Benz RL, Siegfried JW, Teehan BP. Carpal tunnel syndrome in dialysis patients: comparison between continuous ambulatory peritoneal dialysis and hemodialysis populations. *Am J Kidney Dis* 1988;11:473.

762. Cornelia F, Bardin T, Faller B, et al. Rheumatic syndromes and β$_2$-microglobulin amyloidosis in patients receiving long-term peritoneal dialysis. *Arthritis Rheum* 1989;32:785.

763. Cruz A, Gonzalez T, Balsa A, et al. Destructive spondyloarthropathy in long-term CAPD and hemodialysis (letter). *J Rheum* 1989;16:1169.

764. Bicknell JM, Lim AC, Raroque HG, Tzamaloukas A. Carpal tunnel syndrome, subclinical median mononeuropathy, and peripheral polyneuropathy: common early complications of chronic peritoneal dialysis and hemodialysis. *Arch Phys Med Rehab* 1991;72:378.

765. Benhamou CL, Bardin T, Noel LH, et al. Beta-2 microglobulin amyloidosis as a complication of peritoneal dialysis treatment (letter). *Clin Nephrol* 1988;30:346.

766. Athanasou NA, Ayers D, Raine AJ, et al.: Joint and systemic distribution of dialysis amyloid. *Q J Med* 1991;78:205.

767. Jadoul M, Noel H, van Ypersele de Strihou C. β$_2$-microglobulin amyloidosis in a patient treated exclusively by continuous ambulatory peritoneal dialysis. *Am J Kidney Dis* 1990;15:86.

768. Colombi A, Wegmann W. Beta-2 microglobulin amyloidosis in a paitent on long-term continuous ambulatory peritoneal dialysis (CAPD). *Perit Dial Int* 1989;9:321.

769. Feinfeld DA, Verger C, Briscoe AM, et al. Serum myoglobulin in patients on intermittent and continuous ambulatory peritoneal dialysis. *Clin Nephrol* 1987;28:144.

770. Hart PM, Feinfeld DA, Briscoe AM, et al. The effect of renal failure and hemodialysis on serum and urine myoglobulin. *Clin Nephrol* 1982;18:141.

771. Oren A, Husdan H, Cheng PT, et al. Calcium oxalate kidney stones in patients on continuous ambulatory peritoneal dialysis. *Kidney Int* 1984;25:534.

772. Modi KB, Rolton HA, McConnel KN, et al. Comparative study of oxalate in patients on continuous ambulatory peritoneal dialysis and regular haemodialysis. *Perit Dial Bull* 1987;7(suppl 1):S54.

773. Segar WE, Gibson RK, Rhamy R. Peritoneal dialysis in infants and small children. *Pediatrics* 1961;27:603.

774. Chan JCM, Campbell RA. Peritoneal dialysis in children, a survey of its indications and applications. *Clin Pediatr* 1973;12:131.

775. Nolph KD, Sorkin M. Peritoneal dialysis in acute renal failure. In: Brenner BM, Lazarus MJ, eds. *Acute Renal Failure.* Philadelphia: Saunders, 1983:689.

776. Orofino L, Lamoreabe I, Muniz R, et al. Supervivencia del fracaso renal agudo (FRA) sometido a dialisis. *Rev Clin Esp* 1976;141:155.

777. Firmat J, Zucchini A. Peritoneal dialysis in acute renal failure. *Contrib Nephrol* 1979;17:33.

778. Mehl R. Trends during 10 years of dialysis treatment. *Proc Eur Dial Transplant Assoc* 1966;3:330.

779. Stewart JH, Tuckwell LA, Sinnett PF, et al. Peritoneal and haemodialysis: a comparison of their morbidity and of their mortality suffered by dialysed patients. *Q J Med* 1966;35: 406.

780. Mathew TH. Comparison of peritoneal dialysis and haemodialysis in acute renal failure. In: Atkins RC, Thomson NM, Farrell PC, eds. *Peritoneal Dialysis.* Edinburgh: Churchill Livingstone, 1981:80.

781. U. S. Renal Data System: USRDS 1999 Annual Report. *Am J Kidney Dis* 1999;34(suppl 1):S1.

782. Shinzato T, Nakai S, Akiba N, et al. Report on the annual statistical survey of the Japanese society for dialysis therapy in 1996. *Kidney Int* 1999;55:700.

783. Dhingra RK, Young EW, Hulbert-Shearon TE, et al. Type of vascular access predicts mortality in US hemodialysis patients. *J Am Soc Nephrol* 2000;11:182A.

784. Raja RM, Krasnoff SO, Moros JG, et al: Repeated peritoneal dialysis in treatment of heart failure. *JAMA* 1970; 213:2268.

785. McKinnie JJ, Bourjeois RJ, Husserl FE. Long-term therapy for heart failure with continuous ambulatory peritoneal dialysis. *Arch Intern Med* 1985;145:1128.

786. Tormey V, Conlon PJ, Farrell J, et al. Long-term successful management of refractory congestive cardiac failure by intermittent ambulatory peritoneal ultrafiltration. *Q J Med* 1996;89:681.

787. Elhalel-Dranitki M, Rubinger D, Moscovici A, et al. CAPD to improve quality of life in patients with refractory heart failure. *Nephrol Dial Transplant* 1998;13:3041.

788. Stack AG, Molony DA, Rahman NS, et al. Impact of dialysis modality on survival of new ESRD patients with congestive heart failure in the United States. *Kidney Int* 2003;64:1071.

789. Flynn CT. Continuous ambulatory peritoneal dialysis in diabetic patients. In: Legrain M, ed. *Continuous Ambulatory Peritoneal Dialysis.* Amsterdam: Excerpta Medica, 1980: 187.

790. Diaz-Buxo JA. Influence of hypertension on vision in diabetics undergoing peritoneal and hemodialysis. In: Maher JR, Winchester JF, eds. *Frontiers in Peritoneal Dialysis.* New York: Field, Rich, 1986:457.

791. Watanabe Y, Yuzawa Y, Mizumoto D, et al. Long-term follow-up study of 268 diabetic patients undergoing haemodialysis, with special attention to visual acuity and heterogeneity. *Nephrol Dial Transplant* 1993;8:725.

792. Serlie MJM, Struijk DG, de Blok K, Krediet RT. Differences in fluid and solute transport between diabetic and nondiabetic patients at the onset of CAPD. *Adv Perit Dial* 1997; 13:29.

793. Shostak A, Gotloib L. Increased peritoneal permeability to albumin in streptozotocin diabetic rats. *Kidney Int* 1996; 49:705.

794. Krediet RT, Zuyderhoudt FMJ, Boeschoten EW, Arisz L. Peritoneal permeability to proteins in diabetic and non-diabetic continuous ambulatory peritoneal dialysis patients. *Nephron* 1986;42:133.

795. Fried L. Higher membrane permeability predicts poorer patient survival. *Perit Dial Int* 1997;17:387.

796. Nakamoto H, Imai H, Kawanishi H, et al. Effect of diabetes on peritoneal function assessed by personal dialysis capacity test in patients undergoing CAPD. *Am J Kidney Dis* 2002;40:1045.

797. Lin JJ, Wadhwa NK, Suh H, Cabralda T. Comparisons of peritoneal transport between insulin-dependent and non-insulin-dependent diabetic peritoneal dialysis patients. *Perit Dial Int* 1997;17:208.

798. Kim DJ, Kang WH, Kim HJ, et al. The effect of dialysate dwell on gastric emptying time in patients on continuous ambulatory peritoneal dialysis. *Perit Dial Int* 1999;19(suppl 2):S176.

799. U.S. Renal Data System. *USRDS 2003 Annual Data Report: Atlas of End-Stage Renal Disease in the United States.* Bethesda, MD: National Institutes of Health, National Institute of Diabetes and Digestive and Kidney Diseases, 2003.

800. Lee HB, Chung SH, Chu WS, et al. Peritoneal dialysis in diabetic patients. *Am J Kidney Dis* 2001;38(suppl 1):S200.

801. Wang PH, Lau J, Chalmers TC. Meta-analysis intensive blood glucose control on late complications on type I diabetes. *Lancet* 1993;341:1306.

802. Wu MS, Yu CC, Wu CH, et al. Pre-dialysis glycemic control is an independent predictor of mortality in type II diabetic patients on continuous ambulatory peritoneal dialysis. *Perit Dial Int* 1999;19(suppl 2):S179.

803. Crossley K, Kjellstrand CM. Intraperitoneal insulin for control of blood sugar in diabetic patients during peritoneal dialysis. *Br Med J* 1971;1:269.

804. Flynn CT, Nanson JA. Intraperitoneal insulin with CAPD. An artificial pancreas. *Trans Am Soc Artif Intern Organs* 1979;25:114.

805. Flynn CT. The Iowa Lutheran protocol. *Perit Dial Bull* 1981;6:100.

806. Daniels, ID, Markell, MS. Blood glucose control in diabetics II. *Semin Dial* 1993;6:394.

807. Diaz-Buxo, JA, Crawford, TL. Intraperitoneal insulin in diabetic patients on peritoneal dialysis. In: Nissenson A, Fine RN, eds. *Dialysis Therapy.* Philadelphia: Hanley & Belfus, 2002:429.

808. Diaz-Buxo JA. Peritoneal dialysis prescriptions for diabetic patients. *Adv Perit Dial* 1999;15:91.

809. Scarpioni L, Ballocchi S, Scarpioni R, Cristinelli L. Peritoneal dialysis in diabetics. optimal insulin therapy on CAPD: intraperitoneal versus subcutaneous treatment. *Perit Dial Int* 1995;16(suppl 1):S275.

810. Khanna R. Dialysis considerations for diabetic patients. *Kidney Int* 1993;43(suppl 40):S58.

811. Ruotolo G, Micossi P, Galimberti G et al. Effects of intraperitoneal versus subcutaneous insulin administration on lipoprotein metabolism in type I diabetes. *Metabolism* 1990;38:598.

812. Nevalainen P, Lahtela JT, Mustonen J, Pasternack A. The influence of peritoneal dialysis and the use of subcutaneous and intraperitoneal insulin on glucose metabolism and serum lipids in type I diabetic patients. *Nephrol Dial Transplant* 1997;12:145.

813. Nevalainen PI, Lahtela JT, Mustonen J, et al. The effect of insulin delivery route on lipoproteins in type I diabetic patients on CAPD. *Perit Dial Int* 1999;19:148.

814. Balducci A, Slama G, Rottembourg J, et al. Intraperitoneal insulin in uraemic diabetics undergoing continuous ambulatory peritoneal dialysis. *Br Med J* 1981;283:1021.

815. Wideroe TE, Smeby LC, Berg K, et al. Intraperitoneal (IP) insulin absorption during intermittent and continuous peritoneal dialysis. *Adv Perit Dial* 1987;3:369.

816. Seveso M, Galato R, Brando B, et al. Insulin absorption to peritoneal dialysis bags. *Perit Dial Bull* 1987;7(suppl 1): S68.

817. Werb R, Rae A, Taylor P, et al. Intraperitoneal insulin in diabetics on continuous ambulatory peritoneal dialysis. *Perit Dial Bull* 1987;7(suppl 1):S83.

818. Duckworth WC. Insulin degradation: mechanisms, products and significance. *Endocr Rev* 1988;9:319.

819. Colette C, Pares-Herbute N, Monnier L, et al. Effect of different insulin administration modalities on vitamin D metabolism of IDDM patients. *Horm Metab Res* 1989;21:37.

820. Quellhorst E. Insulin therapy during peritoneal dialysis: pros and cons of various forms of administration. *J Am Soc Nephrol* 2002;13(suppl 1):S92.

821. Groop LC, von Bonsdorff MC. Intraperitoneal insulin administration does not promote insulin antibody production

in insulin-dependent diabetes mellitus patients on dialysis. *Diab Nephrol* 1985;4:80.

822. Schneierson SJ. Continuous peritoneal irrigation in the treatment of intractable edema of cardiac origin. *Am J Med Sci* 1949;218:76.

823. Rae AI, Hopper JJ. Removal of refractory edema fluid by peritoneal dialysis. *Br J Urol* 1968;40:336.

824. Cairns KB, Porter GA, Kloster FE, et al. Clinical and hemodynamic results of peritoneal dialysis for severe cardiac failure. *Am Heart J* 1968;76:227.

825. Malach M. Peritoneal dialysis for intractable heart failure in acute myocardial infarction. *Am J Cardiol* 1972;26:61.

826. Chopra MP, Gulati RB, Portal RW, et al. Peritoneal dialysis for pulmonary edema after acute myocardial infarction. *Br Med J* 1970;3:77.

827. Mailloux LU, Swartz CD, Onesti GO, et al. Peritoneal dialysis for refractory congestive heart failure. *JAMA* 1967;199:873.

828. Sears W, Pickering D, Watana W. Cardiac failure due to acute bacterial endocarditis treated with peritoneal dialysis and aortic valve replacement. *Arch Dis Child* 1973;48:322.

829. Raja RM, Krasnoff SO, Moros JG, et al. Repeated peritoneal dialysis in treatment of heart failure. *JAMA* 1970;213:2268.

830. Shapira J, Lang R, Jutrin I, et al. Peritoneal dialysis in refractory congestive heart failure: Part I. Intermittent peritoneal dialysis. *Perit Dial Bull* 1983;3:130.

831. Robson M, Biro A, Knobel B, et al. Peritoneal dialysis in refractory congestive heart failure: Part II. continuous ambulatory peritoneal dialysis. *Perit Dial Bull* 1983;3:133.

832. Mousson C, Tanter Y, Rebibou JM, et al. Treatment of reporting congestive heart failure by continuous peritoneal dialysis. *Perit Dial Bull* 1987;7(suppl 1):S55.

833. Swartz RD. The use of peritoneal dialysis in special situations. *Adv Perit Dial* 1999;15:160.

834. Nolph KD: Replacement of renal function by dialysis. In: Drukker W, Parsons FM, Maher JF, eds. *Peritoneal Dialysis.* Boston: Martinus Nijhoff, 1979:227.

835. Thongboonkerd V, Lumlertgul D, Supajatura V. Better correction of metabolic acidosis, blood pressure control, and phagocytosis with bicarbonate compared to lactate solution in acute peritoneal dialysis. *Artif Organs* 2001;25:99.

836. Freidell HV. Pancreatitis and renal insufficiency. *Am J Gastroenterol* 1960;34:487.

837. Wall AJ. Peritoneal dialysis in the treatment of severe acute pancreatitis. *Med J Aust* 1965;52:281.

838. Bartecchi CE, Mastro ER, Swarts CW. Acute hemorrhagic pancreatitis with hypertriglyceridemia. *Rocky Mt Med J* 1976;73:95.

839. Stone HH, Fabian TC. Peritoneal dialysis in treatment of acute alcoholic pancreatitis. *Surg Gynecol Obstet* 1980;150:878.

840. Glenn LD, Nolph KD. Treatment of pancreatitis with peritoneal dialysis. *Perit Dial Bull* 1982;2:63.

841. Weissberg D, Adam G, Volk H, et al. Acute pancreatitis: a 10-year study. *Am Surg* 1972;38:574.

842. Satake K, Rozmanith JS, Appert HE, et al. Hypotension and release of kinin-forming enzymes into ascitic fluid exudate during experimental pancreatitis in dogs. *Am Surg* 1973;177:497.

843. de Jode LRJ. The management of acute pancreatitis. *Br J Clin Pract* 1980;34:37.

844. Reuler JB. Hypothermia: pathophysiology, clinical setting and management. *Ann Intern Med* 1978;89:519.

845. Gregory RT, Patton JF. Treatment after exposure to cold. *Lancet* 1972;1:377.

846. Zawada ET. Treatment of profound hypothermia with peritoneal dialysis. *Dial Transplant* 1980;9:255.

847. O'Connor J. The treatment of profound hypothermia with peritoneal dialysis. *Perit Dial Bull* 1982;2:171.

848. Henderson LW. Clinical aspects of uremia and dialysis. In: Massry SG, Sellers AL, eds. *Peritoneal Dialysis.* Urbana, IL: Charles C. Thomas, 1976:555.

849. Maher JF. Principles of dialysis and dialysis of drugs. *Am J Med* 1977;62:475.

850. Campion DS, North JDK: Effect of protein binding of barbituates on their rate of removal during peritoneal dialysis. *J Lab Clin Med* 1965;66:549.

851. Etteldorf JN, Dobbins WT, Summitt RL, et al. Intermittent peritoneal dialysis using 5% albumin in the treatment of salicylate intoxication in children. *J Pediatr* 1961;58:226.

852. Knochel JP, Mason AD. Effect of alkalinization on peritoneal diffusion of uric acid. *Am J Physiol* 1966;210:1160.

853. Winchester JF, Gelfand MC, Knepshield JH, et al. Dialysis and hemoperfusion of poisons and drugs—update. *Trans Am Soc Artif Internal Organs* 1977;23:762.

854. Skoutakis VA, Black WD, Acchiardo SR, et al. Peritoneal dialysis in the treatment of acetohexamide induced hypoglycemia. *Am J Hosp Pharm* 1977;34:68.

855. Sidek M, Sieberth HG, Schmitz G, et al. Extrarenal indications for peritoneal dialysis. *Proc Eur Dial Transplant Assoc* 1966;3:355.

856. Twardowski ZJ, Nolph KD, Rubin J, et al. Peritoneal dialysis for psoriasis, an uncontrolled study. *Ann Intern Med* 1978;88:349.

857. Barry KG, Hunter RH, Davis TE, et al. Acute uric acid nephropathy. *Arch Intern Med* 1963;111:452.

858. Maher JF, Rath CE, Schreiner GE. Hyperuricemia complicating leukemia. Treatment with allopurinol and dialysis. *Arch Intern Med* 1969;123:198.

859. Molitoris BA, Alfrey PS, Miller NL, et al. Efficacy of intramuscular and intraperitoneal deferoxamine for aluminum chelation. *Kidney Int* 1987;31:986.

860. Taber T, Hageman T, York S, Miller R. Removal of aluminum with intraperitoneal deferoxamine. *Perit Dial Bull* 1986;6:213.

Infections in Peritoneal Dialysis

Linda F. Fried
Beth M. Piraino

Peritonitis and peritoneal catheter infections cause significant morbidity in peritoneal dialysis (PD) patients,[1–3] accounting for the majority of catheters lost and transfer to hemodialysis, either temporarily or permanently.[4–8] Peritonitis is also a major cause of hospitalization in PD patients.[3] Peritonitis also likely contributes to loss of peritoneal membrane function, particularly in long-term PD patients.[9] Peritonitis is associated with a more rapid decline in residual renal function,[10] an important predictor of survival on PD.[11–13] Peritonitis can result in the death of the patient, either directly from sepsis or indirectly from ensuing complications.[14] Therefore prevention of peritonitis must be a goal of all PD programs. Center protocols can minimize the risk of the development of peritonitis in their patients.[15–17]

Peritonitis should not be viewed as inevitable. Rates have fallen dramatically in the past one to two decades.[18,19] Currently, in any given year, the majority of patients in a well-run PD program will not develop peritonitis (Fig. 17–1). This is in striking contrast to the early era of PD, when peritonitis occurred approximately twice per year.[20]

Advances in the technology of PD connection and appropriate exit-site care have contributed most to the decline in peritonitis risk.[17,21,22] These approaches have resulted in a decrease primarily in infections due to gram-positive organisms: those causing peritonitis via touch contamination ("skin flora," such as coagulase-negative *Staphylococcus*) or via the peritoneal dialysis catheter (*Staphylococcal aureus*).[18,19,21–25] However, there has been little change in the rate of infections due to gram-negative organisms or fungal infections, and these remain serious, frequently requiring hospitalization to manage; they are also associated with an increased frequency of catheter removal and patient death.[3,14,18,19,26]

Programs that have implemented prophylaxis against *S. aureus* have seen a decrement in both catheter infection rates and peritonitis due to this organism.[18,19] However, catheter infection rates due to gram-negative organisms, particularly *Pseudomonas aeruginosa*, have remained relatively constant over time (Fig. 17–2). Consequently the proportion of episodes due to gram-negative organisms relative to gram-positive organisms has increased.[23]

% of patients in the program

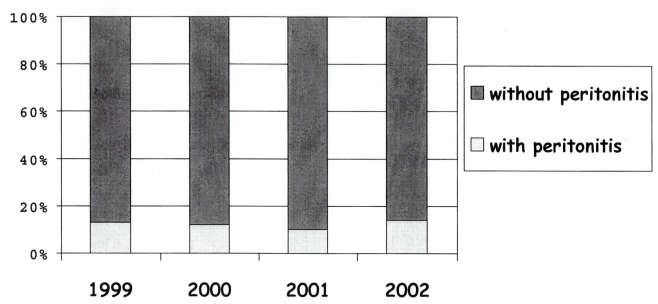

Figure 17–1. Proportion of individuals with and without peritonitis by year in the Dialysis Clinic, Inc. of Oakland PD Registry.

Much remains to be learned about the prevention of peritonitis. Patient training has been rather poorly studied in regard to peritonitis risk, although data from pediatric programs would suggest that this is a very important aspect of maintaining low peritonitis rates.[27] Little is known about either the pathogenesis or prevention of enteric peritonitis. Further research is required in these areas.

CATHETER INFECTIONS

Infections directly involving the peritoneal catheter (exit site and subcutaneous tunnel) are relatively common in PD patients. Rates from centers vary based on the definitions used and on the use of protocols for exit-site care.[28–30] In the era prior to prophylaxis for *S. aureus*, 46 percent of patients

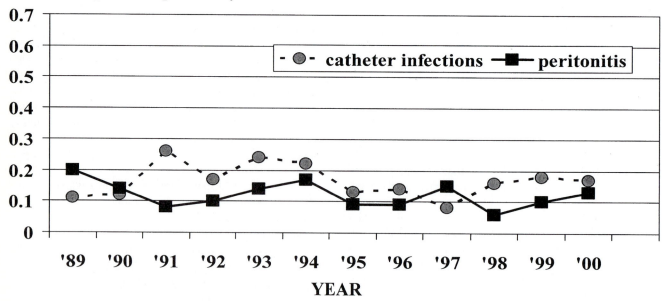

Figure 17–2. Gram-negative peritonitis and catheter infection rates over time in the DCI of Oakland PD Registry.

had an exit-site infection after 1 year on PD; this increased to 78 percent by 3 years.[31] After 1 year on PD, 15 percent of patients had a tunnel infection,[32] although this figure may actually be higher, as many tunnel infections are clinically occult.[33]

Catheter infections are primarily of importance because they can lead to refractory or relapsing peritonitis.[5,33–35] The overall peritonitis rate in patients with catheter infections is more than twice that of patients who do not have catheter infections.[31,33] Approximately 64 percent of those with a history of an exit-site infection developed peritonitis, in contrast to 45 percent of patients without a history of exit-site infection.[5] Prevention of infection, early diagnosis, and treatment are critical for the prevention of peritonitis. If a catheter infection proves refractory to management, catheter replacement should be done to prevent the development of peritonitis. This approach is preferable to waiting until peritonitis ensues, which in this setting is often either refractory or relapsing.[35]

Definitions and Diagnosis

An exit-site infection is defined as purulent drainage at the catheter exit site with or without associated erythema.[36] Erythema alone may represent an exit-site infection as well but alternatively may be due to irritation.[31,37] Purulent exit-site infections are more likely to lead to peritonitis than just erythema at the exit site.[31] Squeezing the exit site while gently pulling on the catheter may identify otherwise occult purulent drainage.[38] Induration and tenderness at the exit site are also abnormal and may represent infection. Bloody drainage generally indicates trauma and may predispose to infection. Crusting and serous drainage do not represent infection but may precede infection.[36,38] It can sometimes be difficult to determine whether serous drainage represents an infectious risk. Culture of drainage is therefore important, since an abnormal-appearing exit site that is culture-positive for serious pathogens—such as *S. aureus* or *P. aeruginosa*—should be treated. In the case of most purulent infections, the culture results are positive, in contrast to cultures of merely erythematous exit sites.

A tunnel infection is an infection of the subcutaneous portion of the catheter. It is clinically present when there is pain, tenderness, erythema, or induration over the subcutaneous pathway.[36] However, studies using ultrasound have found that tunnel infections are often occult.[33] In the presence of a tunnel infection, ultrasound shows decreased echogenicity around the tunnel, indicating a fluid collection.[33,39,40] Tunnel infections most often occur in the presence of an exit-site infection, but they are occasionally found in isolation.[33] Pathologically, the inflammation can involve the outer cuff, intercuff segment, and/or inner cuff. Involvement of the inner cuff is associated with a very high risk of peritonitis with the same organism.[33,41,42] Exit-site

and tunnel infections are often difficult to differentiate and may be collectively referred to as catheter infections.

Organisms Causing Catheter Infections

The most common and serious organisms causing exit-site infections are *S. aureus* and *P. aeruginosa*.[5,30,31,36,43] Skin organisms, such as coagulase-negative *Staphylococcus*, can cause infection, but they are, as a rule, readily treated and rarely lead to peritonitis.[36] Multiple organisms may be cultured from an infected exit site.[44] A positive culture of a normal-appearing exit site does not constitute an infection but represents colonization.[45] Colonization with *S. aureus* is a risk factor for future infections.[46–48] In addition, a negative culture in the presence of an abnormal-appearing exit site does not exclude infection. Exit-site infections which grow *S. aureus* or *P. aeruginosa* should be considered serious and treated aggressively until resolved, as these organisms are often associated with overt or occult tunnel infection and therefore pose a risk for peritonitis.[5,31,49]

The initial choice of antibiotic for an exit-site or tunnel infection should cover *Staphylococcus* unless *Pseudomonas* is suspected or was present in the past.[36] Oral antibiotics are adequate for most catheter infections. Cephalexin, trimethoprim-sulfamethoxazole (TMP-SMX), or penicillinase-resistant penicillins are reasonable first choices. Once culture results have been obtained, the antibiotics can be adjusted. Quinolones are useful for *Pseudomonas* infections, but care must be taken that the medication is not taken with calcium-based phosphate binders or oral iron tablets, which prevent gastrointestinal absorption.

Intensified local care, which may include hypertonic saline compresses to the exit site, may hasten resolution and can be done once or twice daily; it may even be effective without antibiotics[50] (Table 17–1). Treatment should be continued until the exit site is normal.[36] If, after 2 weeks of antibiotics, the infection fails to resolve, repeat cultures should be taken to ensure that there is not a resistant organism. In the case of *S. aureus*, rifampin can be added if there is no contraindication to the use of this drug. Coagulase-negative *Staphylococcus* infections are much more likely to resolve (>90 percent) than infections with *S. aureus* or *Pseudomonas* (40 to 50 percent).[44,49,51,52] A tunnel infection

TABLE 17–1. RECIPE FOR HYPERTONIC SALINE DRESSINGS FOR EXIT SITES

2 tablespoons table salt

1 quart of boiled water

Mix in clean container, keep refrigerated

Pour on 2x2 gauze, heat until warm to touch in microwave oven

Wrap exit site of catheter, allow to sit for 15 minutes

Can do bid or tid

should be suspected for an unresolving infection if the organism is *S. aureus* or *Pseudomonas.*

If deep cuff involvement is not present, externalization and curettage of the external cuff ("cuff shaving") and revision of the tunnel may help to resolve the infection.[53,54] An alternative approach is to replace the external catheter segment, including the superficial cuff, by splicing a new portion to the preexisting catheter and forming a new exit site.[55] If the infection persists, the catheter should be replaced.[56,57] In this way, peritonitis can be avoided.[57] Unless there is extensive subcutaneous tissue involved with the infection, removal and replacement of the catheter can usually be done in the same operation for refractory exit-site and tunnel infections.[56]

Except in the case of coagulase-negative *Staphylococcus* infection, if an exit-site infection is present in the setting of peritonitis with the same organism, successful treatment without removing the catheter is very unlikely.[35,51] Unlike peritonitis in the absence of catheter infections, peritonitis associated with a tunnel infection is generally either refractory to antibiotic therapy or is relapsing.[35] Delay in catheter removal may lead to permanent damage to the peritoneum, precluding future peritoneal dialysis.[57]

Prevention of Catheter Infections

Risk of infection can be minimized by use of appropriate techniques for catheter placement, as shown in Table 17–2. Prophylactic antibiotics at the time of insertion reduce the likelihood of subsequent infection.[58–60] A randomized trial comparing the use of no antibiotics with the administration of cefazolin or vancomycin found the last approach to be most effective[58]: however, because of concern regarding propagation of vancomycin-resistant organisms, vancomycin is generally not recommended for prophylaxis.[61] For this reason, cefazolin is most commonly used.

There are no consistent data that the type of catheter is associated with the catheter infection rate. However, double-cuffed catheters are associated with a lower risk of peritonitis[62]; they are therefore preferred to single-cuff catheters. A downward-directed tunnel also decreases the risk of catheter-related peritonitis and can be achieved with the use of the swan-neck catheter.[36,53,63]

Proper exit-site care is very important (Table 17–3). Until healing occurs (which is variable from patient to pa-

TABLE 17–2. PREVENTION OF CATHETER INFECTIONS: CATHETER PLACEMENT

Double-cuffed catheter

Downward-directed exit site

Prophylactic antibiotics at time of placement

Small exit site and avoidance of hematoma

External cuff at least 0.5 to 1.0 cm below skin opening

TABLE 17–3. CARE OF EXIT SITE

Immediate care after catheter placement (first week)
  Surgical gauze dressing
  Sterile dressing changes by nurse until healed
  No water exposure until healed
Chronic care
  Clean daily with antibacterial soap and water
  Keep exit site clean and dry
  Untreated well water should be avoided
  Catheter should be anchored to avoid trauma
  No swimming in lakes or rivers
  Strict avoidance of hot tubs
  Exit-site antibiotic cream/ointment

tient but generally takes 1 to 3 weeks), dressing changes should be made in a sterile fashion; generally, this is best done by the dialysis nurse.[36] Between dressing changes (often done weekly), the surgical gauze dressing should be left in place unless it becomes blood-soaked. The exit site should not be immersed in water until it is well healed; therefore the patient should not shower for the first week following catheter placement.

Once well healed, the exit site is cleaned daily by the patient using antibacterial soap while showering.[64] At this time the patient can begin applying (Fig. 17–3) an antistaphylococcal antibiotic cream to the exit site with a cotton swab. Several studies have demonstrated the efficacy of this approach in minimizing staphylococcal exit-site infections and thus peritonitis (Fig. 17–4).[65–67] Application of mupirocin to the exit site appears to be more effective in preventing *S. aureus* peritonitis than treatment of the nose with mupirocin.[68] *S. aureus* in the nose is generally the same subtype as that at the catheter exit site.[46,48,69] Perhaps treatment of the nose is less effective than treatment of the exit site with mupirocin because recolonization of the nose

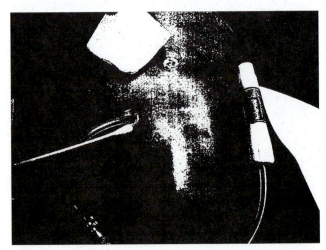

Figure 17–3. Method of applying mupirocin to peritoneal dialysis exit site.

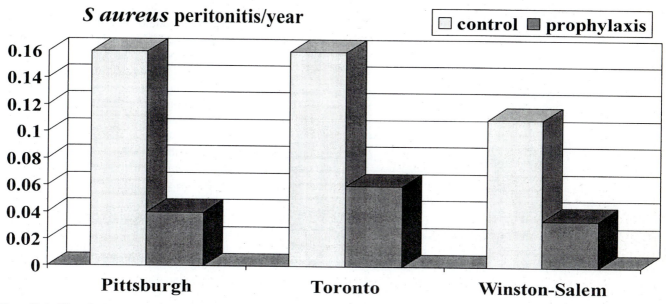

Figure 17–4. Effect of exit-site mupirocin on *Staphylococcus aureus* peritonitis rates. [65-67]

is frequent[70]; therefore intermittent treatment may not be as effective as the daily application of antibiotic cream to the exit site. This approach is an approach well accepted by patients and avoids the need to perform nose cultures.

PERITONITIS

Epidemiology, Rates, and Risk Factors

Rates of peritonitis appear to vary widely from center to center and country to country. This may be due to variations in training methods, connectology, exit-site protocols, and management of relapsing peritonitis. Peritonitis rates (44 episodes, 149 dialysis years) using a double-bag system from Hong Kong are shown in Table 17–4.[71] There is likely a cultural influence, as both the Chinese[71] and Japanese[72]

TABLE 17–4. RATES OF PERITONITIS (EPISODES PER PATIENT YEAR) ON CAPD USING THE DOUBLE BAG SYSTEM[71]

Organism	Rate	Percent
Coagulase negative *Staphylococcus*	0.03	9
Staphylococcus aureus	0.04	14
Streptococcus	0.03	9
Other gram-positive organisms	<0.01	2
Gram-negative organisms	0.10	34
Polymicrobial infections	<.01	2
Fungal	—	0
Sterile	0.07	23
AFB (acid-fast bacilli)	0.02	7
Total	0.30	100

report very low rates of peritonitis. It is also possible that inherited host factors may protect against peritonitis, as Asian patients (from India, Pakistan, Bangladesh, Sri Lanka) trained and cared for in London (21 percent of 325 PD patients) have lower rates of peritonitis than London patients from other ethnic groups.[73]

A number of demographic factors are associated with an increased risk for peritonitis. Children generally have higher rates of infection.[74] The frequency of peritonitis varies strikingly in the pediatric population, with some children having no episodes and others very frequent peritonitis.[74] Older adults (over age 60 or 65) do not appear to have higher rates of peritonitis,[75,76] but the data are conflicting.[77]

African-American patients may have an increased risk of peritonitis.[63,73,78–80] The reasons for this are not clear and not completely explained by differences in socioeconomic status.[73,78–80] Education, or inherited risk factors,[73,80] may play a role,

Immunosuppression, low creatinine generation, and hypoalbuminemia increase the risk of peritonitis.[81–85] A serum albumin level below 2.9 g/dL in particular is associated with increased risk (Fig. 17–5).[85] The mechanism may be related to immunologic impairment associated with malnutrition. HIV-positive patients generally have a high risk of infection and a higher rate of *Pseudomonas*, coagulase-negative staphylococcal, and fungal peritonitis.[83] Steroid therapy increases the risk of *S. aureus* exit-site infections and thus peritonitis.[82] Recently, depressive symptoms have been reported to increase the risk of peritonitis.[86] The reason for this association is unclear, but it might involve the effect of depression on immune function, on technique, or both.

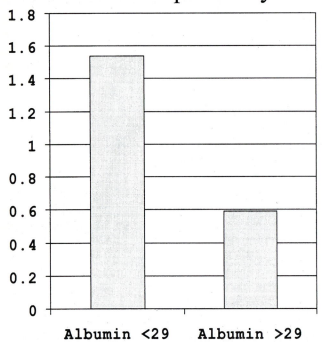

Peritonitis episodes/year

Figure 17–5. Association of low serum albumin (grams per liter) at the start of peritoneal dialysis and subsequent peritonitis rates.[85]

S. aureus carriage increases the risk of both exit-site infections and peritonitis. Compared with noncarriers, carriers have an incidence of *S. aureus* peritonitis that is two to six times higher.[87–90] Patients who are immunosuppressed or diabetic have an increased risk of *S. aureus* exit-site infection, with patients with positive carriage within each group having the higher risk.[82] As is the case with *S. aureus* catheter infections, exit-site prophylaxis decreases the risk of *S. aureus* peritonitis.[65–67,91,92] Exit-site prophylaxis using mupirocin should not be equated with treatment of nasal carriage with mupirocin, as the latter has not been shown consistently to decrease *S. aureus* peritonitis.[68] Health care providers may carry *S. aureus* from one patient to another, so careful hand cleansing during clinic visits is essential to prevent transmission.[93] In children (as opposed to adults), intranasal mupirocin does not decrease exit-site infections or peritonitis,[94] perhaps because of the parents' involvement in caregiving.

The strongest dialysis-related factor associated with peritonitis risk is the type of connection system. The original connection for PD involved a straight spike system with a high risk of contamination at the time of the exchange. With the introduction of disconnect systems, such as the twin bag, peritonitis due to common contaminants declined.[25,72,95] These systems not only eliminate spiking but also provide a flush of approximately 50 mL from the dialysate bag to the drain bag prior to infusion of dialysate. With this system, low-grade touch contamination from the

attachment step is flushed into the drain bag instead of into the patient's abdomen. The addition of a flush to the cycler strikingly reduced peritonitis risk in girls.[96] Although the twin-bag system is more expensive, the higher cost is offset by the savings from reduced peritonitis[25](Fig. 17–6).

While continuous ambulatory peritoneal dialysis (CAPD) is still the most common type of dialysis in some countries, such as Mexico and Hong Kong, continuous cycling peritoneal dialysis (CCPD) is gaining popularity in others. Peritonitis rates with CCPD vs. CAPD is variably reported, likely due to regional differences in the connection methods of the cyclers used. In Europe, cyclers have a Luer-Lok connection system, while in the United States one of the common types of cyclers requires spiking. A modification of the CCPD technique using an assist device to spike the bags may lower peritonitis rates from touch contamination.[97] The flush-before-fill technique with the newer cyclers also decreases the incidence of peritonitis.[96,98]

There appears to be a center effect for peritonitis risk as rates vary significantly from center to center.[85,99] The reason for this is unclear, but it most likely relates to differences in training.[27] Further studies (preferably international) should be done examining the relationship between training (length and content as well as experience of the trainers) and subsequent rates of peritonitis.

Etiology

The routes of entry for peritonitis are summarized in Table 17–5. Contamination at the time of the exchange remains a common cause.[71] This leads to infection with skin flora, often coagulase-negative *Staphylococcus*; however, some patients' skin is colonized with gram-negative organisms.[100] In these patients, touch contamination can lead to gram-negative peritonitis. The Y-set decreases *Acinetobacter* peritonitis, indicating touch contamination as the source of infection for this organism.[101] Other possible causes of contamination are failure to a mask during an exchange, holes in the catheter or tubing, and accidental disconnections.[102,103]

Catheter infections account for 10 to 25 percent of peritonitis episodes if prophylactic protocols against *S. aureus* are not employed.[35,63] Catheter infections can also pro-

	Twin bag (no spiking)	Basic Y (requires spike)
Peritonitis/year	0.26	0.86
Hospitalization days	17	98
Catheter removal	0	4

Figure 17–6. Peritonitis rates, hospitalization, and catheter removal rates on the twin-bag vs. the basic Y-set.[25]

TABLE 17–5. ROUTES OF ENTRY FOR ORGANISMS CAUSING PERITONITIS

Contamination
Catheter related
    Tunnel infection
    Catheter dialysate leak
    Catheter biofilm
Enteric/abdominal source
Bacteremia
Procedure-related
Gynecologic in origin

duce relapsing peritonitis, defined as recurrent peritonitis with the same organism within 4 weeks of stopping antibiotics. This can be due to the presence of a tunnel infection or to a bacterial colonization of a biofilm.[35,104] Recurrent peritonitis in association with a biofilm is most often due to coagulase-negative *Staphylococcus*, while recurrent peritonitis due to a tunnel infection is usually *S. aureus* or *Pseudomonas*.

Gram-negative peritonitis may be caused by intestinal flora. It can result from intraabdominal pathology or severe constipation.[105–110] Gram-negative peritonitis can occur after instrumentation of the gastrointestinal tract, such as colonoscopy with polypectomy, endoscopy with sclerotherapy, or laparoscopic cholecystectomy without prophylactic antibiotics.[111] However, in many cases there is no apparent etiology.[112] It is presumed that the peritonitis occurs because of transmural migration across the gastrointestinal tract,[113] but touch contamination is also a possibility.[108] The presence of multiple gram-negative organisms, especially in combination with anaerobic organisms, suggests perforation (macro or micro). Pneumoperitoneum is relatively common and may be technique-related; but when it occurs in conjunction with peritonitis, visceral perforation must be considered in the differential diagnosis.[114] Diverticulosis in the absence of diverticulitis does not appear to be a risk factor for peritonitis.[115]

Other causes of peritonitis are less common. Transient bacteremia after dental and other procedures may produce peritonitis.[109,111] Rarely, ascending infections from uterine or vaginal sources can lead to peritonitis.[116–118] Similarly, there are reports of gynecologic procedures (uterine biopsy) leading to peritonitis.[111,119]

Presentation and Diagnosis

PD patients with peritonitis generally have cloudy fluid and abdominal pain.[100,120] Approximately 90 percent have pain, often scored as a "10" on a 10-point scale.[120] Severity of pain is a predictor of the need for hospitalization. Aggressive management of pain is appropriate.

Up to 6 percent of adults with peritonitis present with abdominal pain and clear fluid.[121] Usually this represents a delay of leukocytosis, as follow-up cell counts are higher in most cases.[121,122] This delay may be may be secondary to a slower cytokine response to infection. Therefore peritonitis should be considered in all PD patients with abdominal pain, even if the cell count is initially negative.

In patients on automated PD, the early diagnosis of cloudy fluid may be missed in the absence of pain, as patients do not as readily see the effluent. Therefore these patients may present later in the course of the illness. Because of the shortened dwell time, the diagnosis may be more difficult to make.

The presentation can vary from cloudy fluid with no pain to a severe illness associated with clinical signs and symptoms of sepsis.[100,123] Fever may or may not be present. Typically, patients infected with relatively nonvirulent organisms such as coagulase-negative *Staphylococcus* or diphtheroids have cloudy fluid without abdominal pain, fever, or systemic symptoms.[123,124] Thus they are readily treated on an outpatient basis.[125] Conversely, patients infected with more virulent organisms—such as *S. aureus*, *P. aeruginosa*, other gram-negative bacilli or fungi—often have prominent abdominal pain and may also experience diarrhea, nausea, or vomiting and appear acutely ill.[106,126,127] Peritonitis from bowel perforation or other abdominal processes often produces severe symptoms, but the initial presentation may not differ from that of typical peritonitis.[128,129] Patients with peritonitis due to *Streptococcus* are particularly likely to have severe abdominal pain.[127,130–132] Hypotension, while rarely present, is a poor prognostic sign. The pain in PD peritonitis is generally diffuse. Localized abdominal pain may suggest an intraabdominal process.

Tunnel tenderness indicates a tunnel infection, but the sensitivity of the physical examination for tunnel infection is low, especially in the presence of peritonitis.[33] Since tunnel infections are generally associated with exit-site infections, the presence of an exit-site infection in a patient with peritonitis should trigger suspicion of catheter-related peritonitis. Any exit-site drainage in a patient presenting with peritonitis should be cultured.

The presence of peritonitis is confirmed by an effluent dialysate leukocyte count exceeding 100/μL with more than 50 percent polymorphonuclear leukocytes.[133] In general, the effluent in the absence of peritonitis has fewer than 25 leukocytes per microliter and a paucity of neutrophils, with mononuclear cells being the predominant cell type.[121,134,135] A threshold of 50 white blood cells per microliter is used to define peritonitis if the patient is already on antibiotics.[136,137] If the patient is on a form of peritoneal dialysis with short dwell times, as with cycler peritoneal dialysis, or if an aspirate is obtained from a patient on nocturnal peritoneal dialysis with an empty abdomen during the day, then the percentage of neutrophils (>50 percent) is a more sensitive marker than is the total white blood cell concentration.[138]

In the presence of cloudy dialysate, the culture is generally positive for bacteria or fungi. Viral peritonitis is extremely rare.[139] The culture is sterile in approximately 20 percent of episodes that meet the criteria for peritonitis based on cell count.[71] Most of these episodes are due to a microorganism that has not grown in culture. In some cases this may be because the patient was recently taking antibiotics.[140,141] Technical problems with culturing the effluent may also account for many of these episodes.[141]

The method of culturing dialysate also influences the growth of microorganisms. The use of blood culture bottles or concentrating the effluent by filtering increases the yield of positive cultures.[142-144] In general, at least 10 to 20 mL of effluent should be cultured.[145] Bacteremia is rarely present. Therefore routine culturing of the blood is not necessary unless the patient appears septic; the exception is peritonitis due to an intraabdominal process.[106,146] Cultures are generally positive within 24 to 72 hours. Fungal cultures may take longer than the routine time in many labs; therefore a high index of suspicion is needed, especially if the patient is not responding to antibiotics. Gram's stain for earlier diagnosis is predominantly useful in examining for the presence of yeast, which permits an earlier diagnosis of fungal peritonitis.[61,147] Otherwise, the Gram's stain is not very useful, and the antibiotic therapy should not be solely based on it, as culture results can yield more than one organism or a different organism. If both gram-positive and gram-negative organisms are seen, this suggests an intrabdominal process such as a perforated viscus is suggested.

The differential diagnosis for culture-negative cloudy fluid is shown in Table 17–6. Fibrin or blood in the effluent may be mistaken for cloudiness but is usually readily distinguished by an experienced observer. Dialysate eosinophilia occurs early in the course of peritoneal dialysis in some patients, generally resolves spontaneously by 3 months, and is not usually associated with infection.[148-150] However, peritoneal eosinophilia, defined as more than 10 percent of 100

TABLE 17–6. DIFFERENTIAL DIAGNOSIS OF CULTURE-NEGATIVE CLOUDY DIALYSATE

True microorganism-related peritonitis
    Inadequate culture technique
    Antibiotic therapy at the time of culture
    Atypical or slow growing organism—e.g., mycobacteria, fungi
Chemical peritonitis
Pancreatitis
Intraabdominal malignancy
Chyloperitoneum
Culture-negative eosinophilic peritonitis
Ovulation, menstruation

or more leukocytes per microliter in the effluent, can be seen in infectious peritonitis.[151] This is particularly true for peritonitis due to fungi such as *Coccidioides immitis*, *Paecilomyces variotii*, and *Exophiala jeanselmei*.[152-154]

Mycobacterial peritonitis, not rare in countries where tuberculosis is endemic, may be difficult to diagnose. It may present with a predominance of lymphocytes, but neutrophil predominance is more common.[155-158] The use of the polymerase chain reaction (PCR) will greatly hasten the diagnosis.[156,157]

Pancreatitis is another cause of cloudy fluid with sterile cultures. The diagnosis can be confirmed by a serum amylase value greater than three times the upper limit of normal and effluent amylase greater than 100 U/L.[159] Computed tomography (CT) will generally confirm the presence of pancreatitis.[159]

Chemical peritonitis has been reported with some drugs. Intraperitoneal generic vancomycin and amphotericin were formerly reported to cause chemical peritonitis,[160-163] but the current preparations of vancomycin do not seem to cause chemical peritonitis; therefore vancomycin is commonly given via the intraperitoneal route. There are recent cases of culture-negative chemical peritonitis due to icodextrin.[164] The effluent clears on stopping the icodextrin. The cause appears to have been a manufacturing problem that has since been corrected.

The effluent cell count and differential is the key to distinguishing most of the entities mentioned above from infectious peritonitis. In the presence of effluent eosinophilia, a high total dialysate leukocyte count (greater than 1000/μL) and neutrophils more than 50 percent of the total are very suggestive of an infectious etiology.[151] Chemical peritonitis can be difficult to differentiate from infectious peritonitis, since the effluent white cell count is high in both, with a predominance of polymorphonuclear leukocytes.

Treatment

Initial Management. After the cultures are obtained, empiric antibiotics should be started.[61] Antibiotics should not be delayed for culture results. The transfer set should be changed if it appears to be involved in the etiology. If the exit site has drainage, it should be cultured, as well as the effluent dialysate. A decision must be made regarding admission. Historically, outpatient therapy was often feasible, as the most common etiology was touch contamination, resulting in relatively benign peritonitis. Currently, with protocols in place to prevent contamination, many peritonitis episodes are severe. Hospitalization is required if the patient has moderate to severe pain, appears ill, has fever or hypotension, is vomiting and unable to take oral fluids, or if outpatient administration of antibiotics is not feasible. Pain control is important and often neglected.[120]

Peritoneal transport of antibiotics is bidirectional; thus antibiotics may be given intravenously or intraperitoneally.[165,166] In general, intraperitoneal antibiotics are preferred, as this route may be more effective than intravenous and results in higher local levels.[167] The presence of residual renal function requires higher doses or more frequent administration.[165] The dialysis prescription (i.e., higher flow rate requires higher dosing) also affects the pharmacokinetics of commonly used drugs.[166]

Oral antibiotics are generally ineffective. The exception may be the quinolones, but failures with quinolones are common[168–170]; they should not be used as the sole antibiotic for empiric therapy, although they may be useful in addition to other antibiotics.[171,172]

There are many published antibiotic regimens for PD peritonitis. In an effort to standardize the approach, the International Society for Peritoneal Dialysis (ISPD) has published a series of treatment guidelines.[61,173–176] The initial guidelines were published in 1987 and are updated periodically as new information becomes available. The original guidelines emphasized the use of vancomycin, with gram-negative coverage with an aminoglycoside.[173,174] In 1996, the guidelines were changed to recommend curbing the use of vancomycin and using a first-generation cephalosporin with an aminoglycoside as empiric therapy, because of the emergence of vancomycin-resistant organisms.[176] However, concerns were raised about the possible effect on residual renal function of even a short course of aminoglycosides, given the relationship of residual renal function to patient survival. The most recent guidelines, published in 2000, recommended a first-generation cephalosporin with ceftazidime as initial therapy if the patient has significant residual renal function (>100 mL/day).[61] Subsequent therapy is based on the culture results.

These guidelines have been controversial. Some centers have reported high cure rates.[177–180] However, other studies have not found such favorable results or have noted a high proportion of episodes that would not initially be covered by this regimen.[172,181–182] Two randomized trials, which included relatively small numbers of patients, have not completely resolved the issue.[182,183] The ISPD protocol will not cover methicillin-resistant *S. aureus* (MRSA) or enterococcus. Methicillin-resistant coagulase-negative *Staphylococcus* may respond to the first-generation cephalosporin, as the local concentrations of antibiotic are higher than the minimum inhibitory concentration (MIC), but relapsing peritonitis can occur and cure rates may be lower.[184] An increasing proportion of coagulase-negative staphylococci are resistant to methicillin.[19]

Each center must establish a protocol for empiric therapy that is consistent with the local patterns of causative organisms and sensitivities.[172] Centers with a high prevalence of MRSA should continue to use vancomycin, especially in patients sick enough to require hospitalization. Vancomycin

may also be indicated if the patient is a known carrier of MRSA. A drug providing gram-negative coverage—such as an aminoglycoside, aztreonam, or ceftazidime—is also required.[185] Quinolones can be used as part of the initial therapy, but many centers report increasing antimicrobial resistance.[19,168] It is important to evaluate local sensitivities of causative organisms.[172,186]

Antibiotics can be given either as continuous therapy (each CAPD exchange) or intermittently.[61] In CCPD, the antibiotics are given intermittently in the long dwell (at least 4 hours), or the patient may need to be transferred to CAPD temporarily.[61] High systemic levels may be required to reach continuously adequate effluent levels with vancomycin.[166] Therefore, 20 mg/L in each exchange for automated peritoneal dialysis (APD) may be preferable to intermittent dosing.[166] With aminoglycosides, relatively low-dose intermittent administration may be associated with less toxicity. Vancomycin doses need to be higher in individuals with significant residual renal function and possibly in those with more permeable peritoneal membranes.[187] Table 17–7 shows the dosing of commonly used antibiotics for PD peritonitis. In the absence of a tunnel infection, fungal peritonitis, or intraabdominal pathology, 80 to 90 percent of episodes of peritonitis resolve with antibiotics.[123]

Organism-Specific Therapy

Gram-Positive Infections. If a gram-positive organism—especially coagulase-negative *Staphylococcus* or other skin organism—is isolated, the patient should be questioned about a break in technique. Retraining of the patient should be undertaken if contamination is suspected. Specific treatments for various gram-positive organisms are summarized below.

Skin Flora. If the organism isolated is a diphtheroid, *Corynebacterium*, or bacillus, a first-generation cephalosporin for 14 days is generally sufficient, although sensitivities must be checked. The empiric gram-negative coverage can be discontinued. Tunnel infections with these organisms are rare.[57] In the case of coagulase-negative *Staphylococcus*, the course depends on whether the organism is methicillin-resistant. Methicillin-sensitive organisms can be treated with cefazolin for 14 days. The cure rate for methicillin-resistant organisms is lower for cefazolin than for vancomycin,[184] and the patient should be converted to vancomycin if resistance to cephalosporins is reported. Since coagulase-negative *Staphylococcus* can colonize the peritoneal catheter's slime layer, it is important to avoid undertreatment, as this may result in relapsing peritonitis.[188,189] This slime layer, or biofilm, consists of exopolysaccharides within which bacteria reside that are resistant to both host defenses and many antibiotics.[189] Biofilm may play a role in recurrent coagulase-negative staphylococcal episodes of peritonitis.[190] If there is recurrent

TABLE 17–7. DOSING OF INTRAPERITONEAL ANTIBIOTICS FOR PERITONITIS[A]

Intermittent (once a day)	Continuous Dosing
Cephalosporins (continuous preferable)	
Cefazolin or cephalothin	
anuric 15 mg/kg	500 mg load then125mg/L
nonanuric 20 mg/kg	500 mg load, 150 mg/L
Ceftazidime 1–1.5 g/day	250 mg load, then 125 mg/L
Cefotaxime 2 g/day	500 mg load, then 250 mg/L
Ceftriaxone 1 g/day	250 mg load, then 125 mg/L
Aminoglycosides (if nonanuric, increase doses by 25%, intermittent preferable)	
Amikacin 2 mg/kg	25 mg/L
Gentamycin 0.6 mg/kg	8 mg/L
Netilimycin 0.6 mg/kg	8 mg/L
Tobramycin 0.6 mg/kg	8 mg/L
Penicillins	
Amoxicillin Data not available	250–500 mg load, then 50 mg/L
Ampicillin, oxacillin, Data not available nafcillin	125 mg/L
Piperacillin Data not available	4-g load then 250 mg/L
Ampicillin/sulbactam 2 g q 12 h	1-g load, then 100 mg/L
Other antibiotics	

Vancomycin   30 mg/kg up to
    1-g load, then
    30–50 mg/L
	2 g, re-dose
	1 g every 4–5 days

Ciprofloxacin   Data on IP
   not available
   Oral 500 mg bid
	50 mg load then 25 mg/L

Teicoplanin 400 mg bid	400 mg load then 40 mg/L
Aztreonam 1 g	1000 mg load then 250 mg/L

SOURCE: From Keane et al.,[61] with permission.

peritonitis with coagulase-negative *Staphylococcus*, catheter removal/replacement (which can be done as a single procedure) will be highly effective in preventing further episodes.[56,190,191]

Staphylococcus aureus. *S. aureus* peritonitis is generally a more severe form of peritonitis than that caused by coagulase-negative *Staphylococcus*, since it is associated with abdominal pain, which may be accompanied by nausea and vomiting.[126] Approximately one-third of patients with *S. aureus* peritonitis have fever, and a smaller percentage will be hypotensive.[126]

In the majority of cases, *S. aureus* peritonitis is associated with a catheter infection.[5] Catheter removal is often required to resolve the peritonitis or to prevent repetitive episodes.[86,126,190] Relapsing peritonitis after successful treatment is usually due to *S. aureus* or *Staphylococcus epidermidis*.[190,191] Concomitant colonization or infection of the exit site with *S. aureus* is associated with a tenfold increased risk of another episode of *S. aureus* peritonitis.[191] Hospitalization may be prolonged with *S. aureus* peritonitis, and death has been reported.[3,14,126]

If a catheter infection is present, the catheter should be removed, as the chances of resolution are quite small.[35] Attempts to treat refractory peritonitis beyond 5 days with antibiotics without catheter removal result in a high mortality.[192] In addition, a very high proportion of patients will develop subsequent peritoneal membrane failure.[192]

Once the culture results return, the subsequent antibiotic regimen also depends on whether the organism is methicillin-sensitive. If it is, the antibiotics can be changed to an antistaphylococcal penicillin, or a first-generation cephalosporin can be continued if this was the initial regimen. Rifampin can be added at a dose of 600 mg/day.

If the organism is methicillin-resistant, vancomycin should be used. The vancomycin for CAPD should be dosed every 4 to 5 days, with frequency of dosing determined by serum trough levels; the dose should be kept above 10 to 12 mg/L, since dialysate levels will be lower than this and lower trough levels predict treatment failure.[188] More frequent dosing may be needed in individuals with residual renal function.[191]

For patients on APD, it may be preferable to either convert the patient to CAPD, or to add vancomycin, 20 mg/L, to all exchanges.[187] However, a study in children found intermittent dosing to be as effective as continuous therapy.[191] Rifampin should be added to the regimen for MRSA.[61] Treatment failure is more common for MRSA than for methicillin-sensitive staphylococcal infections.[193] The recommended course of treatment with antibiotics is 21 days with or without catheter removal.[61]

Streptococcus and Enterococcus. Streptococcal and enterococcal infections account for 10 to 15 percent of peritonitis episodes.[100,123,127] These are severe infections.[127] Beta-hemolytic streptococcal infections can result in shock and death.[100,130] Patients with cirrhosis seem particularly at risk for streptococcal peritonitis.[127] *Streptococcus viridans* may be related to the connection procedure, as the incidence of peritonitis due to this organism decreases with disconnect systems.[127]

For nonenterococcal *Streptococcus*, penicillins and first-generation cephalosporins can be used and the gram-negative coverage discontinued. The length of recommended therapy is 14 days, but longer courses may be necessary.[61] Relapses are uncommon.[127]

Enterococcal infections are slower to respond to antibiotics. Enterococcal peritonitis should lead to consideration of workup for intraabdominal processes.[107,195] Ampicillin is the preferred therapy, if the organism is sensitive to it.[61] Aminoglycosides may be synergistic. If the organism is resistant to ampicillin, vancomycin should be used. If the organism is a vancomycin-resistant enterococcus, then quinupristin/dalfopristin or linezolide should be used.[61] Vancomycin-resistant enterococcal (VRE) peritonitis is more common in individuals who have received prior antibiotics for peritonitis and in those who have been hospitalized.[196] VRE is relatively uncommon in outpatient PD patients who have not been hospitalized within the preceding year.[197,198]

Gram-Negative Infections. As in the case of gram-positive organisms, once the organism and sensitivities have been determined, the antibiotics should be adjusted. If possible, aminoglycosides should be replaced by other agents. The prolonged use of aminoglycosides can lead to significant oto- and vestibular toxicity and possibly to loss of residual renal function,[199–201] although this does not appear to be the case in children.[191]

The most common organisms isolated in gram-negative peritonitis are *Escherichia coli*, *Klebsiella*, and *Enterobacter.*[112] Gram-negative peritonitis is a serious infection, associated with higher rates of death, hospitalization, catheter loss, and transfer to hemodialysis.[3,14,112,202] This is true even when cases associated with abdominal perforation are excluded. The mortality rate is 4 to 10 percent for gram-negative peritonitis and approaches 50 percent for episodes associated with bowel perforation.[14,106,107,112] This is in con-

trast to <1 percent for coagulase-negative staphylococcal peritonitis.[14] Multiple enteric organisms or the presence of an anaerobe suggests intraabdominal pathology (see below).[114] However, in many cases of peritonitis associated with intraabdominal pathology, only one organism is isolated.[203]

Most gram-negative peritonitis can be treated with one antibiotic for 14 days.[61] Although the ISPD guidelines suggest giving gentamicin as 0.6 mg/kg IP in a single daily dose, several pharmacokinetic studies have subsequently shown that levels are inadequate with this approach.[204–206] Modeling suggests that initial dosing of 1.5 mg/kg in one exchange the first day, followed by 0.5 mg/kg IP once daily subsequently, would be more appropriate.[204]

Some gram-negative infections require two antibiotics. *Pseudomonas, Acinetobacter,* and *Stenotrophomonas* generally require double coverage for 21 days.[61,207,208] Since 1996, increased severity of *E. coli* peritonitis has been reported. Despite double antibiotic coverage, approximately half the patients required catheter removal and/or surgery.[209]

Ceftazidime can be given once daily, 15 mg/kg in one exchange lasting 6 hours, with acceptable levels.[210,211] Cefepime, an attractive option for monotherapy, is generally ineffective against *Pseudomonas.*[212,213]

Pseudomonas. Peritonitis due to *P. aeruginosa* is often the result of a catheter infection with the same organism.[35] Rates of *P. aeruginosa* peritonitis vary from 0.2 to 0.05 patient per year.[51] The rate from center to center is somewhat dependent on the timing of catheter removal: at the time of recalcitrant catheter infection or only after the development of peritonitis. *Pseudomonas* peritonitis is severe and may damage the peritoneum enough to preclude further peritoneal dialysis; therefore prevention is much preferred to treatment.[192,214]

The origin of *Pseudomonas* infections in peritoneal dialysis patients is unknown. This organism is found in water and soil and typically causes infections either in the presence of a foreign body (such as a peritoneal dialysis catheter) or an immunodeficient state (such as renal failure).[215] Of note, HIV-positive CAPD patients have a markedly higher rate of *Pseudomonas* peritonitis than do those who are HIV-negative (1.4 vs. 0.06 per year).[216]

Peritonitis due to *P. aeruginosa* is difficult to treat and can sometimes be fatal.[16,17,51] Therapy with two drugs that are active against *P. aeruginosa* should be implemented.[61,209,217] If a catheter infection is not present, antibiotic therapy may be effective, although long courses may be required to prevent relapse.[51,218,219] If a catheter infection is present, the catheter should be removed without delay.[49]

Polymicrobial Peritonitis. Polymicrobial peritonitis is not inevitably due to bowel pathology; approximately 3 to 9 percent of all peritonitis episodes are due to multiple organisms.[220–222] Combinations of gram-positive organisms alone may account for approximately one-third to one-tenth of episodes of polymicrobial peritonitis.[220–222] Bowel leaks and other intraabdominal pathologies account for only 7 percent of episodes.[221] Catheter removal rates and transfer to hemodialysis are higher in polymicrobial peritonitis than peritonitis due to a single organism.[220,221]

The bowel is a suspected source of peritonitis when two gram-negative bacilli, anaerobes, or a gram-negative bacillus in combination with a fungus grow from the cloudy effluent.[128,222] Fecal peritonitis is associated with severe symptoms, may be associated with bacteremia, and commonly results in transfer of the patient to hemodialysis.[146,223,224] Features helpful in determining whether peritonitis is due to intraabdominal pathology include the growth of multiple enteric organisms, fecal matter in drained dialysate, diarrhea containing dialysate, and a large volume of free air in the abdominal cavity.[106,110] A high mortality is associated with fecal peritonitis, especially if surgery is delayed, so urgent intervention by the surgeon is required if this diagnosis is suspected.[106,110,128,222]

Fungal Peritonitis. Fungal peritonitis occurs in peritoneal dialysis patients at rates of 0.01 to 0.11 per year.[225–227] Abdominal pain may be severe and associated with fever.[228] However, the presentation is similar to that of bacterial peritonitis.[229]

The mortality rate associated with fungal peritonitis in adults is 16 to 45 percent; it is higher when catheter removal is delayed.[225,226,229–231] Prior antibiotic therapy is a risk factor for fungal peritonitis.[230–235] Patients who are HIV-positive have high rates of fungal peritonitis[83,216]—0.94 per year in one series.[216]

Antibiotic therapy of fungal peritonitis without catheter removal in adults is seldom successful and should not be attempted.[236–240] Amphotericin B diffuses poorly from blood into peritoneum[241] and intraperitoneal administration can result in chemical peritonitis.[163,241] Flucytosine, ketoconazole, and fluconazole penetrate the peritoneal cavity readily and are more effective than amphotericin, although catheter removal is still necessary.[236,240–243] The ISPD guidelines recommend the use of flucytosine 1 g orally each day and fluconazole 150 mg per one exchange intraperitoneally every other day, with catheter removal if there is no clinical improvement in 4 to 7 days.[61] Once the diagnosis of fungal peritonitis is confirmed, many investigators favor rapid removal of the peritoneal catheter so as to maintain peritoneal membrane function and allow a return to peritoneal dialysis.[147,234] Therapy is continued for 4 to 6 weeks.

A number of other fungi are rare causes of peritonitis, including *Coccidioides immitis, Cryptococcus neoformans,* Rhizopus species, Aspergillus species, *Alternaria, Fusarium moniliformis, Curvularia lunata, Syncephalastrum, Paecilo-*

myces variotii, Exophiala jeanselmei, Wangiella dermatitidis, Pichia ohmeri, and *Trichoderma.*[152–154,237,244–252] *Aspergillus, Alternaria,* and *C. lunata* can colonize the catheter, leading to peritonitis or catheter obstruction.[250,253–255] Excision of the involved portion of the catheter is advisable if such infections are diagnosed. Coccidioidal peritonitis is associated with previous pulmonary infection and cryptococcal peritonitis with simultaneous meningitis.[256]

Mycobacterial Peritonitis. Mycobacteria are unusual causes of peritonitis; they are more common in Asia than in Europe or the Americas.[155,257,258] The effluent is cloudy and generally has polymorphonuclear predominance.[155–158,258] Acid fast bacilli (AFB) smears are usually negative.[259] Cultures are generally positive,[155,156,258] but ordering them requires an increased risk of suspicion. PCR allows more rapid identification of this infection[156,157,259] than do cultures. Mycobacterial infections are one cause of "culture negative" peritonitis. Both tuberculous and nontuberculous mycobacteria, mainly *Mycobacterium fortuitum,* can cause peritonitis.[155–158,257–261] Both tuberculous and nontuberculous mycobacterial infections appear to respond to appropriate antibiotics; however, ultrafiltration failure may subsequently occur.[155,257,261]

Culture-Negative Peritonitis. If the culture is negative but the patient is improving, a first-generation cephalosporin can be continued for 2 weeks.[61] If the patient is not improving, Gram's stain and culture should be repeated to see whether this reveals an etiology.[262] If the infection remains unresponsive to antibiotics, culture for unusual organisms such as mycobacteria or fungi and removal of the catheter should be considered.

Follow-up of Peritonitis. Clinical response is generally seen in 3 to 5 days. The dialysate leukocyte count in uncomplicated peritonitis normalizes in 4 to 5 days.[124] If there has been no improvement, reevaluation is essential. A repeat culture should be obtained to rule out an organism not covered by the antibiotics. The patient should be assessed for a tunnel infection and for intraabdominal pathology. Ultrasound can be helpful in ruling out an occult tunnel infection.[33,39,40] The normal tunnel is approximately 6 mm in diameter.[41] An increase in size with fluid around the tunnel suggests a tunnel infection. Surgical evaluation should be considered if the organism suggests an abdominal source.[263] A CT scan is often obtained to look for intraabdominal abscess, but this may be unrevealing.[264]

If repeat cultures do not reveal an organism not covered by the administered antibiotics, the catheter must be removed.[263] Catheter removal is indicated at 5 days if there is no response to appropriate therapy; a longer delay poses a significant risk of death or permanent damage to the peritoneum, thus precluding a return to PD.[192,265]

Occasionally, recurrent or unresolving peritonitis is due to abscess formation,[35] which occurs in less than 1 percent of episodes and is more common with gram-negative organisms, fungi, and *S. aureus*.[35,264] CT scan is helpful for diagnosis in these situations. An abscess requires surgical intervention for drainage.

Catheter Removal. The indications for catheter removal are listed in Table 17–8. In general, catheters should be removed for peritonitis that fails to resolve after 5 days of therapy, relapsing peritonitis, peritonitis associated with a catheter infection, fungal peritonitis, peritonitis associated with intraabdominal pathology, and for recalcitrant exit-site/tunnel infections. With delay in catheter removal, as many as half of dialysis patients are unable to return to PD because of damage to the peritoneal membrane.[265] Therefore prevention of peritonitis (as with replacement of any infected catheter that fails to respond to antibiotics) is by far preferable to antibiotic treatment alone.

To prevent peritonitis, simultaneous removal and reinsertion of a catheter is possible in recurrent peritonitis and peritonitis associated with a tunnel infection; this approach should be considered more often than is the current practice.[190,266–271] At the time of the procedure, there should not be evidence of ongoing peritoneal inflammation (peritoneal white blood cell count should be below 300/μm).[190] Therefore this technique should not be used for unresolving peritonitis. Simultaneous replacement should not be done in the face of active or fungal peritonitis.

Prevention of Peritonitis

Given the increased morbidity and mortality associated with peritonitis, centers should focus on prevention. Preventive maneuvers are outlined in Table 17–9. Although there are few data on training, this is undoubtedly central to the low rates of infection seen in some PD programs. Experienced training nurses who are focused on the PD program (and protected from the exigencies of the in-center hemodialysis program) are likely the key to success. A preventative program directed at decreasing infections leads to decreased rates of exit-site infection, peritonitis, and catheter loss.[272]

In terms of patient training, patients should wear masks during exchanges, which should be performed in a

TABLE 17–8. INFECTIOUS INDICATIONS FOR CATHETER REMOVAL

Peritonitis refractory to antibiotics after 5 days
Peritonitis associated with a catheter infection
Recurrent peritonitis with same organism
Fecal peritonitis
Fungal peritonitis
Inadequate drain or no drain associated with peritonitis
Refractory tunnel or exit-site infection

TABLE 17–9. MINIMIZING PERITONITIS RISK

1. Training (contamination)
   Handwashing with antibacterial soap
   Complete drying of hands prior to exchange
   Exchanges done in room without a lot of traffic
   No exposure to dust in the air, fan, open window
   Avoid pets in rooms where exchanges are done
   Mask worn during exchanges
   Training of adequate length
2. Catheter infections
   Prevent catheter infections (see Tables 17–2 and 17–3)
   Replace catheter for refractory catheter infections
3. Connection (contamination)
   Avoidance of spiking
   Flush-before-fill technique
4. Prophylactic antibiotics
   Contamination
   Procedures (endoscopic, uterine biopsy, cholecystectomy, invasive dental work)
   Daily exit-site antibiotic cream
   Antifungal prophylaxis while on long-term antibiotics

private, clean space without exposure to blowing fans, open windows, or animal hair. Pets should be excluded from the room in which exchanges are performed.[273,274] Careful handwashing with antibacterial soap and complete drying of the hands decreases the bacterial count.[275] Alcohol washes may be useful as well.

A twin-bag system should be used for CAPD. For APD, if a cycler that requires spiking is used, a spike assist device may decrease infection rates.[97] Patients must be taught to inspect each dialysate bag prior to use for pinpoint leaks.

The best approach to those high-risk patients with a serum albumin under 2.9 g/dL and/or on immunosuppression (as with failed transplant) is unclear. Aggressive nutritional support has been suggested as a method to decrease peritonitis rates in children[276]; in the absence of data, it would appear reasonable to extrapolate these results to adults.

Historically, prophylactic antibiotics in patients on peritoneal dialysis have not been beneficial. Neither daily cephalexin nor trimethoprim 160 mg plus sulfamethoxazole 800 mg (TMP-SMX), examined during the era of high-risk of peritonitis from contamination, was effective in reducing peritonitis risk.[277,278] However, when analyzed as treatment received (as opposed to intent to treat), TMP-SMX was effective (Fig. 17–7).[278] There are no data on the usefulness of this drug in the prevention of enteric peritonitis.

Prophylactic antibiotics prior to dental, endoscopic, and gynecologic procedures are recommended, since these procedures can lead to peritonitis.[111] Prophylaxis should be

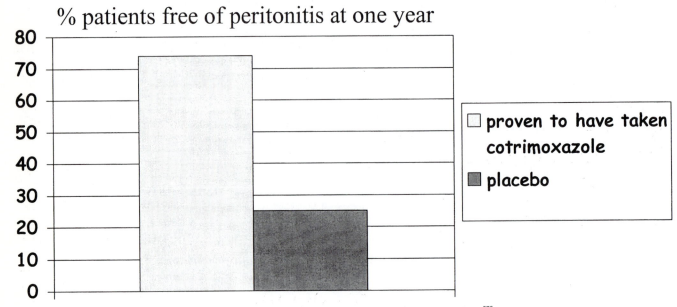

Figure 17–7. Freedom from peritonitis in patients taking cotrimoxazole vs. those given placebo; as-treated analysis.[278]

given for all contaminations. In general, an oral first-generation cephalosporin for 3 to 5 days is sufficient.

There have been a number of studies examining the effect of prophylaxis on preventing *S. aureus* peritonitis.[65–68,91,92] Daily exit-site mupirocin[65–67] (Fig. 17–4) and nasal mupirocin[68,92] decrease the rates of exit-site infection. Exit-site mupirocin can degrade polyurethane and should be avoided with catheters made of this material.[279] There are an increasing number of reports of mupirocin resistance in *S. aureus* infection.[280,281] However, as mupirocin is not used to treat infections, resistance is not as concerning as resistance to vancomycin. Prevention of *S. aureus* infections

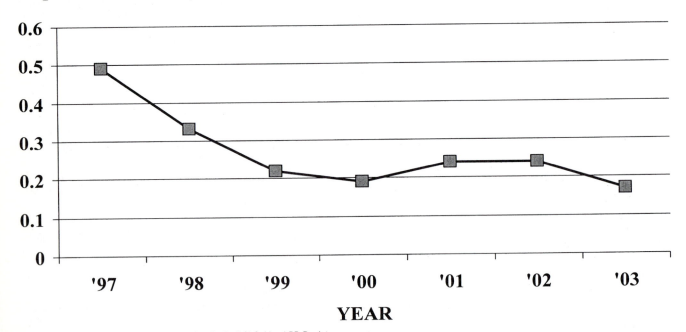

Figure 17–8. Trend in peritonitis rate over time in the DCI Oakland PD Registry.

may decrease the use of vancomycin and the emergence of resistance, so its use appears warranted.

Prior antibiotic use increases the risk of fungal peritonitis,[232,233,237] and this fact identifies a potential target group for prophylaxis. A number of nonrandomized studies or studies with historical controls have shown decreased peritonitis rates with fungal prophylaxis.[282–284] There have been two controlled studies.[285,286] Lo et al. utilized oral nystatin 500,000 U qid with concomitant antibiotic therapy. The nystatin was given regardless of the indication for antibiotic therapy.[285] In this study, nystatin significantly decreased rates of peritonitis due to *Candida*. In contrast, Williams et al. did not find a benefit for nystatin prophylaxis, but their baseline rates were much lower than those of Lo et al.[286]

In summary, rates of peritonitis can be reduced to low levels (Fig. 17–8). Indeed, peritonitis rates can be as low as rates of bacteremia on hemodialysis.[287] To achieve this requires constant surveillance by the PD program, with periodic review of episodes of both peritonitis and exit-site infections. Root-cause analysis should be carried out for every episode of peritonitis to determine the etiology, so that future preventive measures can be implemented. Unfortunately, methods to decrease peritonitis due to enteric organisms or *P. aeruginosa*, which is often secondary to a catheter infection, have not yet been identified. Experienced and dedicated PD nurses are likely important in maintaining a PD program with low infection rates.

REFERENCES

1. Gokal R. Peritoneal dialysis in the 21st century: an analysis of current problems and future developments. *J Am Soc Nephrol* 2002;13:S104–S116.
2. Piraino B. Peritonitis as a complication of peritoneal dialysis. *J Am Soc Nephrol* 1998;9:1956–1964.
3. Fried L, Abidi S, Bernardini J, et al. Hospitalization in peritoneal dialysis patients. *Am J Kidney Dis* 1999;33: 927–933.
4. Weber J, Mettang T, Hubel E, et al. Survival of 138 surgically placed straight double-cuff Tenckhoff catheters in patients on continuous ambulatory peritoneal dialysis. *Perit Dial Int* 1993;13:224–227.
5. Piraino B, Bernardini J, Sorkin M. The influence of peritoneal catheter exit site infections on peritonitis, tunnel infections, and catheter loss in patients on continuous ambulatory peritoneal dialysis. *Am J Kidney Dis* 1986;8:436–440.
6. Piraino B, Bernardini J, Sorkin M. Catheter infections as a factor in the transfer of continuous ambulatory peritoneal dialysis patients to hemodialysis. *Am J Kidney Dis* 1989; 13:365–369.
7. Woodrow G, Turney JH, Brownjohn AM. Technique failure in peritoneal dialysis and its impact on patient survival. *Perit Dial Int* 1997;17:360–364.
8. van Biesen W, Dequidt C, Vijt D, et al. Analysis of the reasons for transfers between hemodialysis and peritoneal dialysis and their effect on survivals. *Adv Perit Dial* 1998; 14:90–94.
9. Davies SJ, Bryan J, Phillips L, et al. Longitudinal changes in peritoneal kinetics: the effects of peritoneal dialysis and peritonitis. *Nephrol Dial Transplant* 1996;11:498–506.
10. Singhal MK, Bhaskaran S, Vidgne E, et al. Rate of decline of residual renal function in patients on continuous ambulatory peritoneal dialysis. *Perit Dial Int* 2000;20:429–438.
11. Paniagua R, Amato D, Vonesh E, et al. Effects of increased peritoneal clearances on mortality rates in peritoneal dialysis: ADEMEX, a prospective, randomized, controlled trial. *J Am Soc Nephrol* 2002;13:1307–1320.
12. Shemin D, Bostom AG, Lambert, et al. Residual renal function in a large cohort of peritoneal dialysis patients: change over time, impact on mortality and nutrition. *Perit Dial Int* 2000;20:439–444.
13. Bargman JM, Thorpe KE, Churchill DN, for the CANUSA Peritoneal Dialysis Study Group. Relative contribution of residual renal function and peritoneal clearance to adequacy of dialysis: a reanalysis of the CANUSA Study. *J Am Soc Nephrol* 2001;12:2158–2162.
14. Fried LF, Bernardini J, Johnston JR, Piraino B. Peritonitis influences mortality in peritoneal dialysis patients. *J Am Soc Nephrol* 1996;7:2176–2182.
15. Prowant B. Nursing interventions related to peritonitis. *Adv Renal Replace Ther* 1996;3:228–231.
16. Borg D, Shetty A, Williams D, et al. Fivefold reduction in peritonitis using a multifaceted continuous quality initiative program. *Adv Perit Dial* 2003;19:202–205.
17. Thomas MC, Harris DC. Management of bacterial peritonitis and exit-site infections in continuous ambulatory peritoneal dialysis. *Nephrology* 2002;7:267–271.
18. Piraino B, Bernardini J, Florio T, Fried L. *S. aureus* prophylaxis and trends in gram-negative infections in peritoneal dialysis patients. *Perit Dial Int* 2003;23:456–459.
19. Zelenitsky S, Barns L, Findlay I, et al. Analysis of microbiological trends in peritoneal dialysis-related peritonitis from 1991–1998. *Am J Kidney Dis* 2000;36:1009–1013.
20. Nolph KD, Sorkin M, Rubin J, et al. Continuous ambulatory peritoneal dialysis: three year experience at one center. *Ann Intern Med* 1980;92:609–613.
21. Mehrotra R, Marwaha, Berman N, et al. Reducing peritonitis rates in a peritoneal dialysis program of indigent ethnic minorities. *Perit Dial Int* 2003;23:83–85.
22. Holley JL, Bernardini J, Piraino B. Infecting organisms in continuous ambulatory peritoneal dialysis patients on the Y-set. *Am J Kidney Dis* 1994;23:569–573.
23. Canadian CAPD Clinical Trials Group. Peritonitis in continuous ambulatory peritoneal dialysis (CAPD): a multi-center randomized clinical trial comparing the Y connector disinfectant system to standard systems. *Perit Dial Int* 1989;9: 159–163.
24. Kiernan L, Kliger A, Gorban-Brennan N, et al. Comparison of continuous ambulatory peritoneal dialysis-related infections with different "Y-tubing" exchange systems. *J Am Soc Nephrol* 1995;5:1835–1838.

25. Harris DCH, Yuill EJ, Byth K, et al. C. Twin-versus single-bag disconnect systems: infection rates and cost of continuous ambulatory peritoneal dialysis. *J Am Soc Nephrol* 1996; 7:2392–2398.

26. Wang AYM, Yu AWY, Li PKT, et al. Factors predicting outcome of fungal peritonitis in peritoneal dialysis: analysis of a 9-year experience of fungal peritonitis in a single center. *Am J Kidney Dis* 2000;36:1183–1192.

27. Holloway M, Mujais S, Kandert M, et al. Pediatric peritoneal dialysis training: characteristics and impact on peritonitis rates. *Perit Dial Int* 2001;21:401–404.

28. Nolph KD. Access problems plague both peritoneal dialysis and hemodialysis. *Kidney Int* 1993;43(suppl 40): S81–S84.

29. Vogt K, Binswanger U, Buchmann P, et al. Catheter related complications during continuous ambulatory peritoneal dialysis: a retrospective study on sixty-two double-cuff Tenckhoff catheters. *Am J Kidney Dis* 1987;10:47–51.

30. Scalamonga A, Castelnovo C, De Vecchi A, et al. Exit site and tunnel infections in continuous ambulatory peritoneal dialysis patients. *Am J Kidney Dis* 1991;18:674–677.

31. Abraham G, Savin E, Ayiomamitis A. Natural history of exit-site infection in patients on continous ambulatory peritoneal dialysis. *Perit Dial Bull* 1988;8:211–216.

32. Holley JL, Bernardini J, Piraino B. Risk factors for tunnel infections in continuous ambulatory peritoneal dialysis. *Am J Kidney Dis* 1991;18:344–348.

33. Plum J, Sudkamp S, Grabensee B. Results of ultrasound-assisted diagnosis of tunnel infections in CAPD. *Am J Kidney Dis* 1994;23:99–104.

34. Zimmerman SW, O'Brien M, Wiedenhoeft FA, et al. *Staphylococcus aureus* peritoneal catheter related infections: a cause of catheter loss and peritonitis. *Perit Dial Bull* 1988; 8:191–194.

35. Gupta B, Bernardini J, Piraino B. Peritonitis associated with exit site and tunnel infections. *Am J Kidney Dis* 1996;28: 415–419.

36. Gokal R, Alexander S, Ash S, et al. Peritoneal catheters and exit-site practices toward optimum peritoneal access: 1998 update (Official report from the International Society for Peritoneal Dialysis). *Perit Dial Int* 1998;18:11–33.

37. Gonthier D, Bernardini J, Holley JL, et al. Erythema: does it indicate infection in a peritoneal dialysis catheter exit site? Adv Perit Dial 1992;8:230–233.

38. Holley JL, Moss AH. Improved diagnosis of CAPD exit site infections with catheter manipulation and the use of a grading system. *Adv CAPD* 1988;4:177–180.

39. Holley JL, Foulks CJ, Moss AF, et al. Ultrasound as a tool in the diagnosis and management of exit-site infections in patients undergoing continuous ambulatory peritoneal dialysis. *Am J Kidney Dis* 1989;14:211–216.

40. Domico J, Warman M, Jaykamur S, et al. Is ultrasonography useful in predicting catheter loss? *Adv Perit Dial* 1993;9: 231–232.

41. Korzets Z, Erdberg A, Golan E, et al. Frequent involvement of the internal cuff segment in CAPD peritonitis and exit site infection: an ultrasound study. *Nephrol Dial Transplant* 1996;11:336–339.

42. Bayston R, Andrews M, Rigg K, et al. Recurrent infection and catheter loss in patients on continuous ambulatory peritoneal dialysis. *Perit Dial Int* 1999;19:550–555.

43. Eisele G, Bailie GR, Lamaestro B. Relationship between peritonitis and exit site infections in CAPD. *Adv Perit Dial* 1992;8:227–229.

44. Piraino B, Bernardini J, Sorkin M. A five year study of the microbiologic results of exit site infections and peritonitis in continuous ambulatory peritoneal dialysis. *Am J Kidney Dis* 1987;4:281–286.

45. Luzar MA. Exit site infection in continuous ambulatory peritoneal dialysis: a review. *Perit Dial Int* 1991;11: 333–340.

46. Amato D, de Jesus Ventura M, Miranda G, et al. Staphylococcal peritonitis in continuous ambulatory peritoneal dialysis: colonization with identical strains at exit site, nose, and hands. *Am J Kidney Dis* 2001;37:43–48.

47. Sesso R, Draire S, Castelo A, et al. *Staphylococcus aureus* skin carriage and development of peritonitis in patients on continuous ambulatory peritoneal dialysis. *Clin Nephrol* 1989;31:264–268.

48. Pignatari A, Pfaller M, Sesso R, et al. *Staphylococcus aureus* colonization and infection on continuous ambulatory peritoneal dialysis. *J Clin Microbiol* 1990;28:1898–1902.

49. Lo CY, Chu WL, Wan KM, et al. *Pseudomonas* exit site infections in CAPD patients: evolution and outcome of treatment. *Perit Dial Int* 1998;18:637–640.

50. Hirsch DJ, Jindal KK. Local care of *Staphylococcus aureus* exit-site infection precludes antibiotic use. *Perit Dial Int* 2002;23: 301–302.

51. Bernardini J, Piraino B, Sorkin M. Analysis of continuous ambulatory peritoneal dialysis-related *Pseudomonas aeruginosa* infections. *Am J Med* 1987;83:829–832.

52. Piraino B. A review of *Staphylococcus aureus* exit-site and tunnel infections in peritoneal dialysis patients. *Am J Kidney Dis* 1990;16:89–95.

53. Swartz RD. Exit-site and catheter care: review of important issues. *Adv Perit Dial* 1999;15:201–204.

54. Suh H, Wadhwa NK, Cabralda T, et al. Persistent exit-site/tunnel infection and subcutaneous cuff removal in PD patients. *Adv Perit Dial* 1997;13:233–236.

55. Cheung A, Wheeler M, Limm W, et al. A salvage technique for CAPD catheters with exit site infections. *Am J Surg* 1995;170:60–61.

56. Swartz R, Messana J, Reynoles J, et al. Simultaneous catheter replacement and removal in refractory PD infections. *Kidney Int* 1991;40:1160–1165.

57. Lo CY, Chu WL, Wan KM, et al. *Pseudomonas* exit-site infections in CAPD patients: evolution and outcomes of treatment. *Perit Dial Int* 1998;18:637–653.

58. Gadallah MF, Ramdeen G, Mignone J, et al. Role of preoperative antibiotic prophylaxis in preventing postoperative peritonitis in newly placed peritoneal dialysis catheters. *Am J Kidney Dis* 2000;36:1014–1019.

59. Bennett-Jones DN, Martin J, Barratt AJ, et al. Prophylactic gentamicin in the prevention of early exit-site infections and peritonitis in CAPD. *Adv Perit Dial* 1988;4:147–150.

60. Katyal A, Mahale A, Khanna R. Antibiotic prophylaxis before peritoneal dialysis catheter insertion. *Adv Perit Dial* 2002;18:112–115.

61. Keane WF, Bailie GR, Boeschoten E, et al. Adult peritoneal dialysis-related peritonitis treatment recommendations: 2000 update. *Perit Dial Int* 2000;20:396–411.

62. Lewis MA, Smith T, Postlethwaite RJ, et al. A comparison of double-cuffed with single-cuffed Tenkhoff catheters in the prevention of infection in pediatric patients. *Adv Perit Dial* 1997;13:264–266.

63. Golper TA, Brier ME, Bunke M, et al. Risk factors for peritonitis in long-term peritoneal dialysis: the Network 9 Peritonitis and Catheter Survival Studies. *Am J Kidney Dis* 1996;38:428–436.

64. Prowant BF, Schmidt LM, Twardowski ZJ, et al. Peritoneal dialysis catheter exit site care. *ANNA J* 1988;15: 219–222.

65. Bernardini J, Piraino B, Holley J, et al. A randomized trial of Stphylococcus aureus prophylaxis in peritoneal dialsis patients: mupirocin calcium ointment 2% applied to exit site versus cyclic oral rifampin. *Am J Kidney Dis* 1996;27: 695–700.

66. Thodis E, Bhaskaran S, Pasadakis P, et al. Decrease in *Staphylococcus aureus* exit site infections and peritonitis in CAPD patient by local application of mupirocin ointment at the catheter exit site. *Perit Dial Int* 1998;18:261–270.

67. Casey M, Taylor J, Clinard P, et al. Application of mupirocin cream at the catheter exit site reduces exit-site infection and peritonitis in peritoneal dialysis patients. *Perit Dial Int* 2000;20:566–568.

68. The Mupirocin Study Group. Nasal mupirocin prevents *Staphylococcus aureus* exit-site infection during peritoneal dialysis. *J Am Soc Nephrol* 1996;7:2403–2408.

69. Kreft B, Eckstein S, Kahl A, et al. Clinical and genetic analysis of *Staphylococcus aureus* nasal colonisation and exit-site infection in patients undergoing peritoneal dialysis. *Eur J Clin Micriobiol Infect Dis* 2001;20:734–737.

70. Perez-Fontan M, Rosales M, Rodriguez-Carmona A, et al. Treatment of *Staphylococcus aureus* nasal carriers in CAPD with mupirocin. *Adv Perit Dial* 1993;9:242–245.

71. Li PKT, Law MCL, Chow KM, et al. Comparison of clinical outcome and ease of handling in two double-bag systems in continuous ambulatory peritoneal dialysis: a prospective, randomized, controlled, multicenter study. *Am J Kidney Dis* 2002;40:373–380.

72. Kawaguchi Y. National comparisons: optimal peritoneal dialysis outcomes among Japanese patients. *Perit Dialysis Int* 1999;19(suppl 3):S9–S16.

73. Crump HA, Raftery MJR, Yaqoob MM. Peritonitis in different racial groups on peritoneal dialysis. *Dial Transplant* 2003;32:142–144.

74. Schaefer F, Kandert M, Feneberg R. Methodological issues in assessing the incidence of peritoneal dialysis-associated peritonitis in children *Perit Dial Int* 2002;22:234–238.

75. Holley JL, Bernardini J, Perlmutter JA, et al. A comparison of infection rates among older and younger patients on continuous peritoneal dialysis. *Perit Dial Int* 1994;14:66–69.

76. Nissenson AR, Diaz-Buxo JA, Adcock A, et al. Peritoneal dialysis in the geriatric patient. *Am J Kidney Dis* 1990;16: 335–338.

77. Perez-Contreras J, Miguel A, Sanchez J, et al. A prospective multicenter comparison of peritonitis in peritoneal dialysis patients aged above and below 65 years. *Adv Perit Dial* 2000;16:267–270.

78. Juergensen PH, Gorban-Brennan N, Troidle L, et al. Racial differences and peritonitis in an urban peritoneal dialysis center. *Adv Perit Dial* 2000; 18:117–118.

79. Farias MG, Soucie JM, McClellan W, et al. Race and the risk of peritonitis: an analysis of factors associated with the initial episode. *Kidney Int* 1994;46:1392–1396.

80. Korbet SM, Vonesh EF, Firanek CA. A retrospective assessment of risk factors for peritonitis among an urban CAPD population. *Perit Dial Int* 1993;13:126–131.

81. Andrews PA, Warr KJ, Hicks JA, et al. Impaired outcome of continuous ambulatory peritoneal dialysis in immunosuppressed patients. *Nephrol Dial Trans* 1996;11:1104–1108.

82. Vychytil A, Lorenz M, Schneider B, et al. New strategies to prevent *Staphylococcus aureus* infections in peritoneal dialysis patients. *J Am Soc Nephrol* 1998;9:669–676.

83. Tebben JA, Rigsby MO, Selwyn PA, et al. Outcome of HIV-infected patients on continuous ambulatory peritoneal dialysis. *Kidney Int* 1993;44:191–198.

84. Wu CH, Huang CC, Wu MS, et al. Total creatinine appearance as indictor of risk of infectious complication in peritoneal dialysis. *Adv Perit Dial* 2000;16:219–222.

85. Wang Q, Bernardini J, Piraino B, et al. Albumin at the start of peritoneal dialysis predicts the development of peritonitis. *Am J Kidney Dis* 2003;41:664–669.

86. Troidle L, Watnick S, Wuerth D, et al. Depression and its association with peritonitis in long-term peritoneal dialysis patients. *Am J Kidney Dis* 2003;42:350–354.

87. Piraino B, Perlmutter JA, Holley JL, et al. *Staphylococcus aureus* peritonitis is associated with *Staphylococcus aureus* nasal carriage in peritoneal dialysis patients. *Perit Dial Int* 1993;13(suppl 2):S332–S334.

88. Wanten GJA, van Oost P, Schneeberger PM, et al. Nasal carriage and peritonitis by *Staphylococcus aureus* in patients on continuous ambulatory peritoneal dialysis: a prospective study. *Perit Dial Int* 1996;16:352–256.

89. Zimakoff J, Pedersen FB, Bergen L, et al. *Staphylococcus aureus* carriage and infections among patients in four haemo- and peritoneal-dialysis centres in Denmark. *J Hosp Infect* 1996;33:289–300.

90. Kingwatanakul P, Warady BA. *Staphylococcus aureus* nasal carriage in children receiving long-term peritoneal dialysis. *Adv Perit Dial* 1997;13:281–284.

91. Zeybel M, Ozder A, Sanlidag C, et al. The effects of weekly mupirocin appliation on infections in continuous ambulatory peritoneal dialysis patients. *Adv Perit Dial* 2003;19: 198–201.

92. Perez-Fontan M, Garcia-Falcon T, Rosales M, et al. Treatment of *Staphylococcus aureus* nasal carriers in continuous ambulatory peritoneal dialysis with mupirocin: long-term results. *Am J Kidney Dis* 1993;22:708–712.

93. Herwaldt LA, Boyken LD, Coffman S, et al. Sources of *Staphylococcus aureus* for patients on continuous ambulatory peritoneal dialysis. *Perit Dial Int* 2003;23:237–241.

94. Araki Y, Hataya H, Ikeda M, Ishikura K, Honda M. Intranasal mupirocin does not prevent exit-site infections in children receiving peritoneal dialysis. *Perit Dial Int* 2002; 23:267–269.

95. Kiernan L, Kliger A, Gorban-Brennan N, et al. Comparison of continuous ambulatory peritoneal dialysis-related infections with different "Y-tubing" exchange systems. *J Am Soc Nephrol* 1995;5:1835–1838.

96. Warady BA, Ellis EN, Fivush BA, et al. "Flush before fill" in children receiving automated peritoneal dialysis. *Perit Dial Int* 2002;23:493–498.

97. Bird M, Dacko C, Miller M, et al. Reducing peritonitis in APD patients. *Perit Dial Int* 1999:19;S29.

98. Smith CA. Reduced incidence of peritonitis by utilizing "flush before fill" in APD. *Adv Perit Dial* 1997;13:224–226.

99. Lupo A, Tarchini R, Cancarini G, et al. Long-term outcome in continuous ambulatory peritoneal dialysis: a 10-year survey by the Italian Cooperative Peritoneal Dialysis Study Group. *Am J Kidney Dis* 1994;24:826–837.

100. Fenton S, Wu G, Cattran D, et al. Clinical aspects of peritonitis in patients on CAPD. *Perit Dial Bull* 1981;1(suppl 6):S4–S7.

101. Dryden MS, McCann M, Wing AJ, et al. Controlled trial of a Y-set dialysis delivery system to prevent peritonitis in patients receiving continuous ambulatory peritoneal dialysis. *J Hosp Infect* 1992;20:185–192.

102. Macia M, Vega N, Elcuaz R, et al. *Neisseria mucosa* peritonitis in CAPD: another case of the "nonpathogenic" *Neisseriae* infection. *Perit Dial Int* 1993;13:72–73.

103. Rubin J, McElroy R. Peritonitis secondary to dialysis tubing contamination among patients undergoing continuous ambulatory peritoneal dialysis. *Am J Kidney Dis* 1989;14:92–95.

104. Dasgupta MK, Costerton JW. Significance of biofilm-adherent bacterial microcolonies on Tenckhoff catheters of CAPD patients. *Blood Purif* 1989;7:144–155.

105. Singharetnam W, Holley JL. Acute treatment of constipation may lead to tansmural migration of bacteria rsulting in gram-negative, polymicrobial, or fungal peritonitis. *Perit Dial Int* 1996;16:423–425.

106. Tzamaloukas AH, Obermiller LE, Gibel LJ, et al. Peritonitis associated with intra-abdominal pathology in continuous ambulatory peritoneal dialysis. *Perit Dial Int* 1993;13:S335–S337.

107. Harwell CM, Newman LN, Cacho CP, et al. Abdominal catastrophe: visceral injury as a cause of peritonitis in patients treated by peritoneal dialysis. *Perit Dial Int* 1997;17: 586–594.

108. Newman LN, Cacho CP, Schulak JA, et al. Abdominal catastrophe: definition and proposal for a new approach. *Adv Perit Dial* 2000;17:93–97.

109. Troidle L, Kliger AS, Goldie SJ, et al. Continuous peritoneal dialysis–associated peritonitis of nosocomial origin. *Perit Dial Int* 1996;16:505–510.

110. Kern EO, Newman LN, Cacho CP, et al. Abdominal catastrophe revisited: the risk and outcome of enteric peritoneal contamination. *Perit Dial Int* 2002;22:323–334.

111. Fried L, Bernardini J, Piraino B. Iatrogenic peritonitis: the need for prophylaxis. *Perit Dial Int* 2000;20:343–345.

112. Bunke CM, Brier ME, Golper TA, for the Academic Subcommittee of the Network 9 Peritonitis Study. Outcomes of single organism peritonitis in peritoneal dialysis: gram-negatives versus gram-positives in the Network 9 Peritonitis Study. *Kidney Int* 1997;52:524–529.

113. Schweinburg FB, Seligman AM, Fine J. Transmural migration of intestinal bacteria: a study based on the use of radioactive *Escherichia coli*. *N Eng J Med* 1976;242:747–751.

114. Chang JJ, Yeun JY, Hasbargen JA. Penumoperitoneum in peritoneal dialysis patients. *Am J Kidney Dis* 1995;25: 297–301.

115. del Peso G, Bajo MA, Gadola L, et al. Diverticular disease and treatment with gastric acid inhibitors do not predispose

116. Swartz RD, Campbell DA, Stone D, et al. Recurrent polymicrobial peritonitis from a gynecologic source as a complication of CAPD. *Perit Dial Bull* 1983;3:32–33.

117. Coward RA, Gokal R, Wise M, et al. Peritonitis associated with vaginal leakage of dialysis fluid in continuous ambulatory peritoneal dialysis. *Br Med J* 1982;284:1529.

118. Stuck A, Seiler A, Fry FJ. Peritonitis due to an intrauterine device in a patient on CAPD. *Perit Dial Bull* 1986;6: 158–159.

119. Maruyama H, Nakamura T, Oya M, et al. Posthysteroscopy *Candida glabrata* peritonitis in a patient on CAPD. *Perit Dial Int* 1997;17:404–405.

120. Piraino B, Bernardini J, Fried L, et al. Pain due to peritonitis. *Perit Dial Int* 1999;19:583–584.

121. Koopmans JG, Boeschoten EW, Pannekeet MM, et al. Impaired initial cell reaction in CAPD-related peritonitis. *Perit Dial Int* 1996;16(suppl 1):S362–S367.

122. Korzets Z, Korzets A, Golan E, et al. CAPD peritonitis—initial presentation as an acute abdomen with clear peritoneal effluent. *Clin Nephrol* 1992;37:155–157.

123. Tranaeus A, Heimburger O, Lindholm B. Peritonitis in continuous ambulatory peritoneal dialysis (CAPD): diagnostic findings, therapeutic outcome and complications. *Perit Dial Int* 1989;9:179–190.

124. Rubin J, Rogers WA, Taylor HM, et al. Peritonitis during continuous ambulatory peritoneal dialysis. *Ann Intern Med* 1980;92:7–13.

125. Fenton SSA, Pei Y, Delmore T, et al. The CAPD peritonitis rate is not improving with time. *ASAIO Trans* 1986;32: 546–549.

126. Kim D, Tapson J, Wu G, et al. Staph aureus peritonitis in patients on continuous ambulatory peritoneal dialysis. *ASAIO Trans* 1984;30:494–497.

127. De Bustillo EM, Aguilera A, Jimenez C, et al. Streptococcal versus *Staphylococcus epidermidis* peritonitis in CAPD. A comparative study. *Perit Dial Int* 1997;17:392–395.

128. Van Reijden HJ, Struijik DG, van Ketel RJ, et al. Fecal peritonitis in patients on continuous ambulatory peritoneal dialysis, an end-point in CAPD? *Adv Perit Dial* 1988;4: 198–203.

129. Wakeen MJ, Zimmerman SW, Bidwell D. Viscus perforation in peritoneal dialysis patients: diagnosis and outcome. *Perit Dial Int* 1994;14:371–377.

130. Borra SI, Chandarana J, Kleinfeld M. Fatal peritonitis due to group B beta-hemolytic *Streptococcus* in a patient receiving ambulatory peritoneal dialysis. *Am J Kidney Dis* 1992;19: 375–377.

131. Cavalieri SJ, Allais JM, Schlievert PM, et al. Group A streptococcal peritonitis in a patient undergoing continuous ambulatory peritoneal dialysis. *Am J Med* 1989;86: 249–250.

132. Yinnon AM, Jain V, Magnussen CR. Group B streptococcus (*Agalactiae*) peritonitis and bacteremia associated with CAPD. *Perit Dial Int* 1993;13:241.

133. Vas SI. The diagnosis and treatment of peritonitis in patients on continuous ambulatory peritoneal dialysis. *Semin Dial* 1995;8:232–237.

134. Keane WF, Peterson PK. Peritonitis during continuous ambulatory peritoneal dialysis: the role of host defense mechanisms. *ASAIO Trans* 1984;30:684–686.

135. Flanigan MJ, Freeman RM, Lim VS. Cellular response to peritonitis among peritoneal dialysis patients. *Am J Kidney Dis* 1985;6:420–424.

136. Riera G, Bushinsky D, Emmanouel DS. First exchange neutrophilia: an index of peritonitis during chronic intermittent peritoneal dialysis. *Clin Nephrol* 1985;24:5–8.

137. Smoszna J, Raczka A, Fuksiewicz A, et al. Prognostic value of different tests in the early diagnosis of peritonitis during standard peritoneal dialysis (SPD). *Adv Perit Dial* 1988;4:194–197.

138. Antonsen S, Pedersen FB, Wang P, and the Danish Study Group on Peritonitis in Dialysis (DASPID). Leukocytes in peritoneal dialysis effluents. *Perit Dial Int* 1991;11:43–47.

139. Struijk DG, Ketel RJ, Krediet RT, et al. Viral peritonitis in a continuous ambulatory peritoneal dialysis patient. *Nephron* 1986;44:384.

140. Eisele G, Adewunni C, Bailie GR, et al. Surreptitious use of antimicrobial agents by CAPD patients. *Perit Dial Int* 1993;13:313–315.

141. Szeto CC, Wong TY, Chow KM, et al. The clinical course of culture-negative peritonitis complicating peritoneal dialysis. *Am J Kidney Dis* 2003;42:567–574.

142. Luce E, Nakagawa D, Lovell J, et al. Improvement in the bacteriologic diagnosis of peritonitis with the use of blood culture media. *ASAIO Trans* 1982;28:259–262.

143. Blondeau JM, Pylypchuk GB, Kappel JE, et al. Comparison of bedside- and laboratory-inoculated Bactec high- and low-volume resin bottles for the recovery of microorganisms causing peritonitis in CAPD patients. *Diagn Microbiol Infect Dis* 1998;31:281–287.

144. Lye WC, Wong PL, Leong SO, et al. Isolation of organisms in CAPD peritonitis: a comparison of two techniques. *Adv Perit Dial* 1994;10:166–168.

145. Sewell DL, Golper TA, Hulman PB, et al. Comparison of large volume culture to other methods for isolation of microorganisms from dialysate. *Perit Dial Int* 1990;10:49–52.

146. Morduchowicz G, van Dyk DJ, Wittenberg C, et al. Bacteremia complicating peritonitis in peritoneal dialysis patients. *Am J Nephrol* 1993;13:278–280.

147. Eisenberg ES, Leviton I, Soeiro R. Fungal peritonitis in patients receiving peritoneal dialysis: experience with 11 patients and review of the literature. *Rev Infect Dis* 1986;8:309–320.

148. Gokal R, Ramos JM, Ward MK, et al. "Eosinophilic" peritonitis in continuous ambulatory peritoneal dialysis (CAPD). *Clin Nephrol* 1981;15:328–330.

149. Piraino BM, Silver MR, Dominguez JH, et al. Peritoneal eosinophils during intermittent peritoneal dialysis. *Am J Nephrol* 1984;4:152–157.

150. Chan MK, Chow L, Lam SS, et al. Peritoneal eosinophilia in patients on continuous ambulatory peritoneal dialysis: a prospective study. *Am J Kidney Dis* 1988;11:180–183.

151. Perez Fontan M, Rodriguez-Carmona A, Galed I, et al. Incidence and significance of peritoneal eosinophilia during peritoneal dialysis-related peritonitis. *Perit Dial Int* 2003;23:460–464.

152. Nankivell BJ, Pacey D, Gordon DL. Peritoneal eosinophilia associated with *Paecilomyces variotii* infection in continuous ambulatory peritoneal dialysis. *Am J Kidney Dis* 1991;18:603–605.

153. Agarwal S, Goodman NL, Malluche HH. Peritonitis due to *Exophiala jeanselmei* in a patient undergoing continuous ambulatory peritoneal dialysis. *Am J Kidney Dis* 1992;21:673–675.

154. Ampel NM, White JD, Varanasi UR, et al. Coccidioidal peritonitis associated with continuous ambulatory peritoneal dialysis. *Am J Kidney Dis* 1988;11:512–514.

155. Lui SL, Lo CY, Choy BY, et al. Optimal treatment and long-term outcome of tuberculous peritonitis complicating continuous ambulatory peritoneal dialysis. *Am J Kidney Dis* 1996;28:747–751.

156. Lye WC. Rapid diagnosis of *Mycobacterium tuberculosis* peritonitis in two continuous ambulatory peritoneal dialysis patients, using DNA amplification by polymerase chain reaction. *Adv Perit Dial* 2002;18:154–157.

157. Abraham G, Mathews M, Sekar L, et al. Tuberculous peritonitis in a cohort of continuous ambulatory peritoneal dialysis patients. *Perit Dial Int* 2001;21(suppl 3):S202–S204.

158. Dunmire RB, Breyer JA. Nontuberculous mcobacterial peritonitis curing continuous ambulatory peritoneal dialysis: case report and review of diagnostic and therapeutic strategies. *Am J Kidney Dis* 1991;18:126–130.

159. Burkart J, Haigler S, Caruana R, et al. Usefulness of peritoneal fluid amyalse levels in the differential of peritonitis in peritoneal dialysis patients. *J Am Soc Nephrol* 1991;1:1186–1190.

160. Charney DI, Gouge SF. Chemical peritonitis secondary to intraperitoneal vancomycin. *Am J Kidney Dis* 1991;17:76–79.

161. Piraino B, Bernardini J, Johnston J, et al. Chemical peritonitis due to intraperitoneal vancomycin (Vancoled). *Perit Dial Bull* 1987;7:156–159.

162. Wong PN, Mak SK, Lee KF, et al. A prospective study of vancomycin- (Vancoled-) induced chemical peritonitis in CAPD patients. *Perit Dial Int* 1997;17:202–204.

163. Coronel F, Martin-Rabadan P, Romero J. Chemical peritonitis after intraperitoneal administration of amphotericin B in a fungal infection of the catheter subcutaneous tunnel. *Perit Dial Int* 1993;13:161–162.

164. MacGinley R, Cooney K, Alexander G, et al. Relapsing culture-negative peritonitis in peritoneal dialysis patients exposed to icodextran solution. *Am J Kidney Dis* 2002;40:1030–1035.

165. Elwell RJ, Bailie GR, Manley HJ. Correlation of intraperitoneal antibiotic pharmacokinetics and peritoneal membrane transport characteristics. *Perit Dial Int* 2000;20:694–698.

166. Manley HJ, Bailie GR. Treatment of peritonitis in APD: pharmacokinetic principles. *Semin Dial* 2002;15:418–421.

167. Bennett-Jones D, Wass V, Mawson P, et al. A comparison of intraperitoneal and intravenous/oral antibiotics in CAPD peritonitis. *Perit Dial Bull* 1987;7:31–33.

168. Bouza P, Falcon TG, Fontan MP, et al. Treatment of CAPD-related peritonitis with ciprofloxacin: results after seven years. *Adv Perit Dial* 1996;12:185–188.

169. Waite NM, Johnson MD, Webster NR, et al. Poor response to oral ciprofloxacin in the treatment of peritonitis in pa-

tients on intermittent peritoneal dialysis. *Perit Dial Int* 1993;13:50–54.

170. Cheng IKP, Chan CY, Wong WT, et al. A randomized prospective comparison of oral versus intraperitoneal ciprofloxacin as the primary treatment of peritonitis complicating continuous ambulatory peritoneal dialysis. *Perit Dial Int* 1993;13(suppl 2):S351–S354.

171. Cheng IKP, Fang GY, Chau PY, et al. A randomized prospective comparison of oral levofloxacin plus intraperitoneal (IP) vancomycin and IP netromycin plus vancomycin as primary treatment of peritonitis complicating CAPD. *Perit Dial Int* 1998;18:371–375.

172. Van Biesen W, Vanholder R, Vogelaers D, et al. The need for a center-tailored treatment protocol for peritonitis. *Perit Dial Int* 1998;18:274–281.

173. Keane WF, Everett ED, Fine RN, et al. CAPD related peritonitis management and antibiotic therapy recommendations. *Perit Dial Bull* 1987;7:55–68

174. Keane WF, Everett ED, Fine RN, et al. Continuous ambulatory peritoneal dialysis (CAPD) treatment recommendations: 1989 update. *Perit Dial Int* 1989;9:247–256.

175. Keane WF, Everett ED, Golper TA, et al. Peritoneal dialysis-related peritonitis treatment recommendations: 1993 update. *Perit Dial Int* 1993;13:14–28.

176. Keane WF, Alexander SR, Bailie GR, et al. Peritoneal dialysis-related peritonitis treatment recommendations: 1996 update. *Perit Dial Int* 1996;16:557–573.

177. Lai MN, Kao MT, Chen CC, et al. Intraperitoneal once-daily dose of cefazolin and gentamicin for treating CAPD peritonitis. *Perit Dial Int* 1997;17:87–89.

178. Goldberg L, Clemenger M, Azadian B, Brown EA. Initial treatment of peritoneal dialysis peritonitis without vancomycin with a once-daily cefazolin-based regimen. *Am J Kidney Dis* 2001;37:49–55.

179. Gucek A, Bren AF, Hergouth V, et al. Cefazolin and netilmycin versus vancomycin and ceftazidime in the treatment of CAPD peritonitis. *Adv Perit Dial* 1997;13:218–220.

180. Fielding RE, Clemenger M, Goldberg L, et al. Treatment and outcome of peritonitis in automated peritoneal dialysis, using a once-daily cefazolin–based regimen. *Perit Dial Int* 2002;22:345–349.

181. Gucek A, Bren AF, Lindic J, et al. Is monotherapy with cefazolin or ofloxacin an adequate treatment for peritonitis in CAPD patients? *Adv Perit Dial* 1994;10:144–146.

182. Flanigan MJ, Lim VS. Initial treatment of dialysis associated peritonitis: a controlled trial of vancomycin versus cefazolin. *Perit Dial Int* 1991;11:31–37.

183. Khairullah Q, Provenzano R, Tayeb J, et al. Comparison of vancomycin versus cefazolin as initial therapy for peritonitis in peritoneal dialysis patients. *Perit Dial Int* 2002;22:339–344.

184. Vas S, Bargman J, Oreopoulos DG. Treatment of PD patients of peritonitis caused by gram-positive organisms with single daily dose of antibiotics. *Perit Dial Int* 1997;17:91–94.

185. Brier ME, Aronoff GR. Initial intraperitoneal therapy for CAPD peritonitis: The Network 9 peritonitis study *Adv Perit Dial* 1994;10:141–143.

186. Agraharkar M, Klevjer-Anderson P, Rubinstien E, Galen M. Use of cefazolin for peritonitis treatment in peritoneal dialysis patients. *Am J Nephrol* 1999;19:555–558.

187. Manley HJ, Bailie GR, Frye RF, McGoldrick MD. Intravenous vancomycin pharmacokinetics in automated peritoneal dialysis patients. *Perit Dial Int* 2001;21:378–385.

188. Mulhern JG, Braden GL, O'Shea MH, et al. Trough serum vancomycin levels predict the relapse of gram-positive peritonitis in peritoneal dialysis patients. *Am J Kidney Dis* 1995;25:611–615.

189. Dasgupta MK, Ulan RA, Bettcher KB, et al. Effect of exit site infection and peritonitis on the distribution of biofilm-encased adherent bacterial microcolonies and Tenckhoff catheters in patients undergoing continuous ambulatory peritoneal dialysis. *Adv CAPD* 1986:6:102–109.

190. Finkelstein ES, Jekel J, Troidle L, et al. Patterns of infection in patients maintained on long-term peritoneal dialysis therapy with multiple episodes of peritonitis. *Am J Kidney Dis* 2002;39:1278–1286.

191. Schaefer F, Klaus G, Muller-Wiefel DE, et al. Intermittent versus continuous intraperitoneal glycopeptide/ceftazidime treatment in children with peritoenal dialysis-associated peritonitis. *J Am Soc Nephrol* 1999;10:136–145.

192. Szeto CC, Chow KM, Wong TYH, et al. Feasibility of resuming peritoneal dialysis after severe peritonitis and Tenkhoff catheter removal. *J Am Soc Nephrol* 2002;13:1040–1045.

193. Swartz RD, Messana JM. Simultaneous catheter removal and replacement in peritoneal dialysis infections: update and current recommendations. *Adv Perit Dial* 1999;15:205–208.

194. Lye WC, Leong SO, Lee EJC. Methicillin-resistant *Staphylococcus aureus* nasal carriage and infections in CAPD. *Kidney Int* 1993;43:1357–1362.

195. Suh H, Wadhwa NK, Cabralda T, et al. Endogenous peritonitis and related outcome in peritoneal dialysis patients. *Adv Perit Dial* 1996;12:192–195.

196. Troidle LK, Kliger AS, Gorban-Brennan N, et al. Nine episodes of CPD-associated peritonitis with vancomycin resistant enterococci. *Kidney Int* 1996;50:1368–1372.

197. Brady JP, Snyder JW, Harsbargen JA. Vancomycin-resistant *Enterococcus* in end-stage renal disease. *Am J Kidney Dis* 1998;32:415–418.

198. Ng R, Zabetakis PM, Callahan C, et al. Vancomycin-resistant *Enterococcus* infection is a rare complication in patients receiving PD on an outpatient basis. *Perit Dial Int* 1999;19:25–28.

199. Shemin D, Maaz D, Pierre DS, et al. Effect of aminoglycoside use on residual renal function in peritoneal dialysis patients. *Am J Kidney Dis* 1999;34:14–20.

200. Lee J, Innes CP, Petyo CM. Vertigo in CAPD patients treated with intraperitoneal gentamicin. *Perit Dial Int* 1989;9: No 97.

201. Gendeh BS, Said H, Gibb AG, et al. Gentamicin ototoxicity in continuous ambulatory peritoneal dialysis. *J Laryngol Otol* 1993;107:681–685.

202. Troidle L, Gorban-Brennan N, Kliger A, et al. Differing outcomes of gram-positive and gram-negative peritonitis. *Am J Kidney Dis* 1998;32:623–628.

203. Miller GV, Bhandari S, Brownjohn AM, et al. "Surgical" peritonitis in the CAPD patient. *Ann R Coll Surg Engl* 1998;80;36–39.

204. Manley HJ, Bailie GR, Frye R, et al. Pharmacokinetics of intermittent intravenous cefazolin and tobramycin in patients treated with automated peritoneal dialysis. *J Am Soc Nephrol* 2000;11:1310–1316.

205. Low CL, Bailie GR, Evans A, et al. Pharmacokinetics of once-daily IP gentamicin in CAPD patients. *Perit Dial Int* 1996;16:379–384.

206. Tosukhowong T, Eiam-Ong S, Thamutok K, et al. Pharmacokinetics of intraperitoneal cefazolin and gentamicin in empiric therapy of peritonitis in continuous ambulatory peritoneal dialysis patients. *Perit Dial Int* 2001;21:587–594.

207. Lye WC, Lee EJC, Leong SO, et al. Clinical characteristics and outcome of *Acinetobacter* infections in CAPD patients. *Perit Dial Int* 1994;14:174–177.

208. Szeto CC, Li PKT, Leung CB, et al. *Xanthomonas maltophilia* peritonitis in uremic patients receiving continuous ambulatory peritoneal dialysis. *Am J Kidney Dis* 1997;29: 91–95.

209. Valdes-Sotomayor J, Cirugeda A, Bajo M, et al Increased severity of *Escherichia coli* peritonitis in peritoneal dialysis patients independent of changes in vitro antimicrobial susceptibility testing. *Perit Dial Int* 2003;23:450–455.

210. Shea S, Bachelor T, Cooper M, et al. Disposition and bioavailability of ceftazidime after intraperitoneal administration in paitents receiving continuous ambulatory peritoneal dialysis. *J Am Soc Nephrol* 1995;7:2399–2402.

211. Graibe DW, Bailie GR, Eisele G, Frye RF. Pharmacokinetics of intermittent intraperitoneal ceftazidime. *Am J Kidney Dis* 1999;33:111–117.

212. Wong KM, Chan YH, Cheung CY, et al. Cefepime versus vancomycin plus netilmicin therapy for continuous ambulatory peritoneal dialysis-associated peritonitis. *Am J Kidney Dis* 2001;38:127–131.

213. Li PK, Ip M, Kaw MC, et al. Use of intraperitoneal cefepime as monotherapy in treatment of CAPD peritonitis *Perit Dial Int* 2000;20:232–241.

214. Szeto CC, Chow KM, Leung CB. Clinical course of peritonitis due to *Pseudomonas* species complicating peritoneal dialysis: a review of 104 cases. *Kidney Int* 2001;59: 2309–2315.

215. Nordbring F. *Pseudomonas*: clinical problems related to virulence factors and development of resistance. *Arch Intern Med* 1982;142:2010–2011.

216. Dressler R, Peters AT, Lynn RI. Pseudomonal and candidal peritonitis as a complication of continuous ambulatory peritoneal dialysis in human immunodeficiency virus-infected patients. *Am J Med* 1989;86:787–790.

217. Leung ACT, Orange G, Henderson IS, et al. Successful use of combined intraperitoneal azlocillin and aminoglycoside in the treatment of dialysis associated *Pseudomonas* peritonitis. *Perit Dial Bull* 1984;4:98–101.

218. Nguyen V, Swartz RD, Reynolds J, et al. Successful treatment of *Pseudomonas* peritonitis during continuous ambulatory peritoneal dialysis. *Am J Nephrol* 1987;7:38–43.

219. Pasadakis P, Thodis E, Eftimimiadou A, et al. Treatment and prevention of relapses of CAPD *Pseudomonas* peritonitis. *Adv Perit Dial* 1993;9:206–210.

220. Holley JL, Bernardini J, Piraino B. Polymicrobial peritonitis in patients on continuous peritoneal dialysis. *Am J Kidney Dis* 1992;19:162–166.

221. Kim GC, Korbet SM. Polymicrobial peritonitis in continuous ambulatory peritoneal dialysis patients. *Am J Kidney Dis* 2000;36:1000–1008.

222. Szeto CC, Chow KM, Wong TYH, et al. Conservative management of polymicrobial peritonitis complicating peritoneal dialysis: a series of 140 consecutive cases. *Am J Med* 2002;113:728–733.

223. Wu G. A review of peritonitis episodes that caused interruption of CAPD. *Perit Dial Bull* 1983;3(suppl 3):S11–S13.

224. Rubin J, Oreopoulos DG, Lio TT, et al. Management of peritonitis and bowel perforation during chronic peritoneal dialysis. *Nephron* 1976;16:220–225.

225. Wang AY, Yu AW, Li PK, et al. Factors predicting outcome of fungal peritonitis in peritoneal dialysis: analysis of a 9-year experience of fungal peritonitis in a single center. *Am J Kidney Dis* 2000;36:1183–1192.

226. TULIP. The rate, risk factors and outcome of fungal peritonitis in CAPD patients: experience in Turkey. *Perit Dial Int* 2000;20:338–341.

227. Vargemezis V, Papadopoulou ZL, Liamos H, et al. Management of fungal peritonitis during continuous ambulatory peritoneal dialysis (CAPD). *Perit Dial Bull* 1986;6:17–20.

228. Holdsworth SR, Atkins RC, Scott DF, et al. Management of *Candida* peritonitis by prolonged peritoneal lavage containing 5-fluorocytosine. *Clin Nephrol* 1975;4:157–159.

229. Bibashi E, Memmos D, Kokolina E, et al. Fungal peritonitis complicating peritoneal dialysis during as 11 year period: report of 46 cases. *Clin Infect Dis* 2003:36:927–931.

230. Goldie SJ, Kiernan-Troidle L, Torres C, et al. Fungal peritonitis in a large chronic peritoneal dialysis population: a report of 55 episodes. *Am J Kidney Dis* 1996;28:86–91.

231. Johnson RJ, Ramsey PG, Gallagher N, et al. Fungal peritonitis in patients on peritoneal dialysis: incidence, clinical features and prognosis. *Am J Nephrol* 1985;5:169–175.

232. Michel C, Courdavault L, Al Khayat R, et al. Fungal peritonitis in patients on peritoneal dialysis. *Am J Nephrol* 1994;14:113–120.

233. Montane BS, Mazza I, Abitbol C, et al. Fungal peritonitis in pediatric patients. *Adv Perit Dial* 1998;14:251–254.

234. Rubin J, Kirchner K, Walsh D, et al. Fungal peritonitis during continuous ambulatory peritoneal dialysis: a report of 17 cases. *Am J Kidney Dis* 1987;10:361–368.

235. Bordes A, Campos-Herrero MI, Fernandez A, et al. Predisposing and prognostic factors of fungal peritonitis in peritoneal dialysis. *Perit Dial Int* 1995;15:275–276.

236. Kleinpeter MA, Butt AA. Non–*Candida albicans* fungal peritonitis in continuous ambulatory peritoneal dialysis patients. *Adv Perit Dial* 2001;17:176–179.

237. Chay BY, Wong SSY, Chan TM, Lai KN. *Pichia ohmeri* peritonitis in a patient on CAPD: response to treatment with amphotericin. *Perit Dial Int* 2000;20:91–94.

238. Chan TM, Chan CY, Cheng SW, et al. Treatment of fungal peritonitis complicating continuous ambulatory peritoneal dialysis with oral fluconazole: a series of 21 patients. *Nephrol Dial Transplant* 1994;9:539–542.

239. Hoch BS, Namboodiri NK, Banayat G, et al. The use of flu-conazole in the management of *Candida* peritonitis in patients on peritoneal dialysis. *Perit Dial Int* 1993;13(suppl 2):S357–S359.

240. Montengro J, Aguirre R, Gonzalez O, et al. Fluconazole treatment of *Candida* peritonitis with delayed removal of the peritoneal dialysis catheter. *Clin Nephrol* 1995;44:60–63.

241. Fabris A, Pellanda MV, Gardin C, et al. Pharmacokinetics of antifungal agents. *Perit Dial Int* 1993;13(suppl 2): S380–S382.

242. Debruyne D, Ryckelynck JP Fluconazole serum, urine, and dialysate levels in CAPD patients. *Perit Dial Int* 1992;12: 328–329.

243. Hoch BS, Namboodiri NK, Banayat G, et al. The use of fluconazole in the management of *Candida* peritonitis in patients on peritoneal dialysis. *Perit Dial Int* 1993;13 (suppl 2):S357–S359.

244. Rota S, Marchesi D, Farina C, de Bievre C. *Trichoderma pseudokoningii* peritonitis in automated peritoneal dialysis patient successfully treated by early catheter removal. *Perit Dial Int* 2000;20:91–92.

245. Smith JW, Arnold WC. Cryptococcal peritonitis in patients on peritoneal dialysis. *Am J Kidney Dis* 1988;11:430–433.

246. Polo JR, Luno J, Menarguez C, et al. Peritoneal mucormycosis in a patient receiving continuous ambulatory peritoneal dialysis. *Am J Kidney Dis* 1989;13:237–239.

247. Prewitt K, Lockard J, Rodgers D, et al. Successful treatment of *Aspergillus* peritonitis complicating peritoneal dialysis. *Am J Kidney Dis* 1989;13:501–503.

248. Vogelgesang SA, Lockard JW, Quinn MJ, et al. *Alternaria* peritonitis in a patient undergoing continuous ambulatory peritoneal dialysis. *Perit Dial Int* 1990;10:313.

249. McNeely DJ, Vas SI, Dombros N, et al. *Fusarium* peritonitis: an uncommon complication of continuous ambulatory peritoneal dialysis. *Perit Dial Bull* 1981;1:946.

250. Brackett RW, Shenouda AN, Hawkins SS, et al. *Curvularia* infection complicating peritoneal dialysis. *South Med J* 1988;81:943–944.

251. Kaplan RA, Alon U, Hellerstein S, et al. Unusual causes of peritonitis in three children receiving peritoneal dialysis. *Perit Dial Int* 1993;13:60–63.

252. Lye WC. Peritonitis due to *Wangiella dermatitidis* in a patient on CAPD. *Perit Dial Int* 1993;13:319–320.

253. DeVault GA, Brown ST, King JS. Tenckhoff catheter obstruction resulting from invasion by *Curvularia lunata* in the absence of peritonitis. *Am J Kidney Dis* 1985;6:165–167.

254. Buchanan WE, Quinn MJ, Hasbargen JA. Peritoneal catheter colonization with *Alternaria*: successful treatment with catheter preservation. *Perit Dial Int* 1994;14:91–92.

255. Wegmann F, Heilesen AM, Horn T. Tenckhoff catheter penetrated by *Aspergillus fumigatus*: a case report. *Perit Dial Int* 1988;8:281–283.

256. Mansoor GA, Ornt DB. Cryptococcal peritonitis in peritoneal dialysis patients: a case report. *Clin Nephrol* 1994;41: 230–232.

257. Cheng IKP, Chan PCK, Chan MK. Tuberculous peritonitis complicating long-term peritoneal dialysis. *Am J Nephrol* 1989;9:155–161.

258. Hussein MM, Mooij JM, Roujouleh H. Tuberculosis and chronic renal disease. *Semin Dial* 2003;16:38–44.

259. Lui SL, Tang S, Li FK. Tuberculous infection in Chinese patients undergoing continuous ambulatory peritoneal dialysis. *Am J Kidney Dis* 2001;38:1055–1060.

260. Mallat SG, Brensilver JM. Tuberculous peritonitis in a CAPD patient cured without catheter removal: case report, reviw of the literature and guidelines for treatment and diagnosis. *Am J Kidney Dis* 1989;13:154–157.

261. White R, Abreo K, Flanagan R, et al. Nontuberculous mycobacterial infections in continuous ambulatory peritoneal dialysis patients. *Am J Kidney Dis* 1993;22:581–587.

262. Bunke M, Brier M, Golper TA. Culture-negative CAPD peritonitis: the Network 9 Study. *Adv Perit Dial* 1994;10: 174–178.

263. Smith JL, Flanigan MJ. Peritoneal dialysis catheter sepsis: a medical and surgical dilemma. *Am J Surg* 1987;154: 602–607.

264. Boroujerdi-Rad H, Juergensen P, Mansourian V, et al. Abdominal abscesses complicating peritonitis in continuous ambulatory peritoneal dialysis patients. *Am J Kidney Dis* 1994;23:717–722.

265. Krishnan M, Thodis E, Ikonomopoulos D, et al. Predictors of outcome following bacterial peritonitis in peritoneal dialysis. *Perit Dial Int* 2002;22:573–581.

266. Schroder CH, Severijnen RSVM, de Jong MCW, et al. Chronic tunnel infections in children: removal and replacement of the continuous ambulatory peritoneal dialysis catheter in a single operation. *Perit Dial Int* 1993;13: 198–200.

267. Majkowski NL, Mendley SR. Simultaneous removal and replacement of infected peritoneal dialysis catheters. *Am J Kidney Dis* 1997;29:706–711.

268. Cancarini GC, Manili L, Brunori G, et al. Simultaneous catheter replacement-removal during infectious complications in peritoneal dialysis. *Adv Perit Dial* 1994;10: 210–213.

269. Fredensborg BB, Meyer HW, Joffe P, et al. Reinsertion of PD catheters during PD-related infections performed either simultaneously or after an intervening period. *Perit Dial Int* 1995;15:374–378.

270. Goldraich I, Mariano M, Rosito N, et al. One-step peritoneal catheter replacement in children. *Adv Perit Dial* 1993;9: 325–358.

271. Posthuma N, Borgstein PJ, Eijsbouts Q, et al. Simultaneous peritoneal dialysis catheter insertion and removal in catheter-related infections without interruption of peritoneal dialysis. *Nephrol Dial Transplant* 1998;13:700–703.

272. Dryden MS, Ludlam HA, Wing AJ, et al. Active intervention dramatically reduces CAPD-associated infection. *Adv Perit Dial* 1991;7:125–128.

273. Joh J, Padmanabhan K, Bastani B. *Pastuerella multocida* peritonitis following cat bite of peritoneal dialysis tubing. With a brief review of the literature. *Am J Nephrol* 1998;18:258–259.

274. Mackay K, Brown L, Hudson K. *Pastuerella multocida* peritonitis in peritoneal dialysis patients: beware of the cat. *Perit Dial Int* 1997;17:608–610.

275. Miller TE, Findon G. Touch contamination of connection devices in peritoneal dialysis–a quantitative microbiologic analysis. *Perit Dial Int* 1997;17:560–567.

276. Dabbagh S, Fassinger N, Clement K, et al. The effect of aggressive nutrition on infection rates in patients maintained on peritoneal dialysis. *Adv Perit Dial* 1991;7:161–164.

277. Low DE, Vas SI, Oreopoulos DG, et al. Prophylactic cephalexin ineffective in chronic ambulatory peritoneal dialysis. *Lancet* 1980;2(8197):753–754.

278. Churchill DN, Taylor DW, Vas SI, et al. Peritonitis in continuous ambulatory peritoneal dialysis (CAPD) patients: a randomized clinical trial of cotrimoxazole prophylaxis. *Perit Dial Int* 1988;8:125–128.

279. Rao SP, Oreopoulos DG. Unusual complication of polyurethane PD catheter. *Perit Dial Int* 1997;17:410–412.

280. Perez-Fontan M, Rosales M, Rodriguez-Carmona A, et al. Mupirocin resistance after long-term use for *Staphylococcus aureus* colonization in patients undergoing chronic peritoneal dialysis. *Am J Kidney Dis* 2002;39:337–341.

281. Annigeri R, Conly J, Vas SI, et al. Emergence of mupirocin-resistent *Staphylococcus aureus* in chronic peritoneal dialysis patients using mupirocin prophylaxis to prevent exit-site infection. *Perit Dial Int* 2001;21:554–559.

282. Wadhwa NK, Suh H, Cabralda T. Antifungal prophylaxis for secondary fungal peritonitis in peritoneal dialysis patients. *Adv Perit Dial* 1996;12:189–191.

283. Zaruba K, Peters J, Jungbluth H. Successful prophylaxis for fungal peritonitis in patients on continuous ambulatory peritoneal dialysis: Six years' experience *Am J Kidney Dis* 1991;17:43–46.

284. Robitaille P, Merouani A, Clermont MJ, et al. Successful antifungal prophylaxis in chronic peritoneal dialysis: a pediatric experience. *Perit Dial Int* 1995;15:77–79.

285. Lo WK, Chen CY, Cheng SW, et al. A prospective randomized control study nystatin prophylaxis for *Candida* complicating continuous ambulatory peritoneal dialysis. *Am J Kidney Dis* 1996;28:549–552.

286. Williams PF, Moncrieff N, Marriott J. No benefit in using nystatin prophylaxis against fungal peritonitis in peritoneal dialysis patients. *Perit Dial Int* 2000;20:349–353.

287. Wang Q, Piraino B, Bernardini J, et al. Comparison of infectious complications between incident hemodialysis and peritoneal dialysis patients: three years experience from a single center. *J Am Soc Nephrol* 2002;13:223A–224A.

Infection and Host Defense in Dialysis Patients

Raymond Vanholder
Annemiere Dhondt

Infection remains among the major causes of morbidity and hospitalization and is the second most common cause of death, after cardiovascular disease, in hemodialysis patients. In recent registries, infectious disease is found to be responsible for 15 to 20 percent of deaths,[1,2] with an annual rate of infection-related hospitalization around 35 percent in the dialysis population.[2] The present mortality rate is, however, lower compared with less recent studies, reporting between 30 and 40 percent.[3] This discrepancy might be attributed to changes in therapeutic approaches to dialysis but also to differences over time in patient characteristics, such as an increase in age, resulting—in the most recent studies—in a relative increase in cardiovascular mortality and a proportional decrease of fatal infection. Bacteria account for most clinical infections, but viral hepatitis also causes substantial problems in hemodialysis patients.

Various predisposing factors for infection are related to the dialysis technique itself, such as the disruption of the protective skin barrier, affinity of bacteria for foreign materials, bioincompatibility of dialysis equipment, and nosocomial transmission of infectious agents. Other pathogenetic factors are the retention of uremic solutes, deficiency and/or resistance to vitamin D, malnutrition, iron overload, bacterial colonization, advanced age, comorbid conditions, and/or the use of immunosuppressive drugs (Table 18–1).

Defense against infection involves a wide cascade of finely tuned mechanisms, including (1) the functional involvement of various circulating (lymphocytes, monocytes, granulocytes) and sessile immune-competent cells (macrophages); (2) the release of humoral substances (cytokines, immunoglobulins, platelet activating factor), eventually resulting in an upgrading of immunocompetence; and

TABLE 18–1. PREDISPOSING FACTORS FOR INFECTION IN PATIENTS ON CHRONIC HEMODIALYSIS

Related to the dialysis technique
 Disruption of the protective skin barrier
 Affinity of bacteria for foreign materials
 Bioincompatibility of dialysis equipment
 Nosocomial transmission of infective agents
Related to renal failure
 Retention of uremic solutes
 Hyperparathyroidism
 Deficiency and/or resistance to vitamin D
Malnutrition
Iron overload
Bacterial colonization
Advanced age
Comorbid conditions
 Diabetes mellitus
 Nephrotic syndrome
 Paraproteinemia
 Liver cirrhosis
 HIV infection
 Urologic anomalies
 Malignancies
Immunosuppressive drugs
 Posttransplantation
 Autoimmune pathology
 Glomerulopathies
Causes of renal failure
 Reflux nephropathy
 Polycystic kidney disease
 Nephrolithiasis

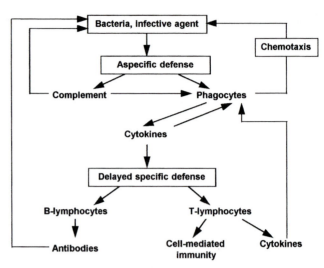

Figure 18–1. Flowchart of events implicated in the immune response against infection.

(3) the attraction of cells toward zones of infection (chemotaxis) (Fig. 18–1). All of these elements interact and eventually lead to the ingestion and destruction of infectious agents by phagocytic cells. Recent evidence suggests that the hemodialysis patient is affected by a baseline activation of host defense mechanisms resulting in inflammation, which contrasts with and mirrors the blunted response of these processes upon activation. The uremic state should hence be considered as an ambivalent condition, where baseline inflammation can lead to malnutrition and atherosclerosis (described as the MIA syndrome),[4] together with a blunted response upon stimulation, possibly leading to an increased propensity for infection. These infections, in return, lead to more inflammation.

In this chapter, we first review the infectious complications related to dialysis and then consider the pathophysiologic mechanisms that are at their origin.

CHARACTERISTICS OF INFECTIOUS DISEASE IN UREMIC AND DIALYSIS PATIENTS

Bacteremia and Sepsis

In recent studies, bloodstream infections are described in western hemodialysis centers with rates between 0.63 and 1.8 per 100 patient-months,[5–9] and a 100- to 300-fold higher annual mortality secondary to sepsis, compared to the general population.[10]

Half of the bacteremic episodes are attributed to infection stemming from the vascular access,[5,9] 22.2 percent from the urinary tract, 6.3 percent from soft tissue, and 4.8 percent from the biliary tract.[5] For the remaining 15.9 percent, no source is identified.[5] *Staphylococcus aureus* and coagulase-negative *Staphylococcus* are responsible for 60 to 70 percent of bloodstream infections.[5–7] In the gram-negative group, *Klebsiella*, *Enterobacter*, and *Escherichia coli* are the dominant infectious agents.[5,7]

Vascular Access–Related Infection

The majority of bacteremias in hemodialysis patients are vascular access–related, with nontunneled catheters being the principal culprit, followed by tunneled cuffed catheters and arteriovenous grafts, native arteriovenous fistulas being the least associated with infection.[11] As bacteria have a particular affinity for foreign materials, synthetic grafts and catheters predispose to infection. In recent publications (Table 18–2), the overall rate of access-related bacteremia is between 1.78 and 1.96 per 100 patient-months,[11–13] with a rate of approximately 0.25 for native fistulas[8,11,13] and 0.52 for grafts,[11–14] respectively. For tunneled cuffed catheters the bacteremia rate varies widely, between 3.3 and 16.5 per 100

TABLE 18–2. RATE OF VASCULAR ACCESS RELATED BACTEREMIA AND INFECTION PER 100 PATIENT-MONTHS

	Overall	Native AV Fistula	AV Graft	Cuffed, Tunneled Catheter	Noncuffed, Nontunneled Catheter
Bacteremia					
Tokars,[11] 2002	1.78	0.25	0.53	4.84	8.73
Stevenson,[13] 2002	1.96	0.26	0.52	7.19	13.8
Taylor,[8] 2002		0.26			
Jean,[15] 2002				3.3	
Marr,[16] 1997				11.7	
Saad,[17] 1999				16.5	
Kairaitis,[18] 1999					19.5
Infection					
Tokars,[11] 2002	3.2	0.56	1.36	8.42	11.98
Stevenson,[13] 2002	5.5	1.18	2.6	15.9	38.2
Saeed,[12] 2002	14.8			13.2	36.9
Minga,[14] 2001			0.68		

patient-months.[11–13,15–17] For noncuffed catheters, the highest described bacteremia rate per 100 patient-months is 19.5.[18]

Preventive measures with aseptic care of catheters are effective in reducing catheter-related infections.[19] In addition, catheter locks with aminoglycosides,[20] taurolidin citrate,[21] citrate, and gentamicin citrate[22] reduce the incidence of catheter infection. Citrate locks can, however, cause symptomatic hypocalcemia if too much of the locking solution escapes into the systemic circulation, whereas the long-term use of aminoglycoside locks can cause ototoxicity[20] and eventually antibiotic resistance.

As carrier status for *S. aureus* is an important risk factor for vascular access–related infection, application of mupirocin ointment at the insertion site of both tunneled cuffed[23] and nontunneled dialysis catheters[24] reduces the risk of catheter-related infection and bacteremia. In addition, Polysporin triple—an ointment composed of bacitracin, gramicidin, and polymyxin B—reduces the infection rate of cuffed tunneled dialysis catheters.[25]

Nasal application of mupirocin eradicates *Staphylococcus* from the nares,[26] resulting in fewer episodes of *S. aureus* infection.[26] The regular use of such ointments is, however, not without risk, as strains of *S. aureus* resistant to mupirocin have been described, especially in patients treated with peritoneal dialysis.[27] Furthermore, the recurrence rate of nasal carriage is considerable if application of the ointment is not sustained.[28] Development of resistance might be reduced by intermittent application.[29] The European Best Practice Guidelines (EBPG) recommend screening for *S. aureus* carrier status in all high-risk patients, such as those with a past history of *S. aureus* infection and those dialyzed with central venous catheters. Intervention to eradicate *S. aureus* nasal carriage should be considered in these high-risk carriers.[30]

Vaccination against *S. aureus* offers no more than partial immunity against bacteremia for approximately 40 weeks[31] and is considered only experimental.

The most important step in the prevention of vascular access–related infection remains the avoidance of dialysis catheters and of vascular grafts in favor of native arteriovenous fistulas.

Infective Endocarditis and Metastatic Infection

In hemodialysis patients endocarditis is a frequently encountered metastatic infection complicating bacteremia, particularly with *S. aureus*.[32] Bacterial seeding to heart valves or distant sites is documented in 16[33] to 44 percent[32] of all *S. aureus* bacteremias, resulting in high mortality.[32]

The mitral valve is most frequently involved in bacterial endocarditis in dialysis patients, followed by the aortic valve and the combined involvement of both.[34] Infective endocarditis is often superimposed upon preexisting valvular abnormalities, which are frequent in hemodialysis patients.[34] The causative organisms for infective endocarditis in dialysis patients are, in decreasing order of frequency, *S. aureus*, *Enterococcus*, *Streptococcus viridans*, coagulase-negative *Staphylococcus*, and other *streptococci*.[35] In a survey by Robinson et al., however, coagulase-negative staphylococci were the second most frequent cause of all infective endocarditis episodes after *S. aureus*.[36] Occasionally, endocarditis with *Corynebacterium* of group JK[37] or with *Flavobacterium odoratum*[38] has been described.

As *S. aureus* is the main culprit, prophylactic measures should aim at the reduction of vascular access–related infections. In addition, prophylactic antibiotic therapy prior to dental procedures is warranted. To reduce mortality from infective endocarditis in hemodialysis patients, it has been suggested to switch patients suffering from endocarditis to peritoneal dialysis.[39]

Besides endocarditis, other metastatic infections such as vertebral osteomyelitis,[32] epidural abscesses,[40] septic arthritis,[14] and multifocal infection[32] have been described in hemodialysis patients.

Bacteremia Related to Dialysis Equipment and Water

Outbreaks of mainly gram-negative bacterial bloodstream infections have been attributed to the use of contaminated dialysis water,[41] dialysis machines,[42] reprocessed dialyzers,[43] and/or intravenously administered medication.[44] Improvements in water treatment systems and in water quality, as recently propagated by the EBPG for hemodialysis, should result in the disappearance of this problem.[45]

Pneumonia

Compared to the general population, the pulmonary infectious mortality is 14- to 16-fold higher among patients on chronic dialysis.[46] In this group, invasive pneumococcal infection is often life-threatening; therefore preventive measures are warranted. It has been demonstrated that at least children and young adults with renal disease produce adequate antibody levels upon vaccination with the 23-valent pneumococcal vaccine.[47] These patients, however, showed a more rapid decline in titers 6 months after vaccination than did the general population. At present, pneumococcal vaccination is recommended in all high-risk patients, including those with renal failure; revaccination is advised provided that at least 5 years have elapsed since the first dose.[48] As antibodies decline faster in renal patients, earlier revaccination could be of benefit in this population. In addition, renal patients with an unknown vaccination status should be vaccinated.[49]

Experimental data on the efficacy of oral immunotherapy against respiratory infection have been published, but without convincing protection being demonstrated.[50]

Urinary Tract Infection

Urinary tract infections are facilitated in hemodialysis patients by oliguria or anuria. Pyocystitis, as observed in patients with urinary diversion procedures, is not infrequent in anuric patients. In addition, anatomic and functional anomalies of the urinary tract causing chronic renal failure—such as polycystic kidney disease, vesicourethral reflux, and neurogenic bladder—also contribute to the frequency and severity of such urinary tract infections.

Clostridial Colitis

Clostridium difficile colitis is described with a higher incidence in patients with chronic renal failure than in the general population[51] and is associated with a high mortality.[51] The liberal use of broad-spectrum antibiotics, especially cephalosporins, for prolonged periods may be responsible for this. In several reports, clusters are described, suggesting nosocomial transmission of *C. difficile*.[51]

Diverticulitis

Because the average age of the dialysis population is progressively increasing, diverticulitis has become a more common problem. In addition, a higher incidence of diverticulitis is found among patients with polycystic kidney disease.[52] Its insidious symptomatology is a major challenge in the renal patient, which may lead to delayed diagnosis and treatment and an adverse outcome.

Periodontitis and Gingivitis

Periodontal disease is at least to some extent present in all dialysis patients.[53] Inadequate dental care can be attributed to financial problems, fear of bleeding complications, or indifference on the part of the patient and nephrologist. Periodontal inflammation can, however, provide entry to organisms causing bacteremia; it can also lead to malnutrition. In addition, periodontal disease has been associated with elevated levels of C-reactive protein (CRP), an indicator of chronic inflammation in hemodialysis patients[54] and of coronary heart disease in the general population.[55]

Antimicrobial Resistance

The prevalence of microorganisms resistant to antimicrobials is high among hemodialysis patients due to the combination of patient-to-patient transmission and the low threshold for initiation of broad-spectrum antibiotics. Hemodialysis patients suspected of having bacteremia are commonly treated with broad-spectrum antibiotics with a prolonged half-life, such as the combination of a glycopeptide (vancomycin or teicoplanin) and ceftazidime, covering both staphylococci and gram-negative organisms. In that way, patient compliance with the intake of oral antibiotics is not an issue and no intravenous infusion is needed in those with already compromised vascular access sites. Unfortunately, this approach may increase the chances of inducing bacterial resistance.

The frequency with which resistant strains are isolated in dialysis patients is highly center- and country-dependent. Methicillin-resistant *S. aureus* (MRSA) is responsible for 1 to 40 percent of all staphylococcal isolates in dialysis patients.[56] Coagulase-negative staphylococci isolated in hemodialysis patients are in the majority of cases methicillin-resistant *S. epidermidis* (MRSE),[56] and even staphylococci with reduced sensitivity to vancomycin have been encountered in the renal unit.[57]

The occurrence of mupirocin-resistant staphylococci is associated with the regular use of mupirocin ointment by peritoneal dialysis patients.[27] Similarly, resistance must be of concern in hemodialysis patients when mupirocin is regularly used.

The reported prevalence of glycopeptide-resistant enterococci (GRE) in patients undergoing chronic hemodialysis varies between 0 to 28 percent.[56] The use of vancomycin is a significant cause of colonization with this organism.

Whereas there is not much debate that MRSA patients should be isolated, the best approach is less clear with regard to GRE. It seems reasonable, however, to separate GRE carriers from other patients as well if feasible.[58] With gram-negative bacteria, resistance to ceftazidime is a serious clinical problem. Recent hospitalization and the liberal use of ceftazidime are two of the responsible factors.

Tuberculosis

Patients with renal failure have a 6.9- to 52.5-fold increased risk of tuberculosis compared to the general population.[59–62] In dialysis centers in the western world, the incidence of the disease is increasing; this is attributed to the immigration of patients from countries where tuberculosis is endemic[63] and, to a lesser extent, to the growing population of HIV-positive patients in the renal unit.

The diagnosis of tuberculosis in dialysis patients is often difficult, as a substantial portion[64] of these patients are anergic, making their tuberculin tests less reliable. In addition, in hemodialysis patients, tuberculosis often presents as extrapulmonary disease, with lymph node, peritoneal, or joint involvement[65,66] accompanied by nonspecific symptoms that could well be attributed to the uremic syndrome per se. Therefore, in order to make a prompt diagnosis, a high level of awareness of the disease is warranted, especially with regard to high-risk patients.

During treatment with antituberculosis drugs, special attention should be paid to potential side effects, as a high incidence of neuropsychiatric, hepatic, and gastrointestinal side effects is noted in the dialysis population.[66]

The EBPG recommend a tuberculin skin test in all high-risk patients, such as those who are immunosuppressed and malnourished.[30] Tuberculosis should, however, not be excluded by a negative test. In the case of a positive test, antibiotic prophylaxis is recommended.[30] All patients with unexplained fever, weight loss, anorexia, hepatomegaly, pulmonary infiltrates, pleural effusion, ascites, or lymphadenopathy should be vigorously evaluated for an active focus of tuberculosis.[30] Preventive therapy should be considered if dialysis patients have been exposed to a patient with clinically active tuberculosis, even if the tuberculin test remains negative.[30]

Concern has recently arisen because of the increasingly frequent emergence of infections with atypical mycobacteria. Due to their multiresistant pattern, it is necessary to treat these with multiple, often toxic antibiotics, including aminoglycosides.

Fungi and Yeast

In parallel with the problems encountered in other immunosuppressed patients, outbreaks of *Aspergillus fumigatus* are described in renal patients,[67] often coincident with construction activities at hospitals, dialysis clinics, or the patient's home.

In an earlier decade, a multitude of mucormycosis infections in dialysis patients had been reported.[68] This is an opportunistic infection caused by fungi of the order Mucorales. In about one-third of these cases, the causative fungus was cultured and always proved to be of the genus *Rhizopus*. This organism manifests itself clinically as a rhinocerebral, pulmonary, gastrointestinal, cutaneous, or widely disseminated infection with a high mortality rate (86 percent). In more than 50 percent of cases, the diagnosis was discovered only postmortem. A major risk factor for the development of mucormycosis in dialysis patients is the treatment of aluminum overload with the chelator deferoxamine.[69]

Infections due to *Candida albicans* are less frequent in hemodialysis than in peritoneal dialysis and transplant patients and are usually related to the vascular access,[70] the presence of comorbid conditions, and/or invasive procedures.

Human Immunodeficiency Virus

HIV infection is becoming a more frequent condition among dialysis patients (1) because the prevalence of HIV is growing in the general population, which is the population at risk to develop renal failure; (2) more importantly, because HIV leads to renal disease, most frequently to collapsing focal glomerulosclerosis; and (3) because of patient-to-patient transmission. This last, however, has only occasionally been reported.[71] The prevalence of positive HIV testing in hemodialysis patients has varied widely between countries and centers, from 0 percent up to 39 percent in some urban centers in the United States during the late 1980s.[72] The majority of the affected patients are black.[73] The EBPG recommend screening for HIV infection in all patients who are starting hemodialysis or transferring from another unit, following informed consent.[30] Once such patients are on routine dialysis, further screening is not recommended.[30] The Centers for Disease Control and Prevention (CDC) do not recommend routine testing for HIV infection of dialysis patients who do not have risk factors for

HIV.[74] False-positive tests are more frequently encountered among renal patients than in the general population.[75]

The choice between hemodialysis and peritoneal dialysis for HIV-positive patients depends on several considerations. Hemodialysis centers without HIV-positive patients and with no isolation facilities may be reluctant to accept infected patients. The CDC, however, does not recommend isolation of HIV-positive patients.[74] With regard to vascular access, it has been reported that HIV-positive patients with synthetic grafts have higher rates of graft infection and failure than HIV-negative patients, whereas infection of endogenous arteriovenous fistulas[76] and of tunneled-cuffed catheters[77] is similar in both HIV-positive and HIV-negative patients.

Because hemodialysis stimulates the production of proinflammatory cytokines, which are known to activate HIV replication, the procedure might lead to an increase in viral load. Conflicting findings about this issue have been published. Fontana et al. observed a doubling of viral load after hemodialysis with dialyzers containing cellulose acetate membranes,[78] whereas Ahuja et al. described a small reduction in plasma HIV levels after dialysis with the same membranes.[79] This discrepancy might be explained by differences in antiretroviral therapeutic approaches between studied populations. The use of polysulfone membranes was associated with only minor changes in viral load.[78]

The prognosis of HIV-infected hemodialysis patients is poor but has improved over the past 15 years, with the cumulative 12-month survival increased from 49 to 74 percent for patients starting hemodialysis in 1991–1992 and 1999–2000, respectively.[80] This improvement in survival is most likely the result of newer antiretroviral treatment protocols. Hemodialysis patients should have full access to the highly active antiretroviral therapy (HAART) in appropriate doses.[81] No difference in mortality was found between HIV-positive patients treated with hemodialysis compared to those on peritoneal dialysis[82]; hence no evidence-based advice can be provided in the choice between these strategies. Health care workers should receive immediate antiviral therapy after needle-stick injury from an infected patient, although the transmission risk is considered to be low, around 0.3 percent.[83]

Hepatitis

Besides the fact that the transmission of hepatitis B between patients is facilitated by the hemodialysis strategy per se, dialysis patients display a high vulnerability to hepatitis B. After an often subclinical acute infection, they are, in contrast to the general population, more prone to become chronic carriers of the hepatitis B virus.[84] In addition, a large proportion of dialysis patients are nonresponders or low responders to vaccination, even after doubling the dose and/or increasing the frequency of hepatitis B vaccine ad-

ministration. These findings are among the most explicit manifestations of the impaired antigen-specific immune function in dialysis patients.

Hepatitis B and C and other causes of dialysis related hepatitis are addressed in Chap. 24.

Influenza

Influenza epidemics cause morbidity and mortality in patients who are older or have chronic illnesses, including dialysis patients. Although the response to influenza vaccine may be lower in dialysis patients, protective antibodies are produced.[85] It has been demonstrated that influenza vaccination in hemodialysis patients is associated with a decreased risk of hospitalization and mortality.[86]

Cytomegalovirus

Cytomegalovirus (CMV) is ubiquitous and subject to easy parenteral transmission. Although symptomatic infection with CMV in healthy adults is generally mild, the virus is known to produce severe symptoms in immunocompromised patients. Despite the prevalence of anti-CMV IgG in 67 percent and of IgM in 25 percent of dialysis patients [hemodialysis and continuous ambulatory peritoneal dialysis (CAPD)][87] and the recognition of a defective immune response in uremic patients, clinical manifestations of CMV infection are uncommon.[88] Frequently, therefore, these infections go unrecognized. The risk for CMV infection has been reduced somewhat since the availability of erythropoietin, with the concomitant decreased need for blood transfusions; nevertheless, many alternative transmission routes remain prevalent. CMV infection must still be considered when there are otherwise unexplained changes in serum transaminases or serious neurologic, respiratory, and/or gastrointestinal symptoms.

Recently, an association has been described between elevated anti-CMV IgG levels and arteriovenous fistula failure,[89] which parallels the association between CMV infection and atherosclerosis suggested in the general population.

Hepatitis Caused by Other Viruses

Several other viral infections (e.g., with Epstein-Barr virus and coxsackie B virus) can secondarily affect the liver and cause an acute hepatitis-like picture in dialysis patients. Herpes simplex virus, varicella zoster virus, and several other viruses that are usually benign in the general population can cause severe disseminated infection, including hepatic involvement, in dialysis patients, especially if they receive immunosuppressive treatment. Frequent reactivations without clinical symptoms have also been described.[90]

ALTERATIONS IN CELLULAR IMMUNE FUNCTION

Lymphocyte Function

Apart from the well-known lymphopenia, a host of disturbances are described in lymphocytes of chronic hemodialysis patients, such as changes in T-cell growth-factor activity, T-cell subset identification, metabolic responsiveness, lymphocyte immune response and/or proliferation, and E rosette–forming capacity. Thymic weight has been shown to decrease in uremic rats, whereas cellular defects point to a maturational impairment of thymic lymphocytes.[91] The proliferative response of peripheral blood mononuclear cells and purified T lymphocytes is inhibited in the presence of uremic serum and is associated with downregulation of IL-2 synthesis.[92] In parallel with this blunted proliferation, Stachowski et al. described a decreased density of TCR1/CD3 receptors on uremic helper-inducer (CD4) T lymphocytes, a diminished binding of cytokines to their receptors, and a decreased density of intercellular adhesion molecule 1 (ICAM-1).[93] In addition to inducing a decrease in the number of T-helper lymphocytes, chronic uremia also impairs the ability of hematopoietic stem cells to increase the erythroid burst-forming units (BFU-E).[94]

Lymphocytes isolated from dialysis patients show increased apoptosis; in addition, serum from dialysis patients promotes lymphocyte apoptosis.[95]

The most striking clinical manifestations of these lymphocyte abnormalities are the blunted response to vaccination against hepatitis B and the propensity for maintaining the carrier state after contact with the hepatitis B virus. As the scrutiny of defective mechanisms evolved, it became clear that most of the described defects could be attributed to disturbances in antigen-presenting cells (APC) and their interplay with T cells via interleukin-2 (IL-2), rather than to T-cell defects per se. Defective IL-2 production[96] and the retention of guanidine compounds[97] have been recognized as potential causative factors. Lymphocyte response to stimulation was disturbed in cultured cells from dialyzed patients.[98] Correction was possible after the addition of IL-2 but not of IL-1. In addition, low-dose IL-2 administered during hepatitis B vaccination stimulated the antibody response.[99] Impaired proliferation of peripheral blood leukocytes and a defect in T-cell activation were attributed to an accessory cell defect in the B7/CD28 pathway.[100] In vitro restoration of this B7/CD28 pathway by the addition of cell lines expressing B7 to uremic mononuclear cells restored leukocytic cellular function of the cells, resulting in stimulation of the B7 IIg and CD28.

Plasma concentration of soluble CD23 levels, a factor identified as a marker of B cell and monocyte activation and possibly involved in T-cell activation, is somewhat increased in nondialyzed uremics and increased to a greater extent in patients on hemodialysis.[101] Dialysis also induces the generation of platelet activating factor (PAF), another mediator of cell interaction.[102]

Conflicting data are found about the balance between T-helper 1 (Th1) and Th2 cells in dialysis patients, Th1 cells being involved in cellular and Th2 cells in humoral immunity. A dominance of Th1 cells was described by Ishuzuka et al. and Sester et al. and attributed to an overexpression of IL-12 by monocytes.[103,104] The dominance of Th2 cells was demonstrated by other groups and attributed to a higher susceptibility of Th1 cells to apoptosis.[105] In addition, Nitta et al. found a skewed Th-cell differentiation toward Th1 cells in hemodialysis patients and toward Th2 cells in peritoneal dialysis patients.[106]

Cytokine Production

Cytokine levels in hemodialysis patients are the result of at least three distinct influences: (1) the chronic impact of uremia, with stimulation of both proinflammatory [tumor necrosis factor alpha (TNF-α), IL-1β, IL-6] and anti-inflammatory (IL-10) cytokine production by monocytes; (2) the retention of cytokines due to decreased renal clearance; and (3) the effect of the hemodialysis procedure with both a stimulation possibly caused by bioincompatibility of the dialysis equipment and a decrease in cytokine concentration due to removal by dialysis, hemofiltration, and/or adsorption on the membrane. In addition, the functional effects of interleukins are often influenced by reactive changes in interleukin receptors and/or their soluble equivalents.

Luger et al. found elevated serum IL-1 levels predialysis compared with normals and postdialysis compared with predialysis.[107] These findings were confirmed by Haeffner-Cavaillon et al.; these authors found two systems of induction: (1) an acute hyperproduction, related to the capacity of the dialyzer to activate complement, and (2) a chronic stimulation by noncomplement factors, possibly lipopolysaccharide (LPS) fragments in the dialysate.[108] In vitro experiments confirmed the accentuation of the dialysis membrane–related monokine synthesis by the contact of leukocytes with LPS.[109] Bingel et al. found differences in intradialytic changes in IL-1 activity depending on the dialyzer membrane used.[110] These differences were related to enhanced IL-1 adsorption and elimination with some membranes (e.g., polyacrylonitrile) compared with others (e.g., regenerated cellulose).[111] In spite of increased baseline cytoplasmic IL-1 activity in the absence of stimulation, response of this activity upon stimulation was suppressed.[112]

Herbelin et al. demonstrated a gradual rise in postdialysis plasma IL-1 in patients on chronic maintenance dialysis starting with the first hemodialysis session.[113] These data suggest a gradual and progressive triggering of the inflammatory response as a consequence of recurrent acute-phase stimulation. Similar results were reported in relation to plasma levels of IL-6.[114] In addition, for Il-6, a further increase in concentration was demonstrated in the posthemodialysis period.[115] Herbelin et al. suggest that factors retained in uremia could be a sufficient signal to initiate basal intracellular IL-1 synthesis and TNF-α release but that a more significant IL-1 release could be triggered during long-term hemodialysis.[116]

Zaoui et al. demonstrated that although baseline IL-2 receptor expression on lymphocytes of patients on chronic complement-activating cuprophan dialyzers was increased, stimulated IL-2 receptor expression by phytohemagglutinin was markedly depressed.[117] These alterations disappeared after a switch to the less complement-activating polymethylmethacrylate membrane. In parallel, a significantly decreased IL-2 activity was detected by Beaurain et al. in the supernatant of stimulated T cells of hemodialyzed patients.[118]

In another study, basal predialysis TNF-values of TNF-α were significantly higher in 69 unselected hemodialysis patients irrespective of the membrane used.[119] While some investigators report that TNF-α is not affected by hemodialysis,[120] others find a rise in TNF-α during dialysis with a cuprophan membrane.[121] The possibility of a discrepancy between free plasma levels and intracellular levels may be one important source for this difference. The role of uremic toxicity in enhanced cytokine production should not be quickly discarded. On the other hand, hemodialysis has been demonstrated to induce gene expression of IL-1β as a marker of inflammation in peripheral blood mononuclear cells.[122] This event was related to the degree of complement activation. Apart from acute effects of the dialysis membrane on cytokine production, cytokine synthesis has been demonstrated to be modulated chronically as well.[123] Van Riemsdijk-van Overbecke et al. found a higher expression of TNF-α receptors on monocytes and lymphocytes of patients on both hemodialysis and peritoneal dialysis compared both to patients with chronic renal failure without renal replacement therapy and to controls.[124]

Thus, most data point to a multifactorial activation of the cytokine system in hemodialyzed uremics. Of interest, then, is to what extent changes in cytokine production will affect the response mechanisms of the host defense system, and in what way. Recently, increasing evidence has been collected that a substantial fraction of uremic and/or dialyzed patients suffer from a hyperinflammatory state, which has been related to overall mortality and morbidity related to malnutrition and atherogenesis.[4] The cytokines as causative agents fit well into this picture of hyperinflammation, although one should not forget that the levels of antiinflammatory cytokines can be elevated in uremia as well[125] and that compounds other than cytokines are probably involved. This hypothesis seems to be in apparent contradiction with the frequently reported blunting of the immune system response upon stimulation in this patient population, but baseline hyperactivity may result in the exhaustion of

the immune system upon stimulation. In possible agreement with this hypothesis, monocyte activation in response to exposure to a cuprophan membrane results in a transient refractoriness of these monocytes to further stimulation with complement factors and formyl-methionine-leucine-phenylalanine (f-MLP).[126] Similarly, but in nonuremic conditions, in an in vitro study, Schleiffenbaum and Fehr demonstrated that preincubation of granulocytes with TNF-α caused functional deactivation of the respiratory burst, corresponding to a downregulation of TNF-α receptors.[127] Interleukin activity may also be counterbalanced by the simultaneous presence of interleukin antagonists, such as anti-IL-1α autoantibodies[128] or IL-1 receptor antagonist (IL-Ra).[129]

Phagocytic Function

The ultimate and essential step in the destruction of infective organisms is their ingestion and killing by phagocytes. It is known that potential disturbances of phagocytosis will result in part from defects at other levels of the immunologic functional cascade, such as lymphocyte function and/or the production of humoral factors such as cytokines, leukotrienes, growth factors, or platelet-activating factor. Phagocytosis, however, occupies a key position and is the endpoint of immune defense.

The response of phagocytic leukocytes to infection is characterized by several steps and aspects of functional capacity: (1) the attraction of phagocytic cells and their movement toward and adhesion at the focus of infection (chemotaxis); (2) the ingestion of bacteria (phagocytosis); and (3) the digestive destruction of ingested bacteria by enzymatic processes (lysozyme and elastase release) and the production of oxygen free radical species (hydrogen peroxide, superoxide, hypochlorite). Functional disturbances may occur at each of these levels.

Impaired chemotaxis is at least in part attributable to (1) an excess of immunoglobulin light chains as a consequence of impaired renal metabolism[130] and (2) the retention of a modified form of ubiquitin with chemotactic inhibiting properties.[131]

Most studies evaluating the response of phagocytic cells to various stimuli[132–136] in ESRD and CAPD patients, and predialysis samples of hemodialyzed patients, demonstrate a decrease in phagocytic functional capacity. These data point to a decreased response of phagocytes to stimulation. Intradialytic response depends on the type of membrane. There is now ample evidence that during dialysis with a cuprophan membrane (first use), the complement cascade is activated,[137] and this is probably the primary reason for the baseline activation of the leukocyte system during dialysis with this type of membrane.[138] Of importance is the question of whether these primarily activated leukocytes are still able to cope with additional natural stimuli, such as microorganisms. In many studies, phagocyte function upon stimulation has been shown to be depressed during dialysis with complement-activating cuprophan as well as with other complement-activating membranes, such as cellulose diacetate.[136,139,140] This functional disturbance, per phagocytic cell, is further intensified by the presence of marked leukocytopenia early after the start of cuprophan dialysis.

In contrast to the data collected during cuprophan dialysis, granulocyte activity remains unaltered during dialysis with other, less complement-activating dialyzer membranes.

Apart from an acute decrease of granulocyte functional capacity during each dialysis with cuprophan, the authors could also demonstrate a progressive decline in basic leukocyte function in predialysis blood samples in patients starting on hemodialysis.[136] A similar decline was not seen with non-complement-activating dialyzers. The nadir in response occurred after 3 to 4 weeks of treatment.

In summary, the majority of studies point to a depression of phagocyte response to stimulation in ESRD patients, which is present before the start of dialysis and is enhanced both acutely and chronically by dialysis with the complement-activating cuprophan membrane. If this functional response is considered the endpoint in the destruction of bacteria causing infection, these abnormalities may play a role in the propensity to infection in nondialyzed and dialyzed uremics. On the other hand, baseline leukocyte activation might be enhanced, and this effect, in its turn, is related to atherogenesis.

Pathophysiology of Phagocytic Dysfunction

Changes in immune cell function may result from alterations in (1) surface molecule and receptor expression and activation; (2) particle ingestion; (3) signal transfer by secondary messengers and target proteins; and (4) enzymatic and metabolic dysfunction (Fig. 18–2).

Surface Molecule and Receptor Expression, Particle Ingestion.

Changes in receptor expression and in particle ingestion have been demonstrated in uremic and/or hemodialyzed patients.[134,141] An intradialytic decrease in receptor expression is described for f-MLP[142] and Fc receptors.[143] In contrast, Roccatello et al. concluded that cuprophan did not affect Fc-receptor expression[141] but only particle interiorization, due to exhaustion of energetic sources. Surface receptor binding of f-MLP and casein was not affected during dialysis with cellulose acetate dialyzers.[144] Skubitz and Craddock[145] described a marked refractoriness of granulocytes to stimulation with C5a during cuprophan hemodialysis, suggesting a downregulation of cellular responses to this chemotactic stimulus. In parallel, Lewis et al.[144] described a suppression of density of surface expression of C5a receptors when normal white blood cells were passed in vitro through cellulosic dialyzers. These changes in complement receptor expression were, however, not confirmed in evalu-

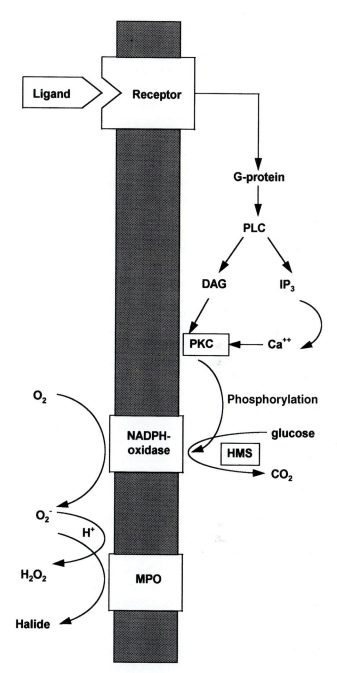

Figure 18–2. Flowchart of the mechanisms involved at the cellular level in the destruction of bacteria by phagocytic leukocytes. Gray area: cell membrane. PLC = phospholipase C; DAG = diacylglycerol; IP$_3$ = inositol-triphosphate; O$_2^-$ = superoxide free radical; HMS = hexose monophosphate shunt; MPO = myeloperoxidase. Binding of ligand to receptor transmits the message via various secondary messengers to protein kinase C, which activates NADPH-oxidase by phosphorylation, resulting in the transformation of O$_2$ to superoxide free radical (O$_2^-$). The energy necessary for this process is delivered by the hexose monophosphate shunt. Superoxide is further transformed to even stronger radicals, such as hydrogen peroxide (H$_2$O$_2$) or hypochlorous acid (the latter through halogenation by an intermediate of myeloperoxidase).

ating the in vivo intradialytic generation of these receptors in uremic patients.

Beta$_2$-integrins (CD11/CD18) have been related to complement activation-dependent release of elastase by neutrophil degranulation.[146] Use of complement-activating dialyzers caused a rapid and prominent increase of MAC-1 (CD11b/CD18) receptors, together with a twofold decrease in selectin LAM-1 receptor expression.[147] Other authors have described a rise in gp 150/95 (CD11c/CD18), whereas no change was observed in the expression of LFA-1 (CD11a/CD18).[148] Spontaneous and stimulated adherence of human monocytes to dialyzer membranes is more pronounced for regenerated cellulose than for AN69.[149] These events may be related to specific activity of PAF as an inducer of monocyte adherence and can be reduced by PAF-receptor antagonists.[149]

In general, the expression of several adhesion molecules has been reported to be enhanced during dialysis with complement-activating membranes. These events may be related to the increased tendency of leukocytes to adhere and to aggregate, eventually resulting in their entrapment in capillary beds, especially of the lungs, and in early dialysis neutropenia. On the other hand, the expression after stimulation of CD14, a lipopolysaccharide receptor, was depressed during hemodialysis with cuprophan but not during dialysis with less complement-activating membranes.[150]

In addition, Jacobson et al. demonstrated that granulocytes from hemodialysis patients require a more intense chemotactic stimulus to upregulate CD11b at the local site of inflammation in the interstitium.[151]

Dysfunction of Metabolic Pathways. A central role in the destruction of ingested bacteria is played by NADPH-oxidase, an enzyme that converts oxygen to superoxide free radicals (Fig. 18–2), which are then transformed to other even more toxic free radicals, such as hydrogen peroxide and hypochlorite. The energy necessary for this process is delivered by the hexose monophosphate shunt (HMS), which converts glucose to CO_2. An inhibition of this process in response to a challenge has been demonstrated both in nondialyzed patients, starting from a creatinine clearance below 15 mL/min, and in stable maintenance hemodialysis patients.[136] That all studied stimuli (including PMA, a direct activator of protein kinase C-dependent metabolism) show a similar suppression, in spite of remarkably different activation mechanisms, suggests that a common distal metabolic pathway is disturbed and that alterations are probably not related to a defect in particle ingestion (Fig. 18–3). Thus, the energy delivery by the HMS for the phagocytic killing of bacteria by NADPH-oxidase is disturbed in uremia.

Changes in Apoptosis. Accelerated apoptosis is seen in uremic neutropils and in cells of healthy donors when incubated with uremic serum.[152] In addition, contact with dia-

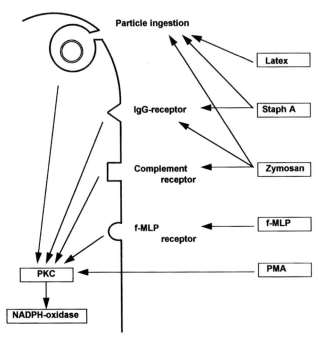

Figure 18–3. Mechanisms of phagocytic activation by various challenging stimuli. F-MLP = formyl-methionine-leucine-phenylalanine; PMA = phorbol myristic acid; PKC = protein kinase C. Latex, zymosan, and Staph A *(Staphylococcus aureus)* are particles. Binding with IgG receptor (zymosan and *S. aureus*) and complement receptor (zymosan) add to the activating capacity of zymosan and *S. aureus*. F-MLP is a small, nonparticle tripeptide, which activates phagocytes by complexing with a specific receptor. PMA is a humoral, nonparticle direct PKC-activator, not working via surface receptors. Because a parallel depression of all these factors is observed in uremia, this suggests a mechanism not related to particle ingestion or to any specific receptor but rather to one of the final metabolic processes at the level of or beyond PKC (see also Fig. 18–2).

lyzer membranes leads to increased apoptosis.[153] In contrast, Cohen et al. found reduced apoptosis in polymorphonuclear cells in relation to elevated concentration of imunoglobulin light chains, as encountered in uremia.[154] Apoptosis could be related to a decrease of the inflammatory response by switching off the involved cells without necrotic release of their potentially inflammatory contents into the surrounding milieu.

CAUSATIVE MECHANISMS

Important changes in immune function in uremia thus affect both general phagocytic and cell-specific defense. Contributing factors are multiple (Fig. 18–4): physical, nutritional, and metabolic conditions and/or anatomic and functional alterations (e.g., of the urinary tract, personal hygiene, underlying chronic infectious disease, socioeconomic factors). Once dialysis is started, additional contributing factors may include the disruption of external cutaneous protective barriers and the affinity of bacteria for foreign polymeric materials. A number of alternative causes

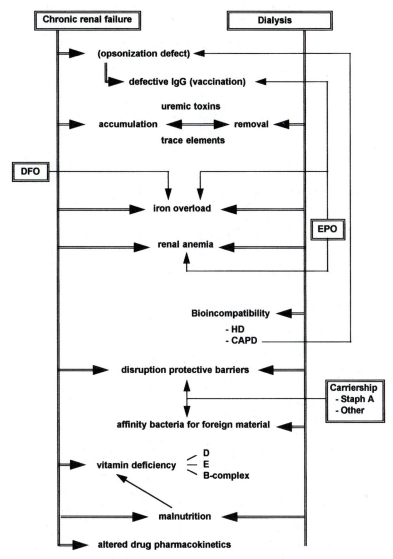

Figure 18–4. Flowchart of the putative factors affecting immune response in hemodialyzed patients. Bold lines: primary events playing a role in virtually all patients, either related to uremia per se (left) or dialysis (right). Thin lines: secondary events, not necessarily operative in all patients. Several factors are interrelated and interact. DFO = deferoxamine; EPO = erythropoietin; HD = hemodialysis; CAPD = continuous ambulatory peritoneal dialysis; Staph A = *Staphylococcus aureus*.

that are not directly related to uremia might be at play as well, such as the use of immunosuppressive agents or other drugs with immunosuppressive characteristics. The contributing factors are multiple and may be influenced by uremia per se, the treatment of uremia by hemodialysis, or both (Fig. 18–4).

Opsonization

A decrease in fibronectin concentration has been implicated as responsible for some defective immunologic mechanisms.[155] In their study, however, Abrutyn et al. considered changes in the quality of opsonization to be pathophysiologically unimportant.[156] Phagocytosis-related CO_2 produc-

tion by phagocytic leukocytes of ESRD patients was not higher for opsonized than for nonopsonized particles (Fig. 18–5), suggesting that opsonization defects, if any, do not affect the intensity of the metabolic response to stimuli in a significant way.

In the peritoneal cavity of CAPD patients, a depletion of opsonins has been demonstrated.[157]

Uremic Toxicity

Immune dysfunction may be caused by depression of one or several steps of the function of leukocytes by uremic toxins. Uremic serum and/or ultrafiltrate have repeatedly been demonstrated to alter aspects of immune function.[133,158]

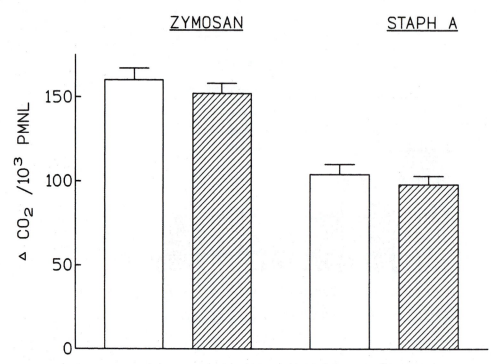

Figure 18–5. Granulocyte CO_2 production in whole blood (expressed as DPM $14CO_2/10^3$ granulocytes for nonopsonized (open bars) and opsonized (hatched bars) zymosan and *Staphylococcus aureus* ($n = 8$). The metabolic response does not improve when opsonized particles are administered (mean ± SEM, opsonized versus nonopsonized: p = not significant by variance analysis).

Hällgren et al. found a negative correlation between serum phosphate and phagocytic activity.[159] However, a myriad of other compounds may be retained together with phosphate, so this correlation does not necessarily point to a causal relationship. Lespier-Dexter et al., in contrast, found no significant correlation of immune function with phosphate but weakly significant correlations with potassium and the potassium/sodium ratio.[160] Glazer et al. added urea to a suspension of normal monocytes up to a final concentration of 200 mg/dL and found a marked suppression of superoxide anion production.[161] Others have found no such suppression of leukocyte function by urea[162]; in general, it is accepted that urea in concentrations currently encountered in uremia is not toxic.[163] According to Wardle and Williams, phenols and phenolic acids depress leukocyte iodination and the activity of myeloperoxidase.[162] Phenols, indoles, and even uric acid may exert their action in part as antioxidants.[164] More recent data show that p-cresol, a lipophilic compound with strong protein binding, markedly inhibits phagocyte functional capacity in concentrations encountered in uremia.[165] Current well-known markers of uremic retention, such as urea or creatinine, have no such effect. Subsequently an inhibitory effect by p-cresol on monocyte excretion of platelet activating factor 1 (PAF-1)[166] and on the cytokine-induced expression of adhesion molecules on endothelial cells and on the adhesion of monocytes to endothelium[167] have been demonstrated as well. According to

Ferrante, human neutrophil locomotion is suppressed by the polyamines spermine and spermidine.[168] Endorphins may also have a suppressive effect on the response of leukocytes to stimuli.[169]

Guanidine compounds have been shown to play a role in the deficiency of B-cell activation and immunoregulation as well as Th-cell dysfunction.[97] Guanidinosuccinic acid inhibits cytokine-induced calcitriol production by monocytic cells.[170] Guanidines depress the functional capacity of phagocytic cells as well.[171] Hörl and coworkers have described a 28,000-Da polypeptide with granulocyte-inhibitory characteristics[172] as well as another moiety, molecular weight of 9500 Da, with similar depressive properties.[173]

Parathyroid hormone (PTH) affects several biochemical functions.[174] According to Esposito et al., phagocytosis is more abnormal in renal patients with a high PTH.[175] Tuma et al. have noted an increased resting-state production of chemiluminescence in hyperparathyroid uremic patients.[176] In addition, Massry et al. observed an enhanced elastase release by granulocytes after in vitro contact with PTH—however, at concentrations exceeding those currently encountered in clinical practice.[177] According to Alexiewicz et al., elevated resting intraphagocytic levels of Ca^{2+} decrease the ATP content of phagocytic cells and cause a smaller rise in cell membrane Ca^{2+} in response to stimulation.[178] All these findings are consistent with the notion that excess PTH may play an important role in the impaired phagocytosis of hemodialyzed patients. Treatment with calcium channel blockers could counteract these PTH-induced disturbances. Nifedipine decreased the elevated intracellular calcium concentration, increased ATP content, and improved impaired phagocytosis.[179] A similar beneficial effect of nifedipine is observed on B lymphocytes with a decrease of intracellular calcium content and a normalization of the inhibited proliferation.[180] In addition, parathyroidectomy results in an increase of immunoglobulin levels in hemodialysis patients.[181]

According to Lewin et al., T-cell proliferation in response to phytohemagglutinin (PHA) stimulation was enhanced in hyperparathyroid but not in parathyroidectomized uremic rats.[182] Hemodialysis patients with high parathyroid levels also had an elevated response to PHA compared to patients with low levels.[183] In addition, CD4-positive cells were higher in patients with high parathyroid hormone levels.[183] Parathyroid hormone increases the cytosolic calcium of thymocytes.[184]

The free radical species produced by immunocompetent cells may generate toxic by-products. The production of hypochlorite may result in the synthesis of organic chloramines by its reaction with organic retention compounds.[185] Because these reagents are lipophilic or have an affinity for cells or intracellular structures (e.g., spermine, spermidine, taurine),[186] the penetration of these organic chloramines into the cell may be facilitated. In addition, organic chloramines may persist longer and/or be metabolized more slowly than their inorganic counterparts, so that their tissue toxicity is protracted in time. Two studies evaluating the role of nitric oxide (NO) in uremic toxicity came to contradictory conclusions, one group pointing to depressed[187] and another to enhanced NO production.[188] Possibly uremia per se depresses NO production due to the accumulation of endogenous inhibitors of NO synthesis, such as asymmetrical dimethylarginine,[187] whereas dialysis, especially with complement-activating membranes, may enhance NO production.[189]

It is thus conceivable that uremic toxins play a primary role in the functional disturbances of leukocytes in uremic patients. The responsible compounds remain, however, largely unknown; probably there are several acting in combination. Most of the compounds claimed to interfere with immune function are larger than urea and creatinine and/or are partly hydrophobic and/or protein-bound. The retention pattern and kinetic behavior of these solutes during dialysis differs from that of urea and of creatinine, the uremic solutes currently determined for estimation of uremic toxicity and dialytic efficiency. If uremic toxins do play a role in the impaired host defense, it could be expected that infection rate would be correlated with dialysis efficiency. Such an inverse relationship between dose of dialysis and infection-related mortality has indeed been demonstrated by

Bloembergen et al. Analysis of cause-specific mortality shows that for each increment of Kt/V by 0.1, the adjusted relative risk of death due to infection decreases by 9 percent.[190] Tokars et al. found that a higher vascular access was related to infection risk in patients with a low urea reduction ratio.[191] However, a relationship between bacteremia and dialysis efficiency or between infection-related mortality and dialysis efficiency or flux could not be confirmed by Hoen et al.[6] or by the HEMO study.[192] The relation between Kt/V and infection could be biased by malnutrition associated with a low distribution volume of urea (V) and hence with an overestimated Kt/V, explaining the lack of correlation between Kt/V and infection rate in some studies.

Iron Overload

It is commonly accepted that, in the general population, both iron overload and deficiency predispose to infection. This ambiguous relation is due to the need for iron of both the metabolism of microorganisms and of host defense components.[193] Bacteria require intracellular iron to support their growth and survival, whereas macrophages need iron as a cofactor for the execution of antimicrobial mechanisms such as the NADPH-dependent oxidative burst and the production of nitrogen radicals.[194] Iron excess, however, impairs the functions of phagocytes and T cells.[195] In hemodialysis patients, the situation is even more complex. Inflammation worsens renal anemia. Hence, in the pre-erythropoietin era, more blood transfusions were needed in patients with frequent infections, and iron load was higher. As previous infection is one of the major risk factors for subsequent infections,[196] an association between iron overload and infection is unavoidable and possibly coincidental rather than causative. In the posterythropoietin era, the relation between iron parameters and infection risk remains equally problematic, since serum ferritin is both a marker of inflammation and of iron reserve.

A host of studies have been published suggesting a relationship between iron load and infection,[5,196,197] including the effect of iron on various aspects of leukocyte function. Patruta et al. describe an association between high serum ferritin levels and impairment of intracellular killing of bacteria and of depressed oxidative burst after stimulation.[198] Polymorphonuclear cells isolated from peritoneal dialysis patients treated with intravenous iron display a decreased killing capacity,[199] and in vitro experiments demonstrate an inhibitory effect of iron on the transendothelial migration of polymorphonuclear cells.[200]

One way to decrease body iron stores is by administering recombinant human erythropoietin (rHuEpO). Having done so in a small group of patients with excessive body iron (average serum ferritin 1860 µg/L), Boelaert et al. found an improvement of phagocytosis together with a decrease of serum ferritin.[201]

Deferoxamine, a natural siderophore, has been successfully used to treat iron overload. Based on theoretical grounds and on in vitro experiments, deferoxamine seems to have protective effects against many bacterial infections.[202] A potential hazard of deferoxamine is, however, the possibility that this siderophore may be utilized by the microorganism itself to acquire iron. The latter has been described with *Rhizopus*, causing mucormucosis in hemodialysis patients treated with deferoxamine.[69] In addition, infections with *Yersinia enterocolitica* and *Listeria monocytogenes* have been described in association with iron chelation.[202]

As a general rule, iron should not be administered to dialysis patients with active infection.

Renal Anemia

Renal anemia may result in inadequate tissue oxygenation and subsequently in a variety of functional disturbances. In chronically hemodialyzed patients, the glycolytic response to stimulation is correlated with the hematocrit (Fig. 18–6). In addition, granulocyte response also improves during treatment with erythropoietin[203] in parallel with better exercise tolerance, as an illustration of metabolic improvement

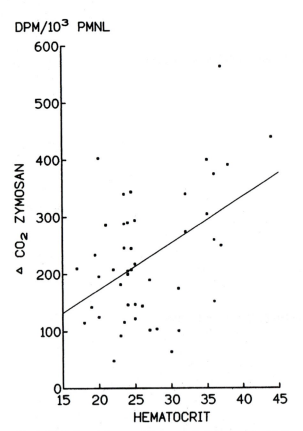

Figure 18–6. Correlation-regression analysis between granulocyte CO_2 production in whole blood in response to zymosan (vertical axis = dependent variable) and hematocrit (horizontal axis = independent variable) ($n = 50$, $r = 0.43$, $p = 0.002$, $y = 7.4x + 30.4$).

with rHuEpO.[204] A beneficial effect of rHuEpO has also been demonstrated on other aspects of the immune system, such as the composition of the subpopulations of lymphocytes, response to vaccination, and immunoglobulin production.[205–208] Improvement of cellular immunity was also observed when rHuEpO was used for other than nephrologic indications.[209]

Trace Elements

Significant changes in concentrations of various trace elements have been demonstrated in renal failure patients.[210] Among the trace element abnormalities that can interfere with immune function are cadmium,[211] mercury,[211] and copper accumulation[212] as well as zinc depletion.[213] Low serum zinc levels are associated with a lower response rate to interferon therapy in children infected with chronic hepatitis B.[214] Zinc therapy may improve impaired cell-mediated immunity in chronically uremic patients.[215] Turk et al., however, found no influence of zinc supplementation on antibody response after influenza vaccination in hemodialysis patients.[216]

Vitamin Deficiency

Cohen et al. reported subnormal vitamin E levels in patients undergoing hemodialysis,[217] although other authors report normal[218] or even elevated levels in ESRD patients.[219] Vitamin E deficiency has been related to a blunted immune response.[220] Supplementation of vitamin E in patients with a decreased blood level resulted in a reduction of the number of OKT^{8+} lymphocytes.[221] In nonsystemically supplemented hemodialysis patients, depletion of folic acid and vitamin C and severe pyridoxine deficiency may occur.[222] Deficiencies in folic acid may impair humoral immune responses.[220] Vitamin C deficiency affects cell immunity.[220] In animal studies, pyridoxine deficiency resulted in depression of antibody response and impaired cellular immunity.[223] Supplementation of these water-soluble vitamins results in normal or greater than normal values of plasma vitamin levels.[224] Since this supplementation is current practice in many dialysis units, deficiencies of these vitamins will rarely play a role in the immune dysfunction of uremia.

Intravenous L-carnitine supplementation in hemodialysis patients had no effect on phagocytic function and viability in vivo.[225]

Receptors for 1,25(OH)$_2$ vitamin D_3 have been identified on human monocytes and T and B lymphocytes.[226] Vitamin D deficiency in chronic uremia may affect immune response, in part because 1,25(OH)$_2$ vitamin D_3 acts as a cytokine,[227] although this effect is mainly restricted to monocytes and macrophages. Chronic renal failure results not only in a deficient renal 1,25(OH)$_2$ vitamin D_3 production, due to a decrease in renal mass with lack of 1α-hydroxylase, but also in changes in calcitriol metabolism (both synthesis and degradation).[228] These effects may at least in part be attributed to a deficient receptor binding affinity for DNA,[229] subsequently impairing the biological actions of calcitriol in renal failure.[230] Hence, vitamin D deficiency and resistance may have important consequences not only on bone and calcium/phosphorus metabolism but also on other vitamin D–dependent metabolic processes, of which immunocompetent mononuclear cell function is one of the most important. Hubel et al. demonstrated that oral calcitriol improved the superoxide generation and bactericidal capacity of monocytes in hemodialysis patients, whereas myeloperoxidase-dependent oxidative metabolism and phagocytic capacity remained unaffected.[231]

Purines are among the potential inhibitors,[229] and the decrease of their concentration may have a beneficial effect, on calcitriol levels and its resultant biological activity.[232] Purines are known, together with other less well defined protein-bound and lipophilic molecules, to depress the expression of lipopolysaccharide receptor CD14 on monocytes in response to calcitriol.[233]

Mononuclear cells are also among the few nonrenal tissue cells that produce $1,25(OH)_2$ vitamin D_3.[234] This production is suppressed by preincubation with guanidinosuccinic acid.[170]

Hemodialysis patients treated with intravenous calcitriol produced a higher percentage of protective antibodies to influenza after vaccination than do patients not treated with calcitriol.[235]

Intravenous administration of paracalcitol to hemodialysis patients converted some anergic patients to reactive patients but was not associated with an improved response to hepatitis B booster vaccine.[236]

Bioincompatibility of Artificial Organ Treatment

The necessity to treat uremia by dialysis has created a new series of pathologies, currently referred to as bioincompatibility-related complications, some of which affect the immune system. Bioincompatibility, as it relates to the immune system, has been emphasized as a complication of the first generation of cellulose membranes, such as cuprophan and cellulose diacetate, which have significant complement- and leukocyte-activating capacity. Newer cellulosic membranes with improved biocompatibility, such as hemophan and cellulose triacetate, have been developed, with biocompatibility comparable to that of the synthetic membranes such as AN69, polysulfone, and polymethylmethacrylate.

Recurrent Complement Activation. Complement-activating dialyzer membranes, such as cuprophan,[237] may have a negative impact on the response of phagocytes in addition to their acute and chronic effect on circulating leukocyte

counts and their activating impact on baseline cell status. The repetitive exposure of blood to bioincompatible cuprophan leads to the recurrent activation of complement, degranulation of neutrophils, and release of oxygen free radical species.[238] Although these reactive oxygen species are bactericidal, their unintended release results in decreased responsiveness to further stimuli.[140] This refractoriness occurs particularly during cuprophan dialysis and is maximal at the nadir of dialysis neutropenia.[140] The reduced response upon stimulation is associated with an increased baseline activity of leukocytes,[139] suggesting exhaustion of the immune system. In addition, the authors described chronic progressive inhibition of immune response during repeated contact with complement-activating dialysis membranes.[136] Hence it is conceivable that the complement system is stimulated in an inappropriate way, decreasing the ability of white blood cells to respond when needed. These findings parallel the poor response to various stimuli of granulocyte function with other chronic inflammatory states—such as acute infection,[239] burns,[240] or trauma [241]—which are also attributed to excess complement activation.[242] Neutrophils preexposed to high concentrations of activated complement are inhibited in their subsequent migratory responses.[243] However, this deactivation is mainly related to locomotion and not to indices of respiratory burst activity.[244] Alternatively, neutrophils activated during passage through the dialyzer may be sequestered in the pulmonary vasculature,[145] probably leading to an increase in the proportion of functionally inactive cells in circulation.[143]

Dialyzer Bioincompatibility and Direct Arguments for Susceptibility to Infection. Although it is clear from the above-mentioned data that dialyzer membrane structure and its effects on various aspects of immune function may cause alterations that eventually result in infectious disease, the ultimate proof of the influence of bioincompatibility on susceptibility to infection will be the demonstration of differences in the incidence of infection, morbidity, and mortality related to the type of membrane used. There are at least two observational clinical studies now available showing a higher mortality due to infection in patients treated by unmodified cellulosic dialyzers.[1,245] In another study, the metabolic response to phagocytic stimuli was depressed in patients treated with cuprophan membranes as opposed to polysulfone.[136] During a follow-up of 6 months, there was also a higher incidence of clinical infection in the patients treated by cuprophan; however, only marginal significance was reached in view of the small number of patients.[136]

Infectious disease may also be induced by the use of foreign materials in vascular access, as for central vein catheters or access grafts. Bacteria have nonspecific affinity for these foreign materials and might induce the formation of biofilm, which is difficult to remove.

Endotoxin Transfer to the Bloodstream

A host of mostly gram-negative organisms have been identified in dialysate circuits.[246] Although bacteria and endotoxins typically are considered not to cross intact dialyzer membranes, they may enter the circulation through microscopic membrane defects. Moreover, endotoxin might be broken down into smaller fragments with macrophage and complement-activating properties, which may cross even small pores.[247] Backfiltration of endotoxin fragments is feared when dialysate pressure within a large-pore dialyzer exceeds the pressure in the blood compartment.[248] Studies by Lonnemann et al. demonstrated, however, that the passage of monocyte-activating material through low-flux regenerated cellulose membranes can also occur.[249] This effect can be attributed to the fact that cellulosic membranes are relatively thin, whereas synthetic membranes are thicker and have strong adsorptive capacity at the dialysate side. In a study by Pereira et al., transfer of monocyte-activating material from the dialysate to the blood side of a dialyzer membrane was higher for small-pore hemophan than for large-pore polyamide,[250] again suggesting that membrane thickness rather than pore size controlled transmembrane transfer of pyrogenic factors.

A criticism of many in vitro studies in this area is that the true in vivo conditions occurring in hemodialysis are rarely accurately mimicked. Moreover, in vivo studies show conflicting results. Several studies demonstrate increasing endotoxin levels in the serum of patients treated with open-membrane dialyzers.[251,252] This transmembrane transfer of LPS or LPS fragments may be responsible for chronic stimulation of IL production.[252] On the other hand, in a study from Powell et al., IL-1β and TNF-α were not elevated during dialysis, in spite of high dialysate endotoxin levels, unless overt pyrogenic reactions occurred.[253] In addition, Grooteman et al. described stable levels of IL-1β, IL-6, and TNF-α during high-flux bicarbonate dialysis with various membranes.[254] In parallel, backfiltrates of *Pseudomonas*-contaminated dialysate did not stimulate monocytes.[255] In two studies by Schouten et al. and van Tellingen et al., there was no difference in acute IL-6 secretion or in chronic C-reactive protein (CRP) expression irrespective of the degree of dialysate purity.[256,257]

Note that the transfer of bacterial products from contaminated water may on occasion cause pyrogenic reactions.[43] On-line dialysate filtration may prevent the bacteria and endotoxins from appearing in dialysate and hence their transfer into the bloodstream.[258]

Acetate Content of Dialysate

Although acetate content in dialysate is currently quite low (4 to 5 mmol/L), negative influences of this moiety on leukocytes are still suspected. It has been demonstrated that acetate-free biofiltration induces less activation of monocytes[259] and neutrophils[260] than does regular bicarbonate dialysis.

Disruption of Protective Barriers

As half of the bacteremic episodes are attributed to infection of the vascular access,[5] the loss of the protective skin barrier at access puncture sites and/or with chronic indwelling catheters is a major potential cause of the elevated infection rate noticed in dialysis patients (both hemodialysis and peritoneal dialysis). In addition to vascular access, direct introduction of infective agents into the bloodstream has been demonstrated with contaminated medications, dialysate, and/or dialysis equipment. In order to limit the disruption of the skin barrier, arteriovenous fistulas, which are punctured three times weekly, are preferred over percutaneous dialysis catheters. If it is impossible to create a fistula, however, alternatives to percutaneous catheters have been developed, such as subcutaneous implantable ports,[261] which at least in theory are protective against infection. In addition, the skin of patients with chronic kidney disease may be dry and atrophic. The nadir in intradialytic immune suppression, if any, is at minute 15, almost immediately after the disruption of the skin barrier.

Affinity of Bacteria for Foreign Material

Polymer surfaces may have an increased affinity for bacteria.[262] In dialyzed patients, the risk of infection is substantial for exogenous vascular access systems composed of foreign material that is present for long periods, such as indwelling central vein catheters[263] or graft material.[264]

Biofilm generation on these materials increases the risk of bacterial adhesion; it is virtually impossible to remove these biofilms from the catheter wall. Prevention of infection can be attempted by the injection of appropriate locks,[21,22] topical application of anti-infective ointment,[23] and/or insertion of specific catheters that prevent bacterial adhesion.[265]

Carrier Status

A risk for recurrent infection is present in nasal carriers of *S. aureus*.[15] Topical and/or oral administration of anti-staphylococcal agents decreases infections due to *S. aureus* in such cases,[266] which might result in overall savings in the cost of treatment,[267] although the development of resistance remains a major area of concern.

The risk of infectious crises may also be increased by the presence of chronic infectious disease (e.g., chronic urinary tract infection).

Time Since Start of Dialysis

It is possible that shifts in granulocyte function occur during the long-term course of dialysis. It has been observed that there is a severe suppression of phagocyte response during the first weeks following the start of dialysis.[136] In a study both cross-sectional and prospective, this functional capacity was shown to improve when dialysis treatment was continued for longer times.[268] Improved immune function after prolonged dialysis was also reported previously in a study using the skin window test as an index of macrophage functional capacity.[269] Hällgren et al. reported a similar nadir in granulocyte uptake of IgG-coated particles during the first 4 months after the start of dialysis.[159]

This functional improvement over time may be attributed to the development of compensatory mechanisms or to the gradual removal of toxic compounds. Alternatively, patients develop a higher degree of baseline inflammatory status. Selection of patients is a less probable explanation for these findings, because a prospective study in a patient group followed for more than 1.5 years also yielded results showing improvement of granulocyte functional capacity over time.[270] Patients have higher values of IL-1 secretion after long-term dialysis than those not yet dialyzed.[116] In addition, the levels of circulating soluble IL-2 receptors are positively correlated with the duration of hemodialysis.[271]

Kessler et al. found no association between the time since the start of dialysis and the risk of bacteremia.[5]

Malnutrition

A substantial number of ESRD patients are clinically malnourished.[272] Parameters of malnutrition are related to delayed wound healing,[273] depression of secretory immunity,[274] impaired macrophage function,[275] reduced natural killer cell activity and IL-2 production,[276] and impaired respiratory burst activity and free radical production in response to phagocytosis.[277] In the series reported by Churchill et al., low serum albumin as an index of malnutrition was associated with an increased risk of infection.[278] Low albumin level is, however, not only a marker of malnutrition but also a sign of inflammation. Hence, it could be argued from such studies that no firm conclusions about the association between malnutrition and infection risk can be drawn. Nevertheless, in the study by Churchill et al., the low albumin at the start of the 12-month observation period was linked with subsequent infection,[278] making it less probable that infection was the cause of hypoalbuminemia in the majority of patients. The use of protein-restricting diets has been associated with nonspecific decreases in circulating leukocyte numbers and in a blunted in vitro response of mononuclear cells to various mitogens.[279]

Drug Treatment

Alternative causes of defective immune function only indirectly related to uremia are the use of immunosuppressive agents in transplant patients with nonfunctioning renal grafts, after liver or heart transplantation followed by progressive renal failure, and in autoimmune disorders such as Wegener's granulomatosis and systemic lupus erythematosus. It has been reported that diabetic patients treated with dialysis while awaiting transplant have fewer infections than after kidney transplantation, which underlines the negative role of immunosuppressive drugs.[280]

Advanced Age

In a prospective study of factors influencing the antibody response to hepatitis B vaccine in hemodialysis patients, age and human leukocyte antigen type were found to be the only factors influencing the response rate.[281] In addition, an increased risk of infectious events[282] and of infection-related death[2] is associated with older age. Others studies however, have failed to demonstrate this relationship.[5]

Diabetes Mellitus

Diabetes mellitus is a risk factor for catheter-related bacteremia in hemodialysis patients,[15] and the presence of diabetes is associated with a higher mortality rate caused by sepsis.[10]

Others studies however, have failed to demonstrate such a relationship.[18]

The Relation of Defective Immune Function to Infection

Are these functional disturbances and the known susceptibility to infection in dialysis patients interrelated? Uremic patients displaying a more defective phagocyte function have a higher incidence of infection than those with a better functional status.[136]

Several studies document a deficient immune response to *S. aureus* infection.[136,283] *S. aureus* is one of the most frequent invading microorganisms causing infection in dialyzed uremic patients.[284,285] Many of these infections are the consequence of bacteremia occurring early in the dialysis procedure, corresponding to a large body of data showing a nadir in responsive capacity early after the start of dialysis. Balakrishnan et al. found a higher frequency of infectious events in dialysis patients with a lower Il-1Ra synthesis upon stimulation with immunoglobulin G.[282]

CONCLUSIONS

Infections remain a frequent problem in dialyzed patients, and they continue to carry a higher morbidity and mortality than in the general population. In spite of significant therapeutic improvements, changes in incidence are not substantial, probably because more and more seriously ill patients are now accepted for chronic dialysis and survive longer. On the other hand, preventive measures are still not applied vigorously enough.

A number of protective measures can be taken to reduce the incidence and the severity of infections in this patient population (Table 18–3). To avoid the migration of pathogens through the cutaneous border and because of the easy fixation of pathogens to foreign material, vascular access systems should be composed as much as possible from endogenous material. When catheters are used, soft catheters for long-term use are preferred. Repeated punctures and other manipulations of the access systems should be avoided. The creation and manipulation of vascular access systems should be confined to appropriate, experienced professionals, and the necessary hygienic measures should be taken. Noncomplement activating dialyzers might reduce infectious risk while optimal solute removal is still pursued.

Carriers of morbid organisms should be isolated. Specific carriers of *S. aureus* should be treated with specific topical unguents. Malnutrition and iron overload should be avoided. Drugs with immunosuppressive effects should be used only when strictly needed.

If these precautions are followed, infectious risk might be reduced in spite of opposing forces—such as increasing resistance to antibiotics, increasing age, and increasing incidence of debilitating comorbid conditions with a negative impact on infections such as diabetes.

TABLE 18–3. CAUSES OF IMMUNE CELL DYSFUNCTION IN UREMIA: PREVENTIVE AND THERAPEUTIC MEASURES

Cause	Preventive and Therapeutic Measures
Dialyzer bioincompatibility	Use non-complement-activating dialyzer membranes
	Use of CAPD dialysate with minimal negative effect on the immune system
Uremic toxicity	Optimum solute removal
	Elimination of both hydrophylic and hydrophobic compounds
	Better definition of responsible toxins
Uremic anemia	Erythropoietin/erythroid stimulaing agents
Interference by medication	Avoid (if possible) immunosuppressive medication
Use immune stimulation?	Interferon?
	Cytokines?
Iron overload	Erythropoietin
	Avoid unnecessary iron and blood transfusions
	Deferoxamine
Deferoxamine	Use carefully; beware of immunosuppressive risks
Infection of dialysis access	Rigid asepsis
	Use materials with a low affinity for bacteria
Chronic infection carrier state	Preventive chronic antibiotics (local or systemic)
Malnutrition	Hyperalimentation
	Growth hormone?
	Erythropoietin/erythroid stimulating agents
Vitamin deficiency	Usual substitution
Resistance to 1,25 (OH)$_2$ vitamin D$_3$	Removal of responsible toxins? Allopurinol?

REFERENCES

1. Bloembergen WE, Hakim RM, Stannard DC, et al. Relationship of dialysis membrane and cause-specific mortality. *Am J Kidney Dis* 1999;33:1–10.
2. Allon M, Depner TA, Radeva M, et al. Impact of dialysis dose and membrane on infection-related hospitalization and death: results of the HEMO Study. *J Am Soc Nephrol* 2003; 14:1863–1870.
3. Mailloux LU, Bellucci AG, Wilkes BM, et al. Mortality in dialysis patients: analysis of the causes of death. *Am J Kidney Dis* 1991;18:326–335.
4. Stenvinkel P, Heimburger O, Paultre F, et al. Strong association between malnutrition, inflammation, and atherosclerosis in chronic renal failure. *Kidney Int* 1999;55:1899–1911.
5. Kessler M, Hoen B, Mayeux D, et al. Bacteremia in patients on chronic hemodialysis. A multicenter prospective survey. *Nephron* 1993;64:95–100.
6. Hoen B, Paul-Dauphin A, Hestin D, Kessler M. EPIBACDIAL: a multicenter prospective study of risk factors for bacteremia in chronic hemodialysis patients. *J Am Soc Nephrol* 1998;9:869–876.
7. Dopirak M, Hill C, Oleksiw M, et al. Surveillance of hemodialysis-associated primary bloodstream infections: the experience of ten hospital-based centers. *Infect Control Hosp Epidemiol* 2002;23:721–724.
8. Taylor G, Gravel D, Johnston L, et al. Prospective surveillance for primary bloodstream infections occurring in Canadian hemodialysis units. *Infect Control Hosp Epidemiol* 2002;23:716–720.
9. Bloembergen WE, Port FK. Epidemiological perspective on infections in chronic dialysis patients. *Adv Renal Replace Ther* 1996;3:201–207.
10. Sarnak MJ, Jaber BL. Mortality caused by sepsis in patients with end-stage renal disease compared with the general population. *Kidney Int* 2000;58:1758–1764.
11. Tokars JI, Miller ER, Stein G. New national surveillance system for hemodialysis-associated infections: initial results. *Am J Infect Control* 2002;30:288–295.
12. Saeed A, I, Al Mueilo SH, Bokhary HA, et al. A prospective study of hemodialysis access-related bacterial infections. *J Infect Chemother* 2002;8:242–246.
13. Stevenson KB, Hannah EL, Lowder CA, et al. Epidemiology of hemodialysis vascular access infections from longitu-

dinal infection surveillance data: predicting the impact of NKF-DOQI clinical practice guidelines for vascular access. *Am J Kidney Dis* 2002;39:549–555.

14. Minga TE, Flanagan KH, Allon M. Clinical consequences of infected arteriovenous grafts in hemodialysis patients. *Am J Kidney Dis* 2001;38:975–978.

15. Jean G, Charra B, Chazot C, et al. Risk factor analysis for long-term tunneled dialysis catheter-related bacteremias. *Nephron* 2002;91:399–405.

16. Marr KA, Sexton DJ, Conlon PJ, et al. Catheter-related bacteremia and outcome of attempted catheter salvage in patients undergoing hemodialysis. *Ann Intern Med* 1997;127:275–280.

17. Saad TF. Bacteremia associated with tunneled, cuffed hemodialysis catheters. *Am J Kidney Dis* 1999;34:1114–1124.

18. Kairaitis LK, Gottlieb T. Outcome and complications of temporary haemodialysis catheters. *Nephrol Dial Transplant* 1999;14:1710–1714.

19. Beathard GA. Catheter management protocol for catheter-related bacteremia prophylaxis. *Semin Dial* 2003;16:403–405.

20. Saxena AK, Panhotra BR, Naguib M. Sudden irreversible sensory-neural hearing loss in a patient with diabetes receiving amikacin as an antibiotic-heparin lock. *Pharmacotherapy* 2002;22:105–108.

21. Allon M. Prophylaxis against dialysis catheter-related bacteremia with a novel antimicrobial lock solution. *Clin Infect Dis* 2003;36:1539–1544.

22. Dogra GK, Herson H, Hutchison B, et al. Prevention of tunneled hemodialysis catheter-related infections using catheter-restricted filling with gentamicin and citrate: a randomized controlled study. *J Am Soc Nephrol* 2002;13:2133–2139.

23. Johnson DW, MacGinley R, Kay TD, et al. A randomized controlled trial of topical exit site mupirocin application in patients with tunnelled, cuffed haemodialysis catheters. *Nephrol Dial Transplant* 2002;17:1802–1807.

24. Sesso R, Barbosa D, Leme IL, et al. *Staphylococcus aureus* prophylaxis in hemodialysis patients using central venous catheter: effect of mupirocin ointment. *J Am Soc Nephrol* 1998;9:1085–1092.

25. Lok CE, Stanley KE, Hux JE, et al. Hemodialysis infection prevention with polysporin ointment. *J Am Soc Nephrol* 2003;14:169–179.

26. Boelaert JR, Van Landuyt HW, Godard CA, et al. Nasal mupirocin ointment decreases the incidence of *Staphylococcus aureus* bacteraemias in haemodialysis patients. *Nephrol Dial Transplant* 1993;8:235–239.

27. Perez-Fontan M, Rosales M, Rodriguez-Carmona A, et al. Mupirocin resistance after long-term use for *Staphylococcus aureus* colonization in patients undergoing chronic peritoneal dialysis. *Am J Kidney Dis* 2002;39:337–341.

28. Holton DL, Nicolle LE, Diley D, Bernstein K. Efficacy of mupirocin nasal ointment in eradicating *Staphylococcus aureus* nasal carriage in chronic haemodialysis patients. *J Hosp Infect* 1991;17:133–137.

29. Boelaert JR, Van Landuyt HW, De Baere YA, et al. Staphylococcus aureus infections in haemodialysis patients: pathophysiology and use of nasal mupirocin for prevention. *J Chemother* 1995;7(suppl 3):49–53.

30. European Best Practice Guidelines for Haemodialysis. Section VI. Haemodialysis-associated infection. *Nephrol Dial Transplant* 2002;17(suppl 7):72–87.

31. Shinefield H, Black S, Fattom A, et al. Use of a *Staphylococcus aureus* conjugate vaccine in patients receiving hemodialysis. *N Engl J Med* 2002;346:491–496.

32. Marr KA, Kong L, Fowler VG, et al. Incidence and outcome of *Staphylococcus aureus* bacteremia in hemodialysis patients. *Kidney Int* 1998;54:1684–1689.

33. Peacock SJ, Curtis N, Berendt AR, et al. Outcome following haemodialysis catheter-related *Staphylococcus aureus* bacteraemia. *J Hosp Infect* 1999;41:223–228.

34. Doulton T, Sabharwal N, Cairns HS, et al. Infective endocarditis in dialysis patients: new challenges and old. *Kidney Int* 2003;64:720–727.

35. McCarthy JT, Steckelberg JM. Infective endocarditis in patients receiving long-term hemodialysis. *Mayo Clin Proc* 2000;75:1008–1014.

36. Robinson DL, Fowler VG, Sexton DJ, et al. Bacterial endocarditis in hemodialysis patients. *Am J Kidney Dis* 1997;30:521–524.

37. Moffie BG, Veenendaal RA, Thompson J. Native valve endocarditis due to *Corynebacterium* group JK. *Neth J Med* 1990;37:236–238.

38. Ferrer C, Jakob E, Pastorino G, Juncos LI. Right-sided bacterial endocarditis due to *Flavobacterium odoratum* in a patient on chronic hemodialysis. *Am J Nephrol* 1995;15:82–84.

39. Fernandez-Cean J, Alvarez A, Burguez S, et al. Infective endocarditis in chronic haemodialysis: two treatment strategies. *Nephrol Dial Transplant* 2002;17:2226–2230.

40. Obrador GT, Levenson DJ. Spinal epidural abscess in hemodialysis patients: report of three cases and review of the literature. *Am J Kidney Dis* 1996;27:75–83.

41. Jackson BM, Beck-Sague CM, Bland LA, et al. Outbreak of pyrogenic reactions and gram-negative bacteremia in a hemodialysis center. *Am J Nephrol* 1994;14:85–89.

42. Block C, Backenroth R, Gershon E, et al. Outbreak of bloodstream infections associated with dialysis machine waste ports in a hemodialysis facility. *Eur J Clin Microbiol Infect Dis* 1999;18:723–725.

43. Vanholder R, Vanhaecke E, Ringoir S. *Pseudomonas* septicemia due to deficient disinfectant mixing during reuse. *Int J Artif Organs* 1992;15:19–24.

44. Grohskopf LA, Roth VR, Feikin DR, et al. *Serratia liquefaciens* bloodstream infections from contamination of epoetin alfa at a hemodialysis center. *N Engl J Med* 2001;344:1491–1497.

45. European Best Practice Guidelines for Haemodialysis. Section IV. Dialysis fluid purity. *Nephrol Dial Transplant* 2002;17(suppl 7):45–62.

46. Sarnak MJ, Jaber BL. Pulmonary infectious mortality among patients with end-stage renal disease. *Chest* 2001;120:1883–1887.

47. Fuchshuber A, Kuhnemund O, Keuth B, et al. Pneumococcal vaccine in children and young adults with chronic renal disease. *Nephrol Dial Transplant* 1996;11:468–473.

48. Rangel MC, Coronado VG, Euler GL, Strikas RA. Vaccine recommendations for patients on chronic dialysis. The Advisory Committee on Immunization Practices and the American Academy of Pediatrics. *Semin Dial* 2000;13:101–107.

49. Sagar S, Pirofski LA. Pneumococcal vaccine with unknown vaccination status. *Semin Dial* 2000;13:207–208.

50. Tielemans C, Gastaldello K, Husson C, et al. Efficacy of oral immunotherapy on respiratory infections in hemodialysis patients: a double-blind, placebo-controlled study. *Clin Nephrol* 1999;51:153–160.

51. Cunney RJ, Magee C, McNamara E, et al. *Clostridium difficile* colitis associated with chronic renal failure. *Nephrol Dial Transplant* 1998;13:2842–2846.

52. Lederman ED, McCoy G, Conti DJ, Lee EC. Diverticulitis and polycystic kidney disease. *Am Surg* 2000;66:200–203.

53. Naugle K, Darby ML, Bauman DB, et al. The oral health status of individuals on renal dialysis. *Ann Periodontol* 1998;3:197–205.

54. Rahmati MA, Craig RG, Homel P, et al. Serum markers of periodontal disease status and inflammation in hemodialysis patients. *Am J Kidney Dis* 2002;40:983–989.

55. DeStefano F, Anda RF, Kahn HS, et al. Dental disease and risk of coronary heart disease and mortality. *BMJ* 1993;306:688–691.

56. Berns JS. Infection with antimicrobial-resistant microorganisms in dialysis patients. *Semin Dial* 2003;16:30–37.

57. Smith TL, Pearson ML, Wilcox KR, et al. Emergence of vancomycin resistance in *Staphylococcus aureus*. Glycopeptide-Intermediate *Staphylococcus aureus* Working Group. *N Engl J Med* 1999;340:493–501.

58. Vanholder R, Van Biesen W. Incidence of infectious morbidity and mortality in dialysis patients. *Blood Purif* 2002;20:477–480.

59. Chou KJ, Fang HC, Bai KJ, et al. Tuberculosis in maintenance dialysis patients. *Nephron* 2001;88:138–143.

60. Hussein MM, Mooij JM, Roujouleh H. Tuberculosis and chronic renal disease. *Semin Dial* 2003;16:38–44.

61. Chia S, Karim M, Elwood RK, FitzGerald JM. Risk of tuberculosis in dialysis patients: a population-based study. *Int J Tuberc Lung Dis* 1998;2:989–991.

62. Simon TA, Paul S, Wartenberg D, Tokars JI. Tuberculosis in hemodialysis patients in New Jersey: a statewide study. *Infect Control Hosp Epidemiol* 1999;20:607–609.

63. Moore DA, Lightstone L, Javid B, Friedland JS. High rates of tuberculosis in end-stage renal failure: the impact of international migration. *Emerg Infect Dis* 2002;8:77–78.

64. Woeltje KF, Mathew A, Rothstein M, et al. Tuberculosis infection and anergy in hemodialysis patients. *Am J Kidney Dis* 1998;31:848–852.

65. Ozdemir FN, Guz G, Kayatas M, et al. Tuberculosis remains an important factor in the morbidity and mortality of hemodialysis patients. *Transplant Proc* 1998;30:846–847.

66. Quantrill SJ, Woodhead MA, Bell CE, et al. Side-effects of antituberculosis drug treatment in patients with chronic renal failure. *Eur Respir J* 2002;20:440–443.

67. Sessa A, Meroni M, Battini G, et al. Nosocomial outbreak of *Aspergillus fumigatus* infection among patients in a renal unit? *Nephrol Dial Transplant* 1996;11:1322–1324.

68. Boelaert JR, Fenves AZ, Coburn JW. Deferoxamine therapy and mucormycosis in dialysis patients: report of an international registry. *Am J Kidney Dis* 1991;18:660–667.

69. Boelaert JR, de Locht M, Van Cutsem J, et al. Mucormycosis during deferoxamine therapy is a siderophore-mediated infection. In vitro and in vivo animal studies. *J Clin Invest* 1993;91:1979–1986.

70. Krishnasami Z, Carlton D, Bimbo L, et al. Management of hemodialysis catheter-related bacteremia with an adjunctive antibiotic lock solution. *Kidney Int* 2002;61:1136–1142.

71. El Sayed NM, Gomatos PJ, Beck-Sague CM, et al. Epidemic transmission of human immunodeficiency virus in renal dialysis centers in Egypt. *J Infect Dis* 2000;181:91–97.

72. Rao TK. Human immunodeficiency virus infection in end-stage renal disease patients. *Semin Dial* 2003;16:233–244.

73. Cooper L. USRDS. 2001 Annual Data Report. *Nephrol News Issues* 2001;15:31,34–35,38.

74. From the Centers for Disease Control and Prevention. HIV and AIDS—United States, 1981–2000. *JAMA* 2001;285:3083–3084.

75. Arnow PM, Fellner S, Harrington R, Leuther M. False-positive results of screening for antibodies to human immunodeficiency virus in chronic hemodialysis patients. *Am J Kidney Dis* 1988;11:383–386.

76. Curi MA, Pappas PJ, Silva MB Jr, et al. Hemodialysis access: influence of the human immunodeficiency virus on patency and infection rates. *J Vasc Surg* 1999;29:608–616.

77. Mokrzycki MH, Schroppel B, von Gersdorff G, et al. Tunneled-cuffed catheter associated infections in hemodialysis patients who are seropositive for the human immunodeficiency virus. *J Am Soc Nephrol* 2000;11:2122–2127.

78. Fontana D, Schut R, Rabb H. Can choice of dialyser membrane have a beneficial effect on HIV load in the HIV-infected dialysis patient? *Nephrol Dial Transplant* 2002;17:529–530.

79. Ahuja TS, Niaz N, Velasco A, et al. Effect of hemodialysis and antiretroviral therapy on plasma viral load in HIV-1 infected hemodialysis patients. *Clin Nephrol* 1999;51:40–44.

80. Ahuja TS, Grady J, Khan S. Changing trends in the survival of dialysis patients with human immunodeficiency virus in the United States. *J Am Soc Nephrol* 2002;13:1889–1893.

81. Izzedine H, Launay-Vacher V, Baumelou A, Deray G. An appraisal of antiretroviral drugs in hemodialysis. *Kidney Int* 2001;60:821–830.

82. Kimmel PL, Umana WO, Simmens SJ, et al. Continuous ambulatory peritoneal dialysis and survival of HIV infected patients with end-stage renal disease. *Kidney Int* 1993;44:373–378.

83. Bell DM. Occupational risk of human immunodeficiency virus infection in healthcare workers: an overview. *Am J Med* 1997;102:9–15.

84. Harnett JD, Parfrey PS, Kennedy M, et al. The long-term outcome of hepatitis B infection in hemodialysis patients. *Am J Kidney Dis* 1988;11:210–213.

85. Cavdar C, Sayan M, Sifil A, et al. The comparison of antibody response to influenza vaccination in continuous ambu-

latory peritoneal dialysis, hemodialysis and renal transplantation patients. *Scand J Urol Nephrol* 2003;37:71–76.

86. Gilbertson DT, Unruh M, McBean AM, et al. Influenza vaccine delivery and effectiveness in end-stage renal disease. *Kidney Int* 2003;63:738–743.

87. Spisni C, Stingone A, Di Vito R, et al. Serum epidemiological trial on the prevalence of the anti-cytomegalovirus antibodies in patients under substitutive treatment with hemodialysis and CAPD. *Nephron* 1992;61:373–374.

88. Esforzado N, Poch E, Almirall J, et al. Cytomegalovirus colitis in chronic renal failure. *Clin Nephrol* 1993;39:275–278.

89. Grandaliano G, Teutonico A, Allegretti A, et al. The role of hyperparathyroidism, erythropoietin therapy, and CMV infection in the failure of arteriovenous fistula in hemodialysis. *Kidney Int* 2003;64:715–719.

90. Smetana Z, Leventon-Kriss S, Broide A, et al. Varicella-zoster virus immune status in CAPD and chronic hemodialysis patients. *Am J Nephrol* 1991;11:229–236.

91. Ikemoto S, Kamizuru M, Hayahara N, et al. Thymus lymphocytes in uraemic rats and the effect of thymosin fraction 5 in vivo. *Clin Exp Immunol* 1992;87:220–223.

92. Donati D, Degiannis D, Raskova J, Raska K Jr. Uremic serum effects on peripheral blood mononuclear cell and purified T lymphocyte responses. *Kidney Int* 1992;42:681–689.

93. Stachowski J, Pollok M, Burrichter H, Spithaler C, Baldamus CA. Signalling via the TCR/CD3 antigen receptor complex in uremia is limited by the receptors number. *Nephron* 1993;64:369–375.

94. Morra L, Moccia F, Gurreri G, et al. Effect of cimetidine on peripheral blood lymphocytes from chronic uremic patients: improvement of burst-promoting activity. *Acta Haematol* 1992;88:109–113.

95. Bhaskaran M, Ranjan R, Shah H, et al. Lymphopenia in dialysis patients: a preliminary study indicating a possible role of apoptosis. *Clin Nephrol* 2002;57:221–229.

96. Langhoff E, Ladefoged J, Odum N. Effect of interleukin-2 and methylprednisolone on in vitro transformation of uremic lymphocytes. *Int Arch Allergy Appl Immunol* 1986;81:5–11.

97. Asaka M, Iida H, Izumino K, Sasayama S. Depressed natural killer cell activity in uremia. Evidence for immunosuppressive factor in uremic sera. *Nephron* 1988;49:291–295.

98. Ladefoged J, Langhoff E. Accessory cell functions in mononuclear cell cultures uremic patients. *Kidney Int* 1990;37: 126–130.

99. Meuer SC, Dumann H, Meyer zum Buschenfelde KH, Kohler H. Low-dose interleukin-2 induces systemic immune responses against HBsAg in immunodeficient non-responders to hepatitis B vaccination. *Lancet* 1989;1:15–18.

100. Girndt M, Kohler H, Schiedhelm-Weick E, et al. T cell activation defect in hemodialysis patients: evidence for a role of the B7/CD28 pathway. *Kidney Int* 1993;44:359–365.

101. Descamps-Latscha B, Herbelin A, Nguyen AT, et al. Soluble CD23 as an effector of immune dysregulation in chronic uremia and dialysis. *Kidney Int* 1993;43:878–884.

102. Tetta C, David S, Biancone L, et al. Role of platelet activating factor in hemodialysis. *Kidney Int Suppl* 1993;39: S154–S157.

103. Ishizuka T, Nitta K, Yokoyama T, et al. Increased serum levels of interleukin-12 may be associated with Th1 differentiation in hemodialysis patients. *Nephron* 2002;90:503–504.

104. Sester U, Sester M, Hauk M, et al. T-cell activation follows Th1 rather than Th2 pattern in haemodialysis patients. *Nephrol Dial Transplant* 2000;15:1217–1223.

105. Moser B, Roth G, Brunner M, et al. Aberrant T cell activation and heightened apoptotic turnover in end-stage renal failure patients: a comparative evaluation between non-dialysis, haemodialysis, and peritoneal dialysis. *Biochem Biophys Res Commun* 2003;308:581–585.

106. Nitta K, Akiba T, Kawashima A, et al. Characterization of TH1/TH2 profile in uremic patients. *Nephron* 2002;91: 492–495.

107. Luger A, Kovarik J, Stummvoll HK, et al. Blood-membrane interaction in hemodialysis leads to increased cytokine production. *Kidney Int* 1987;32:84–88.

108. Haeffner-Cavaillon N, Cavaillon JM, Ciancioni C, et al. In vivo induction of interleukin-1 during hemodialysis. *Kidney Int* 1989;35:1212–1218.

109. Schindler R, Lonnemann G, Shaldon S, et al. Transcription, not synthesis, of interleukin-1 and tumor necrosis factor by complement. *Kidney Int* 1990;37:85–93.

110. Bingel M, Lonnemann G, Koch KM, et al. Plasma interleukin-1 activity during hemodialysis: the influence of dialysis membranes. *Nephron* 1988;50:273–276.

111. Lonnemann G, Koch KM, Shaldon S, Dinarello CA. Studies on the ability of hemodialysis membranes to induce, bind, and clear human interleukin-1. *J Lab Clin Med* 1988;112: 76–86.

112. Blumenstein M, Schmidt B, Ward RA, et al. Altered interleukin-1 production in patients undergoing hemodialysis. *Nephron* 1988;50:277–281.

113. Herbelin A, Nguyen AT, Zingraff J, et al. Influence of uremia and hemodialysis on circulating interleukin-1 and tumor necrosis factor alpha. *Kidney Int* 1990;37:116–125.

114. Herbelin A, Urena P, Nguyen AT, et al. Elevated circulating levels of interleukin-6 in patients with chronic renal failure. *Kidney Int* 1991;39:954–960.

115. Caglar K, Peng Y, Pupim LB, et al. Inflammatory signals associated with hemodialysis. *Kidney Int* 2002;62:1408–1416.

116. Herbelin A, Urena P, Nguyen AT, et al. Influence of first and long-term dialysis on uraemia-associated increased basal production of interleukin-1 and tumour necrosis factor alpha by circulating monocytes. *Nephrol Dial Transplant* 1991;6: 349–357.

117. Zaoui P, Green W, Hakim RM. Hemodialysis with cuprophane membrane modulates interleukin-2 receptor expression. *Kidney Int* 1991;39:1020–1026.

118. Beaurain G, Naret C, Marcon L, et al. In vivo T cell preactivation in chronic uremic hemodialyzed and non-hemodialyzed patients. *Kidney Int* 1989;36:636–644.

119. Roccatello D, Formica M, Cavalli G, et al. Serum and intracellular detection of cytokines in patients undergoing chronic hemodialysis. *Artif Organs* 1992;16:131–140.

120. Tarakcioglu M, Erbagci AB, Usalan C, et al. Acute effect of hemodialysis on serum levels of the proinflammatory cytokines. *Mediators Inflamm* 2003;12:15–19.

121. Ghysen J, De Plaen JF, van Ypersele DS. The effect of membrane characteristics on tumour necrosis factor kinetics during haemodialysis. *Nephrol Dial Transplant* 1990;5: 270–274.

122. Schindler R, Linnenweber S, Schulze M, et al. Gene expression of interleukin-1 beta during hemodialysis. *Kidney Int* 1993;43:712–721.

123. Mege JL, Olmer M, Purgus R, et al. Haemodialysis membranes modulate chronically the production of TNF alpha, IL1 beta and IL6. *Nephrol Dial Transplant* 1991;6:868–875.

124. van Riemsdijk-van Overbeeke IC, Baan CC, Knoop CJ, et al. Quantitative flow cytometry shows activation of the TNF-alpha system but not of the IL-2 system at the single cell level in renal replacement therapy. *Nephrol Dial Transplant* 2001;16:1430–1435.

125. Brunet P, Capo C, Dellacasagrande J, et al. IL-10 synthesis and secretion by peripheral blood mononuclear cells in haemodialysis patients. *Nephrol Dial Transplant* 1998;13: 1745–1751.

126. Himmelfarb J, Lazarus JM, Hakim R. Reactive oxygen species production by monocytes and polymorphonuclear leukocytes during dialysis. *Am J Kidney Dis* 1991;17: 271–276.

127. Schleiffenbaum B, Fehr J. The tumor necrosis factor receptor and human neutrophil function. Deactivation and cross-deactivation of tumor necrosis factor-induced neutrophil responses by receptor down-regulation. *J Clin Invest* 1990;86: 184–195.

128. Sunder-Plassmann G, Sedlacek PL, Sunder-Plassmann R, et al. Anti-interleukin-1 alpha autoantibodies in hemodialysis patients. *Kidney Int* 1991;40:787–791.

129. Pereira BJ, Poutsiaka DD, King AJ, et al. In vitro production of interleukin-1 receptor antagonist in chronic renal failure, CAPD and HD. *Kidney Int* 1992;42:1419–1424.

130. Cohen G. Immunoglobulin light chains in uremia. *Kidney Int Suppl* 2003;63:15–18.

131. Cohen G, Rudnicki M, Horl WH. Isolation of modified ubiquitin as a neutrophil chemotaxis inhibitor from uremic patients. *J Am Soc Nephrol* 1998;9:451–456.

132. Nguyen AT, Lethias C, Zingraff J, et al. Hemodialysis membrane-induced activation of phagocyte oxidative metabolism detected in vivo and in vitro within microamounts of whole blood. *Kidney Int* 1985;28:158–167.

133. Lucchi L, Cappelli G, Acerbi MA, et al. Oxidative metabolism of polymorphonuclear leukocytes and serum opsonic activity in chronic renal failure. *Nephron* 1989;51:44–50.

134. Ruiz P, Gomez F, Schreiber AD. Impaired function of macrophage Fc gamma receptors in end-stage renal disease. *N Engl J Med* 1990;322:717–722.

135. Haag-Weber M, Hable M, Fiedler G, et al. Alterations of polymorphonuclear leukocyte glycogen metabolism and glucose uptake in dialysis patients. *Am J Kidney Dis* 1991;17:562–568.

136. Vanholder R, Ringoir S, Dhondt A, Hakim R. Phagocytosis in uremic and hemodialysis patients: a prospective and cross sectional study. *Kidney Int* 1991;39:320–327.

137. Hakim RM, Fearon DT, Lazarus JM. Biocompatibility of dialysis membranes: effects of chronic complement activation. *Kidney Int* 1984;26:194–200.

138. Lucchi L, Bonucchi D, Acerbi MA, et al. Improved biocompatibility by modified cellulosic membranes: the case of hemophan. *Artif Organs* 1989;13:417–421.

139. Himmelfarb J, Ault KA, Holbrook D, et al. Intradialytic granulocyte reactive oxygen species production: a prospective, crossover trial. *J Am Soc Nephrol* 1993;4:178–186.

140. Vanholder R, Dell'Aquila R, Jacobs V, et al. Depressed phagocytosis in hemodialyzed patients: in vivo and in vitro mechanisms. *Nephron* 1993;63:409–415.

141. Roccatello D, Mazzucco G, Coppo R, et al. Functional changes of monocytes due to dialysis membranes. *Kidney Int* 1989;35:622–631.

142. Cohen MS, Elliott DM, Chaplinski T, et al. A defect in the oxidative metabolism of human polymorphonuclear leukocytes that remain in circulation early in hemodialysis. *Blood* 1982;60:1283–1289.

143. Klempner MS, Gallin JI, Balow JE, Van Kammen DP. The effect of hemodialysis and C5a des arg on neutrophil subpopulations. *Blood* 1980;55:777–783.

144. Lewis SL, Van Epps DE, Chenoweth DE. Leukocyte C5a receptor modulation during hemodialysis. *Kidney Int* 1987; 31:112–120.

145. Skubitz KM, Craddock PR. Reversal of hemodialysis granulocytopenia and pulmonary leukostasis: a clinical manifestation of selective down-regulation of granulocyte responses to C5adesarg. *J Clin Invest* 1981;67:1383–1391.

146. Cheung AK, Parker CJ, Hohnholt M. Beta2 integrins are required for neutrophil degranulation induced by hemodialysis membranes. *Kidney Int* 1993;43:649–660.

147. Himmelfarb J, Zaoui P, Hakim R. Modulation of granulocyte LAM-1 and MAC-1 during dialysis—a prospective, randomized controlled trial. *Kidney Int* 1992;41:388–395.

148. Alvarez V, Pulido R, Campanero MR, et al. Differentially regulated cell surface expression of leukocyte adhesion receptors on neutrophils. *Kidney Int* 1991;40:899–905.

149. David S, Tetta C, Camussi G, et al. Adherence of human monocytes to haemodialysis membranes. *Nephrol Dial Transplant* 1993;8:1223–1227.

150. Dhondt AW, Vanholder RC, Waterloos MA, et al. Leukocyte CD14 and CD45 expression during hemodialysis: polysulfone versus cuprophane. *Nephron* 1996;74:342–348.

151. Jacobson SH, Thylen P, Fernvik E, et al. Hemodialysis-activated granulocytes at the site of interstitial inflammation. *Am J Kidney Dis* 2002;39:854–861.

152. Cendoroglo M, Jaber BL, Balakrishnan VS, et al. Neutrophil apoptosis and dysfunction in uremia. *J Am Soc Nephrol* 1999;10:93–100.

153. Rosenkranz AR, Peherstorfer E, Kormoczi GF, et al. Complement-dependent acceleration of apoptosis in neutrophils by dialyzer membranes. *Kidney Int Suppl* 2001;78: S216–S220.

154. Cohen G, Rudnicki M, Deicher R, Horl WH. Immunoglobulin light chains modulate polymorphonuclear leucocyte apoptosis. *Eur J Clin Invest* 2003;33:669–676.

155. Schena FP, Pertosa G. Fibronectin and the kidney. *Nephron* 1988;48:177–182.

156. Abrutyn E, Solomons NW, St Clair L, et al. Granulocyte function in patients with chronic renal failure: surface adher-

ence, phagocytosis, and bactericidal activity in vitro. *J Infect Dis* 1977;135:1–8.

157. Peterson PK, Matzke G, Keane WF. Current concepts in the management of peritonitis in patients undergoing continuous ambulatory peritoneal dialysis. *Rev Infect Dis* 1987;9: 604–612.

158. Vanholder R, De Smet R, Jacobs V, et al. Uraemic toxic retention solutes depress polymorphonuclear response to phagocytosis. *Nephrol Dial Transplant* 1994;9:1271–1278.

159. Hällgren R, Fjellstrom KE, Hakansson L, Venge P. Kinetic studies of phagocytosis. II. The serum-independent uptake of IgG-coated particles by polymorphonuclear leukocytes from uremic patients on regular dialysis treatment. *J Lab Clin Med* 1979;94:277–284.

160. Lespier-Dexter LE, Guerra C, Ojeda W, Martinez-Maldonado M. Granulocyte adherence in uremia and hemodialysis. *Nephron* 1979;24:64–68.

161. Glazer T, Fishman P, Klein B, et al. Generation of superoxide anions during phagocytosis by monocytes of uremic patients. *Nephron* 1984;38:40–43.

162. Wardle EN, Williams R. Polymorph leucocyte function in uraemia and jaundice. *Acta Haematol* 1980; 64:157–164.

163. Vanholder R, De Smet R. Pathophysiologic effects of uremic retention solutes. *J Am Soc Nephrol* 1999;10: 1815–1823.

164. Wardle EN. Chemiluminescence and superoxide anions generated by phagocytes in uraemia. *Nephron* 1985;40:379.

165. Vanholder R, De Smet R, Waterloos MA, et al. Mechanisms of uremic inhibition of phagocyte reactive species production: characterization of the role of p-cresol. *Kidney Int* 1995;47:510–517.

166. Wratten ML, Tetta C, De Smet R, et al. Uremic ultrafiltrate inhibits platelet-activating factor synthesis. *Blood Purif* 1999;17:134–141.

167. Dou L, Cerini C, Brunet P, et al. P-cresol, a uremic toxin, decreases endothelial cell response to inflammatory cytokines. *Kidney Int* 2002;62:1999–2009.

168. Ferrante A. Inhibition of human neutrophil locomotion by the polyamine oxidase-polyamine system. *Immunology* 1985;54:785–790.

169. Diamant M, Henricks PA, Nijkamp FP, de Wied D. Beta-endorphin and related peptides suppress phorbol myristate acetate-induced respiratory burst in human polymorphonuclear leukocytes. *Life Sci* 1989;45:1537–1545.

170. Gyetko MR, Hsu CH, Wilkinson CC, et al. Monocyte 1 alpha-hydroxylase regulation: induction by inflammatory cytokines and suppression by dexamethasone and uremia toxin. *J Leukoc Biol* 1993; 54:17–22.

171. Hirayama A, Noronha-Dutra AA, Gordge MP, et al. Inhibition of neutrophil superoxide production by uremic concentrations of guanidino compounds. *J Am Soc Nephrol* 2000;11:684–689.

172. Hörl WH, Haag-Weber M, Georgopoulos A, Block LH. Physicochemical characterization of a polypeptide present in uremic serum that inhibits the biological activity of polymorphonuclear cells. *Proc Natl Acad Sci USA* 1990;87: 6353–6357.

173. Haag-Weber M, Mai B, Hörl WH. Isolation of a granulocyte inhibitory protein from uraemic patients with homology of beta 2-microglobulin. *Nephrol Dial Transplant* 1994; 9:382–388.

174. Massry SG. Parathyroid hormone: a uremic toxin. *Adv Exp Med Biol* 1987;223:1–17.

175. Esposito R, Romano-Carratelli C, Lanzetti N, et al. Toxicity in uremia: 2. Correlation between PTH levels and impaired aspecific immunity. *Int J Artif Organs* 1988;11:159–160.

176. Tuma SN, Martin RR, Mallette LE, Eknoyan G. Augmented polymorphonuclear chemiluminescence in patients with secondary hyperparathyroidism. *J Lab Clin Med* 1981;97: 291–298.

177. Massry SG, Schaefer RM, Teschner M, et al. Effect of parathyroid hormone on elastase release from human polymorphonuclear leucocytes. *Kidney Int* 1989; 36: 883–890.

178. Alexiewicz JM, Smogorzewski M, Fadda GZ, Massry SG. Impaired phagocytosis in dialysis patients: studies on mechanisms. *Am J Nephrol* 1991; 11: 102–111.

179. Alexiewicz JM, Smogorzewski M, Klin M, Akmal M, Massry SG. Effect of treatment of hemodialysis patients with nifedipine on metabolism and function of polymorphonuclear leukocytes. *Am J Kidney Dis* 1995; 25:440–444.

180. Alexiewicz JM, Smogorzewski M, Akmal M, Massry SG. A longitudinal study on the effect of nifedipine therapy and its discontinuation on [Ca2+]i and proliferation of B lymphocytes of dialysis patients. *Am J Kidney Dis* 1997;29: 233–238.

181. Yasunaga C, Nakamoto M, Matsuo K, et al. Effects of a parathyroidectomy on the immune system and nutritional condition in chronic dialysis patients with secondary hyperparathyroidism. *Am J Surg* 1999;178:332–336.

182. Lewin E, Ladefoged J, Brandi L, Olgaard K. Parathyroid hormone dependent T cell proliferation in uremic rats. *Kidney Int* 1993;44:379–384.

183. Tzanno-Martins C, Futata E, Jorgetti V, Duarte AJ. Immune response in hemodialysis patients: is there any difference when low and high iPTH levels are compared? *Clin Nephrol* 2000;54:22–29.

184. Stojceva-Taneva O, Fadda GZ, Smogorzewski M, Massry SG. Parathyroid hormone increases cytosolic calcium of thymocytes. *Nephron* 1993;64:592–599.

185. Witko V, Nguyen AT, Descamps-Latscha B. Microtiter plate assay for phagocyte-derived taurine-chloramines. *J Clin Lab Anal* 1992;6:47–53.

186. Thomas EL, Grisham MB, Jefferson MM. Myeloperoxidase-dependent effect of amines on functions of isolated neutrophils. *J Clin Invest* 1983;72:441–454.

187. Vallance P, Leone A, Calver A, et al. Accumulation of an endogenous inhibitor of nitric oxide synthesis in chronic renal failure. *Lancet* 1992;339:572–575.

188. Noris M, Benigni A, Boccardo P, et al. Enhanced nitric oxide synthesis in uremia: implications for platelet dysfunction and dialysis hypotension. *Kidney Int* 1993;44:445–450.

189. Rysz J, Luciak M, Kedziora J, et al. Nitric oxide release in the peripheral blood during hemodialysis. *Kidney Int* 1997;51:294–300.

190. Bloembergen WE, Stannard DC, Port FK, et al. Relationship of dose of hemodialysis and cause-specific mortality. *Kidney Int* 1996;50:557–565.

191. Tokars JI, Light P, Anderson J, et al. A prospective study of vascular access infections at seven outpatient hemodialysis centers. *Am J Kidney Dis* 2001;37:1232–1240.

192. Eknoyan G, Beck GJ, Cheung AK, et al. Effect of dialysis dose and membrane flux in maintenance hemodialysis. *N Engl J Med* 2002;347:2010–2019.

193. Collins HL. The role of iron in infections with intracellular bacteria. *Immunol Lett* 2003;85:193–195.

194. Collins HL, Kaufmann SH, Schaible UE. Iron chelation via deferoxamine exacerbates experimental salmonellosis via inhibition of the nicotinamide adenine dinucleotide phosphate oxidase-dependent respiratory burst. *J Immunol* 2002; 168:3458–3463.

195. Mencacci A, Cenci E, Boelaert JR, et al. Iron overload alters innate and T helper cell responses to *Candida albicans* in mice. *J Infect Dis* 1997;175:1467–1476.

196. Hoen B, Kessler M, Hestin D, Mayeux D. Risk factors for bacterial infections in chronic haemodialysis adult patients: a multicentre prospective survey. *Nephrol Dial Transplant* 1995;10:377–381.

197. Tielemans CL, Lenclud CM, Wens R, et al. Critical role of iron overload in the increased susceptibility of haemodialysis patients to bacterial infections. Beneficial effects of desferrioxamine. *Nephrol Dial Transplant* 1989;4:883–887.

198. Patruta SI, Edlinger R, Sunder-Plassmann G, Hörl WH. Neutrophil impairment associated with iron therapy in hemodialysis patients with functional iron deficiency. *J Am Soc Nephrol* 1998;9:655–663.

199. Deicher R, Ziai F, Cohen G, et al. High-dose parenteral iron sucrose depresses neutrophil intracellular killing capacity. *Kidney Int* 2003;64:728–736.

200. Sengoelge G, Kletzmayr J, Ferrara I, et al. Impairment of transendothelial leukocyte migration by iron complexes. *J Am Soc Nephrol* 2003;14:2639–2644.

201. Boelaert JR, Cantinieaux BF, Hariga CF, Fondu PG. Recombinant erythropoietin reverses polymorphonuclear granulocyte dysfunction in iron-overloaded dialysis patients. *Nephrol Dial Transplant* 1990; 5: 504–517

202. Marx JJ. Iron and infection: competition between host and microbes for a precious element. *Best Pract Res Clin Haematol* 2002;15:411–426.

203. Veys N, Vanholder R, Ringoir S. Correction of deficient phagocytosis during erythropoietin treatment in maintenance hemodialysis patients. *Am J Kidney Dis* 1992;19: 358–363.

204. Robertson HT, Haley NR, Guthrie M, et al. Recombinant erythropoietin improves exercise capacity in anemic hemodialysis patients. *Am J Kidney Dis* 1990;15:325–332.

205. Schaefer RM, Paczek L, Berthold G, et al. Improved immunoglobulin production in dialysis patients treated with recombinant erythropoietin. *Int J Artif Organs* 1992;15: 204–208.

206. Collart FE, Dratwa M, Wittek M, Wens R. Effects of recombinant human erythropoietin on T lymphocyte subsets in hemodialysis patients. *ASAIO Trans* 1990;36:M219–M223.

207. Barany P, Fehrman I, Godoy C. Long-term effects on lymphocytotoxic antibodies and immune reactivity in hemodialysis patients treated with recombinant human erythropoietin. *Clin Nephrol* 1992;37:90–96.

208. Sennesael JJ, Van der NP, Verbeelen DL. Treatment with recombinant human erythropoietin increases antibody titers after hepatitis B vaccination in dialysis patients. *Kidney Int* 1991;40:121–128.

209. Hisatomi K, Isomura T, Galli SJ, et al. Augmentation of interleukin-2 production after cardiac operations in patients treated with erythropoietin. *J Thora Cardiovasc Surg* 1992;104:278–283.

210. Vanholder R, Cornelis R, Dhondt A, Lameire N. The role of trace elements in uraemic toxicity. *Nephrol Dial Transplant* 2002;17(suppl 2):2–8.

211. Daum JR, Shepherd DM, Noelle RJ. Immunotoxicology of cadmium and mercury on B-lymphocytes—I. Effects on lymphocyte function. *Int J Immunopharmacol* 1993;15: 383–394.

212. Pelletier O, Hill I, Birnboim HC. Inhibition by superoxide dismutase-mimetic copper complexes of phorbol ester-induced respiratory burst in human granulocytes. *Biochem Pharmacol* 1992;43:1061–1066.

213. Schlesinger L, Arevalo M, Arredondo S, et al. Effect of a zinc-fortified formula on immunocompetence and growth of malnourished infants. *Am J Clin Nutr* 1992; 56: 491–498.

214. Ozbal E, Helvaci M, Kasirga E, et al. Serum zinc as a factor predicting response to interferon-alpha2b therapy in children with chronic hepatitis B. *Biol Trace Elem Res* 2002;90:31–38.

215. Kimmel PL, Phillips TM, Lew SQ, Langman CB. Zinc modulates mononuclear cellular calcitriol metabolism in peritoneal dialysis patients. *Kidney Int* 1996;49:1407–1412.

216. Turk S, Bozfakioglu S, Ecder ST, et al. Effects of zinc supplementation on the immune system and on antibody response to multivalent influenza vaccine in hemodialysis patients. *Int J Artif Organs* 1998;21:274–278.

217. Cohen JD, Viljoen M, Clifford D, et al. Plasma vitamin E levels in a chronically hemolyzing group of dialysis patients. *Clin Nephrol* 1986;25:42–47.

218. De Bevere VO, Nelis HJ, De Leenheer AP, et al. Vitamin E levels in hemodialysis patients. *JAMA* 1982;247:2371.

219. Stein G, Richter G, Funfstuck R, et al. Serum vitamin E levels in patients with chronic renal failure. *Int J Artif Organs* 1983;6:285–287.

220. Delafuente JC. Nutrients and immune responses. *Rheum Dis Clin North Am* 1991;17:203–212.

221. Taccone-Gallucci M, Giardini O, Ausiello C, et al. Vitamin E supplementation in hemodialysis patients: effects on peripheral blood mononuclear cells lipid peroxidation and immune response. *Clin Nephrol* 1986;25:81–86.

222. Descombes E, Hanck AB, Fellay G. Water soluble vitamins in chronic hemodialysis patients and need for supplementation. *Kidney Int* 1993;43:1319–1328.

223. Axelrod AE. Immune processes in vitamin deficiency states. *Am J Clin Nutr* 1971;24:265–271.

224. Kriley M, Warady BA. Vitamin status of pediatric patients receiving long-term peritoneal dialysis. *Am J Clin Nutr* 1991;53:1476–1479.

225. Thomas S, Fischer FP, Mettang T, et al. Effects of L-carnitine on leukocyte function and viability in hemodialysis patients: a double-blind randomized trial. *Am J Kidney Dis* 1999;34:678–687.

226. Provvedini DM, Tsoukas CD, Deftos LJ, Manolagas SC. 1,25-dihydroxyvitamin D3 receptors in human leukocytes. *Science* 1983;221:1181–1183.

227. Duits AJ, Dimjati W, van de Winkel JG, Capel PJ. Synergism of interleukin 6 and 1 alpha,25-dihydroxyvitamin D3 in induction of myeloid differentiation of human leukemic cell lines. *J Leukoc Biol* 1992;51:237–243.

228. Hsu CH, Vanholder R, Patel S, et al. Subfractions in uremic plasma ultrafiltrate inhibit calcitriol metabolism. *Kidney Int* 1991;40:868–873.

229. Hsu CH, Patel SR, Young EW, Vanholder R. Effects of purine derivatives on calcitriol metabolism in rats. *Am J Physiol* 1991;260:F596–F601.

230. Hsu CH, Patel SR, Young EW, Vanholder R. The biological action of calcitriol in renal failure. *Kidney Int* 1994;46: 605–612.

231. Hubel E, Kiefer T, Weber J, et al. In vivo effect of 1,25-dihydroxyvitamin D3 on phagocyte function in hemodialysis patients. *Kidney Int* 1991;40:927–933.

232. Vanholder R, Patel S, Hsu CH. Effect of uric acid on plasma levels of 1,25(OH)2D in renal failure. *J Am Soc Nephrol* 1993;4:1035–1038.

233. Glorieux G, Hsu CH, De Smet R, et al. Inhibition of calcitriol-induced monocyte CD14 expression by uremic toxins: role of purines. *J Am Soc Nephrol* 1998;9:1826–1831.

234. Reichel H, Recker A, Deppisch R, et al. 25-Hydroxyvitamin D3 metabolism in vitro by mononuclear cells from hemodialysis patients. *Nephron* 1992;62:404–412.

235. Antonen JA, Hannula PM, Pyhala R, et al. Adequate seroresponse to influenza vaccination in dialysis patients. *Nephron* 2000;86:56–61.

236. Moe SM, Zekonis M, Harezlak J, et al. A placebo-controlled trial to evaluate immunomodulatory effects of paracalcitol. *Am J Kidney Dis* 2001;38:792–802.

237. Hakim RM, Breillatt J, Lazarus JM, Port FK. Complement activation and hypersensitivity reactions to dialysis membranes. *N Engl J Med* 1984;311:878–882.

238. Hakim RM. Clinical implications of hemodialysis membrane biocompatibility. *Kidney Int* 1993;44:484–494.

239. Simms HH, Frank MM, Quinn TC, et al. Studies on phagocytosis in patients with acute bacterial infections. *J Clin Invest* 1989;83:252–260.

240. Moore FD Jr, Davis C, Rodrick M, et al. Neutrophil activation in thermal injury as assessed by increased expression of complement receptors. *N Engl J Med* 1986;314:948–953.

241. Solomkin JS, Cotta LA, Ogle JD, et al. Complement-induced expression of cryptic receptors on the neutrophil surface: a mechanism for regulation of acute inflammation in trauma. *Surgery* 1984;96:336–344.

242. Solomkin JS, Jenkins MK, Nelson RD, et al. Neutrophil dysfunction in sepsis. II. Evidence for the role of complement activation products in cellular deactivation. *Surgery* 1981;90:319–327.

243. Nelson RD, McCormack RT, Fiegel VD, et al. Chemotactic deactivation of human neutrophils: possible relationship to stimulation of oxidative metabolism. *Infect Immun* 1979;23: 282–286.

244. Maderazo EG, Woronick CL, Albano SD, et al. Inappropriate activation, deactivation, and probable autooxidative damage as a mechanism of neutrophil locomotory defect in trauma. *J Infect Dis* 1986;154:471–477.

245. Hornberger JC, Chernew M, Petersen J, Garber AM. A multivariate analysis of mortality and hospital admissions with high-flux dialysis. *J Am Soc Nephrol* 1992;3:1227–1237.

246. Klein E, Pass T, Harding GB, et al. Microbial and endotoxin contamination in water and dialysate in the central United States. *Artif Organs* 1990;14:85–94.

247. Takahashi I, Kotani S, Takada H, et al. Structural requirements of endotoxic lipopolysaccharides and bacterial cell walls in induction of interleukin-1. *Blood Purif* 1988;6: 188–206.

248. Ronco C, Feriani M, Chiaramonte S, et al. Backfiltration in clinical dialysis. Nature of the phenomenon and possible solutions. *Contrib Nephrol* 1990;77:96–105.

249. Lonnemann G, Bingel M, Floege J, et al. Detection of endotoxin-like interleukin-1-inducing activity during in vitro dialysis. *Kidney Int* 1988;33:29–35.

250. Pereira BJ, Snodgrass BR, Hogan PJ, King AJ. Diffusive and convective transfer of cytokine-inducing bacterial products across hemodialysis membranes. *Kidney Int* 1995;47: 603–610.

251. Vanholder R, Van Haecke E, Veys N, Ringoir S. Endotoxin transfer through dialysis membranes: small- versus large-pore membranes. *Nephrol Dial Transplant* 1992;7:333–339.

252. Mege JL, Sanguedolce MV, Purgus R, et al. Chronic and intradialytic effects of high-flux hemodialysis on tumor necrosis factor-alpha production: relationship to endotoxins. *Am J Kidney Dis* 1992;20:482–488.

253. Powell AC, Bland LE, Oettinger CW, et al. Lack of plasma interleukin-1 beta or tumor necrosis factor-alpha elevation during unfavorable hemodialysis conditions. *J Am Soc Nephrol* 1991;2:1007–1013.

254. Grooteman MP, Nube MJ, Daha MR, et al. Cytokine profiles during clinical high-flux dialysis: no evidence for cytokine generation by circulating monocytes. *J Am Soc Nephrol* 1997;8:1745–1754.

255. Kumano K, Yokota S, Nanbu M, Sakai T. Do cytokine-inducing substances penetrate through dialysis membranes and stimulate monocytes? *Kidney Int Suppl* 1993;41: S205–S208.

256. Schouten WE, Grooteman MP, Van Houte AJ, et al. Effects of dialyser and dialysate on the acute phase reaction in clinical bicarbonate dialysis. *Nephrol Dial Transplant* 2000;15: 379–384.

257. van Tellingen A, Grooteman MP, Schoorl M, et al. Intercurrent clinical events are predictive of plasma C-reactive protein levels in hemodialysis patients. *Kidney Int* 2002;62: 632–638.

258. Honkanen E, Gronhagen-Riska C, Teppo AM, et al. Acute-phase proteins during hemodialysis: correlations with serum interleukin-1 beta levels and different dialysis membranes. *Nephron* 1991;57:283–287.

259. Carozzi S, Nasini MG, Caviglia PM, et al. Acetate free biofiltration. Effects on peripheral blood monocyte activation and cytokine release. *ASAIO J* 1992;38:52–54.

260. Todeschini M, Macconi D, Fernandez NG, et al. Effect of acetate-free biofiltration and bicarbonate hemodialysis on neutrophil activation. *Am J Kidney Dis* 2002;40:783–793.

261. Schwab SJ, Weiss MA, Rushton F, et al. Multicenter clinical trial results with the LifeSite hemodialysis access system. *Kidney Int* 2002;62:1026–1033.

262. Cowan MM, Taylor KG, Doyle RJ. Role of sialic acid in the kinetics of *Streptococcus sanguis* adhesion to artificial pellicle. *Infect Immun* 1987;55:1552–1557.

263. Vanholder R, Hoenich N, Ringoir S. Morbidity and mortality of central venous catheter hemodialysis: a review of 10 years' experience. *Nephron* 1987;47:274–279.

264. Kherlakian GM, Roedersheimer LR, Arbaugh JJ, et al. Comparison of autogenous fistula versus expanded polytetrafluoroethylene graft fistula for angioaccess in hemodialysis. *Am J Surg* 1986;152:238–243.

265. Bambauer R, Mestres P, Schiel R, et al. Long-term catheters for apheresis and dialysis with surface treatment with infection resistance and low thrombogenicity. *Ther Apher Dial* 2003;7:225–231.

266. Swartz R, Messana J, Starmann B, et al. Preventing *Staphylococcus aureus* infection during chronic peritoneal dialysis. *J Am Soc Nephrol* 1991;2:1085–1091.

267. Boelaert JR, De Baere YA, Geernaert MA, et al. The use of nasal mupirocin ointment to prevent *Staphylococcus aureus* bacteraemias in haemodialysis patients: an analysis of cost-effectiveness. *J Hosp Infect* 1991;19(suppl B):41–46.

268. Vanholder R, Van Biesen W, Van Lanschoot N, et al. Relationship between phagocyte metabolic function and years of maintenance dialysis. *ASAIO Trans* 1990;36:M469–M472.

269. Ringoir S, Van Looy L, Van de HP, Leroux-Roels G. Impairment of phagocytic activity of macrophages as studied by the skin window test in patients on regular hemodialysis treatment. *Clin Nephrol* 1975;4:234–236.

270. Vanholder R, Van Biesen W, Ringoir S. Contributing factors to the inhibition of phagocytosis in hemodialyzed patients. *Kidney Int* 1993;44:208–214.

271. Donati D, Degiannis D, Homer L, et al. Immune deficiency in uremia: interleukin-2 production and responsiveness and interleukin-2 receptor expression and release. *Nephron* 1991;58:268–275.

272. Young GA, Kopple JD, Lindholm B, et al. Nutritional assessment of continuous ambulatory peritoneal dialysis patients: an international study. *Am J Kidney Dis* 1991;17: 462–471.

273. Gherini S, Vaughn BK, Lombardi AV Jr, Mallory TH. Delayed wound healing and nutritional deficiencies after total hip arthroplasty. *Clin Orthop* 1993;188–195.

274. Sullivan DA, Vaerman JP, Soo C. Influence of severe protein malnutrition on rat lacrimal, salivary and gastrointestinal immune expression during development, adulthood and ageing. *Immunology* 1993;78:308–317.

275. Redmond HP, Leon P, Lieberman MD, et al. Impaired macrophage function in severe protein-energy malnutrition. *Arch Surg* 1991;126:192–196.

276. Villa ML, Ferrario E, Bergamasco E, et al. Reduced natural killer cell activity and IL-2 production in malnourished cancer patients. *Br J Cancer* 1991;63:1010–1014.

277. Redmond HP, Shou J, Kelly CJ, et al. Immunosuppressive mechanisms in protein-calorie malnutrition. *Surgery* 1991;110:311–317.

278. Churchill DN, Taylor DW, Cook RJ, et al. Canadian Hemodialysis Morbidity Study. *Am J Kidney Dis* 1992;19: 214–234.

279. Field CJ, Gougeon R, Marliss EB. Changes in circulating leukocytes and mitogen responses during very-low-energy all-protein reducing diets. *Am J Clin Nutr* 1991;54:123–129.

280. Abbott KC, Napier MG, Agodoa LY. Hospitalizations for bacterial septicemia in patients with end stage renal disease due to diabetes on the renal transplant waiting list. *J Nephrol* 2002;15:248–254.

281. Peces R, de la TM, Alcazar R, Urra JM. Prospective analysis of the factors influencing the antibody response to hepatitis B vaccine in hemodialysis patients. *Am J Kidney Dis* 1997;29:239–245.

282. Balakrishnan VS, Schmid CH, Jaber BL, et al. Interleukin-1 receptor antagonist synthesis by peripheral blood mononuclear cells: a novel predictor of morbidity among hemodialysis patients. *J Am Soc Nephrol* 2000;11:2114–2121.

283. Waterlot Y, Cantinieaux B, HarIgA-Muller C, et al. Impaired phagocytic activity of neutrophils in patients receiving haemodialysis: the critical role of iron overload. *Br Med J (Clin Res Ed)* 1985;291:501–504.

284. Nsouli KA, Lazarus M, Schoenbaum SC, et al. Bacteremic infection in hemodialysis. *Arch Intern Med.* 1979;139: 1255–1258.

285. Quarles LD, Rutsky EA, Rostand SG. *Staphylococcus aureus* bacteremia in patients on chronic hemodialysis. *Am J Kidney Dis* 1985;6:412–419.

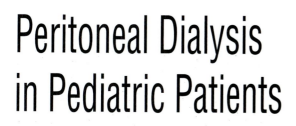

Peritoneal Dialysis in Pediatric Patients

Cornelis H. Schröder

Peritoneal dialysis (PD) can be applied both in acute and chronic renal failure. The choice of dialysis modality in these conditions depends on a number of variables. For HD and the various continuous hemofiltration techniques, an adequate vascular access is required. The advantage of the more rapid removal of fluid and metabolites by these latter modalities counteracts the more complicated technical equipment and procedures. Finally, the experience and preference of the center are important with respect to the choice of dialysis modality. In neonates with inborn errors of metabolism, continuous venovenous hemodiafiltration has largely replaced PD as a treatment modality because of the much more rapid clearance of metabolites with this method.[1,2] If PD is an option for the treatment of chronic renal failure, psychosocial characteristics of the child and his or her family are important determinants. Age, maturation, distance from the dialysis center, and other family characteristics influence the balance of choice between PD and HD.

In recent years the European Paediatric Peritoneal Dialysis Working Group (EPPWG) has prepared several guidelines with respect to the treatment of children on PD.[3–7]

THE PERITONEAL DIALYSIS SYSTEM

PD starts with the insertion of an appropriate catheter. Whereas in the past stiff catheters were popular in the treatment of acute renal failure, these are now replaced by soft polyurethane catheters in most centers. Stiff catheters have the advantage of an easy removal after recovery of renal function but are subject to a number of complications such as leakage and obstruction of outflow. These complications have a considerably lower frequency if cuffed polyurethane catheters are used. In the 1980s an extensive discussion was carried on in the literature about the catheter type to be used. This discussion is not yet completely closed. Most centers adhere to the classic Tenckhoff catheter with two

Dacron cuffs, the one placed just above the peritoneal membrane and the other in the subcutaneous tissue about 1.5 cm from the exit site. The tip of the catheter should be located in Douglas's cavity. Both median and paramedian localization of the catheter can be used. This classic catheter placement results in an upward direction of the catheter tunnel. It was Twardowski's group that drew attention to the fact that upward-directed tunnels would tend more to infection because of the possible accumulation of blood, sweat, and dust as well as the more difficult effluence of eventually present pus.[8] They developed the so-called swan-neck catheter, which is bent between the two cuffs, allowing positioning of the catheter tip in Douglas's cavity as well as the creation of a downward-directed catheter tunnel. This catheter is still widely used, notwithstanding the more difficult surgical implantation technique. More recently swan-neck catheters were advocated in a review on this topic.[9] The difficult surgical technique, together with the fact that, in the younger age group, the relatively low localization of the exit site on the abdominal wall interfered with hygiene and dressing, brought us to the decision to abandon the swan-neck catheter and to return to the simple straight double-cuffed Tenckhoff catheter. According to the 1996 NAPRTCS report, swan-neck catheters were used only 19 percent of time.[10] Many pediatric centers have replaced the straight Tenckhoff catheter with the coil variant, since the latter is reported to reduce infusion pain.[11]

Peritoneal dialysis catheters are available in different sizes. There are adult, pediatric, and neonatal catheters. The adult type can easily be used in all children having a body weight over 10 kg. In smaller ones, the pediatric-type catheters can be applied. Special adaptations are required only in newborns, having a body weight of 3 kg or less. Since our experience with the neonatal type catheter—though limited—has not been positive, a single-cuffed pediatric type Tenckhoff catheter is used in this category of patients. The cuff is localized at the peritoneum/fascia level. A subcutaneous cuff is not placed in these newborns, since this can easily cause erosion through the thin abdominal wall.

All catheters are inserted under general anesthesia in the operating theater by an experienced pediatric surgeon. Patency of the catheter is checked immediately after insertion, and dialysis started as soon as the patient is back on the ward.

Also in children, laparoscopic catheter placement is feasible and has been applied with good results.[12]

Several PD systems are commercially available. There is equipment for both continuous ambulatory PD (CAPD) and automated PD (APD). Since in pediatric PD CAPD has been largely abandoned and replaced by APD, this chapter focuses mainly on the latter. Children are generally treated with nightly intermittent PD (NIPD) or continuous cycling PD (CCPD). Essential are the ways of connecting the tubing to the dialysis bags. Since this connection will be opened several times a day, special attention must be paid to this part of the system so as to prevent infectious complications. Currently, the double-bag Y system for CAPD is universally used. Unfortunately, this system is available only in volumes of 1500 mL and higher. In this system, the draining and the filling bags are connected to each other by Y-shaped tubing. This allows the patient to drain before fill through the same tubing, thus minimizing the chance of infection after unintended contamination. Using this system, an incidence of peritonitis as low as one episode every 37 months has been reported.[13]

The composition of the PD fluid is a matter of debate. The composition of a typical commercially available preparation is given in Table 19–1. All compounds are extensively discussed in the literature. Several authors consider the sodium concentration of these preparations too high for adult overhydrated patients.[14–16] They observe favorable results using sodium concentrations as low as 100 mmol/L. For infants, on the contrary, the sodium concentration of the dialysis fluid appears to be too low, since urinary sodium losses may cause hyponatremia in this group. The calcium concentration of the dialysis fluid may be lowered to allow for the administration of larger amounts of oral phosphate-binding calcium salts, so as to prevent renal osteodystrophy. Although experience with low-calcium (1.25 mmol/L) in children is very limited,[17] the results and experience in studies in adult patients confirm this theory.[18–20] On the other hand, it should be remembered that secondary hyperparathyroidism with long-term low-calcium dialysis may develop even if normocalcemia is obtained.[21–23] Although there is no specific pediatric literature on this topic, it can be assumed that this may also occur in children. A slightly positive calcium balance might be needed in children because of the growing skeleton. With respect to calcium balance in pediatric PD, an individualized strategy avoiding high calcium supply is required.[24]

Most controversy, however, exists regarding the buffer and osmotic agent used. These are responsible for the low pH (5.5) and high osmolarity (340 to 512 mOsm/L) of the dialysis fluid. Cytotoxic effects both on peritoneal macrophages and mesothelial cells have been described.[25,26]

TABLE 19–1. COMPOSITION OF A TYPICAL SOLUTION FOR CONVENTIONAL PERITONEAL DIALYSIS

Sodium (mmol/L)	132–134
Calcium (mmol/L)	1.75
Magnesium (mmol/L)	0.25–0.75
Chloride (mmol/L)	96–104
Lactate (mmol/L)	35–40
Glucose (%)	1.36–4.25
Osmolarity (mOsm/kg)	340–512
pH	5.5

Much research is currently aimed at finding alternative agents for lactate and glucose.

The number of reports of using bicarbonate as a more physiologic buffer is increasing. This can only be applied if a double bag is created, one side containing glucose and calcium and the other sodium bicarbonate. The contents of these bags must be mixed shortly before administration. Bicarbonate-buffered solutions have a more physiologic pH (7.0 to 7.6) than lactate-based solutions (5.5 to 6.5). Most of the studies performed with these solutions report positive results compared with lactate-buffered dialysis solutions.[27–29] In vitro studies have shown markedly better preserved function of both macrophages and human peritoneal mesothelial cells.[30–34] An effective control of acid-base balance is demonstrated by several in vivo studies.[35–39] An interesting property of this solution is the lower incidence of infusion pain.[40] Infusion pain is generally agreed to be due to the acidity of the conventional solutions. Studies in adult patients demonstrate a clear reduction of infusion pain and discomfort. This property is particularly important for children, who are generally treated with short dwell times. Although there is a long experience in the pediatric dialysis centers with the use of custom-made bicarbonate dialysis solutions in patients with lactate acidosis, the experience in chronic PD is still limited. Neutral pH is particularly relevant in children on NIPD, where frequent short cycles continuously expose the peritoneal membrane to a cytotoxic acidic milieu. With the use of a pH-neutral dialysis solution in a peritoneal equilibration test, no differences from the conventional solutions were seen with respect to solute and fluid transport.[41] In addition, a more effective correction of metabolic acidosis and better preservation of peritoneal cell mass (measured by using the marker CA 125) were observed with the use of a pH-neutral bicarbonate-buffered solution.[42] It is known that inflow pain can be treated by pH adjustment of the dialysis fluid with bicarbonate.[40] Recently, it was shown in children that, in addition to the absence of infusion pain, intraperitoneal pressure was lower and vasodilatory effects were reduced with the use of a pH-neutral solution.[43]

The commonly used osmotic agent glucose has the disadvantage of huge absorption, thus impairing ultrafiltration, particularly if long dwell times are applied (as in CCPD). The absorption also gives rise to metabolic disturbances such as hyperlipidemia and the accumulation of toxic glucose degradation products (GDPs) and advanced glycation end products (AGEs). Substances that are absorbed to a lesser degree are being looked for.

Because of the continuous loss of proteins and amino acids during PD, the addition of amino acids to the dialysis fluid has been advocated.[44] Amino acids can contribute as osmotic agents: a 1.1% amino acid solution has a similar ultrafiltration profile as a 1.36% glucose solution.[45] With this approach, the nutritional state of the patient is expected to improve. There are until now, however, no studies proving this positive effect. The few pediatric studies have failed to demonstrate the superiority of amino acid dialysis with respect to nutrition or weight gain.[46–49] From recent guidelines, an uncertain future for amino acid dialysis has been predicted.[4] Other osmotic agents, such as glycerol and polypeptides, have received attention in the literature but are not likely to be applied on a large scale.

An interesting dialysis solution is icodextrin, a mixture of glucose polymers with an average molecular weight of 16 kDa. The 7.5% solution is isosmolar (284 mOsm/L), but it is also acidic (pH 5.2). Polyglucose solutions have been extensively studied in both adults and children. The commercially available polyglucose solution (icodextrin 7.5%) contains glucose polymers with an average molecular weight of 16,200 Da. Because of the low adsorption of these high-molecular-weight substances, ultrafiltration is sustained, making icodextrin very suitable for long dwell times.[50–52] In adult patients, improved ultrafiltration during a daytime dwell was obtained with icodextrin compared to glucose 1.36 percent.[53] De Boer et al. studied the effects of icodextrin in 11 children who were being treated with NIPD.[54] Icodextrin was compared with glucose 1.36% and glucose 3.86% for a 12-hour dwell period. Net ultrafiltration obtained with the icodextrin solution was similar to that obtained with the glucose 3.86% solution and significantly higher than that observed with the glucose 1.36% solution. In these children the daily administration of icodextrin added a mean of 0.52 (standard deviation 0.07) to weekly KT/V urea because of the longer time on dialysis. This increased adequacy was confirmed in a more recent pediatric study showing a mean increase of weekly KT/V of 0.55.[55] The sustained but slow ultrafiltration is illustrated by the absence of a decline in dialysate sodium concentration in the group treated with icodextrin—a phenomenon normally occurring in patients treated with 3.86% glucose, who are presumed to have a normally functioning peritoneal membrane.[56,57] In the 4-hour peritoneal equilibration test net ultrafiltration is much lower than with the use of a 3.86% glucose solution.[58]

The potential toxicity of icodextrin solutions has been studied in both adults and children, yielding similar results.[50,54,59] In a study in which icodextrin was prescribed for the daytime dwell in children on NIPD for 6 weeks, icodextrin blood levels rapidly increased to a steady state, which was reached after 2 weeks.[54] Two weeks after discontinuation of the study, icodextrin was no longer detectable in the blood. Blood levels of the main metabolites of icodextrin (maltose, maltotriose, and maltotetrose) followed a similar pattern. Concentrations were identical to those measured in adult patients.[50,59] Hypersensitivity reactions to icodextrin have been reported in some patients.[60–62] In the one pediatric study, a hypersensitivity reaction was observed in 1 out of 11 patients.[54] In adult patients, long-term experience with icodextrin is increasing; in children, experience is still very limited. An outbreak of sterile peritonitis after icodextrin administration was recently reported[63]; this was caused by contamination of the solution with a peptidoglycan during the manufacturing process, and the problem has now been resolved.[64]

THE PERITONEAL DIALYSIS MODALITY

Essentially a choice between standard manual CAPD and APD must be made. Traditional CAPD consists of four (three to five) daily exchanges of the dialysate, whereas APD represents a number of methods. For pediatric applications, a very attractive mode of APD is NIPD, allowing discontinuation of dialysis during the daytime. Appetite is diminished in PD patients of all ages and may be negatively influenced both by the presence of a considerable amount of fluid in the peritoneal cavity and the absorption of glucose.[65] A case history of dramatic improvement in the nutritional state after conversion from CAPD to NIPD has been presented.[66] Nevertheless, tube feeding is often necessary in young children on PD.[67–69] At present, the placement of a gastrostomy, preferably before PD is started, is preferred by many centers over tube feeding.[70–73] A recently described scoring system may be of help in the decision for more aggressive feeding regimens.[74] APD is the only available PD technique for newborns, since commercially available fluid amounts prohibit the treatment of this age category with CAPD. The application of NIPD may be restricted by the dialysis dose needed: if KT/V urea or weekly creatinine clearances (see below) are unacceptably low, a combination of NIPD and CAPD may be administered, with five to six automated cycles at night, and, for example, two daily exchanges; in many cases one long-time daytime dwell with icodextrin-containing solutions may be sufficient to obtain adequate dialysis. It should be kept in mind that the more complicated dialysis schedules considerably burden family life. One of the main reasons to choose a NIPD regimen is psychosocial: both child and parents are free during the daytime and do not have to worry about dialysis. Their activities are restricted to the assembly of the cycler in the evening, which takes about 20 minutes, and disconnection of the patient in the morning. The child's restlessness during the night may provoke alarms (from lying on the tubing) and may, if excessive, become a contraindication for NIPD. After drainage of the fluid, abdominal pain may sometimes occur; this can be prevented by not completely emptying the abdomen, thus providing a sort of tidal PD.[75]

Several cyclers are available for the performance of APD. Cyclers are portable, hence adding great value to the patients' freedom and comfort.

THE PERITONEAL DIALYSIS PRESCRIPTION

Traditionally, fill volumes of 40 (30 to 50) mL/kg body weight are applied for pediatric PD. There has been much controversy on the volume to be used. Most of this controversy is due to the theoretical basis of peritoneal transport, of which knowledge has been extended in recent years. Since the peritoneal surface area is related to body surface area more than to body weight, it seems logical to relate fluid amounts to body surface area and not body weight.[76] If calculations are based on the standard volume used in adult PD patients (2000 mL), a volume of about 1200 mL/m^2 will have to be administered to children. This leads to large differences in the youngest age group: a newborn baby (3 kg; 0.25 m^2) will receive a fill volume of 120 mL if 40 mL/kg is used but of 300 mL if 1200 mL/m^2 is used. This high volume elicits the apprehension of many pediatric nephrologists, although there are strong recommendations in the literature to use volumes of 800 to 1400 mL/m^2. These recommendations are based on the results of studies of peritoneal equilibration tests as well as on accumulating evidence regarding intraperitoneal pressure. The peritoneal equilibration test (PET) was introduced by Twardowski et al. to characterize peritoneal permeability for solutes in adults.[77] After the infusion of the dialysis fluid, dialysate samples are drawn at 1, 2, 3, and 4 hours and a blood sample at 2 hours to allow calculation of dialysate-to-plasma (D/P) ratios for urea and creatinine and D_t/D_0 ratios for glucose. If a marker molecule is added to the dialysis fluid, water movement (ultrafiltration as well as reabsorption) can also be studied. The PET has been adapted for children by several groups but unfortunately not in a standardized way. This lack of standardization makes it difficult to compare the results of different studies but sheds new light on the problem of the volume to be used. If dialysis volume is scheduled according to body weight, age-dependent differences in the handling of glucose and metabolites are observed.[78–81] Younger children transport glucose and metabolites more rapidly than older ones, and the latter more rapidly than adult patients. If studies are performed using a dialysis volume scaled to body surface area, these differences disappear.[82–88] These findings are supported by studies on fluid transport during pediatric PET. Using dextran 70 as a marker, there was a significant positive correlation between age and transcapillary ultrafiltration when volume was administered according to body weight.[89] This correlation disappeared if tests were performed with a dialysis fluid volume calculated on the basis of body surface area.[90] All these studies provide strong arguments in favor of the scaling of dialysis fluid volume to body surface area instead of body weight. They are supported by studies on intraperitoneal pressure in children. Stable intraperitoneal pressures, within the normal range for adult patients, were measured in children of all ages using volumes up to 1200 mL/m²[91–93] There was a strong negative linear correlation between ultrafiltration volume and intraperitoneal pressure.[94] Thus, intraperitoneal pressure, which under normal basal circumstances is between 5 and 15 cmH₂O, should be used as one of the determinants in prescribing the dialysis volume.[5,95,96]

All results presented lead to the conclusion that dialysis fluid volume should be prescribed based on body surface area and that the younger children will be undertreated if volumes are based on body weight. This is also the experience in daily clinical practice. Nevertheless, caution is needed in neonates, since these large dialysate volumes may exacerbate respiratory difficulties and predispose patients to the development of hernias.[97] Initiation of dialysis should provide small volumes at relatively high frequency. During the first 3 days of treatment a volume of 20 mL/kg may be used.

The dialysis schedule is prescribed on the basis of the results of PET and of measurements of elimination of metabolites (KT/V urea and creatinine clearance) as soon as a stable situation is reached. Until then the dialysis schedule will be based on blood chemistry values.

The results of the PET will mainly determine the dialysis schedule. Since children are generally within the high and high-average transporting categories, short dwell times will allow optimal elimination of metabolites as well as ultrafiltration. Studies of fluid kinetics have shown that maximal net ultrafiltration is generally reached after 1 to 2 hours. Due to decrease of osmolarity and fluid absorption, mainly by the lymphatics, intraperitoneal volume then decreases again (Fig. 19–1). For many children, using a NIPD schedule, five to six nightly cycles of 2 hours (1 1/2 hour dwell time, 1/2 hour inflow and outflow) will provide adequate dialysis. Ultrafiltration can be regulated by the choice of glucose concentration of the dialysis fluid. If underdialysis

occurs using this prescription, a daytime dwell with icodextrin solution can be added. Children having slower transport characteristics are candidates for classic CAPD, with exchanges every 4 to 6 hours. Very low transporting patients, who are rare in the pediatric population, are not suitable for PD and must be treated by HD.

While the PET is a good tool to prescribe the dialysis regimen, it is not useful for prescribing the dialysis dose. Dialysis adequacy is of course partly dependent on the transport characteristics of the peritoneal membrane, but to a larger extent it depends on the quantity of metabolites removed from the body. Of course, there is a close relationship between the function of the peritoneal membrane and the removal rate of metabolites.[98] The amount of metabolites to remove from the body is, in turn, related to the intake of nutrients. Prescription of dialysis dose based only on serum measurements of metabolites, such as urea nitrogen, may be misleading, as patients on dialysis may be catabolic. Kinetic modeling is now an accepted tool for defining the adequacy of the dialysis prescription. KT/V urea represents the urea clearance normalized for distribution volume. The concept of *KT/V*—*K* being the clearance of urea, *T* the duration of dialysis treatment, and *V* the volume of distribution—as developed by Gotch and Sargent,[99] is now used as a model to quantitate therapy prescription based on urea removal. A weekly *KT/V* of 1.7 or more or a creatinine clearance exceeding 50 L/week/1.73 m² was considered sufficient until the DOQI guidelines were published.[100] Presently weekly *KT/V* urea of 2.0 is needed in CAPD, 2.1 in CCPD, and 2.2 in NIPD patients. The accompanying values for weekly creatinine clearances are 60, 63, and 66 L, respectively. If these guidelines are followed, PD will no longer be an option in many adult dialysis patients without residual renal function.[101] For the pediatric population, guidelines are still scarce. In a cross-sectional study, we observed a mean total weekly *KT/V* of 2.31 and a mean total

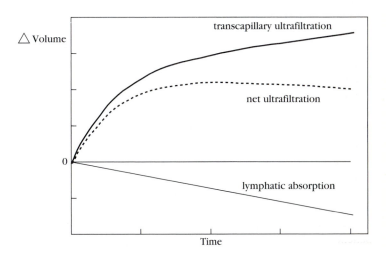

Figure 19–1. Loss of net ultrafiltration as a result of lymphatic absorption.

weekly creatinine clearance of 74 L/week/1.73 m^2.[102] If residual renal function was not taken into account, values were 1.75 and 43, respectively. These data are comparable to those of the other published pediatric studies.[103-106] It is not clear at the moment what should be the objective criteria for optimal *KT/V* urea and creatinine clearance, particularly in light of the ADEMEX study, which showed no relationship between weekly *KT/V* and mortality in a large group of adult patients.[107] It may be difficult to meet the DOQI criteria.[108] Particularly in APD, there may be an important discrepancy between *KT/V* urea and creatinine clearance because of the lower removal rate of creatinine clearance.[5,109] The definition of adequacy of PD is a difficult one. Outcome parameters such as mortality, morbidity, nutritional state, growth, and quality of life are multifactorially determined and not influenced by the adequacy of dialysis alone. The present figures, obtained from the studies cited, should therefore be used only as preliminary guidelines.[5,110] If low *KT/V* urea is combined with clinical signs of underdialysis, the dialysis dose should certainly be increased. This can be reached by increasing the dialysis fluid volume or increasing the number of cycles. The results of the PET can predict the effectiveness of these measures. There are computer programs available to calculate the results.[111]

The studies of PET have provided much information on the function of the peritoneal membrane. It is obvious to use the absorptive properties of this membrane therapeutically. Most experience has been collected with the intraperitoneal administration of insulin in diabetic patients. For pediatric patients, the intraperitoneal administration of the two drugs that must be administered subcutaneously (erythropoietin and growth hormone) can be considered. It has been demonstrated that the resorption of erythropoietin after intraperitoneal administration in a volume of 50 mL after a 12-hour dwell is similar to resorption after subcutaneous administration.[112] If these drugs were administered in the smallest commercially available dialysis bag, containing 250 mL, the resorption was about half. A therapeutic study showed that renal anemia could be effectively treated with intraperitoneal erythropoietin in 250-mL bags for 10 to 12 hours, with a mean dose of 279 U/kg/week.[113] Although this dose is about 30 percent higher than that needed with subcutaneous administration, the advantages with respect to patient and parent acceptance compensate for the somewhat higher cost. Treatment with erythropoietin in 50-mL bags resulted in the need for a lower dose: about 200 U/kg/week.[114,115] Intraperitoneal therapy with erythropoietin is now an accepted modality. Results with the intraperitoneal administration of the recently introduced erythropoietin analogue darbepoietin are not yet available. Intraperitoneal administration of growth hormone is not yet established as a routine procedure. Effective absorption has,

however, been established.[116] The only published therapeutic study was a pilot study in 9 children treated for 2 years.[117] Of these, 5 children had improvement in height standard deviation score, while the others did not demonstrate catch-up growth.

Other medication in children on PD essentially is the same as in chronic renal failure. Because the water-soluble vitamins are removed by dialysis, supplementation with vitamins B and C is mandatory. Since hyperhomocysteinemia, a risk factor for cardiovascular disease in adult patients, is also present in children on PD, additional administration of folic acid is advocated.[118-120] The diet should provide sufficient calories and proteins to allow growth. The concept that the diet in PD can be unlimited is generally not correct. Restrictive measures are often necessary. For infants, pretreatment of formulas with potassium-binding resins can be considered in order to lower the potassium content.[121] Pretreatment with calcium acetate to reduce the phosphate content was not successful.[122]

COMPLICATIONS

Specific complications of PD can occur. Most attention has been paid to the infectious complications. Peritonitis still is an important complication of PD, both in adult patients and children. Notwithstanding the many efforts that have been made to prevent this infectious complication, a frequency of one episode every 12 to 18 months is still reported for adult patients. Generally higher frequencies are reported in children, although recent studies are scarce.[123-125] The most recent figures in a large group of children suggest a frequency of one episode every 13.2 patient-months.[126] The methodologic issues in assessing the incidence of peritonitis in children on PD have been reviewed.[127] Since the distribution of peritonitis in children is non-Gaussian, the assignment of a personal peritonitis risk to each patient provides a better opportunity for risk-factor analysis by routine statistical methods.

Early symptoms of peritonitis are cloudy dialysate, abdominal pain, and fever. The number of leukocytes in the dialysis fluid is elevated. As in adult patients, *Staphylococcus* species are responsible for the largest fraction of episodes: about 50 percent,[128] although there seems to be a tendency toward a higher relative contribution of gram-negative microorganisms, possibly due to better elimination of gram-positives by the widespread prophylactic use of mupirocin (preliminary results from the International Pediatric Peritonitis Registry; unpublished). An advisory committee has recently renewed the guidelines for the treatment of peritonitis.[129] Whereas the guidelines for treatment of peritonitis in adult patients advocate the combination of a first-generation cephalosporin (cephalothin or cephazolin) and a third-generation cephalosporin (ceftazidime), the pediatric guidelines propose the combination of a glycopeptide (vancomycin or teicoplanin) and ceftazidime for a majority of patients. Excellent results have been obtained in children with both regimens,[128,130] but concern for the risk of infection from multiresistant microorganisms—due to widespread administration of glycopeptides—gave rise to a currently unresolved discussion in the literature.[131] Whatever therapy is chosen, its duration should be 14 days; an exception is made for *Staphylococcus aureus*, where a duration of 21 days is advised. Some adjunctive therapy in peritonitis has been recommended. The performance of two or three rapid exchanges of dialysis solution at the start of therapy has been recommended: this may alleviate the symptoms, but it potentially has negative effects on intraperitoneal phagocytes. It is advocated only for severe symptomatic peritonitis.

Next to peritonitis, catheter exit-site and tunnel infections frequently occur. Owing to differing diagnostic criteria, published incidences show a wide range. Exit-site infections generally are treated locally, using betadine-iodine or mupirocine, or systemically with a short course of antibiotics directed against the causative microorganism. Catheter tunnel infections must always be treated systemically. Treatment is initially effective in most cases, but infection generally returns if antibiotics are discontinued. Removal of the catheter should be considered under these circumstances. The catheter may be replaced in a single operative procedure, creating a new tunnel at the contralateral side of the abdomen. Under an antibiotic shield, this regimen was effective in 17 of 21 cases.[132] Fungal infectious complications almost always lead to catheter loss. It is recommended that these patients be treated with HD for at least 4 weeks to cure the infection completely before a new catheter is inserted. The final outcome of fungal peritonitis in children appears to be more favorable than it is in the adult dialysis population.[133]

The complication of sclerosing peritonitis, highly feared in adult patients, is rare in children, since they are treated with PD for a relatively short time. In countries with a low rate of transplantation, such as Japan, several cases have been described, generally occurring after a dialysis period of more than 5 years.[134–136]

After catheter insertion, both leakage and obstruction of the catheter may occur. Leakage can be prevented by delaying the start of PD after placement of the catheter, but this generally will not be possible in acute renal failure. Then, the pericatheter administration of a combination of fibrinogen and thrombin can be used for the treatment of leakage.[137] Obstruction of the catheter will be due to omental wrapping in many cases. Because fibrin may also be the cause of obstruction, an attempt to clear it with intraluminal urokinase or tissue plasminogen activator should always

been undertaken before surgical intervention is considered.[138]

Hernias occur more frequently in children than in adults.[124] These complications are encountered in some 50 percent of pediatric patients. Young age (<4 years) is a clear predisposition. The treatment is always surgical. Hydrothorax, a rare complication, will generally appear toward the end of PD in children.

PD leads to important protein losses. In adult patients, a protein loss of 5 to 10 g/day is observed, but it is much higher during episodes of peritonitis. Together with malnutrition, peritonitis may lead to hypoalbuminemia. A serum albumin < 30 g/L has been associated with an increased mortality in adult patients.[139] In children weighing > 50 kg, protein losses are much the same as in adult patients. In infants, however, a nearly twofold greater peritoneal protein loss was observed.[140] Hypoalbuminemia is associated with an increased incidence of PD failure.[141] The loss of immunoglobulins may lead to a deficiency of IgG_2.[142,143] Possibly these losses may contribute to a severe course of streptococcal peritonitis.[144] Complement and growth factors are also lost into the dialysate.[145,146] In addition, immunity is impaired by a reduced number of B lymphocytes, CD 8[+] T cells, and natural killer cells.[147]

Finally the absorption of glucose from the dialysis fluid leads to an important hyperlipidemia. It is still not clear whether treatment for this condition is indicated.

PROGNOSIS/FUTURE OF PERITONEAL DIALYSIS

It is now proven that PD can be performed for many years. Although on PET, solute transfer increases and ultrafiltration decreases with time on PD, this is not a clinical problem after a period of 4 years.[148] Patients with complications such as multiple episodes of peritonitis are prone to a more rapid deterioration of peritoneal membrane function. Residual renal function, which is reported to be better maintained during treatment by PD than by HD in adult patients, is not different in children in both modalities.[149]

The ultimate goal of dialysis in pediatric patients is renal transplantation. Children on PD are as good candidates for renal transplantation as those on HD.[150] During surgery, the peritoneal membrane should be left intact to allow for postoperative dialysis if needed. The catheter should be left in place until graft function is well established; generally it can be removed after approximately 1 month.[151] After transplantation, ascites occurs in a number of patients. This generally resolves spontaneously.

In recent years many changes in the field of pediatric peritoneal dialysis have been seen. The development of newer cyclers has increased the shift to APD techniques. CAPD has almost completely disappeared as a treatment modality. New dialysis fluids are being developed, and bicarbonate-buffered solutions as well as solutions containing icodextrin are of benefit to patients. Attention to the adequacy of dialysis has led to intensification of the dialysis prescription schedules, although discussion of the needed adequacy is ongoing.

REFERENCES

1. Wong KY, Wong SN, Lam SY, et al. Ammonia clearance by peritoneal dialysis and continuous hemodiafiltration. *Pediatr Nephrol* 1998;12:589–591.
2. Schaefer F, Straube E, Oh J, et al. Dialysis in neonates with inborn errors of metabolism. *Nephrol Dial Transplant* 1999; 14:910–918.
3. Coleman JE, Edefonti A, Watson AR on behalf of the EPPWG. Guidelines by an ad hoc European committee on the assessment of growth and nutritional status in children on chronic peritoneal dialysis. *Perit Dial Int* 2001;21:323.
4. Schröder CH on behalf of the EPPWG. The choice of dialysis solutions in pediatric chronic peritoneal dialysis. Guidelines by an ad hoc European committee. *Perit Dial Int* 2001;21:568–574.
5. Fischbach M, Stefanidis CJ, Watson AR for the EPPWG. Guidelines by an ad hoc European committee on adequacy and the pediatric peritoneal dialysis prescription. *Nephrol Dial Transplant* 2002;17:380–385.
6. Schröder CH on behalf of the EPPWG. The management of anemia in pediatric peritoneal dialysis patients. Guidelines by an ad hoc European committee. *Pediatr Nephrol* 2003; 18:805–809.
7. Strazdins V, Watson AR, Harvey B for the EPPWG. Renal replacement therapy for acute renal failure in children. Guidelines by an ad hoc European committee. *Pediatr Nephrol.* 2004;19:199–207.
8. Twardowski ZJ, Nolph KD, Khanna R, et al. The need for a "swan neck" permanently bent, arcuate peritoneal dialysis catheter. *Perit Dial Bull* 1985;5:219–223.
9. Gokal R, Alexander S, Ash S, et al. Peritoneal catheters and exit-site practices toward optimum peritoneal access: 1998 update. *Perit Dial Int* 1998;18:11–33.
10. Lerner GR, Warady BA, Sullivan EK, Alexander SR. Chronic dialysis in children and adolescents. The 1996 annual report of the North American Pediatric Renal Transplant Cooperative Study. *Pediatr Nephrol* 1999;13:404–417.
11. Harvey EA. Peritoneal access in children. *Perit Dial Int* 2001;21(suppl 3):218–222.
12. Daschner M, Gfrörer S, Zachariou Z, et al. Laparoscopic Tenckhoff catheter implantation in children. *Perit Dial Int* 2002;22:22–26.
13. Lewis J, Abbott J, Crompton K, et al. CAPD disconnect systems UK peritonitis experience. *Adv Perit Dial* 1992;8: 306–312.
14. Imholz ALT, Koomen GCM, Struijk DG, et al. Fluid and solute transport in CAPD patients using ultra low sodium dialysate. *Kidney Int* 1994;45:333–340.
15. Leypoldt JK, Charney DI, Cheung AK, et al. Ultrafiltration and solute kinetics using low sodium peritoneal dialysate. *Kidney Int* 1995;48:1959–1966.
16. Nakayama M, Yokoyama K, Kubo H, et al. The effect of ultra-low sodium dialysate in CAPD. A kinetic and clinical analysis. *Clin Nephrol* 1996;45:188–193.
17. Coulthard MG. Control of hyperparathyroidism in children using peritoneal dialysis solutions with low or zero concentrations of calcium (letter). *Nephrol Dial Transplant* 1992;7: 652–653.
18. Weinreich T, Passlick-Deetjen J, Ritz E, for the Collaborators of the Peritoneal Dialysis Multicenter Study Group. Low dialysate calcium in continuous ambulatory peritoneal dialysis: a randomised controlled multicenter trial. *Am J Kidney Dis* 1995;25:452–460.
19. Hutchison AJ, Were AJ, Boulton HF, et al. Hypercalcaemia, hypermagnesaemia, hyperphosphataemia and hyperaluminaemia in CAPD: improvement in serum biochemistry by reduction in dialysate calcium and magnesium concentrations. *Nephron* 1996;72:52–58.
20. Bro S, Brandi L, Daugaard H, Olgaard K. Calcium concentration in the CAPD dialysate: what is optimal and is there a need to individualize? *Perit Dial Int* 1997;17:554–559.
21. Duncan R, Cochrane T, Bhalla C, et al. Low calcium dialysate and hyperparathyroidism. *Perit Dial Int* 1996; 16(suppl 1):499–502.
22. Buijsen CGM, Struijk DG, Huijgen HJ, et al. Can low-calcium peritoneal dialysis solution safely replace the standard calcium solution in the majority of chronic peritoneal dialysis patients? *Perit Dial Int* 1996;16:497–504.
23. Weinreich T, Ritz E, Passlick-Deetjen J, for the Collaborators of the Multicenter Study Group. Long-term dialysis with low-calcium solution (1.0 mmol/L) in CAPD: effects on bone mineral metabolism. *Perit Dial Int* 1996;16: 260–268.
24. Schröder CH. New peritoneal dialysis fluids: practical use for children. *Pediatr Nephrol* 2003;18:1085–1088.
25. Liberek T, Topley N, Jörres A, et al. Peritoneal dialysis fluid inhibition of phagocyte function: effects of osmolality and glucose concentration. *J Am Soc Nephrol* 1993;3: 1508–1515.
26. Topley N, Coles GA, Williams JD. Biocompatibility studies on peritoneal cells. *Perit Dial Int* 1994;14(suppl 3): 21–28.
27. Jörres A, Williams JD, Topley N. Peritoneal dialysis solution biocompatibility: inhibitory mechanisms and recent studies with bicarbonate-buffered solutions. *Perit Dial Int* 1997; 17(suppl 2):42–46.
28. Feriani M. Use of different buffers in peritoneal dialysis. *Semin Dial* 2000;13:256–260.
29. Passlick-Deetjen J, Lage C. Lactate-buffered and bicarbonate-buffered solutions with less glucose degradation products in a two-chamber system. *Perit Dial Int* 2000;20(suppl 2):42–47.
30. Topley N, Kaur D, Petersen MM, et al. Biocompatibility of bicarbonate buffered peritoneal dialysis fluids: influence on mesothelial cell and neutrophil function. *Kidney Int* 1996; 49:1447–1456.
31. Topley N, Kaur D, Petersen MM, et al. In vitro effects of bicarbonate and bicarbonate-lactate buffered peritoneal dialy-

sis solutions on mesothelial and neutrophil function. *J Am Soc Nephrol* 1996;7:218–224.

32. Rogachev B, Hausmann MJ, Yulzari R, et al. Effect of bicarbonate-based dialysis solutions on intracellular pH (pH$_i$) and TNFα production by peritoneal macrophages. *Perit Dial Int* 1997;17:546–553.

33. Topley N. In vitro biocompatibility of bicarbonate-based peritoneal dialysis solutions. *Perit Dial Int* 1997;17:42–47.

34. Jörres A, Bender TO, Finn A, et al. Biocompatibility and buffers: effect of bicarbonate-buffered peritoneal dialysis fluids on peritoneal cell function. *Kidney Int* 1998;54:2184–2193.

35. Feriani M, Carobi C, La Greca G, et al. Clinical experience with a 39 mmol/L bicarbonate-buffered peritoneal dialysis solution. *Perit Dial Int* 1997;17:17–21.

36. Cancarini GC, Faict D, De Vos C, et al. Clinical evaluation of a peritoneal dialysis solution with 33 mmol/L bicarbonate. *Perit Dial Int* 1998;18:576–582.

37. Feriani M, Kirchgessner J, La Greca G, Passlick-Deetjen J. Randomized long-term evaluation of bicarbonate-buffered CAPD solution. *Kidney Int* 1998;54:1731–1738.

38. Mackenzie RK, Jones S, Moseley A, et al. In vivo exposure to bicarbonate/lactate- and bicarbonate-buffered peritoneal dialysis fluids improves ex vivo peritoneal macrophage function. *Am J Kidney Dis* 2000;35:112–121.

39. Tranæus A for the Bicarbonate/Lactate Study Group. A long-term study of a bicarbonate/lactate-based peritoneal dialysis solution—Clinical benefits. *Perit Dial Int* 2000;20:516–523.

40. Mactier RA, Sprosen TS, Gokal R, et al. Bicarbonate and bicarbonate/lactate peritoneal dialysis solutions for the treatment of infusion pain. *Kidney Int* 1998;53:1061–1067.

41. Schmitt CP, Haraldsson B, Doetschmann R, et al. Effects of pH-neutral, bicarbonate-buffered dialysis fluid on peritoneal transport kinetics in children. *Kidney Int* 2002;61:1527–1536.

42. Haas S, Schmitt CP, Bonzel KE, et al. Improved acidosis correction and recovery of mesothelial cell mass by pH neutral bicarbonate dialysis solution in children on automated peritoneal dialysis. *J Am Soc Nephrol* 2003;14:2632–2638.

43. Fischbach M, Terzic J, Chauvé S, et al. In children, the peritoneal area available for exchange is influenced by the composition of the peritoneal dialysis fluid. *Nephrol Dial Transplant* 2004;19:925–932.

44. Jones MR. Intraperitoneal amino acids: a therapy whose time has come? *Perit Dial Int* 1995;15(suppl 1):67–74.

45. Faller B, Aparicio M, Faict D, et al. Clinical evaluation of an optimized 1.1% amino-acid solution for peritoneal dialysis. *Nephrol Dial Transplant* 1995;10:1432–1437.

46. Canepa A, Perfumo F, Carrea A, et al. Long-term effect of amino-acid dialysis solution in children on continuous ambulatory peritoneal dialysis. *Pediatr Nephrol* 1991;5: 215–219.

47. Honda M, Kamiyama Y, Hasegawa O, et al. Effect of short-term essential amino acid-containing dialysate in young children on CAPD. *Perit Dial Int* 1991;11:76–80.

48. Qamar IU, Levin L, Balfe JW, et al. Effects of 3-month amino acid dialysis compared to dextrose dialysis in children on continuous ambulatory peritoneal dialysis. *Perit Dial Int* 1994;14:34–41.

49. Canepa A, Verrina E, Perfumo F, et al. Value of intraperitoneal amino acids in children treated with chronic peritoneal dialysis. *Perit Dial Int* 1999;19(suppl 2):435–440.

50. Mistry CD, Gokal R, Peers E, MIDAS Study Group. A randomized multicenter clinical trial comparing isosmolar icodextrin with hyperosmolar glucose solutions in CAPD. *Kidney Int* 1994;46:496–503.

51. Woodrow G, Stables G, Oldroyd B, et al. Comparison of icodextrin and glucose solutions for the daytime dwell in automated peritoneal dialysis. *Nephrol Dial Transplant* 1999; 14:1530—1535.

52. Posthuma N, Ter Wee PM, Donker AJM, et al. Assessment of the effectiveness, safety, and biocompatibility of icodextrin in automated peritoneal dialysis. *Perit Dial Int* 2000; 20(suppl 2):106–113.

53. Posthuma N, Ter Wee PM, Verbrugh HA, et al. Icodextrin instead of glucose during the daytime dwell in CCPD increases ultrafiltration and 24-h dialysate creatinine clearance. *Nephrol Dial Transplant* 1997;12:550–553.

54. De Boer AW, Schröder CH, Van Vliet R, et al. Clinical experience with icodextrin in children: ultrafiltration profiles and metabolism. *Pediatr Nephrol* 2000;15:21–24.

55. Van Hoeck KJM, Rusthoven E, Vermeylen L, et al. Nutritional effects of increasing dialysis dose by adding an icodextrin daytime dwell to nocturnal intermittent peritoneal dialysis (NIPD) in children. *Nephrol Dial Transplant* 2003;18:1383–1387.

56. Ho-dac-Pannekeet MM, Schouten N, Langedijk MJ, et al. Peritoneal transport characteristics with glucose polymer based dialysate. *Kidney Int* 1996;50:979–986.

57. Rusthoven E, Willems JL, Monnens LAH, et al. Contribution of transcellular water transport to net ultrafiltration in children using glucose-based and icodextrin dialysate (abstr). *Perit Dial Int* 2000;20:145.

58. Rusthoven E, Krediet RT, Willems HL, et al. Peritoneal transport characteristics with glucose polymer based dialysis fluid in children. *J Am Soc Nephrol.* In press.

59. Posthuma N, Ter Wee PM, Donker AJM, et al. Serum disaccharides and osmolality in CCPD patients using icodextrin or glucose as daytime dwell. Perit Dial Int 1997;17: 602–607.

60. Lam-Po-Tang MKL, Bending MR, Kwan JTC. Icodextrin hypersensitivity in a CAPD patient. *Perit Dial Int* 1997;17: 82–84.

61. Fletcher S, Stables GA, Turney JH. Icodextrin allergy in a peritoneal dialysis patient. *Nephrol Dial Transplant* 1998; 13:2656–2658.

62. Queffeulous G, Bernard M, Vrtousnik F, et al. Severe cutaneous hypersensitivity requiring permanent icodextrin withdrawal in a CAPD patient. *Clin Nephrol* 1999;5 1: 184–186.

63. Boer WH, Vos PF, Fieren MWJA. Culture-negative peritonitis associated with the use of icodextrin-containing dialysate in twelve patients treated with peritoneal dialysis. *Perit Dial Int* 2003;23:33–38.

64. Gokal R. Icodextrin-associated sterile peritonitis. *Perit Dial Int* 2002;22:445–448.

65. Bergström J. Appetite in CAPD patients. *Perit Dial Int* 1996;16 (suppl 1):181–189.

66. Potting CMJ, Schröder CH. CCPD may be the solution for failure of CAPD in some children. *Eur Dial Transplant Nurses Assoc J* 1992;14:26–27.

67. Watson AR, Coleman JE, Taylor EA. Gastrostomy buttons for feeding children on continuous cycling peritoneal dialysis. *Adv Perit Dial* 1992;6:391–395.

68. Geary DF, Chait PG. Tube feeding in infants on peritoneal dialysis. *Perit Dial Int* 1996;16 (suppl 1):517–520.

69. Warady BA, Weis L, Johnson L. Nasogastric tube feeding in infants on peritoneal dialysis. *Perit Dial Int* 1996;16 (suppl 1):521–525.

70. Coleman JE, Watson AR, Rance CH, Moore E. Gastrostomy buttons for nutritional support on chronic dialysis. *Nephrol Dial Transplant* 1998;13:2041–2046.

71. Ramage IJ, Geary DF, Harvey E, et al. Efficacy of gastrostomy feeding in infants and older children receiving chronic peritoneal dialysis. *Perit Dial Int* 1999;19:231–236.

72. Warady BA. Gastrostomy feedings in patients receiving peritoneal dialysis. *Perit Dial Int* 1999;19:204–206.

73. Ledermann SE, Spitz L, Moloney J, et al. Gastrostomy feeding in infants and children on peritoneal dialysis. *Pediatr Nephrol* 2002;17:246–250.

74. Edefonti A, Picca M, Paglialonga F, et al. A novel objective nutritional score for children on chronic peritoneal dialysis. *Perit Dial Int* 2002;22:602–607.

75. Potting CMJ. Alleviation of abdominal pain by adapted tidal peritoneal dialysis. *Eur Dial Transplant Nurses Assoc J* 1994;20:8–10.

76. Esperanca MJ, Collins DL. Peritoneal dialysis efficiency in relation to body weight. *J Pediatr Surg* 1966;1:162–169.

77. Twardowski ZJ, Nolph KD, Khanna R, et al. Peritoneal equilibration test. *Perit Dial Bull* 1987;7:138–147.

78. Schröder CH, Van Dreumel MJ, Reddingius R, et al. Peritoneal transport kinetics of glucose, urea, and creatinine during infancy and childhood. *Perit Dial Int* 1991;11:322–325.

79. Geary DF, Harvey EA, MacMillan JH, et al. The peritoneal equilibration test in children. *Kidney Int* 1992;42:102–105.

80. Geary DF, Harvey EA, Balfe JW. Mass transfer coefficients in children. *Perit Dial Int* 1994;14:30–33.

81. Mendley SR, Majkowski NL. Peritoneal equilibration test results are different in infants, children, and adults. *J Am Soc Nephrol* 1995;6:1309–1312.

82. Kohaut EC, Waldo FB, Benfield MR. The effect of changes in dialysate volume on glucose and urea equilibration. *Perit Dial Int* 1994;14:236–239.

83. Warady BA. The use of the peritoneal equilibration test to modify peritoneal dialysis modality in children. *Semin Dial* 1994;7:403–408.

84. Warady BA, Alexander S, Hossli S, et al. The relationship between intraperitoneal volume and solute transport in pediatric patients. *J Am Soc Nephrol* 1995;5:1935–1939.

85. Warady BA, Alexander SR, Hossli S, et al. Peritoneal membrane transport function in children receiving long-term dialysis. *J Am Soc Nephrol* 1996;7:2385–2391.

86. Warady BA, Fivush B, Andreoli SP, et al. Longitudinal evaluation of transport kinetics in children receiving peritoneal dialysis. *Pediatr Nephrol* 1999;13:571–576.

87. Bouts AHM, Davin J-C, Groothoff JW, et al. Standard peritoneal permeability analysis in children. *J Am Soc Nephrol* 2000;11:943–950.

88. Yoshino A, Honda M, Fukuda M, et al. Changes in peritoneal equilibration test values during long-term peritoneal dialysis in peritonitis-free children. *Perit Dial Int* 2001;21:180–185.

89. Reddingius RE, Schröder CH, Willems JL, et al. Measurement of peritoneal fluid handling in children on continuous ambulatory peritoneal dialysis using dextran 70. *Nephrol Dial Transplant* 1995;10:866–870.

90. De Boer AW, Van Schaijk TCJG, Willems HL, et al. Necessity to adjust dialysate volume to body surface area in pediatric peritoneal equilibration test. *Perit Dial Int* 1997;17: 199–202.

91. Fischbach M, Terzic J, Becmeur F, et al. Relationship between intraperitoneal hydrostatic pressure and dialysate volume in children on PD. *Adv Perit Dial* 1996;12:330–334.

92. Fischbach M, Terzic J, Provot E, et al. Intraperitoneal pressure in children: fill volume related and impacted by body mass index. *Perit Dial Int* 2003;23:391–394.

93. Rusthoven E, Van der Vlugt ME, Van Lingen AJ, et al. Influence of intraperitoneal pressure (IPP) on fluid transport during a peritoneal dialysis equilibration test (PET) in children. *Perit Dial Int.* In press.

94. Fischbach M, Desprez P, Donnars F, Geisert J. Hydrostatic intraperitoneal pressure in children on peritoneal dialysis: practical implications. An 18-month clinical experience. *Adv Perit Dial* 1994;10:294–296.

95. Fischbach M, Terzic J, Menouer S, Haraldsson B. Optimal volume prescription for children on peritoneal dialysis. *Perit Dial Int* 2000;20:603–606.

96. Fischbach M, Terzic J, Laugel V, et al. Measurement of hydrostatic intraperitoneal pressure: a useful tool for the improvement of dialysis dose prescription. *Pediatr Nephrol* 2003;18:976–980.

97. Fischbach M. Peritoneal dialysis prescription for neonates. *Perit Dial Int* 1996;16(suppl 1):512–514.

98. Fischbach M, Haraldsson B, Helms P, et al. The peritoneal membrane: a dynamic dialysis membrane in children. *Adv Perit Dial* 2003;19:265–268.

99. Gotch FA, Sargent JA. A mechanistic analysis of the national cooperative dialysis study (NCDS). *Kidney Int* 1985; 28:526–534.

100. National Kidney Foundation. K/DOQI Clinical Practice Guidelines for Peritoneal Dialysis Adequacy, 2000. *Am J Kidney Dis* 2001;37(suppl 1):65–136.

101. Twardowski ZJ, Nolph KD. Is peritoneal dialysis feasible once a large muscular patient becomes anuric? *Perit Dial Int* 1996;16:20–23.

102. Walk TLM, Schröder CH, Reddingius RE, et al. Adequate dialysis? Measurement of KT/V in a pediatric peritoneal dialysis population. *Perit Dial Int* 1997;17:175–178.

103. Mendley SR, Umans JG, Majkowski NL. Measurement of peritoneal dialysis delivery in children. *Pediatr Nephrol* 1993;7:284–289.

104. Schaefer F, Wolf S, Klaus G, et al. Higher KT/V urea associated with greater protein catabolic rate and dietary protein intake in children treated with CCPD compared to CAPD. *Adv Perit Dial* 1994;10: 310–314.

105. Sliman GA, Klee KM, Gall-Holden B, Watkins SL. Peritoneal equilibration test curves and adequacy of dialysis in children on automated peritoneal dialysis. *Am J Kidney Dis* 1994;24:813–818.

106. Fischbach M, Terzic J, Lahlou A, et al. Nutritional effects of KT/V in children on peritoneal dialysis: are there benefits from larger dialysis doses? *Adv Perit Dial* 1995;11:306–308.

107. Paniagua R, Amato D, Vonesh E, et al. Effects of increased peritoneal clearances on mortality rates in peritoneal dialysis: ADEMEX, a prospective, randomized, controlled trial. *J Am Soc Nephrol* 2002;13:1307–1320.

108. Van der Voort JH, Harvey EA, Braj B, Geary DF. Can the DOQI guidelines be met by peritoneal dialysis alone in pediatric patients? *Pediatr Nephrol* 2000;14:717–719.

109. Nolph KT, Twardowski ZJ, Keshaviah P. Weekly clearances of urea and creatinine on CAPD and NIPD. *Perit Dial Int* 1992;12:298–303.

110. Warady BA. Should the DOQI adequacy guidelines be used to standardize peritoneal dialysis in children? *Perit Dial Int* 2001;21(suppl 3):174–178.

111. Verrina E, Amici G, Perfumo F, et al. The use of the PD Adequest mathematical model in pediatric patients on chronic peritoneal dialysis. *Perit Dial Int* 1998;18:322–328.

112. Reddingius RE, Schröder CH, Koster AM, Monnens LAH. Pharmacokinetics of recombinant human erythropoietin in children treated with continuous ambulatory peritoneal dialysis. *Eur J Pediatr* 1994;153:850–854.

113. Reddingius RE, Schröder CH, Monnens LAH. Intraperitoneal administration of erythropoietin in children on CAPD. *Eur J Pediatr* 1992;151:540–542.

114. Reddingius RE, De Boer C, Schröder CH, et al. Increase of the bio-availability of intraperitoneal erythropoietin in children on peritoneal dialysis by the administration in small dialysis bags. *Perit Dial Int* 1997;17:467–470.

115. Rusthoven E, Van de Kar NCAJ, Monnens LAH, Schröder CH. Long-term effectiveness of intraperitoneal erythropoietin in children on NIPD by administration in small bags. *Perit Dial Int* 2001;21:196–197.

116. Fine RN, Fine SE, Sherman BM. Absorption of recombinant human growth hormone (rhGH) following intraperitoneal instillation. *Perit Dial Int* 1989;9:91–93.

117. Watkins SL. Use of recombinant human growth hormone in children undergoing dialysis. *Semin Dial* 1994;7:421–428.

118. Schröder CH, De Boer AW, Giesen A-M, et al. Treatment of hyperhomocysteinemia in children on dialysis by folic acid. *Pediatr Nephrol* 1999;13:583–585.

119. Feinstein S, Sela B-A, Drukker A, et al. Hyperhomocysteinemia in children on renal replacement therapy. *Pediatr Nephrol* 2002;17:515–519.

120. Kang HG, Lee BS, Hahn H, et al. Reduction of plasma homocysteine by folic acid in children with chronic renal failure. *Pediatr Nephrol* 2002;17:511–514.

121. Schröder CH, Van den Berg AMJ, Willems JL, Monnens LAH. Reduction of potassium in drinks by pre-treatment with calcium polystyrene sulphonate. *Eur J Pediatr* 1993;152:263–264.

122. Schröder CH, Swinkels DW, Verschuur R, et al. Studies with pre-treatment of milk with calcium acetate to reduce the phosphate content (letter). *Eur J Pediatr* 1995;154:689.

123. Neiberger R, Aboushaar MH, Tawan M, et al. Peritonitis in children on chronic peritoneal dialysis: analysis at 10 years. *Adv Perit Dial* 1991;7:272–274.

124. Asseldonk JPM, Schröder CH, Severijnen RSVM, et al. Infectious and surgical complications of childhood continuous ambulatory peritoneal dialysis. *Eur J Pediatr* 1992;151:377–380.

125. Levy M, Balfe JW. Optimal approach to the prevention and treatment of peritonitis in children undergoing continuous ambulatory and continuous cycling peritoneal dialysis. *Semin Dial* 1994;7:442–449.

126. Watkins SL, for the NAPRTCS. Peritoneal dialysis catheter infections and peritonitis in children: a report of the North American Pediatric Renal Transplant Cooperative Study. *Pediatr Nephrol* 2000;15:179–182.

127. Schaefer F, Kandert M, Feneberg R. Methodological issues in assessing the incidence of peritoneal dialysis-associated peritonitis in children. *Perit Dial Int* 2002;22:234–238.

128. Schaefer F, Klaus G, Müller-Wiefel DE, Mehls O, for the MEPPS. Intermittent versus continuous intraperitoneal glycopeptide/ceftazidime treatment in children with peritoneal dialysis-associated peritonitis. *J Am Soc Nephrol* 1999;10:136–145.

129. Warady BA, Schaefer F, Holloway M, et al. Consensus guidelines for the treatment of peritonitis in pediatric patients receiving peritoneal dialysis. *Perit Dial Int* 2000;20:610–624.

130. Rusthoven E, Monnens LAH, Schröder CH. Effective treatment of peritoneal dialysis-associated peritonitis with cefazolin and ceftazidime in children. *Perit Dial Int* 2001;21:386–389.

131. Schröder CH, Rusthoven E, Monnens LAH. Consensus on peritonitis treatment in pediatric patients (with a reply by Warady B). *Perit Dial Int* 2002;22:87–89.

132. Schröder CH, Severijnen RSVM, De Jong MCJW, Monnens LAH. Chronic tunnel infections in children: removal and replacement of the continuous ambulatory peritoneal dialysis catheter in a single operation. *Perit Dial Int* 1993;13:198–200.

133. Warady BA, Bashir M, Donaldson LA. Fungal peritonitis in children receiving peritoneal dialysis: a report of the NAPRTCS. *Kidney Int* 2000;58:384–389.

134. Araki Y, Hataya H, Tanaka Y, et al. Long-term peritoneal dialysis is a risk factor of sclerosing encapsulating peritonitis for children. *Perit Dial Int* 2000;20:445–451.

135. Hoshii S, Honda M, Itami N, et al. Sclerosing encapsulating peritonitis in pediatric peritoneal dialysis patients. *Pediatr Nephrol* 2000;14:275–279.

136. Hoshii S, Honda M. High incidence of encapsulating peritoneal sclerosis in pediatric patients on peritoneal dialysis longer than 10 years. *Perit Dial Int* 2002;22:730–731.

137. Rusthoven E, Van de Kar NCAJ, Monnens LAH, Schröder CH. Fibrin glue successfully used in peritoneal dialysis catheter leakage in children. *Perit Dial Int* 2004;24:287–289.

138. Stadermann MB, Rusthoven E, Van de Kar NCAJ, et al. Local fibrinolytic therapy with urokinase for peritoneal dialysis catheter obstruction in children. *Perit Dial Int* 2002;22:84–86.

139. Struijk DG, Krediet RT, Koomen GCM, et al. The effect of serum albumin at the start of CAPD treatment on patient survival. *Perit Dial Int* 1994;14:121–126.

140. Quan A, Baum M. Protein losses in children on continuous cycler peritoneal dialysis. *Pediatr Nephrol* 1996;10: 728–731.

141. Gulati S, Stephens D, Balfe JA, et al. Children with hypoalbuminemia on continuous peritoneal dialysis are at risk for technique failure. *Kidney Int* 2001;59:2361–2367.

142. Schröder CH, Bakkeren JAJM, Weemaes CMR, et al. IgG2-deficiency in young children treated with CAPD. *Perit Dial Int* 1989;9:261–265.

143. Bouts AHM, Davin J-C, Krediet RT, et al. Immunoglobulins in chronic renal failure of childhood: effects of dialysis modalities. *Kidney Int* 2000;58:629–637.

144. Schröder CH, De Jong MCJW, Monnens LAH. Group B streptococcus: an unusual cause of severe peritonitis in young children treated with continuous ambulatory peritoneal dialysis. *Am J Kidney Dis* 1991;17:231–232.

145. Reddingius RE, Schröder CH, Daha MR, et al. Complement in serum and dialysate in children on continuous ambulatory peritoneal dialysis. *Perit Dial Int* 1995;15:49–53.

146. Van der Kamp HJ, Otten BJ, Swinkels LMJW, et al. Influence of peritoneal loss of GHBP, IGF-1 and IGFBP-3 on serum levels in children with ESRD. *Nephrol Dial Transplant* 1998;14:257–258.

147. Bouts AHM, Out TA, Schröder CH, et al. Characteristics of peripheral and peritoneal white blood cells in children with chronic renal failure, dialyzed or not. *Perit Dial Int* 2000;20: 748–756.

148. Davies SJ, Bryan J, Phillips L, Russell GI. Longitudinal changes in peritoneal kinetics: the effects of peritoneal dialysis and peritonitis. *Nephrol Dial Transplant* 1996;11: 498–506.

149. Feber J, Schärer K, Schaefer F, et al. Residual renal function in children on haemodialysis and peritoneal dialysis therapy. *Pediatr Nephrol* 1994;8:579–583.

150. Nevins TE, Danielson G. Prior dialysis does not affect the outcome of pediatric renal transplantation. *Pediatr Nephrol* 1991;5:211–214.

151. Arbeiter K, Pichler A, Muerwald G, et al. Timing of peritoneal dialysis catheter removal after pediatric renal transplantation. *Perit Dial Int* 2001;21:467–470.

Acid-Base Homeostasis in Dialysis Patients

Jennifer Abbott Hollon
Richard A. Ward

The pH of the body's compartments is constrained within very narrow limits. For example, systemic arterial pH is normally held within the range of 7.35 to 7.43, and excursions outside the range of 6.8 to 7.8 are inconsistent with life. Stringent pH control is necessary because of the strong pH dependence of many of the enzymes that constitute the body's metabolic system. Because acid is continually added to the body as a result of normal metabolic processes, a sophisticated system of checks and balances is required to prevent the pH from drifting outside the desired range. In the first instance, buffers and respiration are responsible for the control of pH. These systems, however, only ameliorate the impact of acid addition on pH. Ultimately, it is the kidneys that are responsible for the elimination of generated acid from the body. The kidneys reclaim the majority of filtered bicarbonate in the proximal tubule and to a lesser degree in the thick ascending limb of the loop of Henle. Regeneration of bicarbonate by the kidney is accomplished in two ways: (1) excretion of ammonium ions through metabolism of glutamate in the proximal tubule and (2) titration of urinary buffers—chiefly HPO_4^-—by hydrogen ions in the collecting duct, a process known as titratable acidity. Replenishment of the bicarbonate supply and excretion of acid are crucial to maintaining normal acid-base balance in the face of daily dietary acid loads.

As functional renal mass decreases, regardless of increased ammoniagenesis and titratable acidity per nephron, hydrogen ion generation eventually exceeds hydrogen ion excretion, leading to metabolic acidosis. Hyperchloremic metabolic acidosis first appears when the glomerular filtration rate (GFR) is 20 to 30 percent of normal, due to diminished excretion of ammonium ions and titratable acid. As the GFR decreases below 15 mL/min, an increased anion gap is also observed due to accumulation of organic acids such as sulfate, urate, and hippurate.[1,2] Decreased intracellular bicarbonate stores and a consequent intracellular acidosis have also been demonstrated in nondialyzed uremic patients with untreated metabolic acidosis.[3] Nevertheless, plasma bicarbonate concentration may remain stable, in the range of 15 mmol/L, although net acid excretion is less than the daily acid load. This observation has given rise to the concept that intracellular buffer systems, such as bone, play a vital role in maintaining acid-base balance under conditions in which normal mechanisms are stressed. Therefore the patient presenting for initiation of dialysis therapy may have a long-standing metabolic acidosis accompanied by depletion of total body buffer stores. While the consequences of acidosis have yet to be fully elucidated, it is increasingly clear that the condition contributes to the pathogenesis of severe chronic kidney disease in at least two ways.

Acidosis and Protein Catabolism

Acidosis has been clearly linked to protein catabolism and may play an important role in the nutritional abnormalities and muscle wasting associated with chronic kidney disease. Chronic kidney disease is associated with abnormal plasma and intracellular amino acid profiles,[4,5] an abnormal amino acid response to a protein meal,[5] increased protein degradation and amino acid metabolism,[6,7] and loss of lean body mass.[8] Many of these abnormalities can be reproduced by metabolic acidosis in the presence of normal renal function.[9–14] Moreover, correction of acidosis decreases serum urea concentrations,[15,16] urinary urea excretion,[15] net protein degradation,[17] and amino acid oxidation[17,18] in patients with chronic kidney disease. Net protein degradation is also decreased when acidosis is corrected by increasing the dialysate bicarbonate concentration in hemodialysis patients[19] or by supplementary oral bicarbonate in patients on peritoneal dialysis.[20]

Two mechanisms by which acidosis increases protein catabolism in uremia have been described. Mitch and colleagues have demonstrated that acidosis resulting from chronic kidney disease increases the activity of the ATP-dependent ubiquitin-proteasome pathway of proteolysis in animal models.[21,22] Correction of the acidosis by feeding bicarbonate reversed these changes in rats,[22] and increasing serum total CO_2 in peritoneal dialysis patients was associated with a reduction in muscle mRNA for ubiquitin.[23] The second mechanism of acidosis-induced protein catabolism is breakdown of branched-chain amino acids. Acidosis is associated with an increase in mRNA and activity of branched-chain ketoacid dehydrogenase, which causes oxidation of branched-chain amino acids.[11,24] Plasma and muscle concentrations of branched-chain amino acids are lower than normal in mildly acidotic hemodialysis patients[25]; these levels increase following the correction of acidosis.[26] How the acidosis of chronic kidney disease activates these proteolytic pathways is not well understood, but the process

may be triggered by glucocorticoids in the presence of insulin resistance.[27,28]

Acidosis and Bone Disease

As discussed later in this chapter, bone is thought to play a role in buffering acid production, as the ability of the kidneys to excrete acid is impaired, thereby contributing to bone disease in chronic kidney disease. This hypothesis is supported by the findings of decreased bone calcium carbonate[29,30] and impaired bone mineralization and osteomalacia[31,32] in patients with chronic kidney disease and moderate to severe acidosis before the institution of dialysis. While these data are suggestive of a role for acidosis in the bone disease of renal failure, its exact contribution remains uncertain.[28,33] Acidosis may also contribute to bone disease indirectly by acting to increase serum levels of parathyroid hormone. In a prospective study, Lefebvre and colleagues randomized 21 stable hemodialysis patients into an experimental group of 11 patients who were given additional bicarbonate via the dialysate and oral administration to correct metabolic acidosis (predialysis serum bicarbonate 24 mmol/L) or a control group of 10 patients who were continued on their standard dialysis prescription (predialysis serum bicarbonate concentration 15 mmol/L). After 18 months, renal osteodystrophy was unchanged in the treatment group but worsened in the control group, as evidenced by an increase in bone osteoid and osteoblastic surfaces and serum PTH.[34] Several other investigators have also reported a decrease in serum PTH concentrations in hemodialysis patients following correction of acidosis.[35-37]

In addition to adverse effects on protein and bone, Lowrie and colleagues have shown that acidosis is a significant risk factor for mortality in hemodialysis patients.[38] Taken together, these observations indicate that correction of acid-base abnormalities is an important goal of dialysis therapy.

THE ACID BURDEN

Sources of Acid

Metabolism of ingested food produces endogenous acid. Protons arise when food is converted to end products of greater electronegativity—as, for example, when the organic sulfur in methionine is converted to sulfate. Conversely, if metabolism results in a more electropositive end product, protons are consumed. The principal reactions contributing to acid production are summarized in Table 20–1. In addition, protons are generated if organic anions formed during the metabolism of neutral substances are excreted before they are completely metabolized to neutral end products. Thus, net acid production results from different reac-

Hydrogen ion production
  1. Oxidation of sulfur-containing amino acids (methionine, cystine, cysteine)
  2. Renal or gastric excretion of metabolizable organic anions
  3. Metabolism of phosphoproteins
  4. Oxidation of organic cations (e.g., lysine, arginine, histidine)
Hydrogen ion consumption
  1. Oxidation of dietary metabolizable anions (e.g., citrate, lactate, and anionic amino acid anions, such as glutamate and aspartate)

tions, the relative magnitudes of which are dependent on the diet consumed.

Magnitude of the Daily Acid Burden

Careful balance studies have demonstrated net acid production to be 0.7 to 1.2 mmol/kg/24 h.[39,40] These studies were performed in normal subjects using a specifically formulated liquid diet. Other studies[41] have shown that acid production varies further as the composition of the diet changes. Goodman[40] found net acid excretion in patients with creatinine clearances between 7 and 29 mL/min to be the same as in normal subjects. Furthermore, when the acidosis in these patients was corrected by bicarbonate administration, acid production did not change. Later, Hood[42,43] and Romeh[44] demonstrated that changes in acid-base status modulate the production of lactic acid and keto acids to protect systemic pH. In patients with chronic kidney disease, similar feedback systems may regulate acid production.

Disposition of the Acid Burden

Newly generated acid is neutralized by the body's buffer systems. An acute acid load is initially buffered 40 percent by extracellular bicarbonate, 10 percent by red blood cells, and 50 percent by intracellular buffers.[45,46] Moreover, Schwartz and colleagues[46] demonstrated that the ratio of intracellular to extracellular buffering remains relatively independent of the degree of acidosis. The acid loads administered in these studies ranged up to 16 mmol/kg in time periods ranging up to 6 hours. In contrast, patients with moderate to severe chronic kidney disease have a net acid accumulation of the order of 19 mmol/24 h, which may persist for weeks or months.[40] In spite of this accumulation, serum bicarbonate remains stable, in the range of 15 to 18 mmol/L.[40] These observations suggest that intracellular buffers become progressively more important as time and the cumulative acid burden increase.

The mechanisms of intracellular buffering are varied and include physicochemical buffering, production or consumption of intracellular acids, transmembrane fluxes of hydrogen ion, and conversion of lactic acid to bicarbonate in the liver.[47] Although skeletal muscle, which represents 30 to 40 percent of body weight, plays a major role in this intracellular buffering, bone buffer stores are thought to have an important role in the long-term buffering of an acid load.[48] Normal subjects with ammonium chloride-induced metabolic acidosis develop a negative calcium balance that matches their net acid retention.[49] The induction of short-term (5 to 10 days) metabolic acidosis in dogs results in a 9.5 percent decrease in bone carbonate.[50] Similar results are obtained in rats rendered acidemic by either acid loading or the induction of diabetes[51] and in cultured bone models of metabolic acidosis.[52] That this mechanism is active in chronic kidney disease is suggested by the finding of a small but significant negative calcium balance[53] and a reduction in bone carbonate[29,30,54] in patients with chronic kidney disease. While Oh[55] has argued that the importance of bone as a buffer source must decrease with the duration of chronic kidney disease because there is a limit to the amount of alkali available in bone, patients may still have substantially depleted bone buffer stores at the initiation of dialysis therapy.

The role of bone buffers following the initiation of dialysis is much less clear. Once dialysis is instituted, the major determinant of acid-base balance becomes the dialysis procedure, and the role of bone becomes predicated on the extent to which the dialysis procedure can deal with the acid load. This subject is considered further in the following sections.

Requirements of Dialysis

One objective of dialysis should be to provide the patient with sufficient base to neutralize the acid burden accrued during the interdialytic period and to replenish any preexisting deficits in total body buffer stores. The National Kidney Foundation's K/DOQI guidelines recommend maintaining a predialysis serum bicarbonate concentration of ≥ 22 mmol/L.[56]

Serum bicarbonate is usually measured as total CO_2. In assessing the serum total CO_2 concentration, care must be taken to avoid artifacts that may lead to a spuriously low value. The use of distantly located central laboratories for routine analysis of blood samples from dialysis units is a common practice. Serum total CO_2 concentrations of samples transported by air to a central laboratory are reported to be 4 to 5 mmol/L less than the values obtained when paired samples are analyzed at a local laboratory.[57,58] The difference does not result from a longer time period between sample collection and analysis[57,58] and only to a small extent on whether the samples are separated by centrifugation or refrigerated.[59] Rather, the decrease in total CO_2 concentration appears to result from loss of CO_2 due to a failure to fill the sample container adequately,[60] to keep the sample capped during storage,[57] or to changes in ambient pressure during air transportation.[61] To minimize false diagnoses of metabolic acidosis, dialysis units should work consistently with one preferably local laboratory and carefully define the values of serum total CO_2 that indicate metabolic acidosis for that laboratory.

In order to develop therapeutic strategies for attaining the goal of a serum bicarbonate concentration ≥ 22 mmol/L, an estimate of the hydrogen ion burden is needed. For routine evaluation of acid-base status in dialysis patients, it is not feasible to perform balance studies of the type described in the previous section. As a first approximation, net acid production can be estimated to be 1 mmol/kg/24 h. Actual acid production can vary appreciably from this figure, both from patient to patient and as an individual patient's diet varies. In an attempt to estimate hydrogen ion production on an individual basis, Gotch and associates[62] developed an empiric correlation between metabolic hydrogen ion generation rate (G_H^+) and protein catabolic rate (PCR). The rationale for their approach was that protein metabolism is the largest contributor to acid production. From a review of published studies in which data on both nitrogen balance and net urinary acid excretion were reported, they found that PCR and G_H^+ could be related by

$$G_H^+ = (0.77 \pm 0.14)(PCR) \qquad (1)$$

where G_H^+ is expressed in mmol/24 h and PCR in g/24 h. PCR can, in turn, be estimated from the net generation rate of urea.[63] In addition to the metabolic generation of hydrogen ions, removal of any organic anions or bicarbonate by dialysis will also effectively generate acid. Thus, the net acid burden presented to the dialysis patient is the sum of metabolic hydrogen ion generation and any dialytic removal of organic anions and bicarbonate. This burden may be modified by the excretion of acid, bicarbonate, or organic anions as a result of any residual renal function.

BASE REPLETION BY DIALYSIS

Hydrogen ions are present in blood at the low concentration of 0.04 µmol/L at a pH of 7.4. Because dialytic mass transfer is diffusive and diffusion relies on a concentration gradient, the accumulated acid burden cannot be disposed of by dialytic removal of hydrogen ions. Even if the clearance of hydrogen ions approached the theoretical maximum of 100 percent of blood flow, only 2 µmol of hydrogen ions would be removed in a 4-hour hemodialysis with a blood flow of 200 mL/min. This removal compares with a daily hydrogen ion burden of approximately 70,000 µmol. Thus, an alternative strategy is required.

As described above, newly generated hydrogen ions initially are neutralized by buffers, predominantly bicarbonate, which in the absence of renal function become depleted. Instead of regenerating these depleted buffer stores by excretion of hydrogen ions, as is done by the natural kidney, dialysis achieves its goal by addition of new buffer to the patient. By including buffers in the dialysate at concentrations greater than those in plasma, diffusive mass transfer results in accrual of new buffer by the patient during dialysis. For this reason, the acid-base status of a patient treated with a typical thrice weekly hemodialysis schedule is characterized by a gradual depletion of buffer stores during the interdialytic periods, interspersed with rapid increases in buffer capacity during dialysis as new buffer is transferred to the patient. This schedule gives rise to the sawtooth pattern typical for many solutes in patients treated with intermittent dialysis. The nature of this pattern means that pH and bicarbonate may lie outside the normal range immediately before and after a dialysis treatment. The amplitude of the swings in acid-base status decreases with more frequent treatments, such as quotidian hemodialysis and continuous ambulatory peritoneal dialysis (CAPD). For a given therapy, the goal of base repletion should be to minimize the excursions in acid-base status and keep body buffers and pH in the normal range.

Base-Repletion Agents

Historically, base repletion by both hemodialysis and peritoneal dialysis was achieved by including sodium bicarbonate in the dialysate.[64,65] The physicochemical properties of bicarbonate led, however, to some practical problems. Chief among these was calcium carbonate precipitation. Solutions containing calcium and bicarbonate ions are metastable with respect to calcium carbonate precipitation at the concentrations and pH required for dialysis, and precipitates will form readily unless scrupulous attention is paid to the elimination of all contaminating carbonate.[66] In the early days of hemodialysis, dialysate was prepared in batch form, with each solute included at its final concentration. The logistics of providing dialysis to an increasing number of patients led to the concept of preparing dialysate on line from a concentrate and water. The preparation of a single concentrate containing all solutes is technically difficult because of the limited solubility of calcium and magnesium in the presence of bicarbonate. In peritoneal dialysis, calcium carbonate precipitation was soon found to be a problem during sterilization and long-term storage of the dialysate. These problems led to a consideration of substitutes for bicarbonate. Acetate had long been known as a source of base,[67] and, in 1964, Mion and coworkers[68] substituted acetate for bicarbonate in hemodialysate. Subsequently, use of acetate became widely accepted, and it essentially replaced bicarbonate in all hemodialysis applications. Acetate, as well as lactate, was also substituted for bicarbonate in peritoneal dialysate.

In the late 1970s, questions began to be raised about the appropriateness of acetate as a dialysate buffer for hemodialysis. The subject was debated over the next several years, with reports appearing both for and against the use of acetate. The principal points of this debate are discussed in subsequent sections. The debate renewed interest in alternatives to acetate and served as an impetus for hemodialysis equipment manufacturers to develop new systems allowing the preparation of bicarbonate-containing dialysate from concentrates. These systems are more complicated than those used for acetate and less forgiving of operator carelessness. Their availability, however, together with the perception that acetate was not the ideal buffer repletion agent, led to almost universal adoption of bicarbonate-containing dialysate for hemodialysis by the early 1990s.

Alternatives to acetate already were being sought for peritoneal dialysis by the early 1970s because of the perceived potential for acetate-containing solutions to irritate the peritoneal membrane. Lactate was the preferred choice of a panel convened in 1973 to make recommendations on the composition of peritoneal dialysis solutions[69] and the use of lactate-containing dialysate became the standard of practice over the ensuing years for both CAPD and automated peritoneal dialysis (APD). However, growing concern about the impact of traditional lactate-containing dialysate on the peritoneal membrane led to the development, in the late 1990s, of new solutions containing bicarbonate or bicarbonate-lactate mixtures. Multicompartment bags are utilized to segregate the bicarbonate from the calcium and magnesium ions until the time of use. These bicarbonate-containing solutions are still not available in the United States.

Base Repletion by Organic Anions

Organic anions achieve buffer addition indirectly. As the negatively charged organic anion is metabolized to the neutral end products carbon dioxide and water, a proton is consumed, and buffer is regenerated. Organic anions such as acetate and lactate enter the blood by virtue of the concentration gradient existing between blood and dialysate. The anion then enters the body's metabolic pathways. Acetate is incorporated into acetyl coenzyme A by acetyl coenzyme A synthetase (EC 6.2.1.1). Subsequently, the acetyl group may have several fates. The major portion enters the Krebs cycle and is oxidized to the neutral end products carbon dioxide and water. Lactate exists as the stereoisomers D(−)-lactate and L(+)-lactate, and the lactate used for peritoneal dialysis consists of a racemic mixture of both. L(+)-lactate is the form normally found in mammalian species and has only one immediate metabolic fate, conversion to pyruvate by L(+)-lactate dehydrogenase. The pyruvate may enter a number of metabolic pathways leading to electroneutral end products. These pathways include oxidation to carbon dioxide and water through the Krebs cycle, conversion to glucose and glycogen via the Embden-Meyerhof pathway, and

conversion to lipids such as cholesterol. The metabolic fate of D(−)-lactate is less well understood. Although D(−)-lactate dehydrogenase does not occur in mammals, D(−)-lactate is metabolized. Two possible pathways have been described, the first through the actions of the enzyme D-2-hydroxyacid dehydrogenase that converts D(−)-lactate to pyruvate[70] and the second through isomerization to L(+)-lactate.[71]

Metabolism to neutral end products requires that a hydrogen ion must be consumed to preserve electroneutrality, thereby generating buffer. Although it is usual to consider this buffer generation in terms of bicarbonate, all body buffer systems are in equilibrium and the hydrogen ion may arise from other sources, such as intracellular protein buffers. For this reason, although oxidation of acetate or lactate will result in the equimolar consumption of hydrogen ions, it should not be expected to result in equimolar bicarbonate generation.

Acetate is readily metabolized under normal conditions,[72-74] primarily by liver and muscle. If, however, insufficient oxaloacetate is available for the formation of citrate, acetyl coenzyme A will be diverted into other metabolic pathways, such as the formation of acetoacetate and β-hydroxybutyrate. This diversion has been demonstrated to occur during the infusion of acetate in the absence of dialysis[75] as well as during dialysis.[76-80] Acetoacetate and β-hydroxybutyrate are univalent anions. Therefore their production from acetate is electroneutral; no hydrogen ion is consumed and no buffer generated. While lactate also enters the Krebs cycle via pyruvate and acetyl coenzyme A, there are no data to support diversion of the acetyl group into acetoacetate and β-hydroxybutyrate during peritoneal dialysis with lactate-containing solutions.

In theory, any organic anion that can be metabolized to neutral end products could be used for buffer repletion during dialysis. For use in dialysis, an anion must demonstrate an adequate rate of buffer generation, possess suitable physicochemical properties, and not be prohibitively expensive. A number of anions such as acetate,[68] succinate,[81] lactate,[75,82,83] and pyruvate[75] were examined over the years for hemodialysis applications. For a variety of reasons, however, only acetate was accepted for routine clinical use. On the other hand, lactate has been widely used for peritoneal dialysis and continuous renal replacement therapies (CRRT). One reason for the use of different organic anions in hemodialysis and peritoneal dialysis is illustrated by the data in Fig. 20–1. These data show that the rate of generation of bicarbonate following lactate infusion is only about 35 percent of that achieved with acetate. In practice, this rate limited the use of lactate to applications in which the rates of mass transfer are relatively slow, such as peritoneal dialysis and CRRT for acute renal failure. In contrast, the data in Fig. 20–1 show that pyruvate infusion increases plasma bicarbonate at a rate almost identical to that achieved with ac-

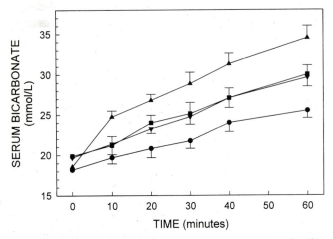

Figure 20–1. Increase in serum bicarbonate following infusions of sodium bicarbonate (▲), sodium acetate (■), sodium pyruvate (▼), and sodium lactate (●) at a rate of 10 mmol/kg/h in the dog. Data are given as mean ± SEM for $n = 6$.

etate infusion. On this basis, pyruvate would be an alternative to acetate. Nevertheless, its instability in solution and its increased cost compared with acetate prevented its use in clinical hemodialysis.

BASE REPLETION IN HEMODIALYSIS

Bicarbonate vs. Acetate

Initially, the debate over whether to continue using acetate for hemodialysis or replace it with bicarbonate focused on an association between the use of acetate and hemodynamic instability but gradually expanded to include a variety of other issues (Table 20–2). The principal areas of dispute were base repletion, hypoxemia, and hemodynamic and central nervous system stability.

Base Repletion. Use of bicarbonate-containing dialysate allows base to be transferred to the patient in a direct and quantitative manner. Bicarbonate is included in the dialy-

sate in a concentration in excess of that in serum and transfer occurs from dialysate to blood down this concentration gradient. The amount of base transferred depends on a variety of factors, which can be manipulated by the clinician depending on the needs of the patient. These factors include the dialysate bicarbonate concentration, the choice of dialyzer, and the blood and dialysate flow rates (see below). The generation of acid secondary to dialytic removal of organic anions is relatively small when bicarbonate-containing dialysate is used. The anion of most concern is lactate, which is present in serum at concentrations in the millimolar range during dialysis against bicarbonate. Gotch and coworkers[62] found dialytic lactate removal to be 9 to 26 mmol per treatment during standard dialysis against a bicarbonate-containing dialysate. Other anions such as acetoacetate and β-hydroxybutyrate remain in the micromolar range and contribute proportionally less to acid generation in these circumstances.

In contrast to the direct base transfer with bicarbonate, base accrual by the patient dialyzed against an acetate-containing dialysate depends on complex metabolic pathways, including the Krebs cycle. Furthermore, because there is no bicarbonate in the dialysate, there is a concentration gradient resulting in a loss of bicarbonate from the blood into the dialysate. When the effective loss of bicarbonate through dialysance of organic anions is also considered, net bicarbonate gain by the patient dialyzed against an acetate-containing dialysate can be seen to be the result of a number of different and competing fluxes (Fig. 20–2).

Using radiotracer techniques, Sigler and associates[84] estimated that only 55 percent of acetate transferred to the patient during dialysis is immediately oxidized to carbon dioxide and water, with 30 percent entering nonoxidative pathways. It is not clear how much of this 30 percent represents anionic species, but the data provide a measure of the potential difference between the rates of acetate metabolism and buffer generation. Acetoacetate and β-hydroxybutyrate are relatively small anions (of the order of 100 Da) and as a result are readily dialyzed. This process creates a short circuit whereby base equivalents enter the blood as acetate and

TABLE 20–2. COMPARISON OF ACETATE- AND BICARBONATE-CONTAINING DIALYSATE

	Acetate	Bicarbonate
1. Base repletion	One concentrate	Two concentrates
	Indirect (relies on metabolism)	Direct
	Zero hydrogen ion balance may not be obtained (may lead to chronic depletion of buffer stores)	Postdialysis alkalemia may occur
2. Physiologic effects	Hypoxemia occurs because of extrapulmonary CO_2 loss	Hypoxemia may occasionally occur in association with alkalemia
	Causes peripheral vasodilation that may lead to hypotension, cramps, etc., if dialysate sodium is too low, or in patients with impaired cardiovascular function	Little effect on cardiovascular system
3. Miscellaneous	May impair dialytic phosphate removal	None known
	May suppress thyroid function and growth hormone	

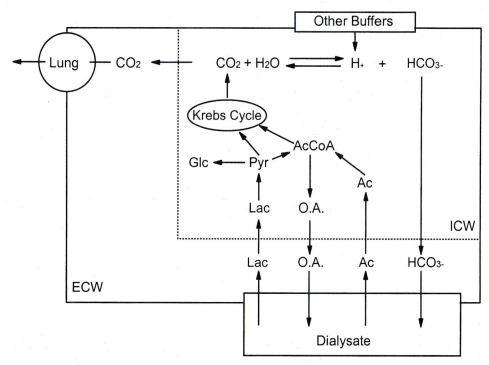

Figure 20–2. Simplified schematic representation of base repletion using acetate- or lactate-containing dialysate. Metabolism of the univalent anions, acetate (Ac) and lactate (Lac), to neutral end products, such as carbon dioxide and water or glucose (Glc), requires the net consumption of a hydrogen ion to preserve electroneutrality; the result is net bicarbonate generation. O.A. represents organic acids, such as acetoacetate and β-hydroxybutyrate. Loss of these univalent anions into the dialysate represents loss of potential bicarbonate from the patient.

then exit into the dialysate in the form of these intermediates. Studies show the dialytic loss of organic acids during standard dialysis against acetate-containing dialysate to be in the range of 40 to 100 mmol.[62,78] Others have estimated that the percentage of transferred acetate ultimately converted to bicarbonate may be as low as 66 percent in some patients[76] and that, from the perspective of base repletion, approximately 10 percent of patients do not adequately metabolize acetate.[85]

Blood acetate levels can vary widely from patient to patient under similar conditions of dialysis. Peak intradialytic acetate levels have been observed to range from less than 2 mmol/L to greater than 15 mmol/L.[76,78,86-88] Under standard dialysis conditions, a normal rate of acetate oxidation results in a low plasma acetate concentration, and blood pH and bicarbonate increase progressively during the treatment. In patients with a reduced capacity for acetate oxidation, blood acetate concentrations are increased and blood pH and bicarbonate may even decrease during dialysis because of the obligatory dialytic loss of bicarbonate associated with the use of acetate. These trends are magnified in highly efficient dialysis generally[76,78,87,89] and in the dialysis of children in particular.[86,90] When dialysis ceases, the demands on metabolism ease and the accumulated acetate, acetoacetate, and β-hydroxybutyrate are metabolized to carbon dioxide and water, with the consequent generation of

buffer. Blood pH and bicarbonate may continue to increase after dialysis as plasma acetate levels decrease.[76,78,87,89,90] Similar fluctuations in acid-base parameters may also occur in other body compartments. Arieff and colleagues[91] have shown that cerebrospinal fluid and brain intracellular pH decrease significantly in experimental dialysis using acetate-containing dialysate. Such changes may be factors in the development of some of the adverse symptoms associated with dialysis.

The limitations placed on bicarbonate generation by metabolism together with the loss of bicarbonate and organic anions into the dialysate have led some to speculate that a zero hydrogen ion balance may not be obtained with acetate-containing dialysate under certain circumstances.[62,92] Ongoing mobilization of bone buffer stores and the development of total body buffer depletion would result. Conclusive evidence for or against this hypothesis is lacking. Use of bicarbonate, however, does result in a greater transfer of base to the patient than is obtained with acetate.[80] Tolchin[76] estimated net bicarbonate gain with acetate-containing dialysate to be in the range of 20 to 60 mmol/day, depending on the dialysis conditions. The hydrogen ion burden to be neutralized by this bicarbonate was, however, not estimated. Vreman and associates[78] found an average net base gain of 74 mmol/day in 31 mass balance studies with acetate-containing dialysate. This value was not different from the patients' estimated average hydrogen ion generation rate of 60 mmol/day. Gotch and coworkers[62] also found that hydrogen ion balance was essentially zero for dialysis against an acetate-containing dialysate. They found, however, a strongly negative (25 mmol/day) hydrogen ion balance when the same patients were dialyzed against a bicarbonate-containing dialysate and speculated[62] that this large negative hydrogen ion balance may have resulted from depletion of bone buffer stores during long-term dialysis against acetate. On the other hand, Gennari[93] has argued that in patients dialyzed long-term against acetate, plasma bicarbonate concentration reaches a new steady state such that hydrogen ion balance remains essentially zero. This aspect of the acetate-bicarbonate debate is likely to remain unresolved now that acetate-containing dialysate is no longer in clinical use.

Hypoxemia. Hypoxemia was commonly observed during the first hour of hemodialysis against acetate-containing dialysate. The decrease in arterial PO_2, which persisted throughout the treatment, was typically in the range of 10 to 20 mmHg. Several mechanisms have been suggested to explain the development of this hypoxemia and the precise etiology remains uncertain.

A major reason for the hypoxemia is hypoventilation induced by a decrease in PCO_2. Two mechanisms have been proposed for the decrease in PCO_2. With acetate-containing dialysate, a concentration gradient exists that results in the loss of dissolved carbon dioxide and bicarbonate into the dialysate. The amount of total carbon dioxide removed is 2 to 3 mmol/min, or about 20 to 30 percent of the patient's metabolic production of carbon dioxide.[94-99] The loss of carbon dioxide is thought to result in a significant reduction in PCO_2, leading to hypoventilation mediated by carbon dioxide-sensitive chemoreceptors, and a consequent decrease in arterial PO_2. The ventilatory response is similar to that found in studies where an extracorporeal membrane lung was used to reduce the carbon dioxide burden to the lungs.[100,101] Some authors[102,103] have argued that loss of bicarbonate and carbon dioxide into the dialysate plays a relatively minor role in decreasing PCO_2. They contend that PCO_2 and ventilation decrease secondary to fixation of metabolic carbon dioxide as bicarbonate during acetate metabolism. If this hypothesis is correct, hypoxemia should occur when acetate is infused into patients with no renal function in the absence of dialysis. Results of such studies have been mixed, with both a decrease[104] and no change[105] in PO_2 being reported. Because carbon dioxide and bicarbonate are dynamically linked through the carbonic acid system and because dialysis against acetate affects this equilibrium in complex ways (Fig. 20–2), it is difficult to separate these two mechanisms and assess their relative importance in reducing ventilation. Whatever the mechanism, the decreased carbon dioxide burden to the lungs

during dialysis against acetate results in a reduced respiratory quotient.[94,96,97-99,106-111] When both dialytic and pulmonary carbon dioxide excretion are taken into account, the total body metabolic quotient remains essentially unchanged,[99,110,111] supporting the argument that removal of carbon dioxide, with consequent hypoventilation, is an important factor in the development of hypoxemia. Substitution of bicarbonate for acetate prevents the loss of carbon dioxide, ventilation is maintained, and arterial PO_2 is sustained at predialysis levels.[96,111] With highly efficient hemodialysis, ventilation may even increase.[112]

Replacement of the acetate in the dialysate by bicarbonate is reported by several groups to ameliorate the hypoxemia,[96,107,108,111,113-115] although this finding has not been universal, and arterial PO_2 has been reported to decrease as much with bicarbonate-containing dialysate as with that containing acetate.[98,99,106] As previously described, pH and serum bicarbonate increase promptly with dialysis against bicarbonate. Alkalemia may result, which, in turn, may serve to decrease ventilation and consequently decrease arterial PO_2.[116] This mechanism is supported by the data of Raja and colleagues,[115] who showed that dialysis-induced hypoxemia was prevented with a dialysate bicarbonate concentration of 29 mmol/L but not with a concentration of 37 mmol/L.

In summary, no single mechanism is likely to be responsible for the observed decrease in arterial PO_2 during hemodialysis. Under different conditions, various processes combine to produce the observed effect. With acetate-containing dialysate, the most important mechanism is changes in ventilation secondary to decreases in carbon dioxide, with transient pulmonary dysfunction and changes in acid-base status acting as secondary modulators. The question of whether dialysis-induced hypoxemia has any clinical consequences remains unanswered. Exacerbation of hypoxemia in patients already hypoxemic because of underlying pulmonary or cardiac disease is clearly undesirable. The situation is less clear for the average patient on dialysis. Ahmad and coworkers[117] have shown that dialysis morbidity was reduced in treatments when nasal oxygen was used to prevent hypoxemia. Heneghan[118] obtained similar results in patients susceptible to severe hypotension.

Vascular and Central Nervous System Stability. In 1976, Novello and coworkers[86] described "acetate intolerance" in three patients. This syndrome was characterized by an increase in plasma acetate concentration to >15 mmol/L postdialysis. Two of the patients also experienced hypotensive episodes. Subsequently, other reports described a greater incidence of symptomatic treatments when acetate was used as the base repletion agent compared with when bicarbonate was used. Differences were reported in the incidence of hypotension[119-127]; general well-being as assessed from a constellation of symptoms including nausea, headache, and fatigue[89,121-123,127-130]; performance test scores[89,121]; ventricular arrhythmias[131]; and ocular dynamics.[132] In contrast, other investigators found little[133] or no[134-136] improvement in symptomatology when bicarbonate was substituted for acetate. Finally, the onset of symptoms is reported both to be correlated[137] and not correlated[88,135] with plasma acetate concentration. These contradictory findings reflect variability in the patients studied and differences in the study design. Moreover, rather than being a cause, high plasma acetate concentrations may be a consequence of hypotension if the hypotension leads to a reduction in tissue perfusion. Nevertheless, close examination reveals a number of factors that seem to predispose to an increased morbidity with acetate dialysis. These factors include the use of a dialysate sodium concentration hyposmolar with respect to serum (<135 mmol/L) and the ability of the patient to mount an appropriate cardiovascular response to the effects of dialysis.

Beginning with the observation of Bergström and coworkers in 1976,[138] considerable evidence has accumulated to suggest that maintenance of serum osmolality during fluid removal protects against the development of hypotension.[139-142] Keshaviah and Shapiro[140] hypothesized that a reduction in extracellular osmolality by diffusive loss of solutes, such as urea and sodium, into the dialysate induces a movement of water from the interstitial to the intracellular space. This movement compromises vascular refilling during ultrafiltration, leading to an excessive decrease in vascular volume and hypotension. The hypothesis is supported by the data of Van Stone and coworkers,[143] who showed that use of a dialysate sodium concentration 7% less than that in serum caused movement of fluid into the intracellular compartment, compounding the reduction in vascular volume caused by ultrafiltration and resulting in hypotension. In contrast, when the concentration of sodium in dialysate exceeded that in serum, water was removed from both the intracellular and extracellular compartments and dialysis was asymptomatic. The benefits derived from maintaining osmolality and substituting bicarbonate for acetate as the base-repletion agent have been compared in studies in which dialysate sodium concentration and the use of acetate or bicarbonate were varied in a four-way crossover design. Velez and colleagues[144] found no difference in the incidence of orthostatic signs and symptoms following dialysis with acetate- and bicarbonate-containing dialysates when the dialysate sodium concentration was 141 mmol/L. Reduction of the dialysate sodium concentration to 130 mmol/L led to a marked increase in postdialysis orthostatic signs and symptoms. The increase was, however, less when bicarbonate was used, particularly in patients with evidence of autonomic insufficiency. This difference may be due to the superior vascular refilling observed with bicarbonate-containing dialysate at low (130 mmol/L)[145] and high dialysate sodium concentrations (140 mmol/L) in

patients with impaired left ventricular function.[146] The results of this and similar studies[147,148] suggest that maintenance of serum osmolality by use of a dialysate essentially isonatremic with respect to serum has a greater impact on hemodynamic stability than does the choice of base-repletion agent.

Sodium acetate has long been known to exert a hypotensive effect when administered intravenously.[149] The mechanism of this action appears to be peripheral vasodilation.[149-153] This action of acetate is nonspecific.[154] The vasoactive agent may be adenosine, which is formed by 5'-nucleotidases from the AMP released during the formation of acetyl coenzyme A.[155,156] Steffen and colleagues infused acetate into the gracilis muscle of dogs and observed a significant increase in tissue concentrations of adenosine, which correlated inversely with changes in vascular resistance,[157] while Carmichael and colleagues found that administration of an adenosine receptor blocker prevented acetate-induced vasodilation in rats.[158] In support of this mechanism, dialysate levels of adenosine metabolites—such as uric acid, inosine, hypoxanthine, and xanthine—are increased during dialysis against acetate vs. dialysis against bicarbonate.[159] Non-adenosine-mediated vasorelaxation has also been described.[160]

Ultimately, a patient's ability to increase heart rate, contractility, and systemic vascular resistance in the face of a decreasing blood volume due to fluid removal will determine whether or not hypotension occurs. Because acetate causes peripheral vasodilation, its use predisposes to hypotension in circumstances when heart rate cannot be increased sufficiently to compensate for a decrease in blood volume in the presence of the vasodilatory agent. Such conditions include long-standing hypertension, which may lead to impaired baroreflex mechanisms,[161] and autonomic insufficiency from diabetes mellitus.[162,163] As seen previously, however, this impact of acetate can be greatly reduced by using a higher dialysate sodium concentration to protect vascular volume. Whether acetate has any direct adverse effects on cardiac function that may predispose to hypotension remains unclear. Several groups[164,165] have shown that cardiac function improves during dialysis with acetate-containing dialysate, independent of volume changes. These studies were performed in patients with apparently normal hearts. In studies using acetate-containing dialysate, myocardial contractility has been reported not to improve during dialysis in patients with preexisting left ventricular hypertrophy,[166] and the frequency of hypotension appears to be greater in patients with hypertrophic cardiomyopathy than in those with normal hearts.[167] In patients with impaired left ventricular function, Leunissen and colleagues[146] reported that the velocity of circumferential fiber shortening improved when bicarbonate-containing dialysate was used but not when acetate-containing dialysate was used. In a similar group of patients, Ruder and colleagues[168] found that the velocity of circumferential fiber shortening improved with both acetate- and bicarbonate-containing dialysates; however, the improvement was significantly greater with bicarbonate than with acetate.

Overall, it is clear that acetate adds to the hemodynamic perturbations induced by dialysis. For some patients, the additional impact of acetate appears to be minor and can be protected against by manipulating the dialysate composition to minimize osmotic shifts during dialysis. Nevertheless, there remain significant subgroups of patients in whom use of acetate is contraindicated because of factors such as autonomic insufficiency or preexisting cardiovascular disease, which compromise the patient's ability to increase cardiac output appropriately.

Other Metabolic Issues. In addition to the questions considered in the preceding sections, acetate has been associated with a number of other potentially adverse consequences for the dialysis patient (Table 20–2).

The metabolism of acetate has a significant impact on body phosphorus. Inorganic pyrophosphate is formed by the cleavage of ATP during the acetylation of coenzyme A, and the increase in Krebs cycle activity also serves to increase phosphorus pool turnover. A redistribution of phosphorus into intracellular pools may result in a reduction in plasma phosphorus[75] and decreased dialytic removal. In contrast, there is no redistribution of phosphorus when bicarbonate is used in the dialysate. Dialytic phosphorus removal is reported to be greater with bicarbonate-containing dialysate than with acetate-containing dialysate,[83,169] and predialysis phosphate concentration is reported to decrease following long-term use of bicarbonate.[127,170] However, even with the use of high-efficiency dialysis and bicarbonate-containing dialysate, only about 1 g of phosphorus is removed per treatment.[83,171] Since this amount is approximately half the daily phosphorus intake, a small difference in phosphorus removal between acetate- and bicarbonate-containing dialysate will have minimal impact on the inability of dialysis alone to control phosphorus balance.

Because acetate enters metabolic pathways through acetyl coenzyme A, concern arose that it may promote lipogenesis through carboxylation of acetyl coenzyme A to malonyl coenzyme A.[172-174] Small amounts of ^{14}C are incorporated into lipids following infusion of ^{14}C-acetate into normal and uremic dogs.[175] It is, however, not clear whether this finding reflects de novo lipid synthesis from acetate or is merely a reflection of entry of ^{14}C into the total carbon pool. Clinical studies[125,176,177] have failed to show any improvement in plasma lipid concentrations following substitution of bicarbonate for acetate in the dialysate, suggesting that acetate plays little if any role in the hyperlipidemia seen in dialysis patients.

Acetate is reported to have a negative impact on some hormonal systems. Long-term sodium acetate administration (0.26 mmol/kg/day) was found to increase circulating levels of thyroid-stimulating hormone in rats,[178] and the secretion of growth hormone has been shown to be suppressed during intravenous acetate infusion and dialysis against acetate-containing dialysate.[179,180] Many hormonal systems are perturbed by uremia per se, and the significance of these findings, if any, is unclear.

Highly Efficient Dialysis. The majority of investigations into the relative merits of acetate and bicarbonate as base-repletion agents were conducted with a combination of dialyzer and blood-flow rate providing a urea clearance of 140 to 200 mL/min and a dialysis time of 4 to 6 hours. The current practice of dialysis involves treatment regimens that provide a significant increase in dialysis efficiency over these more traditional conditions. Dialysis is now characterized by urea clearances in excess of 260 mL/min, obtained by a combination of dialyzers with large surface areas, highly permeable membranes, and increased blood and dialysate flow rates. These dialysis conditions would exacerbate the effects of acetate described in the preceding sections. Early studies[76,78,89] showed that use of large-surface-area dialyzers markedly compromised the patient's ability to maintain acid-base balance, and such treatments were characterized by an increasing acidosis during dialysis. Other crossover studies[181,182] showed that short-time dialysis against acetate, with or without large-surface-area dialyzers, was associated with a decrease in predialysis serum bicarbonate. Urea clearances were <220 mL/min in these studies, and a worsening of this situation must be anticipated as the mass transfer efficiency of the dialyzer is increased. These findings are another reason that bicarbonate is now the base-repletion agent of choice for hemodialysis.

Summary. Although the debate over the relative merits of acetate and bicarbonate stimulated a great deal of research and discussion, the outcome was inconclusive. It is apparent that acetate was a major cause of dialysis-related hypoxemia, primarily because of the obligatory extrapulmonary carbon dioxide removal associated with its use. It is also apparent that acetate can act as a vasodilatory agent in a situation when decreasing vascular volume indicates the desirability of peripheral vasoconstriction. For these reasons, the use of bicarbonate rather than acetate was clearly indicated for the increasing number of patients who initiated dialysis with preexisting pulmonary, cardiovascular, or autonomic insufficiency. The situation regarding hypoxemia and hemodynamic instability was less clear for the average, otherwise healthy patient. The rationale for replacing acetate by bicarbonate in these patients was less compelling when a hemodialysis regimen of modest efficiency was used, particularly if care was taken to minimize osmolar shifts during the dialysis procedure. The question of adequacy of base repletion remains unresolved. Use of bicarbonate results in a greater transfer of base to the patient than was obtained with acetate. While it remains unknown whether use of acetate is associated with a progressive depletion of body buffer stores or merely a lower set point for predialysis serum bicarbonate, bicarbonate appears to be the prudent choice for those patients whose ability to metabolize acetate may be limited—for example, those with small muscle mass or concurrent metabolic disorders. Finally, high-flux and high-efficiency dialysis greatly exaggerate solute fluxes, thereby stressing all the systems involved in acetate metabolism and consequent bicarbonate generation. For this reason, bicarbonate-containing dialysate is indicated for all patients treated with these regimens. The debate over the relative merits of acetate and bicarbonate has become moot. All new dialysis equipment is capable of delivering bicarbonate-containing dialysate and essentially all patients are now treated with bicarbonate-containing dialysate.

Selection of a Dialysate Base Concentration

As discussed earlier, one objective of dialysis is to provide the patient with sufficient bicarbonate to neutralize the acid burden arising from metabolic acid production, the dialytic loss of metabolizable anions, any bicarbonate loss through bicarbonaturia, and—in the case of acetate—bicarbonate loss by dialysis. Historically, this goal was approached by including acetate or bicarbonate in the dialysate at some fixed concentration for all patients. Since the magnitude of the acid burden will clearly vary from patient to patient, a more individualized approach is worthy of consideration. Mathematical models have been developed for the quantitation and individualization of a number of aspects of dialysis therapy.[63]

At first sight, development of a mathematical model for bicarbonate should be straightforward. There is no dependence on metabolism and the flux of base is essentially unidirectional, from dialysate to blood. A mass balance for 1 week of thrice weekly dialysis with a bicarbonate-containing dialysate leads to:

$$10,080 \quad G_{H^+} = 3 \quad \left(J_{Bi} \quad J_{OA} \right)_t \tag{2}$$

where J_{Bi} and J_{OA} are the instantaneous fluxes of bicarbonate and organic anions, respectively, and t is the time of treatment. The fluxes, J_{Bi} and J_{OA}, can be described in terms of the mass transfer properties of the dialyzer, the blood and dialysate flow rates, the ultrafiltration rate, and the blood and dialysate solute concentrations.[63,95] With one exception, all these parameters can be controlled or are known. The exception is the blood solute concentrations of bicarbonate and the organic anions. These concentrations change as dialysis progresses, in a manner dependent on the mass transfer properties of the dialyzer, the dialysate composi-

tion, and the exchange of hydrogen ions between the body's various buffer systems. The usual approach to determining such concentration profiles is to formulate a differential equation expressing the solute concentration as a function of time in terms of parameters that can be measured or estimated by fitting the equation to experimental data. The simple pharmacokinetic approach for bicarbonate assumes distribution in a single pool corresponding to approximately 50 percent of body weight.[183-185] Use of this model leads to the following equation for bicarbonate accumulation during dialysis:

$$\frac{d\left(V_{Bi}C_{PBi}\right)}{dt} = D_{Bi}\left(C_{DBi} - C_{PBi}\right) - G_{H^+} \tag{3}$$

where V_{Bi} is the volume of distribution, D_{Bi} is the dialysance, and C_{PBi} and C_{DBi} are the plasma and dialysate bicarbonate concentrations, respectively. Equation (3) can be solved to yield C_{PBi} as a function of known variables.[63] It is likely, however, that such a model greatly oversimplifies bicarbonate kinetics. Several studies[186-188] have shown that the apparent volume of distribution of bicarbonate is highly variable and dependent on the acid-base status of the subject. These observations are consistent with a bicarbonate distribution volume consisting of two components, an anatomically real volume over which bicarbonate is distributed, and an anatomically imaginary compartment in which bicarbonate is titrated by hydrogen ions from nonbicarbonate buffers, such as phosphates, protein, and bone.[188,189] Based on a consideration of the chemistry and physiology of biological buffers, Fernandez and colleagues[188] have proposed that the bicarbonate distribution space can be described by

$$V_{Bi} = 0.4 = \frac{2.6}{C_{PBi}} \quad \text{body weight} \tag{4}$$

A similar expression has been suggested by Adrogue and colleagues[187] based on studies in dogs. Alternatively, Sargent and Gotch[63] have suggested that variability in the bicarbonate distribution space can be accommodated by using a fixed volume, such as extracellular fluid, and a term, E_{Bi}, that describes the loss of bicarbonate from the fixed volume to other buffer systems. This model gives rise to the following expression for bicarbonate accumulation during hemodialysis:

$$\frac{d\left(V_{Bi}C_{PBi}\right)}{dt} = D_{Bi}\left(C_{DBi} - C_{PBi}\right) - G_{H^+} - E_{Bi} \tag{5}$$

To date, it is unclear what form E_{Bi} should take. We used both zero order and first order approximations for E_{Bi} to examine bicarbonate kinetics in patients previously dialyzed against acetate-containing dialysate and whose predialysis serum bicarbonate concentrations were in the range of 15 to 18 mmol/L. Both approximations gave similar results and yielded values of E_{Bi} in the range of 0.2 to 1.0 mmol/min. These results imply that the quantity of base leaving the extracellular fluid space during a 4-hour dialysis is comparable to the estimated hydrogen ion burden generated in the interdialytic period. This finding is at variance with reports that approximately 40 percent of an acute acid load is buffered by extracellular bicarbonate and the remaining 60 percent by intracellular buffers.[45,46]

A similar approach can be taken for organic anions, such as acetate and lactate, which generate bicarbonate by consuming a hydrogen ion as they are metabolized, but the equations are more complex. In addition to terms for the dialytic fluxes of bicarbonate and organic anions, the equations must include a term for the metabolic elimination rate of the anion, E_A. This term is analogous to E_{Bi} in Eq. (5).

Acetate kinetics in normal humans can be described by a two-compartment model with first-order elimination.[74] The mean metabolic clearance rate has been determined to be 2.31 ± 0.21 L/min or 4.6 mmol/min at a plasma concentration of 2 mmol/L. Similar values have been reported by others.[190] Slightly lower rates have been reported in uremic patients.[84,174,191] Vreman and associates[78] found that acetate kinetics during hemodialysis were best described by a Michaelis-Menten model with a mean K_m of 8.5 mmol/L and a mean V_{max} of 18.1 mmol/min. There was, however, great variability among patients, and the actual peak rate of metabolism during dialysis varied from 1.9 to 7.2 mmol/min. Expression of E_A in terms of Michaelis-Menten kinetics makes the equation complex and not amenable to analytic solution. Furthermore, determination of the Michaelis-Menten constants for an individual patient is difficult. Thus, although a model can be conceptualized, the number of species to be considered, the reliance of buffer generation on metabolism, and the complex nature of the interactions between the various species have precluded development of a practical model for prescribing dialysate containing organic anions for base repletion. The kinetics of lactate in uremia and during renal replacement therapy have not been examined to the same extent as those of acetate.

A different approach to modeling acid-base balance in hemodialysis has been proposed by Thews.[192,193] This approach involves a multicompartment model that is used in a computer simulation to predict the postdialysis plasma bicarbonate concentration from patient-specific data, including the predialysis plasma bicarbonate concentration, and dialysis-specific data, including the dialysate bicarbonate concentration. The model is reported to provide good agreement between the predicted and observed postdialysis plasma bicarbonate concentrations for an individual treatment, although it is sensitive to errors in the predialysis plasma bicarbonate concentration.

To date, no model incorporating the more complex expressions for bicarbonate distribution has achieved widespread use for prescribing dialysate bicarbonate concentrations. Moreover, it is unclear how robust the models will be in patients with chronically depleted buffer stores, whose bicarbonate kinetics might change as their buffer stores are repleted. Further study will be required to identify which, if any, of the models is most appropriate for determining dialysate bicarbonate concentrations and to develop practical methods for determining the model parameters.

Until a quantitative approach to determining dialysate bicarbonate concentrations becomes available, the choice must be made on an empiric basis. Standard clinical practice is to use a nominal dialysate bicarbonate concentration of 35 mmol/L. Given the difference in hydrogen ion generation from patient to patient, this approach is less than ideal, as is evidenced by the wide range of predialysis serum bicarbonate concentrations observed in most patient populations (Fig. 20–3). Moreover, the nominal concentration may not accurately reflect the actual base content of the dialysate. Dialysate containing bicarbonate is formulated from two concentrates. The first contains sodium bicarbonate, and in some cases sodium chloride, whereas the second contains the other cations, such as calcium and magnesium. The second concentrate also contains 2 to 4 mmol of acid/L of final dialysate that, on proportioning, neutralizes an equivalent amount of bicarbonate to create the carbon dioxide necessary to establish the dialysate buffer system. This neutralization reduces the bicarbonate concentration of the final dialysate by an amount equivalent to the added acid. If the acid is present as acetic acid, the final dialysate will contain 2 to 4 mmol/L of sodium acetate, which can enter

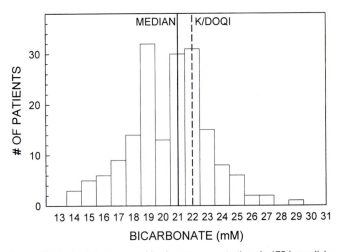

Figure 20–3. Predialysis serum bicarbonate concentrations in 175 hemodialysis patients treated with dialysate containing a nominal 35 mmol/L bicarbonate. The median concentration for the population and the K/DOQI target predialysis serum bicarbonate are shown by the solid and dashed lines, respectively.

the blood and be oxidized with consequent bicarbonate generation. The actual bicarbonate concentration of the dialysate will, however, be less than the nominal value for the concentrate used and may explain why the desired improvement in predialysis serum bicarbonate concentrations has not been obtained in some studies.[125,194,195] An improvement in protein intake, suggested by increases in hydrogen ion generation rates[194] and body weights,[195] with long-term dialysis against bicarbonate may also contribute to this problem. These data suggest that a higher dialysate bicarbonate concentration may be indicated for some patients. Increasing the dialysate bicarbonate concentration can result in improved correction of acidosis, based on predialysis pH and serum bicarbonate concentrations.[34,196-201] However, the effectiveness of this strategy is highly patient-dependent. Leunissen and colleagues[199] adjusted dialysate bicarbonate concentrations in a group of 28 patients in an attempt to correct their acidosis optimally. While they were able to achieve mean values for the group in their target range (predialysis plasma total CO_2 >22 mmol/L, postdialysis total CO_2 in the range of 28 to 32 mmol/L), only 25 percent of individual patients actually met both criteria. Sixteen patients had predialysis total CO_2 values <22 mmol/L and five patients had postdialysis total CO_2 values <28 mmol/L.

In addition to differences in metabolism and rate of hydrogen ion generation, the rest of the dialysis prescription should be considered in choosing a dialysate bicarbonate concentration. The frequency and time of dialysis and the prescribed volume of fluid to be removed during dialysis may influence how well acidosis is corrected with a given dialysate bicarbonate concentration. In general, blood solute concentrations are better controlled by more frequent dialysis treatments.[202] Quotidian nocturnal hemodialysis typically involves six nightly treatments of 8 hours duration per week. Short daily—or hemeral quotidian—dialysis typically involves six treatments of 2 hours duration per week. Although the number of patients studied is small, these therapies appear to provide predialysis plasma bicarbonate concentrations in the normal range.[203] Lower dialysate bicarbonate concentrations of 28 to 35 mmol/L, depending on the patient's protein intake, than are used for standard thrice weekly hemodialysis may be indicated for quotidian nocturnal hemodialysis, while hemeral quotidian hemodialysis may require dialysate bicarbonate concentrations similar to those used for thrice weekly dialysis.

Patients who are poorly compliant with regard to fluid intake make up one group of patients who may benefit from an increased dialysate bicarbonate concentration. Removal of 1 L of ultrafiltrate from plasma with a bicarbonate concentration of 22 mmol/L represents a loss of 22 mmol of buffer by the patient. Thus, a patient requiring 3 L of fluid removal loses 66 mmol of bicarbonate, which approximates

an additional day of metabolic acid production. In addition to loss of bicarbonate via intradialytic fluid removal, excessive base-free water intake during the interdialytic period may also contribute to a low predialysis bicarbonate concentration by dilution.[204] The importance of fluid intake to acid-base balance in hemodialysis patients is supported by clinical observations. Fabris and colleagues found that reducing the intradialytic weight gain by 1 kg increased the predialysis bicarbonate by 1.67 mmol/L,[205] while Agroyannis and associates found significant inverse correlations between pre- and postdialysis plasma bicarbonate concentrations and interdialytic weight gain.[206]

Use of a dialysate bicarbonate concentration of 40 mmol/L or more, without regard to individual patient differences, may result in postdialysis alkalemia (pH >7.5) in some patients,[197,200] with resultant unpleasant side effects. Even at lower dialysate bicarbonate concentrations, there may be a trade-off between achieving a normal predialysis bicarbonate concentration and intradialytic symptoms. In a randomized controlled trial comparing dialysate bicarbonate concentrations of 32 mmol/L and 26 mmol/L, hypotensive episodes occurred in 5.5 percent of dialyses when the higher bicarbonate concentration was used, compared to 1.7 percent with the lower bicarbonate concentration.[207] The incidence of fluid administration for treatment of symptoms was also greater when the higher dialysate bicarbonate concentration was used (21 vs. 14 percent of dialyses).[207] The reasons for this difference are not clear, since the patients were not overtly alkalemic postdialysis.

Supplemental Base

For many patients treated on a standard thrice-weekly dialysis schedule, the goal of minimizing excursions of body pH outside the normal range is not achieved when bicarbonate is provided solely by dialytic transfer. In these patients, dialytic bicarbonate transfer can be supplemented by the use of oral base.[208,209] Leunissen and colleagues[199] were able to correct acidosis optimally in 79 percent of their patients through a combination of increased dialysate bicarbonate concentrations and the administration of 1.5 to 3.0 g/day of sodium bicarbonate. The use of oral calcium carbonate and calcium acetate instead of aluminum hydroxide to reduce dietary phosphate absorption may be one effective means of oral base administration. Anelli and colleagues[210] found that predialysis plasma bicarbonate concentrations increased by an average of 2.2 mmol/L in a group of 11 patients treated with 100 mg/kg calcium carbonate for 2 weeks. In contrast, sevelamer hydrochloride, an effective phosphate binder that is used in patients with hypercalcemia, does not contain alkali and provides no benefit in correcting chronic acidosis compared to calcium acetate or calcium carbonate.[211] In fact, when binding phosphorus, sevelamer releases acid and may aggravate metabolic acidosis.

BASE REPLETION IN PERITONEAL DIALYSIS

Regeneration of depleted buffer stores by peritoneal dialysis is accomplished in a similar manner to that used in hemodialysis—that is, by including buffer in the dialysate in concentrations greater than those in plasma. This buffer then enters the blood by diffusive mass transfer across the peritoneal membrane. With the now obsolete thrice-weekly intermittent peritoneal dialysis (IPD), a sawtooth acid-base pattern similar to that observed in hemodialysis was seen, and the goals for base repletion were the same as those for hemodialysis. The more continuous nature of current therapies, such as CAPD and cycler-based automated peritoneal dialysis (APD), results in less fluctuation in acid-base balance and more nearly steady-state levels of pH and serum bicarbonate.[212] The goal of base repletion by CAPD and APD should be to transfer sufficient base to the patient to maintain pH and serum bicarbonate concentrations in the normal range. A recent report by Mujais indicates that current CAPD and APD therapies achieve this goal for the majority of patients in the absence of comorbidities known to affect acid-base balance.[213] In this survey of 252 patients, the plasma bicarbonate concentration was <22 mmol/L in only 12 percent of patients, although a further 20 percent had a plasma bicarbonate of ≥28 mmol/L. In those patients who do not achieve a normal pH and serum bicarbonate, oral sodium bicarbonate may be used to supplement administration of base through the dialysate.[214]

Base Repletion

As in the case of hemodialysis, use of an organic anion such as lactate for base repletion creates a situation in which a bidirectional flux of base occurs (Fig. 20–2). Lactate moves into the blood, and bicarbonate and other anions move into the dialysate. Peritoneal dialysis is not as efficient as hemodialysis with regard to small molecule transfer and, as a consequence, the magnitudes of these fluxes are much less in peritoneal dialysis than in hemodialysis. At these flux rates, metabolism appears able to handle the burden imposed by dialytic transfer of both D(−)-lactate and L(+)-lactate in most patients, with serum lactate [212,215-219] and pyruvate[212,217,218] remaining essentially in the normal range. The overall ability to metabolize lactate may, however, vary from patient to patient and with other conditions of dialysis. Yamamoto and associates[219] have shown serum lactate concentrations to be increased and lactate uptake decreased when the glucose concentration of the dialysate is increased from 1.36 to 3.86%. These changes presumably reflect the impact of the glucose load on the amount of lactate able to enter the gluconeogenic pathway. Also, hyperlactatemia has

been reported to occur in some patients.[220] Reduced flux rates also aid base repletion in peritoneal dialysis by decreasing the loss of buffers into the dialysate; however, this may also result in insufficient base being transferred to the patient to neutralize metabolic acid production. Mass balance studies indicate that the extent to which acid-base balance is maintained depends on the lactate concentration of the dialysate.[212,215,221] The impetus given by the K/DOQI guidelines to increasing the delivered dose of peritoneal dialysis[222] and the higher exchange volumes used with APD compared to CAPD have also led to better correction of acidosis in peritoneal dialysis patients.

Biocompatibility

Initially, CAPD solutions were available formulated with either acetate or lactate for base repletion. After a number of reports of CAPD patients experiencing pain on inflow, the use of acetate in CAPD solutions was discontinued. The move away from acetate gained further momentum from reports of a progressive decrease in ultrafiltration capacity in some patients[223] and the suggestion[224-226] that acetate played a role in this phenomenon. Later reports[227-229] cast doubt on the existence of a direct association between acetate and loss of ultrafiltration capacity; however, use of acetate for base repletion in peritoneal dialysis ceased. In retrospect, there was little definitive proof that acetate was injurious to the peritoneal membrane, and loss of peritoneal membrane integrity and function continues to be a problem contributing to therapy survival with lactate-containing solutions. Properties of lactate-containing solutions that have been linked to peritoneal membrane damage include an acid pH of 5.2 to 5.5, a lactate concentration of 40 mmol/L, the presence of glucose degradation products, and hyperosmolality.[230,231] In an attempt to mitigate the bioincompatibility of traditional lactate-containing solutions, multicompartment bags have been developed that allow formulation of solutions with neutral pH that contain either bicarbonate or a mixture of lactate and bicarbonate. Randomized trials comparing these solutions with traditional lactate-containing solutions show an equal or improved correction of acidosis,[232-234] an increase in mesothelial cell mass,[234,235] and a reduction in inflammation.[235]

Selection of a Dialysate Base Concentration

Mathematical models have been developed to quantitate solute removal during peritoneal dialysis.[236,237] Comparatively little effort has been made to date, however, to extend these models to encompass acid-base balance. Possible reasons include the difficulty in defining mass transfer across the peritoneal membrane and the fact the pH and serum bicarbonate are generally close to the normal range in patients treated with CAPD and APD. As a consequence, an empiric approach has been used to determine the appropriate dialysate concentration of the base repletion agent for these therapies.

Initially, solutions for CAPD contained 35 mmol/L of lactate. Clinical experience revealed that use of this lactate concentration could result in serum bicarbonate concentrations less than normal in up to 25 percent of patients.[215,221,238] Confirmation was provided by mass balance studies,[215,221] which showed a negative base balance in the range of 10 to 40 mmol/day in some patients. Losses of other anions into the dialysate are small with CAPD, on the order of 4 mmol/day,[221] and the net base gain by the patient is essentially the result of bicarbonate loss and lactate uptake. Bicarbonate loss increases as the target serum bicarbonate concentration is increased. Furthermore, as described previously for hemodialysis, bicarbonate losses will also increase as the volume of fluid to be removed increases. Because the maximum rate of lactate metabolism is apparently not approached in CAPD, any increase in the loss of bicarbonate can be compensated for by slight increases in the dialysate lactate concentration. Solutions with a lactate concentration of 40 mmol/L provide better correction of acidosis in patients treated by CAPD than solutions containing 35 mmol/L of lactate.[239,240] Extended use of a lactate concentration of 40 mmol/L can, however, result in serum bicarbonate concentrations in excess of 30 mmol/L in some patients.[239] Thus, it is reasonable to initiate CAPD with the higher lactate concentration and subsequently change to the lower concentration in those patients who develop alkalemia. A similar strategy can be used for bicarbonate- and bicarbonate/lactate-containing solutions. In general, patients with a higher body weight, body surface area, and protein catabolic rate will benefit from the use of solutions containing higher concentrations of bicarbonate.[241]

BASE REPLETION IN OTHER RENAL REPLACEMENT THERAPIES

Hemofiltration

Unlike hemodialysis and peritoneal dialysis, solute transfer with hemofiltration (HF) is totally dependent on convection. A highly permeable membrane is used to produce a filtrate of plasma water that contains all microsolutes at essentially the same concentration as in plasma. In this respect, HF functions like the glomerulus. Unlike the nephron, however, there are no subsequent tubular functions. The hemofiltrate is discarded and the patient's volume balance maintained by infusing a physiologic electrolyte solution either before or after the hemofilter (predilution or postdilution HF, respectively). Intermittent HF has seen limited use in the treatment of end-stage renal disease, in part because the removal of small molecules is limited in comparison to hemodialysis.[242] However, HF is widely used in continuous renal replacement therapy (CRRT) for the treatment of acute renal failure. CRRT is defined as an extracorporeal blood purification therapy that substitutes for impaired renal function over an extended period of time and is intended to be applied for 24 h/day.[243] In the United States 25 percent of patients with acute renal failure are treated with CRRT; the therapy used most commonly is continuous venovenous hemofiltration (CVVH).

During a typical CVVH treatment, 20 to 40 L of fluid may be exchanged daily, depending on whether the postdilution or predilution configuration is used. With HF, endogenous bicarbonate is lost in the ultrafiltrate and must be replaced. This loss can be 25 to 30 mmol/L. Additional base must be supplied if acidosis is present. The bicarbonate losses in postdilution HF can be calculated from the following:

$$HCO_3^- \text{ loss (mmol/h)} = Q_{UF} \times [HCO_3^-] \times 1.05 \quad (6)$$

Where Q_{UF} is the filtrate flow rate (L/h), $[HCO_3^-]$ is the plasma bicarbonate concentration, and 1.05 is the sieving coefficient of HCO_3^-. Base repletion is effected by including a metabolizable anion in the infusion fluid. Solutions containing acetate, lactate, citrate, and bicarbonate have been used for CRRT. Important differences, which may affect patient management and outcomes, exist between the different anions. As discussed previously, acetate, lactate, and citrate all require metabolism to neutral end products for bicarbonate generation to occur. Acetate is no longer used, for essentially the same reasons it is no longer used in hemodialysis. Citrate can be used for both anion replacement and anticoagulation in cases where heparin is contraindicated. Unlike acetate and lactate, citrate is converted to bicarbonate in a 1:3 ratio rather than 1:1, and alkalosis may develop in as many as 25 percent of cases.[244] Lactate is used most commonly for CVVH and can provide reasonable correction of acidosis if liver function is intact.[245] Increased levels of lactate may occur in patients with liver insufficiency as part of multiorgan failure.[246] These patients lose endogenous bicarbonate during HF and the replacement lactate cannot be metabolized, leading to worsening metabolic acidosis. Thus, bicarbonate should be used instead of lactate in patients with lactic acidosis or liver failure. Critical care patients may exhibit systemic inflammatory response syndrome and are often catabolic. An exogenous lactate load may increase the protein degradation in these patients by stimulating gluconeogenesis via oxidation of amino acids in the liver. Furthermore, lactate may increase intracellular lactate and thereby reduce myocardial contractility. Acute renal failure patients treated with 3 or more days of CVVH with bicarbonate replacement fluid show better correction of acidosis and a significant reduction in the number of hypotensive episodes and cardiovascular events compared to control patients treated with lactate.[247] The serum bicarbonate levels were improved in the bicarbonate-treated group, without significant alkalosis. Extended hemodialysis is another form of CRRT used to treat acute renal failure. It uses bicarbonate-containing dialysate at low flow rates (100 to 200 mL/min) for 12 hours or more daily. In a randomized controlled study comparing extended hemodialysis and CVVH in patients with acute renal failure, arterial blood pH and plasma bicarbonate became normal faster with extended hemodialysis than with CVVH.[248] Continuous venovenous hemodialysis (CVVHD) is similar to extended hemodialysis but uses a lower dialysate flow rate, typically 20 mL/min. Improved control of metabolic acidosis also has been reported for CVVHD when base repletion is accomplished with bicarbonate instead of lactate.[249] Taken together, these data support the use of bicarbonate replacement fluid in CRRT whenever possible.

Hemodiafiltration

Hemodiafiltration (HDF) combines both diffusion and convection in a single therapy.[242] Diffusive solute removal occurs down the concentration gradient between blood and dialysate. Convective solute removal is obtained by using an ultrafiltration rate in excess of that required for net fluid removal. Fluid balance is maintained by infusing a substitution solution in a pre- or postdilution mode. HDF is used both as an intermittent therapy for end-stage renal disease and for CRRT. Originally, intermittent HDF was performed using bicarbonate-containing dialysate and bags of sterile, lactate-containing fluid for the substitution solution. Modern forms of intermittent HDF are performed using systems that prepare the substitution solution on-line by sequential ultrafiltration of bicarbonate-containing dialysate.[250] The dialysate contains bicarbonate at the same concentrations used for hemodialysis and pre- and post-dialysis serum bicarbonate concentrations with postdilution HDF are very similar to those obtained with high-flux hemodialysis.[251] Optimal correction of acidosis with predilution HDF may require higher dialysate and substitution solution bicarbonate concentrations than are needed for postdilution HDF or hemodialysis. Pedrini and colleagues showed that predilution HDF resulted in a 30 percent reduction in net transfer of bicarbonate to the patient compared to postdilution HDF when the same dialysate and substitution solution bicarbonate concentration was used for both therapies.[252]

Sorbent-Based Dialysate Regeneration Systems

Standard hemodialysis therapy requires proximity to a source of purified water able to be delivered at a rate of 30 L/h. To overcome this constraint and provide some portability, Gordon and coworkers[253] introduced a sorbent-based system that utilized a combination of enzymatic degradation, ion exchange, and carbon adsorption to contin-

uously regenerate a small volume (5 to 6 L) of dialysate. A detailed description of the physical chemistry of this system is given in Chap. 38. There are, however, some features having special implications for the maintenance of acid-base balance.

To date, no practical sorbents have been developed for the removal of urea from the spent dialysate. In the absence of a sorbent, urea is removed through enzymatic degradation by immobilized urease. The degradation products are ammonium and carbonate ions. The carbonate ions represent a large potential excess of base that must be neutralized to maintain the pH of the dialysate in the operating range for urease while simultaneously preserving sufficient base for transfer to the patient. This balance is achieved by exchanging the ammonium ions for a mixture of sodium and hydrogen ions. The hydrogen ions then neutralize a portion of the carbonate ions to carbon dioxide. In addition, the anion exchange layer of the sorbent cartridge can be configured to release chloride, acetate, or bicarbonate ions in exchange for the phosphate ions present in the spent dialysate. The result is a complex set of interacting processes influenced by the treatment requirements of the patient: for example, the urea burden to be removed and the extent of metabolic acidosis. The complexity of this system has given rise to some acid-base problems peculiar to the sorbent system.

As the result of enzymatic degradation of urea, large quantities of carbon dioxide enter the dialysate resulting in very high concentrations of dissolved carbon dioxide.[254,255] This carbon dioxide burden can lead to acute hypercapnia. Hence, Hamm and colleagues[256] described a patient who, while being dialyzed with the sorbent regeneration system and mechanically ventilated, developed an arterial PCO_2 and pH of 81 mmHg and 7.0, respectively. The dialysate PCO_2 and pH were 237 mmHg and 6.51, respectively. Similar although less dramatic results have also been reported by Reyes and colleagues.[257] The potential for hypercapnia to occur is clearly increased as the urea burden to the sorbent cartridge is increased. The clinical consequences for the average patient able to excrete the carbon dioxide burden through the lungs are, however, uncertain, and appropriate degassing of the dialysate can eliminate the problem. Of potentially more concern was the observation in early studies that use of the sorbent system did not lead to adequate correction of the patient's metabolic acidosis.[254] These systems exchanged chloride for phosphorus in the anion exchange layer of the sorbent cartridge. Substitution of acetate for chloride as the counter-ion on the anion exchange resin by the manufacturer resulted in a considerable improvement in this situation. Others[258,259] addressed the problem by pre-rinsing the sorbent cartridge with solutions containing sodium bicarbonate. In a small number of patients, long-term use of the latter maneuver was, however, associated with the development of severe osteomalacia that may have been due to release of aluminum from the sorbent cartridge.[259] Similar findings have been reported in patients dialyzed for extended periods with the standard sorbent cartridge,[260] and it was suggested that pH changes may lead to release of aluminum from the sorbent bed. Subsequently, the sorbent cartridge and the procedures for its preparation have been modified to reduce the rate of aluminum release under normal operating conditions.[261,262]

REFERENCES

1. Widmer B, Gerhardt RE, Harrington JT, et al. Serum electrolyte and acid base composition: the influence of graded degrees of chronic kidney disease. *Arch Intern Med* 1979; 139:1099.

2. Lee HY, Joo HY, Han DS. Serum electrolyte and acid base composition in patients with graded degrees of chronic kidney disease. *Yonsei Med J* 1985;26:39.

3. Del Canale S, Fiaccadori E, Coffrini E, et al. Uremic acidosis and intracellular buffering. *Scand J Urol Nephrol* 1986; 20:301.

4. Alvestrand A, Bergström J, Fürst P, et al. Effect of essential amino acid supplementation on muscle and plasma free amino acids in chronic uremia. *Kidney Int* 1978;14:323.

5. Garibotto G, Deferrari G, Robaudo C, et al. Effects of a protein meal on blood amino acid profile in patients with chronic kidney disease. *Nephron* 1993;64:216.

6. May RC, Kelly RA, Mitch WE. Mechanisms for defects in muscle protein metabolism in rats with chronic uremia: influence of metabolic acidosis. *J Clin Invest* 1987;79:1099.

7. Hara Y, May RC, Kelly RA, et al. Acidosis, not azotemia, stimulates branched-chain, amino acid catabolism in uremic rats. *Kidney Int* 1987;32:808.

8. Coles GA. Body composition in chronic kidney disease. *Quart J Med* 1972;41:25.

9. Brenes LG, Brenes JN, Hernandez MM. Familial proximal renal tubular acidosis. A distinct clinical entity. *Am J Med* 1977;63:244.

10. May RC, Kelly RA, Mitch WE. Metabolic acidosis stimulates protein degradation in rat muscle by a glucocorticoid-dependent mechanism. *J Clin Invest* 1986;77:614.

11. May RC, Hara Y, Kelly RA, et al. Branched-chain amino acid metabolism in rat muscle: abnormal regulation in acidosis. *Am J Physiol* 1987;252:E712.

12. Williams B, Layward E, Walls J. Skeletal muscle degradation and nitrogen wasting in rats with chronic metabolic acidosis. *Clin Sci* 1991;80:457.

13. Reaich D, Channon SM, Scrimgeour CM, et al. Ammonium chloride-induced acidosis increases protein breakdown and amino acid oxidation in humans. *Am J Physiol* 1992;263: E735.

14. Cupisti A, Baker F, Brown J, et al. Effects of acid loading on serum amino acid profiles and muscle composition in normal fed rats. *Clin Sci* 1993;85:445.

15. Papadoyannakis NJ, Stefanidis CJ, McGeown M. The effect of the correction of metabolic acidosis on nitrogen and potassium balance of patients with chronic kidney disease. *Am J Clin Nutr* 1984;40:623.

16. Jenkins D, Burton PR, Bennett SE, et al. The metabolic consequences of the correction of acidosis in uraemia. *Nephrol Dial Transplant* 1989;4:92.

17. Reaich D, Channon SM, Scrimgeour CM, et al. Correction of acidosis in humans with CRF decreases protein degradation and amino acid oxidation. *Am J Physiol* 1993;265: E230.

18. Lim VS, Yarasheski KE, Flanigan MJ. The effect of uraemia, acidosis, and dialysis treatment on protein metabolism: a longitudinal leucine kinetic study. *Nephrol Dial Transplant* 1998;13:1723.

19. Graham KA, Reaich D, Channon SM, et al. Correction of acidosis in hemodialysis decreases whole-body protein degradation. *J Am Soc Nephrol* 1997;8:632.

20. Graham KA, Reaich D, Channon SM, et al. Correction of acidosis in CAPD decreases whole body protein degradation. *Kidney Int* 1996;49:1396.

21. Mitch WE, Medina R, Grieber S, et al. Metabolic acidosis stimulates muscle protein degradation by activating the adenosine triphosphate-dependent pathway involving ubiquitin and proteasomes. *J Clin Invest* 1994;93:2127.

22. Bailey JL, Wang X, England BK, et al. The acidosis of chronic kidney disease activates muscle proteolysis in rats by augmenting transcription of genes encoding proteins of the ATP-dependent ubiquitin-proteasome pathway. *J Clin Invest* 1996;97:1447.

23. Pickering WP, Price SR, Bircher G, et al. Nutrition in CAPD: serum bicarbonate and the ubiquitin-proteasome system in muscle. *Kidney Int* 2002;61:1286.

24. England BK, Greiber S, Mitch WE, et al. Rat muscle branched-chain ketoacid dehydrogenase activity and mRNAs increase with extracellular academia. *Am J Physiol* 1995;268:C1395.

25. Bergström J, Alvestrand A, Fürst P. Plasma and muscle free amino acids in maintenance hemodialysis patients without protein malnutrition. *Kidney Int* 1990;38:108.

26. Kooman JP, Deutz NEP, Zijlmans P, et al. The influence of bicarbonate supplementation on plasma levels of branched-chain amino acids in haemodialysis patients with metabolic acidosis. *Nephrol Dial Transplant* 1997;12:2397.

27. Mitch WE, Goldberg AL. Mechanisms of disease: mechanisms of muscle wasting—the role of the ubiquitin-proteasome pathway. *N Engl J Med* 1996;335:1897.

28. Mehrotra R, Kopple JD, Wolfson M. Metabolic acidosis in maintenance dialysis patients: clinical considerations. *Kidney Int* 2003;64(suppl 88):S13.

29. Pellegrino ED, Biltz RM, Rogers PJ. The composition of human bone in uremia: observations on the reservoir functions of bone and demonstration of a labile fraction of bone carbonate. *Medicine* 1965;44:397.

30. Kaye M, Frueh AJ, Silverman M, et al. A study of vertebral bone powder from patients with chronic kidney disease. *J Clin Invest* 1970;49:442.

31. Mora Palma FJ, Ellis HA, Cook DB, et al. Osteomalacia in patients with chronic kidney disease before dialysis or transplantation. *Q J Med* 1983;52:332.

32. Coen G, Manni M, Addari O, et al. Metabolic acidosis and osteodystrophic bone disease in predialysis chronic kidney disease: effect of calcitriol treatment. *Miner Electrolyte Metab* 1995;21:375.

33. Lemann J Jr, Bushinsky DA, Hamm LL. Bone buffering of acid and base in humans. *Am J Physiol* 2003;285:F811.

34. Lefebvre A, de Vernejoul MC, Gueris J, et al. Optimal correction of acidosis changes progression of dialysis osteodystrophy. *Kidney Int* 1989;36:1112.

35. Lu K-C, Shieh S-D, Li B-L, et al. Rapid correction of metabolic acidosis in chronic kidney disease: effect on parathyroid hormone activity. *Nephron* 1994;67:419.

36. Movilli E, Zani R, Carli O, et al. Direct effect of the correction of acidosis on plasma parathyroid hormone concentrations, calcium and phosphate in hemodialysis patients: a prospective study. *Nephron* 2001;87:257.

37. Lin S-H, Lin Y-F, Chin H-M, et al. Must metabolic acidosis be associated with malnutrition in haemodialysed patients? *Nephrol Dial Transplant* 2002;17:2006.

38. Lowrie EG, Lew NL. Death risk in hemodialysis patients: the predictive value of commonly measured variables and an evaluation of death rate differences between facilities. *Am J Kidney Dis* 1990;15:458.

39. Lemann J Jr, Lennon EJ, Goodman D, et al. The net balance of acid in subjects given large loads of acid or alkali. *J Clin Invest* 1965;44:507.

40. Goodman AD, Lemann J Jr, Lennon EJ, et al. Production, excretion, and net balance of fixed acid in patients with renal acidosis. *J Clin Invest* 1965;44:495.

41. Lennon EJ, Lemann J Jr, Litzow JR. The effects of diet and stool composition on the net external acid balance of normal subjects. *J Clin Invest* 1966;45:1601.

42. Hood VL, Tannen RL. pH control of lactic acid and keto acid production: a mechanism of acid-base regulation. *Miner Electrolyte Metab* 1983;9:317.

43. Hood VL. pH regulation of endogenous acid production in subjects with chronic ketoacidosis. *Am J Physiol* 1985;249:F220.

44. Romeh SA, Tannen RL. Amelioration of hypoxia-induced lactic acidosis by superimposed hypercapnea or hydrochloric acid infusion. *Am J Physiol* 1986;250:F702.

45. Swan RC, Pitts RF, Madisso H. Neutralization of infused acid by nephrectomized dogs. *J Clin Invest* 1955;34:205.

46. Schwartz WB, Orning KJ, Porter R. The internal distribution of hydrogen ions with varying degrees of metabolic acidosis. *J Clin Invest* 1957;36:373.

47. Brautbar N. Extrarenal factors in the homeostasis of acid-base balance. *Semin Nephrol* 1981;1:232.

48. Green J, Kleeman CR. Role of bone in regulation of systemic acid-base balance. *Kidney Int* 1991;39:9.

49. Lemann J Jr, Litzow JR, Lennon EJ. The effects of chronic acid loads in normal man: further evidence for the participation of bone mineral in the defense against chronic metabolic acidosis. *J Clin Invest* 1966;45:1608.

50. Burnell JM, Teubner E. Changes in bone sodium and carbonate in metabolic acidosis and alkalosis in the dog. *J Clin Invest* 1971;50:327.

51. Bettice JA. Skeletal carbon dioxide stores during metabolic acidosis. *Am J Physiol* 1984;247:F326.

52. Bushinsky D, Lam BC, Nespeca R, et al. Decreased bone carbonate content in response to metabolic, but not respiratory, acidosis. *Am J Physiol* 1993;265:F530.

53. Litzow JR, Lemann J Jr, Lennon EJ. The effect of treatment of acidosis on calcium balance in patients with chronic azotemic renal disease. *J Clin Invest* 1967;46:280.

54. Pellegrino ED, Biltz RM, Letteri JM. Interrelationships of carbonate, phosphate, monohydrogen phosphate, calcium, magnesium and sodium in uraemic bone: comparison of dialysed and non-dialysed patients. *Clin Sci Mol Med* 1977;53:307.

55. Oh MS. Irrelevance of bone buffering to acid-base homeostasis in chronic metabolic acidosis. *Nephron* 1991;59:7.

56. National Kidney Foundation Kidney Disease Outcomes Quality Initiative. NKF-K/DOQI clinical practice guidelines for nutrition in chronic kidney disease. *Am J Kidney Dis* 2000;35(suppl 2):S38.

57. Bray SH, Tung R-U, Jones ER. The magnitude of metabolic acidosis is dependent on differences in bicarbonate assays. *Am J Kidney Dis* 1996;28:700.

58. Kirschbaum B. Spurious metabolic acidosis in hemodialysis patients. *Am J Kidney Dis* 2000;35:1068.

59. Howse MLP, Leonard M, Venning M, et al. The effect of different methods of storage on the results of serum total CO_2 assays. *Clin Sci* 2001;100:609.

60. Herr RD, Swanson T. Serum bicarbonate declines with sample size in vacutainer tubes. *Am J Clin Pathol* 1992;97:213.

61. Laski ME. Penny wise and bicarbonate foolish. *Am J Kidney Dis* 2000;35:1224.

62. Gotch FA, Sargent JA, Keen ML. Hydrogen ion balance in dialysis therapy. *Artif Organs* 1982;6:388.

63. Sargent JA, Gotch FA. Principles and biophysics of dialysis. In: Maher JF, ed. *Replacement of Renal Function by Dialysis*. Dordrecht, The Netherlands: Kluwer, 1989;87.

64. Pendras JP, Cole JJ, Tu WH, et al. Improved technique of continuous flow hemodialysis. *ASAIO Trans* 1961;7:27.

65. Boen ST. Kinetics of peritoneal dialysis. A comparison with the artificial kidney. *Medicine* 1961;40:243.

66. Klein E, Ward RA, Harding GB. Calcium carbonate precipitation in bicarbonate hemodialysis. *Artif Organs* 1986;10:248.

67. Mudge GH, Manning JA, Gilman A. Sodium acetate as a source of fixed base. *Proc Soc Exp Biol Med* 1949;71:136.

68. Mion CM, Hegstrom RM, Boen ST, et al. Substitution of sodium acetate for sodium bicarbonate in the bath fluid for hemodialysis. *ASAIO Trans* 1964;10:110.

69. Vidt DG. Recommendations on choice of peritoneal dialysis solutions. *Ann Intern Med* 1973;78:144.

70. Cammack R. Assay, purification and properties of a mammalian D-2-hydroxy acid dehydrogenase. *Biochem J* 1969;115:55.

71. Huennekins FM, Mahler HR, Nordmann J. Studies on the cyclophorase system: XVII. The occurrence and properties of an α-hydroxy acid racemase. *Arch Biochem* 1951;30:77.

72. Lipsky SR, Alper BJ, Rubini ME, et al. The effects of alkalosis upon ketone body production and carbohydrate metabolism in man. *J Clin Invest* 1954;33:1269.

73. Skutches CL, Holroyde CP, Myers RN, et al. Plasma acetate turnover and oxidation. *J Clin Invest* 1979;64:708.

74. Richards RH, Vreman HJ, Zager P, et al. Acetate metabolism in normal human subjects. *Am J Kidney Dis* 1982;2:47.

75. Wathen RL, Ward RA, Harding GB, et al. Acid-base and metabolic responses to anion infusion in the anesthetized dog. *Kidney Int* 1982;21:592.

76. Tolchin N, Roberts JL, Hayashi J, et al. Metabolic consequences of high mass-transfer hemodialysis. *Kidney Int* 1977;11:366.

77. Wathen RL, Keshaviah P, Hommeyer P, et al. The metabolic effects of hemodialysis with and without glucose in the dialysate. *Am J Clin Nutr* 1978;31:1870.

78. Vreman HJ, Assomull VM, Kaiser BA, et al. Acetate metabolism and acid-base homeostasis during hemodialysis: influence of dialyzer efficiency and rate of acetate metabolism. *Kidney Int* 1980;18(suppl 10):S62.

79. Desch G, Polito C, Descomps B, et al. Effect of acetate of ketogenesis during hemodialysis. *J Lab Clin Med* 1982;99: 98.

80. Ward RA, Wathen RL, Williams TE, et al. Hemodialysate composition and intradialytic metabolic, acid-base and potassium changes. *Kidney Int* 1987;32:129.

81. Kirkendol PL, Pearson JE, Gonzalez FM. A potential source of fixed base in dialysate solutions: a comparison of the cardiovascular effects of sodium succinate versus bicarbonate and acetate. *ASAIO J* 1980;3:57.

82. Torrente J, Coronel F, Herrero JA, et al. Partial substitution of sodium lactate for sodium acetate in the bath fluid for hemodialysis. *Artif Organs* 1990;14:2.

83. Dalal S, Yu AW, Gupta DK, et al. L-lactate high-efficiency hemodialysis: hemodynamics, blood gas changes, potassium/phosphorus, and symptoms. *Kidney Int* 1990;38:896.

84. Sigler MH, Skutches CL, Teehan BP, et al. Acetate and energy metabolism during hemodialysis. *Kidney Int* 1983; 24(suppl 16):S97.

85. Vinay P, Prud'Homme M, Vinet B, et al. Acetate metabolism and bicarbonate generation during hemodialysis: 10 years of observation. *Kidney Int* 1987;31:1194.

86. Novello A, Kelsch RC, Easterling RE. Acetate intolerance during hemodialysis. *Clin Nephrol* 1976;5:29.

87. Desch G, Oules R, Mion C, et al. Plasma acetate levels during hemodialysis. *Clin Chim Acta* 1978;85:231.

88. Mansell MA, Nunan TO, Laker MF, et al. Incidence and significance of rising blood acetate levels during hemodialysis. *Clin Nephrol* 1979;12:22.

89. Graefe U, Milutinovich J, Follette WC, et al. Less dialysis-induced morbidity and vascular instability with bicarbonate in dialysate. *Ann Intern Med* 1978;88:332.

90. Kaiser BA, Potter DE, Bryant RE, et al. Acid-base changes and acetate metabolism during routine and high-efficiency hemodialysis in children. *Kidney Int* 1981;19:70.

91. Arieff AI, Guisado R, Massry SG, et al. Central nervous system pH in uremia and the effects of hemodialysis. *J Clin Invest* 1976;58:306.

92. Ward RA, Wathen RL. Utilization of bicarbonate for base repletion in hemodialysis. *Artif Organs* 1982;6:396.

93. Gennari FJ. Acid-base balance in dialysis patients. *Kidney Int* 1985;28:678.

94. Sherlock J, Ledwith J, Letteri J. Hypoventilation and hypoxemia during hemodialysis: reflex response to removal of CO_2 across the dialyzer. *ASAIO Trans* 1977;23:406.

95. Sargent JA, Gotch FA. Bicarbonate and carbon dioxide transport during hemodialysis. *ASAIO J* 1979;2:61.

96. Dolan MJ, Whipp BJ, Davidson WD, et al. Hypopnea associated with acetate hemodialysis: carbon dioxide-flow-dependent ventilation. *N Engl J Med* 1981;305:72.

97. Patterson RW, Nissenson AR, Miller J, et al. Hypoxemia and pulmonary gas exchange during hemodialysis. *J Appl Physiol* 1981;50:259.

98. Abu-Hamdan DK, Desai SG, Mahajan SK, et al. Hypoxemia during hemodialysis using acetate versus bicarbonate dialysate. *Am J Nephrol* 1984;4:248.

99. Hunt JM, Chappell TR, Henrich WL, et al. Gas exchange during dialysis: contrasting mechanisms contributing to comparable alterations with acetate and bicarbonate buffers. *Am J Med* 1984;77:255.

100. Kolobow T, Gattinoni L, Tomlinson TA, et al. Control of breathing using an extracorporeal membrane lung. *Anesthesiology* 1977;46:138.

101. Phillipson EA, Duffin J, Cooper JD. Critical dependence of respiratory rhythmicity on metabolic CO_2 load. *J Appl Physiol* 1981;50:45.

102. Oh MS, Uribarri J, Del Monte ML, et al. A mechanism of hypoxemia during hemodialysis. *Am J Nephrol* 1985;5:366.

103. Cardoso M, Vinay P, Vinet B, et al. Hypoxemia during hemodialysis: a critical review of the facts. *Am J Kidney Dis* 1988;11:281.

104. Ikeda T, Hirasawa, Aizawa Y, et al. Effect of acetate upon arterial gases. *J Dialysis* 1979;3:135.

105. Heyrman RM, De Backer WA, Van Waeleghem JP, et al. The effect of acetate on ventilation in haemodialysis patients. *Nephrol Dial Transplant* 1989;4:1060.

106. Eiser AR, Jayamanne D, Kokseng C, et al. Contrasting alterations in pulmonary gas exchange during acetate and bicarbonate hemodialysis. *Am J Nephrol* 1982;2:123.

107. De Backer WA, Verpooten GA, Borgonjon DJ, et al. Hypoxemia during hemodialysis: effects of different membranes and dialysate compositions. *Kidney Int* 1983;23:738.

108. Blanchet F, Kanfer A, Cramer E, et al. Relative contribution of intrinsic lung dysfunction and hypoventilation to hypoxemia during hemodialysis. *Kidney Int* 1984;26:430.

109. Vaziri ND, Wilson A, Mukai D. Dialysis hypoxemia: role of dialyzer membrane and dialysate delivery system. *Am J Med* 1984;77:828.

110. Bouffard Y, Viale JP, Annat G, et al. Pulmonary gas exchange during hemodialysis. *Kidney Int* 1986;30:920.

111. Igarashi H, Kioi S, Geiyo F, et al. Physiologic approach to dialysis-induced hypoxemia. *Nephron* 1985;41:62.

112. Symreng T, Flanigan MJ, Lim VS. Ventilatory and metabolic changes during high efficiency hemodialysis. *Kidney Int* 1992;41:1064.

113. Tolchin N, Roberts JL, Lewis EJ. Respiratory gas exchange by high-efficiency hemodialyzers. *Nephron* 1978;21:137.

114. Nissenson AR. Prevention of dialysis-induced hypoxemia by bicarbonate dialysis. *ASAIO Trans* 1980;26:339.

115. Raja RM, Kramer MS, Rosenbaum JL, et al. Hemodialysis associated hypoxemia: role of acetate and pH in etiology. *ASAIO Trans* 1981;27:180.

116. Heinemann HO, Goldring RM. Bicarbonate and the regulation of ventilation. *Am J Med* 1974;57:361.

117. Ahmad S, Pagel M, Shen F, et al. Effects of oxygen administration on the manifestation of acetate intolerance in dialysis patients. *Am J Nephrol* 1982;2:256.

118. Heneghan WF. Acetate, bicarbonate and hypotension during hemodialysis. *Am J Kidney Dis* 1982;2:302.

119. Iseki K, Onoyama K, Maeda T, et al. Comparison of hemodynamics induced by conventional acetate hemodialysis, bicarbonate hemodialysis and ultrafiltration. *Clin Nephrol* 1980;14:294.

120. Hampl H, Klopp H, Wolfgruber M, et al. Advantages of bicarbonate hemodialysis. *Artif Organs* 1982;6:410.

121. Pagel MD, Ahmad S, Vizzo JE, et al. Acetate and bicarbonate fluctuations and acetate intolerance during dialysis. *Kidney Int* 1982;21:513.

122. Landwehr DM, Okusa MD. The effect of acetate and bicarbonate dialysis on orthostatic blood pressure regulation. *Artif Organs* 1982;6:417.

123. Man NK, Fournier G, Thireau P, et al. Effect of bicarbonate-containing dialysate on chronic hemodialysis patients: a comparative study. *Artif Organs* 1982;6:421.

124. Hakim RM, Pontzer MA, Tilton D, et al. Effects of acetate and bicarbonate dialysate in stable chronic dialysis patients. *Kidney Int* 1985;28:535.

125. Brezin JH, Schwartz AB, Chinitz JL. Switch from acetate (Ac) to bicarbonate (Bi) dialysis: better dialysis tolerance but failure to improve acidosis and hypertriglyceridemia (HTG). *ASAIO Trans* 1985;31:343.

126. Leunissen KML, Hoorntje SJ, Fiers HA, et al. Acetate versus bicarbonate hemodialysis in critically ill patients. *Nephron* 1986;42:146.

127. La Greca G, Feriani M, Bragantini L, et al. Effects of acetate and bicarbonate dialysate on vascular stability: a prospective multicenter study. *Int J Artif Organs* 1987;10:157.

128. Van Stone JC, Cook J. The effect of replacing acetate with bicarbonate in the dialysate of stable chronic hemodialysis patients. *Proc Dial Transplant Forum* 1978;8:103.

129. Uldall PR, Kennedy I, Craske H, et al. A double-blind controlled trial of acetate versus bicarbonate dialysate. *Proc Dial Transplant Forum* 1980;10:220.

130. Thieler VH, Muller K, Schmidt U, et al. Clinical symptomatology during acetate and bicarbonate dialyses: a double-blind study in a group of 25 patients. *Nieren Hochdruckkrankheiten* 1984;13:106.

131. Fantuzzi S, Caico S, Amatruda O, et al. Hemodialysis-associated cardiac arrhythmias: a lower risk with bicarbonate? *Nephron* 1991;58:196.

132. Rever B, Fox L, Christensen R, et al. Adverse ocular effects of acetate hemodialysis. *Am J Nephrol* 1983;3:199.

133. Henrich WL, Woodard TD, Meyer BD, et al. High sodium bicarbonate and acetate hemodialysis: double-blind crossover comparison of hemodynamic and ventilatory effects. *Kidney Int* 1983;24:240.

134. Borges HF, Fryd DS, Rosa AA, et al. Hypotension during acetate and bicarbonate dialysis in patients with acute renal failure. *Am J Nephrol* 1981;1:24.

135. Castellani A, Lonati F, Bigi L, et al. No relationship between acetate and hypotension in a standard dialysis schedule. *Proc Eur Dial Transplant Assoc* 1982;19:340.

136. Van Geelen JA, Woittiez AJJ, Schalekamp MADH. Bicarbonate versus acetate hemodialysis in ventilated patients. *Clin Nephrol* 1987;28:130.

137. Cannella G, Cancarini G, De Marinis S, et al. Interrelationships between blood pressure, blood gases and plasma acetate concentrations during conventional hemodialysis. *Int J Artif Organs* 1982;5:357.

138. Bergström J, Asaba H, Furst P, et al. Dialysis, ultrafiltration, and blood pressure. *Proc Eur Dial Transplant Assoc* 1976; 13:293.

139. Wehle B, Asaba H, Castenfors J, et al. The influence of dialysis fluid composition on the blood pressure response during dialysis. *Clin Nephrol* 1978;10:62.

140. Keshaviah P, Shapiro FL. A critical examination of dialysis-induced hypotension. *Am J Kidney Dis* 1982;2:290.

141. Swartz RD, Somermeyer MG, Hsu C-H. Preservation of plasma volume during hemodialysis depends on dialysate osmolality. *Am J Nephrol* 1982;2:189.

142. Henrich WL. Hemodynamic instability during hemodialysis. *Kidney Int* 1986;30:605.

143. Van Stone JC, Bauer J, Carey J. The effect of dialysate sodium concentration on body fluid compartment volume, plasma renin activity and plasma aldosterone concentration in chronic hemodialysis patients. *Am J Kidney Dis* 1982;2: 58.

144. Velez RL, Woodard TD, Henrich WL. Acetate and bicarbonate hemodialysis in patients with and without autonomic dysfunction. *Kidney Int* 1984;26:59.

145. Hsu CH, Swartz RD, Somermeyer MG, et al. Bicarbonate hemodialysis: influence on plasma refilling and hemodynamic stability. *Nephron* 1984;38:202.

146. Leunissen KML, Cheriex EC, Janssen J, et al. Influence of left ventricular function on changes in plasma volume during acetate and bicarbonate dialysis. *Nephrol Dial Transplant* 1987;2:99.

147. Wehle B, Asaba H, Castenfors J, et al. Influence of dialysate composition on cardiovascular function in isovolaemic haemodialysis. *Proc Eur Dial Transplant Assoc* 1981;18: 153.

148. Bijaphala S, Bell AJ, Bennett CA, et al. Comparison of high and low sodium bicarbonate and acetate dialysis in stable chronic hemodialysis patients. *Clin Nephrol* 1985;23:179.

149. Bauer W, Richards DW Jr. A vasodilator action of acetates. *J Physiol* 1928;66:371.

150. Molnar JI, Scott JB, Frohlich ED, et al. Local effects of various anions and H$^+$ on dog limb and coronary vascular resistances. *Am J Physiol* 1962;203:125.

151. Frohlich ED. Vascular effects of the Krebs intermediate metabolites. *Am J Physiol* 1965;208:149.

152. Olinger GN, Werner PH, Bonchek LI, et al. Vasodilator effects of the sodium acetate in pooled protein fraction. *Ann Surg* 1979;190:305.

153. Steffen RP, McKenzie JE, Haddy FJ. The possible role of acetate in exercise hyperemia in dog skeletal muscle. *Pflugers Arch* 1982;392:315.

154. Daugirdas JT, Nawab ZM, Jain S, et al. Acetate relaxation of isolated vascular smooth muscle. *Kidney Int* 1987;32:39.

155. Liang CS, Lowenstein JM. Metabolic control of the circulation. *J Clin Invest* 1978;62:1029.

156. Żydowo MM, Smoleński RT, Świerczyński J. Acetate-induced changes of adenine nucleotide levels in rat liver. *Metabolism* 1993;42:644.

157. Steffen RP, McKenzie JE, Bockman EL, et al. Changes in dog gracilis muscle adenosine during exercise and acetate infusion. *Am J Physiol* 1983;244:H387.

158. Carmichael FJ, Saldivia V, Varghese GA, et al. Ethanol-induced increase in portal blood flow: role of acetate and A_1- and A_2-adenosine receptors. *Am J Physiol* 1988;255:G417.

159. Tekkanat KK, Port FK, Schmaltz S, et al. Excessive ATP degradation during hemodialysis against sodium acetate. *J Lab Clin Med* 1988;112:686.

160. Nutting CW, Islam S, Ye M, et al. The vasorelaxant effects of acetate: role of adenosine, glycolysis, lyotropism, and pH_i and Ca_i^{2+}. *Kidney Int* 1992;41:166.

161. Tomiyama O, Shiigai T, Ideura T, et al. Baroreflex sensitivity in renal failure. *Clin Sci* 1980;58:21.

162. Kersh ES, Kronenfield SJ, Unger A, et al. Autonomic insufficiency in uremia as a cause of hemodialysis-induced hypotension. *N Engl J Med* 1974;290:650.

163. Daugirdas JT, Nawab ZM, Hayashi JA. Hemodialysis hemodynamics in an animal model: effect of using an acetate-buffered dialysate. *J Lab Clin Med* 1986;107:517.

164. Mehta BR, Fischer D, Ahmad M, et al. Effects of acetate and bicarbonate hemodialysis on cardiac function in chronic dialysis patients. *Kidney Int* 1983;24:782.

165. Nixon JV, Mitchell JH, McPhaul JJ Jr, et al. Effect of hemodialysis on left ventricular function: dissociation of changes in filling volume and in contractile state. *J Clin Invest* 1983;71:377.

166. Madsen BR, Alpert MA, Whiting RB, et al. Effect of hemodialysis on left ventricular performance: analysis of echocardiographic subsets. *Am J Nephrol* 1984;4:86.

167. Klein J, McLeish K, Hodsden J, et al. Hypertrophic cardiomyopathy: an acquired disorder of end-stage renal disease. *ASAIO Trans* 1983;29:120.

168. Ruder MA, Alpert MA, Van Stone J, et al. Comparative effects of acetate and bicarbonate hemodialysis on left ventricular function. *Kidney Int* 1985;27:768.

169. Mastrangelo F, Rizzelli S, De Blasi V, et al. Favourable effects of bicarbonate dialysis on the body pool of phosphorus. *Proc Eur Dial Transplant Assoc* 1984;21:215.

170. Bazzato G, Coli U, Landini S, et al. Removal of phosphate either by bicarbonate dialysis or biofiltration in uremics. *Kidney Int* 1988;33(suppl 24):S180.

171. Lim VS, Flanigan MJ, Fangman J. Effect of hematocrit on solute removal during high efficiency hemodialysis. *Kidney Int* 1990;37:1557.

172. Tsaltas TT, Friedman EA. Plasma lipid studies of uremic patients during hemodialysis. *Am J Clin Nutr* 1968;21:430.

173. Gonzalez FM, Pearson JE, Garbus SB, et al. On the effects of acetate during hemodialysis. *ASAIO Trans* 1974;20:169.

174. Guarnieri GF, Carretta R, Toigo G, et al. Acetate intolerance in chronic uremic patients. *Nephron* 1979;24:212.

175. Davidson WD, Rorke SJ, Guo LSS, et al. Comparison of acetate-1-^{14}C metabolism in uremic and nonuremic dogs. *Am J Clin Nutr* 1978;31:1897.

176. Savdie E, Mahony JF, Stewart JH. Effect of acetate of serum lipids in maintenance hemodialysis. *ASAIO Trans* 1977;23:385.

177. Morin RJ, Srikantaiah MV, Woodley Z, et al. Effect of hemodialysis with acetate vs bicarbonate on plasma lipid and lipoprotein levels in uremic patients. *J Dial* 1980;4:9.

178. Goldman M. Effect of chronic ingestion of sodium acetate on thyroid function. *Experientia* 1981;37:1348.

179. Orskov H, Hansen AP, Hansen HE, et al. Acetate: inhibitor of growth hormone hypersecretion in diabetic and non-diabetic uraemic subjects. *Acta Endocrinol* 1982;99:551.

180. Schmitz O, Hansen AP, Hansen HE, et al. Inhibition of arginine- and hypoglycemia-induced growth hormone release by acetate in dialyzed patients. *Clin Nephrol* 1982;17:70.

181. Ward RA, Farrell PC, Tiller DJ, et al. A clinical evaluation of large-area short-time haemodialysis. *Aust NZ J Med* 1976;6:288.

182. Chapman GV, Mahony JF, Farrell PC. A crossover study of short time dialysis. *Clin Nephrol* 1980;13:78.

183. Swan RC, Axelrod DR, Seip M, et al. Distribution of sodium bicarbonate infused into nephrectomized dogs. *J Clin Invest* 1955;34:1795.

184. Russell CD, Illickal MM, Maloney JV, et al. Acute response to acid-base stress in the dog. *Am J Physiol* 1972;223:689.

185. Uribarri J, Zia M, Mahmood J, et al. Acid production in chronic hemodialysis patients. *J Am Soc Nephrol* 1998;9:114.

186. Garella S, Dana CL, Chazan JA. Severity of metabolic acidosis as a determinant of bicarbonate requirements. *N Engl J Med* 1973;289:121.

187. Adrogue HJ, Brensilver J, Cohen JJ, et al. Influence of steady-state alterations in acid-base equilibrium on the fate of administered bicarbonate in the dog. *J Clin Invest* 1983;71:867.

188. Fernandez PC, Cohen RM, Feldman GM. The concept of bicarbonate distribution space: the crucial role of body buffers. *Kidney Int* 1989;36:747.

189. Poyart CF, Bursaux E, Freminet A. The bone CO_2 compartment: evidence for a bicarbonate pool. *Respir Physiol* 1975;25:89.

190. Lundquist F. Production and utilization of free acetate in man. *Nature* 1962;193:579.

191. Kveim M, Nesbakken R. Utilization of exogenous acetate during hemodialysis. *ASAIO Trans* 1975;21:138.

192. Thews O, Deuber HJ, Hutten H, et al. Theoretical approach and clinical application of kinetic modelling in dialysis. *Nephrol Dial Transplant* 1991;6:180.

193. Thews O. Model-based decision support system for individual prescription of the dialysate bicarbonate concentration in hemodialysis. *Int J Artif Organs* 1992;15:447.

194. Ward RA, Wathen RL, Williams TE. Effects of long-term bicarbonate hemodialysis on acid-base status. *ASAIO Trans* 1982;28:295.

195. Seyffart G, Ensminger A, Scholz R. Increase of body mass during long-term bicarbonate hemodialysis. *Kidney Int* 1987;32(suppl 22):S174.

196. Ahmad S, Pagel M, Vizzo J, et al. Effect of the normalization of acid-base balance on postdialysis plasma bicarbonate. *ASAIO Trans* 1980;26:318.

197. Kobrin SM, Raja RM. Effect of varying dialysate bicarbonate concentration on serum phosphate. *ASAIO Trans* 1989; 35:423.

198. Rault R. Optimal dialysate bicarbonate during hemodialysis. *ASAIO Trans* 1991;37:M372.

199. Leunissen KML, Kooman JP, Waterval PW, et al. Individualization of the dialysate bicarbonate concentration for optimal correction of acidosis. In: Man NK, Botella J, Zuchelli P, eds. *Blood Purification in Perspective: New Insights and Future Trends.* Cleveland, OH: ICAOT Press, 1992:177.

200. Oettinger CW, Oliver JC. Normalization of uremic acidosis in hemodialysis patients with a high bicarbonate dialysate. *J Am Soc Nephrol* 1993;3:1804.

201. Williams AJ, Dittmer ID, McArley A, et al. High bicarbonate dialysate in haemodialysis patients: effects on acidosis and nutritional state. *Nephrol Dial Transplant* 1997;12: 2633.

202. Clark WR, Leypoldt JK, Henderson LW. Quantifying the effect of changes in the hemodialysis prescription on effective solute removal with a mathematical model. *J Am Soc Nephrol* 1999;10:601.

203. O'Sullivan DA, McCarthy JT, Kumar R, et al. Improved biochemical variables, nutrient intake, and hormonal factors in slow nocturnal hemodialysis: a pilot study. *Mayo Clin Proc* 1998;73:1035.

204. Mioni R, Gropuzzo M, Messa M, et al. Acid production and base balance in patients on chronic haemodialysis. *Clin Sci* 2001;101:329.

205. Fabris A, LaGreca G, Chiaramonte S, et al. The importance of ultrafiltration on acid-base status in a dialysis population. *ASAIO Trans* 1988;34:200.

206. Agroyannis B, Fourtounas C, Tzanatos H, et al. Relationship between interdialytic weight gain and acid-base status in hemodialysis by bicarbonate. *Artif Organs* 2002;26:385.

207. Gabutti L, Ferrari N, Giudici G, et al. Unexpected haemodynamic instability associated with standard bicarbonate haemodialysis. *Nephrol Dial Transplant* 2003;18:2369.

208. Van Stone JC. Oral base replacement in patients on hemodialysis. *Ann Intern Med* 1984;101:199.

209. Caruana RJ, Weinstein RS, Campbell HT, et al. Effects of oral base therapy on serum ionized calcium, phosphorus and parathyroid hormone in chronic hemodialysis patients. *Int J Artif Organs* 1989;12:778.

210. Anelli A, Brancaccio D, Damasso R, et al. Substitution of calcium carbonate from aluminum hydroxide in patients on hemodialysis. Effects on acidosis, on parathyroid function, and on calcemia. *Nephron* 1989;52:125.

211. Chertow GM, Burke SK, Raggi P, et al. Sevelamer attenuates the progression of coronary and aortic calcification in hemodialysis patients. *Kidney Int* 2002;62:245.

212. La Greca G, Biasioli S, Chiaramonte S, et al. Acid-base balance in peritoneal dialysis. *Clin Nephrol* 1981;16:1.

213. Mujais S. Acid-base profile in patients on PD. *Kidney Int* 2003;64(suppl 88):S26.

214. Szeto C-C, Wong TY-H, Chow K-M, et al. Oral sodium bicarbonate for the treatment of metabolic acidosis in peritoneal dialysis patients: a randomized placebo-control trial. *J Am Soc Nephrol* 2003;14:2119.

215. Rubin J, Adair C, Johnson B, et al. Stereospecific lactate absorption during peritoneal dialysis. *Nephron* 1982;31:224.

216. Richardson RMA, Roscoe JM. Bicarbonate, L-lactate, and D-lactate balance in intermittent peritoneal dialysis. *Perit Dial Bull* 1986;6:178.

217. Fabris A, Biasioli S, Chiaramonte C, et al. Buffer metabolism in continuous ambulatory peritoneal dialysis: relationship with respiratory dynamics. *ASAIO Trans* 1982;28:270.

218. Dixon SR, McKean WI, Pryor JE, et al. Changes in acid-base balance during peritoneal dialysis with fluid containing lactate ions. *Clin Sci* 1970;39:51.

219. Yamamoto T, Yamakawa M, Kishimoto T, et al. The interrelationship of dialysate glucose and lactate in continuous ambulatory peritoneal dialysis. *ASAIO Trans* 1985;31:595.

220. Lee HA, Hill LF, Hewitt V, et al. Lacticacidemia in peritoneal dialysis. *Proc Eur Dial Transplant Assoc* 1967;4:150.

221. Teehan BP, Schleifer CR, Reichard GA, et al. Acid-base studies in continuous ambulatory peritoneal dialysis. In: Moncrief JW, Popovich RP, eds. *CAPD Update.* New York: Masson, 1981:95.

222. National Kidney Foundation Kidney Disease Outcomes Quality Initiative. NKF-K/DOQI clinical practice guidelines for peritoneal dialysis adequacy: update 2000. *Am J Kidney Dis* 2001;37(suppl 1):S65.

223. Slingeneyer A, Canaud B, Mion C. Permanent loss of ultrafiltration capacity of the peritoneum in long-term peritoneal dialysis: an epidemiological study. *Nephron* 1983;33:133.

224. Faller B, Marichal J-F. Loss of ultrafiltration in continuous ambulatory peritoneal dialysis: a role for acetate. *Perit Dial Bull* 1984;4:10.

225. Nolph KD, Ryan L, Moore H, et al. Factors affecting ultrafiltration in continuous ambulatory peritoneal dialysis. *Perit Dial Bull* 1984;4:14.

226. Faller B, Marichal JF. Evolution of ultrafiltration in CAPD according to the dialysis fluid buffer. In: Maher JF, Winchester JF, eds. *Frontiers in Peritoneal Dialysis.* New York: Springer-Verlag, 1986:274.

227. Nolph K, Ryan L, Moore H, et al. Survey of ultrafiltration in continuous ambulatory peritoneal dialysis. *Perit Dial Bull* 1984;4:137.

228. Kwong MBL, Wu GG, Rodella H, et al. Effect of the peritoneal dialysate buffer on ultrafiltration: studies in normal rabbits. *Perit Dial Bull* 1985;5:182.

229. Katirtzoglou A, Digenis GE, Kontesis P, et al. Is peritoneal ultrafiltration influenced by acetate of lactate buffers? In: Maher JF, Winchester JF, eds. *Frontiers in Peritoneal Dialysis.* New York: Springer-Verlag, 1986:270.

230. Devuyst O, Topley N, Williams JD. Morphological and functional changes in the dialysed peritoneal cavity: impact of more biocompatible solutions. *Nephrol Dial Transplant* 2002;17(suppl 3):12.

231. Hoff CM. In vitro biocompatibility performance of Physioneal. *Kidney Int* 2003;64(suppl 88):S57.

232. Feriani M, Kirchgessner J, La Greca G, et al. Randomized long-term evaluation of bicarbonate-buffered CAPD solution. *Kidney Int* 1998;54:1731.

233. Coles GA, O'Donoghue DJ, Pritchard N, et al. A controlled trial of two bicarbonate-containing dialysis fluids for CAPD: final report. *Nephrol Dial Transplant* 1998;13:3165.

234. Haas S, Schmidt CP, Arbeiter K, et al. Improved acidosis correction and recovery of mesothelial cell mass with neu-

tral-pH bicarbonate dialysis solution among children undergoing automated peritoneal dialysis. *J Am Soc Nephrol* 2003;14:2632.

235. Jones S, Holmes CJ, Krediet RT, et al. Bicarbonate/lactate-based peritoneal dialysis solution increases cancer antigen 125 and decreases hyaluronic acid levels. *Kidney Int* 2001; 59:1529.

236. Spencer PC, Farrell PC. Peritoneal membrane stability and the kinetics of peritoneal mass transfer. In: Nolph KD, ed. *Peritoneal Dialysis.* Boston: Martinus Nijhoff, 1985:581.

237. Teehan BP, Schleifer CR, Sigler MH, et al. A quantitative approach to the CAPD prescription. *Perit Dial Bull* 1985;5: 152.

238. Feriani M. Buffers: bicarbonate, lactate and pyruvate. *Kidney Int* 1996;50(suppl 56):S75.

239. Nolph KD, Prowant B, Serkes KD, et al. Multicenter evaluation of a new peritoneal dialysis solution with a high lactate and a low magnesium concentration. *Perit Dial Bull* 1983;3: 63.

240. Stein A, Moorhouse J, Iles-Smith H, et al. Role of an improvement in acid-base status and nutrition in CAPD patients. *Kidney Int* 1997;52:1089.

241. Feriani M, Passlick-Deetjen J, Jaeckle-Meyer I, et al. Individualized bicarbonate concentrations in the peritoneal dialysis fluid to optimize acid-base status in CAPD patients. *Nephrol Dial Transplant* 2004;19:195.

242. Ledebo I. Principles and practice of hemofiltration and hemodiafiltration. *Artif Organs* 1998;22:20.

243. Kellum JA, Mehta RL, Angus DC, et al. The first international consensus conference on continuous renal replacement therapy. *Kidney Int* 2002;62:1855.

244. Mehta RL, McDonald BR, Ward DA. Regional citrate anticoagulation for continuous arteriovenous hemodialysis. An update after 12 months. *Contrib Nephrol* 1991;93:210.

245. Kierdorf HP, Leue C, Arns S. Lactate- or bicarbonate-buffered solutions in continuous extracorporeal renal replacement therapies. *Kidney Int* 1999;56(suppl 72):S32.

246. Davenport A, Aulton K, Payne RB, et al. Hyperlactatemia and increasing metabolic acidosis in hepatorenal failure treated by hemofiltration. *Renal Failure* 1990;12:99.

247. Barenbrock M, Hausberg M, Matzkies F, et al. Effects of bicarbonate- and lactate-buffered replacement fluids on cardiovascular outcome in CVVH patients. *Kidney Int* 2000;58: 1751.

248. Kielstein JT, Kretschmer U, Ernst T, et al. Efficacy and cardiovascular tolerability of extended dialysis in critically ill patients: a randomized controlled study. *Am J Kidney Dis* 2004;43:342.

249. Leblanc M, Moreno L, Robinson OP, et al. Bicarbonate dialysate for continuous renal replacement therapy in intensive care unit patients with acute renal failure. *Am J Kidney Dis* 1995;26:910.

250. Ledebo I. On-line preparation of solutions for dialysis: practice aspects versus safety and regulations. *J Am Soc Nephrol* 2002;13(suppl 1):S78.

251. Canaud B, Bosc JY, Leray H, et al. On-line hemodiafiltration: state of the art. *Nephrol Dial Transplant* 1998;13 (suppl 2):3.

252. Pedrini LA, De Cristofaro V, Pagliari B. Effects of the infusion mode on bicarbonate balance in on-line hemodiafiltration. *Int J Artif Organs* 2002;25:100.

253. Gordon A, Better OS, Greenbaum MA, et al. Clinical maintenance hemodialysis with a sorbent-based, low-volume dialysate regeneration system. *ASAIO Trans* 1971;17:253.

254. Farrell PC, Mahony JF, Jones BF, et al. Clinical evaluation of a dialysate regeneration system for maintenance hemodialysis. *Aust NZ J Med* 1976;6:292.

255. Pedersen F, Christiansen E. On acid-base problems in REDY dialysis. *Scand J Urol Nephrol* 1976;(suppl 30):28.

256. Hamm LL, Lawrence G, DuBose TD. Sorbent regenerative hemodialysis as a potential cause of acute hypercapnia. *Kidney Int* 1982;21:416.

257. Reyes A, Turchetto E, Bernis C, et al. Acid-base derangements during sorbent regenerative hemodialysis in mechanically ventilated patients. *Crit Care Med* 1991;19:554.

258. Richards CJ, Newhouse CE, Freeman RM. Acetate-free hemodialysis with a sorbent regenerative system. *Proc Dial Transplant Forum* 1977;7:104.

259. Mion C, Branger B, Issautier R, et al. Dialysis fracturing osteomalacia without hyperparathyroidism in patients with HCO$_3$ rinsed REDY cartridge. *ASAIO Trans* 1981;27:634.

260. Pierides AM, Frohnert PP. Aluminum related dialysis osteomalacia and dementia after prolonged use of the REDY cartridge. *ASAIO Trans* 1981;27:629.

261. Curtis JR, Sampson B. Aluminum kinetics during haemodialysis with the Redy 2000 Sorbsystem. *Int J Artif Organs* 1989;12:683.

262. Llach F, Gardner PW, George CRP, et al. Aluminum kinetics using bicarbonate dialysate with the sorbent system. *Kidney Int* 1993;43:899.

Nutrition in Patients with Chronic Kidney Disease and Patients on Dialysis

Marsha Wolfson

Nutritional factors play an important role in the management of patients with end-stage renal disease (ESRD) as well as those with chronic kidney disease (CKD) not yet on dialysis. Nutritional status is important in the morbidity and mortality of patients with CKD[1,2] as well as in their quality of life and ultimate rehabilitative potential. Dietary management has long been an important therapeutic intervention for patients with advanced renal disease, as it has been used to alter the progression of disease[3] and to ameliorate the symptoms and signs of uremia.[4] A large body of evidence demonstrates that patients with uremia suffer from wasting and malnutrition despite seemingly adequate dialysis treatment,[4–8] and many of the metabolic derangements associated with uremia affect nutritional status. The presence of malnutrition can adversely affect survival in patients treated with maintenance hemodialysis.[1,2,9] There has been in-

creased awareness of the role of malnutrition due to inadequate dietary intake and that which may be associated with chronic inflammation and persistent catabolism, which are often present in ESRD patients.[10]

NUTRITIONAL STATUS IN PATIENTS WITH ESRD

Patients with ESRD often display signs and symptoms of wasting and malnutrition. A number of reports demonstrate abnormalities in the same measures of nutritional status used in the evaluation of nonuremic subjects. These abnormalities include reduced anthropometric measurements as well as other measures of body composition, decreased concentrations of many serum or plasma proteins, altered plasma amino acid patterns, and decreased immunologic responsiveness.[2,4–9] However, the evaluation of nutritional status in patients with renal failure does require adaptation of many of these standard measures in order to take into consideration some confounding variables in the renal failure population that may not be present in individuals with normal renal function. The assessment of nutritional status is described in more detail later in this chapter.

Anthropometry provides a simple and direct measure of body composition. Decreased triceps and subscapular skinfold thicknesses have been reported in several studies evaluating nutritional status in patients with CKD and those treated with maintenance dialysis,[4,5] indicating reduced body fat stores. Although body weight is a fairly reliable indicator of body fat in normal subjects, a variety of chronic illnesses as well as fluid overload, which is common among ESRD patients, make accurate body weight measurements difficult. Other anthropometric measurements, such as mid-arm muscle circumference, an indicator of muscle mass, are also reduced in patients with CKD and ESRD when compared with normal subjects of similar age, height, and sex.[4,5] In order to better compare groups of patients with renal failure, norms for anthropometry in patients on maintenance dialysis have been published.[11]

Anthropometric measurements may be less accurate in the presence of edema; therefore, measurements of body composition that can differentiate between body water, body fat, and muscle mass are also used to assess body composition.[12] More recently, computed tomography has been used to determine muscle mass.[13] These measures confirm that body fat stores and muscle mass are often reduced in patients with ESRD.

Although it seems obvious that a severely uremic patient might display signs of malnutrition, it is less clear why patients who are seemingly well dialyzed often appear wasted. Adequate dialysis treatment alone does not seem to be sufficient to prevent wasting.[14] Thunberg and coworkers assessed nutritional status in patients at the onset of hemodialysis treatment and repeated the assessment over 18 months. They found that many patients continued to demonstrate malnutrition throughout the entire 18-month period, suggesting that the institution of maintenance dialysis therapy does not always correct malnutrition.[5]

In addition to abnormal measures of body composition, reduced serum albumin concentration, reduced transferrin levels, and decreased immunoglobulin concentrations are reported in patients with advanced ESRD, suggesting that these patients have protein malnutrition.[4–6,15–18] These abnormalities may also be seen concurrent with inflammation, and malnutrition and inflammation appear to be associated in the patient with ESRD.[13,16,17]

Plasma and muscle amino acid concentrations have been extensively studied in the uremic population. The amino acid profile of uremic patients is uniformly abnormal

in these studies.[19,20] With the exception of renal transplant patients, the amino acid derangements described are similar regardless of the method of renal replacement therapy used. One study demonstrated similar plasma aminograms in patients treated with hemodialysis, hemofiltration, hemoperfusion, intermittent peritoneal dialysis (IPD), or continuous ambulatory peritoneal dialysis (CAPD). Successful renal transplantation resulted in normalization of the plasma amino acid pattern.[20] In a study evaluating plasma amino acid patterns in patients with CKD prior to the institution of renal replacement therapy, there was a direct relationship between the severity of renal failure and the abnormalities in the plasma aminogram.[21]

The plasma amino acid pattern seen in patients with renal failure includes decreased essential amino acids and normal or increased nonessential amino acids, similar to the findings in patients with protein-calorie malnutrition and normal renal function.[22] Several of the changes described are, however, not improved by increased protein intake, suggesting that the absence of kidney function also affects plasma amino acid concentrations. For example N-τ and N-π methylhistidine are increased in renal failure, whereas they are usually decreased in malnutrition. This is because renal excretion of these substances is decreased.[23] Increased citrulline concentrations may be due to decreased conversion to arginine by the diseased kidneys.[24] Impaired conversion of phenylalanine to tyrosine in uremia results in reduced plasma tyrosine levels with normal or increased phenylalanine levels.[25] It should be pointed out, however, that tyrosine concentrations may also be affected by dietary intake and are also low in poorly nourished nonuremic patients. The increased requirement for vitamin B_6 seen in uremia[26] may result in decreased conversion of glycine to serine, leading to an increased glycine-serine ratio.[27] Plasma tryptophan concentrations are reduced in uremia and are related to both decreased protein intake and abnormal binding of tryptophan to plasma proteins.[28]

In summary, amino acid profiles in uremic patients reflect both reduced dietary protein intake and abnormal amino acid excretion and metabolism by the diseased kidneys. In general, there are decreased essential amino acids with increased or normal nonessential amino acids, resulting in a reduced essential to nonessential amino acid ratio. These findings are summarized in Table 21–1.

Despite the importance of plasma amino acid patterns in assessing the development and maintenance of wasting in dialysis patients, measurement of these patterns is not routinely recommended for the assessment of nutritional status in patients with advanced renal failure or ESRD. However, plasma amino patterns may be meaningful given the widespread use of oral and parenteral amino supplements in patients with ESRD. Recent changes in amino acid intake are reflected in amino acid patterns. Several studies have shown

TABLE 21–1. TYPICAL PLASMA AMINO ACID CONCENTRATIONS IN UREMIC PATIENTS

Essential	Histidine	↓
	Isoleucine	↓
	Leucine	↓
	Lysine	↓
	Methionine	N or ↑
	Phenylalanine	N or ↑
	Threonine	↓
	Valine	↓
Total essential		↓
Semiessential	Cystine	N or ↑
	Tyrosine	↓
Nonessential	Alanine	N or ↑
	Arginine	N or ↑
	Asparagine	N or ↑
	Aspartic acid	N or ↑
	Glutamic acid	N or ↑
	Glycine	N or ↑
	Ornithine	N or ↑
	Proline	N or ↑
	Serine	N or ↑
Total nonessential		N or ↑
	Citrulline	↑
	Taurine	N or ↑
	N-π-Methylhistidine	↑
	N-τ-Methylhistidine	↑
Ratio	Essential/nonessential	↓
	Valine/glycine	↓
	Tyrosine/phenylalanine	↓

improvement in nutritional parameters with amino acid supplementation either intravenously in maintenance hemodialysis patients and with amino acid supplementation via peritoneal dialysis.[29–32] However, only one study has shown improvement in the amino acid profile of patients with ESRD in response to nutritional supplementation.[33] Improvement in branched-chain amino acids has also been demonstrated with the correction of metabolic acidosis (see below). Protein-calorie malnutrition is associated with decreased immunologic responsiveness in nonuremic individuals, and similar abnormalities are seen in uremic patients.[6] Both groups demonstrate decreased lymphocyte blastogenesis and delayed cutaneous hypersensitivity.[34–37] In one study, recovery of response to skin test antigens occurred after 3 months of nutritional supplementation.[38]

There is a significant correlation between lymphocyte function and nutritional status in patients treated with maintenance hemodialysis.[6] Interestingly, lymphocyte abnormalities are also reversed when lymphocytes from uremic patients are cultured in sera from normal subjects, suggesting

a role for uremia per se in the reduced immunologic response.[39]

These laboratory abnormalities may have important clinical implications. A recent study in hemodialysis patients found a relationship between serum albumin concentration and measures of protein intake, such as the protein catabolic rate (PCR), as well as with the dialysis dose, as measured by Kt/V. There was also a significant relationship between serum albumin and proinflammatory mediators, with a negative correlation between serum albumin, IL-2 levels, and measures of T-cell function. Increased relative risk of death was associated with higher levels of proinflammatory cytokines, while better immune function was associated with improved survival.[40] These data support an association between nutritional status, serum albumin, and the presence of inflammation; they demonstrate the importance of nutritional status as well as immune status in survival in these patients. It appears that uremia and associated malnutrition may act synergistically to depress immune function in uremic individuals.

From the available data it is apparent that, as a group, patients with ESRD display many of the signs and symptoms of wasting, including depressed serum protein concentrations, reductions in muscle mass, and abnormal plasma amino acid patterns, indicating depletion of protein stores. Dialysis patients also have decreased body weight and skinfold thickness as well as reduced fat mass, suggesting reduced fat stores. Impaired immunologic responsiveness is also common in ESRD. Table 21–2 outlines the nutritional abnormalities associated with uremia. In order to accurately assess nutrition status in patients with renal failure, it is necessary to evaluate a panel of measures. No single measure of nutritional status can be used to determine whether malnutrition is present in these patients. Panels that include

TABLE 21–2. NUTRITIONAL PARAMETERS IN RENAL FAILURE

Anthropometric measurements	
Triceps skinfold thickness	Decreased
Subscapular skinfold thickness	Decreased
Midarm muscle circumference	Decreased
Serum proteins	
Albumin	Decreased
Transferrin	Decreased
IgG	Decreased or normal
IgA	Decreased or normal
IgM	Decreased or normal
C3	Decreased
C4	Normal
Plasma amino acids	
Essential[a]	Decreased
Nonessential	Normal or increased

[a]Histidine is included as an essential amino acid.

measures of body composition, visceral protein pools, protein and energy intake, and functional status identify different aspects of nutritional status. More than one measure is necessary to identify malnutrition with precision.[41] It is also important to understand how the presence of uremia or fluid overload may confound these measures of nutritional status. For example, serum albumin may be lower due to hemodilution or the presence of inflammation.[16,17] Serum prealbumin is elevated in renal failure and therefore the usual normal values are not valid in patients with advanced renal failure and ESRD.[42] Serum transferrin is also impacted by iron stores. Therefore it may be necessary to factor these considerations into the overall assessment of nutritional status.

CAUSES OF MALNUTRITION IN RENAL FAILURE

Reduced Nutritional Intake

Symptoms of uremia include anorexia, nausea, and vomiting. A loss of taste for meat and altered taste in general are common patient complaints. Although these symptoms are somewhat ameliorated by the institution of dialysis therapy, they are usually not completely reversed. The hemodialysis procedure itself is associated with nausea and vomiting, possibly related to rapid fluid and electrolyte shifts during treatment. Hemodialysis patients have delayed gastric emptying,[43] which may exacerbate anorexia. Patients treated with maintenance dialysis have early satiety and consume less food compared with renal failure patients, both predialysis and following a renal transplant.[44,45] CAPD may also result in anorexia in patients with small abdominal cavities filled with dialysis fluid. The glucose load associated with the peritoneal dialysis solution may also reduce appetite.[6,44,46] The required dietary restrictions imposed on patients treated with maintenance dialysis—in particular of sodium, potassium, and fluid—as well as the need for phosphate binders may make food less palatable. Mental depression can also contribute to decreased dietary intake. Diet histories reveal that, as a group, dialysis patients have low energy intake, consuming only about 23 to 27 kcal/kg/day, far less than the 35 kcal/kg/day recommended.[5,41,47] A recent study found that at the initiation of dialysis therapy, a low serum urea nitrogen, creatinine, total protein, albumin, sodium, and phosphate and higher serum potassium were all associated with a significant increase in the relative risk of death. These data suggest that reduced dietary protein intake in the predialysis period—as indicated by the reduced concentrations of serum urea nitrogen, albumin, total protein, creatinine, and phosphate—can contribute to mortality. A lower serum sodium and higher serum potassium further support the increased mortality risk in maintenance dialysis patients associated with overall reductions in dietary intake as renal function deteriorates.[48]

Intercurrent Illness

Patients with ESRD also suffer from frequent episodes of intercurrent illness. Infection, particularly of the vascular access and peritonitis, pulmonary edema, cardiac arrhythmias, and other forms of cardiac disease, as well as gastrointestinal diseases such as peptic ulcers, are frequent complications of uremia.[49] When a patient with renal failure develops a superimposed acute illness there is usually a loss of appetite and a change in eating habits that result in decreased food intake. Hospitalization often results in missed meals due to diagnostic procedures and a reduction in food intake. Serious illness in these patients results in catabolic stress that may lead to negative nitrogen balance and adversely affect nutritional status.[50,51]

Dialysis Losses

A number of studies demonstrate that many nutrients—including amino acids, glucose, and water-soluble vitamins—are removed during hemodialysis.[52,53] Each hemodialysis procedure is associated with the loss of between 4 to 8 g of amino acids.[52,54] There is an even greater loss of amino acids as well as protein losses with peritoneal dialysis,[55] although glucose losses are negligible with this type of dialysis because of the high glucose concentration of peritoneal dialysis solutions. Dialyzer reuse procedures utilizing bleach disinfection may result in changes in dialyzer permeability leading to increased protein losses.[56] When hemodialysis patients do not receive vitamin supplementation, the serum or plasma concentrations of many of the water-soluble vitamins are reduced.[53] The reasons for these findings include losses into dialysate as well as dietary restrictions that may limit vitamin intake along with restrictions on potassium and fluid. The use of phosphate binders may result in the binding of iron as well as phosphate, for example. In addition, there is an increased dietary requirement for vitamin B_6 in patients with renal failure, which is not completely explained by losses into the dialysate or reduced intake.[26] Whether uremia results in an increased requirement for other vitamins has not been adequately studied. Specific recommendations for vitamin replacement are given further on in this chapter.

Acidosis

Acidosis is invariably present in patients with advanced renal failure and those treated with maintenance hemodialysis. Despite the use of bicarbonate-containing dialysate, acidosis is often not adequately corrected by the hemodialysis procedure. The presence of acidosis contributes to malnutrition and wasting because it causes net negative nitrogen and total body protein balance.[57] In addition, recent data suggest that severe metabolic acidosis may be a trigger for chronic inflammation, further impacting nutritional status.[58] In support of the detrimental effects of metabolic acidosis on nutritional status and wasting is evidence that correction of metabolic acidosis is associated with improvement in protein degradation and in nutritional status.[59-62] The correction of metabolic acidosis may also improve amino acid patterns in patients with renal failure. Branched chain amino acid synthesis increases with treatment of metabolic acidosis.[63,64]

EFFECTS OF UREMIA AND DIALYSIS ON NUTRITIONAL STATUS

The dialysis procedure appears to cause increased protein catabolism.[65-67] Hemodialysis treatments cause negative nitrogen balance despite a protein intake of more than 1.5 g/kg/day.[65] Dialysis-related protein catabolism has been demonstrated from studies in which the interdialytic interval was lengthened and protein catabolism decreased with a longer interval between hemodialysis procedures.[67] The contact between blood and the dialysis membrane has also been demonstrated to be associated with increased protein catabolism.[66]

Uremia itself is associated with several metabolic abnormalities that may potentiate malnutrition. These include disturbances of amino acid, protein, carbohydrate, and lipid metabolism.[23-25,68-73] Many of the abnormalities noted in plasma amino acid concentrations cannot be explained by reduced protein intake alone. The kidney is responsible for several amino acid interconversions, and loss of kidney function will alter the rate at which this occurs.[74,75] Because there is resistance to the action of insulin in patients with renal failure, it is possible that reduced insulin-stimulated amino acid uptake by tissues contributes to the abnormal plasma amino acid pattern seen in these patients.[73] Insulin resistance probably also contributes to the mild glucose intolerance and hypertriglyceridemia noted in uremic patients.[70,76-78] The presence of acidosis may further exacerbate insulin resistance in these patients.[79] Other abnormalities of hormonal function such as thyroid, hyperparathyroid, and growth hormone disturbances have been described in patients with renal failure and also contribute to malnutrition in these patients.[71] The causes of malnutrition are summarized in Table 21-3.

INFLAMMATION AND MALNUTRITION

The presence of inflammation has been associated with alterations in several serum measures of nutritional status. Most importantly, the serum albumin is depressed in the presence of inflammation due to the reduction in hepatic albumin synthesis associated with an increased synthesis of acute-phase reactants.[16] This results in hypoalbuminemia,

TABLE 21-3. CAUSES OF POOR NUTRITIONAL STATUS IN UREMIC PATIENTS

1. Altered nutrition:
   Inadequate food intake, dialysis losses, abnormal metabolism of nutrients, catabolic stress of the dialysis procedure
2. Uremia:
   Alteration of enzyme activities, impaired membrane transport, altered protein binding
3. Superimposed illnesses:
   Decreased food intake, increased catabolism, enhanced gluconeogenesis
4. Endocrinopathies:
   PTH, glucagon, insulin, growth hormone, vitamin D_3
5. Altered renal metabolism and degradation of peptides, proteins, insulin, vitamin D, other hormones
6. Acidosis

which is often not responsive to increased dietary protein intake. Acute or chronic inflammation is also associated with increased metabolic stress and can lead to malnutrition and wasting.[80,81] The link between low serum albumin and inflammation, as well as malnutrition is somewhat confounding. It is likely that both catabolic stress induced by chronic inflammation as well as reduced dietary intake both contribute to malnutrition. What is not clear is the relative importance of each in the development of malnutrition. Additional research is needed to more clearly elucidate these relationships.

ASSESSMENT OF NUTRITIONAL STATUS IN PATIENTS WITH RENAL FAILURE

Most patients with renal failure do not appear clinically to be severely malnourished, because many of the manifestations of malnutrition are subtle. In addition, most patients display only a few abnormal parameters of nutritional status at any one time.[5,6] It is important to accurately assess nutritional status regularly in all patients with advanced renal disease in order to identify those patients who may need nutritional intervention and to monitor the effects of any therapeutic regimen.

Most of the methods used to assess nutritional status in subjects with normal renal function can be used in patients with renal disease with minor modifications. The *NKF-K/DOQI Guidelines for Nutrition*, published in 2000, provide excellent guidance for carrying out the nutrition assessment.[41]

History and Physical Examination

The history and physical examination can often provide important clues to the nutritional status of the patient. Complaints of nausea and vomiting or anorexia should be carefully evaluated. The psychosocial history should not be overlooked as the initiation of dialysis treatment is frequently associated with major changes in lifestyle. Depression related to the development of a major illness may affect food intake. Numerous restrictions placed on types of food and fluid may also adversely affect food intake. The history should address other associated diseases that may affect nutritional status, such as chronic alcoholism or diabetes mellitus. A history of recent weight gain or loss should also be elicited.

The physical examination should focus on a careful assessment of body weight, with attention to evaluating the presence of edema. At times, body weight may not appear to change; however, the patient may actually be losing solid weight and gaining fluid weight. This is suspected when blood pressure becomes poorly controlled or the patient develops new congestive heart failure. It is best to weigh patients at the end of dialysis in order to determine the patient's "dry" weight.

A simple tool to evaluate recent changes in nutritional status is the "subjective global assessment" which has been modified from the acute hospital setting to the maintenance dialysis setting.[82]

The method has been validated in dialysis patients and can provide a simple tool to determine whether a patient has developed a change in nutritional status.[83]

Dietary History

Dietary histories should be carried out by a dietician trained to assess food intake. They should be carried out not only to educate patients as to the dietary limitations imposed by renal failure but also on a regular basis to determine whether nutrient intake is adequate. Dietary histories can be obtained from patient recall or through the use of food diaries. Histories are most accurate when the patient weighs all food prior to its consumption. For most clinical needs, a dietary history by recall is, however, sufficient. The food intake records can be reviewed on a regular basis so that if the diet changes, appropriate therapeutic intervention can occur early. In order to improve accuracy, patient recall histories should cover fairly brief periods of time and be representative of the time period. Thus, a 3- to 5-day history including both dialysis and nondialysis days is best. Several dietary histories covering 3 to 5 days are probably more accurate than one covering 7 days. Ethnic food preferences should be noted. The approach of the dietitian in obtaining the dietary history is given in Table 21–4.

From the dietary history, the patient's intake of protein, fat, and carbohydrate can be calculated from standard food tables. Computer programs exist to make this task easier and more accurate. Dietary protein intake can also be calculated using the urea nitrogen appearance (UNA) rate or the urea generation (Gu) rate. UNA is the sum of urinary urea nitrogen (g/day) plus the change in body urea nitrogen (g/day). This is the daily rate of net urea production. Since

TABLE 21–4. DIETITIAN'S APPROACH TO THE IDENTIFICATION OF NUTRITIONAL PROBLEMS

I. Preliminary screening procedures

  A. Initial laboratory values: glucose, BUN, Na^+, K^+, albumin, creatinine, total lymphocyte count and lymphocyte subsets, WBC, hemoglobin, hematocrit

  B. Medications with nutritional implications: e.g., diuretics, insulin, cathartics, MAO inhibitors

  C. Patient interview: weight changes, patterns of eating, changes in appetite, changes in taste, digestive problems, bowel habits, food preferences, food allergies, educational needs

II. In-depth nutritional assessment

  A. Anthropometric measurements: height, weight, arm circumference, triceps skinfold

  B. Evaluation of the skin, hair, mucous membranes

  C. Visceral protein status: MAMC, albumin, transferrin, immunoglobulins

  D. Nitrogen metabolism and balance: UNA, Gu

  E. Calorie expenditure: basal energy expenditure

  F. Calorie requirements: activity level, presence of fever, infection

ABBREVIATIONS: BUN = blood urea nitrogen; WBC = white blood cell (count); MAO = monoamine oxidase; MAMC = midarm muscle circumference; UNA = urea nitrogen appearance (rate); Gu = urea generation (rate).

there is a direct correlation between UNA and total nitrogen output, UNA will reflect nitrogen or protein intake in patients who are in neutral nitrogen balance.[84] For patients who are not yet on dialysis, the formula for calculating UNA is as follows:

$$\text{UNA (gN/day)} = \text{urinary UN (g/day)} + [\text{SUN}f - \text{SUN}i \times (0.6)\ \text{BW}i] + (\text{BW}f - \text{BW}i \times \text{SUN}f)$$

The i and f are initial and final values for the period of measurement. SUN is the serum urea nitrogen (g/L), BW is the body weight (kg), and 0.6 is an estimate of the fraction of body weight that is body water.[84] This formula can be used for patients on hemodialysis but the interdialytic interval should be used for calculation to avoid having to measure the urea in dialysate. To use this method for patients treated with CAPD, one must also measure pooled 24-hour dialysate urea nitrogen concentrations.[85]

Alternatively, one can measure the urea generation rate to determine the protein catabolic rate. Because the protein catabolic rate should equal the dietary protein intake in patients in neutral nitrogen balance, this method can be used to assess dietary protein intake in dialysis patients. This method assumes a singe pool for the volume of distribution of urea. Urea kinetics are described by solving a series of equations using the measurements of SUN concentration at the beginning of a hemodialysis, the end of that hemodialysis, and at the beginning of the subsequent hemodialysis, and the measurement of time from the beginning of the first to the beginning of the next hemodialysis. A computer program is available to aid in the calculations of the various formulas for Gu, PCR, and dietary protein intake (DPI).[86] A full discussion of urea kinetics is given in Chap. 8.

Energy intake should also be estimated from the dietary history and food diary. Standard food tables can be used for these calculations. It should be remembered that glucose is absorbed from dialysate in patients on peritoneal dialysis and this should be included when calculating total energy intake in peritoneal dialysis patients.

Assessment of Body Composition

A measure of body composition is beneficial in the assessment of nutritional status. Measurement of body composition can provide accurate baseline and serial information in dialysis patients in order to better assess nutritional status. The methods most commonly used in dialysis patients include anthropometrics, bioelectrical impedance analysis, and dual x-ray absorptiometry. Other measures, such as the direct measurement total body water, total body potassium, and neutron activation analysis are not readily available except as research tools.

Anthropometric measurements have been in use the longest and are very useful in the nutritional assessment of nonuremic individuals as well as in uremic patients. The technique requires little training and no expensive equipment. Anthropometric measurements can be carried out in the dialysis unit and are used to assess body fat, muscle mass, and body water through measures of skinfold thickness and muscle circumference. Tables standardized for an American population of normal subjects are available,[87,88] making it possible to determine whether any abnormality exists in uremic patients. A number of studies have demonstrated that patients with advanced renal failure have reduced anthropometric measurements of skinfold thickness and arm muscle area, indicating reduced fat and muscle stores.[5,11,18,89] Lange skinfold calipers (Cambridge Instruments, Cambridge, MA) are used to carry out this noninvasive determination. Most dieticians are trained in their use. For arm measurements, the nondominant arm should be used. The presence of a vascular access in the nondominant arm may, however, result in a greater diameter than usual; thus, it is best to use the arm without an arteriovenous fistula for this measurement.

Body fat stores may also be estimated from the relative body weight, which is that percentage of the patient's weight compared with a normal subject of the same age, height, and gender. Relative body weight gives a rapid estimate of whether a patient is overweight, underweight, or normal. Nonetheless, it fails to determine the proportion of body weight that is composed of fat, skeletal muscle, or body water. Therefore other anthropometric measurements should also be carried out.

Muscle mass represents a significant proportion of fat-free body mass and total body protein. In nonuremic subjects, the creatinine-height index is often used to determine the existence of protein depletion.[90] Obviously, this parame-

ter will not be useful in individuals with any degree of renal insufficiency, as creatinine excretion is reduced in these patients.

Anthropometry provides a rapid, noninvasive, and reproducible method for evaluating body fat and protein stores.[5,11,18,85,89] Patients can be followed serially, and decreases in these parameters can result in rapid therapeutic interventions.

A multicenter cooperative study was undertaken to establish anthropometric norms for the dialysis population.[11] Stringent selection criteria were utilized to ensure that only stable maintenance dialysis patients were included in the study. Measurements in male hemodialysis patients (including diabetics) did not differ significantly from data obtained by the second National Health and Nutrition Examination Survey (NHANES II), whereas nondiabetic females were significantly below these levels. Diabetic females were not significantly different from the NHANES II data with the exception of black females above age 55, who had lower triceps skinfold thickness. Measurements of 138 CAPD patients were similar to those of hemodialysis patients. The data from this study provide important information on anthropometric measurements in the "healthy" maintenance dialysis population and provide a good frame of reference. As a general rule, patients whose measurements are greater than 95 percent of normal are considered to be adequately nourished, whereas values between 70 and 90 percent indicate that the patient is at risk for malnutrition and values less than 70 percent represent significant malnutrition.[90] While anthropometry provides a simple and expedient method to assess body fat and muscle mass, there are limitations to its use. The presence of peripheral edema has already been mentioned as limiting the accuracy of the measurement. Skinfold calipers lack precision and there is interoperator variation, making it necessary for serial measurements to be carried out by the same individual. In order to more accurately measure body composition, newer techniques such as bioelectrical impedance and dual x-ray absorptiometry have been used. These methods are dependent on elucidating differences in attenuation by tissues of varying density. A recent study comparing several methods has shown that bioelectrical impedance analysis is a reasonably reliable measure of total body water.[91] Dual energy x-ray absorptiometry can also be used to assess body composition in dialysis patients. It is based on the principle that x-rays passed through body tissues of different composition have different attenuation of the x-ray energy. Using two different levels of energy can better differentiate tissue. This technique has great precision, but it is limited by cost and lack of availability at every center.[92] The dialysis modality has also been felt to affect measures of nutritional status. Body fat has been noted to be higher in the peritoneal dialysis patient as compared to the hemodialysis patient, presumably due to the increased caloric load from dextrose in the dialysis solution. However, one study failed to find a difference between hemodialysis and peritoneal dialysis patients in their percentage of body fat. The authors stressed the importance of using the same method serially to avoid confounding results.[93]

Serum Proteins

Serum proteins are generally reduced as the body's protein stores are depleted. Both serum albumin and transferrin are used to provide information regarding protein status.[90] The indirect correlation between serum albumin concentrations and mortality has generated a great deal of interest in this parameter.[9] Decreased serum albumin levels have been demonstrated to correlate with the depression of other parameters of nutritional status, such as immune function and midarm muscle circumference.[94,95] Often, these nutritional parameters are corrected once nutritional repletion sufficient to raise the serum albumin concentration to normal levels has occurred.[34,90] It has also been shown that serum albumin and transferrin concentrations are correlated in nonuremic individuals.[90] Thus, measurements of serum albumin and transferrin may be useful in assessing protein status in uremic patients. Severe hepatic disease, protein-losing enteropathy, nephrotic syndrome, or other protein-losing disease states, as well as chronic inflammation, may invalidate the serum albumin concentration as a measure of nutritional status. In addition, the effect of uremia on serum albumin concentration is unclear. It should also be remembered that serum albumin levels are reduced with intravascular fluid volume excess, and this should be taken into account when evaluating the serum albumin concentration in patients with excessive interdialytic weight gains. Uremic subjects have alterations in albumin metabolism that may in part be due to uremia and in part related to nutritional status.[17,96] A correlation between serum creatinine and albumin has been reported, suggesting that these parameters may reflect nutritional status in patients treated with maintenance hemodialysis.[6] In that study, albumin also correlated with lymphocyte function, indicating that nutritional status appears to affect these indices in uremic subjects.[6] Many investigators have also demonstrated that serum albumin is depressed in uremic patients who manifest other signs of malnutrition.[4,5,15,89] In addition, serum albumin often improves when nutritional repletion is carried out.[97,98] Finally, improvement in well-being and rehabilitation may be associated with improvement in serum albumin concentrations as well.[6,16] As mentioned earlier, serum albumin concentrations decrease when patients have associated acute or chronic inflammation.[17] Therefore, the serum albumin may not always be a good indicator of nutritional status in these patients. It may be helpful to also measure acute phase reactants in order to determine the presence of acute or chronic inflammation.[80]

Serum transferrin levels have also been used to assess nutritional status in uremic patients. This protein is often depressed in those uremic subjects with other manifestations of protein-calorie malnutrition,[4–6,15,18] and it may also improve with nutritional manipulation.[99]

Serum transferrin levels are increased in patients with severe iron deficiency and may be low in patients with iron overload. As hemodialysis patients often suffer from these abnormalities in iron stores, this may be a confounding variable when transferrin levels are used as an index of nutritional status. For these reasons, at least one study has questioned the value of transferrin determinations in the nutritional assessment of diabetic patients on hemodialysis and peritoneal dialysis.[100] Transferrin levels correlated negatively with serum ferritin, which would be expected if transferrin levels reflected iron stores. Interestingly, there was no correlation between serum albumin and transferrin level. Thus, transferrin may be a poor marker of nutritional status in this setting. These investigators also found that, regardless of nutritional status, serum prealbumin and retinol-binding protein were normal or elevated because of reduced renal excretion,[100] indicating that these may also be poor markers of nutritional status in uremic subjects, although they are useful in nonuremic individuals.

Serum prealbumin levels, on the other hand, may be used to assess nutritional status in patients with renal failure, as long as it is understood that the serum prealbumin concentration is often elevated due to its binding to retinol binding protein, which depends on normal renal function for its excretion.[42] Despite the abnormally elevated levels of prealbumin in hemodialysis patients, serial measurements can be used to assess nutritional status once a baseline level is established for the individual patient.[42] In patients who are felt to be malnourished and in whom a nutritional intervention is undertaken, the serum prealbumin can be used to follow changes in nutritional status. Prealbumin, unlike albumin, has a short half-life and changes rapidly in response to nutritional intervention.[42] Thus, this parameter does seem to be useful in patients with renal failure, if it is monitored serially and changes are compared with the patient's previous levels.[42]

Plasma Amino Acids

Plasma amino acid concentrations are strongly influenced by dietary protein intake and were often used to assess nutritional status.[101] Patients with CKD demonstrate abnormalities in plasma amino acid patterns similar to those seen in protein-calorie malnutrition.[19,21,23,68] These abnormalities may improve toward normal with nutritional supplementation,[68,97–99] further suggesting a relationship between plasma amino acid concentrations and nutritional status. Although measurement of plasma amino acid concentrations is felt to be useful by some investigators in the nutritional assessment of patients with ESRD, it should be remembered that plasma amino acids tend to reflect recent protein intake and thus are of limited value in this regard. The measurement of plasma amino acids also requires special techniques which are not readily available in routine clinical practice, further limiting their value as a routine measure of nutritional status.

The serum cholesterol concentration is reduced in patients with normal renal function and severe malnutrition. In the ESRD patient population, serum cholesterol is reduced when compared with normal subjects. Two studies have demonstrated an inverse relationship between mortality and cholesterol concentrations in ESRD patients.[9,101]

For simplicity, serial measurements of the serum urea nitrogen (SUN) level may be most helpful in monitoring protein intake and nutritional status. Patients who have trends toward reduced SUN levels may be ingesting less protein and becoming wasted. This may lead practitioners to reduce the dialysis prescription, and the wasting may become more severe as decreased dialysis further reduces appetite and protein intake. Low predialysis SUN levels have also been associated with increased mortality.[101] It is important to point out that no one measure of nutritional status can be used for reliable assessments. As previously mentioned, it is important to use a variety of measures in order to more completely evaluate muscle mass, fat mass, and to detect the presence of protein-calorie malnutrition in the maintenance dialysis population.[41]

DIETARY MANAGEMENT OF PATIENTS WITH ESRD

Dietary intervention has been the cornerstone of treatment for patients with renal failure. Many of the clinical disturbances associated with uremia result from an imbalance between ingested nutrients and the capacity of the kidneys to excrete the end products of nutrient metabolism. The accumulation of these metabolic end products leads to many of the clinical disturbances associated with uremia. For certain nutrients, standard intake may be considered excessive. For other nutrients, intake may become inadequate due to dialytic losses or increased requirements in uremia. The goal of dietary management in ESRD is to adjust nutrient intake to meet daily requirements without exceeding excretory capacity. In addition, certain endocrine functions of the kidney are decreased as disease progresses. Although these hormonal alterations cannot be completely corrected by dietary manipulation, the existence of such abnormalities may modify the approach to dietary therapy. With the commencement of dialysis therapy, the problem of excess intake is partially solved. New problems may, however, emerge. Losses of nutrients into dialysate may contribute to further deterioration of nutritional status. Thus, nutritional management in the predialysis patient requires a different approach from nutritional management of the dialysis patient.

Nutritional Management of Patients with CKD

Dietary modification plays an important role in the management of the patient with CKD. Restriction of protein and/or phosphate may slow the progression of renal failure. Protein restriction can also delay the onset of uremic symptoms and associated metabolic disturbances once glomerular filtration rate (GFR) has fallen below 15 mL/min. Abundant evidence from animal and human models suggests that dietary protein intake strongly affects renal and glomerular hemodynamics. Both acute and chronic ingestion of high protein diets result in increased renal blood flow and GFR.[102-106] This hyperfiltration induced by protein feeding may contribute to the progression of underlying renal disease.[107] Experimental models of subtotal renal ablation in rats reveal that reduction of renal mass results in compensatory increases in single-nephron GFR[108,109] and progressive glomerular sclerosis in the remaining kidney tissue.[110] Reduction in protein intake, which lowers GFR in animals with intact renal mass, protects animals from progressive glomerular sclerosis.[111,112] The restriction of dietary protein in patients with all forms of renal disease may retard the progression of ESRD.[3] Several dietary approaches have been investigated. Limitation of protein intake can be achieved by high-quality low-protein diets or mixed-quality low-protein diets supplemented with essential amino acids or their keto analogues.

The Modification of Diet in Renal Disease (MDRD) study was a large multicenter trial to determine the effects of dietary protein restriction and blood-pressure control on the progression of CKD.[113] In the primary efficacy analysis, there was no benefit of low protein diets on the progression of renal disease. This may have been due to the confounding effect of concomitant therapy with angiotensin-converting enzyme inhibitors for blood pressure control in a large cohort of patients in the trial. However, several post hoc analyses indicated that the low-protein diets retarded the progression of renal failure.[4,114,115]

Protein restriction can play a role in ameliorating uremic symptoms in patients with severely diminished renal function, since nitrogen retention is associated with many of the classic signs and symptoms of uremia. Because dietary protein is the major source of nitrogenous wastes, restriction may reduce many of the symptoms of uremia. Protein restriction will initially result in negative nitrogen balance. However, it appears that patients with CKD are capable of adapting to a low-protein diet through suppressing protein degradation.[116] Patients will generally come into neutral balance after about 3 weeks of consuming a diet of

0.6 g/kg protein daily.[117] This quantity of protein is adequate provided that protein requirements are not increased by the existence of increased catabolic stress, heavy proteinuria, gastrointestinal bleeding, or decreased total caloric intake. It is important that protein be of high biologic value in order to permit adequate protein use and avoid increased urea production[118]; that is, the protein consumed should have a high ratio of essential to nonessential amino acids.

Based on the above considerations, the *NKF-K/DOQI Guidelines for Nutrition*[41] recommend that patients with GFR less than 25 mL/min be considered for a diet providing protein at a level of 0.6g/kg/day. If the patient cannot tolerate the diet or if the diet does not provide adequate energy intake, dietary protein intake should be increased to a protein level of 0.75g/kg/day.[41] However, there remains much debate over whether low-protein diets are worth the time and trouble for patients and whether they can meaningfully retard the progression of renal failure.[119,120] It is likely that some patients can benefit from institution of low-protein diets and can delay the need for maintenance dialysis therapy. However, for those patients who cannot comply with dietary restrictions or who cannot consume adequate nutrients with these diets, the timely initiation of dialysis treatment is indicated.

Nutritional Management of Patients Treated with Hemodialysis

When the GFR falls below 10 mL/min, dialysis therapy is usually required to manage fluid and electrolyte balance and control the SUN concentration. Because dialysis therapy is associated with losses of protein and amino acids, the diet should be liberalized and protein intake should be increased to approximately 1.2 g/kg/day.[41] Energy expenditure in the resting state, during controlled exercise, and after a test meal, is the same in chronic hemodialysis patients compared with normal subjects.[1,121–123] Therefore, energy intake should be maintained at 35 kcal/kg/day in order to provide adequate calories and promote protein sparing. This energy intake has been shown to promote positive nitrogen balance in maintenance hemodialysis patients.[41] Careful attention to dietary intake is a critical part of the management of maintenance dialysis patients, because so much of the management of the dialysis therapy itself depends on appropriate nutrient intake. Patients must be educated in order to understand the need to comply with dietary restrictions and still consume adequate intake in order to avoid nutrient deficiencies.

The recommended levels of nutrient intake stated above are probably adequate to maintain nitrogen balance when the patient is in a steady state; however, they may not be adequate to repair nutritional deficiencies that may have occurred in the predialysis period. This may be especially true for patients who have experienced catabolic stress during the predialysis period. Not surprisingly, from 10 to 15 percent of patients on chronic dialysis have severe wasting.

If dietary intake is not adequate or if patients exhibit signs of malnutrition despite adequate dietary intake, other nutritional interventions should be considered. Historically, attempts to improve nutritional status with supplements of essential amino acids administered either orally or intravenously were undertaken.[97,98,124] Although some studies have demonstrated improvement in various nutritional parameters after the institution of such supplement therapy, improvement is not invariable. Hecking and coworkers found no benefit from essential amino acid supplements in their patients.[124] Stable hemodialysis patients who are able to adhere to a 1.2 g/kg/day high biological value protein diet are unlikely to benefit further from amino acid supplementation. For the patient who is malnourished, not eating well, undergoing catabolic stress, or facing major elective surgery, nutritional supplements may be beneficial. Ordinarily, oral supplementation can be used, but many of these patients have nausea and anorexia, and may have difficulty consuming oral supplements. For these patients, the administration of a solution of amino acids and glucose or lipid intravenously during hemodialysis has been advocated.[42,98] Such an infusion results in increased plasma amino acid concentrations during dialysis and prevents the fall in glucose and amino acids associated with hemodialysis. Indeed, as much as 70 percent of the infused amino acids are retained by the patient with this technique.[54] Other investigators have noted improvement in protein and amino acid status, as well as some more general measures of nutritional status, after long-term administration of essential amino acids and glucose to hemodialysis patients, as well as perhaps improvement in mortality.[30,31,42,98] However, this mode of nutrient administration is very costly, and since it can be administered only during the hemodialysis procedure, it may not be as effective as daily oral supplementation. Every effort should be made to encourage compliance with oral supplementation before intradialytic parenteral nutrition is begun. Several newer products that are calorie dense, thus reducing the oral fluid intake, and low in sodium and potassium are available.[125] The use of oral supplements takes considerable effort because of poor patient compliance and often this intervention is not successful. When the dietitian is involved in dietary management, patient compliance often improves. A study by Fedje and coworkers demonstrated improved mortality and morbidity when patients were treated with oral nutritional supplementation.[126]

Because poor appetite may make a significant contribution to the development of malnutrition, several novel interventions have been carried out. Hypoalbuminemic patients with delayed gastric emptying demonstrated increased serum albumin concentrations after treatment with prokinetic agents.[127] Appetite stimulants such as megesterol acetate have also been used to improve appetite.[128,129] Anabolic agents such as recombinant human growth hormone and insulin-like growth factor 1 (IGF-1) have also been used to improve nutritional status in maintenance dialysis patients. [130,131] Recombinant human growth hormone has been shown to be effective when used in conjunction with interdialytic parenteral nutrition.[126] However, side effects, poor compliance with therapy and the cost of these treatments in the face of marginal improvement in nutritional status, have impeded their widespread use. Further study is needed to determine whether these novel interventions have a place in the management of malnutrition in the patient with ESRD.

Hypertriglyceridemia is a common finding in patients with renal failure. As this may be related to insulin resistance, a diet comprising 1.0 to 1.2 g/kg/day of high-biological-value protein, with 35 percent of the calories supplied from carbohydrate, 55 percent supplied from fat, and with a polyunsaturated-saturated fat ratio of 2:1, is recommended for hemodialysis patients.[41,132–134]

Vitamin Therapy

Water-soluble vitamins are lost into dialysate and therefore must be replaced. Vitamins B_1 and B_2 are readily available in adequate concentrations in commercially available multivitamin preparations. Because there is no evidence that nutritional requirements for these vitamins are higher in uremic patients for reasons other than increased dialysate losses, one multivitamin (B complex with ascorbic acid) tablet a day will provide adequate replacement.

Several cases of Wernicke's encephalopathy associated with peritoneal dialysis and hemodialysis have been reported.[135] In three of five patients, the classic triad of ophthalmoplegia, ataxia, and global confusion was absent. All cases were diagnosed only at autopsy. In the setting of prolonged nutritional depletion without vitamin supplements, Wernicke's encephalopathy must be considered. It can present with a grand mal seizure, confusion, loss of memory, or myoclonic jerks and progression to coma.[135]

Vitamin B_{12} stores appear to be adequate in dialysis patients, but they are also usually replaced by the ingestion of a daily multivitamin. Folic acid, 1 mg/day, and ascorbic acid, 100 mg/day, are also recommended for dialysis patients, because blood levels of these vitamins appear to be decreased in the absence of vitamin replacement.[53,136–140] Vitamin B_6 status is abnormal in uremic patients and in those treated with dialysis.[139] A minimum dose of 5 mg of pyridoxine per day will restore B_6 levels to normal.[26] Higher doses may, however, be necessary to correct some of the other abnormalities in uremia that may be related to B_6 deficiency.

The fat-soluble vitamins A, D, and K are not removed by dialysis, and replacement of vitamins A and K is not required in patients with ESRD. Multivitamins containing vitamin A should, in fact, be avoided because of the possibility of vitamin A toxicity. Vitamin D requirements are discussed in Chap. 30.

Trace elements are also important in patients with renal failure. An accumulation of aluminum in the cerebral gray matter of some patients treated with hemodialysis may result in the dialysis encephalopathy syndrome.[141] Aluminum may also accumulate in bone and be associated with renal osteodystrophy.[142] Zinc replacement may be necessary for patients with ESRD. It is unlikely that zinc is removed by dialysis; however, several studies have demonstrated reduced plasma zinc levels in dialysis patients. It is felt that reduced plasma zinc levels may be related to either inadequate dietary intake due to protein-restricted diets or to inhibition of zinc absorption through the gastrointestinal tract. Hypogeusia and sexual impotence are reported to improve when zinc supplements are administered to dialysis patients.[143]

NUTRITION IN PATIENTS TREATED WITH PERITONEAL DIALYSIS

Peritoneal dialysis has emerged as a popular treatment modality for patients with ESRD. The nutritional requirements of peritoneal dialysis patients are unique and deserve special attention. Factors such as protein losses into the dialysate and especially during episodes of peritonitis and glucose absorption from the dialysate may affect the nutritional status and hence dietary management of this group of patients.[83,144–150]

Protein-calorie malnutrition is a significant problem in peritoneal dialysis patients. A cross-sectional multicenter study examined the nutritional status of 224 CAPD patients in six centers in Europe and North America. Some degree of malnutrition was documented in 40 percent of patients, with 8 percent of the total meeting criteria for severe malnutrition.[83] Several studies have documented an association between nutritional status and morbidity and mortality.[146–148] In addition, adequacy of dialysis is becoming recognized as an important factor for maintaining optimal nutritional status.[145] As with hemodialysis patients, markers of nutritional status, particularly serum albumin levels, have been correlated with morbidity and mortality in peritoneal dialysis patients.[147,148]

Protein Losses

Substantial protein losses may occur into the dialysate during PD. On the average, between 5 and 15 g of protein may be lost per day, with albumin comprising approximately two-thirds of the total.[149] Amino acid losses generally range between 1.2 to 3.4 g/day and are proportional to their serum concentrations. Several factors have been shown to influence the quantity of protein lost in the dialysate. In general, the peritoneal clearance of proteins varies inversely with the molecular weight. The peritoneal mass transfer of large molecular weight proteins appears to be continuous throughout an 8-hour dialysis cycle, whereas clearance of low molecular weight substances decreases significantly after the first hour.[55] This may explain why the greatest protein loss occurs during the longer overnight dwell. Protein losses may increase substantially during episodes of peritonitis.[50,149] With successful antibiotic treatment, protein losses generally return to baseline within a day. However, with more severe episodes, protein losses may remain elevated for several weeks. There is large interpatient variability, suggesting that host factors are also important in determining protein losses.[151] One study demonstrated greater protein permeability in diabetics on CAPD.[152] Protein intake does not appear to correlate with protein losses.

Despite large daily protein losses, serum albumin levels are only slightly reduced in the majority of patients on peritoneal dialysis. Kaysen and colleagues[153] studied albumin homeostasis in 16 stable CAPD patients. They demonstrated that albumin synthesis was increased and catabolism decreased as compared with normal controls. As a result, plasma and total albumin mass were preserved regardless of large daily losses.[153]

Glucose Absorption

Glucose absorption during CAPD may contribute significantly to the total caloric intake of an individual patient. Approximately 70 percent of the glucose infused is absorbed from the dialysate and may represent as much as 20 to 30 percent of the daily caloric intake.[44] A strong correlation exists between the amount of glucose instilled per day and the quantity absorbed. The amount absorbed from day to day remains relatively constant in an individual patient, provided the dialysate composition and exchange frequency remain unchanged. The following formula has been suggested for calculating glucose absorption[46]:

$$\text{Glucose absorbed (g/L)} = 11.3$$
$$[\text{average glucose concentration}$$
$$\text{of the dialysate (g/dL/day)}] - 10.9$$

Note that 1.5% dextrose dialysate = 1.30 g glucose/dL; 4.25% dextrose dialysate = 3.76 g glucose/dL.

Nutrient intake of CAPD patients may be altered by the obligatory peritoneal glucose load. Baeyer and coworkers documented an unintentional suppression of oral carbohydrate intake in a group of CAPD patients.[154] This fully compensated for the additional peritoneal carbohydrate load and resulted in a normal overall distribution of nutritional energy sources.

The continuous glucose load imposed by CAPD may have adverse metabolic effects, including hyperlipidemia, weight gain, and glucose intolerance. ESRD is frequently associated with lipoprotein abnormalities, primarily characterized by an increase in very low density lipoprotein (VLDL) levels and a decrease in high-density lipoprotein (HDL) levels.[155] Treatment with CAPD frequently exacerbates these abnormalities. Triglyceride levels often increase further and plasma VLDL cholesterol and low-density cholesterol may also rise.[156–159] Effects on HDL cholesterol levels are inconsistent. More recently, elevated levels of lipoprotein(a), an independent risk factor for atherosclerotic cardiovascular disease, has been documented in CAPD patients.[160,161] Patients utilizing frequent hypertonic exchanges may be at increased risk for developing hyperlipidemia. Although the majority of studies demonstrate a high incidence of hyperlipidemia in CAPD patients, the clinical consequences with regard to cardiovascular risk remain to be determined. Nevertheless, it would seem reasonable to increase the ratio of polyunsaturated to saturated fats in the diet and minimize the number of hypertonic exchanges. Patients with persistent hyperlipidemia regardless of dietary manipulation may require more specific drug therapy.

Mild glucose intolerance is a common finding in patients with CKD.[162] Most studies suggest that CAPD does not cause a further deterioration in glucose tolerance despite the continuous glucose load absorbed from the peritoneum.[154,156–159,163]

Weight gain and the development or exacerbation of obesity are other potential adverse effects of glucose absorption. The average weight gain per patient ranges between 2 to 4 kg over the first year of treatment with peritoneal dialysis. However, this varies markedly from patient to patient and correlates significantly with average daily amounts of glucose absorbed.[164]

Specific Dietary Recommendations

The NKF-K/DOQI guidelines provide specific dietary recommendations for patients treated with peritoneal dialysis.[41] These are outlined in Table 21–5. Although the requirements for peritoneal dialysis have been primarily studied in CAPD patients, it is unlikely that the nutritional requirements for patients on continuous cycling peritoneal dialysis (CCPD) should be significantly different. It should be emphasized that these recommendations may need to be modified during periods of catabolic stress or for patients significantly above or below their ideal body weight.

Metabolic studies in CAPD patients demonstrate that nitrogen balance increases as protein intake rises. Nitrogen balance studies and anthropometric data suggest that patients are anabolic on protein diets of 1.09 g/kg/day or greater.[165] Based on these data, the *NKF-K/DOQI Guidelines for Nutrition*[41] recommend a minimum daily protein allowance of 1.2 to 1.3 g/kg/day for stable CAPD patients. Adequate essential amino acids can be provided from such a diet as long as at least 50 percent of the protein is of high biological value.

TABLE 21–5. DAILY DIETARY ALLOWANCES FOR CAPD PATIENTS

Protein	1.2–1.3 g/kg[a]
Energy (oral and dialysate)	35–42 kcal/kg
Carbohydrate (oral)	35% of ingested calories
Fat	Remainder of ingested nonprotein calories
Polyunsaturated : saturated fatty acid ratio	1.5 : 1.0
Total fiber	20–25 g
Calcium	1000–1400 mg
Phosphorus	800–1200 mg
Magnesium	200–300 mg
Potassium	70–80 meq
Sodium and water	As tolerated by water balance and serum sodium

[a]Per kilogram of mean body weight of normal persons of the same age, height, and gender.

Patients with active infections, peritonitis, concomitant liver disease, or other intercurrent illnesses affecting nutritional status may require more aggressive protein supplementation. Carbohydrate intake should consist of primarily complex carbohydrates and comprise approximately 35 percent of the ingested calories. Total daily caloric requirements generally range between 35 to 45 kcal/kg of ideal body weight.

In general, CAPD patients have fewer restrictions on mineral and fluid intake when compared with hemodialysis patients. In most cases, a liberal intake of fluids and salt can be permitted, as CAPD is efficient in removing water and sodium. Potassium is also effectively removed allowing a fairly liberal intake of 70 to 80 meq/day. In addition, phosphorus control is improved on CAPD; however, in most cases phosphate binders are still required.[166] Calcium uptake from the dialysate is inversely proportional to the serum ionized calcium. Calcium balance is positive in most patients, provided the dietary intake exceeds 700 mg/day.[166]

Vitamin nutrition in CAPD patients may be affected by the loss of water-soluble vitamins into the dialysate. Blumberg and coworkers[167] evaluated vitamin nutrition in 10 stable CAPD patients by measuring blood vitamin levels and obtaining detailed dietary histories. Despite adequate intake of calories and protein, they discovered that many patients had low blood levels of vitamins B_1, B_6, folate, and vitamin C. In contrast, levels of vitamins A and E were frequently elevated. After supplementation of water-soluble vitamins for 7 weeks, vitamins B_6 and C had normalized, whereas vitamin B_1 remained low. Folic acid was markedly elevated after supplementation with 4 mg/day.

Based on the above data, preliminary recommendations for daily vitamin supplementation have been made (Table 21–6). In general, vitamin A should be excluded from daily vitamin supplements in order to prevent excessive accumulation and potential toxicity. On the other hand,

TABLE 21–6. RECOMMENDATIONS FOR DAILY VITAMIN SUPPLEMENTATION IN PATIENTS ON MAINTENANCE DIALYSIS

Vitamin B_1	30–40 mg
Vitamin B_6	10–15 mg
Folic acid	0.5–1 mg
Vitamin C	100–200 mg

Source: Adapted from Blumberg et al.,[167] with permission.

supplementation of water-soluble vitamins should be provided to avoid vitamin deficiency syndromes.

Intraperitoneal Nutrition

Amino acid-containing dialysate provides a unique method of nutritional supplementation for the malnourished CAPD patient.[168,169] In general, this mode of supplementation should be reserved for the patient who demonstrates continued signs of malnutrition despite attempts to enhance oral caloric intake. Approximately 75 to 90 percent of the infused amino acids are absorbed with peak serum levels occurring approximately 30 to 60 minutes after the dwell is started.[151] Usually the dialysate consists of a mixture of essential and nonessential amino acids with an electrolyte composition similar to that of standard glucose-containing solutions. In most cases, one exchange per day is replaced with the amino acid solution. Effects on nutritional status and lipid profiles have been inconsistent, with many studies suffering from relatively small patient numbers and short durations of observation.[170] Nevertheless, the use of amino acid dialysate appears to be a promising nutritional intervention. Further study is needed to identify the patient population that would benefit from this intervention.

In summary, the nutritional requirements of patients treated with CAPD are unique and may be affected by such factors as protein losses and glucose absorption. Most patients do well from a nutritional standpoint and maintain a positive nitrogen balance. It is necessary to assess nutritional status regularly. In this group of patients, avoiding obesity and maintaining adequate intake during episodes of peritonitis and other intercurrent illnesses are also important.

CONCLUSIONS

Most patients with advanced renal failure demonstrate evidence of malnutrition. The long-term clinical consequences of malnutrition in renal disease are not entirely clear. It is possible, however, that morbidity and mortality might be reduced if patients were well nourished.[1,2,6,9] In addition, the ability to recover from catabolic illness and the occurrence of infectious complications might be improved with better nutritional status. Careful systematic evaluation of nutritional status is important for all patients undergoing dialytic therapy. Minimum daily protein requirements may be greater than the routinely prescribed 1.0 g/kg/day. Recent evidence suggests that at least 1.2 to 1.3 g/kg/day of high-biological value protein is needed for dialysis patients.[41] Recent studies also demonstrate that at least 35 kcal/kg/day are required to maintain nitrogen balance.[41]

The role of oral or parenteral nutritional supplementation still remains unclear. There may be a role for oral supplements, in conjunction with very low protein diets, lowering the SUN, and delaying the need for the institution of dialysis therapy. Whether or not this will result in a cost-effective alternative to early dialysis therapy while preserving good nutritional status should be evaluated. Once the patient begins dialysis therapy, careful attention to nutritional factors is required to correct malnutrition that may have developed during the predialysis period or to maintain nutrition in the patient who suffers intercurrent catabolic illness. If oral intake is not adequate, a period of parenteral nutrition or use of gastrointestinal tube feedings should be considered.

Precise requirements for various vitamins remain to be elucidated, although recent work has provided much information in this area. The effect of uremia per se on the metabolism of various nutrients also requires additional study.

The goal in therapy of dialysis patients must be to provide a metabolic milieu that is as normal as possible. Attention to nutrition may help to provide this.

REFERENCES

1. Lowrie EG, Huang WH, Lew NL. Death risk predictors among peritoneal dialysis and hemodialysis patients. A preliminary comparison. *Am J Kidney Dis* 1995;26:220–228.
2. Avram MM, Goldwasser P, Erroa M, et al. Predictors of survival in continuous ambulatory peritoneal dialysis patients: the importance of prealbumin and other nutritional and metabolic markers. *Am J Kidney Dis* 1994;23:91–98.
3. Kasiske BL, Lakatua JD, Ma JZ, et al. A meta-analysis of the effects of dietary protein restriction on the rate of decline in renal function. *Am J Kidney Dis* 1998;31:954–961.
4. Blumenkrantz MJ, Kopple JD. VA cooperative dialysis study participants. Incidence of nutritional abnormalities in uremic patients entering dialysis therapy. *Kidney Int* 1976; 10:514A.
5. Thunberg BJ, Swamy AP, Cestero RVW. Cross-sectional and longitudinal nutritional measurements in maintenance hemodialysis patients. *Am J Clin Nutr* 1981;34:2005–2012.
6. Wolfson M, Strong C, Minturn D, et al. Nutritional status and lymphocyte function in maintenance hemodialysis patients. *Am J Clin Nutr* 1984;37:547–555.
7. Young GA, Kopple JD, Lindholm B, et al. Nutritional assessment of continuous ambulatory peritoneal dialysis pa-

tients: an international study. *Am J Kidney Dis* 1991;17: 462–471.
8. Wolfson M. Nutrition in elderly dialysis patients. *Semin Dial* 2002;15:113–115.
9. Leavey SF, Strawderman RL, Jones CA, et al. Simple nutritional indicators as independent predictors of mortality in hemodialysis patients. *Am J Kidney Dis* 1998;31:997–1006.
10. Pupim LB, Ikizler TA. Uremic malnutrition: new insights into an old problem. Semin Dial 2003;16:224–232.
11. Nelson EE, Hong CD, Pesce AL, et al. Anthropometric norms for the dialysis population. *Am J Kidney Dis* 1990;16: 32–37.
12. Woodrow G, Oldroyd B, Smith MA, et al. Measurement of body composition in CKD: comparison of skinfold anthropometry and bioelectrical impedance with dual energy x-ray absorptiometry. *Eur J Clin Nutr* 1996;50:295–301.
13. Kaizu Y, Ohkawa S, Odamaki M, et al. Association between inflammatory mediators and muscle mass in long-term hemodialysis patients. *Am J Kidney Dis* 2003;42:295–302.
14. Kopple JD. Effect of nutrition on morbidity and mortality in maintenance dialysis patients. *Am J Kidney Dis* 1994;24: 1002–1009.
15. Ooi BS, Darocey AF, Pollack VE. Serum transferrin levels in CKD. *Nephron* 1972;220:1697–1699.
16. Kaysen GA, Rathore V, Shearer GC, et al. Mechanisms of hypoalbuminemia in hemodialysis patients. *Kidney Int* 1995;48: 510–516.
17. Kaysen GA, Stevenson FT, Depner TA. Determinants of albumin concentration in hemodialysis patients. *Am J Kidney Dis* 1997;29:658–668.
18. Young GA, Swanepoel CR, Croft MR, et al. Anthropometry and plasma valine, amino acids and proteins in the nutritional assessment of hemodialysis patients. *Kidney Int* 1982;21: 492–499.
19. Peters JH, Gulyassy PF, Lin SC, et al. Amino acid patterns in uremia: comparative effects of hemodialysis and transplantation. *ASAIO Trans* 1968;14:405–410.
20. Scolari M, Stefoni S, Mosconi G, et al. Effects of renal substitutive programs on amino acid patterns in chronic uremia. *Kidney Int* 1983;24(suppl 16):577–580.
21. Laidlaw SA, Berg RL, Kopple JD, et al. Patterns of fasting plasma amino acid levels in chronic renal insufficiency: results from the feasibility phase of the MDRD study. *Am J Kidney Dis.* 1994;23:504–513.
22. Arroyave G, Wilson D, Defunes C, et al. The free amino acids in blood plasma of children with kwashiorkor and marasmus. *Am J Clin Nutr* 1962;11:514–517.
23. Kopple JD, Jones M, Fukuda S, et al. Amino acid and protein metabolism in renal failure. *Am J Clin Nutr* 1978;31: 1532–1540.
24. Chan W, Wang M, Kopple JD, et al. Citrulline levels and urea cycle enzymes in uremic rats. *J Nutr* 1974;104: 678–683.
25. Pickford JC, McGale EHF, Aber GM. Studies on the metabolism of phenylalanine and tyrosine in patients with renal disease. *Clin Chim Acta* 1973;48:77–83.
26. Kopple JD, Mercurio K, Blumenkrantz MJ, et al. Daily requirement for pyridoxine supplements in CKD. *Kidney Int* 1981;19:694–704.

27. Wolfson M, Laidlaw SA, Flugel-Link RM, et al. Effect of vitamin B_6 deficiency on plasma amino acid levels in chronically azotemic rats. *J Nutr* 1986;116:1865–1872.

28. Fürst P, Alvesstrand A, Bergström J. Effect of nutrition and catabolic stress on intracellular amino acid pools in uremia. *Am J Clin Nutr* 1980;33:1387–1395.

29. Cano N, Labastie-Coeyrehourcq J, Lacombe P, et al. Peridialytic parenteral nutrition with lipids and amino acids in malnourished hemodialysis patients. *Am J Clin Nutr* 1990; 52: 726–730.

30. Chertow GM, Ling J, Lew NL, et al. The association of intradialytic parenteral nutrition administration with survival in hemodialysis patients. *Am J Kidney Dis* 1994;24: 912–920.

31. Capelli JP, Kushner H, Camiscioli TC, et al. Effect of intradialytic parenteral nutrition on mortality rates in end-stage renal disease care. *Am J Kidney Dis* 1994;23:808–816.

32. Li FK, Chan YY, Woo JCY, et al. A 3-year prospective randomized controlled study on amino acid dialysate in patients on CAPD. *Am J Kidney Dis* 2003;42:173–183.

33. Tietze IN, Pedersen EB. Effect of fish protein supplementation on amino acid profile and nutritional status in hemodialysis patients. *Nephrol Dial Transplant* 1991;6:948–954.

34. Law DK, Dudrick SV, Abdon NI. Immunocompetence of patients with protein-calorie malnutrition. *Ann Intern Med* 1973;79:543–550.

35. Bistrian BR, Sherman M, Blackburn GL, et al. Cellular immunity in adult marasmus. *Arch Intern Med* 1977;137: 1408–1411.

36. Huber H, Pastner D, Dittrick P, Braunsteiner H. In vitro reactivity of human lymphocytes in uremia: a comparison with the impairment of delayed hypersensitivity. *Clin Exp Immunol* 1969;5:75–82.

37. Casciani CU, DeSimone C, Bonini S, et al. Immunologic aspects of chronic uremia. *Kidney Int* 1978;13(suppl 8): S49–S54.

38. Hak JL, Leffell M, Lamanna R, et al. Reversal of skin test energy during maintenance hemodialysis by protein and caloric supplementation. *Am J Clin Nutr* 1982;36: 1089–1092.

39. Touraine JL, Touraine F, Revillard JP, et al. T-lymphocytes and serum inhibitors of cell-mediated immunity in renal insufficiency. *Nephron* 1974;14:195–208.

40. Kimmel PL, Phillips TM, Simmens SJ, et al. Immunologic function and survival in hemodialysis patients. *Kidney Int* 1998;54:236–244.

41. Clinical practice guidelines for nutrition in CKD. *Am J Kidney Dis* 2000;35(suppl 2):S17–S104.

42. Cano N, Di Costanzo-Dufetel J, Calaf R, et al. Prealbumin-retinol-binding-protein-retinol complex in hemodialysis patients. *Am J Clin Nutr* 1988;47:664–667.

43. Grodstein G, Harrison A, Roberts C, et al. Impaired gastric emptying in hemodialysis patients. *Kidney Int* 1979;16: 952A.

44. Hylander B, Barkeling B, Rossner S. Eating behavior in continuous ambulatory peritoneal dialysis and hemodialysis patients. *Am J Kidney Dis* 1992;20:592–597.

45. Hylander B, Barkeling B, Rossner S. Changes in patients' eating behavior: in the uremic state, on continuous ambulatory peritoneal dialysis, and after transplantation. *Am J Kidney Dis* 1997; 29:691–698.

46. Grodstein GP, Blumenkrantz MJ, Kopple JD, et al. Glucose absorption during continuous ambulatory peritoneal dialysis. *Kidney Int* 1981;19:564–567.

47. Lorenzo V, de Bonis E, Rufino M, et al. Caloric rather than protein deficiency predominates in stable chronic haemodialysis patients. *Nephrol Dial Transplant* 1995;10: 1885–1889.

48. Iseki K, Uehara H, Nishime K, et al. Impact of the initial levels of laboratory variables on survival in chronic dialysis patients. *Am J Kidney Dis* 1996;28:541–548.

49. Hirschman GH, Wolfson M, Mosimann JE, et al. Complications of dialysis. *Clin Nephrol* 1981;15:66–74.

50. Ikizler TA, Greene JH, Yenicesu M, et al. Nitrogen balance in hospitalized chronic hemodialysis patients. *Kidney Int* 1996; 50(suppl 57):S53–S56.

51. Grodstein GP, Blumenkrantz MJ, Kopple JD. Nutritional and metabolic response to catabolic stress in uremia. *Am J Clin Nutr* 1980;33:1411–1416.

52. Young GA, Parsons FM. Amino nitrogen loss during hemodialysis: its dietary significance and replacement. *Clin Sci Mol Med* 1966;31:299–307.

53. Lasker N, Harvey A, Baker H. Vitamin levels in hemodialysis and intermittent peritoneal dialysis. *ASAIO Trans* 1963;9: 51–56.

54. Wolfson M, Jones MR, Kopple JD. Amino acid losses during hemodialysis with infusion of amino acids and glucose. *Kidney Int* 1982;21:500–506.

55. Bergstrom J, Furst P, Alvestrand A, et al. Protein and energy intake, nitrogen balance and nitrogen losses in patients treated with continuous ambulatory peritoneal dialysis. *Kidney Int* 1993;44:1048–1057.

56. Kaplan AA, Halley SE, Lapkin RA, et al. Dialysate protein losses with bleach processed polysulfone dialyzers. *Kidney Int* 1995;47:573–578.

57. Ballmer PE, McNurlan MA, Hulter HN, et al. Chronic metabolic acidosis decreases albumin synthesis and induces negative nitrogen balance in humans. *J Clin Invest* 1995;95: 39–45.

58. Ulrich C, Kruger B, Kohler H, et al. Effects of acidosis on acute phase protein metabolism in liver cells. *Miner Electrolyte Metab* 1999;25:228–233.

59. Graham KA, Reaich D, Channon SM, et al. Correction of acidosis in hemodialysis decreases whole body protein degradation. *J Am Soc Nephrol* 1997;8:632–637.

60. Kleger GR, Turgay M, Imoberdorf R, et al. Acute metabolic acidosis decreases muscle protein synthesis but not albumin synthesis in humans. *Am J Kidney Dis* 2001;38:1199–1207.

61. Stein A, Moorhouse J, Iles-Smith H, et al. Role of an improvement in acid-base status and nutrition in CAPD patients. *Kidney Int* 1997;52:1089–1095.

62. Verove C, Maisonneuve N, El Azouzi A, et al. Effect of the correction of metabolic acidosis on nutritional status in elderly patients with CKD. *J Ren Nutr* 2002;12:224–228.

63. Kooman JP, Deutz NE, Zijlmans P, et al. The influence of bicarbonate supplementation on plasma levels of branched-chain amino acids in haemodialysis patients with metabolic acidosis. *Nephrol Dial Transplant* 1997;12:2397–2401.

64. Lofberg E, Wernerman J, Anderstam B, et al. Correction of acidosis in dialysis patients increases branched-chain and total essential amino acid levels in muscle. *Clin Nephrol* 1997;48:230–237.

65. Borah MF, Schoenfeld PY, Gotch FA, et al. Nitrogen balance during intermittent dialysis therapy of uremia. *Kidney Int* 1978;14:491–500.

66. Lim VS, Flanigan MJ. The effect of interdialytic interval on protein metabolism: evidence suggesting dialysis-induced catabolism. *Am J Kidney Dis* 1989;14:96–100.

67. Guiterrez A, Alvestrand A, Wahren J, et al. Effect of in vivo contact between blood and dialysis membranes on protein catabolism in humans. *Kidney Int* 1990;38:487–494.

68. Phillips ME, Havard J, Howard JP. Oral essential amino acid supplementation in patients on maintenance hemodialysis. *Clin Nephrol* 1978;6:241–248.

69. Kopple JD, Swendseid ME. Evidence that histidine is an essential amino acid in normal and chronically uremic man. *J Clin Invest* 1975;55:881–891.

70. Reaven GM, Swenson RS, Sanfelippo ML. An inquiry into the mechanism of hypertriglyceridemia in patients with CKD. *Am J Clin Nutr* 1980;33:1476–1484.

71. Horl WH, Heidland A. Glycogen metabolism in muscle in uremia. *Am J Clin Nutr* 1980;33:1461–1467.

72. Quintanilla A, Shambaugh GE, Gilson TP, Craig R. Glucose metabolism in uremia. *Am J Clin Nutr* 1980;33:1446–1450.

73. Arnold WC, Holliday MA. In vitro suppression of insulin-mediated amino acid uptake in uremic skeletal muscle. *Am J Clin Nutr* 1980;33:1428–1432.

74. Pitts RF, Stone WJ. Renal metabolism of alanine. *J Clin Invest* 1967;46:503–538.

75. Fukuda S, Kopple JD. Uptake and release of amino acids by the normal dog kidney. *Miner Electrolyte Metab* 1980;3:237–247.

76. DeFronzo RA, Alvestrand A. Glucose intolerance in uremia: site and mechanism. *Am J Clin Nutr* 1980;33:1438–1445.

77. Mondon CE, Reaven GM. Evaluation of enhanced glucagon sensitivity as the cause of glucose intolerance in acutely uremic rats. *Am J Clin Nutr* 1980;33:1456–1460.

78. DeFronzo RA, Andres A, Edgar P, et al. Carbohydrate metabolism in uremia: a review. *Medicine* 1973;52:469–481.

79. DeFronzo RA, Beckles AD. Glucose intolerance following chronic metabolic acidosis in man. *Am J Physiol* 1979;236:E328–E334.

80. Kaysen GA. Inflammation nutritional state and outcome in end-stage renal disease. *Miner Electrolyte Metab* 1999;25:242–250.

81. Bistrian BR. Interaction between nutrition and inflammation in end-stage renal disease. *Blood Purif* 2000;18:33–36.

82. Detsky AS, McLaughlin JR, Baker J, et al. What is subjective global assessment of nutritional status? *J Parenter Enteral Nutr* 1987;11:8–13.

83. Young GA, Kopple JD, Lindholm B, et al. Nutritional assessment of continuous ambulatory peritoneal dialysis patients: an international study. *Am J Kidney Dis* 1991;17:462–471.

84. Grodstein G, Kopple JD. Urea nitrogen appearance, a simple and practical indicator of total nitrogen output. *Kidney Int* 1979;16:953A.

85. Blumenkrantz MJ, Kopple JD, Gutman RA. Methods for assessing nutritional status of patients with renal failure. *Am J Clin Nutr* 1980;33:1567–1585.

86. Sargent J, Gotch F, Borah M, et al. Urea kinetics: a guide to nutritional management of renal failure. *Am J Clin Nutr* 1978;31:1696–1702.

87. Frisancho AR. Triceps skinfold and upper arm muscle size norms for assessment of nutritional status. *Am J Clin Nutr* 1974;27:1052–1058.

88. Centers for Disease Control. *United States Ten-State Nutrition Survey of 1968–1979*. CDC publication 72–8131. Atlanta: US Department of Health, Education and Welfare, Centers for Disease Control, 1972.

89. Wolfson M, Kopple JD. Nutritional status in apparently healthy hemodialysis patients. *Kidney Int* 1981;19:161A.

90. Blackburn GL, Thornton PA. Nutritional assessment of the hospitalized patient. *Med Clin North Am* 1979;63:1103–1115.

91. Cooper BA, Aslani A, Ryan M, et al. Comparing different methods of assessing body composition in end-stage renal failure. *Kidney Int* 2000;58:408–416.

92. DeVita MV, Stall SH. Dual energy x-ray absorptiometry: a review. *J Renal Nutr* 1999;9:178–181.

93. Stall SH, Ginsberg NS, DeVita MV, et al. Percentage body fat determination in hemodialysis and peritoneal dialysis patients: a comparison. *J Renal Nutr* 1998;8:132–136.

94. Bistrian BR, Blackburn GL, Scrimshaw NS, et al. Cellular immunity in semistarved status in hospitalized adults. *Am J Clin Nutr* 1975;28:1148–1155.

95. White RG, Coward WA, Lunn PG. Serum albumin concentration and the onset of kwashiorkor. *Lancet* 1973;1:63–66.

96. Mariani G, Bianchi R, Pilo A, et al. Albumin catabolism measurement by a double tracer technique in uremic patients during a single dialytic treatment. *Eur J Clin Invest* 1974;4:435–442.

97. Noree LO, Bergström J. Treatment of chronic uremic patients with protein-poor diet and oral supply of essential amino acids. II. Clinical results of long-term treatment. *Clin Nephrol* 1975;3:195–203.

98. Heidland A, Kult J. Long-term effects of essential amino acid supplementation in patients on regular hemodialysis. *Clin Nephrol* 1975;5:238–239.

99. Young GA, Oki JI, Davidson AM, et al. The effects of calorie and essential amino acid supplementation on plasma proteins in patients with CKD. *Am J Clin Nutr.* 1978;31:1802–1807.

100. Miller D, Levine S, Bristrian B. Diagnosis of protein calorie malnutrition in diabetic patients on hemodialysis and peritoneal dialysis. *Nephron* 1983;33:127–132.

101. Degoulet P, Legrain M, Reach I, et al. Mortality risk factors in patients treated by chronic hemodialysis. *Nephron* 1982;103–110.

102. O'Connor WJ, Summerill RA. The effect of a meal of meat on glomerular filtration rate in dogs at normal urine flows. *J Physiol* 1976;256:81–91.

103. Bosch JP, Saccaggi A, Lauer A. Renal functional reserve in humans. Effect of protein intake on glomerular filtration rate. *Am J Med* 1983;75:943–950.

104. Hostetter TH. Renal hemodynamic response to a meat meal in humans. *Kidney Int* 1984;25:168.

105. Meyer TW, Ichikawa I, Zatz R, et al. The renal hemodynamic response to amino acid infusion in the rat. *Trans Assoc Am Phys* 1983;96:76–83.

106. King AJ, Levey AS. Dietary protein and renal function. *J Am Soc Nephrol* 1993;3:1723–1737.

107. Brenner BM, Meyer TW, Hostetter TH. Dietary protein intake and the progressive nature of kidney disease: the role of hemodynamically mediated glomerular injury in the pathogenesis of progressive glomerular sclerosis in aging, renal ablation, and intrinsic renal disease. *N Engl J Med* 1982;307:652–659.

108. Hostetter TH, Olson JL, Rennke HG, et al. Hyperfiltration in remnant nephrons: a potentially adverse response to renal ablation. *Am J Physiol* 1981;241:F85–F93.

109. Kaufman JM, DiMeola HJ, Siegel NJ, et al. Compensatory adaptation of structure and function following progressive renal ablation. *Kidney Int* 1974;6:10–17.

110. Shimamura T, Morrison AB. A progressive glomerulosclerosis occurring in partial five-sixths nephrectomized rats. *Am J Pathol* 1975;79:95–106.

111. Meyer TW, Hostetter TH, Rennke HG, et al. Preservation of renal structure and function by long term protein restriction in rats with reduced nephron mass. *Kidney Int* 1983;23:218.

112. El-Nahas AM, Paraskevakou H, Zoob S, et al. Effect of dietary protein restriction on the development of renal failure after subtotal nephrectomy in rats. *Clin Sci* 1983;65:309–406.

113. Klahr S, Levey AS, Beck GJ, et al. The effects of dietary protein restriction and blood-pressure control on the progression of chronic renal disease. *N Engl J Med* 1994;330:877–884.

114. Levey AS, Adler S, Caggiula AW, et al. Effects of dietary protein restriction on the progression of advanced renal disease in the Modification of Diet in Renal Disease Study. *Am J Kidney Dis* 1996;27:652–663.

115. Levey AS, Greene T, Beck GJ, et al. for the MDRD Study Group: Dietary protein restriction and the progression of chronic renal disease: What have all of the results of the MDRD study shown? *J Am Soc Nephrol* 1999;10:2426–2439.

116. Goodship THJ, Mitch WE, Hoerr RA, et al. Adaptation to low-protein diets in renal failure: leucine turnover and nitrogen balance. *J Am Soc Nephrol* 1990;1:66–75.

117. Kopple JD, Coburn JW. Metabolic studies of low protein diets in uremia. I. Nitrogen and potassium. *Medicine* 1973;52:583–595.

118. Giovanetti S, Maggiore Q. A low-nitrogen diet with proteins of high biologic value for severe chronic uremia. *Lancet* 1964;1:1000–1003.

119. Mehrotra R, Nolph KD. Treatment of advanced renal failure: low protein diets or timely initiation of dialysis? *Kidney Int* 2000;58:1381–1388.

120. Walser M, Mitch WE, Maroni BJ, et al. Should protein intake be restricted in predialysis patients? *Kidney Int* 1999;55: 771–777.

121. Kopple JD, Monteon F, Shaib J. Effect of energy intake on nitrogen metabolism in nondialyzed patients with CKD. *Kidney Int* 1986;29:734–742.

122. Monteon F, Laidlaw S, Shaib J, et al. Energy expenditure in patients with CKD. *Kidney Int* 1986;30:741–747.

123. Slomowitz LA, Monteon FJ, Grosvenor M, et al. Effect of energy intake on nutritional status in maintenance hemodialysis patients. *Kidney Int* 1989;35:704–711.

124. Hecking E, Köhler H, Rainer Z, et al. Treatment with essential amino acids in patients on chronic hemodialysis: a double blind cross-over study. *Am J Clin Nutr* 1978;31: 1812–1826.

125. Cockram DB, Hensley MK, Rodriguez M, et al. Safety and tolerance of medical nutritional products as sole sources of nutrition in people on hemodialysis. *J Renal Nutr* 1998;8(1):25–33.

126. Fedje L, Moore L, McNeely M. A role for oral nutrition supplements in the malnutrition of renal disease. *J Renal Nutr* 1996;6:198–202.

127. Silang R, Regalado M, Cheng TH, et al. Prokinetic agents increase plasma albumin in hypoalbuminemic patients with delayed gastric emptying. *Am J Kidney Dis* 2001;37:287–293.

128. Burrowes JD, Bluestone PA, Wang J, et al. The effects of megesterol acetate on nutritional parameters on nutritional status and body composition in a hemodialysis patient. *J Renal Nutr* 1999;9:89–94.

129. Boccanfuso JA, Hutton M, McAllister B. The effects of megesterol acetate on nutritional parameters in a dialysis population. *J Renal Nutr* 2000;10:36–43.

130. Kotzmann H, Yilmaz N, Lercher P, et al. Differential effects of recombinant human growth hormone therapy in the malnourished hemodialysis patients. *Kidney Int* 2001;60: 1578–1585.

131. Hammerman MR. Insulin-like growth factor I for end-stage renal disease at the end of the millennium. *Curr Opin Nephrol Hypertens* 9:1–3, 2000.

132. Schulman G, Wingard RL, Hutchinson RL, et al. The effects of recombinant human growth hormone and intradialytic parenteral nutrition in malnourished hemodialysis patients. *Am J Kidney Dis* 21:527–534, 1993.

133. Sanfellipo ML, Swenson RS, Reaven GM. Reduction of plasma triglyceride by diet in subjects with CKD. *Kidney Int* 1977;11:54–61.

134. Kopple JD. Nutritional management of CKD. *Postgrad Med* 1978;64:135–144.

135. Jagadha V, Deck J, Halliday W, Smyth H. Wernicke's encephalopathy in patients on peritoneal dialysis or hemodialysis. *Ann Neurol* 1987;21:78–84.

136. Sullivan JF, Eisenstein AB. Ascorbic acid depletion in patients undergoing chronic hemodialysis. *Am J Clin Nutr* 1970;23:1339–1346.

137. Hampers CL, Streiff R, Nathan DG, et al. Megaloblastic hematopoiesis in uremia and in patients on long-term hemodialysis. *N Engl J Med* 1967;276:551–554.

138. Whitehead VM, Comty CH, Posen GA, et al. Homeostasis of folic acid in patients undergoing maintenance hemodialysis. *N Engl J Med* 1968;279:970–974.

139. Stone WJ, Warnock LG, Wagner G. Vitamin B_6 deficiency in uremia. *Am J Clin Nutr* 1975;28:950–957.

140. Dobblestein H, Körner WF, Minpel W, et al. Vitamin B_6 deficiency in uremia and its implications for the depression of immune responses. *Kidney Int* 1974;5:233–239.

141. Alfrey AC, LeGendre GR, Kaehny WD. The dialysis encephalopathy syndrome: possible aluminum intoxication. *N Engl J Med* 1976;294:184–188.

142. Ott SM, Maloney NA, Coburn JW, et al. The prevalence of bone aluminum deposition in renal osteodystrophy and its relation to the response to calcitriol therapy. *N Engl J Med* 1982;307:709–713.

143. Mahajan SK, Prasad AS, Lambujon J, et al. Improvement of uremic hypogeusia by zinc: a double-blind study. *Am J Clin Nutr* 1980;33:1517–1521.

144. Buchwald R, Peña JC. Evaluation of nutritional status in patients on continuous ambulatory peritoneal dialysis (CAPD). *Perit Dial Bull* 1989;9:295–301.

145. Nolph KD, Moore HL, Prowant B, et al. Cross sectional assessment of weekly urea and creatinine clearances and indices of nutrition in continuous ambulatory peritoneal dialysis patients. *Perit Dial Bull* 1993;13:178–183.

146. Jones MR. Etiology of severe malnutrition: results of an international cross-sectional study in continuous ambulatory peritoneal dialysis patients. *Am J Kidney Dis* 1994;23:412–420.

147. Spiegel DM, Anderson M, Campbell U, et al. Serum albumin: a marker for morbidity in peritoneal dialysis patients. *Am J Kidney Dis* 1993;21:26–30.

148. Avram MM, Goldwasser P, Erroa M, et al. Predictors of survival in continuous ambulatory peritoneal dialysis patients: the importance of prealbumin and other nutritional and metabolic markers. *Am J Kidney Dis* 1994;23:91–98.

149. Blumenkrantz MJ, Gahl GM, Kopple JD, et al. Protein losses during peritoneal dialysis. *Kidney Int* 1981;19:593–602.

150. Bannister DK, Acchiardo SR, Moore LW, et al. Nutritional effects of peritonitis in continuous ambulatory peritoneal dialysis (CAPD) patients. *J Am Diet Assoc* 1987;87:53–56.

151. Jones MR, Burkart JM, Hamburger RJ, et al. Replacement of amino acid and protein losses with 1.1% amino acid peritoneal dialysis solution. *Perit Dial Int* 1998;18:210–216.

152. Krediet RT, Zuyderhoudt FMJ, Boeschoten EW, Arisz L. Peritoneal permeability to proteins in diabetic and non-diabetic continuous ambulatory peritoneal dialysis patients. *Nephron* 1986;42:133–140.

153. Kaysen G, Schoenfeld P. Albumin homeostasis in patients undergoing CAPD. *Kidney Int* 1984;25:107–114.

154. Baeyer H, Gahl G, Riedinger H, et al. Adaptation of CAPD patients to the continuous peritoneal energy uptake. *Kidney Int* 1983;23:29–34.

155. Per-Ola A, Samuelsson O, Alaupovic P. Lipoprotein metabolism and renal failure. *Am J Kidney Dis* 1993;21:573–592.

156. Lindholm B, Alvestrand A, Fürst P, et al. Metabolic effects of continuous ambulatory peritoneal dialysis. *Proc EDTA* 1980; 17:283–289.

157. Lindholm B, Norbeck HE. Serum lipids and lipoproteins during continuous ambulatory peritoneal dialysis. *Acta Med Scand* 1986;220:143–151.

158. Boeschoten EW, Zuydergoudt FMJ, Krediet RT, et al. Changes in weight and lipid concentrations during CAPD treatment. *Perit Dial Int* 1988;8:19–24.

159. Morrison G. Metabolic effects of continuous ambulatory peritoneal dialysis. *Annu Rev Med* 1989;40:163–172.

160. Shoji T, Nishizawa Y, Nishitani H, et al. High serum lipoprotein(a) concentrations in uremic patients treated with continuous ambulatory peritoneal dialysis. *Clin Nephrol.* 1992;38:271–276.

161. Thillet J, Faucher C, Issad B, et al. Lipoprotein(a) in patients treated by continuous ambulatory peritoneal dialysis. *Am J Kidney Dis* 1993;22:226–232.

162. Adrogué HJ. Glucose homeostasis and the kidney. *Kidney Int* 1992;42:1266–1282.

163. Lameire N, Matthys D, Matthys E, et al. Effects of long-term CAPD on carbohydrate and lipid metabolism. *Clin Nephrol* 1988;30:S53–S58.

164. Bouma SF, Dwyer JT. Glucose absorption and weight change in 18 months of continuous ambulatory peritoneal dialysis. *J Am Diet Assoc* 1984;84:194–197.

165. Blumenkrantz MJ, Kopple JD, Moran JK, et al. Metabolic balance studies and dietary protein requirements in patients undergoing continuous ambulatory peritoneal dialysis. *Kidney Int* 1982;21:849–861.

166. Delmez JA, Slatapolsky E, Martin KJ, et al. Minerals, vitamin D, and parathyroid hormone in continuous ambulatory peritoneal dialysis. *Kidney Int* 1982;21:862–867.

167. Blumberg A, Hanck A, Sander G. Vitamin nutrition in patients on continuous ambulatory peritoneal dialysis (CAPD). *Clin Nephrol* 1983;244–250.

168. Kopple JD, Bernard D, Messana J, et al. Treatment of malnourished CADP patients with an animo acid–based dialysate. *Kidney Int* 1995;47:1148–1157.

169. Arfeen S, Goodship THJ, Kirkweed A, et al. The nutritional/metabolic and hormonal effects of 8 weeks of continuous ambulatory peritoneal dialysis with a 1% amino acid solution. *Clin Nephrol* 1990;33:192–199.

170. Dibble JB, Young GA, Hobson SM, et al. Amino-acid-based continuous ambulatory peritoneal dialysis (CAPD) fluid over twelve weeks: effects on carbohydrate and lipid metabolism. *Perit Dial Int* 1990;10:71–77.

Nutritional Management of Pediatric Patients on Chronic Dialysis

Alberto Edefonti
Fabio Paglialonga
Marina Picca

Malnutrition can be defined as a nutritional disorder due to a deficient nutrient intake or impaired nutrient metabolism. Protein/calorie malnutrition is a common complication of end-stage renal disease (ESRD) in children and has been linked to a wide range of complications, including growth retardation and death.[1,2] Nutritional management is therefore a fundamental part of the approach to children with ESRD treated with hemodialysis (HD) or peritoneal dialysis (PD).

Because of its multifactorial pathogenesis, and the diagnostic and therapeutic difficulties involved, the treatment of malnutrition in children on dialysis should be multidisciplinary and based on a series of steps: accurate and periodic monitoring of nutritional status, the provision of adequate calorie and protein intake, the optimization of dialysis treatment, drug prescriptions that are specific for each patient,

and continuous psychosocial support for both patient and family. The collaborative efforts of dietitians, nurses, social workers, pediatric nephrologists, and psychologists are essential in order to satisfy the nutritional needs of dialyzed children.[3–7]

ASSESSMENT OF NUTRITIONAL STATUS

Although many methods of assessment and indices of malnutrition have been proposed, there are still many uncertainties concerning the most appropriate diagnostic criteria. Consequently, the published prevalence rates of malnutrition in children with ESRD vary widely from 15 to 58 percent[8–11] and, more importantly, the nutritional management of this population is hampered by the inability to identify malnourished patients clearly, particularly those whose nutritional status is only slightly or moderately altered. As a result, both under- and overtreatment are real risks in clinical practice.

The only consensus that has been reached is the need to use a combination of different nutritional markers when diagnosing malnutrition.[3,4] According to Kopple, the nutritional assessment of adult patients should at least include an index of dietary intake, an index of visceral protein, and an index of body composition[3]; however, there is still no agreement as to which indices should be used, their relative weights, or their differential cutoff points between a normal nutritional status and malnutrition.

What is sure is that we must be able to evaluate the nutritional status of children on dialysis globally by using not only traditional nutritional assessments (such as anthropometry or methods of assessing body mass and composition) but also other factors that can affect the nutritional status of children with ESRD, such as dietary intake and the dialysis dose.

Nutritional status should therefore be evaluated on the basis of 10 partial assessments, the advantages and limitations of which are described in detail below. Because of the need to recognize promptly not only severe nutritional impairment but also mild malnutrition, a multidisciplinary approach is essential.

Medical History

Primary renal disease, prematurity, comorbidities, a history of gastrointestinal disorders or neurologic diseases, episodes of peritonitis, and intercurrent illnesses should all be taken into account and corrected whenever possible because they can influence the various aspects of nutritional assessment and treatment.

Clinical and Physical Examinations

Clinical signs and symptoms comprise changes in appetite; gastrointestinal problems such as nausea, vomiting, diarrhea, and/or constipation; or, in infants, gagging, swallowing difficulties, and an inability to chew solids; energy levels and activity. Physical observations comprise condition of hair, teeth, tongue, skin, nails, breath; the impression of preserved or wasted fat or protein mass; edema and blood pressure. Measurements should be made of urine output for residual renal function, fluid balance and estimated dry weight without edema—if possible also by means of the bioimpedance analysis-derived resistance index. The time spent at the bedside in examining a child cannot be replaced by any of the other partial assessments.

Anthropometry

Anthropometric indices—such as weight (W), height or length (H), height velocity (HV), head circumference (HC), and the body mass index (BMI)—are widely used in clinical practice, but their reliable assessment requires the use of appropriate equipment and techniques. Infants should be weighed naked and older children in light clothing without shoes; the weight should be recorded to the nearest 0.1 kg. Height should be measured with the child standing shoeless on the floor facing away from the wall with heels together, the back as straight as possible and the arms held straight down; the heels, buttocks, shoulders, and head should be touching the wall or the vertical surface of the measuring device. For children aged less than 24 months, recumbent length should be measured using an infant stature board with a fixed headboard and movable footboard. Head circumference should be measured up to 36 months of age using a firm, nonstretch measuring tape.[3]

The anthropometric results should be compared with the corresponding control values, and expressed as standard deviation scores (SDS) according to the following formula:

$$SDS = (X - X_i)/Sd_i$$

where X is the value for the individual patient, X_i the mean value of the normal reference population, and Sd_i the standard deviation for normal controls. The values of children with ESRD could also be compared with the reference percentiles for normal children of the same gender and age.[12,13]

Anthropometric indices are widely employed because they are easy to use, noninvasive, and inexpensive, but they have a number of limitations. Many studies have revealed their lack of sensitivity in detecting mild, early alterations in nutritional status. Although malnutrition is a major determinant of growth impairment in children with ESRD, factors other than nutritional status may be involved, such as age at disease onset, the etiology of the primary renal disease, renal osteodystrophy, water and electrolyte imbalances, metabolic acidosis, anemia, and endocrinologic disturbances.

Measurements of skinfold thicknesses and body diameters require special considerations. Upper arm circumference should be measured midway between the tip of the acromion and the olecranon process, using a steel tape with the right arm hanging loose. Triceps skinfold is measured to the nearest millimeter by means of a skinfold caliper: the measurement is made over the triceps muscle halfway between the elbow and the acromion process of the scapula, using the skinfold parallel to the longitudinal axis of the upper arm.[3]

The direct measurements of triceps skinfold thickness and arm circumference can be used to calculate mid-arm muscle circumference (MAMC), arm muscle area (AMA), and arm fat area (AFA) by means of the following formulas:

$$MAMC = C - (\pi T/10)$$

$$AMA = (10C - \pi T)^2/4\pi$$

$$A = (\pi/4)(10C/\pi)^2$$

$$AFA = A - AMA$$

where C is the midarm circumference (cm), T the tricipital skinfold thickness (mm), and A the area of the arm (mm^2).[14]

The values of children on dialysis can also be compared with the reference percentiles for normal children of the same gender and age.[14]

The main limitations of the parameters derived from skinfold thickness are the poor reproducibility and high interobserver variability of the measurements themselves, because minimal variations in direct measurements lead to large differences in the derived parameters.[15,16] One key recommendation is that all the measurements be made by the same person. Like weight and height, skinfold thickness values can be influenced not only by nutritional status but also other factors such as hydration. Furthermore, as they are not very sensitive, they may identify cases of malnutrition only when this condition is more difficult to reverse.

Various authors have proposed predictive equations for estimating fat mass from the anthropometric measurements, but these do not seem to be useful in pediatric patients. In a study of 98 healthy children, Reilly compared the estimates of body composition obtained using five different equations with those obtained by means of hydrodensitometry and found that the equations were poorly predictive.[17]

In conclusion, when used by trained staff, anthropometric parameters provide a quantitative assessment of nutritional status and play an important role in the follow-up of children on dialysis, particularly if they are integrated in a combined nutritional score.

Dietary Interview and Diary

As malnutrition is frequently associated with reduced protein and caloric intakes, dietary assessment is a key step in evaluating dialysed children: although dietary investigation does not contribute to the final diagnosis of malnutrition, it does allow the prompt recognition of a factor that can determine a progressive decline in nutritional status.

The use of 24-hour dietary recall depends on the ability of parents to remember food details and quantities correctly. A 3-day food record is obviously more precise than a dietary interview but requires the accurate cooperation of the parents, who should be given detailed instructions by a dietitian because a major determinant of the reliability of dietary diaries is the ability of parents to adhere to these instructions. All nutrients should be qualitatively and quantitatively analyzed by computer whenever possible and compared with the recommended daily allowances (RDAs) for children of the same sex and chronological age.[3]

The analysis should include data on calories, proteins, fats, carbohydrates, vitamins, minerals, trace minerals, fluids, and electrolytes; the results should be discussed with the child and his or her family. A written report for the nephrologist and responsible renal nurse is advised.

Medication Check

Given the important role of drugs in controlling the blood chemistry of children with ESRD and the complications of uremia, particular monitoring is required in order to ensure the correct administration and timing of medications. Special attention should be paid to phosphate binders, iron supplementation, diuretics, antihypertensives, antibiotics, growth hormone, erythropoietin, and micronutrient supplements. Noncompliance with drug prescriptions is a common problem in patients on chronic dialysis, particularly adolescents: the administration and timing of medications should therefore be routinely checked.

Biochemical Parameters

Many biochemical parameters have been proposed as a means of evaluating nutritional status in children and adults on chronic PD: some more directly reflect nutritional status (albumin, prealbumin, transferrin, retinol-binding protein, and insulin-like growth factor, or IGF-1), whereas others are indirectly associated with malnutrition, such as the indices of uremia control (urea, creatinine, acid-base balance, calcium, phosphate, electrolytes, hemoglobin, and parathyroid hormone, or PTH) and the indices of inflammation (C-reactive protein, or CRP).[4,18–20]

On the basis of the results of the limited number of published studies, the advantages and limitations of laboratory indices in children are the same as those observed in adults. The most frequently used parameter in pediatric patients is serum albumin. A survey of the prevalence data from the six-state New England area found that more than one-third of the children with ESRD undergoing chronic PD have serum albumin concentrations below 2.9 g/dL.[8] Wong evaluated the association between serum albumin levels at the start of dialysis and the risk of death in 1723 pediatric patients and found that each 1 g/dL difference in serum albumin was associated with a 54 percent higher risk of death, even after adjusting for glomerular causes of the ESRD and other potential confounding variables.[1,21] However, factors other than nutritional status also contribute to low albumin levels, such as fluid overload, urinary and dialysis losses, low hepatic synthesis, and, in children on chronic PD, the hyperpermeable status of the peritoneal membrane.[22–24]

IGF-1 has been proposed as an alternative marker of nutritional status in patients on dialysis. Besbas investigated the correlations between nutritional status as evaluated using anthropometric parameters and that revealed by biochemical indices in a population of hemodialyzed children: the levels of IGF-1 were significantly lower in the patients with malnutrition.[25]

In brief and notwithstanding their limitations (which must be known and taken into account in interpreting the data), biochemical indices of nutritional status represent a powerful tool for the diagnosis of malnutrition and the sub-sequent monitoring of nutritional status.

Dialysis Dose Assessment

Because it has been found that there is a close relationship between the dialysis dose and nutritional status, dialysis prescriptions [dose, dialysis solution(s), ultrafiltration] and residual renal function should be monitored on a monthly basis by the nephrologist and renal nurse.[26–29] In the case of children on PD, more frequent monitoring should take place by telephone or e-mail and the results discussed at team meetings. Dialysis adequacy should be regularly assessed by means of 24-hour PD fluid collections and the peritoneal equilibrium test in order to characterize the permeability of the peritoneal membrane.[4] The Kt/V and/or creatinine clearance data obtained from children on HD or PD should be compared with the dialysis dose requirements established by the DOQI guidelines, which, however, should be used only as rough indicators of prescription adequacy, because many other aspects may be more informative, such as nutrition and growth.

Psychosocial Assessment

As part of the overall nutritional assessment, it is essential that the dietitian and other members of the multidisciplinary team become familiar with each child's psychosocial environment, which includes family/extended family dynamics, lifestyle, activities, exercise patterns, friends, hobbies, nursery/school attendance, and eating patterns at home and elsewhere.

It is recommended that a home visit be made by the dietitian and renal nurse or social worker before a child enters a chronic PD program or at its start.[4] Regular discussions with the psychologist are also needed during the follow-up multidisciplinary team meetings.

Assessment of Protein Metabolism

Nitrogen balance (i.e., the difference between nitrogen intake and nitrogen losses) is among the most powerful indices of metabolic status in patients on chronic dialysis. However, the assessment of nitrogen losses can be complex, because it involves urinary, dialysate, and fecal collections and requires specific nitrogen measurements using Kjeldahl's method or numerous single measurements of nitrogen compounds, including amino acids. We have measured nitrogen losses in the dialysate, urine, and feces of 23 children on chronic PD, and elaborated a mathematical model for estimating nitrogen losses on the basis of the results of easily measurable laboratory dialysate and urine tests and indices, as follows:

$$TNe \text{ (g/day)} = 0.03 + 1.138 \text{ UN urea} + 0.99$$
$$DN \text{ urea} + 1.18 \text{ BSA} + 0.965 \text{ DN protein}$$

where TNe = total estimated nitrogen losses

UN = urine nitrogen urea

DN = dialysate nitrogen urea

BSA = body surface area

DN = dialysate nitrogen protein

The results obtained with these models appeared to be similar to the measured values.[30]

One major limitation of nitrogen balance is that it indicates only the balance between intake and losses at a given time and therefore anabolic or catabolic tendencies rather than nutritional status. However, nitrogen balance studies can support the diagnosis of the early stages of malnutrition, as they take into account both dietary nitrogen intake and the losses due to catabolism.

Although steady-state total nitrogen appearance is the standard means of indirectly assessing dietary protein intake, only urea nitrogen appearance (UNA) is usually readily available. In children treated with chronic PD, UNA can be calculated from the sum of dialysate urea and urinary urea nitrogen corrected for changes in the body urea nitrogen; in steady-state patients, it can be calculated as follows:

$$UNA \text{ (g/day)} = \text{dialysate urea nitrogen (g/day)} + \text{urine urea nitrogen (g/day)}$$

Previous studies of pediatric patients have used UNA as an indicator of dietary protein intake[31,32]; Mendley studied 18 CPD-treated children and defined an age-specific relationship between total nitrogen output and UNA that is very different from that defined for adults.[33]

The protein catabolic rate (PCR), which is also called protein nitrogen appearance (PNA), can be calculated from UNA using various published formulas. Many studies of adults have used the protein catabolic rate as a marker of nutritional status, and it has been shown that there is a positive correlation between PCR and dietary protein intake in children on chronic dialysis.

Brem et al. demonstrated a good correlation between the observed PCR and the PCR values calculated from the urea of peritoneal fluid using Randerson's formula; the PCRs of children treated with PD and HD were similar, and averaged 1.1 ± 0.4 g/kg/day.[8] Goldstein studied four adolescents treated with HD and intradialytic parenteral nutrition and suggested that normalized PCR may be an earlier indicator of a worsening nutritional status than serum albumin.[34]

In conclusion, protein/nitrogen metabolism studies are among the most powerful tools for investigating the metabolic status of patients on chronic dialysis. The use of mathematical models to calculate nitrogen losses makes it possible to obtain nitrogen balance, thus overcoming some practical difficulties, such as time-consuming and costly quantitative determinations of amino acids or the direct measurement of nitrogen in stools. Calculating PCR is advisable, but it depends on individual unit protocols.

Methods of Assessing Body Mass and Body Composition

Many methods have been proposed for the assessment of body composition, including isotope dilution techniques, total body nitrogen, and densitometry; however, most are technically difficult and expensive, and they lead to the risk of exposing children to radiation or invasive procedures. They are thus only suitable for research purposes.

The only two methods of body composition analysis that seem to be useful in the clinical setting are dual-energy x-ray absorptiometry (DXA) and bioelectric impedance analysis (BIA).

Dual-Energy X-ray Absorptiometry. DXA is a noninvasive method of estimating bone mineral content as well as fat and lean body mass; however, it is not widely available and requires operator expertise and patient cooperation. Furthermore, the estimates may be confounded by variations in the hydration of patients on dialysis, and the cost of DXA means that it is not feasible to use it more than once a year.[4]

Bioelectric Impedance Analysis. BIA is a noninvasive, inexpensive, and rapid bedside means of assessing body composition.

Impedance is a measurable property of the electrical ionic conduction of soft tissues, as fat and bone are poor conductors; whole-body impedance is a combination of resistance (R) and reactance (Xc). Resistance (which represents the opposition to flow of an alternating current through intra- and extracellular ionic solutions) is relatively low in lean tissues, which contain large amounts of water and electrolytes, and relatively high in adipose tissue and bone. Reactance is the opposition to flow of and electric current due to capacitance, which is represented in vivo by cell membranes.

The classic method of measurement uses an impedance plethysmograph that emits 800-mcA and 50-kHz alternating sinusoidal currents. After the subject has adopted a supine position, the outer electrodes are placed on the proximal, dorsal surface of the third proximal phalanx of the right hand and foot and the inner electrodes on the wrist and ankle in such a way as to leave 5 cm of free skin around the outer electrodes. Various interpretative models of BIA parameters have been proposed. A first approach used specific predictive equations to estimate body compartments on the basis of the bioelectrical R and Xc indices, but it may have many limitations: (1) the equations are obtained by means of a statistical regression analysis that also considers a num-

ber of independent parameters, such as height, weight and gender, which may account for as much as 80 percent of the result; (2) the validation of these equations is based on statistical correlations that are insufficient to prove the reliability of a system; (3) the equations are strictly population-specific and often not applicable to patients belonging to other populations; and (4) the equations are based on the assumption that the hydration of fat free mass is always 73 percent, which is clearly untrue in pathologic situations and can lead to absurd results unless it is verified directly.

An alternative to conventional BIA is vector BIA (BIVA). Using the R/Xc graph method, the R and Xc measurements are normalized by the stature of the subject, and vectors are plotted as points on the gender-specific 50th, 75th, and 95th tolerance ellipses calculated from the healthy reference population (Fig. 22–1). A number of studies of different populations have shown that changes in hydration are associated with movements of the impedance vector along a line of action lying parallel to the major axis of the reference tolerance ellipses and that alterations in nutritional status are associated with a shift that is parallel to the minor axis of the same ellipses.[35] The reference intervals of the whole-body impedance vector in Italian children have been determined by means of a cross-sectional, multicenter study.[36] However, although vector analysis allows an assumption-free assessment of tissue composition, more experience is necessary in order to confirm its applicability to the pediatric dialyzed population. Furthermore, BIVA is not a quantitative index and therefore seems to be unsuitable for storage in a follow-up nutritional database.

A different approach is based on the directly measured parameters (R and Xc) and the indices directly derived from them: phase angle (PA), which is calculated as the arc tangent of Xc/R, and distance (D), which is calculated as (PA × 10 + Xc)/$2^{1/2}$. PA can vary from 0 degrees if the circuit is only resistive (i.e., a system without cell membranes) to 90

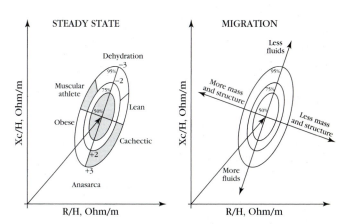

Figure 22–1. R/Xc graph method with 50, 75, and 95 percent tolerance ellipses.

degrees if the circuit is only capacitive (i.e., a system of fluid-free membranes). D is the point at which Xc and PA intersect on a system of Cartesian axes, and the location of D in relation to the origins of the axes can indicate malnutrition. The parameters obtained in a patient can be compared with the standard values measured in reference populations of the same age and gender.[36]

Reactance, phase angle, and distance are all significantly less in malnourished patients than in normal subjects and correlate well with other indices of nutritional status in children and adults. A number of studies of mainly adult patients have demonstrated a good correlation between BIA parameters and morbidity and mortality.[37]

In a study of pediatric patients treated with automated PD, we evaluated the values of anthropometric and BIA parameters during the first 24 months of dialysis and found that the BIA indices Xc, PA, and D were more sensitive than anthropometry in detecting alterations in the body composition of children on PD.[9] These results were confirmed in a subsequent study, which demonstrated that only Xc, PA, and D (and not the predictive equations applied to anthropometry, BIA or DXA measurements) allow the accurate identification of malnourished children on chronic PD.[38]

Alternative multifrequency BIA methods have been proposed but do not offer any clinically significant advantages over standard 50-kHz measurements.

It should be noted that the results in dialyzed patients may be confounded by variations in hydration; therefore BIA should be used only in combination with anthropometric/clinical assessments.

Nutritional Scores. Although many methods of evaluating nutritional status have been proposed, no "gold standard" has yet been established: only the use of different assessments that take into account different aspects of nutritional status can facilitate more precise nutritional monitoring.

The subjective global assessment (SGA), proposed for adult patients, is a widely used nutritional status scoring system based on medical history, a physical examination (including the patient's history of weight loss, anorexia, and vomiting), and the physician's grading of muscle wasting, subcutaneous fat, and edema[39–41]; however, there is no pediatric version.

We have recently proposed a nutritional score based on anthropometry and BIA for PD-treated children: the ABN score. This score is based on nine noninvasive, inexpensive, reliable parameters (if performed by the same operator) that are easy to apply to both ill and healthy children: A1 (height, weight, and BMI); A2 anthropometric parameters (MAMC, AMA, and AFA); and BIA parameters (reactance, phase angle, and distance).[10] All of these indices are expressed as standard deviation scores (SDS) using a five-

point scale: 5 = >0 SDS; 4 = ≤0, and > −1 SDS; 3 = ≤ −1 and > 2 SDS; 2 = ≤ −2 and > −3 SDS; and 1 = < −3 SDS. Average scores were established for each of the A1, A2, and BIA parameters and then summed to obtain the ABN score using a dedicated software program.

In order to establish the cutoff value between a normal nutritional status and malnutrition, the method was first applied to 264 healthy children, and distribution percentiles were calculated for each area and the total ABN score.

The ABN score corresponding to the third percentile (10.33) was considered the limit of normality and then applied to our children on PD: 41.4 percent had ABN scores of more than 10.33 (indicating normal nutrition) and 58.6 percent had scores of less than 10.33 (severe malnutrition was found in only 1.1 percent of the cases). The values of all nine A1, A2, and BIA parameters, as well as serum albumin levels, were significantly higher in the patients with ABN scores above 10.33.[10]

In a large and still ongoing Italian multicenter prospective study, 34 percent of the children on PD were found to be malnourished on the basis of their ABN scores; the major risk factors for malnutrion were identified as being a dialysis duration of more than 2 years and total creatinine clearance values below 60 L/week/1.73 m[2].[29]

In conclusion, the use of global nutritional scores can lead to a more objective assessment of nutritional status, as they take into account the differences between the individual methods. The calculation of ABN scores currently depends on individual unit protocols.

PREVENTION AND TREATMENT OF MALNUTRITION

Before being started on a chronic dialysis program, children require a multidisciplinary nutritional assessment covering various medical, nursing, dietary, and psychosocial factors (Fig. 22–2). Only serial measurements of nutritional parameters allow the early identification of mild alterations in nutritional status. In a study of 18 PD-treated children, we found that the high prevalence of malnutrition at the start of dialysis decreased during the first year but then remained stable.[9] Johansson reported a decrease in total-body potassium (reflecting body cell mass) during long-term PD treatment despite adequate and stable dialysis efficacy.[42] These findings indicate that severe malnutrition is difficult to reverse in children with ESRD and underline the importance of preventing it during the last phase of chronic renal insufficiency as well as of detecting cases of mild malnutrition early, when complete recovery is still possible.

The nutritional follow-up of children on chronic dialysis also requires a multidisciplinary effort based on hospital and home visits and makes use of all the currently available tools, including the latest technologies, such as teledialysis

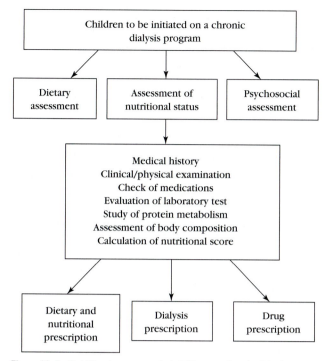

Figure 22–2. Nutritional assessment of children on chronic dialysis.

and audiovideo surveillance, which are particularly useful for children living far from their dialysis center (Fig. 22–3).

There is still no agreement as to the appropriate frequency of nutritional assessments, which clearly depends mainly on the age of the child. According to the DOQI nutritional guidelines, the majority of nutritional parameters should be assessed at least monthly in children below 2 years of age and even more frequently if it is believed that this will benefit the patient. In adolescents, on the other hand, the anthropometric and dietary parameters can be assessed every 3 to 4 months.[3]

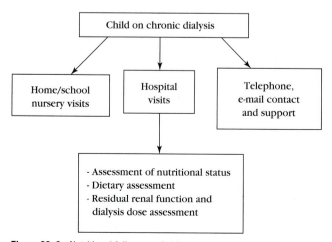

Figure 22–3. Nutritional follow-up of children on chronic dialysis.

Appropriate dietary/nutritional measures, an adequate dialysis prescription, and the correct use of medications are fundamental for the prevention and treatment of malnutrition.

Dietary Measures

The supplements most directly related to nutritional status comprise calories, proteins, and vitamins/trace elements. However, other supplements—such as sodium, potassium, calcium, and phosphate—are also important because they can affect nutrition and growth indirectly. These last aspects have recently been reviewed in DOQI guidelines.[3]

Caloric Intake. A number of studies of infants and children on PD have documented a mean spontaneous caloric intake of less than 75 percent of the RDA.[43–47] The reduction in nutrient intake begins as early as during the predialysis period, together with a decrease in the glomerular filtration rate.[48–50] Anorexia, with nausea and vomiting (which occur when renal insufficiency becomes severe), is the main factor responsible for the decreased nutrient intake. In children with chronic renal failure, anorexia is primarily caused by factors such as the retention of uremic toxins and by metabolic acidosis. Coexisting gastroesophageal reflux and gastrointestinal motility disorders, altered taste perception, anemia, and depression are other aspects of uremic toxicity that can affect food intake. Superimposed comorbidities—such as acute and chronic infections, hypertension or cardiopulmonary disorders, and the administration of multiple medications—all contribute toward making the anorexia worse.

Factors other than anorexia that reduce nutrient intake include unpalatable low-protein/phosphate diets, personal food preferences, and, in some cases, financial constraints. Finally, inadequate dietary prescription may be due to the traditional preference for prescribing nutritional restriction rather than providing nutritional counseling.

There are also some PD-specific factors that may worsen the decreased intake: abdominal distention caused by peritoneal fluid and the absorption of glucose from dialysate as well as sensations of fullness and satiety. Nutrient intake may be severely decreased during episodes of peritonitis and thus contribute to the loss of fat-free mass.

However, the most important factor for children on HD and PD remains the inadequate delivery of dialysis dose as residual renal function declines. A significant correlation between the PCR (a marker of dietary protein intake) and the Kt/V for urea has been demonstrated in adult patients treated with PD,[51,52] and a positive correlation between Kt/V and caloric intake has also been found in PD-treated children.[53] The characteristics of peritoneal membranes assessed by means of the peritoneal equilibration test may also independently influence the growth and nutritional status of children on PD.[54]

On the basis of the considerations outlined above, the first step in preventing malnutrition in dialysed children should clearly be to provide an optimal nutrient intake. However, the optimal nutritional needs of children on chronic dialysis have still not been sufficiently well defined.

We investigated adequate dietary protein and caloric intakes for children treated with automated peritoneal dialysis (APD) on the basis of estimated nitrogen balance studies and found that a caloric intake of 89 percent of the RDA is required to obtain an estimated balance of >50 mg/kg/day, which is considered to provide sufficient nitrogen for all the metabolic and growth needs of uremic children[55]; these values are in line with those suggested by the DOQI guidelines.[3]

According to the DOQI nutritional guidelines for pediatric patients on dialysis, the initial prescribed caloric intake for children treated with maintenance HD or PD should be the RDA for chronological age.[3]

An adequate amount of nonprotein calories should be provided. In a study of 31 children on dialysis, the height velocity SDS correlated positively with total caloric intake and negatively with daily protein intake.[56]

For patients on chronic PD, the calories derived from the glucose in the dialysate should also be considered, as it has been calculated that glucose absorption increases total caloric intake by 7 to 10 kcal/kg.[46]

Except in the case of overt malnutrition, dietary prescriptions exceeding the RDA for age do not seem to be associated with better outcomes in terms of albumin levels, morbidity, or mortality and are currently not justified. Caloric supplementation should be based on height age only if the patient does not gain weight appropriately with a consistent caloric intake at the RDA for chronological age. This recommendation obviously only applies to children whose statural and chronological ages are very different. There are no available data supporting the use of recommendations based on weight age.

The dietary calorie prescription should be adjusted in the follow-up on the basis of the child's response.

Protein Intake. The protein intake of children on dialysis may exceed the recommended levels or may (less frequently) be decreased.[43–47]

No definitive studies of the relationship between protein intake and specific outcome measures such as growth have been published, but, according to the DOQI guidelines, the initial dietary protein intake (DPI) for children treated with maintenance HD should be based on the RDA for chronological age increased by 0.4 g/kg/day.[3] In our study of children on automated PD, we found that a DPI of 144 percent of the RDA is required to obtain an estimated nitrogen balance of >50 mg/kg/day.[55]

DPI should be higher in patients on PD than in those on HD, because PD causes a loss of nitrogenous compounds into the dialysate fluid.[30,57] The majority of the lost protein is represented by albumin, with free amino acids accounting for about 20 percent of total losses; but there is also a loss of other proteins, including immunoglobulins, transferrin, and opsonin. A series of factors can affect the amount of protein loss, including peritoneal membrane permeability and peritoneal surface area. When considered on a milligram-per-kilogram basis, the loss seems to be inversely related to age and size, which means that younger and therefore smaller children have proportionately higher losses.[57] The initial dietary prescription should therefore be at the higher end for infants and toddlers and at the lower end for older children and adolescents.

Protein losses of 100 to 300 mg/kg/day (approximately 10 percent of DPI) have been reported in children on PD regardless of the treatment modality [continuous ambulatory peritoneal dialysis (CAPD), continuous cycling peritoneal dialysis (CCPD), or tidal PD].[57] Episodes of peritonitis can lead to much greater protein and amino acid losses.

Table 22–1 shows the energy and protein intake levels recommended in the DOQI clinical practice guidelines for children on chronic dialysis.[3]

Vitamins and Trace Elements

A few studies have investigated dietary and supplementary vitamin intakes in children receiving chronic dialysis. The spontaneous dietary intake of water-soluble vitamins has been reported to be below the RDA in the majority of children, but the combined dietary and supplementary intake of almost all vitamins is excessive.[47] The serum levels of water-soluble vitamins in children receiving supplementa-

TABLE 22–1. RECOMMENDED ENERGY AND PROTEIN INTAKES FOR CHILDREN ON CHRONIC DIALYSIS, ACCORDING TO THE DOQI GUIDELINES

	Age (years)	Estimated Energy Allowances (kcal/kg/day)	Recommended Dietary Protein Intake (g/kg/day)	
			HD	PD
	0–0.5	108	2.6	2.9–3.0
	0.5–1	98	2.0	2.3–2.4
	1–3	102	1.6	1.9–2.0
	4–6	90	4.6	1.9–2.0
	7–10	70	1.4	1.7–1.8
Males	11–14	55	1.4	1.7–1.8
	15–18	45	1.3	1.4–1.5
	18–21	40	1.2	1.3
Females	11–14	47	1.4	1.7–1.8
	15–18	40	1.2	1.4–1.5
	18–21	38	1.2	1.3

tion have been found to be the same as those of normal children or higher.[58–61]

No published studies have assessed the blood vitamin levels of pediatric patients treated with chronic dialysis in the absence of vitamin supplementation. Combined dietary and supplementary vitamin intake is routinely used in clinical practice. The current recommendations suggest that an intake of 100 percent of the RDA should be considered the starting point for water-soluble vitamins in children on dialysis.[3] Supplementation should be considered if the dietary intake alone fails to meet the daily recommendation, if the measured serum levels are below normal, or in the presence of clinical signs of vitamin deficiency.[3,58]

It has been reported that vitamin A concentrations in serum are high in unsupplemented pediatric patients with ESRD and, despite the loss of vitamin A into PD fluid, chronic renal failure means that dialysis patients are at risk of developing hypervitaminosis A.

Dietary vitamin E intakes above the RDA and serum levels within or above the normal range have been reported in children on PD. As vitamin E excretion in the dialysate is negligible, nutritional supplementation is currently not recommended.

There are few data concerning the vitamin K status of patients with ESRD; supplementation is usually not recommended.

A detailed description of the role of vitamin D metabolites in children with ESRD is beyond the scope of this chapter; supplementation with a vitamin D analogue is clearly recommended in children receiving chronic dialysis in order to prevent or treat hyperparathyroidism and renal osteodystrophy.

Little is known about trace element intakes and needs in children on dialysis. Tamaru first investigated zinc and copper balance in children treated with PD and found poor dietary intakes of both; these patients absorb zinc and lose copper during PD.[62] Coleman reported mean dietary zinc and copper intakes below the RDA, but serum zinc levels were within the normal range before supplementation, and serum copper levels normalized with appropriate supplementation.[60] At present, no routine supplementation of either mineral is recommended. It may be necessary to assess serum levels periodically, and supplementation may be appropriate in patients receiving PD for prolonged periods or those with a poor dietary intake or low serum levels.[3]

Nutritional Supplementation. As many children with ESRD are anorexic, special strategies such as dietary supplements or tube feeding may be required to ensure an adequate nutritional intake; however, these measures are not justified if the spontaneous caloric and protein intakes are adequate in relation to age and the method of dialysis and there are no signs of malnutrition, because increasing nutritional energy

intake would only lead to obesity and not better growth. During infancy, oral supplementation can be achieved by increasing the caloric density of the formula using modular carbohydrate, fat, and protein components. In older children, energy and protein supplementation can be provided by modular components or commercial enteral products in liquid or bar form.

Enteral nasogastric, transpyloric, or gastrostomy tube feeding should be considered in patients who fail to meet their nutritional goals by the oral route alone. Each of these methods has advantages and disadvantages.[63] Nasogastric tubes are well tolerated and easy to insert, but their use is complicated by recurrent episodes of emesis and the need for frequent tube replacement; gastrostomy tubes or buttons are hidden beneath clothing but are also associated with emesis and, in children on PD, exit-site infections, leakage, and peritonitis[64,65]; gastrojejunostomy should be limited to children undergoing enteral tube feeding when severe gastroesophageal reflux is not resolved by medical therapy.

An increasing amount of information concerning the importance of nonnutritive sucking in infants and their difficulties in relearning how to swallow after prolonged enteral feedings is available: when long-term enteral feeding is required, infants should be given opportunities for additional oral stimulation and gratification.

Both nasogastric and gastrostomy tube feeding have led to good results with minimal complications in children. In most cases, they provide some relief to parents and medical personnel frustrated by trying to force an anorectic infant to eat; an additional benefit may be ease of delivering medications to an uncooperative child.[65]

A number of studies have shown that these measures can lead to better growth and an improved nutritional status.[66–70] The approach was first described by Conley,[66] who reported catch-up growth in 5 of 10 dialyzed infants tube fed with 156 to 210 percent of the RDA for proteins and 108 to 134 percent of the RDA for calories; others have reported normal weight gain but no accelerated height velocity.[67] Ledermann used a 30-month enteral feeding program to treat 35 children with chronic renal failure/ESRD (6 on PD), and concluded that long-term enteral feeding prevents or reverses weight loss and growth retardation, with significant catch-up growth if started before the age of 2 years.[68]

Other reports in infants treated with PD suggest that aggressive nutritional therapy is effective in maintaining or improving growth until the time of successful renal transplantation.[71–75] Ledermann has described the results of gastrostomy feeding in 29 children on PD for 11 years[76] and recommends the placement of a percutaneus gastrostomy before starting PD (or open gastrostomy if an antireflux procedure is necessary). The placement of a percutaneous endoscopic gastrostomy (PEG) is contraindicated after the start of PD, but an open gastrostomy (OG) is a safe alternative procedure.[76]

Ramage used gastrostomy feeding to treat 15 infants and older children on PD and concluded that it facilitates weight gain and arrests the decline in height SDS usually observed in infants with ESRD. No significant alteration was observed in the measured biochemical variables, although there was an increase in total protein and albumin.[64]

The findings of the North American Pediatric Renal Transplant Cooperative Study (NAPRTCS) survey of the impact of supplementary feedings on growth and mortality in children below 6 years of age at the start of dialysis were different. Supplements were given to 70 percent of the patients (more frequently to those beginning dialysis before the age of 2 years), with nasogastric tubes being used more commonly in the younger age group and gastrostomy tubes in the group of 2- to 5-year-olds. There were no differences in weight or height SDS after 30 days, 6 months, or 1 year of dialysis between the children who received supplementary feeds and those who did not.[77]

At present it seems advisable to recommend nutritional enteral supplementation in children less than 2 years of age and in older children who are able to meet nutritional goals.

Alternative strategies for achieving the nutritional goals of patients on HD are available, including intradialytic parenteral nutrition (IDPN), which is effective in adult patients with protein-energy malnutrition.[77–80] The DOQI nutritional guidelines provide recommendations for the use of IDPN in adults, but very little is known about its use in children.[34,81–83] Zachwieja treated 10 chronic HD patients 10 to 18 years of age with 0.25 g/kg intravenous amino acid supplementation: 9 of the patients gained weight (a mean increase of 4.5 percent) and 1 lost weight; no improvement in amino acid or albumin levels was observed.[81]

Goldstein used IDPN to treat three malnourished adolescent patients on chronic HD; all showed gains in weight and BMI within 6 weeks of the start of therapy: the mean monthly normalized protein catabolic rate (nPCR) significantly increased, but there was no change in monthly serum albumin levels.[34]

In a recent study, four pediatric HD patients received parenteral nutrition consisting of amino acids (8.5% solution), glucose (10 to 15% dextrose), and 20% fat emulsion at every dialysis session for 7 to 12 weeks; at the end of the study period, the authors observed an increase in oral caloric intake, the percent ideal body weight, BMI, and total lymphocyte count.[82]

At present, it seems advisable to recommend IDPN for a definite period of time in pediatric patients on HD with moderate to severe malnutrition.

Intraperitoneal amino acid supplementation is an alternative for children on PD, although it has been used in only a few pediatric patients and for short periods of time.[84–87] In a Canadian randomized crossover study, seven children were treated for 3 months each with an amino acid–supplemented dialysis solution and a standard dextrose solution:

there were no statistically significant between-period differences in terms of increased weight or height, triceps skinfold thickness, mean arm circumference, total body nitrogen, or questionnaire-based appetite scores.[88] Brew reported the case of a 5-year-old PD patient treated for 1 year with a balanced 1.1% amino acid solution in conjunction with a standard dextrose solution; the serum albumin levels then normalized and the patient showed significant increases in appetite, weight, and linear growth velocity.[89]

The DOQI pediatric nutritional guidelines suggest that the use of amino acid–based PD solutions may be more effective in providing an adequate amino acid or protein load than a sufficient energy intake because the total tolerable osmolality of the dialysate solutions prevents them from providing much energy.[3]

In PD-treated children with severe malnutrition, a trial with an amino acid–based PD solution together with other nutritional measures seems to be advisable.

Optimization of Dialysis

Conventional wisdom suggests that more aggressive dialysis clearance should lead to improvements in appetite and nutrition, but this is not necessarily true. Although early studies suggested a correlation between Kt/V and the normalized protein equivalent of nitrogen appearance (nPNA), the relationship has often been criticized as the mere result of mathematical coupling.[51–53,90,91] However, Aranda et al. found that children on CAPD with a mean total Kt/V of 3.0 ± 0.4 and a mean total weekly creatinine clearance of 80 ± 16 L/1.73 m^2 had a significantly greater nPNA than those with a significantly lower Kt/V and total creatinine clearance.[26] Moreover, Tom et al. monitored 20 children on maintenance HD for an average of 2.2 years and found that the combination of increased dialysis and adequate nutrition (energy intake: 90.6 percent the RDA) significantly improved height SDS (+0.31 SD per year).[27]

A recent study of 15 stable children on HD has demonstrated that adequate dialysis should be achieved in order to ensure a good protein intake. However, nPCR did not increase with a further increase in the delivered HD dose—i.e., Kt/V >1.6; the authors concluded that the nutritional status of children on chronic HD does not seem to benefit from very high dialysis doses.[28]

In the ESRD Clinical Indicators Project, 20 observations were made of 23 children on HD and 43 of 30 pediatric patients on PD. Although serum albumin was not associated with dialysis adequacy in the HD patients, there was a close inverse relationship between albumin levels and Kt/V in the PD patients; the authors concluded that a Kt/V >2.75 in PD-treated children may not improve nutrition per se and could increase albumin losses.[92]

The DOQI guideline recommendations for PD clearance in patients on CAPD are a weekly total Kt/V of at least

2.0 and a weekly total creatinine clearance of at least 60 L/1.73 m^2. The target clearances for patients treated with automated PD are slightly greater: at least 2.1 and 63 L/1.73 m^2 per week.[3,7]

In an Italian prospective multicenter study of 31 children treated with chronic PD, total creatinine clearance of 60 L/week/1.73 m^2 was found to be the most predictive cut-off point for malnutrition: the prevalence of malnutrition was significantly higher in the patients with a total clearance of <60 L/week/1.73 m^2 than in those whose total clearance was >60 L/week/1.73 m^2. This was particularly significant in the children who had been on dialysis for less than 24 months.[29]

A number of authors have stressed the fact that the prevention of malnutrition and its consequences depends not only on the dialysis dose but also on a timely start of treatment, as various studies have shown that malnutrition at the start of dialysis is a strong predictor of subsequent morbidity and mortality in both adult and pediatric patients with ESRD.[93–95]

Data from the United States Renal Data System have shown a positive correlation between low serum albumin and creatinine levels at the start of dialysis and an increased risk of death.[1,2] These results were confirmed in PD-treated patients by Chung and the Canada–U.S.A. (CANUSA) study, which showed that the relative risk of death during PD increased with lower serum albumin and a worse nutritional status as assessed by means of the Subjective Global Assessment and percentage lean body mass.[93,94] Although no prospective randomized clinical trials have been performed, the results of a few observational studies of adult populations suggest that the early start of dialysis may be associated with improved patient outcomes.[96–98]

There is still no clear consensus as to when dialysis should be started in pediatric or adult patients with ESRD, but it is unanimously agreed that the decision to start should be based not only on renal function indices but also on clinical parameters and particularly the indices of nutritional status.[92,99–101] Recently released guidelines on the prescription of PD can be usefully used in clinical practice.[102]

Medications

As dialysis and dietary measures alone cannot completely control uremia, special attention should be given to the prescription of medications aimed at maintaining the body's fluid homeostasis and preventing serious short- or long-term complications such as hydration and serum electrolyte disturbances, acidosis, osteodystrophy, and growth retardation.

The indications, dosages, and side effects of the multiple medications required for children on dialysis can be found elsewhere.[103] However, the need for good biochemical control (which in many cases requires phosphate binders, ion-exchange resins, sodium bicarbonate, calcitriol, and diuretics) is underlined by the results obtained in infants on dialysis, in whom good nutritional status and growth can be achieved only by combining adequate dialysis, nutritional measures, and drug prescriptions.

Two pharmacologic agents merit special comment: recombinant human growth hormone (rhGH) for counteracting malnutrition and sodium bicarbonate for correcting acidosis.

Recombinant human growth hormone is an anabolic hormone that promotes protein synthesis in various tissues. Children with ESRD have high serum GH levels but are characterized by a GH-resistant state that is probably due to reduced hepatic GH-receptor expression and increased IGF-binding protein levels. Both short- and long-term studies have established the safety and efficacy of rhGH in treating growth-retarded children with chronic renal insufficiency at various disease stages.[104–111] GH also has lipolytic and anti-insulin-like effects; thus changes in body composition can be expected during rhGH treatment. However, Vaisman did not find any significant change in lean and fat body mass in chronic renal failure patients treated with rhGH[104]; in another study, muscle mass increased with no change in fat stores or BMI.[105] A study of nine children with chronic renal failure (CRF) treated with rhGH found a significant increase in lean body mass and a decrease in fat body mass.[106]

There are no definitive data concerning the usefulness of rhGH in treating malnutrition in children with ESRD; thus malnutrition per se cannot be considered an indication for rhGH treatment in children on dialysis.

However, according to the DOQI pediatric nutritional guidelines, it should be considered in the case of children with a height or a height velocity for chronological age ≤ –2 SDS and growth potential documented by open epiphyses.[3] It is essential to correct insufficient energy and protein intake, acidosis, hyperphosphatemia, and secondary hyperparathyroidism before starting rhGH treatment.

Metabolic acidosis is due to the inability of an impaired kidney to reabsorb bicarbonate or excrete hydrogen ions. Muscle and bone are degraded to buffer the resulting acidosis and muscle wasting, and defective bone mineralization together with growth impairment may be found in the late phase of chronic renal insufficiency.[112–115]

It is unanimously agreed that a well-controlled acid-base status is necessary in order to prevent and treat malnutrition in children with ESRD. In a recent study, correcting metabolic acidosis improved serum albumin concentrations in patients on HD, and this also induced a decrease in nPCR.[115]

According to the DOQI pediatric nutritional guidelines, if serum bicarbonate levels are less than 22 mmol/L, acidosis should be corrected by means of adequate dialysate NaHCO$_3^-$ concentrations for children on HD, and by oral therapy for children on PD.[3] However, new solutions containing bicarbonate alone or with lactate have recently been introduced for children treated with CAPD and will be soon also be available for children on automated PD.

Compliance to drug prescription is a major concern in children (particularly adolescents) treated with dialysis: 66 percent of adolescents reveal problems with the intake of drugs, 40 percent are occasionally or frequently noncompliant, and 48 percent do not respect the schedule proposed for drug intake. All adolescents with chronic renal failure require discussion with the psychosocial and medical team about noncompliance.

A multidisciplinary approach is the only way to improve noncompliance.

CONCLUSIONS

The diagnosis of (particularly mild to moderate) malnutrition must be made early in children on dialysis in order to increase the probability of reversing the nutritional derangements.

This requires an overall evaluation that is based not only on traditional methods but also on the assessment of all of the factors that can have profound effects on nutritional status.

The approach must be multidisciplinary because 10 different areas must be investigated, and an objective nutritional score devised for children on dialysis may be a useful tool for the diagnosis of malnutrition and the subsequent monitoring of nutritional status.

The prevention and treatment of malnutrition is based on appropriate dietary and nutritional measures, an adequate dialysis prescription, and the correct use of medications.

Diet should be prescribed (and possibly adjusted during follow-up) on the basis of age, residual renal function, and the dialysis modality. Various forms of nutritional supplementation should be considered in the case of a deranged nutritional status or growth impairment, especially in infants. Particular attention should be paid to the medical or surgical treatment of any gastrointestinal, cardiovascular, or other comorbidities and the infectious complications that can affect nutrient intake.

The dialysis dose should initially be prescribed according to the DOQI guidelines and then adjusted on the basis of residual renal function, which should be maintained for as long as possible. This may be one reason for choosing peritoneal rather than HD as the first treatment modality of ESRD.

Regular monitoring of the delivered dialysis dose is of course mandatory, but the DOQI guidelines should only be seen as part of a more complex health assessment, including nutrition, growth, and cardiovascular status.

Compliance to multiple medication prescriptions is a major concern in children (particularly adolescents) on dialysis and also requires a multidisciplinary team approach.

REFERENCES

1. Wong CS, Hingorani S, Gillen DL, et al. Hypoalbuminemia and risk of death in pediatric patients with end-stage renal disease. *Kidney Int* 2002;61:630–637.
2. Wong CS, Gipson DS, Gillen DL, et al. Anthropometric measures and risk of death in children with end-stage renal disease. *Am J Kidney Dis* 2000;36:811–819.
3. National Kidney Foundation. Clinical practice guidelines for nutrition in chronic renal failure II. Pediatric guidelines. *Am J Kidney Dis* 2000;35(suppl l2):S105–S136.
4. Coleman JE, Edefonti A, Watson AR. Guidelines by an ad hoc European Committee on the assessment of growth and nutritional status in children on chronic peritoneal dialysis. *Perit Dial Int* 2001;21;3: www.ispd.org/pdi_journal.html
5. Secker D, Pencharz MB. Nutritional therapy for children on CAPD/CCPD: theory and practice. In: Fine RN, Alexander SR, Warady BA, eds. *CAPD/CCPD in children.* Boston: Kluwer, 1998:567–603.
6. Harvey E, Secker D, Braj B, et al. The team approach to the management of children on chronic peritoneal dialysis. *Adv Renal Replace Ther* 1996;3:3–13.
7. Warady BA, Alexander SR, Watlins S, et al. Optimal care of pediatric end-stage renal disease patients on dialysis. *Am J Kidney Dis* 1999;33:567–583.
8. Brem AS, Lambert C, Hill C, et al. Prevalence of protein malnutrition in children maintained on peritoneal dialysis. *Pediatr Nephrol* 2002;17:527–530.
9. Edefonti A, Picca M, Damiani B, et al. Prevalence of malnutrition assessed by bioimpedance analysis and anthropometry in children on peritoneal dialysis. *Perit Dial Int* 2001;21: 172–179.
10. Edefonti A, Picca M, Paglialonga F, et al. A novel objective nutritional score for children on chronic peritoneal dialysis. *Perit Dial Int* 2002;22:602–607.
11. Canepa A, Perfumo F, Carrea A, et al. Nutritional status in children receiving chronic peritoneal dialysis. *Perit Dial Int* 1996;16(suppl 1): S526–S531.
12. Tanner JM, Whitehouse RH, Takaishi M. Standards from birth to maturity for height, weight, height velocity, and weight velocity: British children, 1965. I. *Arch Dis Child* 1966;41:454–471.
13. Tanner JM, Whitehouse RH, Takaishi M. Standards from birth to maturity for height, weight, height velocity, and weight velocity: British children, 1965. I. *Arch Dis Child* 1966;41:613–635.
14. Frisancho AR. New norms of upper limb fat and muscle areas for assessment of nutritional status. *Am J Clin Nutr* 1981;34:2540–2545.
15. Ulijaszek SJ, Kerr DA. Anthropometric measurement error and the assessment of nutritional status. *Br J Nutr* 1999;82: 165–177.

16. Hall JC, O'Quigley J, Giles GR, et al. Upper limb anthropometry: the value of measurement variance studies. *Am J Clin Nutr* 1980;33:1846–1851.

17. Reilly JJ. Assessment of body composition in infants and children. *Nutrition* 1998;14:821–825.

18. Avram MM, Goldwasser BP, Erroa M, et al. Predictors of survival in continuous ambulatory peritoneal dialysis patients: the importance of prealbumin and other nutritional and metabolic markers. *Am J Kidney Dis* 1996;23:91–98.

19. Chertow GM, Ackert K, Lew NL, et al. Prealbumin is as important as albumin in the nutritional assessment of hemodialysis patients. *Kidney Int* 2000;58:2512–2517.

20. Neyra NR, Hakim RM, Shyr Y, et al. Serum transferrin and serum prealbumin are early predictors of serum albumin in chronic hemodialysis patients. *J Renal Nutr* 2000;10: 184–190.

21. Iseki K, Kawazoe N, Fukiyama K. Serum albumin is a strong predictor of death in chronic dialysis patients. *Kidney Int* 1999;44:115–119.

22. Han DS, Lee SW, Kang SW, et al. Factors affecting low values of serum albumin in CAPD patients. *Adv Perit Dial* 1996;12:288–292.

23. Steinman TI. Serum albumin: its significance in patients with ESRD. *Semin Dial* 2000;13:404–408.

24. Jones CH, Newstead CG, Will EJ, et al. Assessment of nutritional status: serum albumin is not a useful measure. *Nephrol Dial Transplant* 1997;12:1406–1413.

25. Besbas N, Ozdemir S, Saatci U, et al. Nutritional assessment of children on hemodialysis. Value of IGF-I, TNF-alpha and IL-1 beta. *Nephrol Dial Transplant* 1998;13:1484–1488.

26. Aranda RA, Pecoits-Filho RFS, Romao JE Jr, et al. Kt/V in children on CAPD: how much is enough? *Perit Dial Int* 19:588–589.

27. Tom A, McCauley L, Bell L, et al. Growth during maintenance hemodialysis: impact of enhanced nutrition and clearance. *J Pediatr* 1999;134:464–471.

28. Marsenic O, Peco-Antic A, Jovanovic O. Effect of dialysis dose on nutritional status of children on chronic hemodialysis. *Nephron* 2001;88:273–275.

29. Edefonti A, Picca M, Paglialonga F, et al. A multicenter study on the prevalence of malnutrition assessed by the ABN score in children on CPD (abstr). *Nephrol Dial Transplant* 2003;18(suppl 4):824.

30. Edefonti A, Picca M, Damiani B, et al. Models to assess nitrogen losses in pediatric patients on chronic peritoneal dialysis. *Pediatr Nephrol* 2000;15:25–30.

31. Wingen AM, Fabian-Bach C, Mehls O. Evaluation of protein intake by dietary diaries and urea N-excretion in children with chronic renal failure. *Clin Nephrol* 1993;40: 208–215.

32. Orejas G, Santos F, Malaga S, et al. Assessment of protein intake in children with chronic renal insufficiency. *Miner Electrolyte Metab* 1996;22:79–82.

33. Mendley SR, Majkowski NL. Urea and nitrogen excretion in pediatric peritoneal dialysis patients. *Kidney Int* 2000;58: 2564–2570.

34. Goldstein S, Baronette S, Vital Gambrell T, et al. nPCR assessment and IDPN treatment of malnutrition in pediatric hemodialysis patients. *Pediatr Nephrol* 2000;17:531–534.

35. Piccoli A, Rossi B, Pillon L, et al. A new method for monitoring body fluid variation by bioimpedance analysis: the RXc graph. *Kidney Int* 1994;46:534–539.

36. De Palo T, Messina G, Edefonti A et al. Normal values of the bioelectrical impedance vector in childhood and puberty. *Nutrition* 2000;16:417–424.

37. Ott M, Fischer H, Polat H, et al. Bioelectrical impedance analysis as a predictor of survival in patients with human immunodeficiency virus infection. *J AIDS Hum Retrovir* 1995;9:20–25.

38. Edefonti A, Merlotti C, Loi S, et al. Assessment of nutritional status in children treated with automated peritoneal dialysis (APD): comparison between anthropometry, bioimpedance analysis and dual energy x-ray absorptiometry (abstr). *Perit Dial Int* 2001;21(suppl 2):S4.

39. Enia G, Sicuso C, Alati G, et al. Subjective global assessment of nutrition in dialysis patients. *Nephrol Dial Transplant* 1993;8(10):1094–1098.

40. Detsky AS, McLaughlin JR, Baker JP, et al. What is subjective global assessment of nutritional status? *J Parenter Enter Nutr* 1987;11:8–13.

41. Jeejeebhoy KN, Detsky AS, Baker JP. Assessment of nutritional status. *J Parenter Enter Nutr* 1990;14(suppl 5): 193S–196S.

42. Johansson AC, Samuelsson O, Haraldsson B, et al. Body composition in patients treated with peritoneal dialysis. *Nephrol Dial Transplant* 1988;13:1511–1517.

43. MacDonald A. The practical problems of nutritional support for children on continuous ambulatory peritoneal dialysis. *Hum Nutr Appl Nutr* 1986;40:253–261.

44. Canepa A, Perfumo F, Carrea A, et al. Protein and calorie intake, nitrogen losses, and nitrogen balance in children undergoing chronic peritoneal dialysis. *Adv Perit Dial* 1996; 12:326–329.

45. Broyer M, Niaudet P, Champion G, et al. Nutritional and metabolic studies in children on continuous ambulatory peritoneal dialysis. *Kidney Int Suppl* 1983;15:S106–S110.

46. Saluski IB, Fine RN, Nelson P, et al. Nutritional status of children undergoing continuous ambulatory peritoneal dialysis. *Am J Clin Nutr* 1983;38:599–611.

47. Pereira AM, Hamani N, Nogueira PC, et al. Oral vitamin intake in children receiving long-term dialysis. *J Renal Nutr* 2000;10:24–29.

48. Foreman JW, Abitbol CL, Trachtman H, et al. Nutritional intake in children with renal insufficiency: a report of the Growth Failure in Children with Renal Disease study. *J Am Coll Nutr* 1996;15:579–585.

49. Hakim RM, Lazarus JM. Progression of chronic renal failure. *Am J Kidney Dis* 1989;14:396–401.

50. Modification of Diet in Renal Disease Study Group, Kopple JD, Berg R, Houser H, et al. Nutritional status of patients with different levels of chronic renal failure. *Kidney Int* 1989;36(suppl 27):S184–S194.

51. Bergstrom J, Furst P, Alvestrand A, et al. Protein and energy intake, nitrogen balance and nitrogen losses in patients treated with continuous ambulatory peritoneal dialysis. *Kidney Int* 1993;44:1048–1057.

52. Bergstrom J, Lindholm B. Nutrition and adequacy of dialysis. How do hemodialysis and CAPD compare? *Kidney Int* 1993;43(suppl 40):S39–S50.

53. Fischbach M, Terzic J, Lahlou A, et al. Nutritional effects of Kt/V in children on peritoneal dialysis: are there benefits from larger dialysis doses? *Adv Perit Dial* 1995;11:306–308.

54. Schaefer F, Klaus G, Mehls O. Peritoneal transport properties and dialysis dose affect growth and nutritional status in children on chronic peritoneal dialysis. Mid-European Pediatric Peritoneal Dialysis Study Group. *J Am Soc Nephrol* 1999;10:1786–1792.

55. Edefonti A, Picca M, Damiani B, et al. Dietary prescription based on estimated nitrogen balance during peritoneal dialysis. *Pediatr Nephrol* 1999;13:253–258.

56. Zadik Z, Frishberg Y, Drukker A, et al. Excessive dietary protein and suboptimal caloric intake have a negative effect on the growth of children with chronic renal disease before and during growth hormone therapy. *Metabolism* 1998;47:264–268.

57. Quan A, Baum M. Protein losses in children on continuous ambulatory peritoneal dialysis. *Pediatr Nephrol* 1996;10:728–731.

58. Filler G. The DOQI pediatric nutritional guidelines–critical remarks. *Perit Dial Int* 2001;21(suppl 3):S192–S194.

59. Warady BA, Kriley M, Alon U, et al. Vitamin status of infants receiving long-term peritoneal dialysis. *Pediatr Nephrol* 1994;8:354–356.

60. Coleman JE, Watson AR. Micronutrient supplementation in children on continuous cycling peritoneal dialysis (CCPD). *Adv Perit Dial* 1992;8:396–401.

61. Kriley M, Warady BA. Vitamin status of pediatric patients receiving long-term peritoneal dialysis. *Am J Clin Nutr* 1991;53:1476–1479.

62. Tamaru T, Vaughn WH, Waldo FB, et al. Zinc and copper balance in children on continuous ambulatory peritoneal dialysis. *Pediatr Nephrol* 1989;3:309–313.

63. Wassner SJ, Abitbol C, Alexander S, et al. Nutritional requirements for infants with renal failure. *Am J Kidney Dis* 1986;7:300–305.

64. Ramage IJ, Geary DF, Harvey E, et al. Efficacy of gastrostomy feeding in infants and older children receiving chronic peritoneal dialysis. *Perit Dial Int* 1999;19:231–236.

65. Watson AR, Coleman JE, Warady BA. When and how to use nasogastric and gastrostomy feeding for nutritional support in infants and children on CAPD/CCPD. In: Fine RN, Alexander SR, Warady BA, eds. *CAPD/CCPD in Children*. Boston: Kluwer, 1998:281–300.

66. Conley SB, Brewer ED, Gandy S, et al. Normal growth in very small children on peritoneal dialysis: 18 months' experience. *Am J Kidney Dis* suppl1982;(suppl 1):8–12.

67. Warady BA, Weis L, Johnson L. Nasogastric tube feeding in infants on peritoneal dialysis. *Perit Dial Int* 1996;16:S521–S525.

68. Ledermann SE, Shaw V, Trompeter RS. Long-term enteral nutrition in infants and young children with chronic renal failure. *Pediatr Nephrol* 1999;13:870–875.

69. Kohaut EC. Growth in children with end-stage renal disease treated with continuous ambulatory peritoneal dialysis for at least one year. *Perit Dial Bull* 1982;2:159–161.

70. Kuizon BD, Nelson PA, Salusky IB. Tube feeding in children with end-stage renal disease. *Miner Electrolyte Metab* 1997;23:306–310.

71. Brewer ED. Growth of small children managed with chronic peritoneal dialysis and nasogastric tube feedings: 203 month experience in 14 patients. *Adv Perit Dial* 1990;6:245–251.

72. Brewer ED. Supplemental enteral tube feeding in infants undergoing dialysis: indications and outcomes. *Semin Dial* 1994;7:429–434.

73. Qamar IU, Balfe JW. Experience with chronic peritoneal dialysis in infants. *Child Nephrol Urol* 1991;11:159–164.

74. Ellis EN, Pearson D, Champion B, et al. Outcome of infants on chronic peritoneal dialysis. *Adv Perit Dial* 1995;11:266–269.

75. Coleman JE, Watson AR, Rance CH, et al. Gastrostomy buttons for nutritional support on chronic dialysis. *Nephrol Dial Transplant* 1998;13:2041–2046.

76. Ledermann SE, Spitz L, Moloney J, et al. Gastrostomy feeding in infants and children on peritoneal dialysis. *Pediatr Nephrol* 2002;17:246–250.

77. Ellis N, Yiu V, Harley F, et al. The impact of supplemental feeding in young children on dialysis: a report of the North American Pediatric Renal Transplant Cooperative Study. *Pediatr Nephrol* 2001;16:404–408.

78. Korzets A, Azoulay O, Chagnac A, et al. Successful intradialytic parenteral nutrition after abdominal "catastrophes" in chronically hemodialysed patients. *J Renal Nutr* 1999;9:206–213.

79. Smolle KH, Kaufmann P, Holzer H, et al. Intradialytic parenteral nutrition in malnourished patients on chronic haemodialysis therapy. *Nephrol Dial Transplant* 1995;10:1411–1416.

80. Chertow GM, Ling J, Lew NL, et al. The association of intradialytic parenteral nutrition administration with survival in hemodialysis patients. *Am J Kidney Dis* 1994;24:912–920.

81. Zachwieja J, Duran M, Joles JA, et al. Amino acid and carnitine supplementation in haemodialysed children. *Pediatr Nephrol* 1994;8:739–743.

82. Krause I, Shamir R, Davidovits M, et al. Intradialytic parenteral nutrition in malnourished children treated with hemodialysis. *J Renal Nutr* 2002;12:55–59.

83. Brewer ED. Pediatric experience with intradialytic parenteral nutrition and supplemental tube feeding. *Am J Kidney Dis* 1999;33:205–207.

84. Canepa A, Verrina E, Perfumo F, et al. Value of intraperitoneal amino acids in children treated with chronic peritoneal dialysis. *Perit Dial Int* 1999;19(suppl 2):S435–S440.

85. Canepa A, Perfumo F, Carrea A, et al. Long-term effect of amino-acid dialysis solution in children on continuous ambulatory peritoneal dialysis. *Pediatr Nephrol* 1991;11:84–86.

86. Hanning RM, Balfe JW, Zlotkin SH. Effectiveness and nutritional consequences of amino acid-based vs glucose-based dialysis solutions in infants and children receiving CAPD. *Am J Clin Nutr* 1987;46:22–30.

87. Hanning RM, Balfe JW, Zlotkin SH. Effect of amino acid containing dialysis solutions on plasma amino acid profiles in children with chronic renal failure. *J Pediatr Gastroenterol Nutr* 1987;6:942–947.

88. Qamar IU, Levin L, Balfe JW, et al. Effect of 3-month amino acid dialysis compared to dextrose dialysis in children on continuous ambulatory peritoneal dialysis. *Perit Dial Int* 1994;14:34–41.

89. Brew AS, Maaz D, Shemin DG, et al. Use of amino acid peritoneal dialysate for one year in a child on CCPD. *Perit Dial Int* 1996;16:634–636.

90. Schaefer F, Wolf S, Klaus G, et al. Higher Kt/V urea associated with greater protein catabolic rate and dietary protein intake in children treated with CCPD compared to CAPD. Mid-European Pediatric CPD Study Group (MPCS). *Adv Perit Dial* 1994;10:310–314.

91. Walk TLM, Schroder CH, Reddingius RE, et al. Adequate dialysis? Measurement of Kt/V in a pediatric peritoneal dialysis population. *Perit Dial Int* 1997;17:175–178.

92. Brem AS, Lambert C, Hill C, et al. Outcome data on pediatric dialysis patients from the End-Stage Renal Disease Clinical Indicators Project. *Am J Kidney Dis* 2000;36:310–317.

93. Churchill DN. Implications of the Canada-USA (CANUSA) study of the adequacy of dialysis on peritoneal dialysis schedule. *Nephrol Dial Transplant* 1998;13(suppl 6):158–163.

94. Chung SH, Lindholm B, Lee HB. Influence of initial nutritional status on continuous ambulatory peritoneal dialysis patient survival. *Perit Dial Int* 2000;20:19–26.

95. Lowrie EG, Huang WH, Lew NL. Death risk predictors among peritoneal dialysis and hemodialysis patients: a preliminary comparison. *Am J Kidney Dis* 1995;26:220–228.

96. Tattersall J, Greewood R, Farrington K. Urea kinetics and when to commence dialysis. *Am J Nephrol* 1995;15:283–289.

97. Bonomini V, Scolari MP, Coli L, et al. Early, frequent and efficient hemodialysis: a new trend or deja vù from the 1970s? *Home Hemodial Int* 1998;2:3–7.

98. Bonomini V, Feletti C, Scolari MP, et al. Benefits of early initiation of dialysis. *Kidney Int* 1985;28:S57–S59.

99. Churchill DN, Blake PG, Jindal KK, et al. Clinical practice guidelines for initiation of dialysis. Canadian Society of Nephrology. *J Am Soc Nephrol* 10(suppl 13):S289–S291.

100. Obrador GT, Pereira BJG. Initiation of dialysis: current trends and the case for timely initiation. *Perit Dial Int* 20(suppl 2):S142–149.

101. Korevaar JC, Jansen MA, Dekker FW, et al. When to initiate dialysis: effect of proposed US guidelines on survival. *Lancet* 2001;358:1046–1050.

102. Fischbach M, Stefanidis CJ, Watson AR. Guidelines by an ad hoc European committee on adequacy of the paediatric peritoneal dialysis prescription. *Nephrol Dial Transplant* 2002;17:380–385.

103. Hingorani S, Watkins SL. Dialysis for end-stage renal disease. *Curr Opin Pediatr* 2000;12:140–145.

104. Vaisman N, Zadik Z, Duchan R, et al. Changes of body composition of children with chronic renal failure during growth hormone treatment. *Pediatr Nephrol* 1994:8:201–204.

105. Perfumo F, Trivelli A, Delucchi P, et al. Anthropometry and body composition changes in children with chronic renal failure (CRF) treated with recombinant human growth hormone (rhGH). *Pediatr Nephrol* 1995;9:C71.

106. Liponski I, Braillon O, Cochat P. Changes in body composition during recombinant growth hormone treatment in children. *Kidney Int* 1996;50:1775–1777.

107. Feber J, Cochat P, Labl J, et al. Body composition in children receiving recombinant human growth hormone after renal transplantation. *Kidney Int* 1998;54:951–955.

108. Ghio L, Colombo D, Edefonti A, et al. Short-term anabolic effects of recombinant human growth hormone in young patients with a renal transplant. *Transpl Int* 11(suppl 1):1998;S69–S72.

109. Shaefer F, Wuhl E, Haffner D, et al. Stimulation of growth by recombinant human growth hormone in children undergoing peritoneal or hemodialysis treatment. German Study Group for Growth Hormone Treatment in Chronic Renal Failure. *Adv Perit Dial* 1994;10:321–326.

110. Berard E, Crosnier H, Six-Beneton A, et al. Recombinant human growth hormone treatment of children on hemodialysis. French Society of Pediatric Nephrology. *Pediatr Nephrol* 1998;12:304–310.

111. Wuhl E, Haffner D, Nissel R, et al. Short dialyzed children respond less to growth hormone than patients prior to dialysis. German Study Group for Growth Hormone Treatment in Chronic Renal Failure. *Pediatr Nephrol* 1996;10:294–298.

112. Mitch WE, Medina R, Grieber S, et al. Metabolic acidosis stimulates muscle protein degradation by activating the adenosine triphosphate-dependent pathway involving ubiquitin and proteasomes. *J Clin Invest* 1994;93:2127–2133.

113. Ballmer PE, McNurlan MA, Hulter HN, et al. Chronic metabolic acidosis decreases albumin synthesis and induces negative nitrogen balance in humans. *J Clin Invest* 1995;95:39–45.

114. Kang DH, Lee R, Lee HY, et al. Metabolic acidosis and composite nutritional index (CNI) in CAPD patients. *Clin Nephrol* 2000;53;124–131.

115. Brady JP, Hasbargen JA. A review of the effects of correction of acidosis on nutrition in dialysis patients. *Semin Dial* 2000;13:252–255.

Growth and Growth Hormone Treatment in Children with Chronic Renal Insufficiency

Burkhard Tönshoff
Richard N. Fine

The occurrence of growth retardation in children with renal insufficiency has been recognized since the last century[1]; however, the importance of the relationship has been appreciated only for the past two decades. As the treatment of children with end-stage renal disease (ESRD) has advanced and many children's lives have consequently been prolonged by dialysis and renal transplantation, the impact of growth retardation on those with renal insufficiency has emerged. One of the major obstacles to full rehabilitation in children undergoing extended dialysis, as well as those who are successfully transplanted, is persistent growth retardation and failure to obtain optimal adult stature. Disappointingly, optimizing nutritional support and medical care with vitamin D and mineral supplements does not uniformly improve growth in children with chronic renal failure (CRF). A major

breakthrough in the understanding of the pathogenesis of uremic growth failure was achieved only in the last 15 years by a more detailed analysis of the growth hormone (GH)/insulin-like growth factor (IGF) axis in chronic renal disease.[2] The relevance of the impact of alterations of the somatotropic hormone axis is underlined by the therapeutic efficacy of recombinant human (rh) GH therapy in growth-retarded children with CRF, which was introduced in 1988.

PATHOMECHANISM OF GROWTH FAILURE

The pathogenesis of impaired growth in CRF is complex and only partially understood. Although a particular cause can occasionally be found, a combination of several factors is generally responsible for growth impairment (Table 23–1). Furthermore, the patient's age; the type, duration and severity of renal disease; the treatment modality; and the patient's social environment all play important roles.

Protein-Calorie Malnutrition

One of the cardinal abnormalities associated with CRF is a loss of appetite. Spontaneous food intake is usually low when related to the patient's age but normal when adjusted for body mass.[3,4] Thus, it is difficult to know whether low energy intake is the cause or the consequence of impaired growth in children. The same is true for the body protein content of children with CRF and short stature, which is adequate for height but not for age.[5] It is still not clear whether uremia leads to a reduction in anabolism or to an increase in catabolism. Animal studies support both mechanisms, whereas studies in humans suggest increased catabolism as the main alteration of tissue metabolism. At any given level of protein intake, the conversion of dietary to body protein is less efficient in uremic compared with pair-fed control animals.[6] Impaired protein synthesis, resistance to the anabolic effects of insulin, and increased muscle breakdown may all contribute to poor growth. Adequate energy intake is required for anabolism and growth. Energy intake is correlated with growth rate if it is less than 80 percent of the recommended dietary allowance.[7] However, augmentation of energy intake above this level results in obesity rather than in a further stimulation of growth.[7,8] Energy malnutrition is particularly prevalent in uremic infants during the first year of life, when the metabolic rate in relation to body mass is high. Height standard deviation score

TABLE 23–1. ETIOLOGY OF GROWTH IMPAIRMENT IN CHRONIC RENAL FAILURE

- Genetic factors
  - Parent height
  - Gender
  - Syndromal disorder (with kidney disorder as a part)
- Age at start of CRF
- Duration of CRF
- Residual renal function
- Treatment modalities for CRF
- Energy malnutrition
- Water and electrolyte disturbances
- Metabolic acidosis
- Hormonal disorders
  - Disturbance of parathyroid hormone and vitamin D (renal osteodystrophy)
  - Disturbance of the somatotropic hormonal axis
  - Disturbance of the gonadotropic hormonal axis
  - Disturbance of insulin/glucose metabolism
  - Disturbance of other hormones

(SDS) is correlated with body cell mass and serum transferrin or albumin, emphasizing the importance of malnutrition for growth failure in this age group.[9,10] In contrast to deficient calorie intake, protein malnutrition is infrequently seen in children with CRF.[3,4] In a prospective study in which protein intake was limited to the safe levels recommended by the World Health Organization (i.e., 0.8 to 1.1 g/kg per day) but ensuring adequate calorie intake, no impairment of weight and length gain was seen over 3 years.[11]

Disturbances of Water and Electrolyte Metabolism

Many congenital renal diseases that slowly progress toward CRF lead to a loss of electrolytes and a reduced ability of the kidney to concentrate urine. In particular, sodium chloride is lost in patients with obstructive uropathies and renal hypoplasia, and potassium is lost in patients with tubular damage, particularly in nephropathic cystinosis. Polyuria, an expression of the reduced ability of the kidney to concentrate urine, is seen mainly in patients with Fanconi's syndrome and in nephronophthisis.

It is not possible to assess independently the extent to which disturbances in water and electrolyte metabolism contribute to growth retardation in individual patients with CRF. The probability of these factors being significant has, however, been shown by analogous clinical and animal studies. In rats, sodium deficiency decreases protein synthesis and growth, which is only partially reversible by sodium repletion.[12,13] Recently, evidence has been provided that part of the effects previously attributed to sodium deficiency were actually caused by concomitant depletion of chloride. Selective removal of chloride from a sodium-repleted diet caused growth retardation and diminished muscle protein synthesis.[14] In children with Bartter's syndrome, sodium, chloride, and potassium deficits are accepted causes of growth disorders. The same applies both to patients with familial chloride diarrhea and to infants with a reduced chloride diet.[15]

Metabolic Acidosis

Metabolic acidosis is almost inevitably observed in CRF if there is a 50 percent reduction in the normal glomerular filtration rate (GFR). This acidosis is primarily due to the kidney's reduced ability to excrete ammonia. The severity of the acidosis is aggravated by nutritional protein and acid load, catabolism, and altered electrolyte balance. Metabolic acidosis in uremic rats is associated with increased glucocorticoid production and increased protein degradation by activating branched-chain ketoacid catabolism and the ubiquitin-proteasome pathway.[16–20] Moreover, metabolic acidosis has profound effects on the somatotropic hormone axis, downregulating spontaneous GH secretion,[21] the expression of GH receptor and IGF-I mRNA,[22] and both baseline and GH-stimulated serum IGF-I concentrations.[23] Thus, metabolic acidosis per se seems to result in a state of GH insensitivity.

Anemia

Children with CRF develop increasing anemia as a result of erythropoietin (EPO) deficiency. If therapy is not introduced in time, hemoglobin values of around 50 g/L are usual in the terminal stages of renal failure. It is not certain whether or to what extent chronic anemia leads to growth impairment. Children with chronic anemia (e.g., thalassemia major) show retardation of growth and development. When treated with high-frequency transfusion regimens to keep hematocrits close to the normal range, growth rates in these patients may improve.[24] Theoretically, anemia may interfere with growth via various mechanisms, such as poor appetite, intercurrent infections, cardiac complications, and poor oxygenation of cartilage cells in the growth plate. The introduction of recombinant human EPO (rHuEpo) for the treatment of renal anemia has offered the opportunity to study whether changes in growth are induced by the compensation of renal anemia. Whereas short-term stimulatory effects of rHuEPO have been observed in single patients,[25] no persistent effect was observed in prospective trials.[26]

Renal Osteodystrophy

Renal osteodystrophy is caused by a renal disorder in vitamin D metabolism and by secondary hyperparathyroidism. Following unsuccessful prevention or inadequate treatment, osteodystrophy manifests itself clinically as skeletal deformities, muscular hypotension, and occasionally slipped epiphyses. Histologically, the condition presents as a mixture of osteomalacia and osteitis fibrosa, sometimes with one of the components almost completely predominating. In contrast to vitamin D–deficiency rickets, the radiologic changes in epiphyseal joints in renal osteodystrophy are caused by transformation of the primary spongiosa into fibrous tissue and woven bone rather than by the persistence of noncalcified growth cartilage.

Although gross skeletal deformities can contribute to the retardation of a child's growth, the appearance of renal osteodystrophy is not inevitably paralleled by alterations in epiphyseal growth of the long bones. Severe metaphyseal skeletal changes are often detected radiologically in patients with relatively good growth rates. In such cases, osteopathy is unmasked by rapid growth. Growth is arrested completely only when secondary hyperparathyroidism results in severe destruction of the metaphyseal bone architecture.

Whereas treatment with vitamin D and 1,25-dihydroxy-vitamin D_3 [$1,25(OH)_2D_3$] improves growth in uremic rats,[27] equivalent therapeutic success has not been achieved in children with CRF. Treatment with 5000 to 10,000 IU of vitamin D_3 per day did not affect growth in dialyzed children.[28] An early optimistic report in four patients receiving $1,25(OH)_2D_3$ could not be validated in the long term.[29] This therapeutic failure contrasts with the remarkable growth improvement in patients treated for vitamin D-deficiency rickets.

The extent to which secondary hyperparathyroidism contributes to growth impairment is unclear. Parathyroid hormone (PTH) is an anabolic hormone and an intrinsic growth factor, stimulating mitosis in osteoprogenitor cells and growth plate chondrocytes and upregulating the vitamin D receptor.[30,31] Intermittent but not continuous administration of PTH stimulates skeletal growth in normal and uremic rats.[32] However, resistance to the effect of PTH is observed in uremia, characterized by reduced cAMP production in growth plate chondrocytes.[30] Low bone turnover induced by relatively low PTH levels may contribute to growth impairment.[33] At the other end of the spectrum, excessive secretion of PTH can lead to the destruction of growth plate architecture,[34] epiphyseal displacement,[35] and metaphyseal fractures.[36]

Alterations of the Growth Hormone/Insulin-Like Growth Factor Axis in CRF

Growth Hormone. Random fasting serum levels of GH are normal or increased in children and adults with CRF, depending on the extent of renal failure.[37–39] For the interpretation of these data, information about the secretory pattern of GH, such as the specific physiologic regulation of the frequency and amplitude of pulsatile GH secretion and its metabolic clearance, is important. This is particularly the case in patients with CRF, because the kidney accounts for a substantial fraction of the serum turnover of GH.[40] The application of deconvolution analysis has permitted indirect calculation of pituitary GH secretion independent of the metabolic clearance of the hormone. By use of this methodology, the GH secretion rate from the pituitary in CRF was found to be variable between patients and studies. A high-normal calculated GH secretion rate and an amplified number of GH secretory bursts were reported in prepubertal children with ESRD, presumably as a result of attenuated bioactive IGF-I feedback of the somatotropic axis (Fig. 23–1).[41] In adult patients on hemodialysis, the GH secretion rate was clearly elevated,[42] whereas reduced GH secretion rates were observed in pubertal patients with advanced CRF, indicating an altered sensitivity of the somatotropic hormone axis to the stimulatory effect of sex steroids, at least at this developmental stage.[43] The apparent variability in the calculated GH secretion rates in these studies may be due to differences in the age and nutritional status of the study populations, parameters that strongly influence spontaneous GH secretion. A prolonged GH half-life due to a decreased metabolic clearance rate resulting from a reduction in functional renal mass was a consistent finding in all studies.[41–43] The concept that the kidneys account for a sub-

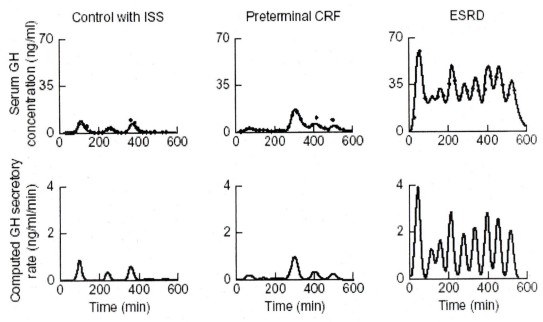

Figure 23–1. Illustrative profiles of pulsatile plasma GH concentrations in one subject with idiopathic short stature, one child with preterminal CRF, and one child with ESRD. The upper panels depict the serial plasma GH concentrations over time, as measured by immunoradiometric assay of plasma derived from blood collected at 20-minute intervals for 10 hours, and the deconvolution-predicted curves, which closely approximate the experimental data points. The lower panels show the deconvolution-calculated GH secretory bursts over a period of 10 hours. Note the presence of an increased number of secretory bursts in the child with ESRD. (From Tönshoff et al.[41] With permission.)

stantial fraction of the serum turnover of GH in humans is supported by data from an infusion study with GH. This demonstrated a 50 percent reduced metabolic clearance rate of GH both in children and adults with CRF, which correlated with the degree of residual renal function (Fig. 23–2).[44]

The apparent discrepancy between normal or elevated GH serum levels and diminished longitudinal growth in children with CRF has led to the concept of insensitivity to the action of GH in the uremic state. It is noteworthy that GH insensitivity is associated with clinical and experimental CRF in the absence of concomitant metabolic acidosis or malnutrition, although these two factors are potentially aggravating. This "uremic" GH insensitivity is due to multiple derangements of distal components of the somatotropic hormone axis, described below.

GH Receptor/Binding Protein. One molecular mechanism for the peripheral insensitivity to the action of GH in CRF is a reduced density of GH receptors in GH target organs. In humans, the circulating high-affinity growth hormone binding protein (GHBP) is thought to reflect GH receptor expression because it is produced by a limited proteolytic cleavage of the GH receptor and release of the extracellular domain into the circulation.[45] Determination of serum GHBP concentrations may be used to assess GH receptor density in tissues, particularly in the liver, because circulating GHBP is believed to derive mainly but not exclusively from liver tissue. GHBP activity in serum is low in children[46,47] and

adults[48–50] with CRF. In a large analysis of 126 children with CRF, serum GHBP concentrations were below the mean for age- and gender-matched controls in 77 percent of CRF patients (Fig. 23–3).[47] The decrease of age- and gender-adjusted serum GHBP levels is related to the degree of renal dysfunction; children with ESRD have the lowest GHBP levels (-2.25 ± 0.22 SDS). In this study,[47] the vast majority (91 percent) of children with CRF had a BMI within the normal range. Nevertheless, BMI, rather than the degree of renal dysfunction, was the prevailing determinant of serum GHBP levels in these children, indicating that variations in nutritional status within the normal range are an important determinant of GH receptor status in tissues.

The decreased GHBP/GH receptor status in children with CRF has functional relevance with respect to growth. Serum GHBP is correlated with both the spontaneous growth rate (Fig. 23–4) and the growth response to GH therapy in children with CRF (Fig. 23–5); baseline GHBP levels predict approximately 30 percent of the growth response to GH treatment in these patients.[47] Hence, GHBP levels serve as an indicator of sensitivity to both endogenous and exogenous GH and may be a useful clinical parameter to predict the growth response to GH. These observations also help to explain the lower growth response to exogenous GH in children with ESRD compared with that in children with residual renal function, because serum GHBP/GH receptor status is suppressed the most in the former group.[47]

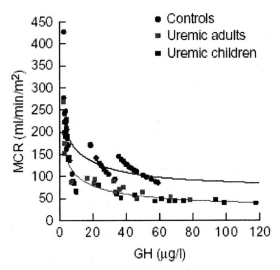

Figure 23–2. Total metabolic clearance rate (MCR) as a function of steady-state plasma GH concentrations in controls and uremic subjects. Total MCR was expressed as a power function of steady-state GH concentrations in controls (solid line) and in uremic patients (dotted line). (From Haffner et al.[44] With permission.)

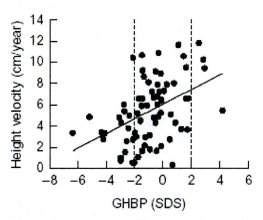

Figure 23–4. Spontaneous height velocity in 75 prepubertal children with CRF as a function of age- and gender-related serum GHBP levels (SD score). The normal range for GHBP (−2 to +2 SDS) is given by a dotted line. There was a significant positive correlation ($r = 0.44$, $p < 0.0001$). (From Tönshoff et al.[47] With permission.)

Is low tissue GH receptor density in CRF the reason or the consequence of high plasma levels of GH in advanced CRF? Most clinical and experimental data argue against direct regulation of GH receptors by endogenous GH in vivo. In the majority of studies, children and adults with GH deficiency have normal serum GHBP levels,[51–53] and these levels do not change during subcutaneous GH replacement therapy.[52,54,55] On the other hand, some patients with idiopathic short stature exhibit clearly decreased serum GHBP levels in the presence of normal GH secretion.[51] These results argue against a direct regulation of GHBP/GH receptors by GH. More likely is a direct suppressive effect of the uremic milieu on tissue GH receptor density, which leads to an adaptive increase in pituitary GH secretion in addition to the diminished feedback downregulation of GH secretion by decreased IGF bioactivity.[41,42]

In concordance with these findings, a significant reduction of hepatic GH receptor mRNA abundance, which was nutrition-independent, has been described in nonacidotic experimental uremia in the 5/6 nephrectomy rat model in most[56,57] but not all[58] studies. These findings suggest that the relative insensitivity to the action of GH in uremia is partially due to a quantitative reduction of GH receptor density in GH target organs, particularly in the liver. The specific metabolic signal of the uremic milieu responsible for

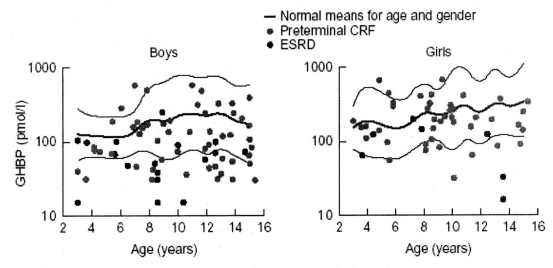

Figure 23–3. Serum GHBP concentrations in 75 boys (left panel) and 51 girls (right panel) with CRF related to the age- and gender-dependent normal range (−2 to +2 SD score). The bold line indicates the normal mean for age and gender. Open symbols represent children with preterminal CRF, closed symbols represent children with ESRD receiving dialysis. (From Tönshoff et al.[47] With permission.)

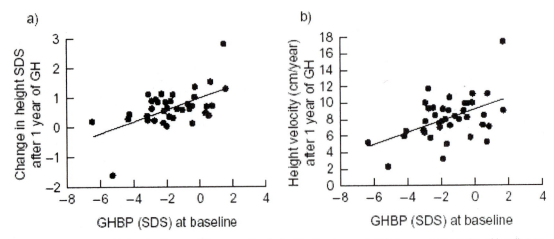

Figure 23–5. Change (Δ) in height SD score (A) and height velocity (B) after 1 year of rhGH therapy as a function of baseline age- and gender-related serum GHBP levels (SD score) in 40 prepubertal children with CRF treated with rh/GH at a dosage of 28 IU/m² body surface area in daily subcutaneous injections. There was a significant positive correlation (A: $r = 0.57$, $p < 0.0001$; B: $r = 0.48$, $p < 0.005$. (From Tönshoff et al.[47] With permission.)

the low GHBP/GH receptor status in CRF remains to be elucidated. Acquired disease states associated with GH insensitivity—such as acute fasting, chronic malnutrition and insulin-dependent diabetes mellitus—also have reduced serum GHBP activity. In experimental uremia, subcutaneous GH treatment altered neither hepatic GH receptor transcript abundance nor serum GHBP levels.[57] Similarly, circulating GHBP levels in children with CRF did not change during rhGH therapy.[47] Hence, the growth-promoting effect of GH, given subcutaneously, is not mediated by hepatic GH receptor upregulation.

Growth Hormone Signaling. Recent evidence indicates that GH resistance in renal failure may be due in part to an acquired defect in the GH-activated Janus kinase 2 (JAK2)-signal transducer and activator of transcription (STAT) pathway.[58] Normally, binding of GH to its receptor induces receptor dimerization, which is followed by autophosphorylation of JAK2, a tyrosine kinase associated with the intracellular domain of the receptor.[59] The activated JAK2, in turn, phosphorylates selective members of the STAT family of proteins, namely STAT1, STAT3, STAT5a, and STAT5b. The phosphorylated STATs form dimers that translocate into the nucleus, bind to specific promoter sequences of GH-dependent genes, and transactivate or repress their transcription (Fig. 23–6). Male mice with STAT5b deficiency and female mice with a combined deletion of STAT5a and STAT5b isoforms are severely growth retarded.[60,61]

In uremic rats, hepatic GH receptor mRNA levels are significantly decreased, but GH receptor protein abundance and GH binding to microsomal and plasma membranes are unaltered. JAK2, STAT1, STAT3, and STAT5 protein abundance are also unchanged. However, GH-induced tyrosine phosphorylation of JAK2, STAT5, and STAT3 was found to be 75 percent lower in the uremic animals. Phosphorylated

STAT5 and STAT3 were also diminished in nuclear extracts.[58]

In the past few years, a family of proteins has been discovered that bind to cytokine receptor–JAK2 complexes and inhibits the kinase activity of JAK2.[62] GH induces the expression of some of these suppressors of cytokine signaling (SOCS), namely SOCS-1, -2, -3, and CIS, through the JAK–STAT signaling pathway. These suppressors, in turn, inhibit activation of the GH receptor–JAK2 complex or STAT5 phosphorylation, thus serving as a negative feedback loop regulating GH activity.[63–65] Deletion of the SOCS2 gene leads to gigantism in mice.[66] In experimental uremia, SOCS2 and SOCS3 mRNA levels increase[58] and, if followed by an increase in protein expression, could be a cause of the depressed JAK2-STAT activity. The mechanism accounting for the increase in SOCS mRNA levels in uremia when GH-activated JAK2-STAT signaling is impaired is somewhat of a puzzle. One potential mechanism could involve the action of cytokines that induce signal transduction through the activation of other members of the JAK family, such as JAK1, JAK3, and Tyk2, that may be unaffected by uremia. It is also possible that the increase in SOCS expression in uremia might be mediated by GH through a non-STAT-mediated pathway.[67] Finally, it should be recognized that uremia affects several biological processes, including gene stability and transcription, interaction between signaling pathways, and the action of a number of hormones and cytokines.

An acquired defect of GH-induced JAK–STAT signaling also occurs in inflammatory states[68,69] that may arise from the overexpression of SOCS. Following administration of endotoxin, phosphorylation of JAK2 is depressed even though GH receptor abundance is unchanged.[68] However, because of an increase in JAK2 protein levels, total phosphorylated JAK2 remains the same. Nevertheless, de-

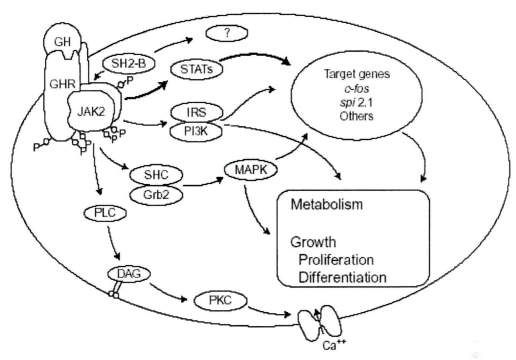

Figure 23–6. Possible signaling pathways initiated by binding of GH. GHR, GH receptor; P, phosphorylated tyrosines; JAK, Janus kinase; ISR, insulin receptor substrate; PI3K, phosphatidylinositol-3-kinase; PLC, phospholipase C; DAG, diacylglycerol; PKC, protein kinase C; MAPK, mitogen-activated protein kinase; STAT, signal transducer and activator of transcription. (From Carter-Su et al.[59] With permission.)

spite this compensation, downstream STAT5 phosphorylation is impaired. These changes are accompanied by an acute increase in SOCS-3 and CIS and, to a lesser degree, SOCS-2 expression. As chronic inflammation is common in patients with advanced kidney disease requiring dialysis treatment, it is conceivable that persistent inflammation with proinflammatory cytokine release may worsen the resistance to GH and thus play a role in the genesis of malnutrition, which is common in these patients.[70]

Insulin-Like Growth Factor (IGF)/IGF Binding Protein (IGFBP) Serum Levels. The effect of GH on longitudinal growth is partially mediated by the IGFs. Serum IGF-I and -II levels in children with preterminal CRF are in the normal range,[71] whereas in ESRD mean age-related serum IGF-I levels are slightly but significantly decreased and IGF-II levels slightly but significantly elevated (Fig. 23–7).[72,73] Hence, total immunoreactive IGF levels in CRF serum are normal but IGF bioactivity, measured by sulfate incorporation into porcine costal cartilage, is markedly reduced.[74,75] Similarly, the level of free IGF-I is reduced by 50 percent in relation to the degree of renal dysfunction.[76] This finding is one of the key abnormalities of the GH/IGF axis in children with CRF.

The discrepancy between normal total immunoreactive IGF levels and decreased IGF bioactivity has been explained by the presence of IGF inhibitors in CRF se-

rum. Uremic serum contains low-molecular-weight (about 1 kDa) IGF inhibitors, the molecular structures of which have not yet been defined.[74] The prevailing inhibitory effect on IGF bioactivity in CRF serum is due to an excess of high-affinity IGFBPs. Six IGFBPs have been distinguished on the basis of their amino acid sequences, which are encoded by different genes.[77,78] The IGFBPs, which are Mr ~30-kDa proteins and are named in the order of their molecular cloning, comprise a unique protein family. The IGFs circulate bound to IGFBPs in complexes of 150 kDa (major) and 35 kDa (minor). The 35-kDa serum fractions contain IGFBP-1, -2, -4, and -6, which are not found in the 150-kDa fractions. IGFBP-1 (28 kDa) is GH-independent, and insulin is the principal suppressive regulator of hepatic IGFBP-1 production.[79] IGFBP-2 (32 kDa) is the second most abundant IGFBP in the circulation. It binds IGF-II with a greater affinity than IGF-I. IGFBP-1 and -2 are major contributors to the unsaturated IGFBP pool found primarily in the 35 kDa serum fraction.[80,81] IGFBP-3, the most abundant serum IGFBP during extrauterine life, has many similarities to IGFBP-5: (1) both can potentiate IGF action, (2) both are upregulated by GH, and (3) both are closely related structurally, sharing among other motifs an 18 amino acid heparin-binding domain that allows them to bind the ALS after binding either IGF-I or IGF-II. The subsequent constituted ternary complex has a molecular weight of approximately 150 kDa.[82] It is thought to act as a reser-

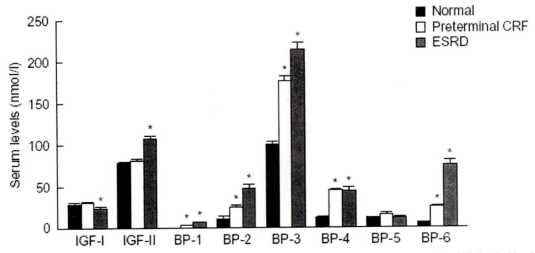

Figure 23–7. Comparison of the molar serum concentrations of IGFs and IGFBPs in children with preterminal CRF (hatched bars) and children with ESRD (filled bars). The respective mean molar concentration in normal age-matched children is given in open bars for comparison. Data are mean + SEM. *Significant vs. control. (From Ulinski et al.[73] With permission.)

voir and a buffer for IGF-I and IGF-II, preventing rapid changes of free IGF levels.

Serum levels of intact IGFBP-1, -2, -4, and -6 are elevated in CRF serum in relation to the degree of renal dysfunction (Figs. 23–8 and 23–9).[73,83–86] These four IGFBPs, which have a high affinity for IGFs, are found in excess in the 35-kDa fractions of CRF sera. In contrast, serum levels of intact IGFBP-3 are normal, but there is an increase in immunoreactive low-molecular-weight fragments of IGFBP-3, in particular a 29-kDa fragment designated IGFBP-3,[29] which has a reduced affinity for IGF peptides.[87] Levels of

immunoreactive IGFBP-5 are not altered in CRF serum, but the majority of IGFBP-5 is fragmented.[73,86]

Figure 23–7 shows the relative contribution of all six IGFBPs to the increased IGF-binding capacity of CRF serum. The relative increase of the respective serum IGFBPs in preterminal CRF ranges from 1.8-fold of control for immunoreactive IGFBP-3 to 4.8-fold for IGFBP-6. Taken together, there is approximately a 25 percent molar excess of IGFBPs over IGFs in the serum of healthy children, whereas in preterminal CRF the molar excess of IGFBPs over IGFs is approximately 150 percent and in ESRD 200

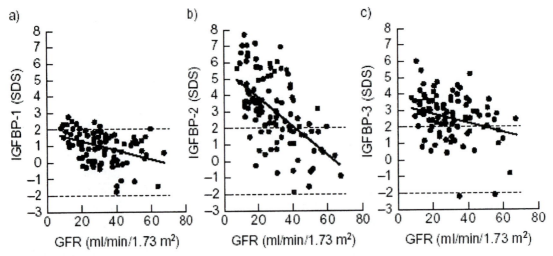

Figure 23–8. Age-related serum IGFBP-1 (panel A), IGFBP-2 (panel B), and IGFBP-3 levels (panel C) as a function of GFR in children with CRF ($n = 94$). A. $r = -0.42$, $p < 0.001$; B. $r = -0.56$, $p < 0.001$; C: $r = -0.28$, $p < 0.005$. The slope of the regression line between GFR and IGFBP-2 SD score was significantly steeper than that observed for IGFBP-1 and for IGFBP-3. (From Tönshoff et al.[71] With permission.)

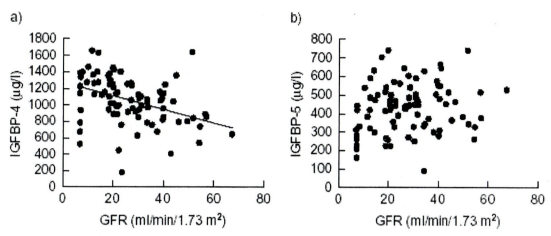

Figure 23–9. Serum IGFBP-4 (panel A) and IGFBP-5 (panel B) as a function of GFR in children with CRF ($n = 89$). There was a significant inverse correlation between GFR and IGFBP-4 ($r = -0.39$, $p < 0.001$) but not IGFBP-5 ($r = 0.16$, $p = 0.14$). From Ulinski et al.[73] With permission.)

percent (Fig. 23–7). This estimation is in good agreement with the finding of a seven- to tenfold increase of free IGF-II binding capacity in the serum of children with preterminal CRF and ESRD, respectively.[75] In summary, these data demonstrate a progressive increase of serum IGFBPs in children with CRF in parallel to the decline of renal function. It is likely that the greater IGFBP excess in ESRD compared with preterminal CRF contributes both to more severe growth retardation and to the reduced response to exogenous GH therapy in these children.[88]

IGF-I Secretion. The pattern of normal immunoreactive IGF serum levels and markedly increased IGFBP levels is unique for CRF. The constellation of increased IGFBP over IGFs also suggests that "normal" IGF-I and IGF-II levels in CRF cannot be interpreted as a consequence of normal production rates of these peptides. In CRF, the binding capacity of IGF capacity is increased by an order of magnitude.[75] Because of the short metabolic half-life of free IGF, one would expect that, under normal conditions, increased IGF binding capacity would be immediately saturated by IGFs produced in the liver. The consequence would be a progressive increase of IGFs concomitantly with the rise in IGFBP as GFR declines. However, this tendency exists only for IGF-II.[71] Hence, the normal serum concentrations of IGF-I in preterminal CRF appear to be inadequately low. This discrepancy is even more pronounced in children with ESRD, in whom slightly decreased serum IGF-I levels are found in the presence of increased IGFBPs and of elevated circulating GH levels.[41,72] Analysis of this complex system using a mathematical model indicated that data from children with CRF are consistent with a markedly reduced IGF-I production rate (Fig. 23–10).[89] Consistent with this hypothesis, he-

patic IGF-I gene expression in experimental uremia is reduced by 50 percent in nonacidotic animals compared with pair-fed controls.[90] This observation adds further evidence to the concept of GH insensitivity in the uremic state.

Mechanism of Increased IGFBP Levels in CRF Serum. Theoretically, increased IGFBP levels in CRF serum could result

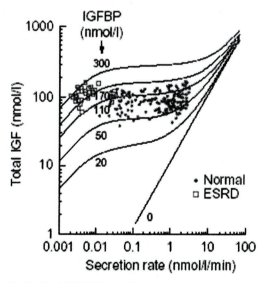

Figure 23–10. Total IGF (IGF-I plus IGF-II) levels as a function of total secretion rate in the presence of various concentrations of IGFBP (0, 20, 50, 110, 170, and 300 nmol/L). The curves were calculated by a kinetic model. Values from normal individuals and from patients with ESRD were added to the graph according to their measured total IGF and IGFBP-3 concentrations. (From Blum.[89] With permission.)

from increased production, reduced transcapillary movement, reduced elimination by the diseased kidneys, or a combination of these factors. The inverse correlation of serum immunoreactive IGFBP-1, -2, -3, -4, and -6 with residual GFR in children with CRF is consistent with the concept that elevated IGFBPs result from impaired renal filtration. Similarly, there is a rapid decline of immunoreactive IGFBP-3 in patients with ESRD after restoration of renal function by a functioning transplant.[72] Notably, increased proteolytic degradation of the IGFBP-3 ternary complex, as described during pregnancy and catabolic states, appears not to be operative in patients with CRF.[91,92] The lack of increase in IGFBP-5 with progressive renal dysfunction has been interpreted as indirect evidence of reduced IGFBP-5 production in advanced CRF, because IGFBP-5 is a GH-responsive IGFBP, the production of which might be reduced as a consequence of GH insensitivity.[73]

Increased hepatic production of IGFBP-1 and -2 appears to contribute to increased IGFBP levels in CRF, as concluded from data in experimental uremia showing a twofold increase of IGFBP-1 mRNA and a fourfold increase of IGFBP-2 mRNA in liver tissue (Fig. 23–11).[90] This alteration is tissue-specific, because IGFBP-2 gene expression in kidney tissue is reduced in CRF. IGFBP-1 regulation is primarily transcriptional, with insulin being the major inhibitor of IGFBP-1 expression. Thus, the insulin resistance of CRF may contribute to high IGFBP-1 levels. The specific metabolic signal responsible for the marked increase of hepatic IGFBP-2 gene expression remains to be elucidated. Because IGFBP-2 mRNA levels are elevated in diabetic[93] and hypophysectomized[94] rats, it has been suggested that insulin and GH are involved in the long-term regulation of hepatic IGFBP-2 gene expression. Insensitivity to the action of GH and insulin in uremic rats might therefore contribute to increased hepatic IGFBP-2 gene expression.

IGFBPs as Modulators of IGF Action in Vitro.   The prevailing inhibitory effect on IGF bioactivity in CRF serum is due to an excess of inhibitory IGFBPs. The removal of these unsaturated IGFBPs from CRF patient sera by affinity chromatography with an IGF-II Sepharose column restores IGF bioactivity in the porcine growth cartilage assay,[75] indicating that unsaturated IGFBPs in CRF serum inhibit the ability of IGFs to act on cartilage tissue in vitro.

To inhibit IGF-mediated linear growth, IGFBPs must accumulate in extravascular fluids in sufficient quantity to block IGF effects on growth plate chondrocytes. IGFBP-1 and -2 and low-molecular-weight forms of IGFBP-3 migrate into lymph fluid and thereby have access to interstitial spaces.[95] Levels of IGFBP-1 and -2 in extravascular fluids, such as lymph and peritoneal dialysate, are 10 percent of serum levels, or 2 nmol/L in the case of IGFBP-1 in the peritoneal dialysate of CRF children.[96] This concentration exceeds the 0.2 nmol IGFBP-1/L needed to inhibit basal growth of chick embryo pelvic cartilage in organ culture.[97] A molar excess of these high-affinity IGFBPs in IGF target tissues can therefore inhibit IGF action through their unsaturated IGF binding sites, thereby preventing the interaction of IGFs with the type 1 IGF receptor.

The biological activity of various intact IGFBPs and their respective fragments from CRF serum has recently been studied systematically in the cartilage model of cul-

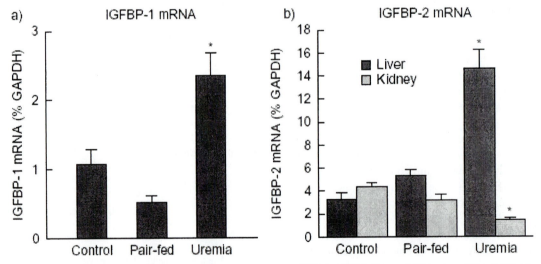

Figure 23–11. Quantification of IGFBP-1 mRNA in liver (panel A) and IGFBP-2 mRNA in liver and kidney (panel B) quantified by Northern blot analysis. Values are expressed as percent of GAPDH expression. *Significant vs. ad libitum–fed controls and pair-fed controls. (From Tönshoff et al.[90] With permission.)

tured growth plate chondrocytes (Table 23–2). IGFBPs-1, -2, and -6 act exclusively as growth inhibitors on IGF-dependent proliferation of growth plate chondrocytes, whereas the biological activity of IGFBP-3 is complex. It has an IGF-independent antiproliferative effect and also inhibits IGF-dependent chondrocyte proliferation under coincubation conditions. Under preincubation conditions, however, IGFBP-3 enhances the IGF-I responsiveness of growth plate chondrocytes by its ability to associate with the cell membrane, where it facilitates IGF-I receptor binding.[100] The IGFBP-3 fragment from CRF serum, IGFBP-3,[29] has limited ability to inhibit IGF-II–mediated mitogenic effects and no ability to inhibit IGF-I–mediated mitogenic effects in cultured osteosarcoma cells, probably due to the low affinity of IGFBP-3 for IGF peptides.[87] IGFBP-4 and -5 have contrasting functions in growth plate chondrocytes.[101] Both intact IGFBP-4 and the fragment IGFBP-4[1–122] have an exclusive inhibitory role in IGF-I-stimulated cells by binding IGF-I in the *N*-terminal domain and preventing or reducing the binding of ligand to its signaling receptor. Intact IGFBP-5, on the other hand, stimulates chondrocyte proliferation, apparently by its association with the cell membrane in the C-terminal domain, thereby better presenting IGF-I to its receptor. However, if accumulated *N*-terminal forms of IGFBP-5 predominate, IGFBP-5 inhibits IGF-I-stimulated proliferation. This action of *N*-terminal IGFBP-5 in chondrocytes contrasts with its stimulatory effect on osteoblast activity and may be important in preserving the cartilage-to-bone developmental sequence that is necessary for normal longitudinal bone growth.

IGFBPs as Modulators of IGF Action in Vivo. There is now direct evidence that circulating IGFBPs are capable of inhibiting growth in nonuremic experimental animals (Table 23–2). Coinjection of IGFBP-1 inhibited the GH- or IGF-I–stimulated weight gain and tibial epiphyseal widening of hypophysectomized rats in a dose-dependent manner.[106] In addition, transgenic mice overexpressing IGFBP-1 in multiple tissues or in liver alone are markedly growth-retarded.[102,103] Similarly, mice overexpressing IGFBP-2 show a reduced postnatal weight gain[104] and inhibition of GH-stimulated growth in giant GH transgenic mice.[107] Overexpression of IGFBP-3 in transgenic mice, leading to a 4.9- to 7.7-fold increase in serum IGFBP-3 levels, produced modest intrauterine and postnatal growth retardation, despite elevated levels of circulating IGF-I.[105] This suggests that, in vivo, the inhibitory effects of excess IGFBP-3 on chondrocyte growth predominate over the modest growth-stimulatory effects observed with IGFBP-3 preincubation.

An important question is whether the imbalance between normal total IGF and the excess of unsaturated IGFBPs contributes to growth failure in the setting of clinical CRF. The normal relationship between circulating IGF-I and relative height is clearly disturbed in CRF (Fig. 23–12).[71] The significantly less steep regression line between height and IGF-I in CRF is consistent with the presence of IGF inhibitors, indicating that the inhibition of IGF bioactivity for stimulation of longitudinal growth is also operative in vivo. Serum levels of IGFBP-1, -2, and -4 correlate significantly and inversely with standardized height in children with CRF, implying that these two IGFBPs con-

TABLE 23–2. INSULIN-LIKE GROWTH FACTOR BINDING PROTEINS[a]

IGFBP	Concentration in CRF Plasma	Correlation to Growth in Clinical CRF	Effect on Growth Plate Chondrocyte Proliferation[A]		Growth in Transgenic Animals
			Intrinsic	IGF-Dependent	
Intact IGFBP-1	Increased (71,85)	Negative (71)	None (100)	↓ (100)	Pre-/postnatally reduced (102,103)
Intact IGFBP-2	Increased (71,85)	Negative (71,85)	None (100)	↓ (100)	Postnatally reduced (104)
Intact IGFBP-3	Normal (84,85)	None[C] (71,85)	↓ (100)	↓ / ↑(100)[B]	Pre-/postnatally reduced (105)
IGFBP-3[29]	Increased (87)	ND	None[D] (87)	↓ (IGF-II)[D] (87)	
Intact IGFBP-4	Increased (73,86)	Negative (73)	None (101)	↓ (101)	ND
IGFBP-4(1–122)	+ (98)	ND	None (101)	↓ (101)	
IGFBP-4(136–237)	+ (98)	ND	None (101)	None (101)	
Intact IGFBP-5	Normal[C] (73,86)	Positive[C] (73,86)	↑ 101)	↑ (101)	ND
IGFBP-5(1–169)	ND	ND	None (101)	↓ (101)	
IGFBP-5(144–252)	+ (99)	ND	None (101)	None (101)	
Intact IGFBP-6	Increased (83)	None (83)	None(100)	↓ (100)	ND

Key: IGFBP, insulin-like growth factor binding proteins; +, fragments present; ND, not done; ↓, inhibitory; ↑, stimulatory; [A]rat growth plate chondrocytes in primary culture; [B]dependent on cell culture conditions; [C]immunoreactive IGFBP levels; [D]human chondrosarcoma cells.

[a] Shown is the concentration of intact insulin-like growth factor binding proteins (IGFBPs) and their respective fragments in CRF plasma, their correlation with parameters of longitudinal growth in children with CRF, their intrinsic and IGF-dependent effect on growth plate chondrocyte proliferation, and the effect of their respective overexpression on growth in transgenic animals. References are in brackets.

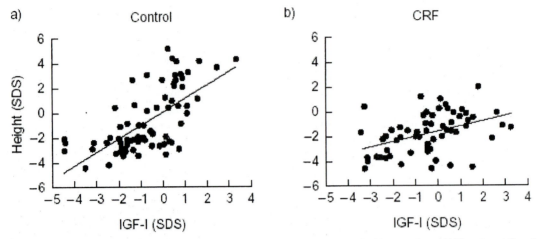

Figure 23–12. Age-related height (SDS) as a function of serum IGF-I levels (SDS) in healthy prepubertal children (panel A) and prepubertal children with CRF (panel B). A. $r = 0.67$, $p < 0.001$; $y = -0.006 + 1.08x$. B. $r = 0.43$, $p < 0.001$; $y = -1.69 + 0.41x$. The slope of the regression in children with CRF was significantly less steep than that in controls. From Tönshoff et al.[71] with permission.)

tribute to the growth failure in these children.[71,73,85] IGF-I (in a positive fashion) and IGFBP-2 (in a negative fashion) contribute independently to the statistical prediction of relative height in children with CRF (Fig. 23–13).[71] The potential role of serum IGFBP-3 in longitudinal growth appears to be more complex. There is neither a positive relationship between immunoreactive IGFBP-3 and standardized height in CRF, as observed under normal conditions in healthy children, nor a negative correlation, which would be expected if IGFBP-3 acted merely as an IGF inhibitor in CRF.[71] On the other hand, GH therapy in CRF induced an increase in serum IGFBP-3 levels. This correlated with im-

proved growth in these children,[85] suggesting a potential growth-stimulatory effect of intact IGFBP-3 in this setting. These discrepant finding are probably due to the molecular heterogeneity of IGFBP-3 in CRF serum, comprising both intact IGFBP-3 and low-molecular-weight fragments, particularly IGFBP-3,[29] with reduced IGF-binding capacity.[87] In contrast, serum IGFBP-5 levels are positively correlated with both standardized height and height velocity among children with CRF, consistent with a potential stimulatory role of this IGFBP on longitudinal growth.[73] Serum IGF-BP-6 levels are not correlated with relative height in children with CRF, suggesting that interactions between serum IGFBP-6 and skeletal growth, if present, are probably complex.[83]

The Impact of GH Therapy on Serum Levels of IGF/IGFBP. If longitudinal growth is stimulated by circulating IGF-I and inhibited by circulating IGFBPs, GH therapy, an effective growth-promoting strategy in CRF, should alter the serum profile of IGF-I and IGFBPs. Supraphysiologic doses of GH induce a rapid and persistent increase in serum IGF-I and, to a lesser extent, IGF-II levels in children with CRF[85,108–110] (Fig. 23–14). During GH treatment, levels of IGF-I and IGF-II correlate positively with the increment in longitudinal growth, suggesting a role for the IGFs in GH-induced catch-up growth.[85] Similarly, levels of "free" or readily accessible IGF-I rise during GH therapy. GH therapy lowers serum levels of the inhibitory binding protein IGFBP-1 by approximately 50 percent (Fig. 23–14) in association with increased serum insulin levels, suggesting that insulin mediates the GH inhibition of IGFBP-1 levels. Levels of IGFBP-2 and -6 are unaffected by GH therapy;

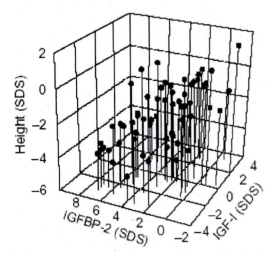

Figure 23–13. Age-related height (SDS) in prepubertal children with CRF as a function of serum IGF-I levels (SDS) and IGFBP-2 levels (SDS). Height could be predicted from a linear combination of the independent variables IGF-I and IGFBP-2 ($r = 0.54$, $p < 0.001$). (From Tönshoff et al.[71] With permission.)

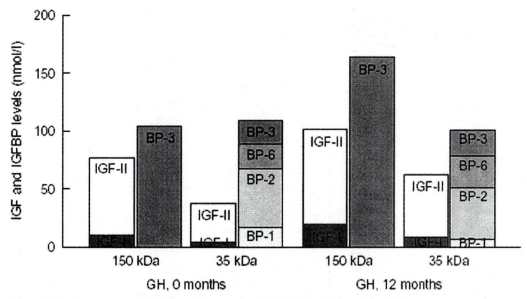

Figure 23–14. Balance between IGFBPs and IGFs in serum of CRF children before and after rhGH treatment. Levels (nanomoles per liter) of IGF-I, IGF-II, IGFBP-1, IGFBP-2, IGFBP-3, and IGFBP-6 in the 150- and 35-kDa fractions of CRF serum are presented. (From Powell et al.[110] With permission.)

IGFBP-4 levels do not change after 3 months of GH[73] but increase slightly after 12 months of therapy.[86] The levels of IGFBP-3, -5, and ALS, all components of the 150-kDa ternary complex, rise with GH treatment and show significant positive correlations with the increment in height.[85] The GH-induced increase in serum IGFBP-3 is confined to the 150-kDa serum fractions.[110] This suggests a role of the ternary complex in GH-induced catch-up growth. IGFs in the ternary complex are probably released by proteolysis of IGFBP-3. This lowers the affinity of IGFBP-3 for IGFs, allowing release of IGFs to proteins with higher affinity, such as IGFBPs in the 35-kDa serum fractions and the type 1 IGF receptor on target tissues. These changes of the serum IGF/IGFBP profile lead to a threefold increase of the initially depressed IGF bioactivity into the normal range.[108] It is also possible that GH-induced increases in serum IGF-BP-3 and -5 are accompanied by increased levels of these IGFBPs in extravascular fluids at target tissues, such as growth plate cartilage. Here, proteolysis of IGFBP-3 and -5 may stimulate growth by releasing bound IGFs in a process that does not involve ALS or the ternary complex.

In summary, GH exerts its stimulatory effect on longitudinal growth not by normalizing increased serum levels of inhibitory IGFBPs, but by increasing serum IGF levels. Some of the GH-induced IGF is bound in new serum ternary complexes, but the majority of stimulated IGF circulates in the 35-kDa serum fractions bound to previously unsaturated excess IGFBPs. This GH-induced rise in levels of IGFs relative to IGFBPs in the 35-kDa fractions of CRF serum presumably leads to an increase of IGFs in extravascular fluids, from whence circulating IGFs have access to

their target tissues (i.e., the growth plate), to interact with the type 1 IGF receptor for stimulation of longitudinal growth.

Summary

Disturbances of the somatotropic hormone axis play an important pathogenic role in growth retardation and catabolism in children with CRF. A simplified overview of the derangements of the somatotropic hormone axis is given in Fig. 23–15. Whereas the GH secretion rate in CRF is variable between patients and studies, a prolonged half-life of GH as a result of a reduced renal metabolic clearance rate is a consistent finding. Accordingly, the serum GH levels in children with CRF are normal or elevated depending on the extent of renal failure. The apparent discrepancy between normal or elevated GH levels and diminished longitudinal growth in CRF has led to the concept of GH insensitivity, which is caused by multiple alterations in the distal components of the somatotropic hormone axis. Serum levels of IGF-I and IGF-II are normal in preterminal CRF, while in ESRD, IGF-I levels are slightly decreased and IGF-II levels slightly increased. In view of the prevailing elevated GH levels in ESRD, these serum IGF-I levels appear as inadequately low. Indeed, there is both clinical and experimental evidence for decreased hepatic production of IGF-I in CRF. This hepatic insensitivity to the action of GH may be partly the consequence of reduced GH receptor expression in liver tissue and partly a consequence of disturbed GH receptor signaling. The action and metabolism of IGFs are modulated by specific high-affinity IGFBPs. CRF serum has a

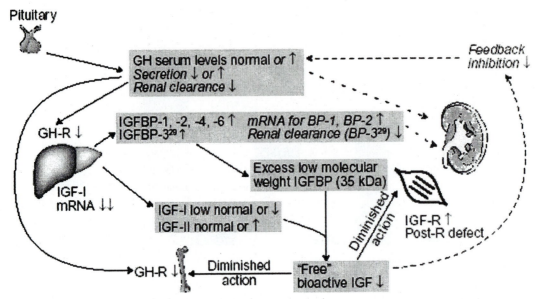

Figure 23–15. Current concept of the derangements of the somatotropic hormone axis in children with CRF.

seven- to tenfold increased IGF-binding capacity that leads to decreased IGF bioactivity of CRF serum despite normal total IGF levels. Serum levels of intact IGFBP-1, -2, -4, -6 and low-molecular-weight fragments of IGFBP-3 are elevated in CRF serum in relation to the degree of renal dysfunction, whereas serum levels of intact IGFBP-3 are normal. Levels of immunoreactive IGFBP-5 are not altered in CRF serum, but the majority of IGFBP-5 is fragmented. Both decreased renal filtration and increased hepatic production of IGFBP-1 and -2 contribute to high levels of serum IGFBP. Experimental and clinical evidence suggests that these excessive high-affinity IGFBPs in CRF serum inhibit IGF action on target tissues by competition with the type 1 IGF receptor for IGF binding. The relevance of the impact of alterations of the somatotropic hormone axis is underlined by the efficacy of GH therapy in growth-retarded children with CRF. The beneficial effect of GH therapy on longitudinal growth in children with appears to be mediated partially by the stimulation of hepatic IGF synthesis, which results in an improved ratio of growth-stimulatory IGFs versus inhibitory IGFBPs in the circulation and, most likely, also in the growth plate.

Growth Plate Disturbances in CRF

Morphology. Longitudinal bone growth results from progressive replacement of growth plate cartilage by osseous tissue at the metaphyseal ends (endochondral ossification) and modeling–remodeling of previously synthesized bone. Physiologically, the rate and extent of growth for a given growth plate is determined by a combination of chondrocyte proliferation, matrix production, and increase of chondrocyte volume.

In experimental uremia in the rat, multiple abnormalities of the growth plate have been described, although the findings regarding the width of the growth plate have been inconsistent. Indeed, growth plate width has been described as increased, reduced or unaltered compared with rats with intact renal function.[111–114] Such divergent findings may be attributable to differences in the severity and duration of CRF and the methodology used. Cobo and coworkers, in their elegant studies in a model of advanced CRF, described how the strict coordination between the processes of cartilage enlargement, cartilage resorption, and osseous tissue formation at the metaphyseal end is disturbed in CRF.[111] Cell proliferation, as assessed by bromodeoxyuridine labeling, did not differ between CRF and control rats, but both the production of cartilage and the ossification were significantly slowed down in uremic rats. However, the two processes were differentially depressed in the sense that cartilage resorption/bone deposition was affected to a higher degree than cartilage formation. This led to a disequilibrium that resulted in an increased growth plate height as a result of accumulation of cartilage at the hypertrophic zone. These changes were associated with an overall decrease in the expression of types II and X collagens, which was particularly marked in the abnormally extended zone of the hypertrophic cartilage.[115] Unlike collagen, the expression of collagenase-3 was not severely disturbed. Electron microscope analysis proved that changes in gene expression were coupled to alterations in mineralization as well as in the collagen fibril architecture at the hypertrophic cartilage. Because the composition and structure of the extracellular matrix have a critical role in regulating the behavior of the growth plate chondrocytes, these results are consistent with the hypothesis that alteration of collagen metabolism in these cells could be a key process underlying growth retardation in uremia.[115]

The degree of secondary hyperparathyroidism may have an impact on the morphology of the growth plate in uremia. A reduced growth plate width and disorganization of the growth plate cartilage of uremic animals with severe secondary hyperparathyroidism have been described.[116] Calcium supplementation in uremic rats to induce biochemical changes consistent with adynamic bone resulted in impaired linear growth associated with marked widening of the growth plate, and disturbances in chondrocyte apoptosis, matrix degradation, and angiogenesis.[117] Thus, both models of high- and low-turnover lesions are associated with growth retardation, but the growth plate abnormalities are markedly different.

PTH/PTH-Related Peptide Receptor. PTH-related peptide (PTHrP), which frequently causes the humoral hypercalcemia of malignancy syndrome, is an autocrine/paracrine regulator of chondrocyte proliferation and differentiation that acts through the PTH/PTHrP receptor (PTH1R). PTHrP is generated in response to Indian hedgehog, which mediates its actions through the membrane receptor patched, but interacts also with hedgehog-interacting protein (Fig. 23–16).[118] Mice lacking PTHrP show accelerated chondrocyte differentiation and thus premature ossification of those bones that are formed through an endochondral process[119]; similar but more severe abnormalities are observed in PTH1R-ablated animals.[120] The mirror image of these skeletal findings (i.e., a severe delay in chondrocyte differentiation and endochondral ossification) is observed in transgenic mice that overexpress PTHrP under the control

of the alpha1(II) procollagen promoter.[121] Severe abnormalities in chondrocyte proliferation and differentiation are also observed in two genetic disorders in humans that are most likely caused by mutations in the PTH1R. Heterozygous PTH1R mutations that lead to constitutive activity were identified in Jansen metaphyseal chondrodysplasia,[122] and homozygous or compound heterozygous mutations that lead to less active or completely inactive receptors were identified in patients with Blomstrand lethal chondrodysplasia.[123] Overall, these results underscore the pivotal role of the PTH/PTHrP in the regulation of chondrocyte differentiation and bone elongation.

Disturbance in the expression of the PTH/PTHrP receptor have been reported in renal failure.[124–127] Gene expression of the PTH/PTHrP receptor is downregulated in kidneys of rats with moderate to severe renal failure.[127] Moreover, reduced expression of the PTH/PTHrP receptor has been reported in osteoblasts of adults with ESRD, particularly in those with low-turnover lesions of bone.[128] In the growth plate, substantial reductions in PTH/PTHrP receptor expression were also found in uremic animals with severe secondary hyperparathyroidism, and treatment with GH appears to modify the expression of the PTH/PTHrP receptor in vivo.[116,126] Interestingly, these disturbances were not observed in nephrectomized rats with lesser degrees of secondary hyperparathyroidism or in those given calcium supplementation to induce adynamic bone.[117] Considering the crucial role of the PTH/PTHrP receptor in the regulation of endochondral bone growth, these findings suggest potential molecular mechanisms by which endochondral bone formation may be altered in renal failure, consequently leading to growth retardation.

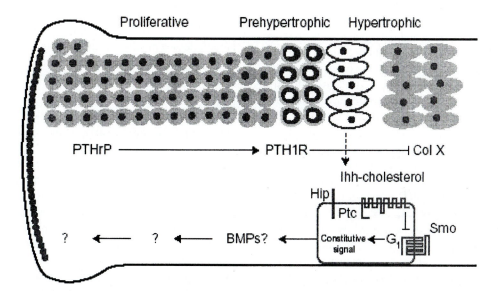

Figure 23–16. Regulation of chondrocyte proliferation and differentiation by PTHrP and Indian hedgehog (*Ihh*). (*Hip* hedgehog-interacting protein; *Ptc* patched; *Smo* smoothened; *Bmps* bone morphogenetic proteins; *Col X* collagen type X). (From Jüppner.[118] With permission.)

In summary, based on the growth plate abnormalities observed in these human disorders and in mice with abnormal expression of either PTHrP or the PTH1R, it appears plausible that impaired expression of PTHrP and/or its receptor contributes to the growth abnormalities in children with ESRD. Mild to moderate renal failure in animals leads to a reduction in PTH1R expression in growth plates and impaired growth, but it remains uncertain whether this contributes to altered chondrocyte growth and differentiation.

GH/IGF System. Little is known regarding alterations in the abundance and actions of the GH/IGF system at the level of the growth plate cartilage in CRF. There is decreased IGF-I gene expression, as demonstrated by in situ hybridization and immunohistochemistry in the growth plates of rats with CRF, and GH therapy increased IGF-I mRNA, particularly in proliferating chondrocytes.[114] Immunohistochemistry has shown that uremic rats have a decreased abundance of GH receptors in the proliferative zone, and only combined therapy with GH and IGF-I could overcome this decrease.[129] These data suggests that growth failure in experimental uremia is, at least in part, due to a decrease in GH receptor abundance in chondrocytes of the proliferative zone of the tibial growth plate. This decreased GH receptor abundance can be overcome by combined GH/IGF-I therapy, thus enhancing generation and proliferation of hypertrophic zone chondrocytes and increasing growth plate width. Metabolic acidosis might contribute to reduced growth factor expression in the growth plate, because murine mandibular condyles cultured in acidic medium exhibited less GH receptor, IGF-I and type 1 IGF receptor expression, and the expected increase in IGF-I mRNA expression with GH stimulation was inhibited in acidotic conditions.[130]

Impact of GH and Calcitriol Therapy on the Growth Plate in CRF. GH and calcitriol have potent and divergent effects on bone and mineral metabolism, and there is limited information on their potential interactions on chondrocyte proliferation and differentiation in renal failure. Dose-dependent inhibitory effects of calcitriol on chondrocyte proliferation have been shown in vitro, and neither GH nor IGF-I can overcome these inhibitory effects.[131,132] *In vivo*, calcitriol doses ranging from 50 to 2000 ng/kg per day impair linear growth.[133-135] Moreover, Kainer and coworkers found that combined therapy with calcitriol and GH abolished the beneficial effects of GH on growth.[136] Calcitriol appears to attenuate the trophic effects of GH therapy on chondrocyte proliferation and differentiation, as judged by reductions in thickness of the growth plate cartilage. In addition, calcitriol appears to offset the GH-induced increases in type X collagen and type II collagen gene expression in animals with advanced secondary hyperparathyroidism.[116] Also, in vitro data indicate that the antiproliferative actions of calcitriol in the growth plate contribute to the reductions in

longitudinal bone growth observed during GH therapy in CRF. High and growth-inhibitory doses of calcitriol blocked the IGF-I-induced cell proliferation in an in vitro cell culture model.[137] These findings support the concept that calcitriol modifies the trophic actions of GH on bone and growth plate cartilage and that it can influence the process of endochondral bone formation.

GROWTH PATTERN IN CHILDREN WITH CRF

The regulatory mechanisms of statural growth during childhood differ in the successive stages of development. During the first 2 years of life, growth is mainly driven by nutritional factors, particularly the intake of energy and protein. In later childhood, growth appears to depend mainly on the somatotropic axis, with nutrition exerting a more permissive influence. During puberty, the growth process is dominated by the gonadotropic hormone axis, which stimulates and finally terminates body growth by a direct action on the growth cartilage and by modulation of the somatotropic axis. In view of these differences in growth regulation, growth in renal disorders will be described separately for the periods of infancy, midchildhood, and puberty.

The first 2 years of life are the most dynamic period of growth. Some 30 percent of total postnatal statural growth is normally achieved during this period. Any disturbance of growth in infancy has a greater impact on growth potential than at later stages of development. Spontaneous growth in children with congenital CRF is characterized by a rapidly increasing height deficit during the first 2 years of life (Fig. 23–17).[138] Thereafter, the growth pattern parallels the normal growth channel observed in mid-childhood. In the late prepubertal period, height velocity again decreases disproportionately, resulting in a further deviation from the normal percentiles. A later pubertal growth spurt of diminished amplitude eventually results in an irreversible loss of growth potential, leading to a stunted adult height (Fig. 23–17).

Infancy

Untreated CRF during early infancy is usually associated with severe growth retardation.[139-143] The loss in relative height is greatest during the first year of life, particularly during the first 6 months. A detailed analysis of the early infantile growth pattern according to the infancy–childhood–puberty model of Karlberg revealed that the infancy growth phase, starting in intra-uterine life and ending during the second year of life, is affected in 50 percent of patients with CRF.[144] Height SDS was already slightly reduced at birth, decreased further during the first 3 postnatal months, stabilized between 3 and 9 months, and decreased again between 10 and 12 months of life. After a transient stabilization of growth rate, a further loss in relative height

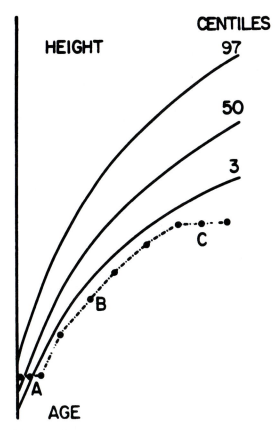

Figure 23–17. Schematic representation of growth in children with renal insufficiency dating from infancy. A, B, and C represent periods of growth. Period A represents the first 2 years of life; period B represents a period of stable renal function from 2 years of age until the onset of puberty; period C represents the development of ESRD at puberty. (From Betts and Macgrath.[138] With permission.)

apparently occurred between 0.75 and 1.5 years of age. In the mechanistic infancy–childhood–puberty model,[144] this period reflects the transition from the infancy to the childhood growth phase (Fig. 23–18). The height deficit acquired during this period may be due either to a delayed onset of the childhood growth phase or to a temporary "offset" of the childhood growth phase. In unselected patients studied by Karlberg and coworkers,[144] a loss of height SDS of nearly 4 SD was observed at the end of the third year of life. The reasons for this secondary deterioration of growth in infancy, which may occur despite adequate nutritional and medical supplementation, are still poorly understood. If the hypothesis is correct that the childhood growth component is mainly driven by the somatotropic axis, the growth patterns during this transitional period could represent changes between periods of normal (infancy and childhood components operative) and impaired GH action (only infancy component intact). With regard to early postnatal life, anorexia, water and electrolyte imbalances caused by uremia, recurrent vomiting, catabolic responses to infections,

and metabolic acidosis have been cited as the main factors compromising this period of growth.

Midchildhood

During the midchildhood period, growth is mainly regulated by endocrine mechanisms. Patients with a reduced renal mass, for example with hypoplastic renal disease, usually grow along the percentile attained at the end of infancy.[145] Patients who develop CRF after the second year of life lose relative height early in the course of the disease and follow the growth percentile after stabilization of the disease process. The degree of renal dysfunction is the principal determinant of the variability in growth during this period. A retrospective analysis in patients with hypoplastic kidney disorders showed a slightly but continuously lower annual growth rate in patients with a glomerular filtration rate (GFR) below 25 mL/min/1.73 m^2 compared with patients above this limit, cumulating in a mean height difference of 6 cm between these subgroups at the age of 10 years[145] (Fig. 23–19). Growth rates were consistently correlated with the patients' average GFR, although only 10 to 15 percent of the variability in growth was actually accounted for by this parameter. The degree of anemia, metabolic acidosis, and malnutrition contributed only marginally to the annual growth rate. It is suggested that catch-up growth is continuously suppressed in the uremic milieu. The percentile-parallel growth pattern during the midchildhood period may therefore reflect a net balance between the growth-suppressive effect of uremia and the inherent tendency for catch-up growth.

Puberty

The onset of puberty is usually delayed in adolescents with CRF. Roughly, two-thirds of adolescents with ESRD enter puberty beyond the normal age range.[146] The early cross-sectional survey published by the European Dialysis and Transplant Association (EDTA) Registry showed that sexual maturation was generally retarded in adolescent boys and girls with ESRD.[147,148] In all, 50 percent of children achieved the subsequent pubertal stages beyond the age when 97 percent of a normal population have passed these maturation hallmarks.[148–150] Later reports confirmed this degree of pubertal delay.[147,151] Late puberty was observed both in children on dialysis and after renal transplantation.

More recently, the Cooperative Study Group for Pubertal Development in CRF followed some 70 patients prospectively through the process of pubertal maturation. In this study the onset of puberty was delayed by an average of 2 to 2.5 years (152). The start of genital maturation (Tanner G2) was delayed by 1.8 years in uremic and 2.5 years in transplanted boys. Full genital maturation was achieved with a delay of 2.2 and 3.2 years, respectively. Thus, once started, puberty appears to proceed at a normal rate. How-

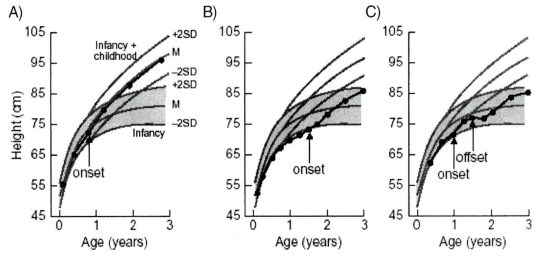

Figure 23–18. Examples of normal and abnormal growth patterns observed in CRF. **A.** normal growth pattern in a CRF patient. Smooth decelerating path during the infancy phase and a smooth transition into the infancy + childhood phase at about 0.75 years of age, representing the age at onset of the childhood component. **B.** CRF patient with normal smooth path of growth in infancy, but with delayed childhood onset (> 1 year of age) seen in 36 percent of all children with congenital CRF. **C.** CRF patient with a childhood onset at 1 year of age followed by a childhood offset period (i.e., a growth curve returning back to the infancy growth pattern seen in 60 percent of these patients). (From Karlberg et al.[144] with permission.)

ever, in individual patients, particularly in those on long-term dialysis, pubertal maturation may be arrested for years.

The age at attainment of pubic hair stage 2 was delayed by 1.3 years in uremic and 1.5 years in transplanted boys compared with healthy controls.[153] At attainment of adult pubic hair phenotype, the uremic boys were 1.9 and the transplanted boys 3.5 years older than the healthy controls. The transplanted boys were the most retarded, despite

cyclosporine-induced hypertrichosis, which may lead to an erroneously early pubic hair staging. According to the EDTA Registry, almost half of the girls treated by dialysis or renal transplantation failed to menstruate before the upper normal age limit of 15 years. Menarche tended to occur later in transplanted than in dialyzed girls.[148,149]

Unlike the development of secondary sexual characteristics, which is delayed but not permanently halted in ure-

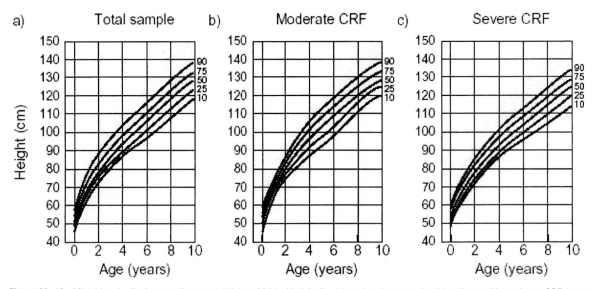

Figure 23–19. Mixed longitudinal percentile curves (10th to 90th) of height for (a) total patient sample, (b) patients with moderate CRF (mean GFR during observation period > 25 mL/min per 1.73 m[2]), and (c) patients with severe CRF (mean GFR < 25 mL/min per 1.73 m[2]). Shaded area represents 3ᵈ to 97th percentiles of height in healthy boys. (From Schaefer et al.[145] With permission.)

mia, reproductive function may be permanently impaired. In autopsy studies in boys with CRF, germ-cell depletion in the testicular tubules has been described.[154] These changes seem not to be reversible by renal transplantation.[155] Persistently reduced sperm counts were observed in 10 of 12 successfully transplanted young adults who had suffered from ESRD during childhood.[155] Erectile dysfunction and decreased libido and fertility are primarily organic in nature and are due to uremia as well as to other comorbid conditions, fatigue, and psychosocial factors.[156]

The frequency of conception is decreased in women with CRF, and pregnancy is very uncommon in adolescents with ESRD. If pregnancy occurs, however, major changes in clinical management, such as prolonged dialysis sessions, are required. The percentage of surviving infants ranges from 70 to 100 percent in women with CRF on conservative treatment or after renal transplantation[155] and from 50 to 80 percent in women on dialysis.[157–159] Intrauterine growth retardation is frequent, and birth weight is reduced by nearly 1 kg.[151,156,157]

The height gain achieved during the pubertal growth spurt is usually reduced.[151,160–163] In a longitudinal analysis of the growth curves of 29 adolescents with various degrees of CRF, the growth spurt started with an average delay of 2.5 years.[152] The degree of the delay was correlated with the duration of CRF. Although a distinct acceleration of growth during puberty occurred, the total pubertal height gain was reduced in both sexes to approximately 50 percent of normal late-maturing children. This reduction was due to a marked suppression of the late prespurt height velocity, a subnormal peak height velocity, and a shortening of the pubertal growth period by 1 year in boys and 1.5 years in girls (Fig. 23–20). Notably, the prolonged prepubertal growth phase, resulting from the delayed onset of the pubertal growth spurt, permitted the patients to grow to an almost normal immediate prespurt height (–1 SDS in boys, +0.1 SDS in girls). Subsequently, relative height was gradually lost during the pubertal growth spurt, resulting in an average relative height of –2.9 SDS in boys and –2.3 SDS in girls.

In prepubertal children with long-standing renal failure, bone maturation is invariably retarded.[147,164–166] In dialysis patients, skeletal maturation is increasingly retarded before the start of puberty and then accelerates dramatically. This observation and the fact that uremic boys respond to exogenous application of testosterone esters by an exaggerated increase in skeletal maturation[166] suggests that the sensitivity of the growth plate to sex steroids is at least conserved. Because proliferation (i.e., growth) cannot keep pace with differentiation (i.e., bone maturation), growth potential may be irreversibly lost during puberty in uremia.

In contrast, in many transplant patients, an apparent standstill of bone maturation is observed, even when the patient is growing and puberty is progressing. This phenomenon is thought to be related to direct interference of corticosteroids with the differentiation of the growth plate. Despite the delayed bone age, late growth is usually not observed.[152,167,168] In fact, the successive stages of the pubertal

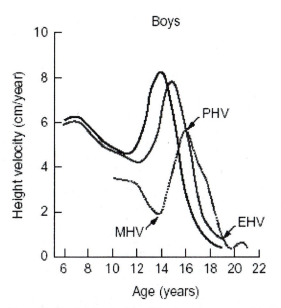

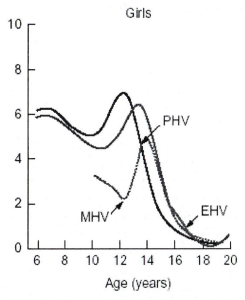

Figure 23–20. Synchronized conditional average curves of height velocity in healthy (a) boys and (b) girls, with average (uninterrupted lines) or late normal (dotted lines) timing of puberty and in patients with end-stage renal failure (dashed lines). The definition of reference points in the growth curve, to which individual height velocity curves are aligned, permits statistical comparisons between normal and pathologic growth patterns. In CRF, minimal height velocity (MHV) at pubertal onset is severely suppressed, a pubertal acceleration occurs, but peak height velocity (PHV) is still reduced and the duration of the growth spurt (distance from PHV to end height velocity (EHV) is diminished. (Adapted from Schaefer et al.[152] With permission.)

growth spurt seem to occur at increasingly earlier bone ages than would be assumed in a normal population.[152]

Final Height

A crucial question in the rehabilitation of children with chronic renal disease is the degree to which final height is compromised. Of the patients with childhood-onset ESRD in the EDTA Registry, 50 percent achieved adult heights below the third percentile. Children with continued dialysis until adulthood reached a lower mean final height than children who received a renal transplant.[167,169–174] Final height appeared to be more severely compromised in boys than in girls. However, this reflects mainly the higher incidence of congenital nephropathies in boys. Final height is most compromised in patients with severe congenital renal disorders, among which nephropathic cystinosis leads to the most obvious growth retardation.[175] However, patients with acquired glomerular diseases usually exhibit a very marked loss in height SDS in the early course of the disease, resulting in the need for growth-promoting treatment in a large proportion of this patient group.

TREATMENT

Conservative Treatment

The therapeutic approach to growth failure in children with CRF should take into account the various contributing pathophysiologic factors. In particular, despite the introduction of rhGH therapy in children with CRF, optimization of permissive factors for normal growth should not be disregarded. Sufficient nutritional support is essential for normal growth in infancy, because height velocity in this phase of rapid growth is related to energy intake. Energy intake should be maintained near 100 percent of the RDA, if necessary by introduction of nasogastric tube feeding.[176] With early initiation of optimal nutritional and medical care, severe growth failure in infants with CRF can be prevented. Even catch-up growth in infants with CRF after correction of nutritional intake has been reported in two studies[177,178] but was not observed in a third study.[179] In midchildhood, during which adequate nutritional support is a permissive prerequisite of normal growth, energy intake should be approximately 100 percent of the RDA, but calorie support in excess of this recommendation results in obesity rather than in increased height gain. Metabolic acidosis should be prevented by treatment with oral bicarbonate preparations, increased renal losses of fluids and electrolytes should be substituted, and the development of renal osteodystrophy and secondary hyperparathyroidism should be prevented by phosphate restriction and 1,25-dihydroxy-vitamin D_3 treatment. However, apart from nutritional support in early infancy, true catch-up growth cannot be obtained by any of these therapeutic interventions. At most, a growth pattern parallel to the growth percentiles can be obtained by optimization of nutritional support and medical treatment.

Dialysis

Hemodialysis. Once children have reached ESRD, growth rates usually deteriorate further. Kleinknecht et al.[180] described the growth of 51 children who underwent hemodialysis for 12 to 111 months. The mean annual loss of relative height was 0.4 SD. One-third of the patients grew "normally" (i.e., along the growth percentile attained at initiation of dialysis), one-third had a slightly retarded growth, and one-third had a severely retarded growth. No specific factor, such as caloric intake, urea production, and duration and modality of dialysis, was delineated to account for the magnitude of growth retardation. The experience that catch-up growth cannot be obtained by hemodialysis treatment was confirmed by other single-center reports[181–184] and the findings of the EDTA registry.[185]

Newer dialysis techniques—such as hemofiltration, hemodiafiltration, and high-flux hemodialysis—were expected to have a more beneficial effect on growth than standard hemodialysis, because they remove "middle molecules," which possibly act as IGF inhibitors, more effectively. Although systematic studies are lacking, these methods do not consistently improve growth in the clinical experience.

Continuous Peritoneal Dialysis. Continuous ambulatory/cycling peritoneal dialysis (CAPD/CCPD) in children has been heralded as a treatment modality that may be associated with an improvement in growth.[186,187] Indeed, growth rates may improve, at least initially, in some children who start CAPD after conservative treatment or prior hemodialysis.[188] This relative improvement in growth has been related to the better nutritional status of patients on CAPD as a consequence of their peritoneal glucose uptake.[189] However, in patients on long-standing CAPD, a gradual decline of relative height is frequently observed, indicating that the impact of the dialysis modality on growth diminishes with time.[190–192] These data temper the initial enthusiasm that CAPD or CCPD has a significant beneficial impact on growth. At best, a centile-parallel growth pattern can be achieved by peritoneal dialysis, certainly not a persistent catch-up growth.

The situation is even more gloomy for infants on CAPD. Growth failure occurs almost inevitably despite sufficient nutritional intake of at least 100 percent of the RDA and maintenance of relative weight and other nutritional indices.[193,194] Warady et al. reported a mean loss of relative height of 0.7 SD during the first year of life in four infants in whom CCPD was initiated during the first month of life.[193] In the report of Kohaut et al., the average loss of height in 10 patients starting CAPD before the third month of life was 1.23 SD.[194] Notably, this loss of relative height was associated with microcephaly in one study, indicating diminished brain growth.[193]

Transplantation

Theoretically, a well-functioning transplant in a child should restore the physiologic conditions required for normal growth. However, growth rates after renal transplantation are highly variable and rarely fulfill the expectations of true catch-up growth. The main contributing factors to growth depression in children with renal transplants are glucocorticoid treatment for immunosuppression and reduced graft function. In addition, the growth response after a successful renal transplant depends on the age of the child and the severity of the growth failure at time of transplantation.

An important determinant of normal growth posttransplant is the function of the renal graft.[195,196] In a report from the North American Pediatric Renal Transplant Cooperative (NAPRTC) Study following 300 children with a functioning graft over 2 years, an increase in the serum creatinine level by 1.0 mg/dL was associated with a decrease in relative height of 0.15 SD.[197] However, it is difficult to assess the impact of glomerular filtration rate (GFR) on growth independently, because patients with poor graft function usually also receive higher amounts of glucocorticoids to suppress chronic graft rejection.

The age of the recipient at the time of transplantation also appears to influence the degree of growth improvement. In the experience of Ingelfinger et al.,[198] only children below the age of 7 years demonstrated true catch-up growth after transplantation. Bosque et al. reported better growth rates in patients with a bone age below 12 years at the time of transplantation.[199] The importance of age-related changes in growth posttransplantation has been emphasized by Tejani et al. with data from the NAPRTC Study.[197] In 300 children with a functioning renal transplant and a baseline height SDS of –2.41 ± 0.09 SD, the average increase in relative height was +0.18 ± 0.06 SD in the first 2 years posttransplantation. However, there were remarkable age-related differences: children in the age group from birth to 1 year, who also had the maximal height deficit, had the maximal improvement in relative height of 0.92 SD over 2 years. For the 2- to 5-year-old group, the change in height SDS was 0.54 SD. No significant improvement in relative height was observed for children 6 to 12 years of age and 13 to 18 years of age. Catch-up growth (defined as a gain of relative height of at least 1 SD in 2 years) occurred in 50 percent of the neonate to 1-year-old, 25 percent of the 2- to 5-year-old, 16 percent of the 6- to 12-year-old, and 6 percent of the 13- to 17-year-old group. The authors drew the gloomy conclusion that growth outcome in children after transplantation has not substantially changed during the past decade.[197]

Other authors also reported excellent growth rates in infants after transplantation, with an average improvement in relative height of 1.4 SD over a period of 2 to 7 years.[200,201] It is noteworthy that this improved longitudinal growth was accompanied by normalized head circumference and cognitive development in these infants. However, renal transplantation in infants below the age of 2 years is still associated with a mortality rate of 16 percent, compared with 4.5 percent in older children.[202]

Certainly, the effect of many of the factors that influence growth post-transplant is interrelated with various other determinants. Hokken-Koelega et al.[203] sought to determine the predictive factors for growth in the first 2 years posttransplant singly and simultaneously in a multiple regression analysis. In their experience, 70 percent of the prepubertal children do not experience appreciable catch-up growth (0.5 SD/year). Patients with the most severe growth retardation at the time of grafting had the most pronounced growth spurt post-transplant but failed to have complete catch-up growth. Alternate-day versus daily prednisone administration had a significant positive influence, whereas a high cumulative dose of prednisone, azathioprine versus cyclosporine A therapy, and a persistently reduced GFR below 50 mL/min/1.73 m^2 had a significantly negative influence on catch-up growth. Other factors, such as gender, chronological and bone age at time of grafting, primary renal disease, duration of former dialysis, repeat transplantation, and target height did not have a significant influence on growth posttransplant.

Glucocorticoids. The cumulative amount of glucocorticoids is certainly a determinant of the growth rates achieved posttransplantation. The introduction of cyclosporine for pediatric transplant patients in 1984 allowed a dose reduction of the concomitant glucocorticoid medication[204]; however, improved growth rates were reported only by some investigators[204,205] and not by others.[206,207] In addition, final height appears not to have been consistently improved by the introduction of cyclosporine in comparison with conventional immunosuppression.[208]

Deflazacort, a prednisolone derivative, causes less suppression of GH secretion and longitudinal growth than conventional glucocorticoids.[209] In response to the substitution of deflazacort in an equivalent immunosuppressive dose for methylprednisolone, nine prepubertal children with renal transplants experienced a moderate increase in height velocity from 1.5 ± 0.3 cm at baseline to 3.2 ± 0.5 cm/year and a reduction in cushingoid appearance. The efficacy and safety of this compound has to be evaluated further in controlled clinical trials.

Alternate-Day Steroids. One possibility to ameliorate steroid-specific side effects in pediatric renal transplant recipients is to administer steroids on an alternate-day basis, because a cumulative dose of corticosteroids has significantly less inhibitory effect on growth velocity when given on alternate days compared with a daily regimen without adversely affecting graft survival or long-term graft function.[210,211] However, the effect on longitudinal growth is only moderate and limited to the first two years posttransplant. For example, in one large-scale study reported from the NAPRTCS registry, relative height increased by 0.50 ± 0.06 SDS in the first two years posttransplant, but no additional height gain was observed in the subsequent years (Fig. 23–21).[211] Currently, only 26 percent of children with functioning renal grafts for more than 4 years posttransplant are on an alternate-day steroid dosing regimen.[212] In a recent report, Qvist et al. investigated the growth, bone age, and renal function of 30 children below 5 years of age at the time of kidney transplantation who were given cyclosporine, azathioprine, and alternate-day corticosteroid treatment. Initially, catch-up growth was observed in 81 percent of all patients, mostly in recipients between 2 and 5 years of age. Nevertheless, in the 5 to 7 posttransplant years, only 35 percent of the children involved showed significantly improved longitudinal growth.[213] Hence an alternate-day medication is thought to ensure catch-up growth in selected pediatric patients in the first few years posttransplant. A comparative study investigating the effect of steroid withdrawal vs. an alternate-day steroid regimen regarding amelioration of steroid-associated side effects and graft function and survival has not been performed so far.

Steroid Withdrawal. Previously, only a few medical centers have studied the effect of glucocorticoid withdrawal on growth and graft function.[214–217] Klare et al.[214] observed a mean increase in relative height of 0.8 ± 0.3 SD in the first year and 0.3 ± 0.2 SD in the second year after grafting in 12 children with a serum creatinine below 2.0 mg/dL. These data indicate that, at least in children with only slightly reduced graft function, cessation of glucocorticoids can in-

duce catch-up growth. However, this regimen was associated with an increased risk of graft rejection with a reported incidence of 50 to 60 percent in the cyclosporine/azathioprine era.[216] To reduce the risk of graft rejection, the patient had to be maintained on higher doses of cyclosporine, which, in turn, increases the risk of cyclosporine nephrotoxicity.

Recent data suggest that the introduction of mycophenolate mofetil (MMF) instead of azathioprine to a cyclosporine-based immunosuppressive regimen in 1996 has significantly increased the safety of steroid withdrawal in pediatric renal transplant recipients. Hoecker et al. recently reported that steroid withdrawal in 20 pediatric renal transplant recipients on cyclosporine and MMF was associated with a marked catch-up growth in the presence of stable graft function, a significant reduction in cushingoid appearance, and a reduced need for antihypertensive medication.[218] The degree of catch-up growth in response to steroid withdrawal in prepubertal children in this study ($+1.47 \pm 0.32$ SDS in 4 years) was remarkable (Fig. 23–22) and appears to be higher than that observed under an alternate-day steroid regimen.[210,211] None of the 20 patients undergoing steroid withdrawal experienced an acute rejection episode throughout the study period of 4 years, and graft function as assessed by creatinine clearances remained stable. It was suggested that these favorable results compared with previous reports in patients on cyclosporine and azathioprine can be ascribed to the higher immunosuppressive potency of MMF than that of azathioprine. A prospective randomized study is currently being performed to assess more reliably the safety of steroid withdrawal on graft function and survival.

An alternative approach to facilitate steroid withdrawal in pediatric renal transplant recipients is a tacrolimus-based immunosuppressive regimen. Shapiro et al. reported that long-term steroid withdrawal was possible in 70 percent of their patients, with 5-year actuarial patient and graft survival rates of 96 and 82 percent, a 39 percent incidence of rejection, and a mean serum creatinine level of 1.2 ± 0.5 mg/dL.[219] In children who were withdrawn from steroids, the mean height SDS at the time of transplantation and at 1 and 4 years were -2.3 ± 2.0, -1.7 ± 1.0, and 0.36 ± 1.5.[220] Eighty six percent of successfully transplanted patients did not take antihypertensive medications. However, the incidence of PTLD in this report (4 to 17 percent) appears to be higher than that observed in children on a CsA/MMF-based immunosuppressive regimen (1 percent).[221]

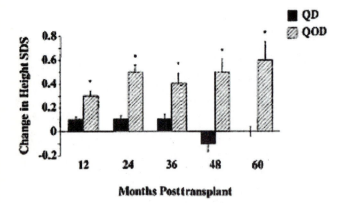

Figure 23–21. Mean change in height SDS from baseline at 30 days after transplantation. The solid bars indicate patients treated continuously on a daily steroid dosing regimen from 12 months after transplantation and the hatched bars indicate patients continuously treated on an every-other-day regimen. * Difference between QD and QOD groups, $p < 0.05$. (From Jabs et al.[211] With permission.)

Steroid Avoidance. An even more promising approach than steroid withdrawal could be the complete avoidance of steroids. It has been argued that a totally steroid-free immunosuppressive milieu from the beginning should not give rise to a steroid-dependent suppression of the immune re-

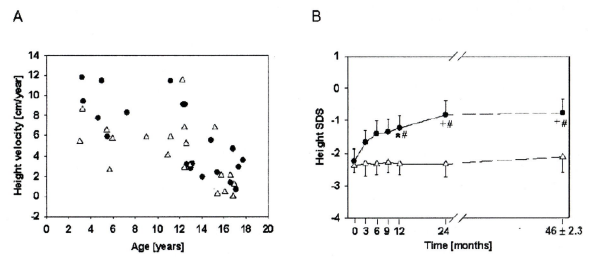

Figure 23–22. Longitudinal growth. **A.** Height velocity in children in the first year after steroid withdrawal (closed symbols, $n = 20$) compared with those remaining on steroids (case controls, open triangles, $n = 20$). **B.** Mean (± SEM) height SDS at baseline, in 3-month intervals for 1 year after study entry, at 2 years, and at 46 ± 2.3 months after study entry in prepubertal patients off steroids (closed symbols, $n = 6$) and controls (open triangles, $n = 6$). Whereas height SDS remained unchanged in patients on steroids, there was a significant increase of height SDS in patients off steroids ($*p < 0.05$ vs. baseline; $^\#p < 0.05$ vs. control, $^+p < 0.01$ vs. baseline). (From Höcker et al.[218] With permission.)

sponse, which makes either steroid withdrawal or alternate-day dosing hazardous for rebound rejection. However, an empirical or experimental proof for this hypothesis is still lacking. Birkeland et al. reported their experience in 14 pediatric renal allograft recipients who received a 10-day initial course of antilymphocyte globulin and surface area–adjusted doses of cyclosporine, 7 of them also receiving MMF as maintenance immunosuppression.[222] One patient died (3 months after transplantation, as a result of a primary Epstein-Barr virus infection-induced lymphoproliferative disorder), another patient's graft never functioned, and a third patient lost his graft after 3 years because of chronic rejection. Three patients experienced early acute cellular rejection, which resolved in two cases with OKT3 and in the third with MMF. There were no late acute rejections. All patients evidenced growth and a growth spurt under this regimen. Even more favorable results have recently been reported by Sarwal et al. in 57 pediatric recipients using a steroid-avoidance immunosuppressive protocol consisting of extended daclizumab use in combination with tacrolimus and MMF.[223] At 12 months' analysis, steroid-free patients experienced a significantly lower clinical acute rejection rate compared with 50 historically matched steroid-based children who served as controls (8 vs. 32 percent). In addition, the known morbid side effects of steroids were avoided without signs of overimmunosuppression. Nevertheless, although prevention of steroid-associated side effects appears to be an even more attractive approach than amelioration by steroid withdrawal, this approach is still experimental and requires further validation.

In summary, catch-up growth in children posttransplant is not regularly observed. Catchup growth is restricted to patients with near-normal graft function and a low-dose, preferably alternate-day glucocorticoid regimen. Recent data indicate that more potent immunosuppressive agents such as MMF and tacrolimus permit steroid withdrawal in a larger proportion of patients, which is associated with spontaneous catch-up growth in the first years posttransplant. However, because not all children grow well despite successful renal transplantation, normalization of growth in the phase before renal transplantation remains an important therapeutic goal.

Treatment with Recombinant Human Growth Hormone

Rationale for rhGH Treatment in Children with CRF. Studies in experimental animals have shown that the relative insensitivity to the action GH can be overcome by supraphysiologic doses of exogenous GH.[224] This observation provided the rationale for the administration of pharmacologic doses of recombinant human GH (rhGH) in an attempt to stimulate growth in children with renal failure.[225]

RhGH acts in uremia by several mechanisms: (1) it reverses the hypercatabolism in the uremic milieu and (2) it increases the bioactivity of circulating insulin-like growth factor (IGF), which may result from the differential action of rhGH on plasma IGFs (significant increase) and inhibitory IGF binding proteins (no major change), with the net result being an increase of IGFs in extravascular fluids. Circulating IGFs have access to their target tissues, i.e., the growth plate, to interact with the type 1 IGF receptor for stimulation of longitudinal growth.[226]

Efficacy of rhGH Treatment

Growth hormone stimulates growth in prepubertal children with CRF, end-stage renal disease (ESRD), and after renal transplantation. It is also effective in infants and growth-retarded pubertal children after renal transplantation.

Prepubertal Children with Preterminal CRF. Recombinant human GH stimulates growth in children with CRF. Several studies demonstrated an approximate twofold increase in mean height velocity, from 4 to 8 cm/year, in the first treatment year.[227–230] This benefit was not attenuated by a strict low-protein/low-phosphate diet (1.0 to 1.2 g protein/kg body weight per day), prescribed in an attempt to slow the progression of the renal disease.[231]

The first multicenter randomized, double-blind, placebo-controlled study in a large group of children with CRF showed a number of positive findings[232]: (1) The mean first-year growth rate was increased (10.7 vs. 6.5 cm/year in the placebo group). (2) The mean growth rate in the second year was also increased (7.8 vs. 5.5 cm/year.) (3) The average increase in relative height in rhGH-treated children increased from 2.94 standard deviation score (SDS) below the mean at baseline to 1.55 SDS below after 2 treatment years; in contrast, relative height decreased 0.2 SDS in the placebo group (Fig. 23–23) (4) The acceleration in growth was not associated with undue advancement of bone age, suggesting

that the height gain during rhGH therapy is likely to be reflected in an actual increase in final height.

Later results from this trial[233] as well as a second study[234] reveal that the efficacy of rhGH in children with CRF continues for those treated for at least 5 years: (1) With the ongoing trial, although the maximum increase in height occurred during the first 2 treatment years, mean standardized height increased each year when compared to the previous year, with a mean increase in standardized height from –2.6 ± 0.8 SDS at baseline to –0.7 ± 0.9 SDS at year 5. Observed side effects included one child with avascular necrosis and elevated plasma insulin concentrations. (2) The second report compared the outcomes of 38 initially prepubertal patients treated with rhGH for a mean period of 5.3 years to that of 50 control children who did not receive rhGH.[234] Children treated with growth hormone had sustained catch-up growth, whereas the control children had progressive growth failure. The mean final heights for boys and girls administered rhGH was 165 and 156 cm, respectively. The mean final adult height of the GH-treated children was 1.6 ± 1.2 SD below normal, which was 1.4 SD above their standardized height at baseline (Fig. 23–24). In contrast, the final height of the untreated children (2.1 ± 1.2 SD below normal) was 0.6 SD below their standardized height at baseline. Furthermore, therapy did not shorten the pubertal growth spurt. 65 percent of these children reached an adult height within the normal range (within 2 SD of normal height). However, mean adult height was still 10.1 and 12.1 cm below genetic target height in boys and girls,

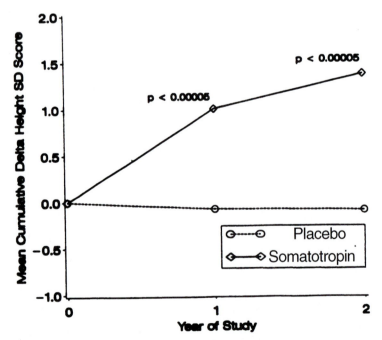

Figure 23–23. Efficacy of GH treatment in children with CRF. Mean cumulative change in relative height in children with preterminal CRF randomized to therapy with GH (*n* = 55) or placebo (*n* = 27). Growth improved only in the children receiving GH. (From Fine et al.[232] With permission.)

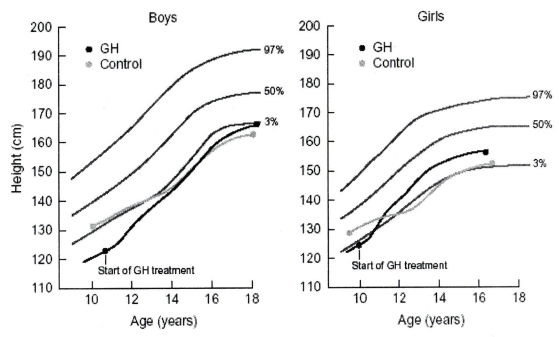

Figure 23–24. Synchronized mean growth curves during GH treatment for 38 children (32 boys and 6 girls) with CRF, compared with 50 control children with CRF not treated with GH, according to sex. Normal values are indicated by the 3rd, 50th, and 97th percentiles. The circles indicate the time of the first observation (the start of GH treatment in the treated children) and the end of the pubertal growth spurt. (From Haffner et al.[234] With permission.)

respectively. In the control boys and girls, adult height was markedly below midparental target height (boys, –15.8 cm; girls, –16.1 cm). Multiple regression analysis revealed that the total height gain during the observation period was positively affected by the duration of rhGH therapy and the initial target height deficit and negatively by the percentage of time spent on dialysis.[234]

In this study, differential analysis of prepubertal versus pubertal growth during GH therapy revealed that GH therapy mainly stimulates prepubertal growth, from a mean of 3.3. to 8.4 cm/year in boys and from 3.7 to 9.7 cm/year in girls (Fig. 23–25). The cumulative prepubertal height gain in the rhGH-treated children was twice that of the untreated controls. Skeletal age advanced faster in the rhGH-treated children (1.1 "years" per year) than in the control group (0.8 "years" per year). However, the onset of the pubertal growth spurt remained similarly delayed in untreated and treated children by approximately 2.5 years.

Pubertal Children. An adequate assessment of the effect of rhGH on pubertal growth requires an analysis of the degree and duration of the pubertal growth spurt. One report demonstrated that the total pubertal height gain was similar in control and GH-treated children with renal failure[234]; the gain was 65 percent of that observed in normal children because of a shorter (by 1.6 years) pubertal growth spurt (Fig. 23–25). After the onset of the pubertal spurt, accelerated bone maturation continued in rhGH-treated boys; this was associated with a shortening of the growth spurt by approxi-

mately 6 months. However, the amplitude of the pubertal growth spurt was slightly higher in the rhGH-treated children (Fig. 23–3), resulting in an unchanged total pubertal height gain in rhGH-treated children. Pubertal height gain was only 65 percent of that observed in healthy children regardless of rhGH treatment, mainly because of the shortened duration of the spurt. These studies demonstrate the potential of rhGH to normalize final height in children with chronic renal failure.

These data differ from promising preliminary results that have been obtained in growth-retarded pubertal children after transplantation: 18 adolescents demonstrated an impressive growth response to rhGH with a mean increment in height after two years of rhGH therapy (15.7 vs. only 5.8 cm in retrospectively matched control patients).[235] This growth response occurred at rhGH doses of either 4 or 8 IU/day per square meter of body surface area.

A comparable increase of height velocity was also noted in the randomized rhGH trial in pubertal children after kidney transplantation.[236] During the first treatment year, there was an increase in standardized height by 0.7 ± 0.5 SDS, compared to 0.1 ± 0.5 SDS in controls; the growth-stimulating effect persisted in the second year, with an increase in standardized height of 0.5 ± 0.6 SDS.[24]

Prepubertal Children with End-Stage Renal Disease. Prepubertal children with ESRD, either on peritoneal dialysis or hemodialysis, also respond to rhGH.[225,230] However, due to the greater degree of uremia in ESRD, the response is generally

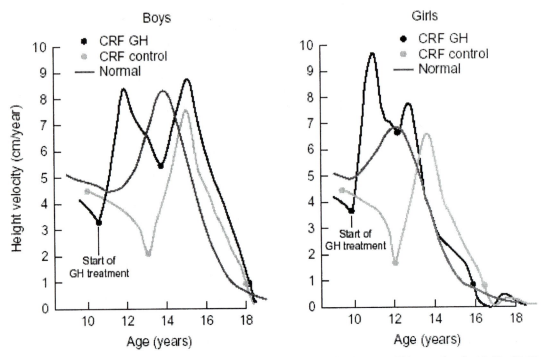

Figure 23–25. Synchronized mean height-velocity curves during GH treatment for the same children as described in Fig. 23–24. The circles indicate the time of the first observation (the start of GH treatment in the treated children), the time of minimal prespurt height velocity, and the end of the pubertal growth spurt. (From Haffner et al.[234] With permission.)

less pronounced and less persistent than that achieved in children with preterminal chronic renal failure. In one study in 17 children on CAPD, for example, height velocity increased from 2.9 to 5.5 cm/year in the first treatment year and then dropped to 3.6 cm/year in the second year of therapy.[237]

In an extended study of 42 children with ESRD on hemodialysis, patients were treated with rhGH for a period of up to 5 years (n = 8).[238] Mean growth velocity increased from 3.5 to 7.0 cm/year and was always over 2.5 cm/year. The mean growth velocity decreased over subsequent years, but remained higher than the prestudy velocity.

Prepubertal Children after Renal Transplantation. Successful renal transplantation reverses the uremic milieu and should theoretically permit normal GH secretion and function. Persistent growth failure in this setting is primarily due to reduced graft function and glucocorticoid therapy. If catch-up growth cannot be achieved by an alternate-day steroid regimen and if discontinuation of steroids appers as an intolerable risk for graft survival, rhGH therapy may be initiated.[239,240]

Exogenous GH reverses the catabolic and growth-depressing effects of glucocorticoids in both experimental and clinical settings.[241] In particular, rhGH can counteract the interference of pharmacologic doses of glucocorticoids with the integrity of the GH/IGF axis. There are two rationales for rhGH administration in short children with renal transplants: (1) rhGH treatment can be considered as substitution therapy in individuals with glucocorticoid-induced GH hyposecretion and (2) rhGH is able to restore IGF bioactivity in children who secrete normal amounts of GH but have decreased biologically available IGF.[239]

The first large randomized study concerning rhGH treatment in children after kidney transplantation has been completed.[236] The following results were reported: (1) During the first year of treatment, growth velocity in the group administered rhGH was significantly increased (7.7 vs. 4.6 cm in the control group). Subsequently, a decrease in growth velocity was noted, with growth of 5.9, 5.5, and 5.2 cm occurring at 2, 3, and 4 years, respectively. These data indicate that GH therapy clearly induces catch-up growth, but the effect becomes limited with time. (2) Biopsy-proven rejection episodes tended to be more frequent during rhGH treatment (20 vs. 9 percent). Compared to those without rejection, the patients who rejected did not differ in age, initial renal function, or immunosuppressive regimen, but history of rejection before initiation of rhGH therapy was discriminatory; 6 of 17 children with two or more rejection episodes had a new rejection during rhGH therapy vs. 1 of 22 with none or only one episode. (3) The mean change in glomerular filtration rate did not differ between the two groups during the first year of the study.

Acute rejection episodes therefore appear to be more frequent during rhGH administration in those patients who have a history of more than one rejection episode. Close monitoring of graft function is therefore recommended.

Nevertheless, rhGH appears to be safe in immunologically low-risk patients with a history of zero or one acute rejection episode.

A second randomized trial of 68 growth-retarded pediatric renal allograft recipients found similar results concerning growth but no increased risk of rejection due to GH therapy.[242] However, more than one acute rejection episode prior to enrollment was predictive of a subsequent rejection following enrollment. There was no difference in adverse events between the two groups.

Hence, the risk of acute rejection episodes in response to GH therapy appears to be less important than initially thought, due perhaps to the use of more potent immunosuppressive drugs in recent years. As an example, an analysis of the 1-year randomized control study of the NAPRTCS in 68 pediatric renal transplant recipients found no increased incidence of acute rejection episodes due to rhGH and no accelerated decline in graft function in the GH-treated group compared to the control group.[242]

Infants with Chronic Renal Failure. Limited data about rhGH therapy in infants are available because most of the previous studies were restricted to children above 2 years of age. An analysis of children below the age of 2.5 years at enrollment into the North-American multicenter placebo-controlled study showed that the relative increase in height was 2.0 SDS in the rhGH-treated group vs. –0.2 SDS in the placebo-treated group.[243] This observation is important clinically, because early initiation of rhGH therapy in this phase of rapid growth might reverse or prevent the otherwise com-

mon irreversible loss of growth potential in infancy. Early initiation of rhGH substitution therapy in GH-deficient children is an important determinant for their later ability to reach their target height. However, adequate energy intake remains an important permissive factor in infants with chronic renal failure. Failure of rhGH treatment has been reported in infants with ESRD and insufficient calorie intake because of frequent vomiting.[230]

Exhaustion of Growth Potential. There is generally an impressive growth response to rhGH in children with renal failure that varies somewhat with the clinical setting. Two issues, however, merit further consideration before therapy can be considered successful.

One of the concerns of rhGH therapy in children with CRF was that the gain in relative height would be lost immediately after successful renal transplantation because the growth potential of these children might have been exhausted. In one report, children with a history of rhGH treatment continued to grow after renal transplantation with a normal growth rate.[244] The degree of their catch-up growth was slightly lower than in those who did not receive rhGH prior to transplantation (Fig. 23–26). Thus, rhGH therapy before transplantation does not obviate but may slightly moderate normal growth after transplantation.

Adult Height. An important related issue has been whether rhGH therapy can augment adult height in children with CRF. Long-term results of children with preterminal CRF treated for five years indicate a positive effect of

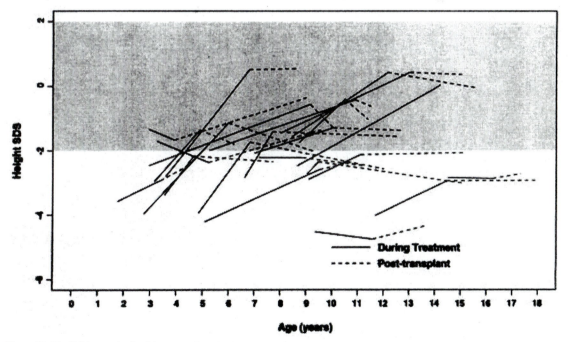

Figure 23–26. Height standardized for age and gender from baseline to last posttransplantation visit for the 30 patients who discontinued rhGH therapy at the time of transplantation. Dashed line denotes the period after transplantation. From Fine et al.[244] With permission.)

rhGH on final height, with frequent attainment of normal height.[233,234]

The efficacy of rhGH to improve final height is mainly affected by the following factors: (1) the total duration of rhGH therapy; (2) the renal failure treatment modality, as ESRD treated by dialysis adversely affects the long-term efficacy of rhGH; and (3) the initial degree of growth retardation as a positive predictor of GH-associated total height gain, indicating that the efficacy of GH therapy appears to depend on the biological "demand" for catch-up growth.

Hokken-Koelega and coworkers[245] followed 45 children (prepubertal at start) with CRF for up to 8 years of GH treatment. Treatment resulted in a sustained and significant improvement in height SDS compared with baseline values. The mean height SDS reached the lower end (–2 SDS) of the normal growth chart after 3 years and even approached genetic target height after 6 years of therapy (Fig. 23–27).

Haffner and coworkers[3] followed 38 initially prepubertal children with CRF treated with GH for a mean of 8 years until they reached their final adult height (Fig. 23–24). The patients were treated with GH during 70 percent of the observation time, mainly due to renal transplantation, at which time GH treatment was stopped. Fifty children with CRF, matched for age and degree of CRF, who did not receive GH because growth was normal served as controls.

The children treated with GH showed sustained catch-up growth, whereas the control children developed progressive growth failure (Fig. 23–24). The mean final adult height of the GH-treated children was 1.6 ± 1.2 SD below normal, which was 1.4 SD (1.5 for boys and 1.2 for girls) above their standardized height at baseline. In contrast, the final height of the untreated children decreased from baseline by a mean of 0.6 SD (0.7 for boys and 0.5 for girls). Calculating the increase in height SDS in treated patients

versus the loss of height SDS in untreated patients, the benefit of GH therapy was 2.2 SD for boys (i.e., 15 cm) and 1.7 SD for girls (i.e., 10.5 cm). The mean total prepubertal height gain was 18.6 cm in boys given GH compared with 9.9 cm in the controls, whereas the total pubertal height gain was only slightly better in the GH-treated group (23.5 vs. 21.0 cm) (Fig. 23–25). The latter finding may be explained, at least in part, by the fact that many children have not been treated with GH during the entire pubertal period because of renal transplantation. The total height gain was positively associated with the initial target-height deficit and the duration of GH therapy, and was negatively associated with the percentage of the observation period spent on dialysis treatment. Table 23–3 summarizes the effects of GH on final height in various studies.

Optimal Time to Initiate rhGH Therapy. Growth hormone therapy should be initiated before transplantation and before puberty, periods for which the available evidence suggests beneficial effects of rhGH on final height. Observational data indicate that rhGH is more successful in these patients when begun at a younger age and early in the course of the renal failure.[251] It therefore appears reasonable to offer rhGH to children with the following characteristics: (1) the patient falls below the third percentile for height; (2) the patient does not show spontaneous catch-up growth even though other factors contributing to uremic growth failure have been adequately stabilized.

It remains uncertain whether a low growth rate (height velocity below the 25th percentile) should also be a treatment criterion in a child with still normal relative height. Such prophylactic therapy might prove to be more effective in increasing adult height than initiation of treatment at the time short stature is established. In addition, children with

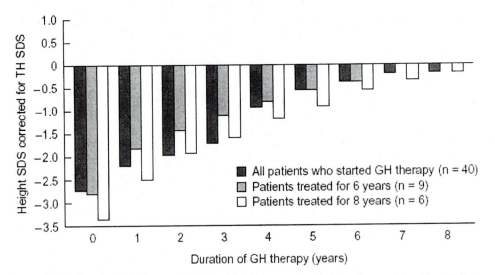

Figure 23–27. Mean height SDS corrected for target height SDS (TH SDS) during 8 years of GH. (From Hokken-Koelega et al.[245] With permission.)

TABLE 23–3. SYNOPSIS OF STUDIES REPORTING ADULT HEIGHT DATA AFTER RECOMBINANT HUMAN GROWTH HORMONE TREATMENT OF GROWTH FAILURE DUE TO CHRONIC RENAL FAILURE[a]

Study	N	CRF Treatment Modalities	Age at Start of rhGH (years)	Pubertal Status at Start of rhGH	Duration of Follow-up (years)	Duration of rhGH (years)	Initial Height SDS	Final Height SDS	Change in height SDS
Dutch (245)	4	Cons. Rx / dialysis	< 11.0	Prepubertal	> 5.0	> 5.0	n.i.	−0.2*	n.i.
KIGS (246)	12	Cons. Rx / dialysis	11.9	Prepubertal	n.i.	5.0	n.i.	n.i.	+1.0
UK (247)	2	Cons. Rx	9.9*	Prepubertal	10.0*	0.4*	−2.2*	−1.1*	+1.1*
	5	Transplant	11.9	Prepubertal	> 6.0	2.9	−3.3	−3.0	+0.3
	6	Transplant	15.6	Pubertal	> 5.0	1.4	−3.4	−2.5	+0.9
NAPRTCS (248)	9	Cons. Rx	n.i.	n.i.	3.2	< 3.2	−3.0	−2.2	+0.7
	22	Dialysis	n.i.	n.i.	4.1	< 4.1	−3.6	−3.2	+0.4
	72	Transplant	n.i.	n.i.	3.7	< 3.7	−3.0	−2.5	+0.5
German (234)	38	47% cons. Rx, 24% dialysis, 29% transplant**	10.4	Prepubertal	7.6	5.3	−3.1	−1.6	+1.4
Belgian (249)	17	Transplant	n.i.	n.i.	n.i.	3.4	−3.0	−1.8	+1.2
Dutch (250)	18	Transplant	15.5	Pubertal	n.i.	n.i.	n.i.	n.i.	Total height gain 19 cm

Key: *, median; **, percentage distribution of patient years spent in each treatment category; Cons. Rx, conservative treatment; rhGH, recombinant human growth hormone; CRF, chronic renal failure;, SDS, standard deviation score; n.i., no information given.

[a]Mean values are given for age, time period, and SDS values unless indicated otherwise.

preterminal CRF appear to respond better to rhGH than those on dialysis. Thus, rhGH therapy should ideally be initiated at a young age with the goal of restoring the level of growth to a normal genetic percentile, well before the need for renal replacement therapy.

Dose of rhGH. The optimal dose and route of administration of rhGH have not been sufficiently studied and current recommendations are largely empiric. The dose of rhGH currently recommend for children with CRF before and after renal transplantation is 0.045 to 0.05 mg/kg body weight per day, given in daily subcutaneous injections. This amount of rhGH corresponds to approximately twice the substitution dose given to GH-deficient children. It is therefore supraphysiologic, and represents pharmacologic therapy rather than replacement therapy. The dose was chosen arbitrarily on the basis of animal experiments showing that high, but not physiologic doses of rhGH were able to overcome the relative insensitivity to rhGH in the uremic state.[224]

Little information is available on different dose regimens of rhGH in children with CRF. The effect of 2 vs. 4 IU rhGH/m[2] body surface area per day was studied in a double-blind, dose-response trial of 23 growth-retarded prepubertal children with preterminal and end-stage CRF.[252] Only the higher dose produced persistent catch-up growth during 2.5 years of treatment, although the short-term growth response (6 months) was comparable between the groups.

Doubling the dose appears to be an adequate therapeutic approach in patients who fail to respond to one year of the initial rhGH regimen. We have observed individual patients in whom such an increase in dose induced sustained catch-up growth over time (Fig. 23–28). However, this procedure may present hazards because a higher dose increases the risk of side effects. The kidney accounts for a substantial fraction (25 to 53 percent) of the total plasma turnover of GH in healthy subjects.[44] Accumulation of rhGH in children with CRF has been excluded in pharmacokinetic studies only for the standard dose of rhGH.[253] Thus, before a higher dose of rhGH can be recommended for nonresponders or those with a diminishing growth response over time, potential accumulation of rhGH in higher doses and other potential side effects must be studied systematically.

Mode of Administration. Daily administration of rhGH is more effective than injections three times weekly in stimulating growth in children with CRF. This is also true for rhGH therapy of children with GH deficiency or Turner's syndrome.

However, subcutaneous injection of rhGH is not well accepted by some children. As a result, attempts have been made to administer rhGH intraperitoneally in children on CAPD by installing it into the dialysis fluid bag, analogous to insulin treatment in diabetic patients. Preliminary data indicate adequate absorption of rhGH via the intraperitoneal route.[254] However, the growth-promoting efficacy of intraperitoneal GH appears to be less consistent than that ob-

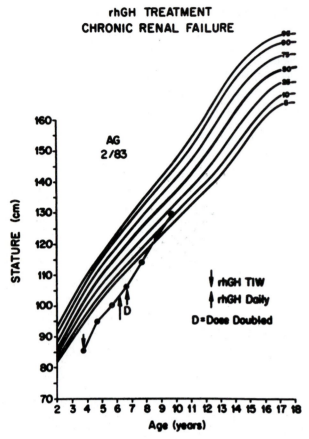

Figure 23–28. Effect of doubling the dose of rhGH (from 0.05 mg/kg/day given subcutaneously to 0.1 mg/kg/day) on growth rate in a child with preterminal CRF.

served with subcutaneous rhGH. In addition, intraperitoneal instillation of rhGH may increase the risk of peritonitis episodes.

Predictors for the Growth Response to rhGH. Parameters that can be used to predict the growth response to rhGH in the individual uremic child are unclear. Factors such as the spontaneous GH secretory patterns are not helpful in this setting.

Whether useful clinical predictors can be identified was directly assessed in a study of 74 children with CRF who were being treated conservatively and 29 dialysis-dependent patients.[251] rhGH was administered for up to five years. Multivariate regression analysis revealed that age, glomerular filtration rate, target height, and prior growth rates were independent predictors of the response to rhGH in the first and second treatment year. During the first year of therapy, for example, the height velocity was negatively correlated with age and positively correlated with the degree of renal function and target height.

Goal and Duration of rhGH Therapy. The ultimate aim of rhGH therapy in children with CRF is "normalization" of final height. There is some debate concerning how this goal is defined. The therapeutic end point could either be attainment of the patient's individual target height (i.e., the 50th percentile of midparental height) or of a normal population-related final height (i.e., greater than the third percentile). Although the former goal is certainly desirable for the individual patient, the latter approach may be economically more acceptable in view of the currently high cost of rhGH therapy (approximately $30,000 per patient per year).

It is uncertain whether rhGH therapy should be discontinued in children with CRF before final height is reached or a well-functioning renal transplant is in place. In a report from the American multicenter trial, a pause in rhGH treatment in children with CRF after attainment of target height led to maintenance of height SDS in 6 of 22 patients (27 percent) and a marked reduction in growth velocity, requiring reinstitution of rhGH therapy in the remaining patients.[249] Thus, cessation of rhGH with assiduous observation of subsequent spontaneous growth may be a therapeutic option in selected patients. The majority of patients require rhGH therapy until the growth rate has fallen below 2 cm/year, which is assumed to be the attainment of final (adult) height.

In contrast, discontinuing rhGH treatment at the time of transplantation does not appear to result in substantive posttransplantation catch-down growth. In the American trial, 30 patients who discontinued rhGH therapy at the time of transplantation and who were followed as long as 68 months after transplantation maintained their relative height at last follow-up.[249]

Side Effects of rhGH Treatment

Children with CRF grow poorly. Although several factors may contribute, including anorexia and metabolic acidosis, near-normal growth can be restored by treatment with rhGH. The major adverse effects that may be associated with prolonged rhGH therapy in these children include (1) carbohydrate intolerance; (2) acceleration of progression of CRF; (3) induction of acute rejection episodes in children after renal transplantation; (4) benign intracranial hypertension; and (5) osseous complications. However, these problems do not appear to represent a significant risk and should not, at present, limit the use of rhGH in children who might benefit.[255]

Carbohydrate Intolerance. Patients with CRF often exhibit relative glucose intolerance, mainly due to an impaired insulin-stimulated glucose disposal into muscle and adipose tissue.[256–258] GH itself is an important regulator of carbohydrate metabolism, the effect being dose- and time-dependent. Long-term exposure to high concentrations of GH in acromegaly, for example, leads to impaired glucose homeostasis in 30 to 60 percent of patients and frank diabetes mellitus in 20 percent.[259] As a result, concern was raised that the preexisting carbohydrate intolerance in children with CRF might be worsened by prolonged rhGH treatment. However, oral glucose tolerance remains unaltered in children with CRF who have been treated with rhGH over up to 5 years before and after renal transplantation.[233,239] In a large data registry, not a single child with CRF developed overt diabetes mellitus during GH therapy.[260]

However, although fasting or stimulated serum glucose concentrations are normal, fasting and glucose-stimulated serum insulin concentrations are significantly elevated during rhGH therapy in children with CRF; the increase is most pronounced in children with functioning renal transplants due to concomitant glucocorticoid therapy.[232,239] This effect persists over 5 years of rhGH administration but is not progressive.[233] The clinical significance of increased insulin secretion over time is uncertain. Insulin resistance and hyperinsulinemia have been implicated as a direct causative factor in the pathogenesis of hypertension and atherosclerosis. However, rhGH is given to children with CRF only until final height has been reached, and normalization of insulin secretion is expected thereafter.

Although GH therapy does not alter glucose tolerance in the vast majority of patients, there are individual cases of the development of diabetes mellitus in children with CRF that is temporally related to the initiation of GH therapy.[261,262] In both cases, diabetes mellitus was reversible after discontinuation of GH therapy. A retrospective analysis of data from an international pharmacoepidemiologic survey of children treated with GH showed a higher than expected incidence of type 2 diabetes mellitus with GH treatment in children without renal disease, whereas the incidence of type 1 diabetes mellitus was not affected.[263]

In summary, GH therapy in the currently recommended dose ranges does not induce overt diabetes mellitus. However, clinical monitoring of glucose homeostasis is recommended, particularly in those patients with additional risk factors, such as concomitant glucocorticoid treatment and familial type 2 diabetes.

Possible Acceleration of Progression of Renal Failure. A number of experimental observations suggest that GH may have an adverse effect on the course of renal disease. As an example, mice overexpressing a GH transgene develop glomerular sclerosis.[264–266] This effect can be prevented by a GH-antagonist transgene.[266] There is evidence, although circumstantial, that glomeruli express another, presently unknown type of receptor with affinity for GH that may transduce signals causing glomerular sclerosis.[265,267,268] The apparent adverse effect of GH does not appear to be mediated

by IGF-I, since IGF-I-transgenic mice do not have accelerated glomerular sclerosis.[264]

The applicability of these experimental findings to children with CRF is uncertain. A controlled trial in which 125 children were followed for as long as 5 years found no evidence of acceleration of CRF.[232,233,255] The mean loss of glomerular filtration rate, as assessed by creatinine clearances, was similar over a period of 2 years in the rhGH and control groups, and the percent of patients who reached ESRD was not different (Fig. 23–29).[232] In another report, the glomerular filtration rate, as assessed by repetitive inulin clearances, remained stable in children with preterminal CRF treated with rhGH over a period of 1 year.[269]

One method by which rhGH may damage the kidney is by raising the glomerular filtration rate; hyperfiltration is thought to be a risk factor for eventual glomerular injury. However, the acute increase of glomerular filtration rate in response to rhGH in healthy subjects is not seen in patients with CRF.[270]

The available clinical data indicate that rhGH therapy does not accelerate the loss of residual renal function in children with preterminal CRF. However, because increases in the plasma creatinine concentration have been observed in individual patients, careful monitoring of renal function is mandatory, and GH therapy should be reconsidered if there is an otherwise unexplained decrease in renal function.

Induction of Acute Rejection in Renal Transplant Recipients. A major concern with the administration of rhGH to short children after renal transplantation is the induction of acute rejection or the aggravation of chronic rejection. GH has

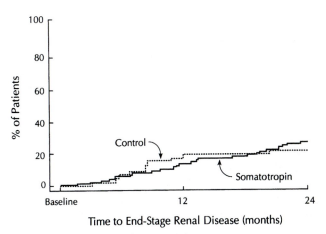

Figure 23–29. Percentage of patients who reached ESRD during 2 years of rhGH therapy (*N* = 55) (solid line) or placebo (*N* = 27) (dotted line). There was no statistically significant difference between the two groups. (From Fine et al.[232] With permission.)

important immunomodulatory properties, such as augmenting antibody synthesis, increasing interleukin-2 synthesis, stimulating proliferation of human lymphoblastoid cells, and increasing the activity of cytotoxic T lymphocytes.[271] There is also experimental and clinical evidence that the immunosuppressive effects of glucocorticoids can be counteracted by exogenous GH.[272]

Open-label rhGH trials in children after transplantation have reported a few unexplained episodes of acute rejection.[273,274] The first large randomized study on rhGH treatment in children after kidney transplantation reported the following results[236]: (1) The mean change in glomerular filtration rate did not differ between the treated and control groups during the first year of the study. (2) The number of acute biopsy-proven rejection episodes tended to be more frequent during rhGH treatment: 9 rejection episodes in 44 GH-treated patients versus 4 in 46 control patients. (3) Compared to those without rejection, the patients who rejected did not differ in age, initial renal function, or immunosuppressive regimen, but history of rejection before initiation of rhGH therapy was discriminatory; 6 of 17 children with two or more rejection episodes had a new rejection during rhGH therapy versus 1 of 22 with none or only one episode.

Two smaller randomized controlled studies.[250,275] and one larger study in 68 patients[242] did not report an increased incidence of acute rejection episodes attributable to rhGH, and there was no accelerated decline in graft function in the GH-treated group compared to the control group.[242] The last study (242) found similar results concerning the risk of rejection as the French study.[236] In the entire study population, an acute rejection episode occurred in 4 of 10 patients with greater than one rejection episode prior to randomization, but in only 4 of 53 with no or one prior rejection.

Thus, greater than one prior acute rejection episode may identify a patient population that is suboptimally immunosuppressed or more immunoreactive. However, the data do not clearly support rhGH treatment as a culprit in precipitating an acute rejection episode. Hence, the risk of acute rejection episodes in GH-treated pediatric renal transplant recipients appears to be lower than initially suspected and may be less relevant given current therapy with potent immunosuppressive drugs. Acute rejection may be more frequent during rhGH administration in those patients who have a history of more than one rejection episode. Close monitoring of graft function is therefore recommended. On the other hand, rhGH appears to be safe in immunologically low-risk patients with a history of no or one acute rejection episode.

Benign Intracranial Hypertension. One survey noted symptoms or signs of intracranial hypertension with papilledema during rhGH therapy in 15 cases of approximately 1670 pa-

tients (0.9 percent) with renal disease.[276] All of the 15 children were using medications which could predispose them to intracranial hypertension; in addition, fluid retention due to chronic renal disease might be another predisposing factor.

The median duration of rhGH treatment before the onset of signs and symptoms was 13 weeks. This temporal relation suggests that rhGH was the precipitating factor. All but two patients were symptomatic; the symptoms generally abated when rhGH therapy was discontinued but two patients had persistent blindness. At least four of these patients had a recurrence of intracranial hypertension after reinitiation of rhGH.

Benign intracranial hypertension is a rare complication (1 percent) in rhGH-treated children with CRF. We recommend routine funduscopic examinations before and during initiation of rhGH therapy and whenever signs or symptoms of intracranial hypertension develop. rhGH should be discontinued when intracranial hypertension is detected and should not be resumed after relief of symptoms because of the risk of recurrence.

Osseous Complications. Data from a multicenter study found no significant difference in radiographic osteodystrophy scores or in serum calcium, phosphorus, or parathyroid hormone levels between the rhGH and control groups.[277] The serum alkaline phosphatase concentration increased transiently.

The risk of slipped capital femoral epiphyses and/or avascular necrosis remains equivocal in children with CRF treated with rhGH. Slipped capital femoral epiphyses were noted in 2 of the 125 patients. The duration of treatment in these children was three months and three year at the time of diagnosis; both had severe renal osteodystrophy. In another review of 103 prepubertal children treated with rhGH, two cases of avascular necrosis were reported.[260]

An aggravation of secondary hyperparathyroidism has been rarely reported.[278,279] This does not appear to be due to a direct stimulation of the parathyroid gland by GH; rather, it may be an indirect consequence of small decreases in ionized calcium. This may be a consequence of GH-stimulated bone apposition or an increase in serum phosphate concentration.

rhGH therapy does not induce or aggravate renal osteodystrophy, but improved growth by rhGH can unmask a preexisting renal osteopathy and thereby induce slipped capital femoral epiphysis, as is also observed in normal children experiencing rapid growth acceleration. We therefore recommend correction of the radiologic and/or serologic abnormalities of renal osteodystrophy prior to initiating GH therapy. Persistent renal osteodystrophy may blunt the response to rhGH as well as predispose to toxicity. It is advisable to obtain bone radiographs of the osseous structures prior to initiating rhGH and to repeat the studies if symptoms occur.

Other. Several other potential side effects have been a concern with rhGH administration to children with CRF. As with other foreign proteins, the development of antibodies against rhGH is theoretically possible. In the placebo-controlled trial, 19 of 82 patients (23 percent) developed low-titer GH antibodies, which were not associated with growth attenuation.[232] The incidence of high-titer antibodies appears to be very low. Nevertheless, testing for antibodies to rhGH is recommended in any patient who fails to respond to therapy.

Other possible untoward effects of rhGH therapy include the following: (1) Subclinical hypothyroidism may be unmasked in a few children, possibly due to the GH-induced stimulation of hypothalamic somatostatin release which inhibits GH as well as TSH secretion.[280] (2) Acromegaloid features are a dose-related phenomenon that should not be troublesome in the context of current rhGH dose ranges in children with CRF. (3) There is no proven increase in the risk of acquiring or getting a recurrence of malignancy following rhGH treatment.[281–283] There have been no definitive reports of leukemia in rhGH-treated children with CRF. However, the need for continued cancer surveillance with the use of rhGH in solid-organ recipients is suggested by a report of two recipients of living-related donor grafts who had received long-term rhGH (approximately 8 years) and developed renal cell carcinoma in the graft 9 to 12 years posttransplant.[284] (4) Acute pancreatitis associated with rhGH therapy for short stature has been reported in a few cases, but not in children with CRF.[285] (5) Retinal changes similar to those seen in patients with diabetic retinopathy were observed in two nondiabetic patients receiving rhGH, but again, not in children with CRF.[286]

SUMMARY

Growth hormone therapy has been shown to stimulate growth significantly in prepubertal children with renal failure and ESRD, and does not appear to exhaust growth potential. We believe that sufficient information is available to recommend the use of rhGH in growth-retarded prepubertal children with renal failure in the following manner: (1) Therapy should be instituted when the patient falls below the third percentile for height and does not show spontaneous catch-up growth after other factors contributing to uremic growth failure have been adequately stabilized. (2) Children with preterminal CRF appear to respond better to rhGH than those on dialysis. Thus, rhGH therapy should be initiated at a young age with the goal of restoring the level of growth to a normal genetic percentile well before the need for renal replacement therapy. (3) The dose of rhGH in children with CRF is 0.045 to 0.05 mg/kg body weight per day; rhGH is given daily via subcutaneous injections. (4) The minimal therapeutic aim should be a height greater than the third percentile of the general population. Therapy is continued until final height is reached or a well-functioning renal transplant is achieved.

REFERENCES

1. Guthrie LG, Oxon MD. Chronic interstitial nephritis in childhood. *Lancet* 1897;1:585.
2. Tönshoff B, Schaefer F, Mehls O. Disturbance of growth hormone-insulin-like growth factor axis in uremia. *Pediatr Nephrol* 1990;4:654.
3. Orejas G, Santos F, Malaga S, et al. Nutritional status of children with moderate chronic renal failure. *Pediatr Nephrol* 1995;9:52.
4. Foreman JW, Abitbol CL, Trachtman H, et al. Nutritional intake in children with renal insufficiency: a report of the Growth Failure in Children with Renal Diseases Study. *J Am Coll Nutr* 1996;15:579.
5. Baur LA, Knight JF, Crawford BA, et al. Total body nitrogen in children with chronic renal failure and short stature. *Eur J Clin Nutr* 1994;48:433.
6. Mehls O, Ritz E, Gilli G, et al. Nitrogen metabolism and growth in experimental uremia. *Int J Pediatr Nephrol* 1980;1:34.
7. Arnold WC, Danford D, Holliday MA. Effects of calorie supplementation on growth in uremia. *Kidney Int* 1983;24:205.
8. Betts PR, Magrath G, White RHR. Role of dietary energy supplementation in growth of children with chronic renal insufficiency. *BMJ* 1977;1:416.
9. Jones RWA, Rigden SP, Barratt TM, et al. The effects of chronic renal failure in infancy on growth, nutritional status and body composition. *Pediatr Res* 1982;16:784.
10. Jones RWA, Dalton RN, Turner C, et al. Oral essential aminoacid and ketoacid supplements in children with chronic renal failure. *Kidney Int* 1983;24:95.
11. Wingen AM, Fabian-Bach C, Schaefer F, et al. Randomised multicentre study of a low-protein diet on the progression of chronic renal failure in children. European Study Group of Nutritional Treatment of Chronic Renal Failure in Childhood. *Lancet* 1997;349:1117.
12. Wassner SJ. Altered growth and protein turnover in rats fed sodium-deficient diets. *Pediatr Res* 1989;26:608.
13. Wassner SJ. The effect of sodium repletion on growth and protein turnover in sodium-depleted rats. *Pediatr Nephrol* 1991;5:501.
14. Heinly MM, Wassner SJ. The effect of isolated chloride depletion on growth and protein turnover in young rats. *Pediatr Nephrol* 1994;8:555.
15. Grossman H, Duggan E, McCamman S, et al. The dietary chloride deficiency syndrome. *Pediatrics* 1980;66:366.
16. Mitch WE, May RC, Kelly RA, et al. Protein metabolism in uremia. In: Davison AM, ed. *Nephrology*. Vol. II. London: Bailliere Tindall 1988:1003.

17. May RC, Hara Y, Kelly RA, et al. Branched-chain amino acid metabolism in rat muscle: abnormal regulation in acidosis. *Am J Physiol* 1987;252:712.

18. May RC, Kelly RA, Mitch WE. Metabolic acidosis stimulates protein degradation in rat muscle by a glucocorticoid-dependent mechanism. *J Clin Invest* 1986;77:614.

19. Williams B, Layward E, Walls J. Skeletal muscle degradation and nitrogen wasting in rats with chronic metabolic acidosis. *Clin Sci* 1991;80:457.

20. Bailey JL, Wang X, England BK, et al. The acidosis of chronic renal failure activates muscle proteolysis in rats by augmenting transcription of genes encoding proteins of the ATP-dependent ubiquitin-proteasome pathway. *J Clin Invest* 1996;97:1447.

21. Challa A, Krieg RJ Jr, Thabet MA, et al. Metabolic acidosis inhibits growth hormone secretion in rats: mechanism of growth retardation. *Am J Physiol* 1993;265:547.

22. Challa A, Chan W, Krieg RJ Jr, et al. Effect of metabolic acidosis on the expression of insulin-like growth factor and growth hormone receptor. *Kidney Int* 1993;44:1224.

23. Brüngger M, Hulter HN, Krapf R. Effect of chronic metabolic acidosis on the growth hormone/IGF1 endocrine axis: new cause of growth hormone insensitivity in humans. *Kidney Int* 1997;51:216.

24. Kattamis CA, Kattamis AC. Management of thalassemias: growth and development, hormone substitution, vitamin supplementation, and vaccination. *Semin Hematol* 1995;32:269.

25. Seidel C, Schaefer F, Walther U, et al. The application of knemometry in renal disease: preliminary observations. *Pediatr Nephrol* 1991;5:467.

26. Schaefer F, André JL, Krug C, et al. Growth and skeletal maturation in dialysed children treated with recombinant human erythropoietin (rhEPO): a multicenter study. *Pediatr Nephrol* 1991;5:C61.

27. Mehls O, Ritz E, Gilli G, et al. Effect of vitamin D on growth in experimental uremia. *Am J Clin Nutr* 1978;31:1927.

28. Mehls O, Ritz E, Gilli G, et al. Role of hormonal disturbances in uremic growth failure. *Contrib Nephrol* 1986;50:119.

29. Chesney RW, Moorthy AV, Eisman JA, et al. Influence of oral 1,25-vitamin D in childhood renal osteodystrophy. *Contrib Nephrol* 1980;18:55.

30. Kreusser W, Weinkauf R, Mehls O, et al. Effect of parathyroid hormone, calcitonin and growth hormone on cAMP content of growth cartilage in experimental uremia. *Eur J Clin Invest* 1982;12:337.

31. Klaus G, von Eichel B, May T, et al. Synergistic effects of parathyroid hormone and 1,25-dihydroxyvitamin D_3 on proliferation and vitamin D receptor expression of rat growth cartilage cells. *Endocrinology* 1994;135:1307.

32. Schmitt CP, Hessing S, Oh J, et al. Intermittent administration of parathyroid hormone (1–37) improves growth and bone mineral density in uremic rats. *Kidney Int* 2000;57:1484.

33. Kuizon BD, Goodman WG, Jüppner H, et al. Diminished linear growth during intermittent calcitriol therapy in children undergoing CCPD. *Kidney Int* 1998;53:205.

34. Krempien B, Mehls O, Ritz E. Morphological studies on pathogenesis of epiphyseal slipping in uremic children. *Virchows Arch* (A) 1974;362:129.

35. Mehls O, Ritz E, Krempien B, et al. Slipped epiphyses in renal osteodystrophy. *Arch Dis Child* 1975;50:545.

36. Mehls O, Ritz E, Oppermann HC, et al. Femoral head necrosis in uremic children without steroid treatment or transplantation. *J Pediatr* 1981;6:926.

37. Samaan NA, Freeman RM: Growth hormone levels in severe renal failure. *Metabolism* 1970;19:102.

38. Pimstone BL, Le Roith D, Epstein S, et al. Disappearance rates of serum growth hormone after intravenous somatostatin in renal and liver disease. *J Clin Endocrinol Metab* 1975;41:392.

39. Davidson M, Fisher M, Dabir-Vaziri N, et al. Effect of protein intake and dialysis on the abnormal growth hormone, glucose, and insulin homeostasis in uremia. *Metabolism* 1976;25:455.

40. Johnson V, Maack T. Renal extraction, filtration absorption, and catabolism of growth hormone. *Am J Physiol* 1977;233:F185.

41. Tönshoff B, Veldhuis JD, Heinrich U, et al. Deconvolution analysis of spontaneous nocturnal growth hormone secretion in prepubertal children with chronic renal failure. *Pediatr Res* 1995;37:86.

42. Veldhuis JD, Iranmanesh A, Wilkowski MJ, et al. Neuroendocrine alterations in the somatotropic and lactotropic axes in uremic men. *Eur J Endocrinol* 1994;131:489.

43. Schaefer F, Veldhuis JD, Jones J, et al. Alterations in growth hormone secretion and clearance in peripubertal boys with chronic renal failure and after renal transplantation. *J Clin Endocrinol Metab* 1994;78:1298.

44. Haffner D, Schaefer F, Girard J, et al. Metabolic clearance of recombinant human growth hormone in health and chronic renal failure. *J Clin Invest* 1944;93:1163.

45. Leung DW, Spencer SA, Cachianes G, et al. Growth hormone receptor and serum binding protein: purification, cloning and expression. *Nature* 1987;330:537.

46. Postel-Vinay MC, Tar A, Crosnier H, et al. Plasma growth-hormone binding is low in uremic children. *Pediatr Nephrol* 1991;5:545.

47. Tönshoff B, Cronin MJ, Reichert M, et al. Reduced concentration of serum growth hormone (GH)-binding protein in children with chronic renal failure: correlation with GH insensitivity. *J Clin Endocrinol Metab* 1997;82:1007.

48. Baumann G, Shaw MA, Amburn K. Regulation of plasma growth hormone-binding proteins in health and disease. *Metabolism* 1989;38:683.

49. Maheshwari HG, Rifkin I, Butler J, et al. Growth hormone binding protein in patients with renal failure. *Acta Endocrinol* 1992;127:485.

50. Kagan A, Zadik Z, Gertler A, et al. Serum concentrations and peritoneal loss of growth hormone and growth-hormone-binding protein activity in older adults undergoing continuous ambulatory peritoneal dialysis: comparison with haemodialysis and normal subjects. *Nephrol Dial Transplant* 1993;8:352.

51. Carlsson LMS, Attie KM, Compton PG, et al. The National Cooperative Growth Study. Reduced concentration of serum

growth hormone-binding protein in children with idiopathic short stature. *J Clin Endocrinol Metab* 1994;78:1325.

52. Ho KYY, Jorgensen JOL, Valiontis E. Different modes of growth hormone (GH) administration do not change GH binding protein activity in man. *Clin Endocrinol* 1993;38:143.

53. Davila N, Alcaniz J, Salto L, et al. Serum growth hormone-binding protein is unchanged in adult panhypopituitarism. *J Clin Endocrinol Metab* 1994;79:1347.

54. Martha PM Jr, Reiter EO, Davila N, et al. Serum growth hormone-binding protein/receptor: an important determinant of growth hormone responsiveness. *J Clin Endocrinol Metab* 1992;75:1464.

55. Tauber M, Portal HB, Sallerin-Caute B, et al. Differential regulation of serum growth hormone (GH)-binding protein during continuous infusion versus daily injection of recombinant human GH in GH-deficient children. *J Clin Endocrinol Metab* 1993;76:1135.

56. Chan W, Valerie KC, Chan JCM. Expression of insulin-like growth factor-1 in uremic rats: growth hormone resistance and nutritional intake. *Kidney Int* 1993;43:790.

57. Tönshoff B, Eden S, Weiser E, et al. Reduced hepatic growth hormone (GH) receptor gene expression and increased plasma GH binding protein in experimental uremia. *Kidney Int* 1994;45:1085.

58. Schaefer F, Chen Y, Tsao T, et al. Impaired JAK-STAT signal transduction contributes to growth hormone resistance in chronic uremia. *J Clin Invest* 2001;108:467.

59. Carter-Su C, Rui L, Herington J. Role of the tyrosine kinase JAK2 in signal transduction by growth hormone. *Pediatr Nephrol* 2000;114:550.

60. Udy GB, Towers RP,. Snell RG, et al. Requirement of STAT5b for sexual dimorphism of body growth rates and liver gene expression. *Proc Natl Acad Sci USA* 1997;94: 7239.

61. Teglund S, McKay C, Schuetz E, et al. Stat5a and Stat5b proteins have essential and nonessential, or redundant, roles in cytokine responses. *Cell* 1998;93:841.

62. Greenhalgh CJ, Hilton DJ: Negative regulation of cytokine signaling. *J Leukoc Biol* 2001;70:348.

63. Davey HW, McLachlan MJ, Wilkins RJ, et al. STAT5b mediates the GH-induced expression of SOCS-2 and SOCS-3 mRNA in the liver. *Mol Cell Endocrinol* 1999;158:111.

64. Ram PR, Waxman DJ: SOCS/CIS protein inhibition of growth hormone-stimulated STAT5 signaling by multiple mechanisms. *J Biol Chem* 1999;275:35553.

65. Tollet-Egnell P, Flores-Morales A, Stavreus-Evers A, et al. Growth hormone regulation of SOCS-2, SOCS-3, and CIS messenger ribonucleic acid expression in the rat. *Endocrinology* 1999;140:3693.

66. Metcalf D, Greenhalgh CJ, Viney E, et al. Gigantism in mice lacking suppressor of cytokine signalling-2. *Nature* 2000;405:1069.

67. Paul C, Seiliez I, Thissen JP, et al. Regulation of expression of the rat SOCS-3 gene in hepatocytes by growth hormone, interleukin-6 and glucocorticoids mRNA analysis and promoter characterization. *Eur J Biochem* 2000;267:5849.

68. Mao Y, Ling PR, Fitzgibbons TP, et al. Endotoxin-induced inhibition of growth hormone receptor signaling in rat liver in vivo. *Endocrinology* 1999;140:5505.

69. Bergad PL, Schwarzenberg SJ, Humbert JT, et al. Inhibition of growth hormone action in models of inflammation. *Am J Physiol Cell Physiol* 2000;279:C1906.

70. Kaysen GA. The microinflammatory state in uremia: causes and potential consequences. *J Am Soc Nephrol* 2001;12:1549.

71. Tönshoff B, Blum WF, Wingen AM, et al. Serum insulin-like growth factors (IGFs) and IGF binding proteins 1, 2, and 3 in children with chronic renal failure: relationship to height and glomerular filtration rate. *J Clin Endocrinol Metab* 1995;80:2684.

72. Tönshoff B, Blum WF, Mehls O. Serum insulin-like growth factors and their binding proteins in children with end-stage renal disease. *Pediatr Nephrol* 1996;10:269.

73. Ulinski T, Mohan S, Kiepe D, et al. Serum insulin-like growth factor binding protein (IGFBP)-4 and IGFBP-5 in children with chronic renal failure: relationship to growth and glomerular filtration rate. *Pediatr Nephrol* 2000;14:589.

74. Phillips LS, Fusco AC, Unterman TG, et al. Somatomedin inhibitor in uremia. *J Clin Endocrinol Metab* 1984;59:764.

75. Blum WF, Ranke MB, Kietzmann K, et al. Growth hormone resistance and inhibition of somatomedin activity by excess of insulin-like growth factor binding protein in uraemia. *Pediatr Nephrol* 1991;5:539.

76. Frystyk J, Ivarsen P, Skjaerbaek C, et al. Serum-free insulin-like growth factor I correlates with clearance in patients with chronic renal failure. *Kidney Int* 1999;56:2076.

77. Baxter RC. Insulin-like growth factor (IGF)-binding proteins: interactions with IGFs and intrinsic bioactivities. *Am J Physiol Endocrinol Metab* 2000;278:E967.

78. Hwa V, Oh Y, Rosenfeld RG. The insulin-like growth factor-binding protein (IGFBP) superfamily. *Endocr Rev* 1999; 20:761.

79. Lee PD, Giudice LC, Conover CA, et al. Insulin-like growth factor binding protein-1: recent findings and new directions. *Proc Soc Exp Biol Med* 1997;216:319.

80. Powell DR, Rosenfeld RG, Sperry JB, et al. Serum concentrations of insulin-like growth factor (IGF)-1, IGF-2 and unsaturated somatomedin carrier proteins in children with chronic renal failure. *Am J Kidney Dis* 1987;10:287.

81. Liu F, Powell DR, Hintz RL. Characterization of insulin-like growth factor binding proteins in human serum from patients with chronic renal failure. *J Clin Endocrinol Metab* 1990;70:620.

82. Baxter RC, Martin JL, Beniac VA. High molecular weight insulin-like growth factor binding protein complex. *J Biol Chem* 1989;264:11843.

83. Powell DR, Liu F, Baker BK, et al. Insulin-like growth factor binding protein-6 levels are elevated in serum of children with chronic renal failure: a report of the Southwest Pediatric Nephrology Study Group. *J Clin Endocrinol Metab* 1997;82:2978.

84. Powell DR, Liu F, Baker BK, et al. Characterization of insulin-like growth factor binding protein-3 in chronic renal failure serum. *Pediatr Res* 1993;33:136.

85. Powell DR, Liu F, Baker BK, et al. Modulation of growth factors by growth hormone in children with chronic renal failure. The Southwest Pediatric Nephrology Study Group. *Kidney Int* 1997;51:1970.

86. Powell DR, Durham SK, Brewer ED, et al. Effects of chronic renal failure and growth hormone on serum levels of insulin-like growth factor-binding protein-4 (IGFBP-4) and IGFBP-5 in children: a report of the Southwest Pediatric Nephrology Study Group. *J Clin Endocrinol Metab* 1997; 84:596.

87. Durham SK, Mohan S, Liu F, et al. Bioactivity of a 29-kilodalton insulin-like growth factor binding protein-3 fragment present in excess in chronic renal failure serum. *Pediatr Res* 1997;42:335.

88. Wühl E, Haffner D, Nissel R, et al. Short dialyzed children respond less to growth hormone than patients prior to dialysis. German Study Group for Growth Hormone Treatment in Chronic Renal Failure. *Pediatr Nephrol* 1996;10:294.

89. Blum WF: Insulin-like growth factors (IGFs) and IGF binding proteins in chronic renal failure: Evidence for reduced secretion of IGFs. *Acta Paediatr Scand Suppl* 1991;379:24.

90. Tönshoff B, Powell DR, Zhao D, et al. Decreased hepatic insulin-like growth factor (IGF)-I and increased IGF binding protein-1 and -2 gene expression in experimental uremia. *Endocrinology* 1996;138:938.

91. Holly JM, Claffey DC, Cwyfan-Hughes et al. Proteases acting on IGFBPs: their occurrence and physiological significance. *Growth Regul* 1993;3:88.

92. Lee DY, Park SK, Yorgin PD, et al. Alteration in insulin-like growth factor-binding proteins (IGFBPs) and IGFBP-3 protease activity in serum and urine from acute and chronic renal failure. *J Clin Endocrinol Metab* 1994;79:1376.

93. Ooi GT, Tseng LYH, Rechler MM. Posttranscriptional regulation of insulin-like growth factor binding protein-2 mRNA in diabetic liver. *Biochem Biophys Res Commun* 1992; 189:1031.

94. Margot JB, Binkert C, Mary JL, et al. A low molecular weight insulin-like growth factor binding protein from rat: cDNA cloning and tissue distribution of its messenger RNA. *Mol Endocrinol* 1989;3:1053.

95. Binoux M, Hossenlopp P: Insulin-like growth factor (IGF) and IGF-binding proteins: comparison of human serum and lymph. *J Clin Endocrinol Metab* 1988;67:509.

96. Kale AS, Liu F, Hintz RL, et al. Characterization of insulin-like growth factors and their binding proteins in peritoneal dialysate. *Pediatr Nephrol* 1996;10:467.

97. Burch WM, Correa J, Shively JE, et al. The 25-kilodalton insulin-like growth factor (IGF)-binding protein inhibits both basal and IGF-I-mediated growth of chick embryo pelvic cartilage in vitro. *J Clin Endocrinol Metab* 1990; 70:173.

98. Standker L, Braulke T, Mark S, et al. Partial IGF affinity of circulating N- and C-terminal fragments of human insulin-like growth factor binding protein-4 (IGFBP-4) and the disulfide bonding pattern of the C-terminal IGFBP-4 domain. *Biochemistry* 2000;39:5082.

99. Standker L, Wobst P, Mark S, et al. Isolation and characterization of circulating 13-kDa C-terminal fragments of human insulin-like growth factor binding protein-5. *FEBS Lett* 1998;441:281.

100. Kiepe D, Ulinski T, Powell DR, et al. Differential effects of IGFBP-1, -2, -3, and -6 on cultured growth plate chondrocytes. *Kidney Int* 2002;62:1591.

101. Kiepe D, Andress DL, Mohan S, et al. Intact IGF-binding protein-4 and -5 and their respective fragments isolated from chronic renal failure serum differentially modulate IGF-I actions in cultured growth plate chondrocytes. *J Am Soc Nephrol* 2001;12:2400.

102. Rajkumar K, Barron D, Lewitt MS, Murphy LJ. Growth retardation and hyperglycemia in insulin-like growth factor binding protein-1 transgenic mice. *Endocrinology* 1995; 136:4029.

103. Gay E, Seurin D, Babajko S, et al. Liver-specific expression of human insulin-like growth factor binding protein-1 in transgenic mice: repercussions on reproduction, ante- and perinatal mortality and postnatal growth. *Endocrinology* 1997;138:2937.

104. Hoeflich A, Wu M, Mohan S, et al. Overexpression of insulin-like growth factor-binding protein-2 in transgenic mice reduces postnatal body weight gain. *Endocrinology* 1999; 140:5488.

105. Modric T, Silha JV, Shi Z, et al. Phenotypic manifestations of insulin-like growth factor-binding protein-3 overexpression in transgenic mice. *Endocrinology* 2001;142:1958.

106. Cox GN, McDermott MJ, Merkel E, et al. Recombinant human insulin-like growth factor (IGF)-binding protein-1 inhibits somatic growth stimulated by IGF-I and growth hormone in hypophysectomized rats. *Endocrinology* 1994; 135:1913.

107. Hoeflich A, Nedbal S, Blum WF. Growth inhibition in giant growth hormone transgenic mice by overexpression of insulin-like growth factor-binding protein-2. *Endocrinology* 2001;142:1889.

108. Tönshoff B, Mehls O, Heinrich U, et al. Growth-stimulating effects of recombinant human growth hormone in children with end-stage renal disease. *J Pediatr* 1990;4:561.

109. Hokken-Koelega AC, Stijnen T, de Muinck Keizer-Schrama SM, et al. Placebo-controlled, double-blind, cross-over trial of growth hormone treatment in prepubertal children with chronic renal failure. *Lancet* 1991;338:585.

110. Powell DR, Durham SK, Liu F, et al. The insulin-like growth factor axis and growth in children with chronic renal failure: a report of the Southwest Pediatric Nephrology Study Group. *J Clin Endocrinol Metab* 1998;83:1654.

111. Cobo A, Lopez JM, Carbajo E, et al. Growth plate cartilage formation and resorption are differentially depressed in growth retarded uremic rats. *J Am Soc Nephrol* 1999;10:971.

112. Cobo A, Carbajo E, Santos F, et al. Morphometry of uremic rat growth plate. *Miner Electrolyte Metab* 1996;22:192–195.

113. Mehls O, Ritz E, Hunziker EB, et al. Improvement of growth and food utilization by human recombinant growth hormone in uremia. *Kidney Int* 1988;33:45.

114. Hanna JD, Santos F, Foreman JW, et al. Insulin-like growth factor-I gene expression in the tibial epiphyseal growth plate of growth hormone-treated uremic rats. *Kidney Int* 1995; 47:1374.

115. Alvarez J, Balbin M, Fernandez M, Lopez JM. Collagen metabolism is markedly altered in the hypertrophic cartilage of growth plates from rats with growth impairment secondary to chronic renal failure. *J Bone Miner Res* 2001;16:511.

116. Sanchez CP, Salusky IB, Kuizon BD, et al. Growth of long bones in renal failure: roles of hyperparathyroidism, growth hormone and calcitriol. *Kidney Int* 1998;54:1879.

117. Sanchez CP, Kuizon BD, Abdella PA, eet al. Impaired growth, delayed ossification, and reduced osteoclastic activity in the growth plate of calcium-supplemented rats with renal failure. *Endocrinology* 2000;141:1536.

118. Jüppner H. Role of parathyroid hormone-related peptide and Indian hedgehog in skeletal development. *Pediatr Nephrol* 2000;14:606.

119. Karaplis AC, Luz A, Glowacki J, et al. Lethal skeletal dysplasia from targeted disruption of the parathyroid hormone-related peptide gene. *Genes Dev* 1994;8:277.

120. Lanske B, Karaplis AC, Lee K, et al. PTH/PTHrP receptor in early development and Indian hedgehog-regulated bone growth. *Science* 1996;273:663.

121. Weir EC, Philbrick WM, Amling M, et al. Targeted overexpression of parathyroid hormone-related peptide in chondrocytes causes chondrodysplasia and delayed endochondral bone formation. *Proc Natl Acad Sci USA* 1996;93:10240.

122. Schipani E, Kruse K, Juppner HA. Constitutively active mutant PTH-PTHrP receptor in Jansen-type metaphyseal chondrodysplasia. *Science* 1995;268:98.

123. Jobert AS, Zhang P, Couvineau A, et al. Absence of functional receptors for parathyroid hormone and parathyroid hormone-related peptide in Blomstrand chondrodysplasia. *J Clin Invest* 1998;102:34.

124. Coen G, Mazzaferro S, Ballanti P, et al. Renal bone disease in 76 patients with varying degrees of predialysis chronic renal failure: a cross-sectional study. *Nephrol Dial Transplant* 1996;11:813.

125. Urena P, Mannstadt M, Hruby M, et al. Parathyroidectomy does not prevent the renal PTH/PTHrP receptor down-regulation in uremic rats. *Kidney Int* 1995;147:1797.

126. Urena P, Ferreira A, Morieux C, et al. PTH/PTHrP receptor mRNA is down-regulated in epiphyseal cartilage growth plate of uraemic rats. *Nephrol Dial Transplant* 1996;11: 2008.

127. Urena P, Kubrusly M, Mannstadt M, et al. The renal PTH/PTHrP receptor is down-regulated in rats with chronic renal failure. *Kidney Int* 1994;45:605.

128. Picton ML, Moore PR, Mawer EB, et al. Down-regulation of human osteoblast PTH/PTHrP receptor mRNA in end-stage renal failure. *Kidney Int* 2000;58:1440.

129. Edmondson SR, Baker NL, Oh J, et al. Growth hormone receptor abundance in tibial growth plates of uremic rats: GH/IGF-I treatment. *Kidney Int* 2000;58:62.

130. Green J, Maor G: Effect of metabolic acidosis on the growth hormone/IGF-I endocrine axis in skeletal growth centers. *Kidney Int* 57:2258.

131. Saggese G, Federico G, Cinquanta L. In vitro effects of growth hormone and other hormones on chondrocytes and osteoblast-like cells. *Acta Paediatr Suppl* 1993;82(suppl 391):54.

132. Scharla SH, Strong DD, Mohan S, et al. 1,25-Dihydroxyvitamin D_3 differentially regulates the production of insulin-like growth factor I (IGF-I) and IGF-binding protein-4 in mouse osteoblasts. *Endocrinology* 1991;129:3139.

133. Silbermann M, Mirsky N, Levitan S, et al. The effect of 1,25-dihydroxyvitamin D_3 on cartilage growth in neonatal mice. *Metab Bone Dis Relat Res* 1983;4:337.

134. Weinreb M Jr, Gazit E, Weinreb MM. Mandibular growth and histologic changes in condylar cartilage of rats intoxi-cated with vitamin D_3 or 1,25(OH)2D_3 and pair-fed (undernourished) rats. *J Dent Res* 1986;65:1449.

135. Silbermann M, von der Mark K, Mirsky N, et al. Effects of increased doses of 1,25 dihydroxyvitamin D_3 on matrix and DNA synthesis in condylar cartilage of suckling mice. *Calcif Tissue Int* 1987;41:95.

136. Kainer G, Nakano M, Massie FS Jr, et al. Hypercalciuria due to combined growth hormone and calcitriol therapy in uremia: effects of growth hormone on mineral homeostasis in 75% nephrectomized weanling rats. *Pediatr Res* 1991; 30:528.

137. Klaus G, Weber L, Rodriguez J, et al. Interaction of IGF-I and 1 alpha, 25(OH)2D_3 on receptor expression and growth stimulation in rat growth plate chondrocytes. *Kidney Int* 1998;53:1152.

138. Betts PR, Macgrath G. Growth pattern and dietary intake of children with chronic renal insufficiency. *Br Med J* 1974; 2:189.

139. Jones RWA, Rigden SP, Barratt TM, et al. The effects of chronic renal failure in infancy on growth, nutritional status and body composition. *Pediatr Res* 1982;16:784–791.

140. Kleinknecht C, Broyer M, Huot D, et al. Growth and development of nondialyzed children with chronic renal failure. *Kidney Int* 1983;24:40.

141. Rizzoni G, Basso T, Setari M. Growth in children with chronic renal failure on conservative treatment. *Kidney Int* 1984;26:52.

142. Warady BA, Kriley MA, Lovell H, et al. Growth and development of infants with end-stage renal disease receiving long-term peritoneal dialysis. *J Pediatr* 1988;112:714.

143. Rees L, Rigden SPA, Ward GM. Chronic renal failure and growth. *Arch Dis Child* 1989;64:573.

144. Karlberg J, Schaefer F, Hennicke M et al. Early age-dependent growth impairment in chronic renal failure. European Study Group for Nutritional Treatment of Chronic Renal Failure in Childhood. *Pediatr Nephrol* 1996;10:283.

145. Schaefer F, Wingen AM, Hennicke M, et al. Growth charts for prepubertal children with chronic renal failure due to congenital renal disorders. European Study Group for Nutritional Treatment of Chronic Renal Failure in Childhood. *Pediatr Nephrol* 1996;10:288.

146. Schärer K, Chantler C, Brunner FP, et al. Combined report on regular dialysis and transplantation of children in Europe, 1975. *Proc Eur Dial Transplant Assoc Eur Renal Assoc* 1976;13:3.

147. Schärer K. Study on pubertal development in chronic renal failure. Growth and development of children with chronic renal failure. *Acta Paediatr Scand Suppl* 1990;366:90.

148. Rizzoni G, Broyer M, Brunner FP, et al. Combined report on regular dialysis and transplantation of children in Europe, XIII, 1983. In: Davison AM, Guillou PJ, eds. *Proceedings of The European Dialysis and Transplant Association—European Renal Association.* Vol 21. London: Pitman Medical, 1984:69.

149. Rizzoni G, Broyer M, Brunner FP, et al. Combined report on regular hemodialysis and transplantation in Europe, 1985. *Proc Eur Dial Transplant Assoc Eur Renal Assoc* 1986; 23:55.

150. Schärer K. *Growth and Endocrine Changes in Children with Chronic Renal Failure.* Basel: Karger, 1989.

151. Ehrich JHH, Rizzoni G, Brunner FP, et al. Combined report on regular dialysis and transplantation in Europe. *Nephrol Dial Transplant* 1991;6(suppl):37.

152. Schaefer F, Seidel C, Binding A, et al. Pubertal growth in chronic renal failure. *Pediatr Res* 1990;28:5.

153. Largo RH, Prader A. Pubertal development in Swiss girls. *Helv Paediatr Acta* 1983;38:229.

154. Burke BA, Lindgren B, Wick M, et al. Testicular germ cell loss in children with renal failure. *Pediatr Pathol* 1989; 9:433.

155. Schaefer F, Walther U, Ruder H, et al. Reduced spermaturia in adolescent and young adult patients after renal transplantation. *Nephrol Dial Transplant* 1991;6:840.

156. Palmer BF. Sexual dysfunction in uremia. *J Am Soc Nephrol* 1999;10:1381.

157. Hou S. Pregnancy in chronic renal insufficiency and end-stage renal disease. *Am J Kidney Dis* 1999;33(2):235.

158. Chan WS, Okun N, Kjellstrand CM. Pregnancy in chronic dialysis: a review and analysis of the literature. *Int J Artif Organs* 1998;21(5):259.

159. Nakabayashi M, Adachi T, Itoh S, et al. Perinatal and infant outcome of pregnant patients undergoing chronic hemodialysis. *Nephron* 1999;82:27.

160. Kleinknecht C, Broyer M, Gagnadoux M, et al. Growth in children treated with long-term dialysis. A study of 76 patients. *Adv Nephrol* 1980;9:133.

161. Offner G, Hoyer PF, Jüppner H, et al. Somatic growth after kidney transplantation. *Am J Dis Child* 1987;141:541.

162. Rees L, Greene SA, Adlard P, et al. Growth and endocrine function after renal transplantation. *Arch Dis Child* 1988; 63:1326.

163. Broyer M, Guest G. Growth after kidney transplantation: a single centre experience. In: Schärer K, ed. *Growth and Endocrine Changes in Children and Adolescents with Chronic Renal Failure. Vol. 20. Pediatric and Adolescent Endocrinology.* Basel: Karger, 1989:36.

164. Betts PR, White RHR. Growth potential and skeletal maturity in children with chronic renal insufficiency. *Nephron* 1976;16:325.

165. Cundall DB, Brocklebank JT, Buckler JMH. Which bone age in chronic renal insufficiency and end-stage renal disease? *Pediatr Nephrol* 1988;2:200.

166. van Steenbergen MW, Wit JM, Donckerwolcke RAG. Testosterone esters advance skeletal maturation more than growth in short boys with chronic renal failure and delayed puberty. *Eur J Pediatr* 1991;150:676.

167. van Diemen-Steenvoorde R, Donckerwolcke RA, Brackel H, et al. Growth and sexual maturation in children after kidney transplantation. *J Pediatr* 1987;110:351.

168. Grushkin CM, Fine RN. Growth in children following renal transplantation. *Am J Dis Child* 1973;125:514.

169. Rizzoni G, Broyer M, Brunner FP, et al. Combined report on regular hemodialysis and transplantation in Europe, 1985. *Proc EDTA* 1986;23:55.

170. Chantler C, Broyer M, Donckerwolcke RA, et al. Growth and rehabilitation of long-term survivors of treatment for end-stage renal failure in childhood. *Proc Eur Dial Transplant Assoc* 1981;18:329.

171. Gilli G, Mehls O, Schärer K. Final height of children with chronic renal failure. *Proc Eur Dial Transplant Assoc* 1984;21:830.

172. Fennell RS III, Love JT, Carter RL, et al. Statistical analysis of statural growth following kidney transplantation. *Eur J Pediatr* 1986;145:377.

173. Schaefer F, Gilli G, Schärer K. Pubertal growth and final height in chronic renal failure. In: Schärer K, ed. *Growth and Endocrine Changes in Children and Adolescents with Chronic Renal Failure. Vol. 22. Pediatric and Adolescent Endocrinology.* Basel: Karger, 1989:59.

174. Hokken-Koelega AC, Van Zaal MA, van Bergen W, et al. Final height and its predictive factors after renal transplantation in childhood. *Pediatr Res* 1994;36:323.

175. Wühl E, Haffner D, Offner G, et al. European Study Group on Growth Hormone Treatment in children with nephropatic cystinosis. Long-term treatment with growth hormone in short children with nephropatic cystinosis. *J Pediatr* 2001; 138:880.

176. Strife CF, Quinlan M, Mears K, et al. Improved growth of three uremic children by nocturnal nasogastric feedings. *Am J Dis Child* 1986;140:438.

177. Kleinknecht C, Broyer M, Huot D, et al. Growth and development of nondialyzed children with chronic renal failure. *Kidney Int* 1983;24:40.

178. Mehls O, Bonzel KE, Wingen A, et al. Normal growth in infants with chronic renal failure (abstr). *Pediatr Nephrol* 1987;1:C90.

179. Abitbol CL, Zilleruelo G, Montane B, et al. Growth of uremic infants on forced feeding regimens. *Pediatr Nephrol* 1993;7:173.

180. Kleinknecht C, Broyer M, Gagnadoux M, et al. Growth in children with long-term dialysis. A study of 76 patients. *Adv Nephrol* 1980;9:133.

181. Broyer M, Kleinknecht C, Loirat C, et al. Growth in children treated with long-term hemodialysis. *J Pediatr* 1974; 84:642.

182. Trachtmann H, Hackney P, Tejani A. Pediatric hemodialysis: a decade's (1974–1984) perspective. *Kidney Int* 1986;30 (suppl):15.

183. Fennel RS III, Orak JK, Hudson T, et al. Growth in children with various therapies for end-stage renal disease. *Am J Dis Child* 1984;138:28.

184. André JL, de Bernardin JM, Martinet M, et al. Evolution staturopondérale des enfants urémiques sous dialyse et aprés transplantation rénale. *Pédiatrie* 1989;44:495.

185. Chantler C, Donckerwolcke RA, Brunner JP, et al. Combined report on regular dialysis and transplantation of children in Europe 1976. In: *Dialysis Transplantation Nephrology.* Tunbridge Wells, UK: Pitman, 1977:70.

186. Kohaut EC. Continuous ambulatory peritoneal dialysis: a preliminary experience. *Am J Dis Child* 1981;135:270.

187. Balfe JW, Vigneux A, Willumsen J. The use of CAPD in the treatment of children with end-stage renal disease. *Periton Dial Bull* 1981;1:35.

188. Stefanidis CJ, Hewitt IK, Balfe JW. Growth in children receiving continuous ambulatory peritoneal dialysis. *J Pediatr* 1983;83:681.

189. Continuous ambulatory and continuous cycling peritoneal dialysis in children. A report of the Southwest Pediatric Nephrology Study Group. *Kidney Int* 1985;27:558.

190. Potter DE, Luis ES, Wipfler JE, et al. Comparison of continuous ambulatory peritoneal dialysis and hemodialysis in children. *Kidney Int* 1986;30(suppl):11.

191. Fine RN, Mehls O. CAPD/CCPD in children: four years' experience. *Kidney Int* 1986;30(suppl):7.

192. von Lilien T, Gilli G, Salusky IB. Growth in children undergoing continuous ambulatory or cycling peritoneal dialysis. In: Schärer K, ed. *Pediatric and Adolescent Endocrinology.* Basel, Switzerland: Karger:27.

193. Warady B, Kriley M, Lovell H, et al. Growth and development of infants with end-stage renal disease receiving long-term peritoneal dialysis. *J Pediatr* 1988;112:714.

194. Kohaut EC, Alexander SR, Mehls O. The management of the infant on CAPD. In: Fine RN, Schärer K, Mehls O, eds. *CAPD in Children.* Berlin: Springer-Verlag, 1985:97.

195. Pennisi AJ, Costin G, Phillips L, et al. Linear growth in long-term renal allograft recipients. *Clin Nephrol* 1977; 8:415.

196. Broyer M, Guest G. Growth after kidney transplantation: a single centre experience. In: Schärer K, ed. *Growth and Endocrine Changes in Children and Adolescents with Chronic Renal Failure,* vol. 20. *Pediatric Adolescent Endocrinology.* Basel: Karger:36.

197. Tejani A, Fine RN, Alexander S, et al. Factors predictive of sustained growth in children after renal transplantation. *J Pediatr* 1993;122:397.

198. Ingelfinger JR, Grupe WE, Harmon WB, et al. Growth acceleration following renal transplantation in children less than 7 years of age. *Pediatrics* 1981;68:255.

199. Bosque M, Munian A, Bewick M, et al. Growth after renal transplants. *Arch Dis Child* 1983;58:114.

200. So S, Chang P, Najaran J, et al. Growth and development in infants after renal transplantation. *J Pediatr* 1987;110:343.

201. Claris-Appiani A, Bianchi ML, Bini P, et al. Growth in young children with chronic renal failure. *Pediatr Nephrol* 1989;3:301.

202. McEnery PT, Stablein DM, Arbus G, et al. Renal transplantation in children. *N Engl J Med* 1992;326:1727.

203. Hokken-Koelega ACS, Van Zaal MAE, De Ridder MAJ, et al. Growth after renal transplantation in prepubertal children: impact of various treatment modalities. *Pediatr Res* 1994;35:367.

204. Offner G, Hoyer PF, Jüppner H, et al. Somatic growth after kidney transplantation. *Am J Dis Child* 1987;141:541.

205. Brodehl J, Offner G, Hoyer PF, et al. Cyclosporin A in pediatric kidney transplantation and its effect on posttransplantation growth. *Nephron* 1986;44:26.

206. Ruder H, Strehlau J, Schaefer F, et al. Low-dose cyclosporin A therapy in cadaver renal transplantation in children. *Transplant Int* 1989;2:203.

207. Broyer M, Guest G, Gagnadoux M. Growth rate in children receiving alternate-day corticosteroid treatment after kidney transplantation. *J Pediatr* 1992;120:721.

208. Bökenkamp A, Brodehl J, Offner G, et al. Long term results in pediatric kidney transplantation: comparison of conventional with cyclosporin A immunosuppression (abstr). *Pediatr Nephrol* 1991;5:C45.

209. Ferraris JR, Day PF, Gutman R, et al. Effect of therapy with a new glucocorticoid, deflazacort, on linear growth and growth hormone secretion after renal transplantation. *J Pediatr* 1992;121:809.

210. Broyer M, Guest G, Gagnadoux MF. Growth rate in children receiving alternate-day corticosteroid treatment after kidney transplantation. *J Pediatr* 1992;120:721.

211. Jabs K, Sullivan EK, Avner ED, et al. Alternate-day steroid dosing improves growth without adversely affecting graft survival or long-term graft function. A report of the North American Pediatric Renal Transplant Cooperative Study. *Transplantation* 1996;61:31.

212. Benfield MR, McDonald R, Sullivan EK, et al. The 1997 Annual Renal Transplantation in Children Report of the North American Pediatric Renal Transplant Cooperative Study (NAPRTCS). *Pediatr Transplant* 1999;3:152.

213. Qvist E, Marttinen E, Rönnholm K, et al. Growth after renal transplantation in infancy or early childhood. *Pediatr Nephrol* 2002;17:438.

214. Klare B, Strom TM, Hahn H, et al. Remarkable long-term prognosis and excellent growth in kidney-transplant children under cyclosporine monotherapy. *Transplant Proc* 1991; 23:1013.

215. Tejani A, Butt KM, Rajpoot D, et al. Strategies for optimizing growth in children with kidney transplants. *Transplantation* 1989;47:229.

216. Reisman L, Lieberman KV, Burrows L, et al. Follow-up of cyclosporine-treated pediatric renal allograft recipients after cessation of prednisone. *Transplantation* 1990;49:76.

217. Hodson EM, Knight JF, Sheil AGR, et al. Cyclosporin A as sole immunosuppressive agent for renal transplantation in children: effect on catch-up growth. *Transplant Proc* 1989; 21:1687.

218. Höcker B, John U, Plank C, et al. Successful withdrawal of steroids in pediatric renal transplant recipients under Cyclosporin A and mycophenolate mofetil treatment: results after four years. *Transplantation* 2004;78;228.

219. Chakrabarti P, Wong HY, Scantlebury VP, et al. Outcome after steroid withdrawal in pediatric renal transplant patients receiving tacrolimus-based immunosuppression. *Transplantation* 2000;70:760.

220. Shapiro R, Scantlebury VP, Jordan ML, et al. Pediatric renal transplantation under tacrolimus-based immunosuppression. *Transplantation* 1999;67:299.

221. Jungraithmayr T, Staskewitz A, Kirste G, et al. Pediatric renal transplantation with mycophenolate mofetil (MMF) based immunosuppression without induction: results after three years. *Transplantation* 2003;75:454.

222. Birkeland SA, Larsen KE, Rohr N. Pediatric renal transplantation without steroids. *Pediatr Nephrol* 1998;12:87.

223. Sarwal MM, Vidhun JR, Alexander SR, et al. Continued superior outcomes with modification and lengthened follow-up of a steroid-avoidance pilot with extended daclizumab induction in pediatric renal transplantation. *Transplantation* 2003;76:1331.

224. Mehls O, Ritz E, Hunziker E, et al. Improvement of growth and food utilization by human recombinant growth hormone in uraemia. *Kidney Int* 1988;33:45.

225. Tönshoff B, Mehls O, Heinrich U, et al. Growth-stimulating effects of recombinant human growth hormone in children with end-stage renal disease. *J Pediatr* 1990;116:561.

226. Powell DR, Durham SK, Liu F, et al. The insulin-like growth factor axis and growth in children with chronic renal failure: a report of the Southwest Pediatric Nephrology Study Group. *J Clin Endocrinol Metab* 1998;83:1654.

227. Rees L, Ridgen SPA, Ward G, et al. Treatment of short stature in renal disease with recombinant human growth hormone. *Arch Dis Child* 1990;65:856.

228. Koch VH, Lippe BM, Nelson PA, et al. Accelerated growth after recombinant human growth hormone treatment of children with chronic renal failure. *J Pediatr* 1989;115:365.

229. Hokken-Koelega ACS, Stijnen T, De Muinck Keizer-Schrama SMPF, et al. Placebo-controlled, double-blind, cross-over trial of growth hormone treatment in prepubertal children with chronic renal failure. *Lancet* 1991; 338:585.

230. Tönshoff B, Dietz M, Haffner D, et al. Effects of two years of growth hormone treatment in short children with renal disease. The German Study Group for Growth Hormone Treatment in Chronic Renal Failure. *Acta Paediatr Scand Suppl* 1991;379:33.

231. van Reenen MJ, Hogg RJ, Sweeney AL, et al. Accelerated growth in short children with chronic renal failure treated with both strict dietary therapy and recombinant human growth hormone. *Pediatr Nephrol* 1992;6:451.

232. Fine RN, Kohaut EC, Brown D, et al. Growth after recombinant human growth hormone treatment in children with chronic renal failure: report of a multicenter randomized double-blind placebo-controlled study. Genentech Cooperative Study Group. *J Pediatr* 1994;124:374.

233. Fine RN, Kohaut E, Brown D, et al. Long-term treatment of growth retarded children with chronic renal insufficiency, with recombinant human growth hormone. *Kidney Int* 1996; 48:781.

234. Haffner D, Schaefer F, Nissel R, et al. Effect of growth hormone treatment on the adult height of children with chronic renal failure. German Study Group for Growth Hormone Treatment in Chronic Renal Failure. *N Engl J Med* 2000; 343:923.

235. Hokken-Koelega ACS, Stijnen T, De Ridder MAJ, et al. Growth hormone treatment in growth-retarded adolescents after renal transplantation. *Lancet* 1994;343:1313.

236. Guest G, Berard E, Crosnier H, et al. Effects of growth hormone in short children after renal transplantation. *Pediatr Nephrol* 1998;12:437.

237. Schaefer F, Wuhl E, Haffner D, et al. Stimulation of growth by recombinant human growth hormone in children undergoing peritoneal or hemodialysis treatment. *Adv Perit Dial* 1994;10:321.

238. Berard E, Crosnier H, Six-Beneton A, et al. Recombinant human growth hormone treatment of children on hemodialysis. French Society of Pediatric Nephrology. *Pediatr Nephrol* 1998;12:304.

239. Tönshoff B, Haffner D, Mehls O, et al. Efficacy and safety of growth hormone treatment in short children with renal allografts: three year experience. *Kidney Int* 1993;44:199.

240. Acott PD, Pernica JM. Growth hormone therapy before and after pediatric renal transplant. *Pediatr Transplant* 2003; 7:426.

241. Tönshoff B, Mehls O. Use of rhGH post transplant in children. In: Tejani AH, Fine RN, eds. *Pediatric Renal Transplantation.* New York: Wiley, 1994:441.

242. Fine RN, Stablein D, Cohen AH, et al. Recombinant human growth hormone post-renal transplantation in children: a randomized controlled study of the NAPRTCS. *Kidney Int* 2002;62:688.

243. Fine RN, Attie KM, Kuntze J, et al. Recombinant human growth hormone in infants and young children with chronic renal insufficiency. *Pediatr Nephrol* 1995;9:451.

244. Fine RN, Brown DF, Kuntze J, et al. Growth after discontinuation of recombinant human growth hormone therapy in children with chronic renal failure. *J Pediatr* 1996;129:883.

245. Hokken-Koelega A, Mulder P, De Jong R, et al. Long-term effects of growth hormone treatment on growth and puberty in patients with chronic renal insufficiency. *Pediatr Nephrol* 2000;14:701.

246. Mehls O, Berg U, Broyer M, Rizzoni G. Chronic renal failure and growth hormone treatment: review of the literature and experience in KIGS. In: Ranke MB, Wilton P, eds. *Growth Hormone Therapy in KIGS – 10 Years Experience.* Heidelberg: Barth, 1999:327.

247. Rees L, Ward G, Rigden SPA. Growth over 10 years following a 1-year trial of growth hormone therapy. *Pediatr Nephrol* 2000;14:309.

248. Fine RN, Sullivan EK, Tejani A. The impact of recombinant human growth hormone treatment on final adult height. *Pediatr Nephrol* 2000;14:679.

249. Janssen F, Van Damme-Lombaerts R, Van Dyck M, et al. Impact of growth hormone treatment on a Belgian population of short children with renal allografts. *Pediatr Transplant* 1997;1:190.

250. Hokken-Kolega A, Stijnen T, De Jong R, et al. A placebo-controlled, double-blind trial of growth hormone treatment in prepubertal children after renal transplant. *Kidney Int* 1996;6:S128.

251. Haffner D, Wühl E, Schaefer F, et al. Factors predictive of the short- and long-term efficacy of growth hormone treatment in prepubertal children with chronic renal failure. *J Am Soc Nephrol* 1998;9:1899.

252. Hokken-Koelega ACS, Stijnen T, De Jong MCJW, et al. Double-blind trial comparing the effects of two doses of growth hormone in prepubertal patients with chronic renal insufficiency. *J Clin Endocrinol Metab* 1994;79:1185.

253. Tönshoff B, Heinrich U, Mehls O. How safe is the treatment of uremic children with recombinant human growth hormone? *Pediatr Nephrol* 1991;5:454.

254. Fine RN, Fine SE, Sherman BM. Absorption of recombinant human growth hormone (rhGH) following intraperitoneal instillation. *Perit Dial Int* 1989;9:91.

255. Yadin O, Fine RN. Long-term use of recombinant human growth hormone in children with chronic renal insufficiency. *Kidney Int Suppl* 1997;58:S114.

256. Schmitz O, Hjollund E, Alberti KGMM, et al. Assessment of tissue sensitivity to insulin in uremic patients on long-term hemodialysis therapy. *Diabetes Res* 1985;2:57.

257. Mak RH, DeFronzo RA. Glucose and insulin metabolism in uremia. *Nephron* 1992;61:377.

258. Adrogué HJ. Glucose homeostasis and the kidney. *Kidney Int* 1992;42:1266.

259. Rizza, RA Mandarino JL, Gerich JE. Effects of growth hormone on insulin action in man. Mechanism of insulin resistance, impaired suppression of glucose production, and impaired stimulation of glucose utilization. *Diabetes* 1982; 31:663.

260. Mehls O, Broyer M, on behalf of the European/Australian Study Group. Growth response to recombinant human growth hormone in short prepubertal children with chronic renal failure with or without dialysis. *Acta Paediatr Suppl* 1994;399:81.

261. Filler G, Franke D, Amendt P, et al. Reversible diabetes mellitus during growth hormone therapy in chronic renal failure. *Pediatr Nephrol* 1998;12:405.

262. Stefanidis CJ, Papathanassiou A, Michelis K, et al. Diabetes mellitus after therapy with recombinant human growth hormone (rhGH). *Br J Clin Pract Suppl* 1996;85:66.

263. Cutfield WS, Wilton P, Bennmarker H, et al. Incidence of diabetes mellitus and impaired glucose tolerance in children and adolescents receiving growth-hormone treatment. *Lancet* 2000;355:610.

264. Doi T, Striker LJ, Gibson CC, et al. Glomerular lesions in mice transgenic for growth hormone and insulin-like growth factor-I: I. Relationship between increased glomerular size and mesangial sclerosis. *Am J Pathol* 1990;137:541.

265. Yang CW, Striker GE, Chen WY, et al. Differential expression of glomerular extracellular matrix and growth factor mRNA in rapid and slowly progressive glomerulosclerosis: studies in mice transgenic for native or mutated growth hormone. *Lab Invest* 1997;76:467.

266. Chen NY, Chen WY, Striker LJ, et al. Co-expression of bovine growth hormone (GH) and human GH antagonist genes in transgenic mice. *Endocrinology* 1997;138:851.

267. Yang CW, Striker LJ, Pesce C, et al. Glomerulosclerosis and body growth are mediated by different portions of bovine growth hormone. Studies in transgenic mice. *Lab Invest* 1993;68:62.

268. Chen NY, Chen WY, Kopchick JJ. Liver and kidney growth hormone (GH) receptors are regulated differently in diabetic GH and GH antagonist transgenic mice. *Endocrinology* 1997;138:1988.

269. Tönshoff B, Tönshoff C, Mehls O, et al. Growth hormone treatment in children with preterminal chronic renal failure: No adverse effect on glomerular filtration rate. *Eur J Pediatr* 1992;151:601.

270. Haffner D, Zacharewicz S, Mehls O, et al. The acute effect of growth hormone on GFR is obliterated in chronic renal failure. *Clin Nephrol* 1989;32:266.

271. Kelley KW. Growth hormone, lymphocytes and macrophages. *Biochem Pharmacol* 1989;38:705.

272. Franco P, Marelli O, Lattuada D, et al. Influence of growth hormone on the immunosuppressive effect of prednisolone in mice. *Acta Endocrinol (Copenh)* 1990;123:339.

273. Tönshoff B, Mehls O. Use of rhGH post transplant in children. In: Tejani AH, Fine RN, eds. *Pediatric Renal Transplantation.* New York: Wiley, 1994:441.

274. Guest G, Berard E, Crosnier H, et al. Effects of growth hormone in short children after renal transplantation. French Society of Pediatric Nephrology. *Pediatr Nephrol* 1998; 12:437.

275. Maxwell H, Rees L. Randomized controlled trial of recombinant human growth hormone in prepubertal and pubertal renal transplant recipients. *Arch Dis Child* 1998;6:481.

276. Koller EA, Stadel BV, Malozowski SN. Papilledema in 15 renally compromised patients treated with growth hormone. *Pediatr Nephrol* 1997;11:451.

277. Watkins SL. Is severe renal osteodystrophy a contraindication for recombinant human growth hormone treatment? *Pediatr Nephrol* 1996;10:351.

278. Kaufman DB. Growth hormone and renal osteodystrophy: a case report. *Pediatr Nephrol* 1998;12:157.

279. Picca S, Cappa M, Rizzoni G. Hyperparathyroidism during growth hormone treatment: a role for puberty? *Pediatr Nephrol* 2000;14:56.

280. Reichlin S. Somatostatin. *N Engl J Med* 1983;309:1495.

281. Boose AR, Pieters R, Delemarre-van de Waal, et al. Growth hormone therapy and leukemia. *Tijdschr Kindergeneeskd* 1992;60:1.

282. Ritzen EM. Does growth hormone increase the risk of malignancies? *Horm Res* 1993;39:99.

283. Guidelines for the use of growth hormone in children with short stature. A report by the Drug and Therapeutics Committee of the Lawson Wilkins Pediatric Endocrine Society. *J Pediatr* 1995;127:857.

284. Tyden G, Wernersson A, Sandberg J, et al. Development of renal cell carcinoma in living donor kidney grafts. *Transplantation* 2000;70:1650.

285. Malozowski S, Hung W, Scott DC, et al. Acute pancreatitis associated with growth hormone therapy for short stature. *N Engl J Med* 1995;332:401.

286. Koller EA, Green L, Gertner JM, et al. Retinal changes mimicking diabetic retinopathy in two nondiabetic, growth hormone-treated patients. *J Clin Endocrinol Metab* 1998; 83:2380.

24

Liver Disease in Dialysis Patients

Fabrizio Fabrizi
Suphamai Bunnapradist
Paul Martin

Liver disease typically is not a frequent management issue in patients on chronic dialysis, although viral hepatitis remains a concern in this population. A short list of the most important causes of liver disease among dialysis patients is shown in Table 24–1; chronic viral hepatitis, both types B and C, is the most frequently recognized etiology of liver disease in the dialysis population.[1] Ethanol-induced liver disease is an infrequent condition among patients with end-stage renal disease (ESRD) on maintenance dialysis. Multisystem disorders, such as lupus, that can result in renal failure generally do not have a major hepatic component.

Hepatitis C (HCV) and to lesser extent B (HBV) viruses are mostly blood-borne. Patients on peritoneal dialysis (PD) have a lower frequency of blood-borne infections than hemodialysis (HD) patients. This is related to various mechanisms: the absence of extracorporeal blood manipulation; the fact that PD takes place in the home, thus avoiding exposure to other patients; and the generally less frequent administration of blood transfusions to PD patients as opposed to HD patients.

This chapter describes the clinical course, diagnosis, and management of liver diseases in patients on dialysis.

HEPATITIS B

HBV is a partially double-stranded, compact DNA virus. It can be recovered from most body fluids and is relatively hardy, permitting protracted survival outside the body. This increases its infectivity. The most common modes of transmission of HBV among adults living in developed countries are sexual contact and intravenous drug use. Vertical transmission from mother to infant is more typical in highly endemic areas, such as Asia and sub-Saharan Africa.[2] The introduction of blood-bank testing has dramatically decreased the risk of transfusion-associated HBV infection. The current estimated risk in the United States of transfusion-related infection with HBV is 1 in 63,000 transfused units.[3]

Currently there are more than 350 million persons with chronic HBV carriage worldwide, of whom over 250,000

TABLE 24–1. CAUSES OF LIVER DISEASE IN DIALYSIS PATIENTS

Hepatitis viruses
Hepatitis B virus (HBV)
Hepatitis C virus (HCV)
Miscellaneous [hepatitis E (HEV), hepatitis A (HAV), hepatitis δ (HDV), cytomegalovirus (CMV), Epstein-Barr virus (EBV), herpes simplex virus (HSV)]
Drug-induced liver disease
Nonalcoholic fatty liver disease
Alcoholic liver disease
Others

die annually from hepatitis B–associated liver disease.[4] HBV infection remains a concern in patients undergoing maintenance dialysis in both industrialized and developing countries.

Interpretation of Diagnostic Tests

Hepatitis B surface antigen (HBsAg) is the first viral marker detectable in serum in acute HBV infection (Table 24–2). By the time clinical and biochemical hepatitis is present, after an incubation period of up to 140 days, other serum markers appear, including antibody to HBV core antigen (anti-HBc). Hepatitis B core antigen (HBcAg) is a marker of viral replication, located in infected hepatocytes, and does not circulate in serum; however, its corresponding antibody, anti-HBc, does. Chronic HBV infection is defined by documented HBsAg positivity in serum for 6 months or more with absence of IgM anti-HBc. IgM anti-HBc serves as a marker of acute or recent HBV infection and is detectable for up to 6 months after infection only, whereas IgG anti-HBc persists indefinitely. If acute HBV infection resolves, neutralizing antibody against HBsAg (anti-HBs) develops. If HBV infection becomes chronic, testing for other serum HBV markers, including HBV DNA and hepatitis B e antigen (HBeAg), should be undertaken. Their

TABLE 24–2. TESTS FOR HEPATITIS B VIRUS (HBV)

Test	Interpretation
HBsAg (hepatitis B surface antigen)	HBV infection
Anti-HBc (Hepatitis B core antibody) IgM anti-HBc	Acute or recent HBV infection
Anti-HBc (hepatitis B core antibody) IgG anti-HBc	Chronic or remote HBV infection
Anti-HBs (hepatitis B surface antibody)	Immunity to HBV (vaccine induced or due to prior infection)
HBeAg (hepatitis B e antigen)	Marker of active viral replication
HBV DNA	Marker of active viral replication

presence implies viral replication and greater infectivity; however, any HBsAg-positive dialysis patient is potentially infectious.[1]

HBV Epidemiology in Dialysis: The Past

Prior to identification of HBV, a number of groups had described hepatitis in dialysis units. In 1966, two cases of fatal hepatitis were observed in HD patients undergoing maintenance dialysis in New York City.[5] Garibaldi et al.[6] prospectively surveyed 65 HD units in the United States in 1967-1970 and reported 355 cases of hepatitis; 260 occurred in dialysis patients and 95 in staff. During this 4-year period, 53 (82 percent) of 65 units reported hepatitis in patients, dialysis staff, or both; 9 (7 percent) of the 136 patients described in detail died as a result of the infection. With the development of diagnostic testing for HBV, more detailed studies became possible. During 1973–1974,[7] a point prevalence survey in 15 U.S. HD centers screened 583 patients and 451 medical personnel for HBV infection; 16.8 percent of the patients and 2.4 percent of the staff were found to be HBsAg-positive. The European Dialysis and Transplant Association reported in a European study published in 1971 that 43 percent of 367 centers had had cases of hepatitis during that year; the case fatality rates from hepatitis were estimated to be 7 percent for patients and 1 percent for staff.[8]

The Centers for Disease Control and Prevention (CDC), in Atlanta, which have been conducting surveillance of viral hepatitis in dialysis centers since 1969, reported that in the period between 1972 and 1974, the incidence of HBsAg seropositivity among patients and staff was 6.2 and 5.2 percent, respectively.[9]

In 1977, the CDC issued recommendations in an effort to limit the spread of HBV within HD units.[10] These guidelines included isolation of HBsAg-positive patients by room, dialysis machine, and staff and routine serologic screening for HBsAg and anti-HBs antibody. The impact of these recommendations was described by Alter and coworkers,[11] who found a decline in the incidence of HBsAg seropositivity from 3 percent (1976) to 0.5 percent (1983) in dialysis patients in the United States; the incidence in staff also decreased from 2.6 to 0.5 percent during those years. Over the same period, the proportion of centers using separation practices increased from 75 to 86 percent, and the proportion of units that screened patients monthly for HBsAg increased from 57 to 84 percent. The highest risk of acquiring HBV for patients was seen in those centers that provided dialysis to HBsAg-positive patients but did not separate these patients by room or machine.

The decrease in HBV prevalence and incidence in HD patients and staff in North America and western Europe[12–14] continued in subsequent years. Various other factors have contributed to this decline in HBV, including screening of blood donors for HBsAg (initiated in 1972) and anti-HBc (initiated in 1987) and the lowered number of blood transfusions received by dialysis patients, most of whom now receive erythropoietin. In addition, vaccination of dialysis patients against HBV (since 1982) plays a role; however, control of spread of HBV in dialysis units (1976–1980) antedated the widespread availability of vaccine against HBV, highlighting the effectiveness of the original CDC recommendations.

Control Practices against the Transmission of Blood-Borne Pathogens in Hemodialysis

Epidemiologic investigations had implicated a number of sources of HBV spread in HD patients, including cross-contamination from surfaces, supplies, or equipment that were not routinely disinfected after use, staff members who simultaneously cared for HBsAg-positive and susceptible patients, intravenous solutions or medication vials that were not exclusively used for one patient, and injections that were prepared in areas adjacent to those where blood samples were handled.[15-18]

To prevent transmission of blood-borne pathogens in general health care settings, "universal precautions" had been initially recommended by the CDC in 1985 and updated in 1988.[19] These procedures are now referred to as "standard precautions" and include (1) handwashing after touching blood and other potentially infectious material, (2) wearing of gloves when touching blood or other potentially infectious material, and (3) use of gowns and face shields when exposure to blood is anticipated.

In addition to these universal precautions, there are now HD unit precautions that are unique to this setting and are even more stringent.[20] These include glove use whenever a patient or HD equipment is touched as well as no sharing of supplies, instruments, or medications between HD patients, including ancillary supply equipment (trays, blood pressure cuffs, clamps, scissors, and other nondisposable items). Further, HD precautions specify the separation of clean areas (used for handwashing and/or the handling and storage of medications) from contaminated areas that serve for the handling of blood samples and HD equipment after use and for the cleaning and disinfection of nondisposable items—such as machines, and environmental surfaces—between uses.

Additional precautions to prevent HBV acquisition in the HD environment are recommended by the CDC[20]: monthly testing for HBsAg of all susceptible patients, prompt review of results, physical separation of HBsAg-positive from susceptible individuals, and cohorting of separate dialysis staff, instruments, supplies, and HD machines for patients with HBsAg positivity.

HBV Epidemiology in Dialysis: Current Status

The National Surveillance of Dialysis-Associated Diseases in the United States conducted by the CDC in 1997 reported a 0.9 percent mean prevalence of HBsAg seropositivity in dialysis patients; the incidence of HBsAg positivity was 0.05 percent.[21] The number of patients who had received at least three doses of hepatitis B vaccine was only 46.7 percent for dialysis patients and 86.6 percent for staff members.

In 2003, a study sample from the Dialysis Outcomes and Practice Patterns Study (DOPPS) including 8433 adult patients selected from 308 dialysis facilities in France, Germany, Italy, Spain, the United Kingdom, Japan, and the United States reported a mean HBsAg facility prevalence of 3.0 percent,[22] which ranged from 0 to 4.6 percent. The seroconversion rate ranged between 0.4 (95 percent CI, 0.2 to 0.6; United States) and 1.8 percent (95 percent CI, 0.6 to 4.9; Germany) per 100 patient-years. A significantly decreased risk for HBsAg seroconversion, which was associated with use of a protocol for patients with HBV, was observed in the statistical model that included all practice patterns simultaneously [risk ratio (RR) = 0.52, p = 0.03]. The majority of facilities (78.1 percent) had a zero seroconversion rate per 100 patient-years.[22] Similar figures of HBV prevalence had been found in prior reports.[23-25]

However, despite the marked decline in transmission of HBV within dialysis centers in the industrialized world, HBV outbreaks in HD units continue to be reported.[26-29] These outbreaks usually reflect the failure to perform screening for HBsAg, to review screening results routinely, or both.[26] In other instances, HBsAg-positive patients shared staff members, equipment, and supplies with susceptible patients.[26] More recently, a cluster of HBV infections occurred in Pennsylvania.[28] An initial patient had HBsAg seroconversion in December 1995; five additional patients seroconverted between March and April 1996. These patients had been dialyzed in two different centers; all had been subsequently transferred between January and February to a third hospital. The transmission from the source patient to the other five patients probably occurred by contaminated multidose vials or supplies shared between patients on HD.

Information about HBV in HD patients in developing countries is less readily available and is mostly based on small series; HBsAg incidence and prevalence are still high in the developing world (Table 24–3).[30-40] An incidence of seroconversion to HBsAg positivity of 0.19 per patient-year was seen in 149 HD patients in Brazil during a median follow-up of 12.9 months.[30] Four cases of acute hepatitis with seroconversion to HBsAg positivity were observed in Moldavia in a population of 169 dialysis patients.[31] Vladutiu et al. observed that in a large unit in Cluj, Romania, the preva-

TABLE 24–3. PREVALENCE OF HBsAG SEROPOSITIVITY AMONG DIALYSIS PATIENTS: RECENT DATA

Country	Prevalence of HbsAG	Reference Year
Croatia	8% (8/100)	1994
Brazil	15.1% (28/285)	1995
Moldavia	17%(29/169)	1999
Brazil	12% (34/282)	1999
Romania	21.8% (23/108)	2000
Italy	4.3%; 95% CI; 3.4, 5.4	2003
France	3.7%; 95% CI; 2.9, 4.7	2003
Japan	2.1%; 95% CI; 1.6, 2.6	2003
United Kingdom	0%; 95% CI; 0, 0	2003
Kenya	8% (8/100)	2003

lence of HBsAg positivity in 1998 (21.6 percent) was higher than that observed in 1993 (17.9 percent) and 1996 (8.2 percent).[32] The authors suspected that sharing of heparin or saline solutions between HD patients or the evacuation of saline solution from the same bottle in successive patients at the beginning of the HD session was the mechanism of HBV spread. Contamination of HD machines was also not excluded. Similar rates of HBsAg incidence and prevalence among chronic HD patients have been observed in other Romanian HD centers.[32] A large outbreak of HBV infection has been recently reported in a Brazilian HD unit.[38]

Clinical Presentation of HBV Infection

Patients on maintenance dialysis with chronic HBV infection typically have mild or absent elevation of alanine aminotransferase (ALT) activity, are anicteric, and rarely develop symptoms of hepatitis. A more marked elevation in ALT may occur at the time of HBsAg acquisition, although typically acute HBV is subclinical in this population, with a high rate of chronicity. Liver biopsy is still the most accurate and reliable method for assessing the severity of liver disease in dialysis patients with HBV, as even cirrhosis may be present with minimal biochemical dysfunction. On the other hand, the relationship between HBsAg seropositivity and ALT activity is stronger than had been appreciated. A recent study in a very large cohort of chronic dialysis patients found that values for aspartate transaminase (AST) and ALT were significantly higher in HBsAg-positive/HBV DNA-positive than HBsAg-negative patients on dialysis; AST, 22.86+/-31.34 vs. 14.19+/9.7 IU/L (p=0.00001); and ALT, 25.07+/-41.59 vs. 13.9+/-41.59 IU/L (p=0.00001),[41] although the degree of elevation was modest. Multivariate analysis demonstrated a strong and independent association between persistent HBsAg positivity and higher levels of ALT. Levels of ALT activity in patients undergoing maintenance dialysis[42–44] or in the predialysis stage[45] are usually depressed, making it more difficult to detect liver disease by

biochemical tests alone. ALT levels in the "normal" range for the general population may be indicative of a pathologic state in the dialysis setting.

Data from the Case Mix Severity Special Study of the U.S. Renal Data System (USRDS) and The Lombardy Dialysis and Transplant Registry (RLDT)[46] have shown that cirrhosis is not a frequent comorbid condition in dialysis populations in the industrialized world [2 percent in the United States and 1.5 percent in northern Italy (Lombardy)]; however, the death rate for dialysis patients with cirrhosis was 35 percent higher than for those without it [mean relative death rate 1.346; 95 percent confidence intervals (CI) 1.030 to 1.758; $p = 0.03$].

A recent international collaborative study from the United States, Europe, Australia, and New Zealand demonstrated that the overall risk of cancer is higher in patients with ESRD treated by dialysis than in the general population. These investigators observed an excess of liver cancer [standardized incidence ratio (SIR) 1.2; 95 percent CI, 1.0 to 1.4] most likely related to greater exposure to hepatitis B and C viruses.[47]

Natural History of HBV Infection

The natural history of HBV in dialysis has not been fully defined, as no large, long-term studies evaluating the course of HBV-related liver disease in dialysis patients are available. A few reports evaluating the histology of HBV-related liver disease in dialysis patients have demonstrated that progression to cirrhosis is not uncommon despite the absence of marked biochemical dysfunction.[48,49] It is possible that reluctance to perform liver biopsies in this population may have prevented recognition of the severity of liver disease.

The most frequent causes of death in patients receiving maintenance dialysis are cardiovascular disease and sepsis.[50] The mean delay to development of HBV-related complications (liver cirrhosis and hepatocellular carcinoma, or HCC) probably exceeds the mean life expectancy of the majority of dialysis patients: many dialysis patients with chronic HBV or HCV will probably die with the infection rather than of it. However, due to improvements in dialysis techniques, the number of dialysis patients with significant liver disease is expected to grow as their life expectancy increases.

Josselson et al.[51] retrospectively evaluated 101 patients on maintenance HD in the United States over a 8-year follow-up period. There was no significant difference between HBsAg-positive and HBsAg–negative patients with regard to age, gender, underlying nephropathy, or race. Time on dialysis was significantly longer in HBsAg-positive than HBsAg–negative patients, 32+/-22 vs. 22.3+/-17.2 months, p<0.01. These investigators did not find significant differences in death rates (50 vs. 34.4 percent), hospitalizations (1.5 vs. 1.2 patients per year), or hospitalized days (18 vs.

11.8 days per year) between HBsAg-positive and HBsAg–negative patients. Similar findings were reported by Harnett and colleagues in 1988[52]: 49 patients on maintenance HD with persistent seropositivity for HBsAg were evaluated over 52 ±5 months. Death due to liver disease was infrequent (2 percent, 1 of 49); spontaneous clearance of HBsAg from serum occurred in 20 percent of patients (10 of 49). Fourteen patients (29 percent) had chronic elevation of serum ALT activity over the follow-up; only one patient was icteric.

Poorer outcomes were observed in a retrospective survey from India. Jha and coworkers[53] followed 424 patients on maintenance HD over a 4-year observation period (1988–1992); de novo HBV infection was lower among patients who received a full course of hepatitis B vaccine than among those who had not completed the vaccination schedule or had not received vaccine at all [4.7 percent (1 of 21) vs. 30 percent (3 of 10) vs. 32 percent (7 of 22), $p<0.05$]. The mortality rate was lower in the first than in the second and third groups [14.2 percent (3 of 21) vs. 30 percent (3 of 10) vs. 50 percent (11 of 22), $p<0.05$]. Patients who became HBsAg-positive had a significantly higher mortality rate than those who remained negative [72.7 percent (8 of 11) vs. 21.4 percent (9 of 42), $p<0.01$]. Death in HBsAg-positive patients was mostly accounted for by apparent fulminant hepatic failure [37 percent (4 of 11) vs. 0 percent (0 of 42), $p<0.01$]. All patients were negative by anti-HCV serologic testing. HBsAg-positive patients did not receive adequate dialysis treatment because of the reuse of dialyzers and other dialysis equipment, which was unavoidable owing to cost constraints. The authors concluded that in financially limited facilities, management of ESRD is apt to be hampered by inadequate dialysis and infections and that these complications may, in turn, aggravate HBV-related liver disease.

Liver-related mortality in patients undergoing dialysis in developed countries is usually low;[50] this supports the notion that aggressive liver disease is rarely present. The course of HBV appears[54] less aggressive in patients remaining on maintenance dialysis than after renal transplantation (RT), as HBV-related liver disease is a major long-term risk of morbidity and mortality after RT.[54] After RT, HBsAg-positive patients with ESRD may have an acceleration in the course of their liver disease; this is related to a number of factors, including an increase in quantitative viremia due to the immunosuppressive therapy given to prevent graft rejection.[55]

Treatment of HBV Infection

There are no clear guidelines indicating which dialysis patients with HBV should receive antiviral therapy. According to generally accepted recommendations in the ESRD population, antiviral therapy should be considered in dialysis patients with HBsAg-positive status for greater than 6 months with persistent presence of HBeAg and/or HBV DNA in serum, elevated ALT activity, and histologic features of chronic hepatitis. However, the long-term advantages of antiviral therapy have been frequently evaluated over years or decades, whereas many dialysis patients typically have a shortened survival due to age and/or comorbid conditions. It seems reasonable to offer antiviral therapy to those HBsAg-positive patients on dialysis who are candidates for RT. HBsAg-positive candidates for RT with signs of active viral replication (i.e., positive HBeAg or HBV DNA) should be placed on antiviral therapy before transplantation in order to slow the progression of liver disease.[54] In fact, all HBV-infected patients must be cautioned that even histologically mild disease has the potential to progress due to immunosuppression after RT. An HBV DNA level > 10^5 copies/mL has been proposed as an appropriate level to confirm the presence of active viral replication. However, in a patient with a lower HBV DNA level in conjunction with other biochemical or histologic evidence of active liver disease, therapy may still be indicated.[56]

At present, evaluation for RT in HBV-infected patients should include a liver biopsy as well as an assessment for markers of replication in serum, both HBV DNA and HBeAg.[54] Extensive fibrosis (stage III) or especially established cirrhosis on biopsy suggests that liver disease is already quite advanced and that RT is best avoided for fear of accelerating the course of liver disease. Nevertheless, the absence in serum of detectable HBV DNA or HBeAg before RT does not preclude reactivation of HBV infection after RT. There are reports indicating that even patients with serologies indicating successful clearance of HBsAg can experience reactivation of HBV following RT.[57–59] Thus, a patient with the presence of hepatitis B core antibody and negative HBsAg should have serial liver chemistries checked during routine post-RT care. If the patient becomes HBsAg-positive, antiviral therapy should be promptly instituted.

Nephrologists have been reluctant to prescribe interferon (IFN) in dialysis patients: it is expensive and associated with many side effects. Numerous trials have shown a generally poorer tolerance of IFN in dialysis patients than in immunocompetent patients with chronic hepatitis. This has been attributed in part to an altered pharmacokinetic profile of IFN in chronic uremia. IFN has been used with limited success in a few patients with chronic HBV infection undergoing chronic HD.[60,61]

Lamivudine (3TC), a second-generation nucleoside analogue, has been shown to be a potent inhibitor of HBV replication.[62–64] Small, uncontrolled trials have described lamivudine use in patients receiving long-term dialysis.[65–68] Recently, Schmilovitz-Weiss and coworkers[65] reported 4 patients on HD who showed a rapid response to lamivudine, administered for a median of 10 months. All were serum

HBsAg- and HBeAg-positive, with median serum HBV DNA 1×10^7 copies per milliliter. Within 4 to 8 weeks of initiation of therapy, HBV DNA became undetectable and serum ALT normalized. Serum HBeAg disappeared in all 4 patients; 3 patients also lost HBsAg. In another clinical trial,[66] 26 HBV-infected RT recipients and 5 HD patients became serum HBV DNA–negative after a median duration of lamivudine treatment of 16.5 (4 to 31) months. Breakthrough, defined by the reappearance of detectable serum HBV DNA, was seen in 8 (31 percent) of kidney recipients and 2 (40 percent) patients on HD. Among HD patients, breakthroughs occurred at the 7th and 18th months after treatment suggesting lamivudine resistance.

Several issues remain to be clarified regarding the use of lamivudine in ESRD, including appropriate duration of therapy. The impact of identified viral factors—such as HBV viral load, presence or absence of routinely occurring HBV mutants, and HBV genotype—will also need clarification. The most significant limitation to lamivudine therapy for chronic HBV has been the emergence of HBV escape mutants relatively resistant to the drug. Adefovir, which is efficacious in lamivudine-resistant HBV, has recently been licensed to treat chronic HBV.[68] As with lamivudine, it must be dose-reduced in patients with chronic kidney disease and those on dialysis.

HBV Vaccine in the Dialysis Population

HBV vaccination is an important tool in preventing the spread of HBV within dialysis units.[69] HBV vaccines, initially plasma-derived (since 1981) and later recombinant (since 1986), are safe and effective. Patients on maintenance dialysis typically show a suboptimal response to HBV vaccination compared to the nonuremic population: the number who develop protective antibody against HBV (anti-HBs) is lower (60 to 70 percent vs. 95 percent in the general population), the antibody titers of those who do mount an antibody response are reduced and decline faster over time.

During the 1980s, three large, controlled, randomized trials with plasma-derived vaccine were conducted in chronic dialysis patients; two of these trials reported a significantly lower rate of HBV infection in study than in placebo patients.[70–72] The protective effect of vaccination against HBV in reducing the risk of HBV acquisition among HD patients has also been demonstrated by the CDC in a case-control study.[73]

Numerous host factors have been identified that contribute to nonresponse to the HBV vaccine. These include older age[74–77]; male gender[70]; body weight[78]; possession of the major histocompatibility complex haplotype HLA-B8, SCOI, or DR3[79–82]; poor nutritional status[83,84]; inadequate dialysis[85]; serologic positivity for anti-HCV antibody[86–88];

history of prior blood transfusion requirement[89];, and abnormal synthesis of interleukin.[90] Failure to complete a full course of HBV vaccination also results in diminished response rates.[91] Finally, it has been reported that PD patients have a lower seroconversion rate than those on HD.[92]

Various strategies have been introduced to enhance response rates in dialysis patients to HBV vaccine: use of double doses,[93–102] administration of multiple vaccine doses,[103–108] and intradermal administration of HBV vaccine.[109–121] Novel approaches have included the administration of adjuvants—levamisole,[122,123] IFN,[124–126] granulocyte-macrophage colony-stimulating factor (GM-CSF),[127–130] thymopentin,[131–136] zinc supplementation,[137,138] and interleukin-2.[139–141] The use of a recombinant pre-S1- and pre-S2-containing HB vaccine has been reported.[142] Vaccinating patients with chronic kidney disease in the predialysis stage is an additional strategy.[143–147] The majority of these approaches have not improved results and are often expensive. HBV vaccination with three double doses (40 µg each dose) of recombinant vaccine by the intramuscular route as early in the course of the kidney disease as possible is currently recommended by the CDC for dialysis patients.[148] From a practical point of view, the yeast-derived vaccine is not more immunogenic than the plasma-derived vaccine and nonresponse to one type is generally not overcome by vaccination with the other.[148]

In the pediatric dialysis population, 60 to 90 percent of children receiving 20 µg of either the three- or four-dose schedule develop protective titers of anti-HBs antibody,[149–154] as in adults. A better response was noted in children with chronic kidney disease not yet on dialysis than in those already on dialysis.[149]

HBV immunization may be a cause of detectable HBsAg among chronic HD patients. In their prospective survey, Ly et al.[155] screened 2400 HD patients monthly between January 1998 and June 2000 and observed that 8 (89 percent) of the 9 patients with de novo HBsAg had transient HBsAg seropositivity, temporally related to HBV immunization. Thus, HD patients should not be tested for HBV infection within a week of immunization and caution should be exercised in interpreting HBsAg seropositivity within 4 weeks of HBV immunization.

The cost-effectiveness of hepatitis B vaccine in dialysis patients has been repeatedly addressed.[156,157] Oddone et al.[157] modeled a decision tree in order to analyze three vaccination strategies for patients with chronic kidney disease: vaccine given prior to dialysis, vaccine given at time of dialysis, and no vaccine. They concluded that the HBV predialysis vaccine strategy was the most clinically effective; however, it was more expensive than the other two approaches. The cost-effectiveness ratios were $25.31 per case of HBV prevented for vaccination at the time of dialysis and $31.11 for the predialysis vaccine.

The duration of natural or acquired immunity against HBV among dialysis patients remains uncertain.[158,159] Both the Advisory Committee on Immunization Practices (ACIP) and the American College of Physicians (ACP) have endorsed postvaccination testing of dialysis patients after a primary vaccination course. The ACIP recommends anti-HBs testing 1 to 2 months after completion of the primary series and annually thereafter.[148] It appears prudent to administer booster doses to those patients with antibody levels <10 U/L. Loss of antibody does not necessarily mean loss of immunity, as immunologic memory may outlast the presence of circulating anti-HBs. Among immunocompetent subjects who respond to vaccination, the risk of acquiring HBV increases as anti-HBs become undetectable, even though the risk of developing clinical hepatitis remains extremely low. However, protection against HBV infection is not maintained when antibody titers fall below protective levels in dialysis patients. Saab et al.[160] compared the strategies to maintain HBV immunity in chronic HD patients who responded to the primary vaccine course. Regular screening of patients for HBV immunity before revaccination (screening strategy) proved to be less costly and associated with fewer HBV infections than the routine, annual administration of the vaccine booster to all HD patients (nonscreening strategy).[160]

HEPATITIS D

The hepatitis D virus (HDV), also known as the delta (δ) agent, is an RNA virus that replicates only in the presence of HBsAg.[161] Thus it can occur only in patients who are HBV-infected. Chronic HDV infection often results in severe liver disease that progresses to cirrhosis in as many as 70 percent of immunocompetent patients. HDV infection may occur simultaneously with acute HBV infection (coinfection). Transmission of HDV is similar to that of HBV, via blood and body fluids containing the virus, although infection most typically is spread by parenteral rather than nonparenteral routes.

The clinical significance of HDV is an increased severity of HBV infection; unlike HBV, HDV is almost invariably associated with clinically important liver damage. Routine serologic diagnosis of HDV infection is currently based on the detection of circulating antibody to HDV antigen (anti-HDV). Information on serologic evidence of delta infection in dialysis patients is limited[162–168]; HDV has been reported very infrequently in patients on maintenance HD. Transmission of HDV between HD patients has, however, been reported in the United States from a patient who was chronically infected with HBV and HDV to an HBsAg-positive patient after a massive bleeding incident; both patients received dialysis at the same station.[166]

HDV infection should be considered mainly in any HBV-infected patient with rapidly deteriorating liver function.

HEPATITIS C

In 1989, the hepatitis C virus (HCV) was identified by cloning and sequencing its genome.[169–171] It is a single-stranded, positive RNA virus with a genome composed of more than 9400 nucleotides, showing organization and sequence homology with the human flaviviruses and animal pestiviruses, all of which are considered members of the family Flaviviridae. Sequence analysis of the viral genome has identified several major HCV genotypes with additional subtypes.[172,173]

HCV is typically spread by parenteral routes and is significantly less infectious than HBV. The most important modes of transmission of HCV in the general population have been blood transfusion and intravenous drug use. HCV infection remains common in ESRD patients undergoing maintenance HD or PD.

Interpretation of Diagnostic Tests

The diagnosis of HCV is routinely made serologically.[174,175] A third-generation assay (enzyme-linked immunosorbent assay 3, or ELISA-3) has recently been introduced, with high sensitivity and specificity even in ESRD patients.[176] Earlier versions of serologic testing were limited by lack of sensitivity, with false-negative results in viremic patients. A variety of tests based on the polymerase chain reaction (PCR) are now available. Quantitative PCR tests measure viral load, whereas the more sensitive qualitative tests can detect even low-level viremia. In interpreting results, it is important to know whether a PCR assay is qualitative or quantitative. The branched-chain DNA assay (bDNA) allows quantitative detection of HCV RNA in serum; it amplifies the signal/probe rather than viral nucleic acid. Although it is less sensitive than PCR, it is a reproducible and reliable technique that has also been used to assess viral load in HCV-infected patients.[54]

The epidemiology of anti-HCV seropositivity by use of the first-,[177–197] second-,[198–222] and third-generation[223–232] ELISA assays has been extensively evaluated in dialysis patients. A PCR test should be considered if there is clinical suspicion of HCV infection despite negative serologies.[233–238]

HCV Epidemiology in Dialysis Centers: Current Status

Patients receiving maintenance dialysis remain at risk of acquiring HCV infection. Screening of blood and blood products for HCV has virtually eliminated the risk of posttransfusion HCV infection in HD; the current risk in the United States of transfusion-related infection with HCV is 1 in 103,000 transfused units.[3]

The CDC has reported that anti-HCV prevalence in chronic HD patients in the United States in 1999 was 8.9 percent.[239] During 1992–1999, national surveillance data indicated that the proportion of centers that tested patients for anti-HCV increased from 22 to 56 percent.[240] Nosocomial transmission of HCV within HD centers has been suggested by numerous epidemiologic findings and has been unequivocally demonstrated by molecular technology.[241–252]

Several findings support the occurrence of nosocomial transmission of HCV within dialysis units: the strong association between prevalence and incidence of HCV in HD,[253,254] the significant and independent relationship between anti-HCV antibody prevalence and time on HD,[255–257] and the higher rate of anti-HCV in patients undergoing center-HD treatment than in patients on PD[258] and those undergoing HD at home.[259] Further, the relative homogeneity of HCV genotypes in some dialysis units is in accordance with the patient-to-patient transmission of HCV in the dialysis setting.[260,261] In addition, a persistent incidence of HCV infection reported in patients on maintenance dialysis in developed countries, despite the elimination of posttransfusion HCV infection, confirms the occurrence of HCV in this setting.[262–268] The prevalence of HCV in dialysis patients in the industrialized world is still very high (Table 24–4).[262–268]

Information on HCV epidemiology among dialysis patients in less developed countries is scarce and based on single-center surveys: prevalence and incidence rates of HCV infection remain very high (Table 24–5).[269–282] This is likely related to various factors, including failure of infection control procedures to prevent the spread of HCV in the HD environment and a high background prevalence of HCV in the general population.

Information on HCV epidemiology among patients on PD is less abundant; a lower frequency of HCV infection in patients on PD compared with those on HD has been repeatedly found,[283–299] no doubt reflecting fewer percutaneous exposures due to the lack of a need for vascular access and management at home rather than in a unit with other patients.

TABLE 24–4. PREVALENCE OF ANTI-HCV AMONG PATIENTS UNDERGOING DIALYSIS IN DEVELOPED COUNTRIES

Authors Reference Year	Anti-HCV Prevalence	Country	
Lombardi M. et al.[262]	22.5% (2.274/10.097)	Italy	1999
Saab S. et al.[263]	7% (172/2.440)	United States	2000
Schneeberger P.M. et al.[236]	3.4% (76/2.286)	Netherlands	2000
Salama G. et al.[264]	16.3% (216/1.323)	France	2002
Hinrichsen H. et al.[233]	6.1% (171/2.796)	Germany	2002

TABLE 24–5. PREVALENCE OF ANTI-HCV AMONG PATIENTS UNDERGOING DIALYSIS IN LESS-DEVELOPED COUNTRIES

Authors	Anti-HCV Prevalence	Country	Reference Year
Todorov V. et al.[277]	65.8% (52/79)	Bulgaria	1998
Covic A. et al.[31]	75% (111/148)	Moldavia	1999
Hassan A.A. et al.[274]	80% (169/210)	Egypt	2000
Djordjevic V. et al.[269]	48.8% (83/170)	Serbia	2000
Taskapan H. et al.[276]	17% (22/129)	Turkey	2001
Jaiswal S.P. et al.[275]	30% (80/265)	India	2002
Valtuille R. et al.[279]	8.5% (7/82)	Argentina	2002
Shaheen F.A. et al.[270]	72.3% (295/408)	Saudi Arabia	2003

Modes of Nosocomial Transmission of HCV in Hemodialysis

A number of mechanisms for the nosocomial spread of HCV within dialysis units have been postulated, including HCV acquisition by a dialysis nurse after a needle-stick injury.[300]

At present, the most important mechanism for nosocomial transmission of HCV within HD units is cross-contamination among patients due to a lack of adherence to infection-control strategies against blood-borne pathogens. Numerous lapses have been identified: sharing of medications (heparin) between HD patients[259]; lack of glove use by the dialysis staff during repositioning of dialysis needles during HD sessions[301]; lack of handwashing before and, less frequently, after activities involving HCV-positive patients on HD.[302,303]

Contamination of dialysis machines has also been implicated by various authors; Simon et al., in Paris,[304] found that 4 of 5 seronegative patients dialyzed on the same machine, with closed circulation of dialysate, seroconverted to HCV positivity within a 2-month period. Chiaramonte and coworkers,[305] during an outbreak of HCV in HD, found that patients using exclusively HD machines with totally disposable dialysate circuits and no ultrafiltration control devices did not acquire HCV infection. Niu and coworkers,[306] during an outbreak of HCV in a HD unit, suspected that the overloading of transducer protectors by increased arterial pressure in the circuit resulted in the reflux of patient blood across the transducer protector to the inside of dialysis machines.

An important potential mode of HCV transmission among HD patients is dialyzer reuse. In Taiwan, a higher frequency of dialyzer reuse in anti-HCV-positive patients than in those who were anti-HCV-negative has been seen [4.2 percent (14 of 145) vs. 1.9 percent (5 of 260), $p = 0.001$].[307] However, this relationship has not been confirmed in other surveys: a Belgian[308] multicenter study reported that the rate of dialyzer reuse was 37.5 percent in patients who had seroconversion for anti-HCV and 40 percent

(158 of 393) in those who did not (NS). A study from the Portuguese Society of Nephrology[309] demonstrated an incidence of HCV infection of 6.1 percent in HD units reprocessing dialyzers and 7.4 percent in units that did not (NS). In units that reprocessed dialyzers from anti-HCV-positive patients compared to those that did not follow any specific precautions in reprocessing dialyzers (incidence, 6.9 percent), centers that used a separate room to reprocess dialyzers and those that did not had significantly lower incidence rates, 0.4 and 2 percent, respectively. Units that reprocessed dialyzers from anti-HCV-positive patients last had a significantly higher incidence of HCV infection, 10.2 percent.[309]

Control of HCV Transmission in Hemodialysis Centers: Current Strategies

The CDC has not mandated designated HD machines or patient isolation for HCV-infected patients; no ban on dialyzer reuse has been mandated for prevention of HCV infection within HD units[20] for several reasons. HCV is present in minute quantities in circulating blood, infectivity of HCV is lower than that of HBV, and HCV is not stable at room temperature. The CDC currently recommends monthly monitoring of serum aminotransferase activity in HD patients; quarterly instead of monthly monitoring of serum ALT activity has been recommended in PD patients. Full implementation of both universal precautions and routine HD unit precautions is necessary to prevent HCV in HD. The CDC has recently included HD patients among those persons who should be tested routinely for HCV based on their risk of infection.[240]

The systematic disinfection of dialysis machines appears a simple and effective way of limiting the spread of HCV infection.[310] Several investigators have been able to eliminate HCV infection by the exclusive enforcement of infection control procedures against blood-borne pathogens.[311] Others have obtained the same result by using universal precautions and dialysis machines with disposable dialysate circuits.[312]

Natural History of HCV Infection

The natural history of HCV infection among patients undergoing long-term dialysis remains undefined. An accurate assessment of the clinical outcomes of HCV in ESRD is hampered by the indolent nature of the disease: its onset is rarely recognized and its course is prolonged.[313]

Liver-related mortality in the dialysis population is very low, as noted earlier. Data from the Registro Lombardo Dialisi e Trapianto (RLDT) have shown that mortality due to liver disease was approximately 2 percent in the 1997 population of the Lombardy Registry.[50] The rate of chronicity of HCV infection after acute hepatitis C is high among

dialysis patients, as it is in the general population. Espinosa et al.[314] followed a large cohort of patients on maintenance dialysis over a 12-year follow-up: 19 cases of acute HCV infection were found. The majority (11 of 19, or 57.8 percent) of these patients had HCV-related liver disease (HCV RNA persistently positive and ALT persistently elevated) over a median follow-up of 3 years (range, 1 to 6 years).

An adequate understanding of the natural history of HCV in the HD population is further hampered by various factors: the age-adjusted death rate of dialysis patients is estimated to be four to five times higher than that of the general population[50]; this clearly prevents observational studies with long follow-up of a liver disease that is typically slowly progressive. Nephrologists are usually reluctant to suggest liver biopsy in HD patients because of concern about bleeding complications, although the degree of fibrosis on liver biopsy is a key and appropriate indicator of progression of chronic liver disease in patients with normal kidney function.[315] The limited information on liver histology in dialysis patients with HCV does show mild histopathologic changes in many cases.[316–326]

Recognition of liver disease on the grounds of biochemical tests is difficult, as serum ALT activity is usually lower among chronic kidney disease patients in the predialysis or dialysis stage than in the general population, as noted earlier. Anti-HCV-positive patients on maintenance dialysis show significantly higher AST/ALT activity than anti-HCV-negative individuals, but these higher AST/ALT values are often in the range considered "normal" for the general population. We have evaluated the pattern of HCV acquisition among HD patients—onset of viral replication associated with a rise in ALT activity and a subsequent decline of HCV RNA levels, with return of ALT to higher preinfection levels but still within the "normal" range for those without ESRD.[327]

Viral, host, and/or environmental factors may influence the outcome of chronic HCV infection, but their precise role in promoting disease progression has yet to be defined in dialysis patients. It has been hypothesized that depressed immunity in chronic uremia is a possible cause of attenuated inflammatory reactions in the liver and, consequently, reduced hepatocyte destruction.

It has also been suggested that HD may exert a hepatic protective activity on the course of HCV, with several mechanisms implicated. A clear relationship between viral load and clinical outcome of hepatitis C has yet to be determined in patients with normal kidney function.[315] HCV viral load in the HD population with HCV infection is typically low and does not increase over time.[328,329] It has been suggested that the HD procedure lowers HCV RNA titers by various mechanisms: the clearance of HCV RNA by the dialysate,[330–333] entrapment of HCV RNA particles by the membrane surface of dialyzers,[334–342] and the production of cytokines and other molecules during HD sessions.[343,344]

Compared to HCV-positive patients with normal renal function, HD patients with HCV infection have prolonged IFN clearance.[345] Rampino et al.[343] have measured enhanced production of hepatocyte growth factors (HGF) during HD sessions; they have suggested a beneficial effect of HGF through hepatocyte proliferation and accelerated liver repair. Badalamenti and coworkers[344] recently observed that levels of IFN-α markedly increase after dialysis using both cellulosic and synthetic membranes; this increase in endogenous IFN could contribute to a reduction in viremia in HCV-positive patients on maintenance dialysis.

Mortality and HCV Infection

Mortality is a reliable endpoint in the natural history of chronic liver diseases in patients with normal kidney function. A significant relationship between HCV status and survival in the dialysis population has been observed in single-center prospective surveys.[346–349] Anti-HCV-positive status was a significant and independent risk factor for mortality among patients on long-term dialysis. Nakayama and coworkers[346] prospectively followed 1470 Japanese patients on chronic HD over a 6-year period (1993 to 1999). Mortality was higher in the anti-HCV-positive group than in the anti-HCV-negative group [33 percent (91 of 276) vs. 23.2 percent (277 of 1193), $p < 0.01$]. Cox proportional hazard examination showed that seropositivity for anti-HCV was one of the risk factors for death, with an adjusted relative risk of 1.57 (95 percent CI, 1.23 to 2.00). As a cause of death, liver cirrhosis and hepatocellular carcinoma (HCC) were significantly more frequent in the anti-HCV antibody-positive than in the anti-HCV antibody-negative patients [8.8 percent (8 of 91) vs. 0.4 percent (1 of 277), $p < 0.001$ and 5.5 percent (5 of 91) vs. 0.0 percent (0 of 277), $p < 0.001$]. Stehman-Breen and coworkers[347] prospectively evaluated 200 patients on chronic HD in the United States over a median 3-year follow-up; the mortality rate was 54.5 percent (24 of 44) in the HCV-antibody-positive and 58 percent (90 of 156) in the HCV-antibody-negative group. However, Cox regression analysis showed that the adjusted relative risk for death was 1.97 (95 percent CI, 1.16 to 3.3, $p < 0.012$) among anti-HCV-positive patients as opposed to those who were negative.

The Japanese Society for Dialysis collected data on 206,314 dialysis patients at the end of the year 2000.[350] For the first time the survey incorporated additional variables including smoking, use of oral antiypertensives, pre- and postdialysis blood pressure, serum HDL cholesterol, and HCV status. The survey showed that a high mortality risk was additionally associated with several parameters, including hepatocellular carcinoma, liver cirrhosis, positive HCV antibody status, and glutamic–pyruvic transaminase levels exceeding 20 IU/L.

Ishida and coworkers[351] investigated the characteristics of 6366 HCV-antibody-positive patients on chronic HD in Japan. HCC was a complication in 114 (1.8 percent) HCV-antibody-positive patients, and cirrhosis was a complication in 536 (8.6 percent). The incidence of both complications was significantly higher in males than in females; no comparison was made with age-adjusted general population members in the same country.

Clinical Presentation of HCV Infection

Patients on maintenance dialysis with HCV infection are usually anicteric and develop few signs or symptoms of hepatitis. Detectable HCV RNA in serum is an important predictor of raised ALT activity among patients undergoing maintenance dialysis, although the levels may still be in the "normal" range for the nonuremic population. In a large cohort of patients ($n=394$) on chronic HD in the Los Angeles area, serum AST and ALT were significantly higher in HCV RNA-positive patients than in individuals with no detectable HCV RNA in serum [23.8 (95 percent CI, 60.8 to 9.3) vs. 17.1 (95 percent CI, 50.4 to 5.8) U/L ($p = 0.009$) and 14.4 (95 percent CI, 48.9 to 4.3) vs. 9.4 (95 percent CI, 37.3 to 2.5) U/L ($p = 0.008$)]. Logistic regression analysis showed an association between HCV viremia, anti-HCV antibody ($p = 0.0001$), and ALT activity ($p = 0.01$).[234]

It has been suggested that the best cutoff point for evaluating HCV should be set at lower levels (<30 IU/L for AST/ALT) to enhance the diagnostic yield of AST/ALT in the dialysis population,[352] where "normal" AST/ALT may be quite low, as discussed above.

Treatment of HCV Infection

The role of antiviral therapy in dialysis patients with hepatitis C remains controversial.[353] At present, it is not clear which dialysis patients with HCV should be treated with IFN. IFN therapy is complex, expensive, and associated with significant side effects; for these reasons nephrologists have been reluctant to offer IFN to their patients. In addition, there is little information about the predictive factors of a sustained virologic response to IFN in dialysis patients. The benefits of IFN therapy have frequently been assessed over years or decades, whereas many dialysis patients have a short expected survival due to age and/or comorbid conditions. Thus, IFN cannot be offered to every dialysis patient with HCV; it seems reasonable to offer IFN to those patients on dialysis considered for RT. Therapy should be offered only after careful discussion of potential benefits and risks of treatment. Expected patient survival must be evaluated in selecting dialysis patients for IFN treatment; patients with a shortened expected survival (i.e., those with diabetes, congestive heart failure, and/or malnutrition) are probably not good candidates for IFN therapy.

Interferon. IFN remains the mainstay of treatment of HCV-related liver disease. It has a variety of antiviral, immunomodulatory, and antiproliferative activities. The available literature on the treatment of hepatitis C with IFN consists predominantly of small and uncontrolled trials.[354–373] Two systematic reviews of the literature have recently been performed with metanalyses of published clinical trials in order to assess the efficacy and safety of initial IFN monotherapy in dialysis patients with chronic hepatitis C.[374,375] Fabrizi et al.[375] identified 14 clinical trials; 2 were controlled studies. The mean overall estimate for sustained virologic response (SVR) and dropout rate were 37 percent (95 percent CI, 28 to 48) and 17 percent (95 percent CI, 10 to 28), respectively. In the subset of clinical trials ($n = 5$) with standard IFN administration [3 million units (UI) thrice weekly, subcutaneous route, 24-week treatment], the overall mean estimate of SVR was 39 percent (95 percent CI, 25 to 56). A recent metanalysis had found that IFN-α at 3 MUI thrice weekly (24 weeks) achieved a SVR of 7 to 16 percent in naive patients with chronic hepatitis C and normal renal function.[376] Several biological mechanisms may be responsible for the relatively higher response to IFN in dialysis patients in spite of immune compromise due to uremia. HD patients with HCV typically have a low viral load, IFN could help to restore the cell-mediated immunity depressed by uremia, and an increase of endogenous IFN activity during HD sessions has also been shown. Importantly, clearance of IFN is lower in dialysis than in nonuremic patients.

The overall mean[375] estimate of dropout rate due to side effects with IFN monotherapy in dialysis patients with chronic hepatitis C (17 percent) was higher than the frequency of side effects requiring IFN discontinuation in nonuremic patients with chronic hepatitis C (5 to 9 percent) with standard IFN doses.[377,378] The altered pharmacokinetic parameters of IFN in the HD population, older age, and high frequency of comorbid conditions in HD patients may to some extent explain the frequency of side effects leading to IFN discontinuation. The profile of side effects during IFN monotherapy in dialysis patients supports this hypothesis: the most frequent side effects requiring interruption of treatment were flu-like symptoms (17 percent), neurologic symptoms (21 percent), and gastrointestinal problems (18 percent). This is different from patients with chronic hepatitis C and normal renal function: the most frequent causes of interruption of IFN monotherapy among them are flu-like syndrome (41 percent), alopecia (16 percent), and depression (7 percent).[379]

Recent reports[380–382] support the use of IFN monotherapy in dialysis patients waiting for a RT because, with suc-

cessful HCV RNA clearance, relapse after RT may not occur despite chronic and aggressive immunosuppressive treatment. IFN therapy in RT recipients is absolutely contraindicated due to frequent and irreversible graft dysfunction.[383–385] Thus therapy of HCV is most appropriately attempted prior to RT with the aim of achieving a sustained viral response even following subsequent RT.

Interferon plus Ribavirin. Therapy for chronic HCV has evolved from IFN-α monotherapy to combination therapy with ribavirin.[377] Bruchfeld and colleagues[386,387] treated 6 HCV-infected patients on chronic dialysis with IFN-α-2b plus ribavirin. In order to distinguish between side effects of the two drugs, IFN-α-2b was given initially as monotherapy at a dose of 3 MUI thrice weekly after dialysis for 4 weeks; thereafter low-dose ribavirin was added, starting at 200 to 400 mg orally once a day for 24 weeks. The SVR was 17 percent (1 of 6). Bruchfeld and coworkers identified three requirements for the safe use of ribavirin in the dialysis population. First, the ribavirin dose must be reduced; second, the plasma concentration of ribavirin should be closely monitored; third, it is necessary to increase the dose of erythropoietin above the standard dose to compensate for ribavirin-associated hemolytic anemia.

A second pilot trial was reported by Tan and colleagues[388] in the Netherlands; five patients with chronic hepatitis C on chronic HD participated in the study. Patients received subcutaneous IFN-α-2b $\times$ 10^6 U three times weekly plus oral ribavirin; the duration of therapy is unclear. Ribavirin was stopped permanently in two patients due to severe anemia; one patient suffered from adverse effects (fever and chills), which resolved after IFN was permanently stopped. Interim analysis showed that, in all patients, serum HCV RNA levels decreased markedly, resulting in a loss of HCV RNA (80 percent) in five patients during treatment. The ribavirin dose in the dialysis patients (200 mg three times weekly) was only one-sixth of the controls' daily ribavirin dose.

PegInterferon. One important reason for the overall poorly sustained response to standard IFN-α is its short half-life. To maintain constant pressure on the virus and reduce the frequency of administration, pegylated formulations of IFN have been developed.[389,390] PegInterferon-α-2a (40 kDa) and PegInterferon-α-2b (12 KDa) have been developed by covalent attachment of a branched 40-kDa polyethylene glycol moiety and a single 12-kDa PEG moiety to IFN-α-2a and IFN-α-2b, respectively. This has resulted in more sustained absorption, reduced clearance, and a smaller volume of distribution, permitting once-weekly dosing.[391] A single-dose study of PegInterferon-α-2a (40 kDa) in 30 patients with stable chronic kidney disease showed no significant changes in pharmacokinetics that would warrant dose adjustment.[392] Regression analyses of pharmacokinetic data from 23 patients with creatinine clearance (CL_{cr}) values ranging from greater than 100 mL/min (normal renal function) to 20 mL/min (severe renal impairment) showed no significant relationship between the pharmacokinetics of PegInterferon-α-2a (40 kDa) and CL_{cr}.[392] The pharmacokinetic profile of PegInterferon-α-2a (40 kDa) in patients on maintenance HD is similar to that in healthy individuals, with only a 30 percent relative reduction in clearance.[393] Multicenter clinical trials with pegylated IFN for the treatment of chronic hepatitis C in dialysis patients are planned.

Liver Dysfunction in Dialysis Patients: Nonviral Agents

There is no evidence that patients on maintenance dialysis are overall more prone to drug hepatotoxicity than nonuremic individuals. However, dialysis patients usually receive multiple medications; thus, drug interactions may play a role in the pathogenesis of drug-induced liver disease in this population. Numerous antibiotics can cause hepatic dysfunction; some cardiovascular drugs, including amiodarone, are hepatotoxic.[394] Monitoring of aminotransferase activity is recommended during treatment of hypercholesterolemia with HMG-CoA reductase inhibitors; however, recent clinical trials have not reported increases in hepatic enzymes during HMG-CoA use in dialysis patients.[395] Allopurinol and anabolic steroids may be hepatotoxic in patients with renal failure. Body aluminum overload due to prolonged exposure to contaminated dialysis fluids and aluminum-containing medications, such as aluminum hydroxyde, can be associated with liver dysfunction.[396–399] Nonsteroidal anti-inflammatory drugs (NSAIDs) rarely cause liver damage. Other causes of obscure liver dysfunction in the dialysis population include steatosis due to obesity, hyperlipidemia, and diabetes mellitus and hepatic congestion due to heart failure. With the advent of erythropoietin treatment, the frequency of iron overload is currently very low; hepatic siderosis due to iron overload was frequent in the past due to multiple transfusions.[400,401]

CONCLUSIONS

Liver disease plays a significant role in morbidity and mortality of patients on maintenance dialysis. The most common forms of dialysis-associated liver diseases are forms of viral hepatitis, which are more frequent in HD than PD patients. The control of spread of HBV infection in dialysis centers has been one of major triumphs in the management of ESRD, but the diffusion of HCV within HD units remains high all over the world. Clinical investigation is under way in order to select the optimal management of HCV-related liver disease in patients on renal replacement therapy.

REFERENCES

1. Martin P, Friedman LS. Chronic viral hepatitis and the management of chronic renal failure. *Kidney Int* 1995;47: 1231–1241.
2. Lee WM. Hepatitis B virus infection. *N Engl J Med* 1997; 337:1733–1745.
3. Schreiber GB, Busch MP, Kleinman SH, Korelitz JJ. The risk of transfusion-transmitted viral infections. *N Engl J Med* 1996;334:1685–1690.
4. Lok ASF. Hepatitis B infection: pathogenesis and management. *J Hepatol* 2000;32(suppl 1):89–97.
5. Friedman EA, Thomson GE. Hepatitis complicating chronic hemodialysis. *Lancet* 1966;2:675–678.
6. Garibaldi RA, Forrest JN, Bryan JA, et al. Hemodialysis-associated hepatitis. *JAMA* 1973;225:384–389.
7. Szmuness W, Prince AM, Grady GF, et al. Hepatitis B infection. A point-prevalence study in 15 US hemodialysis centers. *JAMA* 1974;227:901–906.
8. Parsons FM, Brunner FP, Gurland HJ, Harlen H. Combined report of regular dialysis and transplantation in Europe. *Proc Eur Dial Transplant Assoc* 1971;8:3–17.
9. Snydman D, Bryan J, Hanson B. Hemodialysis-associated hepatitis in the United States, 1972. *J Infect Dis* 1975;132: 109–113.
10. Centers for Disease Control. Hepatitis: control measures for hepatitis type B in dialysis centers. HEW publication no. (CDC) 78–8358 (Viral Hepatitis Investigations and Control Series). Atlanta, GA: US Department of Health, Education, and Welfare, Public Health Services, CDC, 1977.
11. Alter MJ, Favero MS, Maynard JE. Impact of infection control strategies on the incidence of dialysis associated hepatitis in the United States. *J Infect Dis* 1986;153:1149–1151.
12. Decrease in the incidence of hepatitis in dialysis units associated with prevention programme: Public Health Laboratory Service Survey. *Br Med J* 1974;4:751–754.
13. Hepatitis B in retreat from dialysis units in United Kingdom in 1973: Public Health Laboratory Service Survey. *Br Med J* 1976;1:1579–1581.
14. Degos F, Lugassy C, Degott C, et al. Hepatitis B virus and hepatitis B-related viral infection in renal transplant recipients. A prospective study of 90 patients. *Gastroenterology* 1988;94:151–156.
15. Kantor RJ, Hadler SC, Schreeder MT, et al. Outbreak of hepatitis B in a dialysis unit, complicated by false positive HBsAg test results. *Dialysis Transplant* 1979;8:232–235.
16. Carl M, Francis DP, Maynard JE. A common source outbreak of hepatitis B in a hemodialysis unit. *Dialysis Transplant* 1983;12:222–229.
17. Alter MJ, Ahtone J, Maynard JE. Hepatitis B virus transmission associated with a multiple dose vial in a hemodialysis unit. *Ann Intern Med* 1983;99:330–333.

18. Niu MT, Penberthy LT, Alter MJ, et al. Hemodialysis-associated hepatitis B: report of an outbreak. *Dialysis Transplant* 1989;18:542–546.

19. Update: universal precautions for prevention of transmission of human immunodeficiency virus, hepatitis B virus and other blood-borne pathogens in healthcare settings. *MMWR Morb Mortal Wkly Rep* 1988;37:377–382.

20. Kellerman S, Alter MJ. Preventing hepatitis B and hepatitis C virus infections in end-stage renal disease patients: back to basics. *Hepatology* 1999;29:291–293.

21. Tokars JI, Miller ER, Alter MJ, Arduino MJ. National surveillance of dialysis-associated diseases in the United States, 1997. *Semin Dial* 2000;13:75–85.

22. Burdick RA, Bragg-Cresham JL, Woods JD, et al. Patterns of hepatitis B prevalence and seroconversion in hemodialysis units from three continents: The DOPPS. *Kidney Int* 2003;63:2222–2229.

23. Mioli VA, Balestra E, Bibiano L, et al. Epidemiology of viral hepatitis in dialysis centers: a national survey. *Nephron* 1992;61:278–283.

24. Oguchi H, Miyasaka M, Tokunaga S, et al. Hepatitis virus infection (HBV and HCV) in eleven Japanese hemodialysis units. *Clin Nephrol* 1992;38:36–43.

25. Albertoni F, Battilomo A, Di Nardo V, et al. Evaluation of a region-wide hepatitis B vaccination program in dialysis patients: experience in an Italian region. The Latium Hepatitis Prevention Group. *Nephron* 1991;58:180–183.

26. Centers for Disease Control and Prevention. Outbreaks of hepatitis B virus infection among hemodialysis patients— California, Nebraska, and Texas. *JAMA* 1996;275:1394– 1395.

27. Tanaka S, Yoshiba M, Iino S, et al. A common-source outbreak of fulminant hepatitis B in hemodialysis patients induced by precore mutant. *Kidney Int* 1995;48:1972–1978.

28. Hutin YJF, Goldstein ST, Varma JK, et al. An outbreak of hospital-acquired hepatitis B virus infection among patients receiving chronic hemodialysis. *Infect Control Hosp Epidemiol* 1999;20:731–735.

29. Balshaw A, Casey J. One haemodialysis unit's experience of hepatitis B. *EDTNA ERCA J* 2000;26:17–19.

30. Cendoroglo-Neto M, Draibe SA, Silva AE, et al. Incidence and risk factors for hepatitis B and hepatitis C virus infection among haemodialysis and CAPD patients: evidence for environmental transmission. *Nephrol Dial Transplant* 1995; 10:240–246.

31. Covic A, Iancu L, Apetrei C, et al. Hepatitis virus infection in haemodialysis patients from Moldavia. *Nephrol Dial Transplant* 1999;14:40–45.

32. Vladutiu D, Cosa A, Neamtu A, et al. Infection with hepatitis B and C viruses in patients on maintenance dialysis in Romania and in former communist countries: yellow spots on a blank map? *J Viral Hepat* 2000;7:313–319.

33. Lewis-Ximenez LL, Oliveira JM, Mercadante LA, et al. Serological and vaccination profile of hemodialysis patients during an outbreak of hepatitis B virus infection. *Nephron* 2001;87:19–26.

34. Otedo AE, Mc'Ligeyo SO, Okoth FA, Kayima JK. Seroprevalence of hepatitis B and C in maintenance dialysis in a public hospital in a developing country. *S Afr Med J* 2003; 93:380–384.

35. Jankovic N, Cala S, Nadinic B, et al. Hepatitis C and hepatitis B virus infection in hemodialysis patients and staff: a two year follow-up. *Int J Artif Organs* 1994;17:137–140.

36. Teles SA, Martins RMB, Vanderboght B, et al. Hepatitis B virus: genotypes and subtypes in Brazilian hemodialysis patients. *Artif Organs* 1999;23:1074–1078.

37. Cendoroglo-Neto M, Manzano SI, Canziani ME, et al. Environmental transmission of hepatitis B and C viruses within the hemodialysis unit. *Artif Organs* 1995;19:251–255.

38. Teles SA, Martins RM, Gomes SA, et al. Hepatitis B virus transmission in Brazilian hemodialysis units: serological and molecular follow-up. *J Med Virol* 2002;68:41–49.

39. Nemecek V, Reinis M, Konopacova A, et al. Molecular biology and serologic analysis in an epidemic of viral hepatitis B in vaccinated patients on hemodialysis. *Epidemiol Mikrobiol Imunol* 1999;48:160–166.

40. Barton EN, King SD, Douglas LL. The seroprevalence of hepatitis and retroviral infection in Jamaican haemodialysis patients. *West Indian Med J* 1998;47:105–107.

41. Fabrizi F, Mangano S, Alongi G, et al. Influence of hepatitis B virus viremia upon serum aminotransferase activity in dialysis population. *Int J Artif Organs* 2003;26: 1048–1055.

42. Guh JY, Lai YH, Yang CY, et al. Impact of decreased serum aminotransferase levels on the evaluation of viral hepatitis in hemodialysis patients. *Nephron* 1995;69:459–465.

43. Hung KY, Lee KC, Yen CJ, et al. Revised cutoff values of serum aminotransferase in detecting viral hepatitis among CAPD patients: experience from Taiwan, an endemic area for hepatitis B. *Nephrol Dial Transplant* 1997;12:180–183.

44. Yasuda K, Okuda K, Endo N, et al. Hypoaminotransferasemia in patients undergoing long-term hemodialysis: clinical and biochemical appraisal. *Gastroenterology* 1995; 109:1295–1300.

45. Fabrizi F, Lunghi G, Finazzi S, et al. Decreased serum aminotransferase activity in patients with chronic renal failure: impact on the detection of viral hepatitis. *Am J Kidney Dis* 2001;38:1009–1015.

46. Marcelli D, Stanhard D, Conte F, et al. ESRD patient mortality with adjustement for comorbid conditions in Lombardy (Italy) versus the United States. *Kidney Int* 1996;50: 1013–1018.

47. Maisonneuve P, Agodoa L, Gellert R, et al. Cancer in patients on dialysis for end-stage renal disease: an international collaborative study. *Lancet* 1999;354:93–99.

48. Degott C, Degos F, Jungers P, et al. Relationship between liver histopathology changes and HBsAg in 111 patients treated by long-term hemodialysis. *Liver* 1983;3:377–384.

49. Harnett JD, Zeldis JB, Parfrey PS, et al. Hepatitis B disease in dialysis and transplant patients. Further epidemiology and serologic studies. *Transplantation* 1987;44:369–376.

50. Locatelli F, Marcelli D, Conte F, et al. Cardiovascular disease in chronic renal failure: the challenge continues. *Nephrol Dial Transplant* 2000;15(suppl 5):S69–S80.

51. Josselson J, Kyser BA, Weir MR, Sadler JH. Hepatitis B surface antigenemia in a chronic hemodialysis program: lack of

influence on morbidity and mortality. *Am J Kidney Dis* 1987;6:456–461.

52. Harnett JD, Parfrey PS, Kennedy M, et al. The long-term outcome of hepatitis B infection in hemodialysis patients. *Am J Kidney Dis* 1988;11:210–213.

53. Jha R, Kher V, Naik S, et al. Hepatitis B associated liver disease in dialysis patients: role of vaccination. *J Nephrol* 1993;6:98–103.

54. Fabrizi F, Martin P. Hepatitis in kidney transplantation. In: GM Danovitch, ed. *Handbook of Kidney Transplantation*, 3d ed. Philadelphia: Lippincott Williams & Wilkins, 2001: 263–271.

55. Fabrizi F, Martin P, Ponticelli C. Hepatitis B virus and renal transplantation. *Nephron* 2002;90:241–251.

56. Tran T, Martin P. Chronic HBV without e antigen: using HBV DNA to guide management. *Am J Gastroenterol* 2003;98:2115–2117.

57. Nagington J, Cossart YE, Cohen BJ. Reactivation of hepatitis B after transplantation operations. *Lancet* 1977;1: 558–560.

58. Grotz W, Rasenack J, Benzing T, et al. Occurrence and management of hepatitis B virus reactivation following kidney transplantation. *Clin Nephrol* 1998;49:385–388.

59. Blanpain C, Knoop C, Delforge ML, et al. Reactivation of hepatitis B after transplantation in patients with pre-existing anti-hepatitis B surface antigen antibodies: report on three cases and review of the literature. *Transplantation* 1998; 66:883–886.

60. Duarte R, Huraib S, Said R, et al. Interferon-alpha facilitates renal transplantation in hemodialysis patients with chronic viral hepatitis. *Am J Kidney Dis* 1995;25:40–45.

61. Rodrigues A, Morgado T, Areias J, et al. Limited benefits of INF-alpha therapy in renal graft candidates with chronic viral hepatitis B or C. *Transplant Proc* 1997;29:777–780.

62. Dienstag JL, Perrillo RP, Schiff ER, et al. A preliminary trial of lamivudine for chronic hepatitis B infection. *N Engl J Med* 1995;333:1657–1661.

63. Lai CL, Chien RN, Leung NWY, et al for the Asia Hepatitis Lamivudine Study Group. A one-year trial of lamivudine for chronic hepatitis B. *N Engl J Med* 1998;339:61–68.

64. Dienstag JL, Schiff ER, Wright TL, et al for the U.S. Lamivudine Investigator Group. Lamivudine as initial treatment for chronic hepatitis B in the United States. *N Engl J Med* 1999;341:1256–1263.

65. Schmilovitz-Weiss H, Melzer E, Tur-Kaspa R, Ben-Ari Z. Excellent outcome of lamivudine treatment in patients with chronic renal failure and hepatitis B virus infection. *J Clin Gastroenterol* 2003;37:64–67.

66. Fontaine H, Thiers V, Chretien Y, et al. HBV genotypic resistance to lamivudine in kidney recipients and hemodialyzed patients. *Transplantation* 2000;69:2090–2094.

67. Ben-Ari Z, Broida E, Kittai Y, et al. An open-label study of lamivudine for chronic hepatitis B in six patients with chronic renal failure before and after kidney transplantation. *Am J Gastroenterol* 2000;95:3579–3583.

68. Tillmann HL, Bock CT, Bleck JS, et al. Successful treatment of fibrosing cholestatic hepatitis using adefovir dipivoxil in a patient with cirrhosis and renal insufficiency. *Liver Transplant* 2003;9:191–196.

69. Fabrizi F, Martin P. Hepatitis B vaccine and dialysis: current issues. *Int J Artif Organs* 2001;24:683–694.

70. Stevens CE, Alter HJ, Taylor PE, et al. Hepatitis B vaccine in patients receiving hemodialysis. Immunogenicity and efficacy. *N Engl J Med* 1984;311:496–501.

71. Crosnier J, Jungers P, Couroucè AM, et al. Randomised placebo-controlled trial of hepatitis B surface antigen vaccine in French haemodialysis units: II. Haemodialysis patients. *Lancet* 1981;1:797–800.

72. Desmyter J, Colaert J, De Groote G, et al. Efficacy of heat-inactivated hepatitis B vaccine in haemodialysis patients and staff. Double-blind placebo-controlled trial. *Lancet* 1983;2: 1323–1328.

73. Miller ER, Alter MJ, Tokars JI. Protective effect of hepatitis B vaccine in chronic hemodialysis patients. *Am J Kidney Dis* 1999;33:356–360.

74. Steketee RW, Ziarnik ME, Davis JP. Seroresponse to hepatitis B vaccine in patients and staff of renal dialysis centers, Wisconsin. *Am J Epidemiol* 1988;127:772–782.

75. Fraser GM, Ochana N, Fenyves D, et al. Increasing serum creatinine and age reduce the response to hepatitis B vaccine in renal failure patients. *J Hepatol* 1994;21:450–454.

76. Fabrizi F, Di Filippo S, Marcelli D, et al. Recombinant hepatitis B vaccine use in chronic hemodialysis patients. Long-term evaluation and cost-effectiveness analysis. *Nephron* 1996;72:536–543.

77. Peces R, de la Torre M, Alcazar R, Urra JM. Prospective analysis of the factors influencing the antibody response to hepatitis B vaccine in hemodialysis patients. *Am J Kidney Dis* 1997;29:239–245.

78. Vagelli G, Calabrese G, Mazzotta A, et al. More about response to hepatitis B vaccine in hemodialysis patients (letter). *Nephron* 1988;49:171.

79. Pol S, Legendre C, Mattlinger B, et al. Genetic basis of nonresponse to hepatitis B vaccine in hemodialyzed patients. *J Hepatol* 1990;11:385–387.

80. Caillat-Zucman S, Gimenez JJ, Wambergue F, et al. Distinct HLA class II alleles determine antibody response to vaccination with hepatitis B surface antigen. *Kidney Int* 1998;53: 1626–1630.

81. Caillat-Zucman S, Gimenez JJ, Albouze G, et al. HLA genetic heterogeneity of hepatitis B vaccine response in hemodialyzed patients. *Kidney Int* 1993;41:S157–S160.

82. Stachowski J, Pollok M, Barth C, et al. Non-responsiveness to hepatitis B vaccination in haemodialysis patients: association with impaired TCR/CD3 antigen receptor expression regulating co-stimulatory processes in antigen presentation and recognition. *Nephrol Dial Transplant* 1994;9:144–152.

83. Fernandez E, Betriu MA, Gomez R, Montoliu J. Response to the hepatitis B virus vaccine in haemodialysis patients: influence of malnutrition and its importance as a risk factor for morbidity and mortality. *Nephrol Dial Transplant* 1996; 11:1559–1563.

84. Lombardi M, Pizzarelli F, Righi M, et al. Hepatitis B vaccination in dialysis patients and nutritional status. *Nephron* 1992;61:266–268.

85. Kovacic V, Sain M, Vukman V. Efficient haemodialysis improves the response to hepatitis B virus vaccination. *Intervirology* 2002;45:172–176.

86. Navarro JF, Teruel JL, Mateos ML, et al. Antibody level after hepatitis B vaccination in hemodialysis patients: influence of hepatitis C virus infection. *Am J Nephrol* 1996;16: 95–97.

87. Kamel M, El Manialawi, Miller DF. Recombinant hepatitis B vaccine immunogenicity in presence of hepatitis C virus seropositivity (letter). *Lancet* 1994;343:552.

88. Cheng CH, Huang CC, Leu ML, et al. Hepatitis B vaccine in hemodialysis patients with hepatitis C viral infection. *Vaccine* 1997;15:1353–1357.

89. Sennesael JJ, Van der Niepen P, Verbeelen DL. Treatment with recombinant human erythropoietin increases antibody titers after hepatitis B vaccination in dialysis patients. *Kidney Int* 1991;40:121–128.

90. Girndt M, Kohler H, Schiedhelm-Weick E, et al. Production of interleukin-6, tumor necrosis factor alpha and interleukin-10 in vitro correlates with the clinical immune defect in chronic hemodialysis patients. *Kidney Int* 1995;47:559–565.

91. Jibani MM, Heptonstall J, Walker AM, et al. Hepatitis B immunization in UK renal units: failure to put policy into practice. *Nephrol Dial Transplant* 1994;9:1765–1768.

92. Khan AN, Bernardini J, Rault RM, Piraino B. Low seroconversion with hepatitis B vaccination in peritoneal dialysis patients. *Perit Dial Int* 1996;16:370–373.

93. Jilg W, Schmidt M, Weinel B, et al. Immunogenicity of recombinant hepatitis B vaccine in dialysis patients. *J Hepatol* 1986;3:190–195.

94. Bruguera M, Cremades M, Mayor A, et al. Immunogenicity of a recombinant hepatitis B vaccine in haemodialysis patients. *Postgrad Med J* 1987;63:S155–S158.

95. Lelie PN, Reesink HW, de Jong-van Manen ST, Dees PJ, Reerink-Brongers EE. Immune response to a heat-inactivated hepatitis B vaccine in patients undergoing hemodialysis. Enhancement of the response by increasing the dose of hepatitis B surface antigen from 3 to 27 micrograms. *Arch Intern Med* 1985;145:305–309.

96. Benhamou E, Couroucè AM, Jungers P, et al. Hepatitis B vaccine: randomized trial of immunogenicity in hemodialysis patients. *Clin Nephrol* 1984;21:143–147.

97. Bommer J, Ritz E, Andrassy K, et al. Effect of vaccination schedule and dialysis on hepatitis B vaccination response in uraemic patients. *Proc Eur Dial Transplant Assoc* 1983;20: 161–168.

98. Pasko MT, Bartholomew WR, Beam TR Jr, et al. Long-term evaluation of the hepatitis B vaccine (Heptavax-B) in hemodialysis patients. *Am J Kidney Dis* 1988;11:326–331.

99. Kohler H, Arnold W, Renschin G, et al. Active hepatitis B vaccination of dialysis patients and medical staff. *Kidney Int* 1984;25:124–128.

100. Carreno V, Mora I, Escuin F, et al. Vaccination against hepatitis B in renal dialysis units: short or normal vaccination schedule? *Clin Nephrol* 1985;24:215–220.

101. Dentico P, Buongiorno R, Volpe A, et al. Long-term immunogenicity and protective efficacy of recombinant DNA yeast-derived vaccine in hemodialysis patients. *J Nephrol* 1993;6:95–97.

102. Mitwalli A. Responsiveness to hepatitis B vaccine in immunocompromised patients by doubling the dose scheduling. *Nephron* 1996;73:417–420.

103. Marangi AL, Giordano R, Montanaro A, et al. A successful two-step integrated protocol of anti-HBV vaccination in chronic uremia. *Nephron* 1992;61:331–332.

104. van Geelen JA, Schalm SW, de Visser EM, Heijtink RA. Immune response to hepatitis B vaccine in hemodialysis patients. *Nephron* 1987;45:216–218.

105. Guan R, Choong L. Immunogenicity of a recombinant DNA hepatitis B vaccine in patients with chronic renal failure. *Epidemiol News Bull* 1989;15:45–46.

106. Docci D, Cipolloni PA, Mengozzi S, et al. Immunogenicity of a recombinant hepatitis B vaccine in hemodialysis patients: a two-year follow-up. *Nephron* 1992;61: 352–353.

107. Jadoul M, Goubau P. Is anti-hepatitis B virus (HBV) immunization successful in elderly hemodialysis (HD) patients? *Clin Nephrol* 2002;58:301–304.

108. Buti M, Viladomiu L, Jardi R, et al. Long-term immunogenicity and efficacy of hepatitis B vaccine in hemodialysis patients. *Am J Nephrol* 1992;12:144–147.

109. Marangi AL, Giordano R, Montanaro A, et al. Hepatitis B virus infection in chronic uremia: long-term follow-up of a two-step integrated protocol of vaccination. *Am J Kidney Dis* 1994;23:537–542.

110. Waite NM, Thomson LG, Goldstein MB. Successful vaccination with intradermal hepatitis B vaccine in hemodialysis patients previously nonresponsive to intramuscular hepatitis B vaccine. *J Am Soc Nephrol* 1995;5:1930–1934.

111. Charest AF, McDougall J, Goldstein MB. A randomized comparison of intradermal and intramuscular vaccination against hepatitis B virus in incident chronic hemodialysis patients. *Am J Kidney Dis* 2000;36:976–982.

112. Anandh U, Thomas PP, Shastry JC, Jacob CK. A randomised controlled trial of intradermal hepatitis B vaccination and augmentation of response with erythropoietin. *J Assoc Physicians India* 2000;48:1061–1063.

113. Milkowski A, Wyrwicz G, Kubit P, Smolenski O. Comparison of anti-HBV vaccine efficacy given intradermally and intramuscularly in hemodialysis patients. *Przegl Lek* 2000; 57:628–634.

114. Ono K, Kashiwagi S. Complete seroconversion by low-dose intradermal injection of recombinant hepatitis B vaccine in hemodialysis patients. *Nephron* 1991;58:47–51.

115. Mettang T, Schenk U, Thomas S, et al. Low-dose intradermal versus intramuscular hepatitis B vaccination in patients with end-stage renal failure. A preliminary study. *Nephron* 1996;72:192–196.

116. Propst A, Lhotta K, Vogel W, Konig P. Reinforced intradermal hepatitis B vaccination in hemodialysis patients is superior in antibody response to intramuscular or subcutaneous vaccination. *Am J Kidney Dis* 1998;32:1041–1045.

117. Fabrizi F, Andrulli S, Bacchini G, et al. Intradermal versus intramuscular hepatitis B re-vaccination in non-responsive chronic dialysis patients: a prospective randomized study with cost-effectiveness evaluation. *Nephrol Dial Transplant* 1997;12:1204–1211.

118. Chang PC, Schrander-van der Meer AM, van Dorp WT, van Leer E. Intracutaneous versus intramuscular hepatitis B vaccination in primary non-responding haemodialysis patients. *Nephrol Dial Transplant* 1996;11:191–193.

119. Vlassopoulos DA, Arvanitis DK, Lilis DS, et al. Lower long-term efficiency of intradermal hepatitis B vaccine compared to the intramuscular route in hemodialysis patients. *Int J Artif Organs* 1999;22:739–743.

120. Rault R, Freed B, Nespor S, Bender F. Efficacy of different hepatitis B vaccination strategies in patients receiving hemodialysis. *ASAIO J* 1995;41:717–719.

121. Vlassopoulos D, Arvanitis D, Lilis D, et al. Complete success of intradermal vaccination against hepatitis B in advanced chronic renal failure and hemodialysis patients. *Renal Fail* 1997;19:455–460.

122. Kayatas M. Levamisole treatment enhances protective antibody response to hepatitis B vaccination in hemodialysis patients. *Artif Organs* 2002;26:492–496.

123. Deniz Ayli M, Ensari C, Ayli M, et al. Effect of oral levamisole supplementation to hepatitis B vaccination on the rate of immune response in chronic hemodialysis patients. *Nephron* 2000;84:291–292.

124. Quiroga JA, Castillo I, Porres JC, et al. Recombinant gamma-interferon as adjuvant to hepatitis B vaccine in hemodialysis patients. *Hepatology* 1990;12:661–663.

125. Ozener C, Fak AS, Avsar E, et al. The effect of alpha interferon therapy and short-interval intradermal administration on response to hepatitis B vaccine in haemodialysis patients. *Nephrol Dial Transplant* 1999;14:1339–1340.

126. Grob PJ, Joller-Jemelka HI, Binswanger U, et al. Interferon as an adjuvant for hepatitis B vaccination in non- and low-responder populations. *Eur J Clin Microbiol* 1984;3: 195–198.

127. Evans TG, Schiff M, Graves B, et al. The safety and efficacy of GM-CSF as an adjuvant in hepatitis B vaccination of chronic hemodialysis patients who have failed primary vaccination. *Clin Nephrol* 2000;54:138–142.

128. Kapoor D, Agarwal SR, Singh NP, et al. Granulocyte-macrophage colony-stimulating factor enhances the efficacy of hepatitis B virus vaccine in previously unvaccinated haemodialysis patients. *J Viral Hep.* 1999;6:405–409.

129. Anandh U, Bastani B, Ballal S. Granulocyte-macrophage colony-stimulating factor as an adjuvant to hepatitis B vaccination in maintenance hemodialysis patients. *Am J Nephrol* 2000; 20: 53–56.

130. Hess G, Kreiter F, Kosters W, Deusch K. The effect of granulocyte-macrophage colony-stimulating factor (GM-CSF) on hepatitis B vaccination in haemodialysis patients. *J Viral Hepat* 1996;3:149–153.

131. Ervo R, Faletti P, Magni S, Cavatorta F. Evaluation of treatments for the vaccination against hepatitis B + thymopentine. *Nephron* 1992;61:371–372.

132. Donati D, Gastaldi L. Controlled trial of thymopentin in hemodialysis patients who fail to respond to hepatitis B vaccination. *Nephron* 1988;50:133–136.

133. Grob PJ, Binswanger U, Blumberg A, et al. Thymopentin as adjuvant to hepatitis B vaccination. Results from three double-blind studies. *Surv Immunol Res* 1985;4:S107–S115.

134. Zaruba K, Grob PJ, Bolla K. Thymopentin as adjuvant therapy to hepatitis B vaccination in formerly non- or hyporesponding hemodialysis patients. *Surv Immunol Res* 1985;4: 102–106.

135. Palestini M, Messina A, Ciaraffo F, et al. Brief treatment with thymopentin as adjuvant in vaccination for hepatitis B: controlled study in patients on periodic hemodialysis. *Riv Eur Sci Med Farmacol* 1990;12:135–139.

136. Dumann H, Meuer SC, Renschin G, Kohler H. Influence of thymopentin on antibody response, and monocyte and T cell function in hemodialysis patients who fail to respond to hepatitis B vaccination. *Nephron* 1990;55:136–140.

137. Brodersen HP, Holtkamp W, Larbig D, et al. Zinc supplementation and hepatitis B vaccination in chronic haemodialysis patients: a multicentre study (letter). *Nephrol Dial Transplant* 1995;10:1780.

138. Rawer P, Willems WR, Breidenbach T, et al. Seroconversion rate, hepatitis B vaccination, hemodialysis, and zinc supplementation. *Kidney Int* 1987;22:S149–S152.

139. Jungers P, Devillier P, Salomon H, et al. Randomised placebo-controlled trial of recombinant interleukin-2 in chronic uraemic patients who are non-responders to hepatitis B vaccine. *Lancet* 1994;344:856–857.

140. Mauri MJ, Valles M, and the Collaborative Group of Girona. Effects of recombinant interleukin-2 and revaccination for hepatitis B in previously vaccinated, non-responder, chronic uraemic patients. *Nephrol Dial Transplant* 1997;12: 729–732.

141. Boland GJ, de Gast GC, van Hattum J. Effects of interleukin-2 on hepatitis B vaccination in uraemic patients (letter). *Lancet* 1994;344:1368.

142. Haubitz M, Ehlerding G, Beigel A, et al. Clinical experience with a new recombinant hepatitis-B vaccine in previous nonresponders with chronic renal insufficiency. *Clin Nephrol* 1996;45:180–182.

143. Dukes CS, Street AC, Starling JF, Hamilton JD. Hepatitis B vaccination and booster in predialysis patients: a 4-year analysis. *Vaccine* 1993;11:1229–1232.

144. DaRoza G, Loewen A, Djurdev O, et al. Stage of chronic kidney disease predicts seroconversion after hepatitis B immunization: earlier is better. *Am J Kidney Dis* 2002;42: 1184–1192.

145. Seaworth B, Drucker J, Starling J, et al. Hepatitis B vaccines in patients with chronic renal failure before dialysis. *J Infect Dis* 1988;157:332–337.

146. Agarwal SK, Irshad M, Dash SC. Comparison of two schedules of hepatitis B vaccination in patients with mild, moderate and severe renal failure. *J Assoc Physicians India* 1999; 47:183–185.

147. Jungers P, Chaveau P, Couroucè AM, et al. Hepatitis B vaccine in non-dialysed uraemic patients: preliminary results. *Proc EDTA-ERA* 1985;22:1073–1076.

148. Rangel MC, Coronado VG, Euler GL, Strikas RA. Vaccine recommendations for patients on chronic dialysis. The Advisory Committee on Immunization Practices and the American Academy of Pediatrics. *Semin Dial* 2000;13: 101–107.

149. Vazquez G, Mendoza-Guevara L, Alvarez T, et al. Comparison of the response to the recombinant vaccine against hepatitis B virus in dialyzed and nondialyzed children with CRF using different doses and routes of administration. *Adv Perit Dial* 1997;13:291–296.

150. Pillion G, Chiesa M, Maisin A, et al. Immunogenicity of hepatitis B vaccine (HEVAC B) in children with advanced renal failure. *Pediatr Nephrol* 1990;4:627–629.

151. Drachman R, Isacsohn M, Rudensky B, Drukker A. Vaccination against hepatitis B in children and adolescent patients on dialysis. *Nephrol Dial Transplant* 1989;4:372–374.

152. Watkins SL, Alexander SR, Brewer ED, et al for the Southwest Pediatric Nephrology Study Group. Response to recombinant hepatitis B vaccine in children and adolescents with chronic renal failure. *Am J Kidney Dis* 2002;40: 365–372.

153. La Manna A, Polito C, Foglia AC, et al. Normal response to anti-HBV vaccination in children with chronic renal insufficiency. *Child Nephrol Urol* 1991;11:203–205.

154. Callis LM, Clanxet J, Fortuny G, et al. Hepatitis B virus infection and vaccination in children undergoing hemodialysis. *Acta Paediatr* 1985;74:213–218.

155. Ly D, Yee HF Jr, Brezina M, et al. Hepatitis B surface antigenemia in chronic hemodialysis patients: effect of hepatitis B immunization. *Am J Gastroenterol* 2002;97:138–141.

156. Alter MJ, Favero MS, Francis DP. Cost benefit of vaccination for hepatitis B in hemodialysis centers. *J Infect Dis* 1983;148:770–771.

157. Oddone EZ, Cowper PA, Hamilton JD, Feussner JR. A cost-effectiveness analysis of hepatitis B vaccine in predialysis patients. *Health Serv Res* 1993;28:97–121.

158. Rodby RA, Trenholme GM. Vaccination of the dialysis patient. *Semin Dial* 1991;4:102–105.

159. Charest AF, Grand'Maison A, McDougall J, Goldstein MB. Evolution of naturally acquired hepatitis B immunity in the long-term hemodialysis population. *Am J Kidney Dis* 2003; 42:1193–1199.

160. Saab S, Weston SR, Ly D, et al. Comparison of the cost and effectiveness of two strategies for maintaining hepatitis B immunity in hemodialysis patients. *Vaccine* 2002;20: 3230–3235.

161. Fabrizi F, Lunghi G, Martin P. Epidemiology of hepatitis delta virus (HDV) infection in the dialysis population. *Int J Artif Organs* 2002;25:8–17.

162. Pol S, Dubois F, Mattlinger B, et al. Absence of hepatitis delta virus infection in chronic hemodialysis and kidney transplant patients in France. *Transplantation* 1992;54: 1096–1097.

163. Aghanashinikar PN, al-Dhahry SH, al-Marhuby HA, et al. Prevalence of hepatitis B, hepatitis delta, and human immunodeficiency virus infections in Omani patients with renal diseases. *Transplant Proc* 1992;24:1913–1914.

164. Thomas PP, Samuel BU, Jacob CK, et al. Low prevalence of hepatitis D (delta) virus infection in a nephrology unit in south India. *Trans R Soc Trop Med Hyg* 1991;85:652–653.

165. Ashraf SJ, Arya SC, Parande CM. Viral hepatitis markers in patients on haemodialysis in a hyperendemic area. *J Med Virol* 1986;19:41–46.

166. Lettau LA, Alfred HJ, Glew RH, et al. Nosocomial transmission of delta hepatitis. *Ann Intern Med* 1986;104:631–635.

167. Gmelin K, Roggendorf M, Schlipkoter U, et al. Delta infection in a hemodialyzed patient (letter). *J Infect Dis* 1985; 151:374.

168. Marinucci G, Valeri L, DiGiacomo C, Morganti D. Spread of delta infection in a group of haemodialysis carriers of HBsAg. In: Verme G, Bonino F, Rizzetto M, eds. *Viral Hepatitis and Delta Infection*. New York: Liss, 1983:151–154.

169. Choo QL, Kuo G, Weiner AJ, et al. Isolation of a cDNA clone derived from a blood-borne non-A, non-B viral hepatitis genome. *Science* 1989;244:359–362.

170. Alter MJ, Hadler SC, Judson FN, et al. Risk factors for acute non-A, non-B hepatitis in the United States and association with hepatitis C virus infection. *JAMA* 1990;264: 2231–2235.

171. Alter MJ, Margolis HS, Krawczynski K, et al. The natural history of community-acquired hepatitis C in the United States. The Sentinel Counties Chronic non-A, non-B Hepatitis Study Team. *N Engl J Med* 1992;327:1899–1905.

172. Simmonds P. Variability of hepatitis C virus. *Hepatology* 1995;21:570–583.

173. Simmonds P, Alberti A, Alter HJ, et al. A proposed system for the nomenclature of hepatitis C viral genotypes. *Hepatology* 1994;19:1321–1324.

174. Kuo G, Choo QL, Alter HJ, et al. An assay for circulating antibodies to a major etiologic virus of human non-A, non-B hepatitis. *Science* 1989;244:362–364.

175. Aach RD, Stevens CE, Hollinger FB, et al. Hepatitis C virus infection in post-transfusion hepatitis. An analysis with first- and second-generation assays. *N Engl J Med* 1991;325: 1325–1329.

176. Abdel-Hamid M, El-Daly M, El-Kafrawy S, et al. Comparison of second- and third-generation enzyme immunoassays for detecting antibodies to hepatitis C virus. *J Clin Microbiol* 2002;40:1656–1659.

177. Getzug T, Lindsay K, Brezina M, Gitnick G. Hepatitis C virus antibody in hemodialysis patients: prevalence and risk factors (letter). *Lancet* 1990;335:589.

178. Fabrizi F, Di Filippo S, Erba G, et al. Hepatitis C virus infection and hepatic function in chronic hemodialysis patients (letter). *Nephron* 1992;61:119.

179. Moroni GA, Cori P, Marelli F, et al. Indirect evidence for transfusion role in conditioning hepatitis C virus prevalence among dialysis patients (letter). *Nephron* 1991;57: 371–372.

180. Mazzoni A, Innocenti M, Consaga M. Retrospective study on the prevalence of B and non-A, non-B hepatitis in a dialysis unit: 17-year follow-up. *Nephron* 1992;61:316–317.

181. Gubertini G, Scorza D, Beccari M, et al. Prevalence of hepatitis C virus antibodies in hemodialysis patients in the area of Milan. *Nephron* 1992;61:271–272.

182. Pauri P, Salvoni G, Vitolo W, et al. Risk factors and clinical expression of HCV infection in hemodialysis patients. *Nephron* 1992;61:313–314.

183. Conway M, Catterall AP, Brown EA, et al. Prevalence of antibodies to hepatitis C in dialysis patients and transplant recipients with possible routes of transmission. *Nephrol Dial Transplant* 1992;7:1226–1269.

184. Ayoola EA, Huraib S, Arif M, et al. Prevalence and significance of antibodies to hepatitis C virus among Saudi haemodialysis patients. *J Med Virol* 1991;35:155–159.

185. Fujiyama S, Kawano S, Sato S, et al. The prevalence of anti-HCV antibodies in hemodialysis patients. *Gastroenterol Jpn* 1991;26:206–208.

186. Holzberger G, Seidl S, Peschke B, et al. The prevalence of anti-HCV in hemodialysis patients and blood donors in Germany. *Transplant Proc* 1991;23:2658–2659.

187. Jeffers LJ, Perez GO, de Medina MD, et al. Hepatitis C infection in two urban hemodialysis units. *Kidney Int* 1990;38: 320–322.

188. Esteban JI, Esteban R, Viladomiu L, et al. Hepatitis C virus antibodies among risk groups in Spain. *Lancet* 1989;2: 294–297.

189. Kallinowski B, Theilmann L, Gmelin K, et al. Prevalence of antibodies to hepatitis C virus in hemodialysis patients. *Nephron* 1991;59:236–238.

190. Elisaf M, Tsianos E, Mavridis A, et al. Antibodies against hepatitis C virus (anti-HCV) in haemodialysis patients: association with hepatitis B serological markers. *Nephrol Dial Transplant* 1991;6:476–479.

191. Almroth G, Ekermo B, Franzen L, Hed J. Antibody responses to hepatitis C virus and its modes of transmission in dialysis patients. *Nephron* 1991;59:232–235.

192. Mondelli MU, Smedile V, Piazza V, et al. Abnormal alanine aminotransferase activity reflects exposure to hepatitis C virus in haemodialysis patients. *Nephrol Dial Transplant* 1991;6:480–483.

193. Hayashi J, Nakashima K, Kajiyama W, et al. Prevalence of antibody to hepatitis C virus in hemodialysis patients. *Am J Epidemiol* 1991;134:651–617.

194. Huang CS, Ho MS, Yang CS, et al. Hepatitis C markers in hemodialysis patients. *J Clin Microbiol* 1993;31: 1764–1769.

195. Suliman SM, Fessaha S, El-Sadiq M, et al. Prevalence of hepatitis C virus infection in hemodialysis patients in Sudan. *Saudi Med J* 2003;24(suppl 2):S138.

196. Blackmore TK, Stace NH, Maddocks P, Hatfield P. Prevalence of antibodies to hepatitis C virus in patients receiving renal replacement therapy, and in the staff caring for them. *Aust N Z J Med* 1992;22:353–357.

197. Kazi S, Prasad S, Pollak R, et al. Hepatitis C infection in potential recipients with normal liver biochemistry does not preclude renal transplantation. *Dig Dis Sci* 1994;39: 961–964.

198. Vitale C, Tricerri A, Marangella M, et al. Epidemiology of hepatitis C virus infection in dialysis units: first-versus second-generation assays (letter). *Nephron* 1993;64:315–316.

199. Dussol B, Berthezene P, Brunet P, et al. Hepatitis C virus infection among chronic dialysis patients in the south of France: a collaborative study. *Am J Kidney Dis* 1995;25: 399–404.

200. Huraib S, al-Rashed R, Aldrees A, et al. High prevalence of and risk factors for hepatitis C in haemodialysis patients in Saudi Arabia: a need for new dialysis strategies. *Nephrol Dial Transplant* 1995;10:470–474.

201. Golan E, Korzets Z, Cristal-Lilov A, et al. Increased prevalence of HCV antibodies in dialyzed Ashkenazi Jews—a possible ethnic predisposition. *Nephrol Dial Transplant* 1996;11:684–686.

202. Ansar MM, Kooloobandi A. Prevalence of hepatitis C virus infection in thalassemia and haemodialysis patients in north Iran-Rasht. *J Viral Hepat* 2002;9:390–392.

203. Fabrizi F, Martin P, Dixit V, et al. Detection of de novo hepatitis C virus infection by polymerase chain reaction in hemodialysis patients. *Am J Nephrol* 1999;19:383–388.

204. Nakayama E, Liu JH, Akiba T, et al. Low prevalence of anti-hepatitis C virus antibodies in female hemodialysis patients without blood transfusion: a multicenter analysis. *J Med Virol* 1996;48:284–288.

205. Ruffatti A, Bortolotti F, Bianco A, et al. Hepatitis C virus infection in hemodialyzed patients detected by first and second generation assays. *Nephron* 1992;61:344–345.

206. Sakamoto N, Enomoto N, Marumo F, Sato C. Prevalence of hepatitis C virus infection among long-term hemodialysis patients: detection of hepatitis C virus RNA in plasma. *J Med Virol* 1993;39:11–15.

207. Beccari M, Sorgato G, Rizzolo L, Veneroni G. Anti-HCV reactivity in dialysis patients: discrepancies between first and second generation tests (letter). *Nephron* 1993;63:238.

208. Da Porto A, Poli P, Calzavara P, et al. Comparison between first- and second-generation test for anti-hepatitis C virus antibodies in hemodialysis patients. *Nephron* 1992;61: 367–368.

209. Fabrizi F, Raffaele L, Guarnori I, et al. Comparison of second-generation screening and confirmatory assays with recombinant antigens and synthetic peptides against antibodies to hepatitis C virus: a study in renal patients. *Nephron* 1995;69:444–448.

210. Chauveau P, Couroucè AM, Lemarec N, et al. Antibodies to hepatitis C virus by second generation test in hemodialyzed patients. *Kidney Int Suppl* 1993;41:S149–S152.

211. Oliva JA, Ercilla G, Mallafre JM, et al. Markers of hepatitis C infection among hemodialysis patients with acute and chronic infection: implications for infection control strategies in hemodialysis units. *Int J Artif Organs* 1995;18: 73–77.

212. Fabrizi F, Raffaele L, Bacchini G, et al. Antibodies to hepatitis C virus (HCV) and transaminase concentration in chronic haemodialysis patients: a study with second-generation assays. *Nephrol Dial Transplant* 1993;8:744–747.

213. Mondelli MU, Cristina G, Piazza V, et al. High prevalence of antibodies to hepatitis C virus in hemodialysis units using a second generation assay. *Nephron* 1992;61:350–351.

214. al Meshari K, Alfurayh O, Al Ahdal M, et al. Hepatitis C virus infection in hemodialysis patients: comparison of two new hepatitis C antibody assays with a second-generation assay. *J Am Soc Nephrol* 1995;6:1439–1444.

215. de Medina M, Ortiz C, Krenc C, et al. Improved detection of antibodies to hepatitis C virus in dialysis patients using a second-generation enzyme immunoassay. *Am J Kidney Dis* 1992;20:589–591.

216. Pol S, Nousbaum JB, Legendre P, et al. The changing relative prevalence of hepatitis C virus genotypes: evidence in hemodialyzed patients and kidney recipients. *Gastroenterology* 1995;108:581–583.

217. Fujiyama S, Kawano S, Sato S, et al. Changes in prevalence of anti-HCV antibodies associated with preventive measures among hemodialysis patients and dialysis staff. *Hepatogastroenterology* 1995;42:162–165.

218. Dai CY, Yu ML, Chuang WL, et al. Epidemiology and clinical significance of chronic hepatitis-related viruses infection in hemodialysis patients from Taiwan. *Nephron* 2002;90: 148–153.

219. Kolho E, Oksanen K, Honkanen E, et al. Hepatitis C antibodies in dialysis patients and patients with leukaemia. *J Med Virol* 1993;40:318–321.

220. Chan TM, Lok AS, Cheng IK, Chan RT. Prevalence of hepatitis C virus infection in hemodialysis patients: a longitudinal study comparing the results of RNA and antibody assays. *Hepatology* 1993;17:5–8.

221. Dentico P, Volpe A, Buongiorno R, et al. Detection of antibodies to HCV in haemodialysis patients using two second generation ELISA tests. *Ital J Gastroenterol* 1993;25:19–22.

222. El-Shahat YI, Varma S, Bari MZ, et al. Hepatitis C virus infection among dialysis patients in the United Arab Emirates (letter). *Saudi Med J* 2003;24:S134.

223. Fabrizi F, Lunghi G, Raffaele L, et al. Serologic survey for control of hepatitis C in haemodialysis patients: third-generation assays and analysis of costs. *Nephrol Dial Transplant* 1997;12:298–303.

224. Dentico P, Volpe A, Buongiorno R, et al. HCV third generation test in hemodialysis patients. *Ital J Gastroenterol* 1995;27:300–302.

225. Courouce AM, Bouchardeau F, Chauveau P, et al. Hepatitis C virus (HCV) infection in haemodialysed patients: HCV-RNA and anti-HCV antibodies (third-generation assays). *Nephrol Dial Transplant* 1995;10:234–239.

226. Garinis G, Spanakis N, Theodorou V, et al. Comparison of the enzyme-linked immunosorbant assay III, recombinant immunoblot third generation assay, and polymerase chain reaction method in the detection of hepatitis C virus infection in haemodialysis patients. *J Clin Lab Anal* 1999;13:122–125.

227. Courouce AM, Le Marrec N, Girault A, et al. Anti-hepatitis C virus (anti-HCV) seroconversion in patients undergoing hemodialysis: comparison of second- and third-generation anti-HCV assays. *Transfusion* 1994;34:790–795.

228. Othman B, Monem F. Prevalence of antibodies to hepatitis C virus among hemodialysis patients in Damascus, Syria. *Infection* 2001;29:262–265.

229. al Meshari K, al Ahdal M, Alfurayh O, et al. New insights into hepatitis C virus infection of hemodialysis patients: the implications. *Am J Kidney Dis* 1995;25:572–578.

230. Bosmans JL, Nouwen EJ, Behets G, et al. Prevalence and clinical expression of HCV genotypes in haemodialysis patients of two geographically remote countries: Belgium and Saudi Arabia. *Clin Nephrol* 1997;47:256–262.

231. Weinstein T, Tur-Kaspa R, Chagnac A, et al. Hepatitis C infection in dialysis patients in Israel. *Isr Med Assoc J* 2001;3:174–177.

232. Castelnovo C, Lunghi G, De Vecchi A, et al. Comparison of three different tests for assessment of hepatitis C virus in dialysis patients. *Perit Dial Int* 1995;15:241–245.

233. Hinrichsen H, Leimenstoll G, Stegen G, et al and the PHV Study Group. Prevalence and risk factors of hepatitis C virus infection in haemodialysis patients: a multicentre study in 2796 patients. *Gut* 2002;51:429–433.

234. Fabrizi F, Martin P, Dixit V, et al. Quantitative assessment of HCV load in chronic hemodialysis patients: a cross-sectional survey. *Nephron* 1998;80:428–433.

235. Hanuka N, Sikuler E, Tovbin D, et al. Hepatitis C virus infection in renal failure patients in the absence of anti-hepatitis C virus antibodies. *J Viral Hep.* 2002;9:141–145.

236. Schneeberger PM, Keur I, van Loon AM, et al. The prevalence and incidence of hepatitis C virus infections among dialysis patients in the Netherlands: a nationwide prospective study. *J Infect Dis* 2000;182:1291–1299.

237. Dalekos GN, Boumba DS, Katopodis K, et al. Absence of HCV viraemia in anti-HCV-negative haemodialysis patients. *Nephrol Dial Transplant* 1998;13:1804–1806.

238. Bukh J, Wantzin P, Krogsgaard K, et al. High prevalence of hepatitis C virus (HCV) RNA in dialysis patients: failure of commercially available antibody tests to identify a significant number of patients with HCV infection. Copenhagen Dialysis HCV Study Group. *J Infect Dis* 1993;168:1343–1348.

239. Tokars JI, Frank M, Alter MJ. National surveillance of dialysis-associated diseases in the United States, 2000. *Semin Dial* 2002;15:162–171.

240. Centers for Disease Control. Recommendations for preventing transmission of infections among chronic hemodialysis patients. *MMWR* 2001;50(RR-5):1–50.

241. Mizuno M, Higuchi T, Kanmatsuse K, Esumi M. Genetic and serological evidence for multiple instances of unrecognized transmission of hepatitis C virus in hemodialysis units. *J Clin Microbiol* 1998;36:2926–2931.

242. Stuyver L, Claeys H, Wyseur A, et al. Hepatitis C virus in a hemodialysis unit: molecular evidence for nosocomial transmission. *Kidney Int* 1996;49:889–895.

243. Katsoulidou A, Paraskevis D, Kalapothaki V, et al. Molecular epidemiology of a hepatitis C virus outbreak in a haemodialysis unit. Multicentre Haemodialysis Cohort Study on Viral Hepatitis. *Nephrol Dial Transplant* 1999;14:1188–1194.

244. Izopet J, Pasquier C, Sandres K, et al. Molecular evidence for nosocomial transmission of hepatitis C virus in a French hemodialysis unit. *J Med Virol* 1999;58:139–144.

245. Allander T, Medin C, Jacobson SH, et al. Hepatitis C transmission in a hemodialysis unit: molecular evidence for spread of virus among patients not sharing equipment. *J Med Virol* 1994;43:415–419.

246. de Lamballerie X, Olmer M, Bouchouareb D, et al. Nosocomial transmission of hepatitis C virus in haemodialysis patients. *J Med Virol* 1996;49:296–302.

247. Grethe S, Gemsa F, Monazahian M, et al. Molecular epidemiology of an outbreak of HCV in a hemodialysis unit: direct sequencing of HCV-HVR1 as an appropriate tool for phylogenetic analysis. *J Med Virol* 2000;60:152–158.

248. Norder H, Bergstrom A, Uhnoo I, et al. Confirmation of nosocomial transmission of hepatitis C virus by phylogenetic analysis of the NS5-B region. *J Clin Microbiol* 1998;36:3066–3069.

249. Le Pogam S, Le Chapois D, Christen R, et al. Hepatitis C in a hemodialysis unit: molecular evidence for nosocomial transmission. *J Clin Microbiol* 1998;36:3040–3043.

250. McLaughlin KJ, Cameron SO, Good T, et al. Nosocomial transmission of hepatitis C virus within a British dialysis centre. *Nephrol Dial Transplant* 1997;12:304–309.

251. Seme K, Poljak M, Zuzec-Resek S, et al. Molecular evidence for nosocomial spread of two different hepatitis C virus strains in one hemodialysis unit. *Nephron* 1997;77:273–278.

252. Olmer M, Bouchouareb D, Zandotti C, et al. Transmission of the hepatitis C virus in an hemodialysis unit: evidence for nosocomial infection. *Clin Nephrol* 1997;47:263–270.

253. Pujol FH, Ponce JG, Lema MG, et al. High incidence of hepatitis C virus infection in hemodialysis patients in units with high prevalence. *J Clin Microbiol* 1996;34:1633–1636.

254. Petrosillo N, Gilli P, Serraino D, et al. Prevalence of infected patients and understaffing have a role in hepatitis C virus transmission in dialysis. *Am J Kidney Dis* 2001;37:1004–1010.

255. Hardy NM, Sandroni S, Danielson S, Wilson WJ. Antibody to hepatitis C virus increases with time on hemodialysis. *Clin Nephrol* 1992;38:44–48.

256. Schlipkoter U, Oter U, Roggendorf M, et al. Hepatitis C virus antibodies in hemodialysis patients (letter). *Lancet* 1990;335:1409.

257. Schlipkoter U, Gladziwa U, Cholmakov K, et al. Prevalence of hepatitis C virus infections in dialysis patients and their contacts using a second generation enzymed-linked immunosorbent assay. *Med Microbiol Immunol (Berl)* 1992;181:173–180.

258. Chan TM, Lok AS, Cheng IK. Hepatitis C infection among dialysis patients: a comparison between patients on maintenance haemodialysis and continuous ambulatory peritoneal dialysis. *Nephrol Dial Transplant* 1991;6:944–947.

259. Gilli P, Moretti M, Soffritti S, et al. Non-A, non-B hepatitis and anti-HCV antibodies in dialysis patients. *Int J Artif Organs* 1990;13:737–741.

260. Fabrizi F, Lunghi G, Guarnori I, et al. Hepatitis C virus genotypes in chronic dialysis patients. *Nephrol Dial Transplant* 1996;11:679–683.

261. Sampietro M, Badalamenti S, Salvadori S, et al. High prevalence of a rare hepatitis C virus in patients treated in the same hemodialysis unit: evidence for nosocomial transmission of HCV. *Kidney Int* 1995;47:911–917.

262. Lombardi M, Cerrai T, Geatti S, et al. Results of a national epidemiological investigation on HCV infection among dialysis patients. *J Nephrol* 1999;12:322–327.

263. Saab S, Martin P, Brezina M, et al. Serum alanine aminotransferase in hepatitis C screening of patients on hemodialysis. *Am J Kidney Dis* 2001;37:308–315.

264. Salama G, Rostaing L, Sandres K, Izopet J. Hepatitis C virus infection in French hemodialysis units: a multicenter study. *J Med Virol* 2000;61:44–51.

265. Delarocque-Astagneau E, Baffoy N, Thiers V, et al. Outbreak of hepatitis C virus infection in a hemodialysis unit: potential transmission by the hemodialysis machine? *Infect Control Hosp Epidemiol* 2002;23:328–334.

266. Sivapalasingam S, Malak SF, Sullivan JF, et al. High prevalence of hepatitis C infection among patients receiving hemodialysis at an urban dialysis center. *Infect Control Hosp Epidemiol* 2002;23:319–324.

267. Cristina G, Piazza V, Efficace E, et al. A survey of hepatitis C virus infection in haemodialysis patients over a 7-year follow-up. *Nephrol Dial Transplant* 1997;12:2208–2210.

268. Froio N, Nicastri E, Comandini UV, et al. Contamination by hepatitis B and C viruses in the dialysis setting. *Am J Kidney Dis* 2003;42:546–550.

269. Djordjevic V, Stojanovic K, Stojanovic M, Stefanovic V. Prevention of nosocomial transmission of hepatitis C infection in a hemodialysis unit. A prospective study. *Int J Artif Organs* 2000;23:181–188.

270. Shaheen FA, Huraib SO, Al-Rashed R, et al. Prevalence of hepatitis C antibodies among hemodialysis patients in Jeddah area, Saudi Arabia. *Saudi Med J* 2003;2:S125–S126.

271. Broumand B, Shamshirsaz AA, Kamgar M, et al. Prevalence of hepatitis C infection and its risk factors in hemodialysis patients in Tehran: preliminary report from the 'effect of dialysis unit isolation on the incidence of hepatitis C in dialysis patients' project. *Saudi J Kidney Dis Transplant* 2002;13:467–472.

272. Kashem A, Nusarait N, Mohamad M, et al. Hepatitis C virus among hemodialysis patients in Najran: prevalence is more among multi-center visitors. *Saudi J Kidney Dis Transplant* 2002;14:206–211.

273. Al-Shohaib SS, Abd-Elaal MA, Zawawi TH, et al. The prevalence of hepatitis C virus antibodies among hemodialysis patients in Jeddah area, Saudi Arabia. *Saudi Med J* 2003;24:S125–S126.

274. Hassan AA, Khalil R. Hepatitis C in dialysis patients in Egypt: relationship to dialysis duration, blood transfusion, and liver disease. *Saudi J Kidney Dis Transplant* 2000;11:72–75.

275. Jaiswal SP, Chitnis DS, Salgia P, et al. Prevalence of hepatitis viruses among chronic renal failure patients on hemodialysis in Central India. *Dial Transplant* 2002;12:14–20.

276. Taskapan H, Oymak O, Dogukan A, Utas C. Patient to patient transmission of hepatitis C virus in hemodialysis units. *Clin Nephrol* 2001;55:477–481.

277. Todorov V, Boneva R, Ilieva P, et al. High prevalence of hepatitis C virus infection in Bulgaria (letter). *Nephron* 1998;79:222–223.

278. Souqiyyeh MZ, Shaheen FA, Huraib SO, Al-Khader AA. The annual incidence of seroconversion of antibodies to the hepatitis C virus in the hemodialysis population in Saudi Arabia. *Saudi Med J* 2003;24:S122–S123.

279. Valtuille R, Moretto H, Lef L, et al. Decline of high hepatitis C virus prevalence in a hemodialysis unit with no isolation measures during a 6-year follow-up. *Clin Nephrol* 2002;57:371–375.

280. Souza KP, Luz JA, Teles SA, et al. Hepatitis B and C in the hemodialysis unit of Tocantins, Brazil: serological and molecular profiles. *Mem Inst Oswaldo Cruz* 2003;98:599–603.

281. Valtuille R, Frankel F, Gomez F, et al. The role of transfusion-transmitted virus in patients undergoing hemodialysis. *J Clin Gastroenterol* 2002;34:86–88.

282. Souqiyyeh MZ, Shaheen FA, Huraib SO, Al-Khader AA. The annual incidence of seroconversion of antibodies to the hepatitis C virus in the hemodialysis population in Saudi Arabia. *Saudi Med J* 2003;24:S122–S123.

283. Prevalence of hepatitis C virus in dialysis patients in Spain. Spanish Multicentre Study Group. *Nephrol Dial Transplant* 1995;10:78–80.

284. Ng YY, Lee SD, Wu SC, et al. The need for second-generation antihepatitis C virus testing in uremic patients on continuous ambulatory peritoneal dialysis. *Perit Dial Int* 1993;13:132–135.

285. Sayiner AA, Zeytinoglu A, Ozkahya M, et al. HCV infection in haemodialysis and CAPD patients. *Nephrol Dial Transplant* 1999;14:256–257.

286. Krautzig S, Tillmann H, Wrenger E, et al. Hepatitis-C virus (HCV) in peritoneal dialysis (letter). *Clin Nephrol* 1994;41: 120.

287. Gladziwa U, Schlipkoter U, Lorbeer B, et al. Prevalence of antibodies to hepatitis C virus in patients on peritoneal dialysis—a multicenter study. *Clin Nephrol* 1993;40:46–52.

288. Huang CC, Wu MS, Lin DY, Liaw YF. The prevalence of hepatitis C virus antibodies in patients treated with continuous ambulatory peritoneal dialysis. *Perit Dial Int* 1992;12: 31–33.

289. Selgas R, Martinez-Zapico R, Bajo MA, et al. Prevalence of hepatitis C antibodies (HCV) in a dialysis population at one center. *Perit Dial Int* 1992;12:28–30.

290. Hung KY, Shyu RS, Huang CH, et al. Viral hepatitis in continuous ambulatory peritoneal dialysis patients in an endemic area for hepatitis B and C infection: the Taiwan experience. *Blood Purif* 1997;15:195–199.

291. Gorriz JL, Miguel A, Garcia-Ramon R, Perez-Contreras J, et al. Prevalence and risk factors for hepatitis C virus infection in continuous ambulatory peritoneal dialysis patients. *Nephrol Dial Transplant* 1996;11:1109–1112.

292. Lee GS, Roy DK, Fan FY, et al. Hepatitis C antibodies in patients on peritoneal dialysis: prevalence and risk factors. *Perit Dial Int* 1996;16:S424–S428.

293. Durand PY, Chanliau J, Gamberoni J, et al. Prevalence and epidemiology of hepatitis C infection in patients on peritoneal dialysis in France. French PD centers. *Adv Perit Dial* 1996;12:167–170.

294. Akpolat T, Turkish Multicentre CAPD Study Group (TULIP). CAPD: a control strategy to prevent spread of HCV infection in end-stage renal disease. *Perit Dial Int* 2001;21:77–79.

295. Lee HY, Kang DH, Park CS, et al. Comparative study of hepatitis C virus antibody between hemodialysis and continuous ambulatory peritoneal dialysis patients. *Yonsei Med J* 1993;34:371–380.

296. Perez-Fontan M, Moncalian J, Rodriguez-Carmona A, Arrojo F. Prevalence of antihepatitis C antibodies in patients treated with continuous ambulatory peritoneal dialysis and hemodialysis. *Nephron* 1991;58:381–382.

297. Castelnovo C, Sampietro M, De Vecchi A, et al. Diffusion of HCV through peritoneal membrane in HCV positive patients treated with continuous ambulatory peritoneal dialysis. *Nephrol Dial Transplant* 1997;12:978–980.

298. al-Mugeiren M, al-Rasheed S, al-Salloum A, et al. Hepatitis C virus infection in two groups of paediatric patients: one maintained on haemodialysis and the other on continuous ambulatory peritoneal dialysis. *Ann Trop Paediatr* 1996;16: 335–339.

299. Vanderborght BO, Rouzere C, Ginuino CF, et al. High prevalence of hepatitis C infection among Brazilian hemodialysis patients in Rio de Janeiro: a one-year follow-up study. *Rev Inst Med Trop Sao Paulo* 1995;37:75–79.

300. Cariani E, Zonaro A, Primi D, et al. Detection of HCV RNA and antibodies to HCV after needlestick injury (letter). *Lancet* 1991;337:850.

301. Okuda K, Hayashi H, Kobayashi S, Irie Y. Mode of hepatitis C infection not associated with blood transfusion among chronic hemodialysis patients. *J Hepatol* 1995;23:28–31.

302. Arenas Jimenez MD, Sanchez-Paya J, et al. Audit on the degree of application of universal precautions in a haemodialysis unit. *Nephrol Dial Transplant* 1999;14:1001–1003.

303. Arenas Jimenez MD, Sanchez-Paya J. Standard precautions in haemodialysis—the gap between theory and practice (letter). *Nephrol Dial Transplant* 1999;14:823–825.

304. Simon N, Couroucè AM, Lemarrec N, et al. A twelve year natural history of hepatitis C virus infection in hemodialyzed patients. *Kidney Int* 1994;46:504–511.

305. Chiaramonte S, Tagger A, Ribero ML, et al. Prevention of viral hepatitis in dialysis units: isolation and technical management of dialysis. *Nephron* 1992;61:287–289.

306. Niu MT, Alter MJ, Kristensen C, Margolis HS. Outbreak of hemodialysis-associated non-A, non-B hepatitis and correlation with antibody to hepatitis C virus. *Am J Kidney Dis* 1992;19:345–352.

307. Hung KY, Chen WY, Yang CS, et al. Hepatitis B and C in hemodialysis patients. *Dial Transplant* 1995;24:135–139.

308. Jadoul M, Cornu C, van Ypersele de Strihou C. Incidence and risk factors for hepatitis C seroconversion in hemodialysis: a prospective study. The UCL Collaborative Group. *Kidney Int* 1993;44:1322–1326.

309. dos Santos JP, Loureiro A, Cendoroglo et al. Impact of dialysis room and reuse strategies on the incidence of hepatitis C virus infection in haemodialysis units. *Nephrol Dial Transplant* 1996;11:2017–2022.

310. Aucella F, Vigilante M, Valente GL, Stallone C. Systematic monitor disinfection is effective in limiting HCV spread in hemodialysis. *Blood Purif* 2000;18:110–114.

311. Jadoul M, Cornu C, van Ypersele de Strihou C. The Universitaires Cliniques St-Luc (UCL) Collaborative Group. Universal precautions prevent hepatitis C virus transmission: a 54 month follow-up of the Belgian Multicenter Study. *Kidney Int* 1998;53:1022–1025.

312. Gilli P, Soffritti S, De Paoli Vitali E, Bedani PL. Prevention of hepatitis C virus in dialysis units. *Nephron* 1995;70: 301–306.

313. Seeff LB. Natural history of chronic hepatitis C. *Hepatology* 2002;36(suppl 1):S35–S46.

314. Espinosa M, Martin-Malo A, Alvarez de Lara MA, et al. Natural history of acute HCV infection in hemodialysis patients. *Clin Nephrol* 2002;58:143–150.

315. Ghany MG, Kleiner DE, Alter H, et al. Progression of fibrosis in chronic hepatitis C. *Gastroenterology* 2003;124: 97–104.

316. Martin P, Carter D, Fabrizi F, et al. Histopathological features of hepatitis C in renal transplant candidates. *Transplantation* 2000;69:1479–1484.

317. Caramelo C, Ortiz A, Aguilera B, et al. Liver disease patterns in hemodialysis patients with antibodies to hepatitis C virus. *Am J Kidney Dis* 1993;22:822–828.

318. Pol S, Romeo R, Zins B, et al. Hepatitis C virus RNA in anti-HCV positive hemodialyzed patients: significance and therapeutic implications. *Kidney Int* 1993;44: 1097–1100.

319. Glicklich D, Thung SN, Kapoian T, et al. Comparison of clinical features and liver histology in hepatitis C-positive dialysis patients and renal transplant recipients. *Am J Gastroenterol* 1999;94:159–163.

320. Toz H, Ok E, Yilmaz F, et al. Clinicopathological features of hepatitis C virus infection in dialysis and renal transplantation. *J Nephrol* 2002;15:308–312.

321. Alfurayh O, Sobh M, Buali AR, et al. Hepatitis C virus infection in chronic haemodialysis patients, a clinicopathological study. *Nephrol Dial Transplant* 1992;7:327–332.

322. Al-Wakeel J, Malik GH, Al-Mohaya S, et al. Liver disease in dialysis patients with antibodies to hepatitis C virus. *Nephrol Dial Transplant* 1996;11:2265–2268.

323. Cotler SJ, Diaz G, Gundlapalli S, et al. Characteristics of hepatitis C in renal transplant candidates. *J Clin Gastroenterol* 2002;35:191–195.

324. Sterling RK, Sanyal AJ, Luketic VA, et al. Chronic hepatitis C infection in patients with end stage renal disease: characterization of liver histology and viral load in patients awaiting renal transplantation. *Am J Gastroenterol* 1999;94:3576–3582.

325. Ghacha R, Sinha AK, Karkar AM. A clinical and histological study in HCV-reactive hemodialysis patients as a pre-transplant workup. *Dial Transplant* 2001;30:15–18.

326. Ozdogan M, Ozgur O, Gur G, et al. Histopathological impacts of hepatitis virus infection in hemodialysis patients: should liver biopsy be performed before renal transplantation? *Artif Organs* 1997;21:355–358.

327. Fabrizi F, Martin P, Dixit V, et al. Acquisition of hepatitis C virus in hemodialysis patients: a prospective study by branched DNA signal amplification assay. *Am J Kidney Dis* 1998;31:647–654.

328. Fabrizi F, Martin P, Dixit V, et al. Biological dynamics of viral load in hemodialysis patients with hepatitis C virus. *Am J Kidney Dis* 2000;35:122–129.

329. Fabrizi F, Bunnapradist S, Lunghi G, Martin P. Kinetics of hepatitis C virus load during hemodialysis: novel perspectives. *J Nephrol* 2003;16:467–475.

330. Furusyo N, Hayashi J, Ariyama I, et al. Maintenance hemodialysis decreases serum hepatitis C virus (HCV) RNA levels in hemodialysis patients with chronic HCV infection. *Am J Gastroenterol* 2000;95:490–496.

331. Sampietro M, Graziani G, Badalamenti S, et al. Detection of hepatitis C virus in dialysate and in blood ultrafiltrate of HCV-positive patients (letter). *Nephron* 1994;68:140.

332. Valtuille R, Fernandez JL, Berridi J, et al. Evidence of hepatitis C virus passage across dialysis membrane. *Nephron* 1998;80:194–196.

333. Lombardi M, Cerrai T, Dattolo P, et al. Is the dialysis membrane a safe barrier against HCV infection? *Nephrol Dial Transplant* 1995;10:578–579.

334. Mizuno M, Higuchi T, Yanai M, et al. Dialysis-membrane-dependent reduction and adsorption of circulating hepatitis C virus during hemodialysis. *Nephron* 2002;91:235–242.

335. Hayashi H, Okuda K, Yokosuka O, et al. Adsorption of hepatitis C virus particles onto the dialyzer membrane. *Artif Organs* 1997;21:1056–1059.

336. Okuda K, Hayashi H, Yokozeki K, Irie Y. Destruction of hepatitis C virus particles by haemodialysis (letter). *Lancet* 1996;347:909–910.

337. Noiri E, Nakao A, Oya A, et al. Hepatitis C virus in blood and dialysate in hemodialysis. *Am J Kidney Dis* 2001;37:38–42.

338. Angelico M, Morosetti M, Passalacqua S, et al. Low levels of hepatitis C virus RNA in blood of infected patients under maintenance haemodialysis with high-biocompatibility, high-permeability filters. *Dig Liver Dis* 2000;32:724–728.

339. Caramelo C, Navas S, Alberola ML, et al. Evidence against transmission of hepatitis C virus through hemodialysis ultrafiltrate and peritoneal fluid. *Nephron* 1994;66:470–473.

340. Hubmann R, Zazgornik J, Gabriel C, et al. Hepatitis C virus—does it penetrate the haemodialysis membrane? PCR analysis of haemodialysis ultrafiltrate and whole blood. *Nephrol Dial Transplant* 1995;10:541–542.

341. Lindsay KL, El-Shahawy M, Milstein S, et al. HCV RNA levels are lowered during hemodialysis in patients with chronic hepatitis. *Hepatology* 1994;20:239A.

342. Adorati M, Pipan C, Botta G. Membrane compatibility and clearance of hepatitis C virus in chronic dialysis patients (letter). *Nephron* 1999;82:358.

343. Rampino T, Arbustini E, Gregorini M, et al. Hemodialysis prevents liver disease caused by hepatitis C virus: role of hepatocyte growth factor. *Kidney Int* 1999;56:2286–2291.

344. Badalamenti S, Catania A, Lunghi G, et al. Changes in viremia and circulating interferon-alpha during hemodialysis in hepatitis C virus-positive patients: only coincidental phenomena? *Am J Kidney Dis* 2003;42:143–150.

345. Rostaing L, Chatelut E, Payen JL, et al. Pharmacokinetics of alpha IFN-2b in chronic hepatitis C virus patients undergoing chronic hemodialysis or with normal renal function: clinical implications. *J Am Soc Nephrol* 1998;9:2344–2348.

346. Nakayama E, Akiba T, Marumo F, Sato C. Prognosis of anti-hepatitis C virus antibody-positive patients on regular hemodialysis therapy. *J Am Soc Nephrol* 2000;11:1896–1902.

347. Stehman-Breen CO, Emerson S, Gretch D, Johson RJ. Risk of death among chronic dialysis patients infected with hepatitis C virus. *Am J Kidney Dis* 1998;32:629–634.

348. Pereira BJG, Natov SN, Bouthot BA, et al and The New England Organ Bank Hepatitis C Study Group. Effect of hepatitis C infection and renal transplantation in end-stage renal disease. *Kidney Int* 1998;53:1374–1381.

349. Espinosa M, Martin-Malo A, Alvarez de Lara MA, Aljama P. Risk of death and liver cirrhosis in anti-HCV positive long-term haemodialysis patients. *Nephrol Dial Transplant* 2001;16:1669–1674.

350. No authors listed. The current state of chronic dialysis treatment in Japan (as of December 31, 2000). *Ther Apher Dial* 2003;7:3–35.

351. Ishida H, Agishi T, Koyama I, et al. Hemodialysis paradox: survey on the incidence rate of hepatocellular carcinoma in antihepatitis virus C-antibody-positive chronic hemodialysis patients. *Artif Organs* 2001;25:58–60.

352. Espinosa M, Martin-Malo A, Alvarez de Lara MA, et al. High ALT levels predict viremia in anti-HCV-positive HD patients if a modified normal range of ALT is applied. *Clin Nephrol* 2000;54:151–156.

353. Meyers CM, Seeff LB, Stehman-Breen CO, Hoofnagle JH. Hepatitis C and renal disease: an update. *Am J Kidney Dis* 2003;42:631–657.

354. Pol S, Carnot F, Nalpas B, et al. Reversibility of hepatitis C virus-related cirrhosis. *Hum Pathol* 2004;35:107–112.

355. Ozyilkan E, Simsek H, Uzunalimoglu B, Telatar H. Interferon treatment of chronic active hepatitis C in patients with end-stage chronic renal failure. *Nephron* 1995;71:156–159.

356. Pol S, Thiers V, Carnot F, et al. Efficacy and tolerance of alpha-2b interferon therapy on HCV infection of hemodialyzed patients. *Kidney Int* 1995;47:1412–1418.

357. Ellis ME, Alfurayh O, Halim MA, et al. Chronic non-A, non-B hepatitis complicated by end-stage renal failure treated with recombinant interferon alpha. *J Hepatol* 1993; 18:210–216.

358. Casanovas-Taltavull T, Baliellas C, Benasco C, et al. Efficacy of interferon for chronic hepatitis C virus-related hepatitis in kidney transplant candidates on hemodialysis: results after transplantation. *Am J Gastroenterol* 2001;96: 1170–1177.

359. Campistol JM, Esforzado N, Martinez J, et al. Efficacy and tolerance of interferon-alpha(2b) in the treatment of chronic hepatitis C virus infection in haemodialysis patients. Pre- and post-renal transplantation assessment. *Nephrol Dial Transplant* 1999;14:2704–2709.

360. Espinosa M, Rodriguez M, Martin-Malo A, et al. Interferon therapy in hemodialysis patients with chronic hepatitis C virus infection induces a high rate of long-term sustained virological and biochemical response. *Clin Nephrol* 2001;55: 220–226.

361. Benci A, Caremani M, Menchetti D, et al. Low-dose leukocyte interferon-alpha therapy in dialysed patients with chronic hepatitis C. *Curr Med Res Opin* 1998;14:141–144.

362. Hanrotel C, Toupance O, Lavaud S, et al. Virological and histological responses to one year alpha-interferon-2a in hemodialyzed patients with chronic hepatitis C. *Nephron* 2001;88:120–126.

363. Degos F, Pol S, Chaix ML, et al. The tolerance and efficacy of interferon-alpha in haemodialysis patients with HCV infection: a multicentre, prospective study. *Nephrol Dial Transplant* 2001;16:1017–1023.

364. Huraib S, Tanimu D, Romeh SA, et al. Interferon-alpha in chronic hepatitis C infection in dialysis patients. *Am J Kidney Dis* 1999;34:55–60.

365. Huraib S, Iqbal A, Tanimu D, Abdullah A. Sustained virological and histological response with pretransplant interferon therapy in renal transplant patients with chronic viral hepatitis C. *Am J Nephrol* 2001;21:435–440.

366. Raptopoulou-Gigi M, Spaia S, Garifallos A, et al. Interferon-alpha 2b treatment of chronic hepatitis C in haemodialysis patients. *Nephrol Dial Transplant* 1995;10: 1834–1837.

367. Koenig P, Vogel W, Umlauft F, et al. Interferon treatment for chronic hepatitis C virus infection in uremic patients. *Kidney Int* 1994;45:1507–1509.

368. Fernandez JL, Rendo P, del Pino N, Viola L. A double-blind controlled trial of recombinant interferon-alpha 2b in haemodialysis patients with chronic hepatitis C virus infection and abnormal aminotransferase levels. Nephrologists' Group for the Study of HCV infection. *J Viral Hepat* 1997;4:113–119.

369. Uchihara M, Izumi N, Sakai Y, et al. Interferon therapy for chronic hepatitis C in hemodialysis patients: increased serum levels of interferon. *Nephron* 1998;80:51–56.

370. Okuda K, Hayashi H, Yokozeki K, et al. Interferon treatment for chronic hepatitis C in haemodialysis patients: suggestions based on a small series. *J Gastroenterol Hepatol* 1995;10:616–620.

371. Chan TM, Wu PC, Lau JY, et al. Interferon treatment for hepatitis C virus infection in patients on haemodialysis. *Nephrol Dial Transplant* 1997;12:1414–1419.

372. Izopet J, Rostaing L, Moussion F, et al. High rate of hepatitis C virus clearance in hemodialysis patients after interferon-alpha therapy. *J Infect Dis* 1997;176:1614–1617.

373. Tokumoto T, Tanabe K, Ishikawa N, et al. Effect of interferon-alpha treatment in hemodialysis patients and renal transplant recipients with chronic hepatitis C. *Transplant Proc* 1999;31:2887–2889.

374. Russo MW, Goldsweig CD, Jacobson IM, Brown RS. Interferon monotherapy for dialysis patients with chronic hepatitis C: an analysis of the literature on efficacy and safety. *Am J Gastroenterol* 2003;98:1610–1615.

375. Fabrizi F, Dulai G, Dixit V, et al. Meta-analysis: interferon for the treatment of chronic hepatitis C in dialysis patients. *Aliment Pharmacol Ther* 2003;18:1071–1081.

376. Thevenot T, Regimbeau C, Ratziu V, et al. Meta-analysis of interferon randomized trials in the treatment of viral hepatitis C in naive patients: 1999 update. *J Viral Hepat* 2001;8: 48–62.

377. McHutchison JG, Gordon SC, Schiff ER, et al. Interferon alfa-2b alone or in combination with ribavirin as initial treatment for chronic hepatitis C. Hepatitis Interventional Therapy Group. *N Engl J Med* 1998;339:1485–1492.

378. Davis GL, Balart LA, Schiff ER, et al. Treatment of chronic hepatitis C with recombinant interferon alfa. A multicenter randomized, controlled trial. Hepatitis Interventional Therapy Group. *N Engl J Med* 1989;321:1501–1506.

379. Poynard T, Leroy V, Cohard M, et al. Meta-analysis of interferon randomized trials in the treatment of viral hepatitis C. Effects of dose and duration. *Hepatology* 1996;24:778–789.

380. Bunnapradist S, Fabrizi F, Vierling J, et al. Hepatitis C therapy with long term remission after renal transplantation. *Int J Artif Organs* 2002;25:1189–1193.

381. Kamar N, Toupance O, Buchler M, et al. Evidence that clearance of hepatitis C virus RNA after alpha-interferon therapy in dialysis patients is sustained after renal transplantation. *J Am Soc Nephrol* 2003;14:2092–2098.

382. Gonzalez-Roncero F, Gentil MA, Valdivia MA, et al. Outcome of kidney transplant in chronic hepatitis C virus patients: effect of pretransplantation interferon-alpha2b monotherapy. *Transplant Proc* 2003;35:1745–1747.

383. Rostaing L, Modesto A, Baron E, et al. Acute renal failure in kidney transplant patients treated with interferon alpha 2b for chronic hepatitis C. *Nephron* 1996;74:512–516.

384. Magnone M, Holley JL, Shapiro R, et al. Interferon-alpha-induced acute renal allograft rejection. *Transplantation* 1995;59:1068–1070.

385. Ozgur O, Boyacioglu S, Telatar H, Haberal M. Recombinant alpha-interferon in renal allograft recipients with chronic hepatitis C. *Nephrol Dial Transplant* 1995;10:2104–2106.

386. Bruchfeld A, Stahle L, Andersson J, Schvarcz R. Ribavirin treatment in dialysis patients with chronic hepatitis C virus infection—a pilot study. *J Viral Hepat* 2001;8:287–292.

387. Bruchfeld A, Stahle L, Andersson J, Schvarcz R. Interferon and ribavirin therapy in haemodialysis patients with chronic hepatitis C (letter). *Nephrol Dial Transplant* 2001;16:1729.

388. Tan AC, Brouwer JT, Glue P, et al. Safety of interferon and ribavirin therapy in haemodialysis patients with chronic hepatitis C: results of a pilot study. *Nephrol Dial Transplant* 2001;16:193–195.

389. Manns MP, McHutchison JG, Gordon SC, et al. Peginterferon alfa-2b plus ribavirin compared with interferon alfa-2b plus ribavirin for initial treatment of chronic hepatitis C: a randomised trial. *Lancet* 2001;358:958–965.

390. Zeuzem S, Feinman SV, Rasenack J, et al. Peginterferon alfa-2a in patients with chronic hepatitis C. *N Engl J Med* 2000;343:1666–1672.

391. Reddy KR. Controlled-release, pegylation, liposomal formulations: new mechanisms in the delivery of injectable drugs. *Ann Pharmacother* 2000;34:915–923.

392. Martin P, Mitra S, Farrington K, et al. Pegylated (40 KDA) interferon alfa-2a (Pegasys) is unaffected by renal impairment. *Hepatology* 2000;32:370A.

393. Lamb MW, Marks IM, Wynohradnyk L, et al. 40kDA peginterferon alfa-2a (Pegasys) can be administered safely in patients with end-stage renal disease. *Hepatology* 2001;34:326A.

394. Chow T, Galvin J, McGovern B. Antiarrhythmic drug therapy in patients with renal failure, liver failure, and congestive heart failure. *Heart Dis* 1999;1:98–107.

395. Saltissi D, Morgan C, Rigby RJ, Westhuyzen J. Safety and efficacy of simvastatin in hypercholesterolemic patients undergoing chronic renal dialysis. *Am J Kidney Dis* 2002;39:283–290.

396. Alfrey AC, Hegg A, Craswell P. Metabolism and toxicity of aluminum in renal failure. *Am J Clin Nutr* 1980;33:1509–1516.

397. Di Paolo N, Masti A, Comparini IB, et al. Uremia, dialysis and aluminium. *Int J Artif Organs* 1997;20:547–552.

398. Kuruyama H, Kono N, Nakanuma Y, et al. Hepatic granulomata in long-term hemodialysis patients with hyperaluminumemia. *Arch Pathol Lab Med* 1989;113:1132–1134.

399. Arieff AI, Cooper JD, Armstrong D, Lazarowitz VC. Dementia, renal failure, and brain aluminum. *Ann Intern Med* 1979 90:741–747.

400. Pitts TO, Barbour GL. Hemosiderosis secondary to chronic parenteral iron therapy in maintenance hemodialysis patients. *Nephron* 1978;22:316–321.

401. Eschbach JW, Adamson JW. Iron overload in renal failure patients: changes since the introduction of erythropoietin therapy. *Kidney Int* 1999;69:S35–S43.

Gastrointestinal Diseases in Patients with Chronic Kidney Disease

Tam Tran
Pedram Enayati
Rome Jutabha

Gastrointestinal (GI) disorders are common in patients with chronic kidney disease (CKD) and encompass the full spectrum of diseases that affect the general population. This chapter reviews common GI complaints that are referred to gastroenterologists for further evaluation. These diseases merit special consideration in the patient with end-stage renal disease (ESRD) due to their increased incidence and/or severity. The disorders are categorized based on the clinical presentation and symptom complex as reported by the patient. These symptoms include nausea, vomiting, diarrhea, GI bleeding, and abdominal pain.

NAUSEA AND VOMITING

Nausea and vomiting are the most common GI complaints reported by at least 70 percent of patients with ESRD.[1] Nausea and vomiting can be the presenting symptoms of a wide spectrum of diseases. The most commonly encountered causes in patients with CKD include metabolic imbalance, motility disorders, peptic ulcer disease, infection, and side effects of medications (Table 25–1).

Metabolic Disturbances

Patients with CKD frequently suffer from many disturbances in polypeptide hormones (e.g., cholecystokinin, motilin, gastrin) and electrolytes (e.g., uremia, acidosis, hypokalemia, hypercalcemia, hypermagnesemia, byperglycemia) secondary to impaired renal function. These hormonal and metabolic abnormalities are often raised as possible causes of nausea and vomiting, but the pathophysiology remains uncertain.[2]

In dialysis-dependent patients, nausea and vomiting occur most frequently during hemodialysis and are caused by multiple factors. Chronic uremia probably plays a

TABLE 25–1. ETIOLOGIES OF NAUSEA AND/OR VOMITING IN PATIENTS WITH CHRONIC KIDNEY DISEASE

Metabolic abnormalities
   Uremia
   Hyperglycemia
   Hormonal disturbance
   Electrolyte disturbances
   Dysequilibrium syndrome
Gastroparesis
   Diabetes mellitus
   Medications
   Chronic ambulatory peritoneal dialysis
   Dialysis-related GI amyloidosis
   Viral gastroparesis
   Systemic diseases (scleroderma, amyloidosis)
   Neurologic disorders (multiple sclerosis, Parkinsonism, dysautonomias, brainstem tumor)
   Idiopathic
Peptic ulcer disease
Infection/inflammation
   Peritonitis
      Infectious
      Chemical
      Secondary to other intraabdominal infections
      Sclerosing
   Pancreatitis
   Diverticulitis
   Non-GI infections (pyelonephritis, pneumonia)
Medication-related side effects
Bowel obstruction or infarction
   PD-related abdominal hernias
   Ischemic bowel disease
   Sclerosing encapsulating peritonitis
   Beta$_2$-microglobulin amyloidosis

major role in the occurrence of these symptoms. Hypotension due to rapid changes in volume and other mechanisms occurs in 15 to 55 percent of hemodialysis sessions and is highly associated with nausea and vomiting.[3] The incidence of dialysis-related nausea and vomiting has been reported to increase with longer treatment times and a higher rate of urea removal or ultrafiltration.[4] Less commonly, nausea and vomiting may also be the early symptoms of the dysequilibrium syndrome, a neurologic complication of dialysis caused by a shift of water into the brain. This osmotic shift is thought to be induced by urea removal and decreased cerebral intracellular pH during intensive dialysis.[5]

Diagnosis. Initial evaluation of nausea and vomiting should always include serum electrolytes, glucose, pH, hemoglobin A1C, and TSH.

Treatment. Adequate dialysis, timely correction of electrolyte abnormalities, tight glycemic control for diabetic patients, proper nutritional support, and the use of antiemetics for symptomatic relief are effective measures in the management of nausea and vomiting caused by these metabolic disturbances.

Gastroparesis

Nausea and vomiting are the most common clinical features of gastroparesis. There have been conflicting data regarding gastric emptying in patients with CKD. Some studies show a high prevalence of delayed gastric emptying of solid foods,[6,7] while others report no impairment of gastric emptying.[8,9] However, gastroparesis develops in up to 58 percent of patients with diabetes, which is the most common cause of CKD in the United States. Gastric retention in diabetic patients is significantly associated with diabetic neuropathy, hyperglycemia, hypokalemia, and acidosis.[10] Drug-induced gastroparesis is also common in this patient population, who are typically taking multiple medications (see further discussion under "Medications," below). Gastroparesis developing during or after a viral illness has been described in patients infected with rotavirus, Norwalk virus, cytomegalovirus (CMV), and Epstein-Barr virus (EBV).[11,12]

Delayed gastric emptying has been reported in 50 percent of patients on continuous ambulatory peritoneal dialysis (CAPD) when the abdomen is full of dialysate. Intraabdominal pressure therefore may stimulate mechanical or neurogenic pathways that inhibit gastric emptying.[13]

Rarely, patients on long-term dialysis may develop gastric stasis due to neuromuscular infiltration of the GI tract with beta$_2$ microglobulin, which is retained in patients with CKD.[14] In addition, gastroparesis may be the result of underlying systemic or neurologic diseases such as amyloidosis, scleroderma, multiple sclerosis, Parkinsonism, or primary autonomic neuropathy.[15] Unfortunately, an underlying etiology cannot be found in up to one-third of patients with gastroparesis.[16]

Diagnosis. When patients present with clinical evidence suggesting delayed gastric emptying (e.g. nausea, vomiting, early satiety, abdominal pain, pertinent systemic diseases), an EGD or a barium meal should be performed first to exclude mechanical obstruction or mucosal disease. Gastric stasis is highly suspected if undigested solid food is found in the stomach after an overnight fast. The current diagnostic tests of choice for gastroparesis are the [13C]-labeled acetate- and -octanoic acid breath tests which measure expiratory 13-CO_2 concentration or scintigraphic gastric emptying with scans taken immediately after ingestion of the radiolabeled meal and 2 and 4 hours later.[15,17,18]

Treatment. The management of gastroparesis consists of hydration, correction of electrolytes abnormalities, decompression of the dilated upper bowel, meal modification (e.g., frequent small meals, liquid supplements, low-residue diet), tight glycemic control in diabetics, and the use of prokinetics and antiemetics. A small number of patients who remain refractory to all the standard treatments may need total parenteral nutrition or a jejunal feeding tube to bypass the atonic stomach and provide sufficient nutrition.[10] Intrasphincteric botulinum toxin injection into the pylorus and implantable gastric pacing are promising experimental treatments for gastroparesis but further controlled studies are needed.[16,19,20] Surgery is rarely indicated except for total gastrectomy in patients with gastric stasis secondary to previous partial gastrectomy.[15]

Peptic Ulcer Disease

Peptic ulcer disease (PUD) of the esophagus, stomach, or duodenum can result in nausea and vomiting. Pyloric outlet obstruction should be excluded in all patients presenting with a history of PUD and prolonged vomiting. PUD is discussed further under upper GI bleeding.

Infection

Patients with CKD and uremia have increased susceptibility to infection due to impaired cellular function.[21] Nausea and/or vomiting are not uncommon symptoms in some of the prevalent infections in this patient population. In patients undergoing peritoneal dialysis (PD), peritonitis is the most common reason for hospitalization and discontinuation of PD. Infectious peritonitis generally results from intraluminal contamination of the peritoneal catheter and correlates with the duration of PD and frequency of catheter manipulation. *Staphylococcus epidermidis* and *S. aureus* are the most common pathogens. Chemical peritonitis can mimic infectious peritonitis in its presentation and is associated with peritoneal reaction to dialysate. Less frequently, long-term PD may lead to sclerosing peritonitis which is characterized by the deposition of a thick fribrous exudate onto the peritoneal surfaces for unknown reasons. The condition is associated with a reduced efficiency of PD and an increased incidence of infectious peritonitis. Secondary peritonitis from appendicitis, pancreatitis, cholecystitis, or perforated bowel should be also considered. In clinical practice, peritoneal fluid is analyzed and cultured and empiric antibiotics are initiated when dialysate fluid turns cloudy. Infected patients usually have a peritoneal fluid with greater than 100 white cells/mL and >50 percent polymorphonuclear leukocytes. Peritoneal gram stain is positive in less then 40 percent of cases but may be very useful for guiding antibiotic therapy if it is positive. Infectious peritonitis is diagnosed with a positive peritoneal fluid culture.

A peritoneal culture positive for anaerobes or polymicrobial organisms warrants evaluation for secondary peritonitis.[21,22]

Acute pancreatitis has been reported with an increased incidence in patients with ESRD. A majority of the cases has unclear etiology and is associated with PD and polycystic kidney disease (PKD).[23,24] Diverticulitis has been found to be more prevalent among patients with CKD secondary to PKD. Pneumonia and pyelonephritis are non-GI infections that should be kept in mind because of their significant mortality and prevalence in patients with ESRD, respectively.[15]

Medications

Adverse effects of medications are among the most common causes of nausea and/or vomiting. The majority of CKD patients take multiple medications, many of which are known to cause nausea and/or vomiting, and drug accumulation is a contributing factor due to impaired renal excretion. Drug-induced gastric stasis occurs frequently in patients taking TCAs, narcotics, anticholinergics, alpha-2 adrenergic agonists, vincristine and erythromycin.[15] Many ESRD patients develop chronic nausea and vomiting from taking paricalcitol (vitamin D) for secondary hyperparathyroidism.[25] Other medications that often induce nausea and/or vomiting include digitalis, levodopa, bromocriptine, anticancer drugs, NSAIDs, cardiac antiarrhythmic drugs, antihypertensive drugs, diuretics, oral antidiabetic agents, oral contraceptives, and GI medications (e.g., sulfasalazine).[26] Therefore, medications should be reviewed periodically in all patients with the goal of discontinuing nonessential medications and replacing essential ones with substitutes that are not associated with nausea and/or vomiting.

Bowel Obstruction and Infarction

Organic pathology must be first excluded when dialysis patients present with persistent nausea and vomiting that are accompanied by objective signs such as abdominal tenderness and weight loss. Abdominal hernias are a significant complication in patients on PD and occasionally result in small bowel strangulation, incarceration or infarction. Suggested risk factors for developing hernias include CAPD, older age, longer duration of CAPD, previous surgeries and multiparity.[14] Bowel infarction may occur with an increased rate in both HD and PD patients. It is highly associated with the frequency, severity, and duration of dialysis-related hypotension as well as underlying comorbidities such as hypertention, diabetes, and atherosclerosis.[27,28] Bowel obstruction has been reported in sclerosing encapsulating peritonitis in which the developing fibrous layer surrounds the bowel entirely.[22] There are also case reports describing intestinal and colonic pseudo-obstruction in patients with β-2 microglobulin amyloidosis.[29,30]

PHARMACOLOGIC THERAPY OF NAUSEA AND VOMITING

Antiemetics are central to the symptomatic relief of nausea and vomiting while prokinetics are the mainstay in the treatment of gastroparesis (Table 25–2).[10,15,26,31]

Antiemetic Medications

Although there are several families of antiemetics classified by their mechanisms of action, this discussion will focus on the drugs that are most commonly used for metabolic and GI disorders.

Phenothiazines. Phenothiazines produce their antiemetic effect primarily by antagonizing dopamine D_2 receptors in the chemoreceptor trigger zone (CTZ). The two most widely used drugs in this class are prochlorperazine (Compazine) and promethazine (Phenergan). The main adverse effects are extrapyramidal reactions, drowsiness, and hypotension.

Benzamides. The most useful drug in this class is metoclopramide (Reglan), which has multiple antiemetic actions. It antagonizes dopamine D_2 receptors in the chemoreceptor trigger zone (CTZ), enhances acetylcholine release

TABLE 25–2. COMMON MEDICATIONS FOR THE MANAGEMENT OF NAUSEA AND VOMITING

Class	Medication	Primary Mechanisms	Dosing (oral dose first, then intravenous form)	Common Side Effects
Antiemetics	Prochlorperazine (Compazine)	Blocks dopamine D_2 receptors in CTZ	5–10 mg PO, 2.5–10 mg IV, 5–10 mg IM, 25 mg by rectum May be repeated every 6–8 hours PO or every 3–4 hours IV or IM or every 12 hours by rectum until cessation of vomiting	Dystonic reaction (can be treated with diphenhydramine 25–50 mg IM), sedation, lethargy, hypotension
	Promethazine HCl (Phenergan)	Blocks dopamine D_2 receptors in CTZ	12.5–25 mg IV, 25–50 mg IM or by rectum May be repeated every 6 hours until cessation of vomiting	Dystonic reaction (can be treated with diphenhydramine 25–50 mg IM), sedation, dry mouth, dizziness, blurred vision
	Odansetron (Zofran)	Blocks serotonin 5-HT$_3$ receptors in CTZ and peripheral vagal nerve terminals	8 mg IV or 16–24 mg PO once prechemotherapy for acute emesis 8 mg PO bid x 2–3 days for delayed emesis	Mild headache, constipation, diarrhea
Prokinetics	Erythromycin	Stimulates motilin receptors on gastroduodenal smooth muscle to increase antral motility	3mg/kg IV every 8 hours followed by 250 mg PO TID or 7–8 days (30 minutes before meals)	Gastrointestinal upset, pseudomembranous colitis, induction of microbial resistance
	Cisapride (Propulsid)	Stimulates the release of acetylcholine from the myenteric plexus, stimulates antral and duodenal motility, improves antroduodenal coordination, increases lower esophageal lower sphincter pressure	10–20 mg PO 30 minutes before each meal and at bedtime; total dose should not exceed 1 mg/kg or maximal 60–80 mg per day	Abdominal discomfort, dose-dependent diarrhea, headache, cardiac arrhythmias (less than 5% of patients) Available only via limited–access protocol
	Metoclopramide (Reglan)	Blocks dopamine D_2 receptors in CTZ, stimulates acetylcholine release in myenteric plexus, enhances gastric smooth muscle response to acetylcholine, coordinates pyloric relaxation with duodenal peristalsis	10 mg PO 30 minutes before each meal and at bedtime dosing adjustment in renal failure: Ftnt 10–40 mL/min: 50% of normal dose Cl_{cr} < 10 mL/min: 25% of normal dose	Extrapyramidal side effects, restlessness, drowsiness, diarrhea, hyperprolactinemia
	Domperidone (Botilium)	Blocks dopamine D_2 receptors in CTZ and GI tract, increases esophageal and gastric motility and lower esophageal sphincter, enhances gastroduodenal coordination	10–20 mg PO 3–4 times/day, 15–30 minutes before meals dosing adjustment for renal failure: 10–20 mg 1–2 times/day	Rarely hyperprolactinemia Awaiting FDA approval in the United States

ABBREVIATIONS: CTZ = Chemoreceptor trigger zone; Cl_{cr} = Creatinine clearance.

and smooth muscle response to acetylcholine in the upper GI tract, and promotes gastric emptying. However, its clinical use is limited by its ability to cross the blood-brain barrier, with resultant central nervous system (CNS) effects such as drowsiness, restlessness, and extrapyramidal symptoms in up to 20 to 30 percent of patients. Metoclopramide has also been used as an antiemetic to treat chemotherapy-induced emesis. Domperidone is another benzamide with actions and effects similar to those of metoclopramide except that it crosses the blood-brain barrier only minimally and hence lacks CNS adverse effects.

Antiserotoninergics. The serotonin antagonists are the newest and most promising class of antiemetic agents. They have been of great clinical and research interest owing to their superior efficacy in relieving chemotherapy-induced emesis and minimal side-effect profile (e.g.. mild headache, constipation, diarrhea). Ondansetron (Zofran), the most widely used drug in this class, selectively antagonizes 5-HT_3 receptors in the CTZ and in peripheral vagal nerves. It is particularly effective in controlling nausea and vomiting caused by chemotherapy, radiotherapy, anesthesia, and surgery. Its application is being investigated in many other conditions, including uremia and GI motility disorders. The main drawbacks of these medications are their cost.

Prokinetic Medications

Prokinetics promote gastric emptying by acting on various receptors that have been shown to affect GI motility. They are used in gastroesophageal reflux disease, gastroparesis, and pseudoobstruction. The prokinetic agents described below are the most useful in the management of gastroparesis.

Erythromycin. The macrolide antibiotic erythromycin strongly stimulates motilin receptors on gastroduodenal smooth muscle to increase antral propulsive contraction, thereby accelerating gastric emptying. Many small clinical studies have shown that erythromycin improves delayed gastric emptying by 30 to 60 percent and that its efficacy is superior to that of other prokinetic agents including metoclopramide, cisapride, and domperidone. However, whether erythromycin improves symptoms of gastroparesis by accelerating gastric emptying remains controversial and requires well-designed studies.[32] Its use is also limited by tachyphylaxis, induction of bacterial resistance with long-term use, and GI upset.

Cisapride (Propulsid). Cisapride accelerates gastric emptying by stimulating acetylcholine release from postganglionic myenteric neurons via its action on serotonin 5-HT_4 receptors. Cisapride may enhance antral and duodenal motility,

increase lower esophageal sphincter pressure, and improve antral-duodenal coordination. Clinical trials have demonstrated that cisapride improves gastric emptying and associated symptoms in diabetic gastroparesis and intestinal pseudoobstruction for up to 12 months.[33–35] Common side effects of cisapride are abdominal cramping, dose-dependent diarrhea, and headache. In the year 2000, cisapride was withdrawn from the U.S. market because of reported cases of cardiac arrhythmias and sudden death due to QT prolongation. The majority of affected patients took cisapride in conjunction with other drugs metabolized by the cytochrome P450–34A (e.g., macrolide antibiotics, antifungals, and HIV protease inhibitors) or had disorders that may have predisposed them to cardiac arrhythmias (e.g., heart disease, hypomagnesemia, hypokalemia, and liver or renal failure). Therefore cisapride is currently available only to patients who fail other treatment options and meet specific eligibility criteria through the manufacturer's limited-access program. For these reasons, this medication should be avoided in patients with CKD.

Metoclopramide (Reglan). In addition to its antiemetic effect, metoclopramide acts as a prokinetic by stimulating acetylcholine release in the myenteric plexus, enhancing the response of GI tissue to acetylcholine, and coordinating pyloric relaxation with duodenal peristalsis. There are few clinical trials on the efficacy of metoclopramide. Some comparison studies have suggested that metoclopramide is not as effective as erythromycin and cisapride and as effective as domperidone in promoting gastric motility.[36–39] The use of metoclopramide is also limited to short-term treatment because of its CNS side effects.

Domperidone (Botilium). Domperidone also has dual antiemetic and prokinetic effects. It enhances gastric emptying by blocking peripheral dopamine receptor in the GI tract, increasing esophageal and gastric motility, lowering esophageal sphincter pressure, and facilitating gastroduodenal coordination. Several studies have demonstrated the efficacy of domperidone in alleviating gastric stasis, particularly diabetic gastroparesis.[40,41] Because of its mild side-effect profile (e.g., rare incidence of headache, GI upset, and hyperprolactinemia), domperidone is a promising oral prokinetic and is awaiting FDA approval in the United States.

Investigational Medications

Tegaserod and octreotide are thought to hold promise for accelerating bowel transit, but their clinical efficacy has yet to be established. Novel prokinetics undergoing studies are serotonin 5-HT_4 agonists, opiate receptor agonists, macrolides without antibiotic activity, and CCK antagonists.[42,43]

DIARRHEA

Diarrhea is a frequent complaint reported by approximately 25 percent of dialysis patients.[22]

Clostridium difficile–Associated Diarrhea (CDAD)

CDAD has been reported to occur with increased incidence, mortality, and recurrence in patients with CKD.[44,45] Proposed risk factors for recurrent CDAD include advanced age, poor nutrition, antimicrobial therapy, impaired host defenses, intestinal hypermotility, and arteriosclerosis with ischemia involving the gut.

Diagnosis. CDAD is diagnosed by clinical suspicion, stool culture, and cytotoxin test.

Treatment. Eradication of the bacterium and control of the precipitating antibiotics are central to the treatment and prevention of CDAD. Recurrent or refractory cases of CDAD are treated with a second course of metronidazole or vancomycin. Persistent infection despite conventional treatment may benefit from proposed therapies such as tapering and pulsed doses of vancomycin; administration of *Saccharomyces boulardii*, cholestyramine, rifampin; or intravenous immunoglobulins.[46]

Other Causes of Acute Diarrhea

Although the incidence of viral gastroenteritis is not increased in patients with CKD, it is the most common cause of acute diarrhea in all patients. Viral gastroenteritis is usually self-limited and requires only supportive therapy. CMV infection is the most common opportunistic infection following renal transplantation, and CMV antibodies are found in asymptomatic hemodialysis patients with an increased incidence. Symptomatic CMV infection or CMV colitis is rare among nontransplanted CKD patients.[47] Intestinal protozoa—including *Cryptosporidium, Microsporidium, Isospora, Cyclospora,* and *Giardia lamblia*—were detected at a higher incidence in CKD patients with chronic diarrhea.[48,49] Ischemic colitis and bowel infarction should be considered when patients present with bloody diarrhea, hypotension, and sepsis. Dialysis-related peritonitis may also present with acute diarrhea.

Chronic Diarrhea

Chronic diarrhea in CKD patients is often multifactorial (Table 25–3), particularly in those with a long history of diabetes and insulin therapy.

Diabetic Enteropathy

Approximately 8 to 22 percent of diabetics suffer from chronic diarrhea, which is typically painless, watery, and

TABLE 25–3. COMMON CAUSES OF DIARRHEA IN PATIENTS WITH CHRONIC KIDNEY DISEASE

Acute diarrhea
  Infection
    Clostridium difficile
    Viral gastroenteritis
    Protozoa (*Cryptosporidium, Microsporidium, Isopora, Cyclospora, Giardia*)
  Dialysis-related peritonitis
  Bowel ischemia/infarction
Chronic diarrhea
  Diabetic enteropathy
    Autonomic neuropathy
    Anorectal dysfunction
    Intestinal and/or colonic dysmotility
    Exocrine pancreatic insufficiency
    Celiac sprue
    Small bowel bacterial overgrowth
    Bile acid malabsorption
Medications
Clostridium difficile (recurrent)
Fecal impaction (overflow diarrhea)

worse at night.[50] It may alternate with normal bowel movements or constipation and may be associated with fecal incontinence.

Pathogenesis. The pathogenesis of this "diabetic diarrhea" is not fully understood. Studies have suggested that diabetic autonomic neuropathy and resulting intestinal dysmotility, alteration of water and electrolyte absorption in the gut, and anorectal dysfunction play major roles in this condition. Chronic diarrhea in advanced diabetes can also be caused by small-bowel bacterial overgrowth, bile acid malabsorption, celiac sprue, or exocrine pancreatic insufficiency.[51] Abnormalities in small-bowel transit secondary to autonomic neuropathy are postulated to contribute to bacterial overgrowth and bile acid malabsorption. Celiac sprue is more common in patients with type I diabetes, and both diseases have HLA-B8 and HLA-DR3 in common.[10] Exocrine pancreatic insufficiency is secondary to pancreatic atrophy and the GI hormonal disturbances mentioned above.

Management. Due to the multifactorial nature of chronic diarrhea in diabetes, management should be directed at identifying the main causes and treating these underlying conditions.[50] Treatment should be initiated with fluid and electrolyte correction, tight glycemic control, and nutritional support.

Small bowel bacterial overgrowth is diagnosed by a glucose hydrogen breath test and eradicated by a rotating scheme of oral doxycycline, metronidazole, and cefuroxime for 6 to 12 months.

Celiac sprue is diagnosed by small bowel biopsy and treated with a gluten-free diet. The secretin–pancreatic enzyme test is indicated for diagnosing pancreatic insufficiency, which will benefit from pancreatic enzyme supplements.

Fecal incontinence mandates anorectal manometry or sensory testing. Loperamide and biofeedback training are recommended for anorectal dysfunction.

Other Causes of Chronic Diarrhea

Chronic diarrhea can be caused by a variety of medications. Those drugs taken commonly by CKD patients are digoxin, propranolol, lovastatin, metformin, odansetron, magnesium- or aluminum-containing antacids, vitamin D, calcium carbonate, and artificial sweeteners. Fecal impaction is a very common complaint in CKD patients and may lead to chronic diarrhea.

Chronic diarrhea of unclear etiology should be relieved symptomatically with a trial of loperamide, codeine, or diphenoxylate. Clonidine may reduce stool frequency and volume in some refractory cases of chronic diarrhea; however, its use is limited by significant side effects, including orthostatic hypotension, dry mouth, and delayed gastric emptying.[52] Octreotide has been reported to improve intestinal motility and reduce bacterial overgrowth; but treatment with high doses of octreotide should be monitored closely because it may inhibit pancreatic secretion and worsen nutrient malabsorption.[10]

GASTROINTESTINAL BLEEDING

GI bleeding is a common and troublesome complication of ESRD, accounting for as many as 10 to 15 percent of all cases of upper GI bleeding.[53] GI mucosal abnormalities ranging from edema to ulceration occur in two-thirds of patients with CKD. Gastritis, duodenitis, and peptic ulcer disease are often found in adults with CKD on regular hemodialysis and following renal transplantation. Certain risk factors that place ESRD patients at a higher risk for GI bleeding—including cardiovascular disease, current smoking, and risk factors associated with an inability to ambulate independently—place these patients at higher risk. African-American patients and transplant patients were found to have an overall lower risk of upper GI bleeding.[54]

Upper Gastrointestinal Bleeding

Patients with CKD have an increased frequency of recurrent upper GI bleeding (25 percent) compared to those patients without CKD (11 percent). GI inflammation is common in patients on hemodialysis, occurring in 25 to 67 percent.[55,56] Antral gastritis is common, with a prevalence of about 50 percent, whereas duodenitis is less frequent, with a prevalence of 9 to 43 percent.[1,6–10] More recent studies have shown that active peptic ulcer disease (PUD) does not appear to be more common in patients on hemodialysis than in the general population.[57] Esophagogastric varices must be considered in patients with concomitant hepatitis, C-related cirrhosis, and severe upper GI hemorrhage.[58]

Causes. PUD is the most common cause of upper GI bleeding in patients with CKD.[59] Studies have shown that angiodysplasia of the stomach or duodenum is the single most frequent source of bleeding (23 percent) in patients with CKD. Angiodysplasia and erosive esophagitis (Fig. 25–1) were more common causes of upper GI bleeding in the CKD population than in the control group without renal failure (angiodysplasia 5 percent and erosive esophagitis 5 percent).[53]

Endoscopy is the diagnostic method of choice for evaluating bleeding from the upper GI tract. Endoscopic signs of gastroduodenal mucosal inflammation—including erythema, petechiae, and erosions—occur in approximately half of all patients on maintenance dialysis.

Pathogenesis. The association between peptic ulcer disease and renal failure has been a controversial subject since the early days of dialysis. There are several theories as to why CKD patients have a higher rate of hemorrhagic mucosal lesions. Patients with CKD have been found to have persistent hypergastrinemia, and it was assumed that hypersecretion of gastric acids was the cause of gastroduodenal peptic disease. Subsequent studies have shown that despite an increase in the density of gastric parietal, chief, and G cells in patients with CKD, gastric acid secretion is usually decreased rather than increased. This is probably not due to the neutralization of gastric acid by ammonia (acid output inhibition).[60] Therefore the severity of gastroduodenal complications is more related to the removal of acid output inhi-

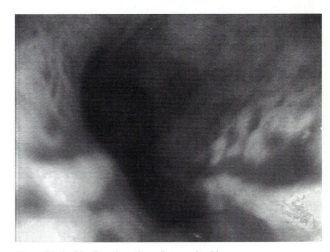

Figure 25–1. Bleeding ulcerative reflux esophagitis.

bition, ammonia, rather than the serum gastrin levels or the amount of acid secretion.[61] Another study, conducted by Itoh et al., concluded that oxygen supply and not blood flow seemed to play an important role in gastric hemorrhages and that oxygen radicals produced during hemodialysis participate in the pathogenesis of mucosal hemorrhage.[62] More recent studies have concluded that the incidence of peptic ulcer in ESRD patients is comparable to that in the general population.[63] Studies evaluating potential physiologic changes in these patients include normal gastric mucosal prostaglandin E_2 levels, normal basal gastric output, and decreased peak acid output in patients with CKD compared to normal subjects.[64]

Initial data seemed to support the hypothesis of an increased prevalence of ulcer disease in the presence of uremia.[65] These theories are supported by physiologic data showing decreased pancreatic and duodenal bicarbonate secretion and elevated gastric cell mass and serum gastrin levels in the presence of ESRD.[66,67] The prevalence of *Helicobacter pylori* in CKD patients has not been systematically assessed. *H. pylori,* a gram-negative bacterium, is considered the most common causative agent of antral gastritis and duodenal ulcer in the normal population.[68] For many years it was assumed that patients with CKD would have a higher incidence of *H. pylori*–induced peptic ulcerations. *H. pylori* has high urease activity and produces ammonia in the presence of urea. Patients with ESRD and *H. pylori* infection have elevated levels of blood urea and ammonia. Elevated ammonia levels are considered an etiologic factor in gastric mucosal disorders. Subsequent studies have found that the prevalence of *H. pylori* in adults with CKD is similar to that of healthy controls, irrespective of upper GI symptoms.[69] Recent studies have found that long-term dialysis patients have a decreased prevalence of *H. pylori* infection. Nakajima et al. found that, in nondialyzed patients, the prevalence of *H. pylori*–positive patients was 56.0 percent, while the percentage was significantly lower in dialyzed patients.[70]

Treatment. Treatments for upper GI bleeding include endoscopic therapy[71,72] (thermal and bipolar coagulation, injection therapy, hemostatic clips, fibrin sealant) and medical management. Medical management of GI bleeding can also be implemented as an adjunct to postendoscopic therapy. Considering the available data, the ideal pharmacologic therapy for patients with acute bleeding appears to be an intravenous proton pump inhibitor (PPI) (e.g., pantoprazole) started immediately after endoscopic therapy. The goal of treatment in these patients, following proper resuscitation, should be directed at achieving acute hemostasis and then healing the ulcers and eliminating precipitating factors such as *H. pylori* and nonsteroidal anti-inflammatory drugs (NSAIDs).

It is very important to identify patients who are at higher risk of hemorrhage, because this knowledge may help in the choice of preventive or therapeutic methods. An acquired platelet dysfunction may develop in uremic patients, and aspirin causes a disproportionate rise in bleeding time. Consequently patients with CKD and angiodysplasia should avoid aspirin.[73] Patients on hemodialysis may also have an increased risk of bleeding from angiodysplasia due to the use of heparin during the procedures.[74] Desmopressin acetate 1-deamino-8-D-arginine vasopressin (DDAVP) successfully reduces the bleeding tendency in patients with CKD for short-term operations or procedures, but the frequency of tachyphylaxis is high and limits the drug's usefulness for major bleeding. Conjugated estrogens shorten bleeding time in uremia and may provide a more sustained hemostatic effect over desmopressin.[75] Pharmacologic treatment with antifibrinolytic agents such as tranexamic acid has been used successfully in the management of both acute and chronic bleeding colonic angiodysplasias.[76]

Thermal coagulation achieves acute hemostasis and prevents rebleeding by coaptive coagulation of the underlying artery at the bleeding site (Fig. 25–2). Injection therapy with absolute alcohol or epinephrine is inexpensive and effective for acute hemostasis. However, the rebleeding rate is high if epinephrine injections alone are used.[77] Another effective method of achieving hemostasis involves the injection of saline, causing a local tamponade. However, in a randomized controlled trial involving 100 patients with high-risk bleeding ulcers, saline injection alone was less effective at preventing recurrent bleeding than bipolar electrocoagulation.[78] Combination therapy with epinephrine injection followed by bipolar electrocoagulation is an effective method for achieving definitive hemostasis for ulcer hemorrhage.[79]

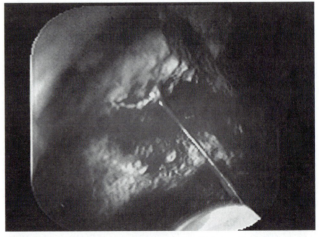

Figure 25–2. Hemostasis of bleeding duodenal ulcer with bipolar electrocoagulation.

Lower Gastrointestinal Bleeding

Lower GI bleeding is usually manifest by bright red blood per rectum. However, hematochezia can also arise from more proximal lesions in the GI tract due to brisk GI bleeding and rapid transit of intraluminal blood.

Angiodysplasia. Angiodysplasia is a very common cause of lower GI bleeding in the elderly. The lesions are usually flat and rarely exceed 5 to 7 mm in diameter. They comprise abnormal microvasculature located in the mucosa and submucosa of the bowel wall (Fig. 25–3). In a study conducted by Marcuard et al., vascular lesions of the GI tract were diagnosed in 32 percent of patients with CKD who presented with GI bleeding. Subsequently, recurrent GI bleeding was a common problem in subjects with angiodysplasia, with 67 percent having a second bleeding episode.[80] The pathogenesis of such lesions in patients with CKD remains to be studied. It has been found that chronic low-grade obstruction of submucosal veins has been implicated in the pathogenesis of vascular ectasias in the elderly.[81] Therefore it is possible that chronic fluid overload in patients with CKD may contribute to the formation of vascular lesions of this kind. A variety of endoscopic treatments can be used to treat angiodysplasia, including electrocoagulation, sclerotherapy, band ligation, and laser therapy (Fig. 25–4). Although acute bleeding can appear to be successfully treated, rebleeding is common and often stems from other lesions. Patients who have multiple lesions or have an underlying bleeding diathesis may be less likely to benefit from endoscopic therapy and are at increased risk of complications. Such patients may benefit from attempts to improve their bleeding tendency.[82] In addition, because angiodysplasia commonly occurs in the small bowel, new technologies such as wireless capsule endoscopy will likely be used in the management of these patients in the future.

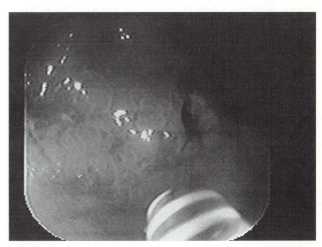

Figure 25–4. Cauterization of gastric vascular ectasia with gold-probe coagulation.

Ischemic Colitis

Mesenteric infarction has become a common complication in patients undergoing dialysis. Although it is more common in patients undergoing hemodialysis, it has been found to occur in patients on CAPD as well. Patients with predisposing factors—such as orthostatic hypoxemia, postural hypotension, and extensive atheromatous changes of the abdominal aorta—were found to be at higher risk of sustaining a mesenteric infarction.[83] It has also been found that the right colon is preferentially involved in the hemodialysis population. Dialysis tends to cause repeated episodes of hypotension; this leads to constriction of the vasa recta in the right colon, which, in turn, may lead to colonic ischemia.[84] Physicians should take into account the possibility of mesenteric ischemia in any uremic patient with arteriooclusive disease, abdominal pain, and leukocytosis, especially if hypotension is the major complication of the hemodialysis session.[85] Ischemic bowel disease should be considered for all patients on chronic dialysis with unexplained abdominal pain or discomfort. Abdominal pain, abdominal distention, and bloody stools are common initial presentations. Early diagnosis and aggressive surgical intervention is the recommended approach for all patients with such a complication.[86]

Diverticular Bleeding

Colonic diverticular disease is common, and its prevalence is age-dependent, increasing from less than 5 percent at age 40, to 30 percent by age 60, to 65 percent by age 85. Among all patients with diverticulosis, 70 percent remain asymptomatic, 15 to 25 percent develop diverticulitis, and 5 to 15 percent develop some form of diverticular bleeding (Fig. 25–5). Traditional treatment of diverticular bleeding that

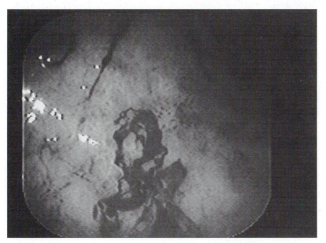

Figure 25–3. Bleeding gastric vascular ectasia.

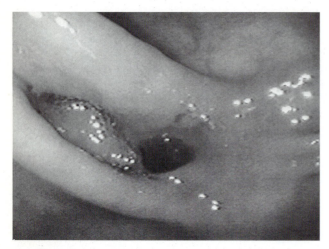

Figure 25–5. Colonic diverticulum with oozing from a visible vessel.

does not stop spontaneously or recurs includes surgery or angiographic embolization. More recently, colonoscopic hemostasis of diverticula with active bleeding or visible vessels has been reported using a combination epinephrine injection and bipolar electrocoagulation (Fig. 25–6).[87]

Small Bowel Bleeding

Bleeding from the small intestine must be suspected in patients with recurrent GI bleeding despite numerous nondiagnostic examinations of the upper and lower GI tract.[88] In these situations, obscure GI bleeding most often originates from the small bowel. It is frequently difficult to establish this diagnosis due to the location (not within reach of standard endoscopes) and nature of the bleeding (slow, intermittent oozing). The most common causes of small bowel bleeding in the CKD population include angiodysplasia, ulcers, and tumors. Diagnostic procedures include tagged red

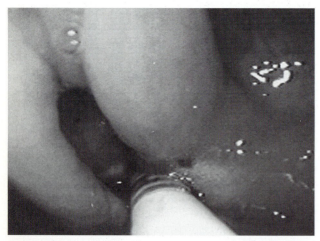

Figure 25–6. Endoscopic electrocoagulation of visible vessel within a colonic diverticulum.

cell scans, mesenteric angiography, push enteroscopy, and—more recently—capsule endoscopy.[89–93] This last modality allows visualization of the entire small bowel via an ingestable device that transmits digital images to an external data recorder over an 8-hour period. Images are then downloaded to a computer work station and analyzed. Therapeutic options for actively bleeding lesions within the small bowel include endoscopic bipolar electrocoagulation via push enteroscopy, angiographic embolization with coils or microbeads, or intraoperative enteroscopy (Table 25–4).

ABDOMINAL PAIN

Abdominal pain is a common complaint that can be caused by a multitude of diseases beyond the scope of this chapter. Several disorders that merit special attention in the CKD patient, due to their increased incidence or severity, are listed in Table 25–5. Organic pathology must be considered first and excluded in any patient presenting with severe abdominal pain. Abdominal pain can be due to various intra- and/or extraluminal causes.

The cause of abdominal pain is primarily elucidated by the clinical presentation and physical findings. For example, a patient with upper abdominal pain and associated nausea, vomiting, and hematemesis should undergo evaluation for suspected upper GI pathology. Mesenteric ischemia should be suspected in a patient with peripheral vascular disease and ESRD due to hypertension and diabetes who has severe postprandial abdominal pain and weight loss. Infarction usually occurs in patients with known cardiovascular, ischemic, or arteriosclerotic disease.

TABLE 25–4. SOURCES OF GASTROINTESTINAL BLEEDING IN PATIENTS WITH END-STAGE RENAL DISEASE

Upper gastrointestinal tract
  Erosive esophagitis
  Erosive gastritis
  Gastroduodenal ulcer
  Gastric angiodysplasia
  Esophagogastric varices[94]
Small bowel
  Angiodysplasia
  Ulcers (related to the use of nonsteroidal anti-inflammatory drugs)
  Tumors[95]
  Varices[96]
Lower gastrointestinal tract
  Colonic neoplasm
  Angiodyplasia
  Diverticular disease
  Ischemic bowel disease
  Rectal ulcer[97]

TABLE 25–5. CAUSES OF ABDOMINAL PAIN IN PATIENTS WITH CHRONIC KIDNEY DISEASE

Intraluminal

Upper GI tract: peptic ulcer disease, perforation

Small bowel: mesenteric ischemia, volvulus, incaceration within an umbilical hernia, adhesions

Colon: ischemic colitis, infectious colitis (*Clostridium difficile*, cytomegalovirus), diverticulitis

Extraluminal

Solid organ: pancreatitis, hepatitis, cholecystitis/choledocholithiasis

Peritoneum: bacterial peritonitis (cirrhotic or patient on chronic ambulatory peritoneal dialysis)

Angiography or magnetic resonance angiography (MRA) of the celiac artery or mesenteric vessels are the diagnostic tests of choice.[100]

Biliary colic is usually caused by contractions of the gallbladder in response to a fatty meal and/or the pressure of a gallstone against the gallbladder outlet or cystic duct opening, leading to increased pressure and pain within the gallbladder. Prolonged or recurrent blockage of the cystic duct can progress to total obstruction, causing acute cholecystitis. Such patients often complain of abdominal pain, most often in the right upper quadrant or epigastrium, with possible radiation to the right shoulder or back.[101] Pancreatitis should be suspected in patients with a history of alcohol abuse or gallstone disease. Almost all patients with acute pancreatitis have acute upper abdominal pain at the onset. Biliary colic, which may herald or progress to acute pancreatitis, may occur postprandially, while acute pancreatitis related to alcohol frequently occurs 1 to 3 days after a binge or cessation of drinking. Patients with fulminant attacks may present in shock or coma.[102]

A patient with hepatitis C cirrhosis and ascites presenting with abdominal pain and tenderness must be evaluated for spontaneous bacterial peritonitis. Patients with peritonitis attempt to minimize their abdominal pain by lying still, often in a supine position, with the knees flexed. The pain may be greatest around the abdomen near the abdominal viscera, where the pain originated, but—as inflammation progresses—it can spread rapidly to involve the entire abdomen.[103] In patients with kidney stones, pain is the most common symptom and varies from a mild and barely noticeable ache to discomfort that is so intense as to require hospitalization and parenteral medications. The site of obstruction determines the location of pain, which may change as the stone migrates, possibly leading the physician to make a false diagnosis. Computed tomography (CT) is the "gold standard" for diagnosis.[101]

Perforation of colonic diverticuli may complicate the clinical course of older patients with ESRD. This problem may arise in part because of the constipating effects of calcium- or aluminum-based phosphate binders. The symptoms of perforation of the colon in elderly dialysis patients may be insidious, as signs of acute peritonitis do not commonly appear until late in the course of the illness. Some of these patients complain of symptoms such as cramping, bloating, flatulence, and irregular defacation.[98] Thus, vague abdominal pain in the elderly patient with low-grade fever may be the only presenting symptom of perforation; such findings should not be ignored. Avoidance of severe, chronic constipation in the long-term dialysis patient is clearly desirable but often difficult to achieve. Stool softeners and osmotic laxatives such as sorbitol are often helpful but are not always effective or safe, especially in patients receiving large quantities of aluminum hydroxide gel. In these patients, overly vigorous use of laxatives, enemas, and parasympathetic agonists may precipitate perforation of the bowel.[99]

Laboratory and imaging studies are used as exclusionary and confirmatory tests to support the clinical diagnosis. Laboratory tests that should be considered in the evaluation of abdominal pain include a complete blood count with differential, amylase, lipase, and liver panel (AST, ALT, bilirubin, GGT, alkaline phosphatase). It is worth noting that both amylase and, to a lesser extent, lipase levels may be falsely elevated in CKD patients. Paracentesis and peritoneal fluid analysis (cell count and differential, Gram's stain, culture, cytology) should be performed for patients with ascites and abdominal pain. Ascitic fluid with a polymorphonuclear neutrophil count greater than 250/mL is diagnostic for spontaneous bacterial peritonitis (SPB). Cultures are sometimes helpful for determining the antibiotic sensitivity of the culprit organism, but cultures are often negative. The results of multiorganism culture suggest a secondary cause for bacterial peritonitis, such as bowel perforation or diverticulitis.[104] Empiric therapy against gram-negative organisms is warranted for suspected SPB pending culture results. Aminoglycoside antibiotics should not be used in cirrhotic patients due to the increased nephrotoxicity in this patient population.

Diagnostic imaging studies to consider include plain films of the abdomen (to rule out obstruction, ileus, perforation), abdominal ultrasound, and abdominal CT scanning (to rule out gallstones, biliary dilatation, and intraabdominal abcesses or mass lesions). CT has reported sensitivities of 96 to 98 percent and specificities of 83 to 89 percent for the detection of appendicitis.[105] On the other hand, right-upper-quadrant ultrasound is the imaging study of choice for patients with pain in the area to rule out cholelithiasis or cholecystitis.[106] Endoscopy and/or colonoscopy is indicated in patients with suspected upper or lower GI tract pathology once perforation and obstruction have been excluded. Surgery consultation should be sought immediately if there are signs or symptoms suggestive of an acute abdomen.

Treatment focuses on the underlying cause of abdominal pain.

CONCLUSION

GI complaints are common in the patient with ESRD. These diseases encompass the full spectrum of disorders that afflict the general population. Certain diseases, however, are more prevalent or more severe in the CKD patient. A high index of suspicion is needed to exclude organic pathology, so as to avoid serious consequences if diagnosis is delayed or missed. Diagnostic tests and treatment strategies can best be formulated in conjunction with the radiologist, gastroenterologist, and surgeon.

REFERENCES

1. Abu Farsakh NA, Roweily E, Rababaa M, et al. Brief report: evaluation of the upper gastrointestinal tract in uremic patients undergoing dialysis. *Nephrol Dial Transplant* 1996;11(5): 847–850.
2. Ravelli AM. Gastrointestinal function in CKD. *Pediatr Nephrol* 1995;9: 756–762.
3. Orofino L, Marcen R, Quereda C, et al. Epidemiology of symptomatic hypotension in hemodialysis: is cool dialysate beneficial for all patients? *Am J Nephrol* 1990;10(3): 177–180.
4. Skroeder NR, Jacobson SH, Lins LE, Kjellstrand CM. Acute symptoms during and between hemodialysis: the relative role of speed, duration, and biocompatibility of dialysis. *Artif Organs* 2003;18(12):880–887.
5. Arieff AI. Dialysis disequilibrium syndrome: current concepts on pathogenesis and prevention. *Kidney Int* 1994; 45(3):629–635.
6. Kao CH, Hsu YH, Wang SJ. Delayed gastric emptying in patients with CKD. *Nucl Med Commun* 1996;17(2):164–167.
7. Van Vlem B, Schoonjans R, Vanholder R, et al. Delayed gastric emptying in dyspeptic chronic hemodialysis patients. *Am J Kidney Dis* 2000;36(5):962–968.
8. Soffer EE, Geva B, Helman C, et al. Gastric emptying in CKD patients on hemodialysis. *J Clin Gastroenterol* 1987; 9:651–653.
9. Wright RA, Clemente R, Wathen R. Gastric emptying in patients with CKD receiving hemodialysis. *Arch Intern Med* 1984;144:495–496.
10. Verne GN, Sninsky CA. Diabetes and the gastrointestinal tract. *Gastroenterol Clin North Am* 1998;27(4):861–vii.
11. Bityutskiy LP, Soykan I, McCallum RW. Viral gastroparesis: a subgroup of idiopathic gastroparesis—clinical characteristics and long-term outcomes. *Am J Gastroenterol* 1997; 92(9):1501–1504.
12. Oh JJ, Kim CH. Gastroparesis after a presumed viral illness: clinical and laboratory features and natural history. *Mayo Clin Proc* 1990;65(5):636–642.
13. Brown-Cartwright D, Smith HJ, Feldman M. Gastric emptying of an indigestible solid in patients with end-stage renal disease on continuous ambulatory peritoneal dialysis. *Gastroenterology* 1988;95:49–51.
14. Johnson WJ. The digestive tract. In: Daugirdas JT, Ing TS, eds. *Handbook of Dialysis,* 2d ed. New York: Little, Brown, 1994:623–634.
15. Camilleri M. Gastroenterology: gastrointestinal motility disorders. In: Dale DC, Federman DD, eds. *Scientific American Medicine*. New York: Web MD, 2003.
16. Lacy BE, Zayat EN, Crowell MD, Schuster MM. Botulinum toxin for the treatment of gastroparesis: a preliminary report. *Am J Gastroenterol* 2002;97(6):1548–1552.
17. Lee JS, Camilleri M, Zinsmeister AR, et al. A valid, accurate, office based non-radioactive test for gastric emptying of solids. *Gut* 2000;46(6):768–773.
18. Thomforde GM, Camilleri M, Phillips SF, Forstrom LA. Evaluation of an inexpensive screening scintigraphic test of gastric emptying. *J Nucl Med* 1995;36(1):93–96.
19. Forster J, Sarosiek I, Delcore R, et al. Gastric pacing is a new surgical treatment for gastroparesis. *Am J Surg* 2003; 182(6):676–681.
20. Horowitz M, O'Donovan D, Jones KL, et al. Gastric emptying in diabetes: clinical significance and treatment. *Diabet Med* 2002;19(3):177–194.
21. Minnaganti VR, Cunha BA. Infections associated with uremia and dialysis. *Infect Dis Clin North Am* 2001;15(2): 385–406, viii.
22. Etemad B. Gastrointestinal complications of renal failure. *Gastroenterol Clin North Am* 1998;27:875–892.
23. Pitchumoni CS, Arguello P, Agarwal N, Yoo J. Acute pancreatitis in CKD. *Am J Gastroenterol* 1996;91(12): 2477–2482.
24. Rutsky EA, Robards M, Van Dyke JA, Rostand SG. Acute pancreatitis in patients with end-stage renal disease without transplantation. *Arch Intern Med* 1986;146(9):1741–1745.
25. Lindberg J, Martin KJ, Gonzalez EA, et al. A long-term, multicenter study of the efficacy and safety of paricalcitol in end-stage renal disease. *Clin Nephrol* 2001;56(4):315–323.
26. Quigley EM, Hasler WL, Parkman HP, Haster WL. AGA technical review on nausea and vomiting. *Gastroenterology* 2001;120(1):263–286.
27. Diamond SM, Emmett M, Henrich WL. Bowel infarction as a cause of death in dialysis patients. *JAMA* 1986;256: 2545–2547.
28. John AS, Tueff SD, Kerstein MD. Nonocclusive mesenteric infarction in hemodialysis patients. *J Am Coll Surg* 2000; 190(1):84–88.
29. Kanai H, Kashiwagi M, Hirakata H, et al. Chronic intestinal pseudo-obstruction due to dialysis-related amyloid deposition in the propria muscularis in a hemodialysis patient. *Clin Nephrol* 2000;535(5):394–399.
30. Bruno M, van Dorp WT, Ferwerda J, et al. Colonic pseudo-obstruction due to beta$_2$-microglobulin amyloidosis after long-term haemodialysis. *Eur J Gastroenterol Hepatol* 1998;10(8):717–720.
31. Marx J. *Rosen's Emergency Medicine: Concepts and Clinical Practice,* 5th ed. St. Louis: Mosby, 2002.
32. Maganti K, Onyemere K, Jones MP. Oral erythromycin and symptomatic relief of gastroparesis: a systematic review. *Am J Gastroenterol* 2003;98(2):259–263.
33. Braden B, Enghofer M, Schaub M, et al. Long-term cisapride treatment improves diabetic gastroparesis but not

glycaemic control. *Aliment Pharmacol Ther* 2002;16(7): 1341–1346.

34. Camilleri M, Alagelada JR, Bell TL, et al. Effect of six weeks of treatment with cisapride in gastroparesis and intestinal pseudoobstruction. *Gastroenterology* 1989;96(3): 704–712.

35. Abell T, Camilleri M, DiMagno EP, et al. Long-term efficacy of oral cisapride in symptomatic upper gut dysmotility. *Dig Dis Sci* 1991;36(5):616–620.

36. Erbas T, Varoglu E, Erbas B, et al. Comparison of metoclopramide and erythromycin in the treatment of diabetic gastroparesis. *Diabetes Care* 1993;16(11):1511–1514.

37. McHugh S, Lico S, Diamant NE. Cisapride vs metoclopramide. An acute study in diabetic gastroparesis. *Dig Dis Sci* 1992;37(7):997–1001.

38. Lux G, Katschinski M, Ludwig S, et al. The effect of cisapride and metoclopramide on human digestive and interdigestive antroduodenal motility. *Scand J Gastroenterol* 1994; 29(12):1105–1110.

39. Patterson D, Abell T, Rothstein R, et al. A double-blind multicenter comparison of domperidone and metoclopramide in the treatment of diabetic patients with symptoms of gastroparesis. *Am J Gastroenterol* 1999;94(5):1230–1234.

40. Silvers D, Kipnes M, Broadstone V, et al. Domperidone in the management of symptoms of diabetic gastroparesis: efficacy, tolerability, and quality-of-life outcomes in a multicenter controlled trial. DOM-USA-5 Study Group. *Clin Ther* 1998;20(3):438–453.

41. Prakash A, Wagstaff AJ. Domperidone. A review of its use in diabetic gastropathy. *Drugs* 1998;56(3):429–445.

42. Horowitz M, Su YC, Rayner CK, Jones KL. Gastroparesis: prevalence, clinical significance and treatment. *Can J Gastroenterol* 2001;15(12):805–813.

43. Rabine JC, Barnett JL. Management of the patient with gastroparesis. *J Clin Gastroenterol* 2001;32(1):11–18.

44. Cunney RJ, Magee CM, McManara C, et al. *Clostridium difficile* colitis associated with CKD. *Nephrol Dial Transplant* 1998;13(11):2842–2846.

45. Yousuf K, Saklayen MG, Markert RJ, et al. *Clostridium difficile*–associated diarrhea and chronic renal insufficiency. *South Med J* 2002;95:681–683.

46. Popoola J, Swann A, Warwick G. Clostridium difficile in patients with renal failure—management of an outbreak using biotherapy. *Nephrol Dial Transplant* 2000;15(5): 571–574.

47. Esforzado N, Poch E, Almirall J, et al. Cytomegalovirus colitis in CKD. *Clin Nephrol* 1993;39(5):275–278.

48. Ali MS, Mahmoud LA, Abaza BE, Ramadan MA. Intestinal spore-forming protozoa among patients suffering from CKD. *J Egypt Soc Parasitol* 2000;30(1):93–100.

49. Turkcapar N, Kutlay S, Nergizoglu G, et al. Prevalence of *Cryptosporidium* infection in hemodialysis patients. *Nephron* 2002;90(3):344–346.

50. Camilleri M. Gastrointestinal problems in diabetes. *Endocrinol Metab Clin* 1996;25(2):361–379.

51. Valdovinos MA, Camilleri M, Zimmerman BR. Chronic diarrhea in diabetes mellitus: mechanisms and an approach to diagnosis and treatment. *Mayo Clin Proc* 1993;68(7): 691–672.

52. Fedorak RN, Field M, Chang EB. Treatment of diabetic diarrhea with clonidine. *Ann Intern Med* 1985;102(2): 197–199.

53. Zuckerman GR, Cornette GL, Clouse RE, Harter HR. Upper gastrointestinal bleeding in patients with CKD. *Ann Intern Med* 1985;102:588–592.

54. Wasse H, Gillen DL, Ball AM, et al. Risk factors for upper gastrointestinal bleeding among end-stage renal disease patients. *Kidney Int* 2003;64(4):1455–1461.

55. Margolis DM, Saylor JL, Geisse G, et al. Upper gastrointestinal disease in CKD. A prospective evaluation. *Arch Intern Med* 1978;138:1214–1217.

56. Musola R, Franzin G, Mora R, Manfrini C. Prevalence of gastroduodenal lesions in uremic patients undergoing dialysis and after renal transplantation. *Gastrointest Endosc* 1984;30:343–346.

57. Ala-Kaila K. Upper gastrointestinal findings in CKD. *Scand J Gastroenterol* 1987;22:372–376.

58. Jutabha R, Jensen DM. Management of upper gastrointestinal bleeding in the patient with chronic liver disease. *Med Clin North Am* 1996;80:1035–1068.

59. Kang JY. The gastrointestinal tract in uremia. *Dig Dis Sci* 1993;38:257–268.

60. Paronen I, Ala-Kaila K, Rantala I, et al. Gastric parietal, chief, and G-cell densities in CKD. *Scand J Gastroenterol* 1991;26:696–700.

61. Ravelli AM. Gastrointestinal function in CKD. *Pediatr Nephrol* 1995;9:756–762.

62. Itoh K. [Gastric haemorrhagic mucosal lesion in uremic patients.] *Nippon Rinsho* 1998;56:2391–2395.

63. Etemad B. Gastrointestinal complications of renal failure. *Gastroenterol Clin North Am* 1998;27:875–892.

64. Margolis DM, Saylor JL, Geisse G, et al. Upper gastrointestinal disease in CKD. A prospective evaluation. *Arch Intern Med* 1978;138:1214–1217.

65. Goldstein H, Murphy D, Sokol A, Rubini ME. Gastric acid secretion in patients undergoing chronic dialysis. *Arch Intern Med* 1967;120:645–653.

66. Dinoso VPJ, Murthy SN, Saris AL, et al. Gastric and pancreatic function in patients with end-stage renal disease. *J Clin Gastroenterol* 1982;4:321–324.

67. Petersen H. The prevalence of gastro-oesophageal reflux disease. *Scand J Gastroenterol Suppl* 1995;211:5–6.

68. Davenport A, Shallcross TM, Crabtree JE, et al. Prevalence of *Helicobacter pylori* in patients with end-stage renal failure and renal transplant recipients. *Nephron* 1991;59: 597–601.

69. Kang JY. Peptic ulcer in hepatic cirrhosis and renal failure. *J Gastroenterol Hepatol* 1994;9(suppl 1):S20–S23.

70. Nakajima F, Sakaguchi M, Amemoto K, et al. Helicobacter pylori in patients receiving long-term dialysis. *Am J Nephrol* 2002;22(5–6):468–472.

71. Gralnek IM, Jensen DM, Kovacs TO, et al. An economic analysis of patients with active arterial peptic ulcer hemorrhage treated with endoscopic heater probe, injection sclerosis, or surgery in a prospective, randomized trial. *Gastrointest Endosc* 1997;46:105–112.

72. Gralnek IM, Jensen DM, Gornbein J, et al. Clinical and economic outcomes of individuals with severe peptic ulcer he-

morrhage and nonbleeding visible vessel: an analysis of two prospective clinical trials. *Am J Gastroenterol* 1998;93: 2047–2056.

73. Navab F, Masters P, Subramani R, et al. Angiodysplasia in patients with renal insufficiency. *Am J Gastroenterol* 1989; 84:1297–1301.

74. Dave PB, Romeu J, Antonelli A, Eiser AR. Gastrointestinal telangiectasias. A source of bleeding in patients receiving hemodialysis. *Arch Intern Med* 1984;144:1781–1783.

75. Heunisch C, Resnick DJ, Vitello JM, Martin SJ. Conjugated estrogens for the management of gastrointestinal bleeding secondary to uremia of acute renal failure. *Pharmacotherapy* 1998;18:210–217.

76. Vujkovac B, Lavre J, Sabovic M. Successful treatment of bleeding from colonic angiodysplasias with tranexamic acid in a hemodialysis patient. *Am J Kidney Dis* 1998;31: 536–538.

77. Llach J, Bordas JM, Salmeron JM, et al. A prospective randomized trial of heater probe thermocoagulation versus injection therapy in peptic ulcer hemorrhage. *Gastrointest Endosc* 1996;43:117–120.

78. Laine L, Estrada R. Randomized trial of normal saline solution injection versus bipolar electrocoagulation for treatment of patients with high-risk bleeding ulcers: is local tamponade enough? *Gastrointest Endosc* 2002;55(1):6–10.

79. Jensen DM, Kovacs TO, Jutabha R, et al. Randomized trial of medical or endoscopic therapy to prevent recurrent ulcer hemorrhage in patients with adherent clots. *Gastroenterology* 2002;123(2):407–413.

80. Marcuard SP, Weinstock JV. Gastrointestinal angiodysplasia in renal failure. *J Clin Gastroenterol* 1988;10:482–484.

81. Boley SJ, Sammartano R, Adams A, et al. On the nature and etiology of vascular ectasias of the colon. Degenerative lesions of aging. *Gastroenterology* 1977;72:650–660.

82. Messmann H. Lower gastrointestinal bleeding—the role of endoscopy. *Dig Dis* 2003;21(1):19–24.

83. Korzets Z, Ben-Chitrit S, Bernheim J. Nonocclusive mesenteric infarction in continuous ambulatory peritoneal dialysis. *Nephron* 1996;74:415–418.

84. Flobert C, Cellier C, Berger A, et al. Right colonic involvement is associated with severe forms of ischemic colitis and occurs frequently in patients with CKD requiring hemodialysis. *Am J Gastroenterol* 2000;95(1):195–198.

85. Fabbian F, Brezzi B, Cavallini L, et al. [Mesenteric ischemia in hemodialysis patients: case report and review of the literature] L'ischemia mesenterica negli emodializzati: descrizione di un caso e revisione della letteratura. *G Ital Nefrol* 2002;19(4):476–478.

86. Hung KH, Lee CT, Lam KK, et al. Ischemic bowel disease in chronic dialysis patients. *Changgeng Yi Xue Za Zhi* 1999; 22:82–87.

87. Jensen DM, Machicado GA, Jutabha R, Kovacs TO. Urgent colonoscopy for the diagnosis and treatment of severe diverticular hemorrhage. *N Engl J Med* 2000;342(2):78–82.

88. Jutabha R, Jensen DM. Diagnosis and treatment of gastrointestinal bleeding of unknown etiology. In: Snape WJ, ed. *Consultations in Gastroenterology*. Philadelphia: Saunders, 1996:155–167.

89. Appleyard M, Glukhovsky A, Swain P. Wireless-capsule diagnostic endoscopy for recurrent small-bowel bleeding. *N Engl J Med* 2001;344(3):232–233.

90. Costamagna G, Shah SK, Riccioni ME, et al. A prospective trial comparing small bowel radiographs and video capsule endoscopy for suspected small bowel disease. *Gastroenterology* 2002;123(4):999–1005.

91. Eliakim R, Fischer D, Suissa A, et al. Wireless capsule video endoscopy is a superior diagnostic tool in comparison to barium follow-through and computerized tomography in patients with suspected Crohn's disease. *Eur J Gastroenterol Hepatol* 2003;15(4):363–367.

92. Hahne M, Adamek HE, Schilling D, Riemann JF. Wireless capsule endoscopy in a patient with obscure occult bleeding. *Endoscopy* 2002;34(7):588–590.

93. Liangpunsakul S, Chadalawada V, Rex DK, et al. Wireless capsule endoscopy detects small bowel ulcers in patients with normal results from state of the art enteroclysis. *Am J Gastroenterol* 2003;98(6):1295–1298.

94. Gralnek IM, Jensen DM, Kovacs TO, et al. The economic impact of esophageal variceal hemorrhage: cost-effectiveness implications of endoscopic therapy. *Hepatology* 1999; 29:44–50.

95. Tang SJ, Jutabha R. Recurrent hemorrhage caused by ileal carcinoid. *Gastrointest Endosc* 2002;55(4):559.

96. Tang SJ, Jutabha R, Jensen DM. Push enteroscopy for recurrent gastrointestinal hemorrhage due to jejunal anastomotic varices: a case report and review of the literature. *Endoscopy* 2002;34(9):735–737.

97. Kanwal F, Dulai G, Jensen DM, et al. Major stigmata of recent hemorrhage on rectal ulcers in patients with severe hematochezia: endoscopic diagnosis, treatment, and outcomes. *Gastrointest Endosc* 2003;57(4):462–468.

98. Lipschutz DE, Easterling RE. Spontaneous perforation of the colon in CKD. *Arch Intern Med* 1973;132:758–759.

99. Adams PL, Rutsky EA, Rostand SG, Han SY. Lower gastrointestinal tract dysfunction in patients receiving long-term hemodialysis. *Arch Intern Med* 1982;142:303–306.

100. Schneider TA, Longo WE, Ure T, Vernava AM III. Mesenteric Ischemia. Acute arterial syndromes. *Dis Colon Rectum* 1994;37:1163.

101. de Dombal FT. Acute abdominal pain in the elderly. *J Clin Gastroenterol* 1994;19:331.

102. Silen W. *Cope's Early Diagnosis of the Acute Abdomen*. Oxford, UK: Oxford University Press, 1990.

103. Bugliosi TF, Meloy TD, Vukov LF. Acute abdominal pain in the elderly. *Ann Emerg Med* 1990;19:1383.

104. Marco CA, Schoenfeld CN, Keyl PM, et al. Abdominal pain in geriatric emergency patients: variables associated with adverse outcomes. *Acad Emerg Med* 1998;5:1163.

105. Balthazar EJ, Birnbaum BA, Yee J, et al. Acute appendicitis: CT and ultrasound correlation in one hundred patients. *Radiology* 1994;190:31.

106. Walsch PF, Crawford D, Crossing FT, et al. The value of immediate ultrasound in acute abdominal conditions: a critical appraisal. *Clin Radiol* 1990;42:47.

Hematologic Aspects of Chronic Kidney Disease

Anatole Besarab
Jason Biederman

The kidney has three major functions: (1) to produce urine and thereby excrete toxic substances and regulate the concentration of solutes in the blood at optimal levels; (2) to produce and secrete hormones that regulate blood flow (renin) and vascular tone (prostaglandins), stimulate RBC production (erythropoietin), and participate in calcium and bone metabolism (1,25-dihydroxycholecalciferol); and (3) to perform a variety of metabolic functions (gluconeogenesis, reabsorption of amino acids, conjugation of drugs). As a result of decline in these functions, chronic kidney disease (CKD) is associated with a variety of disorders resulting from the deleterious effects of solute retention, from the absence of renally produced hormones, particularly erythropoietin, and, in some cases, from the dysfunctional overproduction of renin, resulting in severe hypertension. The most characteristic hematologic abnormality in CKD is anemia, which results primarily from the failure of the kidneys' endocrine function. It persists as a significant problem in many patients receiving adequate dialysis prescriptions. By contrast, dysfunction of the other hematologic elements is less consistent and influenced in large part by the dialysis procedure. This chapter reviews the pathogenesis of the anemia associated with CKD, discusses the diagnosis and therapy of this anemia in patients with CKD, and outlines selected aspects of granulocyte and platelet function in patients with CKD.

THE ANEMIA OF CHRONIC KIDNEY DISEASE: MAGNITUDE OF THE PROBLEM

Several previous reviews on the anemia of CKD and recombinant human erythropoietin (rHuEpo, epoetin) have been published.[1] In this section, we review the pathophysiology of the anemia associated with renal disease; summarize the physiology, structure, and function of erythropoietin; and consider dosing and economic aspects as they relate to the use of epoetin to correct anemia in CKD patients. Although epoetin is now being used to treat a variety of hypoproliferative anemias (chronic infections, inflammatory and malignant diseases), to augment autologous blood donation, and to treat anemia in heart failure, the primary indication for epoetin remains the anemia associated with renal disease. For purposes of further discussion, the five-stage classification of kidney disease severity developed by the Kidney Disease Outcomes Quality Initiative (K/DOQI) is used herein.[2] This nomenclature replaces about 51 synonyms that have been used (e.g., chronic renal or kidney disease, insufficiency, failure, etc). Noting that serum creatinine (SCr) levels are imperfect indicators of the severity of kidney disease, K/DOQI uses a formula developed from and validated within the Modification of Diet in Renal Disease Study[3] to calculate the glomerular filtration rates (GFRs) per 1.73 m^2. It is estimated that up to 25 million people in the United States have CKD of variable degree. Astor and coworkers[4] have estimated that up to 3 million individuals with CKD not requiring renal replacement therapy may have anemia, defined as a Hgb (Hgb) < 12 g/dL in men and < 11 g/dL in women. The prevalence of anemia among Mexican Americans and African Americans with CKD is higher than that among non-Hispanic Caucasians, reaching levels of 16 to 18 percent in stage 4 and 42 to 75 percent in stage 5, respectively.

CLINICAL AND LABORATORY FEATURES

Circulating Blood

Anemia has remained one of the most characteristic and visible manifestations of CKD for over 150 years. Richard Bright[5] first commented on the pallor of patients with renal disease in 1836. Since then, many observers have attempted to characterize and explain the underlying anemia. The severity of anemia that is frequently associated with kidney disease (renal anemia) typically progresses in parallel with the deterioration of renal function[6] and profoundly influences morbidity and mortality, particularly in those with end-stage renal disease (ESRD).[7,8] Even among patients with serum creatinine levels <2 mg/dL, 45 percent have a hematocrit (Hct) <36 percent and 8 percent have a Hct <30 percent.[9] As shown in Fig. 26–1, in the early stages of CKD, the kidney produces erythropoietin in the expected fashion. Therefore, inadequate erythropoietin production is not the initial reason for renal anemia. At this stage, suppression of red blood cell (RBC) synthesis by poorly defined toxins or from shortened RBC survival dominates mechanistically. At more advanced stages of disease, the production of erythropoietin decreases and its levels become lower than those expected for the degree of anemia. At this stage, true erythropoietin deficiency exists. Follow-

ing bilateral nephrectomy, the hematocrit of patients with CKD drops and then stabilizes, indicating that even the end-stage kidney continues to produce some erythropoietin after its excretory function has largely ceased.[10] However, as GFR approaches 20 percent of normal, the great majority of patients become anemic, with Hct <30 vol%.[8] Before the advent of epoetin therapy, a predictable progression of anemia in individual patients could usually be observed as the degree of CKD increased. In late stage 5 CKD, as the individual approaches renal replacement therapy (RRT), either by dialysis or transplantation, the Hct attains a plateau that varies little unless complicating events ensue or epoetin therapy is instituted. Patients with polycystic kidneys frequently have an increased red cell mass prior to the onset of CKD, and their anemia frequently progresses less rapidly as CKD advances than it does in comparably uremic patients with other renal diseases.[11] The uncomplicated anemia of patients with CKD is normocytic and normochromic.[12] Echinocytes or burr cells are the most often observed morphologic RBC change, their frequency correlating with the severity of CKD[13]; this change is considered to be characteristic of CKD. However, even normal cells can undergo a reversible transformation to spiculed, burr cell–like echinocytes when exposed to a glass surface or suspended in incubated plasma.[14] Echinocytes seen in patients with advanced CKD are, at least in part, artifactual and do not circulate as such in blood. Grossly deformed cells, however, such as acanthocytes with a few large spicules or fragmented schistocytes, are undoubtedly formed in the microcirculation in vivo.[15]

Bone Marrow

The bone marrow of patients with end-stage renal disease (ESRD) is usually "normally" cellular, with a normal appearance and maturation sequence of all cellular elements, including the nucleated red cells.[16] The "normality" of the marrow during anemia is misleading, however, because—in the context of anemia—a compensatory increase in erythroid activity is expected. The amount of erythropoiesis in the marrow is actually decreased relative to that expected for the severity of anemia. This is best appreciated by transfusion to near normal Hgb, following which markedly reduced marrow erythropoiesis develops. Following a drop in the Hct due to acute blood loss or after an episode of prolonged hypoxia, the amount of erythropoiesis in the marrow of CKD patients may increase to supernormal levels, although not to the same extent as in comparably affected nonuremic patients. The marrow erythropoiesis can be described as predominantly effective,[17,18] since the corrected reticulocyte count [percentage reticulocyte x (Hct/45)] correlates with the amount of erythroid activity in the bone marrow, and the measured rate of plasma iron turnover is commensurate with the ^{59}Fe incorporated into RBCs. Older

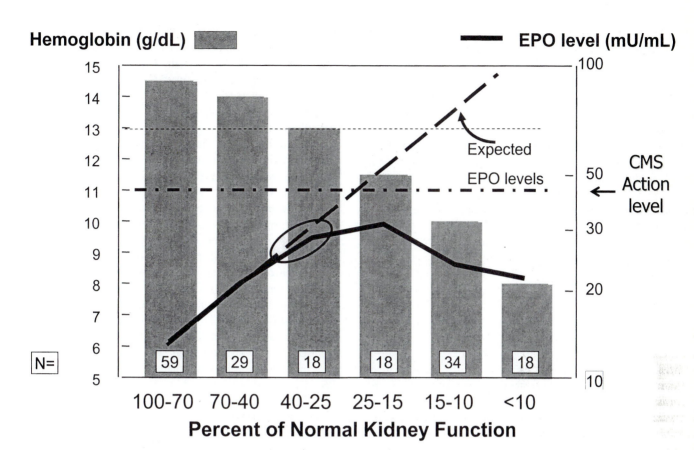

Adapted from Radtke HW et al *Blood* 1979;54:877
and Erslev AJ. *N Engl J Med* 1991;324:1339

Figure 26–1. Anemia in CKD. The mean Hgb levels are provided by the bars. The actual erythropoietin levels in CKD are depicted by the solid line, whereas the expected levels for the degree of anemia are shown by the dashed line. Note that in CKD, inability to produce sufficient erythropoietin for the degree of anemia (oval area) occurs in fairly advanced disease, corresponding to 60 to 75 percent of renal function.

studies suggest a modest decrease in the RBC life span in uremic patients.[19] More recent studies in well-dialyzed patients indicate that the RBC life span can approach normal if blood losses associated with hemodialysis are avoided.[20]

Oxygen Transport

Changes in RBC oxygen-carrying capacity in ESRD subjects have been examined. When measured, the capacity of RBCs to function as oxygen carriers is basically unimpaired.[21] Changes in the oxygen affinity of RBCs in ESRD have been proposed to contribute to some of the asthenic or intradialytic symptoms present in ESRD patients. The changes in the oxygen affinity of RBCs occur as a result of alterations in the concentration of crucial intraerythrocyte organic phosphates.[22,23] The Hgb-oxygen affinity of uremic erythrocytes, however, is decreased to a greater extent than that of erythrocytes from comparably anemic nonuremic patients. In well-dialyzed patients, the intracellular concentration of 2,3-diphosphoglycerate (2,3-DPG) is appropri-

ately increased in response to the level of anemia and the mild hyperphosphatemia,[22] and the affinity of Hgb for oxygen is appropriately decreased.[22] The effect of increased 2,3-DPG in erythrocytes from nonuremic anemic patients is offset by an increase in intracellular pH (mild respiratory alkalosis), but this pH shift does not occur in erythrocytes from uremic patients.[23] Rather, systemic metabolic acidosis from CKD (usually mild) further augments this decrease in oxygen affinity by shifting the oxygen dissociation curve to the right (Bohr effect). These combined effects favor the delivery of oxygen to peripheral tissues even though acidosis also tends to decrease both glycolysis and the concentration of intracellular organic phosphates, both of which tend to increase the oxygen affinity of Hgb.[22] Hgb-oxygen affinity increases only slightly following hemodialysis, as pH increases. Overall, the effect of decreased oxygen affinity on oxygen transport in hemodialysis patients is minimal, delivery of oxygen to peripheral tissues is slightly augmented, and the changes do not explain intra- or interdialytic symptoms.

Iron deficiency and hypophosphatemia are probably of more importance in oxygen delivery and the genesis of any intradialytic or postdialysis symptoms. Iron deficiency has a negative impact on exercise performance independent of the degree of anemia present.[24] The frequent occurrence of iron deficiency in ESRD patients[25] probably contributes directly to the asthenia seen in the dialysis population. Other consequences of ESRD may contribute to altered oxygen delivery. Aggressive use of phosphate binders, defects in enteral phosphate absorption, and hyperalimentation—in concert with dialytic phosphate removal—can result in hypophosphatemia. This reduces the concentration of intracellular organic phosphate compounds,[26] resulting in an increase in the oxygen affinity of Hgb and a temporary decrease in tissue oxygenation.

ERYTHROPOIESIS

Historical Perspective

A relation between tissue hypoxia and the production of RBCs was first proposed in the nineteenth century[27]; at the beginning of the twentieth century, a hypoxia-induced feedback mechanism involving a hematopoietin was proposed.[28] During the next 50 years, this hypothesis gained firm support, with solid experimental data generated by Reissmann[29] and by Erslev.[30] Reismann used parabiotic rats to demonstrate that hypoxia in one animal stimulated erythropoiesis in the normoxic partner.[29] Erslev transfused anemic rabbit plasma into normal recipient rabbits and demonstrated the unequivocal role of "intermediate humoral factor" in erythropoiesis.[30] By 1957, Jacobson and coworkers were able to establish that, in the adult animal, the primary site of erythropoietin production is the kidney.[31] Bilateral nephrectomy virtually abolishes erythropoietin production in humans.[32,33]

Understanding of erythropoiesis progressed before the structure of the erythropoietin molecule was characterized and before the intrarenal site of production was known. Goldwasser and coworkers first purified[34] and then sequenced[35] the amino acids of erythropoietin, making it possible to construct a cDNA library, which allowed the identification and cloning of the erythropoietin gene.[36,37] Transfection of the human gene into Chinese hamster ovary cells allowed mass production of recombinant erythropoietin (epoetin) for clinical use.[37]

Normal Erythropoiesis

Circulating erythropoietin originates predominantly from the kidney (90 percent), with a smaller contribution from the hepatic parenchyma (10 percent). Erythropoietin mRNA has also been detected in the spleen, lung, testis, and brain, but these sites do not secrete erythropoietin under normal conditions. Bilateral nephrectomy virtually abolishes the production of EPO.[31–33] In situ hybridization techniques have localized the mRNA to interstitial cells (also known as type I interstitial cells)[38,39] located near the base of proximal tubular cells, predominantly in the renal cortex.[38] Under conditions of normal oxygenation, interstitial cells positive for EPO mRNA are limited to the deep cortex and outer medulla. With increasing anemia, the positive cells increase in number and spread into the superficial cortex.[39] However, some studies suggest a major role for the cells of the proximal tubule in the production of erythropoietin.[40]

Erythropoietin has its primary effect in the bone marrow. The pluripotent hematopoietic stem cell is capable of forming erythrocytes, leukocytes, and megakaryocytes.[41,42] Under appropriate stimuli, these primitive cells have the capacity for both self-renewal and differentiation into committed progenitor cells. Renewal appears to occur by chance "stochastically"[43] and is initiated primarily by lineage, nonspecific cytokines such as interleukin-3 (IL-3), stem cell factor, insulin-like growth factor 1, and granulocyte-macrophage colony stimulating factor (GM-CSF) (Fig. 26–2).

The transformation of a multipotential stem cell into a mature RBC occurs in two morphologically distinct stages, as depicted in Fig. 26–2.[44] The first stage begins with small mononuclear cells displaying a specific glycophosphoprotein CD34 on their surface,[45] and then sequentially includes the committed erythroid progenitor, the primitive and mature burst-forming unit-erythroid (BFU-E), and the colony-forming unit-erythroid (CFU-E). In the second or precursor stage, the cells appear as morphologically recognizable erythroblasts that mature into pronormoblasts and daughter erythrocytes. Most multipotential committed progenitor cells exist in the resting G_0 stage of the cell cycle[46] and are stimulated into the G_1 stage by IL-1 and IL-6 as well as granulocyte colony-stimulating factor (G-CSF). Under the influence of IL-3 and GM-CSF, they differentiate into primitive BFU-E. Peripheral demands for cellular production can be met only after this transformation of a multipotential stem cell to a unipotential progenitor cell. At this stage, the cells have lost most of their capacity for self-renewal but have gained receptors for erythropoietin, which now becomes essential for the multiplication and differentiation of the BFU-E and CFU-E. There is an increasing dependence on and sensitivity to the effects of erythropoietin with the progressive maturation from primitive BFU-E into CFU-E,[47–49] to the point where the CFU-E will survive and differentiate into a pronormoblast only in the presence of erythropoietin. In mice lacking the erythropoietin and erythropoietin receptor genes, BFU-E and CFU-E are produced to normal levels, indicating that stimulation by erythropoietin is not necessary for commitment to erythroid progenitors; but erythropoietin stimulation is essential for

Normal erythropoiesis

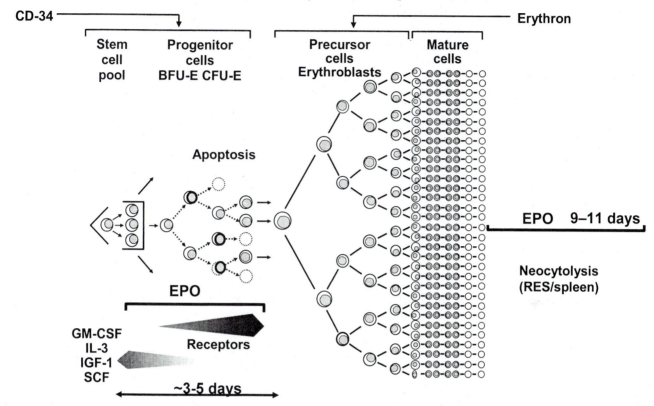

Figure 26–2. Normal erythropoiesis. See text for description. *(Adapted from numerous sources, including Schuster SJ, Caro J.[44])*

CFU-E survival and proliferation. Insulin or insulin-like growth factor 1 (IGF-1) is also required for CFU-E growth.[50] In summary, erythropoietin does not affect division or differentiation of the uncommitted pluripotent stem cell, but its constant presence is critical to the sustenance, multiplication, and differentiation of the committed erythroid progenitors. This concept is key, as discussed further on, with regard to clinical dosing practices and the choice of the optimal route for the administration of epoetin.

Several other factors—such as androgens, thyroid hormone, somatomedin, and catecholamines—appear to augment the growth of CFU-E, but they are not essential.[51] Other cytokines—including IL-1α and 1β, IL-2, tumor necrosis factor alpha (TNF-α), and transforming growth factor beta (TGF-β) have a negative effect on erythropoiesis.[52,53] These cytokines are significant mediators in the anemia of chronic disease, may be activated by certain types of dialysis, and are invariably present during acute infection or inflammation. Their inhibitory effects produce resistance to exogenous erythropoietin in CKD patients.

Erythropoietin exerts its signal through the erythropoietin receptor (p66), a 55-kDa transmembrane protein.[54] Erythropoietin receptors are mainly expressed at the CFU-E

and proerythroblast stages, and receptor number decreases during the final stages of erythroid differentiation, such that reticulocytes and erythrocytes are devoid of erythropoietin receptors.[45–48] Agents are being developed that are not epoetin-like at all, consist of simple polypeptides, but can activate the receptor by molecular mimicry.[55] Once activated, the receptor dimerizes, and tyrosine kinase activity via constitutively expressed JAK2 leads to phosphorylation of intracellular proteins,[56] followed by activation of several signaling pathways (which include STAT, RAS, and phosphoinositol 3-kinase).[57] The signal transducer and activator of transcription (STAT) pathway is the most important. STAT5 is a latent cytoplasmic transcription factor that, once activated via phosphorylation by JAK2, dimerizes, translocates into the nucleus, and binds to specific DNA sequences, allowing transcription of the respective gene products. Additionally, two tyrosine phosphatases, SHP-1 and SHP-2, play a role in erythropoietin-induced signaling and hence in stimulating cell proliferation, the former negatively and the latter positively.[58,59] Erythropoietin has also been shown to modulate calcium influx in erythroid cells through a transient receptor potential channel.[60] Although the exact signals or pathways are still poorly understood, it is unlikely that the ultimate signals are transcription factors for genes involved in the synthesis of globin or other mature erythroid proteins; it is more likely that these signals maintain the viability of progenitor cells.[50] In the absence of erythropoietin, such cells undergo apoptosis and die before they reach the precursor cell stage. The anuclear cells in Fig. 26–2 represent the process of apoptosis when erythropoietin becomes unavailable. In the presence of erythropoietin, they proliferate and eventually transform into precursor cells.

Erythroid progenitor cells exposed to optimal concentration of growth factors and erythropoietin proliferate luxuriously and produce a "burst" of colonies.[61] The kinetics of progenitor cell proliferation in vivo appears very similar but somewhat more restrained than those in vitro. A BFU-E even in the presence of large amounts of erythropoietin will not produce a burst of thousands of CFU-E but merely 50 to 100 CFU-E.[36] In the presence of a normal concentration of erythropoietin (8 to 18 mU/mL) each BFU-E probably makes no more than 4 to 6 CFU-E.

At a certain level of maturation, the CFU-E becomes activated and the cells are transformed into Hgb-synthesizing morphologically recognizable erythroblasts.[61] Further proliferation and maturation of these cells appear to be unaffected by erythropoietin, proceeding at a fixed rate in the presence of adequate supplies of iron, folate, vitamin B_{12}, pyridoxine, ascorbic acid, and trace elements. As shown in Fig. 26–2, each cell that leaves the CFU-E stage ultimately produces 32 daughter cells that leave the marrow as reticulocytes.

Until recently, erythropoietin was believed to have no effect on cells once they were released from the bone marrow. However, another erythropoietin-dependent mechanism affecting circulating cells has been described. Hemolysis of recently formed RBCs occurs when erythropoietin levels fall rapidly, as with descent from altitude, thus permitting rapid adaptation when RBC mass is excessive for the new environment.[62]

Although erythropoietin's main site of action is the bone marrow, several studies have now convincingly shown that epoetin acts on many tissues that express the erythropoietin receptor. Receptors for erythropoietin have been found in the retina, the central nervous system, vascular endothelial and smooth muscle cells, renal tubular cells, and even the heart myocyte. As reviewed recently by Cavillo et al.,[63] erythropoietin markedly reduces the production and release of proinflammatory cytokines and chemokines and dramatically reduces the influx of inflammatory cells into injured tissue in the brain and heart. Erythropoietin markedly prevents the apoptosis of cultured rat cardiomyocytes exposed to prolonged hypoxia. Finally, erythropoietin reduces the size of myocardial infarction produced in rats and therefore helps to preserve myocardial function. No doubt these areas will offer new applications for epoetin.

Already Ehrenreich et al.[64] have shown that erythropoietin improves clinical outcome when given to patients who have suffered acute cerbrovascular events.

Regulation of Erythropoietin Production and Release

While the molecular mechanisms of oxygen sensing remain incompletely understood, in vitro studies with human hepatoma cells in culture have contributed greatly to our present knowledge. One caveat is that these cells respond to hypoxia by a graded increase in erythropoietin gene expression. This is in contrast to the all-or-none rule (recruitment of additional maximally active cells) characteristic of erythropoietin gene expression in the kidney.

The human erythropoietin gene, on the long arm of chromosome 7, consists of five exons and four introns,[52,65] but it is not directly regulated by molecular oxygen. Multiple transcription factors have been proposed, most of which increase gene expression under conditions of hypoxia. GATA-2, a transcription factor that binds upstream to the erythropoietin promoter and represses gene transcription, is unique, as it is the primary candidate causing normoxic erythropoietin gene repression. In response to high partial pressure of oxygen (PO_2), b-type cytochromes produce reactive oxygen species, such as H_2O_2. Human hepatoma cells decrease H_2O_2 production in response to decreased PO_2. It has been proposed that H_2O_2 inhibits erythropoietin gene expression via activation of GATA-2. Other transcription factors have been implemented, including hepatocyte nuclear factor 4 (HNF-4), chicken ovalbumin upstream promoter-transcription factor 1 (COUP-TF1), TNF-a, IL-1b, and NFKB. However, the most important and best studied regulator is HIF-1.

HIF-1 is a 50-bp hypoxia-inducible factor that acts on a hypoxia-responsive element upstream of the gene.[66,67] Studies have shown that hypoxia induces the production of HIF-1,[68-72] which binds to the oxygen-sensitive enhancer to induce gene transcription of mRNA. HIF factors have now been cloned. HIF-1 regulates the expression of many more genes apart from erythropoietin (NO synthase, endothelin 1, adrenomedullin, vascular endothelial growth factor (VEGF), platelet-derived growth factor (PDGF), glucose transporter 1, heme oxygenase, transferrin). These gene products provide adaptation to a reduced oxygen supply. The HIF molecules exist as heterodimers composed of the 120-kDa alpha and 91 to 94-kDa beta subunits. The HIF-1β subunit is permanently present in all nuclei; hence regulation of HIF-1 is accomplished by abundance of the HIF-1α subunit. Hydroxylation of a proline residue within the HIF-1α domain by specific oxidases is a crucial step in the oxygen-sensing mechanism and eventual gene transcription of epoetin and other proteins.[73] Abundance of HIF-1α is determined primarily by degradation via the ubiquitin-proteasome system in response to normoxia.[74] Degradation requires the presence of a normal von Hippel-Lindau gene protein (pVHL), which binds to HIF-1α and permits rapid proteasomic degradation in the presence of oxygen. Cells lacking pVHL are unable to degrade the factor in the presence of oxygen (hypoxia is mimicked).[75] Recently, superoxide (O_2^-) was found to block the accumulation of HIF-1α protein during hypoxia or $CoCl_2$ incubation (an inducer of erythropoiesis) by enhancing its degradation through ubiquitin-proteasome in renal medullary interstitial cells.

Since the primary function of erythropoietin is to regulate the amount of oxygen available to the body by modulating the production of erythrocytes, it is natural that factors influencing its production do so by directly or indirectly affecting oxygen availability. Erythropoietin production is increased by conditions of reduced oxygen delivery and reduced by states of increased oxygen delivery.

The human erythropoietin gene encodes for a 193–amino acid prohormone, the first 27 amino acids being cleaved prior to secretion. Erythropoietin within the kidney exists as a 166–amino acid peptide with two sulfide bridges and four sites of carbohydrate attachment.[76] Arginine, the terminal amino acid at position 166, is removed prior to secretion. The circulating form of human erythropoietin is a glycosylated protein with 165 amino acids. Four complex carbohydrate chains containing high amounts of sialic acids are linked to the protein at four glycosylation sites—three N-linked and one O-linked, and constitute 40 percent of the molecular weight of 30,400 Da (Fig. 26–3). The disulfide cross-links form two loops needed for biological activity.[77]

Analysis of the secondary structure indicates an alpha-helix content of 50 percent; the tertiary structure resembles that of growth hormone, the structural core containing two antiparallel pairs of alpha-helical bundles.[78] Glycosylation is necessary for cellular secretion.[79] The carbohydrate sialic acid moieties are not essential for erythropoietin's action on bone marrow progenitor cells through receptor binding.[80] However, the sialic acid moieties are very important for the hormone's biological activity in vivo, since they allow erythropoietin to circulate long enough to reach the bone marrow, and for biological action in vivo, to prevent rapid liver clearance.[81] Due to rapid uptake via receptor-mediated endocytosis when galactose residues are exposed, desialated erythropoietin has a half-time ($t_{1/2}$) measured in minutes,[82,83] whereas the fully sialated hormone has, in humans, a $t_{1/2}$ varying from 4 to 12 hours.[84] Despite some differences in carbohydrate structure among the available three first-generation epoetin products (epoetin alfa, beta, and omega) resulting from the specific mammalian system used to perform the glycosylation, their biological activity appears to be the similar. The sialoglycoprotein released into the circulation is highly heat- and pH-resistant.

Erythropoietin Blood Levels

Under steady-state conditions in normal individuals, levels of erythropoietin in a given subject are remarkably constant. Diurnal variations do occur but are of relatively low amplitude (about 20 percent around a baseline of 10 to 17

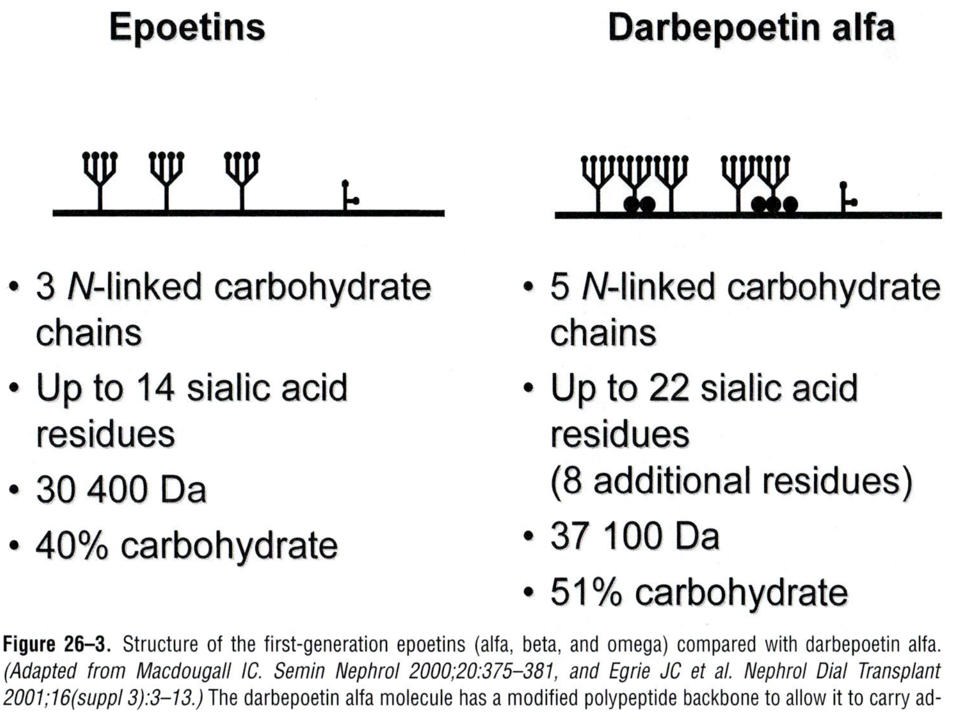

Epoetins

Darbepoetin alfa

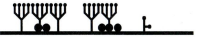

- 3 *N*-linked carbohydrate chains
- Up to 14 sialic acid residues
- 30 400 Da
- 40% carbohydrate

- 5 *N*-linked carbohydrate chains
- Up to 22 sialic acid residues (8 additional residues)
- 37 100 Da
- 51% carbohydrate

Figure 26–3. Structure of the first-generation epoetins (alfa, beta, and omega) compared with darbepoetin alfa. *(Adapted from Macdougall IC. Semin Nephrol 2000;20:375–381, and Egrie JC et al. Nephrol Dial Transplant 2001;16(suppl 3):3–13.)* The darbepoetin alfa molecule has a modified polypeptide backbone to allow it to carry additional carbohydrate side chains and increase the number of sialic acid residues from a maximum of 14 to 22.

mU/mL), with a peak at 1:00 A.M. and a nadir at 1:00 P.M.[85] Individuals with severe obstructive sleep apnea have higher baseline levels and larger amplitude swings, 46 mU/mL and 40 percent, respectively, resulting from prolonged nocturnal hypoxia.[86] Less severe nocturnal hypoxia (shorter duration) does not increase baseline levels.[86] Healthy children appear to have the same levels as healthy adults.[87] Renal erythropoietin production in experimental animals[88] and in humans[89] falls rapidly in response to significant protein deprivation. Hypoxia induces greater erythropoietin production in male than in female rats,[90] and human males excrete more biologically active erythropoietin than do females.[91] However, there are no differences in plasma immunoreactive erythropoietin in male and female humans.[91] The difference in urinary excretion between males and females probably results from differences in renal mass.

Under normal circumstances, plasma levels reflect predominantly renal synthesis of erythropoietin in response to tissue oxygen need. The major site of extrarenal erythropoietin production within the liver is also regulated primarily by the ratio of hepatic oxygen requirements to oxygen supply.[92] In adult animals, the hepatocyte has been identified as the major cell producing erythropoietin.[93,94] Certain factors have a selective effect on extrarenal sites of erythropoietin production. Extrarenal erythropoietin production is increased severalfold following various forms of hepatic injury, such as subtotal hepatectomy[95] and carbon tetrachloride ingestion[96]—effects not seen after nephrectomy or acute tubular necrosis. After hepatic injury, extrarenal erythropoietin production declines immediately but then rises rapidly to supranormal levels during the period of liver regeneration. In acute CKD, whether from tubular necrosis or acute crescenteric glomerulonephritis, deficient production persists; erythropoietin levels do not increase until excretory function recovers and the anemia recovers sluggishly.[97,98]

The most sensitive assay for erythropoietin is a radioimmunoassay (RIA),[98,99] which uses radioiodinated purified erythropoietin as a source of antigen. The results of this assay correlate reasonably well with those of the bioassay. Commercially available RIAs are now widely available to clinicians and have been used to investigate the renal erythropoietin response of a variety of anemias. However, the clinician should be aware that the antisera currently used will measure all immunogenic erythropoietin fragments regardless of their biological or physiologic activity.[100,101]

Integration of the Erythropoiesis Control System

The chief characteristic of the erythropoietin/erythropoiesis growth system is that reduced tissue oxygenation (the error signal) defines the presence of an "inadequate erythron," leading to the production of erythropoietin. The erythron can be viewed as functionally inadequate during chronic hypoxia despite an increase in circulating RBCs (secondary polycythemia). Changes in circulating erythropoietin levels depend almost entirely on hormone synthesis and release.[102,103] The rate of erythropoietin production is determined primarily by the ratio of the oxygen requirements (at or near the site of production) to its oxygen supply.[104,105] As a result, factors that decrease the supply of oxygen to the kidneys (such as decreased renal blood flow, decreased oxygen content of the arterial blood, or increased Hgb oxygen affinity) increase the production of erythropoietin and vice versa (the feedback control loop). Oxygen transport is primarily dependent on the Hgb content of blood. Hgb and Hct are related in a ratio of approximately 1:3. The kidney functions as a "critmeter," since it senses both oxygen tension and extracellular volume.[106] Through erythropoietin, it regulates RBC mass, and through salt and water excretion, it regulates plasma volume. The kidney thus regulates the numerator and denominator of the "crit." It is able to dissociate changes in blood flow from those in oxygenation. The normal Hct of 40 to 50 percent is not random but rather one that maximizes delivery of oxygen to the tissues.

However, the ratio of tissue oxygen demand to supply, through its effects on erythropoietin production, is only a "coarse" regulator of the rate of erythropoiesis. Other modulators are necessary to fine tune the system (the gain of the control system), since without them the RBC mass (total number of erythrocytes) would oscillate due to the prolonged life span of the erythrocytes and the 3- to 5-day lag time between exposure of CFU-E to erythropoietin and the delivery of the mature end product, the erythrocyte, to the bloodstream.

The mechanisms that fine tune erythropoiesis are not well understood. The maximum response of the bone marrow to markedly elevated erythropoietin levels is limited. Although an inverse relationship between the plasma erythropoietin titer and the erythron response to erythropoietin exists, it is not stochiometric. In severe anemias, erythropoietin increases 100- to 1000-fold, yet the maximum RBC production increases only four- to sixfold above the basal rate.[107] Furthermore, a difference in the negative correlations between blood Hgb and the logarithm of erythropoietin concentration is observed in individuals with and without hypoplastic marrows, the levels being significantly higher in those with erythrocytic hypoplasia.[108] These observations have been used as arguments for an additional feedback process independent of tissue PO_2 by which proliferating erythrocytic progenitors lower the blood level of erythropoietin. The rapidity with which these changes in erythropoietin can occur (1 to 2 days) suggests a direct effect on erythropoietin synthesis[109] (see Fig. 26–4) and not merely on consumption by erythrocytic progenitors through the process of internalization and degradation.[110] Furthermore, erythropoietin catabolism appears to be independent of marrow activity.[111]

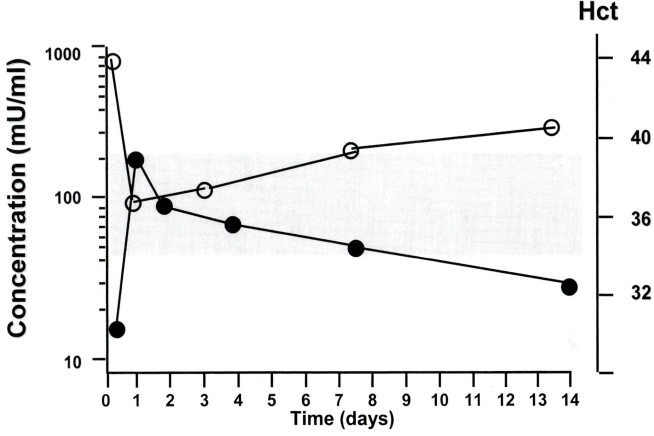

Figure 26–4. Epoetin concentration–time profile following two-unit phlebotomy in normal volunteers. [111.] Erythropoietin scale is logarithmic. Note the rapid decline (threefold) in erythropoietin levels between days 1 and 4 before there is a significant change in Hct.

Nevertheless, in a responsive marrow, the decrease in erythropoietin levels before an increase in RBC mass occurs could result in part from an expansion of progenitors (particularly the CFU-E) and increased removal of erythropoietin by receptor binding. A decrease in erythropoietin levels before a noticeable change in RBC mass does occur in hypoxic rats.[112] Modeling of the kinetics of hematopoietic stem cells during and after hypoxia indicates up to a twofold increase in CFU-E by the fifth day of continuous hypoxia.[113] The decrease in erythropoietin from peak levels is approximately 50 to 70 percent, suggesting that increased consumption could account for this decrease. However, intermittent rather than continuous hypoxia maintains even greater levels, even though the increase in RBC mass (from marrow precursors) is about the same. Jelkmann[114] has suggested that this results from pH-dependent effects on the producing cells themselves or from the weight loss (and therefore the protein deficit) associated with prolonged continuous hypobaric hypoxia. We have also noted rapid (within 24 hours) decreases in erythropoietin levels from peak values in one- and two-unit phlebotomized normal subjects.[115] In these subjects there was no detectable weight loss. Changes in intrarenal oxygen tensions resulting from

intrarenal and systemic hemodynamic changes may therefore explain this rapid return in erythropoietin levels toward normal.

ANEMIA OF CHRONIC KIDNEY DISEASE: PATHOGENESIS

Inadequate Erythropoietin Production

The pathophysiology of the anemia associated with CKD is best understood by considering the homeostatic processes of anemic but otherwise normal individuals. The normal negative biofeedback system induces an increase in erythropoietin production, which is reflected by the plasma erythropoietin concentration (see Fig. 26–5).[107] Autologous blood donors have been studied to determine the response to single or repeated donation of blood. Following donation of 3 to 4 units within a month, plasma erythropoietin levels increase transiently after each donation,[116] with intervening steady-state levels progressively increasing up to twofold baseline and with Hgb decreasing by 2 to 2.5 g/dL from normal values over the same time period.[116,117] As shown in Fig. 26–4, a two-unit phlebotomy, as would occur following acute hemorrhage, reduces Hct from 45 to about 36 percent

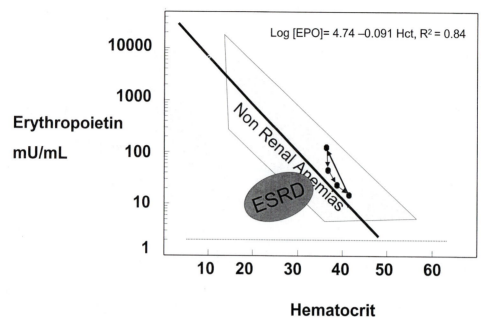

$$\text{Log [EPO]}= 4.74 - 0.091 \, \text{Hct}, \, R^2 = 0.84$$

Figure 26–5. Relationship of serum erythropoietin (EPO) levels to the degree of anemia (Hct). Note that EPO levels can increase a thousandfold in severe anemias and therefore vary inversely with Hct. By contrast, EPO levels in ESRD are shifted to the left but correlate positively with Hct. The solid points and arrows show the response to a two-unit phlebotomy.

within 24 hours and produces a much larger, almost 15-fold increase in plasma erythropoietin levels from 15 to over 200 mU/mL. Rapidly thereafter, however, erythropoietin levels fall, and during correction of the anemia, only two- to three-fold increases in hormone level are needed. Erythropoietin-producing cells are recruited in an on-off fashion[56]; increased production of erythropoietin results from the exponential recruitment of additional erythropoietin-synthesizing cells[118,119] as the hypoxic stimulus increases. This exponential recruitment of erythropoietin-producing cells produces the inverse relationship between circulating erythropoietin levels and Hct. Plasma erythropoietin levels increase from normal values of 5 to 25 to about 100 mU/mL as Hct, a measure of the blood's oxygen-carrying capacity, decreases from values greater than 40 percent to mildly anemic levels of 27 to 33 percent. Levels in excess of 1000 mU/mL are reached at Hcts below 20 percent (Fig. 26–5). Maintenance of "appropriate" plasma levels during severe anemia would require that the kidneys have the capacity to increase erythropoietin production by about 100-fold if metabolic clearance rate were independent of plasma concentration. However, at very high levels, the pharmacokinetics of erythropoietin change and the maximum response of the bone marrow is limited to only a four- to sixfold increase of erythrocyte production (Fig. 26–6).[108] Whole-body clearance of exogenously administered recombinant erythropoietin with increasing doses decreases, which prolongs the half-time of erythropoietin.[120]

During the progression of CKD, the degree of anemia appears to be roughly proportional to the degree of azotemia,[6] but the correlation between the Hct and the GFR as estimated by the blood urea nitrogen (BUN)[6] or creatinine (Cr) is not precise, and particularly so at lower concentrations of BUN or Cr. In nephric ESRD patients on dialysis, the mean baseline values of erythropoietin are marginally higher than normal: 19 to 30 compared with 10 to 17 mU/mL in normals[32,121,122]; but these values are less than 15 to 25 percent of those that would be expected for the level of anemia present. In anephric individuals, the levels are markedly decreased but still measurable by RIA.[32,113,123] The absolute deficiency of erythropoietin in such anephric patients[93] made them blood transfusion–dependent prior to the advent of epoetin.

The steady-state relationship between plasma RIA-erythropoietin levels and Hct (Fig. 26–5) reflects the operation of a negative "feedback" and the homeostatic attempt of normal kidneys to correct the anemia.[123,124] In ESRD patients, this biofeedback mechanism is impaired with the production of erythropoietin by diseased kidneys being inadequate (Fig. 26–5). In nephritic anemic dialysis patients, baseline erythropoietin values are marginally higher than those of normal individuals, but these values are still much lower than those observed in nonuremic patients for similar degrees of anemia. Although there is a considerable degree of dispersion in plasma erythropoietin levels among different ESRD patients, erythropoietin levels within a given pa-

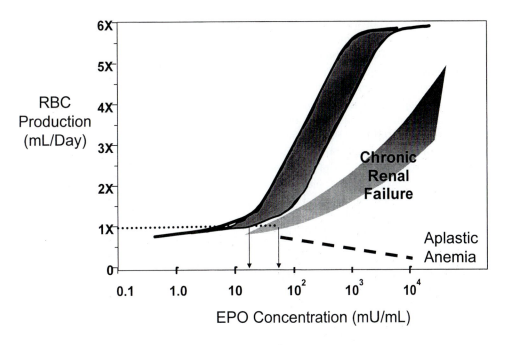

Figure 26–6. Epoetin dose responses.

tient tend to be similar over time. Diseased kidneys are capable of augmenting erythropoietin production in response to appropriate stimuli. Besarab and McCrea[115] and others[125] have shown that ESRD patients with acute blood loss or hemolysis can increase plasma RIA-erythropoietin levels two- to fivefold, but the levels seldom reach those achieved by individuals without renal disease. Diseased kidneys appear incapable of augmenting erythropoietin production chronically in response to an appropriate anemic hypoxic stimulus.[82,126] Patients with autosomal dominant polycystic kidney disease are the exception and typically have higher levels of erythropoietin with less severe anemia.[44] High erythropoietin concentrations have been found in the fluid of cysts originating from proximal tubules with erythropoietin mRNA identified in their interstitial cells.[127]

The amount of erythropoietin that is produced per unit weight of remaining "normal" nonscarred kidney tissue may actually be normal. The importance of adequate renal mass is best illustrated by the correction of anemia following successful kidney transplantation.[124,128] Following such transplantation in ESRD patients, erythropoietin levels increase and are sustained several-fold as excretory function recovers. With increased production of RBCs, anemia corrects and erythropoietin levels progressively decrease.

The above observations indicate that the primary factor in the anemia of CKD is the inadequate production of endogenous erythropoietin by diseased kidneys at CKD stages 3 to 5. The persistent observation of inappropriately low EPO levels in virtually all cases of CKD indicates that the primary factor in the anemia of advanced CKD is inade-

quate production of endogenous erythropoietin by the diseased kidneys. Other factors do play a role but may be more instrumental in the maintenance of anemia, particularly after epoetin therapy. Chief among these are shortened RBC survival (hemolysis or chronic blood loss), iron and other nutritional deficiencies, and the effects of "uremic inhibitors." One should keep in mind that these "other factors" can contribute to the severity of the anemia of ESRD and, if left unattended, will influence the outcome of epoetin treatment.

Shortened Erythrocyte Survival

The life span of RBCs in patients with CKD is usually shorter than normal,[19,129,130] typically decreasing from a normal value of 120 days to average values of 70 to 80 days. Uremic RBCs survive normally when injected into healthy recipients, and normal RBCs may have a shortened life span in uremic recipients.[130,131] In CKD, both metabolic and mechanical factors may produce an unfavorable environment for RBCs. The presence of a metabolic factor is suggested by the normalization of RBC life span after intensive dialysis.[132] However, most RBC enzymes in uremic RBCs are normal or have increased activity, and ATP levels are high.[133] Only the activities of transketolase, active in the hexose monophosphate shunt,[134] and ATPase, which supports the Na^+,K^+ membrane pumps,[135] are decreased. The decreased activity of the Na^+,K^+ pumps influences changes in RBC shape and rigidity, which, in turn, affects RBC life span. This defect has been attributed to either uremic impairment of the enzymatic activity[136] or to decreased synthesis of Na^+,K^+ pump units by uremic reticulocytes.[137] The toxic substances responsible for these metabolic impairments have not been fully identified but are presumably dialyzable, since intensive dialysis corrects the defect. We have noted that RBC life span can approach normal in well-dialyzed patients, with particular attention to minimizing blood sampling for studies.[20] Measurement of RBC life span measures both normal removal of senescent cells by the reticuloendothelial system and extracorporeal premature exit of erythrocytes from the circulation. The latter results from blood losses due to vascular access puncture, residual blood left in dialyzers, occasional blood leaks, phlebotomy for laboratory testing, and clotted dialyzers. Retention of RBCs on the dialysis membranes accounts for a loss of 0.5 to 11 mL of RBCs per dialysis, depending on the type of dialysis membrane used and how carefully the dialyzer is rinsed after dialysis. Such "routine" blood losses associated with hemodialysis typically approximate 60 mL of whole blood per week[138,139] and contribute significantly to the iron deficiency of these patients, resulting in effective iron losses of between 1 and 3 g per year. Such losses are obviously diminished in peritoneal dialysis patients.

Bleeding associated with renal insufficiency[140,141] has been known for decades. Common manifestations include telangiectasia and gastrointestinal angiodysplastic lesions.[142] Functional abnormalities of platelets—characterized by prolonged bleeding times, abnormal platelet aggregation and adhesiveness, and reduced platelet factor 3 release—are well recognized.[143] A reversible abnormality in the activation-dependent binding activity of glycoprotein IIb-IIIa occurs in uremia.[143,144] Other defects include abnormalities in the multimeric structure of von Willebrand factor[145] and acquired platelet storage pool deficiencies of adenosine diphosphate and serotonin.[146] All these notwithstanding, anemia itself appears to be a major factor in sustaining the bleeding tendency, as prolonged bleeding times are corrected by both RBC transfusions[147,148] and the rise in Hct that occurs with therapeutic use of epoetin.[149,150]

Because uremic RBCs survive normally when transfused into healthy recipients,[151] normal RBCs have a reduced life span in uremic individuals,[128,129] and erythrocyte life span can be normalized with intensive dialysis,[132] retention of one or more uremic solutes in the plasma is believed to be responsible for the hemolysis. Levels of C-reactive protein, a marker for inflammation, are elevated in predialysis and more so in dialysis patients.[152] Now that "uremia" has been recognized as an "inflammatory state," the shortened RBC life span may also result from the hemolysis related to inflammation. Unrecognized blood loss will also decrease "apparent" RBC survival. In well-dialyzed patients in whom blood losses are minimized, RBC survival can approach (but not reach) normal.[20]

Iatrogenic Hemolysis

In dialysis patients, decreased activity of the hexose monophosphate shunt renders Hgb and the RBC membrane sensitive to oxidant drugs or chemicals.[153,154] Approximately 25 percent of all uremic patients have defective RBC pentose-phosphate shunt activity as detected by an abnormal ascorbate-cyanide screening test.[154] This reduces NADPH production, thus decreasing available reduced glutathione. Reduced glutathione prevents the formation of unstable oxidized Hgb compounds that precipitate to form Heinz bodies. The administration of substances with strong oxidizing potential—such as primaquine, quinidine, sulfones, furadantin, and nitrofurantoin—should be avoided. Hemolysis with formation of Heinz bodies[155] has been reported in association with inadequate removal of chloramine,[156] coming from city tap water used for dialysate. Although mainly historical, acute hemolysis must also be avoided by removal of copper,[157] zinc,[158] aluminum,[159] and nitrates[160] in the water supply as well as formaldehyde[161] from reprocessed dialyzer equipment. Hypercupremia damages erythrocytes by oxidation of membrane phospholipids and, to a lesser degree, by inhibiting erythrocyte hexokinase. Aluminum and zinc appear to impair erythropoiesis by interfering with heme synthesis.[162,163] Vigorous treatment with nonabsorbable aluminum gels produces hypophosphatemia, which increases the intracellular calcium, in turn resulting in the polymerization of spectrin and making the RBC membrane rigid and susceptible to hemolysis.[164] Hemolysis can be induced by the dialysis process itself even in the absence of an underlying susceptibility of the "uremic" RBC. The factors responsible include exposure to formaldehyde from reprocessed dialyzer equipment,[161] hypotonic dialysate,[165] overheated dialysate,[166,167] malocclusion of the roller pump, and mechanical disruption from dialysis needles.[168] Hypophosphatemia, which increases susceptibility to hemolysis, occurs as a complication of vigorous treatment with nonabsorbable aluminum gels[164] and, on occasion, following the "hungry bone syndrome" that may occur after parathyroidectomy.[169]

Mechanical Fragmentation

Despite data supporting a metabolic basis for hemolysis, some investigators have failed to find a clear-cut correlation between RBC life span and degree of CKD.[6] An alternative mechanism is that RBCs are injured and prematurely destroyed by intravascular mechanical trauma rather than by metabolic alterations.[170] Even normal erythrocytes become deformed when exposed to strong shearing stress and are vulnerable to monocyte-macrophage sequestration, especially at a fibrin interphase.[170] This occurs in some cases of malignant hypertension[171] and in the hemolytic-uremic syndrome, in which the anemia is typically out of proportion to the degree of CKD in the early stages of the disease.[172]

Splenic Dysfunction

A significant number of patients on chronic hemodialysis have splenomegaly.[173,174] These spleens contain hyperplastic lymphoid follicles and increased numbers of macrophages and plasma cells—changes consistent with reaction to chronic antigenic stimulation.[173] One report has described macrophages laden with silicone particles,[175] the silicone perhaps arising from dialysis blood-line tubing stressed by roller pumps. Rosenmund and colleagues[154] have reported that RBCs from dialysis patients with hypersplenism are less filterable than those of other uremic subjects and are more susceptible to oxidative stress. Cells with unstable oxidized Hgb components may be sequestered in the splenic macrophages, which results in hyperplasia of splenic macrophages and splenomegaly. Splenectomy has been performed as a means of prolonging RBC life span in a few patients with splenomegaly and excessive RBC destruction.[176] In general, the results are rarely spectacular and the decision to operate should be carefully weighed, particularly since increasing the dose of epoetin to augment production can be titrated to match the rate of destruction.

Inhibition of Erythropoiesis

Marrow Inhibitors of Erythropoiesis. In the absence of significant overt blood loss, decreases in RBC survival alone do not fully account for the degree of anemia in progressive CKD. If one examines the relationship of erythropoietin levels to Hgb/Hct levels in the earliest stages of kidney disease, erythropoietin levels are appropriately increased for the degree of anemia until renal function drops below 40 percent of normal (Fig. 26–1). Thereafter, erythropoietin levels cannot be sustained and decrease progressively.[6] Numerous in vitro studies have implicated an inhibitory effect of uremic serum on the growth of erythroid precursors or on heme synthesis.[177-180] Intensive dialysis can increase iron utilization and Hct without altering the level of circulating erythropoietin, lending credence to the concept of uremic inhibitors.[131,181]

Older studies tried to identify polar lipids, arsenic, vitamin A, spermine, spermidine, and parathyroid hormone[178,180-183] as specific uremic inhibitors. More recent studies indicate that their role in the genesis of the anemia of CKD is of very minor importance.[184-188] In humans, acute ferrokinetic responses to epoetin do not differ among hemodialysis patients, normal subjects, or patients with CKD restored to normal kidney function by transplantation.[186] The improvement of anemia demonstrated after parathyroidectomy is due to the resolution of marrow fibrosis rather than the removal of erythropoietic inhibition.[188]

Despite clinical experience showing that exogenous erythropoietin easily overcomes the effects of any such putative inhibitors, studies on uremic inhibitors continue because control of such factors could reduce the amount of epoetin needed. Recent studies have focused on the effects of albumin-bound furancarboxylic acid,[189] activated monocytes, and polymorphonuclear leukocyte products[190] on erythropoiesis. Recently, quinolinic acid levels were shown to correlate positively with creatinine concentration and negatively with endogenous erythropoietin levels in uremic rats. Cobalt-stimulated erythropoiesis was suppressed dose-dependently in rats treated chronically with quiniolinic acid. Moreover, quinolinic acid had a dose-dependent inhibitory effect on hypoxia or cobalt induced erythropoietin release and erythropoietin gene expression suggesting disruption of erythropoietin gene activation by HIF-1.[191]

N-acetyl-seryl-lysyl-proline (AcsSDKP) is a physiologic inhibitor of hematopoiesis that is maintained at stable levels in patients without kidney disease. AcsSDKP levels increase almost twofold in patients not on dialysis and more than fivefold in patients on hemodialysis. Use of angiotensin-converting enzyme (ACE) inhibitors increases AcsSDKP levels fourfold. At higher levels, AcsSDKP acts as a uremic toxin producing partial resistance to erythropoietin.[192] ACE inhibitors have also been shown to decrease the levels of insulin-like growth factor 1 (IGF-1), a promoter of erythropoiesis, in studies of posttransplant erythrocytosis.[193] Chronic treatment with angiotensin-receptor blockers (ARBs) were recently shown to suppress BFU-Es in blood isolated from both control and hemodialysis patients—an effect not duplicated by ACE inhibitors.[194] However, the significance of this in vitro finding is uncertain given Wang's report (albeit with only a small cohort of patients) of a lack of benefit of ARBs in the treatment of posttransplant erythrocytosis.[195]

As discussed previously, other cytokines and growth factors influence erythropoiesis in vivo both positively and negatively. Some cytokines—such as IL-1α and β, IL-2, TNF-α, and TGF-β[52,53,196]—have a negative effect on erythropoiesis and appear to participate as significant mediators in the anemia of chronic diseases. Most of the "uremic inhibitor" studies have examined the suppression of the CFU-Es, which are committed erythroid precursors. A further level of complexity has been introduced by experiments to determine whether decreased CFU-E growth can result from a primary defect or deficiency in the BFU-Es or from a reduction in factors stimulating their growth. Abnormalities of in vitro growth of the BFU-E have been demonstrated in patients with ESRD on hemodialysis.[197,198] T lymphocytes harvested from uremic individuals are reported to be unable to promote the growth of BFU-Es in normal or uremic individuals, even in the presence of erythropoietin. This observation suggests that the T lymphocytes of CKD patients fail to produce a certain group of stimulatory factors, collectively providing "burst-promoting activity," which are necessary in the very early stages of erythropoiesis. The specific mechanism is unclear but does not appear to involve a reduction in the BFU-E compartment. This abnormality may arise from the abnormal helper/suppressor T-cell ratio seen in dialysis patients.[200] Hemodialysis with some dialysis membranes is also known to activate two of the putative inhibitors of erythropoiesis, IL-1 and TNF-α.[199,200] Whether or not the anemia of CKD results from such dialysis-related inhibitors or by defective T-lymphocyte function and growth factors,[201] it is clear that such effects can be overcome by epoetin, since the anemia can be corrected almost completely in most patients[202,203]; however, the total amount of erythropoietin needed to maintain a normal Hct may be greater than that endogenously produced in normal individuals. At a Hct of 33 percent, the average plasma erythropoietin level is 35 mU/mL. Assuming no difference in metabolic clearance rate between normals and ESRD subjects, both would require the production of about 45 U/kg/week. Maintenance doses of erythropoietin are significantly higher than this in ESRD, even when administered daily to achieve "relatively" constant levels of circulating erythropoietin.

Decreased RBC production could also result from an imbalance between inhibitory cytokines and growth-factor–promoting substances. The production of both inhibitory cytokines (IL-2, TNF-α, α-interferon) and promoting growth factors (G-CSF) by blood mononuclear cells in anemic hemodialysis patients is decreased. Correction of anemia by transfusion or with epoetin increases production of the inhibitory cytokines.[204] Since IL-2, TNF-α, and α-interferon have negative effects on hematopoiesis, their low production during anemia is an unlikely explanation for the inadequate response of erythropoietic precursors to endogenous erythropoietin.

Nutritional Factors

The patient with CKD or on maintenance dialysis is prone to anorexia, intercurrent illnesses, and dietary restrictions. Dialysis can also produce dialysate nutrient losses. All patients should be observed for malnutrition and vitamin deficiency syndromes. Folate deficiency in dialysis patients is uncommon[205] because routine use of supplements replaces dialysate losses. Most centers supplement their patients with 1 mg/day of folic acid. This is generally safe, as vitamin B_{12} deficiency is uncommon in dialysis patients. More recently, higher-dose folate has been used to reduce homocysteine levels, with variable results. Because of the water solubility of thiamine, pyridoxine, and vitamin B_{12}, deficiencies in one or more of these vitamins could develop from dialytic removal; but no cases have been reported in

dialysis patients. Currently, only pyridoxine supplementation is recommended: 5 mg/day for those with progressive CKD and 10 mg/day for dialysis patients.[206]

Borderline or frank iron deficiency is the most common "nutritional deficiency." It occurs to a lesser extent in conservatively treated patients (pre-ESRD) and in those on CAPD and is a major impediment to the cost-effective use of epoetin. Three factors have been implicated in the pathogenesis of iron deficiency in CKD patients: (1) blood loss caused by retained erythrocytes in dialyzers and blood tubing and on dressings and by frequent phlebotomies for diagnostic testing[139,207]; (2) the bleeding diathesis caused by uremia[208]; and, in the era of aluminum-containing phosphate binders, (3) malabsorption of iron due to such aluminum binders.[209] If the average blood loss within dialyzers and/or following withdrawal of needles is 10 to 15 mL per treatment, then up to 1.5 to 2.25 L of blood can be lost per year. At a Hct of 25 percent, this represents 1 to 2 mg/day of additional elemental iron that must be absorbed and incorporated into RBCs over and above the normal obligatory daily iron losses of 1 to 2 mg/day for the average male and the average childbearing female, respectively. Although iron absorption appears to be unimpaired[210-212] and iron turnover normal in severe renal impairment, iron utilization is regularly decreased, particularly in inflammatory renal disorders.[19] In rare cases of nephrotic syndrome, urinary losses of transferrin can cause low iron-binding capacity, with impairment in the metabolic cycling of iron.[213] Most patients on regular hemodialysis programs require iron supplementation to prevent iron deficiency. Although iron absorption may be decreased in some patients, Eschbach and coworkers[210] have observed that, as expected, the percentage of iron absorbed from the gastrointestinal tract of uremic subjects varies inversely with iron stores. Although they concluded that uremia per se does not interfere with the physiologic regulation of iron absorption, the amount of iron taken orally may not be sufficient to meet the needs of active erythropoiesis, particularly after epoetin administration, and parenteral iron may be necessary.

Of lesser importance now, iron absorption in dialysis patients may also be reduced by the aggressive use of nonabsorbable aluminum gels as phosphate binders within the gastrointestinal tract. These agents chelate iron in the stomach and prevent its absorption in the duodenum.[214] Potentially more dangerous, the presence of iron deficiency augments aluminum absorption.[215] Aluminum toxicity arising from orally ingested aluminum-containing phosphate binders can mimic iron deficiency since it is primarily microcytic.[164,216] Frequently it is seen concomitantly with osteomalacia and may be accompanied by dementia.[217] Aluminum interferes with iron incorporation into the erythroid cell (probably through several enzymes including, aminolevulinic acid dehydratase,[217] a rate-limiting enzyme for heme synthesis), thus reducing sideroblasts in the bone marrow of patients with aluminum-induced microcytosis.[218] Aluminum-induced microcytic anemia can be readily distinguished from iron deficiency by documenting that marrow iron stores are normal or increased.

Decreased serum levocarnitine levels are associated with epoetin hyporesponsiveness; however, replacement therapy has improved the response. Improved RBC survival and decreased Na+,K+-ATPase activity have been proposed as potential mechanisms.[219,220]

DIAGNOSTIC WORKUP AND MONITORING OF ANEMIA IN PATIENTS WITH CHRONIC KIDNEY DISEASE

The initial evaluation of the anemic patient with CKD should include a complete blood count (CBC) with RBC indices, a reticulocyte count, and determination of the serum iron, total iron binding capacity (TIBC), and ferritin (collectively referred to as iron indexes). Recently, the reticulocyte Hgb content (CHr) has received attention as a more reliable predictor of iron sufficiency in hemodialysis patients.[221] Its utility in patients with CKD in stages 3 to 5 is unknown. If the anemia is normochromic and normocytic with a normal or low reticulocyte index, the peripheral smear shows no abnormalities, and the iron-indexes are normal, then no further workup of the anemia is necessary.

Assessment of Iron Status

Controversy exists about the best method of assessing adequate iron stores and iron delivery to the bone marrow in CKD patients, particularly those receiving epoetin. The time-honored tests have been transferrin saturation (TSAT) and serum ferritin, the former reflecting the carrying capacity in blood and the latter reflecting tissue stores of iron. In non-CKD individuals, a ferritin value of less than 30 μg/L has been used as an indication for iron supplementation.[222] This value is too low in patients treated with epoetin. Several studies correlating serum ferritin, TSAT, and stainable bone marrow iron have indicated that ferritin levels as high as 100 to 125 μg/L may indicate iron deficiency in ESRD patients,[222,223] and even these higher levels are unable to detect "functional iron deficiency."[224-228] This condition occurs during epoetin therapy when the erythroid marrow responds to the hormone and iron is removed from transferrin faster than the reticuloendothelial cell can release it to transferrin. As a result, iron delivery becomes limiting and the erythropoietic response lags, or the epoetin dose needed to obtain the desired Hct is higher than it should be. In addition, both ferritin and plasma transferrin are acute-phase reactants. Thus the degree of variation in TSAT and ferritin over time in CKD patients may be quite large and may not

reflect iron delivery or stores. In general, transferrin saturation should be greater than 20 percent and ferritin levels greater than 100 to 200 ng/mL in the iron-replete CKD patient. Low serum iron with elevated ferritin suggests systemic infection, inflammatory disease, or occult malignancy. Normal or high serum iron with normal ferritin but microcytic indexes points to thalassemia or aluminum toxicity. Macrocytosis is unusual in the well-dialyzed patient receiving a vitamin supplement and consuming a recommended protein diet of 1.0 to 1.4 g/kg, but it can occur in elderly patients who limit their dietary intake.

Other techniques have been sought to evaluate functional iron deficiency. These include protoporphyrins[228,229] and the percentage of hypochromic cells.[230] In our opinion, these are probably of no greater use in clinical practice than the combined measurement of both TSAT and ferritin.[231] A new method that measures the Hgb content of reticulocytes (CHr) holds greater promise,[221] as the reticulocyte reflects bone marrow events affecting Hgb synthesis within the preceding several days. This test is in its third generation and was recently found to be quite useful and more sensitive in diagnosing iron deficiency.[232] The CHr is an exciting potential marker of iron sufficiency, as it is inexpensive and more reliable than the ferritin or transferrin saturation.[221] A CHr value below 28 pg has been proposed as a measure of functional iron deficiency, although in practice we have found that trend analysis is more useful to guide iron therapy than any single value.

The Hct level of individual patients remains stable once ESRD has developed and adequate dialysis is delivered. Monitoring of the CBC and RBC indexes as well as the iron indexes monthly in patients on hemodialysis or CAPD should detect variances from the patient's steady-state values. Although a nomogram constructed by Van Wyck[233] can be used to estimate iron needs in correcting the anemia of CKD/ESRD, we prefer to calculate the amount on the basis of 1 mg of iron needed for each 1 mL of packed RBC formed. The increase in packed cells is estimated from the starting and target Hcts and the estimated blood volume of the patient (70 to 80 mL/kg body weight). Patients receiving hemodialysis have significant ongoing weekly blood losses of approximately 40 mg. As a result, unlike patients on CAPD, patients on hemodialysis usually require parenteral iron both during the period of correction of anemia as well as during the long-term maintenance phases.

Serum ferritin levels reflect the iron stores reasonably well in uremic patients,[228] and periodic monitoring of these levels can detect iron deficiency before it becomes severe enough to lower the mean corpuscular volume (MCV) of the RBCs. When the MCV of the RBCs decreases but the serum ferritin remains normal in a patient who has not received intravenous iron dextran, aluminum toxicity should be suspected.

PARADOXICAL ABSENCE OF ANEMIA

In a small cohort of patients not on epoetin, the Hct attains a plateau at a level that exceeds 35 percent, or it stabilizes initially at an anemic level but subsequently rises to normal.[234] Absence of anemia or amelioration of the anemia in patients with CKD requires a search for potential causes. Probable etiologies include (1) decreased plasma volume (particularly prior to dialysis), (2) decreased Hgb-oxygen saturation due to cardiac or pulmonary disease, (3) hereditary or acquired cystic kidneys, and (4) conditions that cause decreased blood flow to the kidneys or liver. The presence of a direct correlation between Hct and erythropoietin levels during steady-state conditions in ESRD patients (Fig. 26–5) suggests that erythropoietin levels are not regulated by "tissue" hypoxia alone (as reflected by the oxygen-carrying capacity of the blood). However, diseased kidneys, even those unable to produce urine, apparently can increase their production of erythropoietin when oxygen saturation falls, tissue hypoxia is increased by cysts, or blood flow to the kidneys is reduced. This is particularly apt to occur in adult polycystic kidney disease, where there is a frequent dissociation between excretory function and Hct.

Several groups have reported that the development of acquired cystic kidney disease (ACKD) associated with increased erythropoietin levels can increase the Hct and accounts for the occasional spontaneous increase in Hct in some patients maintained for years on dialysis.[235,236] Because ACKD is progressive,[237] the associated increase in Hct and erythropoietin levels seen in many patients could result from the progressive development of more cysts over time, with compression of remaining renal tissue. Two mechanisms have been proposed for the increased erythropoietin production in such cases: (1) increasing tissue pressure on remaining renal parenchyma by the cysts, producing worsening local hypoxia, and (2) autonomous production of erythropoietin by proliferating epithelial cells within the cyst wall.[235,236] However, some investigators have not noted a correlation between the presence or absence of cysts and Hct; rather, the Hct appeared to correlate best with age, duration of dialysis, and increased volume of renal tissue.[238] Our experience indicates no correlation between the initial presence or absence of cysts and RIA-erythropoietin levels or between the subsequent development of ACKD and follow-up RIA-erythropoietin levels.[239] Thus the role of cysts per se is still unclear and may depend not only on the number of cysts but also the cell type.[240]

On occasion, Hct increases in an ESRD patient with hepatitis. Kolk-Veghter and colleagues[241] observed a transient increase of Hct in several patients on hemodialysis during episodes of active hepatitis. Others have also noted an increase in the Hct and erythropoietin titer of patients with hepatitis during the period of elevated serum transaminases.[242]

Very rarely, patients with CKD develop polycythemia, either coincidentally due to polycythemia rubra vera or secondary to processes known to cause secondary polycythemia. Those states associated with hypoxemia or reduced renal blood flow may result in an increase in erythropoietin production and improvement in the anemia, but seldom to normal levels. Conditions associated with paraneoplastic erythropoietin production potentially can result in marked increases in the RBC mass. In most instances, high Hcts (>48 percent) in uremics cannot be explained but occur in association with increased erythropoietin levels. Erslev and associates[243] studied two anephric patients whose Hcts gradually rose to more than 30 percent after they had been on chronic hemodialysis for more than a year. In both patients, elevated plasma erythropoietin levels could not be suppressed even after transfusion to Hcts in excess of 40 percent. This suggests that extrarenal erythropoietin production in some patients is regulated differently than renal erythropoietin production—an observation supported by experimental data in transfused uremic rats.[244]

THERAPY OF RENAL ANEMIA

Until the advent of epoetin therapy, anemia was considered a relatively minor problem for patients suffering from the many metabolic consequences of failing kidneys; it was managed with transfusions or androgens. Today, treatment of anemia has assumed greater importance, given the increasing age of the ESRD population; these patients have more frequent and a higher prevalence of ischemic heart and peripheral vascular disease, and they are increasingly diabetics with both microvascular and macrovascular disease. Also, nontransfusion treatment of anemia has assumed more importance because of the risks from transfusion (e.g., HIV, hepatitis C, Nile fever) and the risk of sensitizing potential transplant recipients. Furthermore, many symptoms previously attributed to "uremia"—such as fatigue, cold intolerance, and mental sluggishness—respond to the correction of anemia.

Transfusions

With the advent of epoetin therapy, nonspecific treatments for the management of anemia are of historic interest only; they are therefore dealt with only briefly here. It is still important to provide the basic building blocks for RBC production (iron, vitamins) in all patients and transfusing with packed cells when necessary, since epoetin takes weeks to months to correct anemia. Symptomatic patients, particularly those with ischemic heart or central nervous system (CNS) disease, are candidates for transfusion. Packed RBCs poor in white blood cells are most commonly used for transfusing such patients. The introduction of epoetin for the therapy of the anemia of CKD has virtually eliminated the need for repeated transfusions and the risk of developing hemochromatosis. The major groups still at risk are patients with sickle cell disease[245] or thalassemia,[246] who do not respond to reasonable doses of erythropoietin.

Transfusions should not be withheld from patients with symptomatic or refractory anemia, particularly those with underlying ischemic heart disease, because it takes weeks for epoetin to increase Hct. In situations of gastrointestinal bleeding, postoperative blood loss, or hemolysis, transfusions remain the mainstay of therapy. Given the infection risks of transfusion and the sensitization of potential transplant recipients, transfusions should be used prudently.

Anabolic Steroids

Response to epoetin can be augmented by anabolic androgens, and this approach is sometimes used in countries with limited resources. This therapy consists of blood transfusions with or without the administration of androgenic-anabolic steroids.[247-249] Androgen administration is associated with many unpleasant side effects, such as fluid retention, hirsutism, acne, and cholestasis. The effect is somewhat unpredictable, but—in most nephric uremic patients and in some anephric patients—androgens cause a moderate increase in erythropoietin release and RBC production. Androgenic steroids increase the Hct of uremics by increasing erythropoietin production and, to a lesser extent, stimulating committed bone marrow stem cells. Fluoxymesterone and oxymetholone are given by mouth in doses of 10 to 20 mg/day and 1 to 4 mg/kg/day, respectively. Parenteral preparations, such as nandrolone decanoate or testosterone propionate or enanthate, are presumed to be more effective.[249] They are given in doses of 1 to 4 mg/kg once a week.

Recent studies have explored the use of androgens along with epoetin. One found synergy between epoetin and nandrolone decanoate with few side effects[250]; the other found no synergy and many side effects.[251] A third study found that the use of androgens in men below age 50 was as effective as epoetin and less costly.[252] In view of the known side effects of androgen therapy, particularly in women, its use alone or in combination with epoetin is not encouraged.

Epoetin Administration

Clinical trials with epoetin were initiated in 1985 to 1986, and replacement therapy with epoetin quickly became the most rational therapy for anemia of CKD/ESRD.[202,203,253-255] These initial clinical trials convincingly demonstrated that the Hct could be increased by up to 10 points or more and could be maintained at a level above 30 percent in more than 90 percent of patients. Dialysis-treated patients increase their Hct in a dose-dependent manner,[202] transfusions

are avoided,[253,256] and iron overload is reduced or eliminated; these results have been observed worldwide.[256] Maintenance intravenous doses needed three times a week to maintain steady-state Hcts greater than 31 percent varied significantly among study patients[253]: 15 percent require more than 150 U/kg, 20 percent less than 40 U/kg.

Within a few months of epoetin's general introduction, its dosing levels were much lower than those used in clinical trials.[257-259] The initial reimbursement options contained financial incentives to constrain expenditures.[260] Following a change in the payment method in 1991, dosing increased, but without a corresponding proportional increase in Hct. Payment rewarding additional epoetin use merely produced higher expenditures, not improved management of anemia. This lack of Hct response led the Health Care Financing Administration (HCFA), through the ESRD Networks, to target anemia control as a health care quality-improvement focus.[261] As a result of this program, iron deficiency in epoetin-treated patients has been largely eliminated. Consequently, significant improvement has been made in the management of the anemia of CKD/ESRD. Over 92 percent of hemodialysis patients and about 60 percent of Medicare-eligible patients on continuous ambulatory peritoneal dialysis (CAPD) were receiving epoetin at the end of 1994.[262] Since then, both epoetin dose and mean Hgb have progressively increased, reaching the target range of 33 to 38 percent achieved in clinical trials. As of the last quarter of 2002, mean Hgb had reached 11.7 g/dL and epoetin dose exceeded 7000 U/dose (ESRD CPM Project Report, 2002).[263] In addition, there has been recognition of the need to optimize anemia management before patients reach the stage of kidney failure requiring dialysis.[264]

In CKD patients not yet receiving renal replacement therapy (RRT), the subcutaneous route is effective and permits self-administration. A negative effect of epoetin on renal function has not been noted in clinical human trials or during longer-term follow-up. Studies have shown the safety of subcutaneous injection of epoetin at home once a week. With the development of epoetins with longer circulating half-times, dosing intervals in such patients are being extended out to every 2 to 4 weeks.

RESULTS OF EPOETIN THERAPY

Transfusion Avoidance

Prior to epoetin therapy, up to 25 percent of hemodialysis patients were transfusion-dependent,[265] receiving up to 0.7 units of packed RBCs monthly.[204,205,255,269] These patients were at risk for iron overload and organ dysfunction, although most patients with transfusional iron overload have hemosiderosis,[266] a state with minimal organ dysfunction, and not hemochromatosis.[267] Even livers that contain more than 1000 μg of iron per 100 mg of dry tissue (normal is < 200 μg/100 g dry tissue) show little fibrosis or damage.[172,268] However, iron overload may increase dialysis patients' susceptibility to infection.[269,270]

Since the introduction of epoetin therapy for the anemia of CKD, the need for repeated transfusions has been virtually eliminated and the risk of developing hemochromatosis from transfusions has vanished. Iron-overloaded patients can be treated with higher-dose epoetin to accelerate iron removal through periodic phlebotomies.[271-273] Both magnetic resonance imaging (MRI)[274] and computed tomography (CT)[275] are used to monitor phlebotomy therapy. Thus, we have transitioned from an era in which iron overload was the problem to one in which the major problem for ESRD patients on maintenance epoetin therapy is the development of iron deficiency.

Several studies have demonstrated that the elimination of transfusions produces a marked reduction in the percentage panel reactive antibody (percent PRA)[276] as well as in anti-HLA-specific antibody titers.[277] If blood transfusion cannot be avoided, irradiated packed RBCs should be administered.

Quality of Life

Many of the symptoms attributed to uremia are really the result of anemia. Fatigue, cold intolerance, impotence, and mental sluggishness respond to correction of anemia. In patients with ESRD, correction of anemia with epoetin therapy improves quality of life indexes, including those assessing global well-being and depression in hemodialysis[278] and CAPD patients.[279] CKD patients who do not yet require dialysis also show improvement in quality of life (QOL) indexes following epoetin therapy.[280] Substantial improvements in subjective symptoms were noted in a large, double-blind phase II study.[281] Clinically important improvements were noted in fatigue, perceived strength, and global score of the Sickness Impact Profile; smaller degrees of improvement were noted in relationships and depression[280]; and no change was noted in frustration or sleeping abnormalities. A phase IV trial of over 1000 patients receiving epoetin in clinical practice[282] confirmed these QOL effects even when only a modest mean Hct of 30 percent was achieved. Four of six domains of the Short Form-36 QOL questionnaire showed improvement. The data of Moreno et al.[283] indicate that both the Karnofsky functional scale and the Sickness Impact Profile correlate positively with the Hct between 29 and 35 percent. Whether QOL indicators can be improved further by raising Hct is currently debated. The Canadian Erythropoietin Study Group[284] could not demonstrate an increase in QOL when Hgb was increased from 10.2 to 11.7 g/dL, suggesting that this might be a plateau. Improvement in QOL was one of the few positive results found by Besarab et al.[285] in the normal Hct trial.

Cognition

Improvement in cognition is sensitive to the Hct level and improves when Hcts are increased into the range of 32 to 36 percent.[286-288] Increasing the Hct to 42 percent with epoetin further improves brain and cognitive function,[289] perhaps because maximum delivery of oxygen to the brain occurs within a Hct range of 40 to 45 percent.[290] The reports that neuronal cells carry the erythropoietin receptor[291] and that erythropoietin can be produced within the brain in a paracrine fashion[292] predicted the possible clinical use of epoetin in stoke syndrome.[53] Erythropoietin has effects in many tissues besides the bone marrow[53] and may protect against hypoxia-induced neuronal damage. Certainly the epoetin doses needed for full correction of anemia are two- to threefold higher, and the increased levels may permit erythropoietin to cross into the CNS.

Exercise Tolerance and Rehabilitation

Aerobic work capacity is improved following correction of anemia.[286,293,294] Although some of the benefit accrues from an increase in oxygen-carrying capacity,[294] some of it results from improvement in voluntary muscle function[295] as a result of a possible treatment-induced improvement in muscle oxidative phosphorylation.[296] Improvement in exercise capacity during epoetin therapy also results from increased erythrocyte 2,3 DPG levels,[297] which permit improved oxygen delivery to tissues. A variety of muscle functions improve, including voluntary contractions, force generation, and duration of force contraction. Histologic improvements in architecture and fiber diameter are seen as well.[298] However, increases in maximal uptake of oxygen remain less than in normal subjects; in general, improvements in exercise or cardiopulmonary performance attained initially, when anemia is first corrected, are not augmented further when tested 1-year later.[299] The increase in oxygen-carrying capacity produced by epoetin is accompanied by a significant reduction in peak blood flow to exercising muscle. This limits the gain in oxygen transport. Even after restoration of Hgb, oxygen conductance from the muscle capillary to the mitochondria remains considerably below normal.[300]

Only one study has evaluated work capacity with full correction of anemia (correction of anemia was defined as attainment of a Hct of 40 percent in men and 35 percent in women, with pretreatment Hct averaging about 30 percent).[301] Sixty percent of patients with corrected anemia rated themselves as having increased energy, compared with 42 percent of subjects with uncorrected anemia. Similarly, work capacity scores increased by one or more units in 61 percent of those subjects whose anemia was fully corrected, compared with only 38 percent of the epoetin-treated patients whose anemia was not fully corrected. Changes in work capacity were proportional to epoetin dose. Correction of anemia alone is unlikely to maximize exercise capacity and foster rehabilitation.[302] Optimizing the Hct may be only one component of effective rehabilitation, in conjunction with maintenance or improvement in exercise capacity, maintenance of adequate dialysis, and appropriate changes in socioeconomic and health policies.[303] Other factors such as deconditioning, neuropathy, and cardiovascular disease probably contribute as well, and programs emphasizing exercise training are needed.[312] Poor rehabilitation outcomes in ESRD patients may simply result from initiating therapy for anemia too late in the clinical course of CKD.

Effects on Coagulation

CKD is associated with a bleeding tendency[141,304] attributed to functional platelet abnormalities, characterized by a prolonged bleeding time, abnormal platelet aggregation and adhesiveness, and decreased release of platelet factor 3.[141,305,306] Platelet adhesion to vessel subendothelium is decreased in dialysis patients.[307] This is attributed to a platelet abnormality and a plasma factor that interfere with this process.[308] It has been shown that a reversible abnormality in the activation-dependent binding activity of GP IIb-IIIa occurs in uremia and may be the major cause for the altered platelet function.[143] Additional coagulative abnormalities contribute to prolonged bleeding: the multimeric structure of von Willebrand factor (vWF) in uremia affects the initial interaction with GP Ib and the subsequent activation of GP IIb-IIIa,[144] a reaction crucial for initiation of platelet thrombi; uremic plasma also induces nitric oxide synthesis by cultured endothelial cells that inhibits platelet function.[309]

Many of the hemostatic abnormalities improve following correction of anemia with epoetin. This may result from three effects: (1) a direct effect on megakaryocytes, which, because they have erythropoietin receptors, results in increased platelet counts[310] (as noted in most large series); (2) the migration of platelets radially (to the surface of the blood vessel) as Hct increases; and (3) a change in platelet adhesiveness.[311] Both platelet adhesion and bleeding time, which correlate best with the occurrence of clinical bleeding,[307] are dependent on platelet number, which is usually sufficient in CKD subjects. Platelet adhesion and bleeding time are Hct-dependent. Even before the advent of epoetin, transfusion of washed, filtered RBCs devoid of plasma or other cellular components partially corrected bleeding time and platelet adhesiveness.[148] The therapeutic use of epoetin confirmed that anemia per se was an important cause of the "bleeding abnormalities" in CKD patients. The prolonged bleeding time corrects to normal as Hct increases above 30 percent.[147–159]

Transient increases in platelet count of 25,000 to 40,000[312,313] occur commonly and seldom exceed normal limits. Changes in platelet reactivity and adhesiveness during epoetin therapy are variable.[313,314] Epoetin therapy significantly increases plasma vWF activity, vWF antigen, and fibrinogen, but this effect appears to be indirect.[144] Improvement in platelet function is probably more than a simple correction of the anemia.[152,315] Uremic platelets do have a defect in intracellular calcium[316] that improves in response to epoetin therapy.[317] The improvement in coagulation and increase in viscosity contributes to the increase in heparin requirements during hemodialysis.

Reported changes in various procoagulant and anticoagulant factors following the correction of anemia have been inconsistent. Anemic hemodialysis patients have higher total but lower free protein-S antigen level than normal individuals.[317] Both the antigen and functional activity of antithrombin III (ATIII) of uremic individuals are significantly lower than those of normals. No laboratory evidence of increased thrombogenesis due to reduction of natural coagulation inhibitors has been found in CAPD patients[318] or hemodialysis patients[319] receiving epoetin. Hemodialysis itself seems to activate synthesis of endogenous anticoagulation factors, as levels of protein C increase significantly and progressively.[317,319] An increase in functional protein C reduces thrombosis risk. Partial correction of anemia with erythropoietin does not further effect the levels of this clotting inhibitor during dialysis. During subcutaneous epoetin administered at 20 U/kg twice a week for over a year, bleeding time progressively decreased, vWF antigen or ristocetin cofactor did not change, and fibrinogen and factor VIII clotting activity increased.[320] This last effect could increase clotting risk. However, another study showed no change in fibrinogen levels, ATIII activity, protein-C activity, or protein-S concentration by erythropoietin treatment.[321]

The presence or absence of a procoagulative state following correction of anemia has clinical ramifications. Prior to epoetin therapy and consistent correction of anemia to a Hct greater than 30 percent, bleeding manifestations were a major concern. The feared complications included gastrointestinal bleeding (particularly from telangiectasias), pericarditis, hemorrhagic pleural effusions, spontaneous subcapsular hematomas, and spontaneous retroperitoneal bleeding. Now the concern is whether excessive thrombosis, particularly of vascular accesses, is or is not a major clinical and economic side effect of erythropoietin therapy. An increased propensity to clot vascular accesses has not been unequivocally documented.[254,322,323] In the Canadian multicenter trial[324] and one other clinical trial,[256] an increased risk for thrombosis was noted. This risk appears to be greater in patients with synthetic bridge grafts[324,325] and in those with previously known access dysfunction.[323,326] Native fistulas did not appear to be at risk. However, this whole issue is quite controversial.[327,328] The thrombosis rate can be kept as low as 0.2 events per patient-year with a program of good surveillance of the vascular access. Intraaccess fistula flow does not appear to change during epoetin therapy despite the observed increase in whole-blood viscosity and of Hct into the range of 30 to 36 vol%.[329]

HEMODYNAMIC AND CARDIOVASCULAR EFFECTS

Correction of anemia has major effects on the cardiovascular system. Uncorrected anemia produces a hyperdynamic state that contributes to the development of left ventricular hypertrophy (LVH) in CKD patients.[330] Correction of anemia removes only this component but leaves unaffected any components arising from hypertension, hyperparathyroidism, or other structural abnormalities.[331] Anemia also limits the myocardial oxygen supply, provoking angina pectoris or other ischemic events in those with coronary or peripheral vascular occlusive disease. Anemia and hypertension are therefore the major contributors to left ventricular dysfunction and congestive heart failure.[331] Unfortunately, correction of anemia is frequently associated with de novo or worsening hypertension in epoetin-treated patients.

Left Ventricular Hypertrophy

Cardiovascular disease from hypertension and with LVH is a major risk factor for death.[331] The prevalence of LVH in ESRD patients starting dialysis may be as high as 73 percent.[332] Anemia contributes to the development of LVH.[333] Anemia produces a hyperdynamic state characterized by increased cardiac output and decreased peripheral vascular resistance. The low vascular resistance results from both hypoxic vasodilatation as well as lower blood viscosity. Both left ventricular mass as well as end-diastolic volume increase in response to these compensatory mechanisms in anemia.[334] The increase in cardiac output during anemia correlates well with the degree of anemia and is reversed when the Hct is increased over 30 percent.[335]

During partial sustained correction of anemia in hemodialysis patients with epoetin therapy, incomplete regression of LVH and volume occurs.[333-337] Mean decrease in left ventricular mass among 15 studies averaged 18 percent after a mean treatment time of 45 weeks as Hct was increased from an average of 20 percent to a range of 29 to 35 percent.[338] In general, cardiac output and index decrease, whereas peripheral systemic resistance increases[339] following epoetin therapy unless blood volume increases.[340] In fact, hypervolemia following correction of anemia can produce negative trends on left ventricular ejection fraction and function.[341] To improve cardiac performance, expansion of the blood volume must be diligently prevented by appropriate changes in estimated dry weight (edema-free weight without hypotension) and by blood pressure control.

Cardiovascular disease, particularly in the elderly, is the major cause of death in dialysis patients.[7,342] Hypertension and LVH are the important cardiac risk factors for all dialysis patients.[333,336,337,341] The correction of anemia with epoetin improves exercise-induced ST-segment depression.[298,343] Anemia correlates with mortality 30 days after myocardial infarction in pre-ESRD patients,[344] and correction of anemia is associated with improved New York Heart Association (NYHA) functional class, improved GFR, and improved symptoms in NYHA class III/IV heart failure patients already on "maximal" medical therapy.[345] Foley demonstrated an Hgb <8.8 mg/dL to be associated with higher mortality in ESRD patients.[7] Higher Hct (> 44 percent) in cardiac patients with pre-ESRD is clearly associated with improved survival.[346] Once such patients progress to ESRD, the treatment of cardiac patients with epoetin to higher Hct levels (> 39 percent) was associated with worse outcomes.[285]

Unless hypertension developing during epoetin treatment is refractory to therapy, no CKD patient should remain at an Hct below 27 percent. Despite changes in cardiac output and regional blood flow (e.g., in the calf), peripheral oxygen delivery as measured by transcutaneous Po_2 increases significantly during correction of anemia with epoetin.[347,348]

Hypertension

Worldwide, new or worsening arterial hypertension develops in a subset of 20 to 40 percent of epoetin-treated patients, with the greatest increases affecting daytime systolic and nighttime diastolic pressures.[349,350] Increases in peripheral resistance range from 15 to 100 percent. Concomitant decreases in cardiac output vary from 10 to 35 percent.[348,351-353] This variability may result from such factors as preexisting hypertension, compliance with antihypertensive medication, differences in neurohumoral characteristics, and degree of fluid control. Individuals who become hypertensive or have worsening hypertension are unable to adapt to the increase in peripheral resistance by reducing cardiac output. Hypertension following epoetin therapy is likely to be multifactorial in origin: preexisting hypertension, severe anemia at initiation, rapid increase in Hct, high epoetin doses given intravenously, and the presence of native kidneys. Epoetin-induced hypertension usually develops within several weeks to months of starting epoetin therapy as the Hct is rising[353,354]; it appears to be a time-dependent consequence of long-term epoetin administration. However, increases in blood pressure do not correlate with the increase in Hct, either in humans clinically[348] or in animals,[355] and epoetin-induced hypertension can be dissociated from the rise in erythrocyte mass.[355,356] In animals, epoetin therapy does impair the hypotensive response to nitric oxide (NO) donors, suggesting an impaired vasodilatory response to NO.[355] Other studies show that endogenous NO activity is increased in epoetin-treated rats, perhaps as a counterregulatory mechanism that limits the pressor effect.[357]

These findings have relevance to observations that some patients will exhibit severe hypertension with epoetin administration but not with RBC transfusions that produce identical Hcts.[358] Also, blood pressure remains unchanged in iron-deficient hemodialysis patients whose Hcts are increased from 25 to 32 percent with simple iron repletion.[354] The recent demonstration that erythropoietin can affect both vascular endothelial[359] and vascular smooth muscle[360] cells suggests that part of the hypertensive effect of epoetin results from direct vascular effects independent of changes in Hct. The high concentrations of erythropoietin achieved during intravenous injection (greater than 1000 mU/mL) are capable of increasing endothelin-1 (ET-1) release[359] but leaving prostaglandins unaltered while decreasing plasma atrial natriuretic peptide by 25 percent.[361] In endothelial cell (EC) culture systems, epoetin directly stimulates EC proliferation as a competence factor and also accelerates ET-1 production in association with stimulation of DNA and protein synthesis.[362] Epoetin also produces vascular smooth muscle contraction in renal and mesenteric artery preparations, suggesting a direct pressor effect.[360,363]

The increase in peripheral resistance does not correlate with plasma renin activity or with concentrations of angiotensin I or II.[356] This does not exclude the participation of the renin-angiotensin system, as upregulation at the tissue level through increases in mRNA for renin and its substrate is possible.[364] Catecholamines also do not correlate with mean blood pressure after the administration of epoetin.[365]

Loss of hypoxic vasodilatation[366] and changes in blood viscosity[354,367] following correction of anemia have also been postulated to be mechanisms that increase arterial pressure. Whole-blood viscosity increases appropriately as Hct increases from 29 to 39 percent, whereas plasma viscosity remains normal and unchanged.[368] Erythrocyte deformability (fluidity) also changes over a 30-week epoetin treatment period,[369] first decreasing during the period of rapid correction of anemia but returning to basal levels during the maintenance phase. The epoetin-induced increase in Hgb concentration could theoretically augment vascular resistance by diverting the endogenous vascular relaxation factor, nitric oxide.[355] A number of studies emphasize the important role of adequate control of body fluid and fluid gains in maintaining blood pressure control during epoetin therapy. Maintenance of normal blood pressure requires equivalent decreases in plasma volume as RBC mass is increased so as to avoid changes in preload to the heart. In well-managed patients, measurements of ^{51}Cr-tagged erythrocytes and ^{125}I human serum albumin to measure erythrocyte mass and plasma volume shows that their sum (total blood volume) remains constant during epoetin therapy.[370,371] The importance of blood volume control on blood

pressure is emphasized by the following study: in the absence of adjustments in antihypertensive medication, blood pressure remained unchanged in peritoneal dialysis patients but increased by 8 mmHg in predialysis patients as anemia was corrected.[372] Despite equal expansion of the RBC mass, plasma volume decreased in peritoneal dialysis but not in predialysis patients.

Interestingly, it has been observed that a hypertensive response to epoetin does not occur when it is used to treat other anemias, such as that associated with inflammatory disease[374] or with cancer,[375] or when it is used to treat in anemic pregnant patients without kidney disease[376] for short or long periods of time. Experimental models indicate that epoetin produces hypertension in a remnant model of CKD but not in sham control animals.[377] Thus, renal insufficiency appears to be a prerequisite for the development of hypertension during epoetin therapy.

The greater propensity for hemodialysis patients to develop hypertension has been attributed to result in part from the route of administration. Higher peak erythropoietin levels, and therefore higher ET-1 levels, are achieved in dialysis patients treated with intravenous compared to subcutaneous epoetin.[378] However, other studies have shown that baseline ET-1 levels prior to epoetin therapy are elevated, do not increase during therapy,[365] do not differ between the beginning and end of dialysis, and do not correlate with blood pressure.[365,379] Others have been unable to confirm the original findings of elevated levels following epoetin therapy, finding no changes or decreases in ET-1 levels during chronic epoetin treatment.[380,381] Although, the exact role of vasoactive substances in epoetin-induced hypertension remains undefined, clearly the hormonal profile does influence the blood pressure. Patients switched from intravenous to subcutaneous administration have a reduction of 8 mmHg following the switch.[382]

EFFECTS ON SURVIVAL AND HOSPITALIZATION

Children are most likely to benefit from correction of anemia with epoetin[383,384] through prevention of LVH. In adults, each decrease in Hgb of 1 g/dL below 10 g/dL increases mortality by 18 percent.[385] Yang and coworkers[386] found that each decrease in Hct of 1 percent was associated with a 14 percent increase in mortality over an Hct range of 21 to 31 percent. Lowrie et al.[387] found a stepwise increase in mortality as Hct fell below 30 percent. Others have confirmed the decrease in cardiovascular disease and mortality if Hgb is maintained above 10 g/dL with erythropoietin therapy.[384] Individual analysis of a controlled European multicenter trial of the adverse events, including death, revealed a protective effect of epoetin in high-risk dialysis patients with cardiovascular disease.[388] Some studies indicate that changes in cardiac morphometry and function require up to 1 year of therapy to achieve a maximum result.[389]

In addition to beneficial effects on survival of adult dialysis patients, studies now show a reduction in overall hospitalization in epoetin-treated patients.[390-392] Total costs of care for ESRD patients may thus be reduced in the long term through the use of epoetin.[393]

OTHER EFFECTS OF EPOETIN

Adverse Effects

Adverse effects such as myalgias and seizures (usually resulting from uncontrolled hypertension) do occur[261] but are manageable and in some cases totally preventable by close supervision of the patient. In the initial trials, development of encephalopathy or seizures was not uncommon[202,203,325] and resulted from less than optimal control of blood pressure. This is now much less often observed due to better appreciation of the need to control blood pressure during the ramp-up period. In most cases it is not related to the correction of anemia.

Flu-like reactions have been reported in a minority of patients.[202,203,256,323] The onset is within hours of administration and usually subsides within 12 hours. Slowing the rate of administration[323] can decrease the symptoms. Therapy is discontinued in less than 1 percent of treated patients because of this side effect.

Subcutaneous injection is an effective route of administration. With the use of the original formulation of epoetin alfa, pain resulted from the hypertonic citrate in the formulation.[394] Epoetin beta was better tolerated.[395,396] Addition of benzyl alcohol to the alfa formulation has increased the tolerance to epoetin alfa. Using the highest-concentration solution to minimize the injection volume also minimizes pain.

Correction of anemia to Hcts over 30 percent is associated with painless conjunctival injection.[202,284] This "red eye" is of cosmetic concern only.

Frequency of headache varies from 3 to 33 percent, averaging about 15 percent of treated patients[202,203,253,256,281,284,397]; the incidence does not differ from that among untreated or placebo-treated patients.[284]

Endocrine and Metabolic Effects

Younger uremic men manifest a variety of biochemical hormonal abnormalities as well as sexual dysfunction. In general, sexual function improves with correction of anemia,[398] but the mechanism producing this improvement is not clear. Initial reports suggested that high prolactin was decreased by correction of anemia.[399,399] Correction of anemia also improves responsiveness to thyroid-releasing hormone (TRH) and gonadotrophin-releasing hormone (GnRH) of the thyroidal and gonadal axes, and it is this correction that may be more important than any erythropoietin levels achieved by therapy.[400]

In elderly men, despite a significant erythropoietic response, no significant changes were seen in prolactin, testosterone, luteinizing hormone (LH), follicle-stimulating hormone (FSH), thyroid-stimulating hormone (TSH), free thyroxine, triiodothyronine, or IGF-I levels.[401] Only a small decrease in serum growth hormone concentrations occurred. Advanced age and chronic illness in these patients may have played a role in limiting the hormonal response. In addition, the total immunoreactive levels of gonadotrophins may be misleading, as the correction of anemia is associated with an increased ratio of bioactive to immunoreactive LH.[402]

Several studies have reported a positive nitrogen balance during epoetin therapy,[403,404] but this alone does not improve growth in children or alter the abnormalities in amino acid metabolism.[403] Decreased total cholesterol associated with a fall in apoprotein B and serum triglycerides followed correction of anemia in one study,[405] an important observation in view of the risk of atherosclerotic complications in ESRD patients. Diabetic retinopathy improves with correction of anemia.[406,407] Raising or maintaining RBC mass in the 33 to 36 percent Hct range may be effective adjunctive therapy for correcting hypoxia at the level of the retina.

Dialysis Efficiency

After correction of anemia, serum potassium, phosphate, and creatinine increase,[396,408-411] but the changes are of small magnitude and the major effect on urea kinetic modeling can easily be corrected by changing the dialysis prescription.[410-413] Aside from a change in the patient's appetite, the major reason for the observed (but inconsistent) effects in chemistries is a decrease in solute clearance. In vivo studies have found changes in dialyzer urea clearances because of a decrease in water flow as RBC mass increases. Dialyzer reuse efficiency decreases despite 15 to 50 percent increases in heparin dosing.[408,410] A recent study of high-flux hemodialysis noted an increase in treatment time from a mean of 140 to 169 minutes as Hct increased from 24 to 36 percent.[414] With peritoneal dialysis, clearances of sodium, potassium, and urea and changes in protein loss or glucose absorption do not change after epoetin therapy.[415]

Protection of Kidney Function

There is ample evidence in animal models for the effect of anemia and tissue hypoxia on the progression of kidney disease.[416] Increasingly, epidemiologic evidence supports a role in human disease as well. In the large prospective Canadian data base, Levin et al.[417,418] noted a strong influence of Hgb on the relative risk of needing RRT whether the initial estimated GFR was 30 to 60 mL/min or 10 to 30 mL/min. In the RENAAL study, Keane et al.[419] found that the hazard ratio for the combined endpoint [doubling of serum creatinine (SCr) or reaching ESRD] increased progressively with each lower quartile of Hgb, reference being an Hgb > 13.8 g/dL. In a population study in Japan, Iseki[420] found that anemia increased the risk of ESRD more than threefold in women and almost twofold in men.

The mechanisms of protection are probably multifactorial as illustrated in Fig. 26–7, but revolve around the effects of oxidative stress (OS). OS enhances both tubular damage and interstitial fibrosis. Remaining surviving nephrons increase their oxygen consumption leading to increased production of reactive oxygen species which predisposes them to additional injury.[421] OS stimulates interstitial production of extracellular matrix as well as the production of TGF-β,[422] producing fibrosis. Reactive oxygen species also have proapoptotic effects.[423,424] In vivo, treatment of

rats with antioxidants protects against development of interstitial fibrosis,[422] while deprivation of antioxidants seems to have opposite effects.

The most likely mechanism for renal protection from anemia correction may simply be the increase in erythrocyte mass that increases the antioxidant capacity of blood to combat OS[425] and reduce the effects of tissue hypoxia on tubular damage and interstitial fibrosis. Erythrocytes represent a major antioxidant component of the blood, have a glutathione, superoxide dismutase, and catalase system, and cellular proteins that react with reactive oxygen species (low-molecular-weight proteins of the erythrocyte membrane, vitamin E, or coenzyme Q). In addition RBCs can regenerate consumed redox equivalents through the pentose phosphate pathway and through reduction of oxidized glutathione by glutathione reductase. Thus the antioxidant capacity is a function of the number of cells.

However, recent studies indicate direct effects of erythropoietin on tubular cells, preventing cell death in other tis-

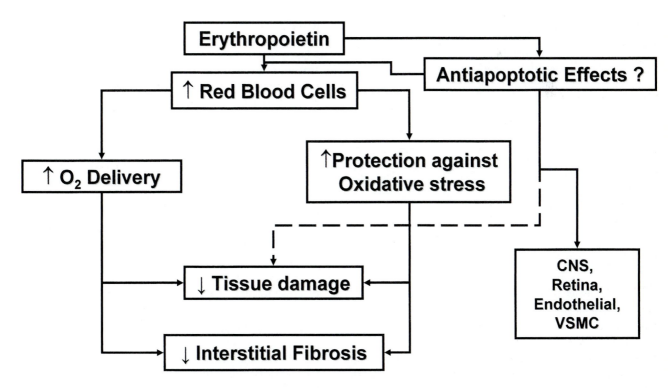

Figure 26–7. Erythropoietin-mechanisms that may modulate the progression of chronic kidney diseases. Solid lines indicate established mechanism. The dashed line represents a possible renal protective effect similar to that present in other systems. CNS = central nervous system, VSMC = vascular smooth muscle cells. (Modified from Rossert et al. *Nephrol Dial Transplant* 2002;17:359–362.

sues besides those of the bone marrow. Epoetin promotes the survival of maturing precursor RBCs by an inhibition of caspase activation[426] and by induction of the expression of antiapoptotic proteins such as Bcl-xL and Bcl-2.[427] Antiapoptotic effects can be observed with other cell types expressing the erythropoietin receptor, such as neuronal cells,[428] endothelial cells,[429] or vascular smooth muscle cells.[430] With the demonstration that proximal tubular cells and medullary collecting duct cells express erythropoietin receptors,[431] epoetin may have a direct effect on renal tubular cells to reduce or prevent apoptosis.

There are now some data that diminished oxygen content due to anemia may itself contribute to interstitial fibrosis and that the progression of CKD can be ameliorated or retarded by treating anemia.[432] There is hope, therefore, that early treatment of anemia can retard progression of CKD through the elimination of tissue hypoxia.[433] Certainly there have been no studies showing any adverse effects of partially correcting anemia in CKD patients.[280,434–436] and invalidating the animal study purporting to demonstrate an adverse effect on kidney function during correction of renal anemia.[437]

Special Considerations in CKD and CHF

Medicare data indicate that the most common cause of hospitalization in elderly patients (> 67 years of age) with CKD prior to the need for dialysis or renal transplantation is congestive heart failure (CHF) (USRDS data; A. Collins, personal communication) occurring in about 23 percent of all patients. It appears that anemia worsens heart failure, which in turn compromises kidney function, producing the cardiorenal-anemia syndrome. Tissue hypoxia is central to the development of CKD and worsening cardiomyopathy as reflex changes in vascular tone and sympathetic activity occur. A vicious cycle ensues that can only be broken by the appropriate management of anemia. Anemia increased the likelihood for death before ESRD during a 2-year follow up of Medicare patients (Medicare 5 percent sample), whether it occurs by itself or in combination with diabetes, CKD, or CHF. Xue et al.[438] analyzed anemia management in over 89,000 Medicare CKD patients who eventually progressed and required dialysis. In those who received no epoetin over 2 years compared to those who received epoetin regularly prior to RRT, the relative risk in the predialysis period was 52 percent greater for cardiac disease, 38 percent greater for hospitalizations due to CHF, and 65 percent greater for mortality within the first year after starting dialysis. Even an effect on the immune system was evident, as there were 41 percent more hospitalizations for infection after starting dialysis in those who were untreated. In their landmark studies, Levin et al.[416,417] showed that the probability of remaining free of RRT was adversely influenced by the presence of cardiovascular disease.

Treatment of anemia with epoetin has been linked to positive cardiac outcomes at earlier stages of CKD.[439,440] In patients with CHF, Silverberg has shown, in an open-label trial, that treatment leading to the amelioration of anemia (from a pretreatment Hgb average of 10.3 g/dL to over 12 g/dL) improved cardiac function and NYHA class and markedly reduced hospitalization.[347] These improvements occurred despite a reduction in diuretic use in the anemia-treated group compared to the untreated group. In summary, anemia is associated with CHF; when anemia is treated, there is improved LVEF and NYHA class status and a decrease in hospitalizations. An additional benefit of treating CHF with CKD is stabilization of kidney function.[441]

Pure Red Cell Aplasia

Pure RBC aplasia (PRCA) is a serious condition with multiple etiologies, including lymphoproliferative disorders, viral infections, autoimmune diseases, drugs, and thymoma. It is characterized by severe anemia, a low blood reticulocyte count with normal white cell and platelet counts, and absence of RBC elements on bone marrow examination. Development of PRCA associated with the presence of neutralizing antierythropoietin antibodies was reported in 13 patients from France treated with epoetin alfa.[442] This complication, requiring transfusion, followed an initial response to epoetin and occurred after a successful duration or epoetin use of 3 to 67 months, with a median of 7 months. Of 9 evaluable patients, 6 recovered some erythropoietic function following discontinuation of epoetin, use of immunosuppressive therapy (immune globulin, plasmapheresis, corticosteroids), and/or renal transplantation. Cross reactivity to other epoetins (epoetin beta and darbepoetin) was noted.

Altered antigenicity of the European product (Eprex, a form of epoetin alfa) due to a difference in manufacturing has been suggested as causal by epidemiologic data. Additional contributing factors may include the product presentation (e.g., prefilled syringes vs. single-dose vials), storage and handling practices, and the subcutaneous route of administration. Over 190 patients with this complication have been noted in Europe, whereas it is rare in the United States.[443,444] The formulation change induced the formation of micelles, which also may have changed the epitopic presentation of sites on the molecule.[445] A definite increase in cases followed the change in formulation in countries using this formulation but not in other countries using other preparations of epoetin alfa, beta, or omega. Almost all cases have been associated with the subcutaneous route of administration. In one patient, wheals developed at the site of subcutaneous injection. Skin responses were evoked at the same site following intravenous epoetin injection, indicating persistence of sensitized cells. The PRCA gradually improved following prednisone treatment.[446] Although recombinant epoetins are known to differ in their carbohydrate content,[447] the neutralizing antibodies identified in the serum of patients with PRCA bind to the protein portion of the epoetin molecule, not to the carbohydrate, and techniques to produce more homogeneous epoetin preparations are not likely to have an effect on PRCA.[448] Regulatory authorities in Europe, Australia, and Canada have limited the use of subcutaneous Eprex in CKD patients, and there has been an apparent decrease in the appearance of PRCA since these policies went into effect. Because the neutralizing antibodies cross-react with other erythropoietic proteins as well as natural erythropoietin, patients with PRCA should not be switched to another erythropoietic agent.

TARGET HGB LEVELS

Currently epoetin therapy in both the United States and Europe can be initiated when the Hgb decreases below 11 g/dL, based on policies of the respective regulatory bodies. This value applies to more than 390,000 patients currently on dialysis in the United States and to millions of people with CKD who do not require dialysis (CKD stages 1 through 4). Currently the recommended upper limit for epoetin therapy is 12 g/dL for CKD and 12.5 g/dL for ESRD patients in the United States. No upper boundary has been set in Europe. Beneficial clinical and economic outcomes associated with Hgb levels of 11 to 12.5 g/dL in dialysis patients have been demonstrated. A number of other studies have demonstrated benefits associated with Hgb levels of 12 g/dL or greater in dialysis patients.

In general, all retrospective, large-scale observational studies show increased QOL, decreased mortality, and a reduced risk of hospitalization with higher Hgb levels, but prospective studies have failed to show much benefit and perhaps risk when Hgb is normalized. The normal Hct trial[285] compared patients whose anemia was treated to an average Hct level of 30 percent versus 42 percent. The prospective study included 1233 patients and required evidence of CHF or ischemic heart disease. The study was terminated because of an increased risk of vascular access thrombosis and a trend toward a higher rate of nonfatal myocardial infarction or death in the normal Hct group when data were assessed using an intent-to-treat analysis (difference did not reach significance at the time of termination). Similarly, the Canadian Normal Hgb trial[449] recruited hemodialysis patients with LVH or LV dilatation (early phase of cardiac disease). Normalizing Hgb in LVH patients produced no regression of hypertrophy but lower rates of progressive LV dilatation. There was no benefit of normalizing Hgb in patients with overt LV dilatation at time of randomization. QOL improved by normalization of Hgb and there was no difference between Hgb groups in access thrombosis, probably due to the use of native arteriovenous fistulas (AVFs) in Canada compared to the use of grafts in the

United States, or in mortality rates. The disappointing effects on LV morphology in the Canadian study made it increasingly apparent that the greater the degree of cardiac damage, the more difficult it is to reverse, even with aggressive anemia treatment.[450] The discrepancy between the results of the U.S. trial and other smaller studies suggest that further studies were needed, especially in patients without heart disease.

Such a study has recently been published. The Swedish study[451] randomized both CKD and ESRD patients to two levels of anemia treatment; partial to 11 g/dL and almost full to 14 g/dL. After 1 year of follow-up, there was no evidence of increased mortality; rather the opposite—although not yet significant. Within each group, mortality risk varied inversely with Hgb level, a finding as well of the Normal Hct trial.[285] This trial indicated that a normal Hgb is safe in CKD patients without heart disease with CKD stages 3 to 5. In addition, QOL was found to be better with normal than with subnormal Hgb.

TREATMENT ISSUES

In the current U.S. health care environment, primary care physicians (PCPs) face a tremendous challenge in identifying, treating, and referring patients with CKD and CKD-related complications and comorbidities. The situation is probably the same for patients with CHF. Anemia is only one aspect of that challenge, albeit one with significant ramifications in terms of cardiac changes and QOL throughout the course of kidney disease or heart failure. The existence of a huge pool of patients who are not receiving the immediate treatment and/or referral they require is clear. As implied by the Arora study,[452] early referral to a nephrologist increases the likelihood of appropriate anemia treatment but does not guarantee it. A survey of 200 European nephrologists revealed a certain reluctance to initiate treatment of anemia in CKD patients prior to ESRD. Although most respondents to the survey regarded epoetin treatment as safe and effective for treating CKD-related anemia, 38 percent administered epoetin to fewer than 10 percent of their CKD patients prior to ESRD. Furthermore, the majority of respondents who administered epoetin did so routinely only when Hgb levels had fallen well below 12g/dL.

The proposed NKF-K/DOQI staging of CKD coupled with the national public awareness initiative, National Kidkey Disease Education Program (NKDEP), may promote a greater sensitivity on the part of PCPs to be alert for CKD and its complications in patients with a GFR <60 mL/min/1.73 m^2 (stage 3). In an optimal health care environment, the PCP plays a key role in patient treatment throughout the progression of CKD. When a patient with

CKD is identified, the PCP monitors and manages the condition and its comorbidities and complications. Accomplishing this may require additional education and interaction with specialist teams. A recent survey of PCPs showed that although most PCPs were confident in their ability to manage hypertension and administer ACE inhibitors in patients with CKD, they were less comfortable with other aspects of CKD care, including treatment of anemia and renal bone disease and educating the patient on nutrition and dialysis.

Definitive recommendations for optimal treatment of CKD- or CHF-related anemia prior to dialysis await prospective, controlled clinical trials. Nevertheless, there currently appears to be an adequate rationale for vigilance, diagnosis, and therapeutic intervention in these patients.

Dosing, Pharmacokinetics, and Route of Administration

All epoetin-treated dialysis patients increase their Hct in a dose-dependent manner. There are two phases, the corrective phase and the maintenance phase, during which the same dose of epoetin is used. The appropriate dose in a given patient is one that permits attainment of the target Hct over the life span of the erythrocyte, as it satisfies both the initiation and maintenance requirements. The response to a given dose of epoetin among patients is quite variable. In part this variability reflects the observation that, even in normal individuals, a tenfold variability in endogenous erythropoietin levels among subjects evidently maintains the same normal RBC mass.[107] The intravenous doses needed to attain a mean Hct of 34 to 35 percent show this same tenfold variation, from 25 to 300 U/kg.

Attempts have been made to use the tools of kinetic modeling to individualize dosing.[84,453] One such attempt by Uehlenger and colleagues[454] involves the use of nomograms to determine a daily marrow RBC production for a given target Hct and then calculate an epoetin dose based on predicted rates of RBC production and marrow sensitivity. The model assumes mean population values for RBC survival, estimated blood volume, and, most importantly, bone marrow sensitivity to epoetin. This procedure does not solve the dilemma of dosage adjustment or the clinical problems resulting from extensive fluctuations around the desired response. However, the model developed does provide considerable insight into the determinants controlling the response to epoetin.

The pharmacodynamic model permits analysis of the effect various factors have on response to a given dose of epoetin. An obvious variable is the RBC survival. The shorter the RBC survival, the lower will be the response to a given dose of epoetin if the other variables are constant. Although RBC survival is generally believed to be short in CKD, averaging about 60 to 80 days,[5] it can also be within the normal range[20] in well-dialyzed nonbleeding patients.

Thus a range of RBC survivals can occur in ESRD patients varying from 40 days to a normal value of 120 days. The patient with a short life span of 40 days, whether due to hemolysis or external blood losses, requires larger amounts of epoetin to reach the target Hct of 33 to 37 percent and also aggressive iron management if bleeding is present. However, the individual with a normal RBC survival may exceed the target Hct of 36 percent even with low doses. These considerations help to explain the wide variation in the amount of epoetin needed to maintain Hct in the range of 32 to 38 percent, varying from 12.5 to over 500 U/kg when epoetin is given three times a week.[253] The modal dose is 75 U/kg. These findings lead to the evidence-based recommendation to initiate therapy with a fixed dose of 50 to 100 U/kg intravenously.[455] When administered subcutaneously, the dose needed is frequently lower (see below); a reasonable starting dosage is 80 to 120 U/kg/week in two to three divided doses.

The response to epoetin is independent of the cause of CKD,[323] although some have suggested that patients with diabetes respond more slowly and need higher doses than nondiabetics.[456] When the bone marrow is examined after 3 or more months of epoetin therapy, the myeloid/erythroid ratio decreases from a baseline of 4.0 to a value of 2.4. Overall, marrow cellularity increases.[457] Importantly, marrow iron seen at baseline decreases markedly. Low pretreatment fibrinogen (no inflammation) and low baseline transferrin receptor (no ineffective RBC production) associated with 20 percent increases in receptor during epoetin therapy were the best predictors of response to treatment and achievement of an Hct greater than 30 percent.[458] These measurements unfortunately are not routinely available. Steady-state levels of transferrin receptor, a quantitative measure of erythropoiesis, increase progressively and double after 6 to 8 weeks of therapy. When epoetin is discontinued, erythropoietic activity decreases.[459]

The response to epoetin in patients on peritoneal dialysis is as good as that in patients on hemodialysis,[460,461] and the dosing frequency is frequently reduced to once a week for convenience.[462,463] Most centers use the subcutaneous route, permitting self-administration at home. CAPD patients respond better than hemodialysis patients to equivalent weekly doses, perhaps because of lower ongoing blood losses.[476] Some centers dose only once a week and obtain good results.[464,465]

Drug dosage should not be drastically lowered after the target Hct is reached, since this produces a "yo-yo" or "ping-pong" effect. The ideal dose would be that which permits attainment of the target Hct over the life span of the erythrocyte, since it satisfies both the initiation and maintenance requirements.[466] During uptitration, we advocate changes in epoetin of 25 to 30 percent of the previous weekly dose or a downtitration of 10 U/kg/dose if Hct rises in excess of 1.5 points per week. The dose should be held only in the very rapid responder whose Hct rises more than 2 points per week or in those who develop difficult-to-control hypertension. In the vast majority of patients, blood pressure can be managed effectively by reducing the dry weight and then adding or increasing an antihypertensive agent if necessary. Only if these approaches fail to control hypertension should one consider holding or markedly reducing the dose. During maintenance therapy, new RBCs should be formed at a rate comparable to the removal rate.

Once a patient reaches the target Hct/Hgb, the frequency of Hct or Hgb monitoring can decrease. We favor monitoring every 2 weeks over monthly because variations in Hct can occur that are unrelated to changes in Hgb or RBC count and because of variations in interdialytic weight gain. In our experience the average patient has a standard deviation of 1.0 g/dL in the Hgb level when measured over the course of a year. Changes in plasma volume change the Hct without changes in RBC mass. Samples should be collected just prior to the dialysis session. End-dialysis samples will show a significant increase in Hct of up to 6 points because plasma volume is decreased at the end of hemodialysis, causing an increase in Hct.[467] Hgb and Hct increase by 1 g/dL and by 3 points, respectively, following dialysis.[468] These increases from predialysis values correlate with percent change in body weight (ultrafiltration). At 24 hours following dialysis, Hct and Hgb levels remain higher, indicating slow reequilibration. The importance of this observation is that patients with predialysis Hct above 38 percent or Hgb levels above 13 g/dL may be at risk from hemoconcentration effects, particularly if they have large interdialytic weight gains. Samples can be collected at any time in peritoneal dialysis patients, as the plasma volume is relatively constant during any given day; however, care should be taken to ensure the same posture.

Epoetin Hyporesponsiveness

Resistance to epoetin is defined by the requirement of either a large dose during initiation or by the development of refractiveness to a previous efficacious dose and dosage escalation to maintain a target Hct. In approximately 10 percent of subjects, a dose >300 U/kg/week will be needed in the absence of any "known" state producing resistance and probably represents differences in epoetin response sensitivity among individuals. Patients requiring more than 450 U/kg/week are considered to be relatively resistant to epoetin. However, biological heterogeneity—variation in intrinsic sensitivity and in RBC survival—accounts for many instances of patients who do require more than 450 U/kg/week to reach and then maintain an Hct greater than 30 percent. This was seen in six patients who required large doses of epoetin to maintain their target Hct but in whom studies of erythroid refractoriness, RBC survival, epoetin pharmacokinetics, parathyroid hormone (PTH), and alu-

minum failed to disclose a reason for their large dosage needs.[469] About 10 percent of our patients need more than 450 U/kg/week of epoetin in the absence of any known state producing resistance. In the remainder, conditions known to produce epoetin resistance must be looked for. At least 10 separate conditions can produce epoetin resistance[470-472]:

1. *Absolute and relative iron deficiency* is the most common condition.[241] Blood loss should always be suspected in those requiring increasing doses or large maintenance doses of intravenous iron. Oral iron is relatively ineffective; we therefore favor intermittent parenteral iron administration (see below).

2. *Infection/inflammation* is the second most common condition, and responsiveness can usually be restored upon recovery. Inflammatory mediators may arise from the underlying process[200,202,473,474] or from hemodialysis.[475] Key mediators are TNF and IL-1.[200,470,476,477] Patients with failed transplants returning to dialysis are frequently resistant to epoetin[478] until the transplant is removed. Peritonitis in CAPD patients usually produces temporary resistance, but on occasion prolonged refractiveness may be seen.[479] Chronic infections may be difficult to diagnose, such as those associated with failed arteriovenous vascular access grafts.[480]

3. *Hyperparathyroidism*[188] is a less common cause, in which the relationship is between the degree of fibrosis and the amount of epoetin needed to maintain a target Hct. Serum levels of PTH do not correlate with epoetin dose.

4. *Aluminum overload* has become a much less common cause of epoetin refractiveness[481,482] as non-aluminum-containing phosphate binders have increasingly replaced aluminum-containing agents.

5. *Hemoglobinopathies* produce relative resistance. Experience in sickle cell disease has been disappointing.[245,483] Therapy of thalassemia requires prolonged high-dose epoetin therapy.[484,485]

6. Patients with *multiple myeloma* on dialysis also require higher-dose epoetin.[486]

7. *Cofactor deficiency* can develop in patients who were initially responsive to epoetin. Evaluation of folate and vitamin B_{12} is needed in select cases.[487,488] Macrocytosis is an inadequate differentiating feature.

8. *Hemolysis* can be induced by residual formaldehyde in dialyzers, producing epoetin refractiveness.[489] Patients with severe hemolysis across heart valves can require transfusions, despite use of large doses of epoetin.[490]

9. The emergence of *erythropoietin antibodies* has been documented.[441-446]

10. *Malnutrition* is associated with low serum albumin levels that, in turn, are associated with low Hcts among dialysis patients. Malnutrition can be quickly worsened by inflammation.[491] Acute-phase reactants correlate with resistance to epoetin.[492]

Iron Therapy

Suboptimal response to epoetin commonly results from failure of an adequate delivery of iron to the erythron. Enhanced iron utilization due to erythropoietin-induced RBC formation can quickly deplete iron stores. Oral iron preparations frequently fail in hemodialysis patients.[493] The USRDS Dialysis Morbidity and Mortality Study showed that 50 percent of patients receiving epoetin were iron deficient.[494] Because erythropoiesis has to be stimulated to a greater than normal degree to compensate for blood losses and or shortened RBC survival, functional iron deficiency frequently develops.

Although a nomogram constructed by Van Wyck[233] can be used to estimate iron needs in correcting anemia, we prefer to calculate the amount on the basis of 1 mg of iron needed for each 1 mL of packed RBC and factor in ongoing RBC losses. The increase in packed cells is estimated from the starting and target Hcts and the estimated blood volume of the patient (70 to 80 mL/kg). Ongoing blood losses during the period of correction are estimated at 600 to 700 mg of additional iron over a 12- to 14-week period. The exact dosing then depends on whether the patient is iron-replete (unusual in most patients starting dialysis) and unlikely to develop relative iron deficiency, using ferritin >800 ng/mL as a cutoff value for the iron-replete state. Iron-replete patients receive only the amount of iron needed to correct the RBC mass as 75 to 125 mg weekly doses until the desired amount is given. Regular monitoring of iron status by measurement of serum ferritin and transferrin saturation (TSAT) is mandatory in the cost-effective management of anemia with epoetin and should be performed monthly.

Once the maintenance period is reached, we have preferred to use a maintenance protocol of 25 to 50 mg of iron intravenously weekly, the dose being adjusted in response to sequential iron indexes. CAPD patients require less iron due to smaller ongoing blood losses. In most cases, administration of 500 or 1000 mg slowly over 4 to 6 hours is sufficient, and adequate response can be maintained for 6 months to 1 year.

In traditional intermittent dosing regimens, intravenous iron is given when TSAT or ferritin fall below 20 percent and 100 ng/mL respectively. A number of studies have indicated that iron-replete patients receiving regular parenteral iron maintain better serum ferritin levels and require less epoetin than patients receiving no parenteral iron supplementation or regular oral iron alone.[224–226,495] Averaged over 7 studies in iron-replete patients (TSAT > 24 percent and ferritin from 200 to 600 ng/mL), administration of a pro-rated weekly dose of iron increased Hct by 14 percent, with a concomitant decrease in epoetin dose of 38 percent.[496] We evaluated a maintenance regimen in which an initial iron dextran dose of 300 to 500 mg was followed by 25 to 100 mg every 1 to 2 weeks (to maintain a transferrin saturation between 30 and 50%) to a traditional intermittent dosing regimen (to maintain a transferrin saturation >20% or a ferritin level >200 ng/mL). The amount of epoetin required in the maintenance group was more than 50 percent lower than that utilized in the intermittent group to achieve the same target Hgb of 10 to 11 g/dL.[497] A more aggressive iron regimen was found to reduce the dosage of epoetin even further.[498] However, this more aggressive regimen produced progressive elevations in serum ferritin level to an average of 730 ng/mL (at month 6) with an average monthly iron administration of 400 mg/month—twice that in the control group.

Until recently, iron dextran was the only available agent used extensively in the United States, although other forms of iron were available in Europe.[225,226,239,499] Administration of sodium ferric gluconate complex, 1.0 g over eight consecutive dialysis days, significantly increased Hgb levels, serum ferritin, and iron saturation in 83 iron-deficient dialysis patients.[500] Many physicians are concerned about the risks of using parenteral intravenous iron dextran. The incidence of severe life-threatening reactions to one or more doses in any patient is quite low, at less than 1 percent.[501,502] The rate per number of injections is even lower at 0.1 percent. Decreasing the infusion rate to less than 10 mg/min minimizes reactions.

Sodium ferric gluconate complex in sucrose may have fewer fatal adverse reactions than iron dextran and its efficacy as good as iron dextran.[503] Similar results have been found with iron sucrose.[504] Both sodium ferric gluconate complex[503] and iron sucrose[505] have been administered to patients allergic to iron dextran. Cost-effectiveness may be the only factor preventing these agents from being preferred over iron dextran, since they are one-third more expensive. They also cannot yet be given as total dose infusion, a practice possible with iron dextran.

The frequency of administration of iron has been evaluated in a few studies only. Administration of 6.25 to 21.3 mg of sodium ferric gluconate complex at every treatment compared to 62.5 mg every 1 to 4 weeks was effective in increasing Hgb levels and prevented an increase in ferritin levels.[506] Administration of iron during each dialysis was also studied using a novel delivery system. Dialysis with a solution containing soluble ferric pyrophosphate, a chelated iron that readily diffuses into the blood compartment, was found to be safe and effective in a preliminary 6-month study of stable hemodialysis patients.[507]

Controversy exists about the best method of assessing adequate iron stores and iron delivery to the bone marrow.

(see Assessment of Iron Status, above). We use CHr and ferritin and have mostly abandoned TSAT.

Iron Overload

Occasionally, patients are clearly iron-overloaded but respond poorly to epoetin and require large doses of it. Several approaches to such patients have been recommended. Ascorbic acid 500 mg given intravenously after hemodialysis one to three times a week can mobilize tissue stores.[508] Although serum ferritin remained unchanged with such a regimen, transferrin saturation increased from 27 to 54 percent and Hct increased from 27 to 32 percent. A control group with normal iron status and without resistance to epoetin showed no changes in TSAT or Hct when challenged in the same manner with ascorbate. An alternative method uses desferrioxamine in patients with iron but without aluminum overload. Epoetin doses decreased dramatically from 400 to 25 U/kg while increasing Hgb levels to and then maintaining them at 11 g/dL.[509] Iron overload has become uncommon with the decrease in transfusions. Persistent blood losses in hemodialysis patients can, over several years of epoetin treatment, produce iron deficiency even in those with initial serum ferritin greater than 5000 ng/mL. It is now rare for any patient to be treated with phlebotomy after overdriving the bone marrow with epoetin.[271,272,510]

NEWER EPOETINS

The current standard of care is to administer epoetin two to three times per week. In practice in patients with CKD, this schedule of administration is achieved mainly in patients receiving hemodialysis because of the thrice-weekly dialysis schedule. In patients receiving peritoneal dialysis and those in the predialysis stage, it is generally given once weekly, due to the less frequent contact between patient and caregiver and the inconvenience of frequent subcutaneous administration. The recommended dosage in all these patient groups is still thrice weekly, however.

Current evidence indicates that efficient erythropoiesis requires the maintenance of erythropoietin above a critical level, below which erythroid cells undergo apoptosis.[511] Frequent dosing, however, places a considerable burden on health care staff as well as on patients. Studies of erythropoietin carbohydrate isoforms in animals have demonstrated a positive relationship between the sialated carbohydrate content of erythropoietin and its half-life (that is, the higher the carbohydrate content, the longer the half-life) and in vivo biological activity.[512] Darbepoetin alfa (Aranesp, Amgen Inc., Thousand Oaks, CA), a novel erythropoiesis-stimulating protein (NESP), was developed as a longer-acting erythropoietic agent using site-directed mutagenesis. It has two additional carbohydrate chains. It has been shown to have a threefold longer terminal elimination half-life compared with epoetin (25 vs. 8.5 hours) when administered intravenously and approximately twice as long (49 hours) when administered subcutaneously.[513] The molecule was approximately 3.6-fold more biologically active than epoetin when each molecule was administered three times per week and 13 to 14 times as active when injected once a week.[514] Darbepoetin does not accumulate over time when given repeatedly. In early clinical trials, dosing frequencies out to every 3 weeks subcutaneously have been reached in CKD patients not on dialysis.[514] An even longer-acting pegylated epoetin-beta preparation is undergoing clinical trials and has a $t_{1/2} > 100$ hours, with the potential for once-monthly dosing.[515]

MISCELLANEOUS CONSIDERATIONS

Angiotensin-Converting Enzyme Inhibitors

Angiotensin-converting enzyme (ACE) inhibitors have been used to control erythrocytosis, particularly that occurring after renal transplantation.[516,517] Although some reports suggest that ACE inhibitors can decrease response to epoetin[518,519] others have not.[520] In view of the importance of ACE inhibitors for cardiac remodeling and antihypertensive treatment in hemodialysis patients, ACE-inhibitor therapy for blood pressure control or heart failure should not be withheld to minimize epoetin dosage. The receptor antagonist losartan does not appear to change any indicator of erythropoiesis in normals and should be studied in ESRD patients receiving epoetin on dialysis.[521]

Malignancy

Malignancy is frequently accompanied by increasing anemia. Larger doses of epoetin should be used, because patients without CKD frequently require larger doses than those received by patients with progressive renal insufficiency.[522]

Intraperitoneal Administration of Epoetin

Intraperitoneal epoetin can be effectively used in small children by the infusion of epoetin in 50 mL of fluid into a "dry" abdomen.[523,524]

Intercurrent Illness or Surgery

Erythropoietic response is reduced during intercurrent illness or surgery. Our policy is to continue the epoetin therapy throughout the intercurrent illness. We generally stop the therapy after renal transplantation. Because erythropoietin production may be delayed, particularly in the presence of delayed graft function, epoetin can reduce the need for postoperative transfusion; however, the amount of epoetin needed to maintain Hct levels is twofold greater than the amount needed prior to transplant.[525]

GRANULOCYTE NUMBER AND FUNCTION IN UREMIC PATIENTS

The changes in granulocyte number and function in uremic patients can be divided into those resulting from the uremic state and those attributable to the hemodialysis procedure. Except for transient episodes of neutropenia during the first 90 minutes of dialysis, the granulocyte counts of uremic patients are normal. Hemodialysis-induced leukopenia begins within minutes of initiating dialysis and is of short duration. The number of circulating granulocytes reaches a nadir within 15 minutes of dialysis onset and is completely restored to normal values within several hours of dialysis.[526] This granulocytopenia is characterized by significant decreases in adhesiveness, aggregability, and surface Fc receptors on circulating leukocytes.[527] Craddock and coworkers[528,529] and Chenoweth and colleagues[530] demonstrated that these effects resulted from activation of C3a and C5a by contact with cellulosic dialysis membranes. Activated C5a triggers adherence of neutrophils to endothelial surfaces and to each other. Recent studies have documented that such neutrophil activation leads to upregulation of adhesion receptors,[531] release of proteinases and other enzymes, production of reactive oxygen species,[190] activation of platelets leading to thromboxane B_2 release,[532] and activation of monocytes leading to cytokine production, specifically IL-1 and TNF-α.[199,200,533,534]

Margination of leukocytes in the pulmonary capillaries is responsible in part for the transient hypoxemia observed during dialysis.[535] This process is self-limited; the rate of complement activation decreases as dialysis proceeds, but the mechanisms for this passivation are not well defined. Complement activation is membrane type–dependent and reduced by the reprocessing of membranes.[529] A number of clinical (double-blind) studies have shown that anaphylatoxin release is related to a variety of clinical symptoms, including chest and back pain and dyspnea; the incidence of these symptoms is reduced by the reprocessing of dialyzer membranes.[536,537] "First-use syndrome" appears to occur in association with new dialyzers of large surface area in a subset of patients (about 5 percent) who appear to activate the complement pathway more vigorously than other patients.[538]

Despite changes in the care of patients with CKD and the development of new antimicrobial agents, the incidence of life-threatening infection in ESRD patients over the past two decades has remained unchanged.[539] Both random and chemoattractant-induced granulocyte mobility, as well as phagocytosis, are reduced in various cohorts of uremic patients.[269,540] Substantial defects in granulocyte chemotaxis, adherence, and expression of receptors involved in phagocytosis are demonstrable in patients dialyzed with cellulosic membranes even when compared with uremic predialysis patients.[541,542] More importantly, chronic hemodialysis with complement-activating membranes attenuates the ability of neutrophils, harvested predialysis, to respond to phagocytic stimuli.[543] The expression of L-selectins, receptors involved in granulocyte-endothelial adhesion, on neutrophils harvested during dialysis is decreased.[530] Granulocyte-endothelial cell adhesion is decreased after dialysis with cellulosic membranes but not after dialysis with more "biocompatible" membranes such as polymethylmethacrylate (PMMA) and polysulfone (PS).

Monocytes, functioning as circulating macrophages, are also activated during hemodialysis with cellulosic membranes. Chronic exposure to such membranes induces refractiveness to further stimuli.[544] Defective monocyte function, such as Fc receptor activity[545] and monocyte-dependent IL-2 production by activated T cells,[546] has been documented.

The dialysis-induced changes in neutrophils and monocytes can result in a wide variety of effects. Proteolytic enzymes released during neutrophil deregulation may contribute to catabolism, while neutrophil elastase release may participate in the pathogenesis of carpal tunnel syndrome. Mononuclear IL-6 and immunoglobulin production is impaired by exposure to certain types of membranes,[547] suggesting that long-term exposure of mononuclear cells to such membranes may contribute to the impaired humoral responses noted in dialysis patients. However, CKD may be the major determinant of the increased plasma IL-6 levels, although the dialysis procedure with cellulosic membranes may contribute to the maintenance of elevated levels.[476] Production of beta2 microglobulin, a substance linked to dialysis amyloidosis, is highly related to IL-6 production.[548]

Lymphocytes are not passive bystanders. The expression of high-affinity IL-2 receptors, crucial to the immune response, is attenuated after chronic exposure to bioincompatible membranes.[549] Changes in T-cell subsets and in vitro immunity become more pronounced in patients with longer durations of maintenance hemodialysis.[550] However, impaired RBC-mediated immunity is present in predialysis CKD patients.[551]

Dysfunction of the host immune system against infection in ESRD patients, particularly those dialyzed with "bioincompatible membranes," is thus not unexpected.[552] In a study of almost 1000 patients, a decrease by one-half was noted in the incidence of infection following a change from a cellulosic to a biocompatible membrane.[553] Similar findings were noted in another study.[554] Nevertheless, no prospective study has yet been performed, nor have any studies documented differences in clinical cellular immunity as a function of membrane type used for hemodialysis. This aspect has become moot with the generalized use of more "biocompatible" membranes.

Interestingly, several reports have indicated that some immune functions improve after correction of anemia with epoetin. Positive effects on the number of natural killer cell and in helper/suppresser T-cell ratios,[555] on immunoglobulin production by peripheral mononuclear cells harvested from epoetin-treated patients,[556] and on phagocytic function[557] have been reported. Although iron overload and correction of this state by epoetin may be responsible for the improvement in phagocytic function,[558] other studies indicate that the effect is unrelated to changes in iron metabolism.[560] Cell-mediated and humoral immune function may also improve. Antibody titers to hepatitis B vaccine are eightfold higher in epoetin-treated patients, although the rate of seroconversion is unaffected.[559] Despite these studies, the effect of epoetin on the overall incidence of infection is difficult to determine, since there has been an explosion of catheter use as vascular access for hemodialysis, which can produce catheter-related bacteremia in an aging dialysis population.

ABNORMALITIES OF HEMOSTASIS IN UREMIA

CKD is associated with a bleeding tendency.[141,304,560] Common manifestations include ecchymoses, purpura, epistaxis, and gastrointestinal bleeding, particularly when associated with telengectasias.[142] Much less common now than previously are hemorrhagic pericarditis,[561] hemorrhagic pleural effusions,[562] spontaneous subcapsular hematomas,[563] and spontaneous retroperitoneal bleeding. A major concern is the development of subdural hematomas.[564] Abnormalities of platelet function in uremic subjects are characterized by prolonged bleeding times, abnormal platelet aggregation and adhesiveness, and decreased platelet factor 3 release.[143,307,309] Changes in the concentrations of circulating clotting factors, when present, are inconsistent and do not contribute significantly to the bleeding tendency.[565] Skin bleeding time, a global test of primary hemostasis, correlates best with the occurrence of clinical bleeding.[307] Both bleeding time and platelet adhesiveness are dependent on platelet numbers. Although statistically the platelet count itself in uremic subjects is lower than in controls, thrombocytopenia of sufficient degree to impair hemostasis is unusual.[566] The platelet count in most patients is above 120,000.

Platelet functional defects are responsible for the abnormalities noted in laboratory studies. Platelet aggregation in response to collagen, adenosine diphosphate (ADP), epinephrine, serotonin, and arachidonic acid is reduced in uremic patients.[567,568] This abnormality begins at a serum creatinine of about 6 mg/dL[569] and is only partially corrected by dialysis[307,556]; it is partially explained by altered cyclooxygenase metabolism.[307] Uremic platelets generate abnormally small amounts of thromboxane A_2 in response to thrombin or arachidonic acid. The metabolism of arachidonic acid also appears to be impaired in uremia at the vessel wall level, as evidenced by increased prostacyclin (PGI_2) formation.[570] Estrogen injection shortens bleeding time,[571] but without changing vascular PGI_2 synthesis.[572]

Platelet adhesion to foreign surfaces and to vessel subendothelium is decreased in uremia[147,309]—an effect that has been attributed to both a platelet abnormality and a plasma factor interfering with this process.[311] Both platelet adhesion and bleeding time are Hct-dependent and were, until the introduction of epoetin, dependent on the degree of anemia. Transfusion of washed, filtered RBCs devoid of plasma or other cellular components has partially corrected these abnormalities.[147,150] Two adhesive proteins, fibrinogen and vWF, and two adhesion receptors, the glycoprotein (GP) Ib-IX-V complex and GP IIb-IIIa complex, are crucial for the initiation of platelet thrombi at the site of vascular injury.[145] It has been shown that a reversible abnormality in the activation-dependent binding activity of GP IIb-IIIa occurs in uremia and may be the major cause for the altered platelet function. Removal of components present in uremic plasma, either in vitro by washing or in vivo by dialysis, markedly improved the GP IIb-IIIa defect.[145] The substance producing this inhibition is believed to be guanidosuccinic acid.[573] The number of GP Ib binding sites on platelets and the binding of vWF to these sites appears to be normal in uremia. Hemodialysis, although removing these substances, may itself affect platelets through their interaction with the membrane surface.[574,575] The defects in aggregation and adhesion may result from the GP IIb-IIIa defect and account for the reduced endothelial coverage by uremic platelets as a consequence of abnormal interaction with vWF.[576]

However, uremic bleeding is likely to result from multiple pathogenic factors. In addition to the defects outlined above, abnormalities in the multimeric structure of vWF have been described.[144] These abnormalities may affect the hemostatic function of platelets by changes in the initial interaction with GP Ib and the subsequent activation of GP IIb-IIIa. Uremic platelets also acquire a storage pool deficiency with decreased concentrations of ADP and serotonin, whereas the ATP/ADP ratio is increased.[146] Uremic platelets have elevated cAMP content[577] and may have disturbed regulation of Ca^{2+} content as well.[318] Finally PTH inhibits in vitro platelet aggregation, perhaps by interfering with Ca^{2+} flux.[578] Remuzzi's group[309] has reported that uremic plasma induces nitric oxide synthesis by cultured endothelial cells. Nitric oxide inhibits platelet function. Nitric oxide formation, in turn, is inhibited by guanosuccinic acid.

Paradoxically, despite these qualitative and quantitative defects in hemostasis, vascular accesses are subject to thromboses,[579] and the incidence of cerebrovascular accidents is significant in both adult and pediatric dialysis populations.[144] Lai et al.[317] have noted that hemodialysis patients had higher total but lower free protein-S antigen levels than normal individuals. Both the antigen and functional activity of antithrombin III (ATIII) was significantly lower than in normals. Neither protein S or ATIII were affected by the dialysis procedure. In contrast, a progressive increase in functional protein C occurred with hemodialysis. These changes in proteins S and C and ATIII reduce thrombosis risk and do not contribute to bleeding. In the CAPD population, significant amounts of proteins are lost in the peritoneal dialysate. Despite documented losses of ATIII and proteins S and C, much greater than those occurring in hemodialysis patients, plasma levels of these procoagulant substances are greater in CAPD than in hemodialysis patients.[318]

The potential usefulness of antiplatelet agents in patients with repeated vascular access thrombosis or external temporary catheters has been evaluated because of the continuous platelet activation by dialysis membranes.[580] However, aspirin, even in relatively low doses, induces a grater prolongation of the bleeding time in uremic than in normal individuals.[581] The bleeding time may remain elevated for a prolonged time in uremics, unrelated to aspirin pharmacokinetics, resulting from blockage of thromboxane A_2 generation.[582] When aspirin is given to patients with CKD with the aim of preventing micro- or macrothrombus formation, one should be cognizant of the major risks taken due to interference with primary hemostasis. Similarly, a multicenter study using clopidrogel bisulfate (Plavix) to reduce vascular access thrombosis was stopped due to excessive bleeding.

Greater understanding of the mechanisms producing uremic bleeding have improved the therapeutic modalities available to prophylactically treat those undergoing invasive or surgical procedures and those who are actively bleeding. Platelet function is significantly improved, although not completely corrected by institution of effective and adequate dialysis. Low-molecular-weight heparins offer advantages in reducing heparin-associated bleeding.[583] PGI_2 has been used as an alternative to heparin in dialysis patients[584] but requires close physician supervision during each dialysis session. In many patients, heparin-free hemodialysis can be performed with the intermittent infusion of 150 to 300 mL of saline every 10 to 30 minutes and the use of high blood flows.[585] Abnormal bleeding time and a defect in platelet adhesion to blood vessel subendothelium are less common in patients with an Hct above 25 to 30 percent, and these parameters are improved by increasing the Hct above this level by transfusion.[150] Accordingly, uremic anemic patients with active bleeding or who require surgery should be transfused to decrease the bleeding tendency. The use of

epoetin is inappropriate in this setting because of the delay in Hct rise, although its nonerythropoietic affects on vascular, neuronal, and cardiac tissue may be beneficial.[586]

The therapeutic use of epoetin proved that anemia was an important cause of the "bleeding abnormalities" noted in CKD patients, since the prolonged bleeding time is corrected to normal during epoetin therapy.[151,153,310,314] An increase in platelet count[312,313] occurs commonly but is usually transient, and total platelet count seldom exceeds normal limits. Changes in platelet reactivity and adhesiveness during epoetin therapy are variable.[311,314,587] Taylor et al.[588] reported that epoetin therapy significantly increased plasma vWF activity, vWF antigen, as well as fibrinogen, but they could not demonstrate a direct effect of epoetin in vitro. Some of the changes noted could increase the risk for thrombosis, particularly during the withdrawal of epoetin. Vascular access function has been studied and thrombosis does not appear to be increased [253,322,589,590] except in patients with previously known access dysfunction.[324] Intraaccess fistula flow remains stable during epoetin therapy despite an increase in whole-blood viscosity.[331] Shand et al.[591] demonstrated that epoetin treatment or renal anemia resulted in the expected changes in RBC mass and blood viscosity, but Doppler assessments of brachial artery flow as well as tests of fistula function and heparin requirements did not differ between epoetin- and placebo-treated subjects. Lai and coworkers[380] found no laboratory evidence of increased thrombogenesis due to reduction of natural coagulation inhibitors in CAPD patients receiving epoetin.

Several other therapeutic modalities have been proposed to treat the patient who is at high risk for invasive interventions or actively bleeding: (1) infusion of cryoprecipitate[592]; (2) injection of 1-deamino-8-D-arginine vasopressin (DDAVP)[593]; and (3) oral or intravenous administration of a conjugated estrogen preparation (Premarin).[594] The rationale for the use of cryoprecipitate and vasopressin is that they increase the circulating titer of high-molecular-weight multimers of vWF, which in turn are required for binding of platelets to subendothelial layers of blood vessels. Cryoprecipitate—a plasma derivative rich in factor VIII, fibrinogen, and fibronectin—will shorten bleeding time in uremic patients. The effect is noticeable within 1 hour and maximal at 4 to 12 hours after infusion.[591] However, the continued risks of transmitting disease with plasma-derived products raises significant concerns about their usage.

Infusion of DDAVP at a dose of 0.3 µg/kg temporarily corrects a prolonged bleeding time without causing appreciable side effects.[592] Intranasal administration at a dose of 3 mg/kg is also effective.[595] Correction of the bleeding time following DDAVP correlates with an increase in the titer of high-molecular-weight vWF multimers in the plasma. This mechanism for its efficacy is confounded, however, by the observation that the blood levels and function of vWF protein (including the percentage of high-molecular-weight multimers) are normal or increased in uremics prior to treatment. Perhaps the GP IIb-IIIa defect can be overcome by increasing vWF. Nevertheless, use of DDAVP is the treatment of choice when rapid onset of hemostatic competence is required. Unfortunately, DDAVP becomes ineffective when administered repeatedly in a short period of time.[596]

When a longer-lasting effect is required, a more promising approach is the use of conjugated estrogens.[570,593] Liu et al.[595] proposed this therapy based on the observation that abnormal bleeding in women with von Willebrand disease improves during pregnancy as blood estrogens increase. A double-blind crossover trial demonstrated that the infusion of conjugated estrogens at a dose of 3 mg/kg for 5 consecutive days effectively shortened the bleeding time in uremic subjects.[570] The effect takes time to develop but may last up to 14 days. In one study, bleeding from gastrointestinal telangiectasias in seven patients with CKD appeared to be controlled by estrogens.[597.]

REFERENCES

1. Besarab A. Recombinant human erythropoietin: physiology, pathophysiology of anemia in CKD, and economic aspects related to dosing. *Am J Nephrol* 1990;10(suppl 2):2–6.

2. Eknoyan G, Levey AS, Levin NW, Keane WF. The national epidemic of chronic kidney disease. What we know and what we can do. *Postgrad Med* 2001;110:23–29.

3. Levey AS, Bosch JP, Lewis JB, et al. A more accurate method to estimate glomerular filtration rate from serum creatinine: a new prediction equation. Modification of Diet in Renal Disease Study Group. *Ann Intern Med* 1999;130: 461–470.

4. Astor BC, Muntner P, Levin A, et al. Association of kidney function with anemia: the Third National Health and Nutrition Examination Survey (1988–1994). *Arch Intern Med* 2002;162:1401–1408.

5. Bright R. Cases and observations, illustrative of renal disease accompanied with the secretion of albuminous urine. *Guys Hosp Rep* 1836;1:338–379.

6. Radtke HW, Claussner A, Erbes PM, et al. Serum erythropoietin concentration in CKD: relationship to degree of anemia and excretory renal function. *Blood* 1979;54:877–884.

7. Foley RN, Parfrey PS, Harnett JD, et al. The impact of anemia on cardiomyopathy, morbidity and mortality in end–stage renal disease. *Am J Kidney Dis* 1996;28:53–61.

8. Levin A. How should anaemia be managed in pre-dialysis patients? *Nephrol Dial Transplant* 1999;14(suppl 2):66–74.

9. Kazmi WH, Kausz AT, Khan S, et al. Anemia: an early complication of chronic renal insufficiency. *Am J Kidney Dis* 2001;38:803–812.

10. Kominami N, Lowrie EG, Lauber LE, et al. The effect of total nephrectomy on hematopoiesis in patients undergoing chronic hemodialysis. *J Lab Clin Med* 1971;78:524–532.

11. Friend D, Hoskins RG, Kirkin MW. Relative erythrocytemia (polycythemia) and polycystic kidney disease with uremia. Report of a case with comments on frequency of occurrence. *N Engl J Med* 1961:264:17–19.

12. Loge JP, Lange RD, Moore CV. Characterization of the anemia associated with chronic renal insufficiency. *Am J Med* 1958;24:4–18.

13. Aherne WA. The "burr" red cell and azotemia. *J Clin Pathol* 1957;10:252–257.

14. Brecher G, Bessis M. Present status of spiculed red cells and their relationship to the discocyte-echinocyte transformation: a critical review. *Blood* 1972;40:333–334.

15. Weed R. The red cell membrane in hemolytic disorders. *Semin Hematol* 1970;7:249–258.

16. Pastermack A, Wahlberg P. Bone marrow in acute CKD. *Acta Med Scand* 1967;181:505–511.

17. Finch CA, Deubelbeiss K, Cook JD, et al. Ferrokinetics in man. *Medicine* 1970;49:17–53.

18. Magid E, Hilden M. Ferrokinetics in patients suffering from CKD and anemia. *Scand J Haematol* 1967;4:33–45.

19. Sutherland DA, McCall S, Jones F, Muirhead EE. The anemia of uremia: hemolytic state measured by the radiochromium method (abstr). *Am J Med* 1955;19:153.

20. Erslev A, Besarab A. The rate and control of baseline red cell production in hematologically stable uremic patients. *J Lab Clin Med* 1995;126:283–286.

21. Mitchell TR, Pegrum GD. The oxygen affinity of haemoglobin in CKD. *Br J Haematol* 1971;21:463–472.

22. Chillar RK, Desforges JF. Red cell organic phosphates in patients with CKD on maintenance haemodialysis. *Br J Haematol* 1974;26:549–556.

23. Lichtman MA, Miller DR. Erythrocyte glycolysis, 2,3-diphosphoglycerate and adenosine triphosphate concentration in uremic subjects: relationship to extracellular phosphate concentration. *J Lab Clin Med* 1970;76:267–279.

24. Finch CA, Miller LR, Inamdar AR, et al. Iron deficiency in the rat: physiological and biochemical studies of muscle dysfunction. *J Clin Invest* 1976;58:447–453.

25. Gokal R, Weatherall DJ, Bunch C. Iron induced increases in red cell size in haemodialysis patients. *Q J Med* 1979;48: 393–401.

26. Lichtman MA, Miller OR, Freeman RB. Erythrocyte adenosine triphosphate depletion during hypophosphatemia in a uremic subject. *N Engl J Med* 1969;280:240–244.

27. Hurtado A, Merino C, Delgado E. Influence of anoxemia on the hematopoietic activity. *Arch Intern Med* 1945;75: 284–323.

28. Erslev AJ. Blood and mountains. In: Wintrobe MM, ed. *Blood, Pure and Eloquent.* New York: McGraw–Hill, 1980: 257–318.

29. Reissmann KR. Studies on the mechanism of erythropoietic stimulation in parabiotic rats during hypoxia. *Blood* 1950;5: 372–380.

30. Erslev AJ. Humoral regulation of red cell production. *Blood* 1953;8:349–357.

31. Jacobson LO, Goldwasser E, Fried W, Plzak L. Role of the kidney in erythropoiesis. *Nature* 1957;179:633–634.

32. Caro J, Brown S, Miller OP, et al. Erythropoietin levels in uremic nephric and anephric patients. *J Lab Clin Med* 1979; 93:449–458.

33. Radtke HW, Erbes PM, Schippers E, Koch KM. Serum erythropoietin concentrations in anephric patients. *Nephron* 1978;22:331–365.

34. Miyake T, Kung CKH, Goldwasser E. Purification of human erythropoietin. *J Biol Chem* 1977;252:5558–5564.

35. Lai P-H, Everett R, Wang FF, et al. Structural characterization of human erythropoietin. *J Biol Chem* 1986;261:3116–3121.

36. Jacobs K, Shoemaker C, Rudersdorf R, et al. Isolation and characterization of genomic and cDNA clones of human erythropoietin. *Nature* 1985;313:806–810.

37. Lin FK, Suggs S, Lin CH, et al. Cloning and expression of the human erythropoietin gene. *Proc Natl Acad Sci USA* 1985;82:7580–7584.

38. Bachmann S, LeHir M, Eckard K-U. Co-localization of erythropoietin mRNA and ecto-5′-nucleotidase immunoreactivity in peritubular cells of rat renal cortex indicates that fibroblasts produce erythropoietin. *J Histochem Cytochem* 1993;41:335–345.

39. Maxwell PH, Osmond MK, Pugh CW, et al. Identification of the renal erythropoietin-producing cells using transgenic mice. *Kidney Int* 1993;44:1149–1162.

40. MacManus MP, Maxwell AP, Abram WP, Bridges JM. The effect of hypobaric hypoxia on misonidazole binding in normal and tumour-bearing mice. *Br J Cancer* 1989;59:349–352.

41. Quesenberg P, Levitt L. Hematopoietic stem cells. *N Engl J Med* 1979;301:755–760.

42. Ogawa M, Porter PN, Hakahata T. Renewal and commitments to differentiation of hematopoietic stem cells: an interpretive review. *Blood* 1983;61:823–829.

43. Ogawa M. Differentiation and proliferation of hematopoietic stem cells. *Blood* 1993;81:2844–2853.

44. Schuster SJ, Caro J. Erythropoietin: physiologic basis for clinical applications. *Vox Sang* 1993;65:169–170.

45. Krause DS, Fackler MJ, Civin CI, May WS. CD34: structure, biology, and clinical utility. *Blood* 1996;87:1–13.

46. Spivak JL, Ferris DK, Fisher J, et al. Cell cycle-specific behavior of erythropoietin. *Exp Hematol* 1996;24:141–150.

47. Gregory CG, Eaves AC. Three stages of erythropoietic progenitor cell differentiation distinguished by a number of physical and biological properties. *Blood* 1978;51:527–537.

48. Kannourakis S, Johnson GR. Fractionation of subsets of BFU-E from normal human bone marrow: responsiveness to erythropoietin, human placental-conditioned medium, or granulocyte-macrophage colony-stimulating factor. *Blood* 1988;71:758–765.

49. Gregory CJ. Erythropoietin sensitivity as a differentiation marker in the hemapoietic system: studies of three erythropoietic colony responses in cell culture. *J Cell Physiol* 1976;9:289–301.

50. Sawada K, Krantz SB, Dessypris EN, et al. Human colony-forming unit-erythroid do not require accessory cells but do require direct interaction with insulin-like growth factors 1 and/or insulin for erythroid development. *J Clin Invest* 1989;83:1701–1709.

51. Krantz SB. Erythropoietin. *Blood* 1991;77:419–433.

52. Faquin WC, Schneider TJ, Goldberg MA. Effect of inflammatory cytokines on hypoxia-induced erythropoietin production. *Blood* 1992;79:1987–1994.

53. Means RT, Krantz SB. Inhibition of human erythroid colony-forming units by tumor necrosis factor requires beta interferon. *J Clin Invest* 1992;91:416–419.

54. D'Andrea AD, Lodish HF, Wong GG. Expression cloning of the murine erythropoietin receptor. *Cell* 1989;57:277–285.

55. Wrighton NC, Farrell FX, Chang R, et al. Small peptides as potent mimetics of the protein hormone erythropoietin. *Science* 1996;273:458.

56. Klingmüller U, Lorenz U, Cantley LC, et al. Specific recruitment of SH-PTP1 to the erythropoietin receptor causes inactivation of JAK2 and termination of proliferative signals. *Cell* 1995;80:729–738.

57. Leyland-Jones B. Evidence for erythropoietin as a molecular targeting agent. *Semin Oncol* 2002;29(suppl 11):145–154.

58. Lacombe C, Mayeux P. The molecular biology of erythropoietin. *Nephrol Dial Transplant* 1999;14(suppl 2):22–28.

59. Jelkmann W, Hellwig-Burgel T. Biology of erythropoietin. *Adv Exp Med Biol* 2001;502:169–187.

60. Chu X, Chueng JY, Barber DL, et al. Erythropoietin modulates calcium influx through TRCP2. *J Biol Chem* 2002;277:34375–34382.

61. Stephenson JR, Axelrod AA, McLeod DL, Shreve MM. Induction of hemoglobin-synthesizing cells by erythropoietin in vitro. *Proc Natl Acad Sci USA* 1971;65:1542–1546.

62. Adamson JW, Torok-Storb B, Lin N. Analysis of erythropoiesis by erythroid colony formation in culture. *Blood Cells* 1978;4:89–103.

63. Calvillo L, Latini R, Kajstura J, et al. Recombinant human erythropoietin protects the myocardium from ischemia-reperfusion injury and promotes beneficial remodeling. *PNAS* 2003;100:4802–4806.

64. Erbayraktar S, Grasso G, Sfacteria A, et al. Asialoerythropoietin is a nonerythropoietic cytokine with broad neuroprotective activity in vivo. *Proc Natl Acad Sci USA* 2003;100(11):6741–6746.

65. Egrie JC, Browne JK. The molecular biology of erythropoietin. In: Erslev AJ, Adamson JW, Eschgbach JW, Winearls CG, eds. *Erythropoietin—Molecular, Cellular, and Clinical Biology*. Baltimore: The Johns Hopkins University Press, 1991:21–40.

66. Beck I, Ramirez S, Weinmann R, Caro J. Enhancer element at the 3′ flanking region controls transcriptional response to hypoxia in the human erythropoietin gene. *J Biol Chem* 1991;266:15563–15566.

67. Semenza GL, Nejfelt MK, Chi SM, Antonarakis SE. Hypoxia-inducible nuclear factors bind to an enhancer element located 3′ to the human erythropoietin gene. *Proc Natl Acad Sci USA* 1991;88:5680–5684.

68. Madan A, Custin PT. A 24-base-pair sequence 3′ to the human erythropoietin gene contains a hypoxia-responsive transcriptional enhancer. *Proc Natl Acad Sci USA* 1993;90:3928–3932.

69. Madan A, Lin C, Hatch SL, Curtin PT. Regulated basal, inducible, and tissue specific human erythropoietin gene ex-

pression in transgenic mice requires multiple cis DNA sequences. *Blood* 1995;85:2735–2741.

70. Semenza GL, Wang GL. A nuclear factor induced by hypoxia via de novo protein synthesis binds to the human erythropoietin gene enhancer at a site required for transcriptional activation. *Mol Cell Biol* 1992;12:5447–5454.

71. Beck I, Weinmann R, Caro J. Characterization of the hypoxia-responsive enhancer in the human erythropoietin gene shows presence of a hypoxia-inducible 120 KD nuclear DNA-binding protein in erythropoietin-producing and non-producing cells. *Blood* 1993;82:704–711.

72. Wang GL, Semenza GL. General involvement of hypoxia-inducible factor 1 in transcriptional response to hypoxia. *Proc Natl Acad Sci USA* 1993;90:4304–4308.

73. Wenger RH. Cellular adaptation to hypoxia: O2-sensing protein hydroxylases, hypoxia-inducible transcription factors, and O_2-regulated gene expression. *FASEB J* 2002;16:1151–1162.

74. Nicola NA, Metcalf D. Subunit promiscuity among hematopoietic growth factor receptors. *Cell* 1991;67:1–4.

75. Wiesner MS, Eckard KU. Erythropoietin tumours and the von-Hippel-Lindau gene: towards identification and mechanism os and dysfunction of oxygen sensing. *Nephrol Dial Transplant* 2002:17:356–359.

76. Recny MA, Scobie HA, Kim Y. Structural characterization of natural human urinary and recombinant DNA-derived erythropoietin. *J Biol Chem* 1987;262:17156–17163.

77. Wang FF, Kung CKF, Goldwasser E. Some chemical properties of human erythropoietin. *Endocrinology* 1985;116:2286–2292.

78. Jelkmann W. Erythropoietin: structure, control of production, and function. *Physiol Rev* 1992;72:449–489.

79. Eckardt KU, Kurtz A. The biological role, site, and regulation of erythropoietin production. *Adv Nephrol Necker Hosp* 1992;21:203–233.

80. Smith Dordal M, Wang FF, Goldwasser E. The role of carbohydrate in erythropoietin action. *Endocrinology* 1985;116:2293–2299.

81. Schuster SJ, Badiavas EV, Costa-Giomi P, et al. Stimulation of erythropoietin gene transcription during hypoxia and cobalt exposure. *Blood* 1989;73:13–16.

82. Dube S, Fisher JW, Powell JS. Glycosylation at specific sites of erythropoietin is essential for biosynthesis, secretion, and biological function. *J Bio Chem* 1988;263:17516–17521.

83. Spivack JL, Hogans BB. The in vivo metabolism of recombinant human erythropoietin in the rat. *Blood* 1989;73:90–99.

84. Besarab A, Flaharty KK, Erslev AJ, et al. Clinical pharmacology and economics of recombinant human erythropoietin in end-stage renal disease: the case for subcutaneous administration. *J Am Soc Nephrol* 1992;2:1405–1416.

85. Cahan C, Decker MJ, Arnold JL, et al. Diurnal variations in serum erythropoietin levels in healthy subjects and sleep apnea patients. *J Appl Physiol* 1992;72:2112–2117.

86. Müller-Wiefel D, Schärer K. Serum erythropoietin levels in children with CKD. *Kidney Int.* 1983; 24(suppl)15:S70–S76.

87. Goldman JM, Ireland RM, Berton-Jones M, et al. Erythropoietin concentrations in obstructive sleep apnea. *Thorax* 1991;46:25–27.

88. Fried W, Heller P, Johnson C. Observations on the regulation of erythropoietin production and of erythropoiesis during prolonged exposure to hypoxia. *Blood* 1970;36:607–616.

89. Catchatourian R, Eckerling G, Fried W. Effect of short term protein deprivation on hemopoietic functions of healthy volunteers. *Blood* 1980;55:625–628.

90. Fried W, Gurney CW. The erythropoietic stimulating effects of androgens. *Ann NY Acad Sci* 1968;149:356–365.

91. Alexanian R. Urinary excretion of erythropoietin in normal men and women. *Blood* 1966;28:344–353.

92. Fried W, Kilbridge T, Krantz S, et al. Studies on extrarenal erythropoietin. *J Lab Clin Med* 1969;73:244–248.

93. Koury ST, Bonurant MC, Koury MJ, Semenza GL. Localization of cells producing erythropoietin in murine liver by in situ hybridization. *Blood* 1991;77:2497–2503.

94. Schuster SJ, Koury ST, Bohrer M, et al. Cellular sites of extrarenal and renal erythropoietin production in anaemic rats. *Br J Haematol* 1992;81:153–159.

95. Anagnostou A, Schade S, Barone J, Fried W. Effects of partial hepatectomy on extrarenal erythropoietin production in rats. *Blood* 1977;50:457–462.

96. Fried W, Barone J, Schade S, Anagnostou A. Effect of carbon tetrachloride on extrarenal erythropoietin production. *J Lab Clin Med* 1979;93:700–705.

97. Nielson OJ, Thaysen JH. Erythropoietic deficiency in acute tubular necrosis. *J Intern Med* 1990;227:373–380.

98. Thaysen JH, Nielson OJ, Brandi L, Szpirt W. Erythropoietin deficiency in acute crescentic glomerulonephritis and in total bilateral renal cortical necrosis. *J Intern Med* 1991;229:363–369.

99. Garcia JF, Sherwood JB, Goldwasser E. Radioimmunoassay of erythropoietin. *Blood Cells* 1979;5:405–409.

100. Sherwood JB, Carmichael LD, Goldwasser E. The heterogeneity of circulating human serum erythropoietin. *Endocrinology* 1988;73:1472–1477.

101. Cotes PM, Tam RC, Reed P, Hellebostad M. An immunologic cross-reactant of erythropoietin in serum which may invalidate EPO radioimmunoassay. *Br J Haematol* 1989;73:265–268.

102. Schooley JC, Mahlmann LJ. Evidence for the de novo synthesis of erythropoietin in hypoxic rats. *Blood* 1972;40: 662–670.

103. Eckard KU, Boutellier U, Kurtz A, et al. Rate of erythropoietin formation in humans in response to acute hypobaric hypoxia. *J Appl Physiol* 1989;66:1785–1788.

104. Erslev AJ, Caro J, Besarab A. Why the kidney? *Nephron* 1985;41:213–216.

105. Tan CC, Eckard K-U, Firth JD, Ratcliffe JP. Feedback modulation or renal and hepatic erythropoietin mRNA in response to graded anemia and hypoxia. *Am J Physiol* 1992; 263:F474–F481.

106. Donnelly S. Why is erythropoietin made in the kidney? The kidney functions as a critmeter. *Am J Kidney Dis* 2001; 38:415–425.

107. Erslev AJ. Erythropoietin. *N Engl J Med* 1991;324:1339–1344.

108. Jelkmann W, Wiedemann G. Serum erythropoietin level: relationship to blood hemoglobin concentrations and erythrocytic activity of the bone marrow. *Klin Wochenschr* 1990;68: 403–407.

109. Birgegard G, Wide L, Simonsson B. Marked erythropoietin increase before fall in Hgb after treatment with cytostatic drugs suggests mechanism other than anemia for stimulation. *Br J Haematol* 1989;72:462–466.

110. Sawyer ST, Krantz SB, Goldwasser E. Binding and receptor-mediated endocytosis of erythropoietin in Friend virus-infected erythroid cells. *J Biol Chem* 1987;262:5554–5562.

111. Piroso E, Flaherty KK, Caro J, Erslev AJ. Erythropoietin half-life in rats with hypoplastic and hyperplastic bone marrows (abstr). *Blood* 1989;74:270A.

112. Fried W, Barone-Varelas J. Regulation of the plasma erythropoietin level in hypoxic rats. *Exp Hematol* 1984;12: 706–711.

113. Loeffler M, Herkenrath P, Wichman HE, et al. The kinetics of hematopoietic stem cells during and after hypoxia. *Blut* 1984;49:427–439.

114. Jelkmann W. Temporal pattern of erythropoietin titers in kidney tissue during hypoxic hypoxia. *Pflügers Arch* 1982;393:988–991.

115. Ross R, McCrea JB, Besarab A. Erythropoietin response to blood loss in hemodialysis patients is blunted but preserved. *ASAIO J* 1994;40:M880–M885.

116. Lorentz A, Jendrissek A, Eckard KU, et al. Serial immunoreactive erythropoietin levels in autologous blood donors. *Transfusion* 1991;31:650–654.

117. Kickler TS, Spivack JL. Effect of repeated whole blood donations on serum immunoreactive erythropoietin levels in autologous donors. *JAMA* 1988;260:65–67.

118. Pugh CW, Tan CC, Jones RW, Ratcliff PJ. Functional analysis of an oxygen-regulated transcriptional enhancer lying 3′ to the mouse erythropoietin gene. *Proc Natl Acad Sci USA* 1991;88:10553–10557.

119. Semenza GL, Koury ST, Nejfelt MK, et al. Cell-type specific and hypoxia-inducible expression of the human erythropoietin gene in transgenic mice. *Proc Natl Acad Sci USA* 1991;88:8725–8729.

120. Flaherty KK, Caro J, Erslev A, et al. Pharmacokinetics and erythropoietic response to human recombinant erythropoietin in healthy men. *Clin Pharmacol Ther* 1990;47: 557–564.

121. Rege AB, Brookins J, Fisher JW. A radioimmunoassay for erythropoietin: serum levels in normal human subjects and in patients with hemopoietic disorders. *J Lab Clin Med* 1982;100:829–843.

122. Naets JP, Garcia JF, Tousaaint CH, et al. Radioimmunoassay of erythropoietin in chronic uraemia of anephric patients. *Scand J Haematol* 1986;37:390–394.

123. Caro J, Schuster S, Besarab A, Erslev AJ. Renal biogenesis of erythropoietin. In: Rich IN, ed. *Molecular and Cellular Aspects of Erythropoietin and Erythropoiesis*. NATO ASI Series. Vol H8. Heidelberg, Germany: Springer–Verlag, 1987:329–336.

124. Besarab A, Caro J, Jarrell BE, et al. Dynamics of erythropoiesis following renal transplantation. *Kidney Int* 1987;32:526–536.

125. Walle AJ, Wong GY, Clemons GK, et al. Erythropoietin–Hct feedback circuit in the anemia of end-stage renal disease. *Kidney Int* 1987;31:1205–1209.

126. Spivak JL. The mechanism of action of erythropoietin. *Int J Cell Cloning* 1986;4:139–166.

127. Eckard K–U, Möllmann M, Neumann R, et al. Erythropoietin in polycystic kidneys. *J Clin Invest* 1989;84:1160–1166.

128. Sun CH, Ward HJ, Wellington LP, et al. Serum erythropoietin levels after renal transplantation. *N Engl J Med* 1989;321:151–157.

129. Eschbach JW, Funk D, Adamson JW, et al. Erythropoiesis in patients with CKD undergoing chronic dialysis. *N Engl J Med* 1967;276: 653–658.

130. Chaplin H, Mollison PL. Red cell life-span in nephritis and in hepatic nephrosis. *Clin Sci* 1953;12:351–360.

131. Ragen PA, Hagedorn AB, Owen CA. Radioisotope study of anemia in CKD. *Arch Intern Med* 1960;105:518–523.

132. Berry ER, Rambach WA, Alt HL, Del Greco F. Effect of peritoneal dialysis on erythrokinetics and ferrokinetics of azotemic anemia. *ASAIO Trans* 1965;10:415–419.

133. Wallas CH. Metabolic studies on the erythrocytes from patients with CKD on haemodialysis. *Br J Haematol* 1974;27: 145–152.

134. Lonergan ET, Semar M, Sterzel RB, et al. Erythrocyte transketolase activity in dialyzed patients: a reversible metabolic lesion of uremia. *N Engl J Med* 1971;284:1399–1403.

135. Cole CH. Decreased ouabain–sensitive adenine triphosphatase activity in the erythrocyte membrane of patients with CKD. *Clin Sci* 1973;45:775–784.

136. Izumo H, Izumo S, DeLuise M, Flier JS. Erythrocyte Na,K pump in uremia: acute correction of a transport defect by haemodialysis. *J Clin Invest* 1984;74:581–588.

137. Cheng JT, Kahn T, Kaji DM. Mechanism of alteration of sodium potassium pump of erythrocytes from patients with CKD. *J Clin Invest* 1984;74:1811–1820.

138. Longnecker RE, Goffinet JA, Hendler ED. Blood loss during maintenance hemodialysis. *ASAIO Trans* 1974;20: 135–140.

139. Lindsay RM, Burton JA, Edward N, et al. Dialyzer blood loss. *Clin Nephrol* 1973;1:29–34.

140. Erslev AJ, Wilson J, Caro J. Erythropoietin titers in anemic nonuremic patients. *J Lab Clin Med.* 1987;109:429–433.

141. Rabiner SF. Uremic bleeding. *Prog Hemost Thromb* 1972; 1:233–250.

142. Clouse RE, Costigan DJ, Mills BA, et al. Angiodysplasia as a cause of upper gastrointestinal bleeding in uremia. *Arch Intern Med* 1985;145:458–461.

143. Benigni A, Boccardo P, Galbusera M, et al. Reversible activation defect of the platelet glycoprotein IIb–IIIa complex in patients with uremia. *Am J Kidney Dis* 1993;22:668–676.

144. Gralnick HR, McKeown LP, Williams SB, Schafer BC. Plasma and platelet von Willebrand factor defects in uremia. *Am J Med* 1988;85:806–810.

145. Savage B, Shattil SJ, Ruggeri ZM. Modulation of platelet function through adhesion receptors. A dual role glycoprotein IIb–IIIa (integrin aIIbb3) mediated by fibrinogen and glycoprotein Ib–von Willebrand factor. *J Biol Chem* 1992;267:11300–11306.

146. Di Minno G, Martinez J, McKean M–L, et al. Platelet dysfunction in uremia. Multifaceted defect partially corrected by dialysis. *Am J Med* 1985;79:552–559.

147. Livio M, Marchesi D, Remuzzi G, et al. Uraemic bleeding: role of anaemia and beneficial effect of red cell transfusions. *Lancet* 1982;2:1013–1015.

148. Fernandez F, Goudable C, Sie P, et al. Low Hct and prolonged bleeding time in uraemic patients: effect of red cell transfusion. *Br J Haematol* 1985;59:139–148.

149. Moia M, Vizzotta L, Cattaneo M, et al. Improvement in the haemostatic defect of uraemia after treatment with recombinant human erythropoietin. *Lancet* 1987;2:1227–1229.

150. Cases A, Escolar G, Reverter JC, et al. Recombinant human erythropoietin treatment improves platelet function in uremic patients. *Kidney Int* 1992;42:668–672.

151. Joske RA, McAlister JM, Prankerd TAJ. Isotope investigations of red cell production and destruction in CKD. *Clin Sci* 1956;15:511–522.

152. Ortega O, Rodriguez I, Gallarp, et al. Significance of high C–reactive proteins levels in pre-dialysis patients. *Nephrol Dial Transplant* 2002;17:1105–1109.

153. Yawata Y, Howe R, Jacob HS. Abnormal red cell metabolism causing hemolysis in uremia: a defect potentiated by tap water hemodialysis. *Ann Intern Med* 1973;79: 362–367.

154. Rosenwund A, Binswanger U, Straub PW. Oxidative injury to erythrocytes, cell rigidity, and splenic hemolysis in hemodialyzed uremic patients. *Ann Intern Med* 1975;82: 460–465.

155. Eaton JW, Kolpin CF, Swofford HS, et al. Chlorinated urban water: a cause of dialysis-induced hemolytic anemia. *Science* 1973;181:463–464.

156. Tipple MA, Schusterman N, Bland LA, et al. Illness in hemodialysis patients after exposure to chloramine contaminated dialysate. *ASAIO Trans* 1991;37:588–591.

157. Manzler AD, Schreiner AW. Copper–induced acute hemolytic anemia: a new complication of home dialysis. *Ann Intern Med* 1970;73:409–412.

158. Petrie JJB, Row PG. Dialysis anaemia caused by subacute zinc toxicity. *Lancet* 1977;1:1178–1180.

159. Short AIK, Winney RJ, Robson JS. Reversible microcytic hypochromic anemia in dialysis patients due to aluminum intoxication. *Proc Eur Dial Transplant Assoc* 1980;17: 233–236.

160. Carlson DJ, Shapiro FL. Methemoglobinemia from well water nitrates: a complication of home dialysis. *Ann Intern Med* 1970;73:757–759.

161. Orringer EP, Mattern WD. Formaldehyde-induced hemolysis during chronic hemodialysis. *N Engl J Med* 1976;294: 1416–1420.

162. Gallery EDM, Blomfield J, Dixon SR. Acute zinc toxicity in haemodialysis. *Br Med J* 1972;4:331–333.

163. Kaiser L, Schwartz KA, Burnatowska-Hledin A, Mayor GH. Microcytic anemia secondary to intraperitoneal aluminum in normal and uremic rats. *Kidney Int* 1984;26: 269–274.

164. Iacob HS, Amsden T. Acute hemolytic anemia with rigid red cells in hypophosphatemia. *N Engl J Med* 1971;285: 1146–1150.

165. Said R, Quintanilla A, Levin N, Ivanovich P. Acute hemolysis due to profound hypo-osmolality: a complication of hemodialysis. *J Dial* 1977;1:447–452.

166. Schuett H, Port FK. Hemolysis in hemodialysis patients. *Dial Transplant* 1980;9:345–347.

167. Berkes SL, Kahn SI, Chazan JA, Garella S. Prolonged hemolysis from overheated dialysate. *Ann Intern Med* 1975;83:363–364.

168. Francos GC, Burke JF, Besarab A, et al. An unsuspected cause of acute hemolysis during hemodialysis. *Trans Am Soc Artif Intern Organs* 1983;24:140–145.

169. Brasier AR, Nussbaum SR. Hungry bone syndrome: clinical and biochemical predictors of its occurrence after parathyroid surgery. *Am J Med* 1988;84:654–660.

170. Bull BS, Rubenberg ML, Dacie JV, Brain MC. Microangiopathic hemolytic anemia: mechanisms of red cell fragmentation. *Br J Haematol* 1968;14:643–652.

171. Capelli JP, Wesson LG, Erslev AJ. Malignant hypertension and red cell fragmentation syndrome. *Ann Intern Med* 1966;64:128–136.

172. Brain MC. The haemolytic-uremic syndrome. *Semin Hematol* 1969;6:162–180.

173. Neiman RS, Bischel MD, Lukes RJ. Hypersplenism in the uremic hemodialyzed patient. *Am J Clin Pathol* 1973;60: 502–511.

174. Platts MM, Anastassiades E, Sheriff S, et al. Spleen size in CKD. *BMJ* 1984;289:1415–1418.

175. Bommer J, Ritz E, Waldherr R. Silicone induced splenomegaly: treatment of pancytopenia by splenectomy in a patient on hemodialysis. *N Engl J Med* 1981;305: 1077–1079.

176. Hartley RA, Morgan TO, Innis MD, Climie GJA. Splenectomy for anemia in patients on regular dialysis. *Lancet* 1971;2:1343–1345.

177. Fisher JW. Mechanism of the anemia of CKD. Editorial review. *Nephron* 1980;25:106–111.

178. Ohne Y, Rege AB, Fisher JW, Barona J. Inhibitors of erythroid colony-forming cells (CFU-E and BFU-E) in sera of azotemic patients with anemia of renal disease. *J Lab Clin Med* 1978;92:916–923.

179. Wallner SF, Vantrin R, Kornick JE, Ward HP. The effect of serum from patients with CKD on erythroid colony growth in vitro. *J Lab Clin Med* 1978;92:370–375.

180. Radtke HW, Rege AB, LaMarche MB, et al. Identification of spermine as an inhibitor of erythropoiesis in patients with CKD. *J Clin Invest* 1980;67:1623–1629.

181. Zappacosta AR, Caro J, Erslev A. The normalization of Hct in end-stage renal disease patients on continuous ambulatory peritoneal dialysis: the role of erythropoietin. *Am J Med* 1982;72:53–57.

182. Segal GM, Stuere T, Adamson JW. Spermine and spermidine are non-specific inhibitors of in vitro hematopoiesis. *Kidney Int* 1987;31:72–76.

183. Wallner SF, Vantrin RM. The anemia of CKD: studies of the affect of organic solvent extraction of the serum. *J Lab Clin Med* 1978;92:363–369.

184. Eschbach JW, Adamson JW, Dennis MB. Physiologic studies in normal and uremic sheep. *Kidney Int* 1980;18: 725–731.

185. Eschbach JW, Mladenovic J, Garcia JF, et al. The anemia of CKD in sheep: the response to erythropoietin-rich plasma in vivo. *J Clin Invest* 1984;74:434–441.

186. Eschbach JW, Haley NR, Eagrie JC, Adamson JW. A comparison of the responses to recombinant erythropoietin in normal and uremic subjects. *Kidney Int* 1992;42: 407–416.

187. Delwechi F, Garrity MJ, Powell JS, et al. High levels of the circulating form of parathyroid hormone do not inhibit in vivo erythropoiesis. *J Lab Clin Med* 1983;102:613–620.

188. Rao DS, Shih M-S, Mohini R. Effect of serum parathyroid hormone and bone marrow fibrosis on the response to erythropoietin in uremia. *N Engl J Med* 1993;328:171–175.

189. Niwa T, Yazawa T, Kodama T, et al. Efficient removal of albumin-bound furancarboxylic acid, an inhibitor of erythropoiesis, by continuous ambulatory peritoneal dialysis. *Nephron* 1990;56:241–245.

190. Himmelfarber J, Lazarus M, Hakim R. Reactive oxygen species production by monocytes and polymorphonuclear leukocytes during dialysis. *Am J Kidney Dis* 1991;3: 271–276.

191. Pawlak D, Koda M, Pawlak S, et al. Contribution of quinolinic acid in the development of anemia in renal insufficiency. *Am J Physiol Renal Physiol* 2003; 284(4):F693–700.

192. Le Meur Y, Lorgot V, Comte L, et al. Plasma levels and metabolism of AcsSDKP in patients with CKD: relationship with erythropoietin requirements. *Am J Kidney Dis* 2001;38: 510–517.

193. Morrone LF, Di Paolo S, Logoluso F, et al. Interference of angiotensin-converting enzyme inhibitors on erythropoiesis in kidney transplant recipients: role of growth factors and cytokines. *Transplantation* 1997; 64(6):913–918.

194. Naito M, Kawashima A, Akiba T, et al. Effects of an angiotensin II receptor antagonist and angiotensin-converting enzyme inhibitors on burst forming units-erythroid in chronic hemodialysis patients. *Am J Nephrol* 2003;23:287–293.

195. Wang AY, Yu AW, Lam CW, et al. Effects of losartan or enalapril on hemoglobin, circulating erythropoietin, and insulin-like growth factor-1 in patients with and without post-transplant erythrocytosis. *Am J Kidney Dis.* 2002;39(3): 600–608.

196. Roodman GD, Bird A, Hatzler D, Montgomery W. Tumor necrosis factor alpha and hematopoietic progenitors: effect of tumor necrosis factor on the growth of erythroid progenitors CFU-E and BFU-E and the hematopoietic cell lines k62, HL60, and HEL cells. *Exp Hematol* 1987;15:928–935.

197. Morra L, Ponassi A, Gurreri G, et al. Alterations of erythropoiesis in chronic uremic patients treated with intermittent hemodialysis. *Biomed Pharmacother* 1987;41:396–399.

198. Morra L, Ponassi A, Guerri G, et al. Inadequate ability of T-lymphocytes from chronic uremic subjects to stimulate the in vivo growth of committed erythroid progenitors (BFU-E). *Acta Haematol* 1988;79:187–191.

199. Kimmel PL, Phillips TM, Phillips E, Bosch JP. Effect of renal replacement therapy on cellular cytokine production in patients with renal disease. *Kidney Int* 1990;38:129–135.

200. Ryan J, Beynon H, Rees AJ, Cassidy MJD. Evaluation of in vitro production of tumor necrosis factor by monocytes in dialysis patients. *Blood Purif* 1991;9:142–147.

201. McGonigle RJS, Husserl F, Wallin JD, Fisher JW. Hemodialysis and continuous ambulatory peritoneal dialysis effects on erythropoiesis in CKD. *Kidney Int* 1984;25: 430–436.

202. Eschbach JW, Egrie JC, Downing MR, et al. Correction of the anemia of end-stage renal disease with recombinant human erythropoietin. Results of combined phase I & II clinical trials. *N Engl J Med* 1987;316: 73–78.

203. Winearls CG, Oliver DO, Pippard MJ, et al. Effect of human erythropoietin derived from recombinant DNA on the anemia of patients maintained by chronic haemodialysis. *Lancet* 1986;2:1175–1177.

204. Gafter U, Kalechman Y, Orlin JB, et al. Anemia of uremia is associated with reduced in vitro cytokine secretion: immunopotentiating activity of red blood cells. *Kidney Int* 1994;45:224–231.

205. Whitehead VM, Comty CH, Posen GA, Kay M. Homeostasis of folic acid in patients undergoing maintenance hemodialysis. *N Engl J Med* 1968;279:970–974.

206. Wolfson M. Use of water-soluble vitamins in patients with CKD. *Semin Dial* 1988;1:28–32.

207. Hocken AG, Marwah PK. Iatrogenic contribution to anemia of CKD. *Lancet* 1971;1:164–165.

208. Castaldi PA, Rozenberg MC, Steward JH. The bleeding disorder of uremia. A qualitative platelet defect. *Lancet* 1966;2:66–68.

209. Elliot HL, Dryburgh F, Fell GS, MacDougall AI. Aluminum toxicity during regular haemodialysis. *Br J Med* 1978;1: 1101–1103.

210. Eschbach JW, Cook JD, Finch CA. Iron absorption in CKD. *Clin Sci* 1970;38:191–201.

211. Milman N. Iron absorption measured by whole body counting and the relation to marrow iron stores in chronic uremia. *Clin Nephrol* 1972;17:77–81.

212. Eschbach JW, Cook JD, Scribner BH, Finch CA. Iron balance in hemodialysis patients. *Ann Intern Med* 1977;87: 710–713.

213. Rifkind D, Kraveti HM, Knight V, Schade AL. Urinary excretion of iron-binding protein in the nephrotic syndrome. *N Engl J Med* 1961;265:115–118.

214. Cannata JB, Alonso-Suarez M, Fernandez-Martin JL, Diaz-Lopez B. Iron deficiency and intestinal aluminum absorption: implications for erythropoietin and desferroxamine therapy. *Semin Dial* 1991;4:224–226.

215. Cannata JB, Fernandez SI, Fernandez MMJ, et al. The role of iron metabolism in absorption and cellular uptake of aluminum. *Kidney Int* 1991;39:799–803.

216. Touam M, Martinez F, Lacour B, et al. Aluminum-induced, reversible microcytic anemia in CKD: clinical and experimental studies. *Clin Nephrol* 1983;19:295–298.

217. Wills MR, Savory J. Aluminum poisoning: dialysis encephalopathy, osteomalacia, and anaemia. *Lancet* 1983;1: 29–34.

218. Eschbach JW, Adamson JW. Anemia of end-stage renal disease (ESRD). *Kidney Int* 1985;28:1–5.

219. Labonia WD. L-carnitine effects on anemia in hemodialyzed patients treated with erythropoietin. *Am J Kidney Dis* 1995; 26(5):757–764.

220. Hurot JM, Cucherat M, Haugh M, Fouque D. Effects of L-carnitine supplementation in maintenance hemodialysis patients: a systematic review. *J Am Soc Nephrol* 2002;13(3): 708–714.

221. Fishbane S, Galgano C, Langley RC Jr, et al. Reticulocyte hemoglobin content in the evaluation of iron status of hemodialysis patients. *Kidney Int* 1997;52(1):217–222.

222. Birgegard G, Nilsson P, Wide L. Regulation of iron therapy by S-ferritin estimations in patients on chronic hemodialysis. *Scand J Nephrol* 1981;15:69–72.

223. Mirahmadi KS, Wellington LP, Winer RL, et al. Serum ferritin level. Determinant of iron requirement in hemodialysis patients. *JAMA* 1977;238:601–603.

224. Fishbane S, Frei GL, Maesaka J. Reduction in recombinant human erythropoietin doses by the use of chronic intravenous iron supplementation. *Am J Kidney Dis* 1995;26: 41–46.

225. Macdougall IC, Tucker B, Thompson I, et al. A randomized controlled study of iron supplementation in patients treated with erythropoietin. *Kidney Int* 1996;50:1694–1699.

226. Silverberg DS, Blum M, Peer G, et al. Intravenous ferric saccharate as an iron supplement in dialysis patients. *Nephron* 1996;72:413–417.

227. Silverberg DS, Iaina A, Peer G, et al. Intravenous iron supplementation for the treatment of the anemia of moderate to severe CKD patients not receiving dialysis. *Am J Kidney Dis* 1996;27:234–238.

228. Moreb J, Popovtzer MM, Friedlaender MM, et al. Evaluation of iron status in patients on chronic hemodialysis: relative usefulness of bone marrow hemosiderin, serum ferritin, transferrin saturation, mean corpuscular volume and red cell protoporphyrin. *Nephron* 1983;35:196–200.

229. Fishbane S, Lynn RI. The utility of zinc protoporphyrin for predicting the need for intravenous iron therapy in hemodialysis patients. *Am J Kidney Dis* 1995;25:426–432.

230. Horl WH, Cavill I, Macdougall IC, et al. How to diagnose and correct iron deficiency during rHuEPO therapy—a consensus rEPOrt (review). *Nephrol Dial Transplant* 1996;11: 246–250.

231. Kalantar-Zadeh K, Hoffken B, Wunsch H, et al. Diagnosis of iron deficiency anemia in CKD patients during the posterythropoietin era. *Am J Kidney Dis* 1995;26:292–299.

232. Fishbane S, Shapiro W, Dutka P, et al. A randomized trial of iron deficiency testing strategies in hemodialysis patients. *Kidney Int* 2001;60:2406.

233. Van Wyck DB, Stivelman JC, Ruiz J, et al. Iron status in patients receiving erythropoietin for dialysis-associated anemia. *Kidney Int* 1989;35:165–170.

234. Charles G, Lundin AP III, Delano BG, et al. Absence of anemia in maintenance hemodialysis. *Int J Artif Organs* 1981;4:277–279.

235. Goldsmith HJ, Ahmad R, Raichura N, et al. Association between rising haemoglobin concentration and renal cyst formation in patients on long term regular dialysis treatment. *Proc Eur Dial Assoc* 1982;19:313–318.

236. Shalhoub RJ, Rajan U, Kim VV, Goldwasser E. Erythrocytosis in patients on long-term hemodialysis. *Ann Intern Med* 1982;97:686–690.

237. Ishikawa I, Saito Y, Onouchi Z, et al. Development of acquired cystic disease and adenomacarcinoma of the kidney

238. Ono K, Kikawa K, Okamoto T, Matsuo H. Normalization of Hct in regular hemodialysis patients: the role of renal cyst formation. *ASAIO Trans* 1985;31:639–643.

239. Besarab A, Caro J, Francos G, et al. Acquired cystic kidney disease (ACKD) and erythropoietin (EPO) in hemodialysis (HD) patients. *Proc 9th Int Congress Nephrol, July, 1987, London, England.* 495.

240. Hughson MD, Hennigar GR, McManus JFA. Atypical cysts, acquired renal cystic disease, and renal cell tumors in end-stage dialysis patients. *Lab Invest* 1980;42:475–480.

241. Kolk Veghter AJ, Bosch E, Van Leeuwen AM. Influence of serum hepatitis on haemoglobin levels in patients on regular haemodialysis. *Lancet* 1971;1:526–528.

242. Pololi–Anagnostou L, Wastenfelder C, Anagnostou A. Marked improvement of erythropoiesis in an anephric patient. *Nephron* 1981;29:277–279.

243. Erslev AJ, McKenna PJ, Capelli JP, et al. Rate of red cell production in two nephrectomized patients. *Arch Intern Med* 1968;122:230–235.

244. Anagnostou A, Vercellotti G, Barone J, Fried W. Factors which affect erythropoiesis in partially nephrectomized and sham operated rats. *Blood* 1976;48:425–433.

245. Thuraisingham RC, MacDougall IC, Cavill I, et al. Improvement in anaemia following renal transplantation but not after erythropoietin therapy in a patient with sickle-cell disease. *Nephrol Dial Transplant* 1993;8:371–372.

246. Neng Lai K, Chiu Wong K, Li PKT, Lui SF. Use of recombinant erythropoietin in thalassemic patients on dialysis. *Am J Kidney Dis* 1992;19:239–245.

247. Adamson JW. Steroid metabolites and hemopoiesis. In: Fisher JW, ed. *Kidney Hormones, Erythropoietin.* London: Academic Press, 1977:437–462.

248. Kalmanti M, Dainiak N, Martino J, et al. Correlation of clinical and in vitro erythropoietic response to androgens in CKD. *Kidney Int* 1982;22:383–391.

249. Neff MS, Goldberg J, Slifkin RF, et al. A comparison of androgens for anemia in patients on hemodialysis. *N Engl J Med* 1981;304:871–875.

250. Ballel SH, Domato DT, Polack DC, et al. Androgens potentiate the effects of erythropoietin in the treatment of anemia of end-stage renal disease. *Am J Kidney Dis* 1991;17: 29–33.

251. Berns JS, Rudnick MR, Cohen RM. A controlled trial of recombinant human erythropoietin and nandrolone decanoate in the treatment of anemia in patients on chronic hemodialysis. *Clin Nephrol* 1992;37:264–267.

252. Teruel JL, Marcen R, Navarro Antolin J, et al. Androgen versus erythropoietin for the treatment of anemia in hemodialyzed patients: a prospective study. *J Am Soc Nephrol* 1996;7:140–144.

253. Eschbach JW, Abdulhadi MH, Browne JK, et al. Recombinant human erythropoietin in anemic patients with end-stage renal disease: results of a phase III multicenter clinical trial. *Ann Intern Med* 1989:111:992–1000.

254. Erslev AJ, Adamson JW, Eschbach JW, Winearls CG, eds. *Erythropoietin: Molecular, Cellular, and Clinical Biology.* Baltimore: Johns Hopkins University Press, 1991.

in glomerulonephritic chronic hemodialysis patients. *Clin Nephrol* 1980;14:1–6.

255. Eschbach JW, Kelly MR, Haley NR, et al. Treatment of the anemia of progressive CKD with recombinant human erythropoietin. *N Engl J Med.* 1989;321:158–163.

256. Sabota JT. Recombinant human erythropoietin in patients with anemia due to end-stage renal disease. *Contrib Nephrol* 1989;76:166–178.

257. Besarab A, McCrea JB. Evolution of recombinant human erythropoietin usage in clinical practice in the United States. *ASAIO J* 1993;39:11–18.

258. Powe NR, Griffiths RI, Greer JW, et al. Early dosing practices and effectiveness of recombinant human erythropoietin. *Kidney Int* 1993;43:1125–1133.

259. Eggers PW, Greer J, Jencks S. The use of Health Care Financing Administration data for the development of a quality improvement project on the treatment of anemia (review). *Am J Kidney Dis* 1994;24:247–254.

260. Sisk JE, Gianfrancesco FD, Coster JM. Medicare payment options for recombinant erythropoietin therapy. *Am J Kidney Dis* 1991;18(suppl 1):93–97.

261. McNamee P, van Doorslaer E, Segaar R. Benefits and costs of recombinant human erythropoietin for end-stage CKD: a review. *Int J Technol Assess Health Care* 1993;9:490–504.

262. United States Renal Data System 1996 Annual Report. *Am J Kidney Dis* 1996;28(suppl 3):S56.

263. ESRD 2002 Report *Am J Kidney Dis*, August 2003.

264. Obrator GT, Roberts T, St Peter WL, et al. Trends in anemia management at initiation of dialysis in the United States. *Kidney Int* 2001;60:1875–1884.

265. Eschbach JW. The anemia of CKD: pathophysiology and the effects of recombinant erythropoietin (review). *Kidney Int* 1989;35:134–148.

266. Pitts TO, Barbour GL. Hemosiderosis secondary to chronic parenteral iron therapy in maintenance hemodialysis patients. *Nephron* 1978;22:316–321.

267. Goldman M, Vangerweghen J-L. Multiple blood transfusions and iron overload in patients receiving haemodialysis. *Nephrol Dial Transplant* 1987:2:316–321.

268. Fleming LW, Hopwood D, Shepherd AM, Stewart WK. Hepatic iron in dialyzed patients given intravenous iron dextran. *J Clin Pathol* 1990;43:119–124.

269. Waterlot Y, Cantinieaux B, Hariga-Muller C, et al. Impaired phagocytic activity of neutrophils in patients receiving hemodialysis: the critical role of iron overload. *BJM* 1985;291:501–504.

270. Boelaert JR, Daneels RF, Schurgers ML, et al. Iron overload in haemodialysis patients increases the risk for bacteremia: a prospective study. *Nephrol Dial Transplant* 1990;5:130–134.

271. McCarthy JT, Johnson WJ, Nixon DE, et al. Transfusional iron overload in patients undergoing dialysis: treatment with erythropoietin and phlebotomy. *J Lab Clin Med* 1989;114:193–199.

272. Lazarus JM, Hakim RM, Newell J. Recombinant human erythropoietin and phlebotomy in the treatment of iron overload in chronic hemodialysis patients. *Am J Kidney Dis* 1990;16:101–108.

273. El-Reshaid K, Johny KV, Hakim A, et al. Erythropoietin treatment in haemodialysis patients with iron overload. *Acta Haematol* 1994;91(3):130–135.

274. Chan PCK, Liu P, Cronin C, et al. The use of nuclear magnetic resonance imaging in monitoring total body iron in hemodialysis patients with hemosiderosis treated with erythropoietin and phlebotomy. *Am J Kidney Dis* 1992;19:484–489.

275. Cecchin E, De Marchi S, Querin F, et al. Efficacy of hepatic computed tomography to detect iron overload in chronic hemodialysis. *Kidney Int* 1990;37:943–950.

276. Grimm PC, Sinai-Trieman L, Sekiya NM, et al. Effects of recombinant human erythropoietin on HLA sensitization and cell mediated immunity. *Kidney Int* 1990;38:12–18.

277. Barany P, Fehrman I, Godoy C. Long term effects on lymphocytotoxic antibodies and immune reactivity in hemodialysis patients treated with recombinant human erythropoietin. *Clin Nephrol* 1992;37:90–96.

278. Evans RW. Recombinant human erythropoietin and the quality of life of end-stage renal disease patients: a comparative analysis. *Am J Kidney Dis* 1991;18(suppl 1):S62–S70.

279. Auer J, Simon G, Stevens J, et al. Quality of life improvements in CAPD patients treated with subcutaneously administered erythropoietin for anemia. *Perit Dial Int* 1992;12:40–42.

280. US Recombinant Human Erythropoietin Predialysis Group. Double-blind, placebo-controlled study of the therapeutic use of recombinant human erythropoietin for anemia associated with CKD in predialysis patients. *Am J Kidney Dis* 1991;14:50–59.

281. Bennett WM. A multicenter clinical trial of epoetin beta for anemia of end-stage CKD. *J Am Soc Nephrol* 1991;1:990–998.

282. Beusterien LM, Nissenson AR, Port FK, et al. The effects of recombinant human erythropoietin on functional health and well-being in chronic dialysis patients. *J Am Soc Nephrol* 1996;7:763–773.

283. Moreno F, Vanderrabano F, Aracil FJ, Perez R. Influence of Hct on the quality of life of hemodialysis patients. *Nephrol Dial Transplant* 1994;9:1034–1037.

284. Canadian Erythropoietin Study Group. Association between recombinant human erythropoietin and quality of life and exercise capacity of patients receiving haemodialysis. *BMJ* 1990;300:573–578.

285. Besarab A, Bolton WK, Browne JK, et al. The effects of normal versus anemic Hct on hemodialysis patients with cardiac disease. *N Engl J Med* 1998;339:584–590.

286. Temple RM, Langan SJ, Deary IJ. Recombinant human erythropoietin improves cognitive function in chronic haemodialysis patients. *Nephrol Dial Transplant* 1992;7:240–245.

287. Nissenson AR. Epoetin and cognitive function. *Am J Kidney Dis* 1992;20(suppl 1):21–24.

288. Marsh JT, Brown WS, Wolcott D, et al. rHuEPO treatment improves brain and cognitive function of anemic dialysis patients. *Kidney Int* 1991;39:155–163.

289. Pickett JL, Theberge DC, Brown WS, et al. Normalizing hematocrit in dialysis patients improves brain function. *Am J Kidney Dis* 1999;33:1122–1130.

290. Kusunoki M, Kimura K, Nakamura M, et al. Effects of Hct variations on cerebral blood flow and oxygen transport on

ischemic cerebrovascular disease. *J Cereb Blood Flow Metab* 1981;1:413–417.

291. Digicaylioglu M, Bichet S, Marti HH, et al. Localization of specific erythropoietin binding sites in defined areas of the mouse brain. *Proc Natl Acad Sci USA* 1995;92:3717–3720.

292. Marti HH, Gassmann M, Wenger RH, et al. Detection of erythropoietin in human liquor: intrinsic erythropoietin production in the brain. *Kidney Int* 1997;51:416–418.

293. Metra M, Cannela G, La Canna G, et al. Improvement in exercise capacity after correction of anemia in patients with end-stage CKD. *Am J Cardiol* 1991;68:1060–1066.

294. McMahon LP, Johns JA, McKenzie A, et al. Hemodynamic changes and physical performance at comparative levels of haemoglobin after long-term treatment with recombinant erythropoietin. *Nephrol Dial Transplant* 1992;7:1199–1206.

295. Davenport A. The effect of treatment with recombinant human erythropoietin on skeletal muscle function in patients with end-stage CKD treated with regular hemodialysis. *Am J Kidney Dis* 1993;22:685–690.

296. Park JS, Kim SB, Park S-K, et al. Effect of recombinant human erythropoietin on muscle energy metabolism in patients with end-stage renal disease: a P-nuclear magnetic resonance spectroscopic study. *Am J Kidney Dis* 1993;21:612–619.

297. Horina JH, Schwaberger G, Brusse H, et al. Increased red cell 2,3-diphosphoglycerate levels in haemodialysis patients treated with erythropoietin. *Nephrol Dial Transplant* 1993;8:1219–1222.

298. Mayer G, Thum J, Graf H. Anaemia and reduced exercise capacity in patients on chronic haemodialysis. *Clin Sci* 1989;76:265–268.

299. Macdougall IC, Lewis NP, Saunders MJ, et al. Long-term cardiopulmonary effects of amelioration of renal anaemia by erythropoietin. *Lancet* 1990;1:489–493.

300. Marrades RM, Roca J, Campistol JM, et al. Effects of erythropoietin on muscle O_2 transport during exercise in patients with CKD. *J Clin Invest* 1996;97:2092–2100.

301. Lim VS. Recombinant human erythropoietin in predialysis patients. *Am J Kidney Dis* 1991;18(suppl 1):34–37.

302. Painter P. The importance of exercise training in rehabilitation of patients with end-stage renal disease. *Am J Kidney Dis* 1994;24:S31–S32.

303. Blagg CR. The socioeconomic impact of rehabilitation. *Am J Kidney Dis* 1994;24(suppl 1):S17–S21.

304. Hassanein AA, McNicol GP, Douglass AS. Relationship between platelet function tests in normal and uraemic subjects. *J Clin Invest* 1970;23:402–406.

305. Steiner RW, Coggins C, Carvalho ACA. Bleeding time in uremia: a useful test to assess clinical bleeding. *Am J Hematol* 1979;7:107–117.

306. Remuzzi G, Penigni A, Dodesini P, et al. Reduced platelet thromboxane formation in uremia: evidence for a functional cyclooxygenase defect. *J Clin Invest* 1983;71:762–768.

307. Castillo R, Lozano T, Escolar G, et al. Defective platelet adhesion on vessel subendothelium in uremic patients. *Blood* 1986;68:337–342.

308. Remuzzi G, Livio M, Marchiaro G, et al. Bleeding in CKD: altered platelet function in chronic uraemia only partially corrected with hemodialysis. *Nephron* 1978;22:347–353.

309. Noris M, Benigni A, Boccardo P, et al. Enhanced nitric oxide synthesis in uremia: implications for platelet dysfunction and dialysis hypotension. *Kidney Int* 1993;44:445–450.

310. Huraib S, Al-Momen AK, Gader AMA, et al. Effect of recombinant human erythropoietin (rHuEPO) on the hemostatic system in chronic hemodialysis patients. *Clin Nephrol* 1991;36:252–257.

311. Akizawa T, Kinugasa E, Kitaoka T, Koshikawa S. Effects of recombinant human erythropoietin and correction of anemia on platelet function in hemodialysis patients. *Nephron* 1991;58:400–406.

312. Vigano G, Benigni A, Mendogni D, et al. Recombinant human erythropoietin to correct uremic bleeding. *Am J Kidney Dis* 1991;18:44–49.

313. Kaupke CJ, Butler GC, Vaziri ND. Effect of recombinant human erythropoietin on platelet production in dialysis patients. *J Am Soc Nephrol* 1993;3:1672–1679.

314. Taylor JE, Belch JJ, Henderson IS, Steward WK. Erythropoietin does not increase whole-blood platelet aggregation. *Nephrol Dial Transplant* 1993;8:1291–1293.

315. Fluck RJ, Roger SD, MacMahon AC, Raine AEG. Modulation of platelet cytosolic calcium during erythropoietin therapy in uraemia. *Nephrol Dial Transplant* 1994;9:1109–1114.

316. Gura V, Creter D, Levi J. Elevated thrombocyte calcium in uremia and its correction by 1 alpha(OH) vitamin D treatment. *Nephron* 1982;30:237–239.

317. Lai K-N, Yin JA, Yuen PMP, Li PKT. Effect of hemodialysis on protein C, protein S, and antithrombin III levels. *Am J Kidney Dis* 1991;27:38–42.

318. Lai K-N, Yin JA, Yuen PMP, Li PKT. Protein C, protein S, and antithrombin III levels in patients on continuous ambulatory peritoneal dialysis and hemodialysis. *Nephron* 1990;56:271–276.

319. Clyne N, Egberg N, Lins LE. Effects of hemodialysis and long-term erythropoietin treatment on protein C, and on free and total protein S. *Thromb Res* 1995;80:161–168.

320. Huraib S, Gader AM, Al-Momen AK, et al. One-year experience of very low doses of subcutaneous erythropoietin in continuous ambulatory peritoneal dialysis and its effect on haemostasis. *Haemostasis* 1995;25:299–304.

321. Maurin N, Fitzner S, Fritz H, et al. Influence of recombinant human erythropoietin on hematological and hemostatic parameters with special reference to microhemolysis. *Clin Nephrol* 1995;43:196–200.

322. Besarab A, Medina F, Musial E, et al. Recombinant human erythropoietin does not increase clotting in vascular accesses. *ASAIO Trans* 1990;36:M749–M753.

323. Sundal E, Kaeser U. Correction of anaemia of CKD with recombinant human erythropoietin: safety and efficacy of one year's treatment in a European multicentre study of 150 haemodialysis-dependent patients. *Nephrol Dial Transplant* 1989;4:979–987.

324. Churchill DN, Muirhead N, Goldstein M, et al. Probability of thrombosis of vascular access among hemodialysis patients treated with recombinant human erythropoietin. *J Am Soc Nephrol* 1994;4:1809–1813.

325. Dy GR, Bloom EJ, Ijelu GK, et al. Effect of recombinant human erythropoietin on vascular access. *ASAIO Trans* 1991;37:M274–M275.

326. Tang I, Vrahos D, Valaitis D, Lau AH. Vascular access thrombosis during recombinant human erythropoietin therapy. *ASAIO Trans* 1992;38:M528–M531.

327. Muirhead N. Erythropoietin is a cause of access thrombosis. *Semin Dial* 1993;6:184–188.

328. Eschbach JW. Erythropoietin is not a cause of access thrombosis. *Semin Dial* 1993;6:180–184.

329. MacDougall IC, Davies ME, Hallett I, et al. Coagulation studies and fistula blood flow during erythropoietin therapy in haemodialysis patients. *Nephrol Dial Transplant* 1991;6:862–867.

330. Silverberg J, Rahal D, Patton R, Sniderman A. Role of anemia in the pathogenesis of left ventricular hypertrophy in end stage renal disease. *Am J Cardiol* 1989;64:222–224.

331. Parfrey PS, Foley RN, Harnett JD, et al. Outcome and risk factors for left ventricular disorders in chronic uraemia. *Nephrol Dial Transplant* 1996;11:1277–1285.

332. Foley RN, Parfrey PS, Harnett JD, et al. Clinical and echocardiographic disease in patients starting end-stage renal disease. *Am J Kidney Dis* 1995;47:186–192.

333. Goldberg N, Lundin AP, Delano B, et al. Changes in left ventricular size, wall thickness, and function in anemic patients treated with recombinant human erythropoietin. *Am Heart J* 1992;124:424–427.

334. Pascal J, Teruel LJ, Moya JL, et al. Regression of left ventricular hypertrophy after partial correction of anemia with erythropoietin in patients on hemodialysis: a prospective study. *Clin Nephrol* 1991;35:280–287.

335. Neff MS, Kim KE, Persoff M, et al. Hemodynamics of uremic anemia. *Circulation* 1971;43:876–883.

336. Silverberg JS, Racine N, Barre PE, Sniderman AD. Regression of left ventricular hypertrophy in dialysis patients following correction of anemia with recombinant human erythropoietin. *Can J Nephrol* 1990;6:26–30.

337. Cannella G, La Canna G, Sandrini M, et al. Reversal of left ventricular hypertrophy following recombinant human erythropoietin of anemic dialyzed uremic patients. *Nephrol Dial Transplant* 1991;6:31–37.

338. Rademacher J, Koch KM. Treatment of renal anemia by erythropoietin substitution. *Clin Nephrol* 1995;44(suppl 1):S56–S60.

339. Fellner SK, Lang RM, Neumann A, et al. Cardiovascular consequences of the correction of the anemia of CKD with erythropoietin. *Kidney Int* 1993;44:1309–1315.

340. Onoyama K, Kumagai H, Takeda K, et al. Effects of human recombinant erythropoietin on anaemia, systemic haemodynamics and renal function in pre-dialysis CKD patients. *Nephrol Dial Transplant* 1989;4:966–970.

341. Schwartz AB, Prior JE, Mintz GS, et al. Cardiovascular hemodynamic effects of correction of anemia of CKD with recombinant erythropoietin. *Transplant Proc* 1991;23:1827–1830.

342. Rostandt SG, Rutsky EA. Cardiac disease in dialysis patients. In: Nissenson AR, Fine RN, Gentile DE, eds. *Clinical Dialysis,* 2d ed. Norwalk, CT: Appleton & Lange, 1990: 409–446.

343. Wizemann V, Kaufman N, Kramer W. Effect of erythropoietin on ischemic tolerance in anemic hemodialysis patients with confirmed coronary artery disease. *Nephron* 1992;62:161–165.

344. Wu WC, Rathore SS, Wang Y, et al. Blood transfusion in elderly patients with acute myocardial infarction. *N Engl J Med* 2001;345(17):1230–1236.

345. Silverberg DS, Wexler D, Sheps D, et al. The effect of correction of mild anemia in severe, resistant congestive heart failure using subcutaneous erythropoietin and intravenous iron: a randomized controlled study. *J Am Coll Cardiol* 2001;37:1775–1780.

346. Horwich TB, Fonarow GC, Hamilton MA, et al. Anemia is associated with worse symptoms, greater impairment in functional capacity and a significant increase in mortality in patients with advanced heart failure. *J Am Coll Cardiol* 2002;39(11):1780–1786.

347. Nonnast-Daniel B, Deschodt G, Brunkhorst R, et al. Long-term effects of treatment with recombinant human erythropoietin on haemodynamics and tissue oxygenation in patients with renal anaemia. *Nephrol Dial Transplant* 1990;5:444–448.

348. Santleben W, Baldamus CA, Bommer J, et al. Blood pressure changes during treatment with recombinant human erythropoietin. *Contrib Nephrol* 1988;66:114–122.

349. Maschio G. Erythropoietin and systemic hypertension. *Nephrol Dial Transplant* 1995;10(suppl 2):4–79.

350. van de Borne P, Tielemans C, Vanherweghem J-L, Degaute J-P. Effect of recombinant human erythropoietin therapy on ambulatory BP and heart rate in chronic hemodialysis patients. *Nephrol Dial Transplant* 1992;7:45–49.

351. Cannella G, La Canna G, Sandrini M, et al. Renormalization of high cardiac output and of left ventricular size following long-term recombinant human erythropoietin treatment of anemic dialyzed uremic patients. *Clin Nephrol* 1990:34:272–278.

352. Abraham PA, Macres MG. Blood pressure in hemodialysis patients during amelioration of anemia with erythropoietin. *J Am Soc Nephrol* 1991;2:927–936.

353. Raine AEG, Roger SD. Effect of erythropoietin on blood pressure. *Am J Kidney Dis* 1991;18(suppl 1):76–83.

354. Stephen HM, Brunner R, Müller R, et al. Peripheral hemodynamics, blood viscosity, and the renin-angiotensin system in hemodialysis patients under therapy with recombinant human erythropoietin. *Contrib Nephrol* 1989;76:292–298.

355. Vaziri ND, Zhou XJ, Naqvi F, et al. Role of nitric oxide resistance in erythropoietin-induced hypertension in rats with CKD. *Am J Physiol* 1996;34:E113–E122.

356. Kaupke CJ, Kim S, Vaziri ND. Effect of erythrocyte mass on arterial blood pressure in dialysis patients receiving maintenance erythropoietin therapy. *J Am Soc Nephrol* 1994;4:1874–1878.

357. del Castillo D, Raij L, Shultz PJ, Tolins JP. The pressor effect of recombinant human erythropoietin is not due to decreased activity of the endogenous nitric oxide system. *Nephrol Dial Transplant* 1995;10:505–508.

358. Edmunds M, Walls J. Blood pressure and erythropoietin. *Lancet* 1988;1:351–352.

359. Carlini R, Dusso AS, Chamberlain I, et al. Recombinant human erythropoietin (rHuEPO) increases endothelin-1 release by endothelial cells. *Kidney Int* 1993;43:1010–1014.

360. Vaziri ND, Zhou XJ, Smith J, et al. In vitro and in vivo pressor effects of erythropoietin. *Am J Physiol* 1995;38:F838–F845.

361. Takayama K, Nagai T, Kinugasa E, et al. Changes in endothelial vasoactive substances under recombinant human erythropoietin in hemodialysis patients. *ASAIO Trans* 1991;37:M187–M188.

362. Nagai T, Akizawa T, Nakashima Y, et al. Effects of rHuEPO on cellular proliferation and endothelin-1 production in cultured endothelial cells. *Nephrol Dial Transplant* 1995;10:1814–1819.

363. Heidenreich S, Rahn KH, Zidek W. Direct vasopressor effect of recombinant human erythropoietin on renal resistance vessels. *Kidney Int* 1991;39:259–265.

364. Eggena P, Willsey P, Jamgotchian L, et al. Influence of recombinant human erythropoietin on blood pressure and renin-angiotensin systems. *Am J Physiol* 1991;261: E642– E646.

365. Torralbo A, Herrero JA, Portoles J, et al. Effects of Hct and vasoactive substance levels on blood pressure of patients treated with erythropoietin (EPO) (abstr). *Kidney Int* 1993;44:1478.

366. Frencken LAM, Wetzels JFM, Sluitter HE, Koene RAP. Evidence for renal vasodilatation in pre-dialysis patients during correction of anemia by erythropoietin. *Kidney Int* 1992;41:384–387.

367. Raine AEG. Hypertension, blood viscosity and cardiovascular morbidity in CKD: implications for erythropoietin therapy. *Lancet* 1988;1:97–99.

368. Brown CD, Kieran M, Thomas LL, et al. Treatment of azotemic, nonoliguric, anemic patients with human recombinant erythropoietin raises whole blood viscosity proportional to Hct. *Nephron* 1991;59:394–398.

369. Linde T, Sandhagen B, Danielson BG, Wikström B. Impaired erythrocyte fluidity during treatment of renal anaemia with erythropoietin. *J Intern Med* 1992;232:601–606.

370. Abraham PA, Opsah JA, Keshaviah PR, et al. Body fluid spaces and blood pressure in hemodialysis patients during amelioration of anemia with erythropoietin. *Am J Kidney Dis* 1990;16:438–446.

371. Lim VS, Kirchner PT, Fangman J, et al. The safety and efficacy of maintenance therapy of recombinant human erythropoietin treatment in patients with renal insufficiency. *Am J Kidney Dis* 1989;14:496–506.

372. Anastassiades E, Howarth D, Howarth J, et al. Influence of blood volume on the blood pressure of predialysis and peritoneal dialysis patients treated with erythropoietin. *Nephrol Dial Transplant* 1993;8:621–625.

373. Cascinu S, Catalano G, Cellerino R. Recombinant human erythropoietin in chemotherapy-associated anemia (review). *Cancer Treat Rev* 1996;21:553–564.

374. Schreiber S, Howaldt S, Schnoor M, et al. Recombinant erythropoietin for the treatment of anemia in inflammatory bowel disease. *N Engl J Med* 1996;334:619–623.

375. Harris SA, Payne G Jr, Putman JM. Erythropoietin treatment of erythropoietin-deficient anemia without renal disease during pregnancy. *Obstet Gynecol* 1996;87:812–814.

376. Poux JM, Lartigue M, Chaisemartin RA, et al. Uraemia is necessary for erythropoietin-induced hypertension in rats. *Clin Exp Pharmacol Physiol* 1995;22:769–771.

377. Carlini R, Russo AS, Obialo I, Rothstein M. Intravenous erythropoietin (rHuEPO) administration increases plasma endothelin and blood pressure in hemodialysis patients. *Am J Hypertens* 1993;6:103–107.

378. Leben M, Grose JH, Kingma I, Langlois S. Plasma immunoreactive endothelin levels in hemodialysis and in CAPD patients with and without erythropoietin therapy (abstr). *Proc XII Int Cong Nephrol,* Jerusalem, Israel. June 1993:358.

379. Brunet P, Lorec AM, Leonetti F, et al. Plasma endothelin in haemodialysis patients treated with recombinant human erythropoietin. *Nephrol Dial Transplant* 1994:9:650–665.

380. Lai KN, Lui SF, Leung JCK, et al. Effect of subcutaneous and intraperitoneal administration of recombinant human erythropoietin on blood pressure and plasma vasoactive hormones in patients on continuous ambulatory peritoneal dialysis. *Nephron* 1991;57:394–400.

381. Navarro JF, Teruel JL, Marcen R, Ortuno J. Improvement of erythropoietin-induced hypertension in hemodialysis patients changing the administration route. *Scand J Urol Nephrol* 1995;29:11–14.

382. Bassi S, Montini G, Edefonti A, et al. Cardiovascular function in a chronic peritoneal dialysis pediatric population on recombinant human erythropoietin treatment. *Perit Dial Int* 1993;13(suppl 2):S267–S269.

383. Martin GR, Ongkingo JR, Turner ME, et al. Recombinant erythropoietin (EPOgen) improves cardiac exercise performance in children with end-stage renal disease. *Pediatr Nephrol* 1993;7(3):276–280.

384. Harnett JD, Kent GM, Foley RN, Parfrey PS. Cardiac function and Hct level. *Am J Kidney Dis* 1995;25:S3–S7.

385. Yang CS, Chen SW, Chiang CH, et al. Effects of increasing dialysis dose on serum albumin and mortality in hemodialysis patients. *Am J Kidney Dis* 1996;17:380–386.

386. Lowrie EC, Huang NL, Lew NL, et al. The relative contributions of measured variables to death risk among hemodialysis patients. In: Friedman EA, ed. *Death on Hemodialysis: Preventable or Inevitable?* Dordrecht: Kluwer, 1995: 121–141.

387. Klinkmann H, Schmidt R, Wieczorek L, Scigalla P. Adverse events of subcutaneous recombinant human erythropoietin. *Contrib Nephrol* 1992;100:127–138.

388. Sikole A, Polenakovic M, Spirovska V, et al. Analysis of heart morphology and function following erythropoietin treatment of anemic dialysis patients. *Artif Organs* 1993; 17(12):977–984.

389. Churchill DN, Muirhead N, Goldstein M, et al. Effect of recombinant human erythropoietin on hospitalization of hemodialysis patients. *Clin Nephrol* 1995;43:184–188.

390. Xia H, Ebben J, Ma JZ, Collins, AJ. Hct levels and hospitalization risks in hemodialysis patients. *J Am Soc Nephrol* 1999;10:1309.

391. Collins AJ, Ma JZ, Ebben J. Impact of Hct on morbidity and mortality. *Semin Nephrol* 2000;20:345.

392. Powe NR, Griffiths RI, Watson AJ, et al. Effect of recombinant erythropoietin on hospital admissions, readmissions, length of stay, and costs of dialysis patients. *J Am Soc Nephrol* 1994;4:1455–1465.

393. Frenken LA, van Lier HJ, Jordan JG, et al. Identification of the component part in an epoetin alfa preparation that causes

pain after subcutaneous injection. *Am J Kidney Dis* 1993;22:553–556.

394. Veys N, Vanholder R, Lemeie N. Pain at the injection site of subcutaneously administered erythropoietin in maintenance hemodialysis patients: a comparison of two brands of erythropoietin. *Am J Nephrol* 1992;12:68–72.

395. Granolleras C, Leskopft W, Shaldon S, Fourcae J. Experience of pain after subcutaneous administration of different preparations of recombinant human erythropoietin: a randomized, double blind cross over study. *Clin Nephrol* 1991; 36:294–296.

396. Acchiardo SR, Quinn BP, Moore LW, et al. Evaluation of hemodialysis patients treated with erythropoietin. *Am J Kidney Dis* 1991;17:290–294.

397. Schaefer RM, Kokot F, Wirnze H, et al. Improved sexual function in hemodialysis patients on recombinant erythropoietin: a possible role for prolactin. *Clin Nephrol* 1989;33:1–5.

398. Steffensen G, Au Aunsholt N. Does erythropoietin cause hormonal changes in haemodialysis patients? *Nephrol Dial Transplant* 1993;8:1215–1218.

399. Ramirez G, Bittle PA, Rabb HA, et al. Effect of haemoglobin and endogenous erythropoietin on hypothalamic-pituitary thyroidal and gonadal secretion: an analysis of anaemic (high EPO) and polycythaemic (low EPO) patients. *Clin Endocrinol* 1995;43:167–174.

400. Carlson HE, Graber ML, Gelato MC, Hershman JM. Endocrine effects of erythropoietin. *Int J Artif Organs* 1995;18:309–314.

401. Schaefer F, van Kaick B, Veldhuis JD, et al. Changes in the kinetics and biopotency of leutinizing hormone in hemodialyzed men during treatment with recombinant human erythropoietin. *J Am Soc Nephrol* 1994;5:1208–1215.

402. Barany P, Petersson E, Ahlberg M, et al. Nutritional assessment in anemic hemodialysis patients treated with recombinant human erythropoietin. *Clin Nephrol* 1991;35:273–279.

403. Garibotto G, Gurreri G, Robaudo C, et al. Erythropoietin treatment and amino acid metabolism in hemodialysis patients. *Nephron* 1993;65(4):533–536.

404. Pollock CA, Wyndham R, Collett PV, et al. Effects of erythropoietin therapy on the lipid profile in end-stage CKD. *Kidney Int* 1994;45:897–902.

405. Friedman EA, Brown CD, Berman DH. Erythropoietin in diabetic macular edema and renal insufficiency. *Am J Kidney Dis* 1995;26:202–208.

406. Berman DH, Friedman EA. Partial absorption of hard exudates in patients with diabetic end-stage renal disease and severe anemia after treatment with erythropoietin. *Retina* 1994;14:1–5.

407. Zehnder C, Glück Z, Descoerdres DE, Blumberg A. Human recombinant erythropoietin in anaemic patients on maintenance haemodialysis. Secondary effects of an increase in haemoglobin. *Nephrol Dial Transplant* 1988;3:657–660.

408. Spinowitz BS, Arsianian J, Charytan C, et al. Impact of epoetin beta on dialyzer clearances and heparin requirements. *Am J Kidney Dis* 1991;18:668–673.

409. Baur T, Lundberg M. Secondary effects of erythropoietin treatment on metabolism and dialysis efficiency in stable hemodialysis patients. *Clin Nephrol* 1990;34:230–235.

410. Veys N, Vanholder R, De Guyper K, Ringoir S. Influence of erythropoietin on dialyzer re-use, heparin needs, and urea kinetics in maintenance hemodialysis patients. *Am J Kidney Dis* 1994;23:52–59.

411. Zehnder E, Pollock M, Ziegenhagen D, et al. Urea kinetics in patients on regular dialysis treatment before and after treatment with recombinant human erythropoietin. *Contrib Nephrol* 1988;66:149–155.

412. Paganni E, Abulhadi M, Garcia J, Magnusson MO. Recombinant human erythropoietin correction of anemia: dialysis efficiency, waste retention, and chronic dose variables. *ASAIO Trans* 1989;35:513–515.

413. Lippi A, Rindi P, Baronti R, et al. Recombinant human erythropoietin and high flux haemodiafiltration. *Nephrol Dial Transplant* 1995;10(suppl 6):51–54.

414. Ksiazek A, Baranowska–Daca E. Hct influence on peritoneal dialysis effectiveness during recombinant human erythropoietin treatment in patients with CKD. *Perit Dial Int* 1993;13(suppl 2):S550–S552.

415. Rossert JA, McClellan WM, Roger SD, et al. Contribution of anaemia to progression of renal disease: a debate. *Nephrol Dial Transplant* 2002;16(suppl 1):60–66.

416. Levin A, Singer J, Thompson CR, et al. Prevalent left ventricular hypertrophy in the predialysis population: identifying opportunities for intervention. *Am J Kidney Dis* 1996;27:347–354.

417. Levin A, Thompson CR, Ethier J, et al. Left ventricular mass index increase in early renal disease: impact of decline in hemoglobin. *Am J Kidney Dis.* 1999;34:125–134.

418. Keane WF, Lyle PA. Recent advances in management of type 2 diabetes and nephropathy: Lessons from the RENAAL study. *Am J Kidney Dis* 2003;41(3 suppl 1):S22–S25.

419. Iseki K, Ikemiya Y, Iseki C, Takishita S. Haematocrit and the risk of developing end-stage renal disease. *Nephrol Dial Transplant* 2003;18(5):899–905.

420. Schrier RW, et al. Increased nephron oxygen consumption: potential role in progression of CKD. *Am J Kidney Dis* 1994;23:176–182.

421. Nath KA et al. Redox regulation of renal DNA synthesis, transforming growth factor–beta 1 and collagen gene expression. *Kidney Int* 1998;53:367–381.

422. Kagedal K, Johansson U, Ollinger K. The lysosomal protease cathepsin D mediates apoptosis induced by oxidative stress. *FASEB J* 2001;15:1592–1594.

423. Yang B et al. Expression of apoptosis-related genes and proteins in experimental chronic renal scarring. *J Am Soc Nephrol* 2001;12:275–288.

424. Grune T, Sommerburg O, Siems WG. Oxidative stress in anaemia. *Clin Nephrol* 2000;53(suppl 1): S18–S22.

425. De Maria R et al Negative regulation of erythropoiesis by caspase-mediated cleavage of GATA-1. *Nature* 1999;401:489–493.

426. Silva M et al. Erythropoietin can promote erythroid progenitor survival by repressing apoptosis through Bcl-XL and Bcl-2. *Blood* 1996;88:1576–1582.

427. Siren AL et al. Erythropoietin prevents neuronal apoptosis after cerebral ischemia and metabolic stress. *Proc Natl Acad Sci* (USA) 2001;98:4044–4049.

428. Carlini RG et al. Effect of recombinant human erythropoietin on endothelial cell apoptosis. *Kidney Int* 1999;55:546–553.

429. Akimoto T et al. Erythropoietin regulates vascular smooth muscle cell apoptosis by a phosphatidylinositol 3 kinase-dependent pathway. *Kidney Int* 2000;58:269–282.

430. Westenfelder C et al. Human, rat, and mouse kidney cells express functional erythropoietin receptors. *Kidney Int* 1999;55:808–820.

431. Kuriyama S, Tomonari H, Yoshida H, et al. Reversal of anemia by erythropoietin therapy retards the progression of CKD, especially in nondiabetic patients. *Nephron* 1997:77:176–185.

432. Fine LG, Bandyopadhay D, Norman JT. Is there a common mechanism for the progression of different types of renal diseases other than proteinuria? Towards the unifying theme of chronic hypoxia. *Kidney Int.* 2000;57(suppl 75): S22–S26.

433. Albertazzi A, Di Liberato L, Daniele F, et al. Efficacy and tolerability of recombinant human erythropoietin treatment in pre-dialysis patients: results of a multicenter study. *Int J Artif Organs* 1998;21:12–18.

434. Kleinman KS, Schweitzer SU, Perdue ST, et al. The use of recombinant human erythropoietin in the correction of anemia in predialysis patients and its effect on renal function: a double-blind, placebo-controlled trial. *Am J Kidney Dis* 1989;14:486–495.

435. Roth D, Smith RD, Schulman G, et al. Effects of recombinant human erythropoietin on renal function in CKD predialysis patients. *Am J Kidney Dis* 1994;24:777–784.

436. Garcia DL, Anderson S, Rennke HG, Brenner BM. Anemia lessens and its prevention with recombinant human erythropoietin worsens glomerular injury and hypertension in rats with reduced renal mass. *Proc Natl Acad Sci USA* 1988;85:6142–6145.

437. Xue JL, St Peter WL, Ebben JP, et al. Anemia treatment in the pre–ESRD period and associated mortality in elderly patients. *Am J Kidney Dis* 2002Dec;40(6):1153–1161.

438. Hayashi T, Suzuki A, Shoji T, et al. Cardiovascular effect of normalizing the hematocrit level during erythropoietin therapy in predialysis patients with chronic renal failure. *Am J Kidney Dis* 2000;35:250–256.

439. Portoles J, Torralbo A, Martin P, et al. Cardiovascular effects of recombinant human erythropoietin in predialysis patients. *Am J Kidney Dis* 1997;29:541–548.

440. Silverberg DS, Wexler D, Blum M, et al. The use of subcutaneous erythropoietin and intravenous iron for the treatment of the anemia of severe, resistant congestive heart failure improves cardiac and renal function and functional cardiac class, and markedly reduces hospitalizations. *J Am Coll Cardiol* 2000;35:1737–1744.

441. Casadevall N, Nataf J, Viron B, et al. Pure red-cell aplasia and antierythropoietin antibodies in patients treated with recombinant erythropoietin. *N Engl J Med* 2002;346(7): 469–475.

442. Gershon SK, Luksenburg H, Cote TR, Braun MM. Pure red–cell aplasia and recombinant erythropoietin. *N Engl J Med* 2002;346:1584.

443. Bunn HF. Drug-induced autoimmune red-cell aplasia. *N Engl J Med* 2002;346:522.

444. Hermeling S, Schellekens H, Crommelin DJ, Jiskoot W. Micelle-associated protein in epoetin formulations: a risk factor for immunogenicity? *Pharm Res* 2003;20(12):1903–1907.

445. Weber G, Gross J, Kromminga A, et al Allergic skin and systemic reactions in a patient with pure red cell aplasia and anti-erythropoietin antibodies challenged with different epoetins. *J Am Soc Nephrol* 2002;13:2381–2383

446. Skibeli V, Nissen-Lie G, Torjesen P. Sugar profiling proves that human serum erythropoietin differs from recombinant human erythropoietin. *Blood* 2001;98:3626.

447. Schlags W, Lachmann B, Walher M, et al. Two-dimensional electrophoresis of recombinant human erythropoietin: a future method for the European Pharmacopeia? *Proteonomics* 2002;2:679–682.

448. Foley RN, Parfrey PS, Morgan J, et al. Effect of hemoglobin levels in hemodialysis patients with asymptomatic cardiomyopathy. *Kidney Int* 2000;58:1325–1335.

449. Levin A, Djurdjev O, Barrett B, et al. Cardiovascular disease in patients with chronic kidney disease: getting to the heart of the matter. *Am J Kidney Dis* 2001Dec;38(6):1398–407.

450. Furuland H, Linde T, Ahlmen J, et al. A randomized controlled trial of haemoglobin normalization with epoetin alfa in pre-dialysis and dialysis patients. *Nephrol Dial Transplant* 2003:353–61.

451. Arora P, Obrador GT, Ruthazer R, et al. Prevalence, predictors, and consequences of late nephrology referral at a tertiary care center. *J Am Soc Nephrol* 1999;10:1281–1286.

452. Salmonson T. Pharmacokinetic and pharmacodynamic studies on recombinant human erythropoietin. *Scand J Urol Nephrol* 1990;129(suppl):166.

453. Uehlenger DE, Gotch FA, Steiner CB. A pharmacodynamic model of erythropoietin therapy for uremic anemia. *Clin Pharmacol Ther* 1992;51:76–89.

454. Muirhead N, Bargman J, Burgess E, et al. Evidence-based recommendations for the clinical use of recombinant human erythropoietin. *Am J Kidney Dis* 1995;26(suppl 1):S1–S24.

455. Muirhead N, Churchill DN, Goldstein M, et al. Comparison of subcutaneous and intravenous recombinant human erythropoietin for anemia in hemodialysis patients with significant comorbid disease. *Am J Nephrol* 1992;12:303–310.

456. Ahn JH, Yoon KS, Lee WI, et al. Bone marrow findings before and after treatment with recombinant human erythropoietin in chronic hemodialyzed patients. *Clin Nephrol* 1995;43:189–95.

457. Beguin Y, Loo M, R'Zik S, et al. Early prediction of response to recombinant human erythropoietin in patients with the anemia of CKD by serum transferrin receptor and fibrinogen. *Blood* 1993;82(7):2010–2016.

458. Beguin Y, Loo M, R'Zik S, et al. Quantitative assessment of erythropoiesis in haemodialysis patients demonstrates gradual expansion of erythroblasts during constant treatment with recombinant human erythropoietin. *Br J Haematol* 1995;89:17–23.

459. Bargmann J. Recombinant human erythropoietin in patient on peritoneal dialysis. *Perit Dial Int* 1989;9:245–246.

460. Hughes RT, Cotes MP, Pippard MJ, et al. Subcutaneous administration of recombinant human erythropoietin to subjects on continuous ambulatory peritoneal dialysis: an erythropoietic assessment. *Br J Haematol* 1990;75:268–273.

461. Besarab A, Golper TA. Response of continuous peritoneal dialysis patients to subcutaneous rHuEPO differs from that of hemodialysis patients. *ASAIO Trans* 1991;37:M395–M396.

462. Lui SF, Law CB, Ting SM, et al. Once weekly versus twice weekly subcutaneous administration of recombinant human erythropoietin in patients on continuous ambulatory peritoneal dialysis. *Clin Nephrol* 1991;36:246–251.

463. Brown CD, Friedman EA. Stable renal function and benign course in azotemic diabetics treated with erythropoietin for one year. *Contrib Nephrol* 1991;88:182–189.

464. Austrian Multicenter Study Group of r–HuEPO in Predialysis Patients. Effectiveness and safety of recombinant human erythropoietin in predialysis patients. *Nephron* 1992;61:399–403.

465. Barany P, Clyne N, Hylander B, et al. Subcutaneous epoetin beta in renal anemia: an open multicenter dose titration study of patients on continuous peritoneal dialysis. *Perit Dial Int* 1995;15:54–60.

466. Nonnast–Daniel B, Schäffer J, Frei U. Hemodynamics in hemodialysis patients treated with recombinant human erythropoietin. *Contrib Nephrol* 1989;76:283–291.

467. Movilli E, Pertica N, Camerini C, et al. Predialysis versus postdialysis Hct evaluation during erythropoietin therapy. *Am J Kidney Dis* 2002;39:850–853.

468. Adamson JW, Egrie JC, Haley NR, et al. Why do some hemodialysis patients (HPD) need large doses of recombinant erythropoietin (rHuEPO)? (abstr). *Kidney Int* 1990;37:235.

469. Danielson B. R–HuEPO hyporesponsiveness—who and why? *Nephrol Dial Transplant* 1995;10(suppl 2):69–73.

470. Drüecke TB. Modulating factors in the hematopoietic response to erythropoietin. *Am J Kidney Dis* 1991;18(suppl 1):87–92.

471. Macdougall IC. Poor response to erythropoietin: practical guidelines on investigation and management. *Nephrol Dial Transplant* 1995;10:607–614.

472. Jongen-Lavrencic M, Peeters HR, Vreugdenhil G, Swaak AJ. Interaction of inflammatory cytokines and erythropoietin in iron metabolism and erythropoiesis in anaemia of chronic disease (review). *Clin Rheumatol* 1995;4:519–525.

473. Muirhead N, Hodsman AB. Occult infection and resistance of anemia to rHuEPO therapy in CKD. *Nephrol Dial Transplant* 1990;5:232–234.

474. Herbelin A, Urena P, Nguyen AT, et al. Elevated circulating levels of interleukin-6 in patients with CKD. *Kidney Int* 1991;39:954–960.

475. Drüecke TB. RHuEPO hyporesponsiveness: who and why? *Nephrol Dial Transplant* 1995;10:62–68.

476. Goicoechea M, Martin J, De Sequera P, et al. Role of cytokines in the response to erythropoietin in hemodialysis patients. *Kidney Int* 1998;54:1337.

477. Almond MK, Tailor D, Marsh FP, et al. Increased erythropoietin requirements in patients with failed renal transplants returning to a dialysis program. *Nephrol Dial Transplant* 1994;9:270–273.

478. Huang TP, Lin CY. Intraperitoneal recombinant human erythropoietin therapy: influence of the duration of continuous ambulatory peritoneal dialysis treatment and peritonitis. *Am J Nephrol* 1995;15:312–317.

479. Nassar GM, Fishbane S, Ayus JC. Occult infection of old nonfunctioning arteriovenous grafts: a novel cause of erythropoietin resistance and chronic inflammation in hemodialysis patients. *Kidney Int* 2002;61(suppl 80):49.

480. Muirhead N, Hodsman AB, Hollomby DJ, Cordy PK. The role of aluminum and parathyroid hormone in erythropoietin resistance in haemodialysis patients. *Nephrol Dial Transplant* 1991;6:342–345.

481. Yaqoob M, Ahmad R, McClelland P, et al. Resistance to recombinant human erythropoietin due to aluminium overload and its reversal by low dose desferrioxamine therapy. *Postgrad Med J* 1993;69(808):124–128.

482. Tomson CR, Edmunds ME, Chambers K, et al. Effect of recombinant human erythropoietin on erythropoiesis in homozygous sickle cell anaemia and CKD. *Nephrol Dial Transplant* 1992;7:817–821.

483. Cheng IKP, Lu H, Wei DCC, et al. Influence of thalassemia on the response to recombinant human erythropoietin in dialysis patients. *Am J Nephrol* 1993;13:142–148.

484. Rachmilewitz EA, Aker M, Perry D, Dover G. Sustained increase in haemoglobin and RBC following long-term administration of recombinant human erythropoietin to patients with homozygous beta-thalassaemia. *Br J Haematol* 1995;90:341–345.

485. Shetty A, Oreopoulos DG. Continuous ambulatory peritoneal dialysis in end-stage renal disease due to multiple myeloma. *Perit Dial Int* 1995;15:236–240.

486. Pronai W, Riegler Keil M, Silberbauer K, Stockenhuber F. Folic acid supplementation improves erythropoietin response. *Nephron* 1995;71:395–400.

487. Zachee P, Chew SL, Daelemans R, Lins RL. Erythropoietin resistance due to vitamin B12 deficiency: case report and retrospective analysis of B12 levels after erythropoietin treatment. *Am J Nephrol* 1992;12:188–191.

488. Ng YY, Chow MP, Lyou JY, et al. Resistance to erythropoietin: immunohemolytic anemia induced by residual formaldehyde in dialyzers. *Am J Kidney Dis* 1993;21:213–216.

489. Evers J. Cardiac hemolysis and anemia refractory to erythropoietin: on anemia in dialysis patients (letter). *Nephron* 1995;71:108.

490. Madour F, Bridges K, Brugnara NL, et al. A population study of the interplay between iron, nutrition, and inflammation in erythropoiesis in hemodialysis patients (abstr). *J Am Soc Nephrol* 1996;7:1456.

491. Gunnell J, Yeun JY, Depner TA, Kaysen GA. Acute-phase response predicts erythropoietin resistance in hemodialysis and peritoneal dialysis patients. *Am J Kidney Dis* 1999;33:63.

492. Wingard RL, Parker RA, Ismail N, Hakim RM. Efficacy of oral iron therapy in patients receiving recombinant human erythropoietin. *Am J Kidney Dis* 1995;25:433–439.

493. US Renal Data Systems. The USRDS Dialysis Morbidity and Mortality Study (Wave 1). In: *U.S. Renal Data Systems Annual Report 1996*. Bethesda, MD: National Institutes of Health, National Institutes of Diabetes and Digestive and Kidney Diseases, 1996:45–67.

494. Sepandj F, Jindal K, West M, Hirsch D. Economic appraisal of maintenance parenteral iron administration in treatment

of the anaemia in chronic haemodialysis patients. *Nephrol Dial Transplant* 1996;11:319–322.

495. Yee J, Besarab A. Iron sucrose: An old therapy becomes new. *Am J Kidney Dis* 2002;40:111–121.

496. Besarab A, Kaiser JW, Frinak S. A study of parenteral iron regimens in hemodialysis patients. *Am J Kidney Dis* 1999; 34:21.

497. Besarab A, Amin N, Ahsan M, et al. Optimization of epoetin therapy with intravenous iron therapy in hemodialysis patients. *J Am Soc Nephrol* 2000;11:530.

498. Taylor JE, Peat N, Porter C, Morgan AG. Regular, low dose intravenous iron therapy improves response to erythropoietin in haemodialysis patients. *Nephrol Dial Transplant* 1996;11:1079–1083.

499. Nissenson AR, Lindsay RM, Swan S, et al. Sodium ferric gluconate complex in surcrose is safe and effective in hemodialysis patients: North American Clinical Trial. *Am J Kidney Dis* 1999;33:471.

500. Hamstra RD, Block MH, Schocket A. Intravenous iron dextran in clinical medicine. *JAMA* 1980;243:1726–1731.

501. Fishbane S. Ungureanu V, Maesaka JK, et al. Safety of intravenous iron dextran in hemodialysis patients. *Am J Kidney Dis* 1996;28:529–534.

502. Fishbane S, Wagner J. Sodium ferric gluconate complex in the treatment of iron deficiency for patients on dialysis. *Am J Kidney Dis* 2001;37:879.

503. Bailie GR, Johnson CA, Mason NA. Parenteral iron use in the management of anemia in end-stage renal disease patients. *Am J Kidney Dis* 2000;35:1.

504. Van Wyck DB, Cavallo G, Spinowitz BS, et al. Safety and efficacy of iron sucrose in patients sensitive to iron dextran: North American Clinical Trial. *Am J Kidney Dis* 2000; 36:88.

505. Bolanos L, Castro P, Falcon TG, et al. Continuous intravenous sodium ferric gluconate improves efficacy in the maintenance phase of rHuEPO administration in hemodialysus patients. *Am J nephrol* 1992;22:67–72.

506. Gupta A, Amin NB, Besarab A, et al. Dialysate iron therapy: infusion of soluble ferric pyrophosphate via the dialysate during hemodialysis. *Kidney Int* 1999;55:1891.

507. Gastaldello K, Vereerstraeten A, Nzame-Nze T, et al. Resistance to erythropoietin in iron-overloaded haemodialysis patients can be overcome by ascorbic acid administration. *Nephrol Dial Transplant* 1995;10(suppl 6):44–47.

508. Goch J, Birgegard G, Danielson BG, Wikstrom B. Treatment of erythropoietin-resistant anaemia with desferrioxamine in patients on haemofiltration. *Eur J Haematol* 1995;55:73–77.

509. Hakim RM, Stivelman JC, Schumann G, et al. Iron overload and mobilization in long-term hemodialysis patients. *Am J Kidney Dis* 1987;10:293–299.

510. Koury MJ, Bondurant MC. Erythropoietin retards DNA breakdown and prevents programmed death in erythroid progenitor cells. *Science* 1990;248:378–381.

511. Egrie JC, Browne JK. Development and characterization of novel erythropoiesis stimulating protein (NESP). *Br J Cancer* 2001;84(suppl 1): 3–10.

512. Macdougall IC, Gray SJ, et al. Pharmacokinetics of novel erythropoiesis stimulating protein compared with epoetin alfa in dialysis patients. *J Am Soc Nephrol*; 1999;10(11): 2392–2395.

513. Jadoul M, Vanrenterghem Y, Foret M, et al. Darbepoetin alfa administered once monthly maintains haemoglobin levels in stable dialysis patients. *Nephrol Dial Transplant* 2004;19: (4):898–903.

514. Fishbane S, Tare N, Pill J, Haselbeck A. Preclinical pharmacodynamics and pharmacokinetics of CERA (Continuous Erythropoietin Receptor Activator), an innovative erythropoietic agent for anemia management of patients with kidney disease. *J Am Soc Nephrol* 2003;14:27A.

515. Shand BI, Bailey RR, Lynn KL, Robson RA. Effect of enalapril on erythrocytosis in hypertensive patients with renal disease. *Blood Press* 1995;4:238–240.

516. Julian BA, Gaston RS, Barker CV, et al. Erythropoiesis after withdrawal of enalapril in post-transplant erythrocytosis. *Kidney Int* 1994;46:1397–1403.

517. Dhondt AW, Vanholder RC, Ringoir SMG. Angiotensin converting enzyme inhibitors and higher erythropoietin requirement in chronic haemodialysis patients. *Nephrol Dial Transplant* 1995;10:2107–2109.

518. Erturk S, Nergizoglu G, Ates K, et al. The impact of withdrawing ACE inhibitors on erythropoietin responsiveness and left ventricular hypertrophy in haemodialysis patients. *Nephrol Dial Transplant* 1999;14:1912.

519. Conlon PJ, Albers F, Butterly D, Schwab S. ACE inhibitors do not affect erythropoietin efficiency in hemodialysis patients (letter). *Nephrol Dial Transplant* 1994;9:1359–1360.

520. Shand BI, Gilchrist NL, Nicholls MG, Bailey RR. Effect of losartan on haematology and haemorheology in elderly patients with essential hypertension: a pilot study. *J Hum Hypertens* 1995;9:233–235.

521. Abels RI. Use of recombinant human erythropoietin in the treatment of anemia in patients who have cancer. *Semin Oncol* 1992;19:29–35.

522. Reddingius RE, Schroder CH. Koster AM, Monnens LAH. Pharmacokinetics of recombinant human erythropoietin in children treated with continuous ambulatory peritoneal dialysis. *Eur J Pediatr* 1994;153:850–854.

523. Bargman JM, Jones JE, Petro JM. The pharmacokinetics of intraperitoneal erythropoietin administered undiluted or diluted in dialysate. *Perit Dial Int* 1992;12:369–372.

524. Loo AV, Vanholder R, Bernaert P, et al. Recombinant human erythropoietin corrects anaemia after renal transplantation: a randomized prospective study. *Nephrol Dial Transplant* 1996;11:1815–1821.

525. Kaplow LS, Goffinet JA. Profound neutropenia during the early phase of hemodialysis. *JAMA* 1968;203:133–135.

526. Spagnuolo PJ, Bass SH, Smith MC, et al. Neutrophil adhesiveness during prostacyclin and heparin hemodialysis. *Blood* 1982;60:924–929.

527. Craddock PR, Fehr J, Dalmasso AP, et al. Hemodialysis leukopenia: pulmonary vascular leukostasis resulting from complement activation by dialyzer cellophane membranes. *J Clin Invest* 1977;58:879–888.

528. Craddock RR, Hammerschmidt D, White JG, et al. Complement (C5A)-induced granulocyte aggregation in vitro: a possible mechanism-complement-mediated leukostasis and leukopenia. *J Clin Invest* 1977;60:260–264.

529. Chenoweth DE, Cheung AK, Ward DM, Henderson LW. Anaphylatoxin formation during hemodialysis: comparison of new and re-used dialyzers. *Kidney Int* 1983;24:770–774.

530. Himmelfarber J, Zaoui P, Hakim R. Modulation of granulocyte LAM-1 and MAC-1 during dialysis—a prospective, randomized controlled trial. *Kidney Int* 1992;41:388–395.

531. Hakim R, Schafer AI. Hemodialysis-associated platelet activation and thrombocytopenia. *Am J Med* 1985;78:575–580.

532. Dinarello CA. Cytokines and biocompatibility. *Blood Purif* 1990;8:208–213.

533. Hakim R. Clinical implications of hemodialysis membrane biocompatibility. *Kidney Int* 1993;44:484–494.

534. De Broe ME, Heyrman RM, De Backer WA, et al. Pathogenesis of dialysis induced hypoxemia: a short overview. *Kidney Int* 1985;33(suppl 24):57–61.

535. Robson MD, Charoenpanich R, Kant KS. Effect of first and subsequent re-use of hemodialyzers on patient well-being. *Am J Nephrol* 1986;6:101–106.

536. Bok DV, Pascal L, Herbenger C, Levin NA. Effect of multiple use of dialyzers on intradialytic symptoms. *Proc Clin Dial Transplant Forum* 1980;10:92–98.

537. Hakim RM, Breilatt J, Lazarus JM, Port FK. Complement activation and hypersensitivity reactions to dialysis membranes. *N Engl J Med* 1984;311:878–882.

538. Mailloux LU, Bellucci AG, Wilkes BM. Mortality in dialysis patients: analysis of the causes of death. *Am J Kidney Dis* 1991;3:326–335.

539. Baum J, Cestero RVM, Freeman RB. Chemotaxis of the polymorphonuclear leukocyte and delayed hypersensitivity in uremia. *Kidney Int* 1975;2(suppl):S147–S153.

540. Ilvento MC, Diez RA, Estevez ME, et al. Hemodialysis decreases spontaneous migration of polymorphonuclears in CKD. *Dial Transplant* 1992;21: 705–708.

541. Descamps-Latscha B, Herbelin A, Nguyen AT, Urena P. Respective influence of uremia and hemodialysis on whole blood phagocyte oxidative metabolism and circulating interleukin-1 and tumor necrosis factor. *Adv Exp Med Biol* 1991;297:183–192.

542. Vanholder R, Ringoir S, Dhondt A, Hakim R. Phagocytosis in uremic and hemodialysis patients: A prospective and cross-sectional study. *Kidney Int* 1991;39:320–327.

543. Roccatello D, Mazzucco G, Coppo R. Functional changes of monocytes due to dialysis membranes. *Kidney Int* 1989;35:622–635.

544. Ruiz P, Gomez F, Schreiber AD. Impaired function of macrophage Fc receptors in end stage renal disease. *N Engl J Med* 1990;322:717–722.

545. Meuer SC, Hauer M, Kurtz P, et al. Selective blockade of the antigen-receptor mediated pathway of T-cell activation in patients with impaired primary immune responses. *J Clin Invest* 1987;80:743–749.

546. Paczek L, Schaefer RM, Teschner M, Heidland A. Suppression of immunoglobulin and interleukin 6 production from peripheral blood mononuclear cells by dialysis membranes. *ASAIO Trans* 1990;34:M459–M461.

547. Memoli B, Libetta C, Rampino T, et al. Hemodialysis related induction of interleukin-6 production by peripheral blood mononuclear cells. *Kidney Int* 1992;42:320–326.

548. Zaoui P, Green W, Hakim R. Hemodialysis with cuprophane membranes modulates interleukin-2 receptor expression. *Kidney Int* 1991;39:1020–1026.

549. Raska K Jr, Raskova J, Shea SM, et al. T cell subsets and cellular immunity in end-stage renal disease. *Am J Med* 1983;75:734–740.

550. Langhoff E, Ladefoged J. In vitro immune functions in patients with minor, moderate, and severe kidney impairment. *APMIS* 1988;96:655–659.

551. Vanholder R, Ringoir S. Infectious morbidity and defects of phagocytic function in end-stage renal disease: a review. *J Am Soc Nephrol* 1993;3:1541–1554.

552. Levin NW, Zasuwa G, Dumler F. Effect of membrane types on causes of death in hemodialysis patients (abstr). *J Am Soc Nephrol* 1991;2:335.

553. Hornberger JC, Chernew M, Petersen J, Garber AM. A multivariate analysis of mortality and hospital admissions with high-flux dialysis. *J Am Soc Nephrol* 1993;3:1227–1237.

554. Collart FE, Dratwa M, Wittek M, Wens R. Effect of recombinant human erythropoietin on T-cell lymphocyte subsets in hemodialysis patients. *ASAIO Trans* 1990;36:M219–M223.

555. Schaefer RM, Paczek L, Berthold G, et al. Improved immunoglobulin production in dialysis patients treated with recombinant erythropoietin. *Int J Artif Organs* 1992;3:71–75.

556. Veys N, Vanholder R, Ringoir S. Correction of deficient phagocytosis during erythropoietin treatment in maintenance dialysis patients. *Am J Kidney Dis* 1992;19:358–363.

557. Boulart JR, Cantineaux BF, Hariga CF, Fondu PG. Recombinant human erythropoietin reverses polymorphonuclear granulocyte dysfunction in iron-loaded dialysis patients. *Nephrol Dial Transplant* 1990;5:504–507.

558. Sennasael JJ, Van der Niepen P, Verbeelen DL. Treatment with recombinant human erythropoietin increases antibody titers after hepatitis B vaccination in dialysis patients. *Kidney Int* 1990;40:121–128.

559. Eknoyan G, Wacksman SJ, Glueck HI, et al. Platelet function in CKD. *N Engl J Med* 1969;280:677–681.

560. Symons HS, Wrong OS. Uremic pericarditis with cardiac tamponade: a report of four cases. *BMJ* 1964;1: 605–607.

561. Nidus BD, Matalon R, Cantacuzino D, et al. Uremic pleuritis—a clinicopathologic entity. *N Engl J Med* 1969;281: 255–256.

562. Borra S, Kleinfeld M. Subcapsular liver hematomas in a patient on chronic hemodialysis. *Ann Intern Med* 1980;93: 574–575.

563. Maher JF, Schreiner GE. Hazards and complications of dialysis. *N Engl J Med* 1965;273:370–377.

564. Panicucci F, Sagripanti A, Pinori E, et al. Comprehensive study of haemostasis in chronic uremia. *Nephron* 1983;33: 5–8.

565. Gafter U, Bessler H, Malachi T, et al. Platelet count and thrombopoietic activity in patients with CKD. *Nephron* 1987;45:207–210.

566. Salzman EW, Neri LL. Adhesiveness of blood platelets in uremia. *Thromb Diath Haemorrh* 1966;15:84–92.

567. Evans EP, Branch RA, Bloom AL. A clinical and experimental study of platelet function in CKD. *J Clin Pathol* 1972;25:745–753.

568. Lindsay RM, Moorthy AV, Koens F, et al. Platelet function in dialyzed and non-dialyzed patients with CKD. *Clin Nephrol* 1975;4:52–57.

569. Remuzzi G, Cavenaghi AE, Mecca G, et al. Prostacyclin-like activity and bleeding in CKD. *Lancet* 1977;2: 1195–1197.

570. Livio M, Mannucci PM, Vigano G, et al. Conjugated estrogens for the management of bleeding associated with CKD. *N Engl J Med* 1986;315:731.

571. Zoja C, Vigano G, Bergamelli A, et al. Prolonged bleeding time and increased vascular prostacyclin in rats with CKD. Effects of conjugated estrogens. *J Lab Clin Med* 1988;112: 380–386.

572. Horowitz HI, Stein IM, Cohen BD, White JG. Further studies on the platelet inhibitory effects of guannidosuccinic acid: its role in uremic bleeding. *Am J Med* 1970;49: 336–345.

573. Hakim RM, Schaefer AI. Hemodialysis-associated platelet activation and thrombocytopenia. *Am J Med* 1985;78: 575–580.

574. Scmitt GW, Moake JL, Rudy CK, et al. Alterations in hemostatic parameters during hemodialysis with dialyzers of different membrane composition and flow design. *Am J Med* 1987;83:411–418.

575. Escolar G, Cases A, Bastida E, et al. Uremic platelets have a functional defect affecting the interaction of von Willebrand factor with glycoprotein IIb-IIIa. *Blood* 1990;76: 1336–1340.

576. Vlachoyannis J, Schoeppe W. Adenylate cyclase activity and cAMP content of human platelets in uraemia. *Eur J Clin Invest* 1982;12:379–381.

577. Benigni A, Livio M, Dodesini P, et al. Inhibition of human platelet aggregation by parathyroid hormone: is cyclic AMP implicated? *Am J Nephrol* 1985;5:243–247.

578. Diskin CJ, Stoke TJ Jr, Pennell AT. Pharmacologic intervention to prevent hemodialysis vascular access thrombosis. *Nephron* 1993;64:1–26.

579. Viener A, Aviram M, Better OS, et al. Enhanced in vitro platelet aggregation in hemodialysis patients. *Nephron* 1986;43:139–143.

580. Livio M, Benigni A, Vigano G, et al. Moderate doses of aspirin and the risk of bleeding in CKD. *Lancet* 1986;1: 414–416.

581. Gaspari F, Vigano G, Orisio S, et al. Aspirin prolongs bleeding time in uremia by a mechanism distinct from platelet cyclooxygenase inhibition. *J Clin Invest* 1987;79:1788–1797.

582. Ljungsber B. A low molecular heparin fraction as an anticoagulant during hemodialysis. *Clin Nephrol* 1985;24:15–20.

583. Zusman RM, Rubin RH, Cato AE, et al. Hemodialysis using prostacyclin instead of heparin as the sole antithrombotic agent. *N Engl J Med* 1981;302:934–939.

584. Sanders PW, Taylor N, Curtis JJ. Hemodialysis without anticoagulation. *Am J Kidney Dis* 1985;5:32–35.

585. Sasaki R. Pleiotropic functions of erythropoietin. *Intern Med* 2003;42(2):142–149.

586. Roger SD, Piper J, Tucker B, et al. Enhanced platelet reactivity with erythropoietin but not following transfusion in dialysis patients. *Nephrol Dial Transplant* 1993;8:213–217.

587. Taylor JE, Belch JJF, McLaren M, et al. Effect of erythropoietin therapy and withdrawal on blood coagulation and fibrinolysis in hemodialysis patients. *Kidney Int* 1993;44: 182–190.

588. Muirhead N, Laupacis A, Wong C. Erythropoietin for anaemia in haemodialysis patients: results of a maintenance study (The Canadian Erythropoietin Study Group). *Nephrol Dial Transplant* 1991;7:811–816.

589. Standage BA, Schuman ES, Ackerman D, et al. Does the use of erythropoietin in hemodialysis patients increase dialysis graft thrombosis rates? *Am J Surg* 1993;165:650–654.

590. Schand BI, Buttimore AL, Hurrell MA, et al. Hemorheology and fistula function in home hemodialysis patients following erythropoietin treatment: a prospective placebo-controlled study. *Nephron* 1993;64:53–57.

591. Janson PA, Jubelirer SJ, Weinstein MJ, Deykin D. Treatment of the bleeding tendency in uremia with cryoprecipitate. *N Engl J Med* 1980;303:1318–1322.

592. Mannucci PM, Remuzzi G, Pusineri F, et al. Deamino-8-D-arginine vasopressin shortens the bleeding time in uraemia. *N Engl J Med* 1983;308:8–12.

593. Liu YK, Kosfield RE, Marcum SG. Treatment of uraemic bleeding with conjugated estrogen. *Lancet* 1984;2:887–890.

594. Shapiro MD, Kellher SP. Intranasal deamino-8-dDAVP shortens the bleeding time in uremia. *Am J Nephrol* 1984;4: 260–261.

595. Canavese C, Salomone M, Pacitti A, et al. Reduced response of uraemic bleeding time to repeated doses of desmopressin (letter). *Lancet* 1985;1:867–868.

596. Bronner MH, Pate MB, Cunningham JY, et al. Estrogen-progesterone therapy for bleeding gastrointestinal telangiectasias in CKD. *Ann Intern Med* 1986;105:371–374.

Cardiac Disease in Dialysis Patients

Robert N. Foley

UREMIA AND THE CARDIOVASCULAR SYSTEM: ANIMAL MODELS

Morphologic and functional models of uremic toxicity provide many clinically relevant insights into the cardiac problems experienced by dialysis patients. Experimental uremia leads to dramatic changes in cardiac morphology, reviewed in detail in Ref.1. A rapid increase in left ventricular mass is seen early in the course of experimental renal failure. This is associated with an increase in the size of cardiomyocytes, which is likely to impose a greater distance for oxygen diffusion. In addition, rates of cardiomyocyte loss through apoptosis are enhanced. Experimental studies show that left ventricular hypertrophy can be partially prevented by angiotensin-converting enzyme (ACE) inhibitors, sympatholytic agents, endothelin-1 receptor blockers, and epoetin. Thickening of the walls of intramyocardial arterioles is another typical feature of experimental renal failure; in parallel with hypertrophy of vascular smooth muscle cells, a pattern suggesting activation of fibrotic processes is seen, including increased expression of vascular endothelial growth factor, platelet-derived growth factor, collagen IV, actin, and integrin-β1. Parathyroid hormone appears to be a permissive factor for these arteriolar changes, which can be abrogated with ACE inhibitors, endothelin-1 receptor blockers, calcium channel blockers, high doses of vitamin E, and a low-phosphate diet. In addition to thickening of the intramyocardial arteriolar wall, a reduction of capillary density is another unattractive morphologic feature of experimental renal failure. Reduced capillary density has not been seen in other types of left ventricular hypertrophy, such as the hypertensive variety. An increase in cardiac interstitial cell and nuclear volume, followed by interstitial fibrosis, is also seen in experimental uremia, which can be prevented by ACE inhibitors, endothelin-1 receptor blockade, vitamin E, and a low-phosphate diet. Thus, morphologic studies suggest that, even in the absence of hemodynamic stress and coronary artery stenosis, the uremic heart is at risk of ischemia, systolic heart failure, and diastolic heart failure.

A classic study examining the functional and metabolic impact of uremia was published in 1993.[2] Cardiac function was studied with the isolated perfused Langendorff preparation, using 31P magnetic resonance imaging (MRI). Uremia led to a lowering of cardiac output, a loss of the normal ability to change cardiac output in response to load changes, and the ability to change contractility with changes in ambient calcium levels. Even with normal oxygen levels in the perfusate, 31P MRI showed that phosphocreatine levels were reduced, as was the ratio of phosphocreatine to adenosine triphosphate (ATP)—a pattern suggesting heightened susceptibility to ischemia.

Thus, functional studies complement morphologic studies and suggest that the uremic heart is at heightened risk from ischemic and hemodynamic stresses.

DIAGNOSTIC TESTS

Coronary Artery Disease

In clinical practice, coronary angiography remains the "gold standard" for diagnosing coronary artery disease in patients on dialysis. The cost and invasiveness of the procedure make it unattractive as a routine test, especially in asymptomatic individuals. Standard exercise stress testing with electrocardiography cannot be advocated on a routine basis because most dialysis patients have impaired exercise capacity and ST-segment abnormalities are so commonly present. Currently, radionuclide and echocardiographic imaging are the noninvasive test techniques most often used, while dipyridamole, dipyridamole plus exercise, or dobutamine are the agents most commonly used to increase cardiac work. It is likely that the accuracy of these tests varies substantially by operator, center, and the background level of coronary artery disease in the population under study. One group showed that combined dipyridamole-exercise thallium imaging was acceptably accurate in dialysis patients; a negative predictive value of 98 percent was observed, implying that a normal test result essentially ruled out significant coronary stenosis.[3] Nuclear cardiology is in a period of great flux; recent advances include the advent of better isotopes, such as technetium-99m (Tc 99m) sestamibi and the use of gated single-photon-emission computed tomography (SPECT), which facilitate quantitative assessment of both myocardial perfusion and left ventricular function. Dobutamine stress echocardiography is logistically easier and cheaper than myocardial perfusion imaging and is thought to be reasonably accurate in the general population and in a limited number of studies in dialysis patients.[4-6] A recent study compared stress echocardiography and stress technetium-99m-tetrofosmin imaging in 66 asymptomatic hemodialysis patients, using a combination of high-dose dipyridamole and symptom-limited exercise to increase cardiac work. Coronary angiography was performed in patients with abnormal noninvasive tests and those considered at high risk for coronary artery disease. In comparison to myocardial perfusion imaging, the sensitivity and specificity of stress echocardiography were 86 and 94 percent, respectively. Stress echocardiography and myocardial perfusion imaging showed similar accuracy, at 84 vs. 91 percent, re-

spectively, for detecting angiographic coronary artery disease.[7]

Several advances have occurred in the approach to coronary artery disease that may have relevance in dialysis populations. First, it has become clear that in most episodes of myocardial infarction, the injury occurs at the site of nonobstructive plaques.[8–10] Second, the overall extent of atherosclerosis, rather than the severity of discrete stenotic lesions, is the most important predictor of outcome.[11] Finally, in distinction to extracoronary arteries, the extent of calcification in coronary arteries closely parallels the extent of atherosclerosis.[12,13] In line with this hypothesis, total coronary artery calcification scores using electron beam tomography outperform standard prediction algorithms for hard coronary events.[14] On a cautionary note, a similar prognostic link has yet to be demonstrated in dialysis patients, a group where extremely high calcification scores are the norm.

Cardiac Morphology and Function

Echocardiography is the most common noninvasive test of cardiac morphology and function in dialysis populations. It provides a reasonable level of accuracy for the study of several aspects of cardiac health, which makes it an attractive first-line investigation of cardiac function. Thus left ventricular cavity volume, mass index, systolic function, diastolic function, valve morphology, valve function, and the presence of nonperfused areas can be evaluated at a single examination. Echocardiography has several undesirable features. It is somewhat subjective and is limited by imperfect test-retest reliability as a longitudinal test within an individual patient.[15] Several factors, such as obesity and emphysema, can make acoustic windows difficult to obtain. Echocardiographic parameters are heavily load-dependent, a particular problem in dialysis populations. For example, it has been shown that estimates of left ventricular mass index are approximately 20 percent higher before dialysis than after dialysis.[16] Ideally, echocardiography should be performed at dry weight, especially when sequential measurements are planned.

Several alternative techniques can be used to assess ventricular structure and function. The use of cardiac biomarkers (such as type B natriuretic peptide) in dialysis patients is likely to remain problematic because of the expected "normal" fluctuations in extracellular fluid volume, the possibility that serum levels reflect renal function, and the possibility of removal during the dialysis procedure. Nuclear techniques include first-pass ventriculography, gated blood pool scanning, and SPECT during myocardial perfusion scanning with thallium-201 or Tc 99m-sestamibi. Cardiac MRI appears to be the current gold standard among minimally invasive tests and exhibits highly impressive test-retest characteristics.[17] One study compared MRI and echocardiography, with studies performed within 24 hours of hemodialysis. Intra- and interobserver variability was higher for echocardiography than for MRI; echocardiographic estimates systematically overestimated left ventricular dimensions in comparison to MRI.[18] Currently, the use of cardiac MRI in routine clinical practice is limited by cost and availability.

DISEASE BURDEN

Prevalence

Cardiovascular disease is a problem of "epidemic" size in end-stage renal disease (ESRD).[19] For example, the 2003 report from the United States Renal Data System showed that 50.6 percent of all new patients starting chronic dialysis had previous cardiovascular disease, with congestive heart failure the most common manifestation, followed by ischemic heart and peripheral vascular disease.[20] A 2003 report from the Dialysis Outcomes and Practice Patterns Study (DOPPS) compared the prevalence of several comorbid conditions in the United States, Europe, and Japan. DOPPS is a prospective observational study of patients in randomly selected, representative hemodialysis units in France, Germany, Italy, Japan, Spain, the United Kingdom, and the United States. The baseline prevalence of coronary artery disease, congestive heart failure, and peripheral vascular disease as well as the mean age, the proportion of diabetic patients, and the mean dialysis vintage are shown in Fig. 27A–1, using data reported in Ref. 21. Echocardiographic abnormalities—such as left ventricular hypertrophy, dilation, systolic dysfunction, and diastolic dysfunction—are common in dialysis patients, with reports dating back to 1978 consistently showing that at least four-fifths of dialysis patients had left ventricular hypertrophy.[22] Few recent studies have systematically assessed the extent of coronary artery disease in representative samples of dialysis patients. One prospective cohort study involved 224 dialysis patients from five hemodialysis centers in Texas in 1998. Of these, 67 volunteered to undergo coronary angiography. Coronary artery disease was found in 42 percent of subjects, with the following distribution of severity: single-vessel disease, 10 percent; two-vessel disease, 15 percent; and three-vessel disease, 16 percent.[23]

Incidence

Less is known about incidence rates of cardiovascular disease in dialysis patients, but these are likely to be high. One prospective study in the early 1990s reported incidence rates of 10 percent per year for both cardiac failure and ischemic heart disease in incident dialysis patients.[24] Another prospective study reported annual rates of first-onset cardiac failure and ischemic heart disease of approximately 7 and 3 percent, respectively.[25,26] The United States Renal Data System has reported rates of incident myocardial infarction, stroke, and peripheral vascular disease of 7.0, 7.1, and 8.4 percent, respectively, in the first year of dialysis therapy.[27] For purposes of comparison, the Framingham Heart Study reported reinfarction rates of 4 percent per year among myocardial infarction survivors, almost half the risk of new myocardial infarction in dialysis patients.[28]

Prognosis

Not unexpectedly, many studies suggest that a previous history of coronary artery disease or congestive heart failure is associated with higher mortality rates in dialysis patients. Mortality rates after new cardiac events are extremely high. In one well-known study, the United States Renal Data System reported mortality rates of 59.3, 73.0, and 89.9 after 1, 2, and 3 years after myocardial infarction in patients on

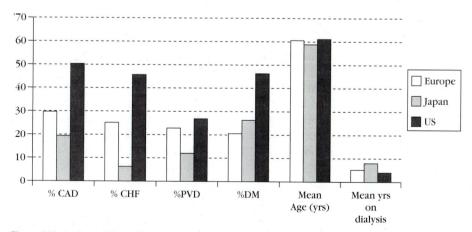

Figure 27A–1. Comorbid conditions at baseline by continent in the Dialysis Outcomes and Practice Patterns Study (DOPPS). (Based on data from Goodkin et al.[21]). CAD, coronary artery disease; CHF, congestive heart failure; PVD, peripheral vascular disease; DM, diabetes mellitus.

renal replacement therapy.[29] Mortality rates after congestive heart failure are similarly high.[25] Left ventricular hypertrophy is associated with higher mortality rates in dialysis patients.[30] Subsequent studies showed that left ventricular morphology and functional status were associated with specific cardiovascular syndromes, such as cardiac failure, myocardial infarction, and congestive heart failure.[31,32] The mortality associations seen in earlier studies have been confirmed in more recent ones.[33,34] Thus, left ventricular hypertrophy appears to represent an intermediate state between cardiac health and advanced cardiac disease. Because of the quantitative nature of cardiac disease, left ventricular mass and cavity volume are useful surrogate measures for epidemiological studies and for interventional trials.

RISK FACTORS, RISK MARKERS, AND BIOMARKERS

The term *risk factor* was coined in the early 1960s. Kannel and colleagues reported a study entitled "Factors of Risk in the Development of Coronary Heart Disease—Six Year Follow-Up Experience. The Framingham Study."[35] In hindsight, purists could argue that the noun *factor* was used prematurely, as it has connotations suggesting causality, and confirmatory controlled trials—the only reliable way to demonstrate causality—had yet to be performed. Similar concerns can be attached to the terms like *reverse causation* and *reverse epidemiology*. Because so few definitive cardiovascular intervention trials have been performed, the term *risk markers* appears preferable. Thus, in recent years, studies examining the prognostic association of serologic factors and genetic polymorphisms have proliferated. While these studies can have clear relevance with regard to biological mechanisms, identifying high-risk groups, and future management, it is often difficult to see how they lead to therapy in the here and now. To date, most studies have examined biomarkers in isolation, which does not readily facilitate identification of the "best" individual biomarker or any combination of biomarkers for clinical and utility.

Smoking

Smoking is a classic example of an avoidable "lifestyle" cardiovascular risk factor.[36] For example, mortality from cardiovascular disease in the Framingham Heart Study dropped by 50 percent over three decades; over half of this decline was explained by changes in modifiable risk factors such as smoking.[37]

Most studies show that the proportion of current smokers is lower in dialysis populations than in the general population, in a pattern suggesting that smokers discontinued smoking after major cardiovascular events had occurred. For example, in the United States Renal Data System Wave 2 study—a prospective cohort study of patients starting dialysis between 1996 and 1997—56.4 percent were lifetime nonsmokers, 3.6 percent were smokers with unknown current status, 20.0 percent had quit for more than 1 year, 5.8 percent had quit within the previous year, and 14.2 percent were current smokers. Patients with previous cardiovascular disease were more likely to be former smokers, less likely never to have smoked, and less likely to be current smokers.[38]

Smoking has been associated with higher death rates in U.S. hemodialysis patients.[39] Smoking may hasten loss of kidney function.[40] More recently, in the Wave 2 study described in the preceding paragraph, smoking was associated with higher rates of congestive heart failure, peripheral vascular disease, and death in a randomly selected prospective cohort of patients starting dialysis.[38]

Glycemic Control

In excess of half of all newly diagnosed patients with ESRD have diabetes mellitus, either as a direct cause of ESRD or a comorbid condition. For example, 59.3 percent of new ESRD patients in 2001 had diabetes mellitus as a primary or secondary condition. Broken down by race/ethnicity, this figure was 48.3 percent for whites, 59.3 percent for African Americans, 79.7 percent for Native Americans, 60.5 percent for Asian Americans, and 72.6 percent for Hispanic Americans.[41] It is probable that this disease burden overwhelmingly represents type 2 diabetes mellitus, although most registry reports do not use accurate methods to differentiate type 2 from type 1 diabetes mellitus.

Only a limited observational literature, specific to dialysis patients, exists to support the belief that excellent metabolic control is a worthwhile aspiration in dialysis patients. One single-center prospective study looked at 150 patients starting hemodialysis between 1989 and 1997. This study found that the 62 percent patients with HbA1c <7.5 percent at dialysis inception had better survival rates, even after adjustment for age and several comorbid factors.[42]

Hypertension

Hypertension in dialysis patients is highly multifactorial, but expansion of the extracellular fluid volume and excessive activity of neurohormonal systems are major contributors.[43–47] Observational studies relating blood pressure levels and survival in dialysis patients have led to many unexpected results. Studies from the general population led to the expectation of a monotonic direct relationship between blood pressure levels and mortality, but this has been seen only in a distinct minority of studies.[48–50] Most studies in dialysis populations have shown associations between low blood pressure and higher mortality rates, or U-shaped or inverted J-shaped association profiles.[51–54] These findings may be an example of reverse causation in a group of patients where coexisting cardiac disease is so common. It is possible, too, that a direct causal relationship exists, with low blood pressure postulated to impair myocardial perfusion. This is a viable postulate when one considers the impaired cardiac bioenergetics, diastolic dysfunction, and decreased capillary density found in animal models[2,55] and the high prevalence of coronary artery disease in dialysis patients.[56]

Arterial stiffening, which is usually present in dialysis patients, is associated with higher mortality rates in the general population.[57] Widening arterial pulse pressure is an expected corollary of arterial stiffening. In contrast to the confusing associations seen when systolic and diastolic blood pressures are studied in isolation, pulse pressure has shown consistent, direct associations with mortality rates in dialysis populations.[58–60]

Surprisingly few observational studies have examined links between blood pressure and cardiovascular syndromes in dialysis patients. One prospective cohort study showed that higher time-averaged blood pressures were associated with progressive left ventricular hypertrophy, ischemic heart disease, and congestive heart failure but also with lower mortality rates.[61] Observational studies have consistently found that higher blood pressures are associated with left ventricular enlargement in chronic kidney disease.[62–64]

Left ventricular hypertrophy and hypertension in dialysis patients partly reflect extracellular fluid volume expansion.[65–67] The improvements in hypertension and left ventricular hypertrophy with daily hemodialysis are likely to reflect a lower extracellular fluid volume.[47–68] Many trials show that ACE inhibitors and angiotensin-receptor blockers help to preserve function in progressive kidney disease[69–75] even after the start of dialysis therapy.[76] On the basis of many trials in nondialysis populations, they are also recommended when low ejection fractions and symptomatic cardiac failure are present.[77–80] Therefore ACE inhibitors or angiotensin-receptor blockers are often recommended as first-line antihypertensive agents in dialysis patients who remain hypertensive after salt and water status have been optimized. No definitive randomized controlled trials underpin these recommendations. In one study, dialysis patients with left ventricular hypertrophy and hypertension were randomly assigned to an ACE inhibitor or nitrendipine, a calcium channel blocker. Although blood pressure reductions were similar with both agents, left ventricular hypertrophy regressed more in the ACE inhibitor group.[81] Beta blockers make theoretical sense because sympathetic overload, sudden death, congestive heart failure, ischemic heart disease, and hypertension are so common in dialysis populations. Beta blockers were associated with lower mortality rates in a retrospective study.[60] A placebo-controlled randomized trial showed longer survival when dialysis patients with dilated cardiomyopathy were treated with carvedilol.[82]

Lipid Abnormalities

Qualitative or quantitative lipid abnormalities are the rule in dialysis patients. Both low[83] and high[84] levels of serum cholesterol have been associated with longer survival in various reports. Low levels of serum cholesterol are likely to reflect malnutrition and inflammation, which clouds mortality associations. Levels of lipoprotein(a) are higher in dialysis patients and have been associated with outcome in observational studies.[85,86] Hydroxymethyl-glutaryl coenzyme A reductase (HMG-CoA) inhibitors ("statins") improve cardiovascular outcomes in high-risk populations.[87–93] Statins appear to be effective and safe at cholesterol reduction in dialysis patients.[94] A recent placebo-controlled study examined fluvastatin in renal transplant recipients. Although no differences in the primary composite outcome were seen, myocardial infarction rates were lower.[95] While ongoing studies are awaited, it seems reasonable to follow ATP III guidelines for treating hypercholesterolemia, with dialysis patients treated as a high-risk population.

Anemia

The physiologic effects of anemia include peripheral vasodilation, increased venous return, and increased cardiac output from the combination of tachycardia and the increased stroke volume associated with cardiac enlargement. Anemia is associated with increasing left ventricular mass, higher hospitalization rates, higher resource consumption, and higher mortality rates in dialysis patients.[96–101] Anemia, however, also reflects ongoing illness—especially the inflammatory, neoplastic, and hemorrhagic varieties—which makes observational studies difficult to interpret. Partial correction of anemia leads to partial regression of left ventricular hypertrophy in dialysis patients.[102–104] The costs and benefits of physiologic hemoglobin targets in dialysis patients remain uncertain. In the U.S. Normal Hematocrit Trial, 1233 hemodialysis patients with preexisting cardiovascular disease were randomly assigned hematocrit targets of 30 or 42 percent. The primary outcome was death or first nonfatal myocardial infarction. Primary outcome rates were similar in both groups, while patients in the normal hematocrit target had higher rates of vascular access loss, suggesting that physiologic hemoglobin targets should not be recommended in hemodialysis patients with known cardiovascular disease.[105] In the Canadian Normalization of Hemoglobin trial, hemodialysis patients with abnormal echocardiographic left ventricular size were randomly treated to hemoglobin levels of 10 or 13.5 g/dL. Higher hemoglobin targets failed to normalize left ventricles that were already enlarged. On the other hand, normal hemoglobin levels seemed to prevent the development of new left ventricular dilation and also improved quality of life, while adverse event rates were similar in both target groups.[106] A randomized double-blind crossover study from Australia showed better peak work rates, VO$_{2max}$, and improvement in left ventricular size and function at hemoglobin levels of 14 g/dL compared to levels of 10 g/dL.[107,108]

Uremia

As discussed above, uremia has dramatic cardiovascular effects in animal models. Short daily hemodialysis in a controlled setting, using a crossover design, has been shown to lead to regression of left ventricular hypertrophy.[86] The HEMO trial, however, showed no survival differences between equilibrated Kt/V values of 1.16 and 1.53, suggesting that current guidelines for dialysis adequacy are pragmatic.[109]

Calcium-Phosphorus-Parathyroid Hormone

Animal studies have shown that parathyroid hormone has toxic effects on cardiac myocytes.[110] Parathyroidectomy may lead to improved left ventricular function in dialysis patients.[111,112] Recent studies suggest that calcium deposition in dialysis patients is a dynamic process.[113] Calcium-phosphate product levels and mortality rates parallel each other in hemodialysis patients.[114] Arterial stiffness in dialysis patients appears to be strongly related to the degree of arterial calcification, which is in turn related to age, dialysis duration, fibrinogen, and the prescribed dose of calcium-based phosphate binders.[115,116] Although sevelamer, a calcium-free phosphorus binder, has been shown to reduce coronary artery calcification scores in hemodialysis patients, it remains to be seen whether this translates into clinical benefit in terms of hard clinical outcomes.

Inflammation

Inflammation, as suggested by the presence of high levels of C-reactive protein, is common in uremic patients and appears to be associated with cardiovascular disease, malnutrition,[117–119] and carotid intima-media thickness.[120] Other inflammatory markers show similar association patterns.[121–124] To date, most of the literature in dialysis patients is limited by cross-sectional research designs; this issue, however, is under intense investigation and shows promise as an area for therapeutic intervention.

Dialysis Access and Bacteremia

The many potential causes of inflammation in dialysis patients are reviewed in Reference 124. Septicemia has dramatic effects on the endothelial, redox, and coagulation systems, overall cardiovascular function, and tissue oxygen availability.[125] Death from sepsis appears to be 30 to 45 times more common in dialysis patients than in the general population.[126] One study, examining patients who began dialysis therapy in 1980s, showed that septicemia was common and associated with a doubling of mortality rates.[127]

Most studies show that septicemia rates in dialysis patients are at least 10 percent per year.[128,129] Septicemia is clearly related to the vascular access used for hemodialysis, with the lowest rates seen with arteriovenous fistulas, followed by synthetic grafts and central venous catheters.[130] Other studies have associated vascular access type with death from any cause, death from infection, and death from cardiovascular causes.[131,132] It is plausible that strategies which lessen reliance on temporary access for dialysis could improve cardiovascular outcomes in dialysis patients.

Endothelial Dysfunction and Oxidative Stress

Patients with renal impairment exhibit endothelial dysfunction and heightened oxidative stress.[133] Asymmetric dimethylarginine (ADMA) is an inhibitor of nitric oxide and is associated with endothelial dysfunction and atherosclerosis in the general population. ADMA levels are elevated in ESRD and, in one study, have been associated with C-reactive protein, carotid intima-media thickness, change in intima-media thickness, and cardiovascular outcome.[134,135] High-dose vitamin E supplementation was found to cut cardiovascular events in half in a placebo-controlled trial of dialysis patients with preexisting cardiovascular disease.[136] Another randomized study, using the antioxidant acetylcysteine, showed similar mortality effects.[137] Trials of antioxidants have been generally[138-141] though not uniformly[142] disappointing in nonuremic populations. Clearly, these data need confirmation in larger groups of patients with renal disease to vouchsafe their generalizability.

Homocysteine

Homocysteine levels and renal function are inversely related.[143] High doses of folic acid or methylated derivates can lead to modest to moderate reductions of homocysteine in dialysis patients.[144–149] Observational studies have produced conflicting conclusions regarding the association between homocysteine levels and cardiovascular outcomes in ESRD.[150,151] To date, no hard-outcome trials of folate therapy have been published. Supersupplementation appears to be a low-risk, cheap strategy. Thus, the somewhat reluctant opinion of this author is to recommend routine supplementation, even in those without overt folate deficiency.

Biomarkers, Troponins

The sheer number of biomarkers reported to be abnormally high or abnormally low in dialysis patients is enormous. Latterly, several of these have been suggested to have prognostic connotations. An in-depth examination of each marker is outside the scope of this chapter with the exception of cardiac muscle enzymes, which are among the best studied, and have clear clinical relevance in the diagnosis of myocardial infarction in dialysis patients.

It has long been known that creatinine kinase-MB isoenzyme levels in asymptomatic dialysis patients often exceed threshold levels indicative of myocardial infarction in the general population.[152–155] Levels of cardiac troponin T (cTn T) are also elevated in approximately 70 percent of dialysis patients.[156] Asymptomatic elevations of cTn I levels are less frequent, and negative tests appear to be useful in ruling out myocardial infarction.[157] In one prospective study, 817 consecutive patients under evaluation for myocardial infarction were tested for myoglobin, cTn I, and CK-MB at 0, 1.5, 3, and 9 hours using a point-of-care device. All markers with the exception of cTn I were correlated with glomerular filtration rates. cTn I appeared to be a reliable test for the diagnosis of myocardial infarction.[23] Many studies show that cTn T and mortality are associated[23,156,158–162] in dialysis patients.[23,156,158,162] The reasons for elevated levels of cardiac enzymes are unknown, but continuous or repetitive injury to cardiomyocytes has been postulated.

RANDOMIZED CONTROLLED TRIALS IN ESRD: 2000 TO 2003

The dialysis community has frequently bemoaned the lack of controlled trials as a basis for rational treatment decisions in such a high-risk patient population. This situation appears to be changing, albeit slowly. This section reviews noteworthy trials published between 2000 and 2003.

Effect of Dialysis Dose and Membrane Flux in Maintenance Hemodialysis

This landmark study[163] involved 1846 hemodialysis patients and used a 2×2 factorial design to assess the impact of high-dose dialysis and high-flux dialyzers. Equilibrated Kt/V values of 1.16 and 1.53 and flux values (based on beta$_2$-microglobulin clearance) of 3 and 34 mL/min were achieved by group assignment. The primary outcome, death from any cause, was not significantly influenced by the dose or flux assignment.

Effect of Fluvastatin on Cardiac Outcomes in Renal Transplant Recipients

This multicenter, randomized, placebo-controlled trial[95] was conducted among renal transplant recipients, a group with obvious similarities to dialysis populations.

It examined the impact of fluvastatin in 2102 patients with total cholesterol levels of 4.0 to 9.0 mmol/L over 5.1 years of follow-up. The primary study outcome was a composite of cardiac death, nonfatal myocardial infarction, or

coronary intervention procedure; fluvastatin did not lead to a statistically significant reduction in the primary outcome, although some components exhibited a positive response, including cardiac deaths and nonfatal myocardial infarction. Clearly, the latter components should be regarded as hypothesis-generating and require confirmation in future studies.

Carvedilol in Dialysis Patients with Dilated Cardiomyopathy

This prospective, placebo-controlled trial[82] found increased 2-year survival in patients with dilated cardiomyopathy a characteristic abnormality in dialysis patients. A placebo-controlled study, it comprised 114 dialysis patients with dilated cardiomyopathy and evaluated the effect of carvedilol in addition to standard therapy. The primary outcome, improvement in left ventricular function on echocardiography, was achieved by carvedilol in an initial study.[164] The current study extends follow-up from 1 to 2 years. In the longer term, carvedilol lowered left ventricular cavity volume and improved ejection fraction as well as the rates of hospitalization, mortality, myocardial infarction, strokes, and worsening heart failure.

Secondary Prevention of Cardiovascular Disease with Antioxidants in Patients with ESRD

Armed with the knowledge that hemodialysis patients are exposed to much greater oxidative stress than most other populations, this single-center, randomized, placebo-controlled trial[136] investigated the effect of high-dose vitamin E supplementation (800 IU/day) in patients with ESRD, specifically with regard to cardiovascular outcomes. It comprised 196 hemodialysis patients known to have cardiovascular disease. The primary study outcome was a composite of myocardial infarction, unstable angina, ischemic stroke, and peripheral vascular disease. A total of 16 percent of the vitamin E group and 33 percent of the placebo group had a primary endpoint ($p = 0.014$), apparently related to a reduction in the myocardial infarction component of the composite outcome. On the negative side, this study was performed in only a single center; therefore its generalizability needs confirmation in a larger study. In addition, the findings run contrary to neutral effects seen in large trials in the general population. On the positive side, the intervention is attractive because it is likely to be safe and inexpensive.

The Use of Acetylcysteine in Patients with ESRD

This randomized, placebo-controlled trial[137] evaluated another antioxidant, twice daily acetylcysteine (600 mg), in 134 hemodialysis patients with ESRD. The primary endpoint was a composite of cardiac events: fatal and nonfatal myocardial infarction, cardiovascular death, coronary artery revascularization, ischemic stroke, and a procedure for peripheral vascular disease. A total of 28 percent of acetylcysteine patients and 47 percent of the control group had a primary endpoint. The pluses and minuses of this study are similar to those of the study previously discussed.

Prevention of Infection with Polysporin Ointment

There has been a growing realization that dialysis via catheter is associated with much higher cardiovascular morbidity and mortality in dialysis patients. Most of this association appears to be driven via the intermediate outcome of bacteremia/septicemia—a state of intense inflammatory activation. This study[165] evaluated whether polysporin triple antibiotic ointment applied to the central venous catheter insertion sites reduces catheter-related infections; it comprised 169 hemodialysis patients over a period of 6 months. The comparative rates of infection (the primary study outcome) were 34 percent in the antibiotic group and 12 percent in the control group ($p = 0.0013$). The number of bacteremias per 1000 catheter days were 2.48 vs. 0.63 ($p = 0.0004$), and the number of deaths were 13 vs. 3 ($p = 0.0041$), respectively.

MANAGEMENT

Risk-factor management in dialysis patients is predicated on their enormous cardiovascular risk. As with all therapies, safety takes precedence over guideline attainment when the

TABLE 27A-1. SELECTED THERAPEUTIC TARGETS

Target	Guideline Body	Comments
Discontinue smoking		
HbA1c <7%	American Diabetes Association[i]	
Euvolemia		
Blood pressure <130/80	Seventh Report of the Joint National Committee on Prevention, Evaluation, and Treatment of High Blood Pressure[ii]	ACE inhibitors or angiotensin-receptor blockers as first-line agents Add beta blockers if coronary artery disease or congestive heart failure present
LDL cholesterol <100 mg/dL	Adult Treatment Panel III[iii]	Statins first-line agents
Hemoglobin 10 to 11 g/dL	National Kidney Foundation K/DOQI[iv]	
Kt/V >1.2 in hemodialysis	National Kidney Foundation K/DOQI[v]	
Kt/V >2.0 per week and	National Kidney Foundation K/DOQI[vi]	
C_{Cr} >60 L/week/1.73 m^2 (high and high-average transporters) or		
C_{Cr} >50 L/week/1.73 m^2 (low-average transporters)		
Fistula for hemodialysis access	National Kidney Foundation K/DOQI[vii]	
Corrected calcium 8.4 to 9.5 mg/dL	National Kidney Foundation K/DOQI[viii]	
Phosphorus 2.7 to 4.6 mg/dL		
Calcium-phosphorus produce <55 mg^2/dL^2		
Parathyroid hormone 150 to 300 pg/mL		
Folic acid		
Vitamin E		
Aspirin	National Kidney Foundation Task Force on Cardiovascular Disease[19]	In the presence of known coronary artery disease

SOURCES:

[i] http://care.diabetesjournals.org/cgi/content/full/27/suppl_1/s15/T6 Accessed January 6, 2004.

[ii] www.nhlbi.nih.gov/guidelines/hypertension/phycard.pdf Accessed January 6, 2004.

[iii] www.nhlbi.nih.gov/guidelines/cholesterol/atp_iii.htm Accessed January 6, 2004.

[iv] www.kidney.org/professionals/doqi/guidelines/doqiupan_ii.html Accessed January 6, 2004.

[v] www.kidney.org/professionals/doqi/guidelines/doqiuphd_ii.html#4 Accessed January 6, 2004.

[vi] www.kidney.org/professionals/doqi/guidelines/doqiuppd_v.html#15 Accessed January 6, 2004.

[vii] www.kidney.org/professionals/doqi/guidelines/doqiupva_i.html#doqiupva1 Accessed January 6, 2004.

[viii] National Kidney Foundation. K/DOQI Clinical practice guidelines for bone metabolism and disease in chronic kidney disease. *Am J Kidney Dis* 2003;42(suppl 3):S1-S202.

latter proves difficult. It is unlikely that definitive trials will be performed in dialysis patients in the near future to support many of the prevention recommendations shown in Table 27A–1. Where possible, guidelines for cardioprotection that have come from national bodies, based on level 1 evidence in the general population, have been used. Two notable exceptions include folate therapy and vitamin E therapy. Folate is recommended because of its modest ability to reduce the greatly elevated homocysteine levels of dialysis patients and because it appears safe and is inexpensive. Vitamin E or acetylcysteine is recommended because of controlled trial evidence of improved outcomes specific to dialysis patients which, although suggestive, needs confirmation in larger studies.[136,137] Aspirin therapy is a difficult management decision in dialysis patients. Although a strong theoretical rationale exists for using it routinely, the risks and benefits of adding another bleeding risk to a group already at risk are unclear. It seems reasonable to suggest using it in patients with known coronary artery disease.

REFERENCES

1. Tyralla K, Amann K. Morphology of the heart and arteries in renal failure (review). *Kidney Int Suppl* 2003;84: S80–S83.

2. Raine AE, Seymour AM, Roberts AF, et al. Impairment of cardiac function and energetics in experimental renal failure. *J Clin Invest* 1993;92:2934–2940.

3. Dahan M, Viron BM, Faraggi M, et al. Diagnostic accuracy and prognostic value of combined dipyridamole-exercise thallium imaging in hemodialysis patients. *Kidney Int* 1998; 54:255–262.

4. Reis G, Marcovitz PA, Leichtman AB, et al. Usefulness of dobutamine stress echocardiography in detecting coronary artery disease in end-stage renal disease. *Am J Cardiol* 1995; 75:707–710.

5. Bates JR, Sawada SG, Segar DS, et al. Evaluation using dobutamine stress echocardiography in patients with insulin-dependent diabetes mellitus before kidney and/or pancreas transplantation. *Am J Cardiol* 1996;77:175–179.

6. Herzog CA, Marwick TH, Pheley AM, et al. Dobutamine stress echocardiography for the detection of significant coronary artery disease in renal transplant candidates. *Am J Kidney Dis* 1999;33:1080–1090.

7. Dahan M, Viron BM, Poiseau E, et al. Combined dipyridamole-exercise stress echocardiography for detection of myocardial ischemia in hemodialysis patients: an alternative to stress nuclear imaging. *Am J Kidney Dis* 2002;40: 737–744.

8. Giroud D, Li JM, Urban P, et al. Relation of the site of acute myocardial infarction to the most severe coronary arterial stenosis at prior angiography. *Am J Cardiol* 1992;69: 729–732.

9. Ambrose JA, Tannenbaum MA, Alexopoulos D, et al. Angiographic progression of coronary artery disease and the development of myocardial infarction. *J Am Coll Cardiol* 1988; 12:56–62.

10. Little WC, Constantinescu M, Applegate RJ, et al. Can coronary angiography predict the site of a subsequent myocardial infarction in patients with mild-to-moderate coronary artery disease? *Circulation* 1988;78:1157–1166.

11. Roberts WC, Jones AA. Quantitation of coronary arterial narrowing at necropsy in sudden coronary death: analysis of 31 patients and comparison with 25 control subjects. *Am J Cardiol* 1979;44:39–45.

12. Rifkin RD, Parisi AF, Folland E. Coronary calcification in the diagnosis of coronary artery disease. *Am J Cardiol* 1979; 44:141–147.

13. Baumgart D, Schmermund A, George G, et al. Comparison of electron beam computed tomography with intracoronary ultrasound and coronary angiography for detection of coronary atherosclerosis. *J Am Coll Cardiol* 1997;30(1):57–64.

14. Budoff MJ. Atherosclerosis imaging and calcified plaque: coronary artery disease risk assessment (review). *Prog Cardiovasc Dis* 2003;46:135–148.

15. Marwick TH. Techniques for comprehensive two dimensional echocardiographic assessment of left ventricular systolic function (review). *Heart* 2003;89(suppl 3):iii2–iii8.

16. Harnett JD, Murphy B, Collingwood P, et al. The reliability and validity of echocardiographic measurement of left ventricular mass index in hemodialysis patients. *Nephron* 1993; 65(2):212–214.

17. Bottini PB, Carr AA, Prisant LM, et al. Magnetic resonance imaging compared to echocardiography to assess left ventricular mass in the hypertensive patient. *Am J Hypertens* 1995; 8:221–228.

18. Stewart GA, Foster J, Cowan M, et al. Echocardiography overestimates left ventricular mass in hemodialysis patients relative to magnetic resonance imaging. *Kidney Int* 1999;56: 2248–2253.

19. Levey AS, Beto JA, Coronado BE, et al. Controlling the epidemic of cardiovascular disease in chronic renal disease: what do we know? What do we need to learn? Where do we go from here? National Kidney Foundation Task Force on Cardiovascular Disease. *Am J Kidney Dis* 1998;32:853–906.

20. U.S. Renal Data System. *USRDS 2003 Annual Data Report: Atlas of End-Stage Renal Disease in the United States.* Bethesda, MD: National Institutes of Health, National Institute of Diabetes and Digestive and Kidney Diseases, 2003:64.

21. Goodkin DA, Bragg-Gresham JL, Koenig KG, et al. Association of comorbid conditions and mortality in hemodialysis patients in Europe, Japan, and the United States: the Dialysis Outcomes and Practice Patterns Study (DOPPS). *J Am Soc Nephrol* 2003;14:3270–3277.

22. Acquatella H, Perez-Rojas M, Burger B, Guinand-Baldo A. Left ventricular function in terminal uremia. A hemodynamic and echocardiographic study. *Nephron* 1978;22: 160–174.

23. deFilippi C, Wasserman S, Rosanio S, et al. Cardiac troponin T and C-reactive protein for predicting prognosis, coronary atherosclerosis, and cardiomyopathy in patients undergoing long-term hemodialysis. *JAMA* 2003;290: 353–359.

24. Churchill DN, Taylor DW, Cook RJ, et al. Canadian Hemodialysis Morbidity Study. *Am J Kidney Dis* 1992;19:214–234.

25. Harnett JD, Foley RN, Kent GM, et al. Congestive heart failure in dialysis patients: prevalence, incidence, prognosis and risk factors. *Kidney Int* 1995;47:884–890.

26. Parfrey PS, Foley RN, Harnett JD, et al. Outcome and risk factors of ischemic heart disease in chronic uremia. *Kidney Int* 1996;49:1428–1434.

27. U.S. Renal Data System. *USRDS 2001 Annual Data Report.* Bethesda, MD: National Institutes of Health, National Institute of Diabetes and Digestive and Kidney Diseases, 2001:153–155.

28. Berger CJ, Murabito JM, Evans JC, et al. Prognosis after first myocardial infarction. Comparison of Q-wave and non-Q-wave myocardial infarction in the Framingham Heart Study. *JAMA* 1992;268:1545–1551.

29. Herzog CA, Ma JZ, Collins AJ. Poor long-term survival after acute myocardial infarction among patients on long-term dialysis. *N Engl J Med* 1998;339:799–805.

30. Silberberg JS, Barre PE, Prichard SS, Sniderman AD. Impact of left ventricular hypertrophy on survival in end-stage renal disease. *Kidney Int* 1989;36:286–290.

31. Parfrey PS, Foley RN, Harnett JD, et al. Outcome and risk factors for left ventricular disorders in chronic uraemia. *Nephrol Dial Transplant* 1996;11:1277–1285.

32. Foley RN, Parfrey PS, Kent GM, et al. Serial change in echocardiographic parameters and cardiac failure in end-stage renal disease. *J Am Soc Nephrol* 2000;11:912–916.

33. London GM, Pannier B, Guerin AP, et al. Alterations of left ventricular hypertrophy in and survival of patients receiving hemodialysis: follow-up of an interventional study. *J Am Soc Nephrol* 2001;12:2759–2767.

34. Zoccali C, Benedetto FA, Mallamaci F, et al—the CREED Investigators. Prognostic impact of the indexation of left ventricular mass in patients undergoing dialysis. *J Am Soc Nephrol* 200;12:2768–2774.

35. Kannel WB, Dawber TR, Kagan A, et al. Factors of risk in the development of coronary heart disease—six year follow-up experience. The Framingham Study. *Ann Intern Med* 1961;55:33–50.

36. Freund KM, Belanger AJ, D'Agostino RB, Kannel WB. The health risks of smoking. The Framingham Study: 34 years of follow-up. *Ann Epidemiol* 1993;3:417–424.

37. Sytkowski PA, D'Agostino RB, Belanger A, Kannel WB. Sex and time trends in cardiovascular disease incidence and mortality: the Framingham Heart Study, 1950–1989. *Am J Epidemiol* 1996;143:338–350.

38. Foley RN, Herzog CA, Collins AJ. Smoking and cardiovascular outcomes in dialysis patients: the United States Renal Data System Wave 2 study. *Kidney Int* 2003;63:1462–1467.

39. Bloembergen WE, Stannard DC, Port FK, et al. Relationship of dose of hemodialysis and cause-specific mortality. *Kidney Int* 1996;50:557–565.

40. Orth SR. Smoking and the kidney. *J Am Soc Nephrol* 2002;13:1663–1672.

41. www.usrds.org/2003/slides/html/03_pt_char_03_files/frame.htm Accessed January 4, 2004.

42. Morioka T, Emoto M, Tabata T, et al. Glycemic control is a predictor of survival for diabetic patients on hemodialysis. *Diabetes Care* 2001;24:909–913.

43. Converse RL Jr, Jacobsen TN, Toto RD, et al. Sympathetic overactivity in patients with chronic renal failure. *N Engl J Med* 1992;327:1912–1918.

44. Orth SR, Amann K, Strojek K, Ritz E. Sympathetic overactivity and arterial hypertension in renal failure. *Nephrol Dial Transplant* 2001;16(suppl 1):67–69.

45. Chan CT, Harvey PJ, Picton P, et al. Short-term blood pressure, noradrenergic, and vascular effects of nocturnal home hemodialysis. *Hypertension* 2003;42:925–931.

46. Charra B, Calemard E, Ruffet M, et al. Survival as an index of adequacy of dialysis. *Kidney Int* 1992;41:1286–1291.

47. Fagugli RM, Reboldi G, Quintaliani G, et al. Short daily hemodialysis: blood pressure control and left ventricular mass reduction in hypertensive hemodialysis patients. *Am J Kidney Dis* 2001;38:371–376.

48. Charra B, Calemard E, Laurent G. Importance of treatment time and blood pressure control in achieving long-term survival on dialysis. *Am J Nephrol* 1997;16:35–44.

49. Fernandez JM, Carbonell ME, Mazzuchi N, Petrucelli D. Importance of blood pressure control in hemodialysis patient survival. *Kidney Int* 2000;58:2147–2154.

50. Lynn KL, McGregor DO, Moesbergen T, et al. Hypertension as a determinant of survival for patients treated with home dialysis. *Kidney Int* 2002;62:2281–2287.

51. USRDS 1992 Annual Data Report. Comorbid conditions and correlations with mortality risk among 3,399 incident hemodialysis patients. *Am J Kidney Dis* 1992;20:32–38.

52. Iseki K, Miyasato F, Tokuyama K, et al. Low diastolic blood pressure, hypoalbuminemia, and risk of death in a cohort of chronic hemodialysis patients. *Kidney Int* 1997;51:1212–1217.

53. Port FK, Hulbert-Shearon TE, Wolfe RA, et al. Predialysis blood pressure and mortality risk in a national sample of maintenance hemodialysis patients. *Am J Kidney Dis* 1999;33:507–517.

54. Zager PG, Nikolic J, Brown RH, et al. "U" curve association of blood pressure and mortality in hemodialysis patients. Medical Directors of Dialysis Clinic, Inc. *Kidney Int* 1998;54:561–569.

55. Amann K, Wiest G, Zimmer G, et al. Reduced capillary density in the myocardium of uremic rats—a stereological study. *Kidney Int* 1992;42:1079–1085.

56. Rostand SG, Brunzell JD, Cannon RO III, Victor RG. Cardiovascular complications in renal failure. *J Am Soc Nephrol* 1991;2:1053–1062.

57. Blacher J, Guerin AP, Pannier B, et al. Impact of aortic stiffness on survival in end-stage renal disease. *Circulation* 1999; 99:2434–2439.

58. Tozawa M, Iseki K, Iseki C, Takishita S. Pulse pressure and risk of total mortality and cardiovascular events in patients on chronic hemodialysis. *Kidney Int* 2002;61:717–726.

59. Klassen PS, Lowrie EG, Reddan DN, et al. Association between pulse pressure and mortality in patients undergoing maintenance hemodialysis. *JAMA* 2002;287:1548–1555.

60. Foley RN, Herzog CA, Collins AJ, United States Renal Data System. Blood pressure and long-term mortality in United

States hemodialysis patients: USRDS Waves 3 and 4 Study. *Kidney Int* 2002;62:1784–1790.

61. Foley RN, Parfrey PS, Harnett JD, et al. Impact of hypertension on cardiomyopathy, morbidity and mortality in end-stage renal disease. *Kidney Int* 1996;49:1379–1385.

62. Levin A, Singer J, Thompson CR, et al. Prevalent left ventricular hypertrophy in the predialysis population: identifying opportunities for intervention. *Am J Kidney Dis* 1996;27:347–354.

63. Tucker B, Fabbian F, Giles M, et al. Left ventricular hypertrophy and ambulatory blood pressure monitoring in chronic renal failure. *Nephrol Dial Transplant* 1997;12:724–728.

64. Foley RN, Parfrey PS, Harnett JD, et al. Clinical and echocardiographic disease in patients starting end-stage renal disease therapy. *Kidney Int* 1995;47:186–192.

65. Rahman M, Dixit A, Donley V, et al. Factors associated with inadequate blood pressure control in hypertensive hemodialysis patients. *Am J Kidney Dis* 1999;33:498–506.

66. Fishbane S, Natke E, Maesaka JK. Role of volume overload in dialysis-refractory hypertension. *Am J Kidney Dis* 1996;28:257–261.

67. Scribner BH. Can antihypertensive medications control BP in haemodialysis patients: yes or no? *Nephrol Dial Transplant* 1999;14:2599–2601.

68. Chan CT, Floras JS, Miller JA, et al. Regression of left ventricular hypertrophy after conversion to nocturnal hemodialysis. *Kidney Int* 2002;61:2235–2239.

69. Lewis EJ, Hunsicker LG, Bain RP, Rohde RD. The effect of angiotensin-converting-enzyme inhibition on diabetic nephropathy. The Collaborative Study Group. *N Engl J Med* 1993; 329:1456–1462.

70. Ruggenenti P, Perna A, Gherardi G, et al. Renal function and requirement for dialysis in chronic nephropathy patients on long-term ramipril: REIN follow-up trial. Gruppo Italiano di Studi Epidemiologici in Nefrologia (GISEN). Ramipril Efficacy in Nephropathy. *Lancet* 1998;352:1252–1256.

71. Maschio G, Alberti D, Janin G, et al. Effect of the angiotensin-converting-enzyme inhibitor benazepril on the progression of chronic renal insufficiency. The Angiotensin-Converting-Enzyme Inhibition in Progressive Renal Insufficiency Study Group. *N Engl J Med* 1996;334:939–945.

72. Agodoa LY, Appel L, Bakris GL, et al—the African American Study of Kidney Disease and Hypertension (AASK) Study Group. Effect of ramipril vs amlodipine on renal outcomes in hypertensive nephrosclerosis: a randomized controlled trial. *JAMA* 2001;285:2719–2728.

73. Parving HH, Lehnert H, Brochner-Mortensen J, et al—the Irbesartan in Patients with Type 2 Diabetes and Microalbuminuria Study Group. The effect of irbesartan on the development of diabetic nephropathy in patients with type 2 diabetes. *N Engl J Med* 2001;345:870–878.

74. Brenner BM, Cooper ME, de Zeeuw D, et al—the RENAAL Study Investigators. Effects of losartan on renal and cardiovascular outcomes in patients with type 2 diabetes and nephropathy. *N Engl J Med* 2001;345:861–869.

75. Lewis EJ, Hunsicker LG, Clarke WR, et al—Collaborative Study Group. Renoprotective effect of the angiotensin-receptor antagonist irbesartan in patients with nephropathy due to type 2 diabetes. *N Engl J Med* 2001;345:851–860.

76. Li PK, Chow KM, Wong TY, et al. Effects of an ACE inhibitor on residual renal function in patients receiving peritoneal dialysis. A randomized, controlled study. *Ann Intern Med* 2003;139(2):105–112.

77. CONSENSUS Trial Study Group. Effects of enalapril on mortality in severe congestive heart failure. Results of the Cooperative North Scandinavian Enalapril Survival Study (CONSENSUS). The CONSENSUS Trial Study Group. *N Engl J Med* 1987;316(23):1429–1435.

78. SOLVD Investigators. Effect of enalapril on survival in patients with reduced left ventricular ejection fractions and congestive heart failure. The SOLVD Investigators. *N Engl J Med* 1991;325:293–302.

79. SOLVD Investigators. Effect of enalapril on mortality and the development of heart failure in asymptomatic patients with reduced left ventricular ejection fractions. The SOLVD Investigators. *N Engl J Med* 1992;327(10):685–691.

80. Cleland JG, Erhardt L, Murray G, et al. Effect of ramipril on morbidity and mode of death among survivors of acute myocardial infarction with clinical evidence of heart failure. A report from the AIRE Study Investigators. *Eur Heart J* 1997; 18:41–51.

81. London GM, Pannier B, Guerin AP, et al. Cardiac hypertrophy, aortic compliance, peripheral resistance, and wave reflection in end-stage renal disease. Comparative effects of ACE inhibition and calcium channel blockade. *Circulation* 1994;90:2786–2796.

82. Cice G, Ferrara L, D'Andrea A, et al. Carvedilol increases two-year survival in dialysis patients with dilated cardiomyopathy: a prospective, placebo-controlled trial. *J Am Coll Cardiol* 2003;41:1438–1444.

83. Lowrie EG, Lew NL. Death risk in hemodialysis patients: the predictive value of commonly measured variables and an evaluation of death rate differences between facilities. *Am J Kidney Dis* 1990;15:458–482.

84. Zoccali C, Benedetto FA, Mallamaci F, et al—the CREED Investigators. Prognostic impact of the indexation of left ventricular mass in patients undergoing dialysis. *J Am Soc Nephrol* 200;12:2768–2774.

85. Cressman MD, Heyka RJ, Paganini EP, et al. Lipoprotein(a) is an independent risk factor for cardiovascular disease in hemodialysis patients. *Circulation* 1992;86:475–482.

86. Goldwasser P, Michel MA, Collier J, et al. Prealbumin and lipoprotein(a) in hemodialysis: relationship with patients and vascular access survival. *Am J Kidney Dis* 1993;22:215–225.

87. 4S investigators. Randomised trial of cholesterol lowering in 4444 patients with coronary heart disease: the Scandinavian Simvastatin Survival Study (4S). *Lancet* 1994;344(8934):1383–1389.

88. Shepherd J, Cobbe SM, Ford I, et al. Prevention of coronary heart disease with pravastatin in men with hypercholesterolemia. West of Scotland Coronary Prevention Study Group. *N Engl J Med* 1995;333:1301–1307.

89. Sacks FM, Pfeffer MA, Moye LA, et al. The effect of pravastatin on coronary events after myocardial infarction in patients with average cholesterol levels. Cholesterol and Recurrent Events Trial investigators. *N Engl J Med* 1996;335:1001–1009.

90. LIPID study group. Prevention of cardiovascular events and death with pravastatin in patients with coronary heart disease and a broad range of initial cholesterol levels. The Long-Term Intervention with Pravastatin in Ischaemic Disease (LIPID) study group. *N Engl J Med* 1998;339(19): 1349–1357.

91. Downs JR, Clearfield M, Weis S, et al. Primary prevention of acute coronary events with lovastatin in men and women with average cholesterol levels: results of AFCAPS/TexCAPS. Air Force/Texas Coronary Atherosclerosis Prevention Study. *JAMA* 1998;279:1615–1622.

92. Sever PS, Dahlof B, Poulter NR, et al—the ASCOT investigators. Prevention of coronary and stroke events with atorvastatin in hypertensive patients who have average or lower-than-average cholesterol concentrations, in the Anglo-Scandinavian Cardiac Outcomes Trial—Lipid Lowering Arm (ASCOT-LLA): a multicentre randomised controlled trial. *Lancet* 2003;361(9364):1149–1158.

93. Heart Protection Study Collaborative Group. MRC/BHF Heart Protection Study of cholesterol lowering with simvastatin in 20,536 high-risk individuals: a randomised placebo-controlled trial. *Lancet* 2002;360(9326):7–22.

94. Harris KP, Wheeler DC, Chong CC—the Atorvastatin in CAPD Study Investigators. A placebo-controlled trial examining atorvastatin in dyslipidemic patients undergoing CAPD. *Kidney Int* 2002;61:1469–1474.

95. Holdaas H, Fellstrom B, Jardine AG, et al—the Assessment of LEscol in Renal Transplantation (ALERT) Study Investigators. Effect of fluvastatin on cardiac outcomes in renal transplant recipients: a multicentre, randomised, placebo-controlled trial. *Lancet* 2003;361(9374):2024–2031.

96. Foley RN, Parfrey PS, Harnett JD, et al. The impact of anemia on cardiomyopathy, morbidity and mortality in end-stage renal disease. *Am J Kidney Dis* 1996;28:53–61.

97. Madore F, Lowrie EG, Brugnara C, et al. Anemia in hemodialysis patients: variables affecting this outcome predictor. *J Am Soc Nephrol* 1997;8:1921–1929.

98. Ma JZ, Ebben J, Xia H, Collins AJ. Hematocrit level and associated mortality in hemodialysis patients. *J Am Soc Nephrol* 1999;10:610–619.

99. Xia H, Ebben J, Ma JZ, Collins AJ. Hematocrit levels and hospitalization risks in hemodialysis patients. *J Am Soc Nephrol* 1999;10:1309–1316.

100. Collins AJ, Li S, Ebben J, et al. Hematocrit levels and associated Medicare expenditures. *Am J Kidney Dis* 2000;36: 282–293.

101. Collins AJ, Li S, St Peter W, et al. Death, hospitalization, and economic associations among incident hemodialysis patients with hematocrit values of 36 to 39%. *J Am Soc Nephrol* 2001;12:2465–2473.

102. London GM, Zins B, Pannier B, et al. Vascular changes in hemodialysis patients in response to recombinant human erythropoietin. *Kidney Int* 1989;36:878–882.

103. Macdougall IC, Lewis NP, Saunders MJ, et al. Long-term cardiorespiratory effects of amelioration of renal anaemia by erythropoietin. *Lancet* 1990;335:489–493.

104. Sikole A, Polenakovic M, Spirovska V, et al. Analysis of heart morphology and function following erythropoietin treatment of anemic dialysis patients. *Artif Organs* 1993; 17:977–984.

105. Besarab A, Kline Bolton W, et al. The effects of normal as compared with low hematocrit in patients with cardiac disease who are receiving hemodialysis and epoetin. *N Engl J Med* 1998;339:584–590.

106. Foley RN, Parfrey PS, Morgan J, et al. Effect of hemoglobin levels in hemodialysis patients with asymptomatic cardiomyopathy. *Kidney Int* 2000;58:1325–1335.

107. McMahon LP, McKenna MJ, Sangkabutra T, et al. Physical performance and associated electrolyte changes after haemoglobin normalization: a comparative study in haemodialysis patients. *Nephrol Dial Transplant* 1999;14:1182–1187.

108. McMahon LP, Mason K, Skinner SL, et al. Effects of haemoglobin normalization on quality of life and cardiovascular parameters in end-stage renal failure. *Nephrol Dial Transplant* 2000;15:1425–1430.

109. Eknoyan G, Beck GJ, Cheung AK, et al—the Hemodialysis (HEMO) Study Group. Effect of dialysis dose and membrane flux in maintenance hemodialysis. *N Engl J Med* 200;347: 2010–2019.

110. Zhang YB, Smogorzewski M, Ni Z, Massry SG. Altered cytosolic calcium homeostasis in rat cardiac myocytes in CRF. *Kidney Int* 1994;45:1113–1119.

111. Drueke T, Fauchet M, Fleury J, et al. Effect of parathyroidectomy on left-ventricular function in haemodialysis patients. *Lancet* 1980;1(8160):112–114.

112. Sato S, Ohta M, Kawaguchi Y, et al. Effects of parathyroidectomy on left ventricular mass in patients with hyperparathyroidism. *Miner Electrolyte Metab* 1995;21: 67–71.

113. Moe SM, O'Neill KD, Duan D, et al. Medial artery calcification in ESRD patients is associated with deposition of bone matrix proteins. *Kidney Int* 2002;61:638–647.

114. Block GA, Hulbert-Shearon TE, Levin NW, Port FK. Association of serum phosphorus and calcium x phosphate product with mortality risk in chronic hemodialysis patients: a national study. *Am J Kidney Dis* 1998;31:607–617.

115. Guerin AP, London GM, Marchais SJ, Metivier F. Arterial stiffening and vascular calcifications in end-stage renal disease. *Nephrol Dial Transplant* 2001;15:1014–1021.

116. Raggi P, Boulay A, Chasan-Taber S, et al. Cardiac calcification in adult hemodialysis patients. A link between end-stage renal disease and cardiovascular disease? *J Am Coll Cardiol* 2002;39(4):695–701.

117. Stenvinkel P. The role of inflammation in the anaemia of end-stage renal disease. *Nephrol Dial Transplant* 2001; 16(suppl 7):36–40.

118. Yeun JY, Levine RA, Mantadilok V, Kaysen GA. C-reactive protein predicts all-cause and cardiovascular mortality in hemodialysis patients. *Am J Kidney Dis* 2000;35:469–476.

119. Foley RN, Parfrey PS, Harnett JD, et al. Hypoalbuminemia, cardiac morbidity, and mortality in end-stage renal disease. *J Am Soc Nephrol* 1996;7:728–736.

120. Zoccali C, Benedetto FA, Maas R—the CREED Investigators. Asymmetric dimethylarginine, C-reactive protein, and carotid intima-media thickness in end-stage renal disease. *J Am Soc Nephrol* 2002;13:490–496.

121. Stenvinkel P, Heimburger O, Paultre F, et al. Strong association between malnutrition, inflammation, and atherosclerosis in chronic renal failure. *Kidney Int* 1999;55(5): 1899–1911.

122. Stenvinkel P, Heimburger O, Wang T, et al. High serum hyaluronan indicates poor survival in renal replacement therapy. *Am J Kidney Dis* 1999;34:1083–1088.

123. Stenvinkel P, Lindholm B, Heimburger M, Heimburger O. Elevated serum levels of soluble adhesion molecules predict death in pre-dialysis patients: association with malnutrition, inflammation, and cardiovascular disease. *Nephrol Dial Transplant* 2000;15:1624–1630.

124. Kaysen GA. The microinflammatory state in uremia: causes and potential consequences. *J Am Soc Nephrol* 12:1549–1557, 2001.

125. Hotchkiss RS, Karl IE. The pathophysiology and treatment of sepsis. *N Engl J Med* 2003;348:138–150.

126. Sarnak MJ, Jaber BL. Mortality caused by sepsis in patients with end-stage renal disease compared with the general population. *Kidney Int* 2000;58:1758–1764.

127. Powe NR, Jaar B, Furth SL, et al. Septicemia in dialysis patients: incidence, risk factors, and prognosis. *Kidney Int* 1999;55:1081–1090.

128. Churchill DN, Taylor DW, Cook RJ, et al. Canadian Hemodialysis Morbidity Study. *Am J Kidney Dis* 1992;19(3): 214–234.

129. Abbott KC, Agodoa LY. Etiology of bacterial septicemia in chronic dialysis patients in the United States. *Clin Nephrol* 2001;56:124–131.

130. Hoen B, Paul-Dauphin A, Hestin D, Kessler M. EPIBACDIAL: a multicenter prospective study of risk factors for bacteremia in chronic hemodialysis patients. *J Am Soc Nephrol* 1998;9:869–876.

131. Pastan S, Soucie JM, McClellan WM. Vascular access and increased risk of death among hemodialysis patients. *Kidney Int* 2002;62:620–626.

132. Dhingra RK, Young EW, Hulbert-Shearon TE, et al. Type of vascular access and mortality in U.S. hemodialysis patients. *Kidney Int* 2001;60:1443–1451.

133. Annuk M, Zilmer M, Lind L, et al. Oxidative stress and endothelial function in chronic renal failure. *J Am Soc Nephrol* 2001 12:2747–2752.

134. Zoccali C, Benedetto FA, Maas R, et al—the CREED Investigators. Asymmetric dimethylarginine, C-reactive protein, and carotid intima-media thickness in end-stage renal disease. *J Am Soc Nephrol* 2002;13:490–496.

135. Zoccali C, Bode-Boger S, Mallamaci F, et al. Plasma concentration of asymmetrical dimethylarginine and mortality in patients with end-stage renal disease: a prospective study. *Lancet* 2001;358(9299):2113–2117.

136. Boaz M, Smetana S, Weinstein T, et al. Secondary prevention with antioxidants of cardiovascular disease in endstage renal disease (SPACE): randomised placebo-controlled trial. *Lancet* 2000;356:1213–1218.

137. Tepel M, van der Giet M, Statz M, et al. The antioxidant acetylcysteine reduces cardiovascular events in patients with end-stage renal failure: a randomized, controlled trial. *Circulation* 2003;107:992–995.

138. Yusuf S, Dagenais G, Pogue J, et al. Vitamin E supplementation and cardiovascular events in high-risk patients. The Heart Outcomes Prevention Evaluation Study Investigators. *N Engl J Med* 2000;342:154–160.

139. Rapola JM, Virtamo J, Ripatti S, et al. Randomised trial of alpha-tocopherol and beta-carotene supplements on incidence of major coronary events in men with previous myocardial infarction. *Lancet* 1997;349(9067):1715–1720.

140. GISSI: Dietary supplementation with n-3 polyunsaturated fatty acids and vitamin E after myocardial infarction: results of the GISSI-Prevenzione trial. Gruppo Italiano per lo Studio della Sopravvivenza nell'Infarto Miocardico. *Lancet* 1999;354(9177):447–455.

141. MRC/BHF Heart Protection Study of antioxidant vitamin supplementation in 20,536 high-risk individuals: a randomised placebo-controlled trial. *Lancet* 2002;360(9326): 23–33.

142. Stephens NG, Parsons A, Schofield PM, et al. Randomised controlled trial of vitamin E in patients with coronary disease: Cambridge Heart Antioxidant Study (CHAOS). *Lancet* 1996;347(9004):781–786.

143. Bostom AG, Culleton BF. Hyperhomocysteinemia in chronic renal disease. *J Am Soc Nephrol* 1999;10:891–900.

144. Bostom AG, Shemin D, Lapane KL, et al. High dose-B-vitamin treatment of hyperhomocysteinemia in dialysis patients. *Kidney Int* 1996;49:147–152.

145. van Guldener C, Janssen MJ, de Meer K, et al. Effect of folic acid and betaine on fasting and postmethionine-loading plasma homocysteine and methionine levels in chronic haemodialysis patients. *J Intern Med* 1999;245:175–183.

146. McGregor D, Shand B, Lynn K. A controlled trial of the effect of folate supplements on homocysteine, lipids and hemorrheology in end-stage renal disease. *Nephron* 2000;85: 215–220.

147. Thambyrajah J, Landray MJ, McGlynn FJ, et al. Does folic acid decrease plasma homocysteine and improve endothelial function in patients with predialysis renal failure? *Circulation* 2000;102:871–875.

148. Ducloux D, Aboubakr A, Motte G, et al. Hyperhomocysteinaemia therapy in haemodialysis patients: folinic versus folic acid in combination with vitamin B6 and B12. *Nephrol Dial Transplant* 2002;17:865–870.

149. Trimarchi H, Schiel A, Freixas E, Diaz M. Randomized trial of methylcobalamin and folate effects on homocysteine in hemodialysis patients. *Nephron* 2002;91:58–63.

150. Mallamaci F, Zoccali C, Tripepi G, et al—the CREED Investigators. Hyperhomocysteinemia predicts cardiovascular outcomes in hemodialysis patients. *Kidney Int* 2002;61: 609–614.

151. Suliman ME, Qureshi AR, Barany P, et al. Hyperhomocysteinemia, nutritional status, and cardiovascular disease in hemodialysis patients. *Kidney Int* 2000;57:1727–1735.

152. Ma KW, Brown DC, Steele BW, From AH. Serum creatine kinase MB isoenzyme activity in long-term hemodialysis patients. *Arch Intern Med* 1981;141:164–166.

153. Martinez-Vea A, Montoliu J, et al. Elevated CK-MB with normal total creatine kinase levels in patients undergoing maintenance hemodialysis. *Arch Intern Med* 1982;142:2346.

154. Green TR, Golper TA, Swenson RD, et al. Diagnostic value of creatine kinase and creatine kinase MB isoenzyme in chronic hemodialysis patients: a longitudinal study. *Clin Nephrol* 1986;25:22–27.

155. Lal SM, Nolph KD, Hain H, et al. Total creatine kinase and isoenzyme fractions in chronic dialysis patients. *Int J Artif Organs* 1987;10:72–76.

156. Apple FS, Sharkey SW, Hoeft P, et al. Prognostic value of serum cardiac troponin I and T in chronic dialysis patients: a 1-year outcomes analysis. *Am J Kidney Dis* 1997;29: 399–403.

157. Morton AR, Collier CP, Ali N, Dagnone LE. Cardiac troponin I in patients receiving renal replacement therapy. *ASAIO J* 1998;44:M433–M435.

158. Ooi DS, Veinot JP, Wells GA, House AA. Increased mortality in hemodialyzed patients with elevated serum troponin T: a one-year outcome study. *Clin Biochem* 1999;32:647–652.

159. Deegan PB, Lafferty ME, Blumsohn A, et al. Prognostic value of troponin T in hemodialysis patients is independent of comorbidity. *Kidney Int* 2001;60:2399–2405.

160. Lowbeer C, Stenvinkel P, Pecoits-Filho R, et al. Elevated cardiac troponin T in predialysis patients is associated with inflammation and predicts mortality. *J Intern Med* 2003; 253:153–160.

161. Scott B, Deman A, Peeters P, et al. Cardiac troponin T and malondialdehyde modified plasma lipids in haemodialysis patients. *Nephrol Dial Transplant* 2003;18:737–742.

162. Choy JB, Armstrong PW, Ulan RA, et al. Do cardiac troponins provide prognostic insight in hemodialysis patients? *Can J Cardiol* 2003;19:907–911.

163. Eknoyan G, Beck GJ, Cheung AK, et al—the Hemodialysis (HEMO) Study Group. Effect of dialysis dose and membrane flux in maintenance hemodialysis. *N Engl J Med* 2002;347:2010–2019.

164. Cice G, Ferrara L, Di Benedetto A, et al. Dilated cardiomyopathy in dialysis patients—beneficial effects of carvedilol: a double-blind, placebo-controlled trial. *J Am Coll Cardiol* 2001;37:407–411.

165. Lok CE, Stanley KE, Hux JE, et al. Hemodialysis infection prevention with polysporin ointment. *J Am Soc Nephrol* 2003;14(1):169–179.

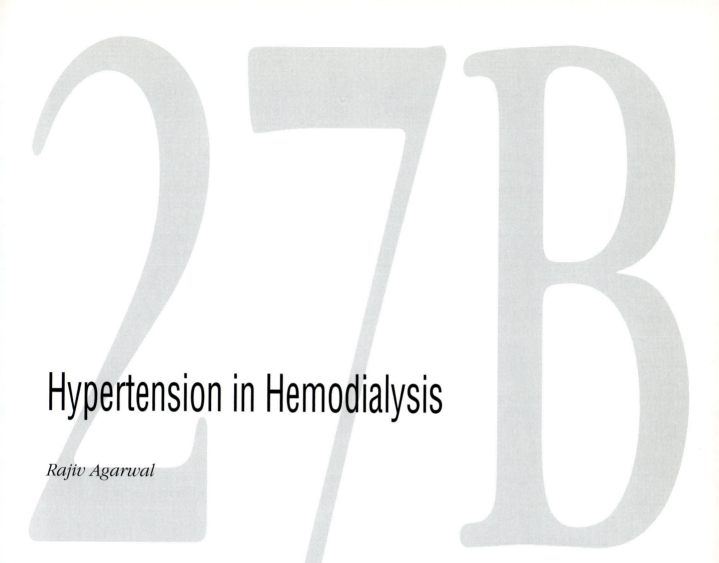

Hypertension in Hemodialysis

Rajiv Agarwal

Hypertension occurs very frequently in chronic kidney disease (CKD) and is nearly universal in patients who reach end-stage renal disease (ESRD). In a survey of 2535 hemodialysis patients from 69 dialysis units in the United States, the prevalence of hypertension was 86 percent.[1] Although many patients received antihypertensive drugs, only 30 percent had well-controlled blood pressure (BP), 58 percent had poorly controlled BP, and 12 percent had untreated hypertension. These findings underscore the appropriate recognition of high BP in hemodialysis patients but poor control despite use of multiple medications.

The purpose of this chapter is to discuss the etiology of hypertension, rationalize the measurement of BP, discuss the relationship between BP and adverse outcomes, and—finally—outline the pharmacologic and nonpharmacologic therapies to control hypertension in this population.

ETIOLOGY OF HYPERTENSION IN DIALYSIS PATIENTS

In hemodynamic terms, hypertension is directly related to cardiac output and systemic vascular resistance. An increase in cardiac output without a concomitant reduction in systemic vascular resistance will therefore elevate BP. Conversely, if systemic vascular resistance is increased without reduction in cardiac output, BP would also increase. Recognition of the symmetry between cardiac output and systemic vascular resistance provides a conceptual framework to analyze the pathophysiology of hypertension in patients on dialysis.

INCREASED CARDIAC OUTPUT DUE TO INCREASED SODIUM AND EXTRACELLULAR FLUID VOLUME

The classic mechanism for hypertension in hemodialysis patients is believed to be sodium and volume overload. Guyton and colleagues have pointed out that the kidneys are critically important in regulating arterial pressure in patients with hypertension.[2,3] They proposed that an initial increase in extracellular fluid volume that occurs in the renoprival state causes an increase in cardiac output but subsequently, through activation of autoregulatory mechanisms, leads to an increase in total vascular resistance with normalization of cardiac output. Guyton et al. proposed that the rise in BP leads to natriuresis, with subsequent normalization of BP.

However, hemodialysis patients cannot reduce BP by renally excreting sodium. Accordingly, a rise in vascular resistance would sustain hypertension in these individuals.

Ultrafiltration dialysis leads to a fall in mean arterial pressure in more than 90 percent of patients, which some have called "volume-dependent hypertension."[4,5] Although there is an unambiguous volume-dependent fall in BP, calling this phenomenon volume-dependent hypertension is erroneous. Volume-dependent hypertension is characterized by a decline in BP in response to sodium and volume restriction that takes several weeks to become manifest. For example, in patients with essential hypertension who are prescribed thiazide diuretics, an initial fall in extracellular fluid (ECF) volume is followed by reduction in vascular resistance, which finally leads to a reduction in BP.[6] Similarly, in patients with stages 3 and 4 CKD who are prescribed loop-diuretics, there is an initial fall in ECF volume associated with a rise in plasma renin activity; subsequently, a reduction in BP is seen.[7] In dialysis patients, reduction in body weight with ultrafiltration, long-duration dialysis coupled with dietary sodium restriction leads to improvement in BP over several weeks to months.[8] The *long-term* changes in BP associated with a reduction in ECF volume are examples of volume-dependent hypertension.

INCREASED SYSTEMIC VASCULAR RESISTANCE

The Renin-Angiotensin System

Although many patients may have plasma renin activity in the normal range, inappropriately increased plasma renin activity in relation to exchangeable sodium has long been recognized in uremic patients with hypertension.[9] That the renin-angiotensin system is activated even in hemodialysis patients is illustrated by the fact that renin is increased with ultrafiltration dialysis,[10] and infusion of saralasin, an angiotensin II antagonist, improves BP. Furthermore, patients treated with the angiotensin-converting enzyme (ACE) inhibitor lisinopril have a dose-dependent increase in plasma renin activity and an improvement in BP.[11]

Sympathetic Nervous System

McGrath[12] has stated that it is an oversimplification to believe that the kidneys are "just bags of renin" as far as BP regulation is concerned. Equally, it cannot be assumed that because arterial pressure can be controlled by sodium and water depletion, that salt and water overload was the original mechanism of the raised BP. Strong evidence has emerged that implicates enhanced sympathetic activity as a cause of hypertension in patients with ESRD.[13] Initial studies provided indirect evidence of increased sympathetic nerve activity. For example, investigators reported diminished vascular response to norepinephrine in animals with

chronic renal failure.[14] This was explained by a chronic increase in sympathetic nerve activity that downregulated adrenergic receptors. However, later studies provided more direct evidence of elevated sympathetic tone in patients with ESRD.[15] This was made possible by direct measurement of efferent sympathetic nerve activity.[16] The latter technique involves microneurography, in which a fine tungsten electrode is placed in the sympathetic nerves that run along the peroneal nerve. Using this technique, investigators have demonstrated that sympathetic activity is increased in those patients on chronic hemodialysis who still have their native kidneys. In contrast, patients with bilateral nephrectomy have reduced sympathetic activity, lower calf vascular resistance, and lower mean arterial pressure.[17] Thus the kidney, although devoid of excretory function, serves as an afferent organ to signal the midbrain region to increase sympathetic activity. The central mechanisms of increased sympathetic activity may involve dopaminergic neuronal transmission. Experiments in hypertensive hemodialysis patients show that administration of the dopamine-releasing drug bromocriptine decreased plasma norepinephrine and other markers of sympathetic outflow and lowered mean arterial pressure.[18] In animals with chronic renal failure, norepinephrine turnover rate is increased in posterior hypothalamic nuclei, and endogenous nitric oxide may be an important regulator of sympathetic activity.[19] Baroreceptor desensitization has also long been recognized in hypertensive patients with ESRD and may contribute to elevated BP.[20]

Circulating Inhibitors of Nitric Oxide

Endothelium-derived nitric oxide plays a critical role in the maintenance and regulation of vascular tone and modulates key processes mediating vascular disease, including leukocyte adhesion, platelet aggregation, and vascular smooth muscle proliferation.[21] Endothelial nitric oxide synthase enzymatically produces nitric oxide from the substrate L-arginine. L-arginine supplementation can partially reverse renal failure–associated endothelial dysfunction.[22] A circulating inhibitor of nitric oxide synthase, asymmetrical dimethyl arginine (ADMA), competes with L-arginine for nitric oxide synthase. In humans with salt-sensitive hypertension, administration of a high-salt diet increases plasma ADMA and BP.[23] Circulating ADMA is increased in subjects with CKD[24] and ESRD[25] and may contribute to endothelial dysfunction and increased BP. In patients with ESRD, ADMA is correlated with increased left ventricular (LV) thickness and reduced ejection fraction, consistent with its ability to increase systemic vascular resistance.[26]

As reviewed by Cooke,[27] of the 300 μmol/day ADMA normally generated, only 50 μmol/day is excreted by the kidneys in normal subjects, whereas the remaining is degraded enzymatically by dimethylarginine dimethylaminohydrolase (DDAH). Pharmacologic inhibition of DDAH with a small molecule, 4124W, causes accumulation of ADMA and generalized vasoconstriction. In contrast, over-expression of DDAH in genetically engineered mice reduces ADMA, improves the bioavailability of nitric oxide and reduces systolic BP. Oxidative stress, which impairs DDAH activity by oxidizing a sulfhydryl moiety critical to enzymatic activity, leads to the accumulation of ADMA and promotes endothelial dysfunction. Inflammation, increased homocysteine levels, reduced antioxidant defenses, and increased free radicals in ESRD may therefore provide an explanation for the relationship between oxidative stress, endothelial dysfunction, and the generation of hypertension. Cohort studies show an association between increased ADMA and cardiovascular events or death in hemodialysis patients.[28]

Erythropoietin

Hypertension is a common adverse effect of erythropoietin therapy.[29–31] It occurs more commonly in those people with preexisting hypertension.[32,33] Although the exact mechanism by which erythropoietin increases BP is not known, it may involve reduced nitric oxide activity due to scavenging by hemoglobin, increase in whole blood viscosity,[34] and increased vascular reactivity to norepinephrine[35] or other mechanisms.[36] Interestingly in animal experiments, hypertension does not track with increase in hemoglobin.[37] If erythropoietin is administered to anemic animals with chronic renal failure but hemoglobin is kept stable by feeding an iron-deficient diet, hypertension still occurs. In blood vessels harvested from these animals treated with erythropoietin, vasodilatory responses to nitric oxide donors were impaired, but response to several vasoconstrictors was normal.

Others

A variety of other substances have been described that can have vasoconstrictive properties. For example, compounds that block the sodium pump, such as digoxin-like immunoreactive substance and ouabain-like compound, can lead to an increase in intracellular calcium, which may elicit vascular smooth muscle contraction.[38] Parathyroid hormone (PTH) can increase intracellular calcium and aggravate hypertension,[39] and parathyroidectomy may improve BP.[40] Conversely, others have reported that elevated PTH levels can reduce the pressor response to norepinephrine in animals with chronic renal failure[41] and parathyroidectomy may not correct hypertension.[42] Loss of medullary prostaglandins and other renally derived vasodilators may also be responsible for hypertension in this population. Plasma concentrations of the vasoconstrictive peptide endothelin are extremely elevated in patients on hemodialysis and much more so than in patients who do not require dialysis.[43] Use of illicit drugs such as cocaine or prescription drugs such as

decongestants containing pseudoephedrine may also contribute to increased BP.

VASCULAR CHANGES AS A BASIS OF SYSTOLIC HYPERTENSION

Data from the National Health and Nutrition Examination Survey III show an increase in systolic BP with age.[44] In contrast, there is an increase in diastolic BP until about age 55 years and then a fall. Accordingly, pulse pressure—that is, the difference between systolic and diastolic BP—widens with age. Structural and functional changes in the arterial circulation that occur with aging are accelerated with hypertension.[45]

In contrast to atherosclerosis that has its origins in the endothelium, arteriosclerosis is an age-related, diffuse process characterized by replacement of elastin by collagen in the walls of large arteries.[46] Fibrosis and hypertrophy of the smooth muscle of the arterial wall results in dilatation and lengthening of the aorta.[47] The elastic properties of the blood vessels hydraulically filter the discontinuous pulsations of the heart to a steady stream in the peripheral vessels, and the age-related changes have important effects on the nature of blood flow through vessels. The modified Windkessel model describes two compliances[48]: the first is proximal, representing the storage capacity of the larger conduit arteries, and the second is distal, representing the elasticity of smaller arteries and branch points involved in reflections and oscillations in the system. As arteries become less distensible, there is a quicker return of the backward pressure wave from the reflection sites toward the heart, boosting pressure during late systole (rather than diastole) by as much as 40 to 50 mmHg in central arteries.[49] The second systolic peak becomes more prominent as arteries stiffen. The lack of aortic distensibility fails to maintain steady flow in diastole and therefore attenuates diastolic pressure. Accordingly, widened pulse pressure is the most robust clinical indicator of arteriosclerosis and cardiovascular risk. Nevertheless, systolic BP, rather than pulse pressure, is considerably simpler to use clinically in the management of hypertensive patients and is the basis of the JNC VII clinical advisory.[50] Among hemodialysis patients who underwent ambulatory BP monitoring,[51] only 3 percent had isolated diastolic hypertension; in the majority of the patients who had untreated or uncontrolled hypertension, systolic hypertension coexisted (Fig. 27B–1).

CARDIOVASCULAR CHANGES IN HEMODIALYSIS HYPERTENSION

Hypertension in hemodialysis patients, as in patients with essential hypertension, is associated with a number of cardiac adaptations and maladaptations (see Chap. 27A).[52]

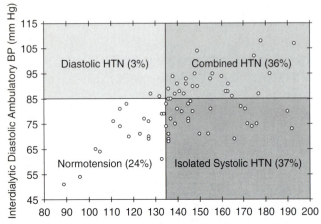

Figure 27B–1. Distribution of ambulatory systolic and diastolic hypertension in patients on chronic hemodialysis. Only 3 percent of these patients had isolated diastolic hypertension. *(From Agarwal and Lewis,[51] with permission.)*

Cardiac changes, such as LV hypertrophy and diastolic dysfunction, go hand in hand with vascular changes such as increased pulse wave velocity (a marker of arteriosclerosis), increased carotid intimal media thickness (a marker of atherosclerosis), and widened pulse pressure.[53]

Both volume and pressure overload are seen in patients with ESRD. The causes of chronic flow overload are well recognized and include the presence of an arteriovenous (AV) access, salt and water overload, and anemia. Pressure overload can occur from hypertension as well as loss of compliance of large arteries and increased reflection from smaller arteries and branch points.

Factors peculiar to uremia that contribute to accelerated vascular stiffening include hyperparathyroidism, increased calcium times phosphorus product, increased circulating endothelin concentration,[54] sympathetic activation,[55] and vascular inflammation; increases in intravascular volume and inappropriately high levels of angiotensin II further augment vascular stiffness.[56] The loss of vessel compliance causes increased LV afterload and impaired coronary perfusion, thus further compromising cardiac function. These pathologic changes in the vascular tree may cause an impairment of circulatory function that is associated with increased cardiovascular morbidity and mortality. The increased vascular stiffness may also affect the assessment and treatment of hypertension, as discussed below.

Assessment of Blood Pressure and the Diagnosis of Hypertension

Ambiguity in the diagnosis of hypertension in hemodialysis patients arises from large swings in BP associated with the dialysis procedure, but the correct assessment of BP is unequivocally important for the management of hypertension.

SOURCES OF ERROR IN THE MEASUREMENT OF BLOOD PRESSURE IN HEMODIALYSIS PATIENTS

Some errors inherent in the assessment of BP in dialysis patients are unique. For example, interdialytic weight gain is associated with increases in BP, the magnitude of which is estimated to be about 1.2 mmHg/lb weight gain.[57] This link between the hydration state and BP is also demonstrated with studies done with ambulatory blood pressure monitoring (ABPM).[58–60] The increase in BP with change in weight appears to be of a greater magnitude in patients with hypertension compared to normotensives.[61] Therefore a variable relationship emerges between BP and volume status that is in part dictated by the characteristics of the patient. Hemodialysis patients often have advanced vascular calcification, which may make indirect sphygmomanometry erroneous.

Very often standard guidelines for the measurement of BP in hemodialysis patients are not followed.[62] For example, due to obesity or large arm size, BP may be taken in the leg or forearm. The recommended practice in patients with essential hypertension requires measurement of BP in both arms and subsequently using the arm with the higher systolic pressure as the reference. However, the arm with the better blood vessels may be the arm with angioaccess, which is not used for the measurement of BP.

Whereas some of these problems with measurement error are remediable, it is clear from the above analysis that patients with ESRD on chronic hemodialysis have certain unique sources of error in the measurement of BP compared to the population with essential hypertension, and an accurate assessment of BP may not be possible by hemodialysis unit readings alone.

INFORMATION PROVIDED BY AMBULATORY BLOOD PRESSURE MONITORING

ABPM has demonstrated that hemodialysis patients do not lower the BP at night—i.e., they have a high prevalence of "nondipping."[63–68] This phenomenon cannot be detected by other methods and provides a more accurate estimate of the BP burden—also called "BP load"—on the cardiovascular system.[69] Whereas in individuals with essential hypertension nondipping is associated with LV hypertrophy, strokes, and cardiovascular morbidity and mortality, in patients on hemodialysis, nondipping is associated with reduced arterial distensibility,[70] and the 24-hour pulse pressure is linked to total mortality.[71]

Because of numerous readings obtained by ABPM and the lack of alerting reactions, there is excellent reproducibility between days when duplicate readings are performed.[72] ABPM is also more sensitive to change with interventions. For example, whereas routine BP monitoring failed to demonstrate changes in BP with the administration of erythropoietin,[73] ABPM was able to detect a rise in overall BP with just 13 patients.[30] When ABPM was compared to home BP monitoring, ABPM was again found to be more sensitive in detecting an increase in BP with erythropoietin.[74] Using only a small number of subjects, we have exploited the reproducibility and sensitivity of ABPM in detecting antihypertensive effects of water-soluble antihypertensive drugs administered to hemodialysis patients three times weekly.[75–77]

ABPM is required for the diagnosis of the "white-coat effect"—that is, an elevation in BP due to alerting reactions in the office setting in patients who have preexisting hypertension. Mitra et al. compared interdialytic ABPM with BP obtained in hemodialysis patients at arrival to the dialysis unit, after 10 minutes of rest in a quiet room, and at other time points.[78] These authors report that the BP on arrival to the hemodialysis unit was higher by 20/10 mmHg than that in the previous 6 hours recorded by ABPM in 15 of 36 (41 percent) patients. Even after resting for 10 minutes, BP was elevated in 19 percent of the patients, suggesting a true white-coat effect. This study suggests that the white-coat effect is common in hemodialysis patients. By comparison, in a population of elderly patients with hypertension but without kidney disease, white-coat hypertension was seen in 13 percent; these patients had a cardiovascular prognosis that was similar to that of patients with well-controlled hypertension.[79] Although home BP monitoring may also be useful for diagnosing the white-coat effect, it has not been studied for this objective in hemodialysis patients.

Cannella and associates have pointed out that "a false normotensive classification to subjects who are actually hypertensive, may possibly cause the link between arterial hypertension and LVH to be missed."[80] Those patients who have normal BP in the dialysis unit, but increased BP outside the dialysis unit as assessed by ambulatory BP monitoring have "masked hypertension." In an elderly population of patients with essential hypertension but without kidney disease, 9 percent were found to have masked hypertension.[81] The cardiovascular prognosis of such patients is similar to that of poorly controlled hypertensives. The causes of masked hypertension in the dialysis population are not known. However, sleep apnea, which commonly occurs in hemodialysis patients, may be an important cause of masked hypertension. Sleep apnea causes a nocturnal increase in BP, the magnitude of which increases with the severity of sleep apnea.[82] The daytime BP in these patients may not be elevated or may not accurately reflect the cardiovascular burden of hypertension; ABPM may be of particular value in assessing cardiovascular risk in such individuals.

ASSESSMENT OF INTERDIALYTIC BLOOD PRESSURE IN HEMODIALYSIS PATIENTS

Numerous studies have analyzed the relationship between BP obtained in the dialysis unit and compared it to the "gold standard" of interdialytic ABPM. Studies using measures of agreement have uniformly concluded that dialysis unit BPs are inadequate surrogates for predicting the precise interdialytic BP.[83–87] Although statistically significant correlation coefficients were found between dialysis unit BP and ABPM in other studies,[63,88] which is unambiguously expected, analysis of the data does not support that BP can be assessed accurately in *individual* patients using dialysis unit BP alone.

Only one of the studies utilizing echocardiography performed a complete interdialytic ABPM[89]; it found that systolic hypertension was present in 25 percent of patients by predialysis BP but in 50 percent of the patients by ABPM, pointing out the high incidence of masked hypertension. Diastolic hypertension was present in 25 percent by predialysis BP and 72.5 percent by ABPM. The best correlation between LV mass index (LVMI) and BP was seen for ABPM (Pearson's correlation coefficients were as follows: Prehemodialysis systolic BP, 0.396; ambulatory BP 0.544; systolic BP load by ambulatory BP, 0.630). A unique and independent predictor of LVMI and interventricular septal thickness, both measures of LV hypertrophy, was systolic BP load; the nighttime ambulatory systolic BP was the best predictor for LV posterior wall thickness. Conlon et al. used only 24-hour BP monitoring but found that predialysis systolic BP overestimated systolic ambulatory BP by 4.7 mmHg ($p = 0.004$) and predialysis diastolic BP underestimated diastolic ambulatory BP by 3.7 mmHg ($p = 0.002$).[90] There was a correlation between systolic ambulatory BP and predialysis systolic BP ($r = 0.67$, $p = 0.0001$) and diastolic ambulatory BP and postdialysis diastolic BP ($r = 0.5$, $p = 0.0021$), but these correlations were not strong enough to replace ambulatory BP. Zoccali et al. used 24-hour ambulatory BP monitoring[91] and concluded that an average of 12 predialysis BPs was as useful as ambulatory BP. Although debatable, it is the present author's opinion that ABPM is a superior tool to assess BP in hemodialysis patients.[92,93] Cannella et al, measured 24-hour ABPM, LV MI, and routine dialysis unit BP averaged over 12 sessions,[94] Predialysis systolic BP was not biased compared to BP obtained in triplicate at 5-minute intervals 15 minutes prior to dialysis, but predialysis diastolic BP overestimated triplicate diastolic readings by 5.3 mmHg, indicating a white-coat effect for diastolic BP. Furthermore, 24-hour ABPM detected 82 percent systolic hypertensives, whereas predialysis systolic readings were hypertensive in only 65 percent, again pointing to the high prevalence of masked hypertension in this population.

Our study, performed in 70 hemodialysis patients, used both qualitative and quantitative methodologies to assess the accuracy of dialysis unit BP monitoring.[95] Compared to 2-week averaged dialysis unit BP there were wide agreement limits between dialysis unit and ambulatory BP (Fig. 27B–2). Thus, predialysis systolic BP could overestimate ABPM by about 50 mmHg or underestimate it by 20 mmHg. Nevertheless, when we compared the sensitivity and specificity of dialysis unit BP by analyzing the receiver operating characteristic curves, we found that hemodialysis unit BPs could be used to predict the control or lack of control of hypertension in a qualitative way (Fig. 27B–3). Thus, a 2-week averaged predialysis BP of >150/85 mmHg or a postdialysis BP of >130/75 mmHg had 80 percent sensitivity in diagnosing hypertension. To individualize treatment thresholds, nephrologists can use various cutoff values. For example, a young, nondiabetic man may benefit from long-term BP lowering, and predialysis BP of >150/85 can be used as a treatment threshold. When the likelihood of false positives must be minimized, as in an

older dialysis patient with underlying coronary artery disease and diabetes, which may confer a much greater mortality risk, thresholds for diagnosing hypertension can be increased by 10/5 mmHg. In other words, predialysis BP of >160/90 mmHg and postdialysis BP of >140/80 mmHg can be used as thresholds for diagnosing hypertension because they have a specificity of at least 80 percent. It is to be emphasized that these thresholds do not predict the level of ABPM with any degree of accuracy; for accurate diagnosis of the level of hypertension, 44-hour interdialytic ABPM must be performed.

Collectively, these studies appear to indicate that hemodialysis unit BP can be used only in a qualitative sense. In many respects BPs obtained in the hemodialysis unit are to ABPM as serum creatinine concentration is to glomerular filtration rate (GFR). Just as an elevated serum creatinine indicates an impaired GFR but cannot accurately predict the GFR, using hemodialysis unit BP can indicate the presence or absence of hypertension but cannot accurately predict the ambulatory BP.

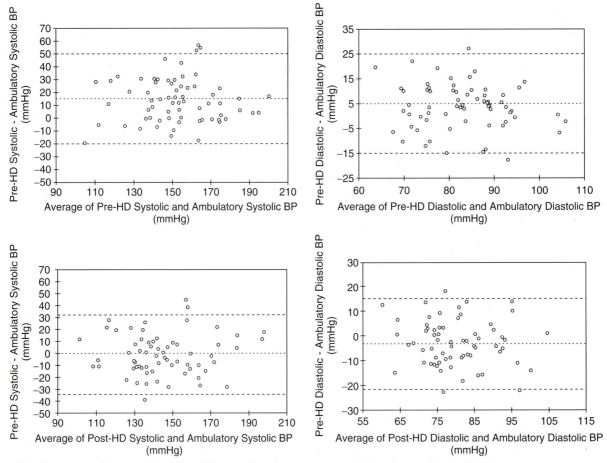

Figure 27B–2. Bland-Altman plots for hemodialysis unit and ambulatory BPs. The horizontal lines, which show the limits of agreement, indicate poor agreement between BPs recorded in the dialysis unit and those obtained by ambulatory BP monitoring. Wide agreement limits preclude the use of dialysis unit BPs for accurate prediction of ambulatory BPs. *(From Agarwal and Lewis,[51] with permission.)*

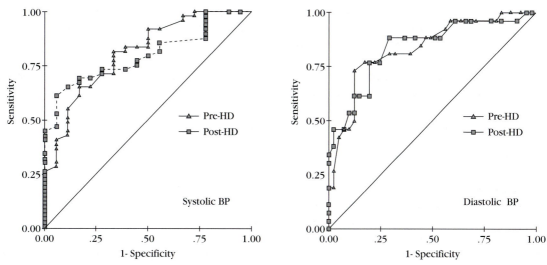

Figure 27B–3. Receiver operating characteristic curves of BPs obtained in the hemodialysis unit and the presence or absence of hypertension as assessed by ambulatory BP monitoring. The diagonal straight line at 45 degrees indicates a hypothetical test with no predictive value. The area under the curve for each of the receiver operating characteristic curves was at least 80 percent, which allows dialysis unit BPs to be used in a qualitative sense. *(From Agarwal and Lewis,[51] with permission.)*

IMPROVING THE ASSESSMENT OF BLOOD PRESSURE IN HEMODIALYSIS PATIENTS

The accuracy of BP measurement in the hemodialysis unit needs urgent attention. Quality control programs should be instituted to more accurately monitor BP in hemodialysis patients. Another source of error commonly overlooked in the hemodialysis population is the white-coat effect, which may be present in 20 percent of hemodialysis patients.[96] This error can be minimized, possibly with home BP monitoring and definitely with ambulatory BP monitoring. Home BP monitoring has been evaluated in a limited number of patients.[97] With this technique, the measurement error can be substantial but still somewhat less than with dialysis unit BP measurements. Nevertheless, home BP monitoring involves the patient in the overall management of BP; in patients with essential hypertension, it has been shown to improve BP control.[98] This technique should therefore be further studied and, until more data become available, should continue to be used for better assessment of hypertension in hemodialysis patients.

As discussed above, hemodialysis unit BPs are useful in a qualitative sense. A predialysis BP of >150/85 mmHg or postdialysis BP of >130/75 mmHg is 80 percent sensitive in diagnosing hypertension. However, if an accurate measurement of BP is needed, there is no substitute for ABPM in the interdialytic period. It can avoid unnecessary therapy in some patients and correctly identify hypertension in others, thus aiding in the delivery of cost-effective care and improving cardiovascular morbidity and mortality in these patients.

Relationship of Hypertension to Adverse Outcomes

While it is amply clear that high BP has a continuous, graded, and etiologically significant relationship with cardiovascular outcomes in the general population,[99] studies in hemodialysis patients have found an inverse relationship between high BPs and outcomes.[100,101] Thus, patients with high BPs have a lower mortality than those with low BPs. It is intellectually troublesome to find such an association, because high BP, which was such an important risk factor for cardiovascular disease prior to onset of dialysis, suddenly becomes a protective factor. In patients with CKD who are not yet on hemodialysis, we strive to lower BP more aggressively than for those with uncomplicated essential hypertension. If these observations—"reverse epidemiology"—are etiologically significant should we be complacent about treating high BP in hemodialysis patients?

POOR ASSESSMENT OF BLOOD PRESSURE: REGRESSION DILUTION BIAS

Assessment of BP in hemodialysis patients is particularly difficult because of large changes during dialysis, poor measurement technique,[102] the white-coat effect,[103] and masked hypertension.[104] Ambulatory BP measurements provide a more accurate reflection of ambient BP[105–107] and are more reproducible[108] than the routine BPs obtained in dialysis units. Routine measurements of BPs would regress toward the mean; that is, those individuals with hypertension would become less hypertensive and those with normotension would become hypertensive, thus diluting the separation between hypertensive and normotensive groups based on routine sphygmomanometry. This phenomenon of "regression dilution bias" would add "noise" to the prognostic variable of interest. It would follow that better precision in the measurement of BP, as through ambulatory BP monitoring, would uncover relationships between hypertension and cardiovascular mortality with smaller sample sizes. Amar et al.,[109] from Toulouse, France, reported 57 treated hypertensive hemodialysis patients who underwent interdialytic ambulatory BP monitoring; cardiovascular death occurred in 10 patients. Although this study had a small number of patients with a relatively short follow-up, it demonstrated that nocturnal systolic BP [risk ratio (RR) 1.41, 95 percent CI 1.08 to 1.84] and 24-hour pulse pressure (RR 1.85, 95 percent CI 1.28 to 2.65) were independent predictors of cardiovascular mortality in treated hypertensive hemodialysis patients.

FACTORS THAT MODIFY THE RELATIONSHIP BETWEEN BLOOD PRESSURE AND MORTALITY

High BP leads to an increase in cardiovascular events, which may be immediately fatal or subsequently increase total mortality. Analyzing a prognostic value of BP in observational cohort studies requires the consideration of various other factors. One such factor that is often ignored in considering hypertension as a prognostic variable in dialysis patients is that of "reverse causation." *Reverse causation* means that the dependent process has a direct or indirect effect on the independent predictor. Consideration of the epidemiologic relationship between high cholesterol and improved survival provides a valuable indication of the existence of other factors that modify the relationship of a risk factor with outcome.

In a recent study of hemodialysis patients[110] who had been on dialysis for less than 1 year, the relationship between total cholesterol and mortality was explored. Since serum cholesterol concentration is influenced by nutritional and inflammatory factors, the investigators measured markers of nutrition and inflammation together with total cholesterol at the outset. As expected, in patients who were inflamed or malnourished or both, serum cholesterol was found to be lower. More importantly, among these patients, an inverse link between total cholesterol and mortality was seen. However, once these patients were excluded, the expected direct relationship between total cholesterol and mortality emerged. Thus, inflammation and malnutrition were important confounding variables in analyzing the relationship between total cholesterol and mortality.

Figure 27B–4 shows the hypothesized relationship between hypertension and mortality when a confounding variable is considered. Long-standing, poorly controlled hypertension may lead to heart failure, which may lower BP—reverse causation. The well-controlled BP in the presence of poor cardiac function is likely to be associated with high cardiovascular mortality (open circles, upper line in Fig. 27B–4). In contrast, poorly controlled BP with intact cardiac function is expected to be associated with increased mortality (solid circles, lower line in Fig. 27B–4). If patients with impaired cardiac function constitute a large part of an observational cohort, a U-shaped relationship between BP and total mortality will be seen (dotted line in the figure). If the confounding variable of heart failure is not considered, the conclusion that lower BP is damaging would be inappropriate.

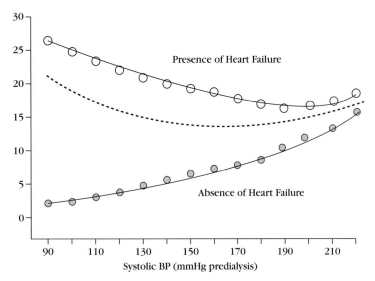

Figure 27B–4. Impact of a confounding variable influencing the relationship between hypertension and mortality. Consideration of confounding variables such as heart failure can help explain the U-shaped relationship between BP and total mortality (dotted line) seen in some studies. See text for details.

Although such a confounding factor has not been explicitly explored in hypertensive dialysis populations, several studies point out that the presence of other diseases modifies the relationship of BP with total mortality in hemodialysis patients. Foley et al.[111] related lower mean arterial pressure with the presence of lower albumin, heart failure, ischemic heart disease, and older age. Japanese investigators[112,113] have reported that if ischemic heart disease is present, higher BP is associated with better survival. In contrast, in healthier patients, systolic hypertension was associated with increased mortality. In a group of 326 French dialysis patients[114] those without diabetes, who had no prior cardiovascular diseases, and those who were younger than 60 years, mean arterial pressure was a predictor of cardiovascular mortality. These analyses were adjusted for adequacy of hemodialysis, serum albumin, conventional cardiovascular risk factors, and prior atherosclerotic disease. In Japanese hemodialysis patients without diabetes, greater total mortality, more strokes, and more myocardial infarctions were seen with higher systolic BP.[115] However, in patients with diabetes, no such effect was seen. In Brazilian hemodialysis patients[116] without prior cardiovascular disease and with 6 1/2 year follow-up, total mortality risk was 2.22-fold higher in hypertensive patients than in normotensives. In Italian dialysis patients[117] below 50 years of age, 31 percent mortality was seen among hypertensive hemodialysis patients compared to 18 percent among normotensives, although no such relationship was seen in the overall cohort. Finally, the link between low BP and increased mortality appears to be due to early deaths. When the relationship between BP and total mortality is analyzed 1 year after the start of hemodialysis, the relationship between low BP and mortality disappears.[118] Early deaths, defined as those occurring during the first 2 years after the onset of dialysis, were associated with withdrawal from dialysis or death from cancers, whereas late deaths were attributable to a higher BP.[119] Similar data have been reported from the Dialysis Outcomes and Practice Patterns Study (DOPPS).[120] In both univariate and multivariate models, a diagnosis of hypertension was associated with reduced mortality (RR 0.74, p <0.0001 in multivariate model). In the first year of dialysis, the survival advantage of a diagnosis of hypertension was large (RR = 0.59), but it failed to retain its protective effect (RR = 0.92, p >0.05) subsequently.

Two studies reported from the United States also suggest the existence of confounding variables. A registry study from the U. S. Renal Data System (USRDS) reported by Port et al.[121] was a cohort analysis of 4499 patients who had been on dialysis for at least 1 year on the last day of 1990. The reference group for systolic BP was 120 to 149 mmHg and for diastolic BP was 70 to 89 mmHg. Deaths due to coronary artery disease, cardiovascular disease, or

"other cardiac diseases" were analyzed. All other deaths were censored. In adjusted analyses, the hazard ratio (HR) for cardiovascular mortality was 1.86 for predialysis systolic BP <110 mmHg and 1.28 for postdialysis systolic BP <110 mmHg. HRs for cardiovascular mortality were 1.32 for postdialysis systolic BP ≥180 mmHg and was of marginal statistical significance (p = 0.06). Diastolic BP was not predictive of cardiovascular deaths except for postdialysis diastolic BP ≥110 mmHg (HR = 2.25, p = 0.04). Predialysis systolic BP <110 mmHg increased the risk of cardiovascular mortality twofold when congestive heart failure was present, with or without coronary artery disease. Coronary artery disease deaths, other cardiac deaths, and noncardiac deaths were all increased with low predialysis systolic BP (<110 mmHg).

Zager et al.[122] reported a cohort of 5433 patients from a large dialysis chain in the United States. Over a mean follow up of 2.6 years, 42 percent of the patients died. An aggregate of 14,126 patient-years of follow-up yielded a crude annual mortality rate of 16.1 percent. BP showed a U-shaped curve with mortality. BP was analyzed as both a fixed and a time-varying covariate in a Cox proportional hazards regression model. Time-varying covariates allow for adjustment of risk exposure such as BP. The effects of low BP were magnified when it was used as a time-varying covariate. For example, total mortality for prehemodialysis BP of <110 mmHg was 64 percent higher when treated as a fixed covariate but increased to 207 percent when treated as a time-varying covariate. When BP is used as a time-varying covariate, it is possible that a risk factor other than hypertension may simultaneously influence BP and mortality; in the latter situation, a fall in BP and cardiovascular mortality may be strongly associated, but this does not prove causation. For example, if a hypertensive patient developed heart failure or an illness that produced a fall in BP, the effect of hypertension when entered as a time-varying covariate would be diluted. A relationship as shown in Fig. 27B–4 would then emerge.

In future analyses of the link between high BP and total mortality, cardiac function and the presence of other parameters—such as malnutrition, inflammation, diabetes, cardiovascular disease, and cancers—should be considered.

WHICH BLOOD PRESSURE PREDICTS RISK: MEAN ARTERIAL, SYSTOLIC, DIASTOLIC, OR PULSE PRESSURE?

CKD is a state of vascular aging. Pulse wave velocity measures vascular stiffness and among hemodialysis patients is a strong predictor of total mortality.[123] With increasing vascular stiffness, augmentation of systolic and attenuation of diastolic pressure occurs, such that the pulse pressure is widened.[124] In observational cohorts, pulse wave velocity is associated with higher systolic BP, and an inverse relationship is seen between total mortality and lower diastolic BP.[125] JNC 7 guidelines designate systolic BP as the primarily target for intervention in people above 50 years of age.[126] Dialysis patients are typically older, but even younger patients may have a vascular age above their chronological age.[127] Directionally opposite changes in systolic and diastolic pressures incurred due to increasing vascular stiffness have a less perceptible effect on mean arterial pressure. Thus it is not surprising that studies seeking an association between mean arterial pressure and total mortality have sometimes failed to find such an association.[128] In contrast, studies have found a direct link between pulse pressure and total mortality.[129] This association between increased pulse pressure and poor long-term outcomes may simply be intrinsic to the poor state of vascular health—reflected by increased vascular stiffness—in patients on hemodialysis. The wisdom of lowering pulse pressure may be questioned in this circumstance. However, therapeutic nihilism is not warranted. In the elderly population with systolic hypertension, a direct link between pulse pressure and long-term cardiovascular outcomes is seen.[130] Furthermore, in randomized controlled trials, improvement of systolic BP with a wide variety of antihypertensive agents—such as thiazide diuretics, beta blockers,[131] angiotensin-receptor blockers,[132] and calcium channel blockers[133]—has led to improved cardiovascular outcomes in this population. Although such trials in hemodialysis patients are sorely lacking, it seems reasonable to extrapolate these findings to this population.

Evidence for considering both systolic and diastolic BP in evaluating total mortality in hemodialysis patients comes from two studies. Tozawa et al. reported a cohort of patients from Okinawa, Japan,[134] where a predialysis BP of 130/80 mmHg was taken as a reference standard to predict total mortality. BP was treated as a continuous variable in the Cox proportion hazards model, where single BPs—systolic and diastolic—or pulse pressures were considered. In addition, conjoint models were developed where the simultaneous effects of systolic and diastolic BP, systolic and pulse pressure, and diastolic and pulse pressure were considered jointly. In the single-BP component model, pulse pressure was the strongest predictor of fatal outcome (HR 1.080 per 10 mmHg increase in pulse pressure). The systolic BP was also a significant predictor (HR 1.040 per 10 mmHg increase) but not as strong. Diastolic BP was not a significant predictor of total mortality. When both the systolic and diastolic BPs were considered *together*, systolic BP was associated with increased total mortality (HR 1.083); but diastolic BP was associated with reduced total mortality (HR 0.886) (Fig. 27B–5).

The second report by Foley et al.[135] from the USRDS used a larger number of patients with a longer follow-up and reported antihypertensive drug use. Over an average follow-up of 3.8 years, 63 percent of the patients died, yielding a median survival of 3.9 years. Thus the crude mortality rate of 166 per 1000 patient-years was similar to that of the overall U.S. hemodialysis population. The authors assessed the value of systolic and diastolic BP separately and conjointly in a Cox proportional hazards model. As expected, when systolic and diastolic BPs were considered separately, there was an inverse relationship between total mortality and BP. However, when systolic and diastolic BPs were considered together, a direct relationship between total mortality and systolic BP but an inverse relationship between diastolic BP and total mortality emerged (Fig. 27B–6). The hazard ratios for total mortality were 1.06/0.79 for predialysis BPs and 3.0/0.87 per 10 mmHg

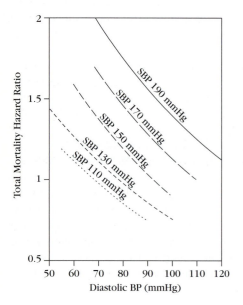

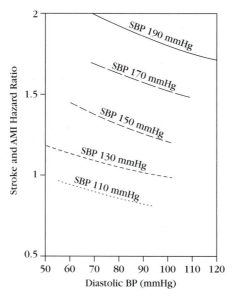

Figure 27B–5. Relationship of systolic and diastolic BP and cardiovascular morbidity and total mortality in hemodialysis patients. High systolic BP predicts increased events, but a low diastolic BP predicts increased mortality, stroke, and acute myocardial infarction (AMI). *(From Tozawa et al.,[134] with permission.)*

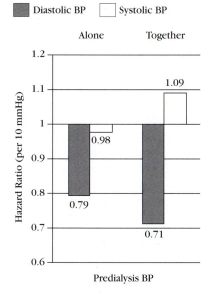
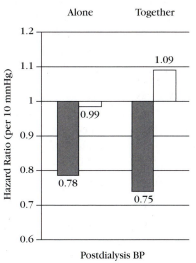

Figure 27B–6. When dialysis unit BPs are considered together in a Cox proportional hazards model, a significant and directionally opposite influence of BP on total mortality is seen. Thus, a low diastolic and a high systolic BP is predictive of mortality. When considered alone, a low diastolic BP is predictive of increased mortality, but no significance is seen for systolic BP. Hazards shown are unadjusted for comorbid factors. *(From Foley et al.,[135] with permission.)*

BP for postdialysis BPs. When the results were adjusted for important confounding variables, the hazard ratios were 0.99/0.95 for predialysis and 1.03/0.94 for posthemodialysis BPs. However, all hazard ratios except the prehemodialysis systolic BPs remained statistically significant. Since the analyses were adjusted for interdialytic weight gain, a higher postdialysis BP when adjusted for the interdialytic weight gain may reflect inadequate achievement of dry weight. These data suggest that inadequate attention to dry weight or the presence of a stiff arterial tree may be independently associated with total mortality in hemodialysis patients.

Finally, Klassen et al.[136] analyzed the relationship between pulse pressure and total mortality in 37,099 patients from a dialysis chain. The interaction between pulse pressure and age, sex, race, diabetes, and level of systolic BP was tested. For any given level of systolic BP, a direct relationship emerged between increasing pulse pressure and death. Each 10 mmHg increase in pulse pressure was associated with a 12 percent increase in hazard of death. Subjects with a prehemodialysis systolic BP <135 mmHg had greater mortality. Pulse pressure in unadjusted analyses had a U-shaped relationship with mortality with the reference pulse pressure of 50 to 59 mmHg. After controlling for the level of systolic BP, there was a direct relationship between a pulse pressure ≥60 mmHg and total mortality. Pulse pressure was predominantly governed by systolic BP (r^2 systolic BP = 0.73, r^2 diastolic BP = 0.057). In further analysis, the authors demonstrated that the pulse pressure–related mortality was driven by those with systolic BP <140 mmHg. There was an important interaction between pulse pressure and age. Pulse pressure in younger patients (<62 years) was twice as likely to be associated with death compared with the effect in older patients (RR 1.24 vs. 1.12)

Taken together, this study implies that those with lower systolic BP, possibly with impaired cardiac systolic function and wide pulse pressure indicating a stiff circulation, have an increased risk of total mortality.

WHAT ABOUT THE J CURVE?

Coronary perfusion occurs during diastole, and it is possible that coronary perfusion may suffer in those individuals in whom diastolic BP is greatly lowered. Although the existence of this relationship has not been determined in hemodialysis populations, evidence in the general population with essential hypertension is lacking. In an analysis of 1 million individuals participating in randomized controlled antihypertensive drug trials, a continuous relationship between BP and long-term mortality was seen,[137] Even among the very old, such as those between 80 and 89 years of age, no J curve was present.

Nevertheless, it is quite likely that a J-shaped relationship between BP and survival exists in dialysis patients.[138] If such a phenomenon truly exists, it can be explained by considering the confounding factors shown in Fig. 27B–4 rather than invoking "reverse epidemiology."

From the above discussion, it is clear that there is a direct relationship between elevated BP and mortality in hemodialysis patients. Increased pulse pressure, which is primarily due to increased systolic pressure, is also associated with cardiovascular morbidity and mortality. The counterintuitive relationship between BP and mortality appears in part to be due to methods of data analysis and the failure to consider confounding variables. Preliminary data suggest that the control of hypertension in hypertensive dialysis patients is associated with improved survival. Furthermore, the use of antihypertensive drug treatment is associated with improved survival regardless of BP control. Low predialysis BP is associated with increased early deaths, particularly in patients with heart failure or other illnesses that lower BP.

Treatment of Hemodialysis Hypertension

For patients with essential hypertension, CKD not yet on dialysis, and those with diabetes mellitus, clear guidelines on BP targets exist. However, there are no such guidelines for patients on hemodialysis. This is because no randomized controlled trials have been performed in such patients to demonstrate the advantages of a given BP target. Very low BP in these individuals may make them intolerant to the hemodynamic stress of hemodialysis. In contrast, high BPs may increase the chances of adverse cardiovascular outcomes.

Clearly there is an emergent need to define goal BPs in hemodialysis patients. However, until such randomized trials are performed, we have to depend on clinical judgment to determine the best BP for our dialysis patients. Operationally, an ideal BP for a dialysis patient is the lowest BP that ensures hemodynamic stability during dialysis as well as orthostatic tolerance immediately postdialysis and is associated with good health-related quality of life. Such a BP should also be associated with the lowest cardiovascular morbidity and mortality. Osmolality and fluid volume–imposed hemodynamic stress during the hemodialysis procedure may have a varying influence on the intradialytic BP. Thus those patients with LV hypertrophy who need a higher filling pressure to maintain cardiac output may have greater declines in BP. Likewise, those patients with a stiff arterial circulation may have a large decline in systolic BP. Accordingly, a single BP target may not be appropriate for all patients. Those with stiff hearts and circulations would either need less hemodynamic stress; for example, by reducing intradialytic weight gain, more frequent dialysis, or prolongation of the dialysis time. Otherwise we may be left with no choice but to accept a higher BP to maintain intradialytic hemodynamic stability and the patient's quality of life. Thus patients who are older, who have vascular disease, and those with underlying diabetes may have different BP goals than those with more pliable circulations and little or no LV hypertrophy.

RESTRICTION OF DIETARY AND DIALYSATE SODIUM AND ACHIEVEMENT OF DRY WEIGHT

The discontinuous nature of the hemodialysis procedure—which is typically performed three times a week—requires that the sodium and water removed during the treatment period must at least match the interdialytic gain of sodium and water. Furthermore, the absolute content of total body water

and sodium must be at a level that does not cause signs and symptoms of volume overload, including hypertension or signs and symptoms of sodium and water depletion, such as dizziness and hypotension. The assessment of total body water and sodium, associated with neither volume overload nor volume depletion, is imperfect; the optimal level is the "dry weight."

Recent data point to the deleterious and expected relationship between excess interdialytic weight gain and poor outcomes in hemodialysis patients. Observational cohort studies in dialysis patients show an association between large interdialytic weight gain and total mortality in patients with diabetes mellitus and poor nutritional status.[139] Foley et al. reported results from a historically prospective study of 11,142 randomly selected patients on hemodialysis on December 31, 1993, from the USRDS Dialysis Morbidity and Mortality Study Waves III and IV. After accounting for multiple comorbid factors, they reported an association of increased mortality with interdialytic weight gain of >4.8 percent.[140]

Dietary salt restriction to limit interdialytic weight gain is a strategy as old as dialysis itself, which would, if practiced diligently, facilitate the achievement of dry weight. However, like many other lifestyle modifications, it is not practiced widely.[141] Nevertheless, centers that have practiced this modality have been rewarded with less use of antihypertensive agents and better BP control.[142,143]

Another strategy to limit interdialytic weight gain and thirst is to lower the dialysate's sodium concentration. Whereas increased dialysate sodium increases interdialytic weight gain,[144,145] the data supporting the reverse phenomenon are not as strong. Nevertheless, in one preliminary study, dialysate sodium was reduced at a rate of 1 meq/L every 3 to 4 weeks—from 140 to 135 meq/L—in combination with the restriction of dietary sodium to <6 g/day.[146] As a result, predialysis BP improved from 147/88 to 136/80 mmHg (a fall in mean arterial pressure from 108 to 98 mmHg, $p = 0.02$) without any change in dry weight. Furthermore, in 4 of the 8 patients, BP medications could be stopped completely. Others, in a study involving 6 hemodialysis patients, have not observed such an improvement.[147] In another study, 15 dialysis patients were sodium-restricted such that their estimated dietary sodium intakes were reduced from 10 to 7 g/day[148] Dialysis parameters and dry weight were kept constant. Predialysis BP decreased with dietary salt restriction from 139/79 to 132/75 mmHg ($p < 0.01$ systolic, $p < 0.05$ diastolic), and mean arterial pressure decreased from 99 to 94 mmHg ($p < 0.01$). Interdialytic weight gain decreased with salt restriction from 2.3 ± 0.73 to 1.8 ± 0.52 kg ($p < 0.001$), whereas postdialysis weight did not change [66.1 ± 11.9 to 66.1 ± 11.8 kg, (normal sodium) NS]. Clearly, these data need to be confirmed in adequately powered larger trials; however, it appears that the restriction of dietary sodium may provide more BP lowering than the lowering of dialysate sodium. However, the latter maneuver is not without problems. In individuals with limited cardiovascular reserve relative to the ultrafiltration rates, a high sodium dialysate confers hemodynamic stability.[144] the lowering of dialysate sodium may cause intradialytic hypotension as well as limited ultrafiltration, thus paradoxically increasing BP.

DRUG THERAPIES FOR HEMODIALYSIS HYPERTENSION

The majority of patients with ESRD on chronic dialysis undergoing standard thrice weekly treatment need antihypertensive drug therapy.[149] However, several authorities have recommended that antihypertensive agents should be withdrawn and patients treated only with nonpharmacologic strategies to achieve BP control.[8,150] This approach, in this author's opinion, has several limitations, discussed below.

Whereas sodium plays an important role in the genesis of hypertension in the anephric state, sodium overload is not the only factor of importance in causing hypertension. If sodium overload were the only causative factor, it would follow that sodium restriction or diuretics would control hypertension in all patients. Clearly this is not the case; diuretics control BP in only half of hypertensive patients or less, because the etiology of hypertension is multifactorial.[151] Even among patients with renal failure, diuretics alone are insufficient in controlling hypertension. In trials of BP control in patients with CKD, multiple drugs are needed to control BP.[152,153] Limiting sodium intake and weight gain in the interdialytic period, although important—much as is glucose control in a patient with diabetes mellitus—this approach appears to be a high-effort, low-reward strategy.[154] The presumption that all hypertensive patients are above dry weight has, in the author's opinion, contributed to the lack of development of pharmacologic antihypertensive strategies in the dialysis population.

Several observational studies have suggested that the use of antihypertensive drugs is associated with improved survival.[155,156] Furthermore, among antihypertensive drugs, beta blockers have been reported to be associated with improved outcomes in observational studies.[157] Therefore it appears that the use of antihypertensive drugs at least does not increase mortality among hemodialysis patients.

Several classes of antihypertensive drugs are available and all except diuretics are effective in controlling hypertension in hemodialysis patients. The selection of these agents should be guided by considering their comorbidities, pharmacokinetics, and hemodynamic effects. For example, in patients with LV hypertrophy, ACE inhibitors may be effective in causing regression, although the trials have been limited in size.[158] Efrati et al. reported their experience from Israel in a retrospective cohort study of 60 patients who had

been treated with ACE inhibitors and 66 patients who had not received the drug.[159] Although BP reduction was not significantly different between the treated and untreated groups, mortality was reduced by 52 percent in the treated individuals (RR 0.48, 95 percent CI 0.25 to 0.91, p <0.002). The relative risk reduction in individuals above 65 years of age was particularly notable (RR 0.21, 95 percent CI 0.08 to 0.58, p = 0.0006). The magnitude of the benefit is such that this would need to be confirmed in randomized controlled trials.

Calcium channel blockers (CCBs) are the most widely prescribed class of drugs in patients on hemodialysis.[160,161] CCBs appear to be more effective when the plasma volume is expanded. Since hypertension in hemodialysis patients is thought to be largely a result of volume expansion, these agents may have a unique advantage in ESRD.[162] Both dihydropyridine[163–165] and nondihydropyridine CCBs have unaltered pharmacokinetics in patients with ESRD on hemodialysis and have little dialyzability.[166,167] Therefore no dose modifications are needed in ESRD. In an observational incident cohort of 2877 treated hypertensive patients starting hemodialysis or peritoneal dialysis followed from 1996 or 1997 until November 2000, nondihydropyridine CCBs were associated with a 22 percent reduction in risk of cardiovascular death.[168] In the subset of patients with preexisting cardiovascular disease, both dihydropyridine and nondihydropyridine CCBs were associated with reduced risk of all-cause and cardiovascular mortality. Kestenbaum et al. analyzed the relationship of CCB use and cardiovascular mortality in a prospective cohort of 4065 patients in the USRDS Morbidity and Mortality Wave II.[169] A total of 51 percent of the 3716 evaluable patients were prescribed a CCB. The use of a CCB was associated with a 21 percent lower risk of total mortality (RR 0.79, 95 percent CI 0.69 to 0.90) and a 26 percent lower risk of cardiovascular-specific mortality (RR 0.74, 95 percent CI 0.60 to 0.91). In patients with preexisting cardiovascular disease, CCB use was associated with a 23 and 22 percent lower risk of total and cardiovascular mortality, respectively.

In a smaller cohort of 188 patients on hemodialysis in Germany who were at high risk of cardiovascular events, administration of CCBs was associated with a striking 67 percent lower mortality.[170] These data dispel the concerns, raised in the past, regarding increased mortality with dihydropyridine CCBs in the general population.[171]

Few studies have examined the efficacy of CCBs for BP control in hemodialysis patients. Although sublingual nifedipine can lower BP in hemodialysis patients,[172] its use should be avoided due to reflex sympathetic activation. The long-acting dihydropyridine CCB, nitrendipine, administered in 40 chronic hemodialysis patients, showed a greater reduction in BP in volume-expanded patients.[173] The distensibility of large conduit vessels was improved with nitrendipine ; this correlated with improvement in LV ejection fraction but not LV mass. Subsequent reports showed that patients with arteriosclerosis (demonstrated by the presence of radiographic aortic calcifications) had a better antihypertensive response to nitrendipine.[174] Sustained-release verapamil controlled BP in 21 of 28 hypertensive ESRD patients.[175] Futhermore, a single dose of oral verapamil 40 mg given before hemodialysis to 10 patients with LV hypertrophy did not aggravate intradialytic hypotension.[176] Preliminary studies with verapamil have even suggested a reduction in intradialytic hypotension.[177]

Several nonhemodynamic benefits of these drugs are possible. For example, diltiazem has been reported to reduce the rate of increase in plasma potassium during the interdialytic period in hemodialysis patients.[178] The reduced rate of rise in plasma potassium was independent of cortisol, aldosterone, or glucose. Sustained-release diltiazem in a dose of 120 mg twice daily was effective in controlling both symptomatic and silent myocardial ischemia in hemodialysis patients.[179] Although lower doses relieved symptomatic angina, they were not effective in relieving silent ischemia. In addition, CCBs may reduce the risk of neointimal hyperplasia and angioaccess thrombosis,[180] neutrophil activation,[181] and cytokine transcription.[182] Thus, CCBs may provide some unique benefits in hemodialysis patients.

ACE inhibitors and beta blockers appear attractive agents due to their independent cardiovascular benefits. We have tested the utility of an antihypertensive agent from each class administered after dialysis in a supervised manner three times weekly to assess the safety and efficacy of these drugs. First we used atenolol, a water-soluble, renally excreted beta blocker, in 8 hemodialysis patients not receiving any antihypertensive drugs.[75] The half-life of atenolol is prolonged in hemodialysis patients, therefore we reasoned that thrice weekly administration would suffice. Since atenolol is removed by hemodialysis, intradialytic hypotension would be mitigated during the time of hemodynamic stress. After confirming hypertension by ABPM, patients were administered atenolol 25 mg following hemodialysis, and the dose of the drug was escalated at weekly intervals to 50 mg and finally 100 mg three times a week. The efficacy of therapy was judged by ambulatory BP monitoring 3 weeks after atenolol therapy was instituted. The mean 44-hour ambulatory BP fell from 144/80 to 127/69 mmHg (p <0.001). The systolic and diastolic BP loads were reduced from 71/30 to 35/11 percent, respectively ($p < 0.001$). There was a persistent antihypertensive effect over 44 hours. The BP reduction was achieved without any increase in intradialytic symptomatic or asymptomatic hypotensive episodes, reduction in delivered dialysis, or statistically significant changes in serum potassium or glucose. In patients on chronic dialysis, the hyperkalemic response to exercise is similar to that seen in normal individuals.[183] However, potassium disposal is associated with a greater norepineph-

rine and insulin response in dialysis patients. It is possible that the response to exercise-induced hyperkalemia may be blunted in situations of exercise in the presence of beta blockade or insulin deficiency. Therefore plasma potassium concentration should be carefully monitored in patients on beta blockers. We have also assessed the antihypertensive effects of lisinopril, a renally excreted ACE inhibitor administered three times weekly following dialysis.[184] Lisinopril was titrated at biweekly intervals at 10-, 20-, or 40-mg doses. If this was not effective after full titration (lisinopril to 40 mg three times weekly), ultrafiltration was added to reduce dry weight. The primary outcome variable was the change in BP from the end of the run-in period to the end of study. No change in mean ambulatory BP was noted during a 2-week run-in period. However, average 44-hour ambulatory BP fell from 149/84 to 127/73 mmHg—a fall of 22/11 mmHg (p <0.001) at final evaluation. Four patients received 10 mg, five 20 mg, and two 40 mg of lisinopril, of whom only one required ultrafiltration therapy. There was a persistent antihypertensive effect over 44 hours. The BP reduction was achieved without any increase in intradialytic symptomatic or asymptomatic hypotensive episodes. Therefore supervised lisinopril therapy was effective in controlling hypertension in patients on chronic hemodialysis. Although some studies have shown little contribution of ACE inhibitors to erythropoietin resistance,[185,186] others have shown that refractory anemia can occur.[187,188] Angiotensin II stimulates erythropoietin release from the kidney. In addition, n-acetyl-seryl-aspartyl-lysyl-proline (AcSDKP), a physiologic inhibitor of hematopoiesis, is degraded by ACE and is partially eliminated in the urine. Accumulation of AcSDKP occurs in ESRD patients and particularly in those treated by ACE inhibitors; this may partly explain erythropoietin hyporesponsiveness in ESRD patients.[189] In patients treated with ACE inhibitors, a high incidence of anaphylactoid reactions has been reported during dialysis with AN69 membranes due to the generation of bradykinin.[190] Thus, ACE inhibitors should not be used in combination with AN69 membranes.

Angiotensin II receptor blockers are also effective in hemodialysis patients. The pharmacokinetics of losartan have been carefully examined and remain unaltered in hemodialysis patients.[191] A multicenter, open label, 6-month study was performed in 406 patients to test the tolerability and efficacy of losartan in patients on hemodialysis.[192] A total of 15 patients discontinued the study due to adverse reactions related to losartan; in 7 of these, the adverse reaction was hypotension. In 2 patients, a possible anaphylactoid reaction was reported after dialysis with an AN69 membrane, necessitating termination of dialysis and losartan in 1 patient. In contrast, 9 patients with a history of previous anaphylactoid reaction with ACE inhibitor and AN69 did not show this complication with losartan and AN69. Thus, losartan is a well-tolerated antihypertensive drug in hemodialysis patients, with a very low incidence of adverse reactions and a lower incidence of anaphylactoid reactions than those detected with ACE inhibitors and AN69.

Several other options are available to control hypertension in hemodialysis patients besides beta blockers, ACE inhibitors, and angiotensin II receptor blockers. For example, transdermal clonidine applied at weekly intervals can improve hypertension control.[193] In addition, minoxidil, a potent vasodilator, is effective for hypertension control.[194] However, it should be used with beta blockers to maintain efficacy. Side–effects—which may include hirsuitism, pericardial effusion, and edema—should be carefully monitored.[195]

INCREASED FREQUENCY AND DURATION OF DIALYSIS

It has long been recognized that the long, slow dialysis (8 hours per session) provided by Charra et al. in Tassin, France, may better control uremia and hypertension instead of simply achieving dry weight. Studies comparing Tassin patients to Swedish patients demonstrate that despite higher ECF volume in Tassin, Tassin patients remained normotensive, a fact that "suggests that normotension may also be achieved in patients with fluid overload provided that the dialysis time is long enough to ensure more efficient removal of one or more vasoactive factors that cause or contribute to hypertension."[196] Therefore these dialysis modalities may be offering better control of uremia, not dry weight alone. More recent studies done in North America show that daily nocturnal dialysis improves BP control and often necessitates discontinuation of antihypertensive drugs.[197]

Chan et al. performed an observational cohort study of 13 dialysis patients treated with conventional hemodialysis and 28 patients treated with nocturnal hemodialysis.[198] BP was reduced significantly from 145/84 to 122/74 mmHg after 2 years in patients receiving nocturnal dialysis, despite reduction in the number of antihypertensive medications from 1.8 to 0.3 per day. In addition, the LV mass index improved from 147 to 114 g/m^2. Those on conventional dialysis did not show any significant change in BP, antihypertensive medications, or LV hypertrophy. No improvement in ECF volume reduction was seen and the improvement in LV hypertrophy was well correlated with improvement in systolic BP.

Fagugli et al. conducted a randomized crossover trial in 12 hemodialysis patients. After 6 months of run in on conventional hemodialysis, patients were randomized to either conventional or daily dialysis for 6 months and then crossed over to the other therapy for an additional 6 months.[199] Weekly Kt/V was held stable in the two groups. The authors reported ambulatory BP in the daily dialysis group improved from 146/78 to 128/73 mmHg and echocardiographic LV mass index improved from 173 g/m^2 to 120

g/m^2. The ECF volume improved from 59 to 48 percent with daily dialysis. Furthermore, a good correlation was seen between ECF volume and LV mass index or ambulatory BP regardless of assignment to daily or conventional dialysis. These data show that the mechanism of BP reduction with daily dialysis may at least in part be due to better ECF volume.

ARE THERE BENEFITS OF TREATING HYPERTENSION?

Long-term, adequately powered studies to discover an association between BP control and cardiovascular outcomes in hemodialysis patients are yet to be published. However, several smaller trials point out the benefits of treating high BP in hemodialysis patients. Foley et al. found a strong link between the LV hypertrophy and heart failure with increasing BP.[200] Cannella et al.[201] found that the treatment of hypertension with ACE inhibitor–based antihypertensive therapy is associated with regression of LV hypertrophy in these patients. Tomita et al., in a long-term follow-up study, found that hypertensive patients had poor outcomes; however, and more importantly, if systolic BP was lowered among hypertensives, patient survival was improved.[202] In the only interventional study, 153 French hemodialysis patients were treated for 54 months with antihypertensive drugs; as a result of dry-weight adjustments and correction of anemia, a BP reduction of 22/12 mmHg (from 169/90 mmHg to 147/78 mmHg) was achieved.[203] This strategy was associated with a reduction in LV mass from 290 ± 80 to 264 ± 86 g ($p < 0.01$). A 10 percent decline in LV mass was associated with a 22 percent improvement in total mortality and a 28 percent improvement in cardiovascular mortality. Although low diastolic BP is associated with increased cardiovascular events in the elderly population with essential hypertension, it is reassuring that treatment of isolated systolic hypertension in the elderly does not increase the risk of cardiovascular morbidity or mortality.[204]

ACKNOWLEDGMENT

The author acknowledges the support of the National Institutes of Health in the form of research grant NIH 5RO1-DK62030–02.

REFERENCES

1. Agarwal R, Nissenson AR, Batlle D, et al. Prevalence, treatment, and control of hypertension in chronic hemodialysis patients in the United States. *Am J Med* 2003; 115:291–297.
2. Guyton AC. The surprising kidney-fluid mechanism for pressure control—its infinite gain! *Hypertension* 1990;16: 725–730.

3. Coleman TG, Guyton AC. Hypertension caused by salt loading in the dog. 3. Onset transients of cardiac output and other circulatory variables. *Circ Res* 1969;25:153–160.

4. Fishbane S, Natke E, Maesaka JK. Role of volume overload in dialysis-refractory hypertension. *Am J Kidney Dis* 1996; 28:257–261.

5. Heidland A, Schaefer RM. Pathophysiology and treatment of hypertension in dialysis patients. *Adv Exp Med Biol* 1989;260:79–91.

6. Conway J, Lauwers P. Hemodynamic and hypotensive effects of long-term therapy with chlorothiazide. *Circulation* 1960;21:21–27.

7. Vasavada N, Agarwal R. Role of excess volume in the pathophysiology of hypertension in chronic kidney disease. *Kidney Int* 2003;64:1772–1779.

8. Charra B, Bergstrom J, Scribner BH. Blood pressure control in dialysis patients: importance of the lag phenomenon. *Am J Kidney Dis* 1998;32:720–724.

9. Kornerup HJ, Schmitz O, Danielsen H, et al. Significance of the renin-angiotensin system for blood pressure regulation in end-stage renal disease. *Contrib Nephrol* 1984;41: 123–127.

10. Henrich WL, Katz FH, Molinoff PB, Schrier RW. Competitive effects of hypokalemia and volume depletion on plasma renin activity, aldosterone and catecholamine concentrations in hemodialysis patients. *Kidney Int* 1977;12:279–284.

11. Agarwal R, Lewis RR, Davis JL, Becker B. Lisinopril therapy for hemodialysis hypertension—hemodynamic and endocrine responses. *Am J Kidney Dis* 2001;38:1245–1250.

12. McGrath BP. Autonomic component in hypertension accompanying renal failure. *Contrib Nephrol* 1984;41:83–89.

13. Converse RL Jr, Jacobsen TN, Toto RD, et al. Sympathetic overactivity in patients with chronic renal failure. *N Engl J Med* 1992;327:1912–1918.

14. Rascher W, Schomig A, Kreye VA, Ritz E. Diminished vascular response to noradrenaline in experimental chronic uremia. *Kidney Int* 1982;21:20–27.

15. Converse RL Jr, Jacobsen TN, Toto RD, et al. Sympathetic overactivity in patients with chronic renal failure. *N Engl J Med* 1992;327:1912–1918.

16. Vallbo AB, Hagbarth KE, Wallin BG: Microneurography: how the technique developed and its role in the investigation of the sympathetic nervous system. *J Appl Physiol* 2004;96: 1262–1269.

17. Converse RL Jr, Jacobsen TN, Toto RD, et al. Sympathetic overactivity in patients with chronic renal failure. *N Engl J Med* 1992;327:1912–1918.

18. Degli Esposti E, Sturani A, Santoro A, et al. Effect of bromocriptine treatment on prolactin, noradrenaline and blood pressure in hypertensive haemodialysis patients. *Clin Sci (Colch)* 1985; 69:51–56.

19. Ye S, Nosrati S, Campese VM. Nitric oxide (NO) modulates the neurogenic control of blood pressure in rats with chronic renal failure (CRF). *J Clin Invest* 1997;99:540–548.

20. Lazarus JM, Hampers CL, Lowrie EG, Merrill JP. Baroreceptor activity in normotensive and hypertensive uremic patients. *Circulation* 1973;47:1015–1021.

21. Furchgott RF. The discovery of endothelium-derived relaxing factor and its importance in the identification of nitric oxide. *JAMA* 1996;276:1186–1188.

22. Hand MF, Haynes WG, Webb DJ. Hemodialysis and L-arginine, but not D-arginine, correct renal failure-associated endothelial dysfunction. *Kidney Int* 1998;53:1068–1077.

23. Fujiwara N, Osanai T, Kamada T, et al. Study on the relationship between plasma nitrite and nitrate level and salt sensitivity in human hypertension: modulation of nitric oxide synthesis by salt intake. *Circulation* 2000;101: 856–861.

24. Vallance P, Leone A, Calver A, et al. Accumulation of an endogenous inhibitor of nitric oxide synthesis in chronic renal failure. *Lancet* 1992;339:572–575.

25. Mallamaci F, Tripepi G, Maas R, et al. Analysis of the relationship between norepinephrine and asymmetric dimethyl arginine levels among patients with end-stage renal disease. *J Am Soc Nephrol* 2004;15:435–441.

26. Zoccali C, Mallamaci F, Maas R, et al. Left ventricular hypertrophy, cardiac remodeling and asymmetric dimethylarginine (ADMA) in hemodialysis patients. *Kidney Int* 2002;62:339–345.

27. Cooke JP. Asymmetrical dimethylarginine: the uber marker? *Circulation* 2004;109:1813–1818.

28. Mallamaci F, Tripepi G, Maas R, et al. Analysis of the relationship between norepinephrine and asymmetric dimethyl arginine levels among patients with end-stage renal disease. *J Am Soc Nephrol* 2004;15:435–441.

29. Abraham PA, Macres MG. Blood pressure in hemodialysis patients during amelioration of anemia with erythropoietin. *J Am Soc Nephrol* 1991;2:927–936.

30. van de Borne P, Tielemans C, Vanherweghem J-L, Degaute J-P. Effect of recombinant human erythropoietin therapy on ambulatory blood pressure and heart rate in chronic hemodialysis patients. *Nephrol Dial Transplant* 1992;7: 45–49.

31. Canadian Erythropoietin Study Group. Effect of recombinant human erythropoietin therapy on blood pressure in hemodialysis patients. *Am J Nephrol* 1991;11:23–26.

32. Ishimitsu T, Tsukada H, Ogawa Y, et al. Genetic predisposition to hypertension facilitates blood pressure elevation in hemodialysis patients treated with erythropoietin. *Am J Med* 1993;94:401–406.

33. Lebel M, Kingma I, Grose JH, Langlois S. Effect of recombinant human erythropoietin therapy on ambulatory blood pressure in normotensive and in untreated borderline hypertensive hemodialysis patients. *Am J Hypertens* 1995;8: 545–551.

34. Koppensteiner R, Stockenhuber F, Jahn C, et al. Changes in determinants of blood rheology during treatment with haemodialysis and recombinant human erythropoietin. *BMJ* 1990;300:1626–1627.

35. Hand MF, Haynes WG, Johnstone HA, et al. Erythropoietin enhances vascular responsiveness to norepinephrine in renal failure. *Kidney Int* 1995;48:806–813.

36. Bode-Boger SM, Boger RH, Kuhn M, et al. Recombinant human erythropoietin enhances vasoconstrictor tone via endothelin-1 and constrictor prostanoids. *Kidney Int* 1996;50: 1255–1261.

37. Vaziri ND, Zhou XJ, Naqvi F, et al. Role of nitric oxide resistance in erythropoietin-induced hypertension in rats with chronic renal failure. *Am J Physiol* 1996;271:E113–E122.

38. Weiler EWJ, Saldanha LF, Khalil-Manesh F, et al. Relationship of Na-K-ATPase inhibitors to blood-pressure regulation in continuous ambulatory peritoneal dialysis and hemodialysis. *J Am Soc Nephrol* 1996;7:454–463.

39. Raine AEG, Bedford L, Simpson AWM, et al. Hyperparathyroidism, platelet intracellular free calcium and hypertension in chronic renal failure. *Kidney Int* 1993;43:700–705.

40. Goldsmith DJA, Covic AA, Venning MC, Ackrill P. Blood pressure reduction after parathyroidectomy for secondary hyperparathyroidism: further evidence implicating calcium homeostasis in blood pressure regulation. *Am J Kidney Dis* 1996;27:819–825.

41. Iseki K, Massry SG, Campese VM. Evidence for a role of PTH in the reduced pressor response to norepinephrine in chronic renal failure. *Kidney Int* 1985;28:11–15.

42. Ifudu O, Matthew JJ, Macey LJ, et al. Parathyroidectomy does not correct hypertension in patients on maintenance hemodialysis. *Am J Nephrol* 1998;18:28–34.

43. Koyama H, Tabata T, Nishzawa Y, et al. Plasma endothelin levels in patients with uraemia. *Lancet* 1989;1:991–992.

44. Franklin SS, Jacobs MJ, Wong ND, et al. Predominance of isolated systolic hypertension among middle-aged and elderly US hypertensives: analysis based on National Health and Nutrition Examination Survey (NHANES) III. *Hypertension* 2001;37:869–874.

45. McVeigh GE, Bratteli CW, Morgan DJ, et al. Age-related abnormalities in arterial compliance identified by pressure pulse contour analysis: aging and arterial compliance. *Hypertension* 1999;33:1392–1398.

46. O'Rourke MF. Wave travel and reflection in the arterial system. *J Hypertens* 1999;17(suppl 5):S45–S47.

47. van Bortel LM, Spek JJ. Influence of aging on arterial compliance. *J Hum Hypertens* 1998;12:583–586.

48. Black HR, Kuller LH, O'Rourke MF, et al. The first report of the Systolic and Pulse Pressure (SYPP) Working Group. *J Hypertens* 1999;17(suppl 5):S3–14.

49. O'Rourke MF. Wave travel and reflection in the arterial system. *J Hypertens* 1999;17(suppl 5):S45–S47.

50. Chobanian AV, Bakris GL, Black HR, et al. The Seventh Report of the Joint National Committee on Prevention, Detection, Evaluation, and Treatment of High Blood Pressure: the JNC 7 report. *JAMA* 2003;289:2560–2572.

51. Agarwal R, Lewis RR. Prediction of hypertension in chronic hemodialysis patients. *Kidney Int* 2001;60:1982–1989.

52. Rostand SG, Brunzell JD, Cannon ROI, Victor RG. Cardiovascular complications in renal failure. *J Am Soc Nephrol* 1991;2:1053–1062.

53. Guerin AP, London GM, Marchais SJ, Metivier F. Arterial stiffening and vascular calcifications in end-stage renal disease. *Nephrol Dial Transplant* 2000;15:1014–1021.

54. Demuth K, Blacher J, Guerin AP, et al. Endothelin and cardiovascular remodelling in end-stage renal disease. *Nephrol Dial Transplant* 1998;13:375–383.

55. Converse RL Jr, Jacobsen TN, Toto RD, et al. Sympathetic overactivity in patients with chronic renal failure. *N Engl J Med* 1992;327:1912–1918.

56. Tycho Vuurmans JL, Boer WH, Bos WJ, et al. Contribution of volume overload and angiotensin II to the increased pulse wave velocity of hemodialysis patients. *J Am Soc Nephrol* 2002;13:177–183.

57. Sherman RA, Daniel A, Cody RP. The effect of interdialytic weight gain on predialysis blood pressure. *Artif Organs* 1993;17:770–774.

58. Dionisio P, Valenti M, Bergia R, et al. Influence of the hydration state on blood pressure values in a group of patients on regular maintenance hemodialysis. *Blood Purif* 1997;15:25–33.

59. Lins RL, Elseviers M, Rogiers P, et al. Importance of volume factors in dialysis related hypertension. *Clin Nephrol* 1997;48:29–33.

60. Lins RL, Elseviers M, Rogiers P, et al. Importance of volume factors in dialysis related hypertension. *Clin Nephrol* 1997;48:29–33.

61. Ventura JE, Sposito M. Volume sensitivity of blood pressure in end-stage renal disease. *Nephrol Dial Transplant* 1997;12:485–491.

62. Rahman M, Griffin V, Kumar A, et al. A comparison of standardized versus "usual" blood pressure measurements in hemodialysis patients. *Am J Kidney Dis* 2002;39:1226–1230.

63. Kooman JP, Gladziwa U, Bocker G, et al. Blood pressure during the interdialytic period in haemodialysis patients: estimation of representative blood pressure values. *Nephrol Dial Transplant* 1992;7:917–923.

64. Baumgart P, Walger P, Gemen S, et al. Blood pressure elevation during the night in chronic renal failure, hemodialysis and after renal transplantation. *Nephron* 1991;57:293–298.

65. Rosansky SJ. Nocturnal hypertension in patients receiving chronic hemodialysis. *Ann Intern Med* 1991;114:96.

66. Jones MA, Sharpstone P, Dallyn PE, Kingswood JC. Reduced nocturnal blood pressure fall is similar in continuous ambulatory peritoneal dialysis to that in hemodialysis and undialysed end-stage renal disease. *Clin Nephrol* 1994;42:273–275.

67. Rosansky SJ. Nocturnal hypertension in patients receiving chronic hemodialysis. *Ann Intern Med* 1991;114:96.

68. Jones MA, Sharpstone P, Dallyn PE, Kingswood JC. Reduced nocturnal blood pressure fall is similar in continuous ambulatory peritoneal dialysis to that in hemodialysis and undialysed end-stage renal disease. *Clin Nephrol* 1994;42:273–275.

69. Cheigh JS, Milite C, Sullivan JF, et al. Hypertension is not adequately controlled in hemodialysis patients. *Am J Kidney Dis* 1992;19:453–459.

70. Amar J, Vernier I, Rossignol E, et al. Influence of nycthemeral blood pressure pattern in treated hypertensive patients on hemodialysis. *Kidney Int* 1997;51:1863–1866.

71. Amar J, Vernier I, Rossignol E, et al. Nocturnal blood pressure and 24-hour pulse pressure are potent indicators of mortality in hemodialysis patients. *Kidney Int* 2000;57:2485–2491.

72. Peixoto AJ, Santos SF, Mendes RB, et al. Reproducibility of ambulatory blood pressure monitoring in hemodialysis patients. *Am J Kidney Dis* 2000;36:983–990.

73. Kaupke CJ, Kim S, Vaziri ND. Effect of erythrocyte mass on arterial blood pressure in dialysis patients receiving maintenance erythropoietin therapy. *J Am Soc Nephrol* 1994;4:1874–1878.

74. Imai Y, Sekino H, Fujikura Y, et al. Pressor effect of recombinant human erythropoietin: results of ambulatory blood pressure monitoring and home blood pressure measurements. *Clin Exp Hypertens* 1995;17:485–506.

75. Agarwal R. Supervised atenolol therapy in management of hemodialysis hypertension. *Kidney Int* 1999;55:1528–1535.

76. Agarwal R, Lewis RR, Davis JL, Becker B. Lisinopril therapy for hemodialysis hypertension—Hemodynamic and endocrine responses. *Am J Kidney Dis* 2001;38:1245–1250.

77. Agarwal R, Lewis RR, Davis JL, Becker B. Lisinopril therapy for hemodialysis hypertension—hemodynamic and endocrine responses. *Am J Kidney Dis* 2001;38:1245–1250.

78. Mitra S, Chandna SM, Farrington K. What is hypertension in chronic haemodialysis? The role of interdialytic blood pressure monitoring. *Nephrol Dial Transplant* 1999;14:2915–2921.

79. Bobrie G, Chatellier G, Genes N, et al. Cardiovascular prognosis of "masked hypertension" detected by blood pressure self-measurement in elderly treated hypertensive patients. *JAMA* 2004;291:1342–1349.

80. Cannella G, Paoletti E, Ravera G, et al. Inadequate diagnosis and therapy of arterial hypertension as causes of left ventricular hypertrophy in uremic dialysis patients. *Kidney Int* 2000;58:260–268.

81. Bobrie G, Chatellier G, Genes N, et al. Cardiovascular prognosis of "masked hypertension" detected by blood pressure self-measurement in elderly treated hypertensive patients. *JAMA* 2004;291:1342–1349.

82. Zoccali C, Benedetto FA, Tripepi G, et al. Nocturnal hypoxemia, night-day arterial pressure changes and left ventricular geometry in dialysis patients. *Kidney Int* 1998;53:1078–1084.

83. Agarwal R, Lewis RR. Prediction of hypertension in chronic hemodialysis patients. *Kidney Int* 2001;60:1982–1989.

84. Mitra S, Chandna SM, Farrington K. What is hypertension in chronic haemodialysis? The role of interdialytic blood pressure monitoring. *Nephrol Dial Transplant* 1999;14:2915–2921.

85. Rodby RA, Vonesh EF, Korbet SM. Blood pressures in hemodialysis and peritoneal dialysis using ambulatory blood pressure monitoring. *Am J Kidney Dis* 1994;23:401–411.

86. Huisman RM, de Bruin C, Klont D, Smit AJ. Relationship between blood pressure during haemodialysis and ambulatory blood pressure in between dialyses. *Nephrol Dial Transplant* 1995;10:1890–1894.

87. Agarwal R, Lewis RR. Prediction of hypertension in chronic hemodialysis patients. *Kidney Int* 2001;60:1982–1989.

88. Coomer RW, Schulman G, Breyer JA, Shyr Y. Ambulatory blood pressure monitoring in dialysis patients and estimation of mean interdialytic blood pressure [see comments]. *Am J Kidney Dis* 1997;29:678–684.

89. Erturk S, Ertug AE, Ates K, et al. Relationship of ambulatory blood pressure monitoring data to echocardiographic findings in haemodialysis patients. *Nephrol Dial Transplant* 1996;11:2050–2054.

90. Conlon PJ, Walshe JJ, Heinle SK, et al. Predialysis systolic blood pressure correlates strongly with mean 24-hour systolic blood pressure and left ventricular mass in stable hemodialysis patients. *J Am Soc Nephrol* 1996;7:2658–2663.

91. Zoccali C, Mallamaci F, Tripepi G, et al. Prediction of left ventricular geometry by clinic, pre-dialysis and 24-h ambulatory BP monitoring in hemodialysis patients: CREED investigators. *J Hypertens* 1999;17:1751–1758.

92. Zoccali C. Prediction of hypertension in hemodialysis patients. *Kidney Int* 2002;61:1179–1184.

93. Agarwal R. Reply from the author. *Kidney Int* 2002;61:1180–1181.

94. Cannella G, Paoletti E, Ravera G, et al. Inadequate diagnosis and therapy of arterial hypertension as causes of left ventricular hypertrophy in uremic dialysis patients. *Kidney Int* 2000;58:260–268.

95. Agarwal R, Lewis RR. Prediction of hypertension in chronic hemodialysis patients. *Kidney Int* 2001;60:1982–1989.

96. Mitra S, Chandna SM, Farrington K. What is hypertension in chronic haemodialysis? The role of interdialytic blood pressure monitoring. *Nephrol Dial Transplant* 1999;14:2915–2921.

97. Agarwal R. Role of home blood pressure monitoring in hemodialysis patients. *Am J Kidney Dis* 1999;33:682–687.

98. Yarows SA, Julius S, Pickering TG. Home blood pressure monitoring. *Arch Intern Med* 2000;160:1251–1257.

99. Chobanian AV, Bakris GL, Black HR, et al. The Seventh Report of the Joint National Committee on Prevention, Detection, Evaluation, and Treatment of High Blood Pressure: the JNC 7 report. *JAMA* 2003;289:2560–2572.

100. Port FK, Hulbert-Shearon TE, Wolfe RA, et al. Predialysis blood pressure and mortality risk in a national sample of maintenance hemodialysis patients. *Am J Kidney Dis* 1999;33:507–517.

101. Zager PG, Nikolic J, Brown RH, et al. "U" curve association of blood pressure and mortality in hemodialysis patients. Medical Directors of Dialysis Clinic, Inc [published erratum appears in *Kidney Int* 1998 Oct;54(4):1417]. *Kidney Int* 1998;54:561–569.

102. Rahman M, Griffin V, Kumar A, et al. A comparison of standardized versus "usual" blood pressure measurements in hemodialysis patients. *Am J Kidney Dis* 2002;39:1226–1230.

103. Agarwal R. Assessment of blood pressure in hemodialysis patients. *Semin Dial* 2002;15:299–304.

104. Erturk S, Ertug AE, Ates K, et al. Relationship of ambulatory blood pressure monitoring data to echocardiographic findings in haemodialysis patients. *Nephrol Dial Transplant* 1996;11:2050–2054.

105. Mansoor GA, White WB. Ambulatory blood pressure monitoring is a useful clinical tool in nephrology. *Am J Kidney Dis* 1997;30:591–605.

106. Agarwal R, Lewis RR. Prediction of hypertension in chronic hemodialysis patients. *Kidney Int* 2001;60:1982–1989.

107. Santos SF, Mendes RB, Santos CA, et al. Profile of interdialytic blood pressure in hemodialysis patients. *Am J Nephrol* 2003;23:96–105.

108. Peixoto AJ, Santos SF, Mendes RB, et al. Reproducibility of ambulatory blood pressure monitoring in hemodialysis patients. *Am J Kidney Dis* 2000;36:983–990.

109. Amar J, Vernier I, Rossignol E, et al. Nocturnal blood pressure and 24-hour pulse pressure are potent indicators of mortality in hemodialysis patients. *Kidney Int* 2000;57:2485–2491.

110. Liu Y, Coresh J, Eustace JA, et al. Association between cholesterol level and mortality in dialysis patients: role of inflammation and malnutrition. *JAMA* 2004;291:451–459.

111. Foley RN, Parfrey PS, Harnett JD, et al. Impact of hypertension on cardiomyopathy, morbidity and mortality in end-stage renal disease. *Kidney Int* 1996;49:1379–1385.

112. Tomita J, Kimura G, Inoue T, et al. Role of systolic blood pressure in determining prognosis of hemodialyzed patients. *Am J Kidney Dis* 1995;25:405–412.

113. Kimura G, Tomita J, Nakamura S, et al. Interaction between hypertension and other cardiovascular risk factors in survival of hemodialyzed patients. *Am J Hypertens* 1996;9: 1006–1012.

114. Charra B. Control of blood pressure in long slow hemodialysis. *Blood Purif* 1994;12:252–258.

115. Tozawa M, Iseki K, Iseki C, et al. Evidence for elevated pulse pressure in patients on chronic hemodialysis: a case-control study. *Kidney Int* 2002;62:2195–2201.

116. De Lima JJ, Vieira ML, Abensur H, Krieger EM. Baseline blood pressure and other variables influencing survival on haemodialysis of patients without overt cardiovascular disease. *Nephrol Dial Transplant* 2001;16:793–797.

117. Duranti E, Imperiali P, Sasdelli M. Is hypertension a mortality risk factor in dialysis? *Kidney Int Suppl* 1996;55: S173–S174.

118. Lynn KL, McGregor DO, Moesbergen T, et al. Hypertension as a determinant of survival for patients treated with home dialysis. *Kidney Int* 2002;62:2281–2287.

119. Mazzuchi N, Carbonell E, Fernandez-Cean J. Importance of blood pressure control in hemodialysis patient survival. *Kidney Int* 2000;58:2147–2154.

120. Goodkin DA, Bragg-Gresham JL, Koenig KG, et al. Association of comorbid conditions and mortality in hemodialysis patients in Europe, Japan, and the United States: the Dialysis Outcomes and Practice Patterns Study (DOPPS). *J Am Soc Nephrol* 2002;14:3270–3277.

121. Port FK, Hulbert-Shearon TE, Wolfe RA, et al. Predialysis blood pressure and mortality risk in a national sample of maintenance hemodialysis patients. *Am J Kidney Dis* 1999; 33:507–517.

122. Zager PG, Nikolic J, Brown RH, et al. "U" curve association of blood pressure and mortality in hemodialysis patients. Medical Directors of Dialysis Clinic, Inc [published erratum appears in *Kidney Int* 1998 Oct;54(4):1417]. *Kidney Int* 1998;54:561–569.

123. Blacher J, Guerin AP, Pannier B, et al. Impact of aortic stiffness on survival in end-stage renal disease. *Circulation* 1999;99:2434–2439.

124. O'Rourke MF. Wave travel and reflection in the arterial system. *J Hypertens* 17(suppl 5):S45–S47.

125. Blacher J, Guerin AP, Pannier B, et al. Impact of aortic stiffness on survival in end-stage renal disease. *Circulation* 1999;99:2434–2439.

126. Chobanian AV, Bakris GL, Black HR, et al. The Seventh Report of the Joint National Committee on Prevention, Detection, Evaluation, and Treatment of High Blood Pressure: the JNC 7 report. *JAMA* 2003;289:2560–2572.

127. Goodman WG, Goldin J, Kuizon BD, et al. Coronary-artery calcification in young adults with end-stage renal disease

128. who are undergoing dialysis. *N Engl J Med* 2000;342: 1478–1483.

128. Salem MM. Hypertension in the haemodialysis population: any relationship to 2 years survival? *Nephrol Dial Transplant* 1999;14:125–128.

129. Klassen PS, Lowrie EG, Reddan DN, et al. Association between pulse pressure and mortality in patients undergoing maintenance hemodialysis. *JAMA* 2002;287:1548–1555.

130. Benetos A. Pulse pressure and cardiovascular risk. *J Hypertens* 1999;17(suppl 5):S21–S24.

131. Black HR. Isolated systolic hypertension in the elderly: lessons from clinical trials and future directions. *J Hypertens* 17(suppl 5):S49–S54.

132. Kjeldsen SE, Dahlof B, Devereux RB, et al. Effects of losartan on cardiovascular morbidity and mortality in patients with isolated systolic hypertension and left ventricular hypertrophy: a Losartan Intervention for Endpoint Reduction (LIFE) substudy. *JAMA* 2002;288:1491–1498.

133. Staessen JA, Fagard R, Thijs L, et al. Randomised double-blind comparison of placebo and active treatment for older patients with isolated systolic hypertension. The Systolic Hypertension in Europe (Syst-Eur) Trial Investigators. *Lancet* 1997;350:757–764.

134. Tozawa M, Iseki K, Iseki C, Takishita S. Pulse pressure and risk of total mortality and cardiovascular events in patients on chronic hemodialysis. *Kidney Int* 2002;61:717–726.

135. Foley RN, Herzog CA, Collins AJ. Blood pressure and long-term mortality in United States hemodialysis patients: USRDS Waves 3 and 4 Study. *Kidney Int* 2002;62: 1784–1790.

136. Klassen PS, Lowrie EG, Reddan DN, et al. Association between pulse pressure and mortality in patients undergoing maintenance hemodialysis. *JAMA* 2002;287:1548–1555.

137. Lewington S, Clarke R, Qizilbash N, et al. Age-specific relevance of usual blood pressure to vascular mortality: a meta-analysis of individual data for one million adults in 61 prospective studies. *Lancet* 2002;360:1903–1913.

138. Zager PG, Nikolic J, Brown RH, et al. "U" curve association of blood pressure and mortality in hemodialysis patients. Medical Directors of Dialysis Clinic, Inc [published erratum appears in *Kidney Int* 1998 Oct;54(4):1417]. *Kidney Int* 1998;54:561–569.

139. Szczech LA, Reddan DN, Klassen PS, et al. Interactions between dialysis-related volume exposures, nutritional surrogates and mortality among ESRD patients. *Nephrol Dial Transplant* 2003;18:1585–1591.

140. Foley RN, Herzog CA, Collins AJ. Blood pressure and long-term mortality in United States hemodialysis patients: USRDS Waves 3 and 4 Study. *Kidney Int* 2002;62: 1784–1790.

141. Shaldon S. Dietary salt restriction and drug-free treatment of hypertension in ESRD patients: a largely abandoned therapy. *Nephrol Dial Transplant* 2002;17:1163–1165.

142. Ozkahya M, Ok E, Cirit M, et al. Regression of left ventricular hypertrophy in haemodialysis patients by ultrafiltration and reduced salt intake without antihypertensive drugs. *Nephrol Dial Transplant* 1998;13:1489–1493.

143. Charra B. "Dry weight" in dialysis: the history of a concept. *Nephrol Dial Transplant* 1998;13:1882–1885.

144. Henrich WL, Woodard TD, McPhaul JJ Jr. The chronic efficacy and safety of high sodium dialysate: double-blind, crossover study. *Am J Kidney Dis* 1982;2:349–353.

145. Oliver MJ, Edwards LJ, Churchill DN. Impact of sodium and ultrafiltration profiling on hemodialysis-related symptoms. *J Am Soc Nephrol* 2001;12:151–156.

146. Krautzig S, Janssen U, Koch KM, et al. Dietary salt restriction and reduction of dialysate sodium to control hypertension in maintenance haemodialysis patients. *Nephrol Dial Transplant* 1998;13:552–553.

147. Kooman JP, Hendriks EJ, van Den Sande FM, Leumissen KM. Dialysate sodium concentration and blood pressure control in haemodialysis patients. *Nephrol Dial Transplant* 2000;15:554.

148. Maduell F, Navarro V. Dietary salt intake and blood pressure control in haemodialysis patients. *Nephrol Dial Transplant* 2000;15:2063.

149. Agarwal R, Nissenson AR, Batlle D, et al. Prevalence, treatment, and control of hypertension in chronic hemodialysis patients in the United States. *Am J Med* 2003;115: 291–297.

150. Shaldon S. Dietary salt restriction and drug-free treatment of hypertension in ESRD patients: a largely abandoned therapy. *Nephrol Dial Transplant* 2000;17:1163–1165.

151. Dickerson JE, Hingorani AD, Ashby MJ, et al. Optimisation of antihypertensive treatment by crossover rotation of four major classes. *Lancet* 1999;353:2008–2013.

152. Klahr S, Levey AS, Beck GJ, et al. The effects of dietary protein restriction and blood-pressure control on the progression of chronic renal disease. Modification of Diet in Renal Disease Study Group. *N Engl J Med* 1994;330: 877–884.

153. Wright JT Jr, Bakris G, Greene T, et al. Effect of blood pressure lowering and antihypertensive drug class on progression of hypertensive kidney disease: results from the AASK trial. *JAMA* 2002;288:2421–2431.

154. Laakso M. Benefits of strict glucose and blood pressure control in type 2 diabetes: lessons from the UK Prospective Diabetes Study. *Circulation* 1999;99:461–462.

155. Zager PG, Nikolic J, Brown RH, et al. "U" curve association of blood pressure and mortality in hemodialysis patients. Medical Directors of Dialysis Clinic, Inc [published erratum appears in *Kidney Int* 1998 Oct;54(4):1417]. *Kidney Int* 1998;54:561–569.

156. Salem MM, Bower J. Hypertension in the hemodialysis population: any relation to one-year survival? *Am J Kidney Dis* 1996;28:737–740.

157. Foley RN, Herzog CA, Collins AJ. Blood pressure and long-term mortality in United States hemodialysis patients: USRDS Waves 3 and 4 study. *Kidney Int* 2002;62: 1784–1790.

158. Paoletti E, Cassottana P, Bellino D, et al. Left ventricular geometry and adverse cardiovascular events in chronic hemodialysis patients on prolonged therapy with ACE inhibitors. *Am J Kidney Dis* 2002;40:728–736.

159. Efrati S, Zaidenstein R, Dishy V, et al. ACE inhibitors and survival of hemodialysis patients. *Am J Kidney Dis* 2002; 40:1023–1029.

160. Agarwal R, Nissenson AR, Batlle D, et al. Prevalence, treatment, and control of hypertension in chronic hemodialysis patients in the United States. *Am J Med* 2003;115:291–297.

161. Griffith TF, Chua BS, Allen AS, et al. Characteristics of treated hypertension in incident hemodialysis and peritoneal dialysis patients. *Am J Kidney Dis* 2003;42:1260–1269.

162. Salvetti A, Bozzo MV, Graziola M, Abdel-Haq B. Acute hemodynamic effect of nifedipine in hypertension with chronic renal failure: the influence of volume status. *J Cardiovasc Pharmacol* 1987;10(suppl 10):143–146.

163. Schonholzer K, Marone C. Pharmacokinetics and dialysability of isradipine in chronic hemodialysis patients. *Eur J Clin Pharmacol* 1992;42:231–233.

164. Buur T, Larsson R, Regardh CG, Aberg J. Pharmacokinetics of felodipine in chronic hemodialysis patients. *J Clin Pharmacol* 1991;31:709–713.

165. Kungys G, Naujoks H, Wanner C. Pharmacokinetics of amlodipine in hypertensive patients undergoing haemodialysis. *Eur J Clin Pharmacol* 59:291–295, 2003

166. Zachariah PK, Moyer TP, Theobald HM, et al. The pharmacokinetics of racemic verapamil in patients with impaired renal function. *J Clin Pharmacol* 1991;31:45–53.

167. Hanyok JJ, Chow MSS, Kluger J, Izard MW. An evaluation of the pharmacokinetics, pharmacodynamics, and dialyzability of verapamil in chronic hemodialysis patients. *J Clin Pharmacol* 1988;28:831–836.

168. Griffith TF, Chua BS, Allen AS, et al. Characteristics of treated hypertension in incident hemodialysis and peritoneal dialysis patients. *Am J Kidney Dis* 2003;42:1260–1269.

169. Kestenbaum B, Gillen DL, Sherrard DJ, et al. Calcium channel blocker use and mortality among patients with end-stage renal disease. *Kidney Int* 2002;61:2157–2164.

170. Tepel M, Giet MV, Park A, Zidek W. Association of calcium channel blockers and mortality in haemodialysis patients. *Clin Sci (Lond)* 2002;103:511–515.

171. Furberg CD, Psaty BM, Meyer JV. Nifedipine. Dose-related increase in mortality in patients with coronary heart disease (see comments). *Circulation* 1995;92:1326–1331.

172. Hannedouche T, Josse S, Godin M, Fillastre JP. Efficacy of sublingual nifedipine in the acute treatment of hypertension in hemodialysis patients. *Curr Ther Res* 1985;38:383–385.

173. London GM, Marchais SJ, Guerin AP, et al. Salt and water retention and calcium blockade in uremia. *Circulation* 1990; 82:105–113.

174. Marchais SJ, Boussac I, Guerin AP, et al. Arteriosclerosis and antihypertensive response to calcium antagonists in end-stage renal failure. *J Cardiovasc Pharmacol* 1991;18 (suppl 5): S14–S18.

175. Beyerlein C, Csaszar G, Hollmann M, Schumacher A. Verapamil in antihypertensive treatment of patients on renal replacement therapy—clinical implications and pharmacokinetics. *Eur J Clin Pharmacol* 1990;39(suppl 1):S35–S37.

176. Sherman RA, Casale P, Cody R, Horton MW. Effect of predialysis verapamil on intradialytic blood pressure in chronic hemodialysis patients. *ASAIO Trans* 1990;36:67–69.

177. Whelton PK, Watson AJ, Kone B, Fortuin NJ. Calcium channel blockade in dialysis patients with left ventricular hypertrophy and well-preserved systolic function. *J Cardiovasc Pharmacol* 1987;10(suppl 10):S185–S186.

178. Solomon R, Dubey A. Diltiazem enhances potassium disposal in subjects with end-stage renal disease. *Am J Kidney Dis* 1992;19:420–426.

179. Cice G, Di Benedetto A, D'Andrea A, et al. Sustained-release diltiazem reduces myocardial ischemic episodes in end-stage renal disease: a double-blind, randomized, crossover, placebo-controlled trial. *J Am Soc Nephrol* 2003; 14:1006–1011.

180. Taber TE, Maikranz PS, Haag BW, et al. Maintenance of adequate hemodialysis access—prevention of neointimal hyperplasia. *ASAIO J* 1995;41:842–846.

181. Haag-Weber M, Schollmeyer P, Horl WH. Granulocyte activation during hemodialysis in the absence of complement activation: inhibition by calcium channel blockers. *Eur J Clin Invest* 1988;18:380–385.

182. Haag-Weber M, Mai B, Horl WH. Normalization of enhanced neutrophil cytosolic free calcium of hemodialysis patients by 1,25-dihydroxyvitamin D_3 or calcium channel blocker. *Am J Nephrol* 1993;13:467–472.

183. Clark BA, Shannon C, Brown RS, Gervino EV. Extrarenal potassium homeostasis with maximal exercise in end-stage renal disease. *J Am Soc Nephrol* 1996;7:1223–1227.

184. Agarwal R, Lewis RR, Davis JL, Becker B. Lisinopril therapy for hemodialysis hypertension— hemodynamic and endocrine responses. *Am J Kidney Dis* 2001;38:1245–1250.

185. Charytan C, Goldfarb-Rumyantzev A, Wang YF, et al. Effect of angiotensin-converting enzyme inhibitors on response to erythropoietin therapy in chronic dialysis patients. *Am J Nephrol* 1998;18:498–503.

186. Cruz DN, Perazella MA, Abu-Alfa AK, Mahnensmith RL. Angiotensin-converting enzyme inhibitor therapy in chronic hemodialysis patients: any evidence of erythropoietin resistance? *Am J Kidney Dis* 1996;28:535–540.

187. Hirakata H, Onoyama K, Hori K, Fujishima M. Participation of the renin-angiotensin system in the captopril-induced worsening of anemia in chronic hemodialysis patients. *Clin Nephrol* 1986;26:27–32.

188. Matsumura M, Nomura H, Koni I, Mabuchi H. Angiotensin-converting enzyme inhibitors are associated with the need for increased recombinant human erythropoietin maintenance doses in hemodialysis patients. Risks of Cardiac Disease in Dialysis Patients Study Group. *Nephron* 1997;77: 164–168

189. Le Meur Y, Lorgeot V, Comte L, et al. Plasma levels and metabolism of AcSDKP in patients with chronic renal failure: relationship with erythropoietin requirements. *Am J Kidney Dis* 2001;38:510–517.

190. Verresen L, Fink E, Lemke HD, Vanrenterghem Y. Bradykinin is a mediator of anaphylactoid reactions during hemodialysis with AN69 membranes. *Kidney Int* 1994;45: 1497–1503.

191. Sica DA, Halstenson CE, Gehr TW, Keane WF. Pharmacokinetics and blood pressure response of losartan in end-stage renal disease. *Clin Pharmacokinet* 2000;38:519–526.

192. Saracho R, Martin-Malo A, Martinez I, et al. Evaluation of the Losartan in Hemodialysis (ELHE) Study. *Kidney Int Suppl* 1998;68:S125–S129.

193. Rosansky SJ, Johnson KL, McConnel J. Use of transdermal clonidine in chronic hemodialysis patients. *Clin Nephrol* 1993;39:32–36.

194. Camel GH, Carmody SE, Perry HM Jr. Use of minoxidil in the azotemic patient. *J Cardiovasc Pharmacol* 2(suppl 2: S173–S180.

195. Campese VM, Stein D, DeQuattro V. Treatment of severe hypertension with minoxidil: advantages and limitations. *J Clin Pharmacol* 1979;19:231–241.

196. Katzarski KS, Charra B, Luik AJ, et al. Fluid state and blood pressure control in patients treated with long and short haemodialysis. *Nephrol Dial Transplant* 1999;14:369–375.

197. Pierratos A, Ouwendyk M, Francoeur R, et al. Nocturnal hemodialysis: three-year experience [see comments]. *J Am Soc Nephrol* 1998;9:859–868.

198. Chan CT, Floras JS, Miller JA, et al. Regression of left ventricular hypertrophy after conversion to nocturnal hemodialysis. *Kidney Int* 2002;61:2235–2239.

199. Fagugli RM, Reboldi G, Quintaliani G, et al. Short daily hemodialysis: blood pressure control and left ventricular mass reduction in hypertensive hemodialysis patients. *Am J Kidney Dis* 2001;38:371–376.

200. Foley RN, Parfrey PS, Harnett JD, et al. Impact of hypertension on cardiomyopathy, morbidity and mortality in end-stage renal disease. *Kidney Int* 1996;49:1379–1385.

201. Cannella G, Paoletti E, Delfino R, et al. Prolonged therapy with ACE inhibitors induces a regression of left ventricular hypertrophy of dialyzed uremic patients independently from hypotensive effects. *Am J Kidney Dis* 1997;30:659–664.

202. Tomita J, Kimura G, Inoue T, et al. Role of systolic blood pressure in determining prognosis of hemodialyzed patients. *Am J Kidney Dis* 1995;25:405–412.

203. London GM, Pannier B, Guerin AP, et al. Alterations of left ventricular hypertrophy in and survival of patients receiving hemodialysis: follow-up of an interventional study. *J Am Soc Nephrol* 2001;12:2759–2767.

204. Somes GW, Pahor M, Shorr RI, et al. The role of diastolic blood pressure when treating isolated systolic hypertension. *Arch Intern Med* 1999;159:2004–2009.

28

Lipoprotein Metabolism and Dyslipidemia in Dialysis Patients

T. M. Chan
M. K. Chan

Death from cardiovascular disease remains a major cause of mortality among dialysis patients.[1–4] Multiple causes—including hyperlipidemia, hypertension, inadequate dialysis, vascular calcification, and subclinical inflammation—all contribute to the pathogenesis of accelerated vascular disease. This chapter presents an overview of the pathogenesis, spectrum, and management of lipid abnormalities in dialysis.

A BRIEF REVIEW OF LIPOPROTEIN METABOLISM

Lipids such as cholesterol and triglycerides are insoluble in water and are transported in the plasma as lipoproteins, with a hydrophobic nonpolar core of cholesteryl esters and triglycerides covered by a hydrophilic coat of apolipoproteins, phospholipids, and unesterified (free) cholesterol. Apart from facilitating the solubilization and transport of lipids, apolipoproteins participate in the metabolism of

lipoproteins and can act as ligands for lipoprotein receptors or cofactors for lipolytic enzymes and lipid transferases. Apolipoproteins follow an alphabetical nomenclature. Increased apo B–containing and decreased apo AI–containing lipoproteins are implicated in atherogenesis. Lipoproteins differ in their relative composition of core lipids and surface apoproteins (Table 28–1) and thus can be classified according to their mobility under an electrical field, or flotation density. Larger lipoproteins contain more core lipids and are less dense than the smaller lipoproteins. Four major classes of lipoproteins are recognized: very low density lipoproteins (VLDLs), intermediate-density lipoproteins (IDLs), low-density lipoproteins (LDLs), and high-density lipoproteins (HDLs).

Chylomicrons are large lipoproteins formed in the lacteal vessels after the adsorption of fat. They transport the "consumed dietary fat" from the intestines to the bloodstream. Triglycerides constitute over 90 percent of the core

TABLE 28–1. COMPOSITION OF LIPOPROTEINS

Lipoprotein Class	Major Lipids	Major Apolipoproteins
Chylomicron	Triglyceride	Apo B48, apo CI, apo CII, apo CIII, apo E
VLDL	Triglyceride	Apo B100, apo CI, apo CII, apo CIII, apo E
IDL	Triglyceride	Apo B100, apo CI, apo CII, apo CIII, apo E
LDL	Cholesterol	Apo B100
Lp(a)	Cholesterol	Apo(a), apo B100
HDL2 and HDL3	phospholipids	Apo AI, apo AII, apo CI, apo CII, apo CIII, apo E

KEY: VLDL, very low density lipoprotein; IDL, intermediate-density lipoprotein; LDL, low-density lipoprotein; HDL, high-density lipoprotein.

of lipids. The apolipoprotein (apo) B48, a truncated form of apo B100, synthesized in the intestine and present in the surface coat of chylomicrons, is involved in the transport process. VLDL, which transports fat of hepatic or endogenous origin, is a relatively large lipoprotein particle synthesized in the liver. The core lipids include triglycerides, which account for about 60 percent of the mass of VLDL; cholesteryl esters; and phospholipids. The major apolipoprotein of VLDL is apo B100, which is synthesized in the liver and is necessary for the hepatic secretion of VLDL. IDL, which contains both triglyceride and cholesterol in similar proportions, is a metabolic product from VLDL and the precursor of LDL.

The liver is the major organ for endogenous cholesterol synthesis, which starts from malonyl-CoA. The rate-limiting step is mediated by 3-hydroxy-3-methylglutaryl coenzyme A (HMG-CoA) reductase. Cholesterol is the main lipid constituent of LDL, which contains little triglyceride. During conversion from VLDL to IDL then LDL, the apo B100 molecule remains attached. The apo B containing lipoproteins can be further classified according to size or density. LDL can be classified by density-gradient centrifugation into large light LDLI (d 1.025 to 1.034 g/mL), LDLII (d 1.034 to 1.044 g/mL), and small dense LDLIII (d 1.044 to 1.063 g/mL). There is increasing evidence for an association between small dense LDL and coronary atherosclerosis,[5,6] and the combination of hypertriglyceridemia, increased small dense LDL, and low HDL are physiologically linked and has been described as the atherogenic lipoprotein phenotype. While reduced hepatic lipase activity and increased LDL buoyancy have been associated with treatment-induced regression of coronary atherosclerosis,[7] whether the LDL particle size alone is a determining factor for atherogenicity remains controversial. VLDL can also be classified into large light triglyceride-rich VLDLI or small dense cholesteryl ester-rich VLDLII, which are under separate regulatory mechanisms, with hypertriglyceridemia and insulin resistance increasing the synthesis of VLDLI and hypercholesterolemia increasing the level of VLDLII.[8] Lipoprotein(a) [Lp(a)] consists of a molecule of LDL linked through a disulfide bridge on apo B to apo (a), a protein homologous to plasminogen. It is speculated that Lp(a) may inhibit the activation of plasminogen to plasmin, thereby reducing fibrinolytic activity.[9] Lp(a) is synthesized in the liver, and its level is inversely related to size polymorphism of apo (a).[10] Lp(a) has been demonstrated as a heritable independent risk factor for premature cardiovascular disease.[11–15]

The core lipids in HDL include cholesteryl ester and some triglyceride, surrounded by phospholipids and apolipoproteins. HDLs may be categorized into those with apo AI as the major apolipoprotein or those containing both apo AI and apo AII. The liver synthesizes both apo AI and apo AII, while the intestine produces only apo AI. HDL can be further classified by ultracentrifugation into subfractions. Thus HDL2 includes larger, more buoyant particles while HDL3 includes smaller, denser particles. Nascent or pre–β HDL includes particles with a higher density than HDL3. Apo AI on the nascent cholesterol-poor HDL particle interacts with the ATP-binding cassette transporter protein ABCA1 on the surface of peripheral cells and macrophages to remove cholesterol from these cells. The cholesterol is then esterified by lecithin-cholesterol acyltransferase (LCAT). The HDL3 thus formed can be converted to the bigger and less dense HDL2 with the further increase in cholesterol content. Variations in the cholesteryl ester content, the transfer of cholesteryl ester or phospholipid with apo B–containing lipoproteins, and remodeling through delipidation all contribute to the heterogeneity of HDL particles, and LCAT plays an important role in the maturation of HDL. HDL transports lipids from the periphery to the liver. Through the interaction between apo AI on HDL particles and BI scavenger receptors, HDL cholesterol is taken up by the liver, which then secretes free cholesterol directly into the bile or converts it into bile acids. Cholesteryl esters in HDL can also be transferred to apo B–containing lipoproteins in exchange for triglyceride through the action of cholesteryl ester transfer protein (CETP). Hepatic and endothelial lipase promote the catabolism of HDL through hydrolysis of their lipid content to generate smaller HDL particles. For example, hydrolysis of the triglyceride in HDL2 by hepatic lipase results in its conversion to the smaller HDL3.[16,17] Apart from the potential beneficial effects of this "reverse cholesterol transport," HDL has been demonstrated to exhibit antioxidant and anti-inflammatory properties.[18–20]

Serum HDL cholesterol concentrations are inversely related to the total body exchangeable cholesterol pool as well as the risk of coronary heart disease. The functional variations in different HDL particles may relate to the heterogeneity of apolipoproteins. In addition, different HDL particles may vary in their biosynthetic or metabolic pathways. For example, HDL2 and increased apo AII content of HDL particles are both linked to higher substrate affinity towards hepatic lipase.[21]

The apolipoprotein moieties of individual lipoproteins serve important physiologic regulatory functions in lipoprotein metabolism. Apo CII activates lipoprotein lipase, while apo CIII does the opposite. Apo AI is the major apolipoprotein in HDL, and it activates LCAT. Apo AII, also found in HDL particles, activates hepatic lipase and may inhibit LCAT. Apo B100 is the major apolipoprotein in LDL and is recognized by specific receptors. Apo B48 serves as a structural protein of chylomicrons, while the other apolipoprotein, apo E, is recognized by hepatic receptors.

With the exception of apo B48, apo B100, and apo (a), all apolipoproteins can freely exchange between different lipoproteins. Such exchange not only enhances the metabolic processing of the individual lipoproteins but also increases the plasma residence time of the apolipoproteins themselves. The metabolism of HDLs is an example. HDLs are synthesized in the liver or derived from chylomicrons and VLDLs through intravascular lipolysis. The liver secretes nascent HDL particles, which are bilayer disks of phospholipids and free cholesterol. These are transformed into spherical particles by the action of LCAT, which esterifies the free cholesterols on the surface of the bilayer and tucks them into the center of the particle. When triglyceride-rich lipoproteins, such as chylomicrons and VLDLs, enter the circulation, they acquire most of their apo C and apo E from HDL. In the further delipidation of these particles, surface components such as apo C and apo E shuttle back to HDL, and cholesteryl esters in HDL are exchanged for triglyceride in the triglyceride-rich lipoproteins, a process facilitated by CETP. The modulatory effect of apolipoproteins on lipid metabolism can be illustrated by apo E, which is a polymorphic glycoprotein serving as a ligand for hepatic lipoprotein receptors, thereby influencing the clearance of the respective lipoprotein particles. In this regard, genetic polymorphism of the apo E gene has been related to serum cholesterol and triglyceride levels and the risk of developing coronary artery disease.[22,23]

Hepatic Lipase and Lipoprotein Lipase

Lipolytic activity may be measured in vivo as intravenous fat tolerance or in vitro as postheparin lipolytic activity.[24] The disappearance of Intralipid emulsion from the plasma follows first-order kinetics. Postheparin lipolytic activity is assayed in plasma obtained after an injection of heparin in doses varying from 20 to 100 U/kg. At least two lipases are released into the circulation by heparin: hepatic lipase and lipoprotein lipase.[25] These two lipases have different antigenic determinants and biochemical profiles.

Hepatic lipase, which is synthesized by the liver, accounts for the major part of total lipolytic activity. Hepatic lipase promotes the catabolism of HDLs through hydrolysis of their lipid content, thereby generating smaller HDL particles. The hydrolysis of the triglyceride in HDL2 by hepatic lipase thus results in its conversion to the smaller HDL3s.[16,17] The action of hepatic lipase can be linked to the apolipoprotein content, as exemplified by the increased propensity of apo AI containing HDL particles to be metabolized by hepatic lipase.[21] IDL particles can be converted into LDL by hepatic lipase, which hydrolyzes the triglyceride content.[26,27] Similarly, hepatic lipase also hydrolyzes the triglyceride molecules in LDL to produce the cholesteryl ester–depleted small dense LDL. Patients with hepatic lipase deficiency have altered HDL mass distribution with grossly elevated HDL triglyceride and dominance of HDL2.[28] The rate at which large VLDLs are converted to smaller VLDLs is unaffected, but subsequent conversion of small VLDLs to IDL is reduced, resulting in an abnormal accumulation of VLDL. Despite this, IDLs accumulate to more than twice their normal level, since their subsequent conversion to LDL is almost totally inhibited. Thus these patients have markedly elevated IDL and reduced LDL.[29,30] Lipoprotein lipase is synthesized in adipose tissue and muscle under the influence of insulin. It is normally located on the endothelial surface and, once activated by apo CII, metabolizes the triglyceride core of VLDLs and chylomicrons. Since apo CII activates and apo CIII inhibits lipoprotein lipase, the characteristic reduction of the ratio of apo CII to apo CIII in renal failure contributes to the suppression of lipoprotein lipase activity.

In summary, lipoprotein lipase hydrolyzes the triglyceride in chylomicrons and VLDL, generating free fatty acids and glycerol, and leads to the formation of denser particles with relatively more cholesteryl esters—namely, chylomicron remnants and VLDL remnants, respectively. The free fatty acids may be consumed in oxidative processes in the mitochondrial matrix, where long-chain fatty acids are transported with the help of carnitine. During caloric excess, free fatty acids may be reesterified with glycerol to form depot fat in adipose tissue, or they may provide the substrate for triglyceride synthesis in the liver. Through the interaction between apo E and LDL-like receptors in the liver, chylomicron remnants are removed from the circulation. Lipoprotein lipase further metabolizes VLDL remnants to IDL. In patients with VLDL overproduction, the triglycerides in the larger VLDL particles can exchange with cholesteryl esters on large LDL particles through the action of CETP, resulting in the production of a triglyceride-enriched LDL. These triglyceride molecules on LDLs are then hydrolyzed by hepatic lipase to produce the cholesteryl ester–depleted small dense LDL. IDL particles can either be removed from circulation through the binding of apo E to the respective receptors in the liver, or they can be converted into LDL by hepatic lipase, which further hydrolyzes the triglyceride. LDL then transports cholesterol to the peripheral tissues. Through the interaction between surface apo B100 and its receptor, LDL is internalized and free cholesterol is generated through lysosomal hydrolysis of the cholesteryl esters.

Apart from being utilized in normal cell functions, the free cholesterol thus released is involved in feedback inhibition of de novo synthesis of cholesterol and high-affinity LDL receptors. The latter is mediated through inhibiting the proteolytic release of the sterol regulatory element binding protein, which normally increases the transcription of both the LDL receptor gene and the gene for HMG-CoA reductase, the rate-limiting enzyme in cholesterol synthesis. In addition to the receptor-mediated LDL catabolic pathway, LDL particles can also undergo oxidation, especially in hypercholesterolemic subjects. With increasing levels of circulating LDL, more LDL particles are channeled to the oxidative pathway. Oxidized LDL is then taken up by macrophages through interaction with surface scavenger receptors.[31] In contrast to the LDL receptor–mediated pathway, this scavenger pathway is not subject to feedback inhibition. Therefore, in hypercholesterolemic subjects, cholesteryl esters can accumulate in macrophages, leading to foam cell formation, inflammation, and atherogenesis. Because of their higher propensity for the scavenger pathway, small dense LDL particles are more susceptible to oxidation and have been ascribed a higher atherogenic potential (Fig. 28–1).

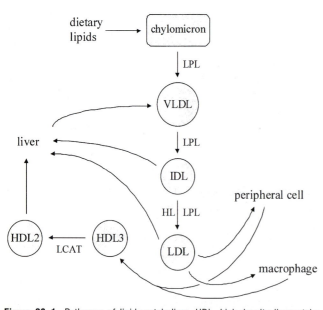

Figure 28–1. Pathways of lipid metabolism. HDL, high-density lipoprotein; HL, hepatic lipase; IDL, intermediate-density lipoprotein; LCAT, lecithin cholesterol acyltransferase; LDL, low-density lipoprotein; LPL, lipoprotein lipase; VLDL, very low density lipoprotein.

LIPOPROTEIN ABNORMALITIES IN UREMIA AND DIALYSIS

Characteristic lipid abnormalities in chronic renal failure include an accumulation of partially catabolized apo B–containing triglyceride-rich particles, in particular the VLDL and IDL classes, while HDL is notably reduced, with decreased relative concentrations of free and esterified cholesterol and increased triglyceride content. The HDL2 subfraction is significantly lower than that found in normal subjects, while the HDL3 level is similar to that in normals.[32–34] LDL concentration may remain normal, but the level of small dense LDLs is increased, the latter conferring a higher atherogenic potential due to their increased susceptibility to oxidation, reduced binding to LDL receptors, and reduced clearance. The relative importance of reduced LDL apo B/E receptor expression and/or function in the genesis of uremic dyslipidemia remains to be defined.[35] The level of Lp(a), another risk factor for atherogenesis, is two to five times normal[36–39] and has been related to reduced renal clearance of Lp(a) and apo(a).[40,41]

In general, the level of triglyceride is increased while that of cholesterol is often normal.[42–55] Lipid abnormalities are clinically evident when the glomerular filtration rate falls below around 40 mL/min; they become more pronounced with increasing severity of renal failure.[56] Characteristic apolipoprotein abnormalities include reduced levels of apo AI and apo AII[57,58] and increased apo B, apo CII, apo CIII, and apo E. The magnitude of decrease in apo AI increases with the severity of renal failure and correlates with hypertriglyceridemia.[32–34,57–70] The increase in apo E may be less than that in nonuremic hypertriglyceridemic subjects[57,59–61,64,65,67,68,71]; this could be related to reduced renal synthesis of apo E. The lipid abnormalities are more pronounced in patients with diabetes mellitus, who exhibit a more than fourfold increase in VLDL, threefold increase in IDL, and reduced HDL[72] (Table 28–2).

Compositional and Qualitative Changes. Compositional changes are most pronounced in IDL and HDL.[73] Cholesterol content is increased in VLDL and IDL, little changed in LDL, and reduced in HDL. Triglyceride levels are increased in all lipoproteins. Apo B is increased in VLDL and IDL, especially in patients with hypertriglyceridemia. Apo CII and apo CIII are increased in VLDL, IDL, and LDL, while apo AI, apo AII, and apo C are reduced in HDL. The distribution of apolipoproteins is altered such that, instead of being found in HDL as in normal subjects, in patients with chronic kidney disease (CKD), 60 to 80 percent of apo CIII and apo E is present in VLDL and LDL due to decreased degradation of triglyceride-rich lipoproteins.[32,53,57,60,74] Decreased apo AI to apo CIII ratio has been considered a hallmark of dyslipidemia in CKD and may be detected when the triglyceride level is still normal.[54] A de-

TABLE 28–2. DYSLIPIDEMIA IN CHRONIC UREMIA/DIALYSIS

Lipids
  Triglyceride level increased
  Total cholesterol and LDL cholesterol often normal but can be increased
    in PD
  HDL cholesterol consistently low, mainly HDL2 subfraction
  Free fatty acid concentration normal
Lipoproteins
  Fasting chylomicronemia common
  VLDL increased, with increased cholesterol content
  IDL increased, with increased cholesterol content
  LDL is enriched with triglyceride; level often normal but can be increased
    in PD
  Lp(a) increased, especially in PD
  HDL usually reduced; enriched with triglyceride but cholesterol content
    decreased
Apolipoproteins
  Apo AI and apo AII reduced
  Apo B, apo CII, apo CIII, and apo E increased
  Apo AI/apo CIII, apo AI/apo B, apo CII/apo CIII ratios reduced
Kinetic parameters
  Lipoprotein lipase and hepatic lipase activity both reduced
  Presence of lipoprotein lipase inhibitors
  Decreased LCAT
  Decreased triglyceride turnover
  Decreased catabolism of VLDL and IDL
  Decreased cholesterol esterification

KEY: apo, apolipoprotein; HDL, high-density lipoprotein; IDL, intermediate-density lipoprotein; lp(a), lipoprotein(a); LCAT, lecithin-cholesterol acyltransferase; LDL, low-density lipoprotein; PD, peritoneal dialysis; VLDL, very low density lipoprotein.

creased ratio of apo AI to apo B is also observed. Since the kidney is an important site for apo AI degradation, there is increased free apo AI (unassociated with lipid) in the plasma of patients with renal failure.[75,76] The ratio of apo CIII to apo CII is increased, although levels of both may be increased, and the increased ratio in VLDL can be observed even in patients with normal triglyceride levels.[71,74] Apo B48, normally found on chylomicrons, is often also present in VLDL.[74] Modifications of apo B—including oxidation, carbamoylation, and glycation or transformation by advanced glycation end products—can occur, which can prolong the half-life of these particles in view of their reduced catabolism through the normal receptor-mediated pathway and their greater propensity for the scavenger receptor pathways, the latter leading to foam cell formation and atherosclerosis.[77] Similarly, decreased paraoxonase activity in renal failure, which normally inhibits HDL oxidation and the lipid peroxidation of LDL, can impair the structure and function of both HDL and LDL.[78]

Hemodialysis vs. Peritoneal Dialysis. Dialysis does not correct the lipoprotein lipase deficiency in uremia owing to the nondialyzable nature of the lipase inhibitor(s). Postheparin lipase activity remains suppressed.[27,79] The adequacy of dialysis, however, plays a pathogenetic role in lipid abnormalities. In this regard, intensive hemodialysis has been reported to increase postheparin lipolytic activity,[80] probably related to reduced insulin resistance.

Hemodialysis (HD). HD involves extracorporeal circulation and repeated heparinization. Heparin has complex effects on lipid metabolism. It releases lipolytic enzymes and hence increases the catabolism of triglyceride-rich lipoproteins. These may be regarded as favorable effects except that, in patients with impaired synthesis of lipoprotein lipase, repeated heparinization may ultimately deplete the enzyme. By increasing triglyceride catabolism, free fatty acid concentrations are acutely raised, which inhibits LCAT activity.[81] The consequent impairment of cholesterol esterification in the presence of increased acute breakdown of triglyceride-rich lipoproteins may impede the disposition of excess cholesterol. Cholesteryl ester transfer from HDL to VLDL and LDL is reduced in HD, irrespective of whether there is hypertriglyceridemia, indicating impaired reverse cholesterol transport.[68,82] The important implications of the latter in atherogenesis can be illustrated by the observation that the combination of low HDL cholesterol and genetic CETP deficiency in HD patients is associated with increased frequency of vascular disease.[83] Amelioration of dyslipidemia after high-flux dialysis with biocompatible membranes has been attributed to the improved clearance of lipase inhibitors.[84,85]

Peritoneal Dialysis (PD). While the caloric contribution by dialysate glucose or acetate in HD is negligible,[86–88] the dextrose content of PD solutions represents a significant load, and contributes to hypertriglyceridemia. In addition, the protein loss in PD stimulates lipoprotein synthesis by the liver, as it does in the nephrotic syndrome.[89] Loss of lipoproteins by the peritoneal route is not significant. Conflicting results have been reported with regard to the relationship between Lp(a) level and albumin loss into the dialysis solution in PD.[90–92]

Uremic dyslipidemia thus persists, but the pattern is modified during dialysis. Lipid abnormalities affect up to 85 percent of dialysis patients, with patients on PD showing a higher prevalence. Hypertriglyceridemia is common in both PD and HD patients, while hypercholesterolemia is more common in PD.[93] Impaired catabolism of triglyceride is the principal abnormality, although increased triglyceride synthesis has been shown in some patients on dialysis.[94–96] Increased caloric intake due to absorption of dextrose from PD solutions leads to increased triglyceride synthesis in PD patients, who already exhibit defective triglyceride catabolism.[97] This can be illustrated by triglyceride turnover studies using labeled glycerol or by fat tolerance tests with or without heparin.[94,98–104] Reduced hepatic lipase and lipoprotein lipase activities are the main causative factors leading to the impaired triglyceride catabolism. Lipoprotein lipase activity in postheparin plasma correlates with the in vivo fractional disappearance rate of Intralipid.[27] While total or LDL cholesterol is not frequently elevated except in some PD patients, small dense LDL is increased.

IDL is usually markedly elevated in uremic plasma, and more than 40 percent of HD patients have elevated levels of IDL. The increase in IDL is attributed in part to reduced catabolism due to lowered hepatic lipase activity.[27] In this context, IDL level has been described as the best lipoprotein predictor of aortic stiffness.[105] Since increased IDL is noted even in patients with normal LDL levels, it has been suggested that target LDL levels should be lower than those in nonuremic subjects in order to minimize vascular complications.[106] The abnormal distribution of apo CIII and apo E between the triglyceride-rich lipoproteins and HDL is also in keeping with the defective catabolism of triglyceride-rich lipoproteins. A reduced ratio of HDL to VLDL and LDL apo CIII is characteristic in uremia.[107] During the catabolism of triglyceride-rich lipoproteins, some cholesterol and apolipoproteins are transferred to HDL.[108] The low HDL cholesterol concentration is therefore at least partly due to the defective triglyceride catabolism. This is supported by the inverse correlation between serum triglyceride and serum HDL cholesterol concentrations and a positive correlation between HDL cholesterol concentrations and lipoprotein lipase activity in postheparin plasma.[27,100,103] Indeed, HDL levels can increase considerably after a heparin-induced increase in lipase activity in HD patients.[27]

Lp(a) is increased in both PD and HD patients, especially in the former.[109–111] Enrichment of apo CIII in VLDL is noted in both PD and HD, while increased free cholesterol, triglyceride, apo B, apo CII, and apo E in VLDL is mainly noted in PD patients. Increased apo CIII with a decreased ratio of apo E to apo CIII persists from the stage of advanced renal failure to HD.[112] IDL from both PD and HD patients demonstrates increased lipid and apolipoprotein mass, with increased free and esterified cholesterol, triglyceride, and elevated levels of apo B, apo CII, apo CIII, and apo E. The content of triglyceride and apo CIII in LDL is increased in both PD and HD patients, while increased apo B content in LDL is mainly noted in PD patients. Thus increased apo CIII content is noted in VLDL, IDL, and LDL. Reduced HDL and the content of free cholesterol and apo AI in HDL are associated with both PD and HD.[113]

The predominant alteration in lipoprotein composition distinguishing PD patients from HD patients is an elevation of apo B in LDL. Increased apo B levels are noted early after the commencement of PD.[69] Consequently, PD patients exhibit higher levels of total cholesterol and apo B, a higher ratio of total to HDL cholesterol, a lower ratio of apo AI to apo B, and higher levels of Lp(a) than do patients on HD.[93,114] While an increased percentage of small dense LDL is noted in patients with advanced renal failure, on PD, or on HD, PD patients are more likely to show increased plasma concentrations of small dense LDL.[115]

Plasma Lipolytic and LCAT Activity

The fractional disappearance of Intralipid emulsion from the plasma is grossly reduced in uremic patients, whether or not they are on dialysis, and is partially improved after heparin injection.[101–104] As renal function approaches zero, there is a progressive decrease in total postheparin lipolytic activity, concomitant with an increase in serum triglyceride concentration.[116] Almost all investigators have reported a reduced total postheparin lipolytic activity in uremic patients.[102,116] In studies in which the two lipases are measured, most investigators concur that lipoprotein lipase activity is reduced.[27,79,117–119] Lipoprotein lipase activities correlate positively with HDL2, while hepatic lipase shows an inverse relationship with HDL3.[120,121] Earlier reports of selective hepatic lipase deficiency in uremic subjects were not confirmed by subsequent studies, which demonstrated that both hepatic lipase and lipoprotein lipase were significantly reduced.[27,122,123] A poorly dialyzable inhibitor of lipoprotein lipase but not of hepatic lipase[119,124] has been demonstrated in uremic plasma, while an association between suppression of hepatic lipase activity and hyperparathyroidism has been reported.[121] The lipase inhibitor activity in uremic plasma has also been attributed to an increased concentration of free apo AI in the nonlipoprotein fraction.[125] Routine hemodialysis, CAPD, or hemofiltration does not return the lipase activities to normal.[27,79,119,126] Instead, the frequent intermittent heparinization of patients on hemodialysis may explain the lower fractional disappearance rate of Intralipid in patients after heparin injection compared with patients on peritoneal dialysis.[101] Since lipoprotein lipase synthesis is stimulated by insulin, in view of the peripheral insulin resistance in uremic patients attributed to a postreceptor defect, it is speculated that the rate of synthesis is inadequate to keep up with the repeated release of lipoprotein lipase following heparinization, thus leading to the reduced level.[127]

Independent investigators have reported on the reduced LCAT activity in uremia.[81,128,129] Heparin given during HD further inhibits LCAT activity by increasing plasma free fatty acid concentrations, and LCAT activity returns to predialysis levels about an hour after stopping HD.[81] The low LCAT activity is not due to low HDL cholesterol or reduced apo AI, which activates the enzyme, but has been linked to hypocalcemia.[121] The low plasma LCAT activity reverts to normal after kidney transplantation due to increased levels of the enzyme.[130]

Metabolic and Hormonal Factors

Insulin Resistance. Insulin resistance due to a post-receptor-binding defect and hyperinsulinemia have been documented in uremic patients irrespective of the type of renal disease.[131] The insulin resistance has been related to relative vitamin D deficiency and anemia.[127,132–134] Lipoprotein lipase activity in uremic subjects is reduced due to insulin resistance and lipase inhibitors such as apo CIII and free apo AI. Lipoprotein lipase is synthesized in adipose tissue and muscle under the influence of insulin, and data from animal studies have demonstrated reduced lipoprotein lipase transcription with increasing severity of uremia.[135] Administration of insulin to nondiabetic uremic rats has been shown to increase lipoprotein lipase activity and decrease VLDL triglyceride concentrations.[136] Insulin resistance in uremia leads to increased hepatic synthesis of triglyceride and VLDLI,[8,80,100] and the fasting glucose level is significantly higher in dialysis patients with a low fractional removal rate of Intralipid.[104]

Parathyroid Hormone. Secondary hyperparathyroidism is common in renal failure, and parathyroid hormone has been regarded as an important uremic toxin. Some investigators have reported improved lipid metabolism and reversal of lipoprotein lipase or hepatic lipase downregulation after parathyroidectomy.[137–140] Others have observed no correlation between lipid and parathyroid hormone levels and that parathyroidectomy could at best ameliorate the lipid abnormalities but not completely correct them.[139–142] In this regard, deficiency of VLDL receptors in uremia has been shown to be independent of parathyroid hormone.[143]

Carnitine Deficiency. The combination of dialysis, dietary restrictions, and low protein intake contributes to the frequent occurrence of tissue carnitine deficiency in dialysis patients. Carnitine is a small, water-soluble, dialyzable molecule.[144] A single HD session reduces the plasma free carnitine concentration by 75 percent, which then returns to the predialysis level after about 8 hours. Carnitine transports long-chain fatty acids across the mitochondrial membrane before they are oxidized.[145] Carnitine deficiency may be responsible for muscle weakness in dialysis patients and may contribute to hyperlipidemia by impairing the oxidation of fatty acids. Carnitine loss in PD effluent appears insufficient to lead to a deficiency state, so that the plasma concentration of total carnitine is at most slightly reduced.[146] Nevertheless, free carnitine is decreased while acylcarnitine levels are increased, resulting in functional deficiency. L-carnitine supplementation has been shown to reduce triglyceride and total cholesterol and to increase HDL cholesterol in dialysis patients.[147]

Thyroid Hormone. Hypothyroidism is associated with reduced triglyceride turnover and increased LDL cholesterol due to downregulation of LDL receptors and thus reduced LDL clearance.[148] Abnormalities in thyroid function tests are common in patients with uremia or on dialysis, but true hypothyroidism is unusual.[149] Serum levels of L-thyroxine and L-triiodothyronine tend to be lower in dialysis patients, with normal TSH levels. Despite this, D-thyroxin treatment has been demonstrated to reduce total cholesterol, LDL cholesterol, and Lp(a) levels in dialysis patients.[150]

Growth Hormone. Growth hormone opposes the peripheral actions of insulin. The paradoxical response of growth hormone to plasma glucose in uremic patients may reduce the synthesis of lipoprotein lipase.[151] Lipoprotein lipase activity is reduced in acromegalics and patients treated with growth hormone.[152,153] However, reductions in triglyceride and apo E levels have been observed after growth hormone therapy in elderly HD patients,[154] while growth hormone therapy in children with renal failure has been associated with an increase in Lp(a).[155] The mechanisms leading to these changes remain to be elucidated.

Glucagon. Glucagon stimulates glycogenolysis, increases hepatic gluconeogenesis, and stimulates the lipolysis of depot fat in adipose tissue by hormone-sensitive lipase. Elevated levels of proglucagon and immunoreactive glucagon have been demonstrated in uremic patients due to altered peritubular uptake and glomerular filtration, respectively, but the consequent effects on lipid metabolism remain obscure.[156,157]

Summary

In summary, reduced lipoprotein lipase activity in uremia leads to decreased catabolism of triglyceride-rich lipid particles and low HDL, and reduced hepatic lipase results in markedly elevated IDL and altered HDL subfractions. While uremic toxins inhibit the activity of lipoprotein lipase, insulin resistance and a paradoxical response of growth hormone to glucose may reduce the synthesis of lipoprotein lipase. Compositional and qualitative changes of lipoproteins interfere with their normal functions as well as their recognition and uptake by receptor-mediated pathways. These particles are then channeled toward alternate routes, such as oxidation and non-receptor-mediated uptake by macrophages. LDL catabolism and clearance are thus altered because of carbamylation and oxidation of lipoproteins in the uremic milieu.[158,159] The clearance of glycosylated LDLs is also decreased.[160] Indeed, cell-interactive properties of LDLs isolated from uremic patients are abnormal.[161]

Dialysis complicates these abnormalities further by introducing other variables. Repeated use of heparin in hemodialysis inhibits LCAT and may deplete the releasable pool of lipoprotein lipase. In addition, substances such as carnitine are dialyzed across hemodialysis membranes.

Peritoneal dialysis causes protein loss and exposes the patient to repeated glucose loads. In the presence of a defective catabolic pathway for triglyceride-rich lipoproteins, increased calories and a tendency for increased hepatic lipoprotein synthesis leads to hyperlipidemia. Hypertriglyceridemia is common in both HD and PD patients. Compared to HD patients, those on PD are more likely to have elevated levels of cholesterol, LDL cholesterol, apo B, a higher ratio of total to HDL cholesterol, and a lower ratio of apo AI to apo B.[114,162] Increased small dense LDL is an established risk factor for cardiovascular disease, and PD patients are more likely to have increased concentrations of small dense LDL.[163] A cross-sectional study has reported elevated small dense LDL in 40 percent of PD patients, 28 percent of HD and predialysis patients, and 2.5 percent of controls.[115] These investigators noted that plasma triglyceride level and hepatic lipase activity were independent predictors of small dense LDL concentration. In vivo clearance studies using radioisotope-labeled LDL have shown that the clearance of LDL is more severely impaired in PD patients than in those on HD.[164] Aggravation of high VLDL and low HDL cholesterol by beta blockers has been observed in patients on PD but not those on HD.[165]

The increased Lp(a) level in patients on dialysis adds further to the atherogenic lipid profile,[37–39,166] and there is an association with the apo(a) phenotype, similar to that found in the general population.[92,167] The cause for the low apo AI and apo AII is still being investigated. Components in the serum of PD patients can inhibit apo AI synthesis, secretion, and mRNA expression by Hep-G2 cells.[168] Most apo AI is metabolized in the liver and the kidney; per gram of tissue, the kidney is the most important site of degradation for apo AI but not HDL cholesterol. This may contribute to the finding of free apo AI in uremic plasma. Stimulation of proximal renal tubular cells with apo AI induces a concentration-dependent secretion of apo AI binding protein, suggesting a role for this protein in the renal tubular degradation or reabsorption of apo AI.[169] PD patients tend to have higher Lp(a) levels than those on HD,[93] and a negative correlation has been observed with serum albumin level.[170] The level of Lp(a) increases in an inflammatory response.[171] While increased mortality, often from vascular complications, has been repeatedly linked to an inflammatory state in dialysis patients,[172–174] it would be of interest to speculate about the role of Lp(a) in pathogenesis.[167] In this regard, associations between C reactive protein, hypoalbuminemia, apo AI, and Lp(a) have been reported.[175–177] There is increasing evidence to show that increased oxidative stress in uremia and dialysis—from contributing factors such as unidentified uremic toxin(s), oxidized LDL, and advanced glycation end products—stimulates IL-6 production, which in turn leads to persistent inflammation.[178–180]

In the assessment and management of lipid disorder in uremic patients, it is important to note that malnutrition, a common complication in dialysis patients, can reduce the level of lipids. For example, a rise in serum cholesterol and triglyceride concentrations may be observed after commencement of dialysis in a malnourished uremic subject.[32,69,181,182] Such rises are often not sustained.[32,51,52] In a longitudinal study, PD patients had higher total cholesterol, apo AI, and apo B than HD patients, and serum albumin correlated directly with apo B and total cholesterol rather than inversely, as occurs in the nephrotic syndrome.[114] Hypoalbuminemia is associated with increased levels of Lp(a), fibrinogen, and platelet aggregability, but its effects on the metabolism of other lipid particles have not been fully elucidated.[183] For both dialysis modalities, patients who died had significantly lower total cholesterol and apo B throughout their entire courses than did survivors.[114]

The overall lipid abnormalities in dialysis patients imply increased atherogenic potential. Increased apo B and reduced HDL cholesterol have been associated with the development of cardiovascular disease in HD patients.[184] Similarly, an increased level of Lp(a) has been shown to be an independent predictor of death due to vascular complications in dialysis patients.[185]

TREATMENT OF LIPID ABNORMALITIES IN DIALYSIS PATIENTS

Cardiovascular mortality is a major cause of death in patients on dialysis. The risk of vascular complications is correlated positively with the level of total cholesterol and LDL cholesterol and negatively with HDL cholesterol level.[186,187] The role of hypertriglyceridemia per se as a separate risk factor is controversial. However, as discussed previously, hypertriglyceridemia is often part of an overall atherogenic lipid profile, especially in patients with renal failure. Together with hypertension, subclinical inflammation, hyperphosphatemia, hyperparathyroidism, and insulin resistance, uremic patients have multiple risk factors for accelerated atherosclerosis and vascular calcification. In the context of HD, low-molecular-weight heparins improve the metabolism of triglyceride-rich lipoproteins and decrease small dense LDL.[188,189] It remains to be investigated whether the overall prevalence of dyslipidemia in HD patients would decrease with increasing popularity of these compounds. Since both dyslipidemia and the increased risk of vascular complications set in when renal function is significantly impaired, the management of dyslipidemia and other measures to reduce the overall vascular risk should start before dialysis.

Reduction of LDL cholesterol and increase of HDL cholesterol levels can reduce the incidence of coronary events.[190,191] The recently published *K/DOQI Clinical Practice Guidelines for Managing Dyslipidemias in Chronic Kidney Disease* state target concentrations of <5.65 mmol/L

(500 mg/dL) and <2.59 mmol/L (100 mg/dL) for triglyceride and LDL, respectively, in adults with CKD,[192] taking into account available data in the literature relating the risk of vascular complications with lipid abnormalities in various forms of kidney disease. Patients with moderate increase in LDL (2.59 to 3.34 mmol/L) may attempt modification of lifestyle and diet before commencing statin therapy. In uremic subjects with hypertriglyceridemia, it is reasonable to inhibit triglyceride synthesis by reducing caloric intake, including that absorbed from peritoneal dialysis solutions, and to increase the catabolism of triglyceride-rich lipoproteins by exercise, adding fish oils to the diet, and treatment with a fibrate. Management of individual patients entails assessment of specific risk factors and contributing causes, including concomitant conditions such as diabetes mellitus, history of smoking, and prior history or family history of vascular events. Nonselective beta-adrenoreceptor blocking agents exert a negative influence on lipoprotein metabolism at least partly by inhibiting post-heparin lipases.[193] It is therefore reasonable to use other agents that may have a beneficial effect on lipid metabolism. It is imperative to exercise caution with dietary restrictions in dialysis patients in view of the high prevalence of malnutrition. In this regard, a low plasma cholesterol concentration may indicate malnutrition, and low serum albumin level is established as a poor prognostic indicator for reduced survival in dialysis patients (Table 28–3).

Lifestyle and Diet

Patients with hyperlipidemia should be advised with regard to appropriate dietary modifications to optimize the quantity of cholesterol and/or energy intake, avoidance of overweight, increased physical activity, abstinence from alcohol, and prevention/treatment of hyperglycemia. Exercise improves lipid abnormalities, and favorable results have been shown in dialysis patients.[194] Programmed exercise in these patients increases lipoprotein lipase activity, increases HDL cholesterol, and decreases serum triglyceride concentrations.

The diet should, in general, consist of about 30 to 35 kcal/kg/day and 1.0 to 1.2 g/kg/day of high-biological-value protein, or 1.2 to 1.5 g/kg/day in the case of CAPD patients to make up for protein loss via the peritoneal route. The caloric distribution should be about one-third each from

TABLE 28–3. TREATMENT OF DYSLIPIDEMIA IN PATIENTS ON DIALYSIS

Lipid-Lowering Agents	Other Measures
Fibrates	Lifestyle: diet and exercise
HMG-CoA reductase inhibitors	Avoidance of excessive calories
Inhibitors of lipid absorption	L-carnitine
Probucol	Low-molecular-weight heparin
Nicotinic acid derivatives	Fish oil

carbohydrates, fat, and protein, respectively, with a polyunsaturated-to-saturated ratio of 1:1 or even 2:1. The caloric contribution from fat can be lower in PD patients, since the dialysate glucose provides supplemental energy. A number of investigators have reported on the efficacy of dietary modifications in ameliorating lipid abnormalities in dialysis patients, especially hypertriglyceridemia.[195–197] Long-term compliance and the prevention of malnutrition remain genuine difficulties.[198] Suboptimal energy intake and malnutrition are established risk factors for increased mortality. A recent clinical trial on lipid-lowering diet showed that HD subjects achieved 18 percent reduction in fat intake, with about 11 percent reduction in LDL cholesterol level, while no significant change was noted in PD patients.[199] Furthermore, 11 percent of recruited subjects could not complete the 14-week study.

Pharmacologic Agents

Treatment of persistent hypertriglyceridemia despite avoidance of excessive caloric intake and appropriate lifestyle modifications often entails the administration of a fibrate. A statin is recommended in patients with predominant hypercholesterolemia, failing which a bile acid sequestrant can be added. In select individuals with severe hypertriglyceridemia despite statin therapy, the latter can be cautiously combined with a fibrate, but the patient should be carefully monitored for the development of rhabdomyolysis. The exact magnitude of benefit resulting from drug treatment is unclear given that these patients usually have long-standing vascular disease before starting dialysis. Prolonged follow-up is required to thoroughly study the effects of lipid-lowering therapy, as has been illustrated by drug trials using cholestyramine or gemfibrozil.[190,191]

Fibrates. The mode of action of fibrates is complex; their most consistent effect is on lipoprotein lipase.[200] Bezafibrate treatment increased hepatic lipase and lipoprotein lipase in uremic patients.[200,201] Gemfibrozil increases both hepatic and lipoprotein lipase in CKD and CAPD patients.[120,202] Both bezafibrate and gemfibrozil reduce gamma-glutaryl-transpeptidase, and may affect the action of HMG-CoA reductase.[203,204] There is usually a 30 to 70 percent reduction in serum triglycerides, and both total cholesterol and LDL cholesterol are reduced. HDL cholesterol is also increased after fibrate therapy,[190] Clinofibrate at a daily dose of 600 mg has been shown to reduce VLDL triglyceride and increase the ratio of apo CII to apo CIII in CAPD patients without increasing postheparin lipases.[205] Fibrate therapy should be beneficial in view of the importance of reduced lipoprotein lipase activity and low HDL cholesterol in the dyslipidemia of dialysis patients. Futhermore, recent data showing an antioxidant effect of the gemfibrozil metabolite on LDL suggest added benefit in addition to its lipid-lowering effect.[206] Clofibric acid and its derivatives may increase creatine phosphokinase, with symptomatic myalgia, if the dose is not reduced in renal failure patients.[207] The dose of bezafibrate used in uremic patients varies from 200 mg every third day in dialysis patients to 100 to 300 mg daily in patients with CKD.[200,201,207,208] A dose not exceeding 300 mg twice daily has been recommended for gemfibrozil in order to prevent a rise in creatinine phosphokinase.[120]

Statins (HMG-CoA Reductase Inhibitors). Statins inhibit HMG-CoA reductase at the rate-limiting step of HMG-CoA conversion to mevalonic acid in cholesterol synthesis. The resulting decrease in hepatic intracellular cholesterol causes upregulation of LDL receptors, which remove both LDL and triglyceride-rich lipoproteins such as VLDL and IDL, thereby reducing LDL cholesterol and triglyceride levels in plasma.[209] Increased apo AI synthesis and decreased CETP-mediated cholesterol transfer from HDL due to a reduction of apo B–containing lipoproteins may contribute to the increase in HDL after statin therapy.[210–213] Recent data indicate that the clinical benefits of statins can also be attributed to their effects on vascular endothelial cell function, coagulation, and inflammation in addition to their lipid-lowering effect.[214] The latter could be of particular relevance to the inflammatory state of patients on dialysis. The efficacy and safety of lovastatin, simvastatin, pravastatin, and atorvastatin in reducing LDL cholesterol, IDL cholesterol, apo B, and triglyceride levels in dialysis subjects have been demonstrated.[215–219] Although the activity of lipoprotein lipase has not been measured, the reduction of VLDL cholesterol suggests an improved clearance of remnant particles.[215] A randomized, prospective, double-blind 24-week study showed that simvastatin was well tolerated and reduced LDL and non-HDL cholesterol by 33 to 36 percent and 25 percent, respectively, in both HD and PD patients.[220] Triglyceride and apo B levels decreased by 6 to 10 percent and 20 percent, respectively; Lp(a) was unchanged; while HDL cholesterol increased by 8 percent in PD patients. Statins are usually well tolerated by patients on dialysis, but it is imperative to monitor for the uncommon occurrence of rhabdomyolysis or abnormal liver function.

Inhibition of Lipid Absorption. Cholestyramine is a polystyrene resin with a bile acid–sequestering action that is useful in lowering serum total cholesterol and LDL cholesterol. It reduces the enterohepatic circulation of cholesterol and increases LDL removal, the latter due to increased synthesis of LDL receptors on hepatocytes.[221] Colestipol has a similar effect. Orally administered activated charcoal can also reduce hyperlipidemia, related to its adsorptive effect.[222] Ezetimibe belongs to a new class of drugs that inhibit intestinal cholesterol absorption by interfering with the putative sterol transport pathway of intestinal epithelial cells. It reduces LDL cholesterol and triglyceride by up to 20 and 15 percent, respectively, and exhibits additive efficacy when used together with a statin.[223] There are few data on its use in patients with renal failure.

Probucol. Probucol has a moderate cholesterol-lowering effect and possesses antioxidant properties.[224] Unfortunately, it may also reduce HDL cholesterol and has been associated with a prolonged QT interval.[225] Nevertheless, promising results on vascular protection and regression of atherosclerosis in animal models have been obtained with probucol or its analogues.[226,227] A study in HD patients showed that probucol at 500 mg/day was well tolerated and reduced plasma triglycerides by 38 percent, total cholesterol by 15 percent, and LDL cholesterol by 19 percent.[228]

Nicotinic Acid and Derivatives. Nicotinic acid decreases hepatic synthesis of VLDL and LDL, and at 3 to 6 g/day significantly reduces LDL cholesterol and increases HDL cholesterol. Plasma triglycerides are also often reduced. However, there is a high incidence of adverse effects, including flushing. There is little information on the efficacy or safety of inositol hexaniacinate in patients with CKD. Acipimox is a derivative with less prominent vasomotor side effects. Conflicting results of acipimox given at 250 mg daily on the triglyceride level of dialysis patients have been reported, while reductions in total cholesterol and LDL cholesterol and an increase in HDL cholesterol have been observed.[229,230]

Carnitine. Carnitine is synthesized from the essential amino acids lysine and methionine. It is involved in the transport of fatty acids to the mitochondria for oxidation. The loss of carnitine in the dialysate, especially in HD, may lead to a marked reduction in free carnitine concentration. Total plasma carnitine levels, which consist of free carnitine and long- and short-chain acylcarnitines, are often within normal limits.[146,231] The characteristic accumulation of lipid droplets in muscle fibers is rare in dialysis patients with carnitine deficiency.[232,233] DL-carnitine has been shown to be effective in the treatment of type IV hyperlipoproteinemia in patients with normal renal function.[234] However, although carnitine supplementation increases the fractional disappearance rate of Intralipid in dialysis patients, its effects on lipid parameters are variable and difficult to predict. Some patients show a paradoxical increase in serum triglycerides, and some may experience a myasthenia-like syndrome.[235–238] In contrast, L-carnitine supplementation in dialysis patients improves muscle symptoms, functional capacity, and the response to erythropoietin.[147,239–241] It also reduces triglyceride and total cholesterol and increases HDL cholesterol in dialysis subjects.[147]

Fish Oil. Fish oils contain eicosapentanoic acid, which is incorporated into thromboxane A3. The latter is less thrombogenic than thromboxane A2. Eicosapentaenoic acid reduces serum triglycerides, albeit by a modest amount. It also improves hypertension and decreases platelet aggregability in dialysis patients.[242–244] The mechanism by which fish oils exert their effect on lipid metabolism is not entirely clear, but inhibition of triglyceride synthesis by the liver has been reported.[245–247] Not only is the dose of fish oil difficult to titrate, but often fish oil can have the paradoxical effect of raising serum cholesterol concentrations.[248,249] The lipid-lowering effect of fish oil supplementation in dialysis patients is not substantial, and some patients develop gastrointestinal intolerance.[250,251]

REFERENCES

1. Lindner A, Charra B, Sherrard DJ, et al. Accelerated atherosclerosis in prolonged maintenance hemodialysis. *N Engl J Med* 1974;290:697–701.

2. Rostand SG, Gretes JC, Kirk KA, et al. Ischemic heart disease in patients with uremia undergoing maintenance hemodialysis. *Kidney Int* 1979;16:600–611.

3. U.S. Renal Data System. *USRDS 2003 Annual Data Report: Atlas of End-Stage Renal Disease in the United States.* Bethesda, MD: National Institutes of Health, National Institute of Diabetes and Digestive and Kidney Diseases, 2003.

4. 2001 Annual Report, European Renal Association – European Dialysis and Transplant Association ERA-EDTA Registy: *ERA-EDTA Registry 2002 Annual Report.* Amsterdam, The Netherlands: Academic Medical Center, May 2004.

5. Krauss RM. Heterogeneity of plasma low-density lipoproteins and atherosclerosis risk. *Curr Opin Lipidol* 1994;5:339–349.

6. Stampfer MJ, Krauss RM, Ma J, et al. A prospective study of triglyceride level, low-density lipoprotein particle diameter, and risk of myocardial infarction. *JAMA* 1996;276:882–888.

7. Zambon A, Hokanson JE, Brown BG, Brunzell JD. Evidence for a new pathophysiological mechanism for coronary artery disease regression hepatic lipase–mediated changes in LDL density. *Circulation* 1999;99:1959–1964.

8. Packard CJ, Shepherd J. Lipoprotein heterogeneity and apolipoprotein B metabolism. *Arterioscler Thromb Vasc Biol* 1997;17:3542–3556.

9. Hajjar KA, Gavish D, Breslow JL, Nachman RL. Lipoprotein(a) modulation of endothelial cell surface fibrinolysis and its potential role in atherosclerosis. *Nature* 1989;339:303–305.

10. Marcovina SM, Koschinsky ML. Lipoprotein(a) as a risk factor for coronary artery disease. *Am J Cardiol* 1998;82:57U–66U.

11. Kostner GM, Kremplere F. Lipoprotein(a). *Curr Opin Lipidol* 1992;3:279–289.

12. Illingworth DR. Lipoprotein metabolism. *Am J Kidney Dis* 1993;22:90–97.

13. Utermann G. Lipoprotein(a). In: Scriver CR, Beaudet AL, Sly WS, et al, eds. *Metabolic and Molecular Basis of Inherited Disease.* New York: McGraw Hill, 1995:1887–1912.

14. Schaefer EJ, Lamon-Fava S, Jenner JL, et al. Lipoprotein(a) levels and risk of coronary heart disease in men—the Lipid Research Clinics Coronary Primary Prevention Trial. *JAMA* 1994;271:999–1003.

15. Cremer P, Nagel D, Labrot B, et al. Lipoprotein Lp(a) as predictor of myocardial infarction in comparison to fibrinogen, LDL cholesterol and other risk factors: results from the prospective Gottingen Risk Incidence and Prevalence Study (GRIPS). *Eur J Clin Invest* 1994;24:444–453.

16. Kuusi T, Saarinen P, Nikkila EA. Evidence for the role of hepatic endothelial lipase in the metabolism of plasma high density lipoprotein 2 in man. *Atherosclerosis* 1980;36:589–593.

17. Patsch JR, Prasad S, Gotto AM, Bengtsson-Olivecrona G. A key role for the conversion of high density lipoprotein-2 into high density lipoprotein-3 by hepatic lipase. *J Clin Invest* 1984;74:2017–2023.

18. Navab M, Berliner JA, Subbanagounder G, et al. HDL and the inflammatory response induced by LDL-derived oxidized phospholipids. *Arterioscler Thromb Vasc Biol* 2001;21:481–488.

19. Xia P, Vadas MA, Rye KA, et al. High density lipoproteins (HDL) interrupt the sphingosine kinase signaling pathway. A possible mechanism for protection against atherosclerosis by HDL. *J Biol Chem* 1999;274:33143–33147.

20. Dimayuga P, Zhu J, Oguchi S, et al. Reconstituted HDL containing human apolipoprotein A-1 reduces VCAM-1 expression and neointima formation following periadventitial cuff-induced carotid injury in apoE null mice. *Biochem Biophys Res Commun* 1999;264:465–468.

21. Mowri HO, Patsch JR, Gotto AM Jr, Patsch W. Apolipoprotein A-II influences the substrate properties of human HDL2 and HDL3 for hepatic lipase. *Arterioscler Thromb Vasc Biol* 1996;16:755–762.

22. Olmer M, Renucci JE, Planells R, et al. Preliminary evidence for a role of apolipoprotein E alleles in identifying haemodialysis patients at high vascular risk. *Nephrol Dial Transplant* 1997;12:691–693.

23. Choi KH, Song HY, Shin SK, et al. Influence of apolipoprotein E genotype on lipid and lipoprotein levels in continuous ambulatory peritoneal dialysis patients. *Adv Perit Dial* 1999;15:243–246.

24. Boberg J, Carlson LA. Determination of heparin-induced lipoprotein lipase in human plasma. *Clin Chim Acta* 1964;10:420–427.

25. LaRosa JC, Levy RI, Windmueller HG, Frederickson DS. Comparison of the triglyceride lipase of liver, adipose tissue and postheparin plasma. *J Lipid Res* 1972;13:356–363.

26. Murase T, Itakura H. Accumulation of an intermediate density lipoprotein in plasma after administration of hepatic triglyceride lipase antibody into rats. *Atherosclerosis* 1981; 39:293–300.

27. Chan MK, Persaud JW, Varghese Z, Moorhead JF. Pathogenic roles of post-heparin lipases in lipid abnormalities in hemodialysis patients. *Kidney Int* 1984;25:812–818.

28. Carlson LA, Holmquist L, Nilsson-Ehle P. Deficiency of hepatic lipase activity in post-heparin plasma in familial hypertriglyceridemia. *Acta Med Scand* 1986;219:435–447.

29. Breckenridge WC, Little JA, Alaupovic P, et al. Lipoprotein abnormalities associated with a familial deficiency of hepatic lipase. *Atherosclerosis* 1982;45:161–179.

30. Demant T, Carlson LA, Holmquist L, et al. Lipoprotein metabolism in hepatic lipase deficiency: studies on the turnover of apolipoprotein B and on the effect of hepatic lipase on high density lipoprotein. *J Lipid Res* 1988;29:1603–1611.

31. Boullier A, Bird DA, Chang MK, et al. Scavenger receptors, oxidized LDL, and atherosclerosis. *Ann NY Acad Sci* 2001; 947:214–222.

32. Parsy D, Dracon M, Cachera C, et al. Lipoprotein abnormalities in chronic hemodialysis patients. *Nephrol Dial Transplant* 1988;3:51–56.

33. Ohta T, Hattori S, Nishiyama S, et al. Quantitative and qualitative changes of apolipoprotein A-I-containing lipoproteins in patients on continuous ambulatory peritoneal dialysis. *Metabolism* 1989;38:843–849.

34. Rubies-Prat J, Espinel E, Joven J, et al. High-density lipoprotein cholesterol subfractions in chronic uremia. *Am J Kidney Dis* 1987;9:60–65.

35. Portman RJ, Scott RC, Rogers DD, et al. Decreased low-density lipoprotein receptor function and mRNA levels in lymphocytes from uremic patients. *Kidney Int* 1992;42: 1238–1246.

36. Cressman MD, Heyka RJ, Paganini EP, et al. Lipoprotein(a) is an independent risk factor for cardiovascular disease in hemodialysis patients. *Circulation* 1992;86:475–482.

37. Murphy BG, Mc Namee P, Duly E, et al. Increased serum apolipoprotein(a) in patients with chronic renal failure treated with ambulatory peritoneal dialysis. *Atherosclerosis* 1992;93:53–57.

38. Irish AB, Simmons LA, Savdie E, et al. Lipoprotein(a) levels in chronic renal disease states, dialysis and transplantation. *Aust NZ J Med* 1992;22:243–248.

39. Kandoussi A, Cachera C, Pagniez D, et al. Plasma level of lipoprotein Lp(a) is high in predialysis or hemodialysis, but not in CAPD. *Kidney Int* 1992;42:424–425.

40. Kronenberg F, Trenkwalder E, Lingenhel A, et al. Renovascular arteriovenous differences in Lp(a) plasma concentrations suggest removal of Lp(a) from the renal circulation. *J Lipid Res* 1997;38:1755–1762.

41. Cauza E, Kletzmaier J, Bodlaj G, et al. Relationship of non-LDL-bound apo(a), urinary apo(a) fragments and plasma Lp(a) in patients with impaired renal function. *Nephrol Dial Transplant* 2003;18:1568–1572.

42. Chan MK, Varghese Z, Moorhead JF. Lipid abnormalities in uremia, dialysis and transplantation. *Kidney Int* 1981;19: 625–637.

43. Papadopoulos NM, Borer WZ, Elin RJ. An abnormal lipoprotein in the serum of uremic patients maintained on chronic hemodialysis. *Ann Intern Med* 1980;92:634–635.

44. Nestel PJ, Fidge NH, Tan MH. Increased lipoprotein-remnant formation in chronic renal failure. *N Engl J Med* 1982; 307:329–333.

45. Kaye JP, Moorhead JF, Wils MR. Plasma lipids in patients with chronic renal failure. *Clin Chim Acta* 1973;44: 301–305.

46. Norbeck HE, Oro L, Carlson LA. Serum lipid and lipoprotein concentrations in chronic renal failure. *Acta Med Scand* 1976;200:487–492.

47. Straprans I, Felts JM, Zacherle B. Apoprotein composition of plasma lipoproteins in uremic patients on hemodialysis. *Clin Chim Acta* 1979;93:135–143.

48. Rapaport J, Avriam M, Chaimovitz C, et al. Defective high density lipoprotein composition in patients on chronic hemodialysis. *N Engl J Med* 1978;299:1326–1329.

49. Felts JM, Zacherle B, Childress G. Lipoprotein spectrum analysis of uremic patients maintained on chronic hemodialysis. *Clin Chem Acta* 1979;93:127–134.

50. Breckenridge WC, Roncari PAK, Khanna R, Oreopoulos DG. The influence of continuous ambulatory peritoneal dialysis on plasma lipoproteins. *Atherosclerosis* 1982;45: 249–258.

51. Ramos JM, Heaton A, McGurk JG, et al. Sequential changes in serum lipids and their subfractions in patients receiving continuous ambulatory peritoneal dialysis. *Nephron* 1983;35:20–23.

52. Lindholm B, Norbeck HE. Serum lipids and lipoproteins during continuous ambulatory peritoneal dialysis. *Acta Med Scand* 1986;220:143–151.

53. Attman PO, Alaupovic P, Gustafson A. Serum apolipoprotein profile of patients with chronic renal failure. *Kidney Int* 1987;32:368–375.

54. Attman PO, Samuelsson O, Alaupovic P. Lipoprotein metabolism and renal failure. *Am J Kidney Dis* 1993;21: 573–592.

55. Rajman I, Harper L, McPake D, et al. Low density lipoprotein subfraction profiles in chronic renal failure. *Nephrol Dial Transplant* 1998;13:2281–2287.

56. Mittman N, Avram MM. Dyslipidemia in renal disease. *Semin Nephrol* 1996;16:202–213.

57. Attman PO, Alaupovic P. Lipid and lipoprotein profiles of uremic dyslipoproteinemia—relation to renal function and dialysis. *Nephron* 1991;57:401–410.

58. Grutzmacher P, Marz W, Peschke B, et al. Lipoproteins and apolipoproteins during the progression of chronic renal disease. *Nephron* 1988;50:103–111.

59. Averna MR, Barbagallo CM, Galione A, et al. Serum apolipoprotein profile of hypertriglyceridemic patients with chronic renal failure on hemodialysis: a comparison with type IV hyperlipoproteinemic patients. *Metabolism* 1989;38: 601–602.

60. Alsayed N, Rebourcet R. Abnormal concentrations of CII, CIII and E apolipoproteins among apolipoprotein B-containing, B-free and AI-containing lipoprotein particles in hemodialysis patients. *Clin Chem* 1991;37:387–393.

61. Lacour B, Roullet J-B, Beyne P, et al. Comparison of several atherogenicity indices by analysis of serum lipoprotein composition in patients with chronic renal failure with or without hemodialysis, and in renal transplant patients. *J Clin Chem Clin Biochem* 1985;23:805–810.

62. Ohta T, Matsuda I. Apolipoprotein and lipid abnormalities in uremic children on hemodialysis. *Clin Chim* 1985;147:145–154.

63. Cassader M, Ruiu G, Tagliaferro V, et al. Lipoprotein and apoprotein levels in different types of dialysis. *Int J Artif Organs* 1989;12:433–438.

64. Bergesio F, Monzani G, Ciuti R, et al. Lipids and apolipoproteins change during progression of chronic renal failure. *Clin Nephrol* 1992;38:264–270.

65. Atger V, Duval F, Frommherz K, et al. Anomalies in composition of uremic lipoproteins isolated by gradient ultracentrifugation: relative enrichment of HDL in apolipoprotein C-III at the expense of apolipoprotein A-I. *Atherosclerosis* 1988;74:75–83.

66. Robert D, Jeanmonod R, Favre H, et al. Changes in lipoproteins induced by the remnant kidney tissue or binephrectomy in chronic uremic patients treated by hemodialysis. *Metabolism* 1989;38:514–521.

67. Sakurai T, Oka T, Hasegawa H, et al. Comparison of lipid, apoproteins and associated enzyme activities between diabetic and non-diabetic end-stage renal disease. *Nephron* 1992;61:409–414.

68. Dieplinger H, Schoenfield PY, Fielding CJ. Plasma cholesterol metabolism in end-stage renal disease. Difference between treatment by hemodialysis or peritoneal dialysis. *J Clin Invest* 1986;77:1071–1083.

69. Sniderman A, Cuanfione K, Kwiterovich PO Jr, et al. Hyperapobetalipoproteinemia: the major dyslipoproteinemia in patients with chronic renal failure treated with chronic ambulatory peritoneal dialysis. *Atherosclerosis* 1987;65:257–264.

70. Senti M, Romero R, Pedro-Botet J, et al. Lipoprotein abnormalities in hyperlipidemic and normolipidemic men on hemodialysis with chronic renal failure. *Kidney Int* 1992;41:1394–1399.

71. Wakabayashi I, Okubo M, Shimade H, et al. Decreased VLDL apoprotein CIII/apoprotein CIII ration may be seen in both normotriglyceridemic and hypertriglyceridemic patients on chronic hemodialysis treatment. *Metabolism* 1987;36:815–820.

72. Attman PO, Knight-Gibson C, Tavella M, et al. The compositional abnormalities of lipoproteins in diabetic renal failure. *Nephrol Dial Transplant* 1998;13(11):2833–2841.

73. Attman PO, Alaupovic P, Tavella M, Knight-Gibson C. Abnormal lipid and apolipoprotein composition of major lipoprotein density classes in patients with chronic renal failure. *Nephrol Dial Transplant* 1996;11(1):63–69.

74. Atger V, Beyne P, Frommherz K, et al. Presence of ApoB-48, and relative Apo-CII deficiency and Apo-CIII enrichment in uremic very-low density lipoproteins. *Ann Biol Clin* 1989;47:497–501.

75. Neary RH, Gowland E. The effect of renal failure and hemodialysis on the concentration of free apolipoprotein AI in serum and the implication for the catabolism of high density lipoproteins. *Clin Chim Acta* 1988;171:239–246.

76. Fuh MMT, Lee CH, Jeng CY, et al. Effect of chronic renal failure on high-density lipoprotein kinetics. *Kidney Int* 1990;37:1295–1300.

77. Quaschning T, Krane V, Metzger T, Wanner C. Abnormalities in uremic lipoprotein metabolism and its impact on cardiovascular disease. *Am J Kidney Dis* 2001;4(suppl 1):S14–S19.

78. Dantoine TF, Debord J, Charmes JP, et al. Decrease of serum paraoxonase activity in chronic renal failure. *J Am Soc Nephrol* 1998;9:2082–2088.

79. Chan MK, Persaud JW, Varghese Z, et al. Post-heparin lipolytic enzymes in patients on CAPD. In: Maher JF, Winchester JF, eds. *Frontiers in Peritoneal Dialysis.* New York: Field, Rich, 1986:437–442.

80. Bagdade JD, Porte D Jr, Bierman EL. Hypertriglyceridemia: a metabolic consequence of chronic renal failure. *N Engl J Med* 1968;279:181–185.

81. Chan MK, Ramdial L, Varghese Z, et al. Plasma lecithin-cholesterol acyl-transferase activity in uremic patients. *Clin Chim Acta* 1982;119:65–72.

82. Hsia SL, Perez Go, Mendez AZ, et al. Defect in cholesterol transport in patients receiving maintenance hemodialysis. *J Lab Clin Med* 1985;106:53–61.

83. Kimura H, Gejyo F, Yamaguchi T, et al. A cholesteryl ester transfer protein gene mutation and vascular disease in dialysis patients. *J Am Soc Nephrol* 1999;10:294–299.

84. Josephson MA, Fellner SK, Dasgupta A. Improved lipid profiles in patients undergoing high flux hemodialysis. *Am J Kidney Dis* 1992;20:361–366.

85. Blankestijn PJ, Vos PF, Rabelink TJ, et al. High-flux dialysis membranes improve lipid profile in chronic haemodialysis patients. *J Am Soc Nephrol* 1995;5:1703–1708.

86. Novarini A, Zuliani U, Bandini L, et al. Observations on lipid metabolism in chronic renal failure during conservative and hemodialysis therapy. *Eur J Clin Invest* 1976;6:473–476.

87. Swamy AP, Cestro RUM, Campbell RG, Freeman RB. Long-term effect of dialysate glucose on the lipid levels of maintenance hemodialysis patients. *ASAIO Trans* 1976;22:54–58.

88. Giocelli G, Dalmasso F, Bruno M, et al. RDT with acetate-free bicarbonate buffered dialysis fluid: long-term effects on lipid pattern, acid-base balance and oxygen delivery. *Proc Eur Dial Transplant Assoc* 1979;16:115–120.

89. Conwill DE, Granger DN, Coole BH, et al. The effect of serum oncotic pressure on serum cholesterol levels: a study in "normal" and nephrotic patients. *South Med J* 1977;70:456–457.

90. Heimburger O, Stenvinkel P, Berglund L, et al. Increased plasma lipoprotein(a) in continuous ambulatory peritoneal dialysis is related to peritoneal transport of proteins and glucose. *Nephron* 1996;72:135–144.

91. Montenegro J, Moina I, Saracho R, et al. Levels of plasma lipoprotein(a) in continuous ambulatory peritoneal dialysis are not related to peritoneal losses of albumin. *Nephron* 1997;76:239–241.

92. Iliescu EA, Marcovina SM, Morton AR, Koschinsky ML. Apolipoprotein(a) phenotype, albumin clearance, and plasma levels of lipoprotein(a) in peritoneal dialysis. *Nephron* 2001;88:168–169.

93. Wheeler DC. Abnormalities of lipoprotein metabolism in CAPD patients. *Kidney Int* 1996;50(suppl 56):S41—S46.

94. Savdie E, Gibson JC, Crawford GA, et al. Impaired plasma triglyceride clearance as a feature of both uremic and post-transplant triglyceridemia. *Kidney Int* 1980;18:774–782.

95. Cramp DG, Tickner TR, Beale DJ, et al. Plasma triglyceride secretion and metabolism in renal failure. *Clin Chim Acta* 1977;76:237–241.

96. Chan PCK, Persaud J, Varghese Z, et al. Apolipoprotein B turnover in dialysis patients: its relationship to pathogenesis of hyperlipidemia. *Clin Nephrol* 1989;31:88–95.

97. Grodstein GP, Blumenkrantz MJ, Kopple JD, et al. Glucose absorption during continuous ambulatory peritoneal dialysis. *Kidney Int* 1981;19:564–567.

98. Cattran DC, Fenton SSA, Wilson DR, et al. Defective triglyceride removal in lipemia associated with peritoneal dialysis and hemodialysis. *Ann Intern Med* 1976;85:29–33.

99. Verschoor L, Lamners R, Birkenhager JC. Triglyceride turnover in severe chronic non-nephrotic renal failure. *Metabolism* 1978;27:879–883.

100. Chan MK, Varghese Z, Persaud JW, et al. Hyperlipidemia in patients on maintenance hemo- and peritoneal dialysis: the relative roles of triglyceride production and triglyceride removal. *Clin Nephrol* 1982;17:183–190.

101. Chan MK, Varghese Z, Persaud JW, et al. Fat clearance before and after heparin in chronic renal failure: hemodialysis reduces post-heparin fractional clearance rates of Intralipid. *Clin Chim Acta* 1980;108:95–101.

102. Ibels LS, Reardon MF, Nestel PG. Plasma post-heparin lipolytic activity and triglyceride clearance in uremic and hemodialysis patients and renal allograft recipients. *J Lab Clin Med* 1976;87:648–658.

103. Chan MK, Varghese Z, Persaud JW, et al. HDL cholesterol and intravenous fat tolerance test in dialysis patients. *Proc Eur Dial Transplant Assoc* 1980;17:247–252.

104. Russell GI, Davies TG, Walls J. Evaluation of the intravenous fat tolerance test in chronic renal disease. *Clin Nephrol* 1980;13:282–286.

105. Shoji T, Nishizawa Y, Kawagishi T, et al. Intermediate-density lipoprotein as an independent risk factor for aortic atherosclerosis in hemodialysis patients. *J Am Soc Nephrol* 1998;9:1277–1284.

106. Shoji T, Ishimura E, Inaba M, et al. Atherogenic lipoproteins in end-stage renal disease. *Am J Kidney Dis* 2001;38:S30–S33.

107. Alaupovic P. The biochemical and clinical significance of the interrelationship between very low density and high density lipoproteins. *Can J Biochem* 1981;59:565–579.

108. Patsch JR, Gotto AM Jr, Olivercrona T, Eisenberg S. Formation of high density lipoprotein 2-like particles during lipolysis of very low density lipoproteins in vitro. *Proc Natl Acad Sci USA* 1978;75:4519–4523.

109. Shoji T, Nishizawa Y, Nishitani H, et al. High serum lipoprotein(a) concentrations in uremic patients treated with contin-

uous ambulatory peritoneal dialysis. *Clin Nephrol* 1992;38:271–276.

110. Thillet J, Faucher C, Issad B, et al. Lipoprotein(a) in patients treated by continuous ambulatory peritoneal dialysis. *Am J Kidney Dis* 1993;22:226–232.

111. Kronenberg F, Konig P, Neyer U, et al. Multicenter study of lipoprotein(a) and apolipoprotein(a) phenotypes in patients with end-stage renal disease treated by hemodialysis or continuous ambulatory peritoneal dialysis. *J Am Soc Nephrol* 1995;6:110–120.

112. Monzani G, Bergesio F, Ciuti R, et al. Lipoprotein abnormalities in chronic renal failure and dialysis patients. *Blood Purif* 1996;14:262–272.

113. Moberly JB, Attman PO, Samuelsson O, et al. Alterations in lipoprotein composition in peritoneal dialysis patients. *Perit Dial Int* 2002;22:220–228.

114. Avram MM, Goldwasser P, Burrell DC, et al. The uremic dyslipidemia: a cross-sectional and longitudinal study. *Am J Kidney Dis* 1992;20:329–335.

115. Deighan CJ, Casiake MJ, McConnell M, et al. Atherogenic lipoprotein phenotype in end-stage renal failure: origin and extent of small dense low-density lipoprotein formation. *Am J Kidney Dis* 2000;35:852–862.

116. McCosh EJ, Karim MS, Solangi K, et al. Hypertriglyceridemia in patients with chronic renal failure. *Am J Clin Nutr* 1976;28:1036–1043.

117. Huttunen JK, Pasternack A, Vanttinen T, et al. Lipoprotein metabolism in patients with chronic uremia. *Acta Med Scand* 1978;204:211–218.

118. Crawford GA, Savdie E, Stewart JH. Heparin-released plasma lipases in chronic renal failure and after renal transplantation. *Clin Sci* 1979;57:155–165.

119. Chan MK, Yeung CK. Lipid metabolism in 31 Chinese patients on three 2–1 exchanges of CAPD. *Perit Dial Bull* 1986;6:12–16.

120. Chan MK. Gemfibrozil improves abnormalities of lipid metabolism in patients on continuous ambulatory peritoneal dialysis. The role of postheparin lipases in the metabolism of high-density lipoprotein subfractions. *Metabolism* 1989;38:939–945.

121. Shoji T, Nishizawa Y, Nishitani H, et al. Impaired metabolism of high-density lipoprotein in uremic patients. *Kidney Int* 1992;41:1653–1661.

122. Mordasini R, Frey F, Flury W, et al. Selective deficiency of hepatic triglyceride lipase in uremic patients. *N Engl J Med* 1977;297:1362–1366.

123. Bolzano K, Krempler F, Sanhoffer F. Hepatic and extrahepatic triglyceride lipase activity in uremic patients on chronic hemodialysis. *Eur J Clin Invest* 1978;8:289–293.

124. Murase T, Cattran DC, Rubinstein B, Steiner G. Inhibition of lipoprotein lipase by uremic plasma. A possible cause of hypertriglyceridemia. *Metabolism* 1975;24:1279–1286.

125. Cheung AK, Parker CJ, Ren K, Iverius PH. Increased lipase inhibition in uremia: identification of pre-beta-HDL as a major inhibitor in normal and uremic plasma. *Kidney Int* 1996;49:1360–1371.

126. Schaefer K, Herrath D, Gullerg CA, et al. Chronic hemofiltration: a critical evaluation of a new method for the treatment of blood. *Artif Organs* 1978;2:386–394.

127. Smith D, De Fronzo RA. Insulin resistance in uremia mediated by post-binding defects. *Kidney Int* 1982;22:54–62.

128. Guarnieri GF, Moracchiello M, Campanacci L, et al. Lecithin-cholesterol acyl-transferase (LCAT) activity in chronic uremia. *Kidney Int* 1978;13(suppl 8):S26–S30.

129. McLeod R, Reeve CE, Frohlich J. Plasma lipoproteins and lecithin: cholesterol acyltransferase distribution in patients on dialysis. *Kidney Int* 1989;25:683–688.

130. Chan MK, Ramdial L, Varghese Z, et al. Plasma LCAT activities in renal allograft recipients. *Clin Chim Acta* 1982;124:187–193.

131. Stefanovic V, Nesic V, Stojimirovic B. Treatment of insulin resistance in uremia. *Int J Artif Organs* 2003;26:100–104.

132. Westervelt FB. Insulin effect in uremia. *J Lab Clin Med* 1969;74:79–84.

133. Mak RH, Wong JH. The vitamin D/parathyroid hormone axis in the pathogenesis of hypertension and insulin resistance in uremia. *Miner Electrolyte Metab* 1992;18:156–159.

134. Mak RH. Correction of anemia by erythropoietin reverses insulin resistance and hyperinsulinemia in uremia. *Am J Physiol* 1996;270(5 Pt 2):F839–F844.

135. Vaziri ND, Liang K. Down-regulation of tissue lipoprotein lipase expression in experimental chronic renal failure. *Kidney Int* 1996;50:1928–1935.

136. Roullet JB, Lacour B, Yvert J-P, Drueke T. Correction by insulin of disturbed TG-rich LP metabolism in rats with chronic renal failure. *Am J Physiol* 1986;250:E373–E376.

137. Drueke T, Lacour B. Parathyroid hormone and hyperlipidemia of uremia. *Contrib Nephrol* 1985;49:12–19.

138. Akmal M, Kasim SE, Soliman AR, Massry SG. Excess parathyroid hormone adversely affects lipid metabolism in chronic renal failure. *Kidney Int* 1990;37:854–858.

139. Vaziri ND, Liang K. Role of secondary hyperparathyroidism in the pathogenesis of depressed lipoprotein lipase expression in chronic renal failure. *Am J Physiol (Renal Physiol)* 1997;273:F925–F930.

140. Klin M, Smogorzewski M, Ni Z, et al. Abnormalities in hepatic lipase in chronic renal failure: role of excess parathyroid hormone. *J Clin Invest* 1996;97:2167–2173.

141. Chan MK. Lipid Metabolism in Renal Replacement Therapy. MD thesis. Hong Kong: University of Hong Kong, 1982.

142. Navarro JF, Teruel JL, Lasuncion MA, et al. Relationship between serum parathyroid hormone levels and lipid profile in hemodialysis patients. Evolution of lipid parameters after parathyroidectomy. *Clin Nephrol* 1998;49:303–307.

143. Liang Liang K, Oveisi F, Vaziri ND. Role of secondary hyperparathyroidism in the genesis of hypertriglyceridemia and VLDL receptor deficiency in chronic renal failure. *Kidney Int* 1998;53:626–630.

144. Bohmer T, Bergren H, Eiklid K. Carnitine deficiency induced by intermittent hemodialysis for renal failure. *Lancet* 1978;1:126–128.

145. Fritz IB, Marquis NR. The role of acylcarnitine esters and carnitine palmityl transferase in the transport of fatty acyl groups across mitochondrial membranes. *Proc Natl Acad Sci USA* 1965;54:1226–1233.

146. Wanner C, Horl WH. Potential role of carnitine in patients with renal insufficiency. *Klin Wochenschr* 1986;64:579–586.

147. Bellinghieri G, Santoro D, Calvani M, et al. Carnitine and hemodialysis. *Am J Kidney Dis* 2003;41(3 suppl 2): S116–S122.

148. Nikkila EA, Kekki M. Plasma triglyceride metabolism in thryroid disease. *J Clin Invest* 1972;51:2103–2114.

149. Fellicetta JV, Green WL, Haas LB. Thyroid function and lipids in patients with chronic renal disease treated by hemodialysis: with comments on the "free thyroxine index." *Metabolism* 1979;28:756–763.

150. Bommer C, Werle E, Walter-Sack I, et al. D-thyroxine reduces lipoprotein(a) serum concentration in dialysis patients. *J Am Soc Nephrol* 1998;9:90–96.

151. Orskov HL, Christensen NJ. Growth hormone in uremia: I. Plasma growth hormone, insulin and glucagon after oral and intravenous glucose in uremic subjects. *Scand J Clin Lab Invest* 1971;27:51–60.

152. Murase T, Yamada N, Ohsawa N, et al. Decline of postheparin lipoprotein lipase in acromegalic patients. *Metabolism* 1980;29:666–672.

153. Asayama K, Amemiya S, Kusano S, Kato K. Growth hormone-induced changes in post-heparin plasma lipoprotein lipase and hepatic triglycerides lipase activities. *Metabolism* 1984;33:129–131.

154. Viidas U, Johannsson G, Mattson-Hulten L, Ahlmen J. Lipids, blood pressure and bone metabolism after growth hormone therapy in elderly hemodialysis patients. *J Nephrol* 2003;16:231–237.

155. Laron Z, Wang XL, Klinger B, et al. Growth hormone treatment increases circulating lipoprotein(a) in children with chronic renal failure. *J Pediatr Endocrinol Metab* 1996;9: 533–537.

156. Kuku SF, Jaspar JB, Emmanuel PS, et al. Heterogeneity of plasma glucagon. *J Clin Invest* 1976;58:742–750.

157. Emmanouel DS, Jaspan JB, Kuku SF, et al. Pathogenesis and characterization of hyperglucagonemia in the uremic rat. *J Clin Invest* 1976;58:1266–1272.

158. Gonen B, Goldberg AP, Harter HR, Schonfield G. Abnormal cell-interactive properties of low-density lipoproteins isolated from patients with chronic renal failure. *Metabolism* 1985;34:10–14.

159. Dasgupta A, Hussain S, Ahmad S. Increased lipid peroxidation in patients on maintenance hemodialysis. *Nephron* 1992;60:56–59.

160. Sasaki J, Cottam GL. Glycosylation of LDL decreases its ability to interact with high-affinity receptors of human fibroblasts in vitro and decreases its clearance from rabbit plasma in vivo. *Biochem Biophys Acta* 1982;713: 199–207.

161. Gonon B, Goldberg AP, Haster HR, Schonfield G. Abnormal cell-interactive properties of low density lipoproteins isolated from patients with chronic renal failure. *Metabolism* 1985;34:10–14.

162. Attman PO, Samuelsson OG, Moberly J, et al. Apolipoprotein B–containing lipoproteins in renal failure: the relation to mode of dialysis. *Kidney Int* 1999;55:1536–1542.

163. O'Neal D, Lee P, Murphy B, Best J. Low-density lipoprotein particle size distribution in end-stage renal disease treated with hemodialysis or peritoneal dialysis. *Am J Kidney Dis* 1996;27:84–91.

164. Horkko S, Huttunen K, Kesaniemi A. Decreased clearance of low-density lipoprotein in uremic patients under dialysis treatment. *Kidney Int* 1995;47:1732–1740.

165. Kontessis PS, Jayathissa SA, Walker JD, et al. Effect of beta-blocker therapy on serum lipoprotein profiles in patients on renal dialysis and in diabetic nephropathy. *Diabetes Res* 1993;23:93–104.

166. Hirata K, Kikuchi S, Saku K, et al. Apolipoprotein(a) phenotypes and serum lipoproteins in maintenance hemodialysis patients with/without diabetes mellitus. *Kidney Int* 1993;44:1062–1070.

167. Bartens W, Nauck M, Schollmeyer P, Wanner C. Elevated lipoprotein(a) and fibrinogen serum levels increase the cardiovascular risk in continuous ambulatory peritoneal dialysis patients. *Perit Dial Int* 1996;16:27–33.

168. Shah GM, Lin ZL, Kamanna VS, et al. Effect of serum subfractions from peritoneal dialysis patients on Hep-G2 cell apolipoprotein A-I and B metabolism. *Kidney Int* 1996;50:2079–2087.

169. Ritter M, Buechler C, Boettcher A, et al. Cloning and characterization of a novel apolipoprotein A-I binding protein, AI-BP, secreted by cells of the kidney proximal tubules in response to HDL or ApoA-I. *Genomics* 2002;79:693–702.

170. Fytili CI, Progia EG, Panagoutsos SA, et al. Lipoprotein abnormalities in hemodialysis and continuous ambulatory peritoneal dialysis patients. *Renal Failure* 2002;24:623–630.

171. Maeda S, Abe A, Seishima M, et al. Transient changes of serum lipoprotein(a) as an acute phase protein. *Atherosclerosis* 1989;78:145–150.

172. Stenvinkel P, Heimburger O, Paultre F, et al. Strong association between malnutrition, inflammation, and atherosclerosis in chronic renal failure. *Kidney Int* 1999;55:1899–1911.

173. Wanner C, Zimmermann J, Schwedler S, Metzger T: Inflammation and cardiovascular risk in dialysis patients. *Kidney Int* 2002;61:S99–S102.

174. Wang AY, Woo J, Lam CW, et al. Is a single time point C-reactive protein predictive of outcome in peritoneal dialysis patients? *J Am Soc Nephrol* 2003;14:1871–1879.

175. Ross EA, Shah GM, Kashyap ML. Elevated plasma lipoprotein(a) levels and hypoalbuminemia in peritoneal dialysis patients. *Int J Artif Organs* 1995;18:751–756.

176. Zimmermann J, Herrlinger S, Pruy A, et al. Inflammation enhances cardiovascular risk and mortality in hemodialysis patients. *Kidney Int* 1999;55:648–658.

177. Sampietro T, Bigazzi F, Dal Pino B, et al. Increased plasma C-reactive protein in familial hypoalphalipoproteinemia: a proinflammatory condition? *Circulation* 2002;105:11–14.

178. Hulthe J, Fagerberg B. Circulating oxidized LDL is associated with subclinical atherosclerosis development and inflammatory cytokines (AIR Study). *Arterioscler Thromb Vasc Biol* 2002;22:1162–1167.

179. Zhang L, Zalewski A, Liu Y, et al. Diabetes-induced oxidative stress and low-grade inflammation in porcine coronary arteries. *Circulation* 2003;108:472–478.

180. Locatelli F, Canaud B, Eckardt KU, et al. Oxidative stress in end-stage renal disease: an emerging threat to patient outcome. *Nephrol Dial Transplant* 2003;18:1272–1280.

181. Avram MM, Fein PA, Anigani A, et al. Cholesterol and lipid disturbances in renal disease. The natural history of uremic dyslipidemia and the impact of hemodialysis and continuous ambulatory peritoneal dialysis. *Am J Med* 1989;87:5-55N–5-60N.

182. Haas LB, Wahl PW, Sherrard DJ. A longitudinal study of lipid abnormalities in renal failure. *Nephron* 1983;33: 145–149.

183. Kim SB, Yang WS, Park JS. Role of hypoalbuminemia in the genesis of cardiovascular disease in dialysis patients. *Perit Dial Int* 1999;19(suppl 2): S144–S149.

184. Koch M, Kutkuhn B, Trenkwalder E, et al. Apolipoprotein B, fibrinogen, HDL cholesterol, and apolipoprotein(a) phenotypes predict coronary artery disease in hemodialysis patients. *J Am Soc Nephrol* 1997;8:1889–1898.

185. Kronenberg F, Neyer U, Lhotta K, et al. The low molecular weight apo(a) phenotype is an independent predictor for coronary artery disease in hemodialysis patients: a prospective follow-up. *J Am Soc Nephrol* 1999;10:1027–1036.

186. Dawber TR. *The Framingham Study: The Epidemiology of Atherosclerotic Disease*. Cambridge, MA: Harvard University Press, 1980.

187. Miller GJ, Miller NE. Plasma high density lipoprotein concentration and development of ischemic heart disease. *Lancet* 1975;1:16–19.

188. Deuber HJ, Schulz W. Reduced lipid concentrations during four years of dialysis with low molecular weight heparin. *Kidney Int* 1991;40:496–500.

189. Wiemer J, Winkler K, Baumstark M, et al. Influence of low molecular weight heparin compared to conventional heparin for anticoagulation during haemodialysis on low density lipoprotein subclasses. *Nephrol Dial Transplant* 2002;17:2231–2238.

190. Helsinki Heart Study: Primary-prevention trial with gemfibrozil in middle-age men with dyslipidemia. Safety of treatment. Changes in risk factors. And incidence of coronary heart disease. *N Engl J Med* 1987;317:1237–1245.

191. Lipid Research Clinics Program: The Lipid Research Clinics Coronary Primary Prevention Trial results: II. The relationship of reduction in incidence of coronary heart disease to cholesterol lowering. *JAMA* 1984;251:365–374.

192. K/DOQI Working Group. K/DOQI Clinicial Practice Guidelines for Managing Dyslipidemias in Chronic Kidney Disease. *Am J Kidney Dis* 2003;4(suppl 3):S39–S58.

193. Tanaka N, Sakaguchi S, Oshige K, et al. Effect of chronic administration of propranolol on lipoprotein metabolism. *Metabolism* 1976;25:1971–1975.

194. Goldberg AP, Hagberg JM, Delmez JA, et al. Metabolic effects of exercise training in hemodialysis patients. *Kidney Int* 1980;18:754–761.

195. Sanfelippo ML, Swenson RS, Reaven GM. Response of plasma triglycerides to dietary changes in patients on hemodialysis. *Kidney Int* 1978;14:180–186.

196. Dornan TL, Gokal R, Pearce JS, et al. Long-term dietary treatment of hyperlipidemia in patients with chronic hemodialysis. *Br Med J* 1980;281:1044.

197. Cattran DC, Steiner G, Fenton SSA, Ampil M. Dialysis hyperlipidemia: response to dietary manipulations. *Clin Nephrol* 1980;13:177–182.

198. DiAmico G, Gentile MG. Influence of diet on lipid abnormalities in human renal disease. *Am J Kidney Dis* 1993;22: 151–157.

199. Saltissi D, Morgan C, Knight B, et al. Effect of lipid-lowering dietary recommendations on the nutritional intake and lipid profiles of chronic peritoneal dialysis and hemodialysis patients. *Am J Kidney Dis* 2001;37:1209–1215.

200. Norbeck HE, Anderson P. Treatment of uremic hypertriglyceridemia with bezafibrate. *Atherosclerosis* 1982;44:125–136.

201. Williams AJ, Baker F, Walls J. The short term effects of bezafibrate on the hypertriglyceridemia of moderate to severe uremia. *Br J Clin Pharmacol* 1984;18:361–367.

202. Pasternack A, Vanttinen T, Solakivi T, et al. Normalization of lipoprotein lipase and hepatic lipase by gemfibrozil results in correction of lipoprotein abnormalities in chronic renal failure. *Clin Nephrol* 1987;27:163–168.

203. Monk JP, Todd PA. Bezafibrate: a review of its pharmacodynamic and pharmacokinetic properties, and therapeutic use in hyperlipidemia. *Drugs* 1987;33:539–576.

204. Berndt J, Gaumert R, Still J. Mode of action of the lipid-lowering agents, clofibrate and BM 15075, on cholesterol biosynthesis in rat liver. *Atherosclerosis* 1978;30:147–152.

205. Nishizawa Y, Shoji T, Nishitani H, et al. Hypertriglyceridemia and lowered apolipoprotein CII/CIII ratio in uremia. Effect of a fibric acid, clinofibrate. *Kidney Int* 1993; 44:1352–1359.

206. Kawamura M, Miyazaki S, Teramoto T, et al. Gemfibrozil metabolite inhibits in vitro low-density lipoprotein (LDL) oxidation and diminishes cytotoxicity induced by oxidized LDL. *Metabolism* 2000;49:479–485.

207. Chan MK. Sustained-release bezafibrate corrects lipid abnormalities in patients on continuous ambulatory peritoneal dialysis. *Nephron* 1990;56:56–61.

208. Williams AJ, Walks J. The pharmakinetics of bezafibrate in patients undergoing continuous ambulatory peritoneal dialysis (CAPD). *Perit Dial Bull* 1986;6:64–71.

209. Alberts AW, Chen J, Kuron G, et al. Mevinolin: a highly potent competitive inhibitor of hydroxy-methyl-glutaryl-coenzyme A reductase and a cholesterol lowering agent. *Proc Natl Acad Sci USA* 1980;77:3957–3961.

210. The Lovastin Study Group II. Therapeutic responses to Lovastatin (Mevinolin) in non-familial hypercholesterolemia. *JAMA* 1986;256:2829–2834.

211. Bonn V, Cheung RC, Chen B, et al. Simvastatin, an HMG-CoA reductase inhibitor, induces the synthesis and secretion of apolipoprotein AI in HepG2 cells and primary hamster hepatocytes. *Atherosclerosis* 2002;163:59–68.

212. Guerin M, Egger P, Soudant C, et al. Dose-dependent action of atorvastatin in type IIB hyperlipidemia: preferential and progressive reduction of atherogenic apoB-containing lipoprotein subclasses (VLDL-2, IDL, small dense LDL) and stimulation of cellular cholesterol efflux. *Atherosclerosis* 2002;163:287–296.

213. Knopp RH. Drug treatment of lipid disorders. *N Engl J Med* 1999;341:498–511.

214. Ridker PM. Connecting the role of C-reactive protein and statins in cardiovascular disease. *Clin Cardiol* 2003; 26(4Suppl3):III39–III44.

215. Wanner C, Horl WH, Luley CH, Wieland H. Effects of HMGCoA reductase inhibitors in hypercholesterolemic patients on hemodialysis. *Kidney Int* 1991;39:754–760.

216. Di Paolo, Bonomini M, Terezio MG, et al. Hypolipidemic effects of simvastatin in CAPD patients with hypercholestolemia. In: Ota K et al, eds. *Current Concepts in Peritoneal Dialysis*. New York: Elsevier, 1992;565–567.

217. Nishizawa Y, Shoji T, Emoto M, et al. Reduction of intermediate density lipoprotein by pravastatin in hemo- and peritoneal dialysis patients. *Clin Nephrol* 1995;43:268–277.

218. Robson R, Collins J, Johnson R, et al. Effects of simvastatin and enalapril on serum lipoprotein concentrations and left ventricular mass in patients on dialysis. The Perfect Study Collaborative Group. *J Nephrol* 1997;10:33–40.

219. Harris KP, Wheeler DC, Chong CC—the Atorvastatin in CAPD Study Investigators. A placebo-controlled trial examining atorvastatin in dyslipidemic patients undergoing CAPD. *Kidney Int* 2002;61:1469–1474.

220. Saltissi D, Morgan C, Rigby RJ, Westhuyzen J. Safety and efficacy of simvastatin in hypercholesterolemic patients undergoing chronic renal dialysis. *Am J Kidney Dis* 2002;39: 283–290.

221. Sheperd JG, Packard CJ, Bicker S, et al. Cholestyramine promotes receptor-mediated low density lipoprotein catabolism. *N Engl J Med* 1980;302:1219–1222.

222. Friedman EA, Saltzman MJ, Delan BG, et al. Reduction in hyperlipidemia in hemodialysis patients treated with charcoal and oxidized starch (oxy-starch). *Am J Clin Nutr* 1978;31:1903–1914.

223. Gagne C, Bays HE, Weiss SR, et al for Ezetimibe Study Group. Efficacy and safety of ezetimibe added to ongoing statin therapy for treatment of patients with primary hypercholesterolemia. *Am J Cardiol* 2002;90:1084–1091.

224. Parthasarathy S, Young SG, Witztum JL, et al. Probucol enhances oxidative modification of low density lipoprotein. *J Clin Invest* 1986;77:641–644.

225. Mellies MJ, Gartside PS, Galtfeleter L, Glueck GJ. Effect of probucol on plasma cholesterol high and low density lipoprotein cholesterol and apolipoprotein A1 and A2 in adults with primary familial hypercholesterolemia. *Metabolism* 1980;29:956–964.

226. Tardif JC. Clinical results with AGI-1067: a novel antioxidant vascular protectant. *Am J Cardiol* 2003; 91 (3A):41A–49A.

227. Sawayama Y, Shimizu C, Maeda N, et al. Effects of probucol and pravastatin on common carotid atherosclerosis in patients with asymptomatic hypercholesterolemia. Fukuoka Atherosclerosis Trial (FAST). *J Am Coll Cardiol* 2002; 39(4):610–616.

228. Fiorini F, Patrone E, Castelluccio A. Clinical investigation on the hypolipidemic effect of simvastatin versus probucol in hemodialysis patients. *Clin Ther* 1994;145:213–217.

229. De Vecchi A, Pini C, Castelnovo C, et al. Low-dose acipimox in type IIb dyslipidemia in CAPD patients. In: Ota K, et al, eds. *Current Concepts in Peritoneal Dialysis*. New York: Elsevier, 1992:555–571.

230. Tzanatos H, Koutsikos D, Agroyannis B, et al. Lipid-lowering effect and safety of acipimox in hemodialysis patients

and renal transplant recipients. *Renal Failure* 1994;16: 391–405.

231. Bertoli M, Battistella PA, Vergani L, et al. Carnitine deficiency induced during hemodialysis and hyperlipidemia: effect of replacement therapy. *Am J Clin Nutr* 1981;34: 1496–1500.

232. Engel AG, Angelini C. Carnitine deficiency of human muscle with associated lipid storage myopathy—a new syndrome. *Science* 1973;179:899–902.

233. Savica V, Bellinghieri G, DiStefano C, et al. Plasma and muscle carnitine levels in hemodialysis patients with morphological and ultastructural examination of muscle samples. *Nephron* 1983;35:232–236.

234. Maebashi M, Kawamura N, Sato M, et al. Lipid lowering effect of carnitine in patients with type IV hyperlipoproteinemia. *Lancet* 1978;2:805–807.

235. Guarnieri GM, Ranieri F, Toigo G, et al. Lipid lowering effect of carnitine in chronically uremic patients treated with maintenance hemodialysis. *Am J Clin Nutr* 1980;33: 1489–1492.

236. Chan MK, Varghese Z, Persaud JW, Moorhead JF. Carnitine in hemodialysis patients. *Lancet* 1980;2:1028–1029.

237. Chan MK, Persaud JW, Varghese Z, et al. Response patterns to DL-carnitine in patients on maintenance hemodialysis. *Nephron* 1982;30:240–243.

238. Lacour B, DiGiulio S, Chanard J, et al. Carnitine improves lipid anomalies in hemodialysis patients. *Lancet* 1980;2: 763–764.

239. Vacha GM, Giocelli G, Siliprandi N, Corsi M. Favorable effects of L-carnitine treatment on hypertriglyceridemia in hemodialysis patients: decisive role of low levels of high density lipoprotein-cholesterol. *Am J Clin Nutr* 1983;38: 532–540.

240. Vacha, GM, Corsi M, Giocelli G, et al. Serum and muscle L-carnitine levels in hemodialysis patients, during and after long-term L-carnitine treatment. *Curr Ther Res* 1985;37: 505–515.

241. Fagher BG, Cederblad M, Erikson M, et al. L-Carnitine and hemodialysis: double blind study on muscle function and metabolism and peripheral nerve function. *Scand J Clin Lab Invest* 1985;45:169–178.

242. Dyeberg J, Mortensen JZ, Nielsan AH, Schmidt EB. n-3 polyunsaturated fatty acids and ischemic heart disease. *Lancet* 1982;2:614.

243. Hamazaki T, Nakazawa R, Tateno S, et al. Effects of fish oil rich in eicosapentaenoic acid on serum lipid in hyperlipidemic hemodialysis patients. *Kidney Int* 1984;26:81–84.

244. Rylance PB, Gordge MP, Sayner R, et al. Fish Oil modifies and reduces platelet aggregability in hemodialysis patients. *Nephron* 1986;43:196–202.

245. Wong SM, Reardon M, Nestel P. Reduced triglyceride formation from long-chain polyenoic fatty acids in rat hepatocytes. *Metabolism* 1985;34:900–905.

246. Nestel P, Conner W, Reardon M, et al. Suppression by diets rich in fish oils of very low density lipoprotein production in man. *J Clin Invest* 1984;74:82–89.

247. Illingworth D, Harris W, Connor W. Inhibition of low density lipoprotein synthesis by dietary omega-3 fatty acids in humans. *Arteriosclerosis* 1984;4:2270–2275.

248. Harris WS. Fish oils and plasma lipid and lipoprotein metabolism in humans. A critical review. *J Lipid Res* 1989;30: 785–807.

249. Kestin M, Clifton P, Belling GB, Nestel P. n-3 fatty acids of marine origin lower systolic blood pressure and triglycerides but raise LDL cholesterol compared with n-3 and n-6 fatty acids from plants. *Am J Clin Nutr* 1990;51:1028–1034.

250. Rolf N, Tenschert W, Lison AE. Results of a long-term administration of omega-3-fatty acids in hemodialysis patients with dyslipoproteinemia. *Nephrol Dial Transplant* 1990;5: 797–801.

251. Donnelly SM, Ali MA, Churchill DN. Effect of n-3 fatty acids from fish oil on hemostasis, blood pressure, and lipid profile of dialysis patients. *J Am Soc Nephrol* 1992;2: 1634–1639.

Endocrine Dysfunction in Chronic Kidney Disease

Mohammad Akmal
Elaine Kaptein

Patients with advanced chronic kidney disease (CKD), whether or not they are receiving maintenance dialysis, may display a wide range of hormonal and metabolic disturbances. There may be abnormalities in both the secretion and metabolism of the endocrine hormones as well as target-organ sensitivity to these hormones. The derangements in parathyroid hormone (PTH), vitamin D, and erythropoietin metabolism are discussed in Chaps. 26 and 30. This chapter details the abnormalities of pancreatic, thyroid, adrenal, and gonadal hormones.

CARBOHYDRATE AND INSULIN METABOLISM

The kidney plays an important role in the regulation of insulin metabolism.[1] In humans, the kidneys' tubular luminal and peritubular uptake of insulin and its subsequent metabolism of the hormone are evidenced by the following: (1)

there is a 30 to 40 percent difference in renal arterial compared to venous insulin concentration[2–4] and (2) insulin clearance is 200 mL/min, significantly higher than the nominal glomerular filtration rate (GFR) of 120 mL/min.[1] These data suggest that one-fourth of daily insulin secretion from the pancreas, or 6 to 8 units of insulin, is degraded by the kidney. A reduction in the metabolic clearance of insulin begins to occur at a GFR of 40 mL/min, and significant prolongation of insulin's half-life ($t_{1/2}$) is observed only after the GFR has decreased to about 15 to 20 mL/min.[1,5] This change in insulin's $t_{1/2}$ is associated with a decrement in insulin requirements in diabetics with progressive chronic kidney disease.[6–8]

Abnormalities of carbohydrate metabolism are commonly observed in patients with CKD[9–12] and are characterized by an abnormal response to an oral or intravenous glucose load. The clinically relevant features of abnormal glucose metabolism in patients with advanced CKD are as follows[12]: (1) normal or mildly elevated fasting blood glucose; (2) spontaneous hypoglycemia; (3) fasting hyperinsulinemia with normal fasting blood glucose levels; (4) variable insulin secretion; (5) a blunted response of plasma glucose to intravenous insulin; (6) decreased peripheral sensitivity to insulin; and (7) reduced insulin requirements in diabetic patients with uremia.

Insulin resistance is almost always present in uremic patients,[9,10,12,13] whereas insulin secretion can be normal,[14] increased,[15] or decreased.[10] The normal response of pancreatic β cells to the presence of insulin resistance is to enhance insulin secretion.[16,17] Glucose intolerance ensues only if impaired tissue sensitivity and inappropriate release of insulin from the β cells coexist.[12,18] Indeed, this phenomenon has been observed both in humans[19] and dogs[20] with uremia.

The toxin(s) that have been postulated to adversely affect glucose metabolism in CKD include creatinine, guanidinosuccinic acid, methylguanidine, growth hormone, glucagon, and parathyroid hormone (PTH).[12] Only for PTH is there substantiated evidence for a role in the genesis of the glucose intolerance of CKD. Support for this contention comes from the finding that patients with primary hyperparathyroidism may display glucose intolerance.[21,22] These patients may have elevated plasma insulin levels both in the fasting state and in response to a glucose load[21,22]; they may also demonstrate resistance to insulin.[22]

It is, therefore, reasonable to suggest that secondary hyperparathyroidism, which is almost a universal finding in patients with advanced CKD,[23–26] may contribute to carbohydrate intolerance in uremia. This hypothesis has been investigated in humans,[19,27] dogs,[20] and rats.[28] The following studies have been performed to investigate the role of PTH in the genesis of carbohydrate intolerance in CKD: intravenous glucose tolerance test (IVGTT) in dogs[20] and rats[28] with CKD; euglycemic insulin clamp and hyperglycemic clamp studies in dogs[20] and humans[19,27]; and insulin release from pancreatic islets during static incubation and dynamic insulin release from perfused pancreatic islets in rats.[28]

IVGTT was performed in two groups of dogs and three groups of rats with CKD, of comparable degree and duration, produced by five-sixths nephrectomy. One group of dogs had intact parathyroid glands (CKD) and hence had secondary hyperparathyroidism; the other underwent thyroparathyroidectomy at the time of induction of CKD (CKD-PTX). The latter group was maintained normocalcemic and euthyroid by a high calcium intake and thyroid supplementation, respectively.[20] The protocol for the rats included three groups: normal controls, rats with chronic kidney disease and intact PTH (CKD), and rats with chronic kidney disease without parathyroid glands (CKD-PTX). The CKD-PTX group was maintained normocalcemic by allowing the rats to freely drink water containing 5 percent calcium. Five-sixths nephrectomy resulted in a significant ($p < 0.01$) decrement in creatinine clearance in both the

CKD (from 56 ± 2 to 12 ± 4) and the CKD-PTX dogs (from 58 ± 3 to 13 ± 3 mL/min), a significant increase in plasma creatinine in rats with CKD but without a significant difference between CKD and CKD-PTX rats, and significantly elevated serum PTH levels in the CKD dogs (from 1.0 ± 0.5 to 37 ± 0.5 μLeq/mL). The serum PTH levels were undetectable in CKD-PTX dogs, and there were no significant differences in plasma concentrations of electrolytes among the animals with CKD with or without PTH before and after induction of chronic renal failure.

The results of IVGTT before and after induction of CKD in CKD and CKD-PTX animals (dogs, rats) are shown in Fig. 29–1. The CKD dogs with secondary hyperparathyroidism displayed glucose intolerance, whereas CKD-PTX dogs did not have glucose intolerance. Similarly, the IVGTT was abnormal only in CKD rats, but glucose tolerance was preserved in CKD-PTX animals.

The rate of decline of plasma concentration of glucose (Kg) decreased significantly ($p < 0.01$) after chronic kidney disease in CKD dogs (from 2.86 ± 0.48 to 1.23 ± 0.18 percent/min), while Kg was not significantly affected in CKD-PTX dogs, with the values being 2.41 ± 0.4 percent/min before and 2.86 ± 0.86 percent/min after CKD (Fig. 29–2).

There was a significant increase in plasma concentrations of insulin during IVGTT in all studies (Fig. 29–3). In the CKD dogs, plasma insulin concentrations increased from 24 ± 2.7 μU/mL to a peak of 105 μU/mL ($p < 0.01$) and remained elevated throughout the study. In CKD-PTX animals, the maximum increase in plasma insulin concentration (from 18 ± 1.2 to 229 ± 19.4 μU/mL) was more than twice that observed in CKD dogs ($p < 0.01$); the levels gradually declined, but they were higher than those in CKD animals for the first 30 minutes ($p < 0.01$) and returned to baseline values by 60 minutes. These differences in plasma insulin were not due to high plasma glucose concentrations in CKD-PTX dogs, since, for any given level of plasma glucose in these dogs during the IVGTT, the plasma insulin values were higher than those observed in CKD animals (Fig. 29–4).

Hyperglycemic and euglycemic insulin clamp techniques[29] have been utilized to quantitate the relative roles of insulin secretion and insulin resistance in the genesis of the glucose intolerance of CKD. In the hyperglycemic clamp technique, the plasma glucose concentration is acutely raised by 125 mg/dL above the basal level. Under the steady-state condition of constant hyperglycemia, the infusion rate of glucose after correction of urinary glucose losses provides a measure of the amount of glucose taken up by all the tissues of the body. In the euglycemic insulin clamp technique, after increasing the plasma insulin concentration by 100 μU/mL, the plasma glucose concentration is maintained constant at the basal level by the periodic adjustment of a variable infusion of 20% glucose. Under this steady-state condition of constant glycemia, all of the in-

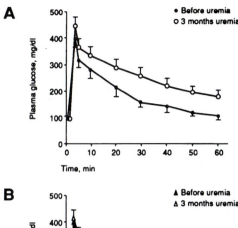

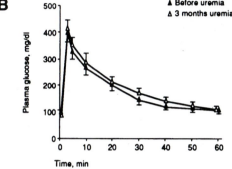

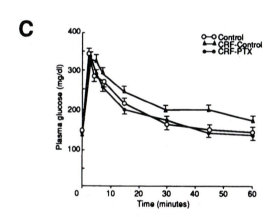

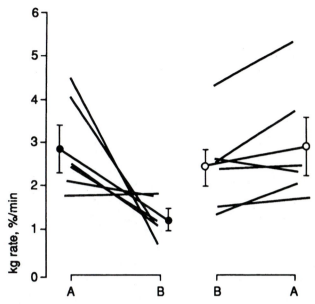

Figure 29–2. The K_g rate before and 3 months after chronic renal failure in dogs with intact PTH (CRF) (left panel), and parathyroidectomized (CRF-PTX) animals (right panel). A denotes before CRF, and B denotes after CRF. Each line represents one animal and the heavy lines depict the mean values with brackets denoting 1 SEM. The K_g rate after CRF was significantly (P = 0.01) lower than before chronic renal failure in CRF dogs. *(From Akmal et al,[21] with permission of The Society for Clinical Investigation.)*

Figure 29–1. Panel A. The changes in plasma glucose concentrations during IVGTT performed before (closed circles) and after (open circles) 3 months of CRF in dogs with intact parathyroid glands. Each data point represents the mean value of six dogs, and the brackets denote 1 SEM. Plasma glucose levels in dogs with CRF were significantly higher ($P < 0.01$) at 20 to 60 minutes. *(From Akmal et al,[21] with permission.)* **Panel B.** IVGTT in parathyroidectomized dogs does not demonstrate any significant differences in glucose concentrations before (closed triangles) and after (open triangles) CRF at all times. *(From Akmal et al,[21] with permission.)* **Panel C.** IVGTT was abnormal only in rats with secondary hyperparathyroidism (CRF-Control). *(From Fadda et al,[28] with permission.)*

fused glucose (M) is taken up by cells and, when added to the rate of residual glucose production measured with tritiated glucose, provides a measure of the amount of glucose metabolized by the entire body in response to the infused insulin.

The results of the studies using the hyperglycemic clamp are shown in Fig. 29–5. The total amount of glucose

metabolized during the 20- to 120-minute period was significantly ($p < 0.01$) lower by 38 percent in the CKD dogs than in the CKD-PTX animals (6.64 ± 1.13 vs. 10.74 ± 1.10 mg/kg/min, $p < 0.025$). The early, late, and total insulin responses were significantly greater in CKD-PTX dogs than in CKD animals. In the early phase (0 to 10 minutes), plasma insulin concentration was 91 ± 7 µU/mL in CKD-PTX animals and 63 ± 10 µU/mL in CKD dogs ($p < 0.05$); in the late phase, the values were 147 ± 31 vs. 72 ± 9 ($p < 0.025$); and the total responses gave values of 143 ± 28 vs. 71 ± 10 µU/mL ($p < 0.01$). There was no significant difference between the M/L ratio in the CKD (9.9 ± 2.66 mg/kg min/µU/mL) and CKD-PTX (8.9 ± 1.30 mg/kg min/µU/mL).

The results of the studies using the euglycemic insulin clamp are presented in Fig. 29–6. The total amount of glucose metabolized during elevated blood levels of insulin in the CKD dogs (5.59 ± 0.71 mg/kg/min) was not different from that in the CKD-PTX animals (5.85 ± 0.47 mg/kg/min). These values were lower than, but not significantly different from, those in the normal dogs (7.75 ± 0.47 mg/kg/min). The M/I ratio was also not different between the two groups (5.12 ± 0.76 vs. 5.18 ± 0.57 mg/kg min/µU/mL,) but both values were significantly lower ($p < 0.01$) than those observed in normal dogs (9.98 ± 1.26 mg/kg min/µU/mL). Thus, these studies suggest that PTH does not affect insulin resistance.

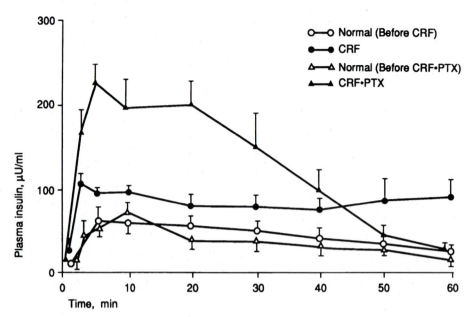

Figure 29–3. The changes in plasma insulin concentrations during intravenous glucose tolerance tests performed before (open symbols) and after 3 months of CRF (closed symbols). Circles represent dogs with CRF and intact parathyroid glands and triangles represent CRF-PTX dogs. *(From Akmal et al,[21] with permission of The Society for Clinical Investigation.)*

The site of insulin resistance has been investigated by Akmal et al. in dogs[20] and by DeFronzo and colleagues[13,18,30,31] and Friedman and associates[32] in uremic subjects. Basal hepatic glucose production was similar in CKD and CKD-PTX dogs (2.33 ± 0.32 vs. 2.38 ± 0.35 mg/kg/min) (Fig. 29–7). These values are not different from those previously reported in normal dogs (2.80 ± 0.20 mg/kg/min).[33] During the insulin clamp, both the time course and magnitude of suppression of hepatic glucose production were similar in both groups of animals. During the 20- to 120-minute period, the hepatic glucose production averaged 0.42 ± 0.22 mg/kg min in CKD dogs and 0.15

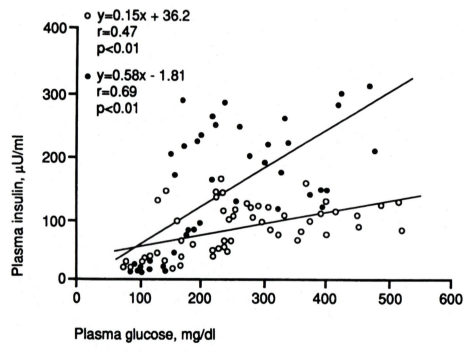

Figure 29–4. The relationship between plasma insulin and glucose concentrations observed during IVGTT performed in CRF (open circles) and CRF-PTX (closed circles). *(From Akmal et al,[21] with permission of The Society for Clinical Investigation.)*

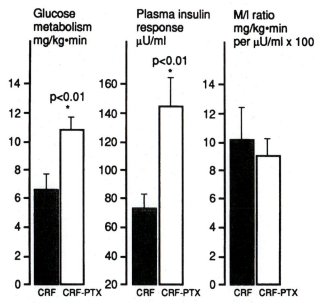

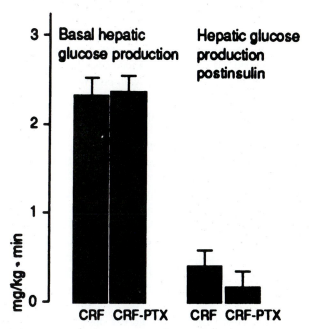

Figure 29–5. Glucose metabolism, total insulin responses, and M/I ratio (total amount of glucose metabolized [M] divided by the total insulin response [I] observed during the hyperglycemic clamp in CRF and CRF-PTX dogs. Each column represents the mean of data from CRF and CRF-PTX dogs. The brackets denote ± 1 SEM. Asterisks indicate significant difference from CRF with P = 0.01. *(From Akmal et al,[21] with permission of The Society for Clinical Investigation)*

Figure 29–7. Basal and postinsulin hepatic glucose production observed during euglycemic insulin clamp in three CRF and three CRF-PTX dogs. The columns represent the mean data and the brackets denote ± 1 SEM. *(From Akmal et al,[21] with permission of The Society for Clinical Investigation.)*

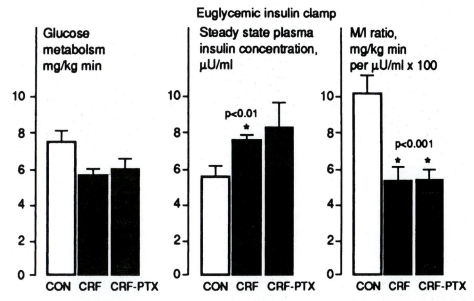

Figure 29–6. Glucose metabolism, steady state plasma insulin concentrations and M/I ratio (total amount of glucose metabolized [M] divided by total insulin responses [I]) observed during euglycemic insulin clamp in normal dogs and in CRF and CRF-PTX dogs. Each column represents the mean of data from six CRF and seven CRF-PTX dogs. The brackets denote ± 1 SEM. CON = Control. Asterisks denote significant difference (P = 0.01) from control. *(From Akmal et al,[21] with permission of The Society for Clinical Investigation.)*

± 0.07 mg/kg/min in CKD-PTX animals. Thus, hepatic glucose production and its suppression in response to hyperinsulinemia are normal. DeFronzo and colleagues[13,18,30,31] also examined the site of insulin resistance by utilizing the clamp technique in combination with both radioisotope (tritiated glucose) turnover methodology and catheterization of the hepatic/femoral veins. From these studies, they found that both suppression of hepatic glucose production and hepatic glucose uptake are normal in uremic patients but the ability of insulin to stimulate glucose uptake by leg tissues is impaired, hence suggesting that the site of insulin resistance is most likely muscle. Similarly, the studies by Friedman et al.[32] have demonstrated that hepatic glucose production in uremic subjects, both before and after insulin infusion, is similar to that in normal controls. These studies—which utilized IVGTI, the hyperinsulinemic euglycemic clamp, and a human skeletal preparation—suggest that insulin resistance does not occur in the liver but rather in muscle.

In dogs with CKD,[20] we did not observe any significant difference in binding affinity, binding-site concentration, and binding capacity of monocytes to insulin among CKD, CKD-PTX, and control dogs. Similarly, Friedman et al. have shown normal insulin receptor binding and kinase activation in uremic subjects.[32]

The results of these studies demonstrate that CKD is associated with glucose intolerance, which results from a combination of insulin resistance and inappropriate release of insulin from the pancreatic islets. Insulin binding to receptors is normal, and the insulin resistance resides in the muscle and not the liver. Furthermore, the state of secondary hyperparathyroidism does not affect insulin resistance but plays a major role in the genesis of the glucose intolerance of CKD by inhibiting appropriate insulin secretion. The normalization of glucose intolerance in CKD in the absence of PTH is due to enhanced insulin secretion from pancreatic β cells, which overcomes the peripheral insulin resistance.

The observations by Mak et al.[19,27] in humans are in agreement with those in dogs[20] and demonstrate that glucose intolerance and insulin resistance exist in adolescents with predialysis CKD or with end-stage renal disease (ESRD) receiving dialytic therapy. After suppression of secondary hyperparathyroidism by dietary phosphate restriction and high doses of phosphate binders in predialysis adolescents,[19] the glucose metabolic rate increased concomitant with an increase in insulin secretion. These investigations also found that correction of secondary hyperparathyroidism by parathyroidectomy in adolescents receiving dialytic therapy was associated with normalization of the glucose metabolic rate and increased insulin secretion, but insulin resistance was not affected.[27] Lu et al.[33] also demonstrated that improvement in secondary hyperparathyroidism utilizing intravenous calcitriol results in an increase in insulin secretion following glucose challenge; they attributed this improvement to intracellular free calcium.

To further elucidate the direct role of PTH in insulin release independent of other factors that may affect insulin metabolism (serum levels of calcium, phosphorus, magnesium, or potassium), we examined insulin secretion by the islets of Langerhans. For these studies, insulin secretion from pancreatic islets was investigated in rats with CKD, parathyroidectomized CKD rats, rats with normal renal function and a state of hyperparathyroidism produced by prolonged administration of PTH, and normal control rats. Two types of protocols were utilized: in one, the rats were studied after 6 weeks of CKD in the presence (CKD) and absence (CKD-PTX) of parathyroid glands; in the other, the normal rats received intraperitoneal injections of 1–84 PTH (Sigma Chemical Company, St. Louis, MO) for 6 weeks. The hormone was dissolved in normal saline and 50 µg was injected in the morning and 50 µg in the late afternoon. The control animals received sham injections of the vehicle only. The insulin release from islets of CKD and CKD-PTX rats was evaluated under static and dynamic conditions. The details of the protocol and methods have been previously reported.[28,32,34]

Insulin release induced by 16.7 mM glucose during static studies in CKD rats was significantly decreased ($p < 0.01$) compared with normal and CKD-PTX animals, but the release of insulin in the latter two groups was not significantly different. In the presence of 16.7 mM glucose, both isobutyl-1-methylxanthine (IBMX) and forskolin significantly ($p < 0.01$) stimulated insulin release in all three groups of animals, but insulin release was significantly lower in CKD rats than in normal and CKD-PTX animals (Fig. 29–8).

Both early (5 minutes) and total (31 minutes) insulin release during the dynamic studies (Fig. 29–9) was significantly lower in CKD rats than in normal and CKD-PTX animals, and the insulin release in the latter two groups was not significantly different. The administration of 1–84 PTH to rats with normal renal function for 6 weeks was also associated with significant impairment in early and total insulin release (Fig. 29–10).

Thus, the reduced release of insulin from pancreatic islets in rats appears to be due to the state of secondary hyperparathyroidism, whether produced by the induction of CKD or by administration of exogenous PTH to rats with normal renal function. This abnormality is prevented by parathyroidectomy prior to the induction of CKD. These observations indicate, therefore, that excess PTH directly suppresses insulin release from pancreatic islets of rats whether or not CKD is present.

The mechanisms through which excess PTH blunts the insulin response to hyperglycemia are not well defined. PTH has been shown to have both acute[35] and chronic[36] effects on insulin secretion. These effects are mediated at

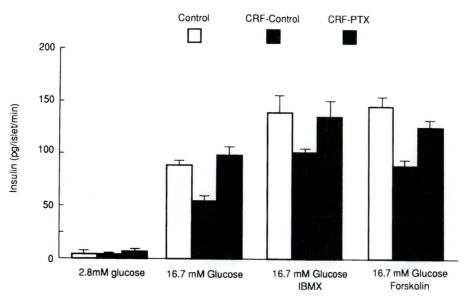

Figure 29–8. Insulin release from pancreatic islets during studies with static incubation in 13 normal rats, six CRF-Control rats, and six CRF-PTX rats. Each column represents mean value and bracket ± 1 SEM. *(Reproduced by permission from Fadda et al.[29])*

least partially through PTH action on cytosolic calcium. Acutely, the hormone increases the cytosolic calcium of the islets and enhances insulin secretion,[35] while the chronic exposure to excess PTH is associated with a sustained increase in cytosolic calcium and a reduced release of insulin.[36] Normally, the increased entry of calcium into the cells is balanced by its extrusion. This balancing effect is achieved directly by the action of Ca^{2+}-ATPase and Na^{+}/Ca^{2+} and indirectly by Na^{+},K^{+}-ATPase.[37] Thus, the sustained elevation of cytosolic calcium in the islets is indica-

tive of suboptimal function of the aforementioned processes to maintain normal resting cytosolic calcium in CKD. Previous studies[38,39] have shown elevated basal cytosolic calcium, decreased levels of ATP content and ATP/ADP ratio in response to glucose, and reduced V_{max} of Ca^{2+}-ATPase in islets from CKD rats. The functional integrity of this enzyme, which requires ATP for its activity, is therefore significantly impaired, resulting in reduced extrusion of calcium from islet cells and subsequent calcium accumulation. This sustained intracellular calcium excess exerts adverse

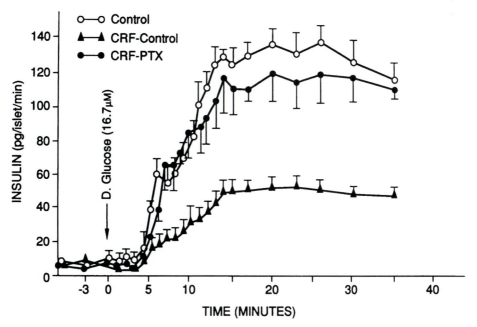

Figure 29–9. Dynamic insulin release from perfused pancreatic islets in five control rats, five CRF-control, and five CRF-PTX rats. Each data point represents the mean value and bracket ± 1 SEM. *(Reproduced by permission from Fadda et al.[29])*

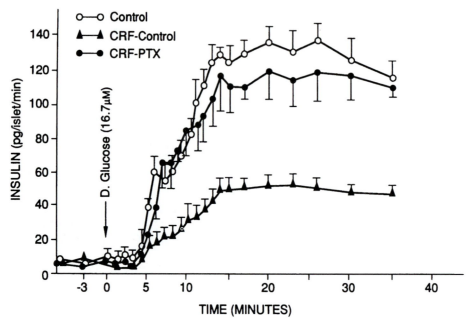

Figure 29–10. Dynamic insulin release from perfused pancreatic islets in four control animals and six PTH-treated rats. Each data point represents the mean value and bracket ± 1 SEM. *(Reproduced by permission from Fadda et al.[29])*

effects on the function of the pancreatic islets. These abnormalities are not observed in parathyroidectomized uremic rats. Furthermore, the initiation of verapamil treatment simultaneously with the induction of CKD prevents the following abnormalities observed in rats with CKD and intact PTH: the rise in cytosolic calcium of pancreatic islets and impairment of insulin secretion[40] and glucose intolerance and impaired insulin secretion.[41] It is also noteworthy that verapamil reverses the glucose intolerance and ameliorates the functional and metabolic abnormalities of pancreatic islets in rats with preexisting chronic renal failure.[42]

In summary, (1) carbohydrate (CHO) intolerance develops in CKD with or without the presence of excess PTH; (2) PTH does not affect insulin resistance and the deranged CHO metabolism is caused by suppression of appropriate release of insulin from pancreatic islets; (3) insulin resistance occurs in skeletal muscle but not in liver; (4) the data from monocyte binding show normal binding affinity, binding-site concentration, and binding capacity of monocytes to insulin in uremic dogs,[30] and there is normal insulin receptor binding and kinase activation in uremic subjects[32]; and (5) the mechanism through which insulin release in CKD is impaired is due to PTH-mediated sustained elevation in cytosolic calcium in pancreatic islets. These abnormalities are not observed in parathyroidectomized uremic rats.

Therapeutic Modalities

Glucose intolerance can be corrected by suppression of secondary hyperparathyroidism or reduction in calcium entry into the pancreatic islets. The former can be achieved by dietary phosphorus reduction, high doses of phosphate binders, oral or intravenous administration of 1,25 vitamin D therapy, and/or parathyroidectomy. Verapamil treatment has also been found to be beneficial in animals. However, it is unusual for patients with CKD to develop overt diabetes unless there is an underlying genetic predisposition. Therefore the aforementioned approaches would not be necessary for abnormal glucose metabolism but are routinely used to correct many complications of end-stage renal disease. Further studies are needed to determine whether verapamil treatment would be of additional benefit in correcting glucose and insulin abnormalities in nondiabetic patients with CKD and those receiving dialytic therapy.

Hypoglycemia

Hypoglycemia has been observed both in diabetic[43,44] and nondiabetic[45–47] patients with ESRD. This abnormality may occur spontaneously or have a specific (nonspontaneous) cause. The mechanisms that may contribute to spontaneous hypoglycemia in such patients are not well defined. These include hyperinsulinemia due to prolonged degradation of endogenous insulin; substrate limitation of gluconeogenesis due to prolonged caloric deprivation and/or loss of alanine during hemodialysis; impaired hepatic gluconeogenesis; and increased glycogenolysis.[48] The presence of sepsis, congestive heart failure, and acidosis may aggravate hypoglycemia.[49,50] Hemodialysis-related hypoglycemia[48] usually occurs in the immediate postdialysis period and has been postulated to be due to a glucose-induced increase in blood insulin levels. Hypoglycemia has also been reported in patients receiving continuous ambulatory peritoneal dialysis.[51]

In the majority of the nonspontaneous episodes of hypoglycemia, a drug or a concomitant disease condition that is known to trigger hypoglycemia is implicated. Nearly half of the hospitalized patients who develop hypoglycemia are diabetics treated primarily with insulin; in these cases the hypoglycemia may be due to insulin itself, or poor caloric intake may contribute to development of this complication.[52] The prolonged duration of insulin action resulting from impaired insulin elimination makes these patients vulnerable to hypoglycemia.[53] Oral hypoglycemic agents,[54] particularly the first-generation sulfonylureas (chlorpropamide, tolbutamide), may also be associated with hypoglycemia because of decreased clearance of sulfonylurea in renal failure, the presence of reduced hepatic clearance and decreased albumin concentration (particularly in elderly patients with renal failure), reduced caloric intake, malnutrition, hepatic failure, alcoholism, or an associated endocrine condition. The most frequent agent of the oral hypoglycemics is chlorpropamide, which accounts for nearly half of the hypoglycemic comas caused by drugs; in one-third of the patients with chlorpropamide-induced hypoglycemia, there is renal impairment.[54] The markedly prolonged half-life of chlorpropamide is due to its exclusive renal excretion.[55,56] Therefore, this oral hypoglycemic agent should not be used in patients with renal failure because of the risk of severe hypoglycemic complications.[57] The half-life of second-generation sulfonylureas (e.g., glyburide) remains unaltered in moderate renal failure because this agent is metabolized by the liver. However, its metabolites do accumulate[58] and are believed to be responsible for prolonged hypoglycemia in diabetic patients with moderate CKD.[59] Thus, glyburide should be avoided in patients with creatinine clearance less than 30 mU/min.[60,61] The renal elimination of glipizide, which is another second-generation sulfonylurea, remains unchanged in patients with renal dysfunction, but the elimination of its metabolites, which probably do not have hypoglycemic activity, is slightly impaired.[62] Therefore hypoglycemia is not a significant risk with glipizide in patients with mild and moderate CKD, but extreme caution should be exercised when using it in patients with advanced renal failure.

Drugs such as sulfonamides, salicylates, phenylbutazone, and anticoagulants like warfarin may also potentiate the hypoglycemic problems of oral hypoglycemic agents, particularly when CKD coexists.[54] The prolonged duration of action of sulfonylureas is often attributed to the impaired hepatic metabolism or abnormal excretion of the drug in the urine.[63,64] The potentiation of the hypoglycemic effect by salicylates, phenylbutazone, and warfarin is observed only with first-generation sulfonylureas. The enhancement of hypoglycemic action by the aforementioned therapeutic agents occurs because of displacement of first-generation sulfonylureas from their binding to albumin, thus increasing their serum concentration and bioavailability.[65] However,

with the second-generation sulfonylureas, such displacement does not occur because binding to albumin for these agents is by nonionic forces and is difficult to displace.[65] The concomitant use of a sulfonamide with a sulfonylurea may be complicated by hypoglycemia because of the prolongation of the half-life of a sulfonylurea.[66–68]

Other drugs—including propoxyphene, propranolol, sulfonamides, salicylates, disopyramide, chlorpromazine, haloperidol, and para-aminobenzoic acid—may enhance or induce hypoglycemia in patients with CKD.[48] The mechanism by which propoxyphene decreases blood sugar is probably due to inhibition of gluconeogenesis,[69] and the blood sugar–lowering effect of this agent has also been observed in a patient with normal renal function.[70] Beta-blocking agents like propranolol and pindolol may be associated with hypoglycemia in diabetic and nondiabetic patients.[71,72] This effect may become more pronounced in the presence of uremia.[73] Angiotensin-converting enzyme inhibitors may induce hypoglycemia by increasing insulin sensitivity[74] and/or by decreasing hepatic glucose production.[75]

Insulin Requirements in Dialysis Patients

Hemodialysis. Hemodialysis has two important effects on insulin metabolism: (1) improvement in tissue sensitivity to insulin, hence lessening the need for insulin treatment,[31] and (2) the return of insulin degradation toward normal, which, in turn, increases the requirement for insulin.[31] Therefore the requirements for insulin may either decrease or increase in diabetic patients receiving hemodialysis.

Continuous Ambulatory Peritoneal Dialysis. Mild to moderate hyperglycemia is common in nondiabetic patients receiving continuous ambulatory peritoneal dialysis (CAPD). The absorption of the glucose from the peritoneal cavity depends on the intraperitoneal instillation of glucose, and CAPD patients derive about 20 percent of their total daily energy intake from this source.[76] However, hyperglycemia is much more common and severe in diabetic patients receiving CAPD, although this problem has been minimized by intraperitoneal insulin administration.[77] Insulin requirements may double or quadruple if insulin is administered intraperitoneally because of the following: (1) enhanced insulin degradation[31]; (2) adherence of the insulin to the peritoneum and mesentery, where it is locally degraded[78]; and (3) extraction of about 50 percent of insulin by the liver, to which the insulin is delivered via the portal vein.[79] It is extremely important to initiate such insulin therapy in the hospital for better glucose control and to avoid hypoglycemia at home.[80]

Carbohydrate Intolerance after Renal Transplantation. Carbohydrate abnormalities after renal transplantation are common. Corticosteroids[81–84] and cyclosporine[85–87] are frequently responsible, but the use of diuretics such as thiazides may also be associated with hyperglycemia.[88] Friedman and associates[89] retrospectively evaluated 1000 renal transplant recipients and reported an incidence of about 15 percent of new-onset diabetes mellitus in previously nondiabetic patients. The postulated mechanisms for steroid-induced diabetes mellitus (DM) include increased hepatic gluconeogenesis and glycogen deposition,[83] hyperglucagonism,[84] and anti-insulin activity.[91] The anti-insulin actions of steroids result from (1) increased production of glucose by these agents for gluconeogenesis and (2) impaired peripheral utilization of glucose.

Postrenal transplant diabetes due to steroid therapy is often observed in older subjects and is more common in black patients. The abnormality is usually mild and self-limiting and is ameliorated by a reduction in dosage or discontinuation of steroid therapy. However, steroid-induced diabetic ketoacidosis may be observed in some patients.[91]

The carbohydrate intolerance in patients receiving cyclosporine therapy is due to the coexistence of insulin resistance and inhibition of insulin release by the pancreatic β cells.[87] Yoshimura et al.[86] have reported a 30 percent higher incidence of diabetes mellitus in renal transplant patients treated with cyclosporine compared with those who received azathioprine therapy. However, in a low-dose steroid therapy (20 mg prednisone/day) study by von Kiparski et al.[91] on 901 transplant recipients, diabetes mellitus was noted in only 4 percent of the patients, and a higher incidence of diabetes was not observed in cyclosporine-treated patients. However, Montori et al.[92] searched databases (MEDLINE, EMBASE, the Cochrane library) including 19 studies with 3611 patients. Twelve-month cumulative incidence of PTDM was lower (<10 percent) than reported three decades ago. Risk factors included older age, nonwhite ethnicity, glucocorticoid therapy for rejection, and immunosuppression with high doses of cyclosporine and tacrolimus. Maes et al.[93] investgated impaired fasting glycemia (IFG) and diabetes mellitus (DM) in 139 transplant recipients without known deranged glucose abnormalities and treated with FK-506 combined with methylprednisolone and mycophenolate mofetil/azathioprine. They found that 15 percent developed IFG and 32 percent DM in the first year after transplantation if American Diabetes Association criteria are used (IFG = at least two fasting plasma glucose levels > 110 mg/dL and DM = at least two blood sugar levels > 126 mg/dL). Risk factors included higher trough levels during the first month posttransplantation (>25 ng/mL), steroid-treated acute rejections, and higher body mass index (BMI).

The incidence of abnormalities in glucose metabolism in transplant recipients are probably underestimated because diagnostic criteria differ between studies and usually the more severe hyperglycemia is reported. The above studies suggest that the risk factors include advancing age, non-white ethnicity, high BMI, and immunosuppressive therapy. Glucocorticoids, tacrolimus, and cyclosporine have been shown to impair the secretion and action of insulin.

THYROID HORMONE AND IODIDE METABOLISM

In patients on chronic dialysis, serum thyroid hormone levels may be abnormal secondary to hypothalamic, pituitary, or thyroid lesions and/or to altered thyroid hormone metabolism due to nonthyroidal illnesses or medications[94] (Table 29–1). For example, free T_4 index values are more frequently reduced by nonthyroidal illnesses in ESRD patients than by hypothyroidism, while values are elevated due to hyperthyroidism and nonthyroidal illness with similar frequency[94] (Table 29–2).

In the absence of hypothalamic, pituitary, or thyroid gland diseases, altered serum thyroid hormone levels reflect

TABLE 29–1. ALTERED THYROID HORMONE METABOLISM IN ESRD PATIENTS

I. Diseases of the hypothalamic-pituitary-thyroid axis
  A. Hypothyroidism
    1. Thyroid gland failure
      a. Permanent—autoimmune thyroiditis, radioiodine, surgical excision
      b. Transient—iodine excess, thyroiditis
    2. Pituitary gland failure
    3. Hypothalamic lesions
  B. Hyperthyroidism
    1. Thyroid gland hyperfunction
      a. Graves' disease
      b. Multinodular toxic goiter
      c. Toxic nodule
      d. Functioning follicular neoplasm (rare)
    2. Thyroiditis
    3. Exogenous thyroid hormone administration
  C. Euthyroid goiter and benign thyroid nodules
  D. Follicular or medullary neoplasms
II. Nonthyroidal factors
  A. End-stage renal disease (ESRD)
  B. Endocrine and metabolic derangements of ESRD
  C. Malnutrition and catabolism
  D. Concurrent systemic nonthyroidal illnesses
  E. Pharmaceutical agents
    1. Dilantin
    2. Beta blockers (high doses)
    3. Glucocorticoids
    4. Iodinated contrast agents—ipodate and Ioponate
    5. Iodine-containing solutions—Povidone
    6. Amiodarone
    7. Lithium
  F. Dialysis therapy

SOURCE: Adapted from Kaptein,[122] with permission.

TABLE 29–2. PREVALENCE OF ALTERED FREE T$_4$ INDEX VALUES DUE TO THYROIDAL AND NONTHYROIDAL DISORDERS IN PATIENTS WITH ESRD

	Increased Free T$_4$ Index		Decreased Free T$_4$ Index	
	Hypothyroid (%)	Sick (%)	Hypothyroid (%)	Sick (%)
Location of Study				
End-Stage Renal Failure				
Michigan	9.5	—	—	—
California[a]	8.3	33.3	0	0
California	2.6	22.5	1.0	0
Maryland	0	—	—	—
Vienna	0	—	—	—
Insulin-Dependent Diabetes Mellitus				
Scotland	3.0	0.7	0	0
Great Britain	2.7	23.0	0	0
General Population				
California	1.1	1.1	0.3	0.9
California	0.6	0.2	0.5	0.2

[a]Children.

Source: Adapted from Kaptein et al.,[100] with permission.

functional disturbances of the hypothalamic-pituitary-thyroid axis and peripheral metabolism, which normalize after the nonthyroidal disorder is alleviated with, for example, treatment of an infection or after renal transplantation.[94] Altered serum thyroxine (T$_4$) and triiodothyronine (T$_3$) metabolism reflects the severity of nonthyroidal disorders, including azotemia, concurrent nonthyroidal illnesses, catabolism, malnutrition, or administration of pharmacologic agents.[94] These changes are not associated with overt clinical manifestations, may be adaptive in nature, and do not benefit from thyroid hormone replacement therapy; thyroid hormone therapy may be harmful.[94] In contrast, coexisting diseases of the hypothalamus, pituitary, or thyroid gland induce significant morbidity in ESRD patients, which is alleviated by specific therapy (Table 29–1).

NORMAL THYROID HORMONE PHYSIOLOGY

The hypothalamic-pituitary-thyroid hormone negative feedback axis controls thyroid gland production of T$_4$ and T$_3$.[95,96] Thyrotropin-releasing hormone (TRH) produced by the hypothalamus stimulates pituitary thyrotrophs to synthesize and release thyroid-stimulating hormone (TSH). Serum TSH concentrations have a diurnal rhythm, with peak levels in the late evening or early morning, as well as pulsatile release.[94,95,96] Circulating TSH stimulates the thyroid gland to synthesize and release T$_4$ and T$_3$, the metabolically active thyroid hormones. The hypothalamic-pituitary-thyroid hormonal axis regulates circulating free T$_4$ levels within a narrow range in euthyroid subjects, and a log-linear relationship exists between serum TSH and free T$_4$ levels when the axis is intact.[95,97] Current TSH assays accu-

rately measure serum TSH levels below the normal range of 0.3 to 0.4 mU/L. Second-generation TSH assays have a sensitivity limit of 0.1 to 0.2 mU/L, third-generation assays have a sensitivity limit of 0.01 to 0.02 mU/L, and fourth-generation assays have a sensitivity limit of 0.001 to 0.002 mU/L, with coefficients of variation of 20 percent.[95] Serum TSH levels below 0.01 mU/L in a third-generation TSH assay and an absent TSH response to TRH occur with excess free T$_4$ or T$_3$ levels, while elevated basal TSH concentrations and an exaggerated TSH response to TRH occur with reduced circulating free T$_4$ but not with decreased free T$_3$ concentrations.[95,96]

Extrathyroidal tissues—including liver, kidney, muscle, and skin—produce 80 percent of T$_3$, the most metabolically active thyroid hormone, and 95 percent of reverse T$_3$, the calorigenically inactive thyroid hormone, via T$_4$ monodeiodination, and they dispose of all thyroid hormones.[95,97] The net contribution of the kidneys to overall thyroid hormone metabolism appears to be small. TSH as well as TRH may be primarily cleared by the kidney, while intact thyroid hormones are filtered, reabsorbed, and secreted by the kidney, and urine is the major route of inorganic iodide elimination.[94]

Thyroid hormones circulate in blood tightly bound to carrier proteins.[97] Thyroid-hormone-binding globulin (TBG) has a high affinity but low binding capacity and binds the majority of T$_4$ and T$_3$; transthyretin (thyroxine binding prealbumin) has a lower affinity and a larger capacity to bind T$_4$ but does not bind T$_3$; while albumin has a very large capacity and low affinity for both thyroid hormones.[98] In normal healthy subjects, 99.97 percent of T$_4$, 99.7 percent of T$_3$, and 99.9 percent of reverse T$_3$ (rT$_3$) are bound to proteins in serum, as determined by the tracer equilibrium dialysis method. Only free thyroid hormones are available to enter tissues and exert a metabolic effect. When TBG capacity and/or affinity is altered by nonthyroidal illnesses or pharmacologic agents, total but not free hormone levels are affected during steady-state conditions.[94]

A variety of in vitro methods are available to estimate free T_4 values in serum.[95] These include (1) direct methods, which include membrane separation methods and direct free T_4 assay methods, and (2) a variety of indirect methods, which utilize total T_4 measurements to estimate free T_4 values (free T_4 estimate methods).[95] In membrane-based methods, semipermeable membranes are used to separate protein-bound from free T_4 by equilibrium dialysis or ultrafiltration, followed by free T_4 measurement in the dialysate. All free T_4 methods provide normal values for healthy euthyroid subjects with normal or modestly increased or decreased TBG concentrations, low levels in hypothyroidism, and high values in hyperthyroidism in otherwise well patients. However, indirect free T_4 estimates may not be accurate in patients with altered hormone-binding states or when inhibitors of hormone binding to serum carrier proteins are present in serum.[95] Thus, low total T_4 levels and low free T_4 estimates are frequently encountered in the absence of hypothalamic, pituitary, or thyroid lesions in patients with moderate to severe nonthyroidal illnesses, including uremia, due to low protein binding of T_4.[94]

UREMIC PATIENTS WITHOUT HYPOTHALAMIC, PITUITARY, OR THYROID DISEASES

In the absence of hypothalamic, pituitary, or thyroid disease, ESRD patients frequently have reduced serum total T_4, free T_4 estimates, and total T3 levels as well as TSH values above the normal range.[94]

Thyrotropin. Elevated basal serum TSH concentrations above the upper normal range of 5 mU/L have been reported in 12 percent of euthyroid patients with ESRD.[94] However, only 1 percent of these elevated TSH values were transiently above 10 mU/L, in association with normal total T_4 and free T_4 index values.[94] All euthyroid ESRD patients with TSH values between 10 and 20 mU/L had repeat TSH values below 10 mU/L. Euthyroid patients with nonrenal nonthyroidal illnesses may have transiently elevated TSH values above 20 mU/L during recovery from acute illnesses. These high TSH levels are associated with normal or rising total T_4 and free T_4 index values, which return to normal with recovery from the nonthyroidal illness.

In contrast, sick uremic patients with primary hypothyroidism have persistently elevated serum TSH values, typically above 20 mU/L, in association with persistently reduced total T_4, free T_4 index, and free T_4 levels by dialysis.[94] Hypothalamic or pituitary causes of hypothyroidism are rare and are usually associated with other endocrine deficiencies, including reduced morning serum cortisol levels as well as reduced growth hormone and/or gonadotropin levels and persistently reduced total and free T_4 levels; TSH values are usually below 15 mU/L.[95] Recent L–thyroxine (L–T_4) withdrawal or treatment of hyperthyroidism can also result in hypothyroidism with normal or low serum TSH concentrations due to persistent central TSH suppression.[98]

On the basis of a second-generation TSH assay, euthyroid ESRD patients undergoing regular maintenance hemodialysis have *not* been reported to have reduced serum TSH values.[94] However, with a second-generation TSH assay, hospitalized patients may have serum TSH values below 0.1 mU/L, more frequently due to nonthyroidal illness (10.3 percent) than to hyperthyroidism (3.3 percent).[94] With a third-generation TSH assay in euthyroid hospitalized patients, 72 percent of serum TSH values below 0.1 mU/L were above 0.01 mU/L in association with normal TSH responses to TRH.[94] In contrast, 97 percent of sick patients with hyperthyroid have TSH values persistently below 0.01 mU/L with absent TSH responses to TRH.[94]

Serum TSH response to exogenous TRH is typically blunted in euthyroid patients with ESRD before as well as after maintenance dialysis therapy[94] and may normalize after correction of anemia with erythropoietin.[94] Serum total T_4 and T_3 concentrations following TRH administration were similar before and after correction of anemia.[94] Interestingly, exogenously administered TRH in ESRD patients receiving maintenance hemodialysis has an increased peak serum TRH concentration, a prolonged half-life, and reduced TRH clearance rate; this may indicate impairment of exogenous TRH degradation and elimination in patients with ESRD receiving hemodialysis therapy.[94]

In ESRD patients receiving chronic hemodialysis therapy, diurnal rhythm of TSH is diminished or absent.[94,99] In addition, the TSH clearance rate is reduced in CKD, possibly reflecting reduced renal clearance; this, in turn, may minimize serum TSH variations.[94] However, a rise in nocturnal TSH is also diminished in patients with a variety of nonrenal, nonthyroidal illnesses and during fasting,[94,95] suggesting that other factors may predominate. The relationship of these changes in TSH secretion to thyroid gland function remains to be determined.

In uremic patients, the increase in serum total T_4 concentrations following exogenous TSH administration was diminished compared to normal subjects, while the increment in serum T_3 concentrations was comparable to that of normal subjects.[94] These findings were interpreted to indicate impaired thyroidal response to TSH. However, thyroidal T_4 production rates are normal in uremic patients.[94]

Thyroxin. In the absence of hypothalamic, pituitary, or thyroid disease, ESRD patients frequently have reduced serum total T_4 and free T_4 index values, primarily due to impaired T_4 binding to TBG, while T_4 production rates in vivo are normal.[94,95] Total T_4 and free T_4 index values were reduced in 21 and 13 percent, respectively, of euthyroid patients with ESRD, and were not related to the presence or duration of dialysis therapy.[100] However, serum albumin levels are significantly lower in dialysis patients with subnormal than in those with normal total T_4 concentrations, suggesting a relationship to malnutrition.[100] These changes are similar to those found in other patients with moderate to severe nonthyroidal illnesses.[95]

T_4 binding to serum carrier proteins is impaired in euthyroid patients with nonthyroidal illnesses to a greater extent than reductions in serum concentrations of TBG, transthyretin, or albumin.[94,95] Free fractions of T_4 and T_3 by equilibrium dialysis are normal or increased in ESRD, while TBG levels are normal or increased, transthyretin concentrations are normal, and serum albumin values may be reduced.[94] Reduced T_4 binding to serum proteins in euthyroid uremic patients may relate to elevated serum levels of 3-carboxy-4-methyl-5-propyl-2-furan propanoic acid (CMPF), indoxyl sulfate, and hippuric acid present in uremic serum.[95] Serum concentrations of indole-3-acetic acid, hippuric acid, and indoxyl sulfate are higher in predialysis than postdialysis sera.[102] Further, addition of indoxyl sulfate and indole acetic acid to normal pooled sera at concentrations similar to those in uremic sera interfered with estimation of free T_4 and free T_3 values by analogue radioimmunoassay, resulting in decreased free hormone estimates.[102] In nonuremic patients, elevated levels of oleic acid, interleukin-6, and tumor necrosis factor-alpha (TNF-α) may reduce serum T_4 binding to carrier proteins, as may elevated bilirubin and nonesterified fatty acids in association with hypoalbuminemia in those with hepatic failure.[94] In addition, exogenous inhibitors of T_4 binding to serum carrier proteins—such as furosemide, nonsteroidal anti-inflammatory drugs, and heparin—may play a role in ESRD patients.[94] Plasma levels of interleukin-1β, TNF-α, and their specific inhibitors are elevated in ESRD patients before as well as during chronic CAPD or hemodialysis therapy.[94]

Serum free T_4 assay values in sera from ESRD patients are highly method-dependent, as they are in patients with nonrenal, nonthyroidal illnesses.[95] Free T_4 levels determined by tracer equilibrium dialysis were normal in 88 to 97 percent of euthyroid ESRD patients, in association with normal thyroidal T_4 production rates and normal extrathyroidal reverse T_3 production rates from circulating T4.[94] However, in one study, free T_4 values by direct dialysis were below the normal range in 31 percent of euthyroid patients with CKD who had normal serum TSH concentrations.[95,102] This high frequency of reduced free T_4 levels by direct dialysis in uremic patients contrasts with the normal or elevated free T_4 values by direct dialysis reported in most

patients with nonrenal nonthyroidal illness even in the presence of reduced total T_4 concentrations.[94,95] The reduced serum free T_4 levels by direct dialysis in uremic sera may be due to in vitro dilution of low-affinity binding inhibitors in uremic sera[94] during the direct dialysis assay, which would increase T_4 binding to serum-binding proteins and spuriously reduce free T_4 levels in the dialysate.[95,98] This may be clinically relevant. For example, to differentiate hypothyroidism from the low total T_4 state of nonthyroidal illness in a severely ill patient with ESRD on antithyroid drug treatment for Graves' disease, we measured a serum TSH, which was suppressed, and then free T_4 by direct dialysis, which was in the hypothyroid range.[98] To determine whether a weakly bound inhibitor of T_4 binding to serum-binding proteins or true hypothyroidism was responsible for the low free T_4 value, this patient's serum was serially diluted using either an ultrafiltrate of the patient's serum, which would contain any unbound inhibitor as well as free T4, or an inert diluent. Free T_4 values were similar with both diluents, providing evidence against the presence of dialyzable and ultrafilterable inhibitor. Thus, this patient was hypothyroid due to antithyroid drug administration, with prolonged central TSH suppression from preexisting hyperthyroidism.[98] Subsequently, the antithyroid drug dose was reduced to restore euthyroidism.[98]

In the general population, elevated free T_4 index values are as frequently due to nonthyroidal illnesses as to hyperthyroidism (Table 29–2) and are frequently associated with mild nonthyroidal illnesses, acute psychiatric disorders, and administration of amiodarone or iodinated contrast agents.[94] However, uremic patients rarely have elevated total T_4 and free T_4 estimate values in the absence of hyperthyroidism (Table 29–2), most likely due to the severity of their nonthyroidal illnesses and malnutrition.[94] In addition, free T_4 assays with the exception of direct dialysis are highly dependent on protein binding of T_4 and frequently provide misleadingly low free T_4 estimates in patients with decreased serum protein binding,[95] as occurs in many ESRD patients. Further, endogenous inhibitors of T_4 binding present in uremic sera may contribute.[94] Elevated free T_4 values in patients with nonrenal, nonthyroidal illnesses may relate to decreased T_4 clearance rates from serum, since T_4 production rates are normal or reduced.[94] In contrast, serum free T_4 values are elevated in hyperthyroidism secondary to increased thyroidal T_4 production rates or to excess L-T_4 administration.

Triiodothyronine. Total and free T3 concentrations are frequently reduced in ESRD patients as with other nonthyroidal illness, malnutrition, and following administration of pharmacologic agents including iodinated contrast agents, amiodarone, propylthiouracil, glucocorticoids, and high dose beta blockers.[94] Total T_3 levels were below 100 ng/dL in 76 percent and free T_3 index values under 100 in 66 percent of 287 euthyroid patients with ESRD.[94] An elevated total T_3 or free T_3 index value in a sick patient is consistent with a diagnosis of hyperthyroidism, while a normal or reduced value does not exclude hyperthyroidism, since extrathyroidal T_3 production may be reduced.

Reduced T_3 levels in nonthyroidal disorders may be due to decreased peripheral tissue conversion of T_4 to T_3, reduced T_3 binding to serum carrier proteins, and underestimation in vitro, while thyroid gland production of T_3 appears to be normal.[94] Malnutrition may be a significant factor inhibiting T4 conversion to T_3, since direct correlations were observed between total T_3 and both serum albumin and transferrin concentrations in uremic patients.[94,100] In addition, CMPF, hippuric acid, and indoxyl sulfate in uremic human sera and bilirubin and nonesterified fatty acids in nonuremic human sera inhibit T_4 uptake and subsequent deiodination of T_4 by rat hepatocytes in vitro and thus may reduce T_3 production from T4 in vivo.[94] In vivo, this may correspond to the reduced transport of T_4 into tissues in patients with ESRD despite normal T_4 binding to serum carrier proteins.[94]

Although T_3 is the most metabolically active thyroid hormone, patients with ESRD are euthyroid, as evidenced by a normal clinical index score, basal metabolic rate, Achilles deep tendon reflex relaxation time, and systolic time interval values.[94] Further, administration of exogenous T_3 in near-physiologic quantities to ESRD patients as well as to nonuremic sick patients or to otherwise healthy fasted subjects increases muscle breakdown.[94] Thus, decreased T_3 production rates and serum free T_3 levels in patients with nonthyroidal illnesses and caloric deprivation are probably adaptive to minimize the catabolic effects of malnutrition and systemic illnesses.[94] Further, L-T_4 treatment of critically ill patients with low serum total T_4 but normal free T_4 concentrations was not beneficial and did not reduce mortality.[94] Thus, thyroid hormone therapy for uremic patients without concurrent hypothyroidism is not recommended, since no beneficial effect can be demonstrated and such therapy may accelerate protein catabolism.

Reverse Triiodothyronine. Patients with ESRD have normal total serum reverse T_3 levels, in contrast to the elevated values observed in the majority of other nonthyroidal disorders.[94] These normal total reverse T_3 levels are associated with elevated serum free reverse T_3 values, normal reverse T_3 production from T_4, and a shift of reverse T_3 from vascular to extravascular sites secondary to an increased rate of reverse T_3 transfer out of serum as well as to enhanced tissue reverse T_3 binding.[94] The clinical significance of these findings remains to be defined.

Iodide Metabolism. Renal iodide excretion normally accounts for the majority of iodide removal from the body, with renal iodide clearance averaging 30 percent of creatinine clearance in normal subjects.[94,103] Ratios of renal iodide to creatinine clearance are higher with severe CKD.[94,103] Serum inorganic iodide levels are four to nine times higher than normal in patients with ESRD, in association with normal or reduced thyroidal radioactive iodine uptake values.[94] Although inorganic iodide is removed by dialysis, serum iodide levels remain elevated in the majority of patients receiving maintenance hemodialysis or CAPD therapy.[94] Discontinuation of povidone for 3 months resulted in modest decreases of serum iodide levels in CAPD patients and no change in serum iodide levels in hemodialysis patients.[94] Elevated levels of serum inorganic iodide may induce goiter formation and/or reversible hypothyroidism in patients with thyroid gland abnormalities who are unable to escape from the inhibition of iodide organification induced by iodide excess (the Wolff-Chaikoff effect).[94]

Effects of Dialysis Therapy. In patients with ESRD, serum total T_4 and T_3, free T_4 and T_3 index, and TSH values were similar in nondialyzed patients and those receiving chronic hemodialysis therapy for 9 hours a week; they were not related to chronicity of hemodialysis therapy.[94,100] However, serum total T_4 and T_3 concentrations were higher in patients receiving 27 hours of maintenance hemodialysis per week than in those receiving 15 or 18 hours, and total T_4 and T_3 levels correlated inversely with serum creatinine values in blood taken immediately before a dialysis treatment.[94] Serum free T_4 by enhanced chemiluminescence immunoassay were 23 percent lower in patients hemodialyzed for 12 hours per week than in undialyzed patients (mean creatinine clearance 15 mL/min), most likely due to the effects of reduced serum albumin binding.[95,99] In addition, free T_4 values were below the normal reference range in 15 percent of these hemodialyzed patients but in none of the undialyzed patients.[99] Lower free T_4 values in the hemodialyzed patients are probably not due to hypothyroidism but to effects of reduced serum albumin binding and/or assay interference by circulating inhibitors of T_4 binding to proteins.[101] Free T_3 and basal TSH values were not different between the two groups.[99] Serum concentrations of total T_4, free T_4 index, total T_3, TBG, TSH, and TSH response to TRH were similar in patients undergoing CAPD and chronic hemodialysis therapy.[94]

Effects of Erythropoietin Therapy. In ESRD patients on maintenance hemodialysis therapy, blunted serum TSH responses to exogenous TRH normalized after correction of anemia with erythropoietin, while serum total T_4 and free T_4 and free T_3 (manufactured by Amersham, Arlington Heights, IL) responses remained blunted.[94] Anemia may induce relative tissue hypoxia, which decreases pituitary responsiveness to TRH; it is reversed by erythropoietin, or erythropoietin could have a direct trophic effect.[94]

Effects of Zinc Supplementation. ESRD patients commonly have zinc deficiency, which has been associated with decreased serum T_4 and T_3 concentrations as well as a blunted TSH response to TRH.[94] Zinc supplementation to patients receiving intermittent peritoneal dialysis therapy increased low basal serum zinc levels toward normal and normalized serum TSH as well as total T_4 and T_3 concentrations.[94] The changes in serum TSH, T_4, and T_3 concentrations correlated with changes in serum zinc levels.[94]

Effects of Renal Transplantation. Within 3 days of renal transplantation, serum T_4 and T_3 concentrations fell and reverse T_3 concentrations rose compared to pretransplant values,[104] presumably due to the acute effects of surgery. In patients with primary graft function, these values returned to preoperative values by day 15 despite therapy with high-dose prednisone. Those with delayed graft function due to acute tubular necrosis had persistently low serum T_3 concentrations, and those with acute graft rejection requiring high doses of prednisone and OKT3 had persistently low serum T_4 and T_3 levels by 15 days as well as reduced TBG concentrations,[104] reflecting the effects of nonthyroidal illness and high doses of prednisone. The T_4/TBG ratio decreased in those with delayed graft function,[104] indicating reduced T_4 binding to TBG. Serum TSH levels fell after transplantation and remained below preoperative levels but not below the normal range, presumably due to the effects of prednisone.[105] In another study, 33 percent of patients evaluated between 2 and 95 months after transplantation receiving prednisolone 15 mg/day had a blunted TSH response to TRH and reduced T_4 and T_3 concentrations.[104] Six months after successful renal transplantation, serum TSH, total T_4, free T_4 index, and total T_3 values as well as T_3 production rates and T_4-to-T_3 conversion rates return to normal.[94] Blunted TSH response to TRH and reduced serum total T_3 concentrations in some transplanted patients may relate to glucocorticoid therapy.[94]

UREMIC PATIENTS WITH HYPOTHALAMIC, PITUITARY, OR THYROID DISEASES

Goiter

ESRD patients have a variably increased prevalence of goiter (up to 58 percent) compared to the general population (Table 29–3).[94] Goiters were present in 43 percent of our 306 ESRD patients compared to 6.5 percent of hospitalized patients without renal disease of similar age, gender, and racial background. Goiter was more frequent in ESRD patients who had received hemodialysis therapy for more than 1 year (50 percent) than in those dialyzed for less than 1

TABLE 29–3. PREVALENCE OF GOITER AND ANTITHYROID ANTIBODY TITERS (PERCENT) IN END-STAGE RENAL DISEASE

	End-Stage Renal Disease		Control Population	
	Goiter	ATA[a]	Goiter	ATA
	%	%	%	%
Denmark	60[b]	7	0	—
Utah	58	0	8	—
California	43	7	6.5	1.4
Illinois	37	0	—	10
South Africa	32	—	—	—
Japan	30	—	6.7	—
Israel	24	—	—	—
Switzerland	20	—	—	—
Belgium	12	0	—	—
Maryland	8	0	—	—
Alberta	2	13	—	—

[a]No thyroid enlargement clinically but increased thyroid gland volume on ultrasonography.
[b]Positive antithyroid antibody titers.
Source: Adapted from Kaptein,[94] with permission.

year or not at all (39 percent).[94] The female-to-male ratio of patients with goiter was 1.4:1 in those with ESRD compared to 2.8:1 in the control group. Goiter frequency did not relate to age, race, presence of DM, elevated TSH or PTH levels, or increased antimicrosomal antibody titers.[94]

Increased serum inorganic iodide levels may block hormone production in patients with preexisting thyroid gland abnormalities such as Hashimoto's thyroiditis, previously treated Graves' disease, or after hemithyroidectomy, as well as in patients with apparently normal thyroid glands, some of whom may have an organification defect.[94] Iodine restriction of patients with elevated nonhormonal iodine levels due to CKD decreased thyroid gland size.[94]

Thyroid gland enlargement is usually evident upon physical examination unless it is substernal. Substernal goiters may be evident on chest x-ray as a superior mediastinal mass and/or as tracheal deviation with or without evidence of compression. Evaluation includes determining whether the patient is euthyroid, hypothyroid, or hyperthyroid; assessing for tracheal compression; and, if a predominant nodule is present, excluding malignancy by a fine-needle-aspiration biopsy.[105] If a euthyroid goiter is associated with compressive symptoms, surgical excision or ablation with iodine 131 (^{131}I) should be considered. The dosage of ^{131}I should be reduced depending pon type, duration and frequency of dialysis (see radioiodine therapy of thyroid carcinoma and hyperthyroidism later in this chapter). Radioiodine therapy may substantially reduce goiter size after one or more dosages but may also induce transient hyperthyroidism as well as permanent hypothyroidism in 25 percent after 5 years and in 100 percent after 8 years.[105]

Since established goiters frequently do *not* decrease in size following L-T$_4$ suppression, a limited trial of L-T$_4$ suppression should be considered only with recent goiter growth if minimal or no adverse effects of L-T$_4$ therapy are anticipated.[106] Risks of mild hyperthyroidism may be significant in patients with overt or subclinical ischemic cardiovascular disease or a predisposition to catabolism and malnutrition. The majority of euthyroid patients with stable goiters require only clinical follow-up and measurement of serum TSH levels every 1 to 2 years.

If L-T$_4$ suppression therapy is elected, the smallest dosage necessary to suppress TSH levels to below normal range should be employed to minimize adverse effects. Overt hyperthyroidism may occur when usual dosages of L-T$_4$ are given to a patient with an autonomous thyroid gland that continues to produce thyroid hormone. Thus, in older patients with known or potential ischemic heart disease, an initial L-T$_4$ dosage of 0.025 mg/day should be given, with serum TSH values monitored in 6 to 8 weeks. If the patient is asymptomatic and the TSH level remains within the normal range, the L-T$_4$ dosage may be increased every 6 to 8 weeks in increments of 0.025 mg/day until TSH is below the normal range. If symptoms of thyroid hormone excess occur, L-T$_4$ therapy should be discontinued and the clinical significance of the goiter reevaluated.

Thyroid Nodules

Thyroid nodules and carcinoma are approximately three times more common in ESRD patients than in the general population. Clinically unsuspected thyroid nodules were found at the time of parathyroidectomy in 64 percent of ESRD patients undergoing maintenance hemodialysis.[94] Further, with the use of a 10-MHz high-frequency sonographic scanner, female patients with ESRD on maintenance hemodialysis were found to have an increased frequency of thyroid nodules (55 percent) compared to normal females (21 percent).[94] Evaluation includes assessment of thyroid function and a fine-needle-aspiration if malignancy is suspected.[106]

Thyroid Cancer

In female chronic dialysis patients in the United States, thyroid malignancy was 2.9 times higher than in a matched population (1.2 times higher in males).[94] In ESRD patients from the United States, Europe, Australia, and New Zealand, thyroid cancer was 2.3 times higher in males and females than in the general population, with the risk being highest in patients less than 34 years of age.[107] Frequency of thyroid malignancy rose with duration of dialysis and may relate to evaluations for secondary hyperparathyroidism.[108] In ESRD patients with secondary hyperparathyroidism, thyroid carcinoma was 3.3 times higher than in an autopsy con-

trol group; half were papillary carcinomas with a diameter of 5 mm or less, which may not be clinically relevant, and serum C-terminal PTH levels were significantly higher in those with thyroid carcinoma.[94]

In renal transplant recipients with preexisting malignancies, 4.5 percent were thyroid carcinomas, with 64 percent of these being papillary, 18 percent follicular, 2.6 percent medullary, and 15 percent unclassified.[94] Only 15 percent of these thyroid carcinomas were incidental findings during parathyroidectomy.[94] The recurrence rate was 7.7 percent and involved patients treated 1 week to 96.5 months before renal transplantation, resulting in one death.[94] In addition, 5 years or more after a functioning renal transplantation, the risk for thyroid carcinoma is increased 6.5- to 7-fold compared to the general population, appearing even higher among patients in Australia and New Zealand.[94]

When a follicular thyroid malignancy is diagnosed, a near-total thyroidectomy is appropriate in patients with an acceptable surgical risk.[106] Subsequent management may include ^{131}I ablation of the thyroid remnant and yearly total body scans in those with follicular malignancy who have a high risk for recurrent or metastatic disease.[106] Serial serum thyroglobulin levels may be useful to evaluate the presence of metastatic lesions, and repeated ^{131}I ablative therapy may be required to treat functioning metastases.[106] Those with medullary carcinoma should be followed with serum calcitonin levels and may require repeated surgical excision of metastases.[106] Patients with follicular neoplasms require lifelong L-T$_4$ suppression therapy, with the extent of suppression depending upon the cardiovascular status.[106]

Preparation of patients for radioiodine therapy should include the avoidance of povidone/iodine for skin cleansing and a low-iodine diet in an attempt to decrease serum iodine levels and increase radioiodine uptake by residual thyroid tissue and functioning metastases. Patients may undergo thyroid hormone withdrawal over 6 weeks to induce hypothyroidism or receive intramuscular human recombinant TSH (Thyrogen) injections to increase radioiodine uptake into residual thyroid tissue and/or functioning metastases.[106,108] Induction of severe hypothyroidism may result in significant morbidity, which will not occur with Thyrogen administration. Uptake of ^{131}I by thyroid remnants and metastases is similar with both methods in patients with normal renal function.[106]

Patients with ESRD require decreased radioiodide dosages in proportion to reduced iodide clearance by native kidneys plus removal by dialysis therapy so as to avoid excess radiation exposure to critical organs such as red marrow.[94,103] Iodide clearance rates during 40 consecutive peritoneal dialysis exchanges, which is rarely used currently, were similar to normal renal clearance.[94] In contrast, CAPD patients receiving three to four 2-L exchanges per day had a total iodide clearance rate by native kidneys plus CAPD that averaged 16 percent of normal, requiring a decrease in the ^{131}I ablative dosage from 150 to less than 30 mCi.[94,103,109] The total body half-time of ^{131}I averaged 40 hours in our CAPD patients, compared to 10 hours in patients without renal disease.[103] In another reported CAPD patient, total body half-time was 44.5 hours.[108] In an additional patient, daily radioiodine removal was only 6 to 10 percent per day by urine plus CAPD, resulting in a total body half-time of 70 hours; this patient received 22 mCi of [131]I.[110] Thus, radioiodine clearance is very low in CAPD patients, requiring reduced dosages of radioiodine for ablative therapy. No data have been reported in patients receiving nightly peritoneal dialysis.

Radioiodide removal by currently available hemodialysis machines and dialyzers is five times higher than native renal clearance.[94] However, ^{131}I clearance by hemodialysis occurs for only 5 to 7 percent of the total week, with minimal ^{131}I clearance between treatments.[94] As a result, total-body half-times of ^{131}I ranged from 20 hours when hemodialysis was initiated immediately after the dosage, to 47 to 56 hours when dialysis was delayed for 24 to 48 hours and then performed triweekly,[94,110] compared to 8 to 10 hours in patients without renal disease.[94] With daily hemodialysis initiated 24 hours after the radioiodine dosage, total body half-times varied from 38 to 52 hours.[111]

Despite four- to sixfold prolonged total-body half-times of radioiodine during the first week after radioiodine is administered, some authors have suggested increased or unchanged radioiodine ablative dosages[110,111] rather than decreased therapeutic radioiodine dosages for hemodialysis patients.[94] These dosages were based on the mistaken assumption that the half-time of inorganic ^{131}I disappearance in athyreotic patients with normal renal function is 3 days or longer; the latter is the half-time of radiolabeled iodothyronines produced by thyroid tissue, not inorganic [131]I. Thus, in the present author's opinion, dosages for radioiodide should be reduced to 40 percent of those for patients with normal renal function if hemodialysis is performed immediately after the dosage and then every 48 hours and to 20 percent if hemodialysis is initiated 24 to 48 hours after the dosage and then repeated triweekly. For example, if 150 mCi of ^{131}I was prescribed for the patient assuming normal renal function, the dosage would be reduced to 30 mCi if the patient was dialyzed 24 to 48 hours after the dosage and then triweekly. Thus, the timing of a dosage of ^{131}I is critical to determine the dosage adjustment necessary to minimize the dose of radiation to the bone marrow in hemodialyzed ESRD patients. Further, in the author's experience, dialysis with sorbent-based dialysis systems, which are still used for patients in isolation rooms at our hospital, removed very little radioiodine, while dialysis with the single-pass machines removes radioiodine effectively, as described in the literature. It should be noted that contamination of equipment was minimal, as was exposure to personnel.

Follow-up for follicular malignancies may require repeated ^{131}I body scans and serum thyroglobulin levels following L-T₄ withdrawal or recombinant TSH intramuscularly to look for functioning metastases. Oral dosages of ^{131}I greater than 2 mCi for total-body scanning in patients with normal renal function result in marked reductions in uptake by the thyroid remnant and metastases of subsequent ablative dosages of [131]I (stunning).[103] For initial remnant ablation, scanning provides minimal information and should not be done. For follow-up total-body scanning to look for functioning metastases, ^{131}I scanning dosages should be appropriately reduced in ESRD patients to minimize stunning.[94]

L-thyroxine suppression therapy is the mainstay of therapy for follicular thyroid cancers, since TSH is believed to stimulate the growth of follicular malignancies. In patients with normal renal function, the dosage of L-thyroxine is titrated so that TSH levels are maintained in the range of 0.4 to 1.0 mU/L, assuming that adverse cardiac manifestations do not occur.[106] Appropriate TSH levels in ESRD patients are unknown.

Hypothyroidism

Primary hypothyroidism has been reported in up to 9.5 percent of patients with ESRD compared to 0.6 to 1.1 percent of the general population[94] (Table 29–2). In our study, 2.6 percent of 306 ESRD patients had primary hypothyroidism. All had TSH values persistently above 20 mU/L and reduced serum total T₄ and free T₄ index values. Of these, 88 percent were female, 75 percent were over the age of 50 years, 50 percent had elevated antimicrosomal antibody titers, 50 percent had goiter, and 50 percent had diabetes mellitus (Table 29–4). In the general population, hypothyroidism is nine times more common in females, occurs in 5 to 10 percent of people over 50 years of age, and induces hypercholesterolemia, hypertension, and cardiac dysfunc-

TABLE 29–4. RISK FACTORS FOR HYPOTHYROIDISM IN PATIENTS WITH END-STAGE RENAL DISEASE

Female gender

Elderly

Autoimmune diseases

Insulin-dependent diabetes mellitus

Systemic lupus erythematosus

Iodine excess[a]

Povidone-iodine and other iodine containing disinfectants

Amiodarone

Iodinated contrast

Other

Interferon therapy for hepatitis C

[a]Potentially reversible causes of hypothyroidism.

tion. Clinical manifestations of hypothyroidism are frequently mimicked or masked by concurrent ESRD, malnutrition, and other nonthyroidal disorders.[94] Thus, a high index of suspicion for hypothyroidism must be present for patients at risk (Table 29–4), and biochemical confirmation must be obtained prior to L-T$_4$ therapy. Biochemical features include persistently elevated TSH values to above 20 mU/L and reduced serum total T$_4$ and free T$_4$ estimate values (Fig. 29–11).[94]

Multiple factors may predispose ESRD patients to develop hypothyroidism (Table 29–2). Serum iodine concentrations are four to nine times higher than normal in ESRD patients.[94] These elevated iodine levels are due to reduced iodine excretion by residual renal function plus minimal removal by dialysis and to increased absorption of topical povodine/iodine.[94] Elevated serum iodine levels may impair the synthesis and release of thyroid hormone in ESRD pa-

tients with underlying thyroid disease, particularly those with an iodide organification defect, concurrent Hashimoto's thyroiditis, previously treated Graves' disease, or after hemithyroidectomy and thus may contribute to the increased frequency of hypothyroidism.[94] In hypothyroid Japanese patients with CKD, elevated serum iodine and TSH levels decreased with iodine restriction in 83 percent of patients; some of these patients had an iodide organification defect.[94] Insulin-dependent diabetic patients without ESRD have an increased frequency of elevated antimicrosomal antibody titers (17 percent) as well as hypothyroidism (3 percent), which may be a factor in some ESRD patients.[94] Interferon therapy for hepatitis C has induced thyroid gland dysfunction in 12 percent of patients, including thyroiditis with transient or permanent hypothyroidism; thus, thyroid peroxidase antibodies and TSH levels should be monitored during and after interferon therapy.[94]

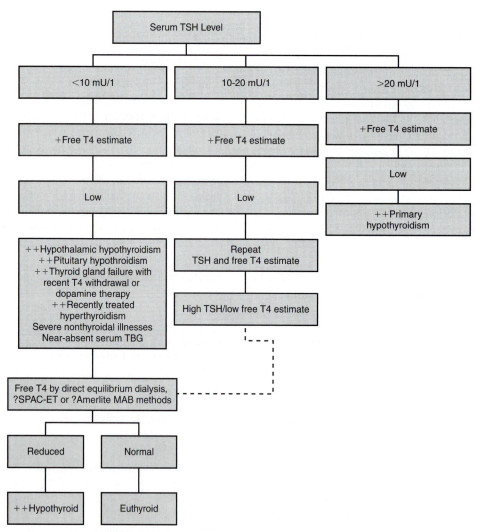

Figure 29–11. Laboratory evaluation for hypothyroidism in ESRD. Note that all free T4 estimates except direct dialysis are dependent on serum protein binding and may provide misleadingly low values in patients with low serum albumin and thyroid-binding globulin concentrations.

Serum TSH is the most effective screening test for hypothyroidism (Fig. 29–11), since reduced total T_4 and free T_4 index values were present in 24 and 13 percent, respectively, of euthyroid ESRD patients, while only 1 percent had TSH values above 10 um/L and all TSH values between 10 and 20 mU/L were transient.[94,95] No ESRD patient with normal free T_4 index values had overt hypothyroidism.[94] A free T_4 estimate using a method that provides normal values in the majority of euthyroid ESRD patients may play a confirmatory role (Fig. 29–11). A serum TSH value below 10 mU/L with a low free T_4 estimate requires exclusion of hypothalamic or pituitary hypothyroidism, recent thyroid hormone withdrawal, or recently treated thyrotoxicosis.[94] Patients with pituitary or hypothalamic hypothyroidism frequently have concurrent hypogonadism, evidenced by loss of axillary and pubic hair and early menopause in women and hypoadrenalism. Adrenal insufficiency can result in profound volume-resistant hypotension with stress—such as that due to hemodialysis, infection, or surgery; this can be confirmed by a reduced morning serum cortisol concentration and requires glucocorticoid replacement therapy. A serum TSH value between 10 and 20 mU/L should be repeated. If the TSH is persistently elevated and the free T_4 estimate is low, primary hypothyroidism is likely and L-T_4 treatment should be initiated. A serum TSH value above 20 mU/L with a reduced free T_4 estimate is diagnostic of thyroid gland failure and warrants L-T_4 therapy. Since clinical symptoms and signs of hypothyroidism are indistinguishable from those of uremia and the prevalence of hypothyroidism is increased, serum TSH values should be measured in high-risk ESRD patients.

When a biochemical diagnosis of hypothyroidism is established, a reversible cause such as iodide excess should be sought; if such is not found, L-T_4 therapy should be initiated.[94] The absorption by the small intestine of exogenous L-T_4 is normally 50 to 80 percent efficient and is unaltered in ESRD and following renal transplantation.[94] The initial dosage regimen for L-T_4 should be based on the clinical status of the patient and adjusted to achieve euthyroidism as determined by clinical symptoms and signs as well as return of serum TSH levels to between 5 and 10 mU/L to avoid inducing hyperthyroidism or hypothyroidism[94] (Tables 29–5 and 29–6). Younger patients without cardiac disease may begin with a dosage of 0.075 to 0.100 mg/day. A small ini-

TABLE 29–5. L-THYROXINE THERAPY OF HYPOTHYROIDISM IN END-STAGE RENAL DISEASE

Initial Dose	Increments	Maintenance
<50 years old, 100–150 mg/day	75–100 µg/day orally	25 µg/day q 6–8 weeks
No cardiac disease		
>50 years old, 75–100 mg/day	25–50 µg/day orally	25 µg/day q 6–8 weeks

TABLE 29–6. DETERMINING MAINTENANCE DOSAGE OF L-T4 FOR HYPOTHYROIDISM

1. Titrate dosage every 6 to 8 weeks until serum TSH is 5 to 10 mU/L.
2. Check TSH in 6 months and then yearly.
3. Do not change L-thyroxine preparations without retitrating dosages.[112]
4. Encourage lifelong compliance.

tial dosage of 0.025 to 0.050 mg/day would be more prudent in elderly patients or in those with known or suspected cardiac disease or autonomous thyroid gland function. Subsequently, the daily L-T_4 dosage may be increased by 0.025 mg every 6 to 8 weeks, assuming that cardiac symptoms do not occur, to return serum TSH levels to between 5 and 10 mU/L—values commonly observed in euthyroid ESRD patients. Since the half-life of T_4 is approximately 7 to 10 days, serum TSH levels should be evaluated and L-T_4 dosage adjusted only every 6 to 8 weeks. Total T_4 and free T_4 estimate values should *not* be normalized, since they may be reduced due to nonthyroidal illness. During therapy with L-T_4, ESRD patients with primary thyroid gland failure may have improvement or resolution of symptoms and signs of hypothyroidism that may have been mistakenly attributed to uremia.

Precise titration of the L-T_4 dosage is necessary to avoid complications of thyroid hormone excess or deficiency. Four synthetic L-T_4 formulations are approved by the U.S. Food and Drug Administration (FDA) and available at this time, including Unithroid, Levoxyl, Synthroid, and generic L-T_4, produced by Mylan Pharmaceuticals.[112] Each preparation must comply with FDA standards for bioavailability but may vary with respect to dissolution and absorption; these preparations are *not* interchangeable.[112] Due to the narrow therapeutic index of L-T_4, changing from one formulation to another may result in increased or decreased L-T_4 absorption, requiring measurement of another TSH levels 6 to 8 weeks after a new steady state is achieved to assure that the TSH concentration is still within the therapeutic range. If the new TSH level is above or below the desired range, the dosage of the L-T_4 preparation will require readjustment and TSH measured repeatedly until the desired level is achieved. Animal preparations, which contain variable quantities of T_4 and T_3, and synthetic L-T_3 are nonphysiologic and are potentially hazardous, particularly in patients with cardiac disease, and should no longer be used.

Failure of serum TSH values to normalize in a patient receiving 1.6 µg/kg body weight or 75 to 100 µg/day of L-thyroxine may indicate noncompliance with the dosage regimen, interference with intestinal absorption of L-T_4, or increased losses or degradation rates of T_4[94] (Table 29–7). In patients taking multiple medications, L-T_4 should be taken at least 1 hour prior to or 2 hours after other medications or food (see Table 29–7). If L-T_4 is taken with other medica-

TABLE 29–7. FAILURE TO RESPOND TO USUAL DOSES OF L-THYROXINE THERAPY

A. Noncompliance with the dosage regimen; commonest

B. Intestinal malabsorption

   1. Mucosal diseases of the small bowel

   2. Jejunoileal bypass and small bowel resection

   3. Diabetic diarrhea

   4. Cirrhosis

   5. Pharmacologic agents

      a. Sucralfate

      b. Aluminum hydroxide

      c. Calcium carbonate[123]

      d. Ferrous sulfate

      e. Kayexalate

      f. Food

      g. Cholestipol

      h. Cholestyramine

      i. Lovastatin?

      j. Activated charcoal

      k. Soy flour

      l. Raloxifene[124]

      m. Dietary fiber supplements[125]

      n. ?Sevelamer[113]

A. Increased hormone losses

   1. Peritoneal dialysis; losses of 8 to 29 μg/day

   2. Nephrotic syndrome; losses of 13 to 69 μg/day

B. Increased degradation rate of T_4[a]

   1. Phenobarbital

   2. Phenytoin

   3. Carbamazepine

   4. Rifampin

   5. Zoloft (probable)

[a]Induce enzymes of the cytochrome P-450 class, which can accelerate thyroxine clearance via pathways that do not lead to the production of T_3.
Source: Adapted from Kaptein and Nelson,[95] with permission.

tions or food, the dosage should be reevaluated whenever medications are altered by measuring serum TSH levels 6 to 8 weeks after the change. Further, in patients with hypothyroidism undergoing renal transplantation, restoration of renal function may result in reduced $L-T_4$ requirements.[113] In patients with ESRD, increased serum iodine levels blocking thyroid hormone release, reduced $L-T_4$ bioavailability, and drug interactions—including reduced intestinal absorption (Table 29–7)—may lead to increased requirements for $L-T_4$ in patients on dialysis.[113] Reversal of these factors after renal transplantation may result in hyperthyroid symptoms and tachyarrthymias due to decreased $L-T_4$ requirements, necessitating dosage reduction.[113]

In contrast to hypothyroidism, euthyroid patients with transiently elevated TSH concentrations or reduced serum total or free T_4 estimates due to nonthyroidal illness should not receive either $L-T_4$ or $L-T_3$ therapy, since neither has been shown to be of benefit and both may be harmful.[94]

Hyperthyroidism

In patients with ESRD, hyperthyroidism due to thyroid gland overproduction occurs with a frequency similar to that in the general population.[94,98,100,115] (Table 29–2). However, hyperthyroidism is infrequently reported in the medical literature[94,98,100,115] and may be difficult to recognize clinically, since the symptoms and signs may be mimicked or masked by concurrent ESRD and other nonthyroidal illnesses.[94,98,100,115] Of 14 reported hyperthyroid patients with ESRD, 12 were female, half were above 60 years of age, and half were below age 40. Hyperthyroidism was due to Graves' disease in 10 and to multinodular toxic goiter in 2 patients. Hyperthyroidism presented with palpitations or weight loss in 78 percent; atrial fibrillation/flutter in 44 percent; weakness, tremor, and/or irritability in 33 percent; and less frequently with nervousness, heat intolerance, confusion, or hypotension during hemodialysis. About 15 percent of elderly patients in the general population with new-onset atrial fibrillation have thyrotoxicosis.[116] Conversely, as many as 25 to 35 percent of elderly patients with thyrotoxicosis will develop atrial fibrillation that is resistant to treatment until the underlying thyroid disorder has been corrected.[116] All ESRD patients with atrial fibrillation should be assessed for hyperthyroidism. Of 12 hyperthyroid patients, 9 had elevated total and/or free T_4 levels; T_3 values were normal or increased in all but one patient. TSH levels were <0.1 mU/L in all 4 reported patients.[98,115] Although serum TSH values may be <0.1 in critically ill patients due to nonthyroidal illnesses, this TSH suppression is transient and values increase to within or even above the normal range with clinical improvement.

Serum TSH values persistently <0.1 mU/L have not been reported in euthyroid patients with ESRD to date in the absence of concurrent or prior hyperthyroidism.[94,98] Thus, a serum TSH concentration measured in a second- or third-generation assay is the most cost-effective screening test for hyperthyroidism, with free T_4 and T_3 estimates and perhaps TSH response to TRH as ancillary tests[94,95,115] (Fig. 29–12). It should be noted that free T4 methods, other than direct equilibrium dialysis, may provide misleadingly low values in patients with reduced serum protein binding of T_4 by albumin and TBG, which is common in ESRD patients.[95] An elevated free T_4 measured by direct dialysis would be consistent with hyperthyroidism and may occasionally be required to substantiate its diagnosis. An elevated free T_3 estimate value is consistent with a diagnosis of hyperthyroidism, while a normal or reduced value does not exclude the diagnosis, since extrathyroidal T_3 production is also reduced in sick patients with hyperthyroidism.[94]

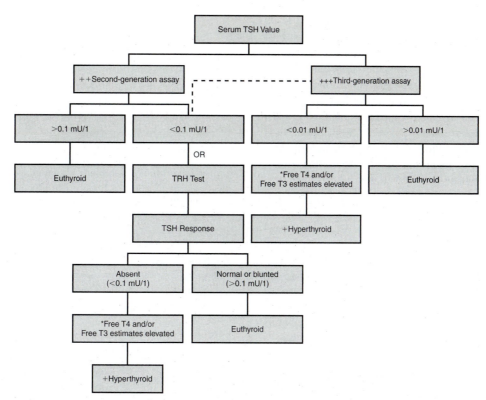

Figure 29–12. Laboratory evaluation for hyperthyroidism in ESRD. Note that all free T_4 estimates except direct dialysis are dependent on serum protein binding and may provide misleadingly low values in patients with low serum albumin and thyroid-binding globulin concentrations.

When hyperthyroidism is diagnosed, the specific-etiology should be determined and appropriate therapy initiated.[94,105,117] The commonest causes of hyperthyroidism are exogenous thyroid hormone administration, Graves' disease, multinodular toxic goiter or toxic adenoma, thyroiditis, and iodide-induced thyrotoxicosis, usually in a patient with multinodular goiter. The etiology of hyperthyroidism is most readily established by performing a a test of iodine-123 (^{123}I) uptake and scan of the thyroid gland prior to initiating or after stopping antithyroid drug therapy assuming the patient has not received an exogenous iodine load. A high uptake with a diffuse pattern is consistent with Graves' disease; a high or normal uptake with a nodular pattern indicates multinodular toxic goiter; and normal or high uptake in a solitary nodule is consistent with toxic adenoma. A radioactive iodide uptake below 2 percent indicates thyroiditis, while an uptake below 10 percent may be associated with exogenous thyroid hormone administration or iodide excess.

Rapid relief of tachycardia, nervousness, and sweating can be achieved by using a beta-blocking agent such as propranolol. For patients with excess thyroid gland production, antithyroid drugs may be administered. Although incompletely defined, the dosages and efficacy of propylthiouracil and methimazole do not appear to be altered in hyperthyroid patients with ESRD.[94] However, since methimazole is not bound to plasma proteins, it should be administered after hemodialysis.[94] These agents usually render the patient with Graves' disease euthyroid in 4 to 6 weeks, while patients with multinodular toxic goiters may require longer to deplete the gland's hormone stores. Sodium ipodate and stable iodide reduce T_4 and T_3 release from the thyroid and can be used in unstable patients with severe thyrotoxicosis or cardiovascular manifestations, but must be administered after antithyroid drugs are initiated to prevent further iodide uptake by the thyroid and further hormone synthesis; they have few side effects. In addition, oral ipodate is a potent inhibitor of T_3 production from T_4, which may shorten the duration of thyrotoxicosis.

Once euthyroidism has been achieved with antithyroid drugs, thyroid ablation with radioactive iodine or surgery should be considered in most patients on chronic dialysis to avoid the cardiovascular consequences of recurrent hyperthyroidism. Radioiodine therapy is appropriate in those with Graves' disease but frequently results in permanent hypothyroidism. For multinodular toxic goiters and toxic adenomas, surgical excision is curative. However, if surgery carries a significant risk, ^{131}I ablation can be used.

In those requiring radioiodine therapy, the appropriate radioiodide dosage depends on thyroidal radioactive iodine uptake and the rate of removal of radioiodide from the body by dialysis and residual renal function.[94] In one patient with

Graves' disease, the administered dose was reduced to 33 percent of the calculated dose and hemodialysis was started 24 hours after the radioiodine was given; radioiodine contamination was minimal.[115] In two other patients given 10 mCi each of ^{131}I followed by hemodialysis 42 and 66 hours later,[118] radioactivity of disposable waste had an effective half-time of 6.3 to 6.6 days, respectively. Effective half-times of ^{131}I clearance from the patients were 6.9 and 7.1 days, respectively, compared to 6.35 days in hyperthyroid patients with normal renal function.[118] These half-times, consistent with a predominance of radiolabeled T_4 and possibly T_3 in the disposable waste as well as in the patients, are derived from new thyroid hormone synthesis incorporating [131]I. After the first one or two dialysis procedures, inorganic ^{131}I levels should be minimal and derived only from the deiodination of T_4 and T_3. Thus, the majority of the radioactivity in the patient and the dialysate is radiolabeled T_4, with a small component of T_3, in contrast to a predominance of inorganic ^{131}I in athyreotic patients with follicular neoplasms. The somewhat longer half-times of radioiodine in the hyperthyroid dialysis patients may be due to impaired excretion of ^{131}I generated from T_4 and T_3 deiodination. Based on these limited data, the radioiodine dosages for patients with Graves' disease receiving hemodialysis therapy should probably be reduced to 33 percent of that calculated for patients with normal renal function.[115] The risk of radiation exposure to personnel would appear to be minimal.[118]

In patients with hyperthyroidism due to accidental or intentional acute ingestion of large quantities of oral L-T_4 or L-T_3, successful treatment may include beta-adrenergic antagonists for tachycardia, decreasing intestinal absorption with activated charcoal or cholestyramine,[119] and/or inhibition of conversion of T_4 to T_3 with the iodinated radiocontrast agent iopanoic acid or ipodate.[120] To date, the efficacy and efficiency of exchange transfusions, hemoperfusion or plasmapheresis, propylthiouracil, and glucocorticoids are unclear.[119,121]

THE HYPOPITUITARY-ADRENAL AXIS IN CHRONIC KIDNEY DISEASE

Cortisol

Although diurnal variation in the secretion of cortisol is well recognized, the secretion is in fact episodic. There are at least 2 to 13 irregular spikes of cortisol secretion interspersed with periods in which no secretion takes place.[126,127] Cortisol and other glucocorticoids are converted to dihydro- and tetrahydro- derivatives in the liver, which are subsequently conjugated to form water-soluble glucocorticoids for excretion in the urine.[128] It is difficult to assess whether or not a state of hypercortisolism exists in renal failure patients for the following reasons:

1. The episodic nature of cortisol secretion[126] yields no insight into the cyclic activity of the pituitary-adrenal system.
2. A valid estimate of the biological activity of cortisol is not available. The accumulated cortisol conjugate in the plasma can react with cortisol antibodies[129] and plasma levels may be overestimated by 50 to 100 percent.[129]
3. The primary route for elimination of 17-hydroxycorticoids is the kidney; therefore the reduction in the urinary excretion of 17-hydroxycorticosteroids cannot be used to investigate the function of the adrenal gland in patients with ESRD.[130,131]

The plasma half-life of cortisol in patients with CKD, whether or not they are receiving dialysis, is consistently prolonged.[130,132–134] However, the circulating plasma levels may be normal[129,132,135–139] or elevated.[132,140–143]

Adrenal Stimulation Tests

Levels of plasma adrenocorticotropic hormone (ACTH) may be normal[144,145] or increased,[136] but the administration of ACTH results in normal secretion of plasma cortisol.[135,136,138–140,144]

Suppression Tests

The reported suppression tests have yielded conflicting results; normal suppression has been reported by Barbour and Servier[135] and impaired suppression by others.[129,140–142] The failure to achieve suppression in circulating cortisol levels is independent of decreased gastrointestinal absorption, as evidenced by when intravenous infusion of dexamethasone[141] or when large oral doses (2 to 8 mg) of this agent are used.[141,142]

The metyrapone test has also been reported to have both normal[135] and abnormal results[140,144] in hemodialysis patients.

These studies suggest that, in ESRD patients, (1) the pituitary-adrenal system cannot be adequately assessed by serum cortisol levels, (2) ACTH stimulation tests are normal, and (3) abnormal dexamethasone and metyrapone tests are often observed. Overall, the data suggest that the pituitary-adrenal axis is deranged in hemodialysis patients.

Aldosterone Secretion in Chronic Kidney Disease

In general, patients with CKD maintain normal potassium (K^+) homeostasis as long as dietary K^+ intake is within normal limits and urine output is adequate. Hyperkalemia is commonly observed in those patients who have severe CKD with a GFR of 5 to 15 mL/min and who develop oligoanuria or ingest excessive amounts of K^+. Two distinct mechanisms that play a role in potassium homeostasis are described. The first maintains external K^+ balance by matching K^+ excretion to dietary K^+ intake.[146] Under the influence of aldosterone, the kidneys play a major role by excreting 90 to 95 percent of the K^+ intake, while the gut may excrete the remaining 5 to 10 percent. The second mechanism, described as extrarenal K^+ "disposal," shifts K^+-ATPase from the extracellular to the intracellular fluid compartment. This mechanism is modulated by a Na^+,K^+-ATPase pump, the activity of which is under the influence of insulin, epinephrine, and other factors such as thyroid status, serum K, and PTH levels.[147–149] With the progression of renal disease, the number of functional nephrons is diminished, so each of the remaining nephrons must adapt and increase K^+ secretory capacity up to 35 meq/day at a GFR as low as 5 mL/min.[150] Colonic adaptation is also demonstrable at this degree of renal impairment when 10 to 20 meq/day of K^+ can be excreted via the enteric route. These adaptive mechanisms are sufficient to prevent hyperkalemia in the presence of normal potassium intake. When potassium intake is increased or potassium is released endogenously, hyperkalemia may develop.

In patients with ESRD, hyperkalemia develops as a result of K^+ retention. However, measured total-body as well as cellular, K^+ concentrations are below normal because of inhibited Na^+,K^+-ATPase pump activity—an abnormality reported to occur in CKD.[146]

In the face of declining renal function, maintenance of K^+ homeostasis is facilitated in part by a high plasma aldosterone level,[150,151] which stimulates K^+ secretion by enhancing the activity of the Na^+,K^+-ATPase pump in the basal lateral membrane of the collecting tubules.[152] The aldosterone level in patients with CKD, whether or not they are receiving dialysis, is reported to be either elevated[153–155] normal,[156–158] or decreased.[159–165] The explanation for these conflicting data, as suggested by Weideman et al.,[157,160] involves multiple factors that include prevailing plasma K^+ level, total K^+ and Na balance, volume status, renin activity, and the effects of medications. Early studies using tritium-labeled aldosterone suggested that aldosterone secretion is increased in patients with CKD.[153–155] However, in a more recent study in patients with CKD, some of whom were maintained on dialysis and some of whom were not, Koshida et al.[166] reported that plasma aldosterone level when measured by radioimmunoassay (RIA) kits without prior extraction may be falsely elevated in some patients. They reported the presence of polar substances in patients with CKD that cross-react with antialdosterone antibody. Extraction or separation of the aldosterone fraction by chromatography procedures before RIA should be carried out in order to obtain a reliable aldosterone measurement. The role of aldosterone secretion in K^+ homeostasis has also been demonstrated in uremic dogs during increases in K^+ intake.[167] In these animals, aldosterone secretion is increased; if this compensatory mechanism is blocked by either intrinsic renal disease or certain drugs, hyperkalemia may develop.

In patients with CKD and hyperkalemia, hyporeninemia is relatively frequent[157,159–165]; this may result in hypoaldosteronism. The syndrome of hyporeninemic hypoaldosteronism (SHH) is commonly found in middle-aged and elderly diabetic patients with unexplained hyperkalemia and some degree of CKD.[168] This syndrome is characterized by hyperkalemia out of proportion to the degree of CKD,[169] hyperchloremic metabolic acidosis (type IV RTA),[170,171] and inappropriately low aldosterone levels. These patients do not have an impairment of cortisol synthesis,[171–176] and the low aldosterone level may be secondary to a deficiency in renin release or activation.[177–180] This syndrome has also been associated with other conditions such as systemic lupus erythematosus, mixed cryoglobulinemia, gout, glomerulonephritis, nephrolithiasis, obstructive uropathy, analgesic nephropathy, interstitial nephropathy, sickle cell disease, renal transplantation,[162,163,181] excess sodium bicarbonate ($NaHCO_3$),[182] and acquired immunodeficiency syndrome (AIDS).[183] The possible mechanisms responsible for a low renin level in this syndrome include structural damage to the renal tubule, a relative block in the processing of prorenin to active renin, reduced adrenergic nerve activity, excess doparninergic tone, volume expansion, low angiotensin II levels, and high K^+.[179] Nadler et al,[184] have suggested that prostacyclin (PGI_2) deficiency plays a role in this syndrome, since PGI_2 is an important regulator of the renin-angiotensin system. Atrial natriuretic peptide, a potent inhibitor of renin,[185] and aldosterone[186] have also been implicated in the etiology of this syndrome. Recently Antonipillai et al.[187] reported that transforming growth factor beta (TGF-β) is increased in the diabetic state; since it can inhibit renin secretion, it may play a role in the low-renin state and therefore may be involved in hyporeninemic hypoaldosteronism. Use of certain medications—such as nonsteroidal antiinflammatory drugs (NSAIDs),[188] angiotensin-converting enzyme (ACE) inhibitors,[189] cyclosporine,[190] and heparin[191]— can also influence aldosterone secretion either directly or indirectly by altering renin production.

Development of hyperkalemia in this syndrome is clear evidence that aldosterone plays an important role in K^+ homeostasis in patients with progressive renal disease.[161–165]

As previously shown, there are a large number of medications used by the patients with renal failure that can influence aldosterone secretion and K homeostasis. Among these are ACE inhibitors, which decrease aldosterone secretion in uremic patients and may induce hyperkalemia,[189] even without any significant changes in plasma creatinine level.[192]

Erythropoietin, frequently used to correct anemia of CKD, has been reported to have conflicting effects on plasma renin activity (PRA) and aldosterone secretion.

Kokot et al.[193] have reported that erythropoietin has a suppressive effect on both PRA and aldosterone secretion in patients on hemodialysis. However, Arik et al.[194] have reported that acute administration of erythropoietin does not have any direct effect on PRA and aldosterone secretion in patients with CKD.

In diabetic patients with or without renal failure, isolated hypoaldosteronism has also been described.[195] It may be associated with normal renin secretion and either normal potassium level or hyperkalemia. In this group of patients, the aldosterone secretion has a normal response to ACTH but not to angiotensin II (Ang II); this is in contrast to patients who have hyporeninemic hypoaldosteronism in which the aldosterone response to both ACTH and Ang II is impaired. In another group of patients with normal plasma renin and without hyperkalemia, the plasma aldosterone level is either normal[157,158,196,197] or elevated.[198,199] Such patients display a normal aldosterone response to provocative stimuli.[156,197] Hene et al.[200] have demonstrated that with a creatinine clearance greater than 50 to 60 mL/min, only a small increase in plasma aldosterone concentration occurred; but with a further reduction in GFR, a progressive rise in plasma aldosterone level was seen.

Aldosterone Secretion in Patients on Dialysis

Conflicting results have been reported in dialysis patients. In nonnephrectomized patients with ESRD receiving maintenance dialysis, plasma aldosterone levels are variable, which reflects the variation in plasma renin activity, K+ levels, and plasma volume.[157,158,161–166] This group of patients has a normal aldosterone response to upright posture or ACTH administration. Sugahara et al.[202] reported that both renin and aldosterone levels increase in parallel with loss of body weight during hemodialysis. Measurement of these hormones seems to be a good indicator for appropriate control of body weight in patients with CKD.[203,204] If plasma K+ level decreases, as occurs during hemodialysis, the volume of induced rise in aldosterone level is frequently altered.[205–208] This phenomenon has also been observed in patients undergoing hemodialysis with intermittent ultrafiltration, when the expected changes in PRA and aldosterone are not present. In these patients, vascular stability in response to reduced blood volume is maintained by the increased release of catecholamines and antidiuretic hormone (ADH), and not by the renin-aldosterone system.[209] In patients who undergo ultrafiltration without dialysis, a procedure that decreases intravascular volume without a change in plasma K+, plasma aldosterone is reported to increase.[205–208] In a recent study,[210] the effect of hemodialysis was found to be different in nondiabetic patients from that observed in diabetic subjects. In the former group, an increase in PRA and a decrease in plasma aldosterone occurred during dialysis, but no significant changes were noted in patients with diabetic nephropathy. This reduced renin response in diabetic patients was considered to be secondary to decreased active renin secretion.

Aldosterone Secretion in Anephric Patients

Most of the studies on plasma aldosterone secretion in dialysis patients were performed in anephric subjects. In these studies, basal plasma aldosterone level was reported to be reduced[138,207,211–213] or normal.[214,215] In these patients, the aldosterone response to different stimuli such as blood volume, ACTH, Ang II, and posture was impaired.[211–213,216] However, in nephrectomized patients receiving CAPD, the aldosterone response to provocative stimuli was maintained.[211] The administration of heparin, which has the potential to inhibit aldosterone biosynthesis, is also considered as a possible cause of altered aldosterone secretion in nephrectomized patients. However, the doses used in these patients during dialysis were unlikely to block aldosterone formation. Therefore serum K+ concentration remains the overriding factor in the regulation of aldosterone secretion in nephrectomized dialyzed patients, and this occurs independent of other factors.[215,217]

Aldosterone Secretion In Postrenal Transplant Patients

In renal transplant patients, immunosuppressive therapy is known to alter the renin-angiotensin-aldosterone system.[218] Some studies suggest that cyclosporine treatment has a stimulatory effect on the renin-angiotensin system,[219] whereas others have failed to show any significant effect.[220] Massry et al.[220] were the first to report the presence of renal tubular acidosis after kidney transplantation. Subsequent studies have confirmed this finding and have shown that these patients develop hyperkalemia secondary to cyclosporine-induced hyporeninemic-hypoaldosteronism.[222] Sugahara et al.[202] have reported that the suppressive effect of cyclosporine on renin secretion occurs within 2 weeks after transplantation, when both renin and aldosterone levels are decreased to the lower limits of normal. These effects of cyclosporine seem to be secondary to a decrease in prostaglandin excretion or expansion of extracellular fluid volume, which occurs during the treatment. The decrease in PRA and aldosterone level occur if body weight changes.

HYPOTHALAMIC-PITUITARY-GONADAL AXIS

Normal sexual function requires the integrity of the hypothalamic-pituitary-gonadal axis. Gonadotropin-releasing hormone (GnRH) is secreted from the hypothalamus and stimulates the production of luteinizing hormone (LH) and follicle-stimulating hormone (FSH) from the pituitary gland. Testosterone is secreted by testicular Leydig cells under the influence of LH and is converted peripherally to estrogen. The inhibitory effect of testosterone on GnRH release and that of estrogen on LH production result in a reduction of LH, with the estrogen having the greatest effect.[223,224] FSH, on the other hand, stimulates production of androgen-binding proteins from Sertoli cells, and this permits these cells to respond to testosterone. FSH also increases the number of LH receptors on Leydig cells and in some manner stimulates spermatogenesis. FSH is controlled by GnRH, as well as by the protein, inhibin, which is synthesized in Sertoli cells.

Abnormalities in spermatogenesis and testosterone production may occur at any level, including the hypothalamus, pituitary, or testes. The hypothalamic and pituitary defects both result in a decrease in FSH, LH, testosterone, and spermatogenesis. However, primary testicular failure is associated with an increase in FSH and LH levels, and a reduction in sperm count and testosterone. Hyperprolactinemia may also be associated with abnormalities similar to primary testicular failure in male dialysis patients.[225–227]

Hypothalamic, Pituitary, and Gonadal Function

Abnormalities of reproductive function may result from derangements of pituitary and gonadal hormones, psychological problems, medications that affect sexual function, anemia, and malnutrition. The easily measurable plasma levels of reproductive hormones are usually utilized to study the sexual abnormalities in patients with CKD.

Sexual Dysfunction in Prepubertal Boys and Men with CKD

Prepubertal Boys. The pubertal development in boys with CKD is frequently delayed and incomplete.[227,228] In prepubertal children, the data on gonadal secretion are controversial. The levels of gonadotropins previously reported in these patients are summarized as follows: normal basal LH and elevated FSH by Ferraris et al.[228]; normal values of both LH and FSH by Perfumo et al.[230]; elevated LH with normal values of FSH and testosterone by Marder et al[229]; and elevated LH and FSH returning to normal values after renal transplantation by Roger et al.[232] The testicular capacity and the biological response to androgens is not impaired in boys.[233] Mean serum FSH 60 minutes after the administration of gonadotropins (GnRH) is significantly lower than in normal controls, suggesting an abnormality of hypothalamic-pituitary function.[233]

Men. Sexual dysfunction related to CKD is particularly evident in over 50 percent of male patients, who usually manifest varying degrees of reduced libido and potency, marked reduction in frequency of intercourse and erectile function, and infertility.[234,235] The sexual dysfunction in uremia is multifactorial but primarily organic in nature, as manifest by abnormal nocturnal penile tumescence.[236] Other factors besides uremic milieu include peripheral neuropathy, autonomic disturbances, peripheral vascular disease, and pharmacologic therapy.[236] In addition, stress and psychological factors commonly present in CKD may also play a role in sexual derangements.[236–239] Steele et al.,[238] who investigated the sexual experience of patients on chronic peritoneal dialysis, found that 63 percent of these patients never had sexual intercourse, 19 percent had intercourse less than or equal to twice a month, and 18 percent had sexual intercourse more than twice a month. The age, amount of dialysis received, and serum albumin concentration were similar among all three groups. Standard psychological evaluation demonstrated that the patients who never had sexual intercourse were more anxious and depressed, with a significantly lower quality of life than the other two groups. These problems may improve but rarely normalize with chronic hemodialysis.[234,235,236]

Spermatogenesis and Testosterone. CKD is accompanied by abnormal spermatogenesis and testicular damage, often with infertility.[226,234] Semen analysis in uremic patients reveals reduced volumes of ejaculate, decreased sperm count and motility, and, not infrequently, azoospermia.[240, 240a,241] Testicular histology shows abnormal spermatogenesis that varies from decreased numbers of mature sperm to complete aplasia of germinal cells. Maturational progression beyond the stage of spermatocytes is unusual,[226,240,240a,241] and hypotestosteronemia is commonly observed in men with CKD.[226,240,240a,241–244] De Krester et al.[243] have reported this abnormality in about 50 percent of uremic males. Hypotestosteronemia (total and free) is a typical finding,[245] even though the binding capacity and concentration of sex hormone-binding globulin are normal.[244–247] Hypotestosteronemia could result from decreased production by Leydig cells and/or increased degradation by the peripheral tissues. The markedly reduced testosterone production rates and normal metabolic clearances in two patients with CKD suggest that hypotestosteronemia is due to reduced production by Leydig cells rather than accelerated degradation by peripheral tissues.[244] Similarly, plasma free testosterone index, a value derived indirectly from the product of total plasma testosterone and the percentage of 3H-testosterone free from binding globulin, is also significantly decreased.[241,248]

Testosterone. Testosterone is 98 percent protein bound, of which 30 percent is bound to plasma β-globulin and the remaining 68 percent to albumin and other proteins because of normal testosterone-binding globulin.[249] Patients with CKD, whether or not they are receiving dialysis, tend to have normal testosterone-binding globulin[244–247] and normal[250,251] to slightly reduced[252] T-albumin levels.

The response of serum testosterone to human chorionic gonadotropins (hCG)—a compound with human luteinizing hormone-like action—is subnormal in the majority of patients,[226,244,253] although it may occasionally be normal.[253] This test does not provide evidence as to whether the Leydig cell failure is of primary or secondary origin, particularly if the test results are not markedly abnormal. The demonstration of downregulation of LH receptors in response to hCG, as shown by some studies,[255,256] suggests that this phenomenon may be partly responsible for the hCG sensitivity in Leydig cells.

Leydig cells are also responsible for the production of most of the estradiol in normal subjects, and estradiol, in turn, is believed to play a significant role in intratesticular regulation of Leydig cell function.[257] Compared to the frequently elevated total plasma estrogen levels,[245,245a] serum estradiol concentration is typically normal in the majority of uremic males,[258,259] but in occasional patients it is found to be elevated.[260]

The mechanisms responsible for testicular damage in uremic males are not well understood. It is possible that plasticizers in dialysis tubing, such as phthalate, may play a role once maintenance hemodialysis is initiated.

Gonadotropins. Serum levels of LH and FSH are variable. They may be normal,[226,241] slightly elevated, or significantly increased.[226,241] Thus, the presence of hypotestosteronemia, impaired spermatogenesis, and elevated gonadotropins in these patients suggests that gonadal dysfunction results from primary end-organ damage. However, studies of Lim et al.[241,242] have shown the following: (1) normal to elevated levels of gonadotropins; (2) low testosterone levels associated with high LH; (3) higher LH levels of LH and testosterone; (4) low FSH associated with azoospermia; and (5) a normal response of increased FSH and LH release following clomiphene administration. These data suggest that the hypothalamic-pituitary axis may also be abnormal in uremia.

Prolactin. This pituitary hormone is frequently elevated in patients with CKD[261]; this may result from either decreased metabolic clearance or autonomous production in uremia. There are conflicting reports about the metabolic clearance of prolactin in uremia. Some studies have reported reduced metabolic clearance in CKD,[262] and Cowden et al.[261] have shown an inverse relation between renal function and serum prolactin levels. There are still others who disagree with the notion that the kidney is an important site for prolactin degra-

dation.[262] The evidence for hyperprolactinemia due to increased production comes from the presence of elevated serum levels of prolactin in dialysis patients[227,264] and uremic sera.[261] Support for the autonomous production of prolactin is provided by the following: (1) failure to suppress prolactin in dialysis patients by dopamine infusion,[245,245a,262] L-dopa,[261,264,265] and acute bromocriptine administration,[226,227,261,266,267] and (2) ineffective stimulation of prolactin secretion by[227,261,264,267] chlorpromazine,[234] and metoclopramide.[265]

The association between hyperprolactinemia and sexual dysfunction has been observed in male patients receiving dialytic therapy.[226,267,269] However, an improvement in libido and potency after normalization of prolactin was seen by some investigators[269] and not by others.[228,270]

The pathogenetic mechanisms for sexual dysfunction in CKD are not well defined. However, several factors may play a role, including secondary hyperparathyroidism, zinc deficiency, vascular insufficiency from arteriosclerosis, autonomic neuropathy from diabetes or uremia, antihypertensive therapy, and psychogenic factors.

Parathyroid hormone is a major uremic toxin; the evidence for its adverse effects on sexual function in CKD patients is provided by the following findings: (1) adequate sexual activity after parathyroidectomy after several years of impotence in two dialysis patients of Massry et al.[271]; (2) the finding of various degrees of impotence in 24 of 33 dialysis patients by Lowe et al.[272] and a significant correlation between the degree of impotence and the magnitude of secondary hyperparathyroidism[273]; and (3) normalization of blood levels of sex hormones and improved potency by suppression of PTH secretion with 1,25-dihydroxycholecalciferol.[271]

Gynecomastia. This abnormality, when unexplained by common factors such as liver disease and medication, is found in about 30 percent of dialysis patients.[241] The postulated mechanisms include the decreased testosterone-estradiol ratio[273] and hyperprolactinemia.[225] However, other investigators have found that estradiol levels and the ratio of estradiol to testosterone are normal, and that hyperprolactinemia is equally distributed among patients with or without gynecomastia.[258,274]

Erectile Dysfunction (ED). ED is the persistent failure to achieve or maintain appropriate erection needed for satisfactory sexual performance; it was found to prevail in 82 percent of hemodialysis (HD) patients.[275] Subjects younger than 50 years had a prevalence of 63 percent of ED (95 percent CI, 53 to 71 percent) but the prevalence of ED was much higher in subjects older than 50 years, occurring in 90 percent (95 percent CI, 84 to 94 percent). In these patients, ED was strongly associated with increasing age and diabetes but was inversely associated with the use of ACE inhibitors.

Sexual Dysfunction In Girls and Adult Females with Chronic Kidney Disease

Prepubertal Girls. Ovarian steroidogenesis is not impaired in prepubertal girls with CKD. Hypothalamic-pituitary function is abnormal in some of these girls. This abnormality is evidenced by failure of LH, FSH, and estradiol to respond normally to GnRH, and is in part attributed to the severe malnutrition observed in some of these patients.[233]

Adult Females. Sexual dysfunction is common in women with CKD.[241,276] This abnormality is characterized by amenorrhea, hypermenorrhea, decreased libido, and infertility. The major clinical manifestation is menstrual dysfunction, which is observed in more than 90 percent of patients, more than half of whom are amenorrheic.[276] In a study of 15 patients reported by Lim et al.,[241] 10 had amenorrhea, 4 had irregular menstrual periods, and 1 had normal menstruation. Amenorrhea is usually observed when the GFR is less than 10 mL/min[277,278] and, in most uremic women including those with normal menstruation, there is an anovular hormonal pattern because plasma progesterone levels are low in most of these patients.[241] Plasma estradiol is also decreased in uremic women.[241]

In menstruating uremic women, the plasma LH levels are not usually abnormal,[281,282] although reduced values have also been reported in rare cases.[279] Variability in basal values of FSH is less frequently observed in such patients, and the majority of premenopausal patients with CKD display normal values.[279] However, in postmenopausal uremic females, both LH and FSH are elevated [274,277,279,280] but estrogen levels are decreased.[274,281]

The secretion of LH and FSH is exhibited either as tonic release or midcycle surge. The tonic release is stimulated by GnRH and inhibited by estrogens, especially estradiol. The regulation of the midcycle surge is achieved by both GnRH and estrogens. The response of gonadotropins to LH-RH is appropriate, and normal negative feedback inhibition by estrogen in female patients with CKD is evidenced by increased secretion of LH and FSH following short-term administration of clomiphene, an antiestrogen agent,[276] and appropriately elevated levels of these hormones in postmenopausal uremic women. The positive estradiol feedback associated with the pulsatile surge of goadotropins, on the other hand, is markedly abnormal in such patients.[276,282] Furthermore, exogenous estrogen administration fails to stimulate the release of LH and FSH as observed in normal women.[276]

These observations suggest that gonadal dysfunction in females with CKD is due to a defect at the gonadal as well as the hypothalamic level.

Therapy. Decreased libido is common in uremic women but generally no treatment is required. Despite anovulation, hot flushes, and sweating—which are associated with menopause—are not present in these patients; therefore, estrogen therapy is not indicated. A topical estrogen application is usually sufficient for a problematic atrophic vaginitis. Dysfunctional uterine bleeding in patients with CKD should be treated with estrogen combined with one of the progesterones in a cyclic fashion, as in nonuremic patients.

Galactorrhea and Hyperprolactinemia

The majority of the uremic women demonstrate elevated levels of prolactin.[244,263,264,264a,276,283] Prolactin secretion fails to respond to stimulatory and inhibitory tests. The role of hyperprolactinemia in the genesis of amenorrhea and/or galactorrhea is suggestive and needs further evaluation. Galactorrhea is usually mild and does not warrant treatment. However, since this abnormality bears a striking resemblance to a prolactin-secreting pituitary tumor, this possibility should be excluded before galactorrhea is ascribed to CKD.

Effect of Dialytic Therapy

Males. The reduced libido and potency found in uremic men usually do not improve with maintenance dialytic therapy.[236,284] Hyperprolactinemia has been reported in 25 percent of male patients with ESRD by Gomez et al.,[227] 57 percent by Lim et al.,[264] and 78 percent in both sexes by Cowden and associates.[261] Patients receiving dialytic therapy continue to have an abnormal hypothalamo-hypophyseal axis in the regulation of PRL, LH, and FSH secretion.[265] Furthermore, there is failure of synthesis and/or release of testosterone.[265] Hyperprolactinemia is observed in 30 percent of dialysis patients and is usually mild in magnitude[267,270]; in HD patients, this abnormality is due to a prolonged half-life, chronic stress, and medications.[227] The pathogenetic mechanisms for the state of hypogonadism in dialysis patients are not well defined. This abnormality occurs even in the absence of zinc deficiency,[285] and the evidence for a mild hyperprolactinemia playing an important role in the genesis of hypogonadism in HD patients is lacking, as normalization of moderate hyperprolactinemia fails to correct serum gonadotropin and testosterone levels.[270] The role of secondary hyperparathyroidism needs further evaluation.

Females. Amenorrhea and infertility are common among dialysis patients.[286] The initiation of HD in some patients may be associated with temporary improvement in menstrual abnormalities, but ultimately the majority of patients develop amenorrhea.[287] Menorrhagia is also observed in women receiving hemodialysis,[288,289]; in some patients, hypermenorrhea may be severe and result in significant blood loss requiring blood transfusion.[276] In patients receiving hemodialysis, PRL, FSH, and LH levels are elevated.[280,290]

The abnormally elevated levels of LH observed in menstruating dialysis patients is deemed an important factor in the genesis of menstrual disturbances.[281] The estradiol levels in hemodialyzed women have been found to be elevated only in those who are menstruating.[281] Overall, dialytic therapy does not correct the abnormalities of gonadal failure observed in patients with CKD. However, successful pregnancies have been reported on occasion in these patients.[234,291]

Effect of Erythropoietin. The correction of anemia with erythropoietin therapy[292] results in (1) the return of gonadotropins and prolactin values to normal and (2) the restoration of FSH response to exogenous GnRH. There is also evidence that treatment of anemia with erythropoietin may be associated with normalization of the pituitary gonadal feedback mechanism, resulting in an increase in testosterone levels and normalization of LH, FSH, and prolactin.[292–296] The correction of anemia to increase the hematocrit to 33 to 36 percent may improve the sexual function[296]; it is likely that such enhancement in sexual activity is secondary to an improvement in quality of life. However, further studies are needed to determine whether improved oxygenation from correction of anemia, a trophic action of erythropoietin per se, improvement in well-being, or some combination of these factors is responsible for the beneficial effects.

Sildenafil. This agent is not often utilized in dialysis patients as first-line therapy for erectile dysfunction due to psychogenic, vascular, or neurogenic causes[297–301] but it can be effective therapy. In a placebo-controlled, randomized, double-blind study of 41 hemodialysis patients, sildenafil was found to be well tolerated and extremely effective in improving erectile function.[298] However, this study excluded a large number of patients such as those above 70 years of age, those receiving nitrates, and/or patients with the diagnoses of diabetes, cirrhosis, angina or severe anemia, history of a recent stroke or myocardial infarction, and an anatomically abnormal penis. To prevent the possibility of hypotension in dialysis patients, some physicians recommend its use on nondialysis days.[302] Current use of sildenafil and nitrates in any form is contraindicated.

Effect of Renal Transplantation

Males. Successful renal transplantation has been reported to normalize both the basal PRL and the PRL stimulation and suppression tests,[235,266,303] improve spermatogenesis,[236,242,304] and restore testicular function and fertility.[303,305] Following renal transplantation, LH, FSH, and the response to GnRH is also restored.[236,242]

Chronic administration of cyclosporine in currently used doses does not appear to prevent the restoration of the hypothalamic-pituitary-testicular axis.[303,305]

Females. Successful renal transplantation in women is followed by near normalization of PRL, amelioration of LH and FSH secretion, and restoration of estrogen secretion.[306] Fertility may be restored in many women,[306] and pregnancies have been reported in some of these patients[306]; these are relatively more common in patients with adequate renal function.[306] However, premature births remain a significant risk, and may be observed in 20 to 50 percent of all pregnancies in renal transplant recipients.[307]

REFERENCES

1. Rubenstein AH, Mako ME, Horowitz DC. Insulin and the kidney. *Nephron* 1975;15:306–326.
2. Katz AI, Rubenstein AH. Metabolism of proinsulin and C peptides in the rat. *J Clin Invest* 1973;52:1113–1121.
3. Rabkin R, Colwell JA. The renal uptake and excretion of insulin in the dog. *J Lab Clin Med* 1969;73:893–900.
4. Zaharko DS, Beck LV, Blankenbaker R. Role of the kidney in the disposal of radioiodinated and nonradioiodinated insulin in dog. *Diabetes* 1966;15:680–685.
5. Rabkin R, Jones J, Kitabchi AE. Insulin extraction from the renal peritubular circulation in the chicken. *Endocrinology* 1977;101:1828–1833.
6. Zubrod CG, Eversole SL, Dana GW. Amelioration of diabetes and striking rarity of acidosis in patients with Kimmelsteil-Wilson lesions. *N Engl J Med* 1951;245:518–525.
7. Kalliomak JL, Markkanen TK, Sourander LB. Correction between insulin requirement and renal retention in diabetic nephropathy. *Acta Med Scand* 1966;166:423–424.
8. Runyan JW, Hurwitz D, Robbins SC. Effect of Kimmelsteil-Wilson syndrome on insulin requirements in diabetes. *N Engl J Med* 1955;252:388–391.
9. Westervelt CG, Schreiner GE. The carbohydrate intolerance of uremic patients. *Ann Intern Med* 1962;57:266–275.
10. Hampers CL, Soeldoner JS, Doak B, Merrill JP. Effect of chronic renal failure and hemodialysis on carbohydrate metabolism. *J Clin Invest* 1966;45:1719–1731.
11. Horton ES, Johnson C, Lebovitz HE. Carbohydrate in uremia. *Ann Intern Med* 1968;68:63–74.
12. DeFronzo RA, Andres R, Edgar P, Walker WG. Carbohydrate metabolism in uremia. A review. *Medicine* 1973;52:469–481.
13. DeFronzo RA, Alverstand A, Smith D, et al. Insulin resistance in uremia. *J Clin Invest* 1981;67:563–568.
14. Saaman NA, Freeman RM. Growth hormone in severe renal failure. *Metab Clin Exp* 1970;19:102–103.
15. Lowrie EG, Soeldner JS, Hampers CL, Merrill JP. Glucose metabolism and insulin secretion in uremia, predialysis, and normal subjects. *Diabetes* 1970;76:603–615.

16. Perley M, Kipnis DM. Plasma insulin responses to glucose and tolbutamide of normal weight and obese diabetic and nondiabetic subjects. *Diabetes* 1966;15:867–874.

18. Beck P, Schalch DS, Parker ML, et al. Corrective studies of growth hormone and insulin plasma concentrations with metabolic abnormalities in acromegaly. *J Lab Clin Med* 1965;66:366–379.

19. DeFronzo RA. Pathogenesis of glucose intolerance in uremia. *Metab Clin Exp* 1978;27:1866–1880.

20. Mak RHK, Bettinelli A, Turner C, et al. The influence of hyperparathyroidism on glucose metabolism in uremia. *J Clin Endocrin Metab* 1985;60:229–233.

21. Akmal M, Massry SG, Goldstein DA, et al. Role of parathyroid hormone in the glucose intolerance of chronic renal failure. *J Clin Invest* 1985;75:1037–1044.

22. Ginsberg H, Olefsky JM, Reaven GM. Evaluation of insulin resistance in patients with primary hyperparathyroidism. *Proc Biol Exp Med* 1975;148:942–945.

23. Kim H, Kalkhoff RK, Costrini NV, et al. Plasma insulin disturbances in primary hyperparathyroidism. *J Clin Invest* 1971;50:2596–2605.

24. Pappenheimer AM, Wilens SL. Enlargement of the parathyroid glands in renal disease. *Am J Pathol* 1935;11:73–91.

25. Roth SI, Marshall RB. Pathology and ultrastructure of the human parathyroid glands in chronic renal failure. *Arch Intern Med* 1969;124:390–407.

26. Berson SA, Yallow R. Parathyroid hormone in plasma in adenomatous hyperparathyroidism, uremia, and bronchogenic carcinoma. *Science* 1968;154:907–909.

27. Massry SG, Coburn JW, Peacock M, Kleeman CR. Turnover of endogenous parathyroid hormone in uremic patients, and those undergoing hemodialysis. *ASAIO Trans* 1972;8: 422–426.

28. Mak RHK, Turner C, Haycock GB, Chantler C. Secondary hyperparathyroidism and glucose intolerance in children with uremia. *Kidney Int* 1983;24:S128–S133.

29. Fadda GZ, Akmal M, Premdas PH, et al. Insulin release from pancreatic islets: effect of CKD and excess PTH. *Kidney Int* 1988;33:1066–1072.

30. DeFronzo RA, Tobin JD, Andres R. Glucose clamp technique: a method for quantifying insulin secretion and resistance. *Am J Physiol* 1979;237:E214–E223.

31. DeFronzo RA, Alverstand A. Glucose intolerance in uremia: site and mechanism. *Am J Clin Nutr* 1980;33:1438–1445.

32. DeFronzo RA, Tobin JD, Rowe JW, Andres R. Glucose intolerance in uremia. Quantification of pancreatic beta cell sensitivity to glucose and tissue sensitivity to insulin. *J Clin Invest* 1978;62:424–435.

33. Friedman JE, Dohm L, Elton CW, et al. Muscle insulin resistance in uremic humans: glucose transport, glucose transporters and insulin receptors. *Am J Physiol* 1991;261(*Endocrinol Metab* 24):E87–E94.

34. Lu KC, Sheih SD, Lin SH, et al. Hyperparathyroidism, glucose tolerance and platelet intracellular free calcium in chronic renal failure. *Q J Med* 1994; 87:359–365.

35. Bevilacqua SE, Barret E, Farranini R, et al. Lack of effect of parathyroid hormone on hepatic glucose metabolism in the dog. *Metab Clin Exp* 1981;30:469–475.

36. Fadda GZ, Akmal M, Lipson LG, Massry SG. Direct effect of parathyroid hormone on insulin secretion from pancreatic islets. *Am J Physiol* 1990;258:E3975–E3984.

37. Perna AF, Fadda GZ, Zhou X-J, Massry SG. Mechanisms of impaired insulin secretion from pancreatic islets. *Am J Physiol* 1990;259:F210–F216.

37. Carafoli E. Intracellular calcium homeostasis. *Annu Rev Biochem* 197;56:395–433.

38. Fadda GZ, Hajjar SM, Perna AF, et al. On the mechanism of impaired insulin secretion in chronic renal failure. *J Clin Invest* 1991;87:255–261.

39. Hajjar SM, Fadda GZ, Thanakitcharu P, et al. Reduced activity of Na$^+$,K$^+$-ATPase of pancreatic islets in chronic renal failure: role of secondary hyperparathyroidism. *J Am Soc Nephrol* 1982;2:1355–1359.

40. Thanakitcharu P, Fadda GZ, Hajjar SM, Massry SG. Verapamil prevents the metabolic and functional derangements in pancreatic islets of chronic renal failure rats. *Endocrinology* 1991;129:1749–1754.

41. Fadda GZ, Akmal M, Soliman AR, et al. Correction of glucose intolerance and the impaired insulin release of chronic renal failure by Verapamil. *Kidney Int* 1990;36:773–779.

42. Thanakitcharu P, Fadda GZ, Hajjar SM, et al. Verapamil reverses glucose intolerance in preexisting chronic renal failure: studies on mechanisms. *Am J Nephrol* 1992;12: 179–187.

42. Block MB, Rubenstein AH. Spontaneous hypoglycemia in diabetic patients with renal insufficiency. *JAMA* 1970;14: 1863–1868.

43. Garber AI, Bier DM, Cryer PE, Pagliara AS. Hypoglycemia in compensated chronic renal insufficiency. Substrate limitation of gluconeogenesis. *Diabetes* 1973;22:493–498.

44. Frizzell M, Larsen PR, Field JB. Spontaneous hypoglycemia associated with chronic renal failure. *Diabetes* 1973;22: 493–498.

46. Rutsky EA, McDaniel HG, Thorpe DL, et al. Spontaneous hypoglycemia in chronic renal failure. *Arch Intern Med* 1978;138:1364–1368.

47. Mansoor GA, Nicholson DM. Hypoglycemia in chronic renal failure. *W I Med J* 1992;41:41–42.

48. Arem R. Hypoglycemia associated with renal failure. *Endocrinol Metab Clin North Am* 1989;18:103–121.

49. Arem R, Garber AJ, Full JB. *Arch Intern Med* 1987; 143(4):827–829.

50. Haviv YS, Sharkia M, Safadi R. Hypoglycemia in patients with renal failure. *Renal Failure* 2000;22(2)219—213.

51. Greenblatt DJ. Fatal hypoglycemia occurring after peritoneal dialysis. *Br Med J* 1972;2:270–271.

52. Fischer KF, Lees JA, Newmann JH. Hypoglycemia in hospitalized patients: causes and outcome. *N Engl J Med* 1986; 315:1245–1250.

53. Corvillain J, Brauman H, et al. Labeled insulin catabolism in chronic renal failure and in the anephric state. *Diabetes* 1971;20:467–475.

54. Seltzer HS. Drug induced hypoglycemia. A review based on 473 cases. *Diabetes* 1972;21:955–966.

55. Jackson IE, Bressler R. Clinical pharmacology of sulfonylurea hypoglycemic agents: Part 1. Drugs. 1981;22:211–245.

56. Petitpierre B, Perrin L, Rudhart M, et al. Comportement de la chlorpropamide et de therapeutiques associees. *Helv Med Arch* 1972;36:245.

57. Appel GB, Nev HC. The use of drugs in renal failure. *Disease-A-Month* 1979;25:1–44.

58. Balant L, Zahnd GR, Weber R, Fabre J. Behavior of glibenclamide, on repeated administration to diabetic patients. *Eur J Clin Pharmacol* 1977;11:19–25.

59. Berger W. 88 Schwere Hypoglykamiezwis-Chenfalle unter der Behandlung mit Sulfonylharnstoffer. *Schweiz Med Wochenschr* 1971;71:1013–1022.

60. Balant L, Fabre JD. Influence of renal insufficiency on the behavior of hypoglycemic sulfonylurea. In: *Gliclazide*. Royal Society of Medicine International Congress and Symposium Series. London: Academic Press, 1975;20:83–93.

61. Pearson JG. Pharmacokinetics of glyburide. *Am J Med* 1985;79:67–71.

62. Balant L, Zahnd G, Georgia A, et al. Behavior of glipizide in renal insufficiency. *Diabetologia* 1973;9(suppl):331–338.

63. Hazard J. Accidents hypoglycemiques provoques par les sulfamides hypoglycemints. Rappel des bases pharmacologiques de leur utilization therapeutique. *Nouv Presse Med* 1976;5:903–905.

64. Laporte J. Au Subject des interactions medicamenteuses. *Nouv Presse Med* 1972;10:361–371.

65. Skillman TG, Feldman JM. The pharmacology of sulfonylureas. *Am J Med* 1981;70:361–372.

66. Cohen BD. Abnormal carbohydrate metabolism in renal disease. Blood glucose unresponsiveness to sulfonylureas, epinephrine and glucagon. *Ann Intern Med* 1962;57:204–213.

67. Dall JLC, Conway H, McAlpine SG. Hypoglycemia due to chlorpropramide. *Scott Med J* 1967;12:403.

68. Soeldner JS, Misbin RI. Hypoglycemia in tolbutamide treated diabetes. *JAMA* 1965;193(5):148–149.

69. Florez LB, Rozansi J, Castro A, Mintz DH. Propoxyphene-induced hypoglycemia. *J Fla Med Assoc* 1977;64(3): 163–164.

70. Wiederholt JC, Genco M, Foley JM. Recurrent episodes of hypoglycemia induced by propoxyphene. *Neurology* 1967; 17:703–706.

71. Bouvenot G, Escande M, Jouve R, Delboy C. Beta bloquants et pathologie gerierale. *Semin Hop Paris* 1977;53(10):639–646.

72. Skinner DJ, Misbin RI. Uses of propranolol. *N Engl J Med* 1975;293(4):1205.

73. Avram MM, Wolf RE, Gan A, et al. Uremic hypoglycemia. Preventable life-threatening complications. *NY State J Med* 1984;84:593–596.

74. Arauz-Pacheco C, Ramirez LC, Rios LM, Raskin P. Hypoglycemia induced by angiotensin converting enzyme inhibitors in patients with non–insulin dependent diabetes receiving sulfonylurea therapy. *Am J Med* 1990;89:811–813.

75. Pollare T, Lithell H, Berne C. A comparison of the effects of hydrochlorthiazide and captopril on glucose and lipid metabolism in patients with hypertension. *N Engl J Med* 1989;321:868–873.

76. Grodstein GP, Blumenkrantz MJ, Kopple JD, et al. Glucose absorption during continuous ambulatory dialysis. *Kidney Int* 1981;19:564–567.

77. Crossley K, Kjellstrand GM. Intraperitoneal insulin for control of blood sugar in diabetic patients during peritoneal dialysis in dogs. *Br Med J* 1971;1:269–270.

78. Shapiro JD, Blumenkrantz MJ, Levin SR, Coburn JW. Absorption and action of insulin added to peritoneal dialysis in dogs. *Nephron* 1979;23:174–180.

79. Biachard WG, Nelson NC. Portal and peripheral vein immunoreactive insulin concentrations before and after glucose infusion. *Diabetes* 1970;19:302–306.

80. Amair P, Khanna R, Leibel B, et al. Continuous ambulatory dialysis in diabetics with end stage renal disease. *N Engl J Med* 1982;306:625–630.

81. Arner P, Gunnarsson R, Blomdahl S, Groth CG. Some characteristic of steroid diabetes: a study in renal transplant recipients receiving high dose corticosteroid therapy. *Diabetes Care* 1983;6:23–25.

82. McGeowen MG, Douglas JF, Brown WA, et al. Advantage of low-dose steroids from the day after renal transplantation. *Transplantation* 1987;29:287–289.

83. Hers HG. Effects of glucocorticoids on carbohydrate metabolism. *Agents Actions* 1985;17:238–245.

84. Marco J, Calle C, Roman D, et al. Hyperglucagonism induced by glucocorticoid therapy in man. *N Engl J Med* 1973;288:128–131.

85. Yagisawa T, Takahashi K, Teraoka S, et al. Deterioration in glucose metabolism in cyclosporine-treated kidney transplant recipients and rats. *Transplant Proc* 1986;18:1548–1551.

86. Yoshimura N, Nakai I, Ohmori Y, et al. Effect of cyclosporine on the endocrine and exocrine pancreas in kidney transplant recipients. *Am J Kidney Dis* 1981;I: 11–17.

87. Yale IF, Chamelian M, Courchesne S, Vigrant C. Peripheral insulin resistance and decreased insulin secretion after cyclosporin A treatment. *Transplant Proc* 1988;20:985–988.

88. Kohner EM, Dollery CT, Lowy C, Schumer B. Effects of diuretic therapy on glucose tolerance in hypertensive patients. *Lancet* 1971;1:986–991.

89. Friedman EA, Shyh TP, Beyer MM, et al. Post-transplant diabetes in kidney transplant recipients. *Am J Nephrol* 1985;5: 196–202.

90. Alalvi JA, Sharma BK, Pillary VKG. Steroid induced diabetic ketoacidosis. *Am J Med Sci* 1971;262:15–23.

91. von Kiparki A, Frei D, Uhlschimdt G, et al. Post transplant diabetes mellitus in renal allograft recipients. A matched pair control study. *Nephrol Dial Transplant* 1990;5:220–225.

92. Montoroi VM, Basu A, Erwin PJ, et al. Posttransplantation diabetes mellitus. *Diabetes Care* 2000;25(3)583–592.

93. Maes BD, Kuypers D, Messiaen T, et al. Post-transplantation diabetes mellitus in FK-506-treated renal transplant recipients: analysis of incidence and risk factors. *Transplantation* 2001;72(10):1655–1661.

94. Kaptein EM. Thyroid hormone metabolism and thyroid diseases in chronic renal failure. *Endocr Rev* 1996;17:45–63.

95. Kaptein EM, Nelson JC. Serum thyroid hormones and thyroid-stimulating hormone. In Korenman JG, ed. *Atlas of Clinical Endocrinology*, Vol. 1: *Thyroid Diseases*. Philadelphia: Current Medicine, Inc. 1999:15–31.

96. Mariotti S. Normal physiology of the hypothalmic-pituitary-thyroidal system and relation to the neural system and other endocrine glands. In: De Groot LJ, Hennemann G, eds. *Thyroid Disease Manager: The Thyroid and Its Diseases.* Endocrine Education, Inc, 2002. www.Thyroidmanager.org

97. Refetoff S. Thyroid hormone serum transport proteins: structure, properties and genes and transcriptional regulation. In: De Groot LJ, Hennemann G, eds. *Thyroid Disease Manager: The Thyroid and Its Diseases.* Endocrine Education, Inc, 2000. www.Thyroidmanager.org

98. Kaptein EM, Wilcox RB, Nelson JC. Assessing thyroid hormone status in a patient with end-stage renal failure: from theory to practice. *Thyroid* 2004;399–402.

99. Yonemura K, Nakajima T, Suzuki T, et al. Low free thyroxine concentrations and deficient nocturnal surge of thyroid-stimulating hormone in haemodialysed patients compared with undialysed patients. *Nephrol Dial Transplant* 2000;15:668–672.

100. Kaptein EM, Quion-Verde H, Chooljian CJ, et al. The thyroid in end-stage renal disease. *Medicine* 1988;67: 187–197.

101. Iitaka M, Kawasaki S, Sakurai et al. Serum substances that interfere with thyroid hormone assays in patients with chronic renal failure. *Clin Endocrinol* 1998;48: 739–746.

102. Okabayashi T, Takeda K, Kawada M, et al. Free thyroxine concentrations in serum measured by equilibrium dialysis in chronic renal failure. *Clin Chem* 1996;42:1616–1620.

103. Kaptein EM, Levenson H, Siegel ME, et al. Radioiodine dosimetry in patients with end-stage renal disease receiving continuous ambulatory peritoneal dialysis therapy. *J Clin Endocrinol Metab* 2000;85:3058–3064.

104. Reinhardt W, Misch C, Jockenhovel F, et al. Triiodothyronine (T3) reflects renal graft function after renal transplantation. *Clin Endocrinol* 1997;46:563–569.

105. Henneman G. Multinodular goiter. In: De Groot LJ, Hennemann G, eds. *Thyroid Disease Manager: The Thyroid and Its Diseases.* Endocrine Education, Inc, 2003. www.Thyroidmanager.org

106. Pacini F, De Groot, LJ. Thyroid cancer. In: De Groot LJ, Hennemann G, eds. *Thyroid Disease Manager: The Thyroid and Its Diseases.* Endocrine Education, Inc, 2003.www.Thyroidmanager.org

107. Maisonneuve P, Agodoa L, Gellert R, et al. Cancer in patients on dialysis for end-stage renal disease: an international collaborative study (comment). *Lancet* 1999;354: 93–99.

108. Mazzaferri EL, Kloos RT: Using recombinant human TSH in the management of well-differentiated thyroid cancer: current strategies and future directions. *Thyroid* 2000;10:767–78.

109. Toubert ME, Michel C, Metivier F, et al. Iodine-131 ablation therapy for a patient receiving peritoneal dialysis. *Clin Nucl Med* 2001;26:302–305.

110. Magne N, Magne J, Bracco J, Bussiere F. Disposition of radioiodine (131)I therapy for thyroid carcinoma in a patient with severely impaired renal function on chronic dialysis: a case report. *Jpn J Clin Oncol* 2002;32:202–205.

111. Jimenez RG, Moreno AS, Gonzalez EN, et al. Iodine-131 treatment of thyroid papillary carcinoma in patients under-going dialysis for chronic renal failure: a dosimetric method. *Thyroid* 2001;11:1031–1034.

112. Klein I, Danzi S. Evaluation of the therapeutic efficacy of different levothyroxine preparations in the treatment of human thyroid disease. *Thyroid* 2003;13:1127–1132.

113. Thomas MC, Mathew TH, Russ GR. Changes in thyroxine requirements in patients with hypothyroidism undergoing renal transplantation. *Ame J Kidney Dis* 2002;39:354–357.

114. Lim VS. Thyroid function in patients with chronic renal failure. *Am J Kidney Dis* 2001;38:580–584.

115. Miyasaka Y, Yoshimura M, Tabata S, et al. Successful treatment of a patient with Graves' disease on hemodialysis complicated by antithyroid drug-induced granulocytopenia and angina pectoris. *Thyroid* 1997;7:621–624.

116. Cooper DS: Hyperthyroidism. *Lancet* 2003;362:459–468.

117. De Groot LJ. Diagnosis and treatment of Graves' disease. In: De Groot LJ, Hennemann C, eds. *Thyroid Disease Manager: The Thyroid and Its Diseases.* Endocrine Education, Inc, 2003. www.Thyroidmanager.org

118. Homer L, Smith AH. Radiation protection issues of treating hyperthyroidism with ^{131}I in patients on haemodialysis. *Nucl Med Commun* 2002;23:261–264.

119. de Luis DA, Duenas A, Martin J, et al. Light symptoms following a high-dose intentional L-thyroxine ingestion treated with cholestyramine. *Horm Res* 2002;57:61–63.

120. Brown RS, Cohen JH III Braverman LE. Successful treatment of massive acute thyroid hormone poisoning with iopanoic acid. *J Pediatr* 1998;132:903–905.

121 Henderson A, Hickman P, Ward G, Pond SM. Lack of efficacy of plasmapheresis in a patient overdosed with thyroxine. *Anaesth Intens Care* 1994;22:463–464.

122. Kaptein EM. Abnormalities of thyroid function in chronic dialysis patients. In: Nissenson AR, ed. *Dialysis Therapy.* Philadelphia: Hanley & Belfus, 2001:361–368.

123. Singh N, Weisler SL, Hershman JM. The acute effect of calcium carbonate on the intestinal absorption of levothyroxine. Thyroid 2001;11:967–971.

124. Siraj ES, Gupta MK, Reddy SS. Raloxifene causing malabsorption of levothyroxine. *Arch Intern Med* 2003;163:1367–1370.

125. Chiu AC, Sherman, SI. Effects of pharmacological fiber supplements on levothyroxine absorption. *Thyroid* 1998;8:667–671.

126. Hellman L, Nakada F, Curti J, et al. Cortisol is secreted episodically by normal man. *J Clin Endocrinol Metab* 1970;30:411–422.

127. Weitzman ED, Fudushima K, Nogeire C. Twenty-four-hour pattern of the episodic secretion of cortisol in normal subjects. *J Clin Endocrinol Metab* 1971;33:14–22.

128. Peterson RE, Wyngaarden JB, Guerra SL, et al. The physiologic disposition and metabolic fate of hydrocortisone in man. *J Clin Invest* 1955;12:1799–1804.

129. Nolan GE, Smith JB, Chavre VJ, Jubiz W. Spurious overestimation of Plasma cortisol in patients with chronic renal failure. *J Clin Endocrinol Metab* 1981;52:1242–1245.

130. Englert E, Brown H, Willardson DG, et al. Metabolism of free and conjugated 17-hydroxycorticosteroids in subjects with uremia. *J Clin Endocrinol Metab* 1958;18:36–48.

131. Blair AJ, Morgan RO, Beck JC. The plasma 17-hydroxy corticosteroids levels in acute and chronic renal failure. *Can J Biochem Physiol* 1961;39:1617–1623.

132. Bacon GE, Kenny PM, Murdaugh HV, Richards C. Prolonged half-life of cortisol in renal failure. *Johns Hopkins Med J* 1973;132:127–131.

133. Mishkin MS, Hsu JH, Walker G, Bledsoe T. Studies on the secretion of cortisol in uremic patients on hemodialysis. *Johns Hopkins Med J* 1972;131:160–164.

134. Deck KA, Seimon G, Dieberth HG, von Bayer H. Cortisol loss and plasma 11 hydroxycorticosteroid profile during hemodialysis. *Verh Dtsch Ges Inn Med* 1968;74:1195–1201.

135. Barbour GL, Siever BR. Adrenal responsiveness in chronic hemodialysis patients. *N Engl J Med* 1979;290:1285.

136. Gilkes JJH, Eady RAJ, Rees LH, et al. Plasma immunoreactive melanotrophic hormones in patients on hemodialysis. *Br Med J* 1975;1:656–657.

137. Gallager BB. The effect of hemodialysis on the plasma cortisol and encephalogram in uremia. *Neurology* 1970;20:975–981.

138. Williams GH, Bailey GL, Hampers CL, et al. Studies on the metabolism of aldosterone in chronic renal failure and anephric man. *Kidney Int* 1973;4:280–288.

139. Weidmann P, Horton R, Maxwell MH, et al. Dynamic studies of aldosterone in anephric man. *Kidney Int* 1973;4:289–298.

140. McDonald WJ, Golper A, Moss RD, et al. Adrenocorticotropin-axis abnormalities in hemodialysis patients. *J Clin Endocrinol Metab* 1979;48:92—95.

141. Rosman PM, Farag A, Peckham R, et al. Pituitary-adrenocortical function in chronic renal failure: blunted suppression and early escape of plasma cortisol levels after intravenous dexamethasone. *J Clin Endocrinol Metab* 1982;54:528–533.

142. Wallace EZ, Rosman P, Toshav N, et al. Pituitary-adrenocortical function in chronic renal failure: studies of episodic secretion of cortisol and dexamethasone suppressibility. *J Clin Endocrinol Metab* 1980;53:528–533.

143. Zumoff G, Fudishima DK, Weitzman ED, et al. The sex difference in plasma cortisol concentration in man. *J Clin Endocrinol Metab* 1974;39:801–805.

144. Akmal M, Manzler AD. Simplified assessment of pituitary adrenal axis in a stable group of chronic renal failure. *ASAIO Trans* 1977;23:703–706.

145. Ramirez G, Etheridge P, Meikle W, Jibiz W. Evaluation of pituitary-adrenal axis in patients with chronic renal failure. *Clin Res* 1978;26:148A.

146. Allon M. Treatment and prevention of hyperkalemia in end stage renal disease. *Kidney Int* 1993;43:1197–1209.

147. Clausen T, Everts ME. Regulation of Na,K pump in skeletal muscle. *Kidney Int* 1989;35:1–13.

148. Sterns RH, Spital A. Disorders of internal potassium balance. *Semin Nephrol* 1987;7:206–222.

149. Soliman AR, Akmal M, Massry SG. Parathyroid hormone interferes with extrarenal disposal of potassium in chronic renal failure. *Nephron* 1989;52:262–267.

150. Tannen LR. Disorders of potassium balance. *Kidney Update* 1989;3:33–55.

151. Weidmann P, Maxwell M, Rowe P, et al. Role of the renin-angiotensin-aldosterone system in the regulation of plasma potassium in chronic renal disease. *Nephron* 1975;15:35–49.

152. Tomita K, Pisano JJ, Knepper MA. Control of sodium and potassium transport in the cortical collection duct of the rat: effects of bradykinin, vasopressin, and deoxycorticosterone. *J Clin Invest* 1985;76:132–136.

153. Cope CL, Pearson J. Aldosterone secretion in severe renal failure. *Clin Sci* 1963;25:331–341.

154. Kleeman CR, Okun R, Heller RJ. The renal regulation of sodium and potassium in patients with chronic renal failure and the effects of diuretics in the excretion of these ions. *Ann NY Acad Sci* 1966;139:520–528.

155. Gold EM, Kleeman CR, Ling S, et al. Sustained aldosterone secretion in chronic renal failure. *Clin Res* 1966;13:135A.

156. Williams GH, Bailey GL, Hampers CL, et al. Studies on the metabolism of aldosterone in chronic renal failure and anephric man. *Kidney Int* 1973;4:280–288.

157. Weidmann P, Maxwell MH, Lupu AN. Plasma aldosterone in terminal renal failure. Ann Intern Med 1973;78: 13–18.

158. Reubi FC, Weidmann P, Gluck Z. Interrelationships between sodium clearance, plasma aldosterone, plasma renin activity, renal hemodynamics and blood pressure in renal disease. *Klin Wochenschr* 1979;57:1273–1285.

159. Saruta T, Nagahama S, Eguchi T, et al. Renin, aldosterone, and other mineralocorticoids in hyperkalemic patients with chronic renal failure showing mild azotemia. *Nephron* 1981;29:128–132.

160. Weidmann P, Maxwell MH, Rowe P, et al. Role of the renin-angiotensin-aldosterone system in the regulation of plasma potassium in chronic renal disease. *Nephron* 1975;15:35–49.

161. Schambelan M, Sebastian A, Biglieri E. Prevalence, pathogenesis, and functional significance of aldosterone deficiency in hyperkalemic patients with chronic renal insufficiency. *Kidney Int* 1980;17:89–101.

162. DeDronzo RA. Hyperkalemia and hyporeninemic hypoaldosteronism. *Kidney Int* 1980;17:118–134.

163. DeFronzo RA, Bia M, Smith D. Clinical disorders of hyperkalemia. *Annu Rev Med* 1982;33:521–524.

164. Phelps KR, Lieberman RL, Oh MS, Carroll HJ. Pathophysiology of the syndrome of hyporeninemic hypoaldosteronism. *Metabolism* 1980;29:186–199.

165. Battle DC. Hyperkalemic hyperchloremic metabolic acidosis associated with selective aldosterone deficiency and distal renal tubular acidosis. *Semin Nephrol* 1981;1:260–274.

166. Koshida H, Miyamori I, Miyazaki R, et al. Falsely elevated plasma aldosterone concentration by direct radioimmunoassay in chronic renal failure. *J Lab Clin Med* 1989;114:294–300.

167. Tuck ML, Davidson MB, Asp N, Schultze RG. Augmented aldosterone and insulin responses to potassium infusion in dogs with renal failure. *Kidney Int* 1986;30:883–890.

168. Williams HD. Hyporeninemic hypoaldosteronism. *N Engl J Med* 1986;314(16):1041–1042.

169. Schambelan M, Sebastian A, Biglieri E. Prevalence, pathogenesis, and functional significance of aldosterone deficiency in hyperkalemic patients with chronic renal insufficiency. *Kidney Int* 1980;17:89–101.

170. Hudson JB, Chobanian AV, Reiman AS. Hypoaldosteronism: a clinical study of a patient with an isolated adrenal mineralocorticoid deficiency, resulting in hyperkalemia and Stokes-Adams attacks. *N Engl J Med* 1957;256:529–536.

171. Jacobs DR, Posner JB. Isolated aldosteronism. II. The nature of the adrenal cortical enzymatic defect, and the influence of diet and various agents on electrolyte balance. *Metabolism* 1964;13:522–531.

172. Gerstein AR, Kleeman CR, Gold EM, et al. Aldosterone deficiency in chronic renal failure. *Nephron* 1968;5:90–105.

173. McGiff JC, Muzzarelli RE, Duffy PA, et al. Interrelationships of renin and aldosterone in a patient with hypoaldosteronism. *Am J Med* 1970;48:247–253.

174. Perez G, Siegel L, Schreiner GE. Selective hypoaldosteronism with hyperkalemia. *Ann Intern Med* 1972;76:757–763.

175. Weidmann P, Reinhart R, Maxwell MH, et al. Syndrome of hyporeninernic hypoaldosteronism and hyperkalemia in renal disease. *J Clin Endocrinol Metab* 1973;36:965–977.

176. Schambelan M, Sebastian A. Hyporeninemic hypoaldosteronism. *Adv Intern Med* 1979;24:385–405.

177. Schambelan M, Stockigt JR, Biglieri EG. Isolated hyperaldosteronism in adults: a renin-deficiency syndrome. *N Engl J Med* 1972;287:573–578.

178. DeLeiva A, Chridtleib AR, Melby JE, et al. Big renin and biosynthesis defect of aldosterone in diabetes mellitus. *N Engl J Med* 1976;295:639–643.

179. Sowers JR, Beck FWJ, Waters BK, Barrett JD, Welch BG. Studies of renin activation and regulation of aldosterone and 18-hydrocorticosterone biosynthesis in hyporeninemic hypoaldosteronism. *J Clin Endocrinol Metab* 1985;61:60–67.

180. Vaamonde CA, Perez GO, Oster JR. Syndromes of aldosterone deficiency. *Min Electrolyte Metab* 1981;5:121.

181. DeFronzo RA. Hyperkalemic states. In: Maxwell MH, Kleeman CR, Narins RG, eds. *Clinical Disorders of Fluid and Electrolyte Metabolism.* New York: McGraw-Hill, 1987:547.

182. Oster FR, Perez GO, Rosen MS. Hyporeninemic hypoaldosteronism after chronic sodium bicarbonate abuse. *Arch Intern Med* 1976;136:1179–1180.

183. Kalin M, Poretsky L, Seres D, Zumoff B. Hyporeninemic hypoaldosteronism associated with the acquired immune deficiency syndrome. *Am J Med* 1987;82:1035–1038.

184. Nadler JL, Lee FO, Hsueh W, Horton R. Evidence of prostacyclin deficiency in the syndrome of hyporeninemic hypoaldosteronism. *N Engl J Med* 1986;314:1015–1020.

185. Obana K, Naruse M, Naruse K, et al. Synthetic rat atrial natriuretic factor inhibits in vitro and in vivo renin secretion in rats. *Endocrinology* 1985;117:1282–1284.

186. Atarashi K, Mulrow PJ, Franco-Saenz R. Effect of atrial peptide on aldosterone production. *J Clin Invest* 1985;76:1807–1811.

187. Antonipillai I, Horton R. Paracrine regulation of the renin aldosterone system. *Biochem Mol Biol* 1993;45:27–31.

188. Corwin HL, Bonventre JB. Renal insufficiency associated with nonsteroidal anti-inflammatory agents. *Am J Kidney Dis* 1984;4:147.

189. Textor SC, Bravo EL, Fouad FM, Tarazi RC. Hyperkalemia in azotemic patients angiotensin-aldosterone system in the regulation of plasma potassium in chronic renal disease. *Nephron* 1975;15:35–49.

190. Foley RJ, Hamner RW, Weinman EJ. Serum potassium concentrations in cyclosporine-and-azathioprine-treated renal transplant patients. *Nephron* 1985;40:280–285.

191. Edes TE, Sunderrajan EV. Heparin-induced hyperkalemia. *Arch Intern Med* 1985;145:1070–1072.

192. Zanella MT, Mattei E, Draibe SA, et al. Inadequate aldosterone response to hyperkalemia during angiotensin converting enzyme inhibition in chronic renal failure. *Clin Pharmacol Ther* 1985;38:613–617.

193. Kokot F, Wiecek A, Grzeszczak W, Klin M. Influence of erythropoietin treatment on plasma renin activity, aldosterone, vasopressin and atrial natriuretic peptide in haemodialyzed patients. *Min Electrolyte Metab* 1990;16:25–29.

194. Arik N, Demirkan F, Erbas B, et al. Acute effect of erythropoietin on plasma renin activity and aldosterone levels in end-stage renal disease. *Nephron* 1992;60:111.

195. Kigoshi T, Morimoto S, Uchida K, et al. Unresponsiveness of plasma mineralocorticoids to angiotensin II in diabetic patients with asymptomatic normoreninemic hypoaldosteronism. *J Lab Clin Med* 1985;105:195–200.

196. Kahn T, Kaji D, Krakoff LR, et al. Potassium transport in chronic renal disease. *Clin Res* 1976;24:403A.

197. Bed T, Katz FH, Henrich WL, et al. Role of aldosterone in the control of sodium excretion in patients with advanced chronic renal failure. *Kidney Int* 1978;14:228–235.

198. Schrier RW, Regal EM. Influence of aldosterone on sodium, water, and potassium metabolism in chronic renal disease. *Kidney Int* 1975;1:156–168.

199. Weidmann P, Maxwell MH, deLima J, et al. Control of aldosterone responsiveness in terminal renal failure. *Kidney Int* 1975;7:351–359.

200. Hene RJ, Boer P, Koomans HA, Mees EJD. Plasma aldosterone concentrations in chronic renal disease. *Kidney Int* 1982;21:98–101.

201. Koshida H, Miyamori I, Miyazaki R, et al. Falsely elevated plasma aldosterone concentration by direct radioimmunoassay in chronic renal failure. *Lab Clin Med* 1989;114:294–300.

202. Sugahara S, Koyama I, Yoshikawa Y, et al. Plasma atrial natriuretic peptide, renin activity, and aldosterone in changes of body fluid volume after renal transplantation. *Transplant Proc* 1992;24(4):1576–1577.

203. Deray G, Maistre G, Cacoub P, et al. Renal and hemodialysis clearance of endogenous natriuretic peptide. A clinical and experimental study. *Nephron* 1990;54:148–153.

204. Tsubakihara Y, Nakanishi I, Yamato E, et al. Remarked hyperaldosteronemia in long-term hemodialysis patients who were recipients of renal transplantation. *J Jpn Soc Dial Ther* 1988;21(2):173–177.

205. Henrich WL, Katz FH, Molinoff PB, Schrier RW. Competitive effects of hypokalemia and volume depletion on plasma renin activity, aldosterone and catecholamine concentrations in hemodialysis patients. *Kidney Int* 1977;12:279–284.

206. Farinelli A, Squerzanti R, Vitali E, et al. Response of plasma aldosterone to sequential ultrafiltration, dialysis, and conventional hemodialysis. *Nephron* 1980;26:274–279.

207. Olgaard K, Madsen S. Regulation of plasma aldosterone in anephric and non-nephrectomized patients during hemodialysis treatment. *Acta Med Scand* 1977;201:457–462.

208. Zager PG, Frey HJ, Gerdes GG, Gaeme PA. Increase plasma levels of 18-hydroxycorticosterone and 18-hydroxy, II-deoxycorticosterone during continuous ambulatory peritoneal dialysis. *Kidney Int* 1982;21:121–128.

209. Mann H, Konigs F, Heintz B, et al. Vasoactive hormones during hemodialysis with intermittent ultrafiltration. *ASAIO Trans* 1990;30:M367–M369.

210. Sasamura H, Suzuki H, Takita T, et al. Response of plasma immunoreactive active renin, inactive renin, plasma renin activity, and aldosterone to hemodialysis in patients with diabetic nephropathy. *Clin Nephrol* 1990;33:288–292.

211. Weidmann P, Horton R, Maxwell MH, et al. Dynamic studies of aldosterone in anephric man. *Kidney Int* 1973;4: 289–298.

212. Boyd GW, Adamson AR, James VHT, Peart WS. The role of the renin-angiotensin system in the control of aldosterone in man. *Proc R Soc Med* 1969;62:1253–1254.

213. Pearl WS. Renin and angiotensin in relation to aldosterone. *Am J Clin Pathol* 1970;54:324–330.

214. Mitra S, Genuth SM, Berman LB, Vertes V. Aldosterone secretion in anephric patients. *N Engl J Med* 1972;286:61–64.

215. Bayard F, Cooke CR, Tiller DJ, et al. The regulation of aldosterone secretion in anephric man. *Clin Invest* 1971;50: 1585–1595.

216. Balikian HM, Brodie AH, Dale SL, et al. Effect of posture on metabolic clearance rate, plasma concentration and blood production rate of aldosterone. *J Clin Endocrinol Metab* 1968;28(11):1630–1640.

217. Cooke CR, Horvath JS, Moore MA, et al. Modulation of plasma aldosterone concentration by plasma potassium in anephric man in the absence of a change in potassium balance. *J Clint Invest* 1973;52:3028–3032.

218. Horl HW, Riegel W, Wanner C, et al. Endocrine and metabolic abnormalities following kidney transplantation. *Klin Wochenschr* 1989;67:907–918.

219. Siegl H, Ryffel B. Effect of cyclosporin on renin–angiotensin-aldosterone system (letter). *Lancet* 1982;2(8310):1274.

220. Gerkewns JF, Bhagwandeen SB, et al. The effect of salt intake on cyclosporine-induced impairment of renal function in rats. *Transplantation* 1984;38:412–417.

221. Massry SG, Preuss HG, Maher JF, Schreiner GE. Renal tubular acidosis after cadaver kidney homotransplantation. *Am J Med* 1967;42:284–296.

222. Battle DC, Mozes MP, Manaligod J, et al. The pathogenesis of hyperchloremic metabolic acidosis associated with kidney transplantation. *Am J Med* 1981;70:786–796.

223. Belchetz PE. Endocrine factors in male gonadal dysfunction. In: Hendry WI, ed. *Recent Advances in Urology/Andrology*. Edinburgh: Churchill Livingstone, 1981:291–323.

224. Santen RJ. Independent effects of testosterone and estradiol on the secretion of gonadotropins in man. In: Troen P, Nankin HR, eds. *The Testis in Normal and Infertile Men*. New York: Raven Press, 1977:197–211.

225. Carter NI, Tyson IE, Tolis G. Prolactin secreting tumors and hypogonadism in 22 men. *N Engl J Med* 1978;299:847–852.

226. Holdsworth S, Atkins RC, de Krester DM. The pituitary-testicular axis in men with chronic renal failure. *N Engl J Med* 1977;296:1245–1249.

227. Gomez F, de la Cuerva R, Wauters IP. Endocrine abnormalities in patients undergoing long-term hemodialysis. The role of prolactin. *Am J Med* 1980;68:522–530.

228. Ferraris I, Saenger P, Levine L, et al. Delayed puberty in males with chronic renal failure. *Kidney Int* 1980;18: 344–350.

229. Sharer K, Chanter C, Brunner FB, et al. Combined report on regular dialysis and transplantation of children in Europe. *Proc Eur Dial Transplant Assoc* 1976;13:59–103.

230. Perfumo F, Giusta M, Gusmaro R, Giordano G. Study of pituitary secretion using the thyrotropic releasing hormone test in uremic prepubertal children. In: Bulls M, ed. *Renal Insufficiency in Children*. New York: Springer-Verlag, 1982: 121.

231. Marder HK, Srivastava L, Burstein S. Hypergonadism in peripubertal boys with chronic renal failure. *Pediatrics* 1983;72:384–389.

232. Roger M, Broyer M, Sharer K, et al. Gonadotropines et androgenes plasmatiques chez les garcans traits pour insufficance renale chronique. *Pathol Biol* 1981;29: 378–379.

233. Castellanos M, Turconi A, Chaler E, et al. Hypothalamic-pituitary-gonadal function in prepubertal boys and girls with chronic renal failure. *J Pediatr* 1993;122:46–51.

234. Palmer BF. Sexual dysfunction in men and women with chronic kidney disease. *Adv Renal Replace Ther* 2003;10(1): 48–60.

235. Diemont WL, Vruggink PA, Meuleman EJ, et al. Sexual dysfunction after renal replacement therapy. *Am J Kidney Dis* 2000;35:845–851.

236. Holdsworth SR, de Krester DM, Atkins RC. A comparison of hemodialysis and transplantation in reversing the uremic disturbances of male reproductive function. *Clin Nephrol* 1978;10:146–150.

237. Charney D, Walton D, Cheung A. Impotence: II. *Semin Dial* 1994;7:22.

238. Steele TE, Wuerth D, Finlelstein S, et al. Sexual disturbance of the peritoneal dialysis patient. *J Am Soc Nephrol* 1996;7: 1165–1168.

239. Toorians Aw, Janssen E, Laan E, et al. Chronic renal failure and sexual functioning: clinical status versus objectively assessed sexual response. *Nephrol Dial Transplant* 1997;12: 2654–2663.

240. Feldman HA, Singer I. Endocrinology and metabolism in uremia and dialysis: a clinical review. *Medicine* 1975;55: 345–376.

240a. Rosas SE, Jaffe M, Franklin E, et al. Association of decreased quality of life and erectile dysfunction in hemodialysis patients. *Kidney Int* 2003;64:232.

241. Lim VS, Kathopalia SC, Herniquez C. Endocrine abnormalities associated with chronic renal failure. *Med Clin North Am* 1978;62:1341–1361.

242. Lim VS, Fang VS. Gonadal dysfunction in uremic men. A study of hypothalamic-pituitary-testicular axis before and after renal transplantation. Am J Med 1975;58:655–662.

243. de Krester DM, Atkins RC, Hudson B, Scott OF. Disordered spermatogenesis in patients with chronic renal failure under-

going maintenance hemodialysis. *Aust NZ J Med* 1974;4:178–181.

244. Stewart-Bentley M, Gans D, Horton R. Regulation of gonadal function in uremia. *Metabolism* 1974;23:1065–1072.

245. Hagen C, OIgaard K, McNeilly AS, Fisher R. Prolactin and pituitary-gonadal axis in male uremic patients on regular dialysis. *Acta Endocrinol* 1976;82:29–38.

245a. Lim VS, Fang VS. Restoration of plasma testosterone levels in uremic men with clomiphene citrate. *J Clin Endocrinol Metab* 1976;43:1370–1377.

246. Cowden EA, Ratcliffe W A, Watcliffe IG, Kennedy AC. Hypothalamic-pituitary function in uremia. *Acta Endocrinol* 1981;98:488–495.

247. Semple CG, Beastall GH, Henderson IS, et al. The pituitary-testicular axis of uraemic subjects on hemodialysis and continuous ambulatory peritoneal dialysis. *Acta Endocrinol* 1981;101:464–467.

248. Lim VS, Auletta F, Kathpalia SC. Gonadal dysfunction in chronic renal failure. An endocrinologic review. *Nephrol Dial Transplant* 1978;7:896.

249. Nishula BC, Dunn IF. Measurement of the testosterone binding parameters for both testosterone-estradiol binding globulin and albumin in individual serum samples. *Steroids* 1979;34:771–791.

250. Kalk WI, Morley IE, Gold CH, Meyers A. Thyroid function tests in patients on regular hemodialysis. *Nephron* 1980;25:173–178.

251. Donaldson P, Newton D, Platt M. Long-term hemodialysis and thyroid. *Br Med J* 1977;1:134–136.

252. Neuhaus K, Baumann G, Walser A, Thalen H. Severe thyroxine and thyroxine-binding proteins in chronic renal failure without nephrosis. *J Clin Endocrinol Metab* 1975;41:395–398.

253. Tourkantonis A, Spiliopolous A, Pharmakiolis A, Settas L. Hemodialysis and hypothalamic-pituitary-testicular axis. *Nephron* 1981;27:271–272.

254. Chen IC, Vidt DG, Zorn EM, et al. Pituitary-Leydig cell function in uremic males. *J Clin Endocrinol Metab* 1970;31:14–17.

255. Saez 1M, Haour F, Cathiard AM. Early hCG-induced desensitization in Leydig cells. *Biochem Biophys Res Commun* 1978;81:552–558.

256. Kirschner MA, Wilder 1A, Ross AT. Leydig cell function in man with gondotropin-producing testicular tumors. *J Clin Endocrinol Metab* 1970;30:504–511.

257. Lipsett ME. Physiology and pathology of the Leydig cells. *N Engl J Med* 1980;303:682–688.

258. Sawin CT, Longcope C, Schmitt GW, Ryan RI. Blood levels of gonadotropins and gonadal hormones in gynecomastia associated with chronic hemodialysis. *J Clin Endocrinol Metab* 1973;36:988–990.

259. Blumberg A, Wildbolz A, Descoeudres C, et al. Influence of 1,25-dihydroxycholecalciferol on sexual dysfunction and related endocrine parameters in patients on maintenance hemodialysis. *Clin Nephrol* 1980;13:208–214.

260. Kawamura J, Daijyo K, Hosokawa S, et al. Hypothalamo-pituitary-testicular axes in men undergoing intermittent hemodialysis. *Int J Artif Organs* 1978;1:224–230.

261. Cowden EA, Ratcliffe W A, Ratcliffe JG, et al. Hyperprolactinemia in renal disease. *Clin Endocrinol* 1978;9:241–248.

262. Sieversten GD, Lim VS, Nakawatase C, Fro LA. Metabolic clearance and secretion rates of human prolactin in normal subjects and in patients with chronic renal failure. *J Clin Endocrinol Metab* 1980;50:845–852.

263. Mollinger RS, Gutkin M. Plasma prolactin in essential and renovascular hypertension. *J Lab Clin Med* 1978;91:693–699.

264. Foulks CJ, Cushner HM. Sexual dysfunction in male dialysis patients. Pathogenesis, evaluation and therapy. *Am J Kidney Dis* 1986;8(4)211–222. (Review)

264a. Lim VS, Auletta F, Kathpalia SC, Frohman LA. Hyperprolactinemia and impaired pituitary response to suppression and stimulation in chronic renal failure: reversal after renal transplantation. *J Clin Endocrinol Metab* 1979;48:101–107.

265. Ramirez G, O'Neil, WM, Bloomer HA, Iubiz W. Abnormalities in the regulation of prolactin in patients with chronic renal failure. *J Clin Endocrinol Metab* 1977;45:658–661.

266. Peces R, Horcajada C, Lopez Novoa JM, et al. Hyperprolactinemia in chronic renal failure: impaired responsiveness to stimulation and suppression. Normalization after transplantation. *Nephron* 1981;28:11–16.

267. Peces R, Casado S, Frutos M, et al. prolactin in chronic renal failure, hemodialysis, and transplant patients. *Proc Eur Dial Transplant Assoc* 1979;16:700–702.

268. Gura V, Weizman A, Maoz B, et al. Hyperprolactinemia: a possible cause of sexual dysfunction in male patients undergoing chronic hemodialysis. *Nephron* 1980;26:53–54.

269. Bommer J, del Pozo, Ritz E, Mommer G. Improved sexual function in male hemodialysis patients on bromcriptine. *Lancet* 1979;2:49–97.

270. Tharandt L, Gruben N, Schafer R, et al. Effects of prolactin suppression on hypogonadism in patients on maintenance hemodialysis. *Proc Eur Dial Transplant Assoc* 1980;17:323–327.

271. Massry SG, Goldstein DA, Procci WR, Kletzky OA. Impotence in patients with uremia. A possible role for parathyroid hormone. *Nephron* 1977;19:305–310.

272. Lowe H, Schultz H, Busch G. Klinische aspekte der Impotenz mannlicher dauerdialyse Patienten. *Med Welt (Stuttg)* 1975;26:1651–1652.

273. Wilson JD, Aiman J, MacDonald PC. The pathogenesis of gynecomastia. *Adv Intern Med* 1980;25:1–32.

274. Nagel TC, Frienkel N, Bell RH, et al. Gynecomastia prolactin, and other peptide hormones in patients undergoing chronic hemodialysis. *J Clin Endocrinol Metab* 1973;36:428–432.

275. Ross SE, Joffe M, Franklin E, et al. Prevalence and determinants of erectile dysfunction in hemodialysis patients. *Kidney Int* 2001;59:2259–2266.

276. Lim VS, Henriquez C, Sievertsen G, Frohman LA. Ovarian function in chronic renal failure. Evidence suggesting hypothalamic anovulation. *Ann Intern Med* 1980;93:21–27.

277. Goodwin NJ, Valenti C, Hall JE, Friedman EA. Effects of uremia and chroni hemodialysis on the reproductive cycle. *Am J Obstet Gynecol* 1968;100:528–535.

278. Rice CG. Hypermenorrhea in the young hemodialysis patient. *Am J Obstet Gynecol* 1973;116:539–543.

279. Zingraff J, Jungers P, Pellisier C, et al. Pituitary and ovarian dysfunction in women on hemodialysis. *Nephron* 1982;30:149–153.

280. Rudolph K, Kunkles RH, et al. Basale an gonadotropin-releasing hormone stimlulierte gonadotropin Sekretion. Sekretin bee patieninna it chronischer Uremie. *Zentralbl Gynacol* 1988;110:683–688.

281. Morley JE, Distiller LA, Pokroy M, et al. Hormonal profiles in renal failure (abstr). *S Afr Med J* 1975;49:474–475.

282. Swamy AP, Woolf PD, Castero RVM. Hypothalamic-pituitary-ovarian axis in uremic women. *J Lab Clin Med* 1979;93:1066–1072.

283. Olgaard K, Hagen C, McNeilly AS. Pituitary hormones in women with chronic renal failure: the effect of chronic intermittent haemo-peritoneal dialysis. *Acta Endocrinol* 1975;80:237–246.

284. Levy NB. Sexual adjustment to maintenance hemodialysis and renal transplantation. National survey by questionnaire: preliminary report. *ASAIO Trans* 1973;29:138–143.

285. Antoniou LD, Shahloub RJ, Sudhakar T, Smith JC. Reversible of uremic impotence by zinc. *Lancet* 1977;11:895–898.

286. Kawashima R, Douchi T, Oki T, et al. Menstrual disturbances in patients undergoing chronic hemodialysis. *J Obstet Gynaecol Res* 1998;24(5):367–373.

287. Soffer O. Sexual dysfunction in chronic renal failure. *South Med J* 1980;73:1599–1600.

288. Newton J, Snowden SA, Parsons V. Control of menstrual bleeding during hemodialysis. *Br Med J* 1976;1:1016–1017.

289. Rice GG. Hypermenorrhea in the young hemodialysis patient. *Am J Obstet Gynecol* 1973;116(4):539–543.

290. Stricker RC, Woolever CA, Goldstein JM, DeVeber G. Serum gonadotropins in patients with chronic renal failure on hemodialysis. *Nephron* 1982;30:149–153.

291. Hou S. Pregnancy and birth control in dialysis patients. *Nephrol Dial Transplant* 1994;23:22–26.

292. Ramirez G, Bittle PA, Sanders H, Bercuu BB. Hypothalamo-hypophyseal thyroid and gonadal function before and after erythropoietin therapy in dialysis patients. *J Clin Endocrinol Metab* 1992;74:517–524.

293. Evans RW, Rader B, Manninen DL, et al. Cooperative multicenter EPO clinical trial group. The quality of life of hemodialysis patients treated with rHuEPO. *JAMA* 1990;263:825–830.

294. Kokot F, Wiecek A, Grzeszczak W, et al. Influence of erythropoietin on foollitropin and lutropin response to luliberin and plasma testosterone levels in hemodialysis patients. *Nephron* 1990;56:126–129.

295. Schaefer RM, Kokot F, Wernze H, et al. Improved sexual function in hemodialysis patients on recombinant erythropoietin: a possible role for prolactin. *Clin Nephrol* 1989;31:1(1):1–50.

296. Delano BG. Improvement in quality of life following treatment with rHuEPO in anemic hemodialysis patients. *Am J Kidney Dis* 1989;14(2 Suppl 1):14–18.

297. Palmer BF. Sexual dysfunction in uremia. *J Am Soc Nephrol* 1999;10:1381–1388.

298. Seibel I, Poli DE, Figueiredo CE, et al. Efficacy of oral sildenafil in hemodialysis patients with erectile dysfunction. *J Am Soc Nephrol* 2002:13;2770–2775.

299. Ifudu O. Care of patients undergoing hemodialysis. *N Engl J Med* 1998;339:1054–1062.

300. Rosas E, Wasserstein S, Kobrin S, Feldman HI. Preliminary observations of sildenafil treatment for erectile dysfunction in dialysis patients. *Am J Kidney Dis* 2001;37:134–137.

301. Turk S, Karalezi G, Tonbul HZ, et al. Erectile dysfunction and the effects of sildenafil treatment in patients on hemodialysis and continuous ambulatory peritoneal dialysis dialysis. *Nephrol Dial Transplant* 2001;16:1818–1822.

302. Mohamed EA, MacDowall P, Coward RA. Timing of sildenafil therapy in dialysis patients—lessons following an episode of hypotension (letter). *Nephrol Dial Transplant* 2000;15:926–927.

303. Samojik E, Kirschner A, Ribot S, Szmel E. Changes in the hypothalamic-pituitary-gonadal axis in men after cadaveric kidney transplantation and cyclosporin therapy. *J Androl* 1992;13:332–336.

304. Phadke AG, Mackinnon KJ, Dosetor JB. Male fertility in uremia. Restoration by renal allograft to recipients. *Can Med Assoc*[AU33] 1970;102:607–608.

305. Handelsman DI, McDowell IF, Caterson ID, et al. Testicular function after renal transplantation: a comparison of cyclosporin A with azathioprine and prednisone combination regimens. *Clin Neurol* 1984;22(3): 144–148.

306. Fine RN. Pregnancy in renal allograft recipients. *Am J Nephrol* 1982;2:117–122.

307. Koutsikos D, Sarandakou A, Agroyannis A, et al. The effects of successful renal transplantation of hormonal studies of female recipients. *Renal Failure* 1990;12:125–132.

Parathyroid Hormone, Vitamin D, and Metabolic Bone Disease in Dialysis Patients

Ziyad Al Aly
Esther A. González
Kevin J. Martin

The kidney is essential for maintaining the homeostasis of divalent ions and the metabolism of vitamin D. Chronic kidney disease leads to disturbances in this homeostatic balance, creating abnormalities in the parathyroid hormone (PTH) and vitamin D systems; it results in a spectrum of bone disorders termed renal osteodystrophy. Over the past decade there have been important advances in the understanding of PTH, divalent ion, and vitamin D metabolism in chronic kidney disease. These advances have led to changes in clinical practice guidelines for the prevention and treatment of renal osteodystrophy.

Renal osteodystrophy comprises a number of skeletal abnormalities. A high state of bone turnover, a manifestation of hyperparathyroidism, leads to osteitis fibrosa, usually characterized by increased osteoclast and osteoblast activity and peritrabecular fibrosis. A low state of bone turnover, associated with relatively low levels of PTH, leads to adynamic bone disease. Another state of low bone turnover, resulting from aluminum accumulation, is termed *osteomalacia* and is characterized by defective mineralization of newly formed osteoid. These disorders may coexist to varying degrees in any given patient, giving rise to *mixed* renal osteodystrophy. In chronic dialysis patients, dialysis-related amyloidosis (DRA), where beta$_2$ microglobulin is a major constituent of amyloid fibrils, has also been implicated in skeletal abnormalities. Chronic metabolic acidosis also influences bone metabolism in patients with chronic kidney disease. The pattern of renal bone disease in any particular patient may also be influenced by factors such as the chronicity and type of kidney disease and its treatment—e.g., corticosteroids.

EPIDEMIOLOGY OF RENAL OSTEODYSTROPHY

Renal osteodystrophy appears to parallel the decline in GFR and is almost a universal phenomenon in patients with stage 5 chronic kidney disease (CKD) who are undergoing any form of renal replacement therapy. The prevalence of different forms of renal osteodystrophy varies among different countries and different time periods mainly due to variable bone aluminum burden and the shift in strategies of therapeutic management of this disease entity.[1-3] Osteitis fibrosa and adynamic bone disease now have approximately an equal prevalence in hemodialysis patients. In contrast, adynamic bone disease appears to be the most prevalent bone lesion in peritoneal dialysis patients.[4] Mixed osteodystrophy is much less frequently observed but is slightly more predominant in the hemodialysis population. Osteomalacia represents only a small fraction of either group but is more common in certain countries such as Brazil, Uruguay, and Argentina, especially before 1990,[5-7] and in certain ethnic groups, particularly Indo-Asians.

PATHOGENESIS OF RENAL OSTEODYSTROPHY

Secondary Hyperparathyroidism (High-Bone-Turnover Renal Osteodystrophy)

Hyperparathyroidism manifest by elevations in the levels of PTH and hyperplasia of the parathyroid glands occurs early in the course of chronic kidney disease.[8,9] In normal individuals, PTH secretion is determined mainly by the concentrations of ionized calcium in serum; however, in the presence of kidney disease, there are a number of abnormalities that contribute to alterations in parathyroid physiology. This is illustrated in Fig. 30–1. Thus there are abnormalities in phosphorus and vitamin D metabolism, intrinsic abnormalities in parathyroid gland function, abnormalities in serum calcium, and an abnormal skeletal response to PTH. All of these factors play important roles in the regulation of calcium homeostasis and mineral metabolism, and although they are considered separately, they are clearly closely interrelated. Different factors may play more important roles at different times in the course of chronic kidney disease, or

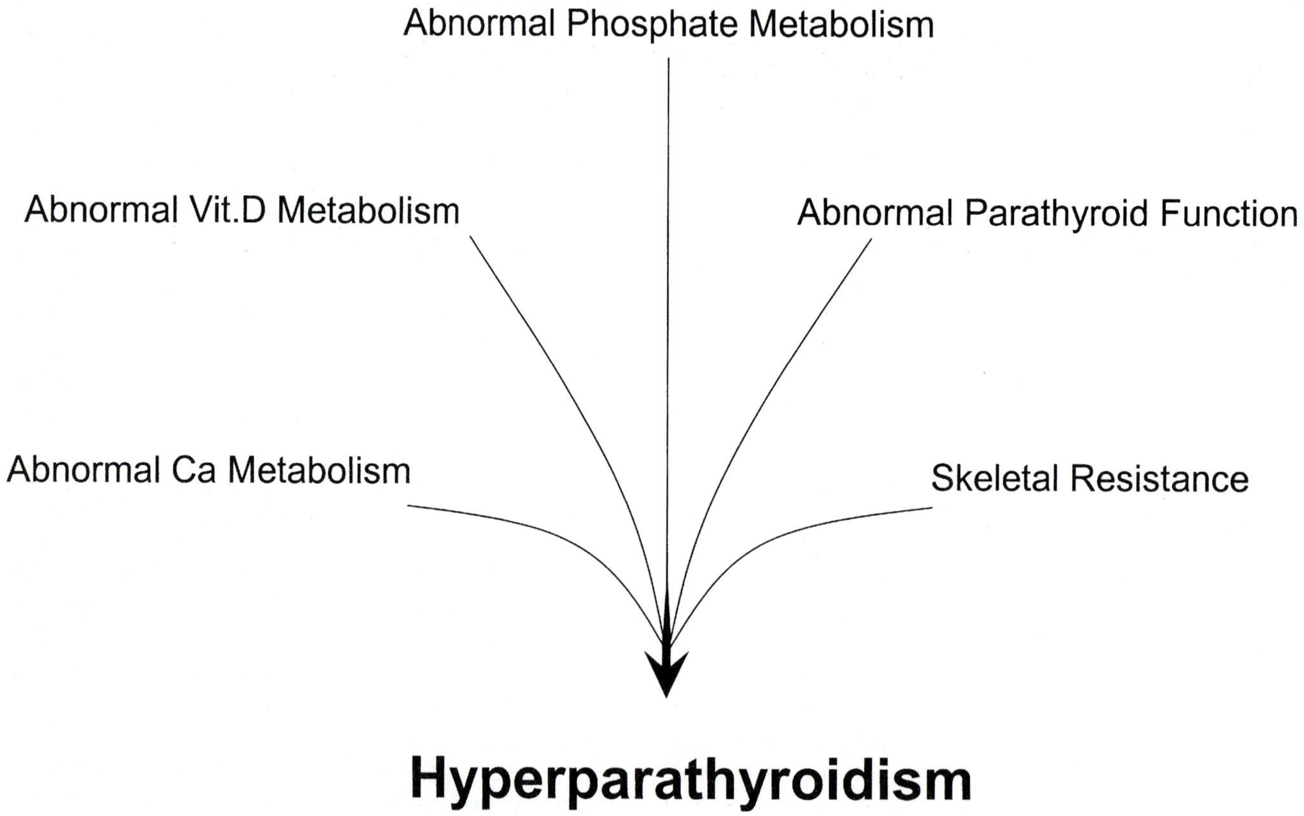

Figure 30–1. The principal factors involved in the pathogenesis of secondary hyperparathyroidism in CKD. All of these factors are closely interrelated and different pathways may dominate according to the type and severity of kidney disease.

they may vary according to the particular nature of kidney disease.

Abnormalities of Phosphorus Metabolism. Many investigators have demonstrated that phosphorus retention in the course of CKD plays an important role in the pathogenesis of secondary hyperparathyroidism.[10–12] While it was initially proposed that phosphate retention would give rise to a decrease in the levels of ionized calcium that would stimulate PTH secretion,[13] additional observations have indicated that hypocalcemia is not necessary for hyperparathyroidism to develop and therefore point to the fact that other consequences of phosphate retention are likely to be important.[14] Nonetheless, it has been clearly demonstrated that if phosphate in the diet is restricted in proportion to the decrease in kidney function, hyperparathyroidism is almost totally prevented.[11] While the observations are clear, the mechanisms involved are not entirely so. It is possible that phosphate retention could serve to decrease the production of calcitriol from the kidney, and the consequences of reduced calcitriol production could certainly contribute to hyperparathyroidism. Recent observations have indicated that this may not be the only mechanism involved, as increased parathyroid growth has been demonstrated to occur within a few days of renal insufficiency, and this process is influenced to an important degree by dietary phosphate content.[15] Studies in vitro have shown that elevations in phosphate concentration stimulate the secretion of PTH independent of changes in the levels of ionized calcium.[16–18] This effect of phosphorus appears to be posttranscriptional and to be mediated by alterations within the parathyroid cell that affect the stability of PTH messenger RNA.[19–21] Additional studies have begun to define the proteins involved in the regulation of PTH mRNA stability. These appear to bind to the 3' untranslated region of PTH messenger RNA and regulate its degradation. Other investigators have demonstrated that alterations in dietary phosphate intake are associated with changes in the sodium-phosphate transporter Pit-1 in the parathyroid gland, but it remains unknown whether such alterations play a part in the regulation of parathyroid function by dietary phosphate.[22] Alterations in dietary phosphate intake have also been shown to regulate the expression of the calcium-sensing receptor in the parathyroid gland and thereby influence the response of the parathyroid to changes in serum calcium.[23] This factor may also contribute to the regulation of parathyroid function by alterations in dietary phosphate intake.

There has been some controversy regarding the role of phosphate retention in the pathogenesis of hyperparathyroidism, since hyperphosphatemia is not present in the course of CKD until GFR reaches very low levels. This absence of hyperphosphatemia has been interpreted to indicate that phosphate retention could not play a significant role. This interpretation is problematic, however, because it is likely that normal levels of serum phosphate are maintained as a result of the increases in serum PTH levels; thus the maintenance of normal phosphatemia is a consequence of the elevated levels of PTH. Therefore the absence of elevations in serum phosphate does not provide any assurance that there is not a disturbance in PTH in CKD and points to the importance of obtaining accurate measurements of PTH to assess disturbances of parathyroid function. Phosphorus also affects parathyroid cell growth. A high-phosphorus diet increases parathyroid cell proliferation, whereas a low-phosphorus diet prevents parathyroid hyperplasia.[24,25] The effect of a low-phosphorus diet to prevent parathyroid hyperplasia has been shown to be associated with increases in the cyclin-dependent kinase inhibitor p21.[24] The stimulation of parathyroid growth by a high-phosphorus diet appears to be associated with increased expression of transforming growth factor alpha (TGF-α), which acts on the epidermal growth factor (EGF) receptor to activate mitogen-activated protein (MAP) kinase and stimulate cell proliferation.[24]

Abnormalities of Vitamin D Metabolism. The kidney is the principal site for the conversion of 25-hydroxyvitamin D to the active metabolite 1,25-dihydroxyvitamin D (calcitriol). Accordingly, in the course of CKD, as renal mass decreases, the ability of the kidney to produce calcitriol becomes limited. Recent studies have shown that the rate-limiting step for the production of calcitriol appears to be due to a megalin-dependent mechanism in the proximal tubule.[26] Thus the precursor, 25-hydroxyvitamin D, which is bound to vitamin D–binding protein, is filtered at the glomerulus. Vitamin D–binding protein then binds to megalin in the brush border of the proximal tubule cell and undergoes endocytosis, which results in the movement of vitamin D–binding protein and its ligand, 25-hydroxyvitamin D, into the cell. Thus, when the associated protein is degraded, 25-hydroxyvitamin D can be delivered to the site of the 1-α-hydroxylase enzyme in the mitochondria, where calcitriol can be produced and returned to the circulation. Accordingly, as GFR falls, the delivery of 25-hydroxyvitamin D to the 1-hydroxylase enzyme progressively decreases and therefore limits the ability of the kidney to produce calcitriol. In clinical kidney disease, levels of calcitriol often remain within the normal range until the GFR falls below 50 percent of normal.[27–30] As in the case of the maintenance of normal phosphatemia, the maintenance of plasma calcitriol in the normal range is facilitated by the development of hyperparathyroidism, which increases the activity of the 1-α-hydroxylase. Thus, even normal levels of calcitriol could be considered inappropriately low for the ambient PTH levels. Low levels of calcitriol can contribute to the development of hyperparathyroidism, since a major action of calcitriol is to decrease transcription of the PTH gene[31,32]; therefore, as calcitriol levels fall, transcription of the PTH gene is increased, contributing to hyperparathyroidism. Calcitriol has also been shown to prevent parathyroid growth in vitro,[33] and findings consistent with this have been demonstrated with calcitriol in experimental models in vivo.[34,35]

In addition to alterations in calcitriol production in the course of CKD, studies have also demonstrated that there may be resistance to the actions of calcitriol in target tissues in uremia. Thus, it has been shown that ultrafiltrates of uremic serum appear to contain substances that result in decreased binding of the vitamin D receptor to the vitamin D response element in DNA.[36] These uremic toxins, then, could be responsible for peripheral resistance to calcitriol by interfering with the normal actions of the vitamin D receptor. The nature of these substances has not been identified, but additional studies have suggested that this effect may be a consequence of reductions in the retinoid X receptor, which is an essential cofactor for vitamin D interaction with DNA.[37]

Abnormalities of Parathyroid Gland Function. In the presence of kidney disease, there appear to be other alterations in the parathyroid gland that do not appear to be explained by the principal regulators of parathyroid function in normal animals or humans, such as the levels of serum calcium, phosphorus, and calcitriol. If hypocalcemia occurs in the course of CKD, it is a powerful stimulus to PTH secretion and parathyroid gland growth. However, hypocalcemia is relatively uncommon in patients with CKD.[38] Again, as in the case of serum phosphorus levels and the levels of calcitriol, it is possible that normal levels of serum calcium are maintained as a consequence of the development of hyperparathyroidism; thus a normal level of serum calcium does not exclude the presence of a disturbance in parathyroid gland function. The parathyroid gland may be less responsive to calcium in the setting of CKD. Studies have shown decreased sensitivity of the enzyme adenylate cyclase to calcium in parathyroid glands from uremic patients.[39] These findings are consistent with studies of PTH secretion showing that the set point for calcium—that is, the calcium concentration at which PTH secretion is decreased by 50 percent—appears to be increased in some cases of advanced hyperparathyroidism in CKD.[40–45] The abnormal set point is not a universal finding, however, and may be influenced by many other factors, including baseline serum calcium, the chronicity of the hyperparathyroidism, the degree of parathyroid hyperplasia, and possibly polymorphisms of the calcium receptor gene.[46–50]

It has been shown that the expression of vitamin D receptors in the parathyroid gland appears to be decreased in the hyperplastic glands from patients and animals with CKD.[51] This decrease in vitamin D receptors may contribute to hyperparathyroidism, since it may limit the ability of circulating calcitriol to decrease PTH gene transcription. A decreased action of calcitriol may also facilitate parathy-

roid growth, since calcitriol negatively regulates parathyroid growth in vivo and in vitro.

Additional studies have also demonstrated that hyperplastic parathyroid glands have decreased expression of the calcium-sensing receptor.[52,53] These observations could indicate a reduced ability to respond to alterations in serum calcium and facilitate hyperparathyroidism. The decreases in calcium-sensing receptor, similar to the decreases in vitamin D receptor described above, appear to be most prominent in nodular areas within the enlarged parathyroid glands. These nodular areas of the parathyroid gland appear to be regions undergoing active proliferation and represent, in some cases, a monoclonal expansion of parathyroid cells.[54] It is likely that the decreased expression of the calcium receptor and vitamin D receptor may be the result rather than the cause of parathyroid hyperplasia, since studies have shown a dissociation in the time course of parathyroid cell growth and the expression of the calcium receptor or vitamin D receptor.[55,56] It should be pointed out, however, that activation of the calcium receptor with a calcimimetic agent has been shown, in experimental animals with CKD, to be effective in the prevention of parathyroid hyperplasia.[57]

Abnormal Skeletal Response to Parathyroid Hormone. An impaired calcemic response to PTH has been known for many years to occur in patients with CKD.[58] This impaired calcemic response to PTH has been termed *skeletal resistance* to the actions of PTH.[59] The pathogenesis appears to be multifactorial, and phosphorus retention, decreased levels of calcitriol, downregulation of the PTH receptor, and N-terminally truncated PTH fragments all appear to play a role. Thus it has been shown that in acute renal failure, prevention of hyperphosphatemia improves the calcemic response to PTH.[60] Decreased levels of calcitriol have also been implicated, although this is somewhat controversial.[61–63] While some investigators have demonstrated that calcitriol can improve the calcemic response to PTH, others have shown no effect of calcitriol. In this regard, studies with calcitriol may be difficult to interpret, since calcitriol may alter the levels of PTH, and parathyroidectomy has been associated with improvement in skeletal resistance to PTH. This latter observation suggests the possibility that PTH-induced downregulation of the PTH receptor might contribute to skeletal resistance to PTH in uremia. Studies have demonstrated that PTH receptor mRNA is decreased in bone from patients with CKD.[64] Studies in animals, however, which confirm that observation, could not demonstrate a restoration of PTH mRNA levels to normal by parathyroidectomy, raising the possibility that other factors may be involved in the regulation of PTH receptor messenger RNA in uremia.[65–67]

More recently, it has been discovered that PTH fragments with a truncated N-terminus, previously considered to have no biological action, may actually be involved in the regulation of skeletal metabolism.[68,69] The actions of such N-terminally truncated PTH fragments appear to oppose the calcemic effects of PTH; their accumulation in the serum in CKD could therefore contribute to skeletal resistance to PTH. Indeed, one such PTH fragment, PTH 7–84, has been shown in vitro to be a potent inhibitor of stimulated bone resorption due to PTH, calcitriol, interleukin-11 (IL-11), or prostaglandin E_2.[70–72] Active studies are in progress to try to elucidate the biological importance of these PTH fragments in vivo.

Adynamic Bone Disease and Osteomalacia (Low-Bone-Turnover Renal Osteodystrophy)

Low-bone-turnover renal osteodystrophy comprises two entities, adynamic bone and osteomalacia.

Adynamic Bone. Adynamic bone is characterized by an extremely slow rate of bone formation in the absence of aluminum. It has been found in increasing frequency in the past decade. Even though it has been reported in patients with CKD prior to starting dialysis therapy,[73,74] it is most prevalent in patients on dialysis therapy and more so in patient on peritoneal dialysis.[4,73–76] Risk factors associated with adynamic bone include advanced age, continuous ambulatory peritoneal dialysis (CAPD), diabetes mellitus, calcitriol therapy, parathyroidectomy, and fluoride and iron intoxication. Patients with adynamic bone commonly have PTH levels lower than those of patients with other forms of renal osteodystrophy.[4,73–78] It is currently believed that this degree of relative hypoparathyroidism plays a role in the pathogenesis of this disease entity. Other factors could also contribute to relative hypoparathyroidism, including the use of calcium-containing phosphate binders, the use of calcitriol, advanced age, and the presence of diabetes. This last has been shown to be associated with low bone turnover even in the absence of renal disease,[79] possibly due to the presence of advanced glycation end products, which may inhibit osteoblastic activity and inhibit PTH secretion in response to hypocalcemia.[80] The pathogenesis of adynamic bone is still unclear. It is possible, however, that many factors in the uremic milieu could affect both osteoblast and osteoclast function.

Osteomalacia. Low-bone-turnover osteomalacia, characterized by an increase in osteoid seams and a slow rate of bone formation with a marked defect in bone mineralization, has been recognized for many years. A wealth of epidemiologic and experimental evidence has linked it to aluminum exposure, either through the use of aluminum-containing phosphate binders or due to the presence of aluminum in dialysate. The decreasing use of aluminum-containing phosphate binders and implementation of better water purification standards have led to a marked decrease in the incidence of low-turnover osteomalacia.[81,82] Studies have shown that aluminum can impair osteoblast growth and activity. Aluminum has also been shown to decrease PTH secretion. In addition to aluminum, other factors have also been implicated in the development of osteomalacia, including vitamin D deficiency, metabolic acidosis, and hypophosphatemia.[83–87] The roles of fluoride and strontium in the development of osteomalacia are still controversial.[88,89]

Other Factors Contributing to Metabolic Bone Disease

Metabolic Acidosis. Metabolic acidosis increases net calcium efflux from bone through physicochemical mechanisms as well as cell-mediated mechanisms. The buffering of hydrogen ions by bone bicarbonate results in the liberation of bone minerals. In addition to bone dissolution, metabolic acidosis has been shown to stimulate osteoclast-mediated bone resorption and inhibit osteoblast-mediated bone formation.[85,90–92] Metabolic acidosis has also been implicated in altering the biological actions of PTH[92–94] and the metabolism of vitamin D.[95,96] Metabolic acidosis has been shown to significantly increase expression of RANKL mRNA, an effect medicated by osteoblastic prostaglandin synthesis, which can be blocked by indomethacin.[97] This may be the mechanism by which metabolic acidosis induces osteoclast-mediated bone resorption. Recently, it has been shown that metabolic acidosis stimulates the response to PTH in osteoblast-like cells by a mechanism that involves an increase in the expression of the PTH/PTHrP receptor mRNA.[98] Therefore the increased levels of PTH/PTHrP receptor may result in an enhanced effect of PTH on bone, leading to increased bone resorption. There is evidence to suggest that the treatment of metabolic acidosis in chronic hemodialysis patients results in improvement in the manifestations of hyperparathyroidism.[99,100]

Corticosteroids. It is well known that corticosteroid use is associated with loss of bone and increased risk of fracture.[101] Corticosteroids cause a decreased rate of bone formation, decreased thickness of the trabeculae, and increased bone resorption. Glucocorticoid treatment results in rapid loss of bone in the first few months, followed by a slower phase of steady bone loss. It has recently been shown that corticosteroids inhibit osteoblastogenesis and promote apoptosis in both osteoblasts and osteocytes.[102,103] These investigators have proposed that glucocorticoid-induced osteocyte apoptosis contributes to the pathogenesis of osteonecrosis, which is a common finding in patients treated with glucocorticoids for renal transplantation.[103] Both cortical and cancellous bone are lost, and the effect of corticosteroid therapy appears to be more pronounced in the axial skeleton leading to vertebral, wrist, femoral, and rib fractures.

Growth Factors and Cytokines. In recent years there have been important advances in our understanding of bone cell biology, and a variety of cytokines and growth factors are now known to be involved in regulating bone remodeling. Alterations in the levels and function of cytokines and growth factors in the uremic milieu might contribute to the pathogenesis of renal osteodystrophy.

Growth Factors. Osteoblast development and differentiation is under the regulation of multiple systemic and local factors including PTH, IGF, bone morphogenetic proteins, fibroblast growth factor, TGF-β, and EGF.[104] The insulin-like growth factor 1 (IGF-1) system is important in osteoblast development and may play a role in the pathogenesis of renal osteodystrophy.[105–108] IGF-1 circulates bound to IGF binding proteins, which modify the effects of IGF-1 on bone. IGF-1 as well as IGFBPs is regulated by a variety of factors, including PTH and calcitriol. Since these hormone systems are altered in uremia, it is possible that abnormalities in the IGF system contribute to the pathogenesis of renal osteodystrophy.[105,109–112] Elevated levels of IGF-1 have been found in patients with CKD and correlate with the rate of bone formation.[113] Others, however, found no correlation between circulating levels of IGF peptides and serologic or histologic markers of renal osteodystrophy.[114] Recent observations have shown low levels of IGFBP-5, a stimulator of IGF actions, in patients with secondary hyperparathyroidism, which correlated with biochemical markers and indices of bone formation.[115]

Bone Morphogenetic Proteins. The bone morphogenetic proteins play an important role in osteoblast development. Bone morphogenetic protein 7 (BMP-7) has been shown to be highly expressed in mouse kidney.[116–122] Therefore it is conceivable that CKD may lead to BMP-7 deficiency, which in turn may result in abnormal bone remodeling. It has been shown in a mouse model of renal bone disease that BMP-7 administration prevented many of the histologic abnormalities characteristic of high-turnover osteodystrophy.[123] In addition, BMP-7 administration prevented the marrow fibrosis that is usually characteristic of hyperparathyroid bone disease.

PTH leads to the increase of EGF receptors on osteoblasts.[124] EGF is known to play an important role in suppressing preosteoblast differentiation.[125,126] Therefore both the increase in PTH levels enhancing the suppressive effects of EGF on osteoblast differentiation and the possible deficiency of BMP-7, deemed important in osteoblast development, may prevent normal osteoblast differentiation, resulting in the accumulation of collagen-producing osteoprogenitor cells and thus giving rise to marrow fibrosis.

Cytokines. There is a wealth of evidence that the uremic state is a state of increased proinflammatory cytokines.[127–129] IL-1, IL-6, and TNF-α, among other proinflammatory cytokines, have been found to be elevated in patients with end-stage renal disease (ESRD) requiring dialysis when compared to normal subjects. These cytokines may modulate bone remodeling through effects on the RANK/RANKL/OPG system. IL-1 and IL-1 receptor antagonist, an inhibitor of IL-1 actions, have been found to be elevated in patients with renal failure who are on dialysis.[128] IL-1 markedly stimulated PGE-2 production and osteoclast formation in mice.[130] Some investigators have demonstrated an inverse relationship between the circulating levels of IL-1 receptor antagonist and osteoblast surface.[131,132] There are also increased levels of IL-6 in patients with CKD. IL-6 levels significantly correlated with markers of bone remodeling in patients with renal osteodystrophy in several recent studies.[133,134] Increased expression of IL-6 receptor mRNA in osteoclasts of patients with CKD correlated with bone-resorbing activity.[135] However, some studies reported an inverse relationship between the ratio of soluble IL-6 receptor (an enhancer of IL-6 actions) to IL-6 (sIL-6R:IL-6 ratio), and osteoclast surface.[129,136,137] TNF-α, which has been shown to be increased in patients with CKD, also plays a role in bone remodeling.[128] Histomorphometric analysis of bone samples showed that increased TNF-α was associated with increased osteoclast surface and decreased osteoid volume and osteoid surface.[138]

PTH appears to modulate the effects of cytokines in renal osteodystrophy. PTH is known to stimulate local IL-6 synthesis in stromal cells.[139] Santos et al. recently reported that there is a marked decrease in the expression of IL-1 beta, TNF-α,, TGF-β, and basic fibroblast growth factor (bFGF) in bone biopsies taken from uremic patients 1 year after parathyroidectomy when compared to results prior to parathyroidectomy.[140]

Circulating osteoprotegerin (OPG) levels have been found to be elevated in patients with CKD requiring dialysis. The OPG concentrations in this category of patients were found to inhibit osteoclast formation in vitro.[141] Circulating OPG levels seem to correlate with the state of bone turnover. Thus, it has been shown that hemodialysis patients with high bone turnover had significantly lower OPG levels than those with low bone turnover.[142]

CLINICAL MANIFESTATIONS OF RENAL OSTEODYSTROPHY

Musculoskeletal Symptoms

Symptoms related to renal osteodystrophy are usually a late manifestation of the disease and are often nonspecific. They are often preceded by biochemical or histologic abnormalities.

Bone pain is the classic symptom of renal osteodystrophy. It is usually nonspecific in nature and may be diffuse or localized to the lower back, hips, knees, and legs. Lower back pain may represent the collapse of a vertebral body, and chest wall pain may represent spontaneous rib fracture. The most debilitating bone pain is seen with osteomalacia, especially when associated with aluminum deposition. Joint pain may be due to periarthritis or arthritis and may result in functional impairment of one or multiple joints. This is often associated with significant hyperparathyroidism. Acute joint pain and swelling may be confused with gout or pseudogout and symptoms are usually responsive to non-steroidal anti-inflammatory drugs; however, attention should be given to underlying secondary hyperparathyroidism. Erosive arthritis and joint effusion may be found in dialysis-related amyloidosis. The joints that are usually involved are the metacarpophalangeal, interphalageal, wrists, shoulders, hips, and knees.

Proximal muscle weakness is usually of gradual onset and may be severe and debilitating in some patients with advanced renal failure. The plasma levels of muscle enzymes are normal and there are no characteristic abnormalities on electromyography. Proximal myopathy and muscle weakness may be related to secondary hyperparathyroidism, phosphate depletion, and vitamin D deficiency.[143,144] Muscle weakness may also arise as a result of peripheral neuropathy, electrolyte disturbances, iron overload, and carnitine deficiency. Spontaneous tendon rupture has been observed in patients with long-standing renal disease on dialysis. It is usually associated with severe secondary hyperparathyroidism.[145–147] The quadriceps, triceps, and Achilles tendons have been most commonly implicated. Involvement of the extensor tendons of the fingers has also been described.

Pruritus or itching is a very common symptom in patients with renal failure. It has been associated with increased levels of PTH, hypercalcemia, and increased calcium phosphorus product. Pruritis has been reported to resolve shortly after parathyroidectomy. Treatment of pruritus is usually symptomatic.

Metastatic and Extraskeletal Calcifications

There are two main forms of extraskeletal or metastatic calcification: amorphous calcium phosphate, found in soft tissues such as heart, lung, and kidney; the second form is hydroxyapatite, similar to that of normally calcifying tissue, which is present in vascular, valvular, joint, and ocular tissues. Metastatic and extraskeletal calcifications are not uncommon in CKD. Extraskeletal calcification can occur in damaged tissue, a phenomenon called *dystrophic calcification*, or in apparently normal tissue. This calcification occurs in a variety of tissues both visceral and nonvisceral, including skin, cartilage, heart, lungs, kidneys, shoulders, limboconjunctival, vascular, and valvular tissues. Recently vascular and cardiac valvular calcification have received

much attention, as they have been linked to cardiovascular mortality in ESRD.[148–151]

Calciphylaxis. Calciphylaxis, also called calcific uremic arteriolopathy, is a devastating complication of ESRD. This disorder is associated with calcium-phosphorus deposition in the subcutaneous arterial vessels, leading to progressive ischemic necrosis of the skin and adipose tissue. Recently, calciphylaxis appears to have become a more prevalent disease, although it is unknown whether the apparent increased prevalence in this disease reflects increased awareness[152] or is related to the increased use of calcium-containing phosphate binders. The skin lesions initially manifest as painful nodules. These may become mottled with violaceous discoloration similar to livedo reticularis and can subsequently ulcerate and become infected. The lesions can be found in the distal extremities, involving the toes, fingers, or ankles or they may be localized in proximal areas such as thighs, buttocks, abdominal wall, and breasts. The proximal lesions appear to be associated with the worst prognosis. Histologically, the lesions are characterized by medial calcification of small- and medium-sized arteries. In his original accounts of calciphylaxis, Seyle described a condition in which tissues, which had been sensitized, responded to a challenge with local calcification and inflammation.[153] Vitamin D and PTH were among the sensitizing agents, while egg white and metallic salts, which included iron dextran, were the challenging agents. Since many patients with hyperparathyroidism are treated with calcium salts and vitamin D, it is important to consider these factors as potential contributors to this problem. While this disorder had typically been associated with severe hyperparathyroidism, many patients with this syndrome now do not have significant hyperparathyroidism at the time of diagnosis. Many of them are obese, and there is a high prevalence of diabetes.[154] Since the lesions are similar to those seen with warfarin skin necrosis, a role for altered coagulation, particularly in the protein C and protein S pathways, in the final manifestations of this problem has been considered.[155–157] Patients on dialysis with calciphylaxis have been noted to have decreased levels of protein C and protein S activity.[156,157] Recent observations suggest that decreased levels of the calcification inhibitor alpha2-Heremans-Schmid glycoprotein (Ahsg, also known as fetuin-A) may play a role in the pathogenesis of calciphylaxis.[158] Although fetuin is now known to be an important inhibitor of ectopic calcification,[159] studies in fetuin knockout mice demonstrate that absence of fetuin alone is not sufficient to result in ectopic calcification, suggesting that additional inhibitors of calcification may be involved.[160] In this regard, osteopontin (OPN) and matrix Gla protein (MGP) were expressed in microvessels at sites of calcification in calciphylaxis models and were absent in normal blood vessels, suggesting a role for these proteins in the pathogenesis of calciphylaxis.[161]

Calcification of the Joints. Articular calcification occurs in renal failure and may result in joint effusion, stiffness, and pain. Periarticular calcification may occur following trauma or in the context of degenerative changes. Calcification may also be implicated in tendon rupture. Tumoral calcinosis represents large areas of calcium and phosphate deposition in the periarticular tissues of large joints such as knees, hips, elbows, and shoulders. It has also been reported in wrists, chest wall, and the cervical spine, causing progressive radiculomyelopathy. It is usually painless in the early stages, but, as the lesion grows in size, it can cause significant symptoms. Tumoral calcinosis usually regresses following parathyroidectomy, renal transplantation, or reduction in calcium and phosphorus product. Surgical excision might be necessary in cases of nerve compression and joint movement limitation.

Cardiovascular Calcification. Cardiovascular calcification is extremely common in patients with ESRD. Goodman et al. showed that coronary artery calcification is common and progressive in young adults with ESRD who are undergoing dialysis.[162] In that study, the prevalence of coronary artery calcification increased progressively with increased dialysis duration. Almost all patients who were on dialysis for more than 20 years had some degree of coronary artery calcification.[162] Vascular and valvular calcification has been associated with increased mortality in both hemodialysis and peritoneal dialysis patients.[148–151,163] A recent study by London et al. in patients on hemodialysis showed an increase in mortality not only in patients with intimal arterial calcification but also in those with medial arterial calcification (Fig. 30–2).[151] Calcification of the cardiovascular system may lead to impaired myocardial function, coronary artery disease, and valvular dysfunction.[164] The mitral and aortic valves often become calcified, and this can be associated with cardiac conduction defects, rupture of the chordae tendineae, and susceptibility to endocarditis. Vascular calcifications are associated with hyperphosphatemia and an elevated calcium phosphorus product.[164–166] Valvular calcifications may be seen on routine chest x-rays or echocardiograms and calcifications of large blood vessels are often manifest on x-rays of the abdomen or extremities. Calcification of coronary arteries is best visualized and quantitated by electron-beam computed tomography (EBCT).[167] High-speed spiral CT is also useful for detecting coronary artery calcification. Ultrasonographic techniques measuring arterial stiffness also appear to be valuable for the assessment of vascular calcification.[168]

Uremic arterial calcification is a significant problem in patients with kidney disease. Recent studies have shown that vascular calcification is an active rather than a passive process. Numerous observations have demonstrated the presence of bone matrix proteins such as osteopontin, osteocalcin, osteonectin, and matrix GLA protein (MGP) in calcified vascular tissue.[169,170] These data are supported by observations in experimental animals in which the MGP-

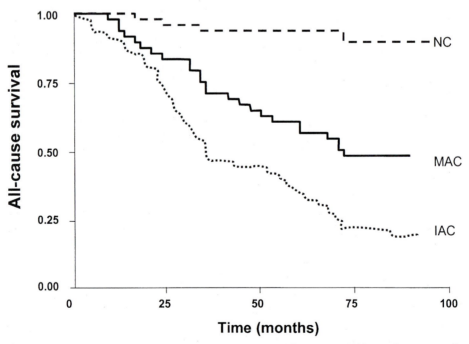

Figure 30–2. The impact of vascular calcification, whether intimal (IAC) or medial (MAC), on all-cause mortality in patients with ESRD. (Modified from London et al.,[151] with permission.)

null mouse,[171] the KLOTHO mouse,[172] the OPG-null mouse,[173] and others show enhanced susceptibility to vascular calcification; these models will facilitate research in this area. The role of the recently identified circulating inhibitor of calcification fetuin/ahsg will need further study.[159,174–177]

Phosphate may be a key regulator of these processes. Thus, phosphorus leads to the expression of the osteoblast differentiating markers, core binding factor α subunit 1 (Cbfa-1) and osteocalcin in human vascular smooth muscle cells; it also increases calcification of vascular smooth muscle cell cultures.[178,179] This process appears to involve the type 3 phosphate transporter Pit-1 (Glvr-1) and can be inhibited by the phosphate transport inhibitor phosphonoformic acid.[178] TNF-α has also been implicated in the calcification process. TNF-α, which is usually elevated in ESRD patients, has been shown to enhance in vitro vascular calcification by promoting osteoblastic differentiation of vascular cells through the cAMP pathway.[180]

Leptin may also be involved in this process. Leptin is a small peptide and is principally cleared by the kidney; serum leptin concentrations are increased in patients with CKD and those undergoing maintenance dialysis.[181] Leptin regulates the osteoblastic differentiation and calcification of vascular cells, and it seems that the arterial wall may be an important peripheral tissue target of its action.[182]

Dialysis-Related Amyloidosis

Dialysis-related amyloidosis (DRA), a condition characterized by the formation and deposition of beta-2-amyloid fibrils in periarticular and articular tissue and resulting in disabling arthropathy, has been described in patients who have been on dialysis for a long period of time.[183–190] The main amyloid deposited is beta$_2$ microglobulin.[191–193] However secondary modifications of the molecule—such as limited proteolysis, conformational changes, and the formation of advanced glycation end products—have also been described.[194,195] Since the manifestations of DRA are confined to articular and periarticular tissue, it has been thought that beta$_2$ microglobulin has a predilection only to those tissues. Recent histologic studies, however, demonstrate the widespread deposition of amyloid.[195] DRA affects more than 50 percent of patients.[196] This entity is basically described in patients with ESRD on hemodialysis, but it also occurs in patients on peritoneal dialysis. Risk factors for developing DRA include the time on dialysis, the type of hemodialysis membrane, and the patient's age at onset of dialysis.[197] Amyloid deposits precede the onset of clinical symptoms by many years. Clinical symptoms usually become evident after 8 to 12 years on hemodialysis.[198] The most common manifestations are carpal tunnel syndrome, shoulder pain, and destructive arthropathy. It appears that patients treated with a biocompatible, highly permeable membrane manifest signs and symptoms of DRA less frequently than patients treated with a less permeable, poorly biocompatible membrane,[199,200] in agreement with the hypothesis that synthesis of beta$_2$ microglobulin may be caused by the release of cytokines following contact of blood with the dialysis membrane. However, a study recently showed that membrane flux, not biocompatibility, is the main determinant of beta$_2$-microglobulin levels.[201] Others have suggested a role for dialysate composition and its microbacteriologic quality.[195]

Carpal tunnel syndrome is a common manifestation of DRA. The differential diagnosis of carpal tunnel syndrome in patients on dialysis includes dialysis-related amyloidosis (DRA), tissue edema secondary to vascular access malfunction, uremic neuropathy, calcification of ligaments, tumoral calcinosis with secondary nerve compression, and vitamin B$_6$ deficiency. Beta$_2$-microglobulin arthropathy is insidious in onset and progressive in nature, sometimes leading to destructive arthropathy.[202,203] Most frequently, it affects the shoulders[204,205]; however, involvement of the hips, knees, elbows, wrists, and fingers has been reported. Beta$_2$-microglobulin arthropathy is usually bilateral; it manifests as chronic arthralgias with or without joint swelling. Shoulder involvement is best demonstrated by magnetic resonance imaging (MRI), which shows thickening of the rotator cuff tendons, the subacromial bursae, or the synovial membrane. A destructive arthropathy has been described in large joints such as hip or knee joints and is characterized by subchondral bone erosions. Destructive spondyloarthropathy, characterized by erosive lesions, is often clinically silent and remains undiagnosed for many years.[202,206–208] The most important risk factor for the development of destructive spondyloarthropathy is duration on dialysis. Destructive spondyloarthropathy is most commonly reported in the cervical spine and may result in spinal cord compression; it is best evaluated by CT or MRI.

The diagnosis of dialysis-related amyloidosis is suspected in dialysis patients with x-ray findings showing subchondral bone cysts that are symmetrical in distribution and increase in number or size over time.[209] The diagnosis is best confirmed by histologic examination using Congo red staining of beta$_2$-amyloid fibrils; this can be followed with the precise typing of amyloid by immunohistochemistry.[209]

DIAGNOSIS OF RENAL OSTEODYSTROPHY

Clinical signs and symptoms of renal osteodystrophy are usually a late manifestation of the disease. Histopathologic examination of undecalcified bone tissue sections obtained through a bone biopsy remains the "gold standard" for the diagnosis of renal osteodystrophy. Its widespread use, however, is limited due to its invasive nature. Thus, the diagnosis of renal osteodystrophy and the implementation of a therapeutic strategy rely on the use of biochemical and radiologic investigations.

Biochemistries

Serum Phosphorus. The level of serum phosphorus remains normal and may even be decreased in the early stages of CKD. Hyperphosphatemia does not usually become evident until the GFR has declined to less than 20 percent of normal. This homeostatic control of serum phosphate level is achieved mainly through the phosphaturic effect of increased PTH,[38,210] although other factors, such as FGF-23, may also play a role. Phosphate is mostly absorbed in the duodenum, the jejunum, and to a smaller extent in the ileum and colon. The majority of phosphate absorption occurs via passive diffusion down a concentration gradient; therefore phosphate absorption is directly related to dietary phosphate intake. Calcitriol is known to increase intestinal absorption of phosphate, and its use may aggravate hyperphosphatemia.

In patients with advanced renal failure, hyperphosphatemia may also be observed in cases of severe hyperparathyroidism as a result of the increased mobilization of phosphorus from bone. Monitoring the serum phosphorus concentration is not very helpful in establishing the diagnosis of a specific type of renal osteodystrophy; however, control of hyperphosphatemia remains a crucial intervention in the setting of CKD, as it may aggravate hyperparathyroidism by decreasing the levels of ionized calcium, decreasing the synthesis of calcitriol, and directly increasing PTH secretion and promoting the growth of parathyroid cells. In addition, it is necessary to control hyperphosphatemia because it is an independent risk factor for death in this patient group and likely plays an important role in vascular calcification.[179]

Serum Calcium. Calcium homeostasis is maintained by the integrated actions of the major calciotropic hormones PTH and calcitriol. This homeostatic control involves the regulation of intestinal calcium absorption, renal calcium reabsorption, and calcium deposition and release from bone. In patients with kidney disease, altered levels of PTH and calcitriol may result in disturbances in this homeostatic balance.

Total serum calcium concentration consists of three fractions: ionized, complexed, and protein-bound. The ionized calcium, approximately 50 percent of total serum calcium, is the physiologically important fraction and can be measured directly. In practice, the total calcium concentration is commonly corrected for changes in serum proteins.

In advanced CKD, hypocalcemia may occur, but this is not a universal finding.[38,210] Hypocalcemia in CKD may result from several mechanisms, including increased serum phosphorus concentration leading to the formation of calcium-phosphorus complexes, impaired calcitriol synthesis leading to decreased intestinal calcium absorption, and

skeletal resistance to the actions of PTH. In advanced renal failure, there may be the retention of various anions resulting in increased complexed fraction and therefore a decreased ionized fraction of total serum calcium. Regardless of the etiology of hypocalcemia, it is important to correct serum calcium concentration during the course of CKD, as it is a very powerful stimulus for PTH secretion.

Hypercalcemia in patients with CKD may be due to several factors. It may be seen with low turnover osteodystrophy such as osteomalacia and adynamic bone disease. In these patients the hypercalcemia often becomes manifest after the administration of low doses of vitamin D compounds or calcium supplements.[211] As a result of the low bone turnover, the excess calcium absorbed from the intestine may not be deposited in the bone, therefore leading to the development of hypercalcemia.[212] Severe secondary hyperparathyroidism may also be associated with hypercalcemia (tertiary hyperparathyroidism). Persistent hyperparathyroidism may also lead to hypercalcemia following successful renal transplantation. Hypercalcemia in CKD may also be the result of therapeutic strategies used in the management of renal osteodystrophy. Thus, the intestinal absorption of calcium may increase following the administration of calcium-containing phosphate binders, since oral calcium administration increases calcium absorption by ionic diffusion. The effect of increasing serum calcium may be more pronounced when calcium salts are administered in conjunction with vitamin D sterols, since these increase calcium transport by the intestinal cells.

Neither the levels of serum phosphorus nor those of serum calcium have diagnostic value with regard to the specific nature of the underlying bone disease; the interpretation of these values in conjunction with measurements of PTH and biological markers of bone turnover may provide important clues as to the nature of the disturbances in mineral homeostasis in kidney disease.

Assay of Parathyroid Hormone. PTH measurement is important in the diagnosis and management of renal osteodystrophy. Understanding of the PTH polypeptide and its metabolites has broadened considerably in the past decade.[213] PTH does not exist solely as an intact 84–amino acid peptide (PTH 1–84) but circulates along with a variety of lower-molecular-weight PTH fragments from the middle and C-terminal regions of the PTH molecule[214,215] that are secreted from the parathyroid gland or generated by PTH metabolism in peripheral organs, especially the liver and kidneys. In advanced CKD, these PTH fragments accumulate in the circulation, since they depend on glomerular filtration for their removal. Accordingly, it is no surprise that assays for PTH directed toward different parts of the PTH molecule yielded different results.[216] PTH assays have evolved considerably since their inception (Fig. 30–3). Refinements of

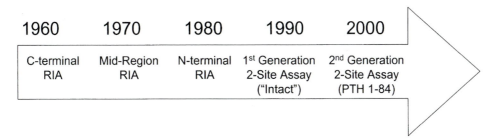

Figure 30–3. Diagrammatic representation of the evolution of PTH assays.

the PTH assay using two-site techniques offered a major improvement over earlier assays; however, it has recently been realized that these first-generation PTH immunometric assays[217–219] detect not only full-length PTH (1–84) but also other amino-terminally truncated PTH fragments such as PTH 7–84.[220] This limitation has led to the development of second-generation two-site immunometric PTH assays that appear to be specific for the full-length PTH 1–84 molecule.[221,222]

The evolution of the PTH assay has generated interest in the amino-terminally truncated PTH fragments, as they may have biological effects. Thus, there is evidence to suggest that PTH 7–84 fragment blunts the calcemic actions of PTH and appears to interact with a PTH receptor, which reacts with the carboxy-terminal region of PTH.[68,69,71] PTH 7–84 infused into experimental animals at high concentrations blunts the effects of PTH 1–84 on bone.[223] Attempts to utilize measurements of PTH 7–84 and a ratio of PTH 1–84 to PTH 7–84 for diagnostic purposes has been suggested but has not been demonstrated uniformly in action by different investigators.[224–226] Further studies are needed to elucidate the biological effects of the PTH peptides, such as PTH 7–84.

Biological Markers of Bone Formation and Bone Resorption

Alkaline Phosphatase. Total alkaline phosphatase activity in serum is the sum of several isoforms: hepatic, skeletal, renal, intestinal, and placental.[227–229] It has been shown that the increased total alkaline phosphatase in uremic patients is often the result of increases in the bone-specific isoform[230]; this has been correlated with histologic findings of hyperparathyroidism. Total alkaline phosphatase may be useful in monitoring the progression of bone disease as well as the response to therapy.[231] However, the most serious limitation of its use is its lack of specificity and sensitivity.

An assay of bone-specific alkaline phosphatase has been developed and its measurement has been suggested to be the most sensitive and specific marker to evaluate the degree of bone remodeling in uremic patients.[232] It has been found that a level of bone-specific alkaline phos-

phatase > 20 ng/mL has a sensitivity and specificity of 100 percent and a positive predictive value of 84 percent for the diagnosis of high-turnover bone disease. In addition, levels of bone-specific alkaline phosphatase > 20 ng/mL combined with PTH levels > 200 pg/mL had a positive predictive value of 94 percent for the diagnosis of high-turnover bone disease. Furthermore, because of the high specificity of the test for high-turnover bone disease, levels of bone-specific alkaline phosphatase > 20 ng/mL allow for the formal exclusion of low-turnover bone disease. Others have found similar results.[233] Thus, measurements of bone-specific alkaline phosphatase may be helpful in the diagnosis of both high- and low-turnover renal osteodystrophy, especially when examined in conjunction with PTH levels.[131,233–238]

Osteocalcin. Osteocalcin—also known as bone Gla protein, BGP, or bone γ-carboxy-glutamic acid–containing protein—is the most abundant noncollagenous protein present in the bone matrix[131,233–238] and is produced only by osteoblasts and odontoblasts. The process of γ-carboxylation of osteocalcin is vitamin K–dependent, and vitamin K deficiency is associated with a decrease in carboxylated osteocalcin, decreased bone mass, and increased fracture risk.[239–242] Although osteocalcin levels have been shown to correlate with histologic parameters of bone formation in patients on hemodialysis as well as those on peritoneal dialysis, they do not appear to add to the predictive value of PTH levels in this regard.[243–246] Although plasma osteocalcin levels have been shown to correlate with bone histomorphometric parameters, the correlations are weaker than those observed with bone-specific alkaline phosphatase and PTH levels.[235,247]

Collagen Peptides and Breakdown Products. Various bone collagen peptides and breakdown products have been measured to obtain a biochemical assessment of bone resorption, but they are not widely used at the present time. Research in this area continues.[232,235,247–250]

Tartrate-Resistant Acid Phosphatase. This bone-specific acid phosphatase, also known as TRAP, has been evaluated as a potential biochemical marker of bone resorption.[251–255] Important limitations to its diagnostic potential include the lack of specificity, as TRAP is produced by many cells lines including but not limited to osteoblasts and osteoclasts.[256] Recent studies have identified TRAP 5b as the osteoclast-specific isoform; future studies involving patients with CKD are needed to evaluate the value of this new marker in the evaluation of renal bone disease.[255,257]

Aluminum Levels and the Deferoxamine Test

The prevalence of aluminum-related bone disease has declined in recent years; however, aluminum overload continues to be a problem in some parts of the world.[6] Serum aluminum levels have a limited diagnostic value and are affected by recent exposure or withdrawal of aluminum-containing products. Serum aluminum is generally not reflective of aluminum tissue stores and is also influenced by iron status.[258] Following cessation of aluminum-containing phosphate binders, serum aluminum levels may fall rapidly over the course of a few months; therefore the incidence of false-negative results of serum aluminum measurement may increase from 30 to 90 percent following cessation of aluminum intake.[259]

The chelator deferoxamine (DFO) has been used to mobilize tissue aluminum in an effort to estimate tissue aluminum stores.[258] However, the DFO test alone is not a reliable indicator of aluminum bone disease; it merely reflects the aluminum burden. When combined with serum PTH, the deferoxamine test has good discriminatory power.[260–262] More recently—in order to minimize the risk for DFO-related cerebral, auditory, and visual side effects and siderophore-mediated opportunistic infections—lower doses of DFO have been used for the evaluation of aluminum bone disease. D'Haese et al. used 5- and 10-mg/kg DFO tests in conjunction with intact PTH (iPTH) levels to identify patients with aluminum-related bone disease, with aluminum overload, or at risk for aluminum toxicity.[260] Using serum aluminum increment above 50 µg/L for the 5-mg/kg DFO test or 70 µg/Lfor the 10-mg/kg test, together with a serum iPTH below 150 ng/L, the test has a sensitivity of 87 percent and a specificity of 95 and 92 percent, respectively, for the identification of aluminum-related bone disease. In addition to the PTH levels, the presence of other metals, such as iron, may affect the results of the test.[261,263] Huang et al. evaluated the influence of body iron stores on the serum aluminum level in hemodialysis patients. Significantly higher basal and peak aluminum levels after DFO infusion were found in patients with serum ferritin less than 300 µg/L.[264] Those patients who were iron replete, however, had lower increases in serum aluminum levels after the challenge with deferoxamine.[264] Similarly, Cannata et al. reported that patients with iron overload (serum ferritin > 1000 µg/L) may have low serum aluminum levels (< 30 µg/L) in the presence of a positive deferoxamine test and significant accumulation of aluminum in bone.[265]

Although random levels of serum aluminum may have low diagnostic yield, the DFO test used in conjunction with PTH and serum ferritin is a useful diagnostic tool. However, because of the potential toxicity of DFO therapy, bone biopsy may still be necessary in patients with borderline values.

Cytokines and Growth Factors

Although a variety of cytokines and growth factors are involved in the regulation of bone remodeling,[266–269] the clinical use of measurements of cytokines or growth factors as diagnostic markers awaits further studies.

Radiographic Investigations

Radiographic screening for bone disease in patients with CKD has a low sensitivity and poor discriminatory ability for the type of bone disease and is therefore of limited value.

Hyperparathyroid Bone Disease. Subperiosteal bone resorption is the classic manifestation of secondary hyperparathyroidism. Subperiosteal bone erosions are initially evident in the middle phalanges of the second or third digits but may also be found in the tibia, femoral neck, humerus, pelvic bones, distal end of the clavicle, and skull. Bone resorption and osteosclerosis in the skull produces a radiographic appearance often referred to as the "pepperpot skull." Cystic lesions of the bone may occur and may represent brown tumors or osteoclastomas, which must be distinguished from malignant tumors. Osteosclerosis of the spine produces a characteristic appearance referred to as the "rugger jersey spine."

Osteomalacia. In adults, pseudofractures or Looser zones are pathognomonic for osteomalacia. These are cortical fractures and may have a poorly mineralizing callus. In children and young adults, characteristic rachitic deformities of the long bones may be seen.

Osteopenia. A decreased bone mineral density may be apparent in renal bone diseases but is nonspecific and may be seen in both high- and low-bone-turnover disease.

Vascular and Extraskeletal Calcification. Extraskeletal calcifications are very common in patients with CKD and may be seen in vascular tissue such as the aortic arch, abdominal aorta, and other large, medium, and small arteries. Valvular calcification may be noted on echocardiograms in patients with CKD on either hemodialysis or peritoneal dialysis. These findings are important, since they have been correlated with cardiovascular mortality. Calcification of other organs and tissues has also been described. Calcification of the subcutaneous tissue may be observed in patients with calciphylaxis. Calcification can also be found around large joints, such as the hip and shoulder joints.

Dialysis-Related Amyloidosis. Bone cysts and periarticular cystic bone lesions may be seen in the wrist, tarsal bone, femoral head, distal radius, acetabulum, pubic symphysis, or tibial plateau and represent dialysis related amyloidosis. A destructive spondyloarthropathy may affect the cervical spine and is manifest as a narrowing of intervertebral spaces with the destruction or sclerosis of adjacent subchondral bones, erosions of vertebral body plates, and cavitations.[270,271] These findings may be similar to those of vertebral osteomyelitis; MRI may be helpful in further evaluation.[272]

Measurements of Bone Mineral Content. Measurements of bone mineral content by dual energy x-ray absorptiometry (DEXA) are not useful for diagnosing the type of renal osteodystrophy. In patients with kidney disease, the role of DEXA as a predictor of fracture risk is also uncertain. It is likely that serial determinations of bone mineral content may have value, but the clinical utility of these determinations requires further study. Osteopenia in this patient group likely requires other detailed evaluation.

Histopathologic Features of Renal Osteodystrophy

Bone biopsy remains the gold standard for the diagnosis and classification of renal osteodystrophy. The widespread use of bone biopsy remains limited mainly because of the invasive nature of the procedure. The histologic features of hyperparathyroidism or osteitis fibrosa show an increased rate of bone formation, increased bone resorption, extensive osteoclastic and osteoblastic activity, and progressive increase in endosteal peritrabecular fibrosis. Unmineralized bone matrix may be increased. In osteitis fibrosa, a disarray in the alignment of collagenous strands in the bone matrix results in an irregular woven pattern that contrasts with the normal parallel alignment of collagenous strands in the lamellar bone. Osteomalacia is characterized by an excess of unmineralized osteoid manifest as wide osteoid seams and a markedly decreased mineralization rate. The presence of increased unmineralized osteoid is not necessarily indicative of a mineralizing defect, since increased quantities of osteoid appear in conditions associated with high rates of bone formation when mineralization lags behind the increased synthesis of the matrix. Other features of osteomalacia include the absence of endosteal fibrosis and markedly reduced cellular activity. Staining for aluminum can demon-

strate that osteomalacic renal bone disease has large deposits of aluminum at the interface between trabecular bone and osteoid. Aluminum content of the mineralization front correlates with the degree of osteomalacia.

Adynamic bone disease is characterized histologically by features similar to those of osteomalacia, a major difference being the absence of osteoid. There is markedly reduced cellular activity and decreased number of both osteoblasts and osteoclasts. Thus, the appearance is of a marked decrease in bone formation which leads to decreased bone mineralization.

Mixed uremic osteodystrophy has features of secondary hyperparathyroidism together with evidence of a mineralization defect. Thus, there is more osteoid than expected, and the tetracycline labeling uncovers a concomitant mineralization defect.

New histologic techniques have recently been examined for their potential to allow a better understanding of the pathobiology of bone disease. The application of such techniques such as immunohistochemistry and in situ hybridization will likely broaden the understanding of bone cell biology in the future.[135]

MANAGEMENT OF RENAL OSTEODYSTROPHY

Recently, new clinical practice guidelines have been introduced for the therapy of renal bone disease.[273] The goals of treatment are to maintain the levels of calcium and phosphorus in blood as close to normal as possible, to take measures to prevent parathyroid hyperplasia, or—if hyperparathyroidism is already present—to take steps to suppress the secretion of PTH. During this therapy, it is necessary to take steps to prevent an excess of calcium burden so as to minimize extraskeletal calcium deposition and to avoid substances that may accumulate and adversely affect the skeleton, such as aluminum. During the course of CKD, the intensity of treatment will vary according to the magnitude of the hyperparathyroidism or existing bone disease.

The recommendations are to begin the assessment and therapy of hyperparathyroidism early in the course of CKD and use a stepped-care approach (Fig. 30–4), since substantial experimental evidence indicates that hyperparathyroidism starts early in the course of CKD. Accordingly, it is necessary to measure the levels of PTH in blood in every patient with a GFR of 60 mL/min or less. If PTH values are substantially above the upper limits of normal for the assay used, several steps need to be taken to bring this level back to the desired range. As emphasized above, the demonstration that serum calcium and phosphorus levels may be normal at these GFRs does not necessarily mean that there is no problem with secondary hyperparathyroidism.

The current recommendations suggest that the first maneuver for the therapy of secondary hyperparathyroidism

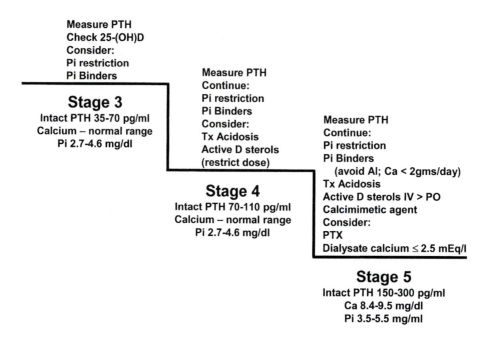

Figure 30–4. A stepped-care approach to the prevention and therapy of renal osteodystrophy in CKD. Evaluation and therapy should begin in stage 3 CKD and be intensified as illustrated as kidney disease progresses.

is to evaluate the vitamin D status of the patient by measurement of 25-hydroxyvitamin D. Many patients with CKD have values that are considered to be low, and this vitamin D deficiency may contribute to hyperparathyroidism. Thus, if 25-hydroxyvitamin D values are less than 30 ng/mL, it is recommended that this should be raised by the administration of ergocalciferol, usually in a dose of approximately 50,000 U once a month. Levels of intact PTH should be followed, and if a satisfactory response is obtained, this treatment can be continued. If hyperparathyroidism persists following the correction of any vitamin D deficiency, the next maneuver is to try to restrict the dietary intake of phosphorus, based on substantial experimental and clinical data. Often this requires a reduction in dietary protein intake, at least to a level of 1 g/kg/day. High-phosphorus foods should be avoided; consultation with dietitians is helpful in this regard. If these maneuvers do not achieve a satisfactory response in PTH levels, phosphate binders should be added. At the present time, it is recommended that calcium-containing phosphate binders such as calcium acetate be given with meals in order to complex phosphorus in the intestine and minimize absorption. These measures may have to be intensified as renal failure progresses. With more advanced kidney disease, one may consider the use of active vitamin D sterols such as calcitriol or 1-α-hydroxy D$_2$; however, caution is required, with limitations of the dosages to avoid toxicity.[274–276]

As kidney disease progresses to stage 5, with GFRs below 15 mL/min or dialysis is required, hyperparathyroidism becomes a significant problem and requires intensification of the measures outlined above. The current recommendations are to maintain calcium concentration within the lower half of the normal range and phosphorus values between 3.5 and 5.5 mg/dL and to try to achieve a target range for intact PTH between 150 and 300 pg/mL, or approximately 75 to 150 pg/mL in the new specific PTH 1–84 assays. The achievement of these goals is somewhat difficult and requires constant monitoring and active intervention. Hyperphosphatemia must be controlled because of the risk of cardiovascular mortality and aggravation of hyperparathyroidism, and several phosphate binders are available. The most commonly used are calcium acetate and calcium carbonate as well as sevelamer hydrochloride, which contains neither calcium nor aluminum. The current recommendations suggest that calcium intake should not exceed 2 g/day, which limits the amount of calcium-containing phosphate binders that can be used. Accordingly, one may have to use sevelamer hydrochloride, which is an effective phosphate binder, and its use is rapidly increasing. These measures directed at phosphorus control alone are often insufficient to control hyperparathyroidism, and the use of active vitamin D sterols is often required in order to suppress the secretion of PTH. Formerly, such therapy utilized calcitriol, usually in injectable form, in patients on hemodialysis[277] and was quite effective in treating hyperparathyroidism. Calcitriol therapy can be limited by its toxicity of hypercalcemia and aggravation of hyperphosphatemia; accordingly, in recent years the trend has been to use vitamin D analogues with lesser calcemic and phosphatemic potential. The most widely used vitamin D analogue in this regard is 19-nor-1,25-dihydroxyvitamin D_2, which is effective at suppressing PTH levels and appears to have less calcemic and phosphatemic effects than the native hormone, calcitriol.[278] Other vitamin D sterols are also in clinical use, and 1-α-hydroxyvitamin D_2 has been used as well.[279] On the basis of studies in animals, there appears to be lesser toxicity of vitamin D_2 compounds when given at very high doses.[280] However, differences between vitamin D_2 and vitamin D_3 sterols at therapeutic doses appear to be minimal,[281] and structural alterations to create vitamin D analogues appear beneficial to minimize toxicity.

Recent studies evaluating the success of current treatment paradigms show that a significant number of patients do not meet the newly recommended targets; in this regard, newer therapies are required. On the horizon are novel phosphate-binding agents such as lanthanum carbonate, which may facilitate phosphorus control. Much additional work needs to be done to evaluate its efficacy in this regard. A novel approach to the treatment of hyperparathyroidism has recently been introduced by targeting the calcium-sensing receptor of the parathyroid gland with a small molecule that can be administered orally. This calcimimetic agent, cinacalcet hydrochloride, has been studied extensively in clinical trials and likely will be available in the near future.[282–284] This agent enhances the effects of calcium on the parathyroid gland and achieves significant suppression of PTH. Unlike other therapeutic strategies, this reduction of PTH is not associated with increases in calcium or phosphorus values. Accordingly, it should be a useful addition to the therapeutic armamentarium for the treatment of hyperparathyroidism.

In the context of treating hyperparathyroidism, it is necessary not to oversuppress PTH, lest low-turnover bone diseases be induced by excessive calcium load or excessive use of vitamin D sterols. This is currently an active area of investigation, and further work will be required to try to refine the therapeutic targets with bone biopsy. Other considerations for the therapy of patients on dialysis would include adjustments of dialysate calcium, efforts to treat any existing acidosis, and potentially using serial evaluations of bone mineral density to ensure that bone does not continue to be lost. Alternate dialysis regimens such as long nocturnal dialysis or daily dialysis may also influence the therapy of hyperphosphatemia. A number of reports have shown that patients on nocturnal dialysis do not require phosphate binders; in fact, many require phosphate supplementation.[285] In contrast, enhanced phosphate removal is not achieved by short daily dialysis, and there is current interest in exploring different dialysis schedules to try to improve patient outcome. Surgical therapy of hyperparathyroidism should also be considered. Current recommendations suggest that failure to lower intact PTH levels to less than 800 pg/mL with medical treatment should prompt consideration of surgical approaches to remove parathyroid tissue. Most commonly, the procedure performed is subtotal parathyroidectomy, either leaving a part of one parathyroid gland in the neck or implanting parathyroid tissue in the forearm. Newer techniques such as minimally invasive parathyroid surgery have not been applied to hyperparathyroidism of CKD. Alternative approaches are ablation of parathyroid tissue by percutaneous injection with ethanol or vitamin D sterols.[286,287] Further follow-up is required to assess the applicability of these less invasive techniques in this field.

REFERENCES

1. Ballanti P, Wedard BM, Bonucci E. Frequency of adynamic bone disease and aluminum storage in Italian uraemic patients—retrospective analysis of 1429 iliac crest biopsies. *Nephrol Dial Transplant* 1996;11:663–667.
2. Malluche HH, Monier-Faugere MC. Risk of adynamic bone disease in dialyzed patients. *Kidney Int Suppl* 1992;38:S62–S67.
3. Monier-Faugere MC, Malluche HH. Trends in renal osteodystrophy: a survey from 1983 to 1995 in a total of 2248 patients. *Nephrol Dial Transplant* 1996;11(suppl 3):111–120.
4. Sherrard DJ, Hercz G, Pei Y, et al. The spectrum of bone disease in end-stage renal failure—an evolving disorder. *Kidney Int* 1993;43:436–442.
5. Cannata-Andia JB. Renal osteodystrophy in Iberoamerica. *Am J Kidney Dis* 1999;34:lviii–lx.
6. Diaz Lopez JB, Jorgetti V, Caorsi H, et al. Epidemiology of renal osteodystrophy in Iberoamerica. *Nephrol Dial Transplant* 1998;13(suppl 3):41–45.
7. Jorgetti V, Lopez BD, Caorsi H, et al. Different patterns of renal osteodystrophy in Iberoamerica. *Am J Med Sci* 2000;320:76–80.
8. Reiss E, Canterbury JM, Kanter A. Circulating parathyroid hormone concentration in chronic renal insufficiency. *Arch Intern Med* 1969;124:417–422.
9. Malluche H, Ritz E, Lange H. Bone histology in incipient and advanced renal failure. *Kidney Int* 1976;9:355–362.
10. Jowsey J, Reiss E, Canterbury JM. Long-term effects of high phosphate intake on parathyroid hormone levels and bone metabolism. *Acta Orthop Scand* 1974;45:801–808.
11. Rutherford WE, Bordier P, Marie P, et al. Phosphate control and 25-hydroxycholecalciferol administration in preventing experimental renal osteodystrophy in the dog. *J Clin Invest* 1977;60:332–341.
12. Slatopolsky E, Caglar S, Pennell JP, et al. On the pathogenesis of hyperparathyroidism in chronic experimental renal insufficiency in the dog. *J Clin Invest* 1971;50:492–499.

13. Bricker NS. On the pathogenesis of the uremic state. An exposition of the "trade-off hypothesis," *N Engl J Med* 1972; 286:1093–1099.

14. Lopez-Hilker S, Galceran T, Chan YL, et al. Hypocalcemia may not be essential for the development of secondary hyperparathyroidism in chronic kidney disease. *J Clin Invest* 1986;78:1097–1102.

15. Denda M, Finch J, Slatopolsky E. Phosphorus accelerates the development of parathyroid hyperplasia and secondary hyperparathyroidism in rats with renal failure. *Am J Kidney Dis* 1996;28:596–602.

16. Slatopolsky E, Finch J, Denda M, et al. Phosphorus restriction prevents parathyroid gland growth. High phosphorus directly stimulates PTH secretion in vitro. *J Clin Invest* 1996;97:2534–2540.

17. Almaden Y, Canalejo A, Hernandez A, et al. Direct effect of phosphorus on PTH secretion from whole rat parathyroid glands in vitro. *J Bone Miner Res* 1996;11:970–976.

18. Almaden Y, Hernandez A, Torregrosa V, et al. High phosphate level directly stimulates parathyroid hormone secretion and synthesis by human parathyroid tissue in vitro. *J Am Soc Nephrol* 9:1845–1852.

19. Moallem E, Kilav R, Silver J, Naveh-Many T. RNA-Protein binding and post-transcriptional regulation of parathyroid hormone gene expression by calcium and phosphate. *J Biol Chem* 1998;273:5253–5259.

20. Yalcindag C, Silver J, Naveh-Many T. Mechanism of increased parathyroid hormone mRNA in experimental uremia: roles of protein RNA binding and RNA degradation. *J Am Soc Nephrol* 1999;10:2562–2568.

21. Kilav R, Silver J, Naveh-Many T. A conserved cis-acting element in the parathyroid hormone 3'-untranslated region is sufficient for regulation of RNA stability by calcium and phosphate. *J Biol Chem* 2001;276:8727–8733.

22. Tatsumi S, Segawa H, Morita K, et al. Molecular cloning and hormonal regulation of PiT-1, a sodium-dependent phosphate cotransporter from rat parathyroid glands. *Endocrinology* 1998;139:1692–1699.

23. Ritter CS, Martin DR, Lu Y, et al. Reversal of secondary hyperparathyroidism by phosphate restriction restores parathyroid calcium-sensing receptor expression and function. *J Bone Miner Res* 2002;17:2206–2213.

24. Dusso AS, Pavlopoulos T, Naumovich L, et al. p21(WAF1) and transforming growth factor-alpha mediate dietary phosphate regulation of parathyroid cell growth. *Kidney Int* 2001;59:855–865.

25. Dusso A, Naumovich L, Pavlopoulos T, et al. Phosphorus regulation of parathyroid cell growth in renal failure: a role for the cyclin-dependent kinase inhibitor p21. *J Am Soc Nephrol* 1998;9:564A.

26. Nykjaer A, Dragun D, Walther D, et al. An endocytic pathway essential for renal uptake and activation of the steroid 25-(OH) vitamin D3. *Cell* 1999;96:507–515.

27. Mason RS, Lissner D, Wilkinson M, Posen S. Vitamin D metabolites and their relationship to azotaemic osteodystrophy. *Clin Endocrinol* 1980;13:375–385.

28. Juttmann JR, Buurman CJ, De Kam E, et al. Serum concentrations of metabolites of vitamin D in patients with chronic kidney disease (CRF). Consequences for the treatment with 1-alpha-hydroxy-derivatives. *Clin Endocrinol* 1981;14: 225–236.

29. Tessitore N, Venturi A, Adami S, et al. Relationship between serum vitamin D metabolites and dietary intake of phosphate in patients with early renal failure. *Miner Electrolyte Metab* 1987;13:38–44.

30. Christiansen C, Christensen MS, Melsen F, et al. Mineral metabolism in chronic kidney disease with special reference to serum concentrations of 1.25(OH)2D and 24.25(OH)2D. *Clin Nephrol* 1981;15:18–22.

31. Silver J, Naveh-Many T, Mayer H, et al. Regulation by vitamin D metabolites of parathyroid hormone gene transcription in vivo in the rat. *J Clin Invest* 1986;78:1296–1301.

32. Russell J, Lettieri D, Sherwood LM. Suppression by $1,25(OH)_2D_3$ of transcription of the pre-proparathyroid hormone gene. *Endocrinology* 1986;119:2864–2866.

33. Kremer R, Bolivar I, Goltzman D, Hendy GN. Influence of calcium and 1,25-dihydroxycholecalciferol on proliferation and proto-oncogene expression in primary cultures of bovine parathyroid cells. *Endocrinology* 1989;125:935–941.

34. Cozzolino M, Lu Y, Finch J, et al. p21WAF1 and TGF-alpha mediate parathyroid growth arrest by vitamin D and high calcium. *Kidney Int* 2001;60:2109–2117.

35. Tokumoto M, Hirakawa M, Kazuhiko T, et al. Diminished expression of cyclin-dependent kinase inhibitor p21 and vitamin D receptor in nodular hyperplasia in secondary hyperparathyroidism. *J Am Soc Nephrol* 2000;11:584A.

36. Patel SR, Ke HQ, Vanholder R, et al. Inhibition of calcitriol receptor binding to vitamin D response elements by uremic toxins. *J Clin Invest* 1995;96:50–59.

37. Sawaya BP, Koszewski NJ, Qi Q, et al. Secondary hyperparathyroidism and vitamin D receptor binding to vitamin D response elements in rats with incipient renal failure. *J Am Soc Nephrol* 1997;8:271–278.

38. Martinez I, Saracho R, Montenegro J, Llach F. The importance of dietary calcium and phosphorous in the secondary hyperparathyroidism of patients with early renal failure. *Am J Kidney Dis* 1997;29:496–502.

39. Bellorin-Font E, Martin KJ, Freitag JJ, et al. Altered adenylate cyclase kinetics in hyperfunctioning human parathyroid glands. *J Clin Endocrinol Metab* 1981;52:499–507.

40. Brown EM, Brennan MF, Hurwitz S, et al. Dispersed cells prepared from human parathyroid glands: distinct calcium sensitivity of adenomas vs. primary hyperplasia. *J Clin Endocrinol Metab* 1978;46:267–275.

41. Felsenfeld AJ, Jara A, Pahl M, et al. Differences in the dynamics of parathyroid hormone secretion in hemodialysis patients with marked secondary hyperparathyroidism. *J Am Soc Nephrol* 1995;6:1371–1378.

42. Felsenfeld AJ, Rodriguez M, Dunlay R, Llach F. A comparison of parathyroid-gland function in haemodialysis patients with different forms of renal osteodystrophy. *Nephrol Dial Transplant* 1991;6:244–251.

43. Goodman WG, Belin T, Gales B, et al. Calcium-regulated parathyroid hormone release in patients with mild or advanced secondary hyperparathyroidism. *Kidney Int* 1995;48: 1553–1558.

44. Malberti F, Corradi B, Pagliari B, et al. The sigmoidal parathyroid hormone-ionized calcium curve and the set

point of calcium in hemodialysis and continuous ambulatory peritoneal dialysis. *Perit Dial Int* 13(suppl 2):S476–479.

45. Ramirez JA, Goodman WG, Gornbein J, et al. Direct in vivo comparison of calcium-regulated parathyroid hormone secretion in normal volunteers and patients with secondary hyperparathyroidism. *J Clin Endocrinol Metab* 1993;76: 1489–1494.

46. De Cristofaro V, Colturi C, Masa A, et al. Rate dependence of acute PTH release and association between basal plasma calcium and set point of calcium-PTH curve in dialysis patients. *Nephrol Dial Transplant* 2001;16:1214–1221.

47. Borrego MJ, Felsenfeld AJ, Martin-Malo A, et al. Evidence for adaptation of the entire PTH-calcium curve to sustained changes in the serum calcium in haemodialysis patients. *Nephrol Dial Transplant* 1997;12:505–513.

48. Indridason OS, Heath H III, Khosla S, et al. Non-suppressible parathyroid hormone secretion is related to gland size in uremic secondary hyperparathyroidism. *Kidney Int* 1996;50: 1663–1671.

49. Yokoyama K, Shigematsu T, Tsukada T, et al. Calcium-sensing receptor gene polymorphism affects the parathyroid response to moderate hypercalcemic suppression in patients with end-stage renal disease. *Clin Nephrol* 2002;57:131– 135.

50. Pahl M, Jara A, Bover J, et al. The set point of calcium and the reduction of parathyroid hormone in hemodialysis patients. *Kidney Int* 1996;49:226–231.

51. Fukuda N, Tanaka H, Tominaga Y, et al. Decreased 1,25-dihydroxyvitamin D3 receptor density is associated with a more severe form of parathyroid hyperplasia in chronic uremic patients. *J Clin Invest* 1993;92:1436–1443.

52. Gogusev J, Duchambon P, Hory B, et al. Depressed expression of calcium receptor in parathyroid gland tissue of patients with hyperparathyroidism. *Kidney Int* 1997;51: 328–336.

53. Kifor O, Moore FD Jr, Wang P, et al. Reduced immunostaining for the extracellulalar Ca^{2+}-sensing receptor in primary and uremic secondary hyperparathyroidism (see comments). *J Clin Endocrinol Metab* 1996;81:1598–1606.

54. Arnold A, Brown MF, Urena P, et al. Monoclonality of parathyroid tumors in chronic kidney disease and in primary parathyroid hyperplasia. *J Clin Invest* 1995;95:2047–2053.

55. Lewin E, Garfia B, Recio FL, et al. Persistent downregulation of calcium-sensing receptor mRNA in rat parathyroids when severe secondary hyperparathyroidism is reversed by an isogenic kidney transplantation. *J Am Soc Nephrol* 2002; 13:2110–2116.

56. Ritter CS, Finch JL, Slatopolsky EA, Brown AJ. Parathyroid hyperplasia in uremic rats precedes down-regulation of the calcium receptor. *Kidney Int* 2001;60:1737–1744.

57. Wada M, Furuya Y, Sakiyama J, et al. The calcimimetic compound NPS R-568 suppresses parathyroid cell proliferation in rats with renal insufficiency. Control of parathyroid cell growth via a calcium receptor. *J Clin Invest* 1997;100: 2977–2983.

58. Evanson JM. The response to the infusion of parathyroid extract in hypocalcaemic states. *Clin Sci* 1966;31:63–75.

59. Massry SG, Coburn JW, Lee DB, et al. Skeletal resistance to parathyroid hormone in renal failure. Studies in 105 human subjects. *Ann Intern Med* 1973;78:357–364.

60. Somerville PJ, Kaye M. Evidence that resistance to the calcemic action of parathyroid hormone in rats with acute uremia is caused by phosphate retention. *Kidney Int* 1979;16: 552–560.

61. Massry SG, Tuma S, Dua S, Goldstein DA. Reversal of skeletal resistance to parathyroid hormone in uremia by vitamin D metabolites: evidence for the requirement of 1,25(OH)2D3 and 24,25(OH)2D3. *J Lab Clin Med* 1979;94: 152–157.

62. Somerville PJ, Kaye M. Resistance to parathyroid hormone in renal failure: role of vitamin D metabolites. *Kidney Int* 1978;14:245–254.

63. Galceran T, Martin KJ, Morrissey JJ, Slatopolsky E. Role of 1,25-dihydroxyvitamin D on the skeletal resistance to parathyroid hormone. *Kidney Int* 1987;32:801–807.

64. Picton ML, Moore PR, Mawer EB, et al. Down-regulation of human osteoblast PTH/PTHrP receptor mRNA in endstage renal failure. *Kidney Int* 2000;58:1440–1449.

65. Urena P, Kubrusly M, Mannstadt M, et al. The renal PTH/PTHrP receptor is down-regulated in rats with chronic kidney disease. *Kidney Int* 1994;45:605–611.

66. Ureña P, Ferreira A, Morieux C, et al. PTH/PTHrP receptor mRNA is down-regulated in epiphyseal cartilage growth plate of uraemic rats. *Nephrol Dial Transplant* 1996;11: 2008–2016.

67. Tian J, Smogorzewski M, Kedes L, Massry SG. PTH-PTHrP receptor mRNA is downregulated in chronic kidney disease. *Am J Nephrol* 1994;14:41–46.

68. Slatopolsky E, Finch J, Clay P, et al. A novel mechanism for skeletal resistance in uremia. *Kidney Int* 2000;58:753–761.

69. Nguyen-Yamamoto L, Rousseau L, Brossard JH, et al. Synthetic carboxyl-terminal fragments of parathyroid hormone (pth) decrease ionized calcium concentration in rats by acting on a receptor different from the pth/pth-related peptide receptor. *Endocrinology* 2001;142:1386–1392.

70. Di Stefano A, Roinel N, de Rouffignac C, Wittner M. Transepithelial Ca^{2+} and Mg^{2+} transport in the cortical thick ascending limb of Henle's loop of the mouse is a voltage-dependent process. *Renal Physiol Biochem* 1993;16:157–166.

71. Divieti P, Inomata N, Chapin K, et al. Receptors for the carboxyl-terminal region of pth(1–84) are highly expressed in osteocytic cells. *Endocrinology* 2001;142:916–925.

72. Divieti P, John MR, Juppner H, Bringhurst FR. Human PTH-(7–84) inhibits bone resorption in vitro via actions independent of the type 1 PTH/PTHrP receptor. *Endocrinology* 143:171–176.

73. Torres A, Lorenzo V, Hernandez D, et al. Bone disease in predialysis, hemodialysis, and CAPD patients: evidence of a better bone response to PTH. *Kidney Int* 1995;47:1434–1442.

74. Hernandez D, Concepcion MT, Lorenzo V, et al. Adynamic bone disease with negative aluminium staining in predialysis patients: prevalence and evolution after maintenance dialysis. *Nephrol Dial Transplant* 1994;9:517–523.

75. Hutchison AJ, Whitehouse RW, Boulton HF, et al. Correlation of bone histology with parathyroid hormone, vitamin D3, and radiology in end-stage renal disease. *Kidney Int* 1993;44:1071–1077.

76. Malluche H, Faugere MC. Renal bone disease 1990: an unmet challenge for the nephrologist. *Kidney Int* 1990;38: 193–211.

77. Cohen-Solal ME, Sebert JL, Boudailliez B, et al. Non-aluminic adynamic bone disease in non-dialyzed uremic patients: a new type of osteopathy due to overtreatment? *Bone* 1992;13:1–5.

78. Coen G, Mazzaferro S, Ballanti P, et al. Renal bone disease in 76 patients with varying degrees of predialysis chronic kidney disease: a cross-sectional study. *Nephrol Dial Transpl*ant 1996;11:813–819.

79. Couttenye MM, D'Haese PC, Verschoren WJ, et al. Low bone turnover in patients with renal failure. *Kidney Int* 1999;56:S70–S76.

80. Yamamoto T, Ozono K, Miyauchi A, et al. Role of advanced glycation end products in adynamic bone disease in patients with diabetic nephropathy. *Am J Kidney Dis* 2001;38: S161–S164.

81. González E, Martin K. Aluminum and renal osteodystrophy: a diminishing clinical problem. *Trends Endocrinol Metab* 1992;3:371–375.

82. Malluche HH, Monier-Faugere MC. Uremic bone disease: current knowledge, controversial issues, and new horizons. *Miner Electrolyte Metab* 1991;17:281–296.

83. Clarke BL, Wynne AG, Wilson DM, Fitzpatrick LA. Osteomalacia associated with adult Fanconi's syndrome: clinical and diagnostic features. *Clin Endocrinol (Oxf)* 43: 479–490.

84. Ghazali A, Fardellone P, Pruna A, et al. Is low plasma 25-(OH)vitamin D a major risk factor for hyperparathyroidism and Looser's zones independent of calcitriol? *Kidney Int* 1999;55:2169–2177.

85. Krieger NS, Sessler NE, Bushinsky DA. Acidosis inhibits osteoblastic and stimulates osteoclastic activity in vitro. *Am J Physiol* 1992;262:F442–F448.

86. Kraut JA, Mishler DR, Singer FR, Goodman WG. The effects of metabolic acidosis on bone formation and bone resorption in the rat. *Kidney Int* 1986;30:694–700.

87. Coen G, Manni M, Addari O, et al. Metabolic acidosis and osteodystrophic bone disease in predialysis chronic kidney disease: effect of calcitriol treatment. *Miner Electrolyte Metab* 1995;21:375–382.

88. Coates T, Kirkland GS, Dymock RB, et al. Cutaneous necrosis from calcific uremic arteriolopathy (see comments). *Am J Kidney Dis* 1998;32:384–391.

89. Cohen-Solal ME, Augry F, Mauras Y, et al. Fluoride and strontium accumulation in bone does not correlate with osteoid tissue in dialysis patients. *Nephrol Dial Transplant* 2002;17:449–454.

90. Frick KK, Bushinsky DA. Chronic metabolic acidosis reversibly inhibits extracellular matrix gene expression in mouse osteoblasts. *Am J Physiol* 1998;275:F840–F847.

91. Frick KK, Bushinsky DA. In vitro metabolic and respiratory acidosis selectively inhibit osteoblastic matrix gene expression. *Am J Physiol* 1999;277:F750–F755.

92. Bushinsky DA, Nilsson EL. Additive effects of acidosis and parathyroid hormone on mouse osteoblastic and osteoclastic function. *Am J Physiol* 1995;269:C1364–C1370.

93. MacDonald PN, Haussler CA, Terpening CM, et al. Baculovirus-mediated expression of the human vitamin D receptor. Functional characterization, vitamin D response element interactions, and evidence for a receptor auxiliary factor. *J Biol Chem* 1991;266:18808–18813.

94. Martin KJ, Freitag JJ, Bellorin-Font E, et al. The effect of acute acidosis on the uptake of parathyroid hormone and the production of adenosine 3',5'-monophosphate by isolated perfused bone. *Endocrinology* 1980;106:1607–1611.

95. Cunningham J, Bikle DD, Avioli LV. Acute, but not chronic, metabolic acidosis disturbs 25-hydroxyvitamin D3 metabolism. *Kidney Int* 1984;25:47–52.

96. Krapf R, Vetsch R, Vetsch W, Hulter HN. Chronic metabolic acidosis increases the serum concentration of 1,25-dihydroxyvitamin D in humans by stimulating its production rate. Critical role of acidosis-induced renal hypophosphatemia. *J Clin Invest* 1992;90:2456–2463.

97. Frick KK, Bushinsky DA. Metabolic acidosis stimulates expression of rank ligand RNA. *J Am Soc Nephrol* 2002;13: 576A.

98. Disthabanchong S, Martin KJ, McConkey CL, Gonzalez EA. Metabolic acidosis up-regulates PTH/PTHrP receptors in UMR 106–01 osteoblast-like cells. *Kidney Int* 2002;62: 1171–1177.

99. Movilli E, Zani R, Carli O, et al. Direct effect of the correction of acidosis on plasma parathyroid hormone concentrations, calcium and phosphate in hemodialysis patients: a prospective study. *Nephron* 2001;87:257–262.

100. Lefebvre A, de Vernejoul MC, Gueris J, et al. Optimal correction of acidosis changes progression of dialysis osteodystrophy. *Kidney Int* 1989;36:1112–1118.

101. Manolagas SC, Weinstein RS. New developments in the pathogenesis and treatment of steroid-induced osteoporosis. *J Bone Miner Res* 1999;14:1061–1066.

102. Weinstein RS, Jilka RL, Parfitt AM, Manolagas SC. Inhibition of osteoblastogenesis and promotion of apoptosis of osteoblasts and osteocytes by glucocorticoids. Potential mechanisms of their deleterious effects on bone. *J Clin Invest* 1998;102:274–282.

103. Weinstein RS, Nicholas RW, Manolagas SC. Apoptosis of osteocytes in glucocorticoid-induced osteonecrosis of the hip. *J Clin Endocrinol Metab* 2000;85:2907–2912.

104. Lian JB, Stein GS, Canalis E, et al. Bone formation: osteoblast lineage cells, growth factors, matrix proteins, and the mineralization process. In: Favous MJ, ed. *Primer on The Metabolic Bone Diseases and Disorders of Mineral Metabolism*. Philadelphia: Lippincott Williams & Wilkins, 1999: 14–29.

105. Conover CA, Rosen C. The role of insulin-like growth factors and binding proteins in bone cell biology. In: Rodan GA, ed. *Principles of Bone Biology*. San Diego, CA: Academic Press, 2002:801–815.

106. Canalis E, McCarthy T, Centrella M. Isolation and characterization of insulin-like growth factor I (somatomedin-C) from cultures of fetal rat calvariae. *Endocrinology* 1988; 122:22–27.

107. Jones JI, Clemmons DR. Insulin-like growth factors and their binding proteins: biological actions. *Endocr Rev* 1995; 16:3–34.

108. Andress DL, Birnbaum RS. Human osteoblast-derived insulin-like growth factor (IGF) binding protein-5 stimulates

osteoblast mitogenesis and potentiates IGF action. *J Biol Chem* 1992;267:22467–22472.

109. Canalis E, Centrella M, Burch W, McCarthy TL. Insulin-like growth factor I mediates selective anabolic effects of parathyroid hormone in bone cultures. *J Clin Invest* 1989; 83:60–65.

110. McCarthy TL, Centrella M, Canalis E. Parathyroid hormone enhances the transcript and polypeptide levels of insulin-like growth factor I in osteoblast-enriched cultures from fetal rat bone. *Endocrinology* 1989;124:1247–1253.

111. McCarthy TL, Centrella M, Canalis E. Cyclic AMP induces insulin-like growth factor I synthesis in osteoblast-enriched cultures. *J Biol Chem* 1990;265:15353–15356.

112. Pfeilschifter J, Laukhuf F, Müller-Beckmann B, et al. Parathyroid hormone increases the concentration of insulin-like growth factor-I and transforming growth factor beta 1 in rat bone. *J Clin Invest* 1995;96:767–774.

113. Andress DL, Pandian MR, Endres DB, Kopp JB. Plasma insulin-like growth factors and bone formation in uremic hyperparathyroidism. *Kidney Int* 1989;36:471–477.

114. Weinreich T, Zapf J, Schmidt-Gayk H, et al. Insulin-like growth factor 1 and 2 serum concentrations in dialysis patients with secondary hyperparathyroidism and adynamic bone disease. *Clin Nephrol* 1999;51:27–33.

115. Jehle PM, Ostertag A, Schulten K, et al. Insulin-like growth factor system components in hyperparathyroidism and renal osteodystrophy. *Kidney Int* 2000;57:423–436.

116. Urist MR. Bone: formation by autoinduction. *Science* 1965; 150:893–899.

117. Gitelman SE, Kobrin MS, Ye JQ, et al. Recombinant Vgr-1/BMP-6-expressing tumors induce fibrosis and endochondral bone formation in vivo. *J Cell Biol* 1994;126: 1595–1609.

118. Reddi AH. Cell biology and biochemistry of endochondral bone development. *Collagen Rel Res* 1981;1:209–226.

119. Thies RS, Bauduy M, Ashton BA, et al. Recombinant human bone morphogenetic protein-2 induces osteoblastic differentiation in W-20–17 stromal cells. *Endocrinology* 1992;130:1318–1324.

120. Gimble JM, Morgan C, Kelly K, et al. Bone morphogenetic proteins inhibit adipocyte differentiation by bone marrow stromal cells. *J Cell Biochem* 1995;58:393–402.

121. Beresford JN, Bennett JH, Devlin C, et al. Evidence for an inverse relationship between the differentiation of adipocytic and osteogenic cells in rat marrow stromal cell cultures. *J Cell Sci* 1992;102(Pt 2):341–351.

122. Ozkaynak E, Schnegelsberg PN, Oppermann H. Murine osteogenic protein (OP-1): high levels of mRNA in kidney. *Biochem Biophys Res Commun* 1991;179:116–123.

123. Gonzalez EA, Lund RJ, Martin KJ, et al. Treatment of a murine model of high-turnover renal osteodystrophy by exogenous BMP-7. *Kidney Int* 2002;61:1322–1331.

124. Drake MT, Baldassare JJ, McConkey CL, et al. Parathyroid hormone increases the expression of receptors for epidermal growth factor in UMR 106–01 cells. *Endocrinology* 1994; 134:1733–1737.

125. Yoneda T. Local regulators of bone. In: Rodan GA, ed. *Principles of Bone Biology*. San Diego, CA: Academic Press, 1996:729–738.

126. Chien HH, Lin WL, Cho MI. Down-regulation of osteoblastic cell differentiation by epidermal growth factor receptor. *Calcif Tissue Int* 2000;67:141–150.

127. Kimmel PL, Phillips TM, Simmens SJ, et al. Immunologic function and survival in hemodialysis patients. *Kidney Int* 1998;54:236–244.

128. Herbelin A, Nguyen AT, Zingraff J, et al. Influence of uremia and hemodialysis on circulating interleukin-1 and tumor necrosis factor alpha. *Kidney Int* 1990;37:116–125.

129. Ferreira A, Simon P, Drueke TB, Deschamps-Latscha B. Potential role of cytokines in renal osteodystrophy (letter). *Nephrol Dial Transplant* 1996;11:399–400.

130. Miyaura C, Inada M, Matsumoto C, et al. An essential role of cytosolic phospholipase A2alpha in prostaglandin E2-mediated bone resorption associated with inflammation. *J Exp Med* 2003;197:1303–1310.

131. Ferreira A. Biochemical markers of bone turnover in the diagnosis of renal osteodystrophy: what do we have, what do we need? *Nephrol Dial Transplant* 1998;13(suppl 3):29–32.

132. Moutabarrik A, Nakanishi I, Namiki M, Tsubakihara Y. Interleukin-1 and its naturally occurring antagonist in peritoneal dialysis patients. *Clin Nephrol* 1995;43:243–248.

133. Herbelin A, Ureña P, Nguyen AT, et al. Elevated circulating levels of interleukin-6 in patients with chronic kidney disease. *Kidney Int* 1991;39:954–960.

134. Montalbán C, García-Unzueta MT, De Francisco AL, Amado JA. Serum interleukin-6 in renal osteodystrophy: relationship with serum PTH and bone remodeling markers. *Horm Metab Res* 1999;31:14–17.

135. Langub MC Jr, Koszewski NJ, Turner HV, et al. Bone resorption and mRNA expression of IL-6 and IL-6 receptor in patients with renal osteodystrophy. *Kidney Int* 1996;50: 515–520.

136. Memoli B, Postiglione L, Cianciaruso B, et al. Role of different dialysis membranes in the release of interleukin-6-soluble receptor in uremic patients. *Kidney Int* 2000;58: 417–424.

137. Le Meur Y, Lorgeot V, Aldigier JC, et al. Whole blood production of monocytic cytokines (IL-1B, IL-6, TNF-a, sIL-6R, IL-1Ra) in hemodialysed patients. *Nephrol Dial Transplant* 1999;14:2420–2426.

138. Siggelkow H, Eidner T, Lehmann G, et al. Cytokines, osteoprotegerin, and RANKL in vitro and histomorphometric indices of bone turnover in patients with different bone diseases. *J Bone Miner Res* 2003;18:529–538.

139. Chiba S, Un-No M, Neer RM, et al. Parathyroid hormone induces interleukin-6 gene expression in bone stromal cells of young rats. *J Vet Med Sci* 2002;64:641–644.

140. Santos FR, Moyses RM, Montenegro FL, et al. IL-1 beta, TNF-alpha, TGF-beta, and bFGF expression in bone biopsies before and after parathyroidectomy. *Kidney Int* 2003; 63:899–907.

141. Kazama JJ, Shigematsu T, Yano K, et al. Increased circulating levels of osteoclastogenesis inhibitory factor (osteoprotegerin) in patients with chronic kidney disease. *Am J Kidney Dis* 2002;39:525–532.

142. Haas M, Leko-Mohr Z, Roschger P, et al. Osteoprotegerin and parathyroid hormone as markers of high-turnover os-

teodystrophy and decreased bone mineralization in hemodialysis patients. *Am J Kidney Dis* 2002;39:580–586.

143. Baker LR, Ackrill P, Cattell WR, et al. Iatrogenic osteomalacia and myopathy due to phosphate depletion. *Br Med J* 1974;3:150–152.

144. Mallette LE, Patten BM, Engel WK. Neuromuscular disease in secondary hyperparathyroidism. *Ann Intern Med* 1975;82:474–483.

145. Lotem M, Berheim J, Conforty B. Spontaneous rupture of tendons. A complication of hemodialyzed patients treated for renal failure. *Nephron* 1978;21:201–208.

146. Lotem M, Robson MD, Rosenfeld JB. Spontaneous rupture of the quadriceps tendon in patients on chronic haemodialysis. *Ann Rheum Dis* 1974;33:428–429.

147. De Franco P, Varghese J, Brown WW, Bastani B. Secondary hyperparathyroidism, and not beta 2-microglobulin amyloid, as a cause of spontaneous tendon rupture in patients on chronic hemodialysis. *Am J Kidney Dis* 1994;24:951–955.

148. Wang AY, Wang M, Woo J, et al. Cardiac valve calcification as an important predictor for all-cause mortality and cardiovascular mortality in long-term peritoneal dialysis patients: a prospective study. *J Am Soc Nephrol* 2003;14:159–168.

149. Salgueira M, Del Toro N, Moreno-Alba R, et al. Vascular calcification in the uremic patient: a cardiovascular risk? *Kidney Int Suppl* 2003;85:5119–5121.

150. Goodman WG. Vascular calcification in end-stage renal disease. *J Nephrol* 2002;15(suppl 6):S82–S85.

151. London GM, Guerin AP, Marchais SJ, et al. Arterial media calcification in end-stage renal disease: impact on all-cause and cardiovascular mortality. *Nephrol Dial Transplant* 2003;18:1731–1740.

152. Angelis M, Wong LL, Myers SA, Wong LM. Calciphylaxis in patients on hemodialysis: a prevalence study. *Surgery* 1997;122:1083–1089; discussion 1089–1090.

153. Seyle H. *Calciphylaxis*. Chicago: University of Chicago Press, 1962.

154. Bleyer AJ, Choi M, Igwemezie B, et al. A case control study of proximal calciphylaxis (see comments). *Am J Kidney Dis* 1998;32:376–383.

155. Comp PC, Elrod JP, Karzenski S. Warfarin-induced skin necrosis. *Semin Thromb Hemost* 1990;16:293–298.

156. Kant KS, Glueck HI, Coots MC, et al. Protein S deficiency and skin necrosis associated with continuous ambulatory peritoneal dialysis. *Am J Kidney Dis* 1992;19:264–271.

157. Mehta RL, Scott G, Sloand JA, Francis CW. Skin necrosis associated with acquired protein C deficiency in patients with renal failure and calciphylaxis. *Am J Med* 1990;88:252–257.

158. Westenfeld R, Heiss A, Ketteler M, et al. Calciphylaxis is linked to systemic deficiency of the calcification inhibitor ahsg/fetuin. *J Am Soc Nephrol* 2002;13:461A.

159. Schafer C, Heiss A, Schwarz A, et al. The serum protein alpha 2-Heremans-Schmid glycoprotein/fetuin-A is a systemically acting inhibitor of ectopic calcification. *J Clin Invest* 2003;112:357–366.

160. Jahnen-Dechent W, Schinke T, Trindl A, et al. Cloning and targeted deletion of the mouse fetuin gene. *J Biol Chem* 1997;272:31496–31503.

161. Canfield AE, Farrington C, Dziobon MD, et al. The involvement of matrix glycoproteins in vascular calcification and fibrosis: an immunohistochemical study. *J Pathol* 2002;196:228–234.

162. Goodman WG, Goldin J, Kuizon BD, et al. Coronary-artery calcification in young adults with end-stage renal disease who are undergoing dialysis. *N Engl J Med* 2000;342:1478–1483.

163. Reslerova M, Moe SM. Vascular calcification in dialysis patients: pathogenesis and consequences. *Am J Kidney Dis* 2003;41:S96–S99.

164. Ganesh SK, Stack AG, Levin NW, et al. Association of elevated serum PO(4), Ca x PO(4) product, and parathyroid hormone with cardiac mortality risk in chronic hemodialysis patients. *J Am Soc Nephrol* 2001;12:2131–2138.

165. London GM, Pannier B, Marchais SJ, Guerin AP. Calcification of the aortic valve in the dialyzed patient. *J Am Soc Nephrol* 2000;11:778–783.

166. Block GA, Port FK. Re-evaluation of risks associated with hyperphosphatemia and hyperparathyroidism in dialysis patients: recommendations for a change in management. *Am J Kidney Dis* 2000;35:1226–1237.

167. Raggi P. Imaging of cardiovascular calcifications with electron beam tomography in hemodialysis patients. *Am J Kidney Dis* 2001;37:S62–S65.

168. London GM, Blacher J, Pannier B, et al. Arterial wave reflections and survival in end-stage renal failure. *Hypertension* 2001;38:434–438.

169. Parhami F, Bostrom K, Watson K, Demer LL. Role of molecular regulation in vascular calcification. *J Atheroscler Thromb* 1996;3:90–94.

170. Giachelli CM. Ectopic calcification: gathering hard facts about soft tissue mineralization. *Am J Pathol* 1999;154:671–675.

171. Luo G, Ducy P, McKee MD, et al. Spontaneous calcification of arteries and cartilage in mice lacking matrix GLA protein. *Nature* 1997;386:78–81.

172. Kuro-o M, Matsumura Y, Aizawa H, et al. Mutation of the mouse klotho gene leads to a syndrome resembling ageing. *Nature* 1997;390:45–51.

173. Bucay N, Sarosi I, Dunstan CR, et al. Osteoprotegerin-deficient mice develop early onset osteoporosis and arterial calcification. *Genes Dev* 1998;12:1260–1268.

174. González EA, Martin KJ. Renal osteodystrophy: pathogenesis and management. *Nephrol Dial Transplant* 1995;10(suppl 3):13–21.

175. Ketteler M, Bongartz P, Westenfeld R, et al. Association of low fetuin-A (AHSG) concentrations in serum with cardiovascular mortality in patients on dialysis: a cross-sectional study. *Lancet* 2003;361:827–833.

176. Ketteler M, Vermeer C, Wanner C, et al. Novel insights into uremic vascular calcification: role of matrix Gla protein and alpha-2-Heremans Schmid glycoprotein. *Blood Purif* 2002;20:473–476.

177. Ketteler M, Wanner C, Metzger T, et al. Deficiencies of calcium-regulatory proteins in dialysis patients: a novel concept of cardiovascular calcification in uremia. *Kidney Int Suppl* 2003;84:S84–S87.

178. Jono S, McKee MD, Murry CE, et al. Phosphate regulation of vascular smooth muscle cell calcification. *Circ Res* 2000;87:E10–17.

179. Giachelli CM, Jono S, Shioi A, et al. Vascular calcification and inorganic phosphate. *Am J Kidney Dis* 2001;38: S34–S37.

180. Tintut Y, Patel J, Parhami F, Demer LL. Tumor necrosis factor-alpha promotes in vitro calcification of vascular cells via the cAMP pathway. *Circulation* 2000;102:2636–2642.

181. Wolf G, Chen S, Han DC, Ziyadeh FN. Leptin and renal disease. *Am J Kidney Dis* 2002;39:1–11.

182. Parhami F, Tintut Y, Ballard A, et al. Leptin enhances the calcification of vascular cells: artery wall as a target of leptin. *Circ Res* 2001;88:954–960.

183. Dzido G, Sprague SM. Dialysis-related amyloidosis. *Minerva Urol Nefrol* 2000;55:121–129.

184. Kenzora JE. Dialysis carpal tunnel syndrome. *Orthopedics* 1978;1:195–203.

185. Bardin T, Zingraff J, Shirahama T, et al. Hemodialysis-associated amyloidosis and beta-2 microglobulin. Clinical and immunohistochemical study. *Am J Med* 1987;83:419–424.

186. Bardin T, Zingraff J, Kuntz D, Drueke T. Dialysis-related amyloidosis. *Nephrol Dial Transplant* 1986;1:151–154.

187. Bardin T, Kuntz D, Zingraff J, et al. Synovial amyloidosis in patients undergoing long-term hemodialysis. *Arthritis Rheum* 1985;28:1052–1058.

188. Bardin T. Dialysis related amyloidosis. *J Rheumatol* 1987; 14:647–649.

189. Drueke TB, Zingraff J, Noel LH, et al. Amyloidosis and dialysis: pathophysiological aspects. *Contrib Nephrol* 1988; 62:60–66.

190. Zingraff JJ, Noel LH, Bardin T, et al. Beta 2-microglobulin amyloidosis in chronic kidney disease. *N Engl J Med* 1990; 323:1070–1071.

191. Connors LH, Shirahama T, Skinner M, et al. In vitro formation of amyloid fibrils from intact beta 2-microglobulin. *Biochem Biophys Res Commun* 1985;131:1063–1068.

192. Campistol JM, Sole M, Bombi JA, et al. In vitro spontaneous synthesis of beta 2-microglobulin amyloid fibrils in peripheral blood mononuclear cell culture. *Am J Pathol* 1992;141:241–247.

193. Ono K, Uchino F. Formation of amyloid-like substance from beta-2-microglobulin in vitro. Role of serum amyloid P component: a preliminary study. *Nephron* 1994;66:404–407.

194. Miyata T, Oda O, Inagi R, et al. beta 2-Microglobulin modified with advanced glycation end products is a major component of hemodialysis-associated amyloidosis. *J Clin Invest* 1993;92:1243–1252.

195. Floege J, Ketteler M. beta2-microglobulin-derived amyloidosis: an update. *Kidney Int Suppl* 2001;78:S164–S171.

196. Kessler M, Netter P, Azoulay E, et al. Dialysis-associated arthropathy: a multicentre survey of 171 patients receiving haemodialysis for over 10 years. The Co-operative Group on Dialysis-associated Arthropathy. *Br J Rheumatol* 1992;31: 157–162.

197. Jadoul M. Dialysis-related amyloidosis: importance of biocompatibility and age. *Nephrol Dial Transplant* 1998; 13(suppl 7):61–64.

198. Stein G, Schneider A, Thoss K, et al. Beta-2-microglobulin-derived amyloidosis: onset, distribution and clinical features in 13 hemodialysed patients. *Nephron* 1992;60:274–280.

199. van Ypersele de Strihou C, Jadoul M, Malghem J, et al. Effect of dialysis membrane and patient's age on signs of dialysis-related amyloidosis. The Working Party on Dialysis Amyloidosis. *Kidney Int* 1991;39:1012–1019.

200. Vandenbroucke JM, Jadoul M, Maldague B, et al. Possible role of dialysis membrane characteristics in amyloid osteoarthropathy. *Lancet* 1986;1:1210–1211.

201. Pickett TM, Cruickshank A, Greenwood RN, et al. Membrane flux not biocompatibility determines beta-2-microglobulin levels in hemodialysis patients. *Blood Purif* 2002;20:161–166.

202. Kuntz D, Naveau B, Bardin T, et al. Destructive spondyloarthropathy in hemodialyzed patients. A new syndrome. *Arthritis Rheum* 1984;27:369–375.

203. Bardin T, Kuntz D. The arthropathy of chronic haemodialysis. *Clin Exp Rheumatol* 1987;5:379–386.

204. Konishiike T, Hashizume H, Nishida K, et al. Shoulder pain in long-term haemodialysis patients. A clinical study of 166 patients. *J Bone Joint Surg Br* 1996;78:601–605.

205. Katz GA, Peter JB, Pearson CM, Adams WS. The shoulder-pad sign—a diagnostic feature of amyloid arthropathy. *N Engl J Med* 1973;288:354–355.

206. Kaplan P, Resnick D, Murphey M, et al. Destructive noninfectious spondyloarthropathy in hemodialysis patients: a report of four cases. *Radiology* 1987;162:241–244.

207. Menard HA, Langevin S, Levesque RY. Destructive spondyloarthropathy in short term chronic ambulatory peritoneal dialysis and hemodialysis. *J Rheumatol* 1998;15:644–647.

208. Cruz A, Gonzalez T, Balsa A, et al. Destructive spondyloarthropathy in long-term CAPD and hemodialysis. *J Rheumatol* 1989;16:1169–1170.

209. Bardin T. Dialysis-associated amyloidosis. In: Drueke T, ed. *The Spectrum of Renal Osteodystrophy*. New York: Oxford University Press, 2001:285–307.

210. Kates D, Sherrard D, Andress D. Evidence that serum phosphate is independently associated with serum PTH in patients with chronic kidney disease. *Am J Kidney Dis* 1997; 30:809–813.

211. Boyce BF, Fell GS, Elder HY, et al. Hypercalcaemic osteomalacia due to aluminium toxicity. *Lancet* 1982;2: 1009–1013.

212. Kurz P, Monier-Faugere MC, Bognar B, et al. Evidence for abnormal calcium homeostasis in patients with adynamic bone disease. *Kidney Int* 1994;46:855–861.

213. Martin KJ, Gonzalez EA. The evolution of assays for parathyroid hormone. *Curr Opin Nephrol Hypertens* 2001; 10:569–574.

214. Canterbury JM, Reiss E. Multiple immunoreactive molecular forms of parathyroid hormone in human serum. 1. *Proc Soc Exp Biol Med* 1972;140:1393–1398.

215. Habener JF, Segre GV, Powell D, et al. Immunoreactive parathyroid hormone in circulation of man. *Nat New Biol* 1972;238:152–154.

216. Martin KJ, Hruska K, Freitag JJ, et al. Clinical utility of radioimmunoassays for parathyroid hormone. *Miner Electrolyte Metab* 1980;3:283–290.

217. Nussbaum SR, Zahradnik RJ, Lavigne JR, et al. Highly sensitive two-site immunoradiometric assay of parathyrin, and its clinical utility in evaluating patients with hypercalcemia. *Clin Chem* 1987;33:1364–1367.

218. Brown RC, Aston JP, Weeks I, Woodhead JS. Circulating intact parathyroid hormone measured by a two-site immunochemiluminometric assay. *J Clin Endocrinol Metab* 1987; 65:407–414.

219. Kao PC, van Heerden JA, Grant CS, et al. Clinical performance of parathyroid hormone immunometric assays. *Mayo Clin Proc* 1992;67:637–645.

220. Lepage R, Roy L, Brossard JH, et al. A non-(1–84) circulating parathyroid hormone (PTH) fragment interferes significantly with intact PTH commercial assay measurements in uremic samples. *Clin Chem* 1998;44:805–809.

221. Brossard JH, Lepage R, Gao P, et al. A new commercial whole-PTH assay free of interference by non-(1–84) parathyroid hormone fragments in uremic samples. *J Bone Miner Res* 1999;14:S444.

222. Gao P, Scheibel S, D'Amour P, et al. Development of a novel immunoradiometric assay exclusively for biologically active whole parathyroid hormone 1–84: implications for improvement of accurate assessment of parathyroid function. *J Bone Miner Res* 2001;16:605–614.

223. Langub MC, Monier-Faugere MC, Wang G, et al. Administration of PTH-(7–84) antagonizes the effects of PTH-(1–84) on bone in rats with moderate renal failure. *Endocrinology* 2003;144:1135–1138.

224. Monier-Faugere MC, Geng Z, Mawad H, et al. Improved assessment of bone turnover by the PTH-(1–84)/large C-PTH fragments ratio in ESRD patients. *Kidney Int* 60:1460–1468.

225. Coen G, Bonucci E, Ballanti P, et al. PTH 1–84 and PTH "7–84" in the noninvasive diagnosis of renal bone disease. *Am J Kidney Dis* 2002;40:348–354.

226. Salusky IB, Goodman WG, Kuizon BD, et al. Similar predictive value of bone turnover using first- and second-generation immunometric PTH assays in pediatric patients treated with peritoneal dialysis. *Kidney Int* 2003;63:1801–1808.

227. Goldstein DJ, Rogers C, Harris H. A search for trace expression of placental-like alkaline phosphatase in non-malignant human tissues: demonstration of its occurrence in lung, cervix, testis and thymus. *Clin Chim Acta* 1982;125:63–75.

228. Seargeant LE, Stinson RA. Evidence that three structural genes code for human alkaline phosphatases. *Nature* 1979; 281:152–154.

229. Weiss MJ, Henthorn PS, Lafferty MA, et al. Isolation and characterization of a cDNA encoding a human liver/bone/kidney-type alkaline phosphatase. *Proc Natl Acad Sci USA* 1986;83:7182–7186.

230. Pierides AM, Skillen AW, Ellis HA. Serum alkaline phosphatase in azotemic and hemodialysis osteodystrophy: a study of isoenzyme patterns, their correlation with bone histology, and their changes in response to treatment with 1alphaOHD3 and 1,25(OH)2D3. *J Lab Clin Med* 1979;93: 899–909.

231. Cannella G, Bonucci E, Rolla D, et al. Evidence of healing of secondary hyperparathyroidism in chronically hemodialyzed uremic patients treated with long-term intravenous calcitriol. *Kidney Int* 1994;46:1124–1132.

232. Urena P, De Vernejoul MC. Circulating biochemical markers of bone remodeling in uremic patients. *Kidney Int* 1999;55: 2141–2156.

233. Coen G, Ballanti P, Bonucci E, et al. Bone markers in the diagnosis of low turnover osteodystrophy in haemodialysis patients. *Nephrol Dial Transplant* 1998;13:2294–2302.

234. Jarava C, Armas JR, Salgueira M, Palma A. Bone alkaline phosphatase isoenzyme in renal osteodystrophy. *Nephrol Dial Transplant* 1996;11:43–46.

235. Urena P, Hruby M, Ferreira A, et al. Plasma total versus bone alkaline phosphatase as markers of bone turnover in hemodialysis patients. *J Am Soc Nephrol* 1996;7:506–512.

236. Goodman WG, Ramirez JA, Belin TR, et al. Development of adynamic bone in patients with secondary hyperparathyroidism after intermittent calcitriol therapy. *Kidney Int* 1994; 46:1160–1166.

237. Couttenye MM, D'Haese PC, Van Hoof VO, et al. Low serum levels of alkaline phosphatase of bone origin: a good marker of adynamic bone disease in haemodialysis patients. *Nephrol Dial Transplant* 1996;11:1065–1072.

238. Pei Y, Hercz G, Greenwood C, et al. Risk factors for renal osteodystrophy: a multivariant analysis. *J Bone Miner Res* 1995;10:149–156.

239. Kohlmeier M, Saupe J, Shearer MJ, et al. Bone health of adult hemodialysis patients is related to vitamin K status. *Kidney Int* 1997;51:1218–1221.

240. Kohlmeier M, Saupe J, Schaefer K, Asmus G. Bone fracture history and prospective bone fracture risk of hemodialysis patients are related to apolipoprotein E genotype. *Calcif Tissue Int* 1998;62:278–281.

241. Szulc P, Chapuy MC, Meunier PJ, Delmas PD. Serum undercarboxylated osteocalcin is a marker of the risk of hip fracture: a three year follow-up study. *Bone* 1996;18: 487–488.

242. Vermeer C, Jie KS, Knapen MH. Role of vitamin K in bone metabolism. *Annu Rev Nutr* 1995;15:1–22.

243. Qi Q, Monier-Faugere MC, Geng Z, Malluche HH. Predictive value of serum parathyroid hormone levels for bone turnover in patients on chronic maintenance dialysis. *Am J Kidney Dis* 1995;26:622–631.

244. Gerakis A, Hutchison AJ, Apostolou T, et al. Biochemical markers for non-invasive diagnosis of hyperparathyroid bone disease and adynamic bone in patients on haemodialysis. *Nephrol Dial Transplant* 1996;11:2430–2438.

245. Malluche HH, Faugere MC, Fanti P, Price PA. Plasma levels of bone Gla-protein reflect bone formation in patients on chronic maintenance dialysis. *Kidney Int* 1984;26:869–874.

246. Coen G, Mazzaferro S, Bonucci E, et al. Bone GLA protein in predialysis chronic kidney disease. Effects of 1,25(OH)2D3 administration in a long-term follow-up. *Kidney Int* 1985;28:783–790.

247. Urena P, Ferreira A, Kung VT, et al. Serum pyridinoline as a specific marker of collagen breakdown and bone metabolism in hemodialysis patients. *J Bone Miner Res* 1995;10: 932–939.

248. Hoshino H, Kushida K, Takahashi M, et al. Short-term effect of parathyroidectomy on biochemical markers in primary and secondary hyperparathyroidism. *Miner Electrolyte Metab* 1997;23:93–99.

249. Parfitt AM, Simon LS, Villanueva AR, Krane SM. Procollagen type I carboxy-terminal extension peptide in serum as a marker of collagen biosynthesis in bone. Correlation with Iliac bone formation rates and comparison with total alkaline phosphatase. *J Bone Miner Res* 1987;2:427–436.

250. Ibrahim S, Mojiminiyi S, Barron JL. Pyridinium crosslinks in patients on haemodialysis and continuous ambulatory peritoneal dialysis. *Nephrol Dial Transplant* 1995;10:2290–2294.

251. Cheung CK, Panesar NS, Haines C, et al. Immunoassay of a tartrate-resistant acid phosphatase in serum. *Clin Chem* 1995;41:679–686.

252. Chamberlain P, Compston J, Cox TM, et al. Generation and characterization of monoclonal antibodies to human type-5 tartrate-resistant acid phosphatase: development of a specific immunoassay of the isoenzyme in serum. *Clin Chem* 1995;41:1495–1499.

253. Kraenzlin ME, Lau KH, Liang L, et al. Development of an immunoassay for human serum osteoclastic tartrate-resistant acid phosphatase. *J Clin Endocrinol Metab* 1990;71:442–451.

254. Halleen J, Hentunen TA, Hellman J, Vaananen HK. Tartrate-resistant acid phosphatase from human bone: purification and development of an immunoassay. *J Bone Miner Res* 1996;11:1444–1452.

255. Halleen JM, Ylipahkala H, Alatalo SL, et al. Serum tartrate-resistant acid phosphatase 5b, but not 5a, correlates with other markers of bone turnover and bone mineral density. *Calcif Tissue Int* 2002;71:20–25.

256. Lau KH, Onishi T, Wergedal JE, et al. Characterization and assay of tartrate-resistant acid phosphatase activity in serum: potential use to assess bone resorption. *Clin Chem* 1987;33:458–462.

257. Halleen JM, Alatalo SL, Suominen H, et al. Tartrate-resistant acid phosphatase 5b: a novel serum marker of bone resorption. *J Bone Miner Res* 2000;15:1337–1345.

258. Milliner DS, Nebeker HG, Ott SM, et al. Use of the deferoxamine infusion test in the diagnosis of aluminum-related osteodystrophy. *Ann Intern Med* 1984;101:775–779.

259. D'Haese PC, Clement JP, Elseviers MM, et al. Value of serum aluminium monitoring in dialysis patients: a multicentre study. *Nephrol Dial Transplant* 1990;5:45–53.

260. D'Haese PC, Couttenye MM, Goodman WG, et al. Use of the low-dose desferrioxamine test to diagnose and differentiate between patients with aluminium-related bone disease, increased risk for aluminium toxicity, or aluminium overload. *Nephrol Dial Transplant* 1995;10:1874–1884.

261. D'Haese PC, Couttenye MM, De Broe ME. Diagnosis and treatment of aluminium bone disease. *Nephrol Dial Transplant* 1996;11:74–79.

262. Pei Y, Hercz G, Greenwood C, et al. Non-invasive prediction of aluminum bone disease in hemo- and peritoneal dialysis patients. *Kidney Int* 1992;41:1374–1382.

263. Cannata JB, Fernandez-Martin JL, Diaz-Lopez B, et al. Influence of iron status in the response to the deferoxamine test. *J Am Soc Nephrol* 1996;7:135–139 .

264. Huang JY, Huang CC, Lim PS, et al. Effect of body iron stores on serum aluminum level in hemodialysis patients. *Nephron* 1992;61:158–162.

265. Vanuytsel JL, D'Haese PC, Couttenye MM, De Broe ME. Higher serum aluminium concentrations in iron-depleted dialysis patients. *Nephrol Dial Transplant* 1992;7:177.

266. Disthabanchong S, Gonzalez EA. Regulation of bone cell development and function: implication for renal osteodystrophy. *J Invest Med* 2001;49:240–249.

267. Hory B, Drüeke TB. The parathyroid-bone axis in uremia: new insights into old questions. *Curr Opin Nephrol Hypertens* 1997;6:40–48.

268. Hruska K. New concepts in renal osteodystrophy. *Nephrol Dial Transplant* 1998;13:2755–2760.

269. Monier-Faugere MC, Malluche HH. Role of cytokines in renal osteodystrophy. *Curr Opin Nephrol Hypertens* 1997;6:327–332.

270. Fiocchi O, Bedani PL, Orzincolo C, et al. Radiological features of dialysis amyloid spondyloarthropathy. *Int J Artif Organs* 1989;12:216–222.

271. Cueto-Manzano AM, Konel S, Hutchison AJ, et al. Bone loss in long-term renal transplantation: histopathology and densitometry analysis. *Kidney Int* 1999;55:2021–2029.

272. Maruyama H, Gejyo F, Arakawa M. Clinical studies of destructive spondyloarthropathy in long-term hemodialysis patients. *Nephron* 1992;61:37–44.

273. Massry S. K/DOQI guidelines released on bone metabolism and disease in CKD. *Nephrol News Issues* 2003;17:38–41, 44.

274. Nordal KP, Dahl E. Low dose calcitriol versus placebo in patients with predialysis chronic kidney disease. *J Clin Endocrinol Metab* 1988;67:929–936.

275. Bianchi ML, Colantonio G, Campanini F, et al. Calcitriol and calcium carbonate therapy in early chronic kidney disease. *Nephrol Dial Transplant* 1994;9:1595–1599.

276. Coen G, Mazzaferro S, Bonucci E, et al. Treatment of secondary hyperparathyroidism of predialysis chronic kidney disease with low doses of 1,25(OH)2D3: humoral and histomorphometric results. *Miner Electrolyte Metab* 1986;12:375–382.

277. Slatopolsky E, Weerts C, Thielan J, et al. Marked suppression of secondary hyperparathyroidism by intravenous administration of 1,25-dihydroxy-cholecalciferol in uremic patients. *J Clin Invest* 1984;74:2136–2143.

278. Martin KJ, González EA, Gellens M, et al. 19-Nor-1-a-25-Dihydroxyvitamin D_2 (Paricalcitol) safely and effectively reduces the levels of intact PTH in patients on hemodialysis. *J Am Soc Nephrol* 1998;9:1427–1432.

279. Maung HM, Elangovan L, Frazao JM, et al. Efficacy and side effects of intermittent intravenous and oral doxercalciferol [1alpha-hydroxyvitamin D(2)] in dialysis patients with secondary hyperparathyroidism: a sequential comparison. *Am J Kidney Dis* 2001;37:532–543.

280. Sjoden G, Smith C, Lindgren U, DeLuca HF. 1 alpha-Hydroxyvitamin D2 is less toxic than 1 alpha-hydroxyvitamin D3 in the rat. *Proc Soc Exp Biol Med* 1985;178:432–436.

281. Weber K, Goldberg M, Stangassinger M, Erben RG. 1 alpha-hydroxyvitamin D2 is less toxic but not bone selective relative to 1 alpha-hydroxyvitamin D3 in ovariectomized rats. *J Bone Miner Res* 2001;16:639–651.

282. Quarles LD, Sherrard DJ, Adler S, et al. The calcimimetic AMG 073 as a potential treatment for secondary hyper-

parathyroidism of end-stage renal disease. *J Am Soc Nephrol* 2003;14:575–583.

283. Lindberg JS, Moe SM, Goodman WG, et al. The calcimimetic AMG 073 reduces parathyroid hormone and calcium x phosphorus in secondary hyperparathyroidism. *Kidney Int* 2003;63:248–254.

284. Goodman WG, Hladik GA, Turner SA, et al. The calcimimetic agent AMG 073 lowers plasma parathyroid hormone levels in hemodialysis patients with secondary hyperparathyroidism. *J Am Soc Nephrol* 2002;13:1017–1024.

285. Mucsi I, Hercz G, Uldall R, et al. Control of serum phosphate without any phosphate binders in patients treated with nocturnal hemodialysis. *Kidney Int* 1998;53:1399–1404.

286. Kitaoka M, Fukagawa M, Ogata E, Kurokawa K. Reduction of functioning parathyroid cell mass by ethanol injection in chronic dialysis patients. *Kidney Int* 1994;46:1110–1117.

287. Fukagawa M, Kitaoka M, Tominaga Y, et al. Selective percutaneous ethanol injection therapy (PEIT) of the parathyroid in chronic dialysis patients—the Japanese strategy. Japanese Working Group on PEIT of Parathyroid, Tokyo, Japan. *Nephrol Dial Transplant* 1999;14:2574–2577.

Neurologic Aspects of Dialysis

Stefano Biasioli

This chapter summarizes the current status of uremic encephalopathy: its pathophysiology, its possible management, and approaches for the future. The neurologic complications of uremia, though identified and described since 1839, have been extensively evaluated only during the past 20 years, primarily as a result of detailed studies on the progression of chronic kidney disease (CKD) and the remarkable survival times of dialyzed patients.[1-4] Two major clinical neurologic syndromes can be observed in uremic patients: (1) uremic encephalopathy (UE), which is closely linked to the progression of kidney disease, and (2) dialysis encephalopathy (DE), resulting from the dialysis treatment itself.[5-9]

UREMIC ENCEPHALOPATHY

Uremic encephalopathy (UE) encompasses the brain dysfunction of uremic individuals and is generally seen prior to the initiation of dialysis. As shown in Table 31–1, uremia is only one of the numerous causes of metabolic encephalopathy (ME). On the other hand, many of the conditions listed can be simultaneously found in uremic patients.

Anemia; impaired glucose metabolism; malnutrition; coenzyme lack; disturbances in fluid, electrolyte, acid-base, and hormonal status; and decreased psychosocial functioning all are present in the "constellation" of neurobehavioral abnormalities of uremia.

Metabolic and toxic disorders of various types produce similar effects on the central nervous system (CNS). Sensorial clouding, dysarthria, tremors, asterixis, asthenia, clumsiness, and seizures are the most common clinical manifestations of metabolic encephalopathies, including uremia. Any one of these may prevail in a given patient, but the fluctuations (daily or hourly) of the neurologic signs in the same patient are unpredictable and typical of this syndrome.

UE may remain subclinical for a long time if renal function decreases gradually, but occasionally it becomes evident in the early stages of renal failure. Thus, the clinical features of UE (Table 31–2) can be divided into early and late disturbances. Four main categories of clinical features are evident: mental function and level of consciousness, neurologic disturbances, motor abnormalities, and hormonal status.

TABLE 31–1. CAUSES OF METABOLIC ENCEPHALOPATHY (ME)

- Respiratory disease
- Infections
- Impaired glucose metabolism
- Anemia
- Nutritional imbalances
- Disturbances in fluid, electrolyte, and acid base balance
- Endocrinopathies
- Liver diseases (necrosis, portal-systemic shunts)
- Uremia
- Body temperature changes
- Intoxications (drugs, etc.)
- Decreased psychosocial adaptation

TABLE 31–2. CLINICAL FEATURES OF UREMIC ENCEPHALOPATHY

Early	Late
• Respiratory disease	• Endocrinopathies
• Infections	• Liver diseases (necrosis,
• Impaired glucose	portal-systemic shunts)
metabolism	• Uremia
• Anemia	• Body temperature changes
• Nutritional imbalance	• Intoxications (drugs, etc.)
• Disturbances in fluid,	• Decreased psychosocial
electrolyte, and acid	adaptation
base balance	

Disturbances of Mental Function

Sensorial Clouding {
• Malaise	• Defective cognition
• Anxiety	• Obtundation
• Loss of recent memory	• Errors of perception
• Impaired concentration	• Illusion
• Insomnia	• Visual hallucinations
• Fatigue	• Agitation
• Apathy	• Delirium
	• Stupor
	• Coma

Neurologic Disturbances

• Dysarthria (slow,	• Myoclonus ⎤ Uremic
slurred, thickened	• Tetany ⎦ Twitching
speech)	
• Tremors	
• Asterixis	

Motor Abnormalities

• Clumsiness	• Limb muscle tone alteration
• Unsteadiness	• Stretch-reflex asymmetry
• Increase of grasp	• Hemiparesis
reflexes	• Convulsions
• Asthenia	

Hormonal Changes

• Altered prolactin	• Hyperprolactinemia
secretion	• Increased PTH
• Increased PTH?	• Hyperhomocysteinemia
• ?	

Disturbances of Mental Function

Mental function changes in UE appear very early. Sensorial clouding (alterations of alertness and awareness of the environment) is typical, together with insomnia, fatigue, apathy, loss of recent memory, and impaired concentration. Episodes of good performance are still possible but short-lived. As renal failure worsens, attention span decreases, and obtundation and malperception appear together with confusion, twitching (the complex of severe asterixis, tremors, and myoclonus), occasionally hallucinations and agitation, seizures, and finally coma.[10] While seizures are relatively uncommon in other MEs, the "curious admixture of clinical signs of cerebral depression and signs of cerebral excitation is distinctive of UE."[11] In the final stage, patients are often catatonic and mute, while deep tendon reflexes often appear to be diminished.

Neurologic Disturbances

Early neurologic disturbances in UE are dysarthria, tremors, and asterixis. Dysarthria is a slow, slurred, thickened speech caused by alterations of fine tongue movements. Tremors (both action and postural) are a sensitive early index of UE, being irregular in amplitude and more apparent during the elicitation of asterixis and during limb movements. They generally occur at a frequency of 8 to 10/s. Asterixis is a sensitive, early sign of UE (and, in general, of ME) and is almost always present once sensorial clouding appears. It is best elicited by hyperextending the upper limbs with the fingers spread apart. After a latency of about 30 seconds, flapping (flexion-extension) movements of the metacarpophalangeal joints and wrist and side-to-side movements of the fingers will appear at irregular intervals. These movements are rapid and arrhythmic, the flexion phase being more rapid than the extension one. It is also possible to demonstrate asterixis in the lower limbs: the recumbent patient dorsiflexes the foot while the leg is elevated and extended. Sudden downward jerking of the foot with a slower return to the previous position occurs. Similar flappings can be elicited in the face, by forced eyelid closure, protrusion of the tongue, and so on. Asterixis is not an involuntary movement disorder but is the result of the inability to maintain a sustained posture (from the Greek: *a* = without, *sterigma* = support). During the downward phase (flap) no muscular activity in the extensors and flexors involved is seen on EMG. There is, thus, electrical silence in the involved muscle during the "flap phase." The precise cause of asterixis is unknown. Malfunction of a hypothetical system in the CNS involved in maintenance of tonic posture has been suggested.

Among the late neurologic disturbances of UE are myoclonus and tetany. Myoclonus is sudden, gross twitching occurring irregularly and asymmetrically in the limbs, trunk, and head. At rest, the muscle contractions are slight (fascicular) and cause no, or only minor, twitching. During movements the contractions become stronger and are described as jerks. In a stuporous patient the movements may appear "ballistic." It has been suggested that myoclonus is mediated by the relaxing of a spino-bulbar-spinal reflex (normally inhibited) due to a functional disturbance of the reticular formation in the lower brain stem. Tetany is frequent in uremia, being mainly associated with other signs. It may be overt (with spontaneous carpopedal spasm) or latent, being manifested by a positive Trousseau sign.[10,11]

Motor Abnormalities

Clumsiness (unsteadiness in walking and performing fine movements) occurs during the early stages of uremia. Some primitive reflexes (e.g., grasp, snout) may be elicited, due to depression of inhibitory mechanisms in the frontal lobes. Limb muscle tone alterations with decorticate posture (lower limbs in extension and upper limbs in flexion) can be seen. Most patients are weak and show focal motor signs, such as stretch-reflex asymmetry and hemiparesis.

Convulsions

Generalized tonic and clonic seizures are frequently seen in advanced untreated uremic patients. They are often a preterminal event.

METHODS OF ASSESSING BRAIN FUNCTION IN UREMIC PATIENTS

To evaluate UE many approaches can be utilized: electroencephalogram (EEG), evoked potentials, psychological testing, cerebrospinal fluid (CSF) analysis, brain density, and amino acid and hormonal studies (Table 31–3).

Electroencephalography

The standard EEG can be considered as a simple and practical brain function test for evaluating uremic encephalopathy.[12–14] EEG changes include disorganization, slowing and loss of α frequency, and a slow background activity together with an excess of θ and δ waves. Specific paroxys-

TABLE 31–3. METHODS FOR EVALUATING UREMIC ENCEPHALOPATHY

- EEG
- Evoked potentials, mainly somatosensory potentials
- Cognitive function testing, mainly the choice reaction time test
- Cerebrospinal fluid studies of commonly measured solutes
- Brain density studies (CT scan)
- Amino acids, mainly neurotransmitter AAs
- Hormones

mal discharges may be seen in the presence of focal seizures. As uremia progresses, the EEG-dominant waves become slower; the EEG equivalent of drowsiness is diffuse slowing. It is possible to grade the degree of the EEG alterations on a scale from 0 to 4 (0 = normal EEG; 4 = EEG of zero waves per second). Various techniques of EEG quantification can be used in uremic patients; the best way is to compare the percentage of EEG power in brain-background rhythm (or α) coming from the frequencies between 3 and 7 Hz and from those between 3 and 13 Hz. Normal individuals exhibit primarily α activity with a low percentage of waveforms from 3 to 7 Hz, while the converse is seen in uremic patients. No relation exists between EEG pattern and any biochemical abnormality except perhaps for blood parathyroid hormone (PTH) levels. Several techniques of EEG analysis can be utilized, including evoked potentials, heuristic techniques, syntactic analysis, photic driving response, and discriminant analysis.[8]

Evoked Potentials. Evoked potentials (EPs) are EEG waveforms that result from the response of the brain to a specific sensory stimulus: auditory, visual, somatosensory, olfactory, or vestibular. It is possible to register accurately the resultant electrical activity following such stimuli (stimulated at various levels on the afferent cortical pathways) using a limited number of electrodes placed on the skin.

Auditory Potentials. Auditory potentials originate from cortical or subcortical (from the level of the cerebral trunk) brain areas. One approach is used to evaluate the auditory potential by means of audiometric techniques. A second approach can be used to identify lesions of the cerebral trunk, helping in the diagnosis of comas of unknown origin. In fact, metabolic disorders do not cause changes of trunk (auditory) potentials, while toxic lesions do.

Visual Potentials. The visual evoked potential represents the cortical response to a flash or pattern stimulus. The most commonly used stimulus is the "pattern reversal" made by a chessboard, where an alteration of appearance and disappearance of a visual stimulus is utilized. In this case a three-phase complex is recorded, the latency of which varies with age. Abnormalities of visual potentials include an increase of latency and decrease of amplitude due to changes in the speed and efficiency of brain function.

Somatosensory Potentials. These are simple to record and very reproducible. The stimuli consist of rectangular impulses (lasting 200 to 500 milliseconds each and being about 15 milliamperes in intensity) conducted through the skin to a large nerve trunk in one arm or leg. The most frequently used is the "median nerve." The electrodes are placed in the "supraclavicular hole" at the level of the second cervical vertebra and on the scalp, in the central-median region. These short-latency potentials are not influenced by the patient's state of alertness or by the effects of toxins. Thus, they can reflect all of the inflammatory, ischemic, and demyelinating lesions that involve the somesthetic trunk of the peripheral nerves. The somatosensory evoked potentials can be divided into the following: (1) early potentials (latency 100 milliseconds), also called far-field potentials; (2) cortical potentials, due to primary cortical response (short-range neurons); and (3) late potentials (similar to early potentials), generated by the activity of long-distance neurons. The somatosensory evoked potentials may or may not be altered in uremia (at least in the early phase), while they usually change after a dialytic session. For example, after an intermittent peritoneal dialysis (IPD) session, the primary cortical response (involving short-range neurons) significantly increases.

Cognitive Function Testing

Several cognitive function tests have been used in uremic patients: trail making, the continuous memory test, the choice reaction time, the continuous performance test, and the "deux barrages" test (or Zazzo's test) for attention levels; Wechsler Adult Intelligence Scale (WAIS) for language, praxis, and visual-perceptive and visual-spatial capacity; and Benton's visual memory test and the Eysenk personality questionnaire (EPI) for personality trait evaluation. According to Arieff, "there appears to be a consensus, based on psychological testing, that CKD results in organic-like losses of intellectual function, particularly information pro-

cessing capacities."[8] On the whole, the choice reaction-time test seems to be best correlated with renal impairment. Major stumbling blocks to the use of cognitive function testing for quantifying the degree of uremic encephalopathy are a patient's lack of motivation and the inexperience of an examiner.

Cerebrospinal Fluid Findings

Few studies on cerebrospinal fluid (CSF) solute content in animals with CKD exist. Values of protein, glucose, and electrolytes are typically normal. According to Arieff et al., in animals with renal failure, "both urea concentration and osmolality are similar in brain, CSF, and plasma" and "half of the increase in brain osmolality is due to the presence of undetermined solutes (idiogenic osmoles)."[5,8,9,15]

Initially, it was thought that these idiogenic osmoles could cause cerebral edema, but, subsequently, Arieff stated that (1) "a cerebral edema is not present in the brain of patients with CKD"[8] and (2) in CKD there is "an increase in brain osmolality, of which at least 40 percent is due to an increase of idiogenic osmoles. . . . Brain water and electrolyte concentration and pHi are normal in CKD, making it unlikely that either brain edema or intracellular acidosis contributes to EEG abnormalities. . . . The identity and the role of idiogenic osmoles in UE remain uncertain."[8,9]

Twenty years ago, La Greca and coworkers[16–18] published studies concerning biochemical, morphologic, and densitometric changes in the uremic brain. In one, they reported CSF values and CSF/plasma ratios of several solutes in 20 subjects (10 with chronic uremia and 10 controls).[18] Table 31–4 (derived from that study) shows that idiogenic

TABLE 31–4.   CEREBROSPINAL FLUID VALUES IN CHRONIC RENAL FAILURE

	CRF (mass units)	Controls (mass units)	CRF (S.I. units)	Controls (S.I. units)
Urea nitrogen	99.0 ± 25.0^a	18.0 ± 6.0	16.4 ± 4.1^a	2.9 ± 0.9
Creatinine	2.8 ± 0.6^a	0.9 ± 0.4	247.5 ± 53.0^a	79.5 ± 35.5
Glucose	61.0 ± 8.0	60.0 ± 15.0	3.3 ± 0.4	3.3 ± 0.8
Ca^{++}	4.3 ± 0.8	5.3 ± 0.5	1.0 ± 0.2	1.3 ± 0.1
PO_4^{22}	2.3 ± 0.2	1.6 ± 0.3	0.7 ± 0.1	0.5 ± 0.1
Na^+	152.0 ± 2.0	149.0 ± 4.0		
K^+	2.9 ± 0.2	3.0 ± 0.1		
Cl^-	119.4 ± 4.1	121.0 ± 3.0		
HCO_3^-	22.0 ± 2.5	23.0 ± 2.0		
pH	7.32 ± 0.03	7.32 ± 0.02		
Anion gap	13.5	8.0		
Osmolality	340 ± 7	300 ± 6		
Idiogeneic osmoles	30	21		

S.I. units: creatinine = μmol/L; other solutes = mmol/L; osmolality = mOsm/kg H_2O. For Na^+, K^+, Cl^-, pH, HCO_3^-, anion gap, osmolality, and idiogenic osmoles, the values–expressed in S.I. units are identical to those expressed in mass units. CKD = chronic kidney disease (10 patients); mean plasma creatinine value = 8.75 ± 0.5 mg%, that is, 773.5 ± 44.2 μmol/L. Controls = 10 subjects with mean plasma creatinine of 0.90 ± 0.06 mg%, that is, 79.5 ± 5.3 μmol/L.
$^aP < 0.01$.

osmoles (calculated as the difference between the increase in osmolality and the increase of measured solutes: urea + Na^+ + K^+ + Cl^-) were higher in CKD than in normal subjects. However, the contribution to the increased osmolality made by urea was about 29 $mOsm/kgH_2O$ (29/40 = 72.5 percent), while that by unmeasured solutes (idiogenic osmoles) was about 9 mOsm/kgH2O (9/40 = 22.5 percent). In addition, although the CSF osmolality of uremic individuals was higher than normal, the CSF/plasma osmolality ratio was similar in uremics (1.02) and in controls (1.00). The same is true for the CSF/plasma ratios of the other solutes (reported in Table 31–4) except for creatinine, the ratio of which was significantly lower in CKD patients (0.32) than in controls (1.00; $p < 0.01$). These data provide indirect evidence against the presence of chronic cerebral edema in uremia.[18]

Abnormalities in Brain Density

The lack of cerebral edema in uremic patients was confirmed by means of computed tomography (CT), which showed that uremic brains had a normal water content.[16,17] Table 31–5 lists densitometric values (in Houndsfield units, or HU) recorded in the white and gray matter in uremic patients. It must be remembered that on the conventional scale, water coincides with zero while bone corresponds to +1000. Therefore a reduction of the densitometric values in comparison with normal individuals means an increased cerebral water content. Densitometric values were normal in uremics and in patients on continuous ambulatory peritoneal dialysis (CAPD). Intermittently dialyzed patients, on the other hand, showed higher predialytic values ("dry" predialytic brain) and normal postdialytic ones ("normal" postdialytic brain water content).[17]

No specific morphologic brain change has been found in UE.[17,19] However, Savazzi and colleagues reported that CT scans of 30 patients under 50 years of age treated by hemodialysis for over 10 years revealed cerebral atrophy in 46.6 percent.[20] All of these observations indicate that in chronic uremia, the genesis of encephalopathy cannot be explained in terms of derangements of commonly measured solutes and/or brain water content or by changes in brain structure.

TABLE 31–5. BRAIN DENSITOMETRICAL VALUES (CT SCAN)

	White Matter (HU)	Gray Matter (HU)
Controls	20–30	35–50
CKD	20–30	35–50
CAPD	20–30	35–50

HU = Houndsfield units; CKD = chronic renal failure; CAPD = continuous ambulatory peritoneal dialysis.

MRI Changes

In case of insufficient peritoneal dialysis (PD) efficiency and severe uremic encephalopathy, cranial magnetic resonance imaging (MRI) may show increased signal intensity bilaterally in the cortical and subcortical areas of the occipital and parietal lobes. These changes are reversible when a normal dialytic efficiency is obtained.[149]

Plasma and CSF Amino Acid Analyses

Plasma (P) and intracellular amino acid (AA) patterns are abnormal in patients with CKD. The intra- and extracellular concentration ratio of some AAs is altered, so that plasma concentrations do not necessarily reflect intracellular values (for example, in muscle).[21–23] The distribution and metabolism of many AAs and proteins are altered in advanced renal failure due to malnutrition, "uremic toxins," calcium and phosphate disorders, endocrine abnormalities, and the reduced ability of the kidneys to metabolize many hormones. Uremia per se may modify the transport of metabolic substrates through the blood-brain barrier (BBB) and CSF-blood barrier and influence cerebral metabolism.[18,22–28] In the last 20 years, it has been pointed out that in uremia, the CSF AA pattern does not reflect P amino acid composition and that the evaluation of the CSF/P ratio, rather than that of CSF alone, may be significant.[18,25,29] It has been shown that in CKD patients, alterations of blood AAs and NH_3 markedly affect the cerebral uptake of some AAs and ammonia:

1. The cerebral uptake of glycine and cystine is increased, that of isoleucine, valine and NH_3 is decreased, while glutamine has no uptake[28] or a decreased[18] uptake. The cerebral extraction of glycine and branched-chain AAs (BCAAs) is correlated with their arterial concentration.

2. A significant increase (both in P and CSF) of glycine/valine and glycine/BCAAs and a nonsignificant increase of glycine/serine and phenylalanine/tyrosine ratios (both in P and in CSF) exists.[18,30]

3. In CKD, the cerebral uptake of glycine is facilitated by decreased concentrations of serine and BCAAs (which compete with glycine for the neutral AA transport system). A similar phenomenon occurs with cystine (the uptake of which is facilitated by low tyrosine values). The defect in cerebral glutamine uptake together with increased NH_3 extraction might be due to decreased transport of glutamine across the BBB and a concomitant reduction in its utilization. It should be remembered that Sullivan et al.[31] showed that patients with uremic encephalopathy have a reduced total plasma tryptophan concentration, high plasma free trypto-

phan, and CSF tryptophan levels with a raised brain 5-hydroxytryptamine (5-HT) turnover.

These observations were partially confirmed and extended by studying not only 5-hydroxyindoleacetic acid (5-HIAA, a metabolite of 5-HT) but also homovanillic acid (HVA, a metabolite of dopamine) in the lumbar CSF of uremic patients. It was found that in CKD, CSF values of 5-hydroxyindoleacetic acid (5-HIAA), homovanillic acid (HVA), and the HVA/5-HIAA ratio are higher than normal (Table 31–6).[30,32] The following have been clearly shown in this regard:[25,26]

1. The CSF concentrations of metabolites mirror those existing in the surrounding nervous tissue.
2. Lumbar CSF HVA levels indicate cerebral metabolism of dopamine, mainly at the nucleus caudatus level.
3. Lumbar CSF 5-HIAA levels represent 5-HT metabolism in the CNS.
4. HVA and 5-HIAA concentrations are higher in ventricular CSF than in lumbar CSF because these metabolites are removed along the CSF axis.
5. The HVA/5-HIAA ratio is lower in lumbar CSF than in ventricular CSF because HVA is more easily reabsorbed than 5-HIAA.

In addition, Biasioli et al. have clearly shown that, in uremia, there is an altered turnover of 5-HT (or serotonin) and of dopamine at the brain level.[30] Glutamine [and the derived gamma-aminobutyric acid (GABA)] and glycine are neurotransmitters (NTs) capable of inhibiting all CNS neurons (GABA) and most spinal neurons (glycine).[31,33–35] HVA and 5-HIAA are the major metabolites of two mono-

amines (dopamine and serotonin) capable of modulating voluntary movements (dopamine) and controlling the sleep-wake cycle, temperature, and behavior (serotonin). The uremic pattern is typical, being characterized by GABA deficiency, glycine excess, altered aromatic AA/BCAA levels, and an altered ratio between dopaminergic and serotoninergic systems.[18,32]

Hormonal Abnormalities

The altered balance between stimulating and depressing neurotransmitters (NTs) may cause several changes of hormone levels and function.[35,36] Few studies in uremic patients[36–38] have evaluated the relationship between monoamines and hormones, such as prolactin (PRL), follicle-stimulating hormone (FSH), luteinizing hormone (LH), and PTH. It has been shown[37] that in mild CKD (serum creatinine levels of about 323 ± 122 μm/L), serum values of 5-hydroxytryptamine (5-HT), PRL, and PTH are significantly increased, while FSH and LH are increased but not significantly. Several correlations have been found between serum creatinine and serotonin; between creatinine and serotonin, PTH or PRL; and between serotonin or PTH and FSH and LH (but only in male patients).[37–40] These findings can be summarized as follows[37]: (1) in CKD, 5-HT synthesis and turnover may be increased and dopamine (DO) synthesis decreased, although its turnover is accelerated; (2) the imbalances between DO and 5-HT could be responsible for some hormonal derangements commonly ascribed to PTH; (3) creatinine, gender, and age may affect PRL levels; (4) 5-HT and PRL are correlated, mainly in men ($r = 0.899$); (5) increased FSH values could be primarily due to 5-HT ($r = 0.744$) and/or PRL ($r = 0.738$) effects rather than to PTH ($r = 0.646$); (6) LH abnormalities could be related to PRL ($r = 0.899$) rather than to PTH ($r = 0.653$); and (7) PTH and 5-HT are possibly correlated, but only in young uremic men ($r = 0.905$).

Thus some hormonal changes observed in uremia may possibly be ascribed to the documented DO/5-HT abnormalities and the decreased inhibitory action of the suppressed DO system. If this is the case, elevated levels of PRL, FSH, LH, and PTH could be avoided by the early use of dopaminergic drugs and/or by drugs that depress 5-HT. In this way, the circadian rhythms of the neurohormones would be safeguarded over a longer period of time and fewer neurologic manifestations would be seen.

PATHOGENESIS OF UREMIC ENCEPHALOPATHY

Many of the factors that contribute to ME can be simultaneously present in uremic patients. Anemia; impaired glucose metabolism; malnutrition; coenzyme lack; disturbances in fluid, electrolyte, acid-base, and hormonal status; increased levels of reactive oxygen species (ROS), and decreased psy-

TABLE 31–6.   MAIN DERANGEMENTS OF AMINO ACIDS AND OF THEIR METABOLITES, IN CSF AND IN PLASMA

	Controls (N = 10)	CRF (N = 10)
CSF/P Glutamine	0.86	0.72[a]
CSF Glycine/Valine	0.29	0.62[a]
CSF Glycine/BCAA	0.14	0.27[a]
CSF Phen/Tyr	1.04	2.00
CSF HVA (ng/mL)	27.8	77.8[b]
CSF 5-HIAA (ng/mL)	23.5	34.6
CSF HVA/5-HIAA	1.18	2.24
P Glycine/Valine	0.82	2.15[a]
P Glycine/BCAA	0.52	1.11[a]
P Phen/Tyr	0.87	1.34

CSF = cerebrospinal fluid; P = plasma; CSF/P = ratio; BCAA = branched chain AA; HVA = homovanillic acid; 5-HIAA = 5-hydroxyindoleacetic acid. In S.I. units (nanomol/L), CSF HVA values were: 166.8 and 466.8 (normal and CRF subjects); while CSF 5-HIAA ones were: 141.0 and 207.6 (for normal and CRF subjects, respectively).
[a]$P < 0.01$
[b]$P < 0.02$.

chosocial adaptation are all characteristic of the uremic syndrome. Table 31–7 summarizes some well-established data concerning UE. As reviewed above, cerebral edema does not result from uremia. In animals (acutely uremic dogs and rats), it has been shown that the decrease in brain metabolic rate and the lower oxygen and energy consumption are the result of a reduced demand and of slowing of the ATPase pump.[51,52] Depressed cerebral oxygen utilization is the rule in uremia, as well as in other MEs, but no correlation exists between the degree of clinical sensorial clouding and this depressed oxygen consumption. This suggests that a generalized impairment of neuronal processes exists in the presence of uremia.[11] In humans, no specific morphologic brain changes have been found[16,17] and no correlation exists between the degree of UE and the abnormalities of the commonly measured solutes (both in CSF and in P).[5,8,18] Brain intracellular pH is also normal in dogs with CKD[8,9]; CSF electrolytes and pH are normal both in patients and in animals with CKD.[5,8,9,42] Despite the extracellular metabolic acidosis and hyperosmolality, the brain seems to exhibit a remarkable homeostatic ability. The identity and role of idiogenic osmoles remain uncertain, but the evidence "lessens the likelihood that idiogenic osmoles are involved in the causation of UE."[9,42] Cerebral glycolysis has been found to be depressed in the acutely uremic brain, but this is not a major point, considering that glycolysis is always depressed by acidosis. Many cerebral enzymes (e.g., ATPase, GOT, GPT, dopadecarboxylase) can be inhibited by uremic dialysate, mainly by phenolic acid and aromatic and aliphatic amines. The clinical importance of these findings

is not yet clear, for they were documented in patients and animals with acute renal failure. The brain content of calcium is significantly elevated in patients with CKD, but not to the extent found in the brains of patients with acute renal failure (ARF).[8] In dogs with CKD, an increased calcium content of the cortical gray matter and hypothalamus was found; this could interfere with many intracellular enzymes and seems to correlate best with the EEG pattern.[9] PTH itself may also cause depression of CNS function.

In CKD, an abnormal P and CSF pattern of AAs has been clearly demonstrated: malnutrition, "uremic toxins," and endocrine disorders can alter the transport of AAs through the BBB, thus playing a major role in changing the CSF concentrations and the CSF/P ratio of several AAs.[8,11,22,23,25,27,28] It is well known that errors in AA metabolism can have neurologic consequences[24] and that, in the presence of liver impairment, the development of encephalopathy is associated with increased entry of aromatic AAs into the brain, increased formation and efflux of glutamine through the BBB (together with impaired efflux of other neutral AAs), and increased synthesis of false neurotransmitters.[33] In CKD, therefore, AA derangements could produce a number of neurologic consequences, as summarized in Table 31–8:

1. Glutamine is the major source for GABA synthesis; glutamine deficiency is a marker of GABA deficiency. Clinical consequences of glutamine deficiency might include low carnitine levels, dyskinesias, and cognitive impairment (early and late disorders).
2. High glycine levels and reduced serine conversion can cause aberrant brain function and pathology (seizures, retardation, abnormal EEG).
3. Because there is no phenylalanine hydroxylase present in the brain, the increased Phen/Tyr ratio (both in plasma and in CSF) makes it likely that a large number of normally minor metabolites will appear. Such metabolites are organic acids including phenylpyruvic, phenyllactic, and phenylacetic acids. Major neurologic abnormalities, both cognitive and motor, can be seen as a result.
4. An increased glycine/BCAA ratio causes a reduced supply of BCAA in brain; that is, a decreased protein and lipid synthesis with a poor "fuel" availability. Neurologic symptoms could consequently appear, as they do in nonuremic children with this condition.
5. The AAA/BCAA + Met + Hist ratio does not change significantly in CKD. This finding is different from that seen after an IPD (intermittent peritoneal dialysis) session. Following IPD, a unique AA pattern is seen, characterized by an altered ratio between the dopamine and serotonin systems.

TABLE 31–7. DISTINCTIVE FEATURES OF UREMIC ENCEPHALOPATHY

- No specific morphological brain change.[16,17]
- No correlation between the degree of UE and CSF or plasma abnormalities of commonly measured solutes.[5]
- No cerebral edema or cellular volume changes.[11,16,17,19]
- Normal CSF concentrations of electrolytes.[5,42,44]
- Normal intracellular pH (pHi) in brain.[8,9]
- Normal CSF pH.[5,8,9,42]
- Increase in brain osmolality due to a rise both of urea and of idiogeneic osmoles. The increase of idiogenic osmoles ranges from 50%[5,41] to 40%[9] or to 22.5%.[25,32]
- Increase in the calcium content in specific brain regions: cortical gray matter and hypothalamus.[9]
- In dogs, a relationship between EEG abnormalities and elevated calcium content in some areas of brain.[4] The role of PTH is debatable.
- Altered AA ratios both in CSF and in plasma (for example, high CSF and P glycine/valine values; high CSF and P phen/tyr ratios; altered DO/5-HT ratios, both in plasma and in CSF).[8,37]
- Increased serum levels of 5-HT, PTH, PRL, FSH, and LH.[37,38]
- Malnutrition (?).
- Nitric oxide (?).
- Anemia is an important contributor.[43–50]

TABLE 31–8. RELATIONSHIP BETWEEN AA AND NEUROLOGIC FUNCTION IN UREMIA

Low CSF Glutamine	⟶ **Low GABA** ⟶	Low carnitine	
		Enhanced release of excitatory ⟶ substances	Excess abnormal involuntary movements (dyskinesias: early
		Cognitive impairment (subcortical dementia: late changes)	changes)
High CSF Glycine	⟶ Aberrant brain function, seizures, retardation		
High Phen/Tyr Ratios	⟶ Increased organic acids ⟶	Mental and motor disturbances	
High Gly/BCAA Ratios	⟶ Reduced supply of BCAAs to the brain Reduced carbohydrate and fat synthesis		
High Serotonin	⟶ Increased { pain threshold / slow-wave sleep / prolactin secretion		
	⟶ Reduced { LRF secretion / CRF secretion		
Low Dopamine	⟶ Decreased irritability, motor activity		
	⟶ Increased prolactin secretion		
Altered DO/5-HT Ratio	⟶ Increased PTH, PRL, FSH, LH		
	⟶ Deranged chronobiology of PRL secretion		

⟶ = causes.

These observations lead to a "unified theory of uremic encephalopathy."[39] The CNS alterations are purely functional but not structural. "Malnutrition" or "AA imbalance" can alter the levels of putative neurotransmitters (such as glutamine, GABA, glycine), of some derived indexes (such as glycine/BCAA ratios), of monoamines (mainly dopamine and serotonin), and, possibly, of neuropeptides. This AA imbalance can give rise directly to many of the clinical features of UE (Table 31–9). The early phase of UE could be attributed to AA derangements and in particular to increased levels of glycine, organic acids (from phenylalanine), and free-tryptophan; to decreased glutamine-GABA

TABLE 31–9. THE "UNIFIED THEORY" OF UREMIC ENCEPHALOPATHY

Early Phase		Late Phase	
Disturbances of Mental Function			
Ataraxia: low dopamine		Obtundation ⎤	
Anxiety: high dopamine		Errors of perception	
Insomnia: high serotonin		Illusions	low GABA
Sensorial clouding: high dopamine, glycine, and organic acids		Hallucinations	
		Agitation	
		Stupor, coma ⎦	
Neurological Disturbances			
Dysarthria ⎤		Myoclonus ⎤	
Tremors ⎬ low GABA, high dopamine		Tetany ⎦ high glycine	
Asterixis ⎦			
Motor Abnormalities			
Clumsiness ⎤		Seizures: high glycine and dopamine	
Unsteadiness ⎬ low GABA, high dopamine			
Grasp reflexes			
Asthenia ⎦			
Hormonal Changes		High PRL α LH ⎤	
Altered prolactin and sleep-wake cycle ⎬ depressed DO/5-HT ratio PTH?		Low LRF α CRF ⎬ high serotonin, low DO	
		Impotence ⎦	
Reduced sexual activity ⎬ high serotonin high PRL-PTH?			

Each abnormality has been linked with a specific change of a given neurotransmitter.

values; and to altered dopamine metabolism. Sensorial clouding, dyskinesias, asthenia, humoral changes, and reduced sexual activity can be explained on this basis. On the other hand, the persistence of very low GABA values and of very high glycine levels and 5-HT/DO ratios could induce the late phase of UE. Subcortical dementia, uremic twitching, seizures, and significant endocrine abnormalities may appear at this stage. In general, the unified theory of UE is based on AA derangements and on the subsequent imbalance of neurotransmitters. The altered "balance" between exciting and depressing neurotransmitters causes disturbances in mental, neurologic, motor, and hormonal functions. If this hypothesis is correct, only a minor role is attributable to the "classic factors" such as PTH, aluminum, and idiogenic osmoles.

It is now evident that a single mechanism cannot explain UE. A number of neurotoxic substances are retained in CKD: among them blood urea nitrogen (BUN) (higher than 200 mg%), ammonia, ROS, cyanide, phenol-like compounds, and middle molecules (MMs). All of these may contribute to UE. There is no evidence supporting a dominant role of MMs in the pathogenesis of UE, even though some studies have found an inverse correlation between EEG abnormalities and middle molecular (B_{12}) clearance.[51,53]

It is well known that in uremia PTH can directly increase the calcium content of the brain and play an indirect role in the wasting syndrome and in the AA imbalance[9,54] contributing to altered prolactin secretion.

UE is not associated with aluminum toxicity; aluminum intestinal absorption per se cannot cause encephalopathy in patients who have not undergone dialysis.[55]

If the hypothesis proposed for the genesis of UE is correct, some well-known small molecules (i.e., certain AAs, their derivatives, and ROS) would take the place of many unknown "middle molecules," sought since the early 1970s but never found. If so, small molecules might yet be implicated in many uremic symptoms, including gastrointestinal (urea), hematologic (guanidines), and hormonal and neurologic (AAs). Many aspects and points need clarification before this hypothesis can be accepted. Is there a relationship between uremic encephalopathy and uremic malnutrition? What is the role of nitric oxide and free radicals in UE? It is well known that glutathione peroxidase (GSHPxP) is decreased in uremia,[56] but there are no conclusive data concerning the relationships existing between GSH (in plasma and red cells), GSHPxP, SOD, and related enzymes in CKD patients.

Finally, recent evidence suggests that the anemia of chronic renal failure may have a direct effect on brain function.[43-50] Abnormalities of cognitive function tests, as well as electrophysiologic data, improve significantly with improvement of anemia with human recombinant erythropoietin (rHuEpo). There are at least three possible explanations for the improved CNS function accompanying the

rising hematocrit level, all probably based on better brain metabolism. First, increased hematocrit will lead to enhanced brain oxygen delivery, with a beneficial effect on brain metabolism. Second, when the hematocrit rises, cerebral blood flow falls, thus correcting localized "brain uremia" because of the decreased delivery to the brain of uremic toxins. Finally, the decrease in cerebral blood flow may decrease intracranial pressure and subtle cerebral edema. CNS function in dialysis patients does not normalize after improvement of anemia with rHuEPO, suggesting that anemia is only one of several factors important in the pathogenesis of UE.

THERAPEUTIC APPROACH TO UREMIC ENCEPHALOPATHY

In order to minimize or prevent the appearance of severe encephalopathy in uremic patients, the following guidelines should be followed: (1) avoid the development of malnutrition; (2) avoid the use of drugs that increase PTH, PRL, and related hormones; (3) ensure an appropriate intake of protein and calories (lower limits = 0.7 to 0.8 g/kg/day and 30 to 35 kcal/kg/day); (4) maintain hematocrit above 30 percent; and (5) start dialytic treatment at a serum creatinine level of about 11 mg%(=973 μm/L) or earlier if there are signs of severe malnutrition and neurologic deterioration. It may be useful to utilize dopaminergic drugs in the presence of mild CKD (i.e., at serum creatinine levels of about 265 μm/L). By doing this, it is usually possible to maintain lower 5-HT, PTH, and PRL levels even though low doses of drugs are used. The prospective use of antioxidant drugs (such as selenium, glutathione, acetylcysteine, vitamins, and L-carnitine) remains to be studied.

Finally, future studies should clarify the role of dialytic treatment in preventing and/or reducing uremic encephalopathy per se.

Peripheral Neuropathy

Neuropathy is frequently present in patients with ESRD, particularly in those with diabetes and/or vascular disease. Paresthesias (of palms and soles), a burning feeling of the distal extremities, and "restless legs syndrome" are the major clinical manifestations. The progression of neuropathy is accompanied by a slowing of motor nerve conduction velocity (MNCV) and sometimes by paralysis due to loss of motor function.[57] The majority of nerve fibers must be severely damaged before a significant slowing of sensory nerve conduction velocity (SNCV) or MNCV measurements is found.[58]

Several morphologic changes in peripheral nerves have been found in uremic patients: decreased density of myelinated fibers, segmental demyelination (mainly in the more distal segments of long axons), and axonal degeneration. The causes of such pathologic alterations have not been found. In this case, too, the MM hypothesis has been abandoned; no relationship between peripheral neuropathy and PTH levels was found in several studies, while in 1985 an association between a decrease in NCV, sodium nerve permeability, and high intracellular calcium content was shown.[59–62]

Autonomic Neuropathy

A number of abnormalities of the autonomic nervous system are seen in uremic patients. They include impaired sweating, impaired baroreceptor function, abnormal Valsalva test, orthostatic hypotension, and bradycardic hypotension.[59] These abnormalities may disappear after the start of dialysis.[60,63]

DIALYSIS-ASSOCIATED ENCEPHALOPATHIES

When uremic patients are started on regular dialytic treatment, UE generally improves. On the other hand, some patients show acute or chronic neurologic signs, as summarized in Table 31–10.[5,8,15,42,64–71]

Acute Neurologic Complications

Among the acute neurologic complications of dialysis, dialysis disequilibrium [or dialytic disequilibrium syndrome (DDS)] is the most frequent. Symptoms suggesting an acute metabolic encephalopathy may develop during a dialysis session or up to 24 hours after dialysis is completed. DDS may occur in a mild form (distress, headache, tremors,

TABLE 31–10. NEUROLOGIC COMPLICATIONS IN DIALYSIS

Acute
  Disequilibrium syndrome (headache, nausea, vomiting, disorientation, visual blurring, tremors, seizures)
  Myoclonus and convulsions (generalized tonic-clonic, focal or multifocal seizures)
  Hyperosmolar coma
  Cranial nerve paralysis
  Epidural and subdural hematomas
  Transient ischemic attacks
Chronic
  Dialysis encephalopathy
    Speech disturbances
    Motor disorders
    Severe mental deterioration
  Dialysis dementia
    Epidemic form
    Sporadic form
  Peripheral neuropathy
    Slight to severe sensitivity
    Motor polyneuropathy
  Autonomic system dysfunction
  Cranial nerve disorders
  Depletion syndrome
  Wernicke-like syndrome

nausea, emesis) or in a more severe form (disorientation, confusion, stupor) which may develop into convulsions and coma.[65–71] Such episodes, rarely fatal, tend to resolve within a few days and usually occur when dialysis therapy is being initiated (i.e., during the early sessions) rather than during chronic treatment. DDS may be prevented if high-efficiency dialysis is avoided. Thus, during the early sessions, it is advisable to use a small dialyzer, low blood flow, and short dialysis time.[5]

Changes in the Water Content in the Central Nervous System

According to a "classic" pathogenetic hypothesis, dialysis disequilibrium is associated with cerebral edema. Urea removal from the blood occurs more rapidly than from the CSF and brain tissue, and a urea osmotic gradient is generated, causing a movement of water into brain cells ("reverse urea effect"). At the same time, hemodialysis (HD) generates a CO_2 gradient between plasma and CSF, lowering the pH both in the CSF and in brain tissue. These changes will be followed by an increase in brain intracellular osmolality, because of the rise of H^+ concentration and the in situ generation of "idiogenic osmoles." These osmoles are primarily acid radicals derived from protein metabolism. This osmotic imbalance causes tissue swelling and cerebral edema. This hypothesis was based on studies performed by Arieff[5] on animals and by Port[66] on some patients. Later on, different pathogenetic theories were proposed based on studies using CT scans in HD patients.[72,73]

A morphologic and densitometric analysis of the brain (before and after the HD session) was performed to address this issue. The finding (after the HD session) of a reduction of parenchymal density was interpreted as cerebral edema. Subsequent studies, performed on a large population [controls, ESRD, HD, intermittent peritoneal dialysis (IPD), and CAPD patients] and using more sophisticated techniques, suggested the following[16,17]:

1. No morphologic modifications linked to dialysis treatment (above all of cerebral tracts, cisternal-ventricular systems, and subarachnoid spaces) were noted. Rare cases of atrophy did not change after dialysis.
2. Cerebral density values in normal subjects range from 35 to 50 Houndsfield units (HU) in the gray matter and from 20 to 30 HU in the white matter. The variability range is about 8 percent.
3. In HD and IPD patients, cerebral density values before dialysis were higher than normal and ranged from 45 to 55 HU in the gray matter and from 30 to 40 HU in the white matter.
4. In HD and IPD patients, cerebral density in both gray and white matter decreased significantly after dialysis, reaching values similar to those recorded in

the normal population. In the interdialytic period, cerebral density increased progressively and reached high values before the subsequent dialysis session.

5. On the contrary, in patients undergoing CAPD and uremic subjects, density values were similar to those seen in the controls.[72,73]

Because cerebral density is inversely correlated to brain water content, it was concluded that, in the postdialytic period, cerebral edema does not occur and brain water content returns to normal values from a predialytic dry status. Since, in continuous dialysis treatment these variations in cerebral density do not occur, it appears that nonphysiologic treatments, such as intermittent treatments, cause the observed modifications of the brain water content. These alterations could be produced by water transport following electrolytic, acid-base, and osmotic changes, but they are not consistent with the hypothesis of postdialytic edema as a primary cause of DDS. In addition, pressure analyses performed before and after the dialytic session did not confirm the presence of CSF hypertension generated by dialysis.

Finally, the continuous and periodic modifications of brain water content—and, therefore, of the metabolic and electrophysiologic activities of the brain cells—could play an important long-term role in the pathogenesis of chronic encephalopathy in dialyzed patients.[73]

Chronic Neurologic Complications

Dialysis Encephalopathy. Dialysis encephalopathy (DE) is a syndrome observed in patients undergoing long-term dialysis, first described by Alfrey in the early 1970s. Since then, several reports have shown similar findings.[69]

DE is a progressive and frequently fatal neurologic disease, with a characteristic set of signs and symptoms. The main patterns include difficulty in communication, cognitive and motor impairment, and alteration of character. DE is first characterized by moderate speech disturbances, central sensorimotor disorders, and mental deterioration to varying degrees.[67] These symptoms may progress to apraxia, alterations of personality, inability to accomplish purposeful movement, and progressive dementia ("dialysis dementia," or DD).[68–71] From a clinical point of view, DE may be divided into two forms: an epidemic form, which develops rapidly, and a sporadic form, which evolves slowly. The *epidemic form* affects a large percentage of patients in the same center or undergoing home dialysis in the same area and seems to be dependent on environmental factors, mainly aluminum intoxication, primarily from contamination of the dialysate with aluminum and a positive aluminum balance (+300 μg per dialysis session). This, however, is now part of the history of dialysis: now it is mandatory to treat tap water either by deionization or by reverse osmosis, before producing the dialysate. *The chronic sporadic form* affects patients undergoing dialytic treatment

for at least 2 years and seems to be linked to individual factors, but not to aluminum intoxication.

Many conflicting hypotheses on the pathogenesis of neurologic alterations have been formulated. Table 31–11 lists some of the factors possibly involved. There is no doubt as to how complex and multifactorial these may be. On the other hand, the unphysiology of the dialytic treatment per se could have several effects on the CNS: changes of brain water content, electrolytic alterations, metabolic changes, and direct toxic effects (see "Aluminum Encephalopathy," below).

Other Information on Dialysis Encephalopathy

During the 1980s, the incidence of DE ranged from 2 to 15 percent (mean 5 percent) at different centers. The frequency later fell, but recent numbers are not available. No racial predilection exists; the male-to-female ratio is 1.4:1; older patients (> 60 years) are more prone to this progressive disease, with most patients dying within 15 to 20 months from the diagnosis.

Even though the main symptoms are included among those shown in Table 31–2 concerning UE, it must be stressed that, in DE, they are intermittent at first and more pronounced in the middle phase; they may worsen acutely during the dialytic session.

Initial symptoms include several difficulties in communication, due both to disturbances of mental function and to neurologic and motor abnormalities. A patient often starts with impairment of memory (loss of recent memory, impaired concentration) and fatigue but then usually progresses to other difficulties, all linked with the Greek prefix "dys." Dysarthria (difficulties with articulation), dysphasia (poor speech coordination), stammering, and stuttering are usually among the first signs of the syndrome. The result is typical: a slow, slurred, thickened speech, occurring in 90 percent of patients with DE.

TABLE 31–11. CAUSES OF DIALYTIC ENCEPHALOPATHY

- Unphysiology of intermittent treatments
- Inadequate removal of "uremic toxins" (urea, MM)
- Trace elements in the brain
- Variations in AA transport/deranged NT
- Alterations of CSF dynamics
- Damage of BBB
- K^+/Ca^{2+} ratio in CSF
- Deficiency of 2-OH-acid dehydrogenase (lactate toxicity)
- Acid-base disorders
- Inhibition of enzymatic system or deficiency of precursors
- Slow viruses (Creutzfeldt-Jakob)
- Malnutrition
- Free radical generation
- Anemia

The progression of the syndrome is associated with more severe disturbances of mental function (depression, affective disorders, agitation, hallucinations), of neuromuscular (myoclonic jerking and seizures) and motor (alteration and/or asymmetry of reflexes, convulsions, hemiparesis) apparatus. Motor disturbances may be seen in 70 percent and seizures (grand mal or focal) in 60 to 90 percent of patients.

Some patients show other "dys" changes: dyslexia (impaired reading, writing and spelling without impairment in the recognition of words); dyscalculia (inability to perform mathematical calculations); dyspraxia (uncoordinated movements); dysgraphia (inability to write).

Initial symptoms appear intermittently but are more pronounced after HD sessions. Patients are frustrated by these symptoms, so they often curtail conversation to avoid embarrassment. But the syndrome progresses, a global dementia usually develops, and in less than 20 months (range 6 to 20) from the onset, the patient usually dies.

The role of other important factors in susceptibility to DD, such as chronic malnutrition, remains to be clarified.

Once DD has appeared, a fatal outcome is the rule. On rare occasions renal transplantation may be curative.[105–107] Reports on the use of barbiturate compounds in the management of the movement disorders associated with DD are purely anecdotal.

On postmortem examination of the brains of patients with DE, some characteristic histopathologic changes have been identified. They include a combination of atrophy, increased gliosis, and cellular deterioration. In some cases, senile plaques and extensive neurofibrillary degenerative tangles in the cerebral cortex, the red nucleus, and in dentato-olivary systems have been found.[64,135]

Aluminum Encephalopathy or the "Aluminum Legend"

Histochemical studies of the brains of patients with DE have shown significant elevation of brain aluminum (Al) content as well as some other heavy metals.[88–104] Even though in these cases the brain Al level is two to three times that of renal patients without DE, this evidence is not conclusive, because Al does not fulfill all of Koch's postulates as an etiologic agent.[135,137]

Elevated brain Al levels have also been found in patients with Alzheimer's disease, metastatic cancer, and hepatic coma.[88–91]

Encephalopathy is not reproducible in animals supplemented with high doses of oral Al. When the dialysate is devoid of Al, the Al balance is usually negative because its removal with waste products can offset its oral gain. Al is present in variable amounts in all foods. In individuals with normal kidney function, the gut is relatively impermeable to Al and the kidneys eliminate the plasma Al in the urine. A positive balance may be obtained only at Al doses of 1000 to 3000 mg/day, while in a normal diet the Al content is usually less than 125 mg/day.

Al toxicity can be precipitated by some gastrointestinal disorders, namely decreased gut motility or the pH of the stomach. Al absorption may be 8 to 50 times higher when Al-containing antacids are taken with orange juice or citric acid.[137]

Al is absorbed from the gut into the blood by two mechanisms: (1) an independent carrier for Al^{3+} (similar to the absorption of Fe^{3+}) and (2) the calcium transport, which is enhanced by calcium channel activators and explains the penetration of Al into the tissues, brain, and bone. Al removal by dialysis is less than that for many other ions due to its strong binding with plasma proteins and its incorporation in tissues. When given orally to patients with elevated tissue Al, deferoxamine, a hexadentate chelator, mobilizes Al from the tissues, increases (from two to four times) the Al plasma levels, and favors Al removal by dialysis.[100–104] In some cases, DE has been stabilized, from weeks to months, using deferoxamine. However, sometimes the increased plasma Al levels can enhance seizure activity in patients with DE.[100–104,138]

Children with ESRD appear to be more prone to DE because of a high absorption of calcium for their growth and of an assimilation of Al higher than that of adults. The question is: If 90 percent of ESRD boys showed elevated plasma levels of Al^{3+}, why is the incidence of DE nonetheless low in this population?[95–96] Evidently, Al is not the unique cause of DE.[90–93] Furthermore it is not clear how Al acts as a toxin in DE or how it enters into brain tissues. Once again, the permeability of the BBB (blood-brain barrier) plays a role. Once it has entered the brain tissue, Al inhibits dihydropteridine reductase (DHPR), an enzyme required for the synthesis of tyrosine, dopa, norepinephrine, and 5-HT.[137] Again, hormonal and neurotransmitter changes appear, altering several neuronal processes and possibly leading to DE.

Cortex samples of patients who have died of DE have shown low levels of choline-acetyltransferase, causing neurotoxic effects on neurons and on the axonal transport system.

The fact that DE is rare in ESRD patients who dialyze in units using bioosmosis but who still take Al phosphate binders together with calcium carbonate and who do not limit the intake of Al in their diet suggests strongly that the water used for dialysate could be the main portal of entry of this element into the body.

On the other hand, the widespread use of reverse-osmosis systems has not eliminated the risk of DE. This fact and the poor ameliorative effect of renal transplantation on DE must be considered.[105–107]

In order to prevent a possible cause of DE, renal units should properly treat tap water; serum Al levels must be monitored on a yearly basis; and Al phosphate binders must be avoided or diminished in favor of other forms of binding agents even if they are more costly. In any case, the certainties of Alfrey and of Arieff have been replaced by many uncertainties and by proper water treatment![89–91,135,139–143]

The precise role of beta amyloid in the pathogenesis of Alzheimer's disease and of the neurologic complications of ESRD is still unknown. But the deposition of beta amyloid in senile plaques in the form of beta-phased sheets is the only characteristic Alzheimer's disease shares with systemic amyloidosis.[141]

Computed EEG and Evoked Potentials in Dialyzed Patients

The electrical activity of the brain and the cortical responses to external stimuli have been investigated and compared in the same patient during the predialytic phase and after the start of chronic HD treatment. As renal failure develops, EEG rhythms become slower. Dialysis improves the EEG, which becomes more rapid and rhythmic. But this finding is absent in patients with DE. The EEG is thus the primary tool for the diagnosis of DE. EEG analysis early in the course of DE shows multifocal bursts of high-amplitude delta activity interspersed with runs of normal background activity. The EEG changes may precede clinical signs and symptoms of DE by several months. As encephalopathy progresses, the EEG may deteriorate to a predominance of slow waves.

If EEGs are performed prior to and after dialysis in patients with ESRD but without DE, some of the following are seen[74,78–81]: wave frequency and rhythmicity generally increase in the postdialysis EEG even though the pattern may include both slow rhythms (a slowing of the basal activity) and some signs of paroxysmal activity, such as spikes, and triphasic bursts.

On the contrary, most patients with DE show peculiar EEGs: a marked slowing of brain background rhythm in association with typical bilateral spikes and wave complexes not usually found in other patients on dialysis. In these patients, the single dialytic session does not significantly ameliorate the predialytic EEG. In DE, the triphasic bursts and slow (frontally predominant) waves mentioned above are less commonly seen. EEG is the main differential diagnostic test used to confirm DE, in conjunction with the typical alterations in the patient's personality.[136]

In summary, the EEG analysis permits the evaluation of the effects of various dialytic techniques on EEGs in a large population, the comparative approach illustrates the pattern of electrical activity of the brain in the same patient over time, and each EEG may be compared with the previous one as a control.[75]

When the behavior of cortical responses to external stimuli (induced by somatosensory or visual evoked potentials) is studied, dialysis seems to ameliorate the evoked responses—that is, to improve the conditions in which neurons act.[78,79]

CSF and Plasma Studies in Dialysis Patients

It is more than likely that water and electrolyte changes induced by a single dialytic session and by chronic dialytic treatment modify the electrical activity of neurons. Thus, when dialytic encephalopathy is studied, the role of multiple solutes and their distribution along the BBB must be taken into account. On the other hand, a change in the permeability of the BBB could play a role in causing DE. The BBB must be divided into a hematoliquoral and a hematoparenchymal part.[81] The latter can be studied only in laboratory animals; the former may be evaluated using CSF/plasma solute ratios.[82] Few studies have assessed change in the CSF/plasma ratios of solutes in dialyzed patients.[27,83] In 1982, Ronco et al. studied these ratios in several groups of subjects: healthy people and ESRD, HD, IPD, and CAPD patients.[84] Urea nitrogen, creatinine, calcium, phosphorous, Na^+, K^+, Cl^-, osmolality, glucose, and acid-base status were determined. It was shown that (1) before the intermittent dialysis session (HD, IPD), the CSF solute concentrations are similar to those in plasma, and (2) after dialysis, CSF urea, creatinine, and osmolality decrease slightly, but their reduction is far less than the plasma values. Thus, an osmolal gradient between CSF and plasma is generated. If this is correct, passage of water from the blood to the brain during the postdialytic period is inevitable. These data confirm the findings obtained by means of CT scanning. On the other hand, in the interdialytic period, plasma concentrations and osmolarity increase gradually (but probably more rapidly than in CSF) resulting in the movement of water out of the brain. The osmotic gradient between plasma and the CSF is maintained by the slow modifications occurring in the latter, accounting for the varying water contents observed in cerebral tissue before and after dialysis.[84]

IPD is less efficient than HD for solute removal, but the glucose absorbed from the peritoneal dialysis solutions contributes to the generation of an osmotic gradient. Conversely, in CAPD patients solute gradients are similar to those observed in undialyzed patients with ESRD.[84]

Amino Acids and Neurotransmission in Dialysis Patients

The synthesis and activity of the common neurotransmitters may be affected by amino acid imbalance and by enzymatic blocks induced by uremia. A change of BBB permeability could alter the uptake of one or more AAs, causing the disruption of some neurotransmitter (NT) systems and possibly explaining the appearance of some symptoms peculiar to DE. It is well known that in hepatic failure several neurologic manifestations can be ascribed to AA disequilibrium, since aromatic AAs pass through the BBB more easily than branched-chain AAs (BCAAs).[13,14,16] McGale and Coll[25,27,83] studied plasma and CSF amino acid patterns in uremic and dialyzed patients (HD sessions of 10 hours); however, they could not obtain conclusive data, probably for technical and methodologic reasons (use of only one lumbar puncture, performed on different patients and at varying times after dialysis). In spite of these limitations, these authors demonstrated that in uremic subjects the evaluation of CSF/P ratio—instead of plasma or CSF concentration alone—is not useful. In 1981, Deferrari and Coll,[28] by measuring the AA gradient between afferent and effluent brain blood, showed that in uremia the cerebral uptake of glycine and cystine increases and that of valine and isoleucine decreases, while glutamine is not substantially taken up by brain.[28] Some of these data were indirectly confirmed by Biasioli et al.[18] Fifteen dialyzed patients (five HD, five IPD, and five CAPD) were studied. Specimens of CSF and venous blood were collected before and after intermittent treatments, while in CAPD patients the samples were collected once, in the middle of the 4-hour exchange. The data confirmed that in uremic patients (dialyzed or not) a cerebral AA disequilibrium does exist. To clarify the degree of this abnormality, the CSF/P ratios of competing AAs in crossing the BBB were calculated. Selective defects in transferring AA precursors of NTs were thus identified. It was shown the following[18,30]:

1. HD causes a significant decrease in CSF/P BCAA ratios and a significant increase in the CSF Gly/Val ratio at the end of each session. These data suggest an augmented brain uptake of glycine and a decrease in the uptake of valine.
2. In IPD, the general trend of Phen + Tyr + BCAA + Met + Hist ratios seems to suggest a preferential transport, through the BBB, of aromatic amino acids and a decreased transport of BCAA.
3. In all the dialytic treatments, a decreased cerebral uptake of glutamine occurs, as shown by the low CSF/P ratio.
4. In CAPD, BCAA values as well as the related indexes are less altered in comparison with IPD or HD.

During continuous treatment, valine CSF values are normal; accordingly, Gly/Val ratios, both in plasma and in CSF, are less altered than in intermittent treatments. This could result in a more efficient neurotransmission linked to glycine concentration. In all dialytic treatments, the behavior of Gly/Val ratios is mainly influenced by valine concentration. This agrees with the conclusions of Alvestrand et al.: "The depletion of valine is the rule in uremic people."[23] This abnormality is worse in HD and IPD patients than in those on CAPD.

A further refinement of this analysis was the measurement of the most important metabolites of aromatic AA in CSF, which represent the final metabolic products of some neurotransmitters.[85] In particular, since only traces of tryptophan are found in CSF (although a certain serotoninergic

activity is registered in some neurons), its main metabolite, 5-hydroxyindoleacetic acid (5-HIAA) was measured in CSF. Furthermore, phenylalanine hydroxylase is lacking in the brain and the consequent transformation of phenylalanine to tyrosine does not occur. Accordingly, tyrosine becomes an essential AA and the only precursor of catecholaminic metabolites (adrenaline, noradrenaline, and dopamine). As the dopaminergic system is the most important in neurotransmission, and in uremia a block of dopamine β-hydroxylase occurs, the main metabolite, homovanillic acid (HVA), was measured in CSF.[30,86,87] In addition, the HVA/5-HIAA ratio was also calculated. A significant difference between HD and IPD can be found here as well. In HD, the low levels of the three indexes suggest a reduced dopaminergic and serotoninergic activity. On the other hand, in IPD the opposite is seen, with increased values of 5-HIAA and HVA, and their ratio suggesting an excessive production or a reduced utilization of these metabolites. These data seem to confirm the hypothesis that the pathogenesis of uremic and dialytic encephalopathy is multifactorial. In HD, the excess of glycine causes an imbalance of inhibitory systems, while the reduced activity of dopaminergic and serotoninergic systems results in the onset of akinesia and of a disorder similar to depression without a manic component ("monopolar component"). In IPD, a preferential passage of aromatic AA across the BBB occurs, leading to an increase in serotonin and dopamine catabolites. This derangement could be responsible for dyskinesias and disorders of the sleep-wake cycle and of the pain threshold.[86,87]

It is possible that many of the neurologic abnormalities observed in dialyzed patients may be due to an alteration of the normal equilibrium existing among the different neurotransmitters.[30,64,86,87] All of these changes could derive from the following phenomena: (1) selective changes of the BBB, altering the uptake of several AAs and the generation of several NTs; (2) enzymatic blocks leading to the synthesis of false NTs; and (3) altered ratios between dopaminergic and serotoninergic systems and among the various enkephalins. Several symptoms peculiar to DE might then appear (Table 31–12).

Medical Care

No uniformly satisfactory treatment for patients with dialysis encephalopathy exists. The condition generally does not improve with increased dialysis frequency or even renal transplantation. Several general treatments may benefit individual patients.

1. Maintenance of adequate dialysis
   a. One should ensure that the patient with dialysis encephalopathy receives adequate dialysis as determined by Kt/V measurements (quantification

TABLE 31–12. MAIN NEUROTRANSMITTERS AND RELATED FUNCTIONS

NT	Function
Glycine	Enhancement of the inhibitory systems
GABA	Inhibitory function
Dopamine	Normal mental activity
Serotonin	Regulation of the brain vascular system; wake-sleep cycle; regulation of vigilance system; pain sensitivity
Acetylcholine Noradrenaline	Common mediators in cortical and subcortical areas; higher mental functions; memory, learning, etc.
Enkephalins β-endorphin Opioid peptides	Neuromodulation; hunger and thirst modulation; behavioral manifestations; control of blood pressure, body temperature sensitivity, and feeding; neuroendocrine activity, etc.

NT = neurotransmitter.

of dose of dialysis therapy; K is the hemodialyzer clearance, t is the duration of the dialysis session, V is the volume of distribution of urea in the body).

   b. A tendency to underdialyze often exists in these patients when the patient asks to end the dialysis sessions early, which is then done.

2. Reduced intake of aluminum

   a. Lowering the dialysate aluminum levels to less than 10 μg/L by deionization and reverse osmosis may be beneficial early in the course of the disease.

   b. Avoiding aluminum-based phosphate binders. In patients with overt disease, eliminating the source of aluminum rarely results in significant clinical improvement.

   c. Improvement in symptoms has been reported in patients treated with deferoxamine, which chelates aluminum and reduces the tissue burden, but this has not been proven to be effective by clinical trials.

3. Treatment of anemia: Anemia should be treated with rHuEPO and iron supplementation as needed to maintain the hematocrit in the range of 33 to 36 percent.

4. Multivitamin supplementation (see below). Avoid malnutrition!

5. Neurologic consultation and mental status monitoring.

6. Motor activity.

7. Drugs: diazepam and clonazepam reduce myoclonus and seizures.

8. When the patient becomes frankly psychotic, hospitalization is mandatory. Afterwards, he or she may require placement in a long-term care setting.

ADDITIONAL NEUROLOGIC ABNORMALITIES IN UREMIC PATIENTS

While UE, DE, DDS, DD, and peripheral neuropathy are unique to dialysis patients, some other neurologic problems, though occurring in the setting of uremia, are not.[108]

Central Nervous System Infection and Hemorrhage

Any infection known to involve the CNS may occur in the dialytic population. Infection of the vascular access, mycotic aneurysm, pulmonary infection, toxoplasmosis, and systemic infection in patients previously transplanted all may involve the CNS, causing the appearance of meningitis, encephalopathy, and hemorrhage.[109–112] Dialysis patients have an increased mortality from cerebral hemorrhage related to hypertension, vascular disease, and exposure to heparin. Headache (although a common sign in HD patients) should be carefully evaluated, especially when appearing at the end of a dialysis session and when associated with a declining neurologic status and fever.

Malnutrition and Encephalopathy

Some 20 to 30 percent of the dialysis population show clear signs of protein-calorie malnutrition. Folate, vitamin C, and water-soluble vitamins are removed during dialysis. Folate deficiency (axonal degeneration, demyelination, and neuronal death), vitamin B_{12} deficiency, and thiamine (B_1) deficiency may present with signs of metabolic encephalopathy (mental slowness, ataxia, and coma). Depletion of trace elements may also be found in dialysis patients. Low blood zinc levels cause hypogeusia, which can be avoided by using zinc supplementation: oral zinc acetate or dialysate zinc.[113–115]

The increase in the concentration ratio of AAAs/BCAAs (similar to that observed during prolonged exercise) can affect neurotransmission in the brain and thereby influence central drive and mood.

Other possible neurologic effects of malnutrition are listed in Table 31–13.

Neurobiology of Aging and Dementia

Thanks to renal transplantation and to prolonged dialytic life, the dialytic population is mainly made up of adults, with a mean age above 65 years (range 20 to 95) and with a mean dialytic age higher than 7 years (84 dialytic months), while the percentage of those who die is about 13 per year (13 percent per year). Thus, the neurologic deficits of aging may be properly considered in this context. A decline in functional efficiency and deterioration of highly specialized neuronal cells is normal in adult life. Involution to senescence is an inevitable physiologic process, possibly acceler-

TABLE 31–13. MALNUTRITION AND ENCEPHALOPATHY

Derangement	Effects
$\uparrow \dfrac{\text{AAAs}}{\text{BCAAs}}$	Damage of central drive and mood
$\downarrow$ Vitamin B_1, B_6, B_{12}	Mental slowness, ataxia, coma
Metabolic acidosis	Impaired muscle contraction, impaired ADP rephosphorylation
Energetic deficiency	Increased inorganic phosphate, decline in muscle force
Decreased physical activity	Altered sympathetic tone ($\downarrow$), hyperlipidemia
Fasting	Ketone body oxidation (in the brain)
$\downarrow$ BMI	BMI $< 14 \rightarrow$ poor psychological state

$\uparrow$ = increase; $\downarrow$ = decrease; $\rightarrow$ = causes; AAAs = aromatic amino acids; BCAAs = branched-chain amino acids; BMI = body mass index (weight [kg]/ht^2[m]).

ated by uremia and by dialytic treatments. Biologically, ESRD patients are older than their normal contemporaries. All their organs (starting with the skin) are prematurely aged, the brain included. The earliest of these changes occurs long before the anagraphic phase of aging, and these effects accumulate (in predictable and unpredictable ways) toward expression late in dialytic life.

If, in the normal population, the probability of death doubles about every 8 years, in ESRD this value must be doubled every 4 years. Senescence—that is, the process of aging—could be defined as a progressive lowering of biological and mental efficiency. In ESRD subjects, this loss of physiologic function may happen early and prematurely and is termed *involution*.

Changes associated with senescence involve skin, hair, teeth, gonads, posture, muscular power, sense of smell, motor activity, reaction time, perception, coordination and agility, cognitive changes (perception, memory, and mental efficiency). Regression is generally linear in normal aging but may be unpredictable in metabolic disorders.

Atrophy of muscles, reduced velocity conduction of nerves (VCN), and diminution of peak power and endurance are the clinical expressions of damage to motor neurons and of skeletal muscle fibers, with atrophy of muscles. Fundamental changes in the nucleus, mitochondria, enzyme content, mitotic proliferation and chromosomes appear. With age, DNA molecules of dividing cells show an increasing number of errors due to several factors, mainly the depletion of enzymes involved in transcription.

Aging Collagen—Loss of Integrity and Function

The pattern of aging is that of a general degenerative disease in which brain damage (more or less severe: shrinkage, loss of weight, cerebral atrophy) is usually present. In the case of diffuse cerebral atrophy, dementia may be seen as well.

In ESRD patients, all of these changes may appear early in life. The question is: How can we slow them down and how can we distinguish a "real" deterioration of aging from a uremic one?

It is well known that sometimes the physician fails to detect the behavioral changes consistent with the diagnosis of "presenile dementia," while the patient's family does spot these mental changes. People with ESRD meet a lot of physicians during the course of treatment, but a baseline psychological test is usually not performed; certainly a periodic screening tool could be useful for detecting slight but progressive mental deterioration. For this purpose, Folstein's Mini-Mental State Examination, requiring only a few minutes, could be used.

About 70 percent of all cases of dementia are due to Alzheimer's disease and about 15 percent are caused by strokes of the multi-infarct type. The remaining 15 percent are caused by more than 20 other diseases, ESRD included, that have dementia as a component.

Finally, supplementation with modest amounts of trace minerals can improve cognitive function in healthy elderly individuals in whom mental status tends to decline with advancing age due to social and economical problems and to the use of medications that interfere with the absorption and utilization of nutrients. In this population, supplementing with a broad spectrum of nutrients can reduce the incidence of mental deterioration.[145] Whether this would be effective in ESRD patients is unclear.

In 16 elderly patients with cerebrovascular disease, supplementation with L-arginine (1.6 g/day for 3 months) improved cognitive function.[146] Arginine, a precursor to nitric oxide, plays a role in learning and memory.

In addition, aerobic exercise could be useful in treating a wide range of medical disorders, including cardiovascular disease, osteoarthritis, diabetes, and depression.

Twenty-Nine Medical Causes of "Schizophrenia"

The term *schizophrenia* is inadequate; *misperceptions of unknown cause* is better. Twenty-nine causes of misperceptions that cause schizophrenia include the following:

1. Well known: dementia paralytica, pellagra, porphyria, hypothyroidism, drug intoxications, homocysteinuria, folic acid and B_{12} deficiency, sleep deprivation, heavy metal toxicity
2. Less well known: hypoglycemia, psychomotor epilepsy, cerebral allergy, wheat-gluten sensitivity, copper excess, Histadyl, pyroluria, Wilson's disease, chronic candidal infection, Huntington's chorea
3. Almost unknown: prostaglandins, dopamine excess, endorphins, serine excess, prolactin excess, dialysis, serotonin imbalance, leucine-histidine imbalance,

interferon and other antiviral drugs, platelets deficient in MAO (monoamine oxidase).

Twenty-nine causes of "schizophrenia"—but, in CKD patients, at least ten may be present simultaneously. A lack of hydrophilic vitamins (thiamine, folic acid, and B_{12}) induces mental symptoms such as confusion, fatigue, poor memory, difficulty in concentrating or learning, mental lethargy, loss of alertness and independence, insomnia, lack of coordination, mania, and paranoia.[144]

Elevated homocysteine levels are usual in CKD patients, being directly responsible for various types of vascular disease, including strokes and coronary artery disease. Prostaglandin deficiency, due to low selenium levels, may contribute to "schizophrenia." Serine excess may produce psychotic effects. Prolactin excess can be associated with extreme mental states. Serotonin and leucine/histidine imbalance can alter mental status. High serotonin levels are connected with a number of severe mental states, such as "paranoid schizophrenia."

In summary, CKD patients could have several concomitant factors, all possibly leading to encephalopathy, besides dialysis and Al intoxication!

Thiamine Deficiency in Dialysis Patients

Dialysis patients are at risk for thiamine deficiency (defined as a thiamine concentration below 50 nmol/L of blood) because of poor nutrition and increased loss of water-soluble vitamins during the dialysis procedure. Thiamine deficiency gives rise to various clinical signs: congestive heart failure, lactic acidosis, and encephalopathy. This latter disorder is characterized by ocular abnormalities, ataxia and mental confusion. If thiamine deficiency is documented, thiamine supplementation (200 mg/day and later 100 mg/day) can bring about a dramatic recovery in mental status.[144]

According to Hung, supplementation with oral thiamine may not be sufficient, since oral thiamine is poorly absorbed. Early recognition and prompt treatment of thiamine deficiency–related encephalopathy may be lifesaving. The present author recommends routine intravenous thiamine supplementation in HD patients with malnutrition in order to prevent encephalopathy.[144]

High Homocysteine: A Risk Factor for Dementia

Plasma total homocysteine (Hcy) has recently emerged as a major vascular risk factor for several diseases: cardiovascular disease, coronary heart disease, atherosclerosis, stroke, poor mental functioning, increased oxidative stress, dementia, and Alzheimer's disease. According to Seshadri, the higher the level of homocysteine above >14 μmol/L, the greater the risk of dementia or Alzheimer's disease.[146] This association was independent of age, sex, plasma vitamin levels, and other risk factors. Vitamin therapy (folic acid alone or with vitamins B_6 and B_{12}) can reduce plasma homocysteine levels. Patients with CKD have very high homocysteine levels (range 30 to 120 μmol/L) and an increased cardiovascular risk.[147] In these subjects too, however, by using proper vitamin supplements (by mouth or intravenously) for more than 8 months, a significant reduction of Hcy may be achieved. That this approach lessens the risk of dementia remains to be proven.[148]

Erythropoietin Encephalopathy

The efficacy of rHuEPO in the treatment of renal anemia is well established. Nevertheless, erythropoietin therapy is associated with serious untoward effects, including increased risk of hypertension, sometimes accompanied by hypertensive encephalopathy and seizures. The pathogenesis may relate to an increase in blood viscosity, a reversal of hypoxic vasodilatation and possibly a direct pressure effect of rHuEPO. The result is cerebral hypoperfusion and focal cerebral edema.

Preexistent atherosclerosis is a possible additional risk factor. Proper guidelines for rHuEPO treatment may prevent such a complication.[150] Use of EPO in the patient with a prior history of seizures is not contraindicated since there is no evidence of an increased risk of seizure in ESRD patients on EPO.

FUTURE TRENDS

DDS is less frequent in peritoneal dialysis patients (IPD, CAPD, CCPD) than in those on HD if the "usual" PD solutions are used. There is no evidence that CAPD patients develop less peripheral neuropathy or UE than HD patients. Even though it was previously shown[116] that, in CAPD patients, the indexes of attention and cognitive processing are better than in HD patients, Teschan demonstrated[117] that 26 patients who had shifted from CAPD to HD did not show any EEG signs of deterioration.

Are nerve conduction studies (NCS) useful for monitoring the adequacy of renal dialysis? In recent years, two different studies came to different conclusions about the value of NCS in dialysis patients. Bolton and Young noted that "NCS are an objective method to measure peripheral nerve function" and "should continue to be regularly utilized in patients receiving chronic hemodialysis."[118] Jennekens and Jennekens-Schinkel, in a standard text on the practice of dialysis, conclude that "according to current opinion, serial measurements of nerve conduction do not offer a reliable index for the adequacy of regular dialysis."[119] According to Phillips,[120] "at present we don't know whether a change of NCS values is sufficiently sensitive to indicate a problem with dialysis." Newer modalities for monitoring peripheral nerve function (such as vibratory and thermal sensation) may be more sensitive than previous tests.[121,122] All tests of neurologic function should be compared with clinical data, other measures of dialysis adequacy *(KT/V)*, and various biochemical tests.[123]

CONCLUSIONS

When the many effects induced by dialysis on the uremic brain are considered, it is apparent that the etiology of uremic neurologic disorders depends on several concomitant events. Each dialytic session per se may acutely modify the conditions in which neurons function. In the long run, each of these "acute" changes (hydroelectrolytic, osmotic, electrical) becomes an important factor in determining the onset and the worsening of the chronic encephalopathy. Malnutrition, anemia, hypertension, atherosclerosis, amino acid imbalance, hormonal disorders, drugs, trace elements, and the unphysiology of dialytic treatments are all factors possibly playing an important role.

The existence of patients (even though subjected to dialysis for more than 20 years) showing no clear sign of dialytic encephalopathy, however, suggests that it is necessary to study patients extensively, starting when mild CKD appears. Only by doing this will it be possible to elucidate all of the possible alterations/causes that may lead to a subclinical (EEG, mental tests, neurohormonal disorders) and eventually a clinical pattern of encephalopathy.

Many aspects of UE still need to be clarified. The roles of free radicals, lipid peroxidation, malnutrition, anemia, and hormonal imbalances are a few of the many areas awaiting clarification. Nuclear magnetic resonance, positron emission transaxial tomography, bioimpedance, computer-aided imaging, and biosensors will probably be utilized by researchers to further elucidate this subject in the near future, as is being attempted by several investigators.[123–130]

In the meantime, it will be possible to try to prevent UE by means of some simple therapeutic interventions: better control of nutritional status, chronic supplementation of hydrosoluble vitamins, aerobic exercise training, and proper dialytic efficiency.[147–149]

REFERENCES

1. Addison T. On the disorders of the brain connected with diseased kidneys. *Guy's Hosp Rep* 1839;4:1–7.
2. Hun H. Nervous symptoms associated with Bright's disease. *Alb Med Ann* 1895;16:139–151.
3. Tyler HR. Neurologic disorders in renal failure. *Am Med* 1968;44:734–748.
4. Tyler HR. Neurologic complications of uremia. In: Strauss MB, Welt LG, eds. *Diseases of the Kidney,* 2d ed. Boston: Little, Brown, 1971:334–342.
5. Arieff AI, Massry SG, Barrientos A, Kleeman GR. Brain water and electrolyte metabolism in uremia: effects of slow and rapid HD. *Kidney Int* 1973;4:177–187.
6. Nissenson AR, Levin ML, Klawans HL, Nausieda PL. Neurological sequelae of end stage renal disease (ESRD). *J Chronic Dis* 1977;30:705–733.
7. Bolton CF, Johnson WJ, Dyck PJ. Neurologic manifestations of renal failure. In: Earley LE, Gottschalk CW, eds. *Strauss and Welt's Diseases of the Kidney,* 3d ed. Boston: Little, Brown, 1979:371–392.
8. Arieff AI. Neurological complications of uremia. In: Brenner BM, Rector FC, eds. *The Kidney,* 2d ed. Philadelphia: Saunders, 1981:2306–2343.
9. Mahoney CA, Arieff AI, Leach WJ, Lazarowitz VC. Central and peripheral nervous systems effects of chronic renal failure. *Kidney Int* 1983;24:170–177.
10. Blagg C. Brain abnormalities and peripheral neuropathy. In: Blagg C, ed. *Textbook of Nephrology.* Baltimore: Williams & Wilkins, 1983:7.15–7.19.
11. Raskin NH, Fishman RA. Neurologic disorders in renal failure. *N Engl J Med* 1976;294:143–148.
12. Kiley JE, Pratt KL, Gisser DG, Schaffer CA. Techniques of EEG frequency analysis for evaluation of uremic encephalopathy. *Clin Nephrol* 1976;5:279–285.
13. Kiley JE, Woodruff MW, Pratt KL. Evaluation of encephalopathy by EEG frequency analysis in chronic dialysis patients. *Clin Nephrol* 1976;5:245.
14. Teschan PE, Ginn HE, Bourne JR, et al. Quantitative indices of clinical uremia. *Kidney Int* 1979;15:676–697.
15. Arieff AI, Lazarowitz VC, Guisardo R. Experimental dialysis disequilibrium syndrome; prevention with glycerol. *Kidney Int* 1978;14:270–278.
16. La Greca G, Dettori P, Biasioli S, et al. Studies on morphological and densitometrical changes in brain after hemo and peritoneal dialysis. *ASAIO Trans* 1981;27:40–44.
17. La Greca G, Biasioli S, Chiaramonte S, et al. Studies on brain density in hemo and peritoneal dialysis. *Nephron* 1982;31:146–150.
18. Biasioli S, Chiaramonte S, Fabris A, et al. Neurotransmitter imbalance in plasma and cerebrospinal fluid during dialytic treatment. *ASAIO Trans* 1983;29:44–49.
19. Olsen S. The brain in uremia. *Acta Psychiatr Scand* 1961; 36(suppl 156):1–10.
20. Savazzi GM, Cusmano F, Degasperi T. Cerebral atrophy in patients on long-term regular hemodialysis treatment. *Clin Nephrol* 1985;23:89–95.
21. Gulyassy PF, Peters JH, Lin SC, Ryan PM. Hemodialysis and plasma amino acid composition in chronic renal failure. *Am J Clin Nutr* 1968;21:565–570.
22. Giordano C, De Pascale C, De Santo NG, et al. Disorder in the metabolism of some amino acids in uremia. In: *Proceedings of the 4th International Congress of Nephrology.* Basel: Karger, 1970:196–205.
23. Alvestrand A, Fürst P, Bergstrom J. Plasma and muscle free amino acids in uremia: influence of nutrition with amino acids. *Clin Nephrol* 1982;18:297–305.

24. Letendre CH, Nagaiah K, Guroff G. Brain amino acids. In: Letendre CH, ed. *Biochemistry of Brain.* Oxford, UK: Pergamon Press, 1980:343–382.

25. McGale EHF, Pye IF, Stonier C, et al. Studies of the interrelationship between cerebrospinal fluid and plasma amino acid concentration in normal individuals. *J Neurochem* 1977;29:291–297.

26. Pardridge WM, Oldendorf WH. Transport of metabolic substrates through the blood brain barrier. *J Neurochem* 1977;5:28–35.

27. Pye IF, McGale EHF, Stonier C, et al. Studies of cerebrospinal fluid and plasma amino acid in patients with steady state chronic renal failure. *Clin Chim Acta* 1979;92:65–72.

28. Deferrari G, Garibotto G, Robaudo C, et al. Brain metabolism of amino acids and ammonia in patients with chronic renal insufficiency. *Kidney Int* 1981;20:505–510.

29. Pauli HG, Vorburger C, Reubi F. Chronic derangement of cerebrospinal fluid acid-base components in man. *J Appl Physiol* 1962;17:993–996.

30. Biasioli S, D'Andrea G, Chiaramonte S, et al. The role of neurotransmitters in the genesis of uremic encephalopathy. *Int J Artif Organs* 1984;7:101–106.

31. Sullivan PA, Murnaghan D, Callaghan N, et al. Cerebral transmitter precursors and metabolites in advanced renal disease. *J Neurol Neurosurg Psychiatry* 1978;41:581–588.

32. Biasioli S, D'Andrea G, Fabris A, et al. The pathogenesis of uremic encephalopathy. *Int J Artif Organs* 1985;8:20–22.

33. Howard JJ, Jeppson, Ziparov V, Fischer JE. Hyperammonaemia, plasma amino acid imbalance and BBB amino acid transport: a unified theory of portal systemic encephalopathy. *Lancet* 1979;2:772–775.

34. Tyler HR, Leavitt S. Asterixis. *J Chronic Dis* 1965;18:409–415.

35. Young SN, Lal S, Sourkes TL, et al. Relationship between tryptophan in serum and CSF and 5-HIAA in CSF of man: effect of cirrhosis of liver and probenecid administration. *J Neurol Neurosurg Psychiatry* 1975;38:322–330.

36. Jellinger K, Irsigler K, Kothbauer P, Riederer P. Brain monoamines in metabolic coma. *Int Congress Series* 1977;427:169–175.

37. Biasioli S, Feriani M, Chiaramonte S, et al. The serotoninergic system in uremia: relationship to hormonal status. In: Friedman E, Beyer M, De Santo N, et al, eds. *Prevention of Progressive Uremia.* New York: Field & Wood, 1989:3:79–82.

38. Biasioli S, D'Andrea G, Micieli G, et al. Hyperprolactemia as a marker of neurotransmitter imbalance in uremic population. *Int J Artif Organs* 1987;10:245–257.

39. Biasioli S, D'Andrea G, Feriani M, et al. Uremic encephalopathy: an updating. *Clin Nephrol* 1986;25:57–63.

40. Biasioli S, Mazzali A, Foroni R, et al. Chronobiological variations of prolactin (PRL) in chronic renal failure (CKD). *Clin Nephrol* 1988;30:86–92.

41. Lowrie EG, Steinberg SM, Galen MA, et al. Factors in the dialysis regimen which contribute to alternations in the abnormalities of uremia. *Kidney Int* 1976;10:409–422.

42. Ronco C, Biasioli S, Borin D, et al. Patologia neurologica in dialisi. *Minerva Nefrol* 1982;4:185–193.

43. Nissenson AR, Marsh JT, Brown WS, Wolcott DL. Central nervous system function in dialysis patients: a practical approach. *Semin Dial* 1991;4(2):115–123.

44. Nissenson AR. Recombinant human erythropoietin: impact on brain and cognitive function, exercise tolerance, sexual potency, and quality of life. *Semin Nephrol* 1989;9 (suppl 2):25–31.

45. Marsh JT, Wolcott DL, Harper R, Nissenson AR. Impairment of brain function by anemia: ameliorative effects on brain and cognitive function of rHuEPO in dialysis patients. *Kidney Int* 1991;29:155–163.

46. Matthew RJ, Rabin P, Stone WJ, Wilson WH. Regional cerebral blood flow in dialysis encephalopathy and primary degenerative dementia. *Kidney Int* 1985;28:64–68.

47. Grotta JC, Manner C, Pettigrew LC, Yatsu FM. Red blood cell disorders and stroke. *Stroke* 1986;17:811–817.

48. Sagales T, Gimeno V, Planella MJ, et al. Effects of rHuEPO on Q-EEG and event-related potentials in chronic renal failure. *Kidney Int* 1993;44:1109–1115.

49. Grimm G, Stockenhuber F, Schneeweiss B, et al. Improvement of brain function in hemodialysis patients treated with erythropoietin. *Kidney Int* 1990;38:480–486.

50. Brown WS, Marsh JT, Wolcott D, et al. Cognitive function, mood and P3 latency: effects of the amelioration of anemia in dialysis patients. *Neuropsychologia* 1991;29:34–45.

51. Mahoney CA, Sarnacki P, Arieff AI. Uremic encephalopathy: role of brain energy metabolism. *Am J Physiol* 1984;247(Renal Fluid Electrolyte Physiol 16):F527–F532.

52. Fraser CL, Sarnacki P, Arieff AI. Altered Na transport in brain of uremic rats: relation to neurotransmission in uremia? *Clin Res* 1984;32:532A.

53. Kiley JE. Residual renal and dialyzer clearance, EEG slowing, and nerve conduction velocity. *ASAIO J* 1981;4:1–8.

54. Massry SG, Procci WR, Goldstein DA, Kletzky OA. Sexual dysfunction. In: *Textbook of Nephrology.* Baltimore: Williams & Wilkins, 1983:7.89–7.92.

55. Gilli P, Fagioli F, Malacarne F. Serum aluminium levels and peritoneal dialysis. *Int J Artif Organs* 1984;7:107–110.

56. Schiavon R, Biasioli S, De Fanti E, et al. The plasma glutathione peroxidase enzyme in hemodialyzed subjects. *ASAIO J* 1994;40:968–971.

57. McGonigle RJS, Bewick M, Weston MJ, Parsons V. Progressive, predominantly motor, uremic neuropathy. *Acta Neurol Scand* 1985;71:379–384.

58. Dyck PJ, Johnson WJ, Lambert EH, et al. Detection and evaluation of uremic peripheral neuropathy in patients on hemodialysis. *Kidney Int* 1975;7:S201–S205.

59. Di Giulio S, Chkoff N, Lhoste F, et al. Parathormone as a nerve poison in uremia. *N Engl J Med* 1978;299:1134–1135.

60. Brismar T, Tegner R. Excitability changes reveal decreased sodium permeability in neuropathy. *Exp Neurol* 1985;87:177–180.

61. Mallamaci F, Zoccali C, Ciccarelli M, Briggs JD. Autonomic function in uremic patients treated by hemodialysis or CAPD and in transplant patients. *Clin Nephrol* 1986;25:175–180.

62. Zoccali C, Ciccarelli M, Mallamaci F, Maggiore Q. Parasympathetic function in hemodialysis patients. *Nephron* 1986;42:285–289.

63. Naik RB, Mathias CJ, Wilson CA. Cardiovascular and autonomic reflexes in hemodialysis patients. *Clin Sci* 1981;60: 165–170.

64. Marsden CD. Basal ganglia disease. *Lancet* 1982;1: 1141–1147.

65. Raju SF, White AR, Barnes TT, et al. Improvement in disequilibrium symptoms during dialysis with low glucose dialysate. *Clin Nephrol* 1982;181:126–129.

66. Port FK, Johnson WJ, Klass DW. Prevention of dialysis disequilibrium syndrome by use of high sodium concentration in the dialysis. *Kidney Int* 1973;3:327–333.

67. Platts MM, Anastassiades E. Dialysis encephalopathy: precipitating factors and improvement in prognosis. *Clin Nephrol* 1981;15:228–233.

68. Smith EC, Mahurkar SD, Mamdani BH, Dunea G. Diagnosing dialysis dementia. *Dial Transplant* 1978;7:1264–1274.

69. Alfrey AC, Mishell JM, Burks J, et al. Syndrome of dyspraxia and multifocal seizure associated with chronic hemodialysis. *ASAIO Trans* 1972;18:257–261.

70. Mahurkar SD, Salta P, Smith EC, et al. Dialysis dementia. *Lancet* 1973;1:1412–1415.

71. Alfrey AC. Dialysis encephalopathy. *Kidney Int* 1986;18: S53–S57.

72. La Greca G, Biasioli S, Chiaramonte S, et al. Brain density studies during hemodialysis. *Lancet* 1980;2:582.

73. Dettori P, La Greca G, Biasioli S, et al. Changes of cerebral density in dialyzed patients. *Neuroradiology* 1982;23: 95–99.

74. Bourne JR, Miezin FM, Ward JW, Teschan PE. Computer quantification of electroencephalographic data recorded from renal patients. *Comput Biomed Res* 1975;8:461–473.

75. Hochman MS. Meperidine associated myoclonus and seizures in long-term hemodialysis patients. *Ann Neurol* 1983;14:593.

76. Mahurkar SD, Meyers L, Cohen J, et al. Electroencephalographic and radionuclide studies in dialysis dementia. *Kidney Int* 1978;13:306–315.

77. Nunez PL. A study of origins of the time dependencies of scalp EEG: 1. Theoretical basis. *Trans Biomed Eng* 1981;28: 271–280.

78. Albertazzi A, Rossini PM, Pirchio M, et al. Checkerboard reversal pattern and flash VEPs in dialyzed and non-dialyzed subjects. *Electroencephalogr Clin Neurophysiol* 1981;52:435–439.

79. Albertazzi A, Di Paolo B, Di Paolo AM, Rossini PM. Modern neurophysiological assessment of uraemic nephropathy. *Proc ESAO* 1982;9:25–29.

80. Marsh JT, Brown WS, Wolcott D, et al. Electrophysiological indices of CNS function in hemodialysis and CAPD. *Kidney Int* 1986;30:957–963.

81. Freeman RB, Sheff MF, Maher JF, Schreiner GE. The blood cerebral fluid barrier in uremia. *Ann Intern Med* 1962;56: 233.

82. Funder J, Wieth JO. Changes in cerebrospinal fluid composition following hemodialysis. *Scand J Clin Lab* 1967;19: 302.

83. McGale EHF, Pye IF, Corston R, et al. The effect of hemodialysis on cerebrospinal fluid and plasma amino acids. *Clin Chim Acta* 1979;92:73.

84. Ronco C, Biasioli S, Chiaramonte S, et al. Modifiche ematoliquorali indotte dalla dialisi extracorporea e peritoneale. In: D'Amico G, ed. *Nefrologia, Dialisis e Trapianto.* Milan: Wichtig, 1982:311–325.

85. Hökfelt T, Johannson O, Ljungdahl A, et al. Peptidergic neurones. *Nature* 1981;284:515–520.

86. La Greca G, Biasioli S, Borin D, et al. Dialytic encephalopathy. *Contrib Nephrol* 1985;3:14–28.

87. Iversen LL. Neurotransmitters and CNS disease. *Lancet* 1982;2:914–918.

88. Sorenson JRJ, Campbell IR, Tepper LB, Lingg RD. Aluminium in the environment and human health. *Environ Health Perspect* 1974;8:3–95.

89. Alfrey AC, Le Gendre GR, Kaenhy WD. The dialysis encephalopathy syndrome: possible aluminium intoxication. *N Engl J Med* 1976;294:184–188.

90. Alfrey AC, Smythe WR. Trace element abnormalities in chronic uremia. *Proc 11th Contractr Conf Artif Kidney Chron Uremia Prog NIAMDD* 1978;11:137–139.

91. Arieff AI, Cooper JD, Armstrong D, Lazarowitz VC. Demential, renal failure, and brain aluminium. *Ann Intern Med* 1979;90:741–747.

92. McDermott JR, Smith AI, Ward MK, et al. Brain aluminium concentration in dialysis encephalopathy. *Lancet* 1978;1: 901–904.

93. Pascoe MD, Gregory MC. Dialysis encephalopathy: aluminium concentration in dialysate and brain. *Kidney Int* 1979;16:90.

94. Dunea G, Mahurkar SD, Mamdami B, Smith EC. Role of aluminium in dialysis dementia. *Ann Intern Med* 1978;88: 502–504.

95. Nathan E, Pedersen SE. Dialysis encephalopathy in a nondialyzed uraemic boy with aluminium hydroxide orally. *Acta Paediatr Scand* 1980;69(6):793–796.

96. Griswald WR, Reznik V, Mendoza SA, et al. Accumulation of aluminium in a nondialyzed uremic child receiving aluminium hydroxide. *Pediatrics* 1983;71:56–58.

97. Slatopolsky E. The interaction of parathyroid hormone and aluminium in renal osteodystrophy. *Kidney Int* 1987;31: 842–854.

98. Slatopolsky E, Weerts C, Lopez-Hilker S, et al. Calcium carbonate as a phosphate binder in patients with chronic renal failure undergoing dialysis. *N Engl J Med* 1986;315: 157–161.

99. Bakir AA, Hryhorczuk DO, Berman E, Dunea G. Acute fatal hyperaluminemic encephalopathy in undialyzed and recently dialyzed uremic patients. *ASAIO Trans* 1986;32: 171–176.

100. Ackrill P, Raltson AJ, Day JP. Role of desferrioxamine in the treatment of dialysis encephalopathy. *Kidney Int* 1986; 18:S104–S107.

101. Sprague SM, Corwin HL, Wilson R, et al. Encephalopathy in chronic renal failure responsive to desferrioxamine therapy: another manifestation of aluminium neurotoxicity. *Arch Intern Med* 1986;146:2063–2064.

102. Hood SA, Clark WF, Hodsman AB, et al. Successful treatment of dialysis osteomalacia and dementia using desferrioxamine infusions and oral 1α hydroxy-cholecalciferol. *Am J Nephrol* 1984;4:369–374.

103. Milne FJ, Sharp B, Bell P, Meyers AM. The effect of low aluminium water and desferrioxamine on the outcome of dialysis encephalopathy. *Clin Nephrol* 1983;20:202–207.

104. Payton CD, Junor BJ, Fell GS. Successful treatment of aluminium encephalopathy by intraperitoneal desferrioxamine. *Lancet* 1984;1:1132–1133.

105. Sullivan D, Murnaghan DJ, Callaghan N. Dialysis dementia, recovery after transplantation. *Br Med J* 1977;2:740.

106. Davison AM, Giles GR. The effect of transplantation on dialysis dementia. *Proc Eur Dial Transplant Assoc* 1979;16: 407–412.

107. Mattern WD, Krigman MR, Blythe NB. Failure of successful renal transplantation to reverse the dialysis-associated encephalopathy syndrome. *Clin Nephrol* 1977;7(6): 275–278.

108. O'Hare JA, Callaghan NM, Murnaghan DJ. Dialysis encephalopathy: clinical, electroencephalographic, and interventional aspects. *Medicine* 1983;62:129–141.

109. Chachati A, Dechenne C, Gordon JP. Increased incidence of cerebral hemorrhage mortality in patients with analgesic nephropathy on hemodialysis. *Nephron* 1987;45:167–168.

110. Isiadinso OA. Early diagnosis of subdural hematoma in hemodialysis patients: use of carotid arteriography. *Angiology* 1976;27:491–493.

111. Lopez RI, Collins GK. Wernicke's encephalopathy: a complication of chronic hemodialysis. *Arch Neurol* 1968;18:248.

112. Jagadha V, Deck JHN, Halliday WC, Smythe HS. Wernicke's encephalopathy in patients on peritoneal dialysis or hemodialysis. *Ann Neurol* 1987;21:78–84.

113. Fornari AJ, Avram MM. Altered taste perception in uremia. *ASAIO Trans* 1978;24:385–388.

114. Mahajan SK, Prasad AS, Lambujon J, et al. Improvement of uremic hypogeusia by zinc. *ASAIO Trans* 1979;25:443–448.

115. Sprenger KB, Bundschu D, Lewis K, et al. Improvement of uremic neuropathy and hypogeusia by dialysate zinc supplementation: a double blind study. *Kidney Int* 1983;16:S315–S318.

116. Tegner R, Lindholm B. Uremic polyneuropathy: different effects of hemodialyzed and continuous ambulatory peritoneal dialysis. *Acta Med Scand* 1985;218:409–416.

117. Teschan PE. Clinical estimates of treatment adequacy. *Artif Organs* 1986;10:201–204.

118. Bolton CF, Young GB. Uremic neuropathy. In: Bolton CF, Young GB, eds. *Neurological Complications of Renal Disease.* Boston, MA: Butterworth, 1990:77–118.

119. Jennekens FGI, Jennekens-Schinkel A. Neurological aspects of dialysis patients. In: Maher JF, ed. *Replacement of Renal Function by Dialysis.* 3d ed. Dordrecht, The Netherlands: Kluwer, 1989:972–986.

120. Phillips LH, Williams FH. Are nerve conduction studies useful for monitoring the adequacy of renal dialysis? *Muscle Nerve* 1993;16:970–974.

121. Tegner R, Lindholm B. Vibratory perception threshold compared with nerve conduction velocity in the evaluation of uremic neuropathy. *Acta Neurol Scand* 1985;71:284–289.

122. Tegner R, Lindhom B. Uremic polyneuropathy: different effects of hemodialysis and continuous ambulatory peritoneal dialysis. *Acta Med Scand* 1985;218:409–416.

123. Hakim RM. Assessing the adequacy of dialysis. *Kidney Int* 1990;37:822–832.

124. Goulon-Goeau C, Said G. Neurologic complications in hemodialysis patients. *Rev Prat* 1990;40(7):644–646.

125. Lipman JJ, Lawrence PL, DeBoer DK, et al. Role of dialysable solutes in the mediation of uremic encephalopathy in the rat. *Kidney Int* 1990;37(3):892–900.

126. Muto Y, Murase M. Metabolic encephalopathy in the aged. *Nippon Naika Gakkai Zasshi* 1990;79(4):468–474.

127. Okada J, Yoshikawa K, Matsuo H, et al. Reversible MRI and CT findings in uremic encephalopathy. *Neuroradiology* 1991;33(6):524–526.

128. Bosch BA, Schlebusch L. Neuropsychological deficits with uraemic encephalopathy. A report of 5 patients. *S Afr Med J* 1991;79(9):560–562.

129. Tattersall JE, Cramp M, Shannon M, et al. Rapid high-flux dialysis can cure uraemic peripheral neuropathy. *Nephrol Dial Transplant* 1992;7(6):539–540.

130. Ogura Y, Chichihara Y. Uremic neuropathy in chronic kidney failure in dialysis. *Nippon Rinsho* 1992;50(suppl): 824–827.

131. Balzer S, Kuttner K. Das fruhe akutisch evozierte Potential. *HNO* 1996;44:559–565.

132. Moe SM, Sprague SM. Uremic encephalopathy. *Clin Nephrol* 1994;42(4):253–260.

133. Bucurescu G. Uremic encephalopathy. *Emedicine.com 2002; topic388.htm: 2–10*

134. Lohr JW, Bashir K. Dialysis encephalopathy. *Emedicine .com 2002; topic665.htm: 1–11*

135. Fuller VL. Dialysis encephalopathy. *Indstate.edn 2002; topic thcme/anderson: 1–8*

136. Hughes JR, Schreeder M. The EEG in dialysis encephalopathy. *Neurology* 1980;30:1148–1154.

137. Wills MR, Savory J. Aluminum and chronic renal failure: sources, absorption, transport and toxicity. *Crit Rev Clin Lab Sci* 1989;27:59–107.

138. Schwartz RD. Deferoxamine and aluminum removal. *Am J Kidney Dis* 1985;6:358–363.

139. Bengtsson T, Sarndahl E, Stendhal O, Andersson T. Toxin-induced blood vessels inclusion caused by the chronic administration of aluminum and sodium fluoride. Their implications for dementia. *Ann NY Acad Sci* 1997;825: 152–166.

140. Jacqmin-Gadda H, Commenges D, Letenneur L, Dartigues JF. Silica and aluminum in drinking water and cognitive impairment in the elderly. *Epidemiology* 1996;7(3):281–285.

141. Crapper MC, Lachlan J. Aluminum and Alzheimer's disease. *Neurobiol Aging* 1986;7:525–532.

142. Lote CJ, Saunders H. Aluminum gastrointestinal absorption and renal excretion. *Clin Sci* 1991;81:289–295.

143. Meiri H, Banin E, Roll M. Aluminum ingestion—is it related to dementia? *Rev Environ Health* 1991;9(4):191–205.

144. Hung SC. Thiamine deficiency and unexplained encephalopathy in HD and PD patients. *Am J Kidney Dis* 2001;38: 941–947.

145. Chandra RK. Effect of vitamin and trace element supplementation on cognitive function in elderly subjects. *Nutrition* 2001;17:709–712.

146. Seshadri S, Beiser A, Selhub J, et al. Plasma homocysteine as a risk factor for dementia and Alzheimer's disease. *N Engl J Med* 2002;400:125–130.

147. Biasioli S, Schiavon R. Homocysteine as a cardiovascular risk factor. *Blood Purif* 2000;18:177–182.

148. Biasioli S, Schiavon R, Petrosino L, et al. Do different dialytic techniques have different atherosclerotic and antioxidant activities? *ASAIO J* 2001;47:516–521.

149. Schmidt M, Sitter TH, Lederer SR, Held E. Reversible MRI changes in a patient with uremic encephalopathy. *J Nephrol* 2001;14:424–427.

150. Dapena F, Tato A, Aguilera A, Delgado R. Posterior leukoencephalopathy caused by EPO. *Nefrologie* 2000; 20(17):87–88.

Diabetes and Dialysis

Frieda Wolf
Mariana S. Markell

Diabetic nephropathy is the leading cause of end-stage renal disease (ESRD) in much of the world at the present time. In the United States, diabetic nephropathy was the leading cause of ESRD listed for new patients funded by Medicare for renal replacement therapy between the years 1997 and 2001, accounting for 45 percent of new cases by primary diagnosis, according to the U.S. Renal Data System (USRDS).[1] The overall burden of diabetes in the ESRD program is 59 percent of all cases, with 80 percent of Native Americans, 73 percent of Hispanics, 61 percent of Asians, 59 percent of blacks, and 58 percent of whites with ESRD being affected. Notably, the highest rates of diabetic nephropathy are in minority populations that have the highest prevalence of type 2 diabetes. The peak incidence of new diabetes in patients with ESRD occurs between the fifth to eighth decades of life. Although USRDS data regarding new-onset ESRD in diabetics do not differentiate between the incidence rates of ESRD in type 1 (insulin-dependent or juvenile diabetes) and type 2 (non-insulin-dependent or maturity-onset diabetes) diabetic patients, other studies suggest that the rates of ESRD are significant for both populations. In the past, approximately 35 percent of type 1 diabetics developed diabetic nephropathy,[2] but recent observational trials have demonstrated a decreasing incidence of nephropathy in more recently diagnosed groups.[3] Although the annual rate of increase of ESRD due to diabetes has declined, the prevalence of diabetes is now 8 percent in the general population, and it continues to rise.[4] Thus, management of the patient with ESRD and diabetes has become more than just a common problem for providers of nephrologic care; it has become a public health crisis of epidemic proportions.

PROGRESSION OF RENAL DISEASE AND CHOICE OF UREMIA THERAPY

For patients with type 1 diabetes, renal disease is believed to progress from microalbuminuria through nephrotic-range proteinuria to ESRD.[5] The time for this progression is variable, but it generally occurs 15 to 25 years following the onset of diabetes.[6] A recent observational trial[3] of type 1 diabetics noted a decline in the incidence of nephropathy in more recently diagnosed cohorts, with approximately 31 percent in the earliest cohort (1965–1969), reduced to 13 percent in the most recent one (1979–1984). This reduction was attributed to improved glycemic and hypertensive control. For type 2 diabetics, the course is less clear, in part because these patients tend to be older and to have concomitant long-standing medical problems, including hypertension and atherosclerosis, which contribute to the development of renal disease and increase morbidity and mortality.[7,8] Furthermore, only 50 percent diabetics are aware of their diagnosis, and many present for the first time with retinopathy after an average of 7 years of undiagnosed, untreated diabetes.

The course of diabetic nephropathy may be slowed by one of several manipulations, including aggressive glycemic control,[9–11] control of hypertension,[12,13] and treatment using angiotensin-converting enzyme (ACE) inhibitors alone or with angiotensin II receptor blockers (ARBs).[14–17] Intensive control of blood glucose in patients with type 1 diabetes may retard glomerular damage. Sustained euglycemia reduces kidney size in patients with previous hyperfiltration[11]; results of the Diabetes Complications and Control Trial[9] (DCCT) suggest that near euglycemia can both decrease the appearance of microalbuminuria and slow the progression of established renal disease. The DCCT cohort was followed prospectively for 8 years[14] after the conclusion of the initial study. During this follow-up period, glycemic levels did not differ significantly between groups, and persistent beneficial effects on albumin excretion and the incidence of hypertension in the group assigned to intensive treatment initially during the DCCT were observed. Unfortunately, it is difficult to achieve the level of glucose control maintained during the DCCT outside a research setting, and there is no therapy certain to halt progression of nephropathic disease once it has been initiated. The United Kingdom Prospective Diabetes Study[10] (UKPDS) followed patients with type 2 diabetes for over 8 years. This multicenter trial included over 4000 people and showed that tight glycemic control significantly decreased the appearance of microalbuminuria and also retarded the progression of microalbuminuria to macroalbuminuria, thereby slowing the progression of nephropathy. Finally, recent prospective trials in type 1[15,16] and type 2[17,18] diabetic patients with nephropathy have demonstrated the usefulness of inhibition of the renin-angiotensin-aldosterone axis with ACE inhibitors and ARBs in conferring renoprotection separate from that of hypertensive control, but not in preventing progression to ESRD completely.

Thus, despite recent advances and in light of the pandemic of type 2 diabetes, new cases of diabetic nephropathy will continue to progress to chronic renal insufficiency and eventually ESRD. As diabetes is a multisystem disorder, patients with diabetic nephropathy present unique problems that must be taken into consideration in initiating treatment with renal replacement therapy.

The nephrotic syndrome is commonly part of the clinical picture of diabetic nephropathy. Patients may lose 4 to 8 g of urinary protein, but daily protein losses may be as high as 20 to 30 g, resulting in impairment of the immune system due to immunoglobulin loss and severe protein malnutrition. Anasarca with leg edema, ascites, and pleural effusions may result from fluid retention of as much as 10 to 30 kg. Dyspnea and fatigue due to massive fluid retention may be difficult to differentiate from symptoms of uremia and may curtail activities of daily living such that transplantation or dialysis must be performed at a glomerular filtration rate (GFR) that is higher than in the nondiabetic person. Diabetic patients whose creatinine clearance falls to about 10 mL/min (serum creatinine concentration of approximately 5 mg/dL) are often too sick to sustain work, home, or school responsibilities without dialytic support, although patients with other forms of renal disease may not need dialysis until the creatinine clearance falls to 5 mL/min (approximately 10 to 15 mg/dL serum creatinine concentration).

The choice of uremia therapy for patients with diabetes is the end result of a number of factors, including nephrologist bias, concomitant extrarenal disease, treatment modality available, and patient's choice. Living related kidney transplantation was the first choice of therapy both in diabetic and nondiabetic ESRD patients in New Zealand/Australia, southern California, and North Carolina in a study of nephrologist preference.[19] When a kidney transplant was not available or was contraindicated for medical reasons, the choice of ESRD therapy differed depending on whether the patient was diabetic or not. Home hemodialysis (HD) was the preferred option for nondiabetic patients in Australia/New Zealand, whereas diabetic patients were referred for peritoneal dialysis (PD). In all three populations surveyed, in-center HD was the least desirable renal replacement modality. In a recent survey of British nephrologists,[20] patient's preference was the foremost reason for choosing a modality, followed by quality-of-life reasons and only then by morbidity/mortality data. Physician or facility reimbursement was the least important determinant. Most nephrologists felt that hospital-based HD and continuous ambulatory PD (CAPD) were overused and that future planning should include increasing the proportion of home HD and PD. This study echoes an American survey of nephrologists,[21] who believe that home therapies are underused. However, in some countries, the choice of ESRD therapy is guided by geography and the availability of the treatment modality. PD is much more widely used in Canada than in the United States, comprising about half of all dialysis. It is no surprise that a Canadian retrospective chart review,[22] which excluded transplant patients, concluded that if an informed patient is given a choice of treatment modality, he or she will more likely choose self-care dialysis.

In helping a diabetic patient with ESRD decide on a specific type of renal replacement therapy, lifestyle considerations must be taken into account, as well as coexisting medical conditions (Table 32–1). Renal transplantation confers the best quality of life and arguably the best survival[23] of the available modalities; however, the risks of anesthesia, major surgery, and subsequent immunosuppression must be taken into consideration prior to referring a diabetic patient for kidney transplantation. Regardless of whether a patient has diabetes, successful use of CAPD is related to patient understanding and compliance. Patient education, autonomy, and strong social support are as important as early pre-ESRD care to the successful use of PD.[24] Unfortunately, there are few data that shed light on which patients will benefit most from PD. Some factors to consider when PD is being offered are patient preference and lifestyle,[25] solute transport characteristics, and residual renal function. A disruptive, unstable, or unsanitary home life will obviate home dialysis of any type as a therapeutic option. Education of the patient by the nephrology team, resulting in an informed decision regarding therapy, is a crucial part of patient preparation for choosing and initiating renal replacement therapy.

TABLE 32–1. VARIABLES THAT AFFECT THE CHOICE OF HOME ESRD THERAPY FOR DIABETIC PATIENTS

ADVANTAGES

Continuous Ambulatory Peritoneal Dialysis
1. Catheter placement does not require major surgery.
2. Minimal "volume" shifts due to continuous nature (good for patients with hypo- or hypertension).
3. Intraperitoneal insulin administration may be more "physiologic."
4. Technique can be taught rapidly.
5. Does not require vascular access.

Home Hemodialysis
1. Does not require major surgery.
2. Excellent patient survival.[a]
3. Excellent rehabilitation[a]; flexible hours make working easier.

DISADVANTAGES

Continuous Ambulatory Peritoneal Dialysis
1. High technique failure rate and mortality.[a]
2. High peritonitis rate.
3. Risk of patient "burnout" because of repetitive nature or technique.
4. Diabetic complications progress.

Home Hemodialysis
1. Must have a committed partner.
2. Some patients experience gradual "failure to thrive."
3. Other complications of diabetes progress.
4. Requires vascular access.

[a]Probable large contribution of selection bias.
Source: Modified from Jassal et al.,[20] with permission.

EXTRARENAL DISEASE

The presence of extrarenal disease complicates decisions regarding initiation of uremia therapy in the patient with diabetes. Disorders of fluid balance, cardiac, or gastric dysfunction may appear to accelerate the course of renal failure by mimicking uremic symptoms, and extrarenal diabetic complications have a tremendous impact on patient survival once dialysis has been initiated.

Cardiovascular disease remains the leading cause of death in diabetic patients[26] on dialysis and following transplantation. It accounts for 40 to 50 percent of all deaths, with cardiovascular mortality being 15 times higher in the ESRD population than in the general population.[27] Only 15 percent of new ESRD patients have normal left ventricular function by echocardiogram. The presence of left ventricular hypertrophy, congestive heart failure, or ischemic heart disease is highly prevalent among chronic kidney failure patients, and having kidney disease by itself increases risk of cardiovascular complications. A recent statement from the American Heart Association[28] indicated that chronic kidney disease (CKD), whether manifest by reduced GFR or proteinuria, is an independent risk factor for cardiovascular disease, and that steps should be taken to slow the progression of nephropathy as well as to control other risk factors. A risk factor–based approach is also recommended by the standards of care (2004) of the American Diabetes Association (ADA), stressing the need to identify coronary heart disease.[29] The accepted risk factors are hypertension, dyslipidemia, smoking, family history of cardiovascular disease, and micro- or macroalbuminuria. According to the ADA's guidelines, patients with increased risk factors should be treated with low-dose aspirin and possibly an ACE inhibitor. Cigarette smoking is a well-known modifiable risk factor for peripheral vascular and cardiovascular disease and has been shown to be an independent risk factor for the progression of renal disease.[30]

The presence of extrarenal disease can influence the choice of renal replacement therapy. Visual impairment or blindness is a common finding that can impair rehabilitation and may limit the patient to in-center HD.

Microaneurysms, the earliest signs of diabetic retinopathy, are present in over 95 percent of people who have had type 1 diabetes for 20 years[31] and 80 percent of those with type 2. Proliferative retinopathy, the presence of new blood vessel growth in the retina, if left untreated, results in vitreous hemorrhage or retinal detachment. It is present in 50 percent of type 1 diabetics after 15 years[32] and in approximately 10 percent of those with type 2.[33,34] The incidence of macular edema is 20 percent in type 1 and 25 percent in type 2 diabetics over a period of 10 years, which contributes to central visual loss. In a survey of 268 diabetic ESRD patients, visual disturbances were noted in 73.1 percent of eyes at initiation of dialysis.[35]

Peripheral neuropathy may limit the choice of ESRD therapy because of "stocking-glove" anesthesia of the extremities, making manipulation of CAPD equipment or setup of HD impossible unless a suitable partner is identified. Autonomic neuropathy, manifest by orthostatic hypotension, may be exacerbated by CAPD or HD, complicating maintenance of appropriate intravascular volume. Autonomic neuropathy may be a contributing cause to intradialytic hypotension, preventing adequate dialysis.[36] Dialytic therapy, whether on HD or PD, fails to improve autonomic/peripheral neuropathy in diabetics[37] unless there is a component of uremic neuropathy as well.

Gastroparesis may complicate the matching of insulin to food intake, and resulting nausea and vomiting may complicate interpretation of uremic symptoms. Small frequent feedings rather than large meals and pharmacologic therapy with metoclopramide, especially in the liquid form, may ameliorate gastroparesis, whereas nausea and vomiting from uremia will be unchanged. Intractable vomiting, after repeated unsuccessful attempts at medical management, is a feature of gastroparesis that may require gastrectomy[38] to improve the quality of life. Symptoms of dyspepsia and gastroparesis, as determined by the carbon-labeled octanoic acid breath test, were more common in patients treated by PD than in those treated by HD[39] in a Belgian study, although prevalence of *Helicobacter pylori* infection by serology was higher in the HD group.

The unpredictable appearance of diarrhea alternating with constipation may cause patients to limit their outside activities to the point of isolation, leading to severe depression. Diarrhea may respond to the use of a psyllium seed derivative such as Metamucil or other treatments that absorb water in the colon, such as Kaopectate. In resistant cases, 1-mg doses of loperamide (Imodium) may be used.[40] As is true for the diabetic patient without kidney disease, diarrhea often remits spontaneously. Constipation, to the point of obstipation, has been observed, especially during the time when dialysis patients were given aluminum hydroxide gels to bind phosphate in the gut. Sorbitol, oil-retention enemas, and daily doses of psyllium seed derivatives are sometimes successful in relieving obstipation.

It is important that comorbid conditions not be forgotten during the initiation and maintenance of a diabetic patient on renal replacement therapy. Amelioration of cardiovascular risk factors, including treatment of hyperlipidemia and cessation of smoking, should be attempted in addition to controlling blood pressure and attempting to maintain euglycemia. These well-known risk factors for cardiovascular disease are emerging as harbingers of the progression of chronic renal disease. Strict control of blood glucose, although theoretically desirable for prevention of coexisting diabetic complications such as neuropathy and retinopathy, is increasingly difficult as renal failure progresses, because 50 to 70 percent of insulin's catabolism occurs through renal routes,[41] and peak insulin action becomes delayed and unpredictable. Uremia exacerbates insulin resistance through secondary hyperparathyroidism, anemia, metabolic acidosis, and possibly, tumor necrosis factor alpha, found in adipose tissue. The use of a nurse-educator who is a specialist both in diabetes and renal disease can facilitate the dose adjustments of insulin and oral hypoglycemic agents, necessary during the initiation of dialysis, by teaching the patient self-monitoring of blood glucose and discussing the results with the patient.

HEMODIALYSIS

Mortality and Comorbid Conditions

HD continues to be the modality by which the majority of diabetic patients with ESRD are treated around the world. The USRDS survey for the year 2001 reports that 109,860 (76.6 percent) of the 142,963 ESRD patients with diabetes by primary diagnosis were dialyzed in center, representing an increase of approximately 10 percent over the preceding decade, concomitant with an increase in the percentage of ESRD patients with diabetic nephropathy.[4] In 2001, CAPD/continuous cyclic PD (CCPD) accounted for 8464 patients (5.9 percent) and renal transplants for 23,625 (17.5 percent) diabetic patients treated for ESRD.

Dialyzed patients with coexistent diabetes continue to have an inferior survival rate when compared with dialyzed patients who do not have diabetes, although the rates have improved substantially over the past 10 years. In the 2000 USRDS survey, 1-year age-, sex-, and race-adjusted survival for patients with diabetic nephropathy was 78 percent, compared with 85.7 percent for patients with ESRD secondary to "glomerulonephritis" and 80.7 percent for patients with ESRD secondary to hypertension, whereas the adjusted 1-year survival for diabetic patients in 1980 was approximately 68 percent. The adjusted 5-year survival, however, a dismal 17.6 percent in 1993, has increased to 31.4 percent in the most recent report.

To further highlight the improved survival of diabetics, in a secondary analysis of mortality data obtained by the Health Care Financing Administration (HCFA) for all patients aged 55 and older and treated by HD between the years 1982 and 1987, patients with diabetes had the worst survival rates.[42] For hemodialyzed diabetic patients above 85 years of age, no patient survived as long as 5 years. At that time there were 1235 diabetic patients over the age of 65 in the USRDS registry,[4] which increased to over 31,000 patients in 1996–1997 and to 40,087 in the last report. In a more recent analysis of mortality trends in the United States,[43] there was a substantial reduction in mortality of patients with ESRD. Although the adjusted 5-year survival probability for diabetics with ESRD over age 65 is only 14 percent for incident patients from 1996 to 1997, the most recent USRDS reports contain 10-year survival probabilities. There seems to be a consensus regarding the decreased survival of diabetics on HD as compared to nondiabetics, which is probably related, among other things, to the burden of comorbidities, deteriorating quality of life, and low serum albumin.[44] However, evidence is accumulating that with better dialysis (increased dialysis dose[45] and anemia management) and attention to comorbidities, overall survival for diabetics on dialysis has improved[46] despite the exponential increase in diabetics with ESRD.[47]

The introduction of PD in the 1970s provided an alternative to HD; PD was and became the preferred method of dialysis for diabetic patients in some countries.[19–21] Comparisons of mortality of patients on PD vs. HD have yielded conflicting and confusing results. In a study of prevalent dialysis patients for the years 1987–1989,[48] PD patients had a 19 percent higher adjusted mortality risk than HD patients. A Canadian study[49] that compared incident dialysis patients from 1990 to 1994 found that PD patients had a 27 percent lower adjusted mortality risk. In an attempt to reconcile these results, incident Medicare patients for the years 1994–1996 were followed for 2 years[50] and Cox regression analysis was performed to assess outcomes. A lower mortality risk was seen in all nondiabetic PD patients as compared to HD and in diabetic women younger than 55 years of age. Diabetic women above age 55 had a higher risk of mortality on HD than with PD. The authors concluded that mortality patterns may change over time, but short-term PD seems to be associated with a superior outcome. Additionally, selection bias must be taken into account when analyzing the results of dialysis modality comparisons. Often the sickest patients are assigned to PD because of its gentler effects in patients with hypotension and cardiac failure.

The leading cause of death in hemodialyzed diabetic patients as well as those treated by PD or transplantation continues to be cardiovascular disease, followed by sepsis.[4] Withdrawal from dialysis was a more common cause of death in the past[51,52] and probably reflected the burden of comorbidities and poor quality of life. For diabetic patients, failure to thrive and medical complications are the most common causes for withdrawal. Overall survival has improved by 17.3 percent on HD and by 28 percent on PD for the incident cohort of patients from 1992 to 1996 as compared with the 1987–1991 cohort of diabetics.

Once dialysis has been initiated, it is important to consider rehabilitation goals for the patient. Rehabilitation should help patients maximize function and optimize quality of life. These goals, in turn, are related in part to the patient's ability to partake in gainful employment or participate in family duties, thus benefiting both the patient and society at large. The USRDS annual data report for the year 2003 included information collected by the Dialysis Morbidity and Mortality Study (DMMS), which comprises patient-reported health and employment status. Only 37 percent of young patients and 16 percent of older patients reported that they were able to work at the start of dialysis; of those, only 60 percent of younger and 40 percent of older patients were actually employed. The level of education correlated closely with both desire to work and actual employment status. Diabetic patients generally reported lower health status than nondiabetics and had lower education status on average than nondiabetic patients.

Vascular Access

Creation of an arteriovenous (AV) fistula utilizing native arteries and veins is the preferred method for establishing access to the vascular system for HD. The excessive mortality noted above for diabetic HD patients with preexisting comorbid conditions may be in part caused by less efficient dialysis secondary to inadequate vascular access blood flow or repeated episodes of hypotension. The emphasis on improving the adequacy of dialysis spawned by NKF-DOQI guidelines for vascular access[53] has renewed interest in increasing the rate of AV fistula placement, especially as evidence began to emerge that synthetic (e.g., polytetrafluoroethylene) vascular grafts were associated with increased risk of thrombosis, stenosis, and infection.[54] Thrombosis is most often secondary to stenosis at the draining vein or at the venous anastomosis, and although prophylactic angioplasty reduces the rate of this complication, surveillance is required in order to detect significant early stenosis; such surveillance is costly and labor-intensive.[55] Creation of an AV fistula may be complicated by the presence of generalized calcification of the vascular system in the long-standing diabetic patient, limiting the patient's choice of access to placement of a prosthetic graft or necessitating insertion of a double-lumen subclavian catheter, both of which, in the patient with diabetes, have been associated with adverse sequelae,[56] including subclavian stenosis or thrombosis and exit-site or tunnel infection. The use of internal jugular catheters carries the same inherent risks. Despite the consensus regarding the superiority of AV fistulas, the high blood flows (400 to 500 mL/min) required to achieve adequate dialysis—along with the increasing age and comorbidities of the ESRD population—have resulted in the decreased use of AV fistulas,[57] which were utilized in only 20 percent of patients in mid-1990s. Survival of fistulas and grafts may be comparable, but in some series grafts require more frequent angioplasty, thrombectomy, and surgical revision, and infections are more common with grafts than with fistulas.[58] Factors associated with a lower likelihood of having a fistula are being female, black, or older, having peripheral vascular disease, or being obese.[59,60]

The most frequently cited reasons for hospitalization in dialyzed diabetic patients used to be complications resulting from placement, thrombosis, or infection of the HD access.[61] In the most recent USRDS report, hospitalization rates due to cardiovascular disease are increasing slightly, but those due to infections increased by 12 to 21 percent. Other causes of hospitalization, including vascular access, have decreased by 9 to 14 percent, which may reflect the trend to having the vascular access created as an ambulatory procedure or to the increased use of temporary dialysis catheters.

Diabetic patients who are not candidates for kidney transplantation should be referred for creation of an AV when the serum creatinine reaches a value between 5 and 8 mg/dL, depending on the patient's symptoms and overall condition, because of potential problems that may be encountered during access maturation. NKF-DOQI guidelines currently recommend the creation of a vascular access when the GFR is below 30 mL/min. If a primary arteriovenous fistula cannot be constructed or fails to mature, there is usually time for a prosthetic graft to be placed prior to the initiation of dialysis, thus avoiding the need for femoral or subclavian cannulation.

Blood Glucose, Hyperlipidemia, Oxidative Stress, and Inflammation

The diabetic patient often develops worsening of blood glucose control and hyperlipidemia following the initiation of HD. Control of blood glucose in the patient with ESRD is complicated by multiple factors (Table 32–2). Hyper-

TABLE 32–2. FACTORS THAT CONTRIBUTE TO BLOOD GLUCOSE ABNORMALITIES IN DIABETIC DIALYSIS PATIENTS

PROBLEM AND CONTRIBUTING FACTORS

Hyperglycemia

Uremia increases peripheral insulin resistance.

Anuria blunts ability to modulate hyperglycemia.

Constant or intermittent exposure to glucose in dialysate.

Poor or inadequate patient follow-up.

Active or occult infection.

Failure to rotate injection site/microvascular disease.

Hypoglycemia

Decreased appetite with poor caloric intake secondary to underdialysis.

Poor glycogen stores secondary to malnutrition.

Prolonged half-life of insulin or oral hypoglycemic agent.

Drugs that interfere with counterregulatory response to hypoglycemia (e.g., beta blocker).

Alternating hypo- and hyperglycemia

Gastroparesis.

Problems with compliance to dietary restrictions.

Timing of peritoneal dialysis exchanges that do not coincide with meals.

Sight impairment, depression.

Frequent hospitalizations for infection; peripheral or cardiovascular disease with disruption of diet and blood glucose regimen.

Source: Modified from Chang and Chou,[36] with permission.

glycemia may be worsened because uremia causes diminished tissue sensitivity to insulin, with resulting peripheral insulin resistance, primarily in muscle and to a lesser degree in adipose tissue.[62] There is also evidence of increased hepatic gluconeogenesis in uremia as well as impaired insulin response to glucose, which is worsened by secondary hyperparathyroidism. These conditions are compounded by the presence of anuria or poor urine output, which impairs or obviates the capacity to lower blood glucose levels by glycosuria.[63] Other factors that exacerbate hyperglycemia include microvascular disease, causing erratic absorption of insulin injected into the subcutaneous tissue, especially if the patient does not rotate injection sites. Prolongation of insulin action—which occurs coincident with the development of renal failure, inanition, and weight loss during the predialytic "uremic" period or due to underdialysis—and the delayed clearance of oral hypoglycemic agents dependent on renal function can lead to severe hypoglycemic episodes.

Hypertriglyceridemia is a well-known cardiovascular risk factor; it is exacerbated by uremia. Hypercholesterolemia and, more often, hypertriglyceridemia—leading to an increase in very low density lipoprotein (VLDL), intermediate-density lipoprotein (IDL), and low-density lipoprotein (LDL)—are commonly encountered in diabetic patients with renal failure and often become more pronounced after the initiation of renal replacement therapy.

Triglyceride-rich apo B100 is increased, predominantly in the VLDL fraction, with minor increases in the IDL and LDL fractions.[64] Plasma apo B100 levels increase in PD but have been reported to remain normal in HD patients.[65] There is also a decrease in apo A lipoproteins associated with HDL. These findings may represent overproduction of apo B100, but the main impairment seems to be the reduced catabolism and clearance of triglyceride-rich lipoproteins.[66]

HD does not significantly alter the "uremic diabetic" lipid profile. PD, however, is associated with worsening of hypertriglyceridemia as well as increased plasma cholesterol and LDL levels. In contrast to HD, there is a more pronounced increase of atherogenic lipoproteins on PD.

The dyslipidemia and hyperglycemia of diabetic nephropathy are believed to act as partners in increasing oxidative and carbonyl stress, leading to microinflammation and accelerated atherosclerosis.[67] The common mechanism by which advanced oxidation protein products, advanced glycation end products, and advanced lipoperoxidation end products—as well as elevated levels of acute-phase reactants such as C-reactive protein (CRP) and fibrinogen, along with oxidative stress—all contribute to endothelial dysfunction[68] is unclear. Endothelial dysfunction and excessive oxidative stress are features of vascular disease common to diabetes, hypertension, dyslipidemia, and cardiovascular disease. In addition, patients with chronic renal failure exhibit endothelial dysfunction, which is worsened by severe oxidative stress, accumulation of oxidized LDL, and chronic inflammation.[69] HD itself, perhaps due to the dialysis membrane, results in a state of microinflammation and uncorrected oxidative and carbonyl stress.

Although the exact mechanism of endothelial dysfunction is unclear, it may be responsible for the excessive mortality from cardiovascular disease that is seen in these patients, which is approximately 20 to 30 times that of the general population. Cardiac mortality in the young dialysis patient is 100 times that of the general population.[70] Pharmacologic strategies to reduce cardiovascular morbidity have been proposed; these involve intake of antioxidant vitamins C and E and folic acid, which reduces plasma homocysteine levels, as well as L-arginine. Smoking cessation and exercise also improve endothelial function.[71]

Control of Intravascular Volume

The rapid volume changes that may occur during HD therapy can cause severe hypotension in patients with diabetic autonomic neuropathy, thus complicating the performance of standard HD and contributing to an insidious form of underdialysis due to reduced access blood flow due to thrombosis or stenosis of the vascular access. In addition, repeated episodes of volume replacement necessitated by hypotension during HD treatment can result in chronic volume overload. Patients with severe neuropathy lose the ability to increase their heart rate as a reflex response to hypotension, even as blood pressure falls below a systolic measurement of 70 mmHg. Use of a "high-conductivity" dialysate bath (with a sodium concentration between 140 and 144 meq/L) may be tried to avoid this complication. Patients treated in this manner often become thirsty during the interdialytic interval, however, and development of volume overload prior to the next treatment is a concern. It may become necessary to switch over to CAPD in the patient with intractable hypotension, as volume changes occur over a longer time period with this technique.

Retinopathy, Vasculopathy

Retinopathy appears to progress or at best stabilize in uremic diabetic patients regardless of the dialytic modality used.[72] As noted above, visual disturbances are present in 73 percent of patients beginning dialysis. Close and frequent ophthalmologic follow-up is imperative, although careful blood pressure control and avoidance of excessive heparinization, which can lead to vitreous hemorrhage, may slow the progression to blindness.

The diabetic with chronic renal failure has a 10 times greater risk for amputation of the lower limbs than diabetics without nephropathy.[73] Complete evaluation includes proper wound care, evaluation of neuropathy and vascular

insufficiency, and vascular surgery, with revascularization when indicated.

CONTINUOUS AMBULATORY PERITONEAL DIALYSIS

Although HD continues to be the leading modality of renal replacement therapy, 50 percent of dialysis patients in Australia and 75 percent of pediatric dialysis patients in Finland are treated with PD.[4] In many nations, including Canada and Mexico, it is the preferred modality for diabetic patients.

Among U.S. dialysis patients, greater use of PD was seen in patients who were younger, employed, married, and living with someone else prior to the start of ESRD; those who were more autonomous and more accomplished educationally[74]; and those who were referred earlier than 4 months prior to initiation of ESRD therapy and had been seen more frequently by a nephrologist prior to ESRD. The highest level of PD use as a dialytic therapy in the United States is in the South and in Nebraska, Kansas, and Texas.[4]

The Canada-USA (CANUSA) Peritoneal Dialysis Study Group[75] examined differences in patient survival between the two countries, where prevalence of PD was 48 percent of units in Canada, as compared with 22 percent in the United States. This cohort of 680 patients was followed for 2 years, and with no significant difference in residual renal function, dialysis adequacy, or comorbidities between the two populations, the relative risk of death was 1.93 in the United States as compared with Canada. The 2-year survival for Caucasians was 77 percent in Canada, compared with 55 percent in the United States.

In many nations—including Australia/New Zealand, England, and Canada—and in some regions of the United States, CAPD is the preferred choice for dialytic treatment in patients with diabetes. The median age of patients on PD is 55, compared with 63 on HD and 47 with functioning transplant. In 2001, a total of 8461 patients in the United States with diabetes were receiving treatment with CAPD or CCPD, accounting for 34.9 percent of all diabetic ESRD patients—a figure that has slowly increased since 1982. In that year, only 835 (9.1 percent) diabetic patients were enrolled in CAPD/CCPD programs.[4]

Most diabetic ESRD patients can be considered candidates for CAPD except those with previous episodes of recurrent peritonitis or severe lower extremity vascular disease.[76] Severe visual impairment or physical disability limiting manual dexterity need not prevent a patient from using CAPD if there is a helper at home. As with home HD, patients whose home lives are unstable or who live in unsanitary conditions should not be considered appropriate candidates for CAPD unless an alternate site for treatment can be established.

Use of CAPD as renal replacement therapy avoids the complications associated with vascular access but requires placement of a permanent intraperitoneal catheter, which can become a source of infection. Peritonitis is a serious complication of catheter infection and is the most important cause of technique failure in PD.[77,78] Overall infection rates do not appear to differ between diabetic and nondiabetic patients. Culture-negative peritonitis, is apparently a result of recent antibiotic therapy or technical problems during dialysate culture[79] and is associated with poor treatment response.

Interpretation of survival comparisons between treatment modalities is confusing, and differences in case mix (underlying comorbid condition) may further complicate interpretation of the literature. An attempt to conduct a meta-analysis of outcome studies[80] yielded inconclusive results. One study[81] that tried to correct for case mix compared 1725 diabetic and 2411 nondiabetic Medicare-funded ESRD incident patients from the late 1980s and analyzed these data using Cox proportional hazards analysis. For nondiabetics, survival was equivalent between modalities. For diabetic patients, higher adjusted mortality was found on PD, RR = 1.26.

In summary, survival appears equivalent overall regardless of whether a patient is treated by HD or PD, with more favorable survival for nondiabetics. The selection of modalities should be based on factors other than concerns regarding patient survival.

Control of Intravascular Volume

CAPD is a continuous process, in which 1.5 to 3 L of commercially prepared dialysate solution are exchanged three to five times per day through a subcutaneously tunneled intraperitoneal catheter. Because the treatment is continuous rather than episodic, as is true of HD, the rapid shifts of water and electrolytes that occur during HD are avoided. Hypotension related to intravascular volume depletion is thus less frequent with CAPD. At the other extreme, control of volume-related hypertension is often easier to achieve by CAPD because of continuous ultrafiltration. For this reason, CAPD is often preferred over HD in ESRD patients with concomitant cardiac failure or severe hypertension.[82]

Blood Glucose, Hyperlipidemia, Oxidative Stress, and PD Solutions

Addition of insulin directly to the peritoneal dialysate allows for a continuous "basal rate" delivery of the hormone. Absorption of intraperitoneal insulin occurs across the visceral peritoneum into the portal circulation (where pancreatic insulin is initially secreted) and across the capsule of the liver,[83] which may allow a more physiologic delivery to the circulation, as suggested by the improved glucose control manifest in patients utilizing this technique.[84] Intraperitoneal administration of insulin has the added advantage that hyperinsulinemia and the formation of anti-insulin antibodies may be prevented,[85] and there is no adverse effect on PD efficiency. In order to establish an appropriate dose, a schedule such as that detailed in Table 32–3 can be used.[86]

As previously mentioned, hyperlipidemia, primarily hypertriglyceridemia, is commonly encountered in diabetic patients with ESRD regardless of therapy. Abnormalities in the lipid profile have been reported to worsen over time in patients treated by CAPD, and despite improved glycemic control with intraperitoneal administration of insulin, there is a significant reduction in HDL and Apo A levels[87] and increased LDL.[88] CAPD patients in general have total cholesterol levels that are higher than those of hemodialyzed patients.

PD therapy is limited by a slow decrease in efficiency over time. Ultrafiltration failure and morphologic changes in the peritoneum are responsible for peritoneal membrane failure.[89] Morphologic alterations include increasing thickness of the collagenous submesothelial layer of parietal peritoneaum, along with surface loss and subendothelial hyalinosis. Advanced glycation end products are found in the peritoneum, especially around vessel walls.[90] These "di-

TABLE 32–3. SAMPLE METHOD FOR DETERMINING INTRAPERITONEAL INSULIN DOSE FOR CAPD PATIENTS

1. Determine previous total daily subcutaneous dose and multiply by 3 for total initial intraperitoneal dose using regular insulin only.
2. Divide dose over four to five exchanges, with the overnight dose at half to two-thirds of the daytime exchange dose—e.g.:

   For a total dose of 120 U of regular insulin

8 A.M., first exchange:	40 U
1 P.M., second exchange:	35 U
6 P.M., third exchange:	30 U
11 P.M., fourth exchange:	15 U

3. Perform exchanges 1/2 hour prior to meals; adjust insulin dose to reflect food intake and activity level.
4. After determining the initial dose, create a "sliding scale" based on blood glucose monitoring, e.g.:

Increase insulin:	2 U for blood glucose 0.200
	4 U for blood glucose 0.400
	6 U for blood glucose 0.600
Decrease insulin:	2 U for blood glucose 0.100

5. Add 2 U for exchange with 2.5% dialysis solution.

   Add 4 U for exchange with 4.25% dialysis solution.
6. For a procedure that requires fasting (e.g., surgery, diagnostic test), decrease insulin dose to half the usual dose in the exchange prior to the procedure. Check blood glucose immediately after the procedure to determine the insulin dose for the next exchange.

Source: From Chang and Chou,[36] with permission.

abetiform" alterations of the peritoneal membrane occur in nondiabetic patients and may be related to bioincompatibility of glucose-containing PD solutions. Newer icodextrin solutions may improve glycemic control further, as was shown in 12 patients, by lowering HbA1c values from 8.9 to 7.9 percent.

SUMMARY OF DIALYSIS OPTIONS

The key disadvantage to CAPD is the substantial risk of infection, specifically peritonitis or "tunnel" (catheter) infection, which limits the utility of therapy and poses the risk of systemic sepsis. Other disadvantages include exhaustion of peritoneal surface exchange area after repeated or indolent peritoneal infection and patient "burnout" following months to years of three to five daily exchanges of peritoneal solution. Comparison of CAPD technique survival with HD is difficult because bias in patient assignment to each treatment influences outcome. In our experience, patients are often assigned to PD because they are "too sick" to undergo HD or have no vascular access. Neither CAPD nor HD offers proven advantages in the management of microvascular disease, and cardiovascular mortality is high in both.

TRANSPLANTATION

Unless contraindications to transplantation exist, living related transplantation is the overwhelming first choice of therapy for diabetic patients with ESRD at most centers, with cadaveric transplants a close second.

Both patient and kidney graft survival for patients with diabetes have improved markedly over the past two decades. The 1-year, age-, sex-, and race-adjusted patient survival rate reported by the USRDS for 2000 for deceased donor recipients was 93 percent. For live donor recipients, it was 97 percent for allografted patients with diabetes, with 1-year death-censored graft survival rates of 93.8 and 96 percent for deceased and living related transplants respectively,[4] similar to the rate for nondiabetic patients.

Interpretation of ESRD mortality statistics according to treatment modality are confounded by selection bias, which tends to cause healthier patients to be referred away from dialysis and toward kidney transplantation. In an attempt to control for this selection bias, mortality of patients awaiting transplantation was compared with that of all patients on dialysis and with those transplanted.[91] The long-term mortality rate was 48 to 82 percent lower among transplant recipients than those on the waiting list, with larger benefits for patients who were younger, white, and diabetic. Those on the waiting list had 38 to 58 percent lower mortal-

ity risk than their cohorts not awaiting transplantation. It appears that survival with renal transplantation is superior to survival on dialysis.

Specific Concerns Pretransplantation

In assessing a living related donor for a patient with diabetes, the increased risk of developing type 1 or 2 diabetes, associated with the presence or absence of several HLA subtypes, must be addressed. At present, there is no accurate way to predict who will develop diabetes later in life, although screening for anti-islet antibodies together with oral glucose tolerance testing, HbA1c levels, and microalbuminuria should be considered prior to acceptance of a first-degree relative as a donor. Regardless of the type of diabetes the patient has, his or her relatives have increased risk of developing diabetes themselves.

Many patients with diabetes have "silent" ischemia of the heart, and, as noted above, not only is cardiovascular disease highly prevalent in renal failure patients but chronic renal failure is a risk factor for cardiovascular disease.[27] It is recommended, therefore, that every prospective diabetic transplant recipient, regardless of whether a living donor or cadaveric transplant is anticipated, undergo cardiac evaluation.

Specific Concerns Posttransplantation

Diabetic nephropathy has been documented to recur in the allograft, and although this problem does not appear to be a major cause of allograft loss, it is associated with higher risk of graft failure and death.[4] The presence of diabetes is also associated with higher risk of fractures posttransplantation. Patients who develop diabetes after transplantation are predisposed to the macro- and microvascular complications of diabetes, such as retinopathy, neuropathy, and cardiovascular disease, as are those whose diabetes antedated the transplant. The major complications of the immunosuppressive agents used in kidney transplantation include worsening of hyperlipidemia, opportunistic infection, posttransplant hypertension, and new-onset diabetes after transplantation. Although calcineurin inhibitors were introduced as steroid-sparing agents, they are associated with the development of diabetes in 10 to 30 percent of patients, especially in populations of Afro-Caribbean or Hispanic descent.[92] Dosage adjustment of insulin or oral hyperglycemic therapy is often required during immunosuppressant therapy, especially during the early posttransplant period, as prednisone, cyclosporine, and tacrolimus alter glucose tolerance. Minimization of immunosupppression dose, diet, weight loss, and treatment of hypertension and dyslipidemia are specific risk-factor-directed strategies to control progressive inflammation and endothelial dysfunction, which may lead to accelerated atherosclerosis and possibly contribute to chronic allograft rejection.

Cardiovascular disease (CVD) accounts for 35 to 50 percent of all-cause mortality in renal transplant recipients; these patients have a twofold risk of cardiovascular death when compared to the general population,[28] which is much lower than the twentyfold risk for the dialysis population. The incidence of CVD is three to five times that of the general population. Risk factors for CVD are similar to those observed in the renal failure population and include hypertension, diabetes, hyperlipidemia, and left ventricular hypertrophy. Screening for microalbuminuria in the post–renal transplant population has not been recommended, as the presence of chronic allograft nephropathy, which also presents with urinary albumin loss, may complicate interpretation of the results.

Pancreatic/Islet Cell Transplantation

A question that is unique to the type 1 diabetic with ESRD is whether pancreatic transplantation should be considered, either concomitantly or after the kidney is transplanted. The timing of the kidney transplant has not been established. In a Swedish study of 92 patients transplanted between 1986 and 1987, 1-year pancreatic graft survival was 72 percent for patients who received a kidney and a pancreas together and 34 percent for those who received a pancreas alone.[93] Detecting rejection and calcineurin toxicity is easier in the patient with a renal transplant, where urine output and serum creatinine can be measured directly, than it is in the patient with only a pancreatic allograft, which may have accounted for survival differences in an earlier era. In one recent retrospective comparison,[94] simultaneous pancreatic and kidney (SPK) transplantation prolonged patient survival significantly: at 8 years posttransplant, survival was 47 percent in kidney-alone vs. 77 percent in the SPK group.

Islet transplantation may present a solution to the complications and morbidity of pancreas transplantation. An Italian study[95] demonstrated similar survival in type 1 diabetic kidney transplant patients who received islet cell transplantation compared with a group who simultaneously received received both kidney and pancreas. They also compared these with a group of renal transplant recipients without islet cell or pancreatic transplant and a group of diabetics on dialysis who had inferior survival. Of interest, the islet cell and pancreatic transplant recipient groups showed better endothelial morphology and fewer signs of endothelial injury than kidney-alone or dialysis patients, and the islet cell group had a less atherothrombotic lipid profile.

Finally, it must be remembered that a large number of diabetic patients with ESRD have type 2 diabetes and, thus would not benefit from pancreatic transplantation, which is at present reserved for type 1 patients.

REHABILITATION

Comparisons of the rehabilitation status of diabetic ESRD patients treated by the different modalities of uremia therapy are difficult because physician bias results in referral of the youngest, healthiest, and most active ESRD patients for kidney transplantation or home dialytic therapy, while the sickest and most physically debilitated remain, by necessity, on in-center HD. In addition, neither observer bias nor patient self-assessment is subject to verification.[96]

In 1989, a study of 459 ESRD patients, using the activities of daily living (ADL) index—which rates items such as self-care (feeding and grooming), mobility (climbing stairs, transferring), and "instrumental" activities such as ability to do housework—found that the lowest scores for independence in ADL, particularly in the ability to perform "instrumental" tasks, were reported for patients with diabetes and/or those who were treated by in-center HD.[97] A more recent study, which evaluated 430 patients from a similar demographic area following the introduction of human recombinant erythropoietin (rHuEPO), reported that 55 percent of patients with diabetes were unable to perform their routine living chores without assistance, compared with 25 percent of patients without diabetes,[98] suggesting that rHuEPO use has not significantly improved rehabilitation in diabetic dialysis patients.

Rehabilitation of diabetic ESRD patients is best in recipients of kidney transplants, and patient satisfaction is evident. The Transplant Learning Center[99] was designed to preserve graft function and improve quality of life after transplantation. Patients may self-refer or be referred by a health care professional. Among the 3676 patients analyzed, sexual dysfunction and headaches had a greater impact on quality of life than the more common changes in face and body shape, hirsutism, and tremor. Greater life satisfaction was strongly associated with being in control of one's health and living a normally active life with satisfying personal relationships.

Because of the increasingly complex options that are now available to the diabetic patient with ESRD, it is important to thoroughly discuss all options for renal replacement therapy and tailor decisions to the needs of each individual. Investigation of the patient's social, familial, and economic situation and education of the patient allows an informed choice to be made regarding treatment for uremia or, at times, regarding the refusal of treatment. A patient who has been coerced into accepting dialysis or kidney transplantation when life seems unbearable because of diabetic complications may actively withdraw from dialysis, as was evidenced by the previously high death rate due to "dialysis withdrawal" among diabetics.[100] Additionally, some patients commit "passive suicide" by noncompliance with dietary, drug, and treatment regimens. Occasionally, however, diabetic patients who are depressed over the loss of kidney function respond to visits by rehabilitated dialysis patients or transplant recipients and reconsider their decision to die.

SUMMARY

Diabetic nephropathy, the leading cause of ESRD in the United States and the world, presents an increasingly complicated management problem from the time that microalbuminuria is first detected, when decisions regarding choice of antihypertensive agent and strictness of metabolic control must be made.

As renal failure progresses, concomitant evaluation medical problems, physical abilities, lifestyle, and social support—together with patient education—should be undertaken in an attempt to retard progression of renal failure and come to an educated decision regarding the ultimate choice of uremia therapy. Although living-donor kidney transplantation is generally considered the optimal choice for the diabetic ESRD patient, those without a suitable donor will by necessity be placed on the cadaveric transplant waiting list and should be referred for the placement of vascular access and/or insertion of a peritoneal catheter early in the course of their disease. In addition, where available and appropriate, the patient may be considered for a simultaneous cadaveric renal and pancreatic or islet cell transplant.

If contraindications to transplantation are present—including chronic infection, recent malignancy, or severe cardiac disease—a decision must be made regarding CAPD vs. HD and whether home or in-center therapy is appropriate. Rehabilitation and survival data for these therapies are similar, although technique survival rates for CAPD decline dramatically as time progresses because of infectious complications. In-center HD has the worst survival and rehabilitation profile, in part because the sickest and most debilitated patients are assigned to that therapeutic modality. Most importantly, extrarenal diabetic complications (urologic, ophthalmologic, neurologic, cardiovascular) must not be forgotten during initial referral and preparation of the patient with ESRD, since maintenance of optimal physical condition allows for better rehabilitation during renal replacement therapy.

REFERENCES

1. United States Renal Data System. *2003 Annual Data Report*. Bethesda, MD: The National Institute of Health, National Institute of Diabetes and Digestive Diseases, November 2003.
2. Krowleswski AS, Warram JH, Christlieb AR, et al. The changing natural history of nephropathy in type I diabetes. *Am J Med* 1985;78:785–794.
3. Hovind P, Tarnow L, Rossing K, et al. Decreasing incidence of severe diabetic microangiopathy in type 1 diabetes. *Diabetes Care* 2003;26(4):1258–1264.
4. United States Renal Data System. *2003 Annual Data Report*. Bethesda, MD: The National Institute of Health, National Institute of Diabetes and Digestive Diseases, November 2003.
5. Steffes MW, Chavers BM, Bilous RW, et al. The predictive value of microalbuminuria. *Am J Kidney Dis* 1989;8(1):25–28.
6. Herman W, Hawthorn BM, Hamman R, et al. Consensus statement: international workshop on preventing the kidney disease of diabetes mellitus. *Am J Kidney Dis* 1989;8(1):2–6.
7. Brenner BM, Cooper ME, de Zeeuw D, et al. Effects of losartan on renal and cardiovascular outcomes in patients with type 2 diabetes and nephropathy. *N Engl J Med* 2001;345:861–869.
8. Wang SL, Head J, Stevens L, et al. Excess mortality and its relation to hypertension and proteinuria in diabetic patients. The World Health Organization multinational study of vascular disease in diabetes. *Diabetes Care* 1996;19:305–312.
9. The DCCT Research Group. Effect of intensive therapy on the development and progression of diabetic nephropathy in the Diabetes Control and Complications Trial. *Kidney Int* 1995;47:1703–1720.
10. United Kingdom Prospective Diabetes Study (UKPDS) Group. Intensive blood-glucose control with sulphonylureas or insulin compared with conventional treatment and risk of complications in patients with type 2 diabetes 9UKPDS 33. *Lancet* 1998;352:837–853.
11. Tuttle KR, Bruton JL, Perusek MC, et al. Effect of strict glycemic control on renal hemodynamic response to amino-acids and renal enlargement in insulin dependent diabetes mellitus. *N Engl J Med* 1991:324;1626–1632.
12. Lewis JB, Berl T, Bain RP, et al. Effect of intensive blood pressure control on the course of type 1 diabetic nephropathy. Collaborative Study Group. *Am J Kidney Dis* 1999;34:809–817.
13. United Kingdom Prospective Diabetes Study Group. Efficacy of atenolol and captopril in reducing risk of macrovascular and microvascular complications in type 2 diabetes: UKPDS 39. *BMJ* 1998;317:713–720.
14. The Writing Team for DCCT and EDIC. Sustained effect of intensive treatment of type 1 diabetes mellitus on development and progression of diabetic nephropathy. *JAMA* 2003;290(16):2159–2167.
15. Lewis EJ, Hunsicker LG, Bain RP, et al. The effect of angiotensin-converting enzyme-inhibition on diabetic nephropathy. *N Engl J Med* 1993;329:1456–1462.
16. Andersen S, Tarnow L, Rossing P, et al. Renoprotective effects of angiotensin II receptor blockade in type 1 diabetic patients with diabetic nephropathy. *Kidney Int* 2000;57:601–606.
17. Brenner BM, Cooper ME, de Zeeuw D, et al. Effects of losartan on renal and cardiovascular outcomes in patients with type 2 diabetes and nephropathy. *N Engl J Med* 2001;345:861–869.

18. Lewis EJ, Hunsicker LG, Clarke WR, et al. Renoprotective effect of the angiotensin-receptor antagonist irbesartan in patients with nephropathy due to type 2 diabetes. *N Engl J Med* 2001;345:851–860.

19. Mattern WD, McGahie WC, Rigby RJ, et al. Selection of ESRD treatment: an international study. *Am J Kidney Dis* 1989;13(6):457–464.

20. Jassal SV, Krishna G, Mallick NP, et al. Attitudes of British Isles nephrologists towards dialysis modality selection: a questionnaire study. *Nephrol Dial Transplant* 2002;17(3): 474–477.

21. Mendelssohn DC, Mullaney SR, Jung B, et al. What do American nephrologists think about dialysis modality selection? *Am J Kidney Dis* 2001;37(1):22–29.

22. Prichard SS. Treatment modality selection in 150 consecutive patients starting ESRD therapy. *Perit Dial Int* 1996; 16(1):69–72.

23. Wolfe RA, Ashby VB, Milford EL. Comparison of mortality in all patients on dialysis, patients on dialysis awaiting transplantation, and recipients of a first cadaveric transplant. *N Engl J Med* 1999;341(23):1725–1730.

24. Stack AG. Determinants of modality selection among incident US dialysis patients: results from a national study. *J Am Soc Nephrol* 2002;13:1279–1287.

25. Wilson J, Nissenson AR. Determinants in APD selection. *Semin Dial* 2002;15(6):388–392.

26. Levin A. Clinical epidemiology of cardiovascular disease in chronic kidney disease prior to dialysis. *Semin Dial* 2003; 16(2):101–105.

27. Foley RN, Parfrey PS, Sarnak MJ, et al. Clinical epidemiology of cardiovascular disease in chronic renal disease. *Am J Kidney Dis* 1998;32:112–119.

28. Sarnak MJ, Levey AS, Schoolwerth AC, et al. Kidney disease as a risk factor for development of cardiovascular disease. *Circulation* 2003;108:2154–2169.

29. American Diabetes Association. Standards of medical care in diabetes. *Diabetes Care* 2004;27(s1):s15–s35.

30. Orth SR. Smoking—a renal risk factor. *Nephron* 2000;86(1): 12–26.

31. Frank, RN. Diabetic retinopathy. *N Engl J Med* 2004;350: 48–58.

32. Klein R, Klein BEK, Moss SE, et al. The Wisconsin Epidemiologic Study of Diabetic Retinopathy: II. Prevalence and risk of diabetic retinopathy when age at diagnosis is less than 30 years. *Arch Ophthalmol* 1984;102:520–526.

33. Klein R, Klein BEK, Moss SE, et al. The Wisconsin Epidemiologic Study of Diabetic Retinopathy: III. Prevalence and risk of diabetic retinopathy when age at diagnosis is 30 or more years. *Arch Ophthalmol* 1984;102:527–532.

34. Kohner EM, Aldington SJ, Stratton IM, et al. UPDDS 30: diabetic retinopathy at diagnosis of non-insulin-dependent diabetes mellitus and associated risk factors. *Arch Opthalmol* 1998;116(3):297–303.

35. Watanabe Y, Yuzawa Y, Mizumotot D, et al. Long-term follow-up study of 268 diabetic patients undergoing hemodialysis, with special attention to visual acuity and heterogeneity. *Nephrol Dial Transplant* 1993;8(8):725–734.

36. Chang MH, Chou KJ. The role of autonomic neuropathy in the genesis of intradialytic hypotension. *Am J Nephrol* 2001;21(5):357–361.

37. Laaksonen S, Voipio-Pulkki L, Erkinjuntti M, et al. Does dialysis therapy improve autonomic and peripheral nervous system abnormalities in chronic uremia? *J Intern Med* 2000;248(1):21–26.

38. Watkins PJ, Buston-Thomas MS, Howard ER. Long-term outcome after gastrectomy for intractable diabetic gastroparesis. *Diabetes Med* 2003;20(1):58–63.

39. Schoonjans R, Van VB, Vandamme W, et al. Dyspepsia and gastroparesis in chronic renal failure: the role of *Helicobacter pylori*. *Clin Nephrol* 2002;57(3):201–207.

40. Markell MS, Friedman EA. Diabetic nephropathy: management of the end-stage patient. *Diabetes Care* 1992;15(9): 1226–1238.

41. Alvestrand A. Carbohydrate and insulin metabolism in renal failure. *Kidney Int Suppl* 1997;(62):S48–S52.

42. Byrne C, Vernon P, Cohen JJ. Effect of age and diagnosis on survival of older patients beginning chronic dialysis. *JAMA* 1994;271(1):34–36.

43. Wolfe RA, Held PJ, Hulbert-Shearon TE, et al. A critical examination of trends in outcomes over the last decade. *Am J Kidney Dis* 1998;32:s9–s15.

44. Merkus MP, Jager KJ, Dekker FW, et al. Predictors of poor outcome in chronic dialysis patients: the Netherlands cooperative study on the adequacy of dialysis. *Am J Kidney Dis* 2000;35(1):69–79.

45. Byrne C, Vernon P, Cohen JJ. Effect of age and diagnosis on survival of older patients beginning chronic dialysis. *JAMA* 1994;271(1):34–36.

46. Held PJ, Port FK, Wolfe RA, et al. the dose of hemodialysis and patient mortality. *Kidney Int* 1996;50:550–556.

47. Wolfe RA, Port FK. Good news, bad news for diabetic versus nondiabetic end-stage renal disease: incidence and mortality. *ASAIO J* 1999;45:117–118.

48. Bloembergen WE, Port FK, Mauger EA, et al. A comparison of mortality between patients treated with hemodialysis and peritoneal dialysis. *J Am Soc Nephrol* 1995; 6:177–183.

49. Fenton S, Schaubel D, et al. Hemodialysis versus peritoneal dialysis: a comparison of adjusted mortality rates. *Am J Kidney Dis* 1997;30:334–342.

50. Collins AJ, Hao W, Xia H, et al. Mortality risks of peritoneal dialysis and hemodialysis. *Am J Kid Dis* 1999;34(6): 1065–1074.

51. Catalano C, Postorino M, Kelly PJ, et al. Diabetes mellitus and renal replacement therapy in Italy: prevalence, main characteristics and complications. *Nephrol Dial Transplant* 1990;5(9):788–796.

52. Julius M, Hawthorne VM, Carpentier-Alting P, et al. Independence in activities of daily living for end-stage renal disease patients: biomedical and demographic correlates. *Am J Kidney Dis* 1989;13(1):61–69.

53. NKF-DOQI clinical practice guidelines for vascular access. *Am J Kidney Dis* 1997;37:s150–s191.

54. Schwab SJ. Vascular access for hemodialysis. *Kidney Int* 1999;55:2078–2090.

55. Hakim R, Himmelfarb J. Hemodialysis access failure: a call to action. *Kidney Int* 1998;54(4):1029–1040.

56. Kairaitis LK, Gottlieb T. Outcome and complications of temporary hemodialysis catheter. *Nephrol Dial Transplant* 1999;14(7):1710–1714.

57. Tokars JI, Miller ER, Alter MJ, et al. National surveillance of dialysis-associated diseases in the United States, 1997. *Semin Dial* 2000;13:75–85.

58. Allon M, Robbin ML. Increasing arteriovenous fistulas in hemodialysis patients: Problems and solutions. *Kidney Int* 2002;62:1109–1124.

59. Allon M, Ornt DB, Schwab SJ, et al. Factors associated with the prevalence of arteriovenous fistulas in hemodialysis patients in the HEMO study. *Kidney Int* 2000;58: 2178–2185.

60. Ifudu O, Macey LJ, Homel P, et al. Determinants of type of initial hemodialysis vascular access. *Am J Nephrol* 1997:17: 425–427.

61. Carlson DM, Duncan DA, Naessens JM, et al. Hospitalization in dialysis patients. *Mayo Clin Proc* 1984;59(11): 769–775.

62. Alvestrand A. Carbohydrate and insulin metabolism in renal failure. *Kidney Int* 1997;52:s48–s52.

63. Daniels ID, Markell MS. Blood glucose control in diabetics: II. *Semin Dial* 1993;6(6):394–397.

64. Prinsen BH, de Sain-van der Velden MG, de Koning EJ, et al. Hypertriglyceridemia in patients with chronic renal failure: possible mechanisms. *Kidney Int Suppl* 2003;(84): S121–S124.

65. Attman PO, Samuelsson OG, Moberly J, et al. Apolipoprotein B–containing lipoproteins in renal failure: the relation to mode of dialysis. *Kidney Int* 1999;55:1536–1542.

66. Attman PO, Samuelsson O, Johansson AC, et al. Dialysis modalities and dyslipidemia. *Kidney Int Suppl* 2003:(84): S110–S112.

67. Kalousová M, Zima T, Tesar V, et al. Relationship between advanced glycoxidation end products, inflammatory markers/acute-phase reactants, and some autoantibodies in chronic hemodialysis patients. *Kidney Int Suppl* 2003;(84): S62–S64.

68. Annuk M, Zilmer M, Fellstrom B, et al. Endothelium-dependent vasodilation and oxidative stress in chronic renal failure: impact on cardioascular disease. *Kidney Int Suppl* 2003;(84): S50–S53.

69. Stenvinkel P, Heimburger O, Paultre F, et al. Strong association between malnutrition, inflammation and atherosclerosis in chronic renal failure. *Kidney Int* 1999;55:1899–1911.

70. Foley RN, Parfrey PS, Sarnak MJ, et al. Clinical epidemiology of cardiovascular disease in chronic renal disease. *Am J Kidney Dis* 1998;32:112–119.

71. Annuk M, Zilmer M, Fellstrom B, et al. Endothelium-dependent vasodilation and oxidative stress in chronic renal failure: impact on cardioascular disease. *Kidney Int Suppl* 2003;(84): S50–S53.

72. Watanabe Y, Yuzawa Y, Mizumotot D, et al. Long-term follow-up study of 268 diabetic patients undergoing hemodialysis, with special attention to visual acuity and heterogeneity. *Nephrol Dial Transplant* 1993;8(8):725–734.

73. Deery HG II, Sangeorzan JA. Saving the diabetic foot with special reference to the patient with chronic renal failure. *Infect Dis Clin North Am* 2001;15(3):953–981.

74. Stack AG. Determinants of modality selection among incident US dialysis patients: results from a national study. *J Am Soc Nephrol* 2002;13:1279–1287.

75. Churchill DN, Thorpe KE, Vonesh EF, et al. Lower probability of patient survival with continuous peritoneal dialysis in the United States compared with Canada. Canada-USA Peritonenal Dialysis Study Group. *J Am Soc Nephrol* 1997; 8(6):965–971.

76. Diaz-Buxo JA. Peritoneal dialysis prescriptions for diabetic patients. *Adv Perit Dial* 1999;15:91–95.

77. Oreopoulos DG, Tzamaloukas AH. Peritoneal dialysis in the next millennium. *Adv Renal Replace Ther* 2000;7: 338–346.

78. Szeto CC, Chow KM, Wong TY, et al. Feasibility of resuming peritoneal diaysis after severe peritonitis and Tenckhoff catheter removal. *J Am Soc Nephrol* 2002;13: 1040–1045.

79. Szeto CC, Wong TY, Chow KM, et al. The clinical course of culture-negative peritonitis complicating peritoneal dialysis. *Am J Kidney Dis* 2003;42(3):567–574.

80. Ross S, Dong E, Gordon M, et al. Meta-analysis of outcome studies in end-stage renal disease. *Kidney Int* 2000; 57(s74): 28–30.

81. Held PJ, Port FK, Turenne MN, et al. Continuous ambulatory peritoneal dialysis and hemodialysis: comparison of patient mortality with adjustment for comorbid conditions. *Kidney Int* 1994;45(4):1163–1169.

82. Abu-Alfa AK, Burkart J, Piraino B, et al. Approach to fluid management in peritoneal dialysis: a practical algorithm. *Kidney Int* 2002;62:s8–s16.

83. Chan E, Montgomery PA. Administration of insulin by continuous ambulatory peritoneal dialysis. *Pharmacotherapy* 1993:13(5):455–460.

84. Scarpioni L, Ballocchi S, Castelli A, et al. Insulin therapy in uremic diabetic patients on continuous ambulatory peritoneal dialysis: comparison of intraperitoneal and subcutaneous administration. *Perit Dial Int* 1994;14(2):127–131.

85. Quellhorst E. Insulin therapy during peritoneal dialysis: pros and cons of various forms of administration. *J Am Soc Nephrol* 2002;13:S92–S96.

86. Daniels ID, Markell MS. Blood glucose control in diaetics: II. *Semin Dial* 1993;6(6):394–397.

87. Nevalainen PI, Lahtela JT, Mustonen J, et al. The effect of insulin delivery route on lipoproteins in type I diabetic patients on CAPD. *Perit Dial Int* 1999;19:148–153.

88. Nevalainen PI, Lahtela JT, Mustonen J, Pasternack A. Subcutaneous and intraperitoneal insulin therapy in diabetic patients on CAPD. *Perit Dial Int* 1996:16:s288—s291.

89. Vardhan A, Zweers M, Gokal R, Raymond T. A solutions portfolio approach in peritoneal dialysis. *Kidney Int* 2003;64:S114–S123.

90. Nakayama M, Kawaguchi Y, Yamada K, et al. Immunohistochemical detection of advanced glycosylation end-products in the peritoneum and its possible pathophysiological role in CAPD. *Kidney Int* 1997;51:182–186.

91. Wolfe RA, Ashby VB, Milford EL. Comparison of mortality in all patients on dialysis, patients on dialysis awaiting transplantation, and recipients of a first cadaveric transplant. *N Engl J Med* 1999;341(23):1725–1730.

92. Markell MS. Post–transplant diabetes: incidence, relationship to choice of immunosuppressive drugs, and treatment protocol. *Adv Renal Replace Ther* 2001;8(1):64–69.

93. Groth CG, Tyden G, Ostman J. Fifteen years experience with pancreas transplantation with pancreatoenterostomy. *Diabetes* 1989;38:13–15.

94. Mohan P, Safi K. Little DM, et al. Improved patient survival in recipients of simultaneous pancreas-kidney transplant compared with kidney transplant alone in patients with type 1 diabetes mellitus and end-stage renal disease. *Br J Surg* 203;90(9):1137–1141.

95. Fiorina P, Folli F, Maffi P, et al. Islet transplantation improves vascular diabetic complications in patients with diabetes who underwent kidney transplantation: a comparison between kidney-pancreas and kidney-alone transplantation. *Transplantation* 2003;75(8):1296–1301.

96. Hutchinson TA, Boyd NF, Feinstein AR, et al. Scientific problems in clinical scales, as demonstrated in the Karnofsky Index of Performance Status. *J Chronic Dis* 1979:32: 661–666.

97. Catalano C, Postorino M, Kelly PJ, et al. Diabetes mellitus and renal replacement therapy in Italy: prevalence, main characteristics and complications. *Nephrol Dial Transplant* 1990;5(9):788–796.

98. Ifudu O, Paul H, Meyers JD, et al. Pervasive failed rehabilitation in center-based hemodialysis patients. *Am J Kidney Dis* 1994;23(3):394–400.

99. Hricik DE, Halbert RJ, Barr ML, et al. Life satisfaction in renal transplant recipients: preliminary results from the Transplant Learning Center. *Am J Kidney Dis* 2001;38 (3):580–587.

100. Mailloux LU, Belluci AG, Napolitano B, et al. Death by withdrawal from dialysis: a 20-year clinical experience. *J Am Soc Nephrol* 1993;3(9):1631–1637.

Drug Usage in Dialysis Patients

Ali J. Olyaei
Angelo M. deMattos
William M. Bennett

End-stage renal disease (ESRD) is a major public health problem worldwide. Factors that account for the increasing prevalence of this condition include the epidemic of diabetes and hypertension as well as the continued occurrence of autoimmune diseases, all coupled with an ageing population.[1-4] Drug therapy is an essential component of the care of patients with ESRD.[5] However, most drugs or their metabolites used in ESRD patients are completely or partially excreted by the kidneys.[6] While the exact burden of drug toxicity in patients with renal failure can be difficult to estimate, observational analysis indicates a higher incidence of adverse drug reactions. In addition to drug excretion, drug metabolism and biotransformation may also be altered by uremia. Therefore, unless proper dosage adjustments are made, patients with compromised renal function are particularly vulnerable to drug accumulation and toxicity. Achieving a proper balance between ensuring efficacy and avoiding toxicity remains a vital issue in patients with ESRD. Most drugs or pharmacologically active metabolites are primarily excreted unchanged through the renal system.

In uremic patients, the active drug moiety may accumulate to a toxic concentration as a result of decreased renal function.[6,7] Knowledge of altered pharmacokinetics and pharmacodynamic variability in renal failure is essential for health care providers, who must make appropriate dosage adjustments to avoid serious adverse drug reactions or ensure therapeutic effectiveness while preventing underdosing. This chapter addresses the principles behind rational drug therapy in patients with chronic kidney disease (CKD) and those on dialysis.

Pharmacokinetics defines drug behavior in the body. An awareness of basic pharmacokinetic principles (absorption, distribution, metabolism, and excretion) is necessary to understand proper drug administration to uremic patients. Pharmacokinetic analysis is useful in explaining drug behavior in each patient and improving the safety and effectiveness of drugs with a narrow therapeutic window. The pharmacodynamic properties of individual agents are related to the free, unbound concentration of drug available at the receptor sites in tissue. Dialysis patients receive an average of 8.4 different drugs. Consequently, the risk of drug–drug interactions is substantially increased in patients with CKD when compared with hospitalized patients without azotemia.[7,8]

PHARMACOLOGIC PRINCIPLES AND ALTERATIONS IN UREMIA

Bioavailability

Bioavailability is defined as the fraction (F) of an active drug moiety reaching the systemic circulation following administration by any route. This concept is clinically important because both the rate and extent of drug absorption influence drug efficacy. The rate of drug absorption is the time it takes to achieve peak plasma concentration and for drug to reach the site of action, while the extent of drug absorption is the quantity of total drug concentration over a given time period (area under the curve, or AUC). *Bioavailability*, therefore, refers to the rate and extent of active drug that reaches the site of pharmacologic activity. Bioavailability is usually determined by measuring the AUC of a drug product divided by a standard AUC plasma concentration rate after a single intravenous dose.[7,9]

$$F = (AUC)_{drug\ product} / AUC_{standard}$$

or

$$F = (AUC)_{PO} / AUC_{IV}$$

Rapid drug absorption is usually desirable for drugs used to treat acute conditions (headache, pain, and insomnia), while more complete drug absorption is desirable for the treatment of chronic conditions. A drug's absorption is affected by the dosage form, site of administration, blood flow at the site of absorption, absorptive surface area, and contact time between the drug and the absorptive surface area. Physicochemical properties of the drug—such as molecular weight, volume of distribution, protein binding, and lipid solubility—are also important.

Because most drugs are administered orally, bioavailability is largely related to gastrointestinal (GI) function. The intravenous route is the preferred form of administration during an acute crisis. However, in many patients with vascular access problems (diabetes, lupus, and so on), it is difficult to establish an intravenous route. The primary problem with oral administration is erratic or/and incomplete absorption. Factors affecting bioavailability of drug absorption through the GI system include membrane permeability, gut luminal metabolism of the drug, metabolism in the gut wall, portal circulation of the liver, and enterohepatic recycling of the drug. The GI membrane is semipermeable, allowing absorption of certain nutrients and retarding the absorption of certain toxic compounds. In patients with renal failure, poor absorption is traced to drug–drug interac-

tions, high pH, and an edematous GI tract. Weak acids such as phenytoin or phenobarbital achieve lower plasma concentrations, while acid-labile drugs (penicillin or ampicillin) may achieve higher plasma concentrations. For most drugs with low molecular weight and high lipid solubility, absorption is passive—that is, characterized by drug movement down an electrochemical or concentration gradient. This movement requires no energy expenditure and is not retarded by metabolic inhibitors.[10,11]

Mesenteric blood perfusion and portal venous circulation play an important role in drug absorption. Following oral absorption, many drugs may undergo a substantial "first-pass" metabolism (presystemic metabolism). In this setting, absorbed drugs may never reach the systemic circulation. For drugs with low hepatic extraction, bioavailability is affected minimally by the first pass through the liver. However, for drugs with a high hepatic extraction ratio, oral administration can profoundly reduce bioavailability. Hepatic first-pass effects are reduced by rectal administration and eliminated by sublingual, transdermal, and parenteral administration.[12]

GI manifestations of uremia (nausea, vomiting, diarrhea, GI tract edema) may contribute to drug malabsorption. Certain medications—for example, low-dose aspirin (81 mg) and other nonsteroidal anti-inflammatory drugs (NSAIDs)—may add to GI symptoms through local irritation. Phosphate-binding aluminum-containing antacids or calcium salts (carbonate or acetate) have a similar effect on the GI pH. Reduction of stomach acidity from H_2 blockers or proton pump inhibitors (PPIs) may further impair absorption of weak acidic drugs. Antacids may also form nonabsorbable chelation products with certain drugs (e.g., digoxin, tetracycline, and many fluoroquinolones).[13,14] These agents should be administered 2 to 4 hours following phosphate-binding agents. In dialysis patients, edema and low muscle-to-body mass may also slow absorption of drugs following intramuscular (IM) administration. In some patients with ESRD, pancreatic exocrine dysfunction has been reported. This may contribute to the malabsorptive syndromes noted in uremic patients. Drug absorption is probably also adversely affected in this setting.[7]

Distribution

Substantial changes in body composition occur as patients with CKD approach the need for dialysis. These changes in protein binding, the ratio of muscle mass to body weight, and extracellular body water may affect drug distribution and plasma drug concentrations. After absorption and equilibration, drugs are distributed throughout the body. Drugs with molecular weights of 500 to 600 Da and low protein binding further rapidly distribute into the interstitial fluid. The apparent volume of distribution (V_d) is the quantity of drug in the body (L/kg body weight) divided by the plasma concentration at steady state.[8] Volume of distribution represents the amount of water in which a drug is dissolved in order to reach an observed plasma concentration. The apparent volume of distribution can be calculated by the amount of drug in the body (dose) divided by the plasma concentration (C) of the drug when plasma and tissue equilibrium is reached:

$$V_d = \text{dose}/C$$

In uremic patients, physiologic changes in body fluid may alter V_d. Lipophilic drugs with a low protein-binding capacity most commonly have large volumes of distribution. In contrast, drugs with high circulating protein binding and water-soluble drugs have small volumes of distribution. Changes in volume of distribution are usually not clinically significant except for those drugs that have a small volume of distribution under normal circumstances (i.e. < 0.7 L/kg). Acidic drugs have a higher affinity for albumin and basic drugs have a higher affinity for alpha-acid glycoproteins. The plasma concentrations and affinity of drugs to both albumin and alpha-acid glycoproteins are altered in uremic patients. In general, intermediate uremic molecules replace both acidic and basic drugs at the site of protein binding, leading to an increased free fraction of drug. Only free drugs or drug metabolites are pharmacologically active. Changes in protein binding may increase or decrease the free or unbound plasma concentration of drugs. Phenytoin is highly protein-bound (98 percent); in uremic patients with low albumin, protein binding is reduced. Therefore, in this setting, free phenytoin levels will rise to toxic levels without any laboratory evidence of phenytoin toxicity. The observed phenytoin plasma concentration should be adjusted for both low albumin and renal failure.[15,16]

Adjusted phenytoin level = observed phenytoin level/(0.1 × albumin + 0.1)

Uremia and albumin abnormalities are not the only conditions affecting drug-protein binding. Alpha-acid glycoproteins bind more commonly to basic drugs such as lidocaine, propranolol, and quinidine. Alpha-acid glycoproteins are low-molecular-weight proteins that are also considered acute-phase reactants. During myocardial infarction, inflammation, and surgery, the concentration of these proteins can be increased, and this reduces the quantity of the unbound active drug at the site of action.[10,11]

Metabolism and Biotransformation

Metabolic transformation is the biochemical conversion of a drug to a more polar, less lipid-soluble, more easily excreted metabolite. Drug biotransformation can be affected by alterations in protein binding, liver enzymes, and liver blood flow. Hepatic biotransformation can be divided into two pathways: phase I and phase II enzymatic systems. In phase I enzymatic systems, a hydroxyl, carboxyl, amino, or sulfur group is added to a drug. These oxidations or reductions make lipophilic agents more polar and water-soluble. In general, renal failure has a limited effect on drugs undergoing hepatic metabolism by the microsomal oxidation pathway. However, new information suggests that CKD can substantially reduce hepatic biotransformation or bioavailability of drugs predominantly metabolized by the liver.[5,17] Animal studies indicate as much as 40 to 80 percent downregulation in hepatic cytochrome P450 metabolism. Cytochrome P450 enzymes are heme-containing proteins located in the endoplasmic reticulum of most cells throughout the body. A high density of cytochrome P450 enzymes is found in the GI tract and liver.[18–20] Cytochrome P450 enzymes are classified into three different families (40 percent homology in amino acid sequence); P450 I, P450 II, and P450 III. Each family is further classified into several subfamilies (70 percent homology in amino acid sequence) and, finally, the individual gene. Greater than 30 cytochrome P450 genes have been reported to be involved in drug metabolism. Approximately 90 percent of all oxidative pathways are believed to use cytochrome P450, 1A2, 2C9, 2C19, 2D6, 2E1, and 3A4. A high incidence of polymorphism for each individual gene has been reported. Race, gender, environment, and other drugs may alter the gene expression of individual cytochrome P450 families and subfamilies.[21–23] Both cytochrome P450 IIIA and 1A2 are highly variable in different individuals, while the variability of cytochrome P450, 2C9, 2C19, and 2D6 is influenced mainly by genetic polymorphism. P-glycoprotein is a membrane-bound transport system responsible for drug transport across cell membranes. P-glycoprotein is an ATP-binding protein, which also acts as a GI barrier for absorption of many xenobiotics. Interestingly, most species display a 60 percent homology in amino acid sequences for p-glycoproteins, suggestive of conservation of xenobiotic trafficking across the cell throughout evolution. P-glycoprotein has two homologous halves and a transmembrane domain arranged into six helices. P-glycoproteins at the site of the GI tract affect the efflux of many drugs and may inhibit drug absorption through the GI tract. As drugs passively diffuse through the GI tract, P-glycoprotein pumps intercept drug penetration into the cell or remove drugs from cytoplasmic areas to the extracellular media.[24]

Elimination/Excretion

Although some drugs are excreted through the biliary-GI system and skin, most are excreted by the kidneys, usually after some metabolic transformation. Obviously this process will not occur in the setting of ESRD. Generally, filtered drugs will be dialyzable to some extent, whereas drugs eliminated in health by tubular secretion may or may not be dialyzable (see below). *Clearance* is defined as the rate of elimination by all routes relative to the concentration of the drug or solute (usually in plasma). Used clinically, *clearance* implies the volume of plasma from which a drug or solute has been completely eliminated per unit time. Clearances by different routes are additive. Systemic or total-body clearance is the sum of regional clearances (e.g., hepatic, renal, respiratory, extracorporeal).[8] Drug clearance by the kidney is a reflection of the usual renal excretory processes—namely, filtration and secretion, countered by reabsorption. Organic acids (uremic toxins) and acidic drugs may compete for the same acid transport system and interfere with each other's secretion. Most drugs are eliminated from the body by first-order kinetics (elimination rate directly proportional to the amount of drug in the body at that time, linear if plotted on semilog graphs, non-saturable).[22] Drug removal rate is conventionally expressed as the elimination half-life ($t_{1/2}$), the time required for the amount of total body drug burden and serum concentration to decrease by 50 percent. The $t_{1/2}$ for any drug is dependent on its clearance and its volume of distribution by the formula

$$t_{1/2} = (0.693/\text{ked}V_d)/\text{clearance}$$

Thus, for a given clearance, the larger the V_d, the longer the half-life. Conversely, a reduction in clearance will prolong $t_{1/2}$. In each half-life, 50 percent of the drug burden is eliminated; therefore only 3 percent remains after five half-lives. For most drugs, total-body clearance is determined by metabolic biotransformation and renal excretion. As mentioned above, for some drugs, metabolism may be enhanced in uremia, increasing clearance and decreasing $t_{1/2}$. In renal impairment, a drug usually cleared by renal mechanisms will have a prolonged $t_{1/2}$. Increases in V_d because of renal dysfunction or decreased protein binding can further complicate this relationship.[9]

APPROACH TO DRUG ADMINISTRATION IN END-STAGE RENAL DISEASE

Assessment of Renal Function

For purposes of this chapter, the creatinine clearance is presumed to be less than 10 mL/min. However, in those patients with substantial residual urine output, a 24-hour creatinine clearance may be helpful. As renal function deteriorates, creatinine clearance becomes increasingly less accurate as a measurement of glomerular filtration rate (GFR). Radioisotope techniques may be preferred in this setting. The drug dosing tables accompanying this chapter

specifically address dosage adjustments for patients whose GFR is low enough to require dialysis.[25]

Determining the Need for Dosage Adjustment

Drugs that have a renal route of elimination or those that are transformed to active metabolites requiring intact renal function for excretion generally require major dosage adjustments in renal failure. Thus, some knowledge of the drug's pharmacology is essential to rational prescribing of these agents. This is especially true for drugs with a low toxic-therapeutic ratio, such as cardiac glycosides, antiarrhythmics, and aminoglycoside antibiotics. In situations where the clinician is in doubt about the need for dosage modification, it is important to review the usual pharmacologic handling of the compound or to follow specific recommendations in a standard reference source.

Loading Doses of Drugs

When patients receive multiple drug doses at established intervals, the plasma concentration rises to a steady state. Ninety percent of this steady-state concentration is achieved in 3.3 elimination half-lives. If dosage is simply adjusted for a prolonged half-life in renal failure, effective therapy may be greatly delayed. Therefore a larger initial dose, or loading dose, is usually required. In practice the usual initial dose used in patients with normal renal function can be administered unless adverse hemodynamic factors (such as volume depletion) supervene. In such cases, it may be prudent to reduce the loading dose to 75 percent of that usually prescribed. In uremia, the V_d of digoxin is decreased; that is the basis for decreasing the digoxin loading dose in this setting.[26,27]

Maintenance Doses

Several methods may be employed to establish a proper dosage regimen in renal failure. The interval extension method lengthens the interval between doses, corresponding to the delayed excretion of the particular drug in the presence of renal failure. This method has the advantages of generating normal drug concentrations, using standard or normal drug quantities, and offering ease of calculation. The major disadvantages are that (1) there may be prolonged periods where the drug concentration may be subtherapeutic and (2) the dosing interval may require an odd dosing schedule. The amount of time when the drug concentration is in the subtherapeutic range may have great importance in the case of bronchodilators and antiarrhythmic drugs. Fortunately, many antimicrobial agents demonstrate a "postantibiotic effect," such that lower drug concentrations following a period of higher concentration are still effective. Using this interval extension method, the amount of time spent above the effective concentration is a function of both drug half-life and the magnitude (height) of the peak concentration (i.e., the area under the drug concentration–time curve). This is, in turn, dependent on the amount given (the normal dose) and the V_d. Thus, the amount of time spent above the effective concentration is dependent on the total dose given. The limiting factor for this approach will be the therapeutic ratio (relationship between effective therapeutic concentration and toxic concentration). The interval extension method is particularly practical for drugs with a relatively long serum half-life.[28,29]

The dosage reduction method is simply the reduction of the size of an individual dose prescribed at the same interval as in health. This method is preferred when a more constant serum concentration is desirable. The advantages of the dosage reduction method are the constancy of drug concentrations, ease of calculation, and convenient dosing intervals. Periods of subtherapeutic concentrations are minimized. The disadvantages are that the unusual quantities administered may lead to medication errors and the stable serum concentrations may not always be desirable (e.g., nephrotoxicity and ototoxicity from aminoglycosides).[29–31]

Drug Concentrations: Role in Drug Administration and Monitoring

Most drug concentrations are determined from serum, but whole-blood and plasma concentrations will occasionally be sought. Differences between these concentrations usually depend on red cell compartmentalization (e.g., cyclosporine). Drug concentrations are generally reported as total drug (protein-bound and free, unbound drug) unless otherwise specifically requested. Drug concentrations can be interpreted only if the dosage schedule is known (e.g., amount, timing, and route of administration). A peak concentration is usually obtained 1 to 2 hours after oral ingestion and 30 to 60 minutes after a parenteral dose. The peak concentration reflects the highest concentration after the rapid distribution phase of a drug, before substantial elimination has begun. The trough concentration is the lowest concentration observed because it is obtained immediately prior to the next dose. The trough concentration is related to the systemic (total-body) clearance of the drug. The peak and trough concentrations can be used to approximate the half-life, assuming first-order kinetics and that the clearance and V_d are constant. On semilog paper, one draws a concentration-vs.-time curve (y axis, log scale; x axis, normal scale), connecting the peak and trough concentration points and extending the line to both intercepts. The time necessary for the drug level to reach half of the peak level is the $t_{1/2}$.

Knowing the $t_{1/2}$ is valuable because, if V_d is constant ($Cl = 0.693 ? V_d/t_{1/2}$), it is used to determine the following: clearance the time required to reach a steady state (three to five half-lives), and the time required to remove the drug completely (more than five half-lives), as well as to estimate dosing intervals. The half-life is an indicator of drug elimination only if V_d is known (not assumed) to be constant. $t_{1/2}$, then, reflects systemic clearance.[32–34]

For drugs where no dosing recommendations are available, the dosing rate can be estimated: it should equal the product of the systemic clearance and the steady-state drug concentration. The dosing rate is the bioavailability (F) times the dose per unit time. As discussed above, clearance is determined from V_d and $t_{1/2}$. Because not all drugs have been tabulated, the clinician should have the information necessary for performing these calculations. All that is needed are the drug concentrations, accurate time recordings, and stable conditions. When the clinician knows what target drug concentration to achieve and which concentrations are associated with toxicity, drug concentration monitoring can be an indispensable tool to individualize therapy. The currently observed concentration (present level) is subtracted from the concentration one wishes to achieve (desired level), leaving the difference level, all in the same units. The difference level times the V_d times the body weight in kilograms will give the amount of drug needed to boost the present level to the desired level. For loading doses, the present level is zero. For maintenance doses, the trough concentration can be used as the present level. This approach can be applied to the administration of any drug for which the concentration is available and the V_d is known. It is particularly suitable in the setting of CKD when the exact drug clearance is not known because of changing conditions (e.g., volatile clinical status, fluctuating hemodynamics, use of dialysis).

Drug Dialyzability

In hemodialysis and peritoneal dialysis, diffusion is the primary method of solute removal; while in continuous arteriovenous hemofiltration (CAVH) and continuous venovenous hemofiltration (CVVH), drug removal occurs through convection and ultrafiltration. In dialysis, since the dialysate is usually free of drugs, there is a concentration gradient from blood to dialysate. Drugs in the blood must be unbound (free) to be dialyzable. In most circumstances the blood-to-dialysate concentration gradient favors net drug removal. The extent of drug removal depends on molecular weight, protein binding, water solubility, volume of distribution, and elimination pathway. For drugs that are mostly metabolized, particularly in the liver, renal failure has a limited effect on drug pharmacokinetics. In addition, the type of dialysis membrane and duration of dialysis can also affect the extent of drug removal.[35–37]

Drug removal is affected by the size of drug and size of permeability of the dialyzer. In general, drugs with a low molecular weight (< 500 Da) will dialyze more easily than drugs with a higher molecular weight. Drugs with a molecular weight between 500 and 20,000 Da can be removed by peritoneal dialysis or high-flux hemodialysis. Highly protein-bound drugs are more likely not to be dialyzable that drugs with limited (less than 70 percent) protein binding. Only free drug (unbound) can pass through the dialysis membrane. However, in patients with CKD, uremic molecules can displace highly protein-bound drugs from the site of attachment and increase the free drug concentration. In this setting, a significant amount of free drug can be removed during dialysis. Another factor that can affect drug removal is the volume of distribution. Drugs with a large volume of distribution (> 250 L) most likely will not be substantially dialyzed. These agents distribute into the tissue compartment and only a small amount circulates in the blood. Therefore the extent of dialyzability of the drug is significantly compromised. Drugs with low water–solubility are usually distributed in the tissue compartment; thus these agents will not dialyze well. In summary, hydrophilic, unbound drugs and those with a low molecular weight are readily cleared during dialysis. However, drugs with a high molecular weight or those that are lipophilic and highly protein-bound are not removed well by dialysis.[31,38,39]

Other factors that may affect drug clearance by dialysis include properties of the dialysate and of the dialyzer membrane. Pore size and the surface area of the dialysis membrane to a large extent affect drug removal by dialysis. For example, during high-flux dialysis, drug removal from plasma is significantly enhanced over conventional dialysis. Vancomycin is not removed extensively by conventional hemodialysis but is removed markedly by the high-flux procedure.

Drugs and Hemofiltration

The use of continuous renal replacement therapy such as CAVH, CVVH, venovenous hemodialysis (CVVHD), or continuous venovenous hemodiafiltration (CVVHDF) is a common practice for the treatment of acute renal failure in critically ill patients who cannot tolerate intermittent dialysis. Hemofiltration is driven by the patient's arteriovenous pressure difference, or pump-driven with CVVHD or CVVHDF. The primary method of solute removal in hemofiltration is convection (solvent drag). CVVH mimics the processes that occur in the kidney. In convection, drug removal occurs along with the solvent in which they are dissolved, and plasma is not exposed to the dialysate solution. The solvent carries the solute through a semipermeable membrane.[31,38,39] The pump creates hydrostatic pressure, which drives the solvent through the membrane. In this setting, the membrane's pore size limits molecular transfer. This method is more efficient in removing drugs with a larger volume distribution and those that are highly protein-bound and less water-soluble. The extent of drug removal during continuous therapies is influenced by the sieving coefficient (SC).

The sieving coefficient defines the ability of drug to move convectively across a membrane:

$$SC = UF/[(A + V)/2$$

where UF = ultrafiltrate
A = arterial concentration
V = venous concentration

The overall rate of ultrafiltration determines drug clearance during CVVH.

$$\text{Rate of drug clearance} = SC \times \text{ultrafiltrate}$$

or

$$\text{Drug removed} = UF \times \text{rate of UF} \times \text{time of procedure}$$

This process is not affected by the concentration gradient across the membrane and is only dependent on membrane pore size. Another form of continuous renal replacement therapy is continuous hemodiafiltration. In this method, about one-third of solute removal is by convection and the remainder by diffusion through "high-flux" membranes. In CVVHDF, solutes are removed by both convection and diffusion, increasing the removal of small molecules more than middle-sized and large molecules. It is important to remember that drug removal during CVVHDF is difficult to predict and will depend on the molecular weight, blood and dialysate flow rates, and membrane used. Therefore patients with renal failure are at risk for drug accumulation and overdosing but also for underdosing, which can be life-threatening in the case of antibiotics.

CONCLUSIONS

The administration of drug therapy in patients with renal failure poses a major dilemma for most practitioners. Unless proper dosage adjustments are made, patients with compromised renal function are particularly vulnerable to drug accumulation and toxicity. Achieving a proper balance between ensuring efficacy and avoiding toxicity remains a vital issue in patients with ESRD. A knowledge of pharmacokinetics and pharmacodynamic variability in renal failure is essential for health care providers, who must make appropriate dosage adjustments to avoid serious adverse drug reactions. In addition, practitioners should understand the factors that affect the extent of drug removal during intermittent or continuous renal replacement therapy.

Tables 33–1 through 33–14, which follow, offer an extensive review of pharmaceutical use in patients with kidney disease.

TABLE 33–1. THERAPEUTIC DRUG MONITORING OF THE MOST COMMONLY USED DRUGS FOR PATIENTS WITH END-STAGE RENAL DISEASE

Drug Name	Therapeutic Range	When to Draw Sample	How Often to Draw Levels
Aminoglycosides (conventional dosing)	Gentamicin and tobramycin: Trough: 0.5–2 mg/L Peak: 5–8 mg/L	Trough: immediately prior to dose Peak: 30-min after a 30-min infusion	Check peak and trough with third dose. For therapy less than 72 h, levels not necessary. Repeat drug levels weekly or if renal function changes
Gentamicin Tobramycin Amikacin	Amikacin: Peak: 20–30 mg/L Trough: < 10 mg/L		
Aminoglycosides (24-h dosing) Gentamicin Tobramycin Amikacin	0.5–3 mg/L	Obtain random drug level 12 hours after dose	After initial dose. Repeat drug level in 1 week or if renal function changes
Carbamazepine	4–12 µg/mL	Trough: immediately prior to dosing	Check 2–4 days after first dose or change in dose.
Cyclosporine	150–400 ng/mL	Trough: immediately prior to dosing	Daily for first week, then weekly
Digoxin	0.8–2.0 ng/mL	12 hours after maintenance dose	5–7 days after first dose for patients with normal renal and hepatic function; 15–20 days in anephric patients
Lidocaine	1–5 µg/mL	8 h after IV infusion started or changed.	
Lithium	Acute: 0.8–1.2 mmol/L Chronic: 0.6–0.8 mmol/L	Trough: Before A.M. dose at least 12 h since last dose	
Phenobarbital	15–40 µg/mL	Trough: Immediately prior to dosing	Check 2 weeks after first dose or change in dose. Follow-up level in 1–2 months
Phenytoin	10–20 µg/mL	Trough: Immediately prior to dosing	5–7 days after first dose or after change in dose
Free phenytoin	1–2 µg/mL		
Procainamide	4–10 µg/mL		
NAPA (n-acetyl procainamide), a procainamide metabolite	Trough: 4 µg/mL Peak: 8 µg/mL 10–30 µg/mL	Trough: Immediately prior to next dose or 12–18 h after starting or changing an infusion Draw with procainamide sample	
Quinidine	1–5 µg/mL	Trough: Immediately prior to next dose	
Sirolimus	10–20 ng/dL	Trough: Immediately prior to next dose	
Tacrolimus (FK-506)	10–15 ng/mL	Trough: Immediately prior to next dose	
Theophylline PO or Aminophylline IV	15–20 µg/mL	Trough: Immediately prior to next dose	
Valproic acid (divalproex sodium)	40–100 µg/mL	Trough: Immediately prior to next dose	Check 2–4 days after first dose or change in dose
Vancomycin	Trough: 5–15 mg/L Peak: 25–40 mg/L	Trough: Immediately prior to dose Peak: 60 min after a 60 min infusion	With 3d dose (when initially starting therapy, or after each dosage adjustment). For therapy less than 72 hours, levels not necessary. Repeat drug levels if renal function changes

TABLE 33–2. ANALGESICS IN RENAL FAILURE

Narcotics and Narcotic Antagonists

	Dosage	Percent of Renal Excretion	Failure			Comments	HD	CAPD	CVVH
			GFR >50	GFR 10–50	GFR <10				
Alfentanil	Anesthetic induction 8–40 μg/kg	Hepatic	100%	100%	100%		N/A	N/A	N/A
Butorphanol	2 mg q3–4h	Hepatic	100%	75%	50%		No data	No data	N/A
Codeine	30–60 mg q4–6h	Hepatic	100%	75%	50%		No data	No data	Dose for GFR 10–50
Fentanyl	Anesthetic induction (individualized)	Hepatic	100%	75%	50%		N/A	N/A	N/A
Meperidine	50–100 mg q3–4h	Hepatic	100%	75%	50%	Normeperidine, an active metabolite, accumulates in ESRD and may cause seizures. Protein binding is reduced in ESRD. 20–25% excreted unchanged in acidic urine.	Avoid	Avoid	Avoid
Methadone	2.5–10 mg q6–8h	Hepatic	100%	100%	50–75%		None	None	N/A
Morphine	20–25 mg q4h	Hepatic	100%	75%	50%	Increased sensitivity to drug effect in ESRD.	None	No data	Dose for GFR 10–50
Naloxone	0.4 mg IV[AU2]	Hepatic	100%	100%	100%		N/A	N/A	Dose for GFR

TABLE 33–3. ANTIBIOTICS IN RENAL FAILURE

Antibiotics	Normal Dosage	Percent of Renal Excretion	Dosage Adjustment in Renal Failure GFR >50	GFR 10–50	GFR <10	Comments	HD	CAPD	CVVH
Aminoglycoside antibiotics									
Streptomycin	7.5 mg/kg q12h (1.0 g q24h for tuberculosis)	60%	q24h	q24–72h	q72–96h	Nephrotoxic. ototoxic. Toxicity worse when hyperbilirubinemic. Measure serum levels for efficacy and toxicity. Peritoneal absorption increases with presence of inflammation.	1/2 normal dose after dialysis	20–40 mg/L/d	Dose for GFR 10–50 & measure levels
Kanamycin	7.5 mg/kg q8h	50–90%	60–90% q12h or 100% q12–24h	30–70% q12–18h or 100% q24–48h	20–30% q24–48h or 100% q48–72h		1/2 full dose after dialysis	15–20 mg/L/d	Dose for GFR 10–50 & measure levels
Gentamicin	1.7 mg/kg q8h	95%	60–90% q8–12h or 100% q12–24h	30–70% q12h or 100% q24–48h	20–30% q24–48h or 100% q48–72h	Concurrent penicillins may result in subtherapeutic aminoglycoside levels. Peak 6–8, trough < 2	1/2 full dose after dialysis	3–4 mg/L/d	Dose for GFR 10–50 & measure levels
Tobramicin	1.7 mg/kg q8h	95%	60–90% q8–12h or 100% q12–24h	30–70% q12h or 100% q24–48h	20–30% q24–48h or 100% q48–72h	Concurrent penicillins may result in subtherapeutic aminoglycoside levels. Peak 6–8, trough < 2	1/2 full dose after dialysis	3–4 mg/L/d	Dose for GFR 10–50 & measure levels
Netilmicin	2 mg/kg q8h	95%	50–90% q8–12h or 100% q12–24h	20–60% q12h or 100% q24–48h	10–20% q24–48h or 100% q48–72h	May be less ototoxic than other members of class. Peak 6–8, trough < 2	1/2 full dose after dialysis	3–4 mg/L/d	Dose for GFR 10–50 & measure levels
Amikacin	7.5 mg/kg q12h	95%	60–90% q12h or 100% q12–24h	30–70% q12–18h or 100% q24–48h	20–30% q24–48h or 100% q48–72h	Monitor levels. Peak 20–30, trough < 5	1/2 full dose after dialysis	15–20 mg/L/d	Dose for GFR 10–50 & measure levels
Cephalosporin						Coagulation abnormalities, transitory elevation of BUN, rash and serum sickness–like syndrome.			

TABLE 33-3. ANTIBIOTICS IN RENAL FAILURE (CONT.)

Antibiotics	Normal Dosage	Percent of Renal Excretion	Dosage Adjustment in Renal Failure GFR >50	GFR 10-50	GFR <10	Comments	HD	CAPD	CVVH
Oral cephalosporin									
Cefaclor	250-500 mg tid	70%	100%	100%	50%		250 mg after dialysis	250 mg q8-12h	N/A
Cefadroxil	500 mg-1 g bid	80%	100%	100%	50%		0.5-1.0 g after dialysis	0.5 g/d	N/A
Cefixime	200-400 mg q12h	85%	100%	100%	50%		300 mg after dialysis	200 mg/d	Not recommended
Cefpodoxime	200 mg q12h	30%	100%	100%	100%		200 mg after dialysis	Dose for GFR <10	N/A
Ceftibuten	400 mg q24h	70%	100%	100%	50%		300 mg after dialysis	No data: Dose for GFR <10	Dose for GFR 10-50
Cefuroxime axetil	250-500 mg tid	90%	100%	100%	100%	Malabsorbed in presence of H_2 blockers. Absorbed better with food.	Dose after dialysis	Dose for GFR <10	N/A
Cephalexin	250-500 mg tid	95%	100%	100%	100%		Dose after dialysis	Dose to GFR <10	N/A
Cephradine	250-500 mg tid	100%	100%	100%	50%		Dose after dialysis	Dose for GFR <10	N/A
IV Cephalosporin									
Cefamandole	1-2 g IV q6-8h	100%	q6h	q8h	q12h		0.5-1.0 g after dialysis	0.5-1.0 g q12h	Dose for GFR 10-50
Cefazolin	1-2 g IV q8h	80%	q8h	q12h	q12-24h		0.5-1.0 g after dialysis	0.5 g q12h	Dose for GFR 10-50
Cefepime	1-2 g IV q8h	85%	q8-12h	q12h	q24h		1 g after dialysis	Dose for GFR <10	Not recommended
Cefmetazole	1-2 g IV q8h	85%	q8h	q12h	q24h		Dose after dialysis	Dose for GFR <10	Dose for GFR 10-50
Cefoperazone	1-2 g IV q12h	20%	No renal adjustment is required			Displaced from protein by bilirubin. Reduce dose by 50% for jaundice. May prolong prothrombin time.	1 g after dialysis	None	None
Cefotaxime	1-2 g IV q6-8h	60%	q8h	q12h	q12-24h	Active metabolite in ESRD. Reduce dose further for combined hepatic and renal failure.	1 g after dialysis	1 g/d	1 g q12h
Cefotetan	1-2 g IV q12h	75%	q12h	q12-24h	q24h		1 g after dialysis	1 g/d	750 mg q12h
Cefoxitin	1-2 g IV q6h	80%	q6h	q8-12h	q12h	May produce false increase in serum	1 g after dialysis	1 g/d	Dose for GFR 10-50

TABLE 33–3. ANTIBIOTICS IN RENAL FAILURE (CONT.)

Antibiotics	Normal Dosage	Percent of Renal Excretion	Dosage Adjustment in Renal Failure GFR >50	GFR 10–50	GFR <10	Comments	HD	CAPD	CVVH
Ceftazidime	1–2 g IV q8h	70%	q8h	q12h	q24h	creatinine by interference with assay.	1 g after dialysis	0.5 g/d	Dose for GFR 10–50
Ceftriaxone	1–2 g IV q24h	50%	No renal adjustment is required				Dose after dialysis	750 mg q12h	Dose for GFR 10–50
Cefuroxime sodium	0.75–1.5 g IV q8h	90%	q8h	q8–12h	q12–24h		Dose after dialysis	Dose for GFR <10	1.0 g q12h
Penicillin						Bleeding abnormalities, hypersensitivity.			
Oral penicillin									
Amoxicillin	500 mg PO tid	60%	100%	100%	50–75%		Dose after dialysis	250 mg q12h	N/A
Ampicillin	500 mg PO q6h	60%	100%	100%	50–75%		Dose after dialysis	250 mg q12h	Dose for GFR 10–50
Dicloxacillin	250–500 mg PO q6h	50%	100%	100%	50–75%		None	None	N/A
Penicillin V	250–500 mg PO q6h	70%	100%	100%	50–75%		Dose after dialysis	Dose for GFR <10	N/A
IV penicillin									
Ampicillin	1–2 g IV q6h	60%	q6h	q8h	q12h		Dose after dialysis	250 mg q12h	Dose for GFR 10–50
Nafcillin	1–2 g IV q4h	35%	No renal adjustment is required				None	None	Dose for GFR 10–50
Penicillin G	2–3 million Units IV q4h	70%	q4–6h	q6h	q8h	Seizures. False-positive urine protein reactions. Six million U/d upper limit dose in ESRD.	Dose after dialysis	Dose for GFR <10	Dose for GFR 10–50
Piperacillin	3–4 g IV q4–6h		No renal adjustment is required						
Ticarcillin/ clavulanate	3.1 g IV q4–6h								
Piperacillin/ tazobactam	3.375 g IV q6–8h								
Quinolones						Photosensitivity, food, dairy products, tube feeding and Al (OH)3 may decrease the absorption of quinolones.			

TABLE 33-3. ANTIBIOTICS IN RENAL FAILURE (*CONT.*)

Antibiotics	Normal Dosage	Percent of Renal Excretion	Dosage Adjustment in Renal Failure			Comments	HD	CAPD	CVVH
			GFR >50	GFR 10–50	GFR <10				
Quinolones									
Cinoxacin	500 mg q12h	55%	100%	50%	Avoid		Avoid	Avoid	Avoid
Fleroxacin	400 mg q12h	70%	100%	50–75%	50%		Dose for GFR <10	400 mg/d	N/A
Ciprofloxacin	200–400 mg IV q24h	60%	q12h	q12–24h	q24h	Poorly absorbed with antacids, sucralfate, and phosphate binders. Intravenous dose 1/3 of oral dose. Decreases phenytoin levels.	250 mg q12h (200 mg if IV)	250 mg q8h (200 mg if IV)	200 mg IV q12h
Lomefloxacin	400 mg q24h	76%	100%	200–400 mg q48h	50%		Dose for GFR <10	Dose for GFR <10	N/A
	400 mg PO/IV q24h	88%	100%	50%	50%				
Levofloxacin	500 mg PO qd	70%	q12h	250 q12h	250 q12h	L-isomer of ofloxacin; appears to have similar pharmacokinetics and toxicities.	Dose for GFR <10	Dose for GFR <10	Dose for GFR 10–50
Moxifloxacin	400 mg qd	20%	No renal adjustment is required				No data	No data	No data
Nalidixic acid	1.0 g q6h	High	100%	Avoid	Avoid		Avoid	Avoid	N/A
Norfloxacin	400 mg PO q12h	30%	q12h	q12–24h	q24h		Dose for GFR <10	Dose for GFR <10	N/A
Ofloxacin	200–400 mg PO q12h	70%	q12h	q12–24h	q24h		100–200 mg after dialysis	Dose for GFR <10	300 mg/d
Pefloxacin	400 mg q24h	11%	100%	100%	100%	Excellent bidirectional transperitoneal movement.	None	None	Dose for GFR 10–50
Sparfloxacin	400 mg q24h	10%	100%	50–75%	50% q48h		No data: Dose for GFR <10	No data	Dose for GFR 10–50
Trovafloxacin	200–300 mg PO q12h	10%	No renal adjustment is required						
Miscellaneous agents									
Azithromycin	250–500 mg PO qd	6%	No renal adjustment is required			No drug–drug interaction with CSA/KF.	None	None	None
Clarithromycin	500 mg PO bid	20%	No renal adjustment is required			Pseudomembranous colitis.	No data: Dose after dialysis	None	None
Clindamycin	150–450 mg PO tid	10%	No renal adjustment is required			Increase CSA/FK level.	None	None	None

TABLE 33-3. ANTIBIOTICS IN RENAL FAILURE (*CONT.*)

Antibiotics	Normal Dosage	Percent of Renal Excretion	Dosage Adjustment in Renal Failure GFR >50	GFR 10–50	GFR <10	Comments	HD	CAPD	CVVH
Dirithromycin	500 mg PO qd		No renal adjustment is required			Nonenzymatically hydrolyzed to active compound erythromycylamine.	None	No data: None	Dose for GFR 10–50
Erythromycin	250–500 mg PO qid	15%	No renal adjustment is required			Increase CSA/FK level, avoid in transplant patients	None	None	None
Imipenem/cilastatin	250–500 mg IV q6h	50%	500 mg q8h	250–500 q8–12h	250 mg q12h	Seizures in ESRD. Nonrenal clearance in acute renal failure is less than in chronic renal failure. Administered with cilastin to prevent nephrotoxicity of renal metabolite.	Dose after dialysis	Dose for GFR <10	Dose for GFR 10–50
Meropenem	1 g IV q8h	65%	1 g q8h	0.5–1g q12h	0.5–1 g q24h		Dose after dialysis	Dose for GFR <10	Dose for GFR 10–50
Metronidazole	500 mg IV q6h	20%	No renal adjustment is required			Peripheral neuropathy, increase LFTs, disulfiram reaction with alcoholic beverages.	Dose after dialysis	Dose for GFR <10	Dose for GFR 10–50
Pentamidine	4 mg/kg/day	5%	q24h	q24h	q48h	Inhalation may cause bronchospasm, IV administration may cause hypotension, hypoglycemia and nephrotoxicity.	None	None	None
Trimethoprim/sulfamethoxazole	1 PO bid	70%	q12h	q18h	q24h	Increase serum creatinine. Can cause hyperkalemia.	Dose after dialysis	q24h	q18h
Vancomycin IV	1 g q12h	90%	q12h	q24–36h	q48–72h	Nephrotoxic, ototoxic, may prolong the neuromuscular blockade effect of muscle relaxants. Peak 30, trough 5–10.			
Vancomycin PO	125–250 mg qid	0%	100%	100%	100%	Oral vancomycin is indicated only for the treatment of *Clostridium difficile.*			
Antituberculosis antibiotics									
Rifampin	300–600 mg PO qd	20%	No renal adjustment is required			Decrease CSA/FK level. Many drug interactions.	None	Dose for GFR <10	Dose for GFR <10

TABLE 33–3. ANTIBIOTICS IN RENAL FAILURE (*CONT.*)

Antibiotics	Normal Dosage	Percent of Renal Excretion	Dosage Adjustment in Renal Failure			Comments	HD	CAPD	CVVH
			GFR >50	GFR 10–50	GFR <10				
Antifungal agents									
Amphotericin B	0.5 mg–1.5 mg/kg/day	<1%	No renal adjustment is required			Nephrotoxic, infusion related reactions, give 250 mL NS before each dose.			
Amphotec	4–6 mg/kg/day	<1%	No renal adjustment is required						
Abelcet	5 mg/kg/day	<1%	No renal adjustment is required						
AmBisome	3–5 mg/kg/day	<1%	No renal adjustment is required						
Azoles and other antifungals						Increase CSA/FK level.			
Fluconazole	200–800 mg IV qd/bid	70%	100%	100%	50%		200 mg after dialysis	Dose for GFR <10	Dose for GFR 10–50
Flucytosine	37.5 mg/kg	90%	q12h	q16h	q24h	Hepatic dysfunction. Marrow suppression more common in azotemic patients.	Dose after dialysis	0.5–1.0 g/d	Dose for GFR 10–50
Itraconazole	200 mg q12h	35%	100%	100%	50%	Poor oral absorption.	100 mg q12–24h	100 mg q12–24h	100 mg q12–24h
Ketoconazole	200–400 mg PO qd	15%	100%	100%	100%	Hepatotoxic.	None	None	None
Miconazole	1200–3600 mg/day	1%	100%	100%	100%		None	None	None
Terbinafine	250 mg PO qd	>1%	100%	100%	100%				
Antiviral agents									
Acyclovir	200–800 mg PO 5x/day	50%	100%	100%	50%	Poor absorption. Neurotoxicity in ESRD. Intravenous preparation can cause renal failure if injected rapidly.	Dose after dialysis	Dose for GFR <10	3.5 mg/kg/d
Amantadine	100–200 mg q12h	90%	100%	50%	25%		None	None	Dose for GFR 10–50
Cidofovir	5 mg/kg weekly x2 (induction); 5 mg/kg every 2 weeks	90%	No data: 50–100%	No data: avoid	No data: avoid	Dose-limiting nephrotoxicity with proteinuria, glycosuria, renal insufficiency; nephrotoxicity and renal clearance reduced with coadministration of probenecid.	No data	No data	Avoid

TABLE 33–3. ANTIBIOTICS IN RENAL FAILURE (*CONT.*)

Antibiotics	Normal Dosage	Percent of Renal Excretion	Dosage Adjustment in Renal Failure GFR >50	GFR 10–50	GFR <10	Comments	HD	CAPD	CVVH
Delavirdine	(maintenance) 400 mg q8h	5%	No data: 100%	No data: 100%	No data: 100%		No data: None	No data	No data: Dose for GFR 1
Didanosine	200 mg q12h (125 mg if <60 kg)	40–69%	q12h	q24h	50% q24h		Dose after dialysis	Dose for GFR <10	Dose for GFR <10
Famciclovir	250–500 mg PO bid to tid	60%	q8h	q12h	q24h	VZV: 500 mg PO tid HSV: 250 PO bid. Metabolized to active compound penciclovir.	Dose after dialysis	No data	No data: Dose for GFR 10–50
Foscarnet	40–80 mg IV q8h	85%	40–20 mg q8–24 h according to ClCr			Nephrotoxic, neurotoxic, hypocalcemia, hypophosphatemia, hypomagnesemia and hypokalemia.	Dose after dialysis	Dose for GFR <10	Dose for GFR 10–50
Ganciclovir IV	5 mg/kg q12h	95%	q12h	q24h	2.5 mg/kg qd	Granulocytopenia and thrombocytopenia.	Dose after dialysis	Dose for GFR <10	2.5 mg/kg q24h
Ganciclovir PO	1000 mg tid	95%	1000 mg tid	1000 mg bid	1000 mg qd	Oral ganciclovir should be used ONLY for prevention of CMV infection. Always use IV ganciclovir for the treatment of CMV infection.	No data: Dose after dialysis	No data: Dose for GFR <10	N/A
Indinavir	800 mg q8h	10%	No data: 100%	No data: 100%	No data: 100%	Nephrolithiasis; acute renal failure due to crystalluria, tubulointerstitial nephritis.	No data: None	No data: Dose for GFR <10	No data
Lamivudine	150 mg PO bid	80%	q12h	q24h	50 mg q24h	For hepatitis B.	Dose after dialysis	No data: Dose for GFR <10	Dose for GFR 10–50
Nelfinavir	750 mg q8h	No data	No data	No data	No data		No data	No data	No data
Nevirapine	200 mg q24h x 14d	< 3	No data: 100%	No data: 100%	No data: 100%	May be partially cleared by hemodialysis and peritoneal dialysis.	No data: None	No data: Dose for GFR <10	No data: Dose for GFR 10–50
Ribavirin	500–600 mg q12h	30%	100%	100%	50%	Hemolytic uremic syndrome.	Dose after dialysis	Dose for GFR <10	Dose for GFR 10–50
Rifabutin	300 mg q24h	5–10%	100%	100%	100%		None	None	No data: Dose for GFR 10–50

TABLE 33–3. ANTIBIOTICS IN RENAL FAILURE (*CONT.*)

Antibiotics	Normal Dosage	Percent of Renal Excretion	Dosage Adjustment in Renal Failure GFR >50	GFR 10–50	GFR <10	Comments	HD	CAPD	CVVH
Rimantadine	100 mg PO bid	25%	100%	100%	50%				
Ritonavir	600 mg q12h	3.50%	No data: 100%	No data: 100%	No data: 100%		No data: None	No data: Dose for GFR <10	No data: Dose for GFR 10–50
Saquinavir	600 mg q8h	<4%	No data: 100%	No data: 100%	No data: 100%		No data: None	No data: Dose for GFR <10	No data: Dose for GFR 10–50
Stavudine	30–40 mg q12h	35–40%	100%	50% q12–24h	50% q24h		Dose for GFR <10 after dialysis	No data	No data: Dose for GFR 10–50
Oseltamivir	75 mg PO bid	10%							
Valacyclovir	500–1000 mg q8h	50%	100%	50%	25%	Thrombotic thrombocytopenic purpura/hemolytic uremic syndrome. Avoid in transplant recipients.	Dose after dialysis	Dose for GFR <10	No data: Dose for GFR 10–50
Vidarabine	15 mg/kg infusion q24h	50%	100%	100%	75%		Infuse after dialysis	Dose for GFR <10	Dose for GFR 10–50
Zanamivir	2 puffs bid x 5 days	1%	100%	100%	100%		None	None	No data
Zalcitabine	0.75 mg q8h	75%	100%	q12h	q24h		No data: Dose after dialysis	No data	No data: Dose for GFR 10–50
Zidovudine	200 mg q8h, 300 mg q12h	8 to 25%	100%	100%	100 mg q8h	Enormous interpatient variation. Metabolite renally excreted.	Dose for GFR <10	Dose for GFR <10	100 mg q8h

TABLE 33–4. ANTIHYPERTENSIVES AND CARDIOVASCULAR AGENTS (*CONT.*)

Antihypertensives and Cardiovascular Agents	Normal Dosage	Percent of Renal Excretion	Dosage Adjustment in Renal Failure GFR >50	GFR 10–50	GFR <10	Comments	HD	CAPD	CVVH
Beta blockers						Decrease HDL, mask symptoms of hypoglycemia, bronchospasm, fatigue, insomnia, depression and sexual dysfunction.			
Acebutolol	400 mg q24h or bid; 600 mg q24h or bid	55%	100%	50%	30–50%	Active metabolites with long half-life.	None	None	Dose for GFR 10–50
Atenolol	25 mg qd; 100 mg qd	90%	100%	75%	50%	Accumulates in ESRD.	25–50 mg	None	Dose for GFR 10–50
Betaxolol	20 mg q24h	80–90%	100%	100%	50%		None	None	Dose for GFR 10–50
Bopindolol	1 mg q24h; 4 mg q24h	< 10%	100%	100%	100%		None	None	Dose for GFR 10–50
Carteolol	0.5 mg q24h; 10 mg q24h	< 50%	100%	50%	25%		No data	None	Dose for GFR 10–50
Carvedilol	3.125 mg PO tid; 25 mg tid	2%	100%	100%	100%		None	None	Dose for GFR 10–50
Celiprolol	200 mg q24h	10%	100%	100%	75%		No data	None	Dose for GFR 10–50
Dilevalol	200 mg bid; 400 mg bid	< 5%	100%	100%	100%		None	None	No data
Esmolol (IV only)	50 µg/kg/min; 300 µg/kg/min	10%	100%	100%	100%	Active metabolite retained in renal failure.	None	None	No data
Labetalol	50 mg PO bid; 400 mg bid	5%	100%	100%	100%		None	None	Dose for GFR 10–50
Metoprolol	50 mg bid; 100 mg bid	< 5%	100%	100%	100%		50 mg	None	No data
Nadolol	80 mg qd; 160 mg bid	90%	100%	50%	25%		40 mg	None	Dose for GFR 0–50
Penbutolol	10 mg q24h; 40 mg q24h	< 10	100%	100%	100%		None	None	Dose for GFR 10–50
Pindolol	10 mg bid; 40 mg bid	40%	100%	100%	100%		None	None	Dose for GFR 10–50
Propranolol	40–160 mg tid; 320 mg/day	<5%	100%	100%	100%	Bioavailability may increase in ESRD. Metabolites may cause increased bilirubin by assay interference in ESRD. Hypoglycemia reported in ESRD.	None	None	Dose for GFR 10–50

TABLE 33–4. ANTIHYPERTENSIVES AND CARDIOVASCULAR AGENTS

Antihypertensives and Cardiovascular Agents	Normal Dosage	Percent of Renal Excretion	Dosage Adjustment in Renal Failure			Comments	HD	CAPD	CVVH
			GFR >50	GFR 10–50	GFR <10				
ACE inhibitors									
Benazepril	10 mg qd	20%	100%	75%	25–50%	Hyperkalemia, acute renal failure, angioedema, rash, cough, anemia and liver toxicity.	None	None	Dose for GFR 10–50
Captopril	6.25–25 mg PO tid	35%	100%	75%	50%	Rare proteinuria, nephrotic syndrome, dysgeusia, granulocytopenia. Increases serum digoxin levels.	25–30%	None	Dose for GFR 10–50
Enalapril	5 mg qd	45%	100%	75%	50%	Enalaprilat, the active moiety formed in liver.	20–25%	None	Dose for GFR 10–50
Fosinopril	10 mg PO qd	20%	100%	100%	75%	Fosinoprilat, the active moiety formed in liver. Drug less likely than other angiotensin-converting enzyme inhibitors to accumulate in renal failure.	None	None	Dose for GFR 10–50
Lisinopril	2.5 mg qd	80%	100%	50–75%	25–50%	Lysine analogue of a pharmacologically active enalapril metabolite.	20%	None	Dose for GFR 10–50
Pentopril	125 mg q24h	80–90%	100%	50–75%	50%		No data	No data	Dose for GFR 10–50
Perindopril	2 mg q24h	<10%	100%	75%	50%		25–50%	No data	Dose for GFR 10–50
Quinapril	10 mg qd	30%	100%	75–100%	75%		25%	None	Dose for GFR 10–50
Ramipril	2.5 mg qd	15%	100%	50–75%	25–50%		20%	None	Dose for GFR 10–50
Trandolapril	1–2 mg qd	33%	100%	50–100%	50%		None	None	Dose for GFR 10–50
Angiotensin II–receptor antagonists									
Losartan	50 mg qd	13%	100%	100%	100%	Hyperkalemia, angioedema (less common than with ACE-inhibitors).	No data	No data	Dose for GFR 10–50
Valsartan	80 mg qd	7%	100%	100%	100%		None	None	None
Candesartan	16 mg qd	33%	100%	100%	50%		None	None	None
Irbesartan	150 mg qd	20%	100%	100%	100%		None	None	None

TABLE 33–4. ANTIHYPERTENSIVES AND CARDIOVASCULAR AGENTS (CONT.)

Antihypertensives and Cardiovascular Agents	Normal Dosage	Percent of Renal Excretion	Dosage Adjustment in Renal Failure GFR >50	GFR 10–50	GFR <10	Comments	HD	CAPD	CVVH
Sotalol	80 bid, 160 mg bid	70%	100%	50%	25–50%		80 mg	None	Dose for GFR 10–50
Timolol	10 mg bid, 20 mg bid	15%	100%	100%	100%		None	None	Dose for GFR 10–50
Calcium channel blockers						Dihydropyridine: headache, ankle edema, gingival hyperplasia and flushing Nondihydropyridine: bradycardia, constipation, gingival hyperplasia and AV block.			
Amlodipine	2.5 PO qd, 10 mg qd	10%	100%	100%	100%	May increase digoxin and cyclosporin levels.	None	None	Dose for GFR 10–50
Bepridil	No data	<1%	No data	No data	No data	Weak vasodilator and antihypertensive.	None	None	No data
Diltiazem	30 mg tid, 90 mg tid	10%	100%	100%	100%	Acute renal dysfunction. May exacerbate hyperkalemia. May increase digoxin and cyclosporin levels.	None	None	Dose for GFR 10–50
Felodipine	5 mg PO bid, 20 mg qd	1%	100%	100%	100%	May increase digoxin levels.	None	None	Dose for GFR 10–50
Isradipine	5 mg PO bid, 10 mg bid	<5%	100%	100%	100%		None	None	Dose for GFR 10–50
Nicardipine	20 mg PO tid, 30 mg PO tid	<1%	100%	100%	100%		None	None	Dose for GFR 10–50
Nifedipine XL	30 qd, 90 mg bid	10%	100%	100%	100%		None	None	Dose for GFR 10–50
Nimodipine		10%	100%	100%	100%		None	None	Dose for GFR 10–50
Nisoldipine	20 mg qd, 30 mg bid	10%	100%	100%	100%		None	None	Dose for GFR 10–50
Verapamil	40 mg tid, 240 mg/day	10%	100%	100%	100%		None	None	Dose for GFR 10–50
Diuretics						Hypokalemia/hyperkalemia (potassium sparing agents), hyperuricemia, hyperglycemia, hypomagnesemia, increase serum cholesterol.			
Acetazolamide	125 mg PO tid, 500 mg PO tid	90%	100%	50%	Avoid	May potentiate acidosis. Ineffective as diuretic in ESRD. May cause neurologic side effects in dialysis patients.	No data	No data	Avoid

909

TABLE 33–4. ANTIHYPERTENSIVES AND CARDIOVASCULAR AGENTS (*CONT.*)

Antihypertensives and Cardiovascular Agents	Normal Dosage	Percent of Renal Excretion	Dosage Adjustment in Renal Failure			Comments	HD	CAPD	CVVH
			GFR >50	GFR 10–50	GFR <10				
Amiloride	5 mg PO qd / 10 mg PO qd	50%	100%	100%	Avoid	Hyperkalemia with GFR <30 mL/min, especially in diabetics. Hyperchloremic metabolic acidosis.	N/A	N/A	N/A
Bumetanide	1–2 mg PO qd / 2–4 mg PO qd	35%	100%	100%	100%	Ototoxicity increased in ESRD in combination with aminoglycosides. High doses effective in ESRD. Muscle pain, gynecomastia.	None	None	N/A
Chlorthalidone	25 mg q24h	50%	q24h	q24h	Avoid	Ineffective with low GFR.	N/A	N/A	N/A
Ethacrynic acid	50 mg PO qd / 100 mg PO bid	20%	100%	100%	100%	Ototoxicity increased in ESRD in combination with aminoglycosides.	None	None	N/A
Furosemide	40–80 mg PO qd / 120 mg PO tid	70%	100%	100%	100%	Ototoxicity increased in ESRD, especially in combination with aminoglycosides. High doses effective in ESRD.	None	None	N/A
Indapamide	2.5 mg q24h	<5%	100%	100%	Avoid		None	None	N/A
Metolazone	2.5 mg PO qd / 10 mg PO bid	70%	100%	100%	100%		None	None	N/A
Piretanide	6 mg q24h / 12 mg q24h	40–60%	100%	100%	100%		None	None	N/A
Spironolactone	100 mg PO qd / 300 mg PO qd	25%	100%	100%	Avoid	Active metabolites with long half-life. Hyperkalemia common when GFR <30, especially in diabetics. Gynecomastia, hyperchloremic acidosis. Increases serum by immunoassay interference.	N/A	N/A	Avoid
Thiazides	25 mg bid / 50 mg bid	>95%	100%	100%	Avoid	Usually ineffective with GFR <30 mL/min. Effective at low GFR in combination with loop diuretic. Hyperuricemia.	N/A	N/A	N/A
Torasemide	5 mg PO bid / 20 mg qd	25%	100%	100%	100%	High doses effective in ESRD. Ototoxicity.	None	None	N/A

TABLE 33–4. ANTIHYPERTENSIVES AND CARDIOVASCULAR AGENTS (*CONT.*)

Antihypertensives and Cardiovascular Agents	Normal Dosage	Percent of Renal Excretion	Dosage Adjustment in Renal Failure			Comments	HD	CAPD	CVVH
			GFR >50	GFR 10–50	GFR <10				
Triamterene	25 mg bid / 50 mg bid	5–10%	q12h	q12h	Avoid	Hyperkalemia common when GFR < 30, especially in diabetics. Active metabolite with long half-life in ESRD. Folic acid antagonist. Urolithiasis. Crystalluria in acid urine. May cause acute renal failure.	Avoid	Avoid	Avoid
Miscellaneous agents									
Amrinone	5 µg/kg/min daily dose <10 mg/kg / 10 µg/kg/min daily dose <10 mg/kg	10–40%	100%	100%	100%	Thrombocytopenia. Nausea, vomiting in ESRD.	No data	No data	Dose for GFR 10–50
Clonidine	0.1 PO bid/tid / 0.6 mg day	45%	100%	100%	100%	Sexual dysfunction, dizziness, postal hypotension.	None	None	Dose for GFR 10–50
Digoxin	0.125 mg qd / 0.25 mg PO qd	25%	100%	50%	25%	Decrease loading dose by 50% in ESRD. Radioimmunoassay may overestimate serum levels in uremia. Clearance decreased by amiodarone, spironolactone, quinidine, verapamil. Hypokalemia, hypomagnesemia enhance toxicity. Vd and total body clearance decreased in ESRD. Serum level 12 h after dose is best guide in ESRD. Digoxin immune antibodies can treat severe toxicity in ESRD.	None	None	Dose for GFR 10–50

TABLE 33–4. ANTIHYPERTENSIVES AND CARDIOVASCULAR AGENTS (*CONT.*)

Antihypertensives and Cardiovascular Agents	Normal Dosage	Percent of Renal Excretion	Dosage Adjustment in Renal Failure			Comments	HD	CAPD	CVVH
			GFR >50	GFR 10–50	GFR <10				
Hydralazine	10 mg PO qid / 100 mg PO qid	25%	100%	100%	100%	Lupus-like reaction	None	None	Dose for GFR 10–50
Midodrine	No data	75–80%	5–10 mg q8h	5–10 mg q8h	No data	Increased blood pressure	5 mg q8h	No data	Dose for GFR 10–50
Minoxidil	2.5 mg PO bid / 10 mg PO bid	20%	100%	100%	100%	Pericardial effusion, fluid retention, hypertrichosis and tachycardia.	None	None	Dose for GFR 10–50
Nitroprusside	1 µg/kg/min	<10%	100%	100%	100%	Cyanide toxicity	None	None	Dose for GFR 10–50
Amrinone	5 µg/kg/min	25%	100%	100%	100%	Thrombocytopenia. Nausea, vomiting in ESRD.	No data	No data	Dose for GFR 10–50
Dobutamine	2.5 µg/kg/min / 15 µg/kg/min	10%	100%	100%	100%	100%	No data	No data	Dose for GFR 10–50
Milrinone	0.375 µg/kg/min / 0.75 µg/kg/min		100%	100%	100%		No data	No data	Dose for GFR 10–50

TABLE 33-5. ANTICOAGULANTS IN RENAL FAILURE

Anticoagulants	Normal Dosage	Percent of Renal Excretion	Dosage Adjustment in Renal Failure			Comments	HD	CAPD	CVVH
			GFR >50	GFR 10–50	GFR <10				
Alteplase	60 mg over 1 hour then 20 mg/h for 2 hours	No data	100%	100%	100%	Tissue-type plasminogen activator (tPa).	No data	No data	Dose for GFR 10–50
Anistreplase	30 U over 2–5 minutes	No data	100%	100%	100%		No data	No data	Dose for GFR 10–50
Aspirin	81 mg/day 325 mg/day	10%	100%	100%	100%	GI irritation and bleeding tendency.			
Clopidogrel	75 mg/day	50%	100%	100%	100%				
Dalteparin	2500 U SQ/day 5000 U SQ/day	Unknown	100%	100%	100%				
Dipyridamole	50 mg tid		No data	100%	100%	100%	No data	No data	N/A
Enoxaparin	20 mg/day 30 mg bid	8%	100%	100%	50%	0.5 mg/kg q12h for treatment of DVT. Check anti-factor Xa activity 4 h after second dose in patients with renal dysfunction. There is some evidence of drug accumulation in renal failure.			
Heparin	75 U/kg load then 0.5 U/kg/min	None	100%	100%	100%	Half-life increases with dose.	None	None	Dose for GFR 10–50
Iloprost	0.5–2.0 ng/kg/min for 5–12h	No data	100%	100%	50%		No data	No data	Dose for GFR 10–50
Streptokinase	250,000 U load then 100,000 U/h	None	100%	100%	100%		N/A	N/A	Dose for GFR 10–50
Sulfinpyrazone	200 mg bid	25–50%	100%	100%	Avoid	Acute renal failure. Uricosuric effect at low GFR.	None	None	Dose for GFR 10–50
Sulotroban	No data	52–62%	50%	30%	10%		No data	No data	No data
Ticlopidine	250 mg bid 250 mg bid	2%	100%	100%	100%	Decrease CSA level and may cause severe neutropenia & thrombocytopenia	No data	No data	Dose for GFR 10–50
Tranexamic acid	25 mg/kg tid–qid	90%	50%	25%	10%		No data	No data	No data
Urokinase	4400 U/kg load then 4400 U/kg qh	No data	No data	No data	No data		No data	No data	Dose for GFR 10–50
Warfarin	5 mg/day Adjust per INR	<1%	100%	100%	100%	Monitor INR very closely. Start at 5 mg/day. 1 mg vitamin K IV over 30 min or 2.5–5 mg PO can be used to normalize INR.	None	None	None

TABLE 33–6. ANTICONVULSANTS IN RENAL FAILURE

Anticonvulsants	Normal Dosage	Percent of Renal Excretion	Dosage Adjustment in Renal Failure — GFR >50	GFR 10–50	GFR <10	Comments	CAPD	HD	CAPD	CVH
Carbamazepine	2–8 mg/kg/day; adjust for side effect and TDM	2%	100%	100%	100%	Plasma concentration: 4–12, double vision, fluid retention, mylosuppression.		None	None	None
Clonazepam	0.5 mg tid; 2 mg tid	1%	100%	100%	100%		100%	None	No data	N/A
Ethosuximide	5 mg/kg/day; adjust for side effect and TDM	20%	100%	100%	100%	Plasma concentration: 40–100, Headache	100%	None	No data	No data
Felbamate	400 mg tid; 1200 mg tid	90%	100%	50%	25%	Anorexia, vomiting, insomnia, nausea,	25%	Dose after dialysis	Dose for GFR <10	Dose for GFR 10–50
Gabapentin	150 mg tid; 900 mg tid	77%	100%	50%	25%	Less CNS side effects compared to other agents	25%	300 mg load, then 200–300 after hemodialysis	300 mg qod	Dose for GFR 10–50
Lamotrigine	25–50 mg/day; 150 mg/day	1%	100%	100%	100%	Autoinduction, major drug–drug interaction with valproate	100%	No data	No data	Dose for GFR 10–50
Oxcarbazepine	300 mg bid; 600 mg bid	1%	100%	100%	100%	Less effect on P450 compared to carbamazepine	100%	No data	No data	No data
Phenobarbitone	20 mg/kg/day; adjust for side effect and TDM	1%	100%	100%	100%	Plasma concentration: 15–40, Insomnia				
Phenytoin	20 mg/kg/day; adjust for side effect and TDM	1%	Adjust for renal failure and low Albumin			Plasma concentration: 10–20, Nystagmus, check free phenytoin level		None	None	None
Primidone	50 mg; 100 mg	1%	100%	100%	100%	Plasma concentration: 5–20	100%	1/3 dose	No data	No data
Sodium valproate	7.5 to 15 mg/kg/day; adjust for side effect and TDM	1%	100%	100%	100%	Plasma concentration: 50–150, weight gain, hepatitis, check free valproate level	100%	None	No data	No data
Topiramate	50 mg/day; 200 mg bid	70%	100%	50%	Avoid		Avoid	No data	No data	Dose for GFR 10–50
Trimethadione	300 mg tid–qid; 600 mg tid–qid	None	q8h	q8–12h	q12–24h			No data	No data	Dose for GFR10–50
Vigabatrin	1 g bid; 2 g bid	70%	100%	50%	25%			No data	No data	Dose for GFR 10–50

TABLE 33–7. ANTIDEPRESSANTS IN RENAL FAILURE

Antidepressants	Normal Dosage	Percent of Renal Excretion	Dosage Adjustment in Renal Failure GFR >50	GFR 10–50	GFR <10	Comments	HD	CAPD	CVVH
Bupropion (immediate release)	100 mg – 250 mg	18%	100%	100%	100%	Hypotension, urinary retention and weakness	No data	No data	N/A
Bupropion (sustained release)	150 mg – 400 mg	<1%	100%	100%	50%	Seizure, no sexual dysfunction	No data	No data	N/A
Citalopram	20 mg – 40 mg	<1%	100%	100%	100%	Less effect on P450			
Clomipramine	25 mg – 250 mg	<1%	100%	100%	100%	Hypotension, urinary retention and weakness	No data	No data	N/A
Desipramine	75 mg – 300 mg	<1%	100%	100%	100%		None	None	N/A
Doxepin	100 mg – 300 mg	<1%	100%	100%	100%		None	None	Dose for GFR 10–50
Fluoxetine	10 mg – 80 mg	2.50%	100%	100%	50%	Active metabolite	No data	No data	N/A
Fluvoxamine	50 mg – 200 mg	<1%	100%	100%	100%	Increase CSA/FK levels, nausea and vomiting	None	No data	N/A
Imipramine	100 mg – 300 mg	<1%	100%	100%	100%		None	None	N/A
Nefazodone	50 mg – 100 mg	<1%	100%	100%	50%	Increase CSA/FK levels, hepatotoxicity	No data	No data	N/A
Nortriptyline	50 mg – 150 mg	<1%	100%	100%	100%	Hypotension, urinary retention and weakness	None	None	N/A
Paroxetine	10 mg – 40 mg	<1%	100%	100%	100%	Weight gain, flu-like syndrome and sedation	No data	No data	N/A
Sertraline	25 mg – 100 mg	<1%	100%	100%	100%	Less effect on P450	No data	No data	N/A
Trazodone	50 mg – 300 mg	<1%	100%	100%	100%	Sexual dysfunction	No data	No data	N/A
Trimipramine	100 mg – 300 mg	<1%	100%	100%	100%	Hypotension, urinary retention and weakness	None	None	N/A
Venlafaxine	75 mg XL – 375 mg XL	<1%	100%	100%	50%	Drug-induced hypertension	None	No data	N/A

TABLE 33–8. HYPOGLYCEMIC AGENTS IN RENAL FAILURE

Dosage Adjustment in Renal Failure is given in the GFR >50 / GFR 10–50 / GFR <10 columns.

Hypoglycemic Agents	Normal Dosage	Percent of Renal Excretion	GFR >50	GFR 10–50	GFR <10	Comments	HD	CAPD	CVVH
Acarbose	25 mg tid, 100 mg tid	35%	100%	50%	Avoid	Avoid all oral hypoglycemic agents on CRRT. Abdominal pain, N/V and flatulence	No data	No data	Avoid
Acetohexamide	250 mg q24h, 1500 mg q24h	None	Avoid	Avoid	Avoid	Diuretic effect. May falsely elevate serum creatinine. Active metabolite has $t_{1/2}$ of 5–8 h in healthy subjects and is eliminated by the kidney. Prolonged hypoglycemia in azotemic patients.	No data	None	Avoid
Chlorpropamide	100 mg q24h, 500 mg q24h	47%	50%	Avoid	Avoid	Impairs water excretion. Prolonged hypoglycemia in azotemic patients.	No data	None	Avoid
Glibornuride	12.5 mg q24h, 100 mg q14h	No data	No data	No data	No data		No data	No data	Avoid
Gliclazide	80 mg q24h, 320 mg q24h	<20%	50–100%	Avoid	Avoid		No data	No data	Avoid
Glipizide	5 mg qd, 20 mg bid	5%	100%	50%	50%		No data	No data	Avoid
Glyburide	2.5 mg qd, 10 mg bid	50%	100%	50%	Avoid		None	None	Avoid
Metformin	500 mg bid, 2,550 mg/day (bid or tid)	95%	100%	Avoid	Avoid	Lactic acidosis	No data	No data	Avoid
Repaglinide	0.5–1 mg, 4 mg tid								
Tolazamide	100 mg q24h, 250 mg q24h	7%	100%	100%	100%	Diuretic effects.	No data	No data	Avoid
Tolbutamide	1 g q24h, 2 g q24h	None	100%	100%	100%	May impair water excretion.	None	None	Avoid
Troglitazone	200 mg qd, 600 mg qd	3%	100%	Avoid	Avoid	Decreases CSA level, hepatotoxic.			
Parenteral agents									
Insulin	Variable	None	100%	75%	50%	Dosage guided by blood glucose levels. Renal metabolism of insulin decreases with azotemia.	None	None	Dose for GFR 10–50
Lispro insulin	Variable	No data	100%	75%	50%	Avoid all oral hypoglycemic agents on CRRT.	None	None	None

TABLE 33–9. ANTIHISTAMINES IN RENAL FAILURE

Antihistamines	Normal Dosage	Percent of Renal Excretion	Dosage Adjustment in Renal Failure			Comments	HD	CAPD	CVVH
			GFR >50	GFR 10–50	GFR <10				
H₁ antagonists									
Acrivastine	8 mg tid or qid	60	100%	50%	50%	May cause excessive sedation in ESRD.	No data	No data	No data
Astemizole	10 mg q24h	None	100%	100%	100%		No data	No data	N/A
Brompheniramine	4 mg q4–6h	3	100%	100%	100%		No data	No data	N/A
Cetirizine	5–20 mg q24h	60–70	100%	50%	25%		None	No data	N/A
Chlorpheniramine	4.0 mg q4–6h	20	100%	100%	100%		None	No data	N/A
Diphenhydramine	25 mg tid–qid	2	100%	100%	100%	Anticholinergic effects may cause urinary retention.	None	None	None
Erbastine	10 mg q24h	40	100%	50%	50%		No data	No data	Dose for GFR 10–50
Fexofenadine	60 mg bid	10	q12h	q12–24h	q24h		No data	No data	Dose for GFR 10–50
Flunarizine	10–20 mg q24h	None	100%	100%	100%		None	None	None
Hydroxyzine	50–100 mg qid	None	100%	50%	50%	Accumulates in ESRD	1	1	1
Orphenadrine	100 mg bid	8	100%	100%	100%		No data	No data	N/A
Oxatomide	No data	None	100%	100%	100%		None	None	N/A
Promethazine	12.5–25 mg qd–qid	None	100%	100%	100%		None	None	1
Terfenadine	60 mg bid	None	100%	100%	100%	Causes torsades de pointes.	None	None	N/A
Tripelennamine	25–50 mg tid–qid	No data	No data	No data	No data		No data	No data	N/A
Triprolidine	2.5 mg q4–6h	No data	No data	No data	No data		No data	No data	N/A
H₂ antagonists									
Cimetidine	400 mg bid or 400–800 mg qhs	50–70	100%	50%	25%	Increases serum creatinine and decreases creatinine clearance by inhibition of creatinine secretion. Mental confusion with renal or hepatic disease. Acute renal failure.	None	None	Dose for GFR 10–50
Famotidine	20–40 mg qhs	65–80	100%	50%	25%		None	None	Dose for GFR 10–50
Nizatidine	150–300 mg qhs	10 to 15	100%	50%	25%		No data	No data	Dose for GFR 10–50
Ranitidine	150–300 mg qhs	80	100%	50%	25%		1/2 dose	None	Dose for GFR 10–50

TABLE 33–10. HYPOLIPIDEMIC AGENTS IN RENAL FAILURE

Hypolipidemic Agents	Normal Dosage	Percent of Renal Excretion	Dosage Adjustment in Renal Failure GFR >50	GFR 10–50	GFR <10	Comments	HD	CAPD	CVVH
Atorvastatin	10 mg/day 80 mg/day	<2%	100%	100%	100%	Liver dysfunction, myalgia and rhabdomyolysis with CSA/FK			
Bezafibrate	200 mg bid–qid 400 mg SR q24h	50%	50–100%	25–50%	Avoid		No data	No data	Dose for GFR 10–50
Cholestyramine	4 g bid 24 g/day	None	100%	100%	100%	Schedule CSA/FK 3 hrs before the dose, N/V and constipation	None	None	Dose for GFR 10–50
Clofibrate	500 mg bid 1000 mg bid	40–70%	q6–12h	q12–18h	Avoid		None	No data	Dose for GFR 10–50
Colestipol	5 g bid 30 g/day	None	100%	100%	100%	Schedule CSA/FK 3 hours before the dose, N/V and constipation	None	None	Dose for GFR 10–50
Fluvastatin	20 mg/day 80 mg/day	<1%	100%	100%	100%	Liver dysfunction, myalgia and rhabdomyolysis with CSA/FK	No data	No data	Dose for GFR 10–50
Gemfibrozil	600 bid	None	100%	100%	100%	Hyperglycemia, rhabdomyolysis, elevation of LFTs	None	No data	Dose for GFR 10–50
Lovastatin	5 mg daily 20 mg/day	None	100%	100%	100%	Liver dysfunction, myalgia and rhabdomyolysis with CSA/FK	No data	No data	Dose for GFR 10–50
Nicotinic acid	1 g tid 2 g tid	None	100%	50%	25%	Toxic reactions frequent in ESRD. Aspirin may attenuate flushing.	No data	No data	Dose for GFR 10–50
Pravastatin	10–40 mg daily 80 mg/day	<10%	100%	100%	100%	Liver dysfunction, myalgia and rhabdomyolysis with CSA/FK	No data	No data	Dose for GFR 10–50
Probucol	500 mg bid	<2%	100%	100%	100%		No data	No data	Dose for GFR 10–50
Simvastatin	5–20 mg daily 20 mg/day	13%	100%	100%	100%	Liver dysfunction, myalgia and rhabdomyolysis with CSA/FK	No data	No data	Dose for GFR 10–50

TABLE 33–11. ANTIPSYCHOTIC AGENTS IN RENAL FAILURE

Antipsychotics	Normal Dosage	Percent of Renal Excretion	Dosage Adjustment in Renal Failure			Comments	HD	CAPD	CVVH
			GFR >50	GFR 10–50	GFR <10				
Phenothiazines									
Chlorpromazine	300–800 mg q24h	Hepatic	100%	100%	100%	Orthostatic hypotension, extrapyramidal symptoms, and confusion can occur.	None	None	Dose for GFR 10–50
Promethazine	20–100 mg q24h	Hepatic	100%	100%	100%		No data	No data	Dose for GFR 10–50
Thioridazine	50–100 mg PO tid. Increase gradually. Maximum of 800 mg/day.	Hepatic	100%	100%	100%	Excessive sedation may occur in ESRD.	None	None	None
Trifluoperazine	1–2 mg bid. Increase to no more than 6 mg.	Hepatic	100%	100%	100%		No data	No data	No data
Perphenazine	8 to 16 mg PO bid, tid, or qid. Increase to 64 mg daily	Hepatic	100%	100%	100%		None	None	None
Thiothixene	2 mg PO tid. Increase gradually to 15 mg daily	Hepatic	100%	100%	100%		No data	No data	No data
Haloperidol	1–2 mg q8–12h	Hepatic	100%	100%	100%		None	None	Dose for GFR 10–50
Loxapine	12.5–50 mg IM q4–6h	Hepatic	100%	100%	100%				
Clozapine	12.5 mg PO. 25–50 daily to 300–450 by end of 2 weeks. Maximum: 900 mg daily	Hepatic	100%	100%	100%	Do not administer drug IV	None	None	None
Risperidone	1 mg PO bid. Increase to 3 mg bid.	Hepatic	100%	100%	100%		No data	No data	No data
Olanzapine	5–10 mg	Hepatic	100%	100%	100%	Potential hypotensive effects.	None	None	None
Quetiapine	25 mg PO bid. Increase in increments of 25–50 bid or tid. 300–400 mg daily by day 4	Hepatic	100%	100%	100%		No data	No data	No data
Ziprasideone	20–100 mg q12h	Hepatic	100%	100%	100%		None	None	None

TABLE 33–12. ARTHRITIS AND GOUT AGENTS IN RENAL FAILURE

Agent	Normal Dosage	Percent of Renal Excretion	Dosage Adjustment in Renal Failure			Comments	HD	CAPD	CVVH
			GFR >50	GFR 10–50	GFR <10				
Allopurinol	300 mg q24h	30	75%	50%	25%	Interstitial nephritis. Rare xanthine stones. Renal excretion of active metabolite with $t_{1/2}$ of 25 h in normal renal function; $t_{1/2}$ one week in patients with ESRD. Exfoliative dermatitis.	1/2 dose	No data	Dose for GFR 10–50
Auranofin	6 mg q24h	50	50%	Avoid	Avoid	Proteinuria and nephrotic syndrome.	None	None	None
Colchicine	Acute: 2 mg then 0.5 mg q6h Chronic: 0.5–1.0 mg q24h	5 to 17	100%	50–100%	Avoid	Avoid prolonged use if GFR < 50 mL/min.	None	No data	Dose for GFR 10–50
Gold sodium	25–50 mg	60–90	50%	Avoid	Avoid	Thiomalate proteinuria; nephrotic syndrome; membranous nephritis.	None	None	Avoid
Penicillamine	250–1000 mg q24h	40	100%	Avoid	Avoid	Nephrotic syndrome.	1/3 dose	No data	Dose for GFR 10–50
Probenecid	500 mg bid	< 2	100%	Avoid	Avoid	Ineffective at decreased GFR.	Avoid	No data	Avoid
Nonsteroidal Anti-Inflammatory Drugs (NSAIDs)						May decrease renal function. Decrease platelet aggregation. Nephrotic syndrome. Interstitial nephritis. Hyperkalemia. Sodium retention.			
Diclofenac	25–75 mg bid	< 1	50–100 %	25–50%	25%		None	None	Dose for GFR 10–50
Diflunisal	250–500 mg bid	< 3	100%	50%	50%		None	None	Dose for GFR 10–50
Etodolac	200 mg bid	Negligible	100%	100%	100%		None	None	Dose for GFR 10–50
Fenoprofen	300–600 mg qid	30	100%	100%	100%		None	None	Dose for GFR 10–50
Flurbiprofen	100 mg bid–tid	20	100%	100%	100%		None	None	Dose for GFR 10–50
Ibuprofen	800 mg tid	1	100%	100%	100%		None	None	Dose for GFR 10–50
Indomethacin	25–50 mg tid	30	100%	100%	100%		None	None	Dose for GFR 10–50
Ketoprofen	25–75 mg tid	< 1	100%	100%	100%		None	None	Dose for GFR 10–50

TABLE 33–12. ARTHRITIS AND GOUT AGENTS IN RENAL FAILURE (*CONT.*)

Agent	Normal Dosage	Percent of Renal Excretion	Dosage Adjustment in Renal Failure			Comments	HD	CAPD	CVVH
			GFR >50	GFR 10–50	GFR <10				
Ketorolac	30–60 mg load then 15–30 mg q6h	30–60	100%	50%	25–50%	Acute hearing loss in ESRD	None	None	Dose for GFR 10–50
Meclofenamic acid	50–100 tid–qid	2 to 4	100%	100%	100%		None	None	Dose for GFR 10–50
Mefanamic acid	250 mg qid	< 6	100%	100%	100%		None	None	Dose for GFR 10–50
Nabumetone	1.0–2.0 g q24h	< 1	100%	50–100%	50–100%		None	None	Dose for GFR 10–50
Naproxen	500 mg bid	< 1	100%	100%	100%		None	None	Dose for GFR 10–50
Oxaproxin	1200 mg q24h	< 1	100%	100%	100%		None	None	Dose for GFR 10–50
Phenylbutazone	100 mg tid–qid	1	100%	100%	100%		None	None	Dose for GFR 10–50
Piroxicam	20 mg q24h	10	100%	100%	100%		None	None	Dose for GFR 10–50
Sulindac	200 mg bid	7	100%	100%	100%	Active sulfide metabolite in ESRD.	None	None	Dose for GFR 10–50
Tolmetin	400 mg tid	15	100%	100%	100%		None	None	Dose for GFR 10–50

TABLE 33–13. ANTITHYROID DRUGS IN RENAL FAILURE

Sedatives	Normal Dosage	Percent of Renal Excretion	GFR >50	Dosage Adjustment in Renal Failure GFR 10–50	Comments GFR <10	HD	CAPD	CVVH
Methimazole	5–20 mg tid	7	100%	100%	100%	No data	No data	Dose for GFR 10–50
Propylthiouracil	100 mg tid	< 10	100%	100%	100%	No data	No data	Dose for GFR 10–50

TABLE 33–14. PSYCHOTROPIC DRUGS IN RENAL FAILURE

Sedatives	Normal Dosage	Percent of Renal Excretion	Dosage Adjustment in Renal Failure			Comments	HD	CAPD	CVVH
			GFR >50	GFR 10–50	GFR <10				
Antidepressants									
Bupropion	100 mg q8h	Hepatic	100%	100%	100%		No data	No data	N/A
Nefazodone	100–600 mg q24h	Hepatic	100%	100%	100%		No data	No data	N/A
Trazodone	150–400 mg q24h	Renal	100%	No data	No data		No data	No data	N/A
Venlafaxine	75–375 mg q24h	Hepatic	75%	50%	50%		None	No data	N/A
Barbiturates						May cause excessive sedation, increase osteomalacia in ESRD. Charcoal hemoperfusion and hemodialysis more effective than peritoneal dialysis for poisoning.			
Pentobarbital	30 mg q6–8h	Hepatic	100%	100%	100%		None	No data	Dose for GFR 10–50
Phenobarbital	50–100 mg q8–12h	Hepatic (renal)	q8–12h	q8–12h	q12–16h	Up to 50% unchanged drug excreted with urine with alkaline diuresis.	Dose after dialysis	1/2 normal dose	Dose for GFR 10–50
Secobarbital	30–50 mg q6–8h	Hepatic	100%	100%	100%		None	None	N/A
Thiopental	Anesthesia induction (individualized)	Hepatic	100%	100%	100%		N/A	N/A	N/A
Benzodiazepines						May cause excessive sedation and encephalopathy in ESRD.			
Alprazolam	0.25–5.0 mg q8h	Hepatic	100%	100%	100%		None	No data	N/A
Clorazepate	15–60 mg q24h	Hepatic (renal)	100%	100%	100%		No data	No data	N/A
Chlordiazepoxide	15–100 mg q24h	Hepatic	100%	100%	50%		None	No data	Dose for GFR 10–50
Clonazepam	1.5 mg q24h	Hepatic	100%	100%	100%		None	No data	N/A
Diazepam	5–40 mg q24h	Hepatic	100%	100%	100%		None	No data	1
Estazolam	1 mg qhs	Hepatic	100%	100%	100%		No data	No data	N/A
Flurazepam	15–30 mg qhs	Hepatic	100%	100%	100%		None	No data	Dose for GFR 10–50
Lorazepam	1–2 mg q8–12h	Hepatic	100%	100%	100%		None	No data	N/A
Midazolam	Individualized	Hepatic	100%	100%	50%		N/A	N/A	N/A
Oxazepam	30–120 mg q24h	Hepatic	100%	100%	100%		None	No data	Dose for GFR 10–50
Quazepam	15 mg qhs	Hepatic	No data	No data	No data		Unknown	No data	N/A
Temazepam	30 mg qhs	Hepatic	100%	100%	100%		None	None	N/A
Triazolam	0.25–0.50 mg qhs	Hepatic	100%	100%	100%	Protein binding correlates with alpha$_1$ acid glycoprotein concentration.	None	None	N/A

TABLE 33–14. PSYCHOTROPIC DRUGS IN RENAL FAILURE (*CONT.*)

Sedatives	Normal Dosage	Percent of Renal Excretion	Dosage Adjustment in Renal Failure			Comments	HD	CAPD	CVVH
			GFR >50	GFR 10–50	GFR <10				
benzodiazepine antagonist									
Flumazenil	0.2 mg IV over 15 seconds	Hepatic	100%	100%	100%	May cause excessive sedation and en-cephalopathy in ESRD.	None	No data	N/A
Miscellaneous sedative agents									
Buspirone	5 mg q8h	Hepatic	100%	100%	100%		None	No data	N/A
Ethchlorvynol	500 mg qhs	Hepatic	100%	Avoid	Avoid	Removed by hemoperfu-sion. Excessive sedation.	Avoid	Avoid	N/A
Haloperidol	1–2 mg q8–12h	Hepatic	100%	100%	100%	Hypertension, excessive sedation.	None	None	Dose for GFR 10–50
Lithium carbonate	0.9–1.2 g q24h	Renal	100%	50–75%	25–50%	Nephrotoxic. Nephrogenic diabetes insipidus. Nephrotic syndrome. Renal tubular acidosis. Interstitial fibrosis. Acute toxicity when serum levels > 1.2 meq/L. Serum levels should be measure periodically 12 h after dose. $T_{1/2}$ does not reflect extensive tissue accumulation. Plasma levels rebound after dialysis. Toxicity enhanced by volume depletion, NSAIDs, and diuretics.	Dose after dialysis	None	Dose for GFR 10–50
Meprobamate	1.2–1.6 g q24h	Hepatic (renal)	q6h	q9–12h	q12–18h	Excessive sedation. Excretion enhanced by forced diuresis.	None	No data	N/A
Selective serotonin-reuptake inhibitors (SSRIs)									
Fluoxetine	20 mg q24h	Hepatic	100%	100%	100%	$T_{1/2}$ of active metabolite is 7–9 days.	No data	No data	N/A
Fluvoxamine	100 mg q24h	Hepatic	100%	100%	100%		None	No data	N/A
Paroxetine	20–60 mg q24h	Hepatic	100%	50–75%	0.5		No data	No data	N/A
Sertraline	50–200 mg q24h	Hepatic	100%	100%	100%		No data	No data	N/A

TABLE 33–14. PSYCHOTROPIC DRUGS IN RENAL FAILURE (*CONT.*)

Sedatives	Normal Dosage	Percent of Renal Excretion	Dosage Adjustment in Renal Failure			Comments	HD	CAPD	CVVH
			GFR >50	GFR 10–50	GFR <10				
Tricyclic antidepressants						Anticholinergic side effects cause urinary retention and orthostatic hypotension. Drug may cause confusion and excessive sedation.			
Amitriptyline	25 mg q8h	Hepatic	100%	100%	100%		None	No data	N/A
Amoxapine	75–200 mg q24h	Hepatic	100%	100%	100%	$T_{1/2}$ of active metabolite is 30 hours	No data	No data	N/A
Clomipramine	100–250 mg q24h	Hepatic	No data	No data	No data		No data	No data	N/A
Desipramine	100–200 mg q24h	Hepatic	100%	100%	100%		None	No data	N/A
Doxepin	25 mg q8h	Hepatic	100%	100%	100%		None	None	Dose for GFR 10–50
Imipramine	25 mg q8h	Hepatic	100%	100%	100%		None	None	N/A
Nortriptyline	25 mg q6–8h	Hepatic	100%	100%	100%		None	None	N/A
Protriptyline	15–60 mg q24h	Hepatic	100%	100%	100%		None	None	N/A
Trimipramine	50–150 mg q24h	Hepatic	100%	100%	100%		None	None	N/A

REFERENCES

1. Sarnak MJ, Levey AS, Schoolwerth AC, et al. Kidney disease as a risk factor for development of cardiovascular disease: a statement from the American Heart Association Councils on Kidney in Cardiovascular Disease, High Blood Pressure Research, Clinical Cardiology, and Epidemiology and Prevention. *Hypertension* 2003;42:1050–1065.

2. Kitiyakara DC, Kopp JB, Eggers DP. Trends in the epidemiology of focal segmental glomerulosclerosis. *Semin Nephrol* 2003;23:172–182.

3. Locatelli F, Pozzoni P, Del Vecchio L. Epidemiology of chronic kidney disease in Italy: possible therapeutical approaches. *J Nephrol* 2003;16:1–10.

4. Pruchnicki MC, Dasta JF. Acute renal failure in hospitalized patients: Part I. *Ann Pharmacother* 2002;36:1261–1267.

5. Winters ME, *Basic Clinical Pharmacokinetics*. Vancouver, British Columbia: Applied Therapeutics, 2003.

6. Olyaei AJ, Bennett WM. The effect of renal failure on drug handling. In: Adrew Webbs, Marc Shapiro, Mervyn Singer, Peter Suter New York, NY *Oxford Textbook of Critical Care*. 1999.

7. Benedetti P, de Lalla F. Antibiotic therapy in acute renal failure. *Contrib Nephrol* 2001;132:136–145.

8. Olyaei AJ, deMattos AM, Bennett WM. Prescribing drugs in renal failure. In: ed. *Brenner and Rector's The Kidney*, 2000 6th edition 2000 "The Kidney" Barry Brenner, WB Sanders Company Philadelphia.

9. Olyaei AJ, deMattos AM, Bennett WM. Drug-drug interaction and most commonly used drug in transplant recipients. In: *Primer on Transplantation*. Norman D, Turka L, eds. 2d ed. University of Pennsylvania, Philadelphia, PA. American Society of Transplantation, 2000.

10. Dager WE. Phenytoin assay errors in uremia. *Ann Pharmacother* 2002;36:939–940.

11. Aweeka FT, Gottwald MD, Gambertoglio JG, et al. Pharmacokinetics of fosphenytoin in patients with hepatic or renal disease. *Epilepsia* 1999;40:777–782.

12. Yuan R, Venitz J. Effect of chronic renal failure on the disposition of highly hepatically metabolized drugs. *Int J Clin Pharmacol Ther* 2000;38:245–253.

13. Schneider V, Henschel V, Tadjalli-Mehr K, et al. Impact of serum creatinine measurement error on dose adjustment in renal failure. *Clin Pharmacol Ther* 2003;74:458–467.

14. Haney SL. Drug use in renal failure. *Crit Care Nurs Clin North Am* 2002;14:77–80.

15. Ibrahim S, Honig P, Huang SM, et al. Clinical pharmacology studies in patients with renal impairment: past experience and regulatory perspectives (see comment). *J Clin Pharmacol* 2000;40:31–38.

16. Swan S, Elliott WJ, Bakris G. "Clinical pharmacology studies in patients with renal impairment: past experience and regulatory perspectives". *J Clin Pharmacol* 2000;40:7–10.

17. Leblond FA, Petrucci M, Dube P, et al. Downregulation of intestinal cytochrome p450 in chronic renal failure. *J Am Soc Nephrol* 2002;13:1579–1585.

18. Clark W. Tacrolimus: immunosuppression following liver and kidney transplant. *J Clin Pharm Ther* 1996;21:135–141.

19. McMaster P, Mirza DF, Ismail T, et al. Therapeutic drug monitoring of tacrolimus in clinical transplantation. *Ther Drug Monit* 1995;17:602–605.

20. Pichette V, Leblond FA. Drug metabolism in chronic renal failure. *Curr Drug Metab* 2003;4:91–103.

21. Pichette V, Leblond FA. Drug metabolism in chronic renal failure. *Curr Drug Metab* 2003;4:91–103.

22. Dreisbach AW, Lertora JJ. The effect of chronic renal failure on hepatic drug metabolism and drug disposition. *Semin Dial* 2003;16:45–50.

23. Guevin C, Michaud J, Naud J, et al. Down-regulation of hepatic cytochrome p450 in chronic renal failure: role of uremic mediators. *Br J Pharmacol* 2002;137:1039–1046.

24. Matheny CJ, Lamb MW, Brouwer KR, Pollack GM. Pharmacokinetic and pharmacodynamic implications of P-glycoprotein modulation. *Pharmacotherapy* 2001;21:778–796.

25. Olyaei AJ, deMattos AM, Bennett WM. Principle of drug usage in dialysis patients. In: *Dialysis Therapy*. Hanley & Belfus, 2001 Nissenson A, Fine R, eds. 3rd ed. Hanley & Belfers Inc./Philadelphia, PA.

26. Mehta RN, Mehta NJ, Gulati A. Late rebound digoxin toxicity after digoxin-specific antibody Fab fragments therapy in anuric patient (see comment). *J Emerg Med* 2002;22: 203–206.

27. Critchley JA, Critchley LA. Digoxin toxicity in chronic renal failure: treatment by multiple dose activated charcoal intestinal dialysis. *Hum Exp Toxicol* 1997;16:733–735.

28. McCormack JP, Cooper J, Carleton B. Simple approach to dosage adjustment in patients with renal impairment. *Am J Health Syst Pharm* 1997;54:2505–2509.

29. Matzke GR, Frye RF. Drug administration in patients with renal insufficiency. Minimising renal and extrarenal toxicity. *Drug Safety* 1997;16:205–231.

30. Lam YW, Banerji S, Hatfield C, Talbert RL. Principles of drug administration in renal insufficiency. *Clin Pharmacokinet* 1997;32:30–57.

31. Taylor CA, III, Abdel-Rahman E, Zimmerman SW, Johnson CA. Clinical pharmacokinetics during continuous ambulatory peritoneal dialysis (review). *Clin Pharmacokinet* 1996;31: 293–308.

32. Olyaei AJ, deMattos AM, Bennett WM. Drug usage in dialysis patients. In: Nissenson AR, Fine RN, Gentile DE, eds. *Clinical Dialysis*. Norwalk, CT: Appleton & Lange, 2001.

33. Bennett WM. Guide to drug dosage in renal failure. In: Speight TM, Holford N, eds. *Avery's Drug Treatment*, 4th ed. Auckland, NZ: ADIS International, 1997:1725–1792.

34. Aronoff GR, Golper TA, Morrison G, et al. *Drug Prescribing in Renal Failure*. Philadelphia: American College of Physicians, 1999.

35. Boxenbaum H, Tannenbaum S, Mayersohn M, Oleson F. Pharmacokinetics tricks and traps: drug dosage adjustment in renal failure. *J Pharm Pharml Sci* 1999;2:2–4.

36. Keller F, Czock D. Pharmacokinetic studies in volunteers with renal impairment. *Int J Clin Pharmacol Ther* 1998;36: 594–598.

37. Subach RA, Marx MA. Drug dosing in acute renal failure: the role of renal replacement therapy in altering drug pharmacokinetics. *Adv Renal Replace Ther* 1998;5:141–147.

38. Joos B, Schmidli M, Keusch G. Pharmacokinetics of antimicrobial agents in anuric patients during continuous venovenous haemofiltration. *Nephrol Dial Transplant* 1996;11: 1582–1585.

39. Keller E. Pharmacokinetics during continuous renal replacement therapy. *Int J Artif Organs* 1996;19:113–117.

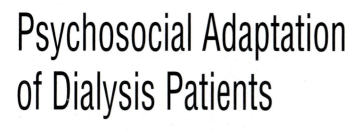

Psychosocial Adaptation of Dialysis Patients

David N. Churchill

Dialysis removes many of the toxins responsible for the uremic syndrome and prolongs survival. However, the dialysis treatment does not fully correct the uremic state and may be associated with treatment-related complications. The residual uremic symptoms and the burden of the treatment itself prevent patients from attaining a state of full health. The perception of a continuous chronic illness combined with the intrusive nature of the dialysis treatments can interfere with many aspects of the patient's life. The degree to which an individual patient can adapt to these medical and psychosocial stresses will determine quality of life.

Alexander and Willems[1] have stated that "the functional basis of quality of life involves continuous functioning reciprocal interactions between persons and their environments." The crucial areas of human life are physical well-being, relations with others, social activities, personal development, recreation, and economic circumstances.

There is an abundant literature addressing the psychological and social problems faced by dialysis patients and the coping styles used in response to these problems. Many of these studies are no longer applicable, as the patient population has changed considerably in recent years. In particular, the dialysis population is older, there is a greater proportion with diabetes mellitus as the cause for end-stage renal disease (ESRD), and these patients have more associated comorbidities. Improvements in dialysis techniques have increased the effectiveness of the therapy and diminished many treatment-related symptoms.

MEASUREMENT ISSUES

The terms *quality of life, health status, functional status,* and *psychosocial adaptation* are often used to address similar concepts. Some have used the term *health-related quality of life* to exclude important aspects of life that are not generally considered related to health (e.g., income, freedom, and quality of the environment).[2]

In order to provide a framework for an understanding of the many questionnaires available for use in this field, a taxonomy has been proposed.[2] Questionnaires can be defined according to their focus, purpose, and methodologic characteristics. Focus is concerned with the construct to be estimated.

The instruments can be classified as generic (global) or specific; the latter category includes disease-specific and function-specific instruments (Table 34–1). A function-specific instrument could address a component of quality of life (e.g., physical function, psychological function, social function, vocational rehabilitation, economic status) or an even more specific function (e.g., neurocognitive or sleep patterns).

The purpose of the questionnaire may be classified as discriminative, predictive, or evaluative (Table 34–1).[3] The objective of a discriminative instrument is to distinguish differences between patients or groups of patients at a single point in time. Predictive instruments are designed to predict future outcomes from current data. The objective of an evaluative instrument is to measure change within patients or groups of patients over time, often in response to a particular intervention. The important methodologic characteristics for a quality-of-life questionnaire are reliability, validity, and responsiveness (Table 34–1).[4,5] Reliability is the extent to which a questionnaire gives the same results on independent repeated occasions under the same conditions. This is particularly important for discriminative instruments. *Validity* refers to the extent to which a questionnaire measures what it claims to measure. If a "gold standard" exists, a comparison of the results from the instrument with those obtained with the gold standard satisfies criterion validity. In the absence of a gold standard for quality of life or for the components of quality of life, other estimates of validity must be used. The most rigorous of these is construct validity, which involves examination of correlations between the new instrument and other questionnaires thought to measure the same domain. An evaluative instrument must be able to detect changes in patients or groups of patients over time. For these instruments, the property of responsiveness must be satisfied. Responsiveness is directly proportional to the change in score that constitutes a clinically important difference and inversely proportional to the between-subject variability of the score in stable patients over time.[5]

Reliability, validity, and responsiveness must be documented for the results of a questionnaire to be considered credible. Ideally, these properties should be established in the population to which the questionnaire will be applied. This is particularly important in the case of psychological tests for dialysis patients. Yanagida and Streltzer[6] have critically reviewed the limitations of psychological tests in this population. Instruments for which reliability and validity have been established in normal populations may not satisfy these methodologic criteria in the dialysis population.

GLOBAL OR OVERALL QUALITY OF LIFE

Hornberger et al.[7] have reported on variability among methods to assess patient well-being or quality of life. The instruments evaluated were the Sickness Impact Profile,[8] Campbell Index of Well-Being,[9] Kaplan-Bush Index of Well-Being,[10] Categorical Scaling,[11] Standard Gamble,[12] and Time Trade-Off.[13] Among 58 hemodialysis patients, the Pearson product-moment correlations were poor and ranged from 0.06 to 0.51. These data suggest that these estimates of quality of life or well-being are not addressing the same construct.

Reliability and validity have been established in the general population and for various disease states for all of these instruments. However, only the Time Trade-Off method and the Sickness Impact Profile have been demonstrated to be reliable and valid for ESRD patients.[14–16]

Sickness Impact Profile

Hart and Evans[15] used the Sickness Impact Profile to evaluate 859 ESRD patients. The Sickness Impact Profile is a standardized instrument containing 136 statements addressing 12 categories of behavior. The overall score may range from 0 to 100 with higher scores indicating a worse health state. The mean scores were 10.0 for home hemodialysis, 12.3 for in-center hemodialysis, 12.2 for continuous ambulatory peritoneal dialysis (CAPD), and 5.5 for transplanted patients. Adjustment for age, sex, and race reduces the difference among the treatment modalities, but the ordering remains unchanged. The Sickness Impact Profile can be considered a generic or global estimate of quality of life in ESRD patients. It is valid and reliable. It is capable of discriminating between renal transplant patients and those treated with various dialysis modalities. It also appears to be responsive in that there are improvements in the quality of life of patients with severe anemia corrected by treatment with recombinant human erythropoietin.[17]

Time Trade-Off

The Time Trade-Off method was used to estimate global quality of life for 194 patients with ESRD.[14] This technique asks the patient, using a standard series of questions with visual aids, to imagine exchanging an improved quality of life for a decreased quantity of life. For example, a patient

TABLE 34–1. MEASUREMENT ISSUES

Focus	Purpose	Properties
Generic	Discriminative	Reliability
Disease specific	Predictive	Validity
Function specific	Evaluative	Responsiveness

with a 10-year life expectancy on dialysis might prefer 5 years of full health followed by death. This would provide a score of 0.50. A score of 0 is equivalent to death and 1.0 is equivalent to full health. Patients with a renal transplant had a mean score of 0.84, followed by CAPD patients at 0.56, home hemodialysis patients at 0.49, and in-center hemodialysis patients at 0.43. In a prospective study, the effect of transplantation on the Time Trade-Off score was evaluated by comparing the score in 27 patients while on dialysis with that determined 3 months after a successful renal transplant.[16] Each patient served as his or her own control. The score increased from 0.41 to 0.74, a mean change score of 0.33 (95 percent confidence interval, 0.26 to 0.40).

However, in the Canadian Multicenter Erythropoietin Study,[17] an increase in hemoglobin value from 74 to 117 g/L improved the Time Trade-Off score only from 0.52 to 0.58, while the Sickness Impact Profile improved from 12.2 to 4.4. If both the Time Trade-Off and the Sickness Impact Profile are reliable, valid, and responsive instruments for an ESRD population, why does one demonstrate an improvement with recombinant human erythropoietin therapy while the other does not? The evidence for responsiveness of the Time Trade-Off in the ESRD population is based on the effect of successful renal transplantation.[16] There is also evidence for responsiveness of the Time Trade-Off in other populations. Patients with hip joint replacement had an increase in score from 0.41 preoperatively to 0.75 at the sixth postoperative month,[18] and patients with intractable ulcerative colitis improved from 0.58 to 0.98 following colectomy.[19] These data indicate that an intervention which improves many of the components of the quality of life will be reflected in the Time Trade-Off score. Treatment with recombinant human erythropoietin improves physical health and some aspects of psychosocial health; this is detected by the Sickness Impact Profile. However, the effect on overall quality of life is not significant. Patients still require the intrusive dialysis treatment with the associated limitations on diet, leisure time, employment, and travel.

Other Generic Instruments

Other investigators have used instruments for estimating quality of life for which there are no established reliability and validity data for patients with ESRD. Publications using the Index of Well-Being,[9] the Life Satisfaction Scale,[20] Cantril's Self-Anchoring Scale,[21] and the EuroQOL[22] exemplify the use of such instruments.

Comparison of Sickness Impact Profile to Time Trade-Off Methods

The Time Trade-Off method must be administered by a skilled interviewer, and there are many potential sources of bias that might affect the responses. This instrument remains useful for research purposes, but it is not applicable to clinical practice. The Sickness Impact Profile, while still valuable, has been replaced by other questionnaires.

Short Form-36

Validity in ESRD. The most widely used and accepted generic or global estimate of health-related quality of life for ESRD patients is the Medical Outcomes Study Short Form-36 (SF-36).[23] This instrument consists of 36 questions, 35 of which are collapsed into eight scales. These scales are physical functioning, role-physical, bodily pain, general health, vitality, social functioning, role-emotional, and mental health. Each scale is scored from 0 to 100, with higher scores being more favorable. The eight scales are compressed into two dimension or summary scores. These are the Physical Component Summary and the Mental Component Summary. The former contains the first five scales; the latter contains the final five scales. General health and vitality are included in both. The summary scores are standardized to have a mean score of 50 in the general U.S. population.[23]

The reliability and validity of SF-36 has been established in diverse patient populations.[24] Despite its widespread use in ESRD studies, there has been limited formal validity testing. Maor and colleagues evaluated the Time Trade-off technique, a visual analogue health-related global quality-of-life questionnaire, and the SF-36 in 56 hemodialysis patients in Israel.[25] The Spearman correlations with the health-related global quality-of-life instrument were 0.38 and 0.40 for the SF-36 physical component and the mental component scores respectively ($p < 0.005$ for each). The Time Trade-off technique correlated with neither the global estimate nor the SF-36. A regression analysis was performed with the SF-36 as the dependent variable and estimates of socioeconomic status, disease severity, comorbidity, depression, social support, and laboratory data as independent variables. The physical and mental component scores of the SF-36 explained 64 and 75 percent of the variance, respectively. These data provide evidence for the construct validity of the SF-36 in hemodialysis patients. The SF-36 has been used to discriminate between patient populations, to predict clinical outcomes, and to evaluate interventions.

Application of SF-36 in End-Stage Renal Disease

SF-36 as a Discriminative Instrument. In 1995, Khan et al.[26] administered the SF-36 to patients with renal transplants and to patients on hemodialysis and peritoneal dialysis. The results were presented by subscale score without calculation of the physical and mental component scores. The perception of health of hemodialysis patients and peritoneal dialysis patients was worse than those with renal transplants and normal controls for six of the eight subscales. Patients were defined as being at low, medium, and high risk according to comorbidity. Analysis of trend showed that four subscale scores were higher with low-risk than with high-risk patients. These data add to the evidence for construct validity for the SF-36 in ESRD patients.

In 2000, Diaz-Buxo and colleagues[27] reported on SF-36 scores for 16,755 hemodialysis and 1260 peritoneal dialysis patients. The unadjusted physical component scores for hemodialysis and peritoneal dialysis patients were 33.3 and 33.7, respectively, compared to a score of 50 for the general U.S. population. The mental component scores were 47.5 and 47.9, respectively. There were differences between CAPD patients and continuous cyclic peritoneal dialysis (CCPD) patients. The former had better and the latter worse physical component scores than the referent hemodialysis patients. With adjustment for case mix and laboratory values, CCPD patients still had significantly lower physical component scores than hemodialysis patients. Conversely, after adjustment for the same variables, CCPD patients had significantly higher mental component scores. The role played by each subscale was explored in detail.

SF-36 as a Predictive Instrument. The role of SF-36 as a predictive instrument was reported by Lowrie and colleagues.[28] The study population comprised 13,952 patients in the Fresenius Medical North America system. The mean physical component score was 33.3; the mean mental component score 47.5. Logistic regression was used to evaluate the associations of the hospitalization rates, as a morbidity surrogate, and mortality with selected independent variables. These included the physical and mental component scores. Each one point increase in the physical component score was associated with a 2 percent reduction in hospitalization and a 2 percent reduction in mortality. Each one point increase in mental component score was associated with a 1 percent decrease in hospitalization and 2 percent decrease in mortality.

In a study of 17,236 patients in the United States, Europe, and Japan,[29] Mapes and colleagues reported similar associations of decreased physical and mental component scores with increased risk of hospitalization and death. Based on the data from the Fresenius Medical Care system[28] and the Dialysis Outcomes and Practice Patterns Study,[29] the SF-36 component summary scores are associated with morbidity and mortality. SF-36, therefore, can be used as a predictive instrument.

SF-36 as an Evaluative Instrument. In 1996, Beusterien et al.[30] reported changes in results of the SF-36 among hemodialysis patients who were given recombinant human erythropoietin for the first time. Their hematocrit values increased from 25.5 to 29.9 percent over a 6-month period. The physical component score increased from 35.3 to 36.5 (NS), while the mental component score increased from 43.4 to 47.3, an increase of 3.7. The latter would be predicted to be

associated with a significant improvement in morbidity and mortality.[28,29]

Summary of Uses for the SF-36 in ESRD Patients

There is evidence for reliability and validity of the SF-36 in patients with ESRD. However, responsivity has not yet been firmly established. This instrument can be used to discriminate among ESRD patient populations, although adjustment for clinical and laboratory status appears important. It can be used to predict clinical outcomes and therefore could be used as a surrogate outcome in clinical trials. It would not replace the need for direct determination of morbidity and mortality. The SF-36 appears to be the best of the currently available questionnaires with which to evaluate global quality of life in ESRD patients.

DISEASE-SPECIFIC QUALITY OF LIFE

Methodology

Generic or global estimates of health-related quality-of-life instruments, however, may not focus adequately on specific clinical problems and may have poor responsiveness. Methodology for the development of disease-specific instruments has been described by Guyatt et al.[31] Items are generated by patients with the disease and by relevant health care professionals. Following item reduction, the reliability, validity, and responsiveness of the instrument must be established.

Kidney Disease Questionnaire (KDQ)

The Kidney Disease Questionnaire developed by Laupacis and colleagues satisfies the criteria described above.[32] It consists of 26 questions in five dimensions (physical symptoms, fatigue, depression, relationships with others, and frustration). Each question is scored on a seven-point ordinal scale, and the unweighted responses are added to give a score for each dimension. The reliability was established by correlations of 0.85 to 0.98 for test-retest reproducibility. The questionnaire demonstrated construct validity when compared with other estimates of quality of life for patients with ESRD. It was more responsive than other measures in detecting improvements associated with increased hemoglobin values for patients treated with recombinant human erythropoietin in a randomized clinical trial.[17] There were improvements in all dimensions except frustration. This instrument is specific for patients with ESRD treated with hemodialysis.

Kidney Disease Quality-of-Life Short-Form (KDQOL-SF)

In an attempt to combine the global quality-of-life estimate provided by the SF-36 with a disease-specific instrument, Hays and colleagues developed the KDQOL.[33] A short form of this instrument, the KDQOL-SF, has been developed as well,[34] a multidimensional validated questionnaire that has a high degree of correlation with the KDQOL. The KDQOL-SF includes the SF-36 and has eight dialysis-targeted dimensions and four additional dimensions. Therefore the entire questionnaire contains 80 items in 20 dimensions, 8 from the SF-36 and the additional 12 noted above. These are well described in the work of Korevaar and colleagues.[35] These authors addressed the reliability and validity of the eight disease-targeted dimensions and found them informative, with a high degree of validity and reliability.[35] The kidney disease–related dimensions are each scored on a scale of 0 to 100, with higher scores indicating better states. The dimensions are dialysis-related symptoms, effects of kidney disease, burden of kidney disease, cognitive function, work status, quality of social interaction, sexual function, and sleep. Carmichael and colleagues applied the KDQOL-SF to 49 hemodialysis patients and 97 peritoneal dialysis patients.[36] In an unadjusted analysis, they found significant differences between dialysis modalities in 8 of the 12 dimensions added to the core SF-36. A larger sample size would be required to evaluate the effect of adjustment for demographic, clinical, and laboratory variables.

KDQ and KDQOL-SF Comparison

In summary, the KDQ remains a simple method for estimating disease-related quality of life for hemodialysis patients. Although it has not been validated for peritoneal dialysis patients, the dimensions are not modality-specific. The KDQ is responsive to change and can be used as an evaluative instrument in clinical trials. The KDQOL-SF has been validated in both hemodialysis and peritoneal dialysis patients. The kidney disease–targeted dimensions appear, in unadjusted analysis, able to discriminate between hemodialysis and peritoneal dialysis patients and could be used to explore the degree to which these dimensions contribute to global quality of life. There is as yet no evidence to support use of the KDQOL-SF as a predictive or evaluative instrument.

NEUROPSYCHOLOGICAL FUNCTION

The clinical observation of improvement in cognitive function associated with dialysis treatment of uremia has generated many studies evaluating the deficits associated with uremia. Detailed descriptions of tests of neuropsychological function and normative data are available.[37] Among patients treated by CAPD, there was an improvement in trails B and digit symbol performance,[38] while those treated with hemodialysis demonstrated improvement in paired associate learning, block design, and the visual retention test.[39] These performance deficits improved to within broad normal limits shortly after the institution of dialysis and thereafter demonstrated little additional improvement. Teshan et al.[40] evaluated the effect on cognitive function of altering the dose of hemodialysis in 10 patients. The weekly clearance of urea was reduced for a period of 3 months and was then returned to the original level. The electroencephalographic discriminant score worsened in all 10 patients and returned to the baseline state with increased dialysis dose. The continuous memory test worsened in all 10 and then improved. In a crossover study of 22 patients comparing the effect of a low- with a high-flux cellulose acetate membrane, no statistically significant difference was found for 23 neuropsychological variables.[41]

Comparison to general adult norms indicated that these patients functioned generally within the low-average range of intelligence. Uremic patients demonstrate mild to moderate impairment on tests that evaluate cognitive flexibility, sustained concentration/attention, perceptual motor speed, learning/memory, and constructional ability. Deficits in verbal intellectual ability tend to be less severe than those in the nonverbal visuospatial sphere. Dialysis rapidly improves performance in these areas. For patients treated with hemodialysis thrice weekly, increasing the proportional clearance of urea *(KT/V)* from 1.27 to 1.42 and using a high-flux dialysis membrane does not further improve performance on these tests.[41]

More intensive dialysis therapies (e.g., daily dialysis, either short or nocturnal) might provide additional cognitive improvement, but formal testing is required to determine this. Of greater concern is the high prevalence of mild and dementia level cognitive impairment in the current dialysis population.[42] Whether this is due to exposure to uremic toxins or heavy metals, progressive vascular disease, or a reflection of the changing demographics of the dialysis population is unclear.

PSYCHOLOGICAL FUNCTION

Patients with ESRD requiring hemodialysis treatment have provided fertile ground for psychological study. The major psychological abnormalities associated with hemodialysis treatment of uremia are dependence-independence conflicts, depression, anger, anxiety, frustration, and denial. The studies addressing psychological function can be divided into those that are descriptive and those that attempt to predict outcomes.

Descriptive Studies

One approach, summarized by Schreiner and Tartaglia,[43] is to analyze the ESRD patient with psychiatric methods and determine feelings, catalogue behavior, test cognitive function, and diagnose psychological symptoms. Depression is considered an important problem for patients with ESRD. The prevalence of depression varies widely and is dependent on the instrument used for diagnosis. The Beck Depression Inventory[44] suggests that there is a high prevalence of depression among hemodialysis patients. This is a 21-item self-report inventory with a scale from 0 to 63. Various cutoff scores have been used to dichotomize patients into depressed and not depressed. Using a score of > 15 defined 45.4 percent of patients as being depressed.[45] However, only 8.1 percent of the patients in that same population met the criteria of the third edition of the American Psychological Association's *Diagnostic and Statistical Manual of Mental Disorders* (DSM-III) for major depressive symptoms. These data are similar to those reported by Smith et al.,[46] who found about half of the hemodialysis patients depressed, according to the Beck Depression Inventory criteria, compared to 5 percent by DSM-III criteria. Many of the symptoms of chronic kidney disease (CKD) are also prominent features of depression. These include fatigue, anorexia, and sleep disorders. Sacks et al.[47] have identified 15 items in the Beck Depression Inventory that reflect cognitive beliefs and eight that reflect somatic symptoms. The former constitute the Cognitive Depression Index, which is considered a better predictor of depression.

The Beck Depression Inventory and the more specific Cognitive Depression Inventory are relatively easy to apply to dialysis patients. They should be considered screening tools and used to identify the 5 to 8 percent patients with major depressive symptoms who might benefit from intensive counseling and appropriate pharmacologic therapy.

Most studies have been performed in Caucasian hemodialysis patients. Although smaller studies have been performed in peritoneal dialysis patients[48] and in those with CKD,[49] the data are inadequate for critical comment. Other patient populations requiring further study are African Americans[50] and Asians.[51] Additional research is required to evaluate the possible interrelations between depression, activation of proinflammatory cytokines, malnutrition, and clinical outcomes.[52,53]

Predictive Studies

Studies that address the association of depression with survival in dialysis patients have yielded contradictory results. These have been reviewed succinctly by Kimmel.[54] Studies suggesting an association between depression and poorer survival[55–58] have methodologic weaknesses. These have included small sample sizes and cross-sectional evaluations that did not adjust for other variables with a possible influence on outcome. More recent studies, using multivariable analytic techniques, have failed to demonstrate such an association.[59–61] In a longitudinal study of chronic hemodialysis patients, Kimmel et al.[62] used the Beck Depression Inventory and the Cognitive Depression Inventory as time-dependent covariates in a Cox regression model and controlled for important medical covariates. They reported

an increase in one standard deviation for depression scores to be associated with an 18 to 32 percent increased risk of mortality. Whether this increase in mortality is due to measurement of constructs other than depression by the questionnaires, a confounder that causes both depression and worse outcome (e.g., chronic inflammation), or is causally related to depression requires further study.

SOCIAL FUNCTIONING

This is a broad but important component of quality of life. It includes social and leisure activities, vocational function, relationships with others, sexual function, and family function. Many questionnaires have been developed to address these contributions to social functioning; few have been validated in the ESRD population. Studies of patients on hospital hemodialysis, home hemodialysis, CAPD, and with successful renal transplantation[63,64] have used an instrument that has been validated in the ESRD population.[65]

Psychosocial Adjustment to Illness Scale (PAIS)

The Psychosocial Adjustment to Illness Scale (PAIS) addresses seven domains that are relevant to adjustment to medical illness.[65] These are health care orientation, vocational function, sexual function, domestic environment, extended family environment, social environment, and psychological distress. This scale has been demonstrated to have internal consistency, reliability, and validity in an ESRD population. The PAIS contains 45 items with a scale from 0 to 4 for each item. Higher scores indicate a more serious problem. The questionnaire is a semistructured clinical interview.

The mean PAIS score for 102 maintenance hemodialysis patients was 36.5, compared with 23.3 for 69 of these patients 18 months later.[63] Although this scale attempts to quantify psychosocial adjustment to illness, not all domains apply to all patients (e.g., vocational function for a retired person). Each domain can be scored individually. The domains with the highest or worst scores were vocational functioning, psychological function, and sexual function. Soskolne and Kaplan de-Nour[64] have used the PAIS to compare home hemodialysis patients, hospital hemodialysis patients, and CAPD patients. There was no difference in any of the seven domains between the hospital- and home-hemodialysis patients. On the other hand, CAPD patients had better scores on the domestic environment domain than did hospital hemodialysis patients.

Clearly, one cannot substitute use of questionnaires for the detailed individualized assessment by skilled social workers. However, the PAIS appears to be capable of discriminating among different ESRD populations and can perhaps detect changes occurring naturally over time or in response to a specific intervention.

FUNCTIONAL STATUS

The Karnofsky Index[66] was originally developed for patients with malignancy. The scale has 10 categories with scores ranging in multiples of 10, from 0 to 100, with higher scores indicating better functional capacity. Hutchinson et al.[67] have aggregated the 10 Karnofsky levels into three alphabetical categories. Level A corresponds to 80 to 100 and describes an individual who is able to carry on normal activity and to work. Level B corresponds to 50 to 70 and is represented by patients who are unable to work but are capable of caring for most of their needs. Level C corresponds to scores of less than 50 and describes patients who are incapable of self-care. These investigators[67] reported unacceptably high interobserver variability in assigning a Karnofsky score. The problem with interobserver variability was ascribed to lack of operational criteria to define the elements of the scale and the nonexhaustive aggregation of the constituent elements of the scale. Despite these methodologic problems, the Karnofsky scale had been extensively used in the evaluation of functional status of ESRD patients.

In 1981, Gutman et al. reported on the functional status of 2481 patients from 17 centers in the United States.[68] Only 60 percent of the nondiabetic and 23 percent of the diabetic patients were in category A (i.e., capable of normal activity and work). With the development of instruments that estimate physical function, either as an independent instrument or as a subscale of a more comprehensive instrument, the Karnofsky Index is less frequently used. The methodologic issues, described by Hutchinson,[67] and the analytic difficulties presented by the noninterval nature of the scale have contributed to the decline in its utilization.

Physical Activity

Johansen and colleagues evaluated several questionnaires to estimate physical activity.[69] The reference standard was an accelerometer[70] with the Human Activity Profile[71] and the Physical Function subscale of the SF-36 correlating well with measured physical activity. These estimates may replace the Karnofsky Index as an estimate of functional ability.

VOCATIONAL REHABILITATION

Gutman et al.[68] observed that the poor functional status of dialysis patients was accompanied by poor vocational rehabilitation. Only 18 percent of the diabetic men and 34 percent of the nondiabetic men were employed. There was less employment outside the home for diabetic than for nondiabetic women: 6 percent compared with 16 percent; and a smaller percentage reporting full-time housework: 18 percent compared with 32 percent. Among working-age males, those with a college education had three times the level of employment as those with less formal education. However, these data are not relevant to the contemporary dialysis population, which is older, more likely diabetic, and with greater comorbidity.

In 1991, Kutner et al.[72] performed a cross-sectional survey of 283 chronic dialysis patients receiving treatment in the southeastern United States. Only 11 percent of the total sample was employed at the time of the survey. Most of those employed held white-collar jobs and tended to have more formal education than those who were unemployed. White males were more likely than white females or blacks of either sex to be employed.

In 1994, Holley and Nespor[73] reported that 33 of 77 (43 percent) hemodialysis patients in Pittsburgh under age 55 were either working full time or attending school. The working patients were better educated and had been on dialysis for a shorter period of time. Blake et al. reported on the employment status of ESRD patients (hemodialysis, peritoneal dialysis, and transplant) in a multicenter study in Ireland.[74] Among those who wished to work, 49 percent were unemployed compared to the national average of 10 percent. Unemployed ESRD patients scored lower than those who were employed on the following SF-36 scales: physical function, physical role, bodily pain, general health, vitality, and emotional role.

In considering vocational rehabilitation, the calculation must exclude those who are retired by virtue of age or who had retired prior to significant ESRD due to comorbidity, such as diabetic complications and cardiovascular disease. The target population should comprise those who cease working as a result of renal failure or dialysis therapy. Dialysis schedules are often a logistic barrier to working, and flexible scheduling may help some of these patients. The recent data from Ireland identifies diminished quality of life, as estimated from the sub-scales of the SF-36, to be associated with unemployment. The impact of correction, if possible, of these factors on employment rates would be an interesting research question.

COMPLIANCE

The issue of compliance for hemodialysis patients has been thoroughly reviewed by Lamping and Campbell.[75,76] The theoretical models of compliance behavior have been reviewed by Wolcott et al.[77] with respect to patients with ESRD treated by dialysis. These models include personality traits, psychodynamics, sociocultural factors, cognitive theory, health belief, and health transactions. However, none of these models explains or predicts compliance in dialysis patients in a satisfactory manner.

Others have examined the relationship between compliance and demographic characteristics. There is no consistent relationship between compliance and race, income, marital status, education, age, or sex.[75] Patients who are employed or do housework either full or part time are more compliant than those who are not.

In order to test these various predictive models, a valid and reliable measure of compliance is required. Lamping and Campbell[74] have classified measures of compliance as objective and subjective.

The most common objective estimates are serum urea, serum potassium, serum phosphorus, and interdialytic weight gain. Objective measures of behavioral compliance (nonattendance for dialysis or shortening dialysis time) were used less often. The serum chemistry values are also influenced by variation in dialysis treatment regimens and by the contribution of residual renal function. The relevance of these indicators for individual patients is uncertain.

Subjective estimations of patient compliance by staff or by patient self-assessment are also subject to bias. For staff evaluation of compliance, ratings may be influenced by perceptions of other patient characteristics that are assumed to be related to compliance. Patient self-reports may overestimate compliance due to the effect of the social desirability bias.[6]

In their detailed review of the hemodialysis compliance literature, Lamping and Campbell[75,76] identified six studies of interventions to improve compliance. Three used token economy programs, two used behavioral contracting, and one used a combination of methods. All interventions produced an increase in compliance, but the effects were temporary. A randomized clinical trial in the United Kingdom in 2003 demonstrated the effectiveness of an educational intervention and one-on-one teaching with a renal dietitian on serum phosphorus levels.[78]

In a review article in 2003, Loghman-Adham noted that factors associated with poor medication compliance included frequent dosing, patient's perception of treatment benefits, poor physician-patient communication, lack of motivation, low socioeconomic background, lack of family support, and younger age.[79] Strategies to improve patient compliance include simplifying the treatment regimen, establishing a partnership with the patient, and increasing awareness through education and feedback.

REFERENCES

1. Alexander JL, Willems EP. Quality of life: some measurement requirements. *Arch Phys Med Rehab* 1981;62:261–265.
2. Guyatt GH, Feeny D, Patrick DL. Measuring health related quality of life. *Ann Intern Med* 1993;118:622–629.
3. Kirschner B, Guyatt GH. A methodologic framework for the evaluation of health indices. *J Chronic Dis* 1985;38:27–36.
4. Carmines EG, Zeller RA. *Reliability and Validity Assessment.* Beverly Hills, CA: Sage Publications, 1979.
5. Guyatt G, Walter S, Norman G. Measuring change over time: assessing the usefulness of evaluative instruments. *J Chronic Dis* 1987;40:171–178.
6. Yanagida EH, Streltzer J. Limitations of psychological tests in a dialysis population. *Psychosom Med* 1979;41:557–567.
7. Hornberger JC, Redelmeier DA, Petersen J. Variability among methods to assess patients' well-being and consequent effect on a cost-effectiveness analysis. *J Clin Epidemiol* 1992;45:505–512.
8. Bergner M, Bobbitt RA, Carter WB, Gilson BS. The sickness impact profile: development and final revision of a health status measure. *Med Care* 1981;19:787–805.
9. Campbell A, Converse PE. *The Quality of American Life: Perceptions, Evaluations and Satisfactions.* New York: Russel Sage Foundation, 1976.
10. Kaplan RM, Bush JW, Berry CC. Health status: types of validity and the index of well-being. *Health Serv Res* 1976; 11:478–507.
11. Froberg DG, Kane RL. Methodology for measuring health state preferences: IV. Progress and a research agenda. *J Clin Epidemiol* 1989;42:675–685.
12. von Neumann J, Morgenstern O. *Theory of Games and Economic Behavior.* Princeton, NJ: Princeton University Press, 1976.
13. Torrance GW, Thomas WH, Sackett DL. A utility maximization model for the evaluation of health care programs. *Health Serv Res* 1972;7:118–133.
14. Churchill DN, Torrance GW, Taylor DW, et al. Measurement of quality of life in end-stage renal disease: the time trade-off approach. *Clin Invest Med* 1987;10:14–20.
15. Hart LG, Evans RW. The functional status of ESRD patients as measured by the sickness impact profile. *J Chronic Dis* 1987;40(suppl 1):S117–S130.
16. Russell JD, Beecroft ML, Ludwin D, Churchill DN. The quality of life in renal transplantation—a prospective study. *Transplantation* 1992;54:656–660.
17. Canadian Erythropoietin Study Group. Association between recombinant human erythropoietin and quality of life and exercise capacity of patients receiving hemodialysis. *Br Med J* 1990;300:573–578.
18. Laupacis A, Wong C, Churchill DN, Canadian Erythropoietin Study Group. The use of generic and specific quality-of-life measures in hemodialysis patients treated with erythropoietin. *Contr Clin Trials* 1991;12:S168–S179.
19. McLeod RS, Churchill DN, Lock AM, et al. Quality of life with ulcerative colitis preoperatively and postoperatively. *Gastroenterology* 1991;101:1307–1313.
20. Morris PLP, Jones B. Life satisfaction across treatment methods for patients with end-stage renal failure. *Med J Aust* 1989;150:428–432.
21. Cantril H. *The Pattern of Human Concerns.* New Brunswick, NJ: Rutgers University Press, 1965.
22. Essink-Bot ML, Stouthard ME, Bonsel GL. Generalizability of valuations on health states collected with the EuroQOL questionnaire. *Health Econ* 1993;2:237–246.
23. Ware JE, Snow KK, Kosinski M, Gandek B. *MOS SF-36 Heath Survey Manual and Interpretation Guide.* Boston: Health Institute, 1993.

24. McHorney CA, Ware JE, Lue JF, Sherbourne CD. The MOS-36 item Short-Form Health Survey (SF-36): III. Tests of data quality, scaling assumptions, and reliability testing across diverse patient groups. *Med Care* 1994;32:40–66.

25. Maor Y, King M, Olmer L, Mozes B. A comparison of three measures: the time trade-off technique, global health related quality of life and the SF-36 in dialysis patients. *J Clin Epidemiol* 2001;54:565–570.

26. Khan IH, Garratt AM, Kumar A, et al. Patients perception of health on renal replacement therapy: evaluation using a new instrument. *Nephrol Dial Transplant* 1995;10:684–689.

27. Diaz-Buxo JA, Lowrie EG, Lew NL, et al. Quality-of-life evaluation using short form 36: comparison in hemodialysis and peritoneal dialysis patients. *Am J Kidney Dis* 2000;35:293–300.

28. Lowrie EG, Curtin RB, LePain N, Schatell D. Medical outcomes study short study form-36: a consistent and powerful predictor of morbidity and mortality in dialysis patients. *Am J Kidney Dis* 2003; 41:1286–1292.

29. Mapes DL, Lopes AA, Satayathum S, et al. Health-related quality of life as a predictor of mortality and hospitalization; the Dialysis Outcomes and Practice Patterns Study (DOPPS). *Kidney Int* 2003;64:339–349.

30. Beusterien KM, Nissenson AR, Port FK, et al. The effects of recombinant human erythropoietin on the functional health and well-being in chronic dialysis patients. *J Am Soc Nephrol* 1996;7:763–773.

31. Guyatt GH, Bombardier C, Tugwell PX. Developing disease specific measures of quality of life. *Can Med Assoc J* 1986;134:889–895.

32. Laupacis A, Muirhead N. Keown P, Wong C. A disease specific questionnaire for assessing the quality of life in patients on hemodialysis. *Nephron* 1992;60:302–306.

33. Hays RD, Kallich JD, Mapes DL, et al. Development of the kidney disease quality of life (KDQOL) instrument. *Qual Life Res* 1994;3:329–338.

34. Hays RD, Kallach JD, Mapes DL. *Kidney Disease Quality of life Short Form (KDQOL-SF); version 1.2.* Santa Monica, CA: Rand Corporation, 1995.

35. Korevaar JC, Merkus MP, Jansen, et al. Validation of the KDQOL-SF: a dialysis-targeted health measure. *Qual Life Res* 2002;11:437–447.

36. Carmichael P, Popoola J, John I, et al. Assessment of quality of life in a single center dialysis population using the KDQOL-SF questionnaire. *Qual Life Res* 2000;9:195–205.

37. Spreen O, Strauss E. *Compendium of Neuropsychological Tests: Administration, Norms and Commentary.* New York: Oxford University Press, 1993.

38. Kenny FT, Oreopoulos DG. Neuropsychological studies of CAPD. Preliminary findings. *Perit Dial Bull* 1981;1:129–133.

39. Hageberg B. A prospective study of patients in chronic hemodialysis, predictive value of intelligence, cognitive deficit and ego defence structures in rehabilitation. *J Psychosom Res* 1974;18:151–160.

40. Teshan PE, Ginn HE, Bourne JR, et al. A prospective study of reduced dialysis. *ASAIO J* 1983;6:108–122.

41. Churchill DN, Bird DR, Taylor DW, et al. Effect of high-flux hemodialysis on quality of life and neuropsychological function in chronic hemodialysis patients. *Am J Nephrol* 1992;12:412–418.

42. Murray AM, Li S, Gibertson S, et al. Prevalence of cognitive dysfunction in hemodialysis patients. *J Am Soc Nephrol* 2003;14:3A.

43. Schreiner GE, Tartaglia C. Uremia: soma or psyche. *Kidney Int* 1978;13(suppl 8):S2–S4.

44. Beck AT, Steer RA, Garbin MG. Psychometric properties of the Beck Depression Inventory: twenty-five years of evaluation. *Clin Psychol Rev* 1988;8:77–100.

45. Craven JL, Rodin GM, Littlefield C. The Beck Depression Inventory as a screening device for major depression in renal dialysis patients. *Int J Psych Med* 1988;18:365–374.

46. Smith MD, Hong BA, Robson AM. Diagnosis of depression in patients with end-stage renal disease. *Am J Med* 1985;79:160–166.

47. Sacks CR, Peterson RA, Kimmel PL. Perception of illness and depression in chronic renal disease. *Am J Kidney Dis* 1990;15:31–39.

48. Jurgensen PH, Wuerth DB, Juergensen DM, et al. Psychological factors and the incidence of peritonitis. *Adv Perit Dial* 1966;13:125–127.

49. Shidler NR, Peterson RA, Kimmel PL. Quality of life and psychosocial relationships in patients with chronic renal insufficiency. *Am J Kidney Dis* 1998;32:557–566.

50. Kimmel PL: Psychosocial factors in dialysis patients. *Kidney Int* 2001;59:1599–1613.

51. Koo J-R, Yoon J-W, Kim G-G, et al. Association of depression with malnutrition in chronic hemodialysis patients. *Am J Kidney Dis* 2003;41:1037–1042.

52. Maes M. Major depression and activation of the inflammatory response system. *Adv Exp Med Biol* 1999;461:25–46.

53. Seidel A, Arolt V, Hunstiger M, et al. Cytokine production and serum proteins in depression. *Scand J Immunol* 1995;41:534–538.

54. Kimmel P. Depression in patients with chronic renal disease. What we know and what we need to know. *J Psychosomatic Res* 2002;53:951–956.

55. Ziarnik JP, Freeman CW, Sherrard DJ, et al. Psychological correlates of survival on renal dialysis. *J Nerv Ment Dis* 1977;164:210–213.

56. Wai L, Richmond J, Burton H, Lindsay RM. Influence of psychosocial factors on survival of home-dialysis patients. *Lancet* 1981;2:1155–1156.

57. Burton HJ, Kline SA, Lindsay RM, Heidenheim AP. The relationship of depression to survival in chronic renal failure. *Psychosom Med* 1986;48:261–269.

58. Schulman R, Price JDE, Spinelli J. Biopsychosocial aspects of long-term survival on end-stage renal disease. *Psychol Med* 1989;19:945–954.

59. Devins GM, Mann J, Mandin H, et al. Psychosocial predictors of survival in end-stage renal disease. *J Nerv Ment Dis* 1990;178:127–133.

60. Husbye DG, Westlie L, Styrovoky TJ, et al. Psychological, social and somatic prognostic indicators in old patients undergoing long term dialysis. *Arch Intern Med* 1987;147: 1921–1924.

61. Christensen AJ, Wiebe JS, Smith TW, Turner CW. Predictors of survival among hemodialysis patients: effect of perceived family support. *Health Psychol* 1994;13:515–521.

62. Kimmel PL, Peterson, Weihs KL, et al. Multiple measures of depression predict mortality in a longitudinal study of chronic hemodialysis patients. *Kidney Int* 2000;57: 2093–2098.

63. Oldenburg B, Macdonald GL, Perkins GJ. Prediction of quality of life in a cohort of end-stage renal disease patients. *J Clin Epidemiol* 1988;41:555–564.

64. Soskolne V, Kaplan De-Nour A. Psychosocial adjustment of home hemodialysis, continuous ambulatory peritoneal dialysis and hospital dialysis patients and their spouses. *Nephron* 1987;47:266–273.

65. Derogatis LR. The psychosocial adjustment to illness scale (PAIS). *J Psychosom Res* 1986;30:77–91.

66. Karnofsky DA, Burchenal JH. The clinical evaluation of chemotherapeutic agents in cancer. In: Macleod CM, ed. *Evaluation of Chemotherapeutic Agents*. New York: Columbia University Press, 1949:191–205.

67. Hutchinson TA, Boyd NF, Feinstein AR, et al. Scientific problems in clinical scales, as demonstrated in the Karnofsky index of performance status. *J Chronic Dis* 1979;32:661–666.

68. Gutman RA, Stead WW, Robinson RR. Physical activity and employment status of patients on maintenance dialysis. *N Engl J Med* 1981;304:309–313.

69. Johansen KL, Painter P, Kent-Braun JA, et al. Validation of questionnaires to estimate physical activity and functioning in end-stage renal disease. *Kidney Int* 2001;59:1121–1127.

70. Meuer G, Westerterp K, Verhoeven P, et al. Methods to assess physical activity with special reference to motion sensors and accelerometers. *IEEE Trans Biomed Eng* 1991;38:221–229.

71. Fix A, Daughton D. *Human Activity Profile (HAP) Manual*. Odessa, FL: Psychological Assessment Resources, 1986.

72. Kutner NG, Brogan D, Fielding B. Employment status and ability to work among working-age chronic dialysis patients. *Am J Nephrol* 1991;11:334–340.

73. Holley JL, Nespor S: An analysis of factors affecting employment of chronic dialysis patients. *Am J Kidney Dis* 1994;23: 681–685.

74. Blake C, Codd MB, Cassidy A, O'Meara YM. Physical function, employment and quality of life in end-stage renal disease. *J Nephrol* 2000;13:142–149.

75. Lamping DL, Campbell KA. Hemodialysis compliance: assessment, prediction and intervention; Part I. *Semin Dial* 1990;3:52–56.

76. Lamping DL, Campbell KA. Hemodialysis compliance: assessment, prediction and intervention: Part II. *Semin Dial* 1990;3:105–111.

77. Wolcott DL, Maida CA, Diamond R, Nissenson AR. Treatment compliance in end-stage renal disease patients on dialysis. *Am J Nephrol* 1986;6:329–338.

78. De Brito Ashurst I, Dobbie H. A randomized controlled trial of an educational intervention to improve phosphate levels in hemodialysis patients. *J Renal Nutr* 2003;13:267–274.

79. Loghman-Adham M. Medication non-compliance in patients with chronic disease: issues in dialysis and renal transplantation. *Am J Managed Care* 2003;9:155–171.

Psychosocial Care of Children on Dialysis

Hilary Lloyd
Robert J. Postlethwaite

Clinical practice in pediatric nephrology bears out the recurrent findings of methodologically robust epidemiologic studies: psychiatric disorders and psychosocial difficulties are frequent in children and adolescents with renal failure.[1]

This makes it particularly important that pediatric nephrology teams have good awareness of the issues and problems and that they can offer or find appropriate assistance for their patients so affected.

It is far more than an issue of quality of life, although this is, of course, important in the most basic of humanitarian sense. Preventative strategies and early intervention should not be neglected in children's mental health.

Priorities for psychosocial care are as follows:

1. Enhancing the general quality of care by paying attention to psychosocial issues and mental health needs
2. Developing a ward/team ethos where the mental health issues facing sick children and their families are understood
3. Identifying patients and families at especially high risk of psychological difficulties that may complicate and compromise their medical treatment
4. Identifying mental health problems at an early stage, where possible, so that intervention can be delivered
5. Recognizing patients with more severe mental health problems that may need involvement of a specialist child mental health clinical team

The evidence base for treatment of mental health problems in children and adolescents is growing. Effective evidence-based treatments for both common and less common mental health problems have been developed (e.g., for oppositional defiant disorder, attention deficit hyperactivity disorder, obsessive compulsive disorder, depression, psychosis, anorexia nervosa).

All members of the nephrology clinical team have a role in psychosocial care. Dietitians, play workers, physiotherapists, and hospital teachers as well as social workers, nurses, and doctors may be the first (and sometimes only) recipients of highly important information about the psychological well-being of children and their families and may be especially well placed to play a part in the management of psychological difficulties.

Psychological problems can cause physical symptoms that may obfuscate evidence of the progress of renal disease (e.g., anorexia nervosa, depression, somatoform disorders). These conditions may have a serious impact on compliance with treatment and adherence to prescribed regimens and thereby on morbidity and mortality. Physical debility, metabolic disturbances, and some prescribed medicines (e.g., steroids) can all affect mental states and directly cause frank psychiatric disorders (e.g., acute and subacute confusional states, mood disorders).

After reviewing what is known about the epidemiology of psychosocial problems in children and adolescents with renal disease and on dialysis in particular, this chapter discusses general issues of concern in the psychosocial domain with respect to child nephrology and dialysis patients. Some specific issues and problems that have particular relevance are discussed. A proposed model of psychosocial care is described, and key points highlighted.

The arguments for a holistic approach in all areas of pediatric medicine are well rehearsed and acknowledged and are not reiterated here. The increasingly sophisticated specialization within medicine can pull against a holistic approach. None of us can know it all. This chapter argues for a team approach, not just to the medical and surgical aspects of pediatric nephrology but to the psychosocial aspects as well.

Nowadays, the best way of ensuring good psychosocial care is by having a team that includes nephrologists, nurses, a dietitian, hospital teacher, social worker, and mental health professionals.

Like pediatrics and nephrology, child mental health is becoming an increasingly specialized area with effective treatments and an increasingly robust evidence base. Nephrologists cannot be expected to correctly diagnose all mental health problems in their patients, let alone treat them. However, a functional psychosocial team should be able to recognize when children have significant mental health problems, seek appropriate advice, and make appropriate referrals for specialist mental health assessment and intervention. Good team communication is the key.

PSYCHOSOMATIC RELATIONSHIPS

Experienced clinicians will be well aware that there are high rates of psychological problems in children and adolescents with chronic disease. High-quality epidemiologic research has repeatedly found that children with chronic physical illness are at increased risk of psychological prob-

lems.[2,3] The multifactorial nature of causation of psychological problems will also be evident to experienced clinicians.

Despite the complex interactive nature of risk factors in child mental health problems, and the multi-factorial nature of causation in many, it is worth considering certain key relationships between psyche and soma in attempting to formulate the difficulties that present in a particular case.

1. Even minor illnesses can have an effect on mental state. Lethargy, avolition, frustration, and fear are all common reactions to acute illnesses. Lethargy and avolition may be systemic somatic effects. Minor degrees of lowering of mood (dysphoria) may be understandable psychological reactions to physical illness, disability, and hospitalization. Low mood can also be the result of a biological mechanism in a systemic illness. Psychotic illnesses (schizophreniform or affective) can be symptomatic of brain pathology. Confusional states may have infective, metabolic, anoxic, or traumatic etiology, or may be caused by drugs. Steroids regularly produce mild to moderate psychological effects and may cause frank mood disorders and/or disinhibited behavior.

2. The acute or repeated experience of pain, unpleasant treatments, limitations, disability, disruption to school life, and/or lifestyle constraints may precipitate psychological reactions including low mood, adjustment reactions (including disturbed conduct), and anxiety disorders. Adolescents may be particularly concerned about future prospects, including medical prognosis, career, marriageability, and fertility.

3. Psychiatric conditions may have significant somatic effects. For example, although they are seen less often in children and adolescents than in adults, the biological symptoms of depression include changes in sleep, appetite, bowel function, and energy. Anorexia nervosa, in addition to weight loss, may lead to cold extremities, bradycardia, peripheral cyanosis, lanugo hair, and, as a late effect, osteoporosis. Anxiety disorders may present with urinary frequency, gastrointestinal disturbances, palpitations, and tremor. Secondary nocturnal enuresis may be symptomatic of an adjustment reaction.

4. Somatoform disorders present with symptoms initially suggestive of physical disease, but in fact the primary cause is psychological. Symptoms may be loss of function, such as incontinence, or positive symptoms such as pain. Somatic complaints other than those mentioned above may also be the marker for other common psychiatric disorders, such as anxiety or depression. Psychopathology in

the patient may be strikingly inapparent. Family dysfunction is variable, but secondary gains of the illness role are common though not necessarily obvious.

5. Occasionally, physical symptoms in children may be induced by the malevolent act of another (abuse due to Munchausen syndrome by proxy).

RENAL FAILURE AS A RISK FACTOR FOR PSYCHIATRIC DISORDER IN CHILDREN

The epidemiology literature contains a wealth of evidence that chronic physical illness and disability are risk factors for mental health problems in children and adolescents.

In the Isle of Wight study,[2] psychiatric disorders were found in 17 percent of chronically ill children, compared with 7 percent of health children. Comparable rates were found in the Ontario Child Health Study[3] and by Pless.[4] Cadman et al.[3] found greater degrees of social isolation in children with physical illness and disability, thus raising the possibility that this may be a contributory mechanism for mental health problems.

Renal failure is like all other chronic illnesses—it is linked to a two- to threefold increase in the rate of psychiatric disorder.

Garralda et al.[1] found that 32 percent of children on hemodialysis showed a definite mental health problem and a further 41 percent a mild problem.

Markers of social disadvantage are also risk factors for child psychiatric disorder (e.g., poverty, poor housing, educational failure, family instability, being looked after by the social services). On the whole, boys are at greater risk of disruptive behavioral disorders (e.g., attention-deficit hyperactivity disorder, conduct disorder, oppositional defiant disorder), while older girls experience an excess of emotional disorders (e.g., depression) and eating disorders.

Where physical illness befalls a child with preexisting mental health problems, these are likely to be exacerbated and treatment of the physical illness to be compromised by them.

Some psychiatric conditions, have high population base rates. In attention deficit hyperactivity disorder, the population base rate is of the order of 2 to 5 percent. Children with renal disease may therefore present with ADHD without any suggested causal link. Untreated ADHD could be a major problem in a child hospitalized on a pediatric ward, and, of course, especially when treatment such as dialysis demands that he or she move relatively little while treatment is patiently and passively received. Preexisting oppositionality and defiance or conduct disorder are also likely to be relatively common. Children with oppositional defiant disorder and conduct disorder are likely to play out conflicts and issues via problems with treatment adherence.

Family history of depression and major mental illness may be relevant risk factors in adolescents, and there may be some heritable disposition toward anxiety disorders.

Awareness of these issues may help pediatric nephrology teams to identify those children at particularly high risk of developing mental health problems in the wake of chronic illness and disability.

Examples of possible mechanisms of the risk of mental health problems in children with renal failure are adjustment to debility or disability, anxiety about prognosis, anxiety about treatment and procedures, effects on family or carers, mood effects of physical debility, disruption to schooling (and thereby peer relationships), repeated hospitalizations, growth impairment (and its effect on self-image), and occasionally iatrogenic effects of medications.

GENERAL ISSUES IN THE PSYCHOSOCIAL CARE OF CHILDREN

Breaking Bad News

All doctors sometimes have to give bad news. It must be understood that breaking bad news should be a process and not an event that is over after the first conversation. News that a child who has chronic renal failure has reached the stage for dialysis can be difficult for parents to grasp because it marks advancement of the disease and underscores the severity of the condition, and bringing all the demands and disruptions the treatment entails.

Breaking bad news can tax the communication skills of even the most experienced and sensitive of clinicians. Books and courses are available that are aimed at teaching those aspects of communication skills that can be taught, and the interested or inexperienced may find these of great assistance.[5,6] Arguably, time, respect, and listening are the most vital aspects of successful communication with parents and children. The clinician must also ensure that there is a shared, mutual understanding of the language used by all parties.

Those who are breaking the news must be able to deal sensitively with the emotional reactions that may sometimes be provoked. It is helpful to clarify for parents and children whom they may approach for clarification and when; reiteration or questioning may be needed later.

What, how, and when to tell the child may be a source of considerable anxiety to parents, and they may welcome discussion about this with a clinician. A flexible approach that takes account of the child's developmental stage and previous experiences is called for.

Coping Behaviors and Psychological Defenses

Despite the fact that chronic illness and disability significantly increase the risk of mental health problems, the majority of children with physical illness and disability do not have substantial mental health problems. Consideration of how such children and parents cope with their predicaments may assist in both recognizing when others are not coping and in planning interventions to assist them in developing coping strategies.

Coping is the means of adaptive psychological management of an adverse, stressful situation or predicament such as chronic illness or disability. Models of conscious cognitive and behavioral strategies or "coping behaviors" have been described by Hamburg and Hamburg,[7] as succinctly outlined by Graham.[8]

Hamburg and Hamburg have a usefully identified some of the characteristics of children and parents who deal successfully with stress. They tend to

1. Have a "day-to-day outlook"; they ration the amount of stress to be coped with at any one time (e.g., think only about the next stage of treatment, such as an operation or starting dialysis, and not further ahead)
2. Seek information about their condition and treatment
3. Rehearse what is going to be difficult (e.g., prepare responses to expected teasing)
4. Try a variety of ways of dealing with a problem rather than persisting with one unsatisfactory, unsuccessful approach
5. Construct buffers against disappointment—e.g., prepare for failure of an operation and not just for its success

Coping depends on physical resources (money and employment), social resources (support from friends, family, social services), and psychological resources such as beliefs, problem-solving skills, and personality. Eiser[9] gives a detailed and comprehensive review of other models of coping.

The other psychological ingredient of adaptation to stress is generally considered to be defense mechanisms. This acknowledges a model of unconscious psychological process. Defense mechanisms relevant to adaptation to physical illness and disability are also described by Graham[8]; the reader who wishes to know more is referred to this resource. Defense mechanisms are an important and essential aspect of adaptation but can become maladaptive. In addition, it is not uncommon, in clinical experience, to find that coping children "compartmentalize" areas of their lives. That is to say, they do not allow the illness to intrude into some arenas in which they operate and in which they are, to all intents and purposes, healthy and normal. For example, a young person may attend a regular social activity without allowing other participants to know of his or her medical condition. Such compartmentalization was apparent in the Manchester pediatric hemodialysis study, although not described in the publications.

Defense mechanisms are also used by professionals in helping them to cope with the emotional stress of dealing with sick, disabled, and dying children. That is, the defense mechanisms of professionals, too—not only those of parents and children—can become maladaptive.

Care of the Dying Child

The principles of breaking bad news are outlined above. The various identifiable phases of grief are available elsewhere.[10,11] Such general patterns lend an understanding to the overall process of grief but do not form a rigid model, and, of course, individual families respond in different ways to the anticipated and actual death of a child.[12,13] Each parent does not necessarily progress in their grief at the same rate, and the grief of individual family members may make them less able to support each other. Staff may become the target of a parent's anger, which is a manifestation of grief. Siblings may also need support.

Parents' views on what to tell the child patient are important. Although it is usually agreed that openness about outcome with reassurance about palliative care are important principles, some children make it clear that they are not ready to confront the realities of their illness; therefore a flexible approach is needed. Children come to understand the finality of death between the ages of 5 and 8 years. Older dying children may try to avoid distressing their already upset parents further, thus failing to express their own fears and anxieties. Children may be highly sensitive to their parents' anxieties and anger; they may be angry themselves and may direct this anger toward parents or staff. In such situations, parents and staff may be helped by recognizing and understanding this displacement.

The support of a key worker from among the hospital staff may be valuable to families. Teams must consider how and when requests for autopsies or donation of organs should be made. Postbereavement appointments with the consultant and sometimes other staff are now routine in many hospital units. Some hospitals offer postbereavement counseling or bereavement groups as an option for families.

While grief is an essentially normal process, atypical and complicated grief reactions occur in both adults and children and may warrant specialist mental health consultation or intervention.

Hospital staff may also be emotionally affected by the anticipated or actual death of a patient, and thought should be given to how staff can be supported. Clinical supervision provides some opportunities for nursing staff. Psychosocial meetings of the team, described in greater detail below, may provide useful opportunities for such support.

Awareness of the likely and actual effects on other patients of the death of a patient—one with whom they may may have developed a relationship over weeks, months, or even years of meeting in clinic, ward, or dialysis unit—is also needed. Again, psychosocial team meetings provide a useful forum in which to discuss such issues and formulate a considered approach.

LESSONS FROM THE MANCHESTER PSYCHOSOCIAL STUDIES OF PEDIATRIC NEPHROLOGY PATIENTS

Pediatric nephrology has not been neglected in psychosocial research. Beginning in the mid 1980s, the psychiatric nephrology liaison teams in Manchester have produced perhaps the most substantial series of publications examining psychological effects and adjustment at the various stages of renal disease and treatment from infancy through adulthood. Their work includes a set of studies of the impact of growth hormone in the chronic renal failure (CRF) arena, an audit of psychological risk factors, and a paper examining appropriate psychological research methodologies.[14] The early papers reflect the management of renal disease, which has since undergone radical changes.

Renal teams now work with a group of children facing more severe illness and carrying greater physical and cognitive handicaps, thus limiting the extent to which conclusions from the earlier work can be extrapolated to the present day. Nevertheless, these studies still provide substantial information, and some of which merits repeating.

Among these findings are the following. Psychiatric morbidity is increased in children with end-stage renal failure (ESRF), when compared with controls, whatever the stage of illness. Most of these problems are short-lived adjustment disorders or minor symptoms that are not seriously deleterious to the child's emotional state or quality of life. For children in the predialysis stage, these minor psychiatric problems are manifested primarily in the school setting and through mood changes, but no deleterious effects on the child's self-concept were found. Children on hemodialysis (no children were on peritoneal dialysis when these studies were carried out) manifested prominent mood changes, lowered self-esteem, and problems seen primarily at home rather than at school. After transplantation, mood and self-concept improved, paralleled by parental perceptions of improvements in their child's physical and psychological health. However, psychiatric morbidity was still greater than in healthy controls—a finding likely to be marked currently because of the inclusion of more children diagnosed in utero and with many very severe physical and other problems. Social development—measured by having a special friend—showed a clear gradient according to severity of illness.

The young adult survivors of ESRF in the late 1980s did not have increased psychiatric morbidity compared with healthy controls: if there was continuity of findings between child and young adult, it was for those with mood disorders. However lower self-esteem was found in adults with earlier onset of illness and lower educational attainments: both are commoner today. In the young adults there was evidence of more limited and later independence from families, but generally these young people had adjusted their expectations as well as their lifestyles. Parental mental health problems and family stress were closely related to stage of illness, with more problems in the families of severely affected children: this risk factor too is likely to have increased proportionally. Parental mental health improved after transplantation but increased behavior problems were still reported.

SPECIFIC ISSUES FOR THE PSYCHOSOCIAL CARE OF CHILDREN WITH END-STAGE RENAL DISEASE

In renal disease and in dialysis itself there are some specific characteristics that may, in individual patients, be potent contributors to psychological problems:

1. The emphasis on diet and weight. This may be sensitizing for young people at risk for eating disorders, such an anorexia and bulimia nervosa.
2. Shunts, catheters, fistulas, which may have an impact on body image.
3. Dialysis regimens. Hemodialysis, by disrupting normal life and especially life at school, with the restriction of activities even for a short time three times a week week in and week out, may be more difficult for some children to tolerate. The same issues may be problematic for children on peritoneal dialysis, although to a lesser degree for most.
4. Nonadherence. The demands of adherence to diet, fluid intake, dialysis regimen, and medication offers a whole matrix of possible contention to children and families, where compliance/oppositionality are already or are becoming issues.
5. Medication. Steroids by their effects on mood or body, and cyclosporine, by causing hirsutism.
6. Growth impairment.
7. Traumatic procedures.
8. Complexity of syndromes. Syndromes that, in addition to causing renal failure, cause deformity, affect intellectual functioning, and cause other disabilities.
9. Stages of illness. Parental morbidity and family stress are related to stage of illness. There are increased problems in the families of more severely affected children. Successful transplants tend to be associated with improved parental mental health and better psychosocial adjustment in the children.

Burden of Dialysis Treatment and Care

Generally, the burden of care in dialysis is added to the general psychological and practical burden of caring for a child with a chronic, life-threatening disease (see above); this context needs to be understood.

While dialysis treatments and regimens have become more effective and less incapacitating over the course of the last decade, they remain very tiring for both patient and family and disruptive to the lives of all concerned.

While peritoneal dialysis is generally not as disruptive to normal life as hemodialysis,[15] not least because it takes less time and is generally done at home, it is a major intrusion in a child's life.

Of course, children on dialysis are also taking medication and are fluid- and diet-restricted. Medication frequently involves regular injections, and feeding may be by nasogastric tube or gastrostomy. As noted above, shunts, fistulas, catheters, and changing girth may bring body image issues to the fore for some children and adolescents.

Individual children and families are likely to vary in their perception and experience of the burden of illness and treatment; debility is not the only dimension.

Disrupted school attendance is a major issue for children. The disruption of peer activities and relationships is also important.

While the issues posed by illness in examination years are readily understood, sometimes those caused by missing the rites of passage, such as leaving primary school, starting high school, or finishing high school are overlooked.

Practical consequences of the care and treatment of children with renal disease may be a major source of strain in families—e.g., dietary restrictions; the child's subjection to unpleasant, distressing procedures "for his or her own good"; limitations on holidays; time off work for appointments; and restrictions on social life and career development. Parents whose young child is on continuous ambulatory peritoneal dialysis (CAPD) must be sufficiently organized and able to find the time for weighing, taking blood pressure, caring for the catheter, and sometimes giving nasogastric or gastrostomy feedings by day and by night. Younger couples tend to have greater difficulties in mobilizing the support of friends and relatives.

Complexity of Syndromes

To the practitioner new to pediatric nephrology, whether pediatrician or psychiatrist, the complexity of the syndromes and conditions of children with CRF may be striking. For those who have been immersed in the field for some time, there may be an understandable tendency for the focus to become very fixed on the specialty system. But these are not simply children with renal disease nor children with simple renal disease. Within a CRF population, there is a high proportion of children with multisystem disease or complex syndromes affecting other organs, often including the brain. These complexities may interact as risk factors for emotional and behavioral problems as well as increasing the burden of care on families and staff. In a review of a case series by North and Eminson,[16] 50 percent had specific or global learning disability and 25 percent had a dysmorphic syndrome or neurologic condition.

Early Adjustment of the Child Patient

According to individual circumstances, the child dialysis patient may be adjusting to any or all of the following: illness and debility, diagnosis, prognosis, the stress of uncertainty, disruption to school and social life, and dialysis itself.

There is a wide spectrum of normal responses and adjustment. Severe responses, known as "adjustment disorders," include elements of maladjustment and give rise to increased impairments, which may be emotional, behavioral, or social. Such adjustment disorders are described in greater detail below.

Stages of Illness

Parental morbidity and family stress are related to stage of illness. There are increased problems with more severely affected children. Successful transplants tend to be associated with improved parental mental health and better psychosocial adjustment in children.

Nonadherence

Nonadherence to treatment is a major cause of morbidity in CRF. It is a significant cause of loss of transplanted organs.

In the dialysis patient, nonadherence may be focused on all or any aspect of treatment. Nonadherence to diet and fluid restriction seriously compromise dialysis by making it difficult to define exchanges.

Some child patients become nonadherent after a period of adherence. In clinical practice, this usually occurs after a change of treatment, or a like/family event. Such sudden nonadherence is not difficult to pick up and usually resolves rapidly with a transparent, understanding, firm educational approach.

Where the nonadherence is a reaction to a sense of lack of control, many children and adolescents will respond positively to being given some appropriate, limited control over treatment.

In other children and adolescents, nonadherence is chronic and habitual. Such children and adolescents often have preexisting psychological problems, especially conduct and/or relationship problems or high levels of risk factors.

Nonadherence may become a tool used by adolescents to demonstrate their defiance, rebellion, and despair. In some it becomes a metaphor for suicide.

In managing nonadherence, it has been shown in children with renal transplants that the most important issue is to recognize and understand the underlying causes, issues, and precipitants so that a useful ameliorative approach can be devised.[17] There is little doubt that this holds true for children on dialysis, as illustrated by the following vignette.

Vignette: Nonadherence

Patient X was 6 years of age when he presented with renal failure after a sudden illness. He was an only child of a single mother and had a sensitive, strong-willed temperament. X refused medication, protested against his CAPD, refused to attend school without great protest, and became noncompliant with his mother's attempts to bathe him, wash his hair, and brush his teeth. Once at school, after the severe protest that left his mother fatigued and demoralized, X settled in and was his usual self with his peers and teachers. X refused to talk to the therapist from the mental health team.

The situation was unlocked by a meeting between dialysis nursing staff, play specialist, mother, and psychiatrist, in which the psychiatrist offered an understanding of the child's behavior as being a manifestation of anger, fear, and maladaptive attempts to exert control over a situation where he felt he had none.

A plan was agreed to that rewarded compliance and appropriate behavior and that offered appropriate limited choices in treatment (e.g., involvement in a "venipuncture plan"—deciding how he would like to sit when blood was taken).

Other Complications of Treatment

A number of treatments for renal disease can have noxious effects on mental functioning, whether via a direct effect on the brain or through a psychological reaction to side effects involving appearance. Steroids can lead to behavioral problems because of irritability and mood disorders. Children and particularly adolescents may be very distressed by their cushingoid appearance. Similarly, cyclosporine can cause hypertrichosis, which can be very distressing, especially to adolescent girls. Operative procedures may cause worrying scarring and disfigurement.

EARLY DETECTION OF MENTAL HEALTH PROBLEMS

As in most of medicine, interventions for mental health problems are more likely to be successful early in the course of the disorder. Awareness of the manifestations of child mental health problems should lead to their early identification, with prompt referral or consultation. In addition, identification of high-risk cases (i.e., those with other, preexisting risk factors such as social disadvantage, impaired parental mental health, previous history of emo-

tional/behavioral difficulties, and/or learning disability) and awareness of high-risk situations (treatment failures, life-threatening complications, aversive procedures) are necessary.

SOME SPECIFIC PSYCHIATRIC DISORDERS

The whole range of child psychiatric disorders may be seen in children with renal disease, but the following deserve particular mention.

Adjustment Disorders. Adjustment disorders are a group of psychiatric disorders that are defined by virtue of their onset in the period of adaptation to a significant life change or to the consequences of a stressful life event. The life-change or consequences of the life event are regarded as the sufficient and necessary causes of the adjustment disorder, although individuals have greater or lesser degrees of predisposition and vulnerability. In renal disease, the precipitating life event may be the diagnosis, understanding (or misunderstanding) of prognosis, the illness itself, or a particular treatment, the consequences of which may be varied and in any one or several of the spheres of physical debility, lifestyle restrictions, treatment regimens, and disruption to social relationships, education, and family functioning. Adjustment disorders may be predominantly manifest in conduct problems or emotional difficulties or a mixture of the two. Younger children may regress (e.g., start to speak less maturely, return to sucking thumbs or fingers, resume bedwetting). In addition to the clear onset within a month or so of the adverse life change or event, adjustment disorders virtually all resolve within 6 months, although this will inevitably depend to some degree on what the future holds. It seems likely that adjustment disorders are more likely to occur when circumstances have prevented preparation for the precipitating event.

Depressive adjustment disorders are characterized by persistently low mood (although this may fluctuate in the course of a day), often accompanied, according to severity, by poor concentration, sleep disturbances (e.g., early morning awakening—typical in adult depressive disorders but less common in young people), irritability, reduced appetite, and weight loss. Occasionally appetite and weight may increase in depression. Depressive adjustment disorders may be severe and prolonged and should be referred to child and adolescent psychiatric teams.

Some adjustment disorders may be very acute and severe. Young children may appear regressed and withdrawn or become extremely noncompliant toward their parents over everyday matters, not just treatment.

Depression. Depression is not uncommon in adolescents but less so in younger children; bipolar (manic-depressive) illness is increasingly recognized in adolescents. Both are illnesses with a genetic component. The symptoms are, of course, those of depressive adjustment disorders (see above) but may also include intense self-criticism and guilt, with distorted perceptions about the future and the risks of renal illness or treatment. Severe biological symptoms of depression, including psychomotor retardation, are uncommon in children.

Depressive cognitions may include suicidality and hopelessness (which may not necessarily be apparent and may need to be inquired about) and may be linked to nonadherence. Depression in children and adolescents is easily missed or attributed to normal "moods" or to an understandable response to the renal disease or treatment. Depression may seem "understandable," which can tend to make clinicians ignore it, but the issue is one of severity and impairment. It is responsive to psychiatric treatment (usually cognitive therapy and in more severe cases, antidepressants) and carries an increased risk of relapse and recurrence in adulthood. A low threshold for referral to child psychiatrists should be firmly maintained.

Eating Disorders. Whether there is any overall increased risk of eating disorders with CRF is unknown. As only 1 percent of 18-year-old girls suffer from anorexia nervosa and it is still more rare in boys and in younger adolescents, a very large study would have to be done to investigate this possibility. Clinical practice, however, suggests that there may be a link. The continued focus on the female form and the media's premise that thinness is desirable are powerful societal pressures for vulnerable youngsters. Shunts, catheters, hypertrichosis from medication, fluid retention, cushingoid facies, dietary restrictions, frequent weighings of CRF patients, those dialyzed as well as those who have had transplants—may key into the sensitivities of adolescence. When a young person begins to control his or her weight because of an eating disorder (anorexia or bulimia nervosa), the treatment and control of the renal condition, most particularly when dialysis is involved, may be rapidly jeopardized. It is worth thinking about the possibility of an eating disorder in any young person, but particularly in a teenage girl whose weight is fluctuating unexpectedly and inexplicably. Again, referral to a child psychiatrist who is able to maintain a close liaison with the pediatric team will be essential, and physicians should not be deceived by bland reassurances from patients that they are not trying to lose weight.

Anorexia nervosa and bulimia nervosa can seriously compromise dialysis, particularly by the obfuscation of the cause of loss of weight, abnormal dietary restriction, and the rapid fluctuations in body weight associated with these conditions.

Posttraumatic Stress Disorder. This is a delayed and/or protracted response to an exceptionally threatening or cata-

strophic situation. Unfortunately, such situations can be medical and can happen either as a direct result of acute illness or as a consequence of treatment. Virulent, serious disease and emergency situations may severely constrain or completely preclude, the psychological preparation that would otherwise have been offered. Posttraumatic stress disorder should be suspected in children who have enduring, intense maladaptive reactions following intrusive medical procedures, catastrophes, or complications, particularly if they also manifest low mood, poor concentration, and sleep disturbance. People with posttraumatic stress disorder are often clinically depressed and have intense anxiety symptoms, nightmares, and intrusive memories of the adverse events ("flashbacks"). Posttraumatic stress disorder calls for skilled psychiatric intervention that may involve psychotherapy, cognitive behavioral therapy, and/or psychotropic medication.

Postoperative, Infective, or Metabolic Confusional States. These may be especially difficult to recognize in younger children. Signs of impaired or fluctuating consciousness may be subtle. Children so affected will not be registering new information. Visual misinterpretations and hallucinations tend to be exacerbated by poor light, and such children may have to be nursed with lights on at night.

Fear of Procedures. Most doctors learn early in their careers not to put questions to children if they are unprepared for the answer or unable to modify their behavior in response. One learns to avoid such pitfalls as asking, "May I take some blood please?" What is surprising is not why some children show extreme fear of procedures but that so few do. Children who appear to enjoy procedures or are too readily compliant are a source of concern because it is unusual to deny fear, pain, and distress so strongly; a high cost may be paid later, in psychological terms, for such repression of normal reactions. Most children manage to put up with procedures with proper preparation, attention to pain, and discomfort during the procedure and praise thereafter for bravery, but some become frankly phobic. Parents cannot always manage to be supportive of their children in respect of procedures. Finding out the parent's own attitudes, views, and fears may be useful. Children will be reassured about procedures only if they are properly educated in the first place. Developmentally appropriate explanations should be offered where possible. Lies such as "it won't hurt" are likely to damage the child's fragile trust and to make future compliance waver. An understanding, calm, patient, and firm attitude is usually the most successful. Clinical team members should let each other know when a child is intensely fearful. It is much easier to deal with a panic-stricken child when one has been forewarned. Dealing with frightened children demands judgment and a mixture of firmness and flexibility that is not contradictory. Play specialists can offer very useful distraction or guided imagery. Child mental health teams may be able to assist in situations where children have become phobic about procedures (most commonly termed "needle phobia").

OTHER COMPLICATIONS OF RENAL FAILURE WITH POTENTIAL MENTAL HEALTH CONSEQUENCES

Separations. Attachment is the infant's predisposition to seek proximity to certain people and to be more secure in their presence. It is a process fundamental to the development of secure, meaningful social relationships. Separation anxiety is the anxiety and distress shown by small children when they are separated from their primary attachment figure(s). Separation anxiety is a normal phenomenon in young children and may be intensified or prolonged in response to stress. Although increased separation anxiety is common as a response of young children to enforced separation and hospitalization, there is little to suggest that serious illness and its consequences have a significant effect on attachment, especially now that parents are encouraged to room in and admissions are generally short.

As described by Graham,[8] the short-term effects of hospitalization depend on the age of the child (above 1 year, the younger the child, the more severe the distress), the social circumstances of the family (financial and parental relationship), the adequacy of preparation for hospitalization, the child's condition (the greater the degree of discomfort and distress, the greater the degree of disturbance), the frequency of painful procedures,[18] the presence of familiar figures (rooming-in facilities), the child's previous experience of hospitalization, the parent-child relationship, the temperament or personality of the child, the coping style of the child, the provision of play and education facilities of the ward, the attitudes of hospital staff, and the degree to which the ward is child-centered.

Children who have been repeatedly admitted to hospital in early and later childhood are slightly more likely to develop behavioral and emotional disturbances in adolescence.[19] These effects are particularly likely if admissions are for long periods and if the children come from disadvantaged homes. The reasons for this are unclear and it is possible that, with improvements in hospital practice, this adverse effect may be minimized or may disappear entirely.[20]

Parents may be taken aback by the fact that their young child becomes more oppositional on discharge home, but this may be related to the separation experiences or other aspects of treatment. Preparation for these reactions should be routine (rather than an assumption that everything will be "plain sailing" once the onerous phase of hospital admission is over); if introduced carefully, such explanations will be perceived as useful.

Short Stature. Many of the chronic renal conditions or their treatment affect growth, sometimes so severely that comparison with "normal" short stature seems ridiculous for those who are six or seven standard deviations below it. Nevertheless, there is little literature relating specifically to the psychological effects of growth limitation in the context of renal disease. Even when selected because of short stature and in the context of treatment trials, short stature has a lower priority than other issues in the minds of parents and children with renal failure.[21] This probably reflects appropriate priority setting. However, this study did identify a group of children who had linked physical and psychological vulnerability. Such patients were more likely to be on dialysis. They showed a trend toward more depression, lower self-esteem, and more maternal mental distress, and their concern about growth increased when interventions failed to improve it.[21]

Because of the limited literature specifically relating to short stature in renal failure, some generalizations from other sources and from clinical studies are in order.

In early childhood, the problem of short stature demands practical adaptations at home and school and affects mainly parents and other adults in the child's orbit, who may be overprotective. This is a good time, however, to prepare parents for the difficulties ahead, with discussions about why overprotectiveness is bad for children (it has demonstrable negative effects on their self-esteem and confidence) and about ways in which parents can make sure that their children are included in a range of age- and developmentally appropriate activities, even though others may think that these children are too small to participate.

In middle childhood, as the self-concept develops, the child's own self-image becomes more relevant and peer-group issues begin to arise, although not always negatively at this stage. Being treated as a "baby" in big girls' games is not to everyone's taste, however. Smallness and quickness may be joined in children's minds, so that smaller ones are sometimes perceived as useful and "cute"; such perceptions may convey benefits. For those with learning difficulties, short stature may be protective, signaling greater youth and therefore fewer demands from the outside world. Parents can help their children to deal with practical difficulties and to become used to demonstrating their true age with a variety of identity cards and passes.

It is in adolescence that, for boys particularly, clear social and peer-group advantages are conveyed by early physical development; being the tallest increases a boy's popularity with both sexes and signals maturity. Thus short boys are disadvantaged in all these areas. For girls, it seems that being "average" in development is more important that being first; therefore short-statured adolescent girls may be less severely affected than boys their age and may indeed be advantaged by the protectiveness they attract.

Preparations for the practical difficulties and the problem-solving approach to peer-group issues can always be improved, but it is hard to prepare for the intensity of feelings of some adolescents or the reactions to an unpleasant or bullying peer group. These should obviously be tackled through the school system as well as individually. Interventions depend on the strength and nature of the young person's distress, but brief cognitive and behavioral inputs in relation to teasing, confidence, and "acting tall" have been demonstrated to be effective.[22] Frank anxiety or depression should be treated aggressively by Child and Adolescent Mental Health Services (CAMHS) professionals and not rationalized as normal reactions to an abnormal predicament. Firm parental approaches to well-meaning infantilization by other adults may be necessary. Where group sessions are held by the renal and psychosocial team with the young people themselves, peer-group talk about the problems and sharing of reactions and solutions may be very supportive.

MILIEU ISSUES

Children on dialysis are likely to spend considerable time in hospital, be it in the initial stages of their illness, when complications set in, or on the hemodialysis unit. The milieu of the ward or unit is likely to be especially important for those spending the most time there. Many wards and units have to cater to both children and adolescents, posing questions about how to best provide an environment and milieu appropriate to the needs of both age groups. Where possible, discrete areas for the two age groups will offer advantages. Not all teenagers will welcome spending time in units decorated with cartoon characters. Involving adolescents in devising "house rules" for the hemodialysis unit and in designing and decorating the unit can help to reduce alienation. Adolescents need to have a say in their management and treatment (according to competence). All these factors stem from a recognition of the importance of facilitating an empowering attitude and ethos in what is generally a disempowering predicament.

LIAISON CHILD MENTAL HEALTH

To be effective, liaison mental health services need to be responsive. Some situations require consultation (discussion with professionals, case not seen). Others require planned mental health referral and assessment. Still others need rapid assessment and advice (e.g., Is this low mood due to intracranial pathology in systemic lupus erythematosus? Could this be this anorexia nervosa?). Children treated in regional centers but living at home may ultimately be best served by their local mental health service rather than the center's liaison service (especially if intensive outpatient intervention is needed or liaison with other local agencies such as the school is required). In other cases it is the liaison advice to the nephrology team that is most important. Any part of the whole range of mental health services may be needed for individual patients. Nephrology services need access to an experienced and skilled psychiatrist or psychologist who can be the gateway to other child and adolescent mental health resources as appropriate. With good liaison psychiatry/psychology, pediatric teams will develop some expertise in recognizing mental health problems and in managing the less severe and more common of these. Teams will be able to identify those children for whom more specialist mental health input is required. The whole range of assessment and therapeutic resources of specialist mental health services may be needed by renal patients who have significant mental health problems, but in particular the following are likely to be most frequently needed: child and adolescent psychiatry, child clinical psychology, (for behavioral skills and the elucidation of complex cognitive deficits), play therapy, and social work.

We advocate a model that includes all of the following liaison activities:

1. Emergency/urgent response: confusional states, severe mood disorders, severe adjustment disorders; rapid response for serious psychiatric problems in inpatients
2. Planned nonurgent case assessment/intervention (outpatient)
3. Case-by-case liaison with care team
4. Regular psychosocial liaison meetings (some case-related functions, but also looking at general issues for team and/or ward)

Resources and professional relationships may well be limiting factors in the structure of a psychosocial team. We suggest that one identified senior mental health professional (usually a psychiatrist or psychologist) be nominated as the key liaison person who can involve other members of mental health services as appropriate.

As outlined above, psychiatric disorders and less severe psychological problems are many and varied. Effective, evidence-based treatments are increasingly available for mental health problems (e.g., cognitive behavior therapy, behavioral treatments, parent management training, psychotropic medications). There is a spectrum of treatability from cure through remitting and relapsing conditions to palliation and prevention of deterioration and secondary impairments, but this certainly does not, in our view, compare unfavorably with the medical and surgical treatment of renal failure and its causes.

The advantages of regular psychosocial liaison meetings are that the mental health specialist becomes known to—and, hopefully, trusted by—the renal or pediatric team. In this way, the culture of considering and discussing psychosocial issues as a matter of course is promoted and the appropriateness of referring cases can be clarified. A team used to recognizing, rather than denying, and reflecting on and considering sympathetically the psychosocial aspects of illness is likely to do a better job of meeting the mental health needs of all of its patients, not just those who have major difficulties. Well-functioning mental health–nephrology liaison should empower members of the nephrology team to recognize and deal with the commoner and less severe mental health problems encountered by their child patients, while referring the more complex and severe cases for specialist mental health attention.

We would suggest that psychosocial meetings offer a more efficient and effective model of liaison than joint clinics.

REFERENCES

1. Garralda ME, Jameson RA, Reynolds JM, et al. Psychiatric adjustment in children with chronic renal failure. *J Child Psychol Psychiatry* 1988;29(1):79–90.
2. Rutter M, Tizard J, Whitmore K. *Education, Health and Behaviour*. London: Longman Press, 1970.
3. Cadman D, Boyle M, Szatmari P, Offord DR. Chronic illness, disability and mental and social well-being: findings of the Ontario Child Health Study. Pediatrics 1987;795: 805–813.
4. Pless IB, Roghman KJ. Chronic illness and its consequences: observations based on three epidemiologic surveys. *J Pediatr* 1971;79:351–359.
5. Lloyd M, Bor R, eds. *Communication Skills for Medicine*. New York: Churchill Livingstone, 1996.
6. Billings A, Stoeckle JD. *The Clinical Encounter*. St. Louis: Mosby, 1998.
7. Hamburg D, Hamburg B. A life-span perspective on adaptation and health. In: Kaplan B, Ibrahim M, eds. *Family and Health: Epidemiological Approaches*. Chapel Hill, SC: University of South Carolina Press, 1980.
8. Graham P, Turk J, Verhulst F. *Child Psychiatry: A Developmental Approach*, 3d ed. Oxford, UK: Oxford University Press, 1999.
9. Eiser C. *Growing up with a Chronic Disease: The Impact on Children and Their Families*. London: Jessica Kingsley, 1993.
10. Lindeman E. The symptomatology and management of acute grief. *Am J Psychiatry* 1994;151(6 suppl):155–160.
11. Parkes CM. *Bereavement: Studies of Grief in Adult Life*. New York: Penguin Books, 1972.
12. Burton L. *Care of the Child Facing Death*. London: Routledge & Keegan Paul, 1975.
13. Gyulay JE. *The Dying Child*. New York: McGraw-Hill, 1978.
14. Postlethwaite RJ, Garralda ME, Eminson DM, Reynolds JC. Lessons from psychosocial studies of chronic renal failure. *Arch Dis Child* 1996;75:455–459.
15. Moghal NE, Wittich E, Milford DV. The impact of renal replacement therapy on toddler time. *ANNA J* 1999;26: 331–335.
16. North C, Eminson DM. A review of a psychiatry-nephrology liaison service. *Eur J Child Adolesc Psychiatry* 1998;7: 235–245.
17. Wolff G, Strecker K, Vester U, et al. Non-compliance following renal transplantation in children and adolescents. *Pediatr Nephrol* 1998;12:703–708.
18. Saylor C, Pallmeyer TP, Finch AJ, et al. Predictors of psychological distress in hospitalized pediatric patients. *J Am Acad Child Adolesc Psychiatry*, 1987;26,(2):232–236.
19. Quinton D, Rutter M. Early admissions and later disturbances of behaviour: an attempted replication of Douglas' findings. *Dev Med Child Neurol* 1976;18:447–459.
20. Shannon FT, Fergusson DM, Dimond ME. Early hospital admissions and subsequent behaviour problems in 6 year olds. *Arch Dis Child* 1984;59:815–819.
21. Postlethwaite RJ, Eminson DM, Reynolds JM, et al. Growth in renal failure: a longitudinal study of emotional and behavioural changes during trials of growth hormone treatment. *Arch Dis Child* 1998;78(3): 222–229.
22. Eminson DM, Powell RP, Hollis S. Cognitive behavioural interventions with short statured boys. In: Stabler B, Underwood L, eds. *Growth, Stature and Adaptation*. Chapel Hill, NC: University of North Carolina, 1994.

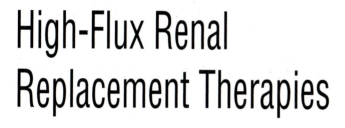

High-Flux Renal Replacement Therapies

Bernard Canaud
Detlef H. Krieter

Renal replacement therapy (RRT) by hemodialysis is a fully established and routinely performed treatment for end-stage renal disease (ESRD). Conventional hemodialysis (HD) (e.g., three sessions per week lasting 3 to 4 hours each) remains the major modality of life-supporting therapy in patients with chronic kidney disease. Long-term HD has become, over the last three decades, the basic option in the therapeutic armamentarium of the nephrologist, representing a temporary or sometimes permanent alternative to renal transplantation (the latter in those patients where transplantation is contraindicated or not available).

RRT has some intrinsic limitations due to both the conditions of use (nonselective semipermeable artificial membrane, blood-flow limits, treatment duration limits) and the intermittency (three times a week) of HD sessions. Whatever the technical options applied (highly permeable membrane, prolonged time, more frequent sessions, enhanced dialysis performance), RRT will never be able to mimic native kidney function. The homeostasis of the "internal milieu" is periodically and incompletely restored by HD sessions. Uremic toxins, which include a wide spectrum of substances of varying molecular weight (from 60 Da to more than 20 kDa), are incompletely removed during an HD session.[1,2] Moreover, middle- or higher- molecular-weight albumin-bound toxic substances are virtually unaffected by HD. The periodicity of HD sessions creates an "unphysiologic" condition wherein the patient's solute status varies alternatively between high concentrations (peak values in the predialysis period) and low concentrations (nadir values in the postdialysis period), never reaching a state of fluid and solute equilibrium. Moreover, the lack of selectivity of the dialysis membrane leads to the removal of beneficial nutrient substances. Repeated blood/HD interaction (membrane and dialysate) exposes the patient to periodic activation of circulating blood cells (i.e., leukocytes, platelets) and protein cascades (i.e., coagulation, complement), which, in turn, can trigger the release of proinflammatory and tissue-injuring mediators.

On the other hand, the success of long-term HD is clearly illustrated by two objective facts: first, the lives of a million ESRD patients worldwide are maintained by an artificial form of random response technique (RRT); second, the survival of HD patients is usually evaluated in term of decades. This very positive view of HD must be weighed against the increasingly reported incidence of dialysis-related pathology in long-term HD, including beta$_2$-microglobulin amyloidosis, accelerated atherosclerosis and ageing, left ventricular hypertrophy, vascular and valvular calcifications, and malnutrition. Dialysis-related pathology clearly marks the limits of the conventional HD approach in the long term—namely over 10 years. Inasmuch as nephrologists are concerned both with the mortality (quantity of life) and morbidity (quality of life) of ESRD patients, they must acknowledge that conventional HD is not satisfactory as a long-term form of supportive therapy. It is clear, therefore, that there is a need to improve both quantity and quality of life delivered by RRT. Several technical options and/or treatment strategies have been developed to improve overall treatment efficacy. High-flux and high-efficiency dialysis methods look appealing in this context. By enhancing the various components of solute clearance (diffusion, convection and adsorption), high-flux HD improves overall solute removal capacity and enlarges the spectrum of removable substances. In brief, diffusive clearance enhances small solute removal, convective clearance favors medium- and high-molecular-weight solute removal, and adsorptive clearance facilitates removal of reactive solutes according to their electrostatic and/or chemical reactivity independently from their molecular weight.[4]

HIGH-FLUX RENAL REPLACEMENT THERAPIES: DEFINITION AND TERMINOLOGY

Over the last decade, the use of high-flux therapies using synthetic highly permeable membranes has steadily increased, while the use of conventional cellulosic low-flux membranes has declined. Today, synthetic high-flux dialyzers are used in 40 to 60 percent of ESRD patients. Interestingly, the increased use of high-flux dialyzers is usually associated with clinical beneficial effects, including reduced morbidity and mortality and improved well-being.[3]

From the literature, however, one must recognize that the terms high-efficiency and high-flux dialysis are still very confusing. In addition to this confusion, such terminology does not facilitate the ability of individuals to read or interpret clinical HD trials. Therefore, in an attempt to help clinicians in their choice of dialyzers and their understanding of the relevant literature, this chapter is intended to review and clarify this nomenclature by discussing two areas:

1. Dialyzer clearance, K_D, versus body clearance, K_{BD}
2. High-efficiency vs. high-flux dialysis

Dialyzer clearance (K_D) is the instantaneous blood purification capacity that is achieved in the extracorporeal exchanger device according to the operational conditions (blood flow, dialysate flow). K_D evaluates the solute exchange capacity of the device for a panel of selected solutes characterized by increasing molecular weights (e.g., urea, creatinine, phosphate, and beta$_2$ microglobulin). K_D obtained at fixed operational conditions (blood, dialysate and ultrafiltration flows) is expressed in milliliters per minute.[4,5]

K_oA is the mass transfer coefficient per unit surface of a given solute and reflects the maximum clearance achieved at conditions of infinite blood and dialysate flow rates. It is a more precise "bioengineering" way of expressing solute membrane permeability, since it reflects a property of the membrane not affected by operational conditions.[4,5]

The product of $K_D \times t_{HD}$ represents the total cumulative clearance of the extracorporeal device achieved after a certain time of application. This cumulative extracorporeal clearance does not necessarily represent the effective patient clearance.

Body clearance (K_{BD}) stands for the effective delivered clearance and reflects the true clearing capacity of the patient's body. K_{BD} integrates all limiting factors resulting from the complex patient/dialysis interaction (e.g., solute tissue or cell sequestration, protein-binding capacity, recirculation, compartmentalization). In vivo, effective clearance relies on dialyzer performances and solute access (blood solute concentration) which result from intracorporeal kinetics and body permeability.

High-efficiency dialysis is defined as comprising a treatment schedule that delivers high urea clearance whatever type of membrane is used (cellulosic or synthetic, low-or high-flux) or technical option is applied [HD or hemodiafiltration (HDF)]. Urea clearances higher than 210 mL/min and K_oA values above 600 mL/min are accepted threshold values of high-efficiency dialysis. In this case, urea body clearance ($K_{BD} \times t_{HD}$) in a 70-kg patient will be above 50 L and normalized body clearance ($K_{BD} \times t_{HD}/V$) will be higher than 1.4.

High-flux dialysis is defined as dialysis based on high ultrafiltration rates whatever the type of membrane or technical option used. Dialyzers fitted with membranes having an ultrafiltration coefficient (K_{UF}) higher than 20 mL/h/mmHg are defined as high-flux dialyzers.[5a] Using this definition, flux is considered as the rate of water crossing the dialysis membrane. By extension and because of the generally positive correlation between water flux and the clearance of medium-molecular-weight molecules (e.g., beta$_2$ microglobulin, 11.8 kDa), the term *high-flux membrane* has been used as a synonym for *highly permeable membrane*. A new confounding factor has recently been introduced into the HD field with the term *mid-flux permeable dialyzer*.

It would, therefore, be of value to clarify and adopt a standard terminology qualifying hemodialyzer and HD performance, clearly articulating that the function of the hemodialyzer is to clear uremic toxins. We propose to restrict use of the term *flux* to dialyzer solute permeability while abandoning water-flux considerations based on the ultrafiltration coefficient. The aim of each HD session is to clear the maximum amount of uremic toxins. We propose to use the term *efficiency* to qualify the *dialysis dose* delivered by means of body urea Kt/V. Accordingly, the nomenclature could be simplified by dividing dialysis dose into three levels of efficiency:

1. Low-efficiency dialysis: *Kt/V* less than 1.2 per session
2. Mid-efficiency dialysis: *Kt/V* between 1.2 and 1.4 per session
3. High-efficiency dialysis: *Kt/V* above 1.4 per session

Solute flux permeability related to middle molecules can be divided into four levels of flux (Table 36–1):

1. Low-flux hemodialyzer: beta$_2$-microglobulin clearance below 20 mL/min (or beta$_2$-microglobulin K_oA lower than 30 mL/min)
2. Mid-flux hemodialyzer: beta$_2$-microglobulin clearance higher than 20 mL/min (or beta$_2$-microglobulin K_oA greater than 30 mL/min)
3. High-flux hemodialyzer: beta$_2$-microglobulin clearance higher than 40 mL/min (or beta$_2$-microglobulin K_oA greater than 50 mL/min)
4. Super-flux hemodialyzer: beta$_2$-microglobulin clearance above 60 mL/min (or beta$_2$-microglobulin K_oA greater than 100 mL/min)

TECHNICAL PREREQUISITES FOR HIGH-FLUX THERAPIES

High-flux modalities require specific technical options and careful clinical surveillance to ensure safety and optimal performance. These requirements are as follows:

Patients must have a functioning high-flow vascular access able to deliver an effective extracorporeal blood flow ranging between 350 and 450 mL/min on a regular basis. Native or polytetrafluoroethylene (PTFE)-grafted arteriovenous fistulas with flow rates of 900 to 1500 mL/min are usually adequate to sustain such high extracorporeal blood flows.

A high-flux dialyzer is a basic component required to perform high-flux therapy. Several high-flux dialyzers now available have nominal performances satisfying the requirements for high-efficiency HD. All high-flux dialyzers have a dialysis membrane with high hydraulic permeability ($K_{UF} \geq 50$ mL/h/mmHg), high solute permeability (K_oA urea > 600 and beta$_2$ microglobulin > 60 mL/min), and a large surface area of exchange (1.50 to 2.10 m^2). High-flux membranes usually consist of hollow fibers made of synthetic polymers (i.e., polysulfone, polyarylethersulfone, polyacrylonitrile, polyamide).

Appropriate HD machines (blood monitoring and dialysate proportioning systems) are needed that are specifically designed to carry out the dialysis treatment safely and to monitor treatment parameters. Blood pump speed must be adequate to achieve high flow rates up to 500 mL/min. It should be possible to increase dialysate fluid production, conventionally set at 500 mL/min, up to 1000 mL/min if desired. Bicarbonate-based dialysate solution must be used and is generally available for modern dialysis machines. Ef-

TABLE 36-1 PROPOSAL FOR A DIALYZER CLASSIFICATION AND ITS APPLICATION IN DIFFERENT TREATMENT MODES

		Low-Flux Low-Efficiency	Mid-flux	High-Flux High-Efficiency	Super-Flux
Ultrafiltration	K_{uf}, mL/mmHg/h	<20	>20 <30	[3]30 <50	[3]50
Urea	K_d, mL/min	<180	>180 <200	[3]200 <220	[3]220
	K_oA, mL/min	<500	[3]500 <600	[3]600 <700	[3]700
	Kt/V	<1.2	[3]1.2 <1.4	[3]1.4 <1.6	[3]1.6
β$_2$-Microglobulin	K_d, mL/min	<20	>20 <40	[4]40 <60	[3]60
	K_oA, mL/min	<30	>30 <50	[3]50 >100	[3]100
Albumin leak	Grams per session	0	0	<2	[3]2 <5
Modality		LF-HD	MF-HD HDF off line HF off line	HF-HD HDF on line HF on line	HF-HD HDF on line HF on line

^{a}Operational conditions: Qb 350–450 mL/min; Qd 600–800 mL/min; Quf 100–200 mL/min.

K_{uf}, ultrafiltration coefficient; K_d, dialyzer clearance; K_oA, mass transfer coefficient per unit surface of a given solute; Kt/V, dialysis dose delivered by means of body urea; LF-HD, low-flux hemodialysis; MF-HD, medium-flux hemodialysis; HF-HD, high-flux hemodialysis; HDF, hemodiafiltration.

fective blood-flow monitoring is calculated by new dialysis monitors by measuring the blood pressure drop within the pump segment from arterial and venous pressure gauges. The ultrafiltration rate is controlled by means of a fluid-balancing module (volumetric by a fluid-balancing chamber or flowmetric by a flow-rate equalizer module) installed on the dialysate inlet and outlet. The dialysis monitor regulates the transmembrane pressure (TMP) according to the membrane's hydraulic permeability by means of the ultrafiltration pump in order to keep the filtration rate constant. The temperature of the dialysate is usually set manually. Modules that monitor blood temperature, implemented on new dialysis machines, make it possible to maintain a neutral thermal balance in order to improve the patient's tolerance of dialysis. Dialysate composition may be modified to satisfy each patient's specific needs regarding electrolyte and mineral metabolism. Ultrafiltration and sodium profiling systems may be used to facilitate extracellular fluid removal and vascular refilling during the dialysis session.

Ultrapure dialysate is desirable and available on most newer high-flux dialysis machines. The production of sterile and nonpyrogenic dialysis fluid is achieved by on-line "cold sterilization" of the dialysate. Sterilizing ultrafilters interposed on the inlet dialysate line are part of the dialysis machine. The ultrafilters, usually two in series, are disinfected together with the machine and replaced periodically to prevent supersaturation and release of endotoxins.[6]

On-line production of substitution fluid for HDF and hemofiltration (HF) is a fully recognized process. Several European Community–certified on-line HDF (and/or HF) machines are currently available on the European market. "On-line machines" benefit from specific recommendations of the European Renal Association (European Best Practice Guidelines). On-line HDF/HF machines are equipped with an infusion module including a filtration module (two ultrafilters in series) and an adjustable infusion pump (0 to 250 mL/min). A fraction of fresh dialysate produced by the dialysis machine is diverted by the infusion module. This fraction is converted to infusate by "cold sterilization" through the filtration module and then infused into the patient's blood via the venous (postdilution mode) or arterial bubble trap (predilution mode). The dialysate fraction diverted from the dialyzer inlet is then directly recovered by enhanced ultrafiltration of the patient's blood via the fluid-balancing module of the dialysate proportioning machine. Dialysate flow production in HDF machines is usually about 800 mL/min. The flow of dialysate is usually not adjusted for the infusion rate; i.e., the effective dialysate flow through the dialyzer equals the set dialysate flow minus the infusion flow rate. Typical infusion rates are 100 mL/min in the postdilution and 200 mL/min in the predilution HDF mode to keep a comparable clearance capacity of small solutes.

Water used in high-flux therapies, including on-line HDF/HF methods, should comply with very stringent criteria of purity. Such high refinement in water purification has led to the concept of "ultrapure water," a virtually sterile and nonpyrogenic water.[6] Technical aspects of water treatment systems and water distribution piping systems are detailed in Chap. 4. Basic technical options required to produce ultrapure water consist of a pretreatment system (microfiltration, softeners, activated charcoal, down-sizing microfiltration) followed by two reverse-osmosis modules in series. Ultrapurified water is then delivered to dialysis machines via a distribution loop (with or without microfiltration technique), ensuring its permanent recirculation. A quality assurance process is required to ensure the quality of the water produced on a regular basis.[6]

Dialysis schedule and prescription must be applied in order to provide the most efficient dialysis dose delivery both for small solutes and high-molecular-weight substances. The conventional treatment schedule is based on three dialysis sessions per week of 4 hours each (12 hours per week).[7] In this short treatment HD program, it is of paramount importance to ensure high blood flows (400 mL/min) coupled with high dialysate and/or infusate flow rates in order to remove a sufficiently large mass of uremic toxins to correct the extracellular fluid overload and restore the composition of the "internal milieu." Innovative treatment schedules are designed to improve the overall efficacy of extracorporeal renal replacement therapies. It has been suggested that increasing the frequency and/or duration of sessions in order to achieve a more physiologic and effective treatment session might be of value.[7]

TECHNICAL OPTIONS

Conventional Methods

High-Flux Hemodialysis (HF-HD). High-flux HD relies on the use of high-flux hemodialyzers and high blood and dialysate flow rates using a standard HD machine. Due to the high hydraulic permeability of the dialysis membrane (ultrafiltration coefficient >20 mL/h/mmHg), a dialysis fluid–balancing module on the dialysis machine (ultrafiltration controller) is clearly mandatory. The pressure equilibrium regime required for maintaining the zero net fluid balance in the body of a high-flux hemodialyzer results in ultrafiltration that occurs in the first part of the dialyzer module, being built up by dialysate backfiltration. This beneficial internal filtration exchange is a surrogate for "internal HDF."[8] High-flux HD combines diffusive and convective clearance in the same dialyzer. Interestingly, for some middle-molecular substances, the internal convective clearance may contribute up to 25 percent of the total clearance[8] (see Chap. 4). Introduced in the early 1970s, the first high-flux membrane for clinical use was the synthetic polyacrylonitrile membrane, AN69.[9] Several synthetic high-flux dialysis membranes with specific permeability characteristics are now available (Table 36–2). Initially, higher costs for dialyzers and the increased technical requirements for the dialysis equipment hampered the widespread use of high-flux dialysis. However, 30 years after the introduction of hemodialysis, more than 60 percent of ESRD patients worldwide were being treated with this type of therapy.[10]

Hemofiltration. Hemofiltration is a purely convective method that relies on the use of a high-flux hemofilter with an optimal blood flow and negative pressure gradient generating high plasma filtration rates. Dissolved solutes are carried out in the bulk flow of the ultrafiltrate (solute drag) generated by the pressure gradient applied across the membrane (TMP). Small solutes pass freely through the filter (sieving coefficient = 1), while larger solutes above the cutoff limit of the membrane are restricted from transport (sieving coefficient = 0). Ultrafiltration flow is volumetrically compensated by continuous infusion of substitution fluid in order to keep volume status constant. Any weight loss required to restore euvolemia is achieved by altering the ultrafiltration/infusion balance as necessary. The substitution fluid (infusate) is a sterile and pyrogen-free physiologic solution. Initially, the infusate was provided in disposable plastic bags (5 L). Currently, the substitution fluid is prepared by cold sterilization (sterilizing ultrafiltration) of dialysis fluid with on-line hemofiltration machines during the treatment. Such machines are capable of performing the entire range of standard extracorporeal RRT.

The infusion site defines the type of hemofiltration modality. The substitution fluid can be infused either before the hemofilter (predilution hemofiltration), after the hemofilter (postdilution hemofiltration), or at both pre- and postfilter sites (mixed hemofiltration) (Fig. 36–1).[11] Postdilutional HF is the more efficient method in terms of solute removal for both low- and mid-molecular-weight substances. Due to patient characteristics or hemorrheologic conditions (e.g., normal hematocrit, high protein concentration), it is sometimes advisable to adjust the postdilution infusion rate or to select a premixed- or mixed-dilution mode. As a simple and practical recommendation to prescribing the substitution volume in HF, the target Kt/V per session must be multiplied by the patient's water volume (55 percent of body weight or urea distribution volume) in the postdilution HF mode and by twice the patient's water volume in the predilution HF mode.[12] Total ultrafiltrate volume is thus the sum of infusate volume and weight loss.[12]

Hemodiafiltration (HDF). HDF is based on the combination of diffusive and forced convective solute clearance in the same dialyzer module. HDF requires the use of a high-flux dialyzer, high blood (350 to 450 mL/min) and dialysate (600 to 800 mL/min) flows, and a simultaneous ultrafiltration/infusion flow exchange. By combining diffusive and convective clearances, HDF represents the most efficient form of blood purification over a wide spectrum of solutes and molecular weights. Ultrafiltration flow is achieved by exerting a high negative TMP on the blood through the dialysate circuit. Substitution fluid (infusate) is a sterile nonpyrogenic physiologic solution that is infused into the patient's blood to compensate volumetrically for the ultra-

TABLE 36-2 HIGH-FLUX DIALYZERS AVAILABLE FOR THE DIFFERENT CONVECTIVE TREATMENT PROCEDURES (INCOMPLETE SELECTION)

DIALYZER	MEMBRANE MATERIAL	MANUFACTURER	STERILIZATION MODE	SURFACE AREA (m²)	K_{UF} (mL/h/mmHg)	UREA CLEARANCE (mL/min)	TREATMENT MODE
HF80S	Polysulfone	FMC	In-line steam	1.8	55	192	HD/HDF/HF
FX80	Helixone	FMC	In-line steam	1.8	59	197	HD/HDF/HF
Optiflux F180 NR	Polysulfone	FMC	ETO	1.8	55	196	HD/HDF/HF
Polyflux 170H	Polyamix	Gambro	Steam	1.7	48	195	HD/HDF/HF
APS-900	APS	Asahi	Gamma	1.8	75	192	HD/HDF/HF
Tricea 190G	CTA	Baxter	Gamma	1.9	37	198	HD
BLS 819G	DIAPES	Bellco	Gamma	1.9	80	192	HD/HDF/HF
HI PS 18	Polysulfone	B. Braun	Gamma	1.8	55	192	HD/HDF/HF
FLX-18GWS	PEPA	Nikkiso	Gamma	1.8	47	197	HD/HDF/HF
Surelyzer PES-190DH	DIAPES	Nipro	Gamma	1.9	55	198	HD/HDF/HF
Sureflux-190FH	CTA	Nipro	Gamma	1.9	85	199	HD
BS-1.8	Toraysulfone	Toray	Gamma	1.8	52	198	HD/HDF/HF
H9	Arylane	Hospal	Gamma	2.0	88	194	HD/HDF/HF
Nephral ST 500	AN69 ST	Hospal	Gamma	2.2	65	195	HD/HDF/HF

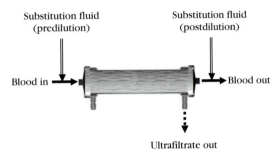

Figure 36–1. Schematics of hemofiltration.

filtered fluid. Weight loss required to establish euvolemia is accomplished by increasing the ultrafiltration volume according to the patient needs. Depending on the site of fluid substitution, several HDF modalities are routinely practiced, including postdilution HDF (infusion after hemodiafilter), predilution HDF (infusion before hemodiafilter), or mixed HDF (simultaneous pre- and posthemodiafilter infusion) (Fig. 36–2). As in hemofiltration, substitution fluid was provided initially in disposable plastic bags (5 L). Currently, the substitution fluid is prepared by on-line cold sterilization of the dialysis fluid. Specifically designed HDF machines are required to perform on-line HDF safely. Typical infusion flows are 100 mL/min (24 L for a 4-hour session) in postdilution HDF and 200 mL/min (48 L for a 4-hour session) in the predilution HDF mode. To prevent excessive alarms from abnormal TMP, it is recommended that the infusion rate be coupled to the effective blood flow. A simple rule for prescribing infusion flow is to use one-third of the inlet blood flow in postdilution HDF and half of the inlet blood flow in predilution HDF.

Unconventional Methods

Several technical variations of high-flux HDF have been described over the past decade. All claim to be associated with some advantages over standard procedures.

Middilution Hemodiafiltration.
Middilution HDF differs from standard HDF in comprising two high-flux dialyzers in series while the substitution fluid is infused into the blood

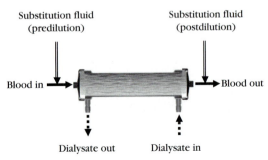

Figure 36–2. Schematics of hemodiafiltration.

between the two dialyzers. This arrangement results in a postdilution stage followed by a predilution stage (Fig. 36–3). Because of the use of two dialyzers, the technical requirements of the method are complicated and costly. Very recently, a middilution HDF technology has been introduced that integrates the two high-flux dialyzers into a single-fiber-bundle cartridge (Fig. 36–4).[13] This hemodiafilter (Nephros OLpūr MD 190) has overcome the previously mentioned disadvantages, facilitating its clinical use. In this configuration, a high infusion rate (200 mL/min) performed on the distal head of the module between the two dialyzer stages makes it possible to increase convective clearance. In a first prospective clinical study, this hemodiafilter has demonstrated its clinical feasibility and enhanced performance compared to conventional HDF.[13]

Mixed Hemodiafiltration.
Mixed pre- and postdilution on-line HDF represents a recently introduced technical variation that ensures safer rheologic and operating conditions than postdilution HDF.[14] In this procedure one fraction of the substitution fluid is infused into the posthemodiafilter infusion site while the other fraction is infused into the prehemodiafilter infusion site, resulting in a mixed infusion (Fig. 36–5). The ratio of pre- to postinfusion flow is feedback-controlled by the HDF monitor to maintain the TMP in a safe range (250 to 300 mmHg). It has been shown that with this technique, significantly higher beta$_2$-microglobulin clearances can be achieved.[15]

Programmed Filtration.
Programmed filtration is an adaptation of on-line HDF designed to reduce albumin leakage while enhancing the removal of middle molecules. In this case, the ultrafiltration profile of the HDF machine is programmed to downregulate the filtration flow or the transmembrane pressure during the initial phase of the HDF session so as to reduce albumin loss. With this method, significantly higher beta$_2$-microglobulin removal and lower albumin loss can be achieved.[16]

Push/Pull Hemodiafiltration.
Push/pull HDF is the Japanese version of on-line high-flux HDF. It is actually a form of high-flux HD, which maximally exploits the internal filtration of the dialyzer. The main feature of this technique is a double-cylinder piston pump (push/pull pump) integrated with one cylinder in the functionally closed dialysate circuit and, in the pressure-controlled version, with the other via an air column and a partition chamber in the venous part of the extracorporeal blood circuit. In this configuration, about 25 alternate repetitions of ultrafiltration (pull) and backfiltration (push) are performed in the hemodialyzer during one single blood passage, resulting in more than 120 L of ultrafiltered plasma water being replaced by backfiltered dialysate in a 4-hour treatment.[17] To avoid pyrogen transfer to the patient during the backfiltration phase, a cold steril-

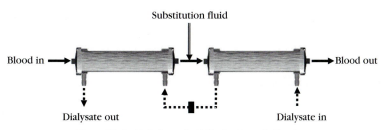

Figure 36–3. Technique of middilution hemodiafiltration.

ization of the fresh dialysis fluid is performed by sterilizing ultrafilters. Due to the high volume of ultrafiltered plasma water, push/pull HDF has demonstrated a higher beta$_2$-microglobulin reduction rate than is achieved by conventional postdilution hemodiafiltration. Despite the same highly permeable dialyzer, the albumin loss with this method is significantly lower.[18]

Double High-Flux Hemodialysis. Double high-flux HD is a simple modification of conventional high-flux HD in which two high-flux dialyzers are assembled in series and dialysis fluid irrigates countercurrently in the two hemodiafilters. An adjustable clamp restriction on the dialysis circuit between the two dialyzers is used to favor ultrafiltration in the first dialyzer and backfiltration in the second dialyzer. Due to cost and handling issues, this technique has not been widely adopted.

Acetate-Free Biofiltration (AFB). AFB is a conventional low-flow postdilution HDF technique (Fig. 36–2) in which a sterile isotonic bicarbonate solution is infused as substitution fluid while at the same time a buffer-free standard dialysate is used.[19] The infusion rate of the bicarbonate sub-

stitution fluid is adjusted individually with respect to the correction of acidosis. Substitution volumes below 10 L per 4 hours of treatment—e.g., 1.6 to 1.8 L/h—are usually needed.[20]

Paired Hemofiltration (PHF). PHF is a double-chamber HDF technique developed in the early 1980s that has been modified to achieve high-flux HDF.[21] The system is based on the association of two hemodiafilters in series, one with a small surface (e.g., 0.4 m^2) that permits the infusion of substitution fluid (backfiltration) and the second a high-flux hemodialyzer (1.8 m^2) that allows convective and diffusive exchange from dialysate. The ultrafiltrate is replaced by a sterile substitution fluid produced on line by cold sterilization of the fresh dialysis fluid.

Hemodiafiltration with Endogenous Reinfusion (HFR). HFR is a method derived directly from the paired hemofiltration technique. The main feature of HFR is the on-line regeneration of ultrafiltrate, accomplished by passing it through an adsorbing device. The regenerated ultrafiltrate is thus reinfused as an endogenous substitution fluid (Fig. 36–6).[22,23]

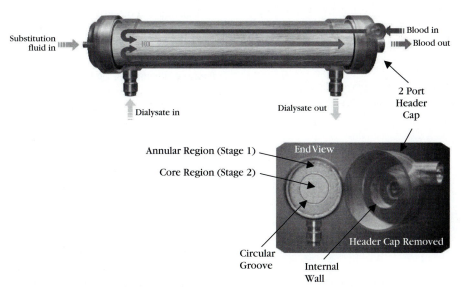

Figure 36–4. Middilution hemodiafiltration in a single cartridge: the Nephros Olpūr.

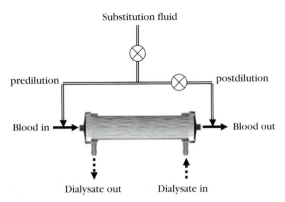

Figure 36–5. Schematics of mixed hemodiafiltration.

Adsorption Columns. Specific adsorption of uremic toxins is a very difficult approach, since it remains unclear at which proteins it should be targeted. Beta$_2$ microglobulin plays a significant role in dialysis-related amyloidosis and may represent a good candidate. Some attempts have been made to develop specific adsorbers to increase removal of beta$_2$ microglobulin during high-flux dialysis. A specific adsorbent hemoperfusion column for the removal of beta$_2$ microglobulin (Lixelle) has been developed and evaluated in Japan.[24,25] This column, used in series with a high-flux dialyzer (Fig. 36–7), has been shown to significantly decrease beta$_2$-microglobulin levels and improve dialysis-related amyloid symptoms.[25]

CLINICAL RESULTS

High-flux therapies were developed in recent years to improve the overall quality and efficiency of dialysis in order to correct or to prevent the development of dialysis-related complications (DRCs) such as atheromatosis, inflammation, malnutrition, and beta$_2$-microglobulin amyloidosis in long-term ESRD patients. DRCs are putatively due to the accumulation of toxic middle molecules (> 500 Da) in uremic patients; it was speculated that the use of large-pore membranes would have the potential to reduce the inci-

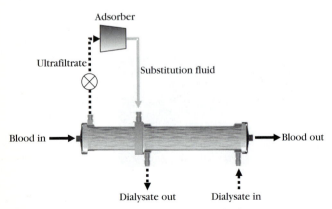

Figure 36–6. Schematics of hemodiafiltration with endogenous reinfusion.

dence of these complications. Over the last decade, dialyzer manufacturers and physicians have made tremendous efforts to enhance the removal of middle molecules. Dialyzer design has been optimized to increase instantaneous solute clearances (low- and mid-molecular-weight solutes). At present, treatment strategy is focused on increasing overall body clearances of solutes (longer dialysis duration and/or more frequent sessions).

Indeed, the scientific literature remains quite confusing in this area and is not very helpful to the physician regarding the beneficial effects of high-flux therapies. In this section, we summarize our present knowledge. Three aspects are discussed:

1. Confounding and confusing factors that may restrict the interpretation of data
2. Positive effects of high-flux therapies in acute and/or short-term studies
3. Clinical benefits of high-flux therapies in mid- and long-term studies

Confounding and Confusing Factors

Several factors complicate the interpretation of scientific studies related to the application of high-flux therapies to patients with ESRD. These have been repeatedly discussed in the scientific literature. However, it is necessary to recall some of them in order to underline the fact that evidence-based medicine is far from being easily applied in the dialysis field. To illustrate this difficulty, we focus on some particularly important examples:

Synthetic vs. Cellulosic Dialysis Membranes. Most reports have compared high-flux therapies (HD, HF, HDF) using highly permeable synthetic membranes to low permeability cellulosic membrane. In this context, one would agree that it is difficult to discern the benefits of increased solute permeability apart from the advantages of more biocompatible membranes.

Purity of Bicarbonate Dialysate. High-flux therapies must be used with bicarbonate buffered dialysate and microbiologically safe dialysis fluid solutions. Due to the high porosity of membranes exposing the patient to backtransport phenomena and pyrogen reactions, most reports on high-flux therapies have involved systems using ultrapure dialysis fluid. By improving the overall biocompatibility of the dialysis system, the regular use of highly purified dialysate has certainly contributed to reduced activation of circulating cells and proteins and to the prevention of inflammation.[6]

Synthetic Highly Permeable Membranes. Synthetic membranes are the basis of high-flux therapies. Due to the chemical composition and electric charge requirements of such membranes, they have a certain bioreactivity that con-

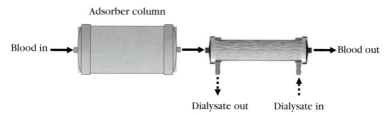

Figure 36–7. Schematics of beta$_2$-microglobulin adsorption using the Lixelle adsorber for direct hemoperfusion in series with a high-flux dialyzer.

tributes to their enhanced blood clearing capacity by adsorption of reactive species such as beta$_2$-microglobulin and cytokines.[26] The true contribution of this component of solute removal is difficult to quantify in clinical studies assessing high-flux dialyzer performance.

Acute and Short-Term Clinical Studies.

Most of the published studies on high-flux therapy have been performed either in acute settings (over a limited number of sessions) or over a short term (less than 6 months). It is difficult to transpose results reported in such circumstance to long-term treatment. Solute kinetics within the body may be affected over time by changes in blood solute concentration. In addition, long-term studies have been performed comparing ESRD treated with high-flux dialysis with those undergoing low-flux treatment, using information from historical databases. It is obviously difficult to compare historical and prospective groups of patients, since many components of the treatment change over time, which can confound the results significantly.

Impact of Dialyzer Reuse.

Several studies have compared the impact of high-flux and low-flux membranes on dialysis performance and patient outcomes where dialyzer reprocessing and reuse was practiced. The reuse process may seriously alter both dialyzer permeability and dialyzer bioreactivity.[27,28] Again, this confounding of results makes interpretation of outcomes data difficult.

Operational Conditions.

High-flux therapies require high blood and dialysate flows in order to to optimize dialyzer performance. Flow conditions used for high-flux therapies vary considerably between studies. This variation renders comparison difficult if not impossible. The contribution of convective clearance may also complicate the complexity of the analysis.

Effects of High-Flux Therapies on Solute Removal

The enhanced efficiency of high-flux therapies is one of the best-documented aspects of the method. Almost all acute and short-term studies have demonstrated the higher middle-molecule removal rates of high-flux sessions and have reported a positive impact, with a significant decline of

middle-molecule concentrations over time. It is important to note that HDF provides significantly greater instantaneous clearance of both low- and middle-molecular-weight solutes than does high-flux HD. Acute or short-term comparative studies confirm the superiority of high-flux therapies using a high convective clearance, such as on-line HDF, in removing middle-molecular solutes. A typical figure comparing the solute removal rate (percentage of reduction) of several molecular weight solutes in high-flux HD and HDF is presented in Fig. 36–8. As shown, the reduction rate for solutes ranging in the middle-molecular range, of up to 13.4 kDa, averages 75 percent in on-line postdilution HDF and is significantly lower in high-flux HD.

Phosphate removal is increased with HDF methods, reaching 30 to 35 mmol per session. Based on three sessions weekly, phosphate removal in HDF (90 to 105 mmol/week) is clearly still not adequate to restore phosphate balance in the uremic patient. Accordingly, control of phosphatemia requires the use of oral phosphate binders even if a dose reduction might be possible.[29] Beta$_2$-icroglobulin is effectively removed by high-flux therapies. Convective modalities, such as on-line HDF, are, however,

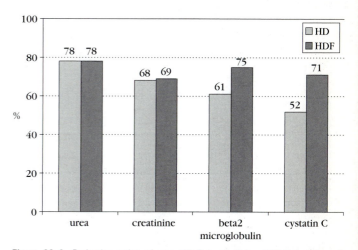

Figure 36–8. Reduction ratios of urea (60 Da), creatinine (113 Da), beta$_2$ microglobulin (11,800 Da), and cystatin C (13,400 Da) in HD and postdilution on-line HDF. Data derive from a controlled study on 10 ESRD patients using a high-flux polysulfone dialyzer (1.8 m^2), a blood flow of 350 mL/min, dialysate flows of 500 (HD) and 800 (HDF) mL/min, and an infusion flow rate of 100 mL/min in HDF. Middle-molecule reduction is significantly higher in HDF vs. HD.

significantly more effective than high-flux HD in removing beta$_2$-microglobulin. The reduction ratio of beta$_2$-microglobulin is close to 70 to 80 percent in HDF, as compared to 40 to 50 percent in HD. Beta$_2$-microglobulin mass removal per session is between 180 and 220 mg, while it is 70 to 100 mg in high-flux HD.[30,31] Several prospective controlled studies have confirmed that the enhancement of beta$_2$-microglobulin clearance resulting from a change in the dialysis mode was accompanied by a significant decline of blood beta$_2$-microglobulin concentrations during a midterm period.[30,32] It is, however, not possible to link this observation to a reduced incidence of beta$_2$-microglobulin amyloidosis in long-term dialysis patients treated with high-flux therapies.

Complement factor D, a proinflammatory mediator with a larger middle-molecular weight, is removed effectively by on-line HDF.[33] The clinical importance of reduced factor D levels in the antibacterial response in ESRD patients is currently not proven.

Elevated leptin (16 kDa) levels in uremia are suspected to be associated with an enhanced frequency of malnutrition. Leptin concentrations are known to decrease after HDF sessions. Predialysis leptin concentrations were reduced to a lower level in patients regularly treated by HDF,[34] but the impact on nutritional status is unclear.

Cytokine removal has been repeatedly reported with high-flux therapies in both acute and chronic ESRD patients.[35] The benefits of cytokine removal remain debatable even in septic patients and are being intensively studied.

A protein-bound erythropoietic inhibitor, 3-carboxy-4-methyl-5-propyl-2-furanpropionic acid (CMPF), can be reduced with protein-leaking high-flux membranes.[36] HD with such dialysis membranes seems to ameliorate renal anemia to a greater extent than conventional dialysis.[37]

Several circulating advanced glycation end products (AGEs) and AGE precursors, which are suspected to be involved in DRC, are effectively reduced in diabetic and nondiabetic ESRD patients treated with high-flux and super-flux HD membranes.[38] Once again, the clinical benefits of this remain to be proven.

Elevated levels of homocysteine in plasma, an established cardiovascular risk factor in healthy subjects, have been significantly reduced with super-flux HD in two preliminary studies.[39-41] Due to the almost complete protein binding of homocysteine, its reduction has been attributed to the removal of higher-molecular-weight inhibitors of homocysteine metabolism. Whether lower homocysteine levels will improve cardiovascular outcomes in ESRD patients is unknown.

Clinical Benefits of High-Flux Therapies

Several published reports have documented that the regular use of high-flux therapies has beneficial effects in long-term dialysis patients. In this section we update current knowledge in this field.

Clinical Tolerance of Dialysis Sessions. Improved tolerance of the dialysis session is consistently reported with convective high-flux modalities (HDF/HF). The incidence of hypotensive episodes is reduced with HDF/HF compared to conventional dialysis despite equivalent weight loss. This is particularly valuable in patients prone to cardiovascular and hypotensive events. Although not completely understood, the positive effect of these modalities has been related to vasomodulation involving several factors, including a negative thermal balance,[41] a high sodium concentration of the substitution fluid, and the removal of vasodilating mediators.

Postdialysis fatigue is reduced with high-flux therapies. This is particularly useful in the elderly, diabetics, and other high-risk patients. HD intolerance symptomatology (e.g., nausea, vomiting, cramps, headache) is reduced with high-flux HDF/HF compared to conventional HD.[42]

Blood Pressure Control and Cardiac Consequences. Better control of arterial blood pressure has been reported with high-flux therapies. This is particularly true with HDF/HF. This beneficial effect is mainly due to the intradialytic hemodynamic stability that permits patients to reach "dry weight" and to restore sodium fluid balance adequately. The duration of sessions and compliance to dietary sodium restriction contribute as well to achieving this primary objective of dialysis treatment. Regular use of high-flux therapies has been associated with a reduction of left ventricular hypertrophy, contributing to better preservation of cardiac function. This positive effect is also associated with the correction of anemia and adequate blood pressure control, suggesting that the effect is due not only to high-flux treatment.[43,44]

Maintenance of Residual Renal Function. Residual renal function, when present, is an important contributor to improved outcomes in ESRD patients by reducing interdialytic weight gain and enhancing treatment efficiency by removing middle molecules.[45] Although there is still some debate, recent studies have shown that high-flux therapy is associated with a longer and better preservation of residual renal function than conventional HD. This positive effect of high-flux therapy appears to be comparable to that observed in peritoneal dialysis patients.[46] This phenomenon, not completely understood, might be linked to the reduction in kidney inflammation seen when membranes with improved biocompatibility are used, and/or to the reduction of kidney insults associated with a lower frequency of hypotensive events.

Inflammation and Hemocompatibility. High-flux therapies offer a clear benefit in ameliorating the inflammatory state of HD patients. Several prospective studies have shown that sensitive markers of the acute-phase reaction (such as C-reactive protein, interleukins-1 and 6, IL1 and IL6-RA, albumin), remain stable over time in high-flux therapies, while they steadily worsen with conventional HD.[47] This result has also been observed with on-line HDF despite the large amounts of intravenous infusion of substitution fluid (20 to 50 L).[48] Note that this positive effect results from the combined use of synthetic biocompatible membranes and ultrapure dialysis fluid. Preventing inflammation is a crucial objective in order to reduce the incidence of dialysis-related complications in long-term dialysis patients.[49]

Malnutrition. Calorie and/or protein malnutrition is observed in about one-third of dialysis patients. Several recent studies have shown that the use of high-flux membranes has a positive impact on the nutritional state as compared to that of low-flux membranes.[50] High-flux membranes reduce the protein catabolic effect induced by low-flux cellulosic membranes. Serum albumin tends to increase when patients are treated with high-flux membranes. Anthropometric parameters, such as dry weight and body-mass index, tend to improve over time in patients treated with high-flux therapies. This is corroborated by an increase in dietary protein intake derived from the rate of urea generation.[50] Indeed, one must recognize that this positive effect of high-flux therapies might result from the beneficial combination of high-flux membranes and ultrapure dialysate and associated decreased inflammation, or, more speculatively, with the removal of anorexia-inducing uremic toxins.[51]

Dyslipidemia and Oxidative Stress. The abnormal lipid profile, increased oxidative stress and high levels of AGEs consistently found in dialysis patients are important contributors to the severe complications of atheromatosis that are seen. The regular use of high-flux membranes has been shown to improve the lipid profile[52] and to reduce oxidative stress and AGEs in these patients.[53] Indeed, although not completely understood, this beneficial effect may be partly due to the biocompatibility of the dialysis membrane and the ultrapurity of the dialysate.[54] Note that the increased loss of natural antioxidant substances (e.g., vitamin C, vitamin E, selenium) may abolish part of the beneficial effect of high-flux therapies, particularly with high-flux convective modalities.[55] To prevent the enhancement of oxidative stress by high-flux modalities, it is highly desirable to supplement patients with natural antioxidant substances.

Uremic Neuropathy. Currently, neuropathy has become rare in patients undergoing standard dialysis treatments. Neuropathy should be considered as a marker of dialysis inadequacy that requires correction. It has been reported that intensification of treatment by the application of high-flux therapies is capable of reversing neuropathy.[56]

Correction of Anemia. Renal anemia, present in the vast majority of ESRD patients, has been successfully treated with recombinant human erythropoietin (rHuEPO). High-flux therapies have been reported to improve anemia control and to reduce the need for rHuEPO treatment in HD patients. This positive effect has been particularly noted when patients were switched from low-flux HD to high-flux HDF or to HD with protein-leaking high-flux membranes.[31,37] These observations suggest that high-flux methods might remove a protein-bound erythropoietic inhibitor substance.[36] Note that the correction of anemia in this context is associated with improved biocompatibility of the dialysis system and a reduced inflammatory state in the patient.

Beta$_2$-Microglobulin Amyloidosis. Beta$_2$-microglobulin amyloidosis has become a major complication of long-term HD therapy. Using carpal tunnel syndrome as a crude and typical first manifestation of beta$_2$-microglobulin amyloidosis in HD patients, it is commonly accepted that the incidence of this complication reaches 50 percent after 10 years and 100 percent after 20 years of conventional HD treatment. Several large studies have shown that the extended use of high-flux membranes has a beneficial impact on the development of beta$_2$-microglobulin amyloidosis, reducing its incidence by 50 percent.[57] Interestingly, it has been reported that the regular use of ultrapure water was also responsible for a significant reduction of carpal tunnel syndrome in HD patients.[58] Most of the recent studies are epidemiologic in nature and do not take into account potential confounding factors. Indeed, almost all studies report a significant reduction in the incidence of carpal tunnel syndrome (by 50 percent) with the use of high-flux methods and ultrapure dialysis fluid, but these findings are difficult to interpret because several confounding factors are present, including high-flux membrane type, enhanced convective clearance, ultrapure dialysate, and reduced inflammation.

Morbidity and Mortality. Morbidity and mortality are objective and measurable endpoints of renal replacement therapy. In this context, *morbidity* refers to the hospitalization rate and duration.

Interestingly, several studies have demonstrated the positive impact of high-flux therapies in terms of morbidity and mortality. Large cohort studies [e.g., the U.S. Renal Data System (USRDS) studies] have shown a significant reduction of morbidity and mortality in patients treated with high-flux methods as compared to those treated with low-flux dialyzers.[3,57] Unfortunately, these positive results were not confirmed in the large prospective and controlled HEMO study, recently reported.[5a] Indeed, it must be emphasized that in the HEMO study, dialyzer reuse may have altered hemodialyzer performance and blunted the beneficial effects of high-flux methods. Although it is difficult to prove that high-flux therapies have a true beneficial effect on morbidity or mortality per se, it is more easily supportable to claim that high-flux therapies are not harmful to patients. In addition, it has also been shown convincingly that high-flux modalities improve the quality of life of dialysis patients.

RISKS AND HAZARDS OF HIGH-FLUX THERAPIES

Pyrogen Permeability of Dialysis Membranes

The passage of bacterial products (e.g., endotoxins, exotoxins, fragments of endotoxin, lipopolysaccharides, lipid A, muramyl dipeptides) from dialysate to the patient's blood is a common risk of all HD methods. Due to their larger pore size, the use of high-permeability membranes is associated with a theoretically higher risk of pyrogen passage than low-permeability membranes. Patients, therefore, are exposed to a variety of reactions, both acute clinical and chronic subclinical reactions.

Acute reactions are typically observed when a massive passage through the dialysis membrane of pyrogenic substances (endotoxins or their fragments) occurs. The endotoxins' passage results in a severe pyrogenic reaction that can lead to endotoxic shock. In this case, the reaction is clinically symptomatic, comprising various degrees of febrile reactions, severe hypotension, tachycardia, breathlessness, cyanosis, and general malaise. Symptoms related to the patient's comorbid conditions—such angina pectoris or abdominal pain—may be associated. Fever recedes within a few hours. Leukopenia is usually present. Blood cultures remain negative. Because of improvement in the microbiological purity of dialysis fluid, such pyrogenic reactions have become rare.

Chronic reactions are observed with low and/or repeated passage of bacterial products through the dialysis membrane into the patient's blood.[59] These do not produce clinical symptoms. In such cases, the repeated passage of pyrogenic substances results in a periodic activation of blood cells and circulating protein cascades. Activated cells (e.g., macrophages/ monocytes) subsequently induce the production and release of several mediators, including proinflammatory substances such as cytokines (interleukins-1 and 6 and TNF).[59] The resulting chronic microinflammation is frequently reported in HD patients and may contribute to the dialysis-related complications seen in long-term dialysis patients.[59]

In this scenario, the role of several components should be considered:

    Permeability characteristics of the hemodialyzer
    Microbiological dialysate purity
    Backtransfer phenomena resulting from the dialysis-fluid-balancing module

Hemodialyzer Permeability. A variety of in vitro studies have evaluated the permeability of dialysis membranes to bacterial substances. Depending on the methods employed, the results may differ significantly; therefore extrapolation to clinical conditions should be done cautiously. From in vitro testing, it can be stated that dialysis membranes are permeable to bacterial substances, but to different degrees depending on the membrane material.[60]

Several in vivo studies have confirmed the safe barrier of high-flux synthetic dialyzers against endotoxins and other pyrogenic substances. This property has been confirmed in spite of very unfavorable clinical conditions, such as high levels of dialysate contamination and increased backtransport phenomena. Synthetic high-flux membranes show more favorable results than cellulosic low-flux membranes in terms of the capacity to retain pyrogens.[60] This interesting property has been attributed to the high pyrogen adsorptive capacity of synthetic membrane polymers. One must keep in mind, however, that, under favorable conditions, some low-molecular-weight bacterial substances have the capacity to pass through the dialyzer membrane. It is noteworthy that synthetic membranes are not equal in terms of the capacity to retain pyrogens.[60] Significant differences may exist in the virtually same polymer materials (e.g., polysulfone) according to manufacturer, brand type, and batch number.

Microbiological Dialysate Purity. The use of ultrapure dialysis fluid is a basic prerequisite to reduce the risk of dialysate contamination and improve the overall biocompatibility of the dialysis system. To achieve this goal, we refer the interested reader to articles and textbooks covering this topic. Briefly, it is recommended that one use ultrapure water on a regular basis, employ HD machines equipped with ultrafilters that sterilize the dialysis fluid, and perform frequent disinfection procedures of the dialysis system.[6,59]

Backtransfer Phenomena. Backdiffusion and backfiltration are part of the hemodialyzer exchange occurring when a dialysis-fluid balancing module is employed. To protect patients against the risks and hazards associated with contaminated dialysis fluid, it is highly desirable to use ultrapure dialysis fluid on a routine basis.

Protein Loss

High-flux HD can be associated with increased albumin loss. The use of highly permeable membranes to enhance middle molecule clearance tends to increase albumin loss. This phenomenon is clearly related to the dialysis modality used. The same type of highly permeable dialyzer used in high-flux HD will induce an albumin loss of 2 to 4 g per session, while its use in high-flux convective modalities will increase albumin loss by a factor of two or even more. This is enhanced when postdilution modalities are employed. The use of certain brands of high-flux dialyzers and some super-flux dialyzers tends to aggravate the albumin loss, which can reach 7 to 20 g per session.[61] The clinical and biological consequences of albumin loss must be evaluated with a focus on the nutritional status of long-term HD patients. This is particularly important in malnourished and elderly patients.

Deficiency Syndromes

Enhanced loss of nutrients is a theoretical risk of high-flux modalities. Soluble vitamins, trace elements, small peptides, and proteins may be lost during high-flux HD.[55] The total amount of nutrients lost per session is, however, sufficiently low to be easily compensated by adequate oral intake. Such detrimental effects of high-flux modalities may be accentuated in malnourished and elderly patients. Adequate replacement should be provided orally in a timely, appropriate fashion.

CONCLUSIONS

At present, high-flux modalities offer the most effective RRT for the patient with ESRD. By enhancing the contribution of convective clearance, hemodiafiltration and/or hemofiltration enlarge the spectrum of uremic toxins cleared, thus optimizing the overall efficacy of the extracorporeal RRT. By combining the use of ultrapure dialysis fluid and synthetic hemocompatible membranes, these high-flux modalities considerably improve the hemocompatibility profile of the HD system. Preliminary clinical studies indicate that these technical improvements reduce dialysis-related morbidity in long-term-treated patients. Now, it remains to be proven that tailoring the dialysis schedule to the patient's needs, either by increasing session frequency (e.g., daily hemodiafiltration) or lengthening treatment duration (longer dialysis sessions), will have an additive beneficial effect on outcome.

REFERENCES

1. Vanholder R, Glorieux G, De Smet R, et al. New insights in uremic toxins. *Kidney Int Suppl* 2003;84:S6.
2. Vanholder R, Glorieux GL, De Smet R. Back to the future: middle molecules, high flux membranes, and optimal dialysis. *Hemodial Int* 2003;7:52.
3. Port FK, Wolfe RA, Hulbert-Shearon TE, et al. Mortality risk by hemodialyzer reuse practice and dialyzer membrane characteristics: results from the USRDS dialysis morbidity and mortality study. *Am J Kidney Dis* 2001;37:276.
4. Hoenich NA, Woffindin C, Ronco C. Haemodialysers and associated devices. In: Jacobs C, Kjellstrand CM, Koch KM, Winchester JF, eds. *Replacement of Renal Function by Dialysis*, 4th ed. Dordrecht/Boston/London: Kluwer, 1996:188.
5. Sargent JA, Gotch FA. Principles and biophysics of dialysis. In: Jacobs C, Kjellstrand CM, Koch KM, Winchester JF, eds. *Replacement of Renal Function by Dialysis*, 4th ed. Dordrecht/Boston/London: Kluwer, 1996:34.
5a. Eknoyan G, Beck GJ, Cheung AK, et al. Effect of dialysis dose and membrane flux in maintenance hemodialysis. *N Engl J Med* 2002;19:347.
6. Canaud B, Bosc JY, Leray H, et al. Microbiologic purity of dialysate: rationale and technical aspects. *Blood Purif* 2000; 18:200.
7. European Best Practice Guidelines Expert Group on Hemodialysis, European Renal Association. Section II. Haemodialysis adequacy. *Nephrol Dial Transplant* 2002; 17(suppl 7):16.
8. Schmidt M, Baldamus CA, Schoeppe WA. Backfiltration in hemodialyzers with highly permeable membranes. *Blood Purif* 1984;2:108.
9. Man NK, Granger A, Rondon-Nucete M, et al. One year follow up of short dialysis with a membrane highly permeable to middle molecules. *Proc Eur Dial Transplant Assoc* 1973; 10:236.
10. Goodkin DA, Mapes DL, Held PJ. The dialysis outcomes and practice patterns study (DOPPS): how can we improve the care of hemodialysis patients? *Semin Dial* 2001;14(3): 157–159.
11. Hillion D, Haas T, Pertuiset N, et al. Pre-/postdilution hemofiltration. *Blood Purif* 1995;13:241.
12. Ledebo I: Principles and practice of hemofiltration and hemodiafiltration. *Artif Organs* 1998;22:20.
13. Krieter DH, Leray Moragues H, Collins G, et al. Novel middilution dialyzer "Nephros MD 190": first clinical performance data (abstr). *Nephrol Dial Transplant* 2003;18(suppl 4):756.
14. Pedrini LA, De Cristofaro V, Pagliari B, et al. Mixed predilution and postdilution online hemodiafiltration compared with the traditional infusion modes. *Kidney Int* 2000;58: 2155.
15. Pedrini LA, De Cristofaro V. On-line mixed hemodiafiltration with a feedback for ultrafiltration control: Effect on middle-molecule removal. *Kidney Int* 2003;64:1505.
16. Kim ST, Yamamoto C, Taoka M, et al. Programmed filtration, a new method for removing large molecules and regulating albumin leakage during hemodiafiltration treatment. *Am J Kidney Dis* 2001;38(4 suppl 1):S220.
17. Miwa M, Shinzato T. Push/pull hemodiafiltration: technical aspects and clinical effectiveness. *Artif Organs* 1999;23: 1123.
18. Shinzato T, Miwa M, Nakai S, et al. Alternate repetition of short fore- and backfiltrations reduces convective albumin loss. *Kidney Int* 1996;50:432.
19. Zucchelli P, Santoro A, Ferrari G, et al. Acetate-free biofiltration: hemodiafiltration with base-free dialysate. *Blood Purif* 1990;8:14.
20. Schrander-v d Meer AM, ter Wee PM, Donker AJM, et al. Dialysis efficacy during acetate-free biofiltration. *Nephrol Dial Transplant* 1998;13:370.
21. Ghezzi PM, Frigato G, Fantini GF, et al. Theoretical model and first clinical results of the paired filtration-dialysis (PFD). *Life Support Syst* 1983;1(suppl 1):271.
22. Ghezzi PM, Botella J, Sartoris AM, et al. Use of the ultrafiltrate obtained in two-chamber (PFD) hemodiafiltration as replacement fluid. Experimental ex vivo and in vitro study. *Int J Artif Organs* 1991;14:327.
23. Ghezzi PM, Gervasio R, Tessore V, et al. Hemodiafiltration without replacement fluid. An experimental study. *ASAIO J* 1992;38:61.
24. Furuyoshi S, Nakatani M, Tamin J, et al. New adsorption column (Lixelle) to eliminate β_2-microglobulin for direct hemoperfusion. *Ther Apher* 1998;2:13.

25. Abe T, Uchita K, Orita H, et al. Effect of β2-microglobulin adsorption column on dialysis-related amyloidosis. *Kidney Int* 2003;64:1522.

26. Yanai M, Higuchi T, Kawano K, et al. Elution identification of proteins adsorbed onto dialysis membranes during clinical use. *Nihon Univ J Med* 2001;43:277.

27. Cheung AK, Agodoa LY, Daugirdas JT, et al. Effects of hemodialyzer reuse on clearances of urea and beta$_2$-microglobulin. The Hemodialysis (HEMO) Study Group. *J Am Soc Nephrol* 1999;10:117.

28. Klinkmann H, Grassmann A, Vienken J. Dilemma of membrane biocompatibility and reuse. *Artif Organs* 1996;20:426.

29. Zehnder C, Gutzwiller JP, Renggli K. Hemodiafiltration—a new treatment option for hyperphosphatemia in hemodialysis patients. *Clin Nephrol* 1999;52:152.

30. Lornoy W, Becaus I, Billiouw JM, et al. On-line haemodiafiltration. Remarkable removal of beta$_2$-microglobulin. Long-term clinical observations. *Nephrol Dial Transplant* 2000;15(suppl 1):49.

31. Maduell F, del Pozo C, Garcia H, et al. Change from conventional haemodiafiltration to on-line haemodiafiltration. *Nephrol Dial Transplant* 1999;14:1202.

32. Locatelli F, Mastrangelo F, Redaelli B, et al. Effects of different membranes and dialysis technologies on patient treatment tolerance and nutritional parameters. The Italian Cooperative Dialysis Study Group. *Kidney Int* 1996;50:1293.

33. Ward RA, Schmidt B, Hullin J, et al. A comparison of on-line hemodiafiltration and high-flux hemodialysis: a prospective clinical study. *J Am Soc Nephrol* 2000;11:2344.

34. Widjaja A, Kielstein JT, Horn R, et al. Free serum leptin but not bound leptin concentrations are elevated in patients with end-stage renal disease. *Nephrol Dial Transplant* 2000;15: 846.

35. Tetta C, Bellomo R, D'Intini V, et al. Do circulating cytokines really matter in sepsis? *Kidney Int Suppl* 2003;84:S69.

36. Niwa T, Asada H, Tsutsui S, et al. Efficient removal of albumin-bound furancarboxylic acid by protein-leaking hemodialysis. *Am J Nephrol* 1995;15:463.

37. Kawano Y, Takaue Y, Kuroda Y, et al.: Effect of alleviation of renal anemia by hemodialysis using the high flux dialyzer BK-F. *Kidney Dial* 1994;200.

38. Stein G, Franke S, Mahiout A, et al. Influence of dialysis modalities on serum AGE levels in end-stage renal disease patients. *Nephrol Dial Transplant* 16:999.

39. Van Telligen A, Grooteman MPC, Bartels PCM, et al. Long-term reduction of plasma homocysteine levels by super-flux dialyzers in hemodialysis patients. *Kidney Int* 2001;59:342.

40. Galli F, Benedetti S, Buoncristiani U, et al. The effect of PMMA-based protein-leaking dialyzers on plasma homocysteine levels. *Kidney Int* 2003;64:748.

41. Van der Sande FM, Kooman JP, Konings CJ, et al. Thermal effects and blood pressure response during postdilution hemodiafiltration and hemodialysis: the effect of amount of replacement fluid and dialysate temperature. *J Am Soc Nephrol* 2001;12:1916.

42. Chanard J, Brunois IP, Melin JP, et al. Long-term results of dialysis therapy with a highly permeable membrane. *Artif Organs* 1982;6:261.

43. Drueke TB, Eckardt KU, Frei U, et al. Does early anemia correction prevent complications of chronic renal failure? *Clin Nephrol* 1999;51:1.

44. Horl MP, Horl WH. Hemodialysis-associated hypertension: pathophysiology and therapy. *Am J Kidney Dis* 2002; 39:227.

45. Catizone L, Cocchi R, Fusaroli M, et al. Relationship between plasma beta 2-microglobulin and residual diuresis in continuous ambulatory peritoneal dialysis and hemodialysis patients. *Perit Dial Int* 1993;13(suppl 2):S523.

46. McKane W, Chandna SM, Tattersall JE, et al. Identical decline of residual renal function in high-flux biocompatible hemodialysis and CAPD. *Kidney Int* 2002;61:256.

47. van Tellingen A, Grooteman MP, Schoorl M, et al. Intercurrent clinical events are predictive of plasma C-reactive protein levels in hemodialysis patients. *Kidney Int* 2002;62:632.

48. Canaud B, Wizemann V, Pizzarelli F, et al. Cellular interleukin-1 receptor antagonist production in patients receiving on-line haemodiafiltration therapy. *Nephrol Dial Transplant* 2001;16:2181.

49. Deppisch RM, Beck W, Goehl H, et al. Complement components as uremic toxins and their potential role as mediators of microinflammation. *Kidney Int Suppl* 2001;78:S271.

50. Lindsay RM, Spanner E, Heidenheim AP, et al. A multicenter study of short hour dialysis using AN69S. Preliminary results. *ASAIO Trans* 1991;37:M465.

51. Schiffl H, Lang SM, Stratakis D, et al. Effects of ultrapure dialysis fluid on nutritional status and inflammatory parameters. *Nephrol Dial Transplant* 2001;16:1863.

52. Blankestijn PJ, Vos PF, Rabelink TJ, et al. High-flux dialysis membranes improve lipid profile in chronic hemodialysis patients. *J Am Soc Nephrol* 1995;5:1703.

53. Chun-Liang L, Chiu-Ching H, Chun-Chen Y, et al. Reduction of advanced glycation end products levels by on-line hemodiafiltration in long-term hemodialysis patients. *Am J Kidney Dis* 2003;42:524.

54. Ward RA, McLeish KR. Oxidant stress in hemodialysis patients: what are the determining factors? *Artif Organs* 2003; 27:230.

55. Morena M, Cristol JP, Bosc JY, et al. Convective and diffusive losses of vitamin C during haemodiafiltration session: a contributive factor to oxidative stress in haemodialysis patients. *Nephrol Dial Transplant* 2002;17:422.

56. Tattersall JE, Cramp M, Shannon M, et al. Rapid high-flux dialysis can cure uraemic peripheral neuropathy. *Nephrol Dial Transplant* 1992;7:539.

57. Locatelli F, Manzoni C, Di Filippo S. The importance of convective transport. *Kidney Int Suppl* 2002;80:115.

58. Lonnemann G, Koch KM. Beta(2)-microglobulin amyloidosis: effects of ultrapure dialysate and type of dialyzer membrane. *J Am Soc Nephrol* 2002;13(suppl 1):S72.

59. Lonnemann G. The quality of dialysate: an integrated approach. *Kidney Int Suppl* 2000;76:S112.

60. Lonnemann G, Koch KM. Replacement of renal function by dialysis. In: Jacobs C, Kjellstrand CM, Koch KM, Winchester JF, eds. *Replacement of Renal Function by Dialysis*, 4th. ed. Dordrecht/Boston/London: Kluwer, 1996:726.

61. Hillion D, Terki NH, Savoiu C, et al. Albumin loss with high-flux dialysers is underestimated (abstr). *J Am Soc Nephrol* 1999;10:283A.

Quality, Safety, and Accountability in Dialysis

Jay B. Wish

"A substantial number of ESRD facilities do not achieve minimum patient outcomes;...serious deficiencies...included medication errors, contamination of water used for dialysis, and insufficient physician involvement in patient care." – United States General Accounting Office, October 2003.[1]

The problems found in ESRD facilities in the United States mirror fundamental shortcomings in the American health care system in general, as described in the Institute of Medicine's (IOM) 2001 report "Crossing the Quality Chasm: A New Health Care System for the 21st Century."[2] The IOM concludes that "the American health care delivery system is in need of fundamental change." The concepts contained in this report apply equally well to the delivery of complex medical services such as renal replacement therapy throughout the developed world. It contrasts the current approach to health care with 10 "simple rules for the 21st century health care system," as summarized in Table 37–1. A common theme for these "simple rules" is the paradigm shift from health care system–centered care to patient-centered care. The IOM proposes six key aims for the twenty-first-century health care system, which are summarized in Table 37–2. The IOM points out that much of the quality "chasm" that currently exists in health care delivery is due to misaligned incentives between health care systems, payers, medical professionals, patients, technology, education, and legal liability. The IOM places responsibility for the fundamental restructuring of the health care delivery system to realign these incentives at the highest levels of the federal government, including Congress and the Department of Health and Human Services, with ongoing input from all stakeholders. Public and private purchasers, health care organizations, clinicians, and patients will have to work together to achieve the fundamental changes in organizational structure, information technology, education, reimbursement, accountability, and liability that will be required to conform with the 10 simple rules for health care delivery. As the IOM report makes very clear, multiple interrelated

TABLE 37–1. SIMPLE RULES FOR THE TWENTY-FIRST-CENTURY HEALTH CARE SYSTEM[2]

Current Approach	New Rule
Care is based primarily on visits.	Care is based on continuous healing relationships.
Variations in care are based on professional autonomy.	Variation in care, when it exists, is consequent to patient needs and values.
Professionals control care.	The patient is the source of control.
Information is a record.	Knowledge is shared and flows freely.
Decision making is based on training and experience.	Decision making is evidence-based.
"Do no harm" is an individual responsibility.	Safety is a system property.
Secrecy is necessary.	Transparency is necessary.
The system reacts to needs.	Needs are anticipated.
Cost reduction is sought.	Waste is continuously decreased.
Preference is given to professional roles over system.	Cooperation among clinicians is a priority.

dimensions of health care delivery must be addressed, improved, and aligned to shrink the quality chasm. Several of these dimensions have immediate relevance to the care of dialysis patients and include quality, safety, and accountability. Patient safety, which is a subset of health care quality, is defined as freedom from accidental injury stemming from the processes of health care.[3] Although patient safety is often equated with the reduction of medical errors, it actually emerges from the interaction of the components of the system and does not reside in a single process of care. Medical errors, both those of omission and commission, are a subset of safety, but patient safety also includes the establishment of an environment that is designed to minimize adverse events that may be unrelated to medical errors. Quality, in turn, can be seen as a subset of a larger universe of

TABLE 37–2. AIMS FOR THE TWENTY-FIRST-CENTURY HEALTH CARE SYSTEM[2]

Safety: Avoiding injuries to patients from the care that is intended to help them.

Effectiveness: Providing services based on scientific knowledge to all who could benefit and refraining from providing services to those not likely to benefit (avoiding underuse and overuse, respectively).

Patient-centeredness: Providing care that is respectful of and responsive to individual patient preferences, needs, and values and ensuring that patient values guide all clinical decisions.

Timeliness: Reducing waits and sometimes harmful delays for both those who receive and those who give care.

Efficiency: Avoiding waste, including waste of equipment, supplies, ideas, and energy.

Equitableness: Providing care that does not vary in quality because of patients' personal characteristics such as gender, ethnicity, geographic location, and socioeconomic status.

health care delivery attributes that Woolf[4] has termed "caring" in Fig. 37–1. This would include not only the traditional domains of quality but also patient experiences that are less easily measured and might include feelings of being unheard, rushed, inconvenienced, humiliated, or being unable to acquire desired information, instruction, or reassurance. Margaret Washington, the former executive director of an ESRD Network, surveyed over 1400 patients and 900 physicians to ascertain which "caring" issues are of foremost concern to patients and physicians and found, not surprisingly, that most of these hinge on improved patient-physician communication.[5] Patients wish that their physicians would have more flexible office hours, speak in terms they could better understand, give them undivided attention during their encounters, exhibit a less condescending attitude, and show more interest in the patient as a person rather than as a "case." In particular, dialysis patients wish their doctors would visit the dialysis unit more often, give them more regular feedback regarding their progress, and be more understanding when they are unable to be compliant with medications, diet, or dialysis scheduling. The IOM's strong recommendation regarding a shift to a patient-centered approach in health care delivery has led to the recent publication of a number of patient-centered approaches to ambulatory care access,[6] satisfaction,[7] and complaint resolution.[8,9] Of particular relevance to the dialysis population, with its high percentage of minority patients, are the findings of Cooper et al.[10] that racial concordance between patient and physician is associated with longer interactions, higher patient ratings of care, and improved

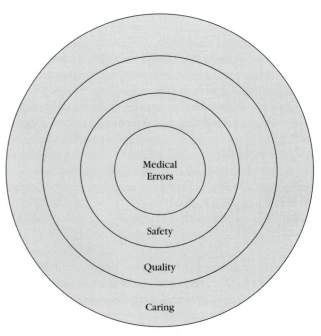

Figure 37–1. Domains of health care delivery. (Adapted from Woolf,[4] with permission.)

communication. This suggests that racial and ethnic discordance between dialysis patients and nephrologists may be an additional barrier to patient satisfaction, compliance, and favorable outcomes.

QUALITY

Quality in health care has taken on increased importance over the past decade, as payers, regulators, and patients have all demanded an improved product from health care providers. In the 1980s and early 1990s, the emphasis was on *quality assurance*. However, traditional quality assurance activities were never embraced by physicians because quality assurance departments in hospitals were generally staffed by nurses involved in risk management and utilization review, which fostered the concept that quality assurance was a burdensome, intrusive function with little impact on patient outcome. Although industry had successfully applied the principles of quality improvement for many years because of the opening of worldwide markets that forced manufacturers to focus on quality, American health care providers had been immune from competitive pressures until the increased penetration of capitated payment plans forced health care providers to lower costs and improve quality. In 1992, Medicare introduced the Health Care Quality Improvement Project (HCQIP), which redirected oversight organizations, such as peer review organizations and ESRD Networks, from a quality assurance to a quality improvement model. The successful application of this model at the dialysis provider level has led to a continuous

improvement in the processes of care, such as adequacy of dialysis and anemia management, as demonstrated by the ESRD Clinical Performance Measures Project[11,12] (Fig. 37–2).

The principles of quality improvement are so intuitive that it is difficult to understand why physicians have been so resistant to embracing them. Table 37–3 summarizes the benefits of quality improvement.[13] Quality improvement is similar to the differential diagnosis of a medical problem. First, one rules out a list of possible etiologies ("rule outs"). Then one initiates testing or therapy to rule out each possibility until the diagnosis is confirmed. Finally, one checks the patient for evidence of improvement to validate that the diagnosis and choice of therapy were correct. In quality improvement, a multidisciplinary team at the provider level examines an issue in which there is an opportunity for improvement. This might be a structural issue such as staffing ratios or the water treatment system, a process issue such as the drawing of postdialysis BUN levels or the administration of influenza vaccine, or an outcome issue such as a high percentage of patients with low *Kt/V* or with dialysis catheters. The team then brainstorms to list the "differential diagnosis," classified by category, such as procedures, equipment, policies, staff factors, and patient factors. The team then votes on which one or more of these causes might be responsible for the suboptimal performance and then develops and implements a change in process to test whether this improves performance. Data collected before and after the process change are compared; if significant improvements in performance occur following the change, then the process change is incorporated more widely.

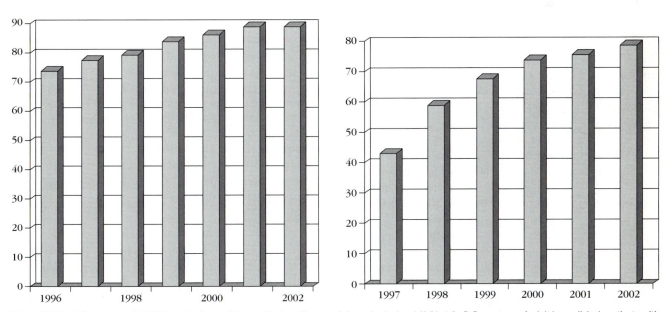

Figure 37–2. *A.* Percentage of adult in-center hemodialysis patients with mean delivered calculated *Kt/V* ≥1.2. *B.* Percentage of adult hemodialysis patients with mean hemoglobin ≥11 g/dL. (From 2003 Annual Report, ESRD Clinical Performance Measures Project.[12])

TABLE 37–3. BENEFITS OF QUALITY IMPROVEMENT

Improved patient outcomes
    Decreased morbidity and mortality
    Improved quality of life
    Improved satisfaction
Improved facility outcomes
    Increased patient census
        fewer absences for hospitalization
        decreased mortality
        increased market share
    Decreased costs
        increased efficiency
        improved employee retention and productivity
        improved risk management
        fewer regulatory hassles
Improved systemwide outcomes
    Decreased hospitalization expenses
    More cost-effective care
    Improved rehabilitation
    Contribution to evidence-based literature

Thus, the fundamental principles underlying quality improvement are as follows: (1) all work can be described as a process, (2) variation exists in every process, (3) the performance of processes can be measured, (4) measurement requires comparison, and (5) the goal is to reduce variation within acceptable limits by testing and validating the processes that will produce the best results. Although the advancement of evidence-based medicine and the proliferation of clinical practice guidelines have begun to clarify which care processes are likely to produce the best clinical outcomes, all providers face unique barriers to process improvement that must be identified at the facility level by those who know the processes best. For example, Sehgal et al.,[14,15] in a study of 29 hemodialysis facilities in northeastern Ohio, found that the three major barriers to adequacy of hemodialysis were low dialysis prescription, catheter use, and shortened treatment time, and that the individual facilities varied widely with regard to the percentage of patients with inadequate dialysis having each of these barriers. Quality improvement efforts to improve adequacy of dialysis had to be customized to the individual facility's unique barriers, and the authors concluded that a "one size fits all" approach to quality improvement by hemodialysis facilities, dialysis chains, or regulators is doomed to failure.

Ultimately, care represents a linkage of many processes and the success of quality improvement initiatives requires the empowerment of those individuals who are "in the trenches." An obstacle to the successful implementation of a quality improvement culture is management failing to relinquish power to its employees and to trust its employees to effectively use the resources that have been put at their disposal to improve processes of care and patient outcomes. Quality improvement has been described as both "bottom up" and "top down." The top-down aspect means that management must commit itself at the highest level (e.g., board of directors, chief executive officer) to a quality improvement culture and to allocate the resources necessary for a quality improvement program to succeed. This includes the data management infrastructure necessary to track processes and outcomes; education and training of staff in the principles and application of quality improvement techniques; providing employees with the protected time necessary to attend quality improvement meetings and to manage quality improvement data; and individuals in leadership positions, emphasizing their commitment to quality improvement through their own actions and words. The bottom-up aspect of quality improvement means that it is ultimately the workers, who execute the care processes on a daily basis, who are best qualified to examine which processes of care are most effective, identifying the barriers to improve outcomes, and ultimately implementing changes in processes to overcome those barriers and to benefit the patients. W. Edwards Deming, considered by many to be the "godfather" of continuous quality improvement methodology, articulated 14 areas of cultural change that are necessary for an institution to succeed in its quality improvement efforts.[16,17] These are summarized in Table 37–4.

Although the IOM[18] has developed a somewhat arcane definition of health care quality ("the degree to which health services for individuals and populations increase the likelihood of desired health outcomes and are consistent with current professional knowledge"), many health care providers, including physicians, may find it easier to relate to health care quality as a product delivered by a provider to a customer. This customer could be identified as the patient or the payer and, as in other markets, the customer can and should articulate whether or not the product meets expecta-

TABLE 37–4. DEMING'S FOURTEEN POINTS

1. Create constancy of purpose for the improvement of product or service.
2. Adopt the new philosophy.
3. Cease dependence on mass inspection.
4. End the practice of awarding business on price tag alone.
5. Improve constantly and forever the system of production and service.
6. Institute training and retraining.
7. Institute leadership.
8. Drive out fear.
9. Break down barriers between staff areas.
10. Eliminate slogans, exhortations, and targets for the work force.
11. Eliminate numerical quotas.
12. Remove barriers to pride of workmanship.
13. Institute a vigorous program of education and retraining.
14. Take action to accomplish the transformation.

tions. The expectations of a payer such as Medicare are very clear and are contained in the conditions for coverage for dialysis facilities. However, satisfying these conditions for coverage is merely meeting a minimum standard of care required of all dialysis providers and is quality assurance, not quality improvement. Because the ultimate goal of quality improvement is to improve outcomes for patients, the patient's perspective must be considered, and the use of patient satisfaction and quality-of-life instruments has become increasingly important to identify opportunities for process improvement, especially in the context of the ongoing paradigm shift to a more patient-centered health care delivery environment.[19]

The development of a data management infrastructure is essential to compare a provider's own performance to others and to itself over time. Data are a cornerstone of quality improvement. An adequate data management infrastructure is essential to enable repeated measurement of indicators over time and to permit inferences about causality and the improved decision making that is ultimately based on evidence.

Another cornerstone of quality improvement culture is the respect for the individual. Quality improvement projects succeed because they are owned and championed at the process level rather than at the executive level. The culture of quality improvement requires a paradigm shift from management to leadership, from control to coaching, from resistance to openness to change, from suspicion to trust, from an internal focus to a customer focus, and to seeing people as resources rather than commodities.

Physicians have traditionally resisted quality activities as second guessing by nonexperts and have almost invariably delegated quality activities to a head nurse or quality assurance coordinator. Quality improvement cannot be delegated; all individuals, especially those in leadership positions, must embrace it for it to succeed. The commitment of the nephrologist is particularly vital for quality improvement to succeed in the dialysis facility because the physician is a respected leader who sets an example by his or her own actions, and because the physician is a central figure for many of the care processes that ultimately affect patient outcomes. The failure of physician buy-in is a common barrier to the successful deployment of quality improvement at the provider level. Table 37–5 summarizes some of the other barriers.[13] It is easy to become discouraged about quality improvement because it does not always work on the first try. In a differential diagnosis of a medical problem, sometimes many negative tests are performed before a positive test ultimately identifies the nature of the problem. The same is true for quality improvement. The physicians, in particular the medical director of the dialysis facility, must have the patience to champion the quality improvement approach through several unsuccessful cycles until its inevitable success converts the skeptics and is integrated into

TABLE 37–5. BARRIERS TO QUALITY IMPROVEMENT

- Management does not allocate sufficient resources for data infrastructure, employee training, and protected staff time.
- Management behavior is not consistent and sends mixed message to employees.
- Management fears employee empowerment.
- Physician buy-in is not possible.
- There is no effort to identify and train effective team leaders.
- There is failure to identify a "champion" for a specific project.
- Discouragement or impatience regarding an unsuccessful project is readily expressed.
- Blame is readily assigned.

the facility's culture. Improvement of physician buy-in to quality improvement can be achieved by giving physicians their own individual data (they are scientists and they love data); by giving physicians comparative data (they are competitive and love to "win"); and by inducing physicians to attend quality improvement meetings by providing refreshments (physicians are busy and most likely to attend meetings if they are concurrent with meals). The medical director of a dialysis facility should provide leadership for staff physicians by identifying their individual interests and recruiting them as champions for specific quality improvement projects. The medical director is also in the best position to provide liaison between a dialysis facility's management, its staff, and the medical staff, providing advocacy leadership for the quality agenda and access to the evidence-based literature that may provide a template for process improvement.

The design and implementation of a quality improvement project (QIP) is relatively straightforward. The leadership of the facility must first make a commitment to adopting a quality improvement culture and providing the data, personnel, and educational resources that are necessary for its implementation. This could be a clinical outcome such as anemia management, a patient satisfaction issue such as waiting time to begin dialysis, an internal cost-effectiveness issue such as low dialyzer reuse, or a regulatory issue such as hepatitis testing. Next, a multidisciplinary team is constituted with interest and expertise in the project. Any literature regarding the issue should be gathered and shared among team members. The team should ascertain whether standards for this issue already exist and whether these can be used as a template for process improvement. The next step is to determine the scope of the data collection activity, including the sources of data, data collection tools, logistics of data collection, and methods of data analysis. The data are then managed to analyze the processes involved and to identify sources of variation. After the analysis of process has been completed, causes of process variation are identified and an intervention opportunity is selected. An improvement trial is designed and implemented, and follow-up data are collected and analyzed to determine whether the process change resulted in decreased variation and improved outcomes. Ultimately, the results of the project are reported back to team members and, if the intervention was successful, process change is implemented on a wider scale with continued cycles of follow-up for validation. Many of the tools used for quality improvement activities are summarized in Tables 37–6[20,21] and 37–7.[22]

It is essential that there be no assignment of blame throughout this quality improvement process. When a problem is identified, it should be determined how this system failed the individual rather than how the individual failed the system. Improvements to the system almost invariably lead to improvements in individual performance, and the "ownership" of the process by those responsible for implementing the process improves consistency, employee morale, and employee retention. The key features of quality improvement in health care are summarized in Table 37–8.

A successful QIP may lead to the discovery of a process improvement that can be applied more widely within the dialysis community. As such, the establishment of such a "benchmark" or "best practice" would constitute "generalizable knowledge," which is one of the defining attributes of research. Recently, the Office of Human Research Protection (OHRP) within the Department of Health

TABLE 37–6. TOOLS FOR QUALITY IMPROVEMENT

Task	Tool or Resource
Define opportunity for improvement	Examine existing data (statistical process control charts)
	Survey staff and patients
	Triggers from oversight bodies
Determine whether standards exist	National Kidney Foundation's Kidney Disease Outcomes Quality Initiative (K/DOQI) guidelines
	Benchmark facilities from ESRD network or corporate chain
Take a systematic approach to improvement	Plan-do-check-act cycle (Shewart)
	FOCUS-PDCA cycle (see Table 37–7)
Implement process analysis	Cause-and-effect diagrams ("fishbone")
	Flowcharts
	Process analysis diagrams
Employ data analysis	Check sheets
	Pareto diagrams
	Run charts
	Control charts
	Histograms
	Scatter diagrams
Implement change	New protocols
	Champion and team
	Behavioral change theory
Sustain change	Periodically repeat all of above
	Avoid complacency

Source: Adapted from McClellan and Goldman[20] and Wish,[21] with permission.

TABLE 37–7. FOCUS-PDCA APPROACH TO PROCESS IMPROVEMENT

F = Find a process to improve
O = Organize a quality improvement project team
C = Clarify the current process
U = Understand process variations
S = Select the process improvement strategy
P = Plan the improvement
D = Do (carry out the planned change)
C = Check the results
A = Act to adopt more widely

Source: Model recommended by the Joint Commission on Accreditation of Healthcare Organizations.[22]

and Human Services determined that because quality improvement activities are "a systematic investigation, involving the collection on identifiable private information and data through intervention or interaction, designed to develop or contribute to generalizable knowledge," they meet the definition of research specified in the U.S. Code of Federal Regulations and are therefore required to undergo review by an Institutional Review Board (IRB). Since a QIP involves a process change which is designed to improve an outcome but which could conceivably result in an adverse outcome, the intent of the OHRP ruling is to offer patients involved in QIPs the same protection they would receive if they were involved in a more traditional clinical research project. In most cases, the IRB will determine that patients involved in a QIP are not at risk and that the QIP is exempted from further IRB review and informed patient consent. It has been proposed that institutional or regional quality improvement boards, operating in parallel to the current IRBs, be established as a means of ensuring that patients participating in QIPs are protected. This would prevent the current IRB system from being overwhelmed with QIP reviews and would be designed to expedite review and exemption of QIPs in which patients are not at risk.[23]

TABLE 37–8. KEY FEATURES OF HEALTH CARE QUALITY

Methods
Internally and externally customer-driven
Management by fact
Respect for people
Teamwork
Disciplined problem-solving process
Results
Appropriateness: balancing benefit and risk
Effectiveness: ability of intervention to achieve desired outcome in population
Efficiency: ability to provide effective care at lowest possible cost
Safety: minimizing adverse effects of interventions
Consistency: minimize variability of process and outcome
Patient satisfaction: ability to meet or exceed expectations

Despite the published success of quality improvement activities in dialysis facilities[24,25] and in the Medicare population,[26,27] there remains considerable skepticism regarding the business case for quality in health care, especially in dialysis, where high up-front costs for data management infrastructure, personnel, and education are less likely to be offset by increased revenues because of the high mortality rate of the patient population. A glaring example of this lack of alignment between quality and economics was experienced by Children's Hospital and Health Center in San Diego, California where, as a result of 92 percent adherence to its 62 clinical pathways, the facility reduced treatment costs by $5.2 million over 6 years and increased its market share of the area's pediatric population of patients (14 years old and under) from 46 to 70 percent. This increase in market share was achieved with fewer staff because the pathways provided increased clinical efficiency, effectiveness, and care coordination as well as improved communication. But because the pathways lowered the average length of stay per hospital admission and payers typically reimburse pediatric hospitals on a per-diem basis, the hospital experienced a $19.1 million operating loss in 2002 (compared to a $12.4 million operating loss in 2001).[28] In a review of other studies that examined strategies to improve patient care—such as physician education, provider feedback on performance, delegation of tasks, reminders, improved data infrastructure, continuous quality improvement, and patient-oriented interventions—Grol[29] found that physician-oriented strategies were of limited or mixed effectiveness, patient-oriented strategies were more effective, and combined strategies, especially those that incorporate information systems to align financial incentives, were most effective. Grol recommended a more widespread application of integrated methods and comprehensive programs that combine, for instance, evidence-based guidelines, clinical pathways, indicators for continuous assessment, and quality improvement projects embedded within a wider quality system. He noted the success of some disease management programs in the United States, where quality and financial incentives are aligned to benefit the patient, health plan, and disease management organization. Only by crossing borders between professional pride and self-regulation, external accountability, payer profit, organizational development, and pleasing and involving patients can we overcome the obstacles to optimal medical care.[29]

PATIENT SAFETY

In 2000, the Institute of Medicine published its landmark report, *To Err is Human: Building a Safer Health System*,[3] which noted that between 44,000 and 98,000 patients in America die each year as a result of medical errors. This makes medical errors the eighth leading cause of death and

results in additional national costs of $17 to $29 billion, of which health care costs represent over half. In addition to the economic costs, morbidity, and mortality, medical errors result in a loss of trust in the health care system by patients, loss of morale by health care professionals, loss of worker productivity by employers, and reduced school attendance by children. The authors note that the decentralized and fragmented nature of the health care delivery system contributes to unsafe conditions for patients, yet licensing and accreditation processes have focused limited attention on the issue. Health care organizations and providers have not focused on patient safety because of issues regarding liability risk exposure when efforts to uncover and learn from errors are successful. Medical errors can be of omission or of commission; the types of medical errors are summarized in Table 37–9.[30]

The IOM report noted that health care services are a complex and technologic industry prone to accidents, especially because many of its components are not well integrated. Nonetheless, much can be done to make systems more reliable and safe, as the failure of large systems is due to multiple faults that occur together. One of the greatest contributions to accidents in any industry, including health care, is human error. Humans commit errors for a variety of known and complicated reasons, but most human errors are induced by system failures. Redesigning the system to prevent human errors is more productive than assigning blame. Latent areas are more insidious because they are difficult for people working in the system to identify, as they may be hidden in computers or layers of management, and people become accustomed to working around the problem. Latent

TABLE 37–9. TYPES OF MEDICAL ERRORS

Diagnostic
Error or delay in diagnosis
Failure to employ indicated tests
Use of outmoded tests
Failure to act on results of tests

Therapeutic
Error in performance of an operation, procedure, or test
Error in administering a treatment
Error in the dose or method of using a drug
Use of outmoded therapy
Avoidable delay in treatment or in responding to an abnormal test result
Inappropriate (not indicated) treatment

Preventive
Failure to provide prophylactic treatment
Inadequate monitoring or follow-up of treatment

Other
Failure of communication
Equipment failure
Other system failure

SOURCE: Adapted from Leape et al.,[30] with permission.

errors can and should be identified long before an active error, and these pose the greatest threat to safety in a complex system because they lead to operator errors. Current error reporting and response systems tend to focus on active errors, but discovering and fixing latent errors and decreasing their duration is more likely to have a greater effect on building safer systems because this will prevent active errors before they occur.

The IOM report made a number of recommendations to federal agencies and health care providers to improve patient safety.[3] These are summarized in Table 37–10.

Following the release of the IOM report on patient safety, the Renal Physicians Association, Forum of ESRD Networks, and National Patient Safety Foundation cosponsored a consensus conference of stakeholders in end-stage renal disease (ESRD) to establish a patient safety agenda for the ESRD community. One of the first steps was to agree on a glossary of patient safety terms, which are summarized in Table 37–11.[3,31] Representatives of five of the six largest dialysis chains in the United States ranked their most problematic patient safety issues; these were compiled at the stakeholders meeting and are listed in Table 37–12. Note that although many of these patient safety issues are related to medical errors, some, such as patient falls and access cannulation problems, may respond to improved systems of care, which is why the concentric circle for patient safety encompasses that for medical errors in Fig. 37–1.

The collaborative effort between the Renal Physicians Association, Forum of ESRD Networks, and the National Patient Safety Foundation led to the articulation of 47 action options to improve ESRD patient safety,[32] many of which parallel those of the IOM in the *To Err is Human* report.[3] Many of these action options are national efforts that will require further funding if they are to be tackled. At the individual provider level, however, efforts will be required to raise awareness about the magnitude of the patient safety issue and the need for change, along with a change in the culture of the provider to a blameless one in which staff regularly report "near misses" without fear of retribution. Systems must be implemented to track errors and adverse events such that patterns can be identified and systems can be improved. Since medical errors occur at the operator level, it is essential that a dialysis unit's staff be trained in the safety sciences and that errors and adverse events are viewed as opportunities for prevention rather than as evidence of individual failure. Patient safety officers should be designated to stay current with the patient safety literature, which is expanding rapidly, so that proven safety practices can be implemented in the facility without delay. In their review of patient safety in ESRD, Kliger and Diamond[33] use real case studies to illustrate how near misses can alert a facility to the presence of systemic problems, which, when corrected, will prevent future injury. In one case, a patient was dialyzed with another patient's dialyzer and suffered no harm, but this alerted the facility to the fact that its procedures for pairing a patient with a reprocessed dialyzer were not followed due to short staffing and led to a system change which matched patients to their dialyzers based on bar coding. In another case, a patient was treated in a hospital emergency room with an antibiotic that prolonged the effect of warfarin, leading to prolonged bleeding from his needle puncture sites after the dialysis treatment. This underscored the system failure for data sharing among the patient's health care providers, as the physician who prescribed the antibiotic was unaware that the patient was taking warfarin. The dialysis facility, hospital, and nursing home caring for the patient subsequently implemented a shared data system for patient pharmaceuticals along with a computer-driven system to alert clinicians about potential drug–drug interactions.

As with quality improvement, the key to success in improving patient safety is the cultural change at the organizational level to promote a blameless environment. Health care providers must receive education in the safety sciences particularly with regard to the importance of error detection and reporting, and a data collection and reporting infrastructure must be developed to track and eliminate latent errors and near misses before they become active errors and adverse events.

The tensions between the tort system and patient safety demand that the adversarial dispute resolution paradigm in health care be reexamined.[34] Although it is possible that appeals to physicians' ethical commitments to patient welfare and the demonstrated successes of industry-based models of systemic quality improvement may gradu-

TABLE 37–10. RECOMMENDATIONS OF THE INSTITUTE OF MEDICINE TO IMPROVE PATIENT SAFETY

Establish a Center for Patient Safety within the Agency for Healthcare Research and Quality

Establish a mandatory nationwide reporting system for the most serious medical errors and a voluntary nationwide reporting system for less serious medical errors

Extend peer-review protections to safety data used for improving safety and quality

Focus greater attention on patient safety by regulators and purchasers of health care services

Improve performance standards and expectations of health care professionals regarding patient safety through education and credentialing

Improve FDA oversight of drug packaging, labeling, and naming to minimize medication errors

Define executive responsibility for patient safety and institute patient safety programs at the health care organization and professional levels

Implement proven medication safety practices

SOURCE: Adapted from Kohn et al.[3]

TABLE 37–11. BASIC PATIENT SAFETY GLOSSARY

Accident: An event that involves damage to a defined system that disrupts the ongoing or future output of the system.

Active error: An error that occurs at the level of the front-line operator, the effects of which are felt almost immediately.

Adverse event: Untoward, undesirable, and usually unanticipated event directly associated with care or services provided within the jurisdiction of a medical center, outpatient clinic, or other facility. Examples of common adverse events include patient falls, medication errors, unexpected reactions or complications, procedural errors or complications, completed suicides, parasuicidal behaviors (attempts/gestures/threats), and missing patient events. Note that although not all adverse events are due to errors, they still represent safety issues.

Bad outcome: Failure to achieve a desired outcome of care.

Error: The failure of a planned action to be completed as intended or the use of a wrong plan to achieve an aim. Errors can include problems in practice, products, procedures, and systems.

Genotype: The characteristic collection of factors that lead to the surface, phenotypical appearance of the event.

Latent error: Errors in design, organization, training, or maintenance that lead to operator errors and whose effects typically lie dormant in the system for long periods of time.

Microsystem: Organization built around the definition of repeatable core service competencies. Elements of a microsystem include (1) a core team of health care professionals, (2) a defined population of patients, (3) carefully designed work processes, and (4) an environment capable of linking information on all aspects of work and patient or population outcomes to support ongoing evaluation of performance.

Near miss: An event or situation that could have resulted in an accident injury or illness, but did not, either by chance or through timely intervention. Also known as a close call or near hit.

Patient safety: Freedom from accidental injury stemming from the processes of health care. Safety emerges from the interaction of the components of the system; it does not reside in a person, device or department. Improving safety depends on learning how safety emerges from the interactions of the components and processes that minimize the likelihood of errors and maximize the likelihood of intercepting them before they occur. Patient safety is a subset of health care quality.

Phenotype: What happens in an incident; what people actually do or what they do wrong; what you can observe. This is specific to the local situation and context; it is the surface appearance of the incident.

Quality of care: Degree to which health services for individuals and populations increase the likelihood of desired health outcomes and are consistent with current professional knowledge.[18]

Risk management: Clinical, administrative, and manufacturing activities undertaken to identify, evaluate, and reduce the risk of injury to patients, staff, and visitors and the risk of loss to the organization itself. Risk containment is a subset of immediate actions taken to safeguard patients from the repetition of an unwanted occurrence.

Root cause: The most fundamental reason an event has occurred.

Sentinel events: An unexpected occurrence involving death or serious physical or psychological injury or the risk thereof. Serious injury specifically includes loss of limb or function. The phrase "risk thereof" includes any process variation for which a recurrence would carry a significant chance of a serious adverse outcome. Such events are called "sentinel" because they signal the need for immediate investigation and response.

Standard: A minimum level of acceptable performance or results, *or* excellent levels of performance, *or* the range of acceptable performance or results.

System: Set of interdependent elements interacting to achieve a common aim. These elements may be both human and nonhuman (equipment, technologies, etc.).

SOURCE: Adapted from Kohn et al.,[3] with permission, National ESRD Patient Safety Initiative, Phase II Report.[31]

---

ally yield buy-in to safety initiatives, the success of this approach is doubtful, because the conflicts between the tort system and error reduction programs are fundamental and severe, and physicians' concerns about being sued and losing their liability insurance have escalated considerably in recent years. A tort reform strategy may allay some of these concerns by health care providers, but while reducing economic exposure, tort reform does not create a more efficient system. In a no-fault system, an injured patient would only have to demonstrate that a disability was caused by medical management as opposed to the disease process; there would be no need to prove negligence. Such an approach would be better aligned with the blameless philosophy of patient safety and quality improvement, which emphasizes evidence-based analysis of systems of care. A no-fault approach to patient injury would also align incentives for risk reduction, especially if hospitals and their medical staffs are insured by the same entity and all efforts to prevent medical errors are undertaken jointly. Blame and economic punishment for errors that are made by well-intentioned people working in the health care system drives the problem of patient safety underground and alienates people who are best placed to prevent such problems from recurring. On the other hand, failure to assign blame when it is due is also undesirable as it erodes trust in the medical profession. Although it is important to meet society's needs to blame and extract retribution when appropriate, this should not be a prerequisite for compensation as the current tort system requires. The business case for patient safety is much more clear-cut than that for quality improvement. Although the litigation losses associated with medical errors are relatively low, preventable adverse events are likely to result in substantial personnel, regulatory and marketing costs that may impair profitability and compromise organizational perfor-

TABLE 37–12. SAFETY ISSUES INVOLVING DIALYSIS PATIENTS

1. Falls
2. Medication errors, including
   Deviation from prescription
   Allergic or other adverse reactions
   Omissions
3. Access-related events, including
   Clots
   Infiltrates
   Difficult cannulation
   Poor blood flow
4. Dialysis errors
   Incorrect dialyzer
   Incorrect line
   Incorrect dialysate
   Dialyzer or dialysis-equipment-related sepsis
5. Excessive blood loss
   Separation of blood lines
   Improper hookup
   Prolonged bleeding from needle sites

Source: Adapted from National ESRD Patient Safety Initiative Phase II Report.[31]

mance.[36] In addition, marketing costs of adverse events, in terms of lost public confidence and tarnished reputation, could threaten organizational survival. Ultimately, for patient safety efforts to succeed, patients, health care providers, and the legal system must understand the distinction between blameworthy behavior and the inevitable human errors that result from the systemic factors that underlie most failures and complex systems.

ACCOUNTABILITY

Even if an ideal blameless culture for patient safety and quality improvement were achieved, there must be accountability. There is a hierarchy of accountability within each dialysis unit organization, between chain facilities and their corporate parent, and between dialysis providers (including nephrologists), payers, regulators, and patients. Since Medicare funds are used to pay for most ESRD services in the United States and these funds are appropriated by Congress, Congress holds the Centers for Medicare and Medicaid Services (CMS) accountable for assuring that the dialysis services purchased with these funds is of high quality. The 2003 report by the General Accounting Office[1] cited at the beginning of this chapter is not the first to suggest that the quality of dialysis services in the United States falls short of Congressional expectations. In 1991, the Institute of Medicine reported "It is time to establish an advisory group of nephrology professionals and experts in quality as-

sessment and design to develop ESRD-specific quality assessment and quality assurance systems."[37] In 1994, a national expert panel examining quality of care in the United States ESRD program recommended "The Federal government needs to develop a far more comprehensive and coordinated strategy for quality improvement in the ESRD program than it has to date."[38] The mortality rate for ESRD patients in the United States has consistently been higher than that in Europe, Japan, and Australia and, although some argue that this is caused by differences in case mix,[39] data from the United States Renal Data System (USRDS)[40] and from the Dialysis Practice Patterns and Outcomes Study (DOPPS)[41,42] suggest that this is not entirely the case. The progressive consolidation of dialysis interests in the United States, dominated by the for-profit dialysis chains, has raised concerns that quality of care has been compromised to maximize stockholder returns. In June 2000, the Office of the Inspector General (OIG) issued a report[43] recommending that CMS hold individual dialysis facilities more fully accountable for the quality of care delivered to ESRD patients and that CMS use facility-specific performance measures to encourage facilities to improve the quality of care and ensure that facilities meet minimum standards of operation. The OIG report indicated that the current system of oversight of ESRD patients falls short in several respects, including the following: (1) standardized performance data are rarely used to hold individual facilities accountable; (2) the complaint system serves as an unreliable means for identifying and resolving quality of care concerns, (3) Medicare certification surveys play a limited role in ensuring facilities meet minimum standards, and (4) medical injuries are not systematically monitored. The OIG recommended that CMS revise the Medicare conditions for coverage for dialysis facilities so that they serve as a more effective foundation for accountability; that CMS use facility-specific performance measures to encourage facilities to improve the quality of care and to help facilities meet minimum standards; that CMS strengthen the complaint system for dialysis patients and staff; that CMS enhance the role of Medicare on-site certification surveys; and that CMS facilitate the development of publicly accountable means for identifying serious medical injuries and analyzing their causes.

In June 2000, the GAO also released a report[44] that was particularly critical of the relative infrequency of onsite inspections by state survey agencies, pointing out that in 1999 only 11 percent of facilities were surveyed. At this survey rate, once the dialysis facility receives its initial certification, it is not likely to be resurveyed for about 9 years. The GAO also reported that the percentage of surveyed facilities with conditions for coverage deficiencies increased from 6 percent in 1993 to 15 percent in 1999. The GAO report observed that CMS lacked enforcement tools for facilities that failed to comply with the Medicare conditions of coverage. The GAO recommended that the frequency of onsight inspections by state surveys be increased by the allocation of additional congressional funds for this purpose.

Despite the allocation of those additional funds, the follow-up GAO report in 2003[1] noted that CMS's goal to resurvey 33 percent of ESRD facilities annually had not been achieved on a consistent basis. Fifteen states failed to meet this goal in either fiscal year 2001 or 2002, and the percentage of facilities nationwide that went nine or more years without an inspection increased from 1.6 percent in fiscal year 1998 to 5.4 percent in fiscal year 2002. The 2003 GAO report also noted an unacceptably high frequency of a number of deficiencies noted by state surveyors which could adversely affect patient outcomes, including failure to monitor laboratory values and medication supply, failure to administer medication as prescribed, failure to administer dialysis treatments as prescribed, failure to monitor concentration of chemicals in the water system, and failure to involve a transplant surgeon in the review of the patient's long-term care plan.[1]

It should be pointed out that both the OIG and the GAO reports endorse the dual oversight model of the ESRD program, with the 18 ESRD Networks facilitating a quality improvement approach to patient care processes and outcomes through a confidential and collegial relationship with dialysis providers and with the state survey agencies continuing to take a quality assurance approach to investigate and enforce compliance with Medicare's condition for coverage, which are the minimum standards for operation of a dialysis facility designed to minimize patient harm. These two contrasting approaches are summarized in Table 37–13. Both the OIG and GAO reports recommended that there be increased information sharing between the ESRD Networks and state survey agencies to identify and target for intervention those facilities with the greatest opportunities for improvement.

TABLE 37–13. DUAL OVERSIGHT MODEL OF THE ESRD PROGRAM

Quality Improvement	Quality Assurance
ESRD networks	State survey agencies
Collegial mode	Regulatory mode
Educate and elevate	Investigate and enforce
Cooperative	Challenging
Flexible	Rigid
Foster process improvements	Enforce minimums
Guidance	Directive
Trusting	Skeptical
Professional accountability	Public accountability
Confidentiality	Public disclosure
Systems focus	Outlier focus
Improve patient outcomes	Minimize preventable harm

Source: Adapted from the Department of Health and Human Services.[43]

The 1997 Balanced Budget Act (BBA) enacted by Congress requires the Secretary of Health and Human Services to develop and implement a method to measure and report on the quality of dialysis services provided under Medicare. CMS contracted with a peer review organization in 1998 to develop scientifically validated clinical performance measures derived from the National Kidney Foundation's Kidney Disease Outcomes Quality Initiative (NKF-K/DOQI) clinical practice guidelines. These clinical performance measures—which address dialysis adequacy, anemia management, and nutrition—are currently applied to random sample hemodialysis and peritoneal dialysis patients on an annual basis to generate a "snapshot" cross-sectional analysis of regional and national outcomes. The outcomes for Kt/V and hemoglobin in adult hemodialysis patients for 2002 and previous years are illustrated in Fig. 37–2. Although the national trend of continuous improvement in these parameters is favorable, the 2003 GAO report (1) observed that in 512 of the 3158 hemodialysis facilities for which data were available, 20 percent or more patients had inadequate dialysis [urea reduction ratio (URR) less than 65 percent], and in nearly 1700 of 3325 dialysis facilities for which data were available, 20 percent or more patients had inadequate anemia management as defined as a hematocrit less than 33 percent. At 135 facilities, more than 50 percent of patients had a hematocrit less than 33 percent. The GAO report noted that research has shown variation in such patient outcomes as dialysis adequacy is largely attributable to factors at the facility such as its policies governing patient care, associated practice patterns, and attention to individual patient outcomes, as opposed to patient-specific causes.[45] The ESRD Clinical Performance Measures Project[12] does not currently collect facility-specific outcome data. The data cited in the 2003 GAO report[1] were from Medicare billing data, as a dialysis facility is required to provide the hematocrit of each patient when it bills Medicare for erythropoietin and to indicate a range within which each patient's URR falls when it submits a bill to Medicare for the dialysis composite rate.

Facility-specific hematocrit and URR data, along with facility-specific standardized ratios for mortality, hospitalization, and transplantation, are compiled each year by the Kidney, Epidemiology and Cost Center (KECC) at the University of Michigan for every dialysis facility under contract with CMS. The facility-specific profiles are sent to the respective ESRD Networks for distribution to the individual facilities, to state surveyor agencies, and posted in a "consumer-friendly" form on Medicare's "Dialysis Facility Compare" website (www.medicare.gov/Dialysis/Home.asp). The standardized ratios for dialysis patients were developed in the early 1980s by Wolfe et al. at the USRDS using multivariate analysis case mixed adjustment methodologies that had been previously applied to other populations. The standardized mortality ratio (SMR) for a facility is the observed number of deaths in a given year divided by the expected number of patient deaths in that year. The expected number of patient deaths is calculated by adding up the individual death rates for each of the patients in the cohort, corrected for days at risk. The expected death rate for an individual patient was originally determined by his or her age, gender, race and the presence or absence of diabetes as the cause of the ESRD. More recently, the KECC has further adjusted the expected death rate by the number of years the patient has been on dialysis as well as by a facility comorbidity index, facility body-mass index (BMI), and population death rates. The facility co-morbidity index is derived from the comorbidities of the facility's patients as indicated on the CMS End Stage Renal Disease Medical Evidence Form (2728), which is completed by a patient's nephrologist when the patient initiates renal replacement therapy. The methodology for deriving the facility comorbidity index was described by the KECC in an abstract in 2001[46]; but, as of this writing, it has not undergone the scrutiny of publication in a peer-reviewed journal.

Lacson et al.[47] examined some of the limitations of the facility-specific SMR for profiling health care quality in dialysis. The authors used four distinct statistical methods—USRDS, Poisson, logistic, and Cox regression—to compute facility-specific SMRs and found that the different methods produced statistically different differences in SMR distribution. Of the SMR methods used, the USRDS - method, the one being employed by CMS to trigger intervention activities by state survey and certification agencies and to classify facilities for consumer awareness on the Dialysis Facility Compare website, produced the least stable SMR-based ranking of facilities over time. Although facility-specific SMR may be useful as an epidemiologic research tool or to drive internal quality improvement activities, Lacson et al. cautioned that regulatory monitoring, actions, and/or performance recognition based on the SMR should be avoided.

Krumholz et al.[48] also concluded that hospital ratings based on mortality data poorly discriminated between any two individual hospitals' processes of care. They concluded that limitations in discrimination may undermine the value of health care quality ratings based on mortality and may lead to misperceptions of hospitals' performance. The ESRD Network of Texas Medical Review Board (MRB) noted a poor correlation between the USRDS-method SMR and deficiencies noted in state licensure surveys. In a June 2000 position paper,[49] the MRB specifically recommended against the use of the SMR to target dialysis facility surveys for state survey and certification activities. The MRB found that the model was weak due to lack of validation and was not predictive. In fact, the MRB found that random selection of dialysis facilities for survey and certification activity was preferable to SMR targeting as numerous serious deficiencies related to health and safety were discovered in fa-

cilities that had superior SMR data and thus would not have been selected based on such a trigger. The SMR also fails to meet several of the key attributes of a clinical performance measure as specified by the IOM,[50] which are listed below:

1. Have a solid evidence basis.
2. Measure clinical performance (not cost or utilization).
3. Be actionable by a provider or professional.
4. Cover the domains of interest.
5. Specify methodologic considerations.
6. Be biometrically tested for validity, sensitivity, specificity, reliability, and reproducibility.

The KECC facility-specific profiles also provide a standardized hospitalization ratio and standardized transplantation ratio which uses a similar methodology to the SMR, adding up the individual patients' hospitalization rates and transplantation events for each of the patients in the cohort, corrected for days at risk. The facility-specific hospitalization and transplant data are not currently posted on the Dialysis Facility Compare website for consumer consideration, but are distributed to the respective state Departments of Health to trigger survey activities and to the individual facilities to drive internal quality improvement.

The use of the same data for internal quality improvement activities and for external quality oversight and consumer choice raises several concerns. Traditionally, quality data shared between a health care provider and its respective peer-review organization, or specifically between a dialysis facility and its ESRD Network, have been confidential and nondiscoverable, so that there is the highest probability that the data will be valid and free of "gaming." Such data can be used to drive internal quality improvement processes at the facility level and allow the respective ESRD Network to target the outlier facilities for confidential and collegial quality improvement intervention activities. As soon as quality data become public, either through their release to Medicare state survey and certification agencies, to the Dialysis Facility Compare website or other patient-accessible media, there is inevitably a gaming, which undermines the effective use of these same data for internal quality improvement activities. This effect was demonstrated in a comparison by ESRD Networks 9 and 10 of confidential quality improvement hematocrit and urea reduction ratio (URR) data collected from facilities for quality improvement purposes with hematocrit and URR data submitted to Medicare on billing forms by those same facilities over the same time period. Although the hematocrit data provided for quality improvement represented the first blood draw of the month and the hematocrit data provided for Medicare billing represented the last blood draw of the month, there were significant differences between the two data sets that could not be explained by random variation alone. Not surprisingly, the quality improvement hematocrit data tended to show higher hematocrits, which might be rewarded through Network recognition, while the billing hematocrit data tended to be lower, which would minimize the likelihood of a facility having its erythropoietin billings challenged by the local fiscal intermediary.[51] The URR data for internal quality improvement collected by the network was a much larger data set than the URR data collected by Medicare on the billing forms. As the Medicare billing forms did not require the entry of a URR code for dialysis reimbursement, there was a self-censoring of lower URRs on the Medicare billing forms when those data were compared with the more complete data set that was collected by the Network for quality improvement purposes.[52]

Another major concern regarding the public release of performance data is that of "cherry picking" of the most compliant and healthiest patients to make a facility's performance measure profile appear more favorable, masking process deficiencies and undermining the quality improvement process.[39] This phenomenon has already been observed in Texas, where a unique relationship existed between the ESRD Network and the state Department of Health with increased sharing of quality data to trigger state survey and licensure activities. Texas has experienced a growth of patients discharged from their dialysis facility due to noncompliance issues, which far exceeds that observed in other parts of the country. Although most of the community recognizes the need for public accountability by health care providers, there is considerable evidence that patients do not use these data consistently to make choices among health care providers and health care plans. Nonetheless, the public reporting of quality data has sensitized health care providers to their opportunities for process and outcomes improvements and, in that sense, has improved the overall quality of health care delivery.[53]

The use of physician "report cards" for quality improvement, accountability, and patient choice also is controversial. ESRD Networks 9 and 10 concluded that its use of confidential, nephrologist-specific outcomes reports on dialysis adequacy, anemia management, vascular access, and nutrition was effective in improving the rate of improvement in these parameters in the Network's four-state area as compared to the rate of improvement of these same parameters in the nation.[54] In a randomized controlled trial comparing the use of physician-specific outcomes feedback with an identical outcomes feedback plus achievable benchmark feedback among 70 community physicians caring for almost 3000 diabetic Medicare patients in Alabama, Kiefe et al.[55] found that the use of achievable benchmarks significantly enhanced the effectiveness of physician performance feedback as compared to profiling alone. However, in another study of 232 physicians caring for 3642 patients with type 2 diabetes, the use of physician report cards was unable to reliably detect practice differences and was shown to

result in the deselecting of patients with high prior costs, poor adherence, or poor response to treatments (cherry picking).[56] Landon et al.[57] emphasize that in order for performance measures to be successful, they must be evidence-based, have agreed on standards for satisfactory performance (benchmarking), have standardized specifications, provide adequate sample size for reliable estimate of individual physician performance, have appropriate adjustment for confounding patient factors (case mix), allow for care to be attributable to the individual physician, be feasible to collect, and be representative of the activities of the specialty. In a more complete report, *Physician Clinical Performance Assessment: The State of the Art. Issues, Possibilities, and Challenges for the Future*,[58] these same authors make the important distinction between the attributes of performance measures used for quality improvement and those used for accountability (credentialing, financial incentives, and selection). As the purpose of quality improvement measures is to improve quality and decrease variation, statistical ability to discriminate between providers, performance level cutoffs, and statistical modeling are unnecessary. On the other hand, these same attributes are absolutely essential if performance measures are to be used for accountability, and a much higher level of statistical robustness and evidence basis is required for quality measures used for accountability vs. quality improvement. These authors observe that currently used physician performance measures are not sufficiently robust to use for assessing physician competence, to reward physician outcomes, or to use for selection by patients and families. The authors conclude that current state-of-the-art physician clinical performance assessment is best suited to promote continuous clinical quality improvement within the physician's practice environment. Although measurement of physician clinical performance is possible, use of this information for reporting external to the physicians' practice environment for purposes of physician competence assessment, patient choice, and rewarding physician excellence is limited by concerns that most of these performance measures do not meet the criteria outlined above. Premature or inappropriate use of physician performance measures for external accountability or selection may stifle quality improvement activities, lead to manpower shifts and patient access to care issues as opportunity costs for compliance, lead to data gaming, which inaccurately depicts the data quality and, most unfortunately, lead to cherry picking of patients.

Such concerns notwithstanding, the ESRD program in the United States is under increasing scrutiny by Congress and Medicare as the cost of the ESRD program continues to escalate both in terms of absolute dollars and as a percentage of total Medicare expenditures,[40] as quality of care issues linger based on the most recent GAO report,[1] and because of the focus on chronic kidney disease as one of the target areas in the blueprint for the federal government's next decade of health care quality improvement efforts, *Healthy People 2010*.[59] Specific recommendations within the *Healthy People 2010* document with relevance to ESRD include the goal to increase the proportion of new hemodialysis patients who use arteriovenous fistulas as the primary mode of vascular access, to increase the proportion of dialysis patients registered on the waiting list for transplantation, to increase the proportion of patients with chronic kidney failure who receive a transplant within 3 years of registration on the waiting list, and to reduce deaths from cardiovascular disease in patients with chronic kidney failure. To provide more detailed oversight of process and outcome at the dialysis provider level, CMS is developing a "core data set" that will include data elements, standardized data definitions, and specifications for the frequency of collection. It is anticipated that the core data set will include all of the data elements currently collected by the national ESRD Clinical Performance Measures Project but will be expanded to include all patients rather than a random sample and will include many elements not currently captured by the ESRD Clinical Performance Measures Project. CMS is also developing a data collection infrastructure which will require electronic transmission of patient-specific data from dialysis providers and corporate chains to the ESRD Networks and to CMS. This data collection infrastructure will capture the core data set, but will also replace the paper forms currently used by dialysis facilities such as the Medical Evidence Form (2728), the Death Report (2746), and the Annual Facility Survey (2744). Patient tracking among renal replacement therapy modalities will also be included in this new electronic data system named VISION (Vital Information Structure for Improvement of Outcomes in Nephrology). Individual dialysis facilities will enter the required data through a secure website and large corporate chains will submit data on behalf of all of their facilities through a periodic data "dump." Ultimately, the facility and patient-specific data acquired through VISION and its Network to CMS data transmission counterpart SIMS (Standard Information Management System) will be integrated with ESRD data from other sources including Medicare billing data, USRDS data, United Network for Organ Sharing (USOS) data and additional data collected through special studies or other sources. This integrated data system is named CROWN (consolidated renal operations in a web-enabled network) and will be used by CMS and other health care planners in the federal government to formulate policy regarding quality and reimbursement issues. The core data set collected through VISION will replace the hematocrit and URR data currently collected through the billing process, and provider-specific profiles derived from the core data set will be used by individual Networks to target quality improvement activities on a confidential basis. Of more concern is whether facility or physician-specific pro-

files derived from the core data set will be used prematurely or inappropriately for public accountability and patient choice. CMS has announced plans to expand the facility-specific data available on the Dialysis Facility Compare website to include additional quality elements to be derived from the core data set and also, perhaps, to report the results of patient satisfaction surveys. It should also be noted that the Medicare Prescription Drug, Improvement, and Modernization Act of 2003 contains a section (238) that directs the IOM to conduct an evaluation of leading health care performance measures in the public and private sectors and options to implement policies that align performance with payment under the Medicare program. The availability of a large set of provider-specific process and outcome measures within the ESRD program makes it likely that the IOM will examine this data set as a potential model for linking performance with payment and that, ultimately, nephrologists and dialysis facilities will be financially rewarded or penalized based on their respective performance data.

The availability to CMS of many new domains of provider-specific data through VISION makes it imperative that performance measures be developed for ESRD that meet the IOM criteria outlined above. As with the structural, process, and outcomes issues addressed with internal quality improvement methodologies, performance measures are also classified as structural, process, or outcome. Structural measures refer to the organizational characteristics that provide the infrastructure for quality care. These are the basis for most regulations (such as Medicare's conditions for coverage for dialysis facilities) and are generally the target for survey and certification activities as ensuring minimal capacity for quality. Although Jarr et al.[60] found a poor correlation between dialysis facility survey deficiencies (which focus mostly on structural measures) and patient outcomes, an internal quality improvement focus on structural measures may be beneficial to patients and the organization.[61] Process measures quantify the delivery of recommended procedures or services that are correlated with desired outcomes. These form the basis of many of the measurement sets used for public accountability of health plans, such as the Health Plan Employer Data and Information Set (HEDIS), but the appropriate data collection infrastructure must be in place to adequately capture process measure information. Outcome measures are used to capture the effect of an intervention on health status or patients' perceptions of care. Although outcome data are often much easier to capture (though a system like VISION) than process data, analysis of outcome data and use of outcome data as performance measures requires much more statistical sophistication, such as case-mix adjustment, than process data.[62]

It must be recognized that health care delivery is not subject to the same specifications and tolerances that will be applied to a supplier of an industrial product. Therefore, given the complexity of health care delivery in general and the variability and unpredictability of patient outcomes in particular, it is unrealistic for payers and oversight agencies to set rigid standards of performance by providers, especially when no clear unanimity exists regarding many processes of care. The renal community shares CMS's and Congress's goals to increase dialysis provider accountability and to improve patient outcomes. This includes the GAO goal[1] that every dialysis facility be reviewed at least on a tri-annual basis, with more frequent reviews for facilities with compliance problems. The renal community supports the continued development and application of validated clinical performance measures derived from evidence-based clinical practice guidelines, such as those currently being used to assess anemia management, adequacy of dialysis, and vascular access in hemodialysis patients. Nonetheless, many providers fear the advent of "cookbook" medicine in which the training and experience of the practitioner are devalued. Evidence-based clinical practice guidelines, which are designed as clinical decision-making tools, have a misguided tendency to evolve into standards of care. Quality oversight activities then become inappropriately oppressive and cross the line to become the practice of medicine by the regulator. This is a scenario that ESRD payers, providers, and the patient community must avoid at all costs because it stifles the innovation that leads to quality improvement, returns to the outlier focus of quality assurance, and may ultimately limit access to care as providers begin to cherry-pick patients to avoid the perception of underperformance. The development of a national data infrastructure to allow for provider-specific data collection and provider-specific profiling to drive internal quality improvement activities holds great promise for process and outcome improvement. However, the use of these same data for public accountability carries many concerns that must be addressed and may undermine the success of the quality improvement partnership between the ESRD Networks and dialysis providers. A system of public accountability implemented by CMS must include case mix adjustment strategies to minimize patient selection bias and encourage facilities to accept high-risk patients without fear that their adverse outcomes may inversely impact on their public facility profiles.

"A major redesign of the health care sector is needed. This redesign can occur only in an environment that fosters and rewards improvement. All parties should recognize that problems will be encountered along the way with data, measures and reports, necessitating continuous improvement and refinement. There must also be rewards and benefits to providers taking part in these efforts in the form of reduced regulatory burden, feedback of information useful for quality improvement, and public recognition and rewards for exemplary performance." —Institute of Medicine, *Leadership by Example, 2003.*[62]

REFERENCES

1. U.S. General Accounting Office Report to the Chairman, Committee on Finance, U.S. Senate. Dialysis facilities: problems remain in ensuring compliance with Medicare quality standards. GAO-04–63. Washington, DC: U.S. GAO, October 2003.
2. Institute of Medicine. *Crossing the Quality Chasm. A New Health System for the 21st Century.* Washington, DC: National Academy Press, 2001.
3. Institute of Medicine Errors in health care. In: Kohn LT, Corrigan JM, Donaldson MS, eds. *To Err is Human. Building a Safer Health System.* Washington, DC: National Academy Press, 2000.
4. Woolf SH. Patient safety is not enough: targeting quality improvements to optimize the health of the population. *Ann Intern Med* 2004;140:33.
5. Washington MS. *Doctor, Can You Hear Me? Patient, Are You Listening?* Pittsburgh, PA: Washington Associates, 2003.
6. Berry LL, Seiders K, Wilder SS. Innovations in access to care: a patient-centered approach. *Ann Intern Med* 2003;139:568.
7. Aragon SJ. Commentary: a patient-centered theory of satisfaction. *Am J Med Quality* 2003;18:225.
8. Pinchert JW, Miller CS, Hollo AH, et al. What health professionals can do to identify and resolve patient satisfaction. *J Quality Improvement* 1998;24:303.
9. Garbutt J, Bose D, McCawley BA, et al. Soliciting patient complaints to improve performance. *Joint Comm J Quality Safety* 2003;29:103.
10. Cooper LA, Roter DL, Johnson RL, et al. Patient-centered communication, ratings of care, and concordance of patient and physician race. *Ann Intern Med* 2003;139:907.
11. McClellan WM, Frankenfield DL, Frederick PR, et al. Improving the care of ESRD patients: a success story. *Health Care Fin Rev* 2003;24:89.
12. Centers for Medicare and Medicaid Services. *2003 Annual Report, ESRD Clinical Performance Measures Project.* Baltimore, MD: Department of Health and Human Services, Centers for Medicare and Medicaid Services, Center for Beneficiary Choices, December 2003.
13. Wish JB. Improving outcomes in dialysis patients. In: Nissenson AR, Fine RN, eds. *Dialysis Therapy,* 3d ed. Philadelphia: Hanley & Belfus, 2002.
14. Sehgal AR, Snow RJ, Singer ME, et al. Barriers to adequate delivery of dialysis. *Am J Kidney Dis* 1998;31:593.
15. Sehgal AR, Leon JB, Siminoff LA, et al. Improving the quality of hemodialysis treatment. A community-based randomized controlled trial to overcome patient-specific barriers. *JAMA* 2002;287:1961.
16. Deming WE: *Out of the Crisis.* Cambridge, MA: Massachusetts Institute of Technology, 1989.
17. Walton M: *The Deming Management Method.* New York: Putnam, 1986.
18. Lohr KN, ed. *Medicare: A Strategy for Quality Assurance.* Washington, DC: National Academy Press, 1990.
19. DeOreo PB. The use of patient-based instruments to measure, manage, and improve quality of care in dialysis facilities. *Adv Renal Replace Ther* 2001;8:125.

20. McClellan WM, Goldman RS. Continuous quality improvement in dialysis units: basic tools. *Adv Renal Replace Ther* 2001;8:95.

21. Wish JB. Assuring quality of care in dialysis patients. In: Nissenson AR, Fine RN, Gentile DE, eds. *Clinical Dialysis,* 3d ed. Norwalk, CT: Appleton & Lange, 1995.

22. Joint Commission on Accreditation of Healthcare Organizations (JCAHO). *An Introduction to Quality Improvement in Healthcare.* Oakbrook Terrace, IL: JCAHO, 1991.

23. Diamond LH, Kliger AS, Goldman RS, et al. Commentary: quality improvement projects: how do we protect patients' rights? *Am J Med Quality* 2004;19:25.

24. VanValkenburgh DA. Implementing continuous quality improvement at the facility level. *Adv Renal Replace Ther* 2001;8:104.

25. Goldman RS. Improving serum albumin levels in hemodialysis patients by a continuous quality improvement project. *Adv Renal Replace Ther* 2001;8:114.

26. Jencks SF, Cuerdon T, Burwen DR, et al. Quality of medical care delivered to Medicare beneficiaries. A profile at state and national levels. *JAMA* 2000;284:1670.

27. Jencks SF, Huff ED, Cuerdon T. Change in the quality of care delivered to Medicare beneficiaries, 1998–1999 to 2000–2001. *JAMA* 2003;289:305.

28. Evans EA. Thinking out loud: Questions of quality, cost, and unintended consequences. *Dialysis Transplant* 2003;32:582.

29. Grol R. Improving the quality of medical care. Building bridges among professional pride, payer profit, and patient satisfaction. *JAMA* 2001;286:2578.

30. Leape L, Brennan AG, Troyen A, et al. Preventing medical injury. *Qual Rev Bull* 1993;19:144.

31. Forum of End Stage Renal Disease Networks, National Patient Safety Foundation, Renal Physicians Association. *National ESRD Patient Safety Initiative. Phase II Report.* December 2001. Accessed at www.renalmd.org/downloads/ESRDreport2/pdf

32. Renal Physicians Association, Forum of ESRD Networks. *Collaborative Leadership for ESRD Patient Safety. Phase 1 Report of the National Patient Safety Consensus for the Community of Stakeholders in End Stage Renal Disease.* January 2001. Accessed at www.renalmd.org/publications/downloads/ESRDFinalReport/pdf

33. Kliger AS, Diamond LH. Patient safety in end-stage renal disease: how do we create a safe environment? *Adv Renal Replace Ther* 2001;8:131.

34. Runciman WB, Merry AF, Tito F. Error, blame and the law in heath care—an antipodean perspective. *Ann Intern Med* 2003;138:974.

35. Brennan TA, Mello MM. Patient safety and medical malpractice: a case study. *Ann Intern Med* 2003;139:267.

36. Weeks WB, Bagian JP. Making the business case for patient safety. *Joint Comm J Quality Safety* 2003;29:51.

37. Levinsky NG, Retig RA. The Medicare end-stage renal disease program: a report from the Institute of Medicine. *N Engl J Med* 1991;324:1143.

38. Schrier RW, Burrows-Hudson, Diamond L, et al. Measuring, managing, and improving quality in the end-stage renal disease setting: Committee statement. *Am J Kidney Dis* 1984;24:383.

39. Friedman EA. Selection bias impacts results of uremia therapy. *Am J Kidney Dis* 2000;36:208.

40. *U.S. Renal Data System 2003 Annual Report.* Bethesda, MD: National Institutes of Health, National Institute of Diabetes and Digestive and Kidney Diseases, 2003.

41. Mapes DL, Lopes AA, Satayathum S, et al. Health-related quality of life as a predictor of mortality and hospitalization: the Dialysis Outcomes and Practice Patterns Study (DOPPS). *Kidney Int* 2003;64:339.

42. Rayner HC, Pisoni RL, Gillespie BM, et al. Creation, cannulation and survival of arteriovenous fistulae—data from the Dialysis Outcomes and Practice Patterns Study (DOPPS). *Kidney Int* 2003;63:323.

43. Department of Health and Human Services, Office of the Inspector General: *External Review of Dialysis Facilities: A Call for Greater Accountability.* OEI-01–00050, June 2000.

44. United States General Accounting Office Report to Special Committee on Aging, U.S. Senate. *Oversight of Kidney Dialysis Facilities Needs Improvement.* GAO/HEHS-00–114. Wahsington, DC: U.S. Government Printing Office, June 2000.

45. Fink JC, Blahut SA, Briglia AE, et al. Effect of center- versus patient-specific factors on variation in dialysis adequacy. *J Am Soc Nephrol* 2001;12:164.

46. Wolfe RA, Ashby VB, Port FK. 1993 DMMS comorbidity index validated by Medical Evidence Form data. *J Am Soc Nephrol* 2001;11:247A.

47. Lacson E Jr, Teng M, Lazarus M, et al. Limitations of the facility-specific standardized mortality ratio for profiling health care quality in dialysis. *Am J Kidney Dis* 2001;37:267.

48. Krumholz HM, Rathore SS, Chen J, et al. Evaluation of a consumer-oriented internet health care report card. *JAMA* 2002;287:1277.

49. Medical Review Board of ESRD Network 14. *Position Paper on the Use of Outcomes for Survey Selection Purposes.* Dallas: ESRD Network of Texas, June 2000.

50. Field MJ, Lohr KN, eds. Institute of Medicine, Committee on Clinical Practice Guidelines: *Guidelines for Clinical Practice: From Development to Use.* Washington, DC: National Academy Press, 1992.

51. Brier ME. Medical Review Board of ESRD Networks 9 and 10: validation of HCFA hematocrit data with network data. *J Am Soc Nephrol* 2000;11:140A.

52. Brier ME, Aronoff GR. The public release of dialysis facility specific quality assurance data. Comparing HCFA's Dialysis Facility Compare to The Renal Network Data System (TRNDS). *J Am Soc Nephrol* 2001;12:192A.

53. Marshall MN, Shekelle PG, Leatherman S, et al. The public release of performance data. What do we expect to gain? A review of the evidence. *JAMA* 2000;283:1866.

54. Paganini EP, Stark S, Wish J, et al. Physician activity reporting: is it worthwhile? *J Am Soc Nephrol* 1999;10:252A.

55. Kiefe CI, Allison JJ, Williams OD. Improving quality improvement using achievable benchmarks for physician feedback. A randomized controlled trial. *JAMA* 2001;285:2891.

56. Hofer TP, Hayward RA, Greenfield S, et al. The unreliability of individual physician "report cards" for assessing the costs and quality of care of a chronic disease. *JAMA* 1999;281:2098.

57. Landon BE, Normand ST, Blumenthal D, et al. Physician clinical performance assessment: prospects and barriers. *JAMA* 2003;290:1183.

58. Daley J, Vogeli C, Blumenthal D, et al. *Physician Clinical Performance Assessment: The State of the Art. Issues, Possibilities, and Challenges for the Future.* Boston, MA: Institute for Health Policy, Massachusetts General Hospital, 2002.

59. U.S. Department of Health and Human Services. *Healthy People 2010,* 2d ed. Washington, DC: U.S. Government Printing Office, 2000.

60. Jarr BG, Hwang W, Fink NE, et al. The relation between dialysis facility survey deficiencies and patient outcomes. *J Am Soc Neprhol* 1999;10:244A.

61. Meyer GS, Massagli MP. The forgotten component of the quality triad: can we still learn something from "structure"? *J Quality Improvement* 2001;27:484.

62. Institute of Medicine Executive Summary. In: Corrigan JM, Eden J, Smith BM, eds. *Leadership by Example. Coordinating Government Roles in Improving Health Care Quality.* Washington, DC: The National Academies Press, 2003.

Sorbent Dialysis

Warren B. Shapiro

Despite recent advances in hemodialysis efficiency brought about by improvements in both dialyzers and equipment, the need still remains for a portable hemodialysis system that can be used within the hospital setting; in adverse circumstances where there are limitations of space, utilities and water; or in the home setting. Hemodialysis requires large amounts of pure water for the preparation of dialysis fluid. In many areas of the world, high-quality water and adequate drainage are not available, and even the most modern hemodialysis machines are delicate and difficult to move. It was in response to this need for portability that sorbent systems designed to regenerate dialysate were first developed.

In order to regenerate dialysis fluid, metabolic and nitrogenous waste products must be removed and, throughout the years, many schemes have been developed for this purpose. Sorbents are compounds that selectively or nonselectively bind or remove some chemicals from solution while allowing others to remain untouched. There are two main groups of sorbents: *ad*sorbents, which attract and bind chemicals to their outer surfaces, and *ab*sorbents, which bind chemicals to their inner surfaces. Sorbents can be non-specific or specific. Specific sorbents such as those that have tailored ligands or antibodies on their surface have been used to bind antibodies and to remove lipids directly from blood.[1] Nonspecific sorbents include activated charcoal and resins, which can also be manipulated by altering their pore size, leading to a greater selectivity of species removal according to molecular size and ability to penetrate the porous network of the sorbent.[2]

It has been known for more than 100 years that activated carbon (charcoal) can remove nitrogenous waste products such as uric acid and creatinine, as well as color and odor, from urine.[3] However, activated carbon is inefficient at binding significant amounts of urea. It requires 10 to 20 kg of activated carbon to remove the average daily production of urea.[4] Another drawback to activated carbon that limits its usefulness as a single agent for dialysate detoxification is its inability to alter the concentrations of electrolytes such as sodium (Na), chloride (Cl), calcium (Ca), phosphorus (P), hydrogen (H), and magnesium (Mg). Attempts to increase the efficiency of activated carbon as a urea binder or to use it in direct contact with blood (hemoperfusion) have proven impractical for the treatment of uremia.[5] Other approaches, such as electrolysis of urea, have been developed, but to date none has been commercially available.[6]

THE REDY SORBENT SYSTEM

Only one practical dialysis regeneration system has been marketed and continues to be supported; the recirculating dialysis (REDY 2000) system previously manufactured by Organon Teknika Corporation and currently supported by Renal Solutions, Inc., of Warrendale, PA. The REDY 2000 sorbent system, unlike other hemodialysis machines, can be used in any location where hemodialysis is indicated. It is not necessary to have pure water or drainage available, since spent dialysate (dialysis solution that has passed through the dialyzer and now contains urea, creatinine, and other "uremic toxins") is regenerated by means of a sorbent cartridge instead of being discarded. Because dialysate is cleansed and reused, only a small volume (6 L) of dialysate is re-

quired for a complete treatment, compared with 120 L or more for a standard single-pass system.

The Dialysis Machine

The REDY 2000 sorbent system is made up of two components: a dialysis machine and a sorbent cartridge. The dialysis machine (Fig. 38–1) has a 6-L reservoir from which dialysate is pumped through the sorbent cartridge (at a rate of 250 mL/min) to regenerate the dialysate. The maximum rate of blood flow rate through the dialyzer with the REDY sorbent system is 350 mL/min. The dialysis machine also contains an infusate pump, which controls the addition of a solution consisting of the acetate salts of Ca, Mg, and K to the dialysate as replacement for those ions adsorbed by passage through the sorbent cartridge. Dialysate flow, pressure, temperature, blood leak, conductivity detectors, infusate and ultrafiltration alarms, as well as a system for measuring dialysate volume are included.

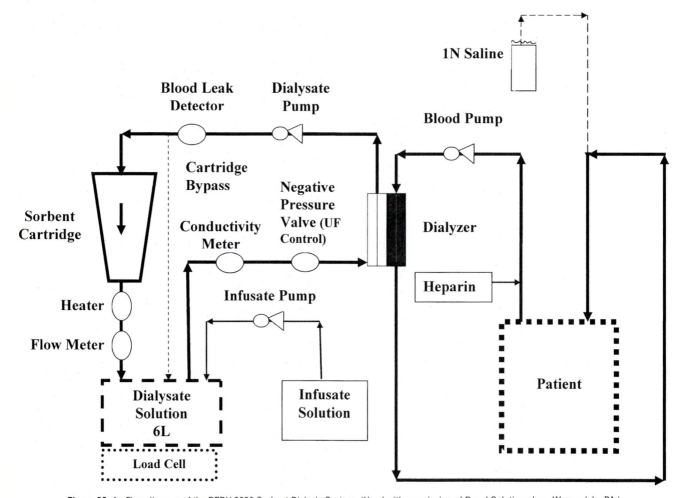

Figure 38–1. Flow diagram of the REDY 2000 Sorbent Dialysis System. (Used with permission of Renal Solutions Inc., Warrendale, PA.)

The REDY 2000 contains a negative pressure valve to increase transmembrane pressure resulting in movement of fluid from the patient's blood into the dialysate.[7] Any ultrafiltrate removed from the patient enters the dialysis reservoir and is regenerated by the sorbent cartridge. Because this is a closed system, all ultrafiltrate removed from the patient remains in the reservoir and can be accurately measured as an increase in dialysate weight.

The Sorbent Cartridge

The sorbent cartridge is the key component of the REDY sorbent system. It is composed of five layers (Fig. 38–2) through which the spent dialysate passes in a retrograde fashion: (1) the purification layer; (2) the enzyme layer (urease); (3) the cation exchange layer (zirconium phosphate); (4) the anion exchange layer (zirconium oxide); and (5) the adsorbent layer (activated carbon).

The first layer contacted by the effluent dialysate is the purification layer, which consists of activated carbon to remove particulate matter, heavy metals (such as copper, mercury, and lead), and oxidizing agents (such as chlorine, chloramines, and hypochlorite). These substances may be present in the water used to prepare dialysate or as contaminants from cleaning the machine and must be removed, since they could denature the urease in the next layer.

The second layer is composed of urease (bound to aluminum oxide), which catalyzes the conversion of urea into ammonia and carbamic acid (NH_2COOH). Carbamic acid in turn breaks down into ammonium and bicarbonate (HCO_3) ions. The hydrolysis of urea by urease may be summarized by the following equation[8]:

$$(NH_2)_2CO + 3\ H_2O \rightarrow 2\ NH_4^+ + HCO_3^- + OH^- \qquad (1)$$

The third layer consists of zirconium phosphate (ZP), a cation exchanger loaded with H and Na. For each mole of urea hydrolyzed in the second layer, two moles of ammonium carbonate are generated, and the ammonium is then exchanged for H and 0.4 moles of Na:

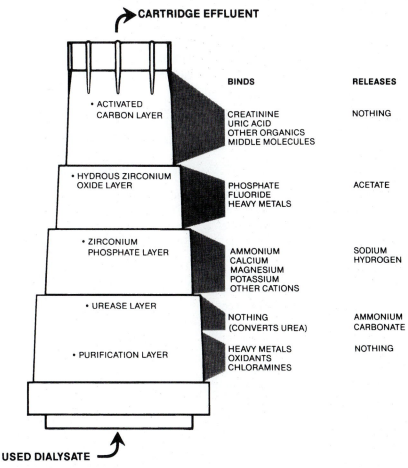

CARTRIDGE EFFLUENT

	BINDS	RELEASES
• ACTIVATED CARBON LAYER	CREATININE URIC ACID OTHER ORGANICS MIDDLE MOLECULES	NOTHING
• HYDROUS ZIRCONIUM OXIDE LAYER	PHOSPHATE FLUORIDE HEAVY METALS	ACETATE
• ZIRCONIUM PHOSPHATE LAYER	AMMONIUM CALCIUM MAGNESIUM POTASSIUM OTHER CATIONS	SODIUM HYDROGEN
• UREASE LAYER	NOTHING (CONVERTS UREA)	AMMONIUM CARBONATE
• PURIFICATION LAYER	HEAVY METALS OXIDANTS CHLORAMINES	NOTHING

USED DIALYSATE

Figure 38–2. Diagram of the REDY sorbent cartridge showing the layers and how they function. (Used with permission of Renal Solutions Inc., Warrendale, PA.)

$$NH_4^+ + OH^- + ZP\text{-}H \rightarrow ZP\text{-}NH_4 + H_2O \qquad (2)$$

$$NH_4 + HCO_3^- + ZP\text{-}H \rightarrow ZP\text{-}NH_4 + H_2O + CO_2 \qquad (3)$$

$$NH_4 + ZP\text{-}Na \rightarrow ZP\text{-}NH_4 + Na^+ \qquad (4)$$

In addition to ammonium ions, zirconium phosphate also exchanges Ca, Mg, and K for Na.[8] These ions are completely removed from the dialysate by the cartridge and must be replaced, which is accomplished by a continuous infusion of the acetate salts of these ions (infusate) into the dialysate reservoir, as described above.

Zirconium phosphate is both a cation exchanger and a buffer. Therefore the relative amounts of Na and H exchanged by the zirconium phosphate layer depends on the pH and anions (HCO_3 and acetate) present in the effluent dialysate. If HCO_3 is present in dialysate, either initially (HCO_3 buffered dialysate) or from the patient's blood via the dialyzer, the zirconium phosphate layer will absorb it (to form carbon dioxide and water). Initially, ammonium ions are exchanged for H ions, leading to the production of carbonic acid which then dissociates into carbon dioxide and water [Eq. (2) and (3)]. Because of this initial exchange of ammonium for H ions, the pH in the dialysate falls markedly during the first hour of treatment. Later in the course of treatment, the zirconium phosphate buffer pair releases more Na (in the form of HCO_3) than H, resulting in an increase in the dialysate pH. It should be noted that the release of H, Na, and HCO_3 ions is linked to urea breakdown and exchange for ammonium ions and results in a steady increase in dialysate Na and HCO_3 during the treatment.[10]

The fourth layer is composed of hydrated zirconium oxide in the acetate form. This layer is an anion exchanger and releases acetate in exchange for anions such as fluoride and phosphorus. Zirconium oxide will also absorb ionic, aluminum, mercury, and lead but not sulfate. Patients who are chronically treated with the REDY sorbent system have been shown to have higher levels of blood sulfate compared with patients treated with single-pass dialysis systems (see below).[11]

The fifth layer contains activated carbon, which removes creatinine, uric acid, and other nitrogenous waste products. The activated carbon layer absorbs glucose from the dialysate, decreasing the glucose concentration in regenerated dialysate by one-third at the start of the treatment. Later in the treatment, as glucose is metabolized by the patient and the dialysate glucose level falls, previously adsorbed glucose will be released from the sorbent cartridge. Approximately 30 g of glucose is transferred during an "average" REDY sorbent dialysis, about the same amount as with a single-pass system.[7]

Sorbent Cartridge Urea Removal

Currently two types of sorbent cartridges are available: the SORB cartridge D-3160, which has a urea nitrogen capacity of 20 ± 3 g, and the HISORB D-3260, which has a capacity of 30 ± 3 g (Table 38–1). The HISORB is usually used for patients who weigh >80 kg or who have a pretreatment serum urea nitrogen of >100 mg/dL.[10] At present, the Renal Solutions Corporation is in the process of developing four new and improved sorbent cartridges. The metabolism of urea in the sorbent cartridge results in the production of ammonium, which must be adsorbed by the zirconium phosphate layer (see above). If the patient has a large urea load, it is possible that the ammonium adsorption capacity of the zirconium phosphate layer may be exceeded, allowing free ammonia to enter the blood. If this occurs, ammonium toxicity could result, which is clinically manifest by nausea and/or vomiting. The amount of urea removed during a dialysis treatment (in grams), and therefore the determination of which sorbent cartridge to use, may be ascertained by multiplying the estimated pre- to posttreatment decrease in urea nitrogen (grams per kilogram of body weight) by the total body water (body weight x 0.6).[10] One may test for the presence of ammonium by using ammonium test papers (available from the SORB Technology division of Renal Solutions, Inc.) placed into the sorbent cartridge effluent stream at 30-minute intervals in the third hour and every 15 minutes thereafter. However, for very large or very catabolic patients the manufacturer recommends that testing be performed at 15-minute intervals after the first hour. If the test becomes positive, the cartridge should be changed or the treatment terminated.

Sorbent Cartridge Creatinine and Uric Acid Removal

The carbon layer can remove up to 10 g of creatinine and up to 7.5 g of uric acid.[12,13]

Sorbent Cartridge Acid-Base Balance

Three different dialysate bath compositions can be used with the REDY system for routine treatment and for the

TABLE 38–1. SPECIFICATIONS OF THE REDY SORBENT SYSTEM (MODEL 2000)

Dialysate capacity	6 L
Dialysate flow rate	250 mL/min
Blood flow rate	350 mL/min maximum
Urea removal	
D3160 sorbent cartridge	20 g urea nitrogen
D3260 sorbent cartridge	30 g urea nitrogen
Creatinine removal	10 g/treatment
Uric acid removal	7.5 g/treatment
Na added to the dialysate in a 4-hour treatment	360–480 meq

treatment of acid-base disturbances; two different HCO_3-plus-acetate combinations (kits 1 and 2) and one chloride-containing bath (with a small amount of acetate) to treat patients with alkalosis. The chemical composition and clinical indications for the use of the four HCO_3 and chloride-containing baths are shown in Table 38–2.

DIALYSATE BATHS

Bicarbonate/Acetate Baths

The amount of acetate to which a patient is exposed during a REDY sorbent system dialysis is relatively small; it should be readily metabolized during a 4-hour treatment. Therefore the likelihood that a patient treated with the REDY system would develop symptoms of high blood acetate levels (such as hypotension, headache, and depressed myocardial contractility) is minimal.[14] However, it has been shown that the use of a dialysis bath containing bicarbonate (HCO_3) and acetate with the REDY system does result in fewer episodes of hypotension.[15] In addition, by altering the amount of HCO_3 in the initial dialysis bath, it is possible to customize the dialysate for the treatment of varying degrees of metabolic acidosis. The manufacturer has developed two premixed bicarbonate (HCO_3)-containing kits for the treatment of mild or moderate metabolic acidosis (Table 38–2). As can be seen in the table, the initial HCO_3 levels drop by about half after 15 minutes of recirculation through the REDY sorbent cartridge (titration). This bath titration is necessary to decrease the initial alkaline pH of the dialysis bath (pH 8.2) in order to prevent precipitation of Ca and Mg (as the carbonate salts). An alternate method of titrating or neutralizing the initial alkaline pH of the dialysis bath is to use 1 N HCl to lower the pH. Either method will result in a decrease in the dialysate HCO_3, as shown in Table 38–2.

Chloride Baths (with and without Acetate)

The REDY system can also be used to treat metabolic alkalosis by employing a bath that contains a combination of chloride and 8 to 15 meq/L acetate in the infusate for the treatment of severe alkalosis. There is little or no HCO_3 in these dialysis solutions. When they are used, therefore, there is a significant concentration gradient from blood to dialysate with respect to HCO_3, leading to a decrease in blood HCO_3.[16] When the all-chloride bath is used, an arterial blood gas should be obtained when plasma and dialysate equilibrate (2 to 3 hours) to determine the degree of correction obtained. If correction is not sufficient, the dialysate can be drained and replaced with fresh sodium chloride dialysate to restore the concentration gradient for HCO_3.[9] Use of the REDY 2000 sorbent system is a relatively simple way to correct metabolic alkalosis in the dialysis patient.

SODIUM BALANCE DURING SORBENT DIALYSIS

As discussed above, the sorbent cartridge's zirconium phosphate layer adds Na to the dialysate in exchange for urea, resulting in a steady increase in the dialysate Na level throughout the dialysis treatment. In order to balance this rise, it is necessary to start treatment with a dialysate Na that is lower than that of the patient's serum (i.e., 110 to 120 meq/L). (For a discussion of Na kinetics with HCO_3- or Cl-containing baths, the reader is referred to *The Guide to Custom Dialysis* from the SORB Technology Division, Renal Solutions, Inc., Warrendale, PA.) At the end of a 4-hour treatment, the dialysate Na will be 155 to 160 meq/L. The sources of Na are as follows[17]: (1) 50 meq for the first passage of dialysate through the sorbent cartridge; (2) 150 meq/mole of urea nitrogen exchanged; (3) 18 to 30 meq from the saline used to prime the dialyzer; (4) 200 meq in exchange for Ca and Mg in the infusate; and (5) 50 meq in exchange for each meq of K in the infusate.

The actual amount of Na produced varies with the amount of urea, Ca, Mg, and K absorbed by the cartridge. Because of the difference in volume between the patient's total body water and the dialysate bath (42 L for a 70-kg patient versus 6 L of dialysate), the slower dialysate flow rate (250 vs. 500 mL/min in a single-pass system) and the time required for distribution of Na throughout the larger volume of the patient, only about half of the Na generated by the sorbent cartridge enters the patient. This amounts to an increase in the patient's serum Na of about 1 meq/L/h.[18]

TABLE 38–2. CHEMICAL COMPOSITION OF DIALYSATE AND CLINICAL INDICATION FOR THE USE OF CUSTOM DIALYSIS KITS

Kit	NaHCO₃	NaCl (g)	Dextrose (g)	Infusate Ion	Initial NaHCO₃ (meq)	Initial NaCl (meq)	Posttitration NaHCO₃ (meq)	Posttitration NaCl (meq)	Posttitration NaAc[a] (meq)	Clinical Indications
1	10	42	48	Acetate	20	120	10	120	10	Mild metabolic acidosis
2	30	21	48	Acetate	60	60	30	60	30	Moderate metabolic acidosis
	-	42	48	Acetate	-	120	-	120	-	Mild metabolic alkalosis

[a]Sodium acetate.

ADJUSTMENT OF THE PATIENT'S SERUM ELECTROLYTES USING THE REDY SORBENT SYSTEM

With the REDY 2000 sorbent system, it is relatively easy to manipulate the patient's blood electrolytes by varing the composition of the dialysate and infusate.

Adjustment of the Serum Na

Usually an initial dialysate bath Na of 110 to 120 meq/L is sufficient to maintain the body Na levels of patients with normal or near-normal serum Na at the start of treatment. Because of the addition of Na from the saline used for dialyzer priming plus initial cartridge equilibration (as discussed above), the dialysate Na will have increased from baseline, so that it will be about 130 meq/L when the patient starts treatment.[17] Depending on the patient's serum Na level, an adjustment of the initial dialysate Na concentration may be required, which can be accomplished by varying the volume of concentrate used to make the dialysate or by adding water or hypertonic saline to the dialysate as needed during the treatment.

In order to decrease the patient's serum Na in cases of hypernatremia, the dialysate Na should be maintained at the patient's serum Na minus 10 meq/L by removing 500 to 1000 mL of dialysate periodically and replacing it with water until the desired dialysate Na is achieved (as indicated by conductivity measured by the REDY machine).[19,20]

It is important to remember that rapid changes in serum Na can be dangerous, resulting in permanent brain damage. Therefore, both hyper- and hyponatremia should be corrected slowly.[21]

Adjustment of the Serum Ca

Both hypo- and hypercalcemia can be corrected with the REDY 2000 by altering the concentration of infusate Ca. The usual infusate Ca concentration is 3.0 meq/L, which can be increased to 4.5 meq/L for the treatment of hypocalcemia or decreased to 2 or even 0 meq/L for the treatment of hypercalcemia.[19]

Adjustment of the Serum K

As it comes from the manufacturer, the infusate does not contain any K. Therefore it is possible to treat the patient with hyperkalemia with a zero-K bath (no K in the infusate) if necessary. The K can be adjusted upward in increments of 1 meq/L by adding premixed packets of potassium acetate to the infusate. For the patient with hypokalemia, an infusate K concentration of 3 to 4 meq/L can be used. During the treatment of severe hypo- or hyperkalemia, the serum K should be measured about halfway through the dialysis procedure and the infusate K readjusted up or down as necessary.[19]

IMPORTANT INFORMATION FOR THE REDY 2000 SORBENT SYSTEM USER

Prevention of Possible Hyponatremia and/or Acidosis

As discussed above, the production of both Na and HCO_3 by the REDY sorbent cartridge is linked to urea removal. Therefore if the urea load is small, as is seen with a small patient or one who does not have a very high level of blood urea nitrogen (BUN) (<50 mg/dL), it is possible that not enough Na and HCO_3 will be generated during the dialysis, possibly resulting in hyponatremia and/or inadequate correction or actual worsening of existing acidosis. Once this possiblity is recognized, hyponatremia can be prevented by raising the initial dialysate Na to 130 to 135 meq/L from the usual level of 110 to 120 meq/L. Acidosis can be prevented by adding extra bicarbonate to the dialysis bath or giving intravenous HCO_3 supplementation to the patient.[21]

Prevention of Possible Respiratory Acidosis

Carbon dioxide (CO_2) is produced in the sorbent cartridge when urea is broken down to carbonate and the carbonate converted to HCO_3. This HCO_3, initially present in the dialysate or from the patient's blood, will react with hydrogen released from the zirconium phosphate layer to form CO_2 and water. The CO_2 dissolved in the dialysate (PCO_2 in the open dialysis tank equals 250 mmHg) enters the dialyzer, where some of it crosses the membrane into the patient's blood. For this reason, the blood in the venous line will have a higher CO_2 content (and thus will be slightly darker in color) than during single-pass dialysis. If this excess CO_2 is not excreted by the lungs in patients with pulmonary disease who are not on a respirator or who are on a respirator at a fixed respiratory rate, CO_2 excretion may be limited and respiratory acidosis due to hypercapnia may result.[22,23] Therefore, the REDY 2000 should be used with caution in patients with severe repiratory disease; if it is used, blood gases should be drawn every half hour during dialysis.

Citrate Anticoagulation

It has been reported that the use of citrate as an anticoagulant during sorbent dialysis may lead to a loss of the integrity of the sorbent cartridge with resultant leakage of aluminum and ammonia.[24] Therefore the manufacturer advises against using citrate anticoagulation during sorbent dialysis.

Sulfate Removal

Although the sorbent cartridge is able to remove most uremic toxins from the dialysate and thus from the patient's blood, it does not efficiently remove sulfate. Thus, patients chronically treated with the REDY sorbent system have been reported to have sulfate levels higher those of patients treated with single-pass dialysis.[11] One study attempted to link the elevated sulfate levels seen in a group of patients with elevated alkaline phosphatase levels, but no bone histology, parathormone, vitamin D, or aluminum levels were obtained, and the elevation of alkaline phosphate returned to normal after treatment with vitamin D.[25]

Dialyzer Clearance with Sorbent Dialysis Compared with Single-Pass Treatment

The clearance of a solute by the dialyzer is determined by the blood flow rate, the dialysate flow rate, and the mass transfer coefficient area product, which, in turn, is dependent on the individual dialyzer characteristics and the molecular weight of the particular solute.[26] Because of the internal configuration of the sorbent cartridge, the dialysate flow rate is limited to 250 mL/min, compared with 500 mL/min for conventional single-pass dialysis systems and as high as 800 to 1000 mL/min for the newer, high-efficiency machines. Lowering the dialysate flow rate from 500 to 250 mL/min (with no change in the blood flow rate) results in a decrease in the clearance of urea of about 10 percent.[27] In order to compensate for this, the dialysis time, the blood flow, the dialyzer mass transfer coefficient area product, or a combination of all three must be increased.[7]

It should also be noted that the REDY 2000 cannot accommodate the newer, high-flux dialyzers because the system has no volumetric ultrafiltration control.

Zirconium Leakage

Zirconium, present in the zirconium phosphate and oxide layers of the sorbent cartridge, has been demonstrated to be present in the bones of patients chronically treated with the sorbent dialysis system. Zirconium transfer to the patient has been confirmed by measurements of zirconium levels in arterial and venous plasma, as well as inlet and outlet dialysate.[26] The toxicity of zirconium is not known, and although it has been suggested that zirconium may produce bone disease (osteomalacia), rats with chronic renal failure loaded with zirconium acetate failed to show any differences in bone morphology compared with controls not receiving zirconium.[28,29]

Aluminum Leakage

In the original REDY sorbent cartridge, aluminum oxide (alumina) was used as a space filler in the zirconium phosphate and oxide layer as well as a binder for urease, since it was thought that alumina was nontoxic. Subsequent studies showed that when this original sorbent cartridge (no longer manufactured) was used with HCO_3 dialysate, the aluminum was rendered soluble, resulting in elevated dialysate and eventually plasma aluminum levels and clinical aluminum toxicity in chronically treated patients.[30–32]

The manufacturer subsequently removed all aluminum from the REDY cartridge with the exception of that used to bind urease. The space formerly occupied by the alumina was filled with a polystyrene spacer and later with glass beads. When the redesigned sorbent cartridge (D-3160) was studied, after rinsing with HCO_3, it was found that the post-cartridge dialysate aluminum levels were in the acceptable range (<10 μg/L) both in vivo and in vitro.[33] When this cartridge was used in a hemofiltration mode in humans, it was shown to remove aluminum from the patient's plasma.[33] Other workers confirmed that the new sorbent cartridge no longer leaked aluminum, whether used with acetate- or HCO_3-containing dialysate.[34,35] However, a report by Drury et al. noted a wide variation in dialysate aluminum in the postsorbent cartridge effluent. In addition, when aluminum was added to the dialysate, 50 minutes on average was required before the dialysate aluminum level was reduced to <30 μg/L.[36]

A study by Llach et al. showed, in vitro and in vivo, that the REDY sorbent cartridge can remove aluminum from water in which the level is as high as 470 μg/L. Under these circumstances, the post-sorbent-cartridge aluminum was <10 μg/L. In vivo, when REDY sorbent was compared to single-pass dialysis, it was shown that there was no difference in the pre- and posttreatment plasma aluminum concentrations between the two types of dialysis treatment, and dialysate aluminum remained below 4 μg/L at all times with both treatments.[37]

This study by Llach et al. confirms the sorbent cartridge's ability to remove aluminum from dialysate containing as much as 470 μg/L. In addition, Llach et al. showed that during a 4-hour dialysis with the REDY system utilizing bicarbonate dialysate, the sorbent cartridge does not release aluminum.[37] Thus, the "aluminum problem" with the sorbent cartridge should be laid to rest at long last. Of course, it would be best if the manufacturer could eliminate all aluminum from the sorbent cartridge, but to date no other urease binder but alumina has been found. However, despite the fact that aluminum is still within the cartridge, it appears safe to use with either acetate- or bicarbonate-containing dialysates. Plasma aluminum levels should be drawn periodically in any chronic dialysis patient whether treated with the REDY sorbent system or single-pass dialysis.

CONCLUSIONS

The REDY 2000 sorbent system is a unique method of providing dialysis for patients with acute or chronic renal failure in almost any location where electricity is available. When used properly, this system is capable of correcting a wide variety of acid-base and electrolyte disorders, which would otherwise be difficult or impossible to accomplish with conventional single-pass dialysis. Based upon the data from Llach et al., it appears that the aluminum problem has been solved and the REDY sorbent system can be used safely provided that the user is familiar with the workings of the system.

THE ALLIENT SORBENT SYSTEM

The Dialysis System

The Allient is a new sorbent dialysis system being developed by Renal Solutions, Inc., for hemodialysis treatments at alternate sites such as a patient's home or an acute or subacute setting. As with previously described sorbent-based devices, this dialysate purification system is a completely self-contained, transportable unit (110 pounds); however, the Allient is more flexible in the range of treatments that it can perform than previous sorbent systems, such as the REDY 2000.

The Allient also uses dialysate regeneration. Initial dialysate is made by dissolving dry dialysate powders in 6 L of tap water. The dialysate, after passing through the dialyzer, is pumped through newly redesigned sorbent cartridges, which are the heart of the Allient system. Four reformulated cartridges have been developed that provide higher dialysate flow rates (up to 400 mL/min), improved sodium balance, more consistent bicarbonate and pH dynamics, and increased urea capacity (9.5 to 35 g urea) compared with the original cartridge. Otherwise the new cartridges function identically to the SORB and HISORB cartridges. The new cartridges vary from each other primarily in the amount of material in each layer to ensure appropriate urea nitrogen capacity for a particular range of dialysate and blood flow rates. If the ammonium adsorption capability of a cartridge is exceeded during a treatment, the Allient's ammonium monitor will trigger an alarm eliminating the need for manual ammonia testing, which was necessary with previous sorbent dialysis systems.

Total fluid balance is automatically tracked with the Allient and will allow the system to achieve prescribed dry weight directly for a patient with this closed, recirculating system even if numerous saline boluses are given. The Allient measures the increase in dialysate weight and adjusts the differential speed of the dialysate pumps accordingly to attain the desired ultrafiltration rate. This results in true ultrafiltration control, which allows the use of high flux dialyzers.

The Allient uses a dual-diaphragm, pressure-activated blood-pumping system rather than the traditional roller-type of blood pump. This new Pulsar Blood Movement System uses a pressure-actuated diaphragm pump, which applies the desired pressure gradient to the blood entering and leaving the system and can be utilized in single- or dual-needle modes.

CONCLUSIONS

The Allient sorbent system will be a unique method for providing hemodialysis in almost any location where electricity is available. By updating proven technology, the Allient has the potential to address many of the limitations of current dialysis methods and products.

CONTINUOUS WEARABLE PERITONEAL-BASED ARTIFICIAL KIDNEY

An automated wearable artificial kidney could provide "dialysis on the go" and free patients from the chores of hemodialysis three to six times weekly or exchanging peritoneal dialysate, thereby allowing them to resume normal living activities. However, a major obstacle to developing a wearable kidney is the large volume of dialysate or replacement solution required. The use of sorbents to regenerate the dialysate solves this problem.

Roberts et al. have proposed a wearable artificial kidney based on the use of peritoneal dialysis.[38] Using a dialysate flow rate of 2 to 4 L/h produced by a small rechargeable battery-powered pump and performing continuous flow peritoneal dialysis (CFPD) 24 hours a day, 7 days a week, the weekly Kt/V is estimated to be 6.5, greater than that obtained by standard peritoneal dialysis and most thrice-weekly hemodialysis.[39] They have demonstrated, in vitro, that the spent dialysate (including the protein) can be regenerated with a modified, sterile mini-REDY cartridge.[40–41] Recirculating the protein-containing regenerated dialysate could minimize protein loss, enhance the removal of protein-bound toxins, and increase ultrafiltration.[42–44] The main requirement would be for the patient to exchange the sorbent cartridge and replace the infusate solution (containing Ca, Mg, K acetate, and glucose) every 4 hours daily and 8 hours overnight.

This device is now in a prototype form. The concepts are sound and have been tested by in vitro and in vivo experiments. We look forward to further developments in this interesting sorbent application.

REFERENCES

1. Bosch T, Lennertz A, Kordes B, et al. Low density lipoprotein hemoperfusion by direct adsorption of lipoproteins from whole blood (DALI apheresis): clinical experience from a single center. *Ther Apher* 1999;3:209.
2. Ash S, Winchester J. Introduction: sorbents in extracorporeal blood therapy. *Adv Renal Replace Ther* 2002;9:1.
3. Bosch J. A study of a decolorizing carbon. *J Am Chem Soc* 1980;42:1564.

4. Wing A, Parsons F, Drukker W. Dialysate regeneration. In: Drukker W, Parsons F, Maher J, eds. *Replacement of Renal Function by Dialysis,* 2d ed. Boston:, Martinus Nijhoff, 1983:323.

5. Giordano C, Esposito R, Bello P. A cold charcoal depurator for adsorption of high quantities of urea. *Kidney Int* 1973;10: (suppl 16):S284.

6. Kolff N, Gregonis D, Wisniewski S, et al. A membrane system to remove urea from dialysate. *Contractors Conference Artificial Kidney Chronic Uremia Program NIAMDD.* 1979; 12:215.

7. Roberts M, Daugardis J. REDY sorbent hemodialysis. In: Daugardis J, Ing T, eds. *Hand Book of Dialysis,* 2d ed. Boston: Little, Brown, 1994:198.

8. Kelleher S, Nolan C. Complications of sorbent regenerative hemodialysis. *Dial Transplant* 1987;16:323.

9. Shapiro W. The current status of sorbent hemodialysis. *Semin Dial* 1990;3:40.

10. Cobe Renal Care, Inc. *Sorbent Dialysis Primer,* 4th ed. Lakewood, CO: Cobe Renal Care, 1993:44.

11. Freeman R, Richards C. Studies on sulphate in end-stage renal disease. *Kidney Int* 1979;15:167.

12. Kelleher S, Nolan C. Complications of sorbent regenerative hemodialysis. *Dial Transplant* 1987;16:323.

13. Cobe Renal Care, Inc. *Sorbent Dialysis Primer,* 4th ed. Lakewood, CO: Cobe Renal Care, 1992:22.

14. Veech R. The untoward effects of the anions of dialysis fluids. *Kidney Int* 1988;34:587.

15. Raja R, Henriquez M, Kramer M, et al. Improved dialysis tolerance using REDY sorbent system with bicarbonate dialysate in critically ill patients. *Dial Transplant* 1979;8:241.

16. Cobe Renal Care, Inc. *Guide to Custom Dialysis,* rev ed. Lakewood, CO: Cobe Renal Care, 1993:8.

17. Cobe Renal Care, Inc. *Sorbent Dialysis Primer,* 4th ed. Lakewood, CO: Cobe Renal Care, 1993:16.

18. Cobe Renal Care, Inc. *Sorbent Dialysis Primer,* 4th ed. Lakewood, CO: Cobe Renal Care, 1993:15.

19. Shapiro W. REDY sorbent hemodialysis system. In: Nissenson A, Fine R, eds. *Dialysis Therapy,* 2d ed. Philadelphia: Hanley & Belfus, 1993:146.

20. Cobe Renal Care, Inc. *Sorbent Dialysis Primer,* 4th ed. Lakewood, CO: Cobe Renal Care, 1993:19.

21. Cobe Renal Care, Inc. *Guide to Custom Dialysis,* rev ed. Lakewood, CO: Cobe Renal Care, 1993:12.

22. Drukker W, Van Doom W. Dialysate regeneration. In: Maher J, ed. *Replacement of Renal Function by Dialysis.* Boston: Martinus Nijhoff, 1989:41.

23. Hamm L, Lawrence G, DuBose T Jr. Sorbent regeneration hemodialysis as a potential cause of acute hypercapnia. *Kidney Int* 1992;21:416.

24. Suki W, Bonuelous D, Yocum S, et al. Citrate for regional anticoagulation. *ASAIO Trans* 1988;34:524.

25. Whalan J, Freeman R, Richards C. Elevated serum alkaline phosphatase in patients receiving sorbent cartridge hemodialysis. *ASAIO J* 1981;4:9.

26. Odell R, Sorbent dialysis. In: Nissenson A, Fine R, Gentile D, eds. *Clinical Dialysis,* 2d ed. Norwalk, CT: Appleton & Lange, 1990:714.

27. Christopher T, Camhi V, Jarker L, et al. A study of hemodialysis with lowered dialysate flow. *ASAIO Trans* 1971;17:92.

28. Odell R, Farrell P, Brown D, et al. The kinetics of chelation of Al, Fe and Zr by DFO (abstr). *Kidney Int* 1985;26:234.

29. Rodriguez M, Felsenfeld A, Samara S, et al. Zirconium does not produce osteomalacia in rats with chronic renal failure. *ASAIO Trans* 1985;31:655.

30. Gracek E, Babb A, Uveli D, et al. Dialysis dementia. The role of dialysate pH in altering the dialysis of aluminum. *ASAIO Trans* 1979;25:409.

31. Mion C, Branger B, Issautier R, et al. Dialysis fracturing osteomalacia without hyperparathyroidism in patients treated with HCO_3 rinsed REDY cartridge. *ASAIO Trans* 1981;27: 634.

32. Shapiro W, Schilb T, Waltrous C, et al. Aluminum leakage from the REDY sorbent cartridge. *Kidney Int* 1983;23:536.

33. Shapiro W, Shilb T, Porush J. Sorbent recycling of ultrafiltrate in man-45 week crossover study. *Clin Nephrol* 1986; 26(suppl 1):S47.

34. Culpepper C, Cummings R, Westervelt F, et al. Aluminum kinetics of the REDY system. A study of the impact of deferoxamine therapy. *ASAIO Trans* 1981;29:6.

35. Mourad G, Roura R, Misse P, et al. Bicarbonate dialysis using a modified sorbent regeneration system with low aluminum release (abstr). *Eur Dial Transplant Assoc Eur Renal Assoc* 1983;20:89.

36. Drury P, Harston G, Ineson P, et al. Aluminum release from the Sorbsystem D-3160 and D-3260 cartridges. *Life Support Syst* 1986;4:211.

37. Llach F, Gardner P, George C, et al. Aluminum kinetics using bicarbonate dialysate with the sorbent system. *Kidney Int* 1993;43:899.

38. Roberts M, Lee, D. A proposed peritoneal-based wearable artificial kidney. *Home Hemodial Intern* 1999;3:65.

39. Roberts M, Ash SR, Lee D. Innovative peritoneal dialysis: flow-thru and dialysate regeneration. *ASAIO J* 1999;45:372.

40. Roberts M, Capparelli AW, Lee D. An automated wearable artificial kidney (AWAK) based upon sorbent regeneration of peritoneal dialysate (PD) (abstr). *Fifth Annual Spring Clinical Nephrology Meetings of the National Kidney Foundation.* A-14, 1996.

41. Roberts M, Dinovo E, Yanagawa N, et al. Can peritoneal protein be regenerated and reused for binding toxins (abstr)? *J Am Soc Nephrol* 1999;10:228.

42. Bosch JP, Lauer A, Constaniner A, Glabman S. Filtration peritoneal dialysis: a method to eliminate protein loss. *Blood Purif* 1983;1:154.

43. Ettidorf J, Dobbins W, Summitt R, et al. Intermittent peritoneal dialysis using 5 percent albumin in the treatment of salicylate intoxication in children. *J Pediatr* 1961;58:226.

44. Park M, Heimburger O, Bergstrom J, et al. Albumin-based solutions for peritoneal dialysis: investigations with a rat model. *Artif Organs* 1995;19:307.

Continuous Renal Replacement Therapy

Paul M. Palevsky

Continuous renal replacement therapy (CRRT) was initially described as a means for fluid removal in volume-over-loaded patients who were resistant to diuretic therapy.[1] Over the course of the more than two decades since its initial description, modifications of the original technique have resulted in the development of a spectrum of related therapies for the management of hemodynamically unstable patients with acute renal failure (ARF). As a result, it is not appropriate to speak of CRRT as a single treatment. Rather, CRRT represents a family of related therapies designed to provide uninterrupted renal support to critically ill patients over a period of days. It is this feature that distinguishes CRRT from conventional hemodialysis and more recently described extended duration variants that are prescribed on an intermittent basis.

Continuous therapies have gained increasing acceptance for the management of critically ill patients with acute renal failure, although with wide regional variation.[2,3] The increasing utilization of these therapies has occurred despite the lack of objective evidence that they are associated with improved survival. Nevertheless, there is a strong sense among many nephrologists and intensivists that these therapies provide advantages over more traditional forms of dialysis in the management of critically ill patients, particularly in patients in whom ARF is a component of the multisystem organ failure syndrome. These advantages include more stable control of fluid, electrolyte, and solute balance; improved cardiovascular stability; and greater ability to maintain fluid balance despite the administration of large volumes of hyperalimentation solution and other obligatory fluids.[4]

HISTORY OF CRRT

Although the techniques of continuous hemodialysis and isolated ultrafiltration had been described years earlier,[5,6] the first practical application of CRRT was described by Kramer et al. in 1977.[7] Using a high-flux hemofilter interposed in an arteriovenous (AV) circuit between the femoral artery and femoral vein, an ultrafiltration rate of 200 to 600 mL/h could be achieved. By combining the removal of large volumes of uremic ultrafiltrate with intravenous administration of balanced electrolyte solutions, this technique of continuous AV hemofiltration (CAVH) was able to achieve control of the biochemical and clinical manifestations of uremia.[8,9] At approximately the same time, Paganini and Nakamoto described the technique of slow continuous ultrafiltration (SCUF).[10] Their technique used a similar AV circuit but with lower ultrafiltration rates and permitted the management of volume overload in patients with diuretic-unresponsive oliguria with or without uremia. The lower ultrafiltration rates used with this technique did not permit sufficient solute removal for the management of uremia. The clinical utility of CAVH for the management of ARF in critical illness was ultimately established following the publication of larger case series by Lauer et al. in 1983[11] and Kaplan et al. in 1984.[12]

Limitations to the technique of CAVH led to continued innovation. In highly catabolic patients, especially those with severe sepsis, the ability to control marked azotemia was limited. Solute removal in CAVH was limited by the maximally achievable ultrafiltration rate, which rarely exceeded 15 L/day. A variety of strategies to optimize clearance were employed, including modifications of catheter, tubing, and hemofilter design to minimize resistance of the extracorporeal circuit and increase blood flow; application of negative pressure at the filter outlet to increase ultrafiltration rates; prefilter administration of replacement fluid to alter the rheologic properties of the perfusing blood; and even the use of blood pumps to augment the blood's flow rate.[11-14] Ultimately, however, solute clearance with CAVH remained limited.

Continuous AV hemodialysis (CAVHD) and continuous AV hemodiafiltration (CAVHDF) were developed to further augment the clearance of urea and other low-molecular-mass solutes.[15-17] In these modalities, dialysate was perfused through the hemofilter ultrafiltrate compartment, combining the diffusive solute transport of dialysis with the convective transport of hemofiltration. This modification permitted a doubling of the effective urea clearance achievable with continuous therapy.

The final step in the evolution of CRRT was the conversion from AV to venovenous extracorporeal circuits. Using an AV circuit, blood flow—and hence treatment efficiency—is limited by the gradient between mean arterial pressure and central venous pressure, a limitation that is greatest in hemodynamically unstable patients. In addition, the need for an arterial cannula is associated with a high complication rate, including arterial bleeding, thromboembolization, and infection. This combination of restricted treatment efficiency and complications of arterial cannulation led multiple investigators to develop venovenous

pump-driven techniques.[18-21] The initial technology for venovenous therapy was primitive, primarily utilizing jury-rigged equipment. Over the course of the past decade, however, increasingly sophisticated equipment specifically designed for the performance of continuous venovenous therapies has become available. With the advent of this technology, continuous therapy has matured from a treatment used by a small number of nephrologists for the most desperately ill patients to a mainstream therapy for the management of ARF.[2,22]

NOMENCLATURE

The use of a common nomenclature in the description of the various modalities of CRRT is of great importance. Prior to efforts to develop a common nomenclature in the mid-1990s, there was considerable inconsistency in terminology; multiple terms were use to describe treatments that were essentially similar, while similar terms were used to describe different therapies. A consensus set of definitions was developed at the International Conference on Continuous Renal Replacement Therapy in 1995[23] and was further refined as part of the Acute Dialysis Quality Initiative.[24]

Continuous Renal Replacement Therapy

Continuous Renal Replacement Therapy (CRRT) is defined as any extracorporeal blood-purification technique intended to substitute for impaired renal function over an extended period of time and intended to be utilized 24 hours a day. The various modalities included in the CRRTs are listed in Table 39–1 and illustrated schematically in Fig. 39–1. These treatments are usually divided, on the basis of vascular access, into AV and venovenous therapies. In the AV therapies, the extracorporeal circuit originates from an artery and terminates in a vein. Flow through the AV circuit is usually dependent upon the pressure gradient between the arterial circulation (mean arterial pressure) and central venous pressure, although pump-assisted AV circuits have been described. In the venovenous (VV) therapies, the extracorporeal circuit originates from and terminates in a vein with pump-driven blood flow through the circuit.

Slow Continuous Ultrafiltration

Slow continuous ultrafiltration (SCUF) is a form of CRRT used for the management of refractory edema with or without renal failure. In SCUF, an ultrafiltrate is generated across a semipermeable membrane at a volume that is constrained not to exceed the volume necessary for the safe and effective management of fluid overload. Replacement fluids are not utilized. SCUF may be provided using either an AV or venovenous circuit.

TABLE 39–1. MODALITIES OF CONTINUOUS RENAL REPLACEMENT THERAPY

Modality of CRRT	Abbreviation	Mechanism of Solute Removal	Replacement Fluid	Dialysate
Arteriovenous therapies				
Slow continuous ultrafiltration	SCUF	Minimal convection	No	No
Continuous arteriovenous hemofiltration	CAVH	Convection	Yes	No
Continuous arteriovenous hemodialysis	CAVHD	Predominantly diffusion	No	Yes
Continuous arteriovenous hemodiafiltration	CAVHDF	Mixed convection and diffusion	Yes	Yes
Venovenous therapies				
Slow continuous ultrafiltration	SCUF	Minimal convection	No	No
Continuous venovenous hemofiltration	CVVH	Convection	Yes	No
Continuous venovenous hemodialysis	CVVHD	Predominantly diffusion	No	Yes
Continuous venovenous hemodiafiltration	CVVHDF	Mixed convection and diffusion	Yes	Yes

Continuous Hemofiltration

Continuous hemofiltration (CH) is a form of CRRT in which a volume of ultrafiltrate in excess of that required for volume management is generated across a semipermeable membrane by the transmembrane pressure gradient. The volume of ultrafiltrate is in excess of that required for the treatment of fluid overload; the excess ultrafiltrate is replaced intravenously with a balanced electrolyte solution in order to achieve the desired fluid balance. Solute removal in CH occurs primarily by convection. Continuous hemofiltration may be performed using either an AV circuit (continuous AV hemofiltration, or CAVH) or venovenous circuit (continuous venovenous hemofiltration, or CVVH).

Continuous Hemodialysis

Continuous hemodialysis (CHD) is a form of CRRT characterized by the slow countercurrent flow of dialysate through the ultrafiltrate-dialysate compartment of the membrane. Solute removal occurs primarily by diffusion across the semipermeable membrane down a solute concentration gradient. Ultrafiltration is restricted to the volume necessary for the management of volume overload, and intravenous replacement fluids are not required. Continuous hemodialysis may be performed using either an AV circuit (continuous AV hemodialysis, or CAVHD) or venovenous circuit (continuous venovenous hemodialysis, or CVVHD).

Continuous Hemodiafiltration

Continuous hemodiafiltration (CHDF) is a technique of CRRT that combines the diffusive solute removal of CHD with the convective clearance of CH. Blood and dialysate are circulated through the extracorporeal circuit as in CHD, permitting diffusive solute clearance. In addition, an ultrafiltrate volume in excess of that necessary to achieve targeted fluid removal is generated and the excess ultrafiltrate is replaced intravenously with a balanced electrolyte solution in order to achieve the desired fluid balance. Continuous hemodiafiltration may be performed using either an AV circuit (continuous AV hemodiafiltration, or CAVHDF) or venovenous circuit (continuous venovenous hemodiafiltration, or CVVHDF).

Two additional terms have been proposed to describe variants of CH and CHD[25]: *continuous high-volume hemofiltration* (HVHF) and *continuous high-flux dialysis* (CHFD). In HVHF, ultrafiltrate volumes may be in excess of 6 to 10 L/h. It has been proposed that such high volumes of ultrafiltrate may be of benefit in removal of inflammatory mediators in patients in whom ARF occurs in the setting of sepsis.[26] Such a benefit has not, however, been demonstrated in clinical trials, and the use of HVHF should be reserved for experimental protocols. CHFD is CHD performed with high-flux synthetic membranes. It has been hypothesized that use of such membranes would be associated with increased convective solute transport within the membrane due to augmented filtration from the blood into the dialysate compartment and associated backfiltration from the dialysate into the blood.[27,28] On theoretical grounds, this would be associated with increased convective solute transport; however, clinical data to support this modality as distinct from CHD are not available.

MECHANISMS OF SOLUTE TRANSPORT IN CRRT

The modalities of CRRT differ with regard to their biophysical mechanisms of solute transfer across the hemodialyzer/hemofilter membrane. In continuous hemofiltration, regardless of whether blood access is obtained using an AV (CAVH) or a venovenous (CVVH) circuit, all solute mass transfer occurs by convection.[29,30] In contrast, solute transport during continuous hemodialysis (CAVHD, CVVHD) occurs primarily by diffusion, although ultrafiltration for volume management results in a smaller component of convective solute movement.[29,30] Continuous hemodiafiltration (CAVHDF, CVVHDF) provides a balance between convective and diffusive solute transport.

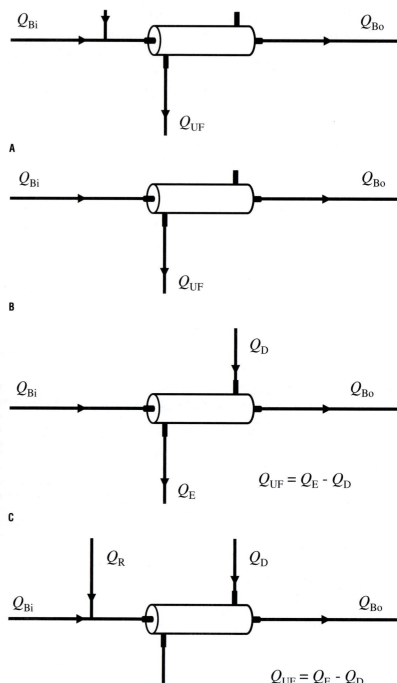

Figure 39–1. Schematic representation of modalities of CRRT. In each schematic, blood flow is from left to right with inflow designated Q_{Bi} and outflow Q_{Bo}. Each modality may be provided as an arteriovenous (AV) or venovenous (VV) therapy. In AV therapies, blood flow will be driven by the pressure gradient between the arterial and venous circulations. In VV therapies, blood flow will be pump-driven. *A.* Slow continuous ultrafiltration (SCUF). In SCUF, the ultrafiltrate rate (Q_{UF}) is equal to the desired rate of fluid removal. No replacement fluid is administered and no dialysate is utilized. *B.* Continuous hemofiltration (CH). In CH, the ultrafiltrate (Q_{UF}) volume exceeds the need for fluid removal and the excess ultrafiltrate is replaced with intravenous fluids (Q_R). *C.* Continuous hemodialysis (CHD). In CHD, dialysate is perfused through the ultrafiltrate compartment of the membrane. Ultrafiltration (Q_{UF}) is equal to the difference between effluent outflow (Q_E) and dialysate inflow (Q_D). The ultrafiltration rate equals the desired rate of fluid removal and no replacement fluid is administered. *D.* Continuous hemodiafiltration (CHDF). In CHDF, dialysate is perfused through the ultrafiltrate compartment of the membrane. Ultrafiltration (Q_{UF}) is equal to the difference between effluent outflow (Q_E) and dialysate inflow (Q_D). As in CH, the ultrafiltration rate (Q_{UF}) exceeds the desired rate of fluid removal, and the excess ultrafiltrate is replaced with intravenous fluids (Q_R).

Convection

Convection describes the bulk transfer of solute across a semipermeable barrier as the result of filtration across the membrane. Solutes are entrained in the flow of plasma water during ultrafiltration, a process referred to as "solvent drag," and passively cross the membrane in the absence of concentration gradients. The ultrafiltration rate (Q_{UF}) is determined by the product of the hydraulic permeability of the membrane (k_M) the membrane surface area (A) and the transmembrane pressure gradient. The transmembrane pressure gradient is determined by the difference between the hydrostatic gradient (ΔP), favoring ultrafiltration, and the oncotic pressure produced by plasma proteins (Π), restraining ultrafiltration.

$$Q_{UF} = k_M A(\Delta P - \Pi) \tag{1}$$

In AV therapies, transmembrane hydrostatic pressure is limited and oncotic pressure plays a significant restraining effect on ultrafiltration, to the point of filtration pressure equilibrium.[11] In venovenous therapies, the transmembrane hydrostatic pressures are higher and oncotic pressure is less significant as a determinant of ultrafiltration.

The propensity for individual solutes to cross a semipermeable membrane by convection is a function of the relationship between the charge and molecular radius of the solute and the structure of the pores in the hemofilter membrane. This propensity is quantified by the membrane reflection coefficient σ, with values ranging from 0, for solutes that are not restricted by the membrane, to 1, for impermeant solutes. In clinical practice, it is more common to use the sieving coefficient S, where $S = 1-\sigma$, which can be calculated from the ratio of solute concentrations in ultrafiltrate (C_{UF}) and blood (C_B):

$$S = C_{UF}/C_B \tag{2}$$

The sieving coefficients of some clinically relevant solutes are listed in Table 39–2. Small solutes, such as urea, have values near unity, while large molecules, such as albumin, which are retained by hemofiltration membranes, have values near zero.[12,31]

The convective flux of a solute across the membrane (J_C) is expressed as

$$J_C = Q_F S C_B \tag{3}$$

Since clearance (K) equals J/C_B, the convective clearance of a solute may be expressed as

TABLE 39–2. OBSERVED SIEVING COEFFICIENTS IN CONTINUOUS HEMOFILTRATION

Solute	Sieving Coefficient
Sodium	0.99
Potassium	0.99
Chloride	1.05
Bicarbonate	1.24
Urea	1.05
Creatinine	1.02
Glucose	1.04
Phosphate	1.04
Calcium	0.64
Uric acid	1.02
Creatinine phosphokinase	0.68
Bilirubin	0.03
Total protein	0.02
Albumin	0.01

Source: From Kaplan et al.[12]

$$K_C = Q_F S \tag{4}$$

From this equation, it is apparent that the convective clearance of low-molecular-mass solutes, such as urea, with sieving coefficients $\cong 1$, approximates the ultrafiltration rate.

Diffusion

Diffusion is the movement of solute across a semipermeable membrane down a concentration gradient. Diffusion is described by Fick's law, which states that diffusive flux (J_D) is equal to the product of the coefficient of diffusion (k_D), the surface area of the membrane (A), and the concentration gradient across the membrane ($\Delta C/\Delta x$):

$$J_D = - k_D A(\Delta C/\Delta x) \tag{5}$$

The rate of diffusion of a solute is inversely related to its molecular radius. Thus, low-molecular-mass solutes will diffuse faster than species with higher molecular mass.

The differing biophysical mechanisms of solute transport in different modalities of CRRT have clinical implications. Diffusive therapies, such as continuous hemodialysis, are relatively more efficient for the removal of low- vs. higher-molecular-mass species. In contrast, in convective therapies, the relative removal of low- and intermediate-mass solutes will be similar; only as the solute's molecular radius approaches the pore size of the membrane will the transfer of the solute across the membrane diminish. Thus, as illustrated in Fig. 39–2, convective therapies, such as continuous hemofiltration, will provide greater removal of intermediate-mass solutes (MW 1000 to 10,000 Da) as compared to pure diffusive therapies.

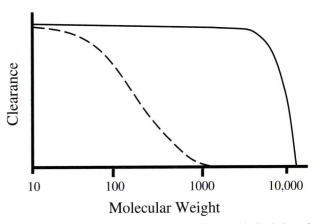

Figure 39–2. Convective and diffusive solute clearance. Idealized plots of convective (solid line) and diffusive (broken line) clearance as a function of solute molecular mass. Convective clearance remains relatively constant as molecular mass increases until the solute molecular size approaches that of the membrane pores. In contrast, diffusional clearance is inversely related to molecular mass, and rapidly declines as molecular mass increases. Convective therapies provide higher clearances for solutes in the range of 1000 to 10,000 Da than primarily diffusive therapies.

DETERMINANTS OF SOLUTE CLEARANCE

Calculation of Solute Clearance

Mathematical statements of clearance in CRRT can be derived from analyses of solute mass balance across the hemodialyzer/hemofilter based on either blood-side disappearance or dialysate-side appearance.[17] Blood-side clearance is calculated based on the disappearance of solute from the blood compartment over the length of the hemodialyzer/hemofilter and may be calculated as

$$K = (Q_{Bi}C_{Bi} - Q_{Bo}C_{Bo})/C_{Bi} \qquad (6)$$

where Q_B and C_B represent the blood flow rate and solute concentration in the blood, respectively, and the subscripts i and o designate the inlet and outlet of the hemodialyzer/hemofilter, respectively.

Since the ultrafiltration rate (Q_{UF}) is equal to the difference between inlet (Q_{Bi}) and outlet (Q_{Bo}) blood flow, Eq. (6) can be rewritten as

$$K = Q_{Bi}(C_{Bi} - C_{Bo})/C_{Bi} + Q_{UF}C_{Bo}/C_{Bi} \qquad (7)$$

The first term in this equation, $Q_{Bi}(C_{Bi} - C_{Bo})/C_{Bi}$ represents diffusive clearance in the absence of ultrafiltration, while the second term, $Q_{UF}C_{Bo}/C_{Bi}$, represents convective clearance in the absence of diffusion.

Since the change in solute concentration in the blood over the length of the dialyzer tends to be small, it is more common to calculate clearance based on solute appearance in the hemofilter/hemodialyzer effluent:

$$K = (Q_E C_E - Q_D C_D)/C_B \qquad (8)$$

where Q_D and Q_E are the dialysate inflow and effluent outflow rates, respectively, and C_B, C_D, and C_E are the solute concentrations in the blood, dialysate, and effluent, respectively. Since the ultrafiltration rate (Q_{UF}) is equal to the difference between the effluent outflow and dialysate inflow rates ($Q_{UF} = Q_E - Q_D$), Eq. (8) may be rewritten as

$$K = Q_D(C_E - C_D)/C_B + Q_{UF}C_E/C_B \qquad (9)$$

The first term of this equation, $Q_D(C_E - C_D)/C_B$, approximates the diffusive component of clearance, or that amount of clearance which would occur in the absence of ultrafiltration. For solutes such as urea, which are not present in fresh dialysate ($C_D = 0$), this term simplifies to $Q_D C_E/C_B$, or the product of the dialysate flow rate and the equilibration between dialysate and blood (C_E/C_B). The second term, $Q_{UF}C_E/C_B$, represents convective solute clearance in the absence of dialysate flow ($Q_D = 0$). Since in pure convective therapy C_E/C_B is equal to the sieving coefficient (S), this term may be rewritten as $K_C = Q_{UF} S$ [Eq. (4)].

It must be recognized, however, that these terms are mathematical descriptions of clearance and do not physically describe the actual diffusive and convective processes.

In particular, this analysis does not take into consideration the component of convective flux that may occur during continuous hemodialysis as the result of filtration/backfiltration over the length of the hemodialyzer. When membranes with high hydraulic permeability ("high-flux" membranes) are utilized, this component of convective transport which may occur in the absence of net ultrafiltration may substantially augment diffusive clearance.[27] In addition, this analysis does not take into consideration interactions between diffusive and convective solute flux, as discussed below.

Determinants of Diffusive Clearance

Continuous hemodialysis is operationally different from conventional intermittent hemodialysis in that the dialysate inflow rate (Q_D) is much less than the blood flow rate (Q_{Bi}). In conventional intermittent hemodialysis, blood flow rates are typically in the range of 300 to 500 mL/min, with dialysate flow rates between 500 and 800 mL/min. At these flow rates, equilibration between blood and dialysate does not occur, and solute clearance increases with increasing blood flow rates. In contrast, in continuous hemodialysis, dialysate flow rates are usually less than 50 mL/min (3000 mL/h) with blood flow rates of 50 to 150 mL/min in AV therapy and 100 to 250 mL/min in venovenous therapy. At these flow rates, near complete equilibration between blood and dialysate is present for low-molecular-mass solutes.[17,32,33] Brunet et al. have systematically evaluated solute clearances during CRRT at various combinations of dialysate and ultrafiltration flow rates.[32] Using a 0.6-m^2 AN69 membrane and a blood flow rate of 150 mL/min, they demonstrated essentially complete equilibration between blood and dialysate for urea, creatinine, phosphate, and uric acid at a dialysate flow rate of 1000 mL/h. At higher dialysate flow rates, equilibration was less complete, ranging from 0.96 for urea to 0.76 for uric acid.[32] More complete equilibration was observed with a 1.0-m^2 membrane.[32] As shown in Fig. 39–3, despite the incomplete equilibration at higher flow rates, there is a strong dependence between dialysate flow and small solute clearance. In contrast, the clearance of higher-molecular-mass solutes, such as β_2 microglobulin, is limited by a slow rate of diffusion, and exhibits minimal dependence on dialysate flow.[32] It is likely that the clearance of this and other intermediate-molecular-mass species during continuous hemodialysis actually occurs through convective flux, as no augmentation of clearance is observed when diffusive therapy is added to convection in CVVHDF.[32,34]

The other implication of the operational conditions in continuous hemodialysis is the relative independence of clearance on blood flow rate. Sigler and Teehan demonstrated that diffusive clearance was independent of blood flow for $Q_B > 60$ mL/min during CAVHD when dialysate

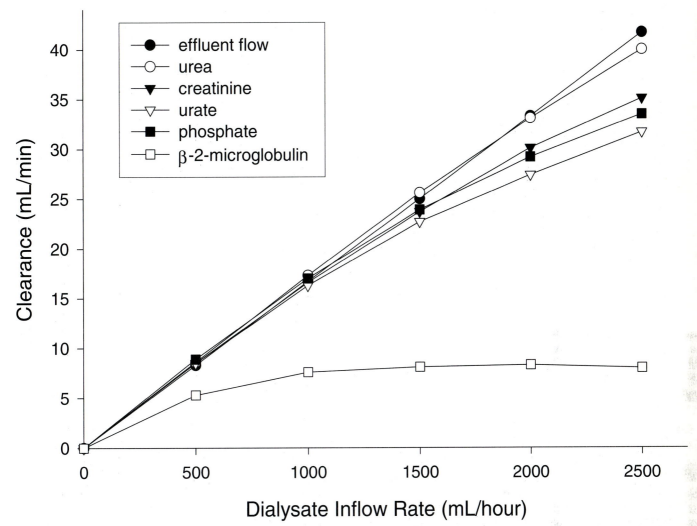

Figure 39–3. Solute clearance during CVVHD. Relationship between clearance and dialysate flow during CVVHD. Measurements were made using a 0.6-m² AN69 membrane at a blood flow rate of 150 mL/min with no net ultrafiltration at dialysate flow rates between 500 and 2500 mL/h. Effluent flow represents the line of identity for dialysate flow. (Adapted from Brunet et al.,[32] with permission.)

flow was 16.7 mL/min.[17] Similarly, Relton et al. demonstrated that urea clearance increased only minimally when blood flow was increased above 100 mL/min during CVVHD with a dialysate flow of 33.3 mL/min.[33]

Determinants of Convective Clearance

As predicted by Eq. (4), solute clearance in continuous hemofiltration is proportional to the ultrafiltration rate. As shown in Fig. 39–4, for low-molecular-mass solutes and sieving coefficients (S) of approximately 1, solute clearance is equal to the ultrafiltration or effluent flow rate.[32] A more complex pattern is observed for higher-molecular-mass species, such as β_2 microglobulin, which exhibit a nonlinear relationship between clearance and ultrafiltration rate. As shown in Fig. 39–4, as transmembrane water flux increases, the sieving coefficient for β_2 microglobulin also increases.[32]

The mechanism for this phenomenon is poorly understood and may be related to either a local accumulation of molecules at the surface of the membrane by reflexion, resulting in a subsequent increase in convective flux, or to the recruitment of additional pores or alteration in pore geometry associated with changes in transmembrane pressure and increased fluid flux across the membrane.[32]

The site of infusion of replacement fluid is also an important determinant of convective clearance (Fig. 39–5). In CAVH, hemoconcentration and increased plasma oncotic pressure when filtration fraction exceeds 20 percent of extracorporeal plasma flow may significantly limit ultrafiltration rates.[11,12] Administration of replacement fluid into the extracorporeal circuit prior to the hemofilter diminishes hemoconcentration, attenuates the increase in oncotic pressure, and increases solute clearance.[14,35] The benefit of predilution in CVVH has been controversial. Administra-

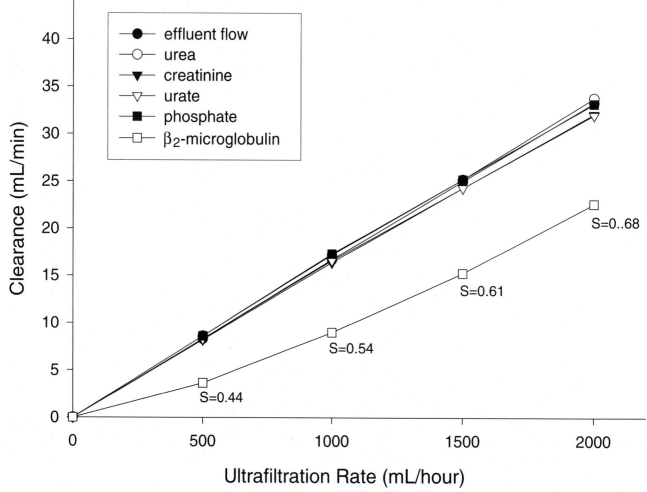

Figure 39–4. Solute clearance during CVVH. Relationship between clearance and ultrafiltration rate during CVVHD. Measurements were made using a 0.6-m² AN69 membrane at a blood flow rate of 150 mL/min with ultrafiltration rates between 500 and 2000 mL/h without predilution. Effluent flow represents the line of identity for ultrafiltrate flow. Observed sieving coefficients (S) for β₂ microglobulin are shown. (Adapted from Brunet et al.,[32] with permission.)

tion of replacement fluid in pumped systems helps minimize the filtration fraction, but at the expense of reducing the solute concentration in the hemofilter, thereby reducing effective solute clearance. The reduction in solute concentration is a function of the blood flow rate (Q_{Bi}) and the infusion rate of the replacement fluids (Q_R):

$$K = Q_{UF}\, S\, Q_{Bi}/(Q_{Bi} + Q_R) \qquad (10)$$

The impact of predilution administration of replacement fluid on solute clearance during CVVH is illustrated in Fig. 39–6. At a blood flow rate of 150 mL/min, predilution administration of replacement fluids at an infusion rate of 2000 mL/h resulted in a reduction in clearance of approximately 15 percent.[32] Although predilution decreases solute clearance, Uchino et al. have demonstrated a counterbalancing improvement in hemofilter patency.[36] As a result of decreased time off therapy associated with predilution, they

observed no change in overall treatment efficiency with predilution administration of replacement fluids.[36]

Interaction between Diffusive and Convective Clearance

Initial observations reported minimal interaction between the convective and diffusive components of solute flux during CAVHDF.[17] This observation, shown in Fig. 39–7, is in contrast to observations in intermittent high-volume hemodiafiltration, in which total clearance is recognized to be less than the sum of dialytic (diffusive) and hemofiltration (convective) clearances occurring separately.[37–39] The mechanism for this interaction is complex and is thought to relate to alterations in the unstirred layer along the membrane surface, resulting in a relative reduction in the solute concentration gradient across the membrane. When higher ultrafiltration rates are utilized in CRRT, a similar interaction can be observed.[32,34] As shown in Fig. 39–8, the magnitude of this interaction is a function of the solute, the membrane

Predilution

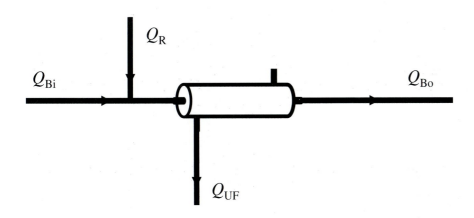

Postdilution

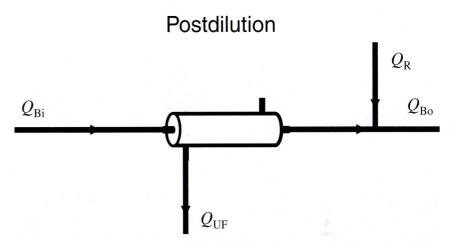

Figure 39–5. Schematic representation of pre- and postdilution administration of replacement fluid in CVVH. Schematic representation of pre- and postdilution administration of replacement fluid in CVVH. In predilution, replacement fluid is infused into the extracorporeal circuit prior to the hemofilter. In postdilution, the infusion is distal to the hemofilter.

surface area, and the dialysate flow rate (Q_D). While the observed urea clearance was within 10 percent of predicted values, the interaction between convection and diffusion resulted in a reduction in urate clearance in excess of 15 percent.[32]

TECHNICAL CONSIDERATIONS

Vascular Access

Performance of CRRT requires adequate access to the circulation for creation of the extracorporeal circuit. In the AV therapies, access is achieved utilizing separate arterial and venous cannulas with perfusion of the circuit driven by the arteriovenous pressure gradient. In the venovenous therapies, vascular access is obtained using two venous cannulas

(or a single double-lumen cannula) with circulation through the extracorporeal circuit driven by a mechanical blood pump.

Arteriovenous Access. Vascular access for AV therapies is accomplished most commonly by the use of wide-bore arterial and venous catheters, although external AV shunts have also been utilized.[40] Catheter access provides better blood flow than AV shunts, especially in the setting of hypotension, and generally is the preferred mode of vascular access.[41] The design and placement of the catheters is critical for minimizing circuit resistance and optimizing extracorporeal blood flow. The arterial catheter should be nontapered, should be no smaller than 8F, and should have a single end hole for blood inflow.[40] Catheter length should be minimized to reduce resistance. The femoral artery is the

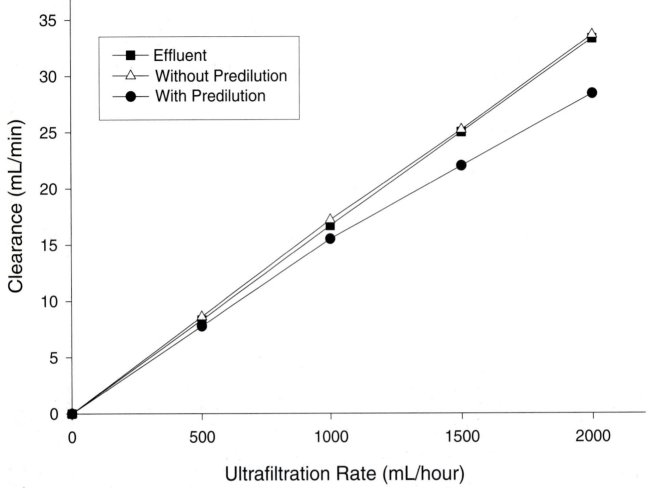

Figure 39–6. Effect of predilution on urea clearance during CVVH. Urea clearance in the presence or absence of prefilter administration of replacement fluid. Measurements were made using a 0.6-m^2 AN69 membrane at a blood flow rate of 150 mL/min with ultrafiltration rates between 500 and 2000 mL/h. Replacement fluid was administered to match the ultrafiltration rate. Effluent flow rate represents the line of identity for ultrafiltrate flow. (Adapted from Brunet et al.,[32] with permission.)

most convenient site for cannulation, providing the highest flow rates; however, other large-bore vessels, such as the brachial and axillary arteries, may be used. The venous catheter should also be large bore and nontapered so as to not increase intrinsic circuit pressure.

The use of AV access is associated with more numerous and more serious complications than are seen with venovenous therapies.[42] The majority of these complications are associated with the arterial catheter and include hemorrhage, distal thromboembolism, arterial aneurysm formation, AV fistula formation, and infection. Extreme caution must be used at the time of catheter placement to ensure adequate distal circulation. The catheter site and distal extremity should be continuously monitored for evidence of vascular injury while the catheter remains in place. Catheter removal should be performed only after systemic anticoagulation has been reversed. Prolonged pressure must be applied to the catheter site after removal to obtain hemostasis.

Venovenous Access. Venovenous access may be obtained either by cannulating two veins or by cannulating a single vein using a double-lumen catheter. Standard hemodialysis catheters may be utilized in the subclavian, internal jugular, or femoral positions. The subclavian position is associated with the lowest rate of infectious complications[43] but may result in the development of central venous stenosis, complicating long-term vascular access in patients whose ARF does not resolve and who remain dialysis-dependent.

Extracorporeal Circuit

AV circuits can be viewed as consisting of five resistors arranged in series: the arterial access, arterial blood tubing, hemodialyzer/hemofilter, venous blood tubing, and venous catheter. Since the driving pressure for extracorporeal blood flow is fixed by the AV pressure gradient, optimization of blood flow is dependent upon minimization of circuit resis-

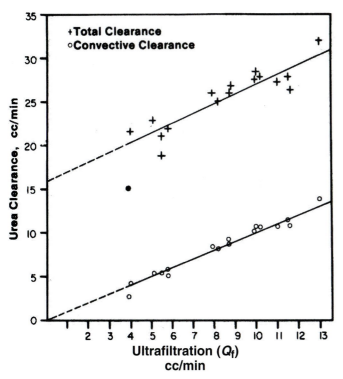

Figure 39–7. Urea clearance during CAVHDF. Whole-blood urea clearance vs. ultrafiltration rate. Each total clearance point (+) has its corresponding convective component (o) plotted directly under it on the lower line. Each set of points represents either an individual patient ($n = 12$) or a repeat study on the same patient done at least 1 day apart ($n = 5$). One point (•) was not included in the regression analysis because of a very low blood flow and lack of membrane equilibration. The distance between the lines represents diffusional clearance. (From Sigler et al.,[17] with permission.)

tance. Issues relating to the arterial and venous catheters were discussed above. In order to further minimize resistance, the arterial and venous blood lines should be as short as possible, without sites of constriction. These concerns are eliminated in pumped venovenous systems that are not dependent upon the limited AV pressure gradient. The use of a blood pump, however, requires increased complexity of the circuit. In order to provide adequate safety monitoring, pressure transducers and an air detector are mandatory. The increased circuit length and the introduction of air-blood interfaces results in increased circuit thrombogenicity.[44]

Hemofilters/Hemodialyzers

There are a wide variety of membranes available for use in CRRT. Hemofilters used for primarily convective therapies (CAVH and CVVH) require high hydraulic permeability to sustain adequate ultrafiltration. In contrast, the hydraulic permeability of hemodialyzers used for diffusive therapies is less critical. Hemodialyzer efficiency is dependent upon the membrane's coefficient of diffusion, which is a function

of membrane composition, thickness, and surface area. Membranes that are optimized for convective therapy may provide inadequate diffusive clearance.[33]

The geometry of hemofilter and hemodialyzer design contributes to treatment efficiency in AV therapies. The hemofilter is the major site of resistance in the CAVH extracorporeal circuit. The use of hollow-fiber hemofilters with large cross-sectional area and short axial length minimizes resistance and maximizes blood flow at a fixed AV pressure gradient.[45] In addition, the resistance across the axial length of the hemofilter can be decreased by increasing the inner diameter of the individual hollow fibers.[45] In CAVHD, diffusive solute clearance is enhanced by the use of parallel-plate hemodialyzers as compared to hollow-fiber membranes of equal or greater surface area.[46] These design concerns lose importance in pumped venovenous systems in which extracorporeal blood flow is independent of arterial blood pressure.

Conflicting data exist regarding the impact of hemodialysis membrane biocompatibility on the outcomes of ARF.[47–51] Metanalyses of this data have also yielded conflicting results; one analysis concluded that synthetic membranes conferred a survival advantage over unsubstituted cellulosic (e.g., cuprophan) membranes,[52] while a second metanalysis found no survival advantage with either membrane type.[53] The relevance of these data to CRRT is uncertain since all of the data were derived from studies of intermittent hemodialysis. From the pragmatic standpoint, this issue may be of only marginal significance, since the majority of hemodialysis membranes available for CRRT are of synthetic composition. In addition, cellulosic membranes are not appropriate for hemofiltration-based therapies, as they do not provide sufficient hydraulic permeability.

Pumps

Early descriptions of the venovenous modalities of CRRT utilized nonproprietary systems created at individual institutions. These systems generally comprised a peristaltic blood pump to obtain blood flow and volumetric intravenous infusion pumps to regulate ultrafiltration and the flow of dialysate and/or replacement fluid. Safety monitors were limited, frequently consisting only of an air detector on the venous return line. The linear peristaltic pumps used to regulate ultrafiltration were error-prone, leading to poor regulation of fluid balance.[54]

This early technology has now been supplanted by integrated machines specifically designed for the management of CRRT.[55] These machines are equipped with fluid-balancing controls, to ensure delivery of prescribed fluid management, and integrated safety alarms including air detectors and pressure monitors. The incorporation of user-friendly operator interfaces allows for more efficient nursing management.

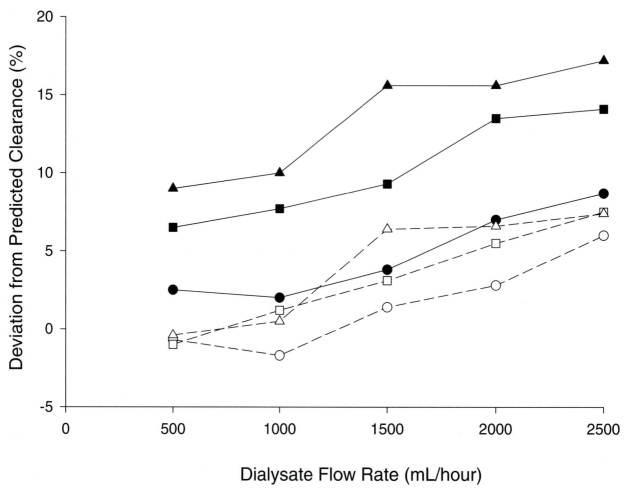

Figure 39–8. Deviation between observed and expected clearance during CVVHDF. Deviation between observed and expected clearance of urea (■), creatinine (⊠), and urate (△) during CVVHDF at a blood flow of 150 mL/min and an ultrafiltration rate of 2000 mL/h using either a 0.6-m² (solid line) or 1.0-m² (broken line) AN69 membrane. Percent deviation was calculated from the difference between the actual measured clearance under the specified conditions and the arithmetic sum of CVVH clearance at an ultrafiltration rate of 2000 mL/h and CVVHD clearance with no net ultrafiltration. (Data from Brunet et al.,[32] with permission.)

Dialysate and Replacement Fluids

The requirement for intravenous replacement solutions and/or dialysate during CRRT is dependent upon the modality of therapy utilized. In continuous hemofiltration, intravenous replacement fluids are required to restore excess ultrafiltrate losses and maintain extracellular fluid volume. In continuous hemodialysis, dialysate is perfused through the dialysate compartment to provide diffusive clearance, while ultrafiltration is limited to that required for management of volume overload, thus eliminating the need for replacement fluids. In hemodiafiltration, both replacement fluids and dialysate are required.

Similar considerations guide the composition of dialysate and replacement fluids. Both must ensure the maintenance of normal extracellular electrolyte composition while achieving satisfactory removal of metabolic waste products and control of extracellular volume. The precise composition of these fluids should be individualized in order to compensate for specific electrolyte and acid-base disturbances.

Dialysate. As previously described, equilibration of low-molecular-weight solutes between blood and dialysate is nearly complete during continuous hemodialysis. Thus, the composition of dialysate should approximate the desired plasma composition. Initial descriptions of continuous hemodialysis utilized peritoneal dialysis fluid as dialysate.[17,56,57] Although this fluid is readily available, it does not have an optimal composition for this application. In particular, its high glucose content resulted in high rates of glucose absorption and hyperglycemia.[58] Hemofiltration fluid was modified from peritoneal dialysate to provide a more optimal glucose and electrolyte composition (Table 39–3).

Until recently, bicarbonate-buffered dialysis solutions have not been commercially available. Bicarbonate-buffered solutions had to be compounded by hospital pharmacies or prepared at the point of use. Preparation of bicarbonate-buffered dialysate by collection of dialysate from a conventional dialysis machine has also been described.[59,60] Filtration of this nonsterile dialysate is required, as this fluid is an excellent growth medium for bacteria, and bacterial growth and endotoxin production may occur during storage. More recently, several commercially available bicarbonate-buffered dialysis solutions have become available (Table 39–3).

Replacement Fluid. The composition of the ultrafiltrate generated during continuous hemofiltration and hemodiafiltration approximates that of plasma water. The optimal replacement solution should also approximate normal plasma water composition, replacing the electrolytes and minerals lost through ultrafiltration without replacing the metabolic solutes (e.g., urea) which accumulate in renal failure. Early descriptions of CAVH utilized modified saline solutions to which buffer—such as bicarbonate, acetate, or lactate—had been added.[11,12,31] Supplemental potassium, calcium, and magnesium were also added to replace their losses in the ultrafiltrate. There is no specific need for glucose in replacement fluids; ultrafiltrate glucose losses can readily be replaced through adjustments in the prescription of nutritional support. If glucose is added, supraphysiologic concentrations should be avoided, as they pose a risk of carbohydrate overfeeding and may result in significant hyperglycemia.[61]

No commercially prepared fluids are licensed in the United States for use as replacement fluid for CRRT. Lactated Ringer's solution,[12,62] peritoneal dialysis fluid,[61,63] and hemodiafiltration fluid[19] are lactate-buffered fluids that have been utilized for this purpose in an off-label use. As shown in Table 39–3, lactated Ringer's solution and peritoneal dialysis fluid are both hyponatric and may result in the development of hyponatremia. In addition, the glucose load in peritoneal dialysis fluid is associated with the development of hyperglycemia.[61]

Until recently, no bicarbonate-buffered fluids were commercially available. As a result, a variety of strategies to compound bicarbonate-buffered fluids at the point of use have been developed.[12,21,31,57,64] Because of concern over the stability of fluids containing bicarbonate and calcium salts, these strategies included multibag formulations in which the bicarbonate and divalent ions were infused separately through a tubing manifold or infused sequentially. More recently, several sterile, bicarbonate-buffered dialysis solutions for CRRT have become available. Although these fluids are not approved in the United States for intravenous administration as replacement fluid, they have been utilized in this manner.[65] Use of these solutions avoids the risk of potentially dangerous compounding errors, which may occur when complex solutions are prepared on small scale at an individual pharmacy or at the point of use.[65]

Selection of Buffer. Lactate, acetate, and bicarbonate have all been used as buffer in replacement fluids and dialysate for CRRT. Although studies have demonstrated satisfactory correction of metabolic acidosis with lactate-buffered fluids,[66] multiple concerns have been raised regarding the use of a nonphysiologic buffer. Lactate is rapidly metabolized by the liver; however, elevations in blood lactate levels are observed when infusion rates exceed metabolic clearance.[67,68] During CRRT with lactate-buffered fluids, modest elevations in blood lactate concentration are common[33]; however, marked elevations in blood lactate levels are generally seen only in patients with lactic acidosis or impaired hepatic metabolism.[69] Whether the modest hyperlactatemia seen in most patients treated with CRRT is associated with

TABLE 39–3. COMPOSITION OF COMMERCIALLY AVAILABLE FLUIDS FOR CRRT

	Lactated Ringer's Solution	Peritoneal Dialysis Fluid[a]	Hemofiltration Fluid[a]	Prismasate[b]		Normocarb[c]
				BGK2	BK0	
Sodium (mmol/L)	130	132	140	140	140	140
Potassium (mmol/L)	4	-	2	2	-	-
Bicarbonate (mmol/L)	-	-	-	32	32	35
Lactate (mmol/L)	28	40	30	3	3	-
Calcium (mmol/L)	1.35	1.75	1.75	-	1.75	-
Magnesium (mmol/L)	-	0.25	0.75	0.5	0.5	0.75
Glucose (mg/dL)	-	1,360	100	110	-	-

[a]Baxter Healthcare Corporation, Deerfield, IL.
[b]Gambro, Lakewood, CO.
[c]Dialysis Solutions Inc, Richmond Hill, Ontario, Canada.

morbidity is not clear. Elevations in blood lactate alter the pyruvate:lactate ratio, increase protein catabolic rate, and may contribute to myocardial depression. Several recent studies have suggested that lactate-buffered fluids are less effective in controlling metabolic acidosis and are associated with greater hemodynamic instability than bicarbonate-buffered fluids.[70–72] Thirty-eight percent of patients treated using lactate-buffered fluids sustained cardiovascular complications as compared to only 15 percent of patients receiving bicarbonate-buffered fluids.[70] Similarly, there were 0.6 episodes of hypotension per 24 hours in patients treated using lactate-buffered fluids as compared to 0.26 episodes per 24 hours with bicarbonate-buffered fluids.[70] Use of lactate-buffered fluids was associated with a fall in mean arterial pressure of 2.7 mmHg, as compared to a 5.8 mmHg rise in pressure with lactate-free fluids.[72] Although these studies were not adequately powered to detect an impact on survival, they suggest that use of bicarbonate-buffered fluids may be preferable, particularly in hemodynamically unstable patients, even in the absence of underlying lactic acidosis or liver dysfunction.

Anticoagulation

Clotting of the extracorporeal circuit is the most common reason for interruption of CRRT treatment.[73] Multiple anticoagulation regimens have been developed for prevention of circuit clotting (Table 39–4). The goal of all of these strategies is to balance the risk of clotting of the CRRT circuit with the risk of bleeding, particularly in patients who have underlying coagulopathies or are in the immediate postoperative period.

The most widely utilized anticoagulant for CRRT is unfractionated heparin.[74] Heparin is infused into the prefilter blood line as close to the access catheter as possible. Low dose infusions are usually sufficient to inhibit clotting of the extracorporeal circuit without systemic effect. Multiple infusion regimens have been proposed including weight based dosing (e.g., 10 IU/kg/h) or dosing based on circuit blood flow rate (e.g., 0.15 IU/mL/min).[59] In general, these regimens provide infusion rates of between 250 and 750 IU/h. Therapy may be monitored with frequent testing of the patient's partial thromboplastin time (PTT), with a goal of a PTT approximately 1.5 times control in the return line with a normal systemic PTT. Alternatively, the activated clotting time in the return line may be monitored, with a target prolongation of 1.5 to 2 times control. Regional heparin anticoagulation has been advocated for patients with active bleeding or at high risk for bleeding complications.[75] This technique involves neutralization of the heparin infused into the prefilter limb through the infusion of protamine sulfate into the return line. Major complications of heparin include excessive anticoagulation and the development of heparin-induced thrombocytopenia (HIT). This latter condition requires the immediate cessation of heparinization due to increased risks of both bleeding and paradoxical thrombosis.

A variety of other anticoagulation techniques have been proposed as an alternative to heparin. Fractionated, low-molecular-weight heparinoids have been tried as alternative therapy. Dalteparin demonstrated no better efficacy or safety than unfractionated heparin and was more expensive.[76] Danaparoid, a less sulfated low-molecular-weight heparin, has been proposed as an alternative anticoagulant in patients with HIT and has recently been shown to be safe and effective for anticoagulation during CRRT.[77,78] Given the erratic clearance of low-molecular-weight heparinoids in renal insufficiency, factor Xa levels must be monitored during treatment. Prostacyclin (prostaglandin I_2),[79,80] hirudin,[81,82] and argatroban[83] have also been utilized as alternative anticoagulants. All are more costly than heparin but may be of benefit in patients with HIT. The use of prostacyclin is also limited by its narrow therapeutic margin between anticoagulant and hypotensive effects.

Regional citrate anticoagulation is also effective for anticoagulation. Citrate chelates calcium, thereby inhibiting the coagulation cascade. Citrate is infused into the proximal prefilter blood line; calcium is infused either into the venous return line or peripherally to maintain a normal systemic ionized calcium concentration. The original protocol for citrate anticoagulation used high concentrations of citrate and necessitated the use of specialized dialysate and replacement solutions.[84] Multiple additional protocols have now been published, providing simplified management of citrate anticoagulation.[65,85–88] Although these regimens are reported to be highly effective, no randomized comparisons with heparin anticoagulation have been published. Complications associated with citrate anticoagulation include hypocalcemia and metabolic alkalosis.

Performance of CRRT in the absence of anticoagulation has also been reported.[89] Anticoagulation-free management is most likely to be successful in patients with underlying coagulopathies or thrombocytopenia. Prefilter administration of replacement fluids has been suggested to decrease clotting risk; however, periodic saline flushes provided no benefit in prolonging system patency.[89]

TABLE 39–4. ANTICOAGULATION STRATEGIES

Heparin
  Standard infusion
  Regional infusion
Low-molecular-weight heparin
Prostacyclin
Hirudins
Citrate
Anticoagulant-free

DOSING OF CRRT

As previously discussed, the urea clearance during convective therapies is approximately equal to the ultrafiltration rate (corrected for prefilter fluid administration), and equilibration of urea between blood and dialysate is essentially complete during continuous hemodialysis. Thus, urea clearance during the continuous therapies approximates effluent flow rate (Q_E). There is, however, no validated method for normalizing clearance values between patients. In conventional hemodialysis, dose is commonly expressed as the fractional clearance of urea, Kt/V, where K is urea clearance, t is duration of therapy, and V is the volume of distribution of urea. Daily Kt/V can be estimated based on the 24-hour effluent volume ($V_E = Q_E t \cong Kt$) divided by the estimated volume of distribution of urea (V). Since this latter value cannot be reliably predicted,[90] normalization of clearance to body surface area, as used for assessment of glomerular filtration rate, or body mass (e.g., mL/kg/h) has been suggested.[91]

There is increasing evidence of a relationship between dose of renal replacement therapy and outcome in ARF.[92-94] Prospective studies evaluating the impact of CRRT dose on outcome are limited. Ronco et al. evaluated outcomes in 425 critically ill patients with ARF randomized to treatment with CVVH at doses of 20, 35, or 45 mL/kg/h.[94] Survival 15 days after stopping CVVH was 41 percent in the low-dose arm compared to 57 and 58 percent in the 35- and 45-mL/kg/h arms, respectively (Fig. 39–9). In contrast, Bouman et al. compared high-volume continuous hemofiltration (72 to 96 L/day) initiated within 12 hours after fulfilling criteria for ARF ($n = 35$) to low-volume hemofiltration (24 to 36 L/day) initiated either within 12 hours ($n = 35$) or after meeting conventional criteria for initiation of renal replacement therapy (BUN > 112 mg/dL, potassium > 6.5 meq/L or severe pulmonary edema) ($n = 36$).[95] No difference in survival was observed in the three groups; however, overall survival was 72.6 percent, suggesting that this study population had different characteristics than the population studied by Ronco et al. While these data suggest that higher doses of CRRT may be of benefit in high-risk patients, further investigation is required to establish dosing recommendations for CRRT.

SELECTION OF MODALITY

Arteriovenous vs. Venovenous Therapies

Venovenous therapy has largely supplanted AV therapy at most centers performing CRRT. Advantages of AV therapies include greater ease of setup and operation, lower extracorporeal blood volumes, and the absence of blood pumps with the associated need for pressure monitors and air detectors. Disadvantages include the need for prolonged arterial cannulation, with attendant risks of arterial injury, hemorrhage, and thrombosis, as well as the reliance of extracorporeal blood flow on mean arterial pressure. Given the restrictions on blood flow inherent in an AV circuit, these therapies are not able to provide the higher solute clearances that are routinely obtained using pumped venovenous therapies.[20,21,42] Based on these considerations, a consensus conference held in 2000 concluded that venovenous therapies are preferred to AV modalities of CRRT and that the latter should be reserved for settings in which venovenous therapy cannot be provided due to the absence of adequate equipment or trained personnel.[96, 97]

Convective vs. Diffusive Therapies

Achievable clearances of low-molecular-weight solutes are essentially similar for the convective and diffusive therapies.[32,33,98] In general, however, the convective therapies (continuous hemofiltration and hemodiafiltration) provide higher clearances for solutes with molecular weights greater than 500 to 1000 Da.[32,98] It has been postulated that enhanced clearance of inflammatory mediators, particularly in patients whose ARF occurs in the setting of sepsis, may provide a benefit of convective as opposed to diffusive therapies.[99] Animal models have suggested that cytokine clearance can be enhanced using high volume hemofiltration.[26,100,101] In one trial comparing CVVH to CVVHD in patients with ARF and severe systemic inflammatory response syndrome (SIRS), CVVH was associated with decreased plasma tumor necrosis factor-alpha (TNF-α) levels as compared to CVVHD, however levels of other cytokines, including interlukin-6 (IL-6) and interleukin-10 (IL-10)

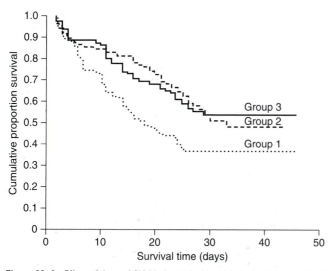

Figure 39–9. Effect of dose of CVVH on survival in ARF. Kaplan-Meier survival curves of patients treated at doses of CVVH of 20 mL/kg/h (group 1), 35 mL/kg/h (group 2) and 45 mL/kg/h (group 3). Survival in group 1 was significantly lower than in groups 2 and 3 (p <0.05). There was no difference in survival between groups 2 and 3. (From Ronco et al.,[94] with permission.)

were not different.[98] In trauma patients without renal failure, CVVH was associated with decreases in both TNF-α and IL-6[102] and was associated with improved hemodynamic stability.[103] It is uncertain, however, whether the cytokine clearance is achieved by convective removal or membrane adsorption.[104] The clinical relevance of the cytokine clearance that has been observed has also been questioned, as the clearances that are achievable with CRRT are markedly lower than the biological turnover of these mediators.[105] In the absence of outcome data, it is not possible to make recommendations regarding the use of predominantly convective modalities as compared to diffusive therapies.[97] Randomized clinical trials to address this question need to be performed.

DRUG DOSING DURING CRRT

Drug clearance by CRRT is a function of multiple factors including the molecular weight of the drug, the degree of protein binding, the composition of the membrane, and the drug concentration in the blood.[106–108] For low-molecular-weight drugs, clearance by convection and diffusion will be similar. As molecular weight increases, drug removal by diffusion declines to a greater extent than convective clearance. The majority of published data on drug clearance during CRRT are derived from an era when most therapy was provided using AV circuits and dialysate and ultrafiltration rates were relatively low as compared to current treatment protocols.[109–112] During this earlier era, drug clearances with CRRT were relatively low and the differences between drug removal by diffusion and convection were small. Now that higher-volume therapy is more widely used, the differences between convective and diffusive clearance take on greater clinical importance.[113] In addition, many studies assume nonrenal drug clearance based on observations in patients with chronic kidney disease. There is substantial evidence that nonrenal clearances are substantially higher in ARF than in chronic kidney disease, which could result in inappropriate dosing.[114,115] In the absence of adequate data to guide drug therapy, it is critical that careful pharmacokinetic monitoring be performed to ensure adequate and nontoxic plasma levels of administered agents.

COMPARISON OF CRRT WITH OTHER MODALITIES OF RENAL SUPPORT FOR ARF

Dose Equivalence with Intermittent Therapies

There are no reliable methods for relating the dose of CRRT to the dose of intermittent hemodialysis delivered on a three-time per week or more frequent schedule. In end-stage kidney disease, the outcomes achieved with continuous ambulatory peritoneal dialysis provided at a weekly Kt/V of 1.7 to 2.0 are similar to the outcomes associated with thrice-weekly hemodialysis dosed to provide a single-pool Kt/V of 1.2 per treatment.[116–118] This equivalence occurs despite the fact that the arithmetic sum of the weekly delivered dose of hemodialysis is substantially greater than the "equivalent" weekly dose of peritoneal dialysis.

There are many possible reasons for this lack of arithmetic equivalency. In intermittent hemodialysis, urea concentration fluctuates in a sawtooth pattern, with a rapid fall during treatment and a slow rise during the intradialytic interval. Since the quantity of urea removed during each unit of time is proportional to the blood urea concentration, the absolute rate of urea elimination is greatest at the start of treatment and falls continuously throughout the treatment. Thus, during the latter portion of a conventional hemodialysis treatment, urea removal becomes relatively inefficient. A higher dose of therapy is required to compensate for this inefficiency.[119] In addition, the mechanism of toxicity in uremia is poorly understood. To the extent that toxicity correlates with the peak blood urea concentration, the efficiency of treatment increases as the interval between treatments decreases, with maximal efficiency achieved by continuous therapy.[120] In addition, the exclusive use of urea kinetic modeling in assessing the dose of therapy discounts the contribution of higher-molecular-weight solutes to the toxicity of uremia. The clearance of these solutes correlates better with duration of therapy than with urea kinetics.[119]

Three mathematical models have been proposed for correlating the doses of continuous and intermittent renal replacement therapies. These models differ with regard to how they correlate the steady-state urea concentration achieved by continuous therapy with the pattern of peak and trough urea concentrations observed with intermittent hemodialysis. In the first model, the target steady-state urea concentration is equal to the peak predialysis urea concentration[120]; in the second model, this concentration is set to equal the mean predialysis urea concentration[121]; and in the third model, it is equal to the time-averaged urea concentration.[122,123] At the present time, all three of these equivalency models must be considered theoretical, as none have been rigorously validated in clinical practice.

Comparison with Intermittent Hemodialysis

Advocates for CRRT suggest that it is a better therapy for the management of ARF, particularly in hemodynamically unstable patients. They posit that the slower, more gradual removal of fluid and solute during CRRT enhances hemodynamic stability and that increased net salt and water removal permits better treatment of volume overload, permitting more aggressive nutritional management. The data supporting these opinions is primarily anecdotal.

The majority of studies comparing intermittent hemodialysis and CRRT have been nonrandomized or retrospective studies.[124–128] Swartz et al. analyzed the survival data of 349 patients with ARF who received either CRRT or intermittent hemodialysis at a single center.[129] Although the initial univariate analysis showed the odds of death for patients receiving CRRT to be more than twice that of patients receiving intermittent hemodialysis, multivariate risk adjustment to control for severity of illness yielded an adjusted risk of death of 1.09 (95 percent CI: 0.67 to 1.80) for CRRT as compared to intermittent hemodialysis.[129]

In a small, randomized, prospective study that has been published only in abstract form, Sandy et al. compared the outcome of 39 patients with ARF treated with continuous venovenous hemodialysis (CVVHD) to 40 patients treated with intermittent hemodialysis.[130] The two groups were well matched in terms of acuity of illness. Mortality was 71.4 percent in the continuous therapy group versus 60 percent in the intermittent therapy group.

Mehta et al. performed a multicenter prospective randomized trial comparing CRRT to intermittent hemodialysis in 166 patients with ARF.[131] An intention-to-treat analysis found a 28-day all-cause mortality of 59.5 percent in patients randomized to CRRT as compared to 41.5 percent in patients randomized to hemodialysis and an in-hospital mortality of 65.5 vs. 47.6 percent. This study was flawed, however, by unbalanced randomization, resulting in significantly higher APACHE III scores and a significantly greater percentage of patients with liver failure in the CRRT group. Using multivariable stepwise logistic-regression analysis, hepatic failure, APACHE III score, and organ system failure (OSF) score were all independently related to ICU mortality. Based on this analysis, the adjusted odds of death associated with CRRT was 1.58 (95 percent CI: 0.7 to 3.3). Similarly, a time-to-event analysis using a Cox proportional hazards model demonstrated an adjusted hazard ratio associated with CRRT of 1.35 (95 percent CI: 0.89 to 2.06; $p = 0.16$). Despite the higher mortality in the CRRT group, patients initially treated with CRRT had higher rates of recovery of renal function than patients treated with intermittent hemodialysis.[131]

Two metanalyses have been published analyzing the impact of dialysis modality on mortality and renal recovery in ARF.[132,133] Kellum et al. analyzed 13 studies encompassing a total of 1400 patients with ARF comparing continuous to intermittent renal replacement therapy.[132] Only 3 of the 13 were prospective, randomized studies. Overall there was no difference in mortality; however, the quality of the analyzed studies was poor, with only 6 of the studies comparing groups with equal severity of illness at baseline. Attempting to adjust for study quality and severity of illness, the authors calculated a relative risk of death in patients treated with CRRT of 0.72 (95 percent CI: 0.60 to 0.87). In the six studies with similar baseline severity of illness, unadjusted relative risk of death with CRRT was 0.48 (95 percent CI: 0.34 to 0.69). The authors concluded that, given the

weakness in study quality, the current evidence was insufficient to draw strong conclusions regarding the mode of renal support in critically ill patients with ARF, but that the data suggests a potential benefit of continuous as compared to intermittent therapy.[132] In the second metanalysis, Tonelli et al. included 5 randomized studies, only 3 of which were included in the prior analysis.[133] In this analysis, no difference was found in either survival (relative risk for death for IHD: 0.96; 95 percent CI: 0.85 to 1.08) or recovery of renal function.[133] Thus, there remain insufficient data to favor the use of either continuous or intermittent therapy in patients who are hemodynamically stable enough to tolerate intermittent hemodialysis.

Comparison with Peritoneal Dialysis

Peritoneal dialysis is an alternative modality for providing continuous renal replacement therapy. A single study has been published comparing outcomes in patients with ARF managed with peritoneal dialysis to outcomes in patients managed with CVVH.[134] The study included a total of 70 patients with infection-associated ARF, 48 of whom had *falciparum* malaria. The mortality rate in the patients treated with peritoneal dialysis was 47 percent, as compared with 15 percent in the patients managed using CVVH. Although this data suggests that peritoneal dialysis is less effective than CRRT in the management of ARF, the generalizabilty of this study to the general population of patients with ARF is uncertain.

REFERENCES

1. Kramer P, Matthias C, Matthaei D, Scheler F. Elimination of cardiac glycosides through hemofiltration. *J Dial* 1977;1(7): 689–695.
2. Mehta R, Letteri J. Current status of renal replacement therapy for acute renal failure. A survey of US nephrologists. *Am J Nephrol* 1999;19(3):377–382.
3. Bellomo R, Cole L, Reeves J, Silvester W. Renal replacement therapy in the ICU: the Australian experience. *Am J Kidney Dis* 1997;30(5 Suppl 4):S80–S83.
4. Manns M, Sigler MH, Teehan BP. Continuous renal replacement therapies: an update. *Am J Kidney Dis* 1998;32(2): 185–207.
5. Scribner BH, Caner JEZ, Buri R, Quinton W. The technique of continuous hemodialysis. *Trans Am Soc Artif Intern Organs* 1960;6:88–103.
6. Silverstein ME, Ford EA, Lysaght MJ, Henderson LW. Treatment of severe fluid overload by ultrafiltration. *N Engl J Med* 1974;291:747–750.
7. Kramer P, Wigger W, Rieger J, et al. [Arteriovenous haemofiltration: a new and simple method for treatment of over-hydrated patients resistant to diuretics]. *Klin Wochenschr* 1977;55(22):1121–1122.

8. Kramer P, Schrader J, Bohnsack W, et al. Continuous arteriovenous haemofiltration. A new kidney replacement therapy. *Proc Eur Dial Transplant Assoc* 1981;18:743–749.

9. Kramer P, Kaufhold G, Grone HJ, et al. Management of anuric intensive-care patients with arteriovenous hemofiltration. *Int J Artif Organs* 1980;3:225–230.

10. Paganini EP, Nakamoto S. Continuous slow ultrafiltration in oliguric acute renal failure. *Trans Am Soc Artif Intern Organs* 1980;26:201–204.

11. Lauer A, Saccaggi A, Ronco C, et al. Continuous arteriovenous hemofiltration in the critically ill patient. Clinical use and operational characteristics. *Ann Intern Med* 1983;99(4): 455–460.

12. Kaplan AA, Longnecker RE, Folkert VW. Continuous arteriovenous hemofiltration. A report of six months' experience. *Ann Intern Med* 1984;100(3):358–367.

13. Kaplan AA, Longnecker RE, Folkert VW. Suction-assisted continuous arteriovenous hemofiltration. *Trans Am Soc Artif Intern Organs* 1983;29:408–413.

14. Kaplan AA. Predilution versus postdilution for continuous arteriovenous hemofiltration. *Trans Am Soc Artif Intern Organs* 1985;31:28–32.

15. Geronemus R, Schneider N. Continuous arteriovenous hemodialysis: a new modality for treatment of acute renal failure. *Trans Am Soc Artif Intern Organs* 1984;30: 610–613.

16. Ronco C. Arterio-venous hemodiafiltration (A-V HDF): a possible way to increase urea removal during CAVH. *Int J Artif Organs* 1985;8:61–62.

17. Sigler MH, Teehan BP. Solute transport in continuous hemodialysis: a new treatment for acute renal failure. *Kidney Int* 1987;32(4):562–571.

18. Ing TS, Purandare VV, Daugirdas JT, et al. Slow continuous hemodialysis. *Int J Artif Organs* 1984;7:53.

19. Wendon J, Smithies M, Sheppard M, et al. Continuous high volume venous-venous haemofiltration in acute renal failure. *Intens Care Med* 1989;15(6):358–363.

20. Storck M, Hartl WH, Zimmerer E, Inthorn D. Comparison of pump-driven and spontaneous continuous haemofiltration in postoperative acute renal failure. *Lancet* 1991;337(8739): 452–455.

21. Macias WL, Mueller BA, Scarim SK, et al. Continuous venovenous hemofiltration: an alternative to continuous arteriovenous hemofiltration and hemodiafiltration in acute renal failure. *Am J Kidney Dis* 1991;18(4):451–458.

22. Hyman A, Mendelssohn DC. Current Canadian approaches to dialysis for acute renal failure in the ICU. *Am J Nephrol* 2002;22(1):29–34.

23. Bellomo R, Ronco C, Mehta RL. Nomenclature for continuous renal replacement therapies. *Am J Kidney Dis* 1996; 28(suppl 3):S2–S7.

24. Gibney RT, Kimmel PL, Lazarus M. The Acute Dialysis Quality Initiative. Part I: definitions and reporting of CRRT techniques. *Adv Renal Replace Ther* 2002;9(4):252–254.

25. Ronco C, Bellomo R. Continuous renal replacement therapy: evolution in technology and current nomenclature. *Kidney Int Suppl* 1998;66:S160–S164.

26. Grootendorst AF, van Bommel EF, van Leengoed LA, et al. High volume hemofiltration improves hemodynamics and survival of pigs exposed to gut ischemia and reperfusion. *Shock* 1994;2(1):72–78.

27. Ronco C, Bellomo R. Continuous high flux dialysis: an efficient renal replacement. In: Vincent JL, ed. *Yearbook of Intensive Care and Emergency Medicine.* Heidelberg, Germany: Springer-Verlag, 1996:690–696.

28. Ronco C, Ghezzi P, Bellomo R, Brendolan A. New perspectives in the treatment of acute renal failure. *Blood Purif* 1999;17(2–3):166–172.

29. Ronco C, Bellomo R. Basic mechanisms and definitions for continuous renal replacement therapies. *Int J Artif Organs* 1996;19(2):95–109.

30. Garred L, Leblanc M, Canaud B. Urea kinetic modeling for CRRT. *Am J Kidney Dis* 1997;30(5 Suppl 4):S2–S9.

31. Golper TA. Continuous arteriovenous hemofiltration in acute renal failure. *Am J Kidney Dis* 1985;6(6):373–386.

32. Brunet S, Leblanc M, Geadah D, et al. Diffusive and convective solute clearances during continuous renal replacement therapy at various dialysate and ultrafiltration flow rates. *Am J Kidney Dis* 1999;34(3):486–492.

33. Relton S, Greenberg A, Palevsky PM. Dialysate and blood flow dependence of diffusive solute clearance during CVVHD. *ASAIO J* 1992;38(3):M691–M696.

34. Golper TA, Cigarran-Guldris S, Jenkins RD, Brier ME. The role of convection during simulated continuous arteriovenous hemodialysis. *Contrib Nephrol* 1991;93:146–148.

35. Kaplan A. Enhanced efficiency during continuous arteriovenous hemofiltration: the use of predilution. *Int J Artif Organs* 1986;9(3):139–142.

36. Uchino S, Fealy N, Baldwin I, et al. Pre-dilution vs post-dilution during continuous veno-venous hemofiltration: impact on filter life and azotemic control. *Nephron Clin Pract* 2003;94(4):c94–c98.

37. Jaffrin MY, Gupta BB, Malbrancq JM. A one dimensional model of simultaneous hemodialysis and ultrafiltration with a highly permeable membrane. *J Biomech Eng* 1981;108: 261–266.

38. Husted FC, Nolph KD, Vitale FC, Maher JF. Detrimental effects of ultrafiltration on diffusion in coils. *J Lab Clin Med* 1976;87:435–442.

39. Granger A, Vantard G, Vantelon J, Perrone B. A mathematical approach to simultaneous dialysis and filtration. *Proc Eur Soc Artif Organs* 1978;5:174–177.

40. Uldall R. Vascular access for continuous renal replacement therapy. *Semin Dial* 1996;9(2):93–97.

41. Olbricht CJ, Haubitz M, Habel U, et al. Continuous arteriovenous hemofiltration: in vivo functional characteristics and its dependence on vascular access and filter design. *Nephron* 1990;55(1):49–57.

42. Bellomo R, Parkin G, Love J, Boyce N. A prospective comparative study of continuous arteriovenous hemodiafiltration and continuous venovenous hemodiafiltration in critically ill patients. *Am J Kidney Dis* 1993;21(4): 400–404.

43. O'Grady NP, Alexander M, Dellinger EP, et al. Guidelines for the prevention of intravascular catheter-related infections. Centers for Disease Control and Prevention. *MMWR Recomm Rep* 2002;51(RR–10):1–29.

44. Baldwin I, Tan HK, Bridge N, Bellomo R. Possible strategies to prolong circuit life during hemofiltration: three controlled studies. *Renal Failure* 2002;24(6):839–848.

45. Ronco C. Continuous renal replacement therapies in the treatment of acute renal failure in intensive care patients. Part 1: theoretical aspects and techniques. *Nephrol Dial Transplant* 1994;9(suppl 4):191–200.

46. Yohay DA, Butterly DW, Schwab SJ, Quarles LD. Continuous arteriovenous hemodialysis: effect of dialyzer geometry. *Kidney Int* 1992;42(2):448–451.

47. Schiffl H, Lang SM, Konig A, et al. Biocompatible membranes in acute renal failure: prospective case-controlled study. *Lancet* 1994;344(8922):570–572.

48. Hakim RM, Wingard RL, Parker RA. Effect of the dialysis membrane in the treatment of patients with acute renal failure. *N Engl J Med* 1994;331(20):1338–1342.

49. Himmelfarb J, Tolkoff Rubin N, et al. A multicenter comparison of dialysis membranes in the treatment of acute renal failure requiring dialysis. *J Am Soc Nephrol* 1998;9(2):257–266.

50. Jorres A, Gahl GM, Dobis C, et al. Haemodialysis-membrane biocompatibility and mortality of patients with dialysis-dependent acute renal failure: a prospective randomised multicentre trial. International Multicentre Study Group. *Lancet* 1999;354(9187):1337–1341.

51. Albright RC Jr, Smelser JM, McCarthy JT, et al. Patient survival and renal recovery in acute renal failure: randomized comparison of cellulose acetate and polysulfone membrane dialyzers. *Mayo Clin Proc* 2000;75(11):1141–1147.

52. Subramanian S, Venkataraman R, Kellum JA. Influence of dialysis membranes on outcomes in acute renal failure: a meta-analysis. *Kidney Int* 2002;62(5):1819–1823.

53. Jaber BL, Lau J, Schmid CH, et al. Effect of biocompatibility of hemodialysis membranes on mortality in acute renal failure: a meta-analysis. *Clin Nephrol* 2002;57(4):274–282.

54. Roberts M, Winney RJ. Errors in fluid balance with pump control of continuous hemodialysis. *Int J Artif Organs* 1992;15(2):99–102.

55. Ronco C, Bellomo R, Kellum JA. Continuous renal replacement therapy: opinions and evidence. *Adv Renal Replace Ther* 2002;9(4):229–244.

56. Bellomo R, Ernest D, Love J, et al. Continuous arteriovenous haemodiafiltration: optimal therapy for acute renal failure in an intensive care setting? *Aust N Z J Med* 1990;20(3):237–242.

57. Bellomo R, Parkin G, Love J, Boyce N. Use of continuous haemodiafiltration: an approach to the management of acute renal failure in the critically ill. *Am J Nephrol* 1992;12(4):240–245.

58. Bellomo R, Colman PG, Caudwell J, Boyce N. Acute continuous hemofiltration with dialysis: effect on insulin concentrations and glycemic control in critically ill patients. *Crit Care Med* 1992;20(12):1672–1676.

59. Tam PY, Huraib S, Mahan B, et al. Slow continuous hemodialysis for the management of complicated acute renal failure in an intensive care unit. *Clin Nephrol* 1988;30(2):79–85.

60. Leblanc M, Moreno L, Robinson OP, et al. Bicarbonate dialysate for continuous renal replacement therapy in intensive care unit patients with acute renal failure. *Am J Kidney Dis* 1995;26(6):910–917.

61. Monaghan R, Watters JM, Clancey SM, et al. Uptake of glucose during continuous arteriovenous hemofiltration. *Crit Care Med* 1993;21(8):1159–1163.

62. Ronco C, Brendolan A, Bragantini L, et al. Continuous arteriovenous hemofiltration with AN69S membrane: procedures and experience. *Kidney Int Suppl* 1988;24:S150–S153.

63. Bonnardeaux A, Pichette V, Ouimet D, et al. Solute clearances with high dialysate flow rates and glucose absorption from the dialysate in continuous arteriovenous hemodialysis. *Am J Kidney Dis* 1992;19(1):31–38.

64. Golper TA, Price J. Continuous venovenous hemofiltration for acute renal failure in the intensive care setting. Technical considerations. *Asaio J* 1994;40(4):936–939.

65. Bunchman TE, Maxvold NJ, Brophy PD. Pediatric convective hemofiltration: Normocarb replacement fluid and citrate anticoagulation. *Am J Kidney Dis* 2003;42(6):1248–1252.

66. Thomas AN, Guy JM, Kishen R, et al. Comparison of lactate and bicarbonate buffered haemofiltration fluids: use in critically ill patients. *Nephrol Dial Transplant* 1997;12(6):1212–1217.

67. Davenport A, Will EJ, Davison AM. Hyperlactataemia and metabolic acidosis during haemofiltration using lactate-buffered fluids. *Nephron* 1991;59(3):461–465.

68. Clasen M, Bohm R, Riehl J, et al. Lactate or bicarbonate for intermittent hemofiltration? *Contrib Nephrol* 1991;93:152–155.

69. Hilton PJ, Taylor J, Forni LG, Treacher DF. Bicarbonate-based haemofiltration in the management of acute renal failure with lactic acidosis. *Q J Med* 1998;91(4):279–283.

70. Barenbrock M, Hausberg M, Matzkies F, et al. Effects of bicarbonate- and lactate-buffered replacement fluids on cardiovascular outcome in CVVH patients. Kidney Int. 2000;58(4):1751–1757.

71. Barenbrock M, Schaefer RM. Cardiovascular outcome in critically ill patients treated with continuous haemofiltration—beneficial effects of bicarbonate-buffered replacement fluids. *Edtna Erca J* 2002;Suppl 2:4–6.

72. McLean AG, Davenport A, Cox D, Sweny P. Effects of lactate-buffered and lactate-free dialysate in CAVHD patients with and without liver dysfunction. *Kidney Int* 2000;58(4):1765–1772.

73. Venkataraman R, Kellum JA, Palevsky P. Dosing patterns for continuous renal replacement therapy at a large academic medical center in the United States. *J Crit Care* 2002;17(4):246–250.

74. Davenport A, Mehta S. The Acute Dialysis Quality Initiative, Part VI: access and anticoagulation in CRRT. *Adv Renal Replace Ther* 2002;9(4):273–281.

75. Kaplan AA, Petrillo R. Regional heparinization for continuous arterio-venous hemofiltration (CAVH). *ASAIO Trans* 1987;33(3):312–315.

76. Reeves JH, Cumming AR, Gallagher L, et al. A controlled trial of low-molecular-weight heparin (dalteparin) versus unfractionated heparin as anticoagulant during continuous

venovenous hemodialysis with filtration. *Crit Care Med* 1999;27(10):2224–2228.

77. Davenport A. Management of heparin-induced thrombocytopenia during continuous renal replacement therapy. *Am J Kidney Dis* 1998;32(4):E3.

78. Lindhoff-Last E, Betz C, Bauersachs R. Use of a low-molecular-weight heparinoid (danaparoid sodium) for continuous renal replacement therapy in intensive care patients. *Clin Appl Thromb Hemost* 2001;7(4):300–304.

79. Ponikvar R, Kandus A, Buturovic J, Kveder R. Use of prostacyclin as the only anticoagulant during continuous venovenous hemofiltration. *Contrib Nephrol* 1991;93:218–220.

80. Fiaccadori E, Maggiore U, Rotelli C, et al. Continuous haemofiltration in acute renal failure with prostacyclin as the sole anti-haemostatic agent. *Intens Care Med* 2002;28(5):586–593.

81. Schneider T, Heuer B, Deller A, Boesken WH. Continuous haemofiltration with r-hirudin (lepirudin) as anticoagulant in a patient with heparin induced thrombocytopenia (HIT II). *Wien Klin Wochenschr* 2000;112(12):552–555.

82. Vargas Hein O, von Heymann C, Lipps M, et al. Hirudin versus heparin for anticoagulation in continuous renal replacement therapy. *Intens Care Med* 2001;27(4):673–679.

83. Dager WE, White RH. Argatroban for heparin-induced thrombocytopenia in hepato-renal failure and CVVHD. *Ann Pharmacother* 2003;37(9):1232–1236.

84. Mehta RL, McDonald BR, Aguilar MM, Ward DM. Regional citrate anticoagulation for continuous arteriovenous hemodialysis in critically ill patients. *Kidney Int* 1990;38(5):976–981.

85. Palsson R, Niles JL. Regional citrate anticoagulation in continuous venovenous hemofiltration in critically ill patients with a high risk of bleeding. *Kidney Int* 1999;55(5):1991–1997.

86. Kutsogiannis DJ, Mayers I, Chin WD, Gibney RT. Regional citrate anticoagulation in continuous venovenous hemodiafiltration. *Am J Kidney Dis* 2000;35(5):802–811.

87. Tolwani AJ, Campbell RC, Schenk MB, et al. Simplified citrate anticoagulation for continuous renal replacement therapy. *Kidney Int* 2001;60(1):370–374.

88. Tobe SW, Aujla P, Walele AA, et al. A novel regional citrate anticoagulation protocol for CRRT using only commercially available solutions. *J Crit Care* 2003;18(2):121–129.

89. Prasad GVR, Palevsky PM, Burr R, et al. Factors affecting system clotting in continuous renal replacement therapy: results of a randomized, controlled trial. *Clin Nephrol* 2000;53(1):55–60.

90. Himmelfarb J, Evanson J, Hakim RM, et al. Urea volume of distribution exceeds total body water in patients with acute renal failure. *Kidney Int* 2002;61(1):317–323.

91. Paganini EP, Depner T, Wensley D. The Acute Dialysis Quality Initiative. Part III: solute control (treatment dose). *Adv Renal Replace Ther* 2002;9(4):260–264.

92. Paganini EP, Tapolyai M, Goormastic M, et al. Establishing a dialysis therapy/patient outcome link in intensive care unit acute dialysis for patients with acute renal failure. *Am J Kidney Dis* 1996;28(suppl 3):S81–S89.

93. Schiffl H, Lang SM, Fischer R. Daily hemodialysis and the outcome of acute renal failure. *N Engl J Med* 2002;346(5):305–310.

94. Ronco C, Bellomo R, Homel P, et al. Effects of different doses in continuous veno-venous haemofiltration on outcomes of acute renal failure: a prospective randomised trial. *Lancet* 2000;356(9223):26–30.

95. Bouman CS, Oudemans-Van Straaten HM, Tijssen JG, et al. Effects of early high-volume continuous venovenous hemofiltration on survival and recovery of renal function in intensive care patients with acute renal failure: a prospective, randomized trial. *Crit Care Med* 2002;30(10):2205–2211.

96. Kellum JA, Mehta RL, Angus DC, et al. The first international consensus conference on continuous renal replacement therapy. *Kidney Int* 2002;62(5):1855–1863.

97. Palevsky PM, Bunchman T, Tetta C. The Acute Dialysis Quality Initiative. Part V: operational characteristics of CRRT. *Adv Renal Replace Ther* 2002;9(4):268–272.

98. Kellum JA, Johnson JP, Kramer D, et al. Diffusive vs convective therapy: effects on mediators of inflammation in patient with severe systemic inflammatory response syndrome. *Crit Care Med* 1998;26(12):1995–2000.

99. Ronco C, Tetta C, Mariano F, et al. Interpreting the mechanisms of continuous renal replacement therapy in sepsis: the peak concentration hypothesis. *Artif Organs* 2003;27(9):792–801.

100. Grootendorst AF, van Bommel EF, van der Hoven B, et al. High volume hemofiltration improves right ventricular function in endotoxin-induced shock in the pig. *Intens Care Med* 1992;18(4):235–240.

101. Grootendorst AF, van Bommel EF. The role of hemofiltration in the critically-ill intensive care unit patient: present and future. *Blood Purif* 1993;11(4):209–223.

102. Sanchez-Izquierdo JA, Perez Vela JL, Lozano Quintana MJ, et al. Cytokines clearance during venovenous hemofiltration in the trauma patient. *Am J Kidney Dis* 1997;30(4):483–488.

103. Sanchez-Izquierdo Riera JA, Alted E, et al. Influence of continuous hemofiltration on the hemodynamics of trauma patients. *Surgery* 1997;122(5):902–908.

104. Bouman CS, van Olden RW, Stoutenbeek CP. Cytokine filtration and adsorption during pre- and postdilution hemofiltration in four different membranes. *Blood Purif* 1998;16(5):261–268.

105. Sieberth HG, Kierdorf HP. Is cytokine removal by continuous hemofiltration feasible? *Kidney Int Suppl* 1999;72:S79–S83.

106. Matzke GR, Frye RF, Joy MS, Palevsky PM. Determinants of ceftriaxone clearance by continuous venovenous hemofiltration and hemodialysis. *Pharmacotherapy* 2000;20(6):635–643.

107. Matzke GR, Frye RF, Joy MS, Palevsky PM. Determinants of ceftazidime clearance by continuous venovenous hemofiltration and continuous venovenous hemodialysis. *Antimicrob Agents Chemother* 2000;44(6):1639–1644.

108. Joy MS, Matzke GR, Frye RF, Palevsky PM. Determinants of vancomycin clearance by continuous venovenous hemofiltration and continuous venovenous hemodialysis. *Am J Kidney Dis* 1998;31(6):1019–1027.

109. Golper TA, Pulliam J, Bennett WM. Removal of therapeutic drugs by continuous arteriovenous hemofiltration. *Arch Intern Med* 1985;145(9):1651–1652.

110. Golper TA, Wedel SK, Kaplan AA, et al. Drug removal during continuous arteriovenous hemofiltration: theory and clinical observations. *Int J Artif Organs* 1985;8(6):307–312.

111. Golper TA, Bennett WM. Drug removal by continuous arteriovenous haemofiltration. A review of the evidence in poisoned patients. *Med Toxicol Adverse Drug Exp* 1988;3(5): 341–349.

112. Golper TA. Drug removal during continuous hemofiltration or hemodialysis. *Contrib Nephrol* 1991;93:110–116.

113. Mueller BA, Pasko DA, Sowinski KM. Higher renal replacement therapy dose delivery influences on drug therapy. *Artif Organs* 2003;27(9):808–814.

114. Mueller BA, Scarim SK, Macias WL. Comparison of imipenem pharmacokinetics in patients with acute or chronic renal failure treated with continuous hemofiltration. *Am J Kidney Dis* 1993;21(2):172–179.

115. Macias WL, Mueller BA, Scarim SK. Vancomycin pharmacokinetics in acute renal failure: preservation of nonrenal clearance. *Clin Pharmacol Ther* 1991;50(6):688–694.

116. NKF-K/DOQI Clinical Practice Guidelines for Peritoneal Dialysis Adequacy: update 2000. *Am J Kidney Dis* 2001; 37(1 suppl 1):S65–S136.

117. Paniagua R, Amato D, Vonesh E, et al. Effects of increased peritoneal clearances on mortality rates in peritoneal dialysis: ADEMEX, a prospective, randomized, controlled trial. *J Am Soc Nephrol* 2002;13(5):1307–1320.

118. Burkart JM. The ADEMEX study and its implications for peritoneal dialysis adequacy. *Semin Dial* 2003;16(1):1–4.

119. Gotch FA, Sargent JA, Keen ML. Wither goest Kt/V. *Kidney Int* 2000;58(Supplement 76):S3–S18.

120. Keshaviah PR, Nolph KD, Van Stone JC. The peak concentration hypothesis: a urea kinetic approach to comparing the adequacy of continuous ambulatory peritoneal dialysis (CAPD) and hemodialysis. *Perit Dial Int* 1989;9(4): 257–260.

121. Gotch FA. The current place of urea kinetic modelling with respect to different dialysis modalities. *Nephrol Dial Transplant* 1998;13(suppl 6):10–14.

122. Casino FG, Lopez T. The equivalent renal urea clearance: a new parameter to assess dialysis dose. *Nephrol Dial Transplant* 1996;11(8):1574–1581.

123. Liao Z, Zhang W, Hardy PA, et al. Kinetic comparison of different acute dialysis therapies. Artif Organs 2003;27(9): 802–807.

124. van Bommel EF, Ponssen HH. Intermittent versus continuous treatment for acute renal failure: where do we stand? *Am J Kidney Dis* 1997;30(5 Suppl 4):S72–S79.

125. Lameire N, Van Biesen W, Vanholder R. Dialysing the patient with acute renal failure in the ICU: the emperor's clothes? *Nephrol Dial Transplant* 1999;14(11):2570–2573.

126. Bellomo R, Boyce N. Acute continuous hemodiafiltration: a prospective study of 110 patients and a review of the literature. *Am J Kidney Dis* 1993;21(5):508–518.

127. Bellomo R, Farmer M, Parkin G, et al. Severe acute renal failure: a comparison of acute continuous hemodiafiltration and conventional dialytic therapy. *Nephron* 1995;71(1): 59–64.

128. van Bommel E, Bouvy ND, So KL, et al. Acute dialytic support for the critically ill: intermittent hemodialysis versus continuous arteriovenous hemodiafiltration. *Am J Nephrol* 1995;15(3):192–200.

129. Swartz RD, Messana JM, Orzol S, Port FK. Comparing continuous hemofiltration with hemodialysis in patients with severe acute renal failure. *Am J Kidney Dis* 1999;34(3): 424–432.

130. Sandy D, Moreno L, Lee JC, Paganini EP. A randomized, stratefied, dose equivalent comparison of continuous venovenous hemodialysis (CVVHD) vs intermittent hemodialysis (IHD) support in ICU acute renal failure (ARF) patients. *J Am Soc Nephrol* 1998;9:225A.

131. Mehta RL, McDonald B, Gabbai FB, et al. A randomized clinical trial of continuous versus intermittent dialysis for acute renal failure. *Kidney Int* 2001;60(3):1154–1163.

132. Kellum JA, Angus DC, Johnson JP, et al. Continuous versus intermittent renal replacement therapy: a meta-analysis. *Interns Care Med* 2002;28(1):29–37.

133. Tonelli M, Manns B, Feller-Kopman D. Acute renal failure in the intensive care unit: a systematic review of the impact of dialytic modality on mortality and renal recovery. *Am J Kidney Dis* 2002;40(5):875–885.

134. Phu NH, Hien TT, Mai NT, et al. Hemofiltration and peritoneal dialysis in infection-associated acute renal failure in Vietnam. *N Engl J Med* 2002;347(12):895–902.

Pediatric Hemofiltration

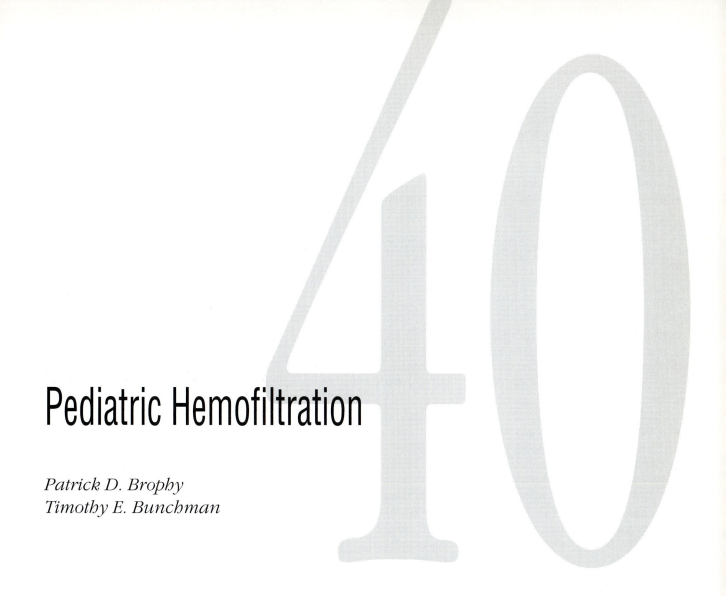

Patrick D. Brophy
Timothy E. Bunchman

TREATMENT: DIALYTIC THERAPY

The complex metabolic abnormalities associated with acute renal failure (ARF) may require dialysis to restore fluid and electrolyte balance. Currently three dialysis modalities are in common use for ARF: peritoneal dialysis (PD), hemodialysis (HD), and hemofiltration (HF). The choice of dialysis modality is best determined based on the local standard of care. With this determination, a variety of considerations must be taken into account.[1] The first of these is experience with the modality. A great deal of preparation and planning is required in order to introduce a new dialysis therapy during the care of a complex, acutely sick patient. The second consideration is access. If the peritoneal membrane is disrupted or no vascular access can be obtained, the choices are obvious. The third consideration is the patient's hemodynamic stability. Patients who are hemodynamically unstable will often not tolerate the fluid shifts associated with intermittent HD as opposed to more continuous modalities such as PD or HF. The fourth consideration is the goal of the dialysis. When the goal is fluid removal, any

of these modalities can work effectively. However when acute solute clearance is necessary, HD is more efficient; yet any of the three modalities will achieve this goal.[1,2]

Other chapters in this book have concentrated on PD and HD for chronic and acute dialysis. This section focuses on hemofiltration as a mode of renal replacement therapy for the pediatric patient in the intensive care unit setting.

CONTINUOUS RENAL REPLACEMENT THERAPY

Continuous renal replacement therapy (CRRT) is a term coined to describe a continuous mode of dialysis at the bedside. Historically this has included PD or HF, but it is now used almost interchangeably with HF. Continuous hemofiltration can be accomplished either via an arteriovenous or venovenous access. The major difference between the two is that arteriovenous HF uses an arterial access and the blood pressure to pump blood through the circuit, and venovenous HF uses a machine to pump blood through the system. Studies have shown that arteriovenous HF provides inadequate solute clearance compared to venovenous HF, and is associated with a more frequent need to change to other modalities.[3,4] Because of this, arteriovenous HF has largely fallen from use. Therefore the major focus of discussion here is venovenous HF.

Venovenous HF can be utilized in any of three modalities. These include continuous venovenous HF (CVVH), continuous venovenous HF with dialysis (CVVHD), and continuous venovenous hemodiafiltration (CVVHDF). The major difference between CVVH and CVVHD is that the former provides convective and the latter diffusive clearance.[5]

CONTINUOUS VENOVENOUS HEMOFILTRATION

CVVH is based on the concept of convective clearance. This is a process whereby blood runs along a porous membrane enabling the removal of an ultrafiltrate, which is replaced with either a pre- or postfilter sterile infusate in the vascular space. Based on concepts of convective clearance, solute is removed in the ultrafiltrate of serum and replaced with a solution free of this solute. Over time, solute is removed, and any remaining solute is diluted to achieve clearance. Small and middle molecules are convectively cleared based on the concentration of the solute in the vascular space and the rate of ultrafiltration; this is related to its sieving coefficient. The sieving coefficient of a solute is dependent on its molecular weight, the "charge" of the HF membrane, and the degree to which the solute is protein-bound.

CONTINUOUS VENOVENOUS HEMOFILTRATION WITH DIALYSIS

CVVHD is based on employing a dialysis solution in a countercurrent fashion to the blood flow across a dialysis membrane, thereby allowing diffusive clearance. This is more comparable to HD. Because dialysate may have some backfiltration into the vascular space, sterile and physiologic dialysate is necessary. The constituents of the dialysate create a solute gradient and allow solute to move from the blood compartment to the dialysate compartment, achieving clearance. The clearance of solute across the membrane is again related to the sieving coefficient (diffusive coefficient) of the solute as well as the charge and pH of the membrane and finally the concentration gradient across the membrane. Low-molecular-weight compounds (e.g., urea) have a sieving (diffusive) coefficient approaching 1, and their clearance is similar with either convective or diffusive clearance. With solutes of middle and larger molecular weight, the sieving (diffusive) coefficient becomes less than 1, and better clearance is achieved by convective therapies. Work by Maxvold et al. has shown that urea clearance (low molecular weight) is equal with either CVVH or CVVHD.[6]

CONTINUOUS VENOVENOUS HEMODIAFILTRATION

CVVHDF is a modality that combines both convective and diffusive therapies. To achieve clearance, this method employs a combination of both a pre- or postfilter replacement fluid and a dialysis fluid. In theory this combination of diffusive and convective clearance may improve clearance that exceeds either the convective or diffusive method alone. However, data thus far have not shown a significant increase in solute clearance, indicating that this technique may do little to improve clearance of solute. As there has been no demonstrable benefit of this "additive" effect to date, most programs use one or the other method so as to minimize complications at bedside.

ULTRAFILTRATION

Ultrafiltration in the setting of HF is based on the concept of net fluid removal. As opposed to PD, where ultrafiltration is controlled by osmolar fluid shifts, ultrafiltration in HF is achieved by a transmembrane pressure. Ultrafiltration can be increased either by increasing the venous return pressure, thus creating a higher pressure across the membrane, or by increasing the pull across the membrane by increasing the pressure at the ultrafiltration site. The newer generation of HF machinery provides computerized control of UF that is accurate to 1 to 2 percent (personal communication, Timothy Kudelka, RN).

EQUIPMENT

In the late twentieth century, all equipment related to HF was adapted from existing blood pumps, intravenous pumps, and/or HD machines. Adapted machinery had the beauty of being easy to use at bedside, but it was without such technical safeguards such as air-leak detectors, blood warmers, and ultrafiltration controllers. These adaptive devices allowed for continuous therapy at bedside but also increased the work of the nursing staff as well as the potential error rate associated with thermic control and ultrafiltration error.[2,7]

Newer machinery has taken the historical benefits of adaptive machinery at bedside and added a thermic warmer for replacement or dialysis fluid as well as very accurate ultrafiltration devices and air-leak detectors. These additional three components have made this therapy much safer at bedside. This machinery has incorporated computer models that will allow for a continuous readout of therapies at bedside. In North America, companies that provide this newer machinery include B-Braun Diapact System, Gambro Prisma System, Edwards Life Science Aquarius System, Baxter BM-25, and—in the future—Accura System, as well as the CRRT option of the hemodialysis machine by the Fresenius 2008H and 2008K machines. Outside North America, HF machines include the Hygieia Plus, Medica EQUASmart, and Rand Performer. All of these machines have in common blood flow rates from 10 to 300 mL/min; dialysis flow rates from as little as 0 to 3 L/h; replacement flow rates from 0 to 5 L/h; various ultrafiltration rates, with accurate ultrafiltration controllers, with the range of ± 1 percent; as well as accurate thermic control. Additionally, all these machineries have air-leak detectors as well as venous and arterial pressure monitors.

The B-Braun (Edwards Life Sciences, Baxter), as well as the Fresenius System allow the user to pick the dialysis membrane. The membrane can be any of the commercially available membranes associated with or independent of the manufacturer's product. The Gambro Prisma System has a cassette system that enhances the ease of administration and commencement of HF but requires the user to employ the specific membrane associated with the cassette. No matter which company is utilized, these new-generation machines have a number of advantages over historic options. as noted above.

MEMBRANES

Membranes for HF are similar to those for HD. They vary based on the components of the membranes, sieving coefficient, as well as surface area. The two major types of membranes available for HF are made of polysulfone or acrylonitrile. Both have the advantage of being mildly negatively charged and possessing a high sieving coefficient, thereby allowing for adequate solute clearance and ultrafiltration either by convective or diffusive modalities; they are considered "biocompatible." Although either is a reasonable choice, septic animal models have demonstrated a superior benefit of the acrylonitrile membrane over the polysulfone membrane when used in a convective mode.[8] Human studies are needed to further delineate membrane impact upon CRRT outcome. Table 40–1 lists the various membranes available.

The acrylonitrile (AN69) membrane has unique features that are problematic in acidotic patients. In those with a metabolic acidosis, when the acidotic plasma interacts with the membrane, the production of bradykinin occurs. When this "activated plasma" is infused back into the patient, it can cause an anaphylactic-like response. This is accentuated in small patients who require blood priming during the onset of HF. The pH of blood-bank blood ranges from 6.2 to 6.4 and is very high in potassium and very low in calcium. A number of programs have reported anaphylaxis in patients during blood priming with the AN69 membrane. This is easily preventable by either dialyzing the

TABLE 40–1. PEDIATRIC CIRCUIT VOLUMES AND HEMOFILTER PROPERTIES

Patient Size (kg)	Hemofilter	Properties/ Surface Area	Priming Volume	Arterial/Venous Line Volumes (total circuit volume = TCV)
< 10	AMICON Minifilter Plus	Polysulfone 0.07 m^2	15 mL	3 mL/3mL (TCV = 21 mL)
>10	RENAFLO II HF 400	Polysulfone 0.3 m^2	28 mL	7 mL/7 mL TCV = 42 mL
	700	0.7 m^2	53 mL	TCV = 67 mL
	1200	1.25 m^2	83 mL	TCV = 97 mL
>10	HOSPAL Multiflow 60	Acrylonitrile and sodium methallyl sulfonate copolymer 0.6 m^2	48 mL	6.5 mL/13.8 mL (TCV= 67.3 mL)
	ASAHI PAN	Polyacrylonitrile		
	0.3	0.3 m^2	33 mL	
	0.6	0.6 m^2	63 mL	
	1.0	1.0 m^2	87 mL	

Note: Venovenous HF requires a larger circuit volume depending on the pumps utilized. For the nonadapted systems such as the PRISMA, the filter is the Multiflow 60 and the circuit volume is fixed at around 100 mL.

blood for a period of time prior to initiating therapy or by using a bypass maneuver.[9] This first option brings the pH up and the potassium down, and it normalizes the calcium.

TUBING

Tubing for HF is available from several companies. At present the Edwards Life Sciences (Aquarius) and Baxter (Accura) have plans for "low volume" and adult tubing to be used with their machines. The Fresenius HD machine, which can be adapted for CRRT, utilizes tubing used for HD. This includes neonatal and pediatric tubing as well as adult tubing. Gambro, for their Prisma System (in the United States), is in the process of developing a system that is 50 percent smaller. The B-Braun has both low-volume and adult tubing, allowing for membranes of various sizes. The current Baxter BM-25 has both low- and high-volume tubing.

Historically, many nephrologists have been told that if a patient has greater than 10 percent of blood volume outside the body, blood priming is necessary to maintain hemodynamic stability. This experience has been extrapolated to the critical care unit, and the same 10 percent rule has been applied for HF. This is an invalid approach, because one is taking a principle that applies to a stable, chronically treated outpatient population and applying it to an unstable inpatient population. Therefore blood priming should no longer be based on the extracorporeal blood volume but rather on the combination of the extracorporeal blood volume and the hemodynamic stability or instability of a given patient. Except for the bradykinin risk associated with blood priming in the AN69 membrane, blood priming should be considered necessary for any patient who is hemodynamically unstable at the time when the need for HF first arises. Therefore the volume of tubing in association with the blood volume of the HF membrane may determine the need for priming.

ACCESS

Access for HD can be either cuffed or noncuffed. In most settings, a noncuffed catheter is placed for acute dialysis. Table 40–2 provides a list of access types for both HD and HF patients. A noncuffed access can be placed in the internal jugular or subclavian vein or the femoral space. Many nephrologists prefer to avoid the use of subclavian catheters, as some of these patients may develop end-stage renal disease (ESRD) and thus may require the creation of a fistula at a future time. Placement of an IJ vs. a femoral catheter is debated by many programs with regard to the preferred site. The advantage of the IJ catheter is that it is independent of the patient's motion and appears to provide adequate blood flow with insignificant resistance in recirculation. The disadvantage of the IJ catheter is the increased risk of both pneumothorax and hemothorax at the time of placement. The advantage of a femoral line is that it poses

less risk at the time of placement as compared to a "high" line. The disadvantage of the femoral line, although not borne out by the literature, is that, in theory at least, it may be more likely to lead to infection. Further, the disadvantage of the femoral site in those patients who are moving during this therapy may affect blood flow, causing intermittent inhibition of dialysis.

SOLUTIONS

In considering solutions for HF, solutions for convective (replacement) as well as diffusive (dialysis) therapies must be taken into account. Both lactate- and bicarbonate-based solutions are available. The rationale for using lactate-based solutions is not that lactate is physiologic; rather, it has to do with permeability of the plastic bags. When bicarbonate is placed directly in the plastic bags, the bicarbonate will leach out as CO_2 over a short period of time and lose its buffering capacity. Therefore, while lactate is clearly not physiologic, it is stable in solution and does not leach out of the bag.

In the setting of a lactate-based solution, as lactate is delivered to the patient, there may be an associated rise in the patient's lactate levels, making it difficult at bedside to tell whether this is related to lactate from the patient (such as bowel ischemia or low cardiac output) or to lactate from the solution. One can easily determine this by differentiating between an "L" and a "D" isomer lactate level, but in the vast majority of most institutions these are sendouts that will involve a 3- to 4-week turnaround time for results. Obviously, this slow turnaround time does not allow for proper determination of the underlying cause and can lead to erroneous decision making.

Comparison data thus far have shown that a bicarbonate solution is not only more physiologic but also associated with improved outcome, poses fewer problems of hemodynamic instability, and involves less need for vasopressors or bicarbonate replacement. These data reinforce the idea that lactate should no longer be used in HF.[10]

In the fall of 2000, Normocarb (Dialysis Solutions, Inc., Richmond Hills, Ont.) became the first bicarbonate-based solution for HF. Normocarb comes as a 240-mL concentrate that, when mixed with a 3-L bag of sterile water, has 140 meq/L sodium, 35 meq/L HCO_3^-, 1.5 meq/L magnesium, and 108 meq/L CL. The solution does not contain calcium, glucose, phosphorus, or potassium. This product has been used successfully for both pediatric and adult HF both as a dialysate and a physiologic replacement fluid.[11–13] Subsequent to the availability of Normocarb, Gambro has released Prismasate, which was approved only for dialysis. This comes as a 5-L bag with a specialized chamber that, when opened, has constituents similar to those of Normocarb.

TABLE 40–2. SUGGESTED SIZE AND SELECTION OF HF VASCULAR ACCESS FOR PEDIATRIC PATIENTS

Patient Size	Catheter Size and Source	Site of Insertion
Neonate	Single-lumen 18-,16-, 14-gauge (Cook)	Femoral artery or vein
	Single-lumen 5F (Medcomp)	Femoral artery, vein, or umbilical vein
	Dual-lumen 7F (Cook/Medcomp)	Internal/external- jugular, subclavian, or femoral vein
3–6 kg	Dual-lumen 7F (Cook/Medcomp)	Internal/external- jugular, subclavian, or femoral vein
	Triple-lumen 7F (Medcomp, Arrow)	Internal/external- jugular, subclavian, or femoral vein
6–30 kg	Dual-lumen 8F (Kendall, Arrow)	Internal/external- jugular, subclavian, or femoral vein
>25 kg	Dual-lumen 9F (Medcomp)	Internal/external- jugular, subclavian, or femoral vein
>40 kg	Triple-lumen 12.5F (Arrow, Kendall)	Internal/external- jugular, subclavian, or femoral vein

ANTICOAGULATION

Anticoagulation for HF may be approached generally in three distinct ways. The first approach would be no coagulation, the second is to use heparin, and the third involves citrate.

The use of no anticoagulation has been shown time and again to be fraught with a shorter circuit lifetime as well as a high risk of clotting in general. The approach of no anticoagulation is typically used in a patient with disseminated intravascular coagulation who has a low platelet count. Many of these patients, however, have a paradoxical hypercoaguability requiring some anticoagulation to prevent the system from clotting. Further, many of these patients are on continuous fresh frozen plasma replacement as well as platelet infusions that will correct the underlying anticoagulation problem, at the same time promoting coagulation of the system.

Historically, many programs have used heparin. Heparin is infused in the system prefilter and is used to anticoagulate the system. Heparin's anticoagulation effect is measured by taking a postfilter PTT or an activated clotting time (ACT). The advantage of doing an ACT is that it can be monitored at bedside. Many institutions have not been allowed to use ACT monitoring at bedside because this would violate Clinical Laboratory Improvement Amendments (CLIA) guidelines.[14] Therefore many institutions have been required to send a PTT to the coagulation lab, with a prolonged turnaround time.[15]

When heparin is used as an anticoagulant, the target ACT is between 180 to 220 seconds or a PTT between 11/2 and 2 times normal.[2,15] The advantage of heparin is that it has long been used and most nephrologists are familiar with it. Its disadvantage is that it is infused into the patient and is associated with systemic anticoagulation within the patient. Further, heparin can be associated with heparin-induced thrombocytopenia (HIT), further increasing the risk of bleeding. In many patients with multi-organ-system failure (MOSF) who require renal replacement therapy, systemic heparinization may be an additional risk factor and should be avoided.

Citrate anticoagulation began to be utilized by adult programs in the early 1990s and more recently by pediatric programs.[11–13,16–18] Citrate anticoagulation is carried out by infusing citrate postpatient and prefilter into the system. Citrate then binds to the serum calcium, making the system hypocalcemic and decreasing the chance for clotting, as clotting is a calcium-dependent process. In order to avoid citrate toxicity and systemic hypocalcemia, calcium is infused back into the patient independent of the dialysis system. Therefore there are two processes to monitor with citrate anticoagulation. The first is to titrate the citrate anticoagulation into the system to target the system of ionized calcium between 0.25 and 0.4 mmol/L. The second is to infuse calcium back into the patient to target the patient's ionized calcium between 1.1 and 1.3 mmol/L.[11–13,16–18]

The use of citrate anticoagulation may cause citrate toxicity or a metabolic alkalosis. Citrate toxicity occurs when its delivery rate exceeds its clearance rate. The clearance rate of citrate is related to both the clearance of the dialysis membrane (either convective or diffusive) as well as hepatic metabolism. Citrate is converted into bicarbonate by the normally functioning liver. Therefore one sign of excessive citrate exposure is that of a metabolic alkalosis.[11]

The second sign or symptom of citrate excess is related to the "citrate gap." This is seen when the patient manifests a rising total calcium with a drop in ionized calcium. This phenomenon is related to the binding of the citrate to the calcium. This is again a sign and symptom of excessive citrate delivered to the patient independent of the clearance. The correction of citrate gap can be easily done by stopping the citrate exposure for 20 to 30 minutes or 1 or 2 hours and restarting the citrate at 70 percent of the previous rate.

Metabolic alkalosis can easily be corrected by decreasing the citrate exposure, increasing the dialysate rate by clearance of citrate, or by infusing an acidotic solution back to the patient. Many programs use citrate anticoagulation with a bicarbonate-based solution such as Normocarb, which can result in metabolic alkalosis. By using replacement fluid of normal saline, one can easily correct this metabolic alkalosis. The pH in normal saline is 5 to 5.4; therefore this is a low-grade acid exposure back to the patient, which will correct the metabolic alkalosis. A newer generation of Normocarb is currently being readied for FDA review. Normocarb-25 (NC-25) will have a total bicarbonate base of 25 meq/L instead of 35 meq/L, thus reducing the occurrence of metabolic alkalosis.

NUTRITION IN CONTINUOUS RENAL REPLACEMENT THERAPY

A luxury of CRRT is continuous delivery of nutrition. Implementation of nutrition to patients with ARF should encourage the use of enteral means due to the potential benefit of enteral immunity and the longer-term risks of total parenteral nutrition (TPN). In prescribing nutrition, it is important to consider the nutrition losses that occur due to clearance across the HF membrane.

A prospective crossover study by Maxvold et al. demonstrated that a standard CVVH or CVVHD prescription with a delivery of 1.5 g/kg/day of protein will result in approximately 20 percent of amino acids being cleared by CRRT.[6] This causes a negative nitrogen balance in the child, worsened by the fact that many of the parenteral formulas lack glutamine, which is preferentially cleared on HF. Therefore patients are not only patients in a negative nitrogen balance but further are in a negative glutamine balance, placing them at risk for impaired protein synthesis (which is controlled in part by glutamine).

More recent work by Bellomo et al. has demonstrated that when protein is delivered at 2.5 g/kg/day in adults with MOSF, nitrogen balance in some patients remains negative, while it becomes positive in others.[19]

These data have helped guide our practice, which is presently to delivery 2 to 3 g/kg/day of protein to the patient then adjust to a target a BUN of 40 to 50 mg/dL as a "crude" marker of nutrition.

DRUG CLEARANCE

A frequent discussion at bedside is the proper dosing of medications based upon the balance of clearance/accumulation of the medication in regard to the CRRT prescription. Whereas data exists on CAVH, little information is available on the more aggressive prescriptions now being delivered with CRRT. An understanding of the factors that affect clearance will help the bedside clinician give a reasonable estimate of medication losses.[20]

1. Convective prescriptions (CVVH) will give greater clearance of solutes of the middle and larger molecular size when compared to diffusive clearance (CVVHD).
2. Protein binding will affect clearance; greater binding (e.g., carbamazepine with 75 percent protein binding) results in less clearance than with drugs that are less protein-bound.
3. The molecular weight of the solute will affect clearance. The pore size of some of the newer membranes approaches 50 kDa and will give high clearance of these larger particles.
4. The type of membrane and the charge of the membrane (negative or positive) affect adherence of the particle to the membrane as well as the clearance by the membrane.
5. Finally the overall prescription (i.e., amount of replacement fluid or dialysate per hour) will enhance clearance of solute.

Therefore, in determining the clearance of medications, all of the above factors must be considered. In the setting of a septic child on CRRT, many err by placing the child at risk for overtreatment instead of undertreatment.

PRESCRIPTION FOR CONTINUOUS RENAL REPLACEMENT THERAPY

The proper prescription for HF is based on the clinician's perception. The initial consideration is modality; convection (CVVH) or diffusion (CVVHD). For low-molecular-weight solutes (e.g., blood urea nitrogen), there is no difference. For higher-molecular-weight solutes (e.g., vancomycin, "cytokines"), there may be a benefit from convective clearance.

For CVVHD, the optimal amount of dialysate is unclear. Maxvold et al. used 2000 mL/h/1.73 m^2 (based upon extrapolation of adult data of 2 L/h) and demonstrated a urea clearance of ~ 30 mL/min/1.73 m^2.[6] While Ronco et al. have demonstrated improved outcomes with increasing replacement fluid volume (convective clearance),[21] neither pediatric nor adult data examining the effects of incremental increases in dialysate for optimal outcome exist. In the light of lack of data on incremental increase and in the face of data on acceptable urea clearance, 2000 mL/1.73 m^2/h of dialysis seems reasonable.

Blood flow rate (BFR) and membrane choice are also prescription considerations. The BFR is usually determined and limited by the vascular access and alarms. Essentially the amount of BFR is often prescribed to prevent either high- or low-pressure alarms. Further, as discussed the section on membranes, the HF machine often dictates the choice of membrane. As HF is a continuous therapy, the issue of too small a dialyzer is less a concern in CRRT as opposed to HD. In very catabolic patients (e.g., those with rhabdomyolysis, or burn patients), it may be necessary to maximize the surface area of the membrane to effect clearance.

Data do exist in adults for CVVH prescription. The sentinel article by Ronco demonstrates that with increasing dose of convective clearance there was a significant increase in survival. Similar data do not exist for the pediatric population. However, in reviewing Maxvold's data, many pediatric patients receiving a CRRT dose of 2000 mL/h/1.73 m^2 are in the same dosing range of 35 mL/kg/h, which corresponds with Ronco's findings in adults.[6,21]

COMPLICATIONS OF HEMOFILTRATION

The complications of HF include overanticoagulation associated with heparin, citrate toxicity, citrate hypocalcemia, as well as metabolic alkalosis associated with citrate. All these are easily identifiable and correctable.

Excessive ultrafiltration can occur in patients on HF. This has happened more commonly when patients were on older systems, when intravenous pumps were used as a way to inhibit ultrafiltration rates. Intravenous pumps have been used historically as a way to measure ultrafiltration but have been found to have up to a 30 percent error rate for measurement. Therefore the newer machinery allows for an accurate ultrafiltration rate within about a 1 percent error rate.[3,7]

Thermic control (both hypothermia and hyperthermia) issues can be seen in HF. Close bedside observation is necessary as a cool patient may falsely be assigned a diagnosis of sepsis or alternately a fever may be masked by the cooling effect of HF. Therefore, one must have a high index of suspicion and not use the presence or absence of a patient's fever as a sole determination of worsening sepsis.

TIMING OF BEGINNING CONTINUOUS RENAL REPLACEMENT THERAPY

To date no prospective data exist on when to initiate CRRT or CRRT vs. other RRT therapies. Ronco et al. showed that in adults, increasing doses of replacement fluid statistically improves outcome.[21] Both prescriptions of 35 and 45 mL/kg/h showed superior survival rates when compared to 25 mg/kg/h. Further, in this paper, they showed that there was a statistical improvement in survival when patients were started on CRRT when BUN was at or below 80 mg/dL. This suggests that early intervention based on solute clearance improves outcome.

Goldstein et al. showed, in a series of children on CRRT, that the amount of fluid overload (percent FO) at the time of commencing CRRT affected outcome. Survivors had an average FO of 16 percent, whereas nonsurvivors had an average FO of 32 percent.[22] These data suggest that early intervention from an ultrafiltration perspective affects survival.

A prospective multicenter pediatric database demonstrates similar findings (personal communication, Stuart Goldstein, MD).

OUTCOME IN ACUTE RENAL FAILURE

The outcome of children with ARF is as varied as their reasons for developing ARF/MOSF. Outcome data have been established using predominately single-center studies.[1,2,4,22] Work by Fleming et al. showed that the use of CRRT was superior to that of PD in the postoperative cardiac population, resulting in improved clearance and improved delivery of nutrition, yet there was no difference in survival. This observation was perhaps influenced by the small numbers of children in this study.[4] As noted above, Goldstein et al. showed that the amount of fluid overload (percent FO) at the time of CRRT initiation affected outcome, with survivors having an average FO of 16 percent and nonsurvivors an average FO of 32 percent.[22] In this population, neither PRISM score at the time of admission to the intensive care unit (ICU) nor this score at the time of commencing CRRT correlated with outcome. This was expanded upon by Goldstein's presentation at the Second International Conference on Pediatric Renal Replacement Therapy in June 2002. He presented data on 50 children from five separate centers, showing that his use of this model of FO at the time of com-

mencing CRRT demonstrated that survivors had an average FO of 8 percent while nonsurvivors had an FO of 16 percent, with an overall survival rate of 60 percent. In contrast to these single-center data, PRISM score at the time of beginning CRRT (but not at the time of ICU admission) did correlate with survival (personal communication, Stuart Goldstein). Work by these authors looked at a large series of children with ARF treated by PD, HD, or CRRT and identified the underlying disease and the use of vasopressor agents as factors predicting outcome.[2]

Concern over the utilization of CRRT in smaller children has been well addressed by Zobel et al., who showed that CVVHD in infants provided a more effective solute clearance than CAVHD.[23] Symons et al. showed in 86 infants < 10 kg who required CVVHD that there was no difference in survival when compared to the older children until the child's size was < 3 kg.[24]

Recently, Clermont et al. looked at four groups of adults in ICUs that had an overall incidence of ARF of 17 percent of 1530 admissions.[25] They looked at survival in patients without ARF, those with ARF that did not "require" dialysis, those with ARF that "required" dialysis, and those with ESRD already (and continued) on dialysis. ICU mortality was 5 percent in those without renal disease, 11 percent in those with ESRD, 23 percent in the nondialysis ARF population, and 57 percent in those with ARF on acute dialysis. The authors point out that the severity score (APACHE III) predicted outcome only in those without ARF but was less predicative of mortality.

In essence, the outcome of children is superior to that of adults, yet the outcome appears to be correlated best with the reason for initiating RRT. Current scoring systems (APACHE, PRISM) do not adequately capture or predict these confounding variables.

SUMMARY

CRRT is effective for the treatment of fluid and solute management in ARF/MOSF. Prospective studies are looking at anticoagulation, impact of replacement/dialysis, effect of bicarbonate vs. lactate based solutions, as well as nutritional and medication clearance. Speculation and bias exists with regard to when to begin CRRT and for what indications to begin. Clinical experience coupled with work by Ronco and Goldstein would support that early initiation is better. If minimal risk is evident and possible benefit maximal, early CRRT initiation should be considered as standard practice.

Taking into account both a critical care and nephrology perspective, our collective experience suggests that early intervention with CRRT characterized by aggressive replacement/dialysis fluid parameters as well as the use of citrate anticoagulation results in superior patient outcomes. With the advent of Ronco's recent paper on sepsis with filtration and plasma absorption, the indication for CRRT use in MOSF becomes more evident regardless of the presence or absence of ARF.[26]

REFERENCES

1. Lowrie L. Renal replacement therapies in pediatric multiorgan dysfunction syndrome. *Pediatr Nephrol* 2000;14:6–12.

2. Bunchman TE, McBryde KD, Mottes TE, et al. Pediatric acute renal failure: outcome by modality and disease. *Pediatric Nephrol* 2001;16:1067–1071.

3. Bunchman TE, Maxvold NJ, Kershaw DB, et al. Continuous venovenous hemodiafiltration in infants and children. *Am J Kidney Dis* 1995;25:17–21.

4. Fleming F, Bohn D, Edwards H, et al. Renal replacement therapy after repair of congenital heart disease in children: a comparison of hemofiltration and peritoneal dialysis. *J Thorac Cardiovasc Surg* 1995;109:322–331.

5. Palevsky P, Bunchman T, Tetta C: The acute dialysis quality initiative: Part V. operational characteristics of CRRT. *Adv Renal Replace Ther* 2002;9(4):268–272.

6. Maxvold NJ, Smoyer WE, Custer JR, et al. Amino acid loss and nitrogen balance in critically ill children with acute renal failure: a prospective comparison between classic hemofiltration and hemofiltration with dialysis. *Crit Care Med* 2000; 28:1161–1165.

7. Jenkins R, Harrison H, Chen B, et al. Accuracy of intravenous infusion pumps in continuous renal replacement therapies. *Trans Am Soc Artif Intern Organs* 1992;38:808.

8. Rogiers P, Zhang H, Pauwels D, et al. Comparison of polyacrylonitrile (AN69) and polysulphone membrane during hemofiltration in canine endotoxic shock. *Crit Care Med* 2003; 31(4):1219–1225.

9. Brophy PD, Mottes TA, Kudelka TL, et al. AN-69 membrane reactions are pH-dependent and preventable. *Am J Kidney Dis* 2001;38:173–178.

10. Barenbrock M, Hausberg M, Matzkies F. Effects of bicarbonate and lactate buffered replacement fluids and cardiovascular outcome in CVVH patients. *Kidney Int* 2000;58:1751–1757.

11. Bunchman TE, Maxvold NJ, Barnett J, et al. Pediatric hemofiltration: Normocarb dialysate solution with citrate anticoagulation. *Pediatr Nephrol* 2002;17:150–154.

12. Tobe S, Aujla P, Walele A, et al. A novel regional citrate anticoagulation protocol for CRRT using only commercially available solutions. *J Crit Care* 2003;18(2):121–129.

13. Bunchman TE, Maxvold, NJ Brophy PD. Pediatric convective hemofiltration: Normocarb replacement fluid and citrate anticoagulation. *Am J Kidney Dis* 2003;42(6):1248–1252.

14. Hansen K, Lavanty D. CLIA regulations updated. *Clin Lab Sci* 2003;15:68–69.

15. Geary D, Gajaria M, Freyer-Keene S, et al. Low-dose and heparin-free hemodialysis in children. *Pediatr Nephrol* 1991; 5(2):220–224.

16. Mehta RL, McDonald BR, Aguilar MM, et al. Regional citrate anticoagulation for continuous arteriovenous hemodialysis in critically ill patients. *Kidney Int* 1990;38:976–981.

17. Tolwani A, Campbell R, Schenk M, et al. Simplified citrate anticoagulation for continuous renal replacement therapy. *Kidney Int* 2001;60:370–374.

18. Chadha V, Garg U, Warady BA. Citrate clearance in children receiving continuous venovenous renal replacement therapy. *Pediatr Nephrol* 2002;17:819–824.

19. Bellomo R, Tan H, Bhonagiori S, et al. High protein intake during continuous hemodiafiltration: impact on amino acids and nitrogen balance. *Int J Artif Organs* 2002;25:263–268.

20. Schetz M, Ferdinade P, Van den Berghe G, et al. Pharmacokinetics of continuous renal replacement therapy. *Intens Care Med* 1995;21:612–620.

21. Ronco C, Bellomo R, Homel P, et al. Effects of different doses in continuous venovenous hemofiltration on outcomes of acute renal failure: a prospective randomized trial. *Lancet* 2000;356:26–30.

22. Goldstein S, Currier H, Graf J, et al. Outcome in children receiving continuous venovenous hemofiltration. *Pediatrics* 2001;107:1309–1312.

23. Zobel G, Ring E, Zobel V. Continuous arteriovenous renal replacement systems for critically ill children. *Pediatr Nephrol* 1989;3:140–143.

24. Symons JM, Brophy PD, Gregory MJ, et al. Continuous renal replacement therapy in children up to 10 kg. *Am J Kidney Dis* 2003;41(5):984–989.

25. Clermont G, Acker CG, Angus DC, et al. Renal failure in the ICU: comparison of the impact of acute renal failure and endstage renal disease on ICU outcomes. *Kidney Int* 2002;62(3): 986–996.

26. Ronco C, Brendolan A, Lonnemann G, et al. A pilot study of coupled plasma filtration and absorption in septic shock. *Crit Care Med* 2002;30:1250–1255.

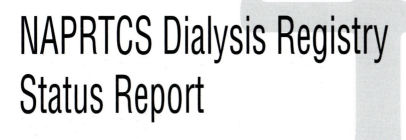

NAPRTCS Dialysis Registry Status Report

Donald Stablein
Lynya Talley

CHRONIC PEDIATRIC RENAL FAILURE

End-stage renal disease (ESRD) refers to severe kidney failure that necessitates the initiation of dialysis therapy or kidney transplantation to maintain life and is a source of significant morbidity for those affected. In order to better understand factors associated with progression to ESRD in children, the North American Pediatric Renal Transplant Cooperative Study Group (NAPRTCS)[1] was founded in 1987.

HISTORY OF THE NAPRTCS

The NAPRTCS was established with the purpose of studying renal transplantation in children and adolescents in North America. The NAPRTCS comprises four functional components, including the Clinical Coordinating Center (CCC), the Data Coordinating Center (DCC), the Affiliated Laboratory Center (ALC), and the Participating Centers Committee (PCC). These four components are governed by a board of directors and are supported by an external advisory committee. In the beginning, the operational objective of this group was to obtain voluntary participation of all renal transplant centers in the United States and Canada in which four or more pediatric patients received renal allografts annually. The scientific objectives included capture of information regarding current practice and trends in immunosuppressive therapy with the ultimate goal of improving the care of pediatric renal allograft recipients in North America. In 1992, the registry was expanded to include subjects receiving maintenance dialysis. In in 1994, it was again expanded to capture chronic renal insufficiency (CRI), defined as Schwartz-calculated creatinine clearance <75 mL/min/1.73 m^2. As a result of its efforts, the NAPRTCS hopes to elucidate the clinical course and nat-

TABLE 41–1. DIALYSIS PATIENT DEMOGRAPHICS

	N	%
Total	5392	100.0
Gender		
Male	3022	56.0
Female	2370	44.0
Age groupings		
0–1	683	12.7
2–5	550	10.2
6–12	1678	31.1
13–17	2067	38.3
>17	413	7.7
Race		
White	2663	49.4
Black	1290	23.9
Hispanic	1104	20.5
Other	335	6.2

ural history of patients with renal dysfunction and to continue following these patients as they move among the end-stage renal disease (ESRD) therapeutic modalities.

Recruitment of Centers and Subjects

Initially the participating centers were identified by information from the U.S. Health Care Finance Administration Medical Information Service, the End Stage Renal Disease Networks, and the Canadian Renal Failure Register of Pediatric Renal Transplants. Because the goal of the NAPRTCS

has been to register and follow children with renal failure, centers with pediatric nephrologists and surgeons were targeted. There are 154 participating medical centers in the United States, Mexico, Costa Rica, and Canada who have registered to participate. Initially, in order to be included in the registry, subjects had to have not yet reached their 18th birthday at the time of their index transplant. However, upon expanding the registry in 1992, the age criterion was changed to include subjects who had not yet attained their 21st birthday at the time of index transplant or at the time of index initiation of dialysis (whichever came first). This report contains data submitted through February 2004.

PATIENT CHARACTERISTICS

Demographic Characteristics and Nephrologic History

The characteristics of patients registered in the dialysis component of NAPRTCS are shown in Table 41–1. The majority of registrants were male (56 percent). Nearly half of the patients identified themselves as white and 24 percent as black. Forty-six percent of the registrants were 13 years of age and older at the time of dialysis initiation. Specifically, 12.7 percent were infants under 2 years of age, 10.2 percent were between 2 and 5 years of age, 31.1 percent were between 6 and 12 years of age, and the remainder were over age 13. In addition, Table 41–2 shows the distribution of age groups according to type of modality: peritoneal dialysis (PD) or hemodialysis (HD). A larger proportion of PD patients (30 percent) are less than 6 years old compared to HD patients (9 percent). Detailed in Table 41–3 are the

TABLE 41–2. NUMBER AND PERCENT DISTRIBUTIONS OF PATIENT RACE/ETHNICITY, BY DIALYSIS MODALITY AND AGE AT INITIATION

		Peritoneal Dialysis							
		0–1		2–5		6–12		>12	
	Total	N	%	N	%	N	%	N	%
PD Patients	3513	642	18.3	429	12.2	1123	32.0	1319	37.5
White	1878	413	22.0	240	12.8	578	30.8	647	34.5
Black	697	97	13.9	64	9.2	206	29.6	330	47.3
Hispanic	734	103	14.0	91	12.4	280	38.1	260	35.4
Other	204	29	14.2	34	16.7	59	28.9	82	40.2
		Hemodialysis							
		0–1		2–5		6–12		>12	
	Total	N	%	N	%	N	%	N	%
HD patients	1877	42	2.2	121	6.4	553	29.5	1161	61.9
White	785	23	2.9	62	7.9	231	29.4	469	59.7
Black	593	7	1.2	25	4.2	153	25.8	408	68.8
Hispanic	370	10	2.7	23	6.2	123	33.2	214	57.8
Other	129	2	1.6	11	8.5	46	35.7	70	54.3

TABLE 41–3. PATIENT DIAGNOSES

	N	%
Total	5392	100.0
Diagnosis		
Aplasia / hypoplasia / dysplasia	785	14.6
Focal segmental glomerulosclerosis	763	14.2
Obstructive uropathy	708	13.1
SLE nephritis	189	3.5
Reflux nephropathy	188	3.5
Chronic glomerulonephritis	174	3.2
Hemolytic uremic syndrome	172	3.2
Polycystic disease	153	2.8
Congenital nephrotic syndrome	135	2.5
Medullary cystic disease	117	2.2
Idiopathic crescentic glomerulonephritis	115	2.1
Prune belly	110	2.0
Membranoproliferative glomerulonephritis type I	104	1.9
Familial nephritis	94	1.7
Pyelonephritis / interstitial nephritis	84	1.6
Renal infarct	80	1.5
Cystinosis	80	1.5
Berger's (IgA) nephritis	69	1.3
Henoch-Schönlein nephritis	64	1.2
Membranoproliferative glomerulonephritis type II	52	1.0
Wilms tumor	39	0.7
Other systemic immunologic disease	37	0.7
Drash syndrome	34	0.6
Wegener's granulomatosis	31	0.6
Oxalosis	26	0.5
Membranous nephropathy	24	0.4
Sickle cell nephropathy	19	0.4
Diabetic glomerulonephritis	5	0.1
Other	520	9.6
Unknown	421	7.8

most common diagnoses: aplastic/hypoplastic/dysplastic kidneys, focal segmental glomerulosclerosis, and obstructive uropathy.

Modality Initiation and Termination

Two types of dialysis modalities are used with pediatric patients and both have their advantages and disadvantages. Peritoneal dialysis (PD) is typically the modality of choice in the pediatric patient due to the flexibility it allows. PD can be performed at home while hemodialysis (HD) requires 3- to 4-hour sessions three to four times a week. In NAPRTCS, a patient may be reentered in the dialysis component every time a new chronic dialysis modality is initiated. Changes of access or changes between peritoneal dialysis subtypes are reported within the modality course.

Patients entered on January 1, 1992, had ongoing dialysis and no prior information was collected; we restrict many analyses to the incident cohort where the patient's dialysis history is known.

Information on modality initiations and terminations among registrants in the NAPRTCS dialysis registry is shown in Table 41–4. An independent course of dialysis therapy is defined to have occurred when a patient is maintained on a given modality for 30 or more days. The registry currently has data on 6028 independent courses of dialysis therapy among the incident cases: 4655 had one course, and as detailed in the table, 973 had two or more courses. Of the 6028, a total of 3609 (59.9 percent) were on PD and 2419 (40.1 percent) on HD. There have been 4379 modality terminations. Most terminations were due to the patient being transplanted (63.6 percent) or a change of modality (22.9 percent), with the remainder of terminations due to death (3.1 percent) and the return of native kidney function (2.6 percent). Modality changes, when a surviving patient was not transplanted and there was no return of native function, were due primarily to excessive infection (35 percent), patient or family choice (22.1 percent), or other medical reasons (13.7 percent).

TABLE 41–4. MODALITY INITIATION AND TERMINATION

	N (6028)	% (100)
Dialysis course		
First	4655	77.2
Second	973	16.1
Third	276	4.6
Fourth	87	1.4
Fifth or more	37	0.6
Modality		
PD	3609	59.9
HD	2417	40.1
Terminations		
Reasons for dialysis termination	4379	100.0
Patient transplanted	2786	63.6
Change of modality	1002	22.9
Death	137	3.1
Native kidney function returned	116	2.6
Other	1	0.0
None reported	337	7.7
Reasons for change of modality	1002	100.0
Excessive infection	289	28.8
Patient/family choice	221	22.1
Access failure	104	10.4
Inadequate ultrafiltration	50	5.0
Inadequate solute clearance	21	2.1
Excessive hospitalization (dialysis-related)	21	2.1
Other (medical)	137	13.7
Other (nonmedical)	159	15.9

PERITONEAL DIALYSIS

Means of Access

The majority of catheters used to provide access in PD were of the Tenckhoff curled configuration (N=2553, 63 percent); Table 41–5. Other configurations were Tenckhoff straight (N=1169, 28.9 percent), Toronto western (N=33, 0.8 percent), presternal (N=281, 6.9 percent), and other (N=15, 0.4 percent). About 57 percent of catheters had a single cuff and 73.6 percent had a straight tunnel. The most common exit site orientation was lateral (44.2 percent).

The First Year of Dialysis

The follow-up data for peritoneal dialysis were compiled for 1 month (N=3161), 6 months (N=2497), and 12 months (N=1674) after initiation (Table 41–6). Most patients use automated peritoneal dialysis (APD) at each follow-up time point rather than continuous ambulatory peritoneal dialysis (CAPD) or intermittent peritoneal dialysis (IPD). The proportion of registrants using APD varied between 67.9 and 71.3 percent at the follow-up time points. CAPD was used by 20.8 percent of patients at 1-month follow-up, decreasing to 17.1 percent at 12 months.

At 1 month postinitiation, 86.3 percent of patients were receiving recombinant human erythropoietin (rHuEPO) and 9.7 percent were receiving recombinant human growth hormone (rHGH; at 6 months, 90.9 percent were receiving rHuEPO and 14.2 percent rHGH. At 1 year, these proportions increased to 91.3 percent and 19.1 percent, respectively.

The combined percentage of patients entered on the cadaver waiting list or with a workup in progress was simi-

TABLE 41–5. PERITONEAL DIALYSIS ACCESS

	N (4051)	% (100)
Catheter		
Tenckhoff straight	1169	28.9
Tenckhoff curled	2553	63.0
Toronto western	33	0.8
Presternal	281	6.9
Other	15	0.4
Cuffs		
One	2309	57.0
Two	1742	43.0
Tunnel		
Swan neck	1071	26.4
Straight	2980	73.6
Exit-site orientation		
Up	539	13.3
Down	1302	32.1
Lateral	1791	44.2
Unknown	419	10.3

TABLE 41–6. PERITONEAL DIALYSIS AT FOLLOW-UP

	1 Month		6 Months		12 Months	
	N	%	N	%	N	%
Total	3161	100.0	2497	100.0	1674	100.0
Current modality						
CAPD	657	20.8	462	18.5	286	17.1
APD	2145	67.9	1765	70.7	1193	71.3
IPD	215	6.8	154	6.2	78	4.7
Missing/unknown	144	4.6	116	4.6	117	7.0
EPO Therapy						
Yes	2729	86.3	2269	90.9	1528	91.3
No	384	12.1	183	7.3	77	4.6
Missing/unknown	48	1.5	45	1.8	69	4.1
Human growth hormone therapy						
Yes	307	9.7	355	14.2	320	19.1
No	2806	88.8	2092	83.8	1282	76.6
Missing/unknown	48	1.5	50	2.0	72	4.3
Seizures						
Yes	117	3.7	124	5.0	57	3.4
No	2966	93.8	2307	92.4	1529	91.3
Missing/unknown	78	2.5	66	2.6	88	5.3
Exit-site infections						
Yes	314	9.9	557	22.3	373	22.3
No	2762	87.4	1871	74.9	1215	72.6
Missing/unknown	85	2.7	69	2.8	86	5.1
Transplant status						
On cadaver list	438	13.9	627	25.1	547	32.7
Workup in progress	1195	37.8	785	31.4	447	26.7
Medical reasons	1159	36.7	728	29.2	369	22.0
Family/personal preference	303	9.6	290	11.6	234	14.0
Missing/unknown	66	2.1	67	2.7	77	4.6
Number of peritonitis episodes						
0	2708	85.7	1752	70.2	1184	70.7
1	403	12.7	500	20.0	320	19.1
2	50	1.6	158	6.3	102	6.1
>2	-	-	87	3.5	68	4.1
Type of infection						
Fungal	40	6.2	19	2.0	8	1.3
Gram-positive	283	44.2	462	49.4	299	50.1
Gram-negative	133	20.8	224	24.0	142	23.8
Gram-positive and negative	24	3.7	11	1.2	12	2.0
Other	137	21.4	184	19.7	119	19.9
Cultured, no growth	6	0.9	18	1.9	3	0.5
No culture	18	2.8	17	1.8	14	2.4

lar at 1 and 6 months of follow-up. At 6 months, one-fourth of the patients (25 percent) were on the cadaver waiting list; another 31 percent had transplant preparation workup in progress. Other reasons given for not being on the list after 6 months include medical (29 percent) and family or patient preference (12 percent).

Data have been reported on cases of catheter access revision (Table 41–7). Catheter accesses were revised due to catheter malfunction (44 percent), peritonitis (18 percent), exit-site tunnel inflections (20 percent), dialysis leaks (4 percent), and other causes (13 percent).

Peritonitis Infections

The number of peritonitis episodes reported to date are shown in Table 41–6, along with characterization of organism culture results. One or more peritonitis episodes was experienced by 14.3 percent ($N = 453$) PD patients in the first month. In months 1 to 6, a total of 29.8 percent had one or more peritonitis infections; in the next 6-month period, the percentage was similar, 29.3 percent ($N=490$).

Figure 41–1 demonstrates the time to first peritonitis infection by catheter access characteristics. The proportion of patients who remain infection-free over the course of 30 months after dialysis initiation is higher for those utilizing other catheter types than for those using either Tenckhoff or curled catheters ($p = 0.005$). Also, patients with only one cuff acquire their first peritonitis infection faster than patients with two cuffs ($p <0.001$). Also those with straight tunnels remain infection-free longer than patients with swan

neck catheters ($p = 0.027$). In addition, patients with either downward or unknown exit sites of orientation take longer to acquire their first peritonitis infection than those patients with upward or lateral exit sites.

HEMODIALYSIS

Means of Access

Information about HD access locations and devices can be found in Table 41–8. HD access approaches included the following: external percutaneous catheters ($N=1899$, 79 percent), of which 1174 (62 percent), 629 (33 percent), and 80 (4 percent) were located in the subclavian, jugular, and femoral veins, respectively, and 62 (3 percent) were of single-lumen configuration. Others included internal arteriovenous fistulas ($N=281$, 11.7 percent), internal arteriovenous grafts ($N=206$, 8.6 percent), and external arteriovenous shunts ($N=7$, 0.3 percent). The majority of shunts, fistulas, and grafts were located in the lower arm (63.8 percent).

The First Year of Dialysis

Follow-up data on HD access were reviewed for 1, 6, and 12 months (Table 41–9). Most patients (87 percent) received three treatments per week, with 10 percent receiving fewer than three weekly treatments and 1 percent reporting home-based dialysis. The median treatment duration is 9 hours (mean = 9.8 hours) weekly with quartiles of 9 and 12 hours. More HD patients than PD patients received

TABLE 41–7. PERITONEAL ACCESS REVISION

| | Number of Accesses | Number of Revisions | Revision/ Access Ratio | Reasons for Access Revision (%) | | | | | | | | | |
| | | | | Infection | | Leak | | Malfunction | | Peritonitis | | Other | |
				N	%	N	%	N	%	N	%	N	%
All revisions	3719	790	21.2	103	20	23	4	228	44	94	18	68	13
Catheter													
Tenckhoff straight	1033	228	22.1	26	17	6	4	72	48	30	20	17	11
Tenckhoff curled	2318	490	21.1	67	21	15	5	135	42	57	18	46	14
Toronto western	28	6	21.4	-	-	-	-	3	75	1	25	-	-
Other	274	52	19.0	8	24	1	3	16	47	6	18	3	9
Cuffs													
One	2040	479	23.5	50	17	17	6	129	43	66	22	36	12
Two	1611	301	18.7	52	25	6	3	95	45	28	13	31	15
Tunnel													
Swan necked/curved	1013	191	18.9	34	23	7	5	60	41	24	17	20	14
Straight	2617	584	22.3	68	19	15	4	163	45	70	19	45	12
Exit-site orientation													
Up	490	143	29.2	15	19	5	6	30	38	21	27	7	9
Down	1196	241	20.2	34	20	8	5	78	46	24	14	25	15
Lateral	1585	305	19.2	44	22	9	4	88	44	36	18	24	12

Note: Table does not show missing values.

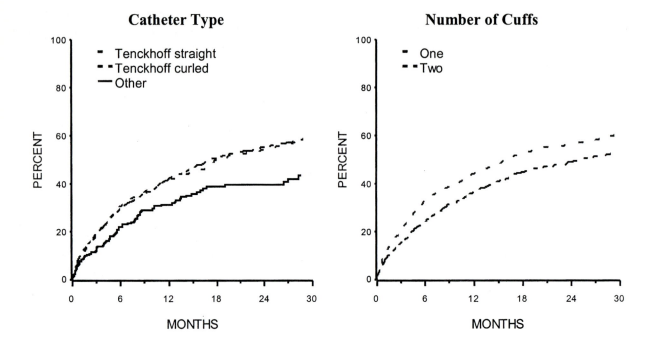

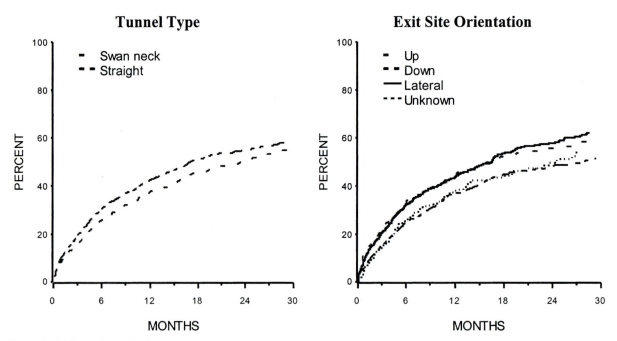

Figure 41–1. Time to first peritonitis infection, by catheter access characteristics.

TABLE 41–8. HEMODIALYSIS ACCESS

	N (2393)	% (100)
External percutaneous catheter	1899	79.4
Subclavian vein	1174	
Jugular vein	629	
Femoral vein	80	
Single lumen	62	
Double lumen	1821	
External arteriovenous shunt	7	0.3
Internal arteriovenous fistula	281	11.7
Internal arteriovenous graft	206	8.6
Autologous vein	7	
Bovine graft	1	
Polytetrafluoroethylene (PTFE) graft	190	
Other graft	4	
Locations of shunts, fistulas, and grafts		
Total known	152	100.0
Upper arm	36	23.7
Lower arm	97	63.8
Thigh	19	12.5

rHuEPO. Among HD patients, 90.9 percent (*N*=1786) received rHuEPO at 1 month and a similar percentage were treated with this therapy at the later time points. Regarding transplant status, at 1 month of follow-up, 15 percent of HD patients were on a cadaver waiting list, a proportion that increased during follow-up to 38 percent at 12 months. At 1 month, 37 percent had a workup in progress, a proportion that declined during follow-up to 18 percent at 12 months. Other reasons given for not being on the list included medical (34.7 percent at 1 month, 27.0 percent at 6 months, and 25.2 percent at 12 months) and family or patient preference (9.4 percent at 1 month, 11.3 percent at 6 months, and 12.3 percent at 12 months).

HD access revision data are shown in Table 41–10. Accesses were revised because of infection (15 percent), clotting (27 percent), malfunction (25 percent), or to create more permanent access (25 percent). The access revision ratio varied by the type of access, with the greatest ratio seen for external percutaneous catheters and the lowest for internal arteriovenous fistulas.

TABLE 41–9. HEMODIALYSIS AT FOLLOW-UP

	1 Month		6 Months		12 Months	
	N	%	N	%	N	%
Total	1965	100.0	1361	100.0	937	100.0
EPO therapy						
Yes	1786	90.9	1233	90.6	848	90.5
No	115	5.9	54	4.0	33	3.5
Missing	64	3.3	74	5.4	56	6.0
Human growth hormone therapy						
Yes	186	9.5	143	10.5	109	11.6
No	1714	87.2	1143	84.0	770	82.2
Missing	65	3.3	75	5.5	58	6.2
Seizures						
Yes	1778	90.5	1155	84.9	803	85.7
No	96	4.9	112	8.2	56	6.0
Unknown	22	1.1	17	1.2	16	1.7
Missing	69	3.5	77	5.7	62	6.6
Exit-site infections						
Yes	194	9.9	231	17.0	128	13.7
No	1668	84.9	1024	75.2	724	77.3
Missing	103	5.2	106	7.8	85	9.1
Transplant status						
CD waiting list	295	15.0	403	29.6	355	37.9
CD or LD workup in progress	731	37.2	356	26.2	171	18.2
Medical reason	682	34.7	367	27.0	236	25.2
Family/patient preference	184	9.4	154	11.3	115	12.3
Missing	73	3.7	81	6.0	60	6.4

TABLE 41–10. HEMODIALYSIS ACCESS REVISION

	Number of Accesses	Number of Revisions	Reasons for Access Revisions									
			Infection		Clot		Malfunction		Reaccess		Other	
			N	%	N	%	N	%	N	%	N	%
Total	3985	10,535	344	15	616	27	577	25	584	25	187	8
HD access												
External	3188	8784	306	16	410	21	527	27	538	28	154	8
Shunt	14	31	1	8	6	46	1	8	4	31	1	8
Fistula	375	512	8	7	67	56	20	17	15	13	10	8
Graft	376	1166	27	12	130	57	25	11	26	11	20	9

PD/HD Differences in Modality Changes

There are striking differences (p <0.001) in the reasons given for changing modalities according to type of dialysis received (PD vs. HD). Table 41–11 shows that excessive infection was reported as the reason for change in 43.4 percent of PD patients vs. 7.8 percent of HD patients. The most common reason given among HD patients was patient/family choice (41.8 percent). This reason was given by only 8.3 percent of PD patients.

DIALYSIS DOSE

In 2003, NAPRTCS initiated collection of dialysis dose measurements with capture, at each reporting time point, of the most recent single-pool Kt/V and urea reduction ratio (URR) for HD patients and the most recent weekly Kt/V for PD patients. Table 41–12 displays initial reported Kt/V by age grouping, race, visit timing since initiation, and baseline body-mass index (BMI) standardized score for 151

TABLE 41–11. REASONS FOR CHANGE OF MODALITY AMONG PATIENTS WHO WERE NOT TRANSPLANTED

	Hemodialysis Patients		Peritoneal Patients	
	N	%	N	%
Reasons for change of modality	409	100.0	592	100.0
Excessive infection	32	7.8	257	43.4
Patient/family choice	171	41.8	49	8.3
Access failure	56	13.7	48	8.1
Inadequate ultrafiltration	3	0.7	47	7.9
Inadequate solute clearance	-	-	21	3.5
Excessive hospitalization (dialysis-related)	10	2.4	11	1.9
Other (medical)	61	14.9	76	12.8
Other (nonmedical)	76	18.6	83	14.0

TABLE 41–12. _KT/V_ BY MODALITY, AGE, RACE, VISIT AND BASELINE BMI

		_KT/V_		
		N	Mean	SE
Modality				
Peritoneal dialysis	Age	151		
	0–1	20	2.0	0.1
	2–5	17	2.7	0.4
	6–12	53	2.6	0.2
	>12	61	2.2	0.1
	Race			
	Nonblack	112	2.5	0.1
	Black	39	2.1	0.2
	Visit month			
	1	38	2.2	0.1
	6	36	2.7	0.3
	12	27	2.5	0.3
	>12	50	2.3	0.1
	BMI Z-score			
	<0	65	2.6	0.2
	>0	86	2.2	0.1
Hemodialysis	Age	75		
	0–1	2	1.2	0.2
	2–5	6	1.8	0.4
	6–12	31	1.6	0.1
	>12	36	1.7	0.2
	Race			
	Nonblack	40	1.7	0.1
	Black	35	1.6	0.1
	Visit month			
	1	25	1.7	0.2
	6	8	1.4	0.3
	12	14	1.6	0.1
	>12	28	1.8	0.1
	BMI Z-score			
	<0	23	1.8	0.2
	>0	52	1.6	0.1

peritoneal dialysis and 75 hemodialysis patients. Within modality, dialysis dose is similar in all subgroups except for a trend ($p = 0.03$) toward higher PD dose in nonblack patients. Thus dose appears to be delivered similarly across multiple subgroups. For peritoneal dialysis, the median Kt/V was 2.1, the lower quartile was 1.7, and the lowest decile was 1.4. PD strategies (CAPD vs. APD vs. IPD) did not differ significantly in Kt/V values, but the 7 IPD patients had a mean of 1.7. Kt/V percentiles (50th, 25th, and 10th) for HD patients are 1.6, 1.3, and 1.1.

Mean URR values for selected hemodialysis patient subgroups are presented in Table 41–13. As with Kt/V, statistically significant differences between the subgroups are not detected. For the 60 hemodialysis patients with both measures, a strong rank correlation was observed ($r = 0.85$, $p < 0.001$) between Kt/V and URR values.

TEMPORAL TRENDS

We contrast patients initiating dialysis in 1999 and later with those from earlier years to examine changes in patient characteristics and practices. Initial modality type (PD vs. HD) is similar in both eras, as are presenting demographic characteristic of age and sex. A trend towards increased percentage of minority patients in the registry is observed, with white patients declining 3 percentage points to 47 percent and the proportion of black patients increasing to 26 percent in the more recent cohort. Patient sensitization has im-

TABLE 41–14. PERITONITIS INFECTION-FREE SURVIVAL BY TIME PERIOD AND PERITONEAL DIALYSIS TYPE

	3 Months		6 Months		1 Year		2 Years	
	%	SE	%	SE	%	SE	%	SE
CAPD								
< 1999	76.7	2.0	64.3	2.3	49.7	2.6	40.0	2.9
1999–2004	80.6	3.4	75.4	3.9	69.0	4.7	50.4	7.8
APD								
< 1999	80.9	1.1	69.4	1.3	57.3	1.5	44.7	1.8
1999–2004	83.2	1.6	74.8	1.9	62.1	2.4	44.0	3.3

proved substantially, with the proportion of patients having baseline PRA levels of zero moving from 66 percent to 88 percent from the earlier to later cohort. Cadaver wait-listing strategies appear similar in both periods.

Peritonitis-free survival was compared for both CAPD and APD by time period. Results in Table 41–14 demonstrate that among CAPD and APD patients, improvements in delaying the time to peritonitis infections have been made during recent years. For example, among the early CAPD cohort (<1999), by 1 year, at least 50 percent had had a peritonitis infection. Conversely, among the later CAPD cohort (1999–2004), half remained infection-free until 2 years postdialysis ($p = 0.028$). Among the APD group, the proportion ultimately acquiring a peritonitis in-

TABLE 41–13. URR FOR HEMODIALYSIS PATIENTS BY AGE, RACE, VISIT AND BASELINE BMI

		URR	
	N	Mean	SE
All	77	73.4	1.1
Age			
0–1	2	59.0	9.0
2–5	7	74.9	3.1
6–12	30	74.0	1.5
>12	38	73.4	1.6
Race			
Nonblack	42	73.5	1.6
Black	35	73.3	1.4
Visit month			
1	28	69.8	1.9
6	6	69.8	4.4
12	14	75.4	1.5
>12	29	76.6	1.6
BMI Z-score			
<0	25	73.6	2.0
>0	52	73.3	1.3

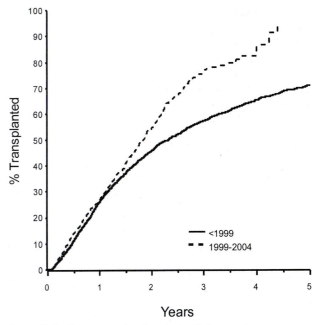

Figure 41–2. Time to transplant, by cohort period.

fection remained the same for the early cohort and the later cohort at 2 years postdialysis (44.7 percent vs. 44.0 percent, respectively; $p = 0.261$). However, the rate of progression was much slower for the 1999–2004 cohort. At 1 year post-dialysis for the early APD cohort, the proportion infection-free was 57.3 percent. For the 1999–2004 cohort, the proportion infection-free at 1 year was 62.1 percent.

For HD patients, a small lengthening of weekly dialysis duration is observed. Current HDs patients experience a 3 percent longer (0.3 h/week) increase to a mean of 10 hours of HD per week.

Importantly, as depicted in Fig. 41–2, despite the limited availability of organs, time from dialysis to transplant has not worsened in recent years. In this analysis, cases are considered "events" if transplanted and "censored" otherwise. Shorter times are observed in both eras if the analysis is restricted to wait-listed patients (data not shown). The median time to transplant in the early cohort was 2.3 years, vs. 1.8 years in the recent cohort ($p < 0.001$).

REFERENCE

1. NAPRTCS 2004, NAPRTCS online; www.naprtcs.org.

Preemptive Kidney Transplantation in Infancy

Richard A. Cohn
Timothy E. Bunchman

The year 2004 marked the 50th anniversary of the first successful kidney transplant in the United States.[1] While advances in both hemodialysis and peritoneal dialysis for children continue to occur, it is more apparent than ever that kidney transplantation is the preferred mode of renal replacement therapy (RRT) for children with end-stage renal disease (ESRD). Over the past decade, since the previous edition of this textbook, the number of successful outcomes in pediatric kidney transplantation has risen dramatically. The specific reasons are discussed later in this chapter. As a result, infants beyond their first birthday and all children should proceed to kidney transplantation in a preemptive fashion or after a minimal period of time on dialysis. It can be argued that transplanted children resume a more normal growth and development pattern than their counterparts on dialysis, thus making transplant the most attractive opportunity for infants who are at the period of most rapid height and brain growth. Moreover, because "catch-up growth" may be difficult to achieve, it seems prudent to prevent growth retardation as much as possible. The goal of this chapter, then, is to outline indications for RRT in infancy, review the available modalities, and compare the advantages and disadvantages of each.

INDICATIONS FOR RENAL REPLACEMENT THERAPY IN INFANCY

Published data on chronic renal failure (CRF) or ESRD in infants identifies that approximately 50 percent of these infants have renal disease associated with high-output renal failure[2-6] (Table 42–1). This group includes those with obstructive or reflux uropathies, renal dysplasia, and hypoplasia. This contrasts with older children, who have ESRD much more commonly from glomerular disorders, collagen vascular disease, and hereditary renal diseases,[7,8] which are

TABLE 42–1. ETIOLOGY OF CHRONIC RENAL FAILURE/END-STAGE RENAL DISEASE IN CHILDREN < 4 YEARS OF AGE

Study	Hypoplasia/ Dysplasia	Obstructive Uropathy	Oxalosis	Congenital Nephrotic Syndrome	Other	Ref
NAPRTCS	29%	20%				2
Najarian et al.	33%	20%	11%	8%	29%	3
Salusky et al.		75%	13%		12%	4
Kohaut et al.	33%	45%			22%	5
Briscoe et al.	38%	5%		19%	38%	6

commonly associated with oligoanuria and thus may preclude these children from preemptive transplantation. In addition, other causes of ESRD—such as primary hyperoxaluria, bilateral Wilms' tumor (as in patients with Drash syndrome), bilateral renal vein thrombosis, and cortical necrosis—can occur in infants.

Another indication for RRT, which accounts for 10 to 25 percent of transplanted infants in various reports, is the congenital nephrotic syndrome.[6,9] This disorder results in steroid-resistant nephrotic syndrome, placing these patients at high risk of recurrent potentially serious infections and thrombotic phenomena. Since heavy proteinuria usually persists with relatively preserved glomerular function, bilateral nephrectomy, and subsequent anuric renal failure is required to reverse the nephrotic state prior to transplantation. In order to discuss RRT options, an understanding of the unique complications of ESRD in infants is first needed. The modes of RRT are reviewed in the next several sections, with referral to the diseases where it is most relevant.

Kidney Failure in Infancy

There are numerous complications of kidney failure in adults, but those that are unique to pediatrics pertain to growth and development. These issues are magnified in infants who are at the age of most rapid growth and neurologic development. This chapter focuses on these areas in the infant with CRF/ESRD.

Growth in Infants with Renal Failure. In healthy children, 50 percent of final adult height is attained by age 2. In addition, the brain's volume increases more than twofold in the first 2 years of life, achieving about 80 percent of its total size.[10] Therefore, attention to and correction of the factors that inhibit growth in the infant has effects throughout the child's life. Growth failure in patients with ESRD is multifactorial; major contributing factors include chronic metabolic acidosis, renal osteodystrophy, suboptimal caloric intake, and anemia (Fig. 42–1). Additional factors—including age of onset of CRF, salt and water balance (in renal dysplasia), primary renal disease, and alterations in growth hormone binding proteins—may further influence growth. We

believe that the condition of the patients prior to dialysis and transplantation has a major impact on how quickly they "catch up" to their peers with regard to growth and development.

Recent pharmacologic advances have accompanied a better understanding of the pathophysiology of growth failure. This has resulted in the availability of a number of medical supplements with which to provide improved treatment of the factors associated with growth failure in children with ESRD. Such medical treatments include active vitamin D metabolites, recombinant human erythropoietin (rHuEPO), and recombinant human growth hormone (rhGH).[11,12]

Additional gains in the treatment of growth have come from stricter attention to caloric intake and its effect on weight gain, linear growth, and brain growth. One method

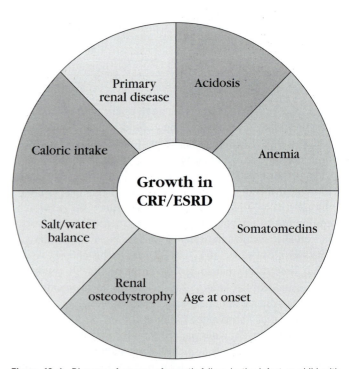

Figure 42–1. Diagram of causes of growth failure in the infant or child with chronic renal failure or end-stage renal disease.

used to optimize caloric intake is to override the anorexia seen in many uremic children by using force feedings via a nasogastric or gastrostomy tube. Some centers choose to use the recommended dietary allowance (RDA) for protein and calorie intake as a starting point for nutritional needs of the infant with CRF/ESRD. It should be remembered, though, that the RDA is a recommendation for normal, healthy populations.[13] Since the caloric needs of children with ESRD are unknown, strict adherence to these recommendations may lead to malnourishment, which would add to the growth impairment in these patients.

Rizzoni et al. reported on the linear growth velocity of five infants with CRF [mean glomerular filtration rate (GFR) 14 mL/min/1.73 m^2; range 4 to 21 mL/min/1.73 m^2] managed conservatively.[14] Growth during periods of caloric intake $\geq$100 percent of the RDA averaged 97 percent of that predicted (range 61 to 130 percent); whereas that during periods of intake $\leq$100 percent averaged 53 percent of the predicted growth (range 10 to 72 percent). It was also noted that the stunting of linear growth during infancy can be profound—as high as 0.6 SD/month; it was thus emphasized that aggressive attention to growth during infancy is essential to prevent marked height growth failure later in childhood.

Work by Parekh et al. looked at 23 infants treated with "specified findings" without the use of growth hormone. They demonstrated that with a focus of ~120 to 140 cal/kg/day and ~200 to 220 mL/kg/day of fluid in infants with dysplasia, normal growth is attainable.[15] Van Dyck and colleagues found similar results in 20 infants, noting that attention to specific components of nutrition was needed to obtain growth.[16] Recent work by Ledermann et al. in the United Kingdom, Ramage et al. in Canada, and Brewer et al. in Texas showed similar improvement in growth.[17–19] Work by Davies et al. noted that when G tubes have been in place for more than 1 year and are no longer needed, surgical closure is recommended.[20] Our protocol has been to institute enteral tube feedings within the first week or two of life in infants with kidney failure so as to ensure adequate caloric intake. We begin with 120 kcal/kg/day as a starting goal and aim for 30 g/day weight gain and an increase in head circumference of 0.5 cm/week in the first 3 months of life. With meticulous attention to these growth parameters, we can achieve near normal growth in these patients. We have been able to tailor the formula used in infants with ESRD to their nutritional needs and urine output. In the infant with polyuria, frequent or continuous hypo- or isosmolar formulas are utilized. These include commercially available full-strength (0.67 cal/mL) Similac PM 60/40 (Ross Labs, Columbus, Ohio), or one-third (0.67 cal/mL) to one-half (1 cal/mL) strength Suplena (Ross) or Nepro (Ross). In the anuric infant, concentrated (1 cal/mL) PM 60/40 or full-strength (2 cal/mL) Suplena or Nepro can be utilized. Both Suplena and Nepro have been associated with hypermagne-

semia; therefore serum magnesium levels should be measured in the infant receiving these formulas. Water-soluble vitamin supplements are necessary in the infant on dialysis and may be needed in the infant with CRF.

Metabolic acidosis can begin to be seen in patients whose GFR is less than 50 percent of normal.[10] Because it is well known from patients with isolated acidosis (e.g., renal tubular acidosis) that growth impairment is common, acidosis must be monitored and treated aggressively once renal insufficiency is diagnosed. Predialysis patients in our center are typically placed on sodium bicarbonate (or sodium citrate) at an initial dose of 2 meq/kg/day; this is titrated to maintain plasma HCO_3 levels between 22 and 26 meq/L and venous pH values above 7.30. Once patients reach dialysis, the standard dialysate bath contains 40 meq/L of base (lactate or bicarbonate); supplemental bicarbonate by mouth is usually not required. Anemia is usually apparent when GFR falls below 25 percent of normal, even sooner in patients with renal dysplasia. While the role of anemia is questioned by some as a cause of growth failure in patients with ESRD, it is generally agreed that children feel better when their hematocrit is closer to normal.[15] This means they are likely to have more energy and be more active, thus engaging with their environment more fully. Attention to keeping the hematocrit between 32 and 36 percent with the use of rHuEPO potentially gives today's infants with renal failure a level of energy not previously seen in these patients, who in the past were transfused to hematocrits of 20 to 25 percent. Dabbagh et al. showed improved caloric intake in four children on dialysis treated with rHuEPO who were managed without a gastrostomy tube (52 to 94 percent RDA), with a resultant increase in growth rate (4.4 to 7.1 cm/year). These investigators concluded that rHuEPO did have a positive effect on linear growth, but it was more likely due to better nutritional intake than a direct effect of the drug itself.[21]

The use of rHuEPO in children has been studied; Brandt reported that over 80 percent of the 44 children with CRI/ESRD who received it responded within 8 weeks of initial therapy to targeted hemoglobin levels. Side effects included hypertension and hyperkalemia; as expected, iron deficiency developed with its continued use.[22] Lerner et al. recently reported experience with darbopoetin in children with chronic kidney disease and, as expected, the half-life of this compound was two- to fourfold longer than that reported for rHuEPO in pediatric patients.[23] The effectiveness of rHuEPO has been enhanced by the use of intravenous iron infusions.[24] Prescribing the longer-acting form of rHuEPO (Aranesp, Amgen, Thousand Oaks, CA) may improve anemia by affecting compliance.

Correction of the anemia may have positive effects on the neurologic development of infants, although no controlled study to date has adequately addressed this issue. A huge advantage to rHuEPO therapy is that it eliminates the need for transfusions, reducing human leukocyte antigen sensitization and making eventual transplantation easier, as well as avoiding exposure to viral diseases.[26]

We initiate rHuEPO therapy at 150 to 300 U/kg/week dosed once per week and titrated to a hematocrit of 32 to 36 percent. Iron studies (serum iron, total iron-binding capacity, and serum ferritin) are also obtained prior to starting rHuEPO, as it is well known that once the erythropoietic response begins, iron stores will rapidly be depleted. It is important to maintain a transferrin saturation level above 20 percent. Iron supplementation is thus begun very soon after starting rHuEPO so as to ensure a continuous bone marrow response. RHuEPO nonresponsiveness may occur in infants with chronic inflammatory states, severe hyperparathyroidism, aluminum toxicity, and the aforementioned iron deficiency. Therefore, in the infant who does not respond appropriately to rHuEPO, we will often measure C-reactive protein and parathyroid hormone level as well as repeating the iron studies.

Secondary hyperparathyroidism is a large component of the renal osteodystrophy that contributes to poor growth in infants with ESRD. Stimuli leading to parathyroid gland hyperplasia in these patients are hyperphosphatemia and low levels of calcitriol, both of which result in a decreased ionized calcium. Calcitriol has an effect that occurs before the hypocalcemic stimulation of the parathyroid gland takes place, however. Receptors on the parathyroid gland for 1,25-dihydroxy vitamin D_3 [1,25(OH)$_2$ vitamin D_3] modulate the feedback and alter the set point for parathyroid hormone (PTH) release resulting in hyperparathyroidism when 1,25(OH)$_2$ vitamin D_3 levels are low.

Salusky et al. emphasize that PTH is elevated in patients with renal failure, and a goal of intact PTH level should be two to three times normal, since values in this range have been associated with a normal bone histology.[27] Elevated PTH values have been shown to correlate with poor linear growth in peritoneal dialysis patients.[28,29] In addition, it has been shown that low PTH values can result in adynamic bone disease, which leads to poor growth as well.[27]

On the basis of these data, we tend to aim for intact PTH values in infants of 150 to 300 pg/mL in order to optimize bone growth. After a few weeks of life, we begin following intact PTH levels and use this as a guide to titrate our vitamin D supplementation. 1,25(OH)$_2$ vitamin D_3, or calcitriol, is the treatment of choice for vitamin D replacement therapy. It should be pointed out that because the growth equation in infants with renal failure is complex, patients who are compliant with their calcitriol, resulting in ideal PTH values, may also be those who are more compliant with their rHuEPO, sodium bicarbonate, diet, and dialysis, making it difficult to isolate individual factors.

Other hormonal factors have been implicated as causes of the growth impairment in patients with ESRD and these are primarily linked to growth hormone and its mediators, such as insulin-like growth factor 1 (IGF-1). Although growth hormone (GH) levels in serum have been measured and found to be elevated in some patients, there appears to be overall resistance to this hormone. There is reduced GH receptor expression in renal failure in addition to elevated IGF-binding proteins, which appear to inhibit the "free," bioactive IGF-1.[30,31] This has led to the popularity of treating children with recombinant human growth hormone (rhGH). The improved growth from this agent is felt to be due to an increase in IGF-1 that exceeds the increase in IGF-binding proteins, resulting in a net increase in the bioactivity of IGF-1.

Over the past decade we have seen a dramatic improvement in linear growth both in children with chronic renal insufficiency as well as those on dialysis treated with rhGH (Nutropin; Genentech, South San Francisco, CA). Fine et al. reported significant increases in growth velocity in children with chronic renal failure as compared with untreated controls, without a concomitant decline in glomerular filtration fate (GFR). While adverse effects must be monitored—especially intracranial hypertension, slipped capital femoral epiphysis, avascular necrosis, and worsening hyperparathyroidism—use of rhGH in this population was deemed safe.[32] One must be careful not to implement rhGH therapy until hyperparathyroidism, acidosis, and inadequate calorie intake have been satisfactorily corrected. Last, two unique causes of CRF/ ESRD that occur in infancy are cystinosis and angiotensin-converting enzyme (ACE) fetopathy.[33] Infants with these diseases may not respond to the previously described therapy and may benefit from rhGH therapy.

Neurologic Development in Infants with Renal Failure

It is known that 50 percent of postnatal brain growth occurs in the first year of life.[34] The period of postnatal brain growth that is most vulnerable to insults occurs 25 to 30 weeks after birth, when glial proliferation is occurring. One type of glial cell, the oligodendrocyte, is responsible for central nervous system (CNS) myelin synthesis. The period of most rapid myelination occurs between the time just before birth and 6 to 8 months of life. Simply put, anything interfering with the process of myelination will inhibit normal brain development.[35]

In the first year of life, both total brain weight and total brain protein increase at a greater rate than does head circumference. Winick and Rosso found a linear relationship between brain DNA content, a measure of brain cell number, and head circumference.[36] It has also been shown that head circumference correlates with intelligence in children with microcephaly alone.[37] Hence, microcephaly in an infant with renal failure portends a poor prognosis for neurologic development.

Neurologic development in infants with CRF/ESRD has been noted to be markedly impaired by a number of authors. Early reports, such as the retrospective analysis by Rotundo et al., revealed a number of severe neurologic abnormalities in 20 of 23 infants who presented with chronic renal insufficiency before 1 year of age.[38] Neurologic findings listed were developmental delay in 19 infants, microcephaly in 15 infants, seizures in 13, hypotonia in 13, and dyskinesia in 11. The head circumference, despite being normal at birth in all infants, was >2 SD below normal in 15 infants and >3 SD below normal in 12 of these. Two of the three others who were unaffected neurologically had head circumferences within normal limits. Rotundo et al. point out that the clinical and electroencephalographic (EEG) findings in these patients looked much like the dialysis dementia syndrome that had been described in adults and attributed to aluminum toxicity. In fact, 16 of 20 affected infants were given aluminum-containing phosphate binders prior to the detection of their neurologic findings. Also of note is the authors' statement that "oral alkali" was used to treat acidosis; because it is not specified, one could speculate whether or not citrate was used as this alkali. It is well known that citrate enhances aluminum absorption in the gastrointestinal (GI) tract by altering tight junctions in the intestinal epithelium; this would make even a stronger case for aluminum toxicity in these infants.[11,19] McGraw and Haka-Ikse studied 12 children with onset of CRF in infancy and also found a high incidence of neurologic developmental sequelae.[34] The majority of these patients had microcephaly, seizures, and cerebral atrophy [based on computed tomography (CT) findings]. Most, too, had evidence of moderate to severe gross motor and language delay. One patient developed a severe progressive neurologic disorder at 17 months of age featuring seizures, choreoathetosis, progressive hypotonicity, and loss of developmental milestones. A well-functioning renal allograft placed at 22 months of age failed to improve his neurologic status. These authors concluded that the poor neurologic outcome in their study was due to a number of factors including malnutrition, aluminum toxicity, psychosocial deprivation, and the toxic effects of uremia. They point out that other disease states in infancy that can lead to malnutrition and recurrent hospitalizations (e.g., congenital heart disease and malabsorption syndromes) fail to develop the permanent CNS damage that had been reported in infants with renal failure. They also noted that older children who acquire renal failure are not affected in the same manner as infants, thus stating that we need to intervene aggressively with infants, since they are very vulnerable even to minor insults that can have long-lasting sequelae in the future.

More recently, better outcomes in infants with renal failure have been reported.[35,36] Polinsky et al. discussed five patients with onset of progressive renal insufficiency within the first 4½ months of life.[35] Four of five had creatinine clearance (Ccr) <15 mL/min/1.73 m^2, the other had a Ccr of 37.6 mL/min/1.73 m^2. The weight-to-height ratios ranged from 84 to 95 percent, indicating only mild malnutrition at best. The head circumferences fell over the first 12 to 18 months of life but remained within 2 SD of the mean in all but one patient. Also noted was the much sharper decline of the linear growth curve over this same time period, suggesting a "brain-sparing" effect during this period of rapid brain growth. Development was assessed in these infants using both the Bayley Scales of Infant Development (in 3 infants) and the Gesell Developmental Schedules (in all 5 infants). With the exception of one patient (with a Ccr = 37.6), most scores were within 2 SD of the mean and considered normal. An additional patient had scores more than 2 SD below the mean in language and personal-social functioning, but these improved when reassessed 6 months later on continuous cycling peritoneal dialysis (CCPD). The investigators felt that their data were much more encouraging than previous infant reports and attributed it to good nutrition, good psychosocial backgrounds in four of five families, and limited usage of aluminum-containing phosphate binders.[35] Only the patient with "relatively good" renal function and head growth but a poor psychosocial situation tested poorly in all aspects. This led the authors to conclude that the poor social situation affected the development of this one child negatively. This study was one of the first to shed favorable light on the long-term neurologic outcome of infants with ESRD.

An additional study by Warady et al. of four patients treated with aggressive nutrition and peritoneal dialysis in the first month of life also reported encouraging results.[39] This study differed from previous ones in that no patient received aluminum-containing phosphate binders and all were on multivitamins with iron. In addition, all patients received calcitriol. Some actually required phosphate supplements and three of four received sodium chloride to keep the serum sodium normal. Caloric intake via oral or nasogastric feedings ranged from 83 to 111 percent of the RDA; protein intake ranged from 2.3 to 3.4 g/kg/day (107 to 163 percent RDA). All had weights above the fifth percentile, and three of four had head circumferences within 2 SD of the mean. Most importantly, with regard to developmental assessments, motor delay was common (hypotonia in three of four, with an abnormal primitive reflex profile and gross motor delay in all). However, none of these patients had seizures, and the EEG and CT scans done on select patients were normal. While unable to exclude the contributions of dialysis (as all patients were on CCPD), the authors concluded that aggressive nutrition in infancy and avoidance of the neurotoxic effects of aluminum produced these favorable results.

With regard to the "direct" effects of uremia on CNS function, Fennell et al. have shown that older children with ESRD manifest lower verbal, visual, perceptual, memory, and especially visual motor skills when compared with controls.[40,41] Also, immediate recall and memory were found to worsen with worsening renal function. Additionally, the verbal performance scores in children ages 6 to 11, but not those of children >12 years, fell with increasing duration of renal failure. This was attributed to the greater susceptibility of the the 6- to 11-year-olds, since they were of the age of rapid acquisition of new language skills. Equally important are the earlier findings of Fennell et al. that performance skills, while not differing between predialysis and dialysis subjects, did show improvement after renal transplantation. Although difficult to assess objectively in the younger children, this has obvious implications for infants with CRF/ESRD who clearly have rapid development of language and performance skills. Any factor(s) that can affect their immediate recall and memory negatively will have a negative impact on the acquisition of new skills. If indeed these patients improve with transplantation, this would make a strong argument for early transplantation, so as to allow development to proceed as normally as possible. Work in the latter 1990s to the present illustrates that aggressive nutrition, early intervention with vitamin D, treatment of anemia, as well as focus on development results in significant improvement in neurodevelopment.[42–44]

DIALYSIS IN INFANTS

Peritoneal dialysis (PD) and hemodialysis (HD) are two dialytic modalities used in infants and children with ESRD. Discussion of the advantages and disadvantages of both modalities follows. It should be mentioned here that the mortality of children undergoing dialysis appears to correlate inversely with age (Table 42–2). Therefore the factors that affect the mortality of infants on dialysis are addressed below.

Peritoneal Dialysis in Infancy

Both continuous ambulatory peritoneal dialysis (CAPD) and CCPD are modalities used frequently in children and infants. Since these are reviewed in detail elsewhere in this text, we focus on those aspects of PD in infants that are unique to this age group. In addition, we consider the growth and development of patients on PD vs. other modalities while also looking at the costs and complications of this therapy.

PD is now the most commonly used modality for ESRD in the United States, Canada, and the United Kingdom for children below 15 years of age.[45] Data from the North American Pediatric Renal Transplant Cooperative Study (NAPRTCS) dialysis patient database, which began in January 1992, suggest that PD is preferred far above HD for infants below 2 years of age who need dialysis. A total of 94 percent (621 of 660) of infants were treated with PD, while 6 percent (39 of 660) were receiving HD. This was substantially different from the dialysis breakdown of all registered patients below 21 years of age in the same study: 65 percent PD vs. 35 percent HD.[7]

PD in infants can be done as CAPD or CCPD. Those on CAPD require a system capable of accurately handling small volumes. Most infants are begun on fill volumes of 10 mL/kg and slowly advanced up to 30 mL/kg per dwell. A 5-kg infant will be started at volumes as low as 50 mL; thus, even a small dead-space volume in the circuit can be quite significant. Infants can also be dialyzed via a CCPD system, but this often requires adjustment of the volume return alarms, especially in those infants who maintain a high urine output.

The advantages to PD in infants include ease of access to the peritoneal cavity, avoidance of systemic heparinization, and continuous solute clearance and fluid removal. This more physiologic form of RRT provides blood pressure control superior to that seen on HD.[46,47] In addition, because continuous fluid removal occurs, nutritional formulas can be given in an essentially unrestricted manner so as to optimize caloric intake for growth.

Equally important is the fact that the parents can be trained to perform PD at home, allowing the family a degree of independence from the hospital while also giving them some control over the care of their child. These parents, who may be disappointed by not having "the perfect child," understandably become frustrated at their inability to feed and care successfully for their frequently hospitalized infant. This can lead to inconsistent care and often a withdrawal of emotional support, which further contributes to developmental delay in these children. Thus, PD gives the family a refuge from the hospital, which helps restore a semblance of order to the household while giving them more confidence in caring for their child. The risk of intensive home therapy stems from the associated stress.[48]

When compared with HD, the primary drawbacks of PD are infection and the need for a competent, caring family capable of carrying out PD at home. One could argue that if the family is not caring and competent, the prognosis for eventual renal transplantation, where compliance with immunosuppressive medicines is vital, may be bleak.[49]

TABLE 42–2. AGE-BASED MORTALITY RATES OF INFANTS AND CHILDREN ON DIALYSIS

Study	Dialysis Modality	Recipient Age	1-Year Mortality	Reference
NAPRTCS	PD/HD	0–1	16%	7
NAPRTCS	PD/HD	2–5	14%	7
NAPRTCS	PD/HD	> 5	3%	7
Kohaut et al.	PD	< 2	22%	5

Another negative aspect of PD in children is receiving subcutaneous human recombinant erythropoietin (rHuEPO). Due to the painful administration of this product, compliance with its use is a problem for patients on PD. While patients on HD who receive rHuEPO intravenously are devoid of the pain from these subcutaneous injections, new hope for patients on PD appears to be in sight. A report showed an effective response to intraperitoneal rHuEPO when given in higher dosages (300 U/kg/week). This method of administration would eliminate the patient/parent struggles that normally occur when the drug is given subcutaneously.[50]

Additional disadvantages of PD include protein losses into the dialysate.[51] The significant albumin losses that occur can be counteracted by the use of high-protein formulas. It is not uncommon for a growing infant on PD to require as much as 3 to 4 g/kg/day of dietary protein. Brewer et al. reported a positive impact on linear growth in six infants who received enteral feedings.[52] The caloric intake in this study ranged from 60 to 140 percent of the RDA, with a mean protein intake of 3.8 g/kg/day. These findings support the idea of "catch-up" growth in infants on PD who are aggressively fed with high-protein formulas during this period of rapid growth.

A potential advantage of this protein removal on PD is improved clearance of growth inhibitors that accumulate in the "uremic" patient. Insulin-like growth factor binding protein 3 (IGFBP-3) is known to accumulate in patients with renal failure, which may interfere with the bioactivity of IGF-1. We have demonstrated that IGFBP-3 is partially cleared by PD, with a potential improvement of IGF-I bioactivity.[53] Ongoing studies are in progress to assess the impact of this finding further.

Complications of Peritoneal Dialysis in Infancy. Infectious complications of PD include peritonitis and exit-site infections. Peritonitis occurs quite frequently in the PD population, which greatly affects the overall care of these patients. Stone et al. reviewed a 5-year experience of 93 children (20 children <5 years old) on CAPD and CCPD and found that 61 percent of these patients developed exit-site infections and 59 percent developed peritonitis.[54] This calculates to one episode every 11.6 and 11.8 patient-months, respectively. It should be noted that 39 percent of the 154 peritonitis episodes were sterile. Fungal peritonitis occurred in three (2 percent) of these patients, necessitating catheter removal with a change to HD in all three. In total, six patients required a change to HD as a result of membrane failure consequent to peritonitis, and 29 catheters needed replacement for recurrent or persistent peritonitis.

A report by the North American Pediatric Renal Transplant Cooperative Study (NAPRTCS) revealed an incidence of peritonitis at one episode every 7.1 patient-months in the 534 children on PD. The definition of peritonitis differed somewhat in this study: all "apparent" peritoneal infections requiring antibiotics regardless of cell count or culture were used. Nonetheless, only about 16 percent of their cultures were sterile, so this more frequent incidence of peritonitis seems to be real and independent of the differences in the definitions. As in the previous study, fungal peritonitis accounted for a small number (3 percent) of all cases.[7]

While most reports deal with children in general, the few reports on infant PD suggest that complications in infancy may be even greater. A report by Kohaut et al.[5] revealed an incidence of peritonitis as one episode every 4.5 patient-months in nine infants who began CAPD before 3 months of age. Other reported complications included the death of two infants in this study, resulting in a mortality rate of 22 percent, or one death every 48 patient-months, which was significantly higher than that in older children (1 in every 185 patient-months).

Salusky et al reported an incidence of peritonitis of only one episode every 11.6 patient-months in eight infants (2.5 to 8.5 months old) managed on CCPD.[4] This difference from that reported by Kohaut et al. may be due in part to the difference in technique used, since it has been well established that the incidence of peritonitis will increase in proportion to the number of "breaks" introduced into the system. Thus, CCPD appears to be advantageous based on its lower apparent rates of infection and hospital admission compared with those reported with CAPD in infants.

Additionally, Kohaut et al. noted that a significantly greater number of infants had hypotension and hyponatremia when compared with older children on CAPD. This was attributed to the polyuria in several of the infants with dysplasia and obstructive uropathy, accompanied by their inherent inability to access salt and water. This may have been additionally affected by sodium losses into the dialysate.[55]

Other reported complications of PD include hernias (ventral—near the catheter insertion site, inguinal, and umbilical) ranging from 42 percent in children to 75 percent in infants.[4,54] In addition, further complications in children include dialysate leakage in 14 percent, external cuff extrusion in 11 percent, catheter obstruction in 7 percent, catheter migration in 2 percent, and temporary hydrothorax in 2 percent. While the hernias often required surgical repair, the other complications required a decrease in the dialysate volume, catheter replacement, or, in a few instances, a temporary change in dialysis modality.

Immunologic Effects of Peritoneal Dialysis in the Infant. Immunologic abnormalities have been described in adults with ESRD, but only recently have they been evaluated in pediatrics. Two separate reports have shown that both B- and T-cell function in children on dialysis (CAPD and HD) appear to be normal.[56,57] Serum IgG in children on CAPD, although normal, was depressed slightly when compared with controls. Further, antibody responses to the mumps and combined measles, mumps, and rubella (MMR) vaccines were normal.

Other studies assessing response to vaccines have been reported by Moxey-Mims et al., who demonstrated seroconversion to the hepatitis B vaccine (Hepta-vax-B Merck, Sharp and Dohme) in 15 of 17 patients on PD and 5 of 6 patients on HD.[58] All three nonconverters had systemic lupus erythematosus (SLE) and were being treated with corticosteroids. Although the authors could not conclude definitely, they felt that the low-dose immunosuppression was probably insufficient and that the vasculitis itself was the most likely cause.

Other studies have shown an inadequate protective antibody response in one patient and a waning antibody response to subtherapeutic levels in another when eight children on PD were evaluated after being immunized with the *Haemophilus influenzae* type b vaccine.[59] In addition, it was found that 5 of 16 of these children who were more than 5 years old and thus not immunized lacked protective antibody.

A retrospective study by Schulman et al. in young children confirmed a poor seroconversion rate in dialysis patients (9 of 10 on PD) to MMR.[60] Only 3 of 10 children seroconverted to all three vaccines, compared with 91 percent of the control children. The Schulman report suggests that infants (median age 17 months in this study) may have more problems with seroconversion to MMR than do the older children (mean 9.7 years) reported by Hisano et al.[57] These more recent studies of vaccine responsiveness in young children on PD suggest a need to follow antibody titers in these patients.

Hypogammaglobulinemia in infants and children on PD has been noted by several authors.[61,62] While it is well known that patients lose immunoglobulins in the PD effluent, adult studies have shown no drop in serum levels. In fact, it has been suggested that the immunodeficiency present in the uremic state is improved in patients on PD when compared with those on HD, possibly due to the improved removal of immunosuppressive middle molecules with PD.[51,63] Fivush et al. noted 5 of 7 of their patients on CAPD to have serum IgG levels >2 SD below the mean.[61] Interestingly of those with hypogammaglobulinemia that were immunized, 4 of 4 had protective antibody to diphtheria and tetanus, while 3 of 4 manifested protective antibodies to rubella. The authors also point out that the rate of IgG loss in the dialysis effluent correlated with the length of time that the patient was on dialysis.

Katz et al. found 12 of 13 patients <2 years of age on PD had low (>2 SD below the mean) IgG levels as opposed to 2 of 8 age-matched patients with ESRD managed conservatively.[62] It should be noted that diet/protein intake and creatinine clearance were matched in these patients as well.

Serious bacterial infections occurred in 3 of 8 children on PD with IgG <100 mg/dL, resulting in one infant's death. These authors, too, found that the IgG losses in the PD effluent of these infants were no greater than those of adults; when corrected for body surface area, they were actually less than those of older children and adults. The authors concluded that uremia may impair immunoglobulin synthesis in infancy. This impaired production combined with PD losses of IgG results in clinically significant hypogammaglobulinemia in infants.

Neu et al. reported the death of an 11-month-old PD patient with panhypogammaglobulinemia (low IgG, IgA, and IgM) and polymicrobial gram-negative sepsis.[64] They emphasized the need to screen for hypogammaglobulinemia in the infant on PD, with the consideration of gamma globulin treatment for those with low IgG.

Schroeder et al. reported two patients (15 months and 5 years of age) with severe group B streptococcal peritonitis, which was attributed to IgG subclass 2 deficiency.[65] This pathogen, the most common bacterial cause of sepsis in the first 2 months of life, essentially becomes nonexistent after the infant reaches 6 months of age. Previous studies have revealed that mothers of newborns with this infection have likewise been deficient in IgG subclass 2.

Despite these drawbacks, PD can be successfully carried out in the infant with ESRD. Warady et al. point out that only those patients with an inadequate peritoneal cavity—such as infants with abdominal wall defects, a diaphragmatic hernia, or a history of extensive abdominal surgeries resulting in adhesions—are unlikely candidates for PD.[45]

Our dialysis access consists of a surgically placed single-cuffed Tenckhoff curled catheter. These infants are maintained on CCPD with a target urea clearance of 225 mL/kg/day, which can usually be accomplished with peritoneal volumes of 30 mL/kg per dwell. Because many patients live 2 to 3 hours away from the medical center, most families prefer PD, since uncomplicated delivery of this dialytic therapy requires far fewer hospital visits than would be needed on HD. Holtta et al. showed in 34 infants that PD at home is effective with a low peritonitis rate, improved growth, and a low (6 percent) mortality rate.[66] In a large series of 20 infants, Ledermann et al. demonstrated similar outcomes with excellent growth leading to transplantation.[67]

Hemodialysis in Infancy

HD is usually regarded as a second-line mode of dialysis in infants. While it is still reported to be used in one-third of pediatric dialysis treatments, it probably accounts for no more than 10 percent of those treatments in infancy.[7] The need for specialized infant-specific vascular access, dialyzers, HD machines, and HD blood lines—as well as physicians and nursing staff experienced in infant HD—makes this modality less frequently utilized.[68,69] The techniques of HD are discussed elsewhere in this book, but the aspects of HD specific to infants are addressed below.

In many centers, HD is used either as a short-term "bridge" from nephrectomy to transplantation (as in the congenital nephrotic syndrome) or as the "last-ditch effort" after peritoneal membrane failure. Infants on chronic HD need the same attention to prevention of renal osteodystrophy, anemia, infections, and growth impairment, as well as malnutrition, as infants undergoing other modalities of RRT.

Difficulties with infant HD begin and end with vascular access. The use of Gore-Tex grafts or AV fistulas is rare in this population due to the small caliber of the infant's vessels. Therefore externalized access is usually the access of choice. This may include a single-lumen Hickman, which can be utilized for single-needle HD, or a dual-lumen access, of which supplies are limited.[70,71] We utilize either a cuffed or uncuffed catheter in this population, depending upon the duration of need. Infant access ideally consists of a catheter of short length and wide caliber, resulting in minimal flow resistance.[72] Blood flow rates may range from 20 to 120 mL/min, and recirculation rates should not exceed 5 percent.

Many companies make HD machines that can be adapted (with neonatal blood lines) to accommodate small extracorporeal circuits. This is usually accomplished by excluding the arterial drip chamber (and arterial pressure monitor) and by using a small (2- to 4-mL) venous drip chamber.[68] These lines can be combined by commercially available infant dialyzers to have a total extracorporeal circuit as small as 30 to 38 mL (Table 42–3). Therefore, if one uses the "10 percent rule" (where no more than 10 percent of the blood volume of the patient is extracorporeal), this circuit can be utilized in a 4.5-kg infant without blood priming. In infants weighing less than 4.5 kg, attention to the infant's hemodynamics and the hematocrit will dictate the need for blood priming. The obvious problems with blood priming include inherent risks of infection, hyperkalemia, and an increase in the viscosity of the circuit, with a potential increase in heparin requirements. In addition, as mentioned previously, the HLA sensitization that occurs with blood transfusion can have a negative impact on the outcome of the future kidney transplant.

TABLE 42–3. DIALYZERS AVAILABLE FOR INFANTS

Dialyzer	Composition	SA (m²)	Priming Volume (mL)
Asahi AM 0.3	Cuprammonium	0.3	30
Fresenius F3	Polysulfone	0.4	30
Gambro CA-50	Cellulose acetate	0.5	38
Cobe HG-100	Hemophan	0.22	18

Once the circuit is "strung," attention to ensure occlusion at the pump head and calibration of the blood pump is imperative prior to commencing HD. A typical blood-flow rate in a pediatric patient is 3 to 5 mL/kg/min. Therefore, in a 5-kg infant, a blood-flow rate of no more than 15 to 25 mL/min is required. Blood-flow rates in excess of that may increase the risk of dialysis disequilibrium secondary to osmolar shifts due to urea clearance. The presence of an ultrafiltration controller is preferred in order to have an accurate and reliable rate of ultrafiltration. Most ultrafiltration controllers have an error rate as high as +50 mL/h; therefore continual reassessment of the infant's volume status (heart rate and blood pressure variability) is required. Some centers prefer to have the infant placed on a continuous reading bed scale as a way to follow the ultrafiltration rate. The weights on the bed scale are influenced by the movement of the child and the unidentified placement or removal of objects from the scale. Therefore strict attention to these factors is mandatory during infant HD.

Because the RDA for caloric intake is 115 kcal/kg/day in the first 6 months of life and 105 kcal/kg/day for the second 6 months of life, the volume of feedings consumed in infancy to achieve adequate growth far exceeds that taken by older children and adults. Because the nutrition of infants is largely formula-based, ultrafiltration is the primary indication for frequent HD treatments (4 to 6 days per week).

At the end of an HD treatment, attention to the extracorporeal blood return is necessary. Some infants will tend toward hypertension or even congestive heart failure as this 5 to 7 mL/kg of extracorporeal blood is rapidly transfused into the infant. In anuric infants, we frequently utilize an "air" return, which negates the need for additional saline back into the infant. This is done by disconnecting the "arterial" line and returning the blood via the "venous" line without a normal saline flush. This is a potentially hazardous technique and is best done with two persons in order to avoid an air embolus.

In centers that utilize a single-needle HD approach, issues identical to those mentioned above exist. Additionally, attention to arterial and venous times is necessary to balance adequate dialysis with ultrafiltration.

Heparin requirements in infants are similar to those in older children. The utilization of a bedside activated clotting time (ACT) machine is preferred. Maintaining an ACT between 150 and 200 seconds is adequate for most treatments.[73] This is usually easily achieved by an initial bolus of 10 to 20 U/kg of heparin at the onset of HD with 10 to 20 U/kg/h throughout the treatment in a patient with normal coagulation. If reversal of heparin is needed at the end of the treatment, a slow infusion of 1 mg of protamine for each 200 U of heparin infused during the treatment will usually normalize the heparin effect. Because the half-life of heparin is longer than that of protamine, additional protamine may be required.

In infants on chronic HD, the complications of CRF should be anticipated and avoided. Anemia associated with ESRD is treated with the use of intravenous rHuEPO, which can be administered during the HD treatment. Center preference will dictate dosage amount and frequency, although the range is usually between 50 and 300 U/kg/dose per HD treatment for a target posttreatment hematocrit of 32 to 36 percent. Intravenous iron can easily be administered during HD treatments, obviating the need for oral iron. Further, attention to the return of all of the blood in the extracorporeal circuit is necessary to avoid ongoing blood and iron loss. Renal osteodystrophy is preventable by normalizing the serum phosphorus, avoiding aluminum-containing compounds, and administering adequate active vitamin D. Phosphorus can be normalized by the use of specialized formulas containing minimal phosphorus or binding of phosphorus with calcium carbonate or acetate. In the older population, increased phosphorus clearance can be obtained with the use of a high efficiency dialyzer. At present, no infant-sized high-efficiency membrane exists. In practical terms, due to the increased frequency of HD treatments needed in infants, hyperphosphatemia is rare. Intravenous calcitriol can be administered as an alternative to oral vitamin D during the HD treatment in order to minimize the need for additional oral medications. Malnutrition is a preventable problem associated with HD in the infant population. Infant formula selection should be dictated by the urine output as well as the infant's serum chemistries, as previously described.[74]

The external catheter utilized for HD is associated with its own inherent risk of "line infections," as is any external access. Meticulous attention to the prevention of infection while maintaining thorough "site care" is mandatory in order to minimize this risk. General opinion is that an exit-site or line infection presents less of a potential risk of morbidity in the well-nourished patient.

Other factors that make HD less appealing include inferior blood pressure control.[46] Since much of the hypertension in ESRD is volume-related, euvolemia is achieved at best for just a few hours of the day. This is especially problematic in the infant whose nutrition is primarily fluid-based, thereby necessitating frequent dialysis treatments.

Growth on chronic HD is thought to be less than that which occurs on chronic PD.[75] This is thought to be due to less liberal dietary intake, larger fluctuations in serum chemistries, an increased association of hypertension with HD, and potentially less clearance of growth inhibitors, which appears to be enhanced in PD.

Unlike those on PD, infants on HD are closely tied to a medical center. Even if the patient lives near the hospital, this degree of dependency on the hospital system can put a great strain on the nuclear family.

Outcome in HD in infants and small children can be similar to that seen with PD. Programs dedicated to the use of HD as a primary modality have reported >90 percent survival rates with this modality, using it as the bridge to transplantation.[76,77] The need for dedicated staff, delivery systems, and experience make this a reasonable therapy in children who cannot be on PD for physical or social reasons.

KIDNEY TRANSPLANTATION IN INFANCY

It is agreed that a kidney transplant is the definitive form of RRT for children because it provides a quality of life superior to that offered by any mode of dialysis.[78] With regard to the question of infant transplantation, most would not ask whether to transplant an infant but rather *when*. Is it harmful to keep an infant on dialysis for months to years before deciding to pursue a kidney transplant? We begin by reviewing kidney transplantation in infancy before presenting the pros and cons of this mode of therapy.

Preemptive Kidney Transplantation in Infancy

Transplantation as the primary mode of RRT *without dialysis* is referred to as preemptive transplantation. The advantage of this mode of therapy is that the patients are relatively healthy as they approach transplantation, making for a less complicated postoperative course. It eliminates the need for insertion of dialysis access, either vascular or peritoneal, and thus reduces the number of exposures to general anesthesia. In addition, it avoids the need to spend considerable hours in training families to care for a dialysis patient optimally, perform exchanges, etc. Patient and graft survival rates for all pediatric patients under the age of 21 have improved significantly over the past decade (Table 42–4).

Comparisons of preemptive transplantation to transplantation after the onset of dialysis have been reported.[79–81] In all pediatric studies reported, not a single survival advantage was noted in any age group that received dialysis or with any dialysis modality as compared with no dialysis

TABLE 42–4A. PEDIATRIC PATIENT SURVIVAL RATES AMONG INDEX TRANSPLANTS (1997–2003)

	1 Year		2 Years		3 Years	
	%	SE	%	SE	%	SE
No dialysis, $n = 661$	99.1	.42	98.8	.48	98.5	.58
HD only, $n = 734$	99.1	.39	98.7	.50	98.0	.72
PD only, $n = 984$	98.6	.40	97.4	.61	96.1	.84
HD + PD, $n = 133$	98.1	1.4	98.1	1.4	98.1	1.4
Total, 2512	98.9	.23	98.2	.32	97.4	.43

TABLE 42–4B. PEDIATRIC GRAFT SURVIVAL RATES AMONG INDEX TRANSPLANTS (1997–2003)

	1 Year		2 Years		3 Years	
	%	SE	%	SE	%	SE
No dialysis	94.7	.91	93.5	1.1	91.1	1.4
HD only	94.5	.91	90.8	1.3	86.0	1.8
PD only	93.5	.82	90.6	1.1	86.8	1.4
HD + PD	94.3	2.1	93.0	2.4	87.8	3.7
Total	94.2	.50	91.6	.63	87.8	.84

prior to kidney transplantation. Therefore preemptive transplantation is the optimal choice whenever feasible. Studies in adults have been even more dramatic. Mange et al. reported that preemptive kidney transplantation was associated with a reduction of 52 percent in the rate of graft failure during the initial posttransplant year and a reduction of 86 percent during subsequent years; all recipients had received a kidney from a live donor.[82] Centers experienced in infant transplantation often report better results than smaller centers that perform few transplants per year; as a result, it is these experienced centers that often speak loudest for infant transplantation. A report from the University of Minnesota has stated that "The optimal therapy for patients under five is preemptive, living related donor transplantation."[83]

Preparation for Infant Transplantation

All patients with congenital urologic abnormalities must undergo a pretransplant evaluation of the urinary tract with kidney/bladder ultrasonography and contrast voiding cystourethrogram (VCUG) so that anatomy and physiology of the lower urinary tract is delineated. Since at least 25 percent of infants <2 years of age with CRF/ESRD have obstructive or reflux uropathy as the cause, knowing the urologic anatomy and function is imperative prior to proceeding to transplant. If evidence for a small, noncompliant bladder or a large bladder with a high-pressure system (as evidenced by high-grade reflux or hydronephrosis) exists on VCUG, urodynamic studies are performed. Video urodynamics has become popular in recent years, combining contrast cystography with urodynamics to fully assess bladder function. Some patients require pretransplant urologic surgery if the bladder is not suitable for transplantation. Such procedures may include an "augmentation" procedure using intestine so as to improve the capacitance of the bladder. Drawbacks of intestinal (usually ileum) augmentation procedures include those of systemic acidosis and bladder colonization, which increases the potential for future urinary tract infections (UTI). This can be traced to the pH of the secretions of the intestinal lining, since alkaline secretions from the native ileum may result in bicarbonate losses in the urine, leading to metabolic acidosis and increased bacterial overgrowth in

the bladder. Also, the intestinal tract tends to secrete a great deal of mucus, making urinary outflow obstruction another problem seen in these patients. If urethral drainage is inadequate, a stoma for catheterization sometimes is created at the time of reconstructive surgery. This is usually done using an appendiceal stoma connecting the bladder to the anterior abdominal wall, often in close proximity to the umbilicus. Investigators state that the principal goals of surgery are to provide "a sterile, nonrefluxing content reservoir" that can be emptied easily.[84] Kidney transplantation into an uncorrected urologic system risks allograft injury due to high bladder pressures transmitted to the transplanted kidney. Therefore a thorough urologic evaluation is done on transplant candidates who have abnormalities of the genitourinary system as assessed by the screening tests noted above.

Correction of a refluxing system should be addressed prior to transplantation. In the face of a chronically infected kidney, nephrectomy is mandated. If a refluxing system that is not associated with urinary infection is present, however, preservation of the native kidney (via native ureter reimplantation) would preserve native kidney urine output in the posttransplant period. This may be especially helpful in the event of primary nonfunction or allograft loss. This native urine output would allow for ease of dialysis or potentially continuation of conservative care without dialysis.

With regard to getting the infant "ready" for transplant, the immunization record is reviewed. Since patients on immunosuppressive medications should not receive live virus vaccines, those transplanted in the first year of life may be incompletely immunized to varicella, measles, mumps, and rubella.[85] We generally delay transplantation until all live immunizations have been administered and positive titers to specific viruses are documented. Varicella is associated with a higher mortality in the transplant recipient.[86] Varicella vaccine is a live attenuated virus, and, according to the Committee on Infectious Diseases of the American Academy of Pediatrics, is unacceptable for administration to transplant patients.[85] Not only must the transplant recipient be immunized but all siblings and close friends should receive the vaccine, thus diminishing the likelihood of exposing the transplant patient to this highly infectious organism.[87] A vaccine against cytomegalovirus, once thought to be on the horizon for transplant patients,[88] has not reached clinical utility.

A number of studies support living donor transplants in infants.[2,3,6,89–91] Our bias is to educate families about transplantation at the pretransplant evaluation of their infants and to encourage donation if early transplantation is desired by the family. ABO and tissue typing are sent on both the infant and parents. If a suitable donor is available, further workup in the infant is pursued. If a suitable donor is not found in the immediate family, a search to extended family members and friends is made. Once a potential donor is located, a complete history and physical is performed by an internist; if the donor passes this step, screening laboratory tests of kidney function, liver function, blood sugar, electrocardiogram, and 24-hour urine collection are performed. A preoperative CT angiogram is then done and evaluated by the transplant surgeon. Thus, there are a number of checkpoints that a potential donor must pass through before a transplant is undertaken. Twenty-year follow-up on living donors suggest that the risk to the donor is minimal.[92]

Factors Affecting Infant Transplantation

Several factors appear to influence the outcome of kidney transplantation in the infant. Immunologic responsiveness is heightened in the infant[93] making factors such as allograft source and immunosuppression protocols more important in this age group. In addition, technical factors at the time of transplantation appear to play a larger role in this high-risk population.

Donor Source. Although kidney transplantation in infants was reported as early as 1971, the initial results utilizing pediatric or anencephalic cadaveric (CAD) donors were quite poor, causing most transplant physicians to shy away from infants.[3] Others reported good outcomes 1 year posttransplant in infants, which made transplant physicians more optimistic.[94] It was the report of Miller et al., that infants as small as 5.4-kg could tolerate transplantation of an adult kidney, which had a major impact on allograft survival and the way infant transplantation would later be performed.[95] Nevins reported on 44 infants below 2 years of age.[96] In this report, actuarial patient and allograft survival rates at 4 years of follow-up were 95 and 80 percent, respectively. The author reported that 3 of 13 infants below 1 year of age received a kidney transplant before the initiation of dialysis and concluded that there was no contraindication to preemptive transplantation and that obligatory dialysis was not necessary in infants with CRF.

So et al. published encouraging results on 9 infants (2 to 7.5 years posttransplant) being evaluated for growth and development after renal transplantation.[97] Their pretransplant patient population included 6 of 9 with height and head circumferences >2 SD below the mean; 5 of these patients had seizures, 4 had abnormal cognitive development, and 6 had abnormal motor development. Posttransplant evaluation revealed normal head circumference (within 2 SD of the mean) in all 9 infants; normal height scores in 5 of 9 infants; normal cognitive development in all 9; normal motor development in 5 of 7 tested; and freedom from seizures in all. The authors concluded that kidney transplantation should be considered a treatment option even in the first year of life for children with ESRD, especially those showing signs of poor growth and development on dialysis.

While the number of authors supporting infant transplantation continued to grow, others remained skeptical.

Fine stated that infants with renal failure with accompanying delayed growth and development should be maintained on dialysis until 2 years of age.[98] He felt this would alleviate the guilt burden on the family to provide a living donor and would optimize growth that would otherwise be hampered by "the catabolic consequences of transplantation." Moreover, Arbus et al. published discouraging results for CAD donor transplant survival in young children (predicted 1-year graft survival of 57 percent in children <2 years old receiving an adult CAD kidney). They recommended maintaining children on dialysis until their third birthday, at which time their chances of a successful CAD donor transplant would have improved.[91] However, they recommended that if a suitable living donor (LD) were available, a transplant should be reconsidered, since LD success rates in infants are superior.

Najarian et al. found similar results to those above in 75 children below 2 years of age.[3] They found 1-year CAD graft survival to be 25 percent in CAD transplants done in infants <1 year of age and 50 percent in CAD transplants in infants 1 to 2 years of age. In marked contrast, LD survival rates at 1 year posttransplant were 94 and 83 percent, respectively, in these age groups. Data such as these lead most pediatric transplant nephrologists and surgeons to prefer a LD transplant when kidney transplants in infants and young children are being arranged.

A single-center study that analyzed the outcome of kidney transplantation in 21 children <2 years old confirmed some of the previous pessimism regarding CAD transplant outcome in small infants.[6] The actuarial 5-year patient survival was 86 percent LD and 70 percent CAD. The graft survival data were 93 percent at 1 year and 86 percent at 5 years for LD, while those for CAD were 38 percent at both 1 and 5 years. The 1-year mortality rate was 7 percent following LD and 30 percent following CAD, compared with the 22 percent mortality rate for infants on PD.[5] Thus, the authors concluded that, while both LD and CAD transplants are possible in infants, the outcome is superior in the LD recipient. In addition, they concluded that, since the mortality rates of infant transplantation and dialysis were similar, the decision to transplant the infant should be based on the infant's size, growth, and development. These data have been substantiated by data from national infant dialysis registries and NAPRTCS (Talley and Stablein, personal communication)[2,7,8] (Tables 42–5 and 42–6). The NAPRTCS data are from years 1997 through 2003 and thus reflect the use of more current immunosuppressive regimens. They contain important information in a few respects. First, 3-year *patient* survival after kidney transplantation for all children under 5 years of age is superb, averaging 96.2 percent. Even for children under 2 years of age, patient survival is excellent, averaging 92.8 percent. Second, 3-year graft survival for children under 5 years of age is similarly excellent, averaging 89.7 percent. For children under 2 years of age,

TABLE 42–5A. PATIENT SURVIVAL RATES AMONG INDEX TRANSPLANTS AGES < 2 YEARS (1997–2003)

	1 Year		2 Years		3 Years	
	%	SE	%	SE	%	SE
No dialysis (n = 30)	100	0	100	0	100	0
HD only (n = 22)	86.7	8.8	86.7	8.8	86.7	8.8
PD only (n = 74)	98.3	1.7	91.0	4.3	91.0	4.3
HD + PD (n = 9)	100	0	100	0	100	0
Total (n = 135)	96.8	1.8	92.8	2.9	92.8	2.9

TABLE 42–5C. PATIENT SURVIVAL RATES AMONG INDEX TRANSPLANTS AGES < 5 YEARS (1997–2003)

	1 Year		2 Years		3 Years	
	%	SE	%	SE	%	SE
No dialysis (n = 113)	98.9	1.1	98.9	1.1	98.9	1.1
HD only (n = 100)	96.1	2.2	96.1	2.2	93.6	3.3
PD only (n = 265)	99.2	.58	96.5	1.5	95.4	1.8
HD + PD (n = 40)	100	0	100	0	100	0
Total (n = 518)	98.6	.60	97.2	.89	96.2	1.1

graft survival is not only superb, averaging almost 89 percent at 3 years, but is similar to that in children 2 to 5 years old. Third, children under 2 years of age who received their initial kidney transplant *without* prior dialysis had 100 percent patient survival and 97 percent graft survival at 3 years. These values were superior to any of the data from the dialyzed groups. Patient and graft survival rates at 3 years for children 2 to 5 years of age were similarly excellent, remaining slightly better in the preemptive group than in children who required dialysis.

Immunosuppression Effect. Two other studies published from UCLA and the University of Minnesota shed light on the prospects of CAD transplant in infants and young children when both aggressive immunosuppression is instituted and young donor kidneys are avoided.[99,100] Ettenger et al. showed, in children under 6 years of age, that the 1-year actuarial CAD allograft survival was 33 percent in those who received either azathioprine/prednisone or cyclosporine/prednisone alone, compared with 90 percent in those on "quadruple" therapy (antithymocyte globulin, azathioprine, cyclosporine, and prednisone). There may be confounding

variables here because the former group were transplanted from 1980 to 1985, when the use of young donor kidneys was more frequent; moreover, the cause of graft loss was "technical" in one case, thrombosis in two others, and rejection in the remainder. If one corrects for published technical/thrombotic losses, there still appears to be an immunologic benefit of quadruple therapy in the infant receiving a CAD donor allograft.[99]

Donor Age. McLorie et al. were among the first to report on the effect of donor age on graft survival, noting that transplant recipients under 6 years of age had improved graft survival when the donor was more than 6 years of age.[100] Ettenger et al. also noted that the calculated GFR for CAD allografts in recipients below 6 years of age was significantly higher at 4 and 8 months posttransplant in those receiving a donor allograft >6 years of age.[99] This effect was not significant at 1 year of age, but that may have been due to the very few patients followed out to 1 year in this study. Interestingly, data from NAPRTCS show that cold-storage time of >24 hours and donor age of <5 years negatively affect the allograft survival.[2,101] Analysis of CAD transplants

TABLE 42–5B. PATIENT SURVIVAL RATES AMONG INDEX TRANSPLANTS AGES 2 TO 5 YEARS (1997–2003)

	1 Year		2 Years		3 Years	
	%	SE	%	SE	%	SE
No dialysis (n = 83)	98.5	1.5	98.5	1.5	98.5	1.5
HD only (n = 78)	98.4	1.6	98.4	1.6	95.1	3.6
PD only (n = 191)	99.5	.52	98.4	1.2	97.0	1.9
HD + PD (n = 31)	100	0	100	0	100	0
Total (n = 383)	99.1	.53	98.6	.72	97.2	1.20

TABLE 42–6A. GRAFT SURVIVAL RATES AMONG INDEX TRANSPLANTS AGE < 2 YEARS (1997–2003)

	1 Year		2 Years		3 Years	
	%	SE	%	SE	%	SE
No dialysis (n = 30)	96.7	3.3	96.7	3.3	96.7	3.3
HD only (n = 22)	88.6	7.8	88.6	7.8	88.6	7.8
PD only (n = 74)	97.3	1.9	87.4	5.0	83.9	5.9
HD + PD (n = 9)	100	0	100	0	100	0
Total (n = 135)	95.9	1.8	90.5	3.2	88.7	3.6

TABLE 42–6B. GRAFT SURVIVAL RATES AMONG INDEX TRANSPLANTS AGES 2 TO 5 YEARS (1997–2003)

	1 Year		2 Years		3 Years	
	%	SE	%	SE	%	SE
No dialysis (n = 83)	94.2	2.8	94.2	2.8	91.9	3.6
HD only (n = 78)	93.1	3.0	91.2	3.5	88.5	4.3
PD only (n = 191)	93.5	1.8	92.5	2.1	88.8	2.9
HD + PD (n = 31)	93.6	4.4	93.6	4.4	93.6	4.4
Total (n = 383)	93.6	1.3	92.8	1.4	90.0	1.9

allocated to infants revealed that allografts from donors <5 years of age were associated with a 50 percent 1-month acute rejection rate and an allograft failure rate of 38 percent at 1 year. It was noted that the "ideal" age of the transplant donor is 20 to 25 years.[101] It has been consistently reported that high failure rates in infant CAD transplantation occur with the use of young donor kidneys; therefore, if successful CAD transplantation is to be achieved in infancy, the use of adult kidneys is imperative. In the 1970s and 1980s, when the impact of donor age on infant transplant outcome was not appreciated, it made the most sense to allocate the infant organs to infants. However, based on current knowledge, maintaining the infant on dialysis while awaiting an LD or adult CAD kidney is ideal.

Immunologic Responsiveness and Rejection Incidence. Another reason for decreased graft survival in small infants is the infants' increased propensity for allograft rejection. This may stem from increased immunogenicity of infants. Ettenger et al. showed that uremic children below 5 years of

TABLE 42–6C. GRAFT SURVIVAL RATES AMONG INDEX TRANSPLANTS AGES ≤ 5 YEARS (1997–2003)

	1 Year		2 Years		3 Years	
	%	SE	%	SE	%	SE
No dialysis (n = 113)	94.8	2.3	94.8	2.3	93.1	2.8
HD only (n = 100)	92.2	2.9	90.7	3.2	88.6	3.7
PD only (n = 265)	94.5	1.4	91.2	2.0	87.5	2.7
HD + PD (n = 40)	95.0	3.5	95.0	3.5	95.0	3.5
Total (n = 518)	94.2	1.1	92.2	1.3	89.7	1.7

age on PD had an increased total T-cell number, increased T-helper/suppressor ratio, and a higher rate of spontaneous blastogenesis, all of which argue for the younger transplant candidate being at higher risk for allograft rejection.[102,103] In addition, the "typical" signs of fever, hypertension, allograft tenderness, and oliguria are rarely seen in infants, making it very difficult to detect early rejection in this patient population.[104] Thus, infants may be at risk for severe rejection not only because they appear to be more immunogenic but also because the diagnosis of acute rejection may be more difficult and thereby delayed in this age group. Since rejection can account for a large percentage of graft losses in children, methods to prevent rejection or identify early diagnosis in these patients should result in a positive long-term impact on allograft survival.

Technical Factors. An additional reason for the decreased success of infant transplantation is the long anastomosis times needed to perform this technically challenging surgery.[105] This long "cross clamp" time can lead to early delay in graft function. In fact, primary nonfunction accounted for 13 percent of all allograft failures in children as reported by NAPRTCS.[2] They also showed that CAD graft survival at 2 years was 74 percent in those children who did not need dialysis in the first week posttransplant vs. 52 percent in those who did as a result of delayed graft function from acute tubular necrosis (ATN). The proportional hazards model looking to isolate factors associated with graft failure in recipients less than 1 year of age found only ATN as a risk factor in LD transplants. One can appreciate how the long anastomosis times required for a good surgical outcome can lead to postoperative problems such as ATN, which can impair long-term allograft function in these infants.[105]

Hemodynamic Considerations. Hemodynamic causes of ATN can be influenced by the perioperative management of the transplanted infant.[3,106] Strict attention to the maintenance of adequate intravascular volume is imperative. Because the adult allograft placed into the infant necessitates a "steal" phenomenon with regard to blood flow, it is mandatory that the anesthesiologist push the central venous pressure up to 15 to 18 cmH$_2$O just prior to allograft perfusion. This expanded intravascular volume is very transient, because once the arterial and venous cross clamps are released, the central venous pressure (CVP) falls rapidly. In an 8-kg infant receiving an adult kidney, approximately 25 percent of the infant's blood supply will be infused into the adult kidney at the time of allograft perfusion. Again, maintaining the CVP at 10 to 12 cmH$_2$O for the first 2 to 3 postoperative days will provide adequate perfusion to the allograft assuming that the cardiac function is otherwise normal. Once urine output is established, we replace urine milliliter for milliliter every hour with D_5 1/2 NS with 10 meq/L of sodium bicarbonate. Close monitoring of physical findings, including peripheral pulses and perfusion in conjunction with the heart rate and blood pressure, is mandatory so as to correctly assess intravascular volume in these challenging infants.

Despite improving patient and graft survival data in infants, one must always prepare for the worst by making sure that dialysis access exists before the patient leaves the operating room. The CCPD patients in our center have a peritoneal catheter in place, which we use with small (10-mL/kg) volumes for postoperative dialysis. Our infants on HD already have vascular access, which is also sufficient. It is the preemptive transplant population, however, that lacks dialysis access and therefore may require placement of a temporary HD catheter at the time of transplantation. This HD access can also be used for CVP monitoring, immunosuppressive infusions, and phlebotomy.

Allograft thrombosis also appears to occur more frequently in younger transplant recipients.[91] Harmon et al. found that graft thrombosis accounted for 22.7 percent of all graft failures in infants <2 years of age.[107] In LD recipients <6 years old, the thrombosis rate was 12.5 percent (4 of 32) in those not having received pretransplant dialysis vs. 2.8 percent (3 of 109) in those receiving dialysis. Also, patient age was associated with allograft thrombosis in LD recipients; children <6 years of age receiving LD transplants lost 7 of 24 allografts from graft thrombosis, compared with 1 of 43 in those >6 years of age. In the CAD transplants, however, age of recipient was not found to be a factor, but cold ischemia time and donor age were both strongly associated with thrombosis in the transplant. Cold-storage time of >24 hours was found to put patients at a 3.6-fold greater risk of thrombosis.[2,101]

Posttransplant Complications

Beyond the perioperative period, complications of kidney transplantation include patient mortality, graft failure, infection, and hypertension. Najarian et al. reported 16 deaths in their 75 infants.[3] Of these, 9 were infection-related (including 4 from sepsis in splenectomized patients), 3 were due to recurrent oxalosis, and 4 were from miscellaneous causes (liver failure 16 years posttransplant in autosomal recessive polycystic kidney disease, aspiration of tube feeds, "acute metabolic disturbance" after acute loss of graft, and a postoperative coagulopathy). In addition, 30 grafts were lost: 10 from chronic rejection, 5 from acute rejection, 5 from recurrent disease, and 3 from technical problems. Seven others were considered lost when a patient died with a functioning graft.

Because immunosuppressive medications are required to prevent rejection, kidney transplant recipients face a higher risk of infection. Although a thorough discussion of this subject is beyond the scope of this chapter, we can briefly mention those infections that are both common or life-threatening in this patient population.

Viruses of the herpes group are very important in kidney transplantation. These include cytomegalovirus (CMV), Epstein-Barr virus (EBV), varicella zoster virus (VZV), and the herpes simplex viruses (HSV). One virus that is potentially problematic after kidney transplantation is CMV. This virus is seen in nearly 60 percent of people 16 to 20 years of age.[78,107] Because of the frequent use of adult kidneys (>90 percent of live donor kidneys and a growing majority of CAD kidneys), the most common situation is an allograft from a seropositive kidney donor transplanted into a seronegative recipient, especially if the recipient is below 6 years of age. It is the seronegative CMV recipient who receives a seropositive allograft who is at high risk for primary CMV infection. Infection from CMV classically occurs between the first and sixth months posttransplant. Symptomatic CMV disease may consist of fever, hepatitis, pneumonitis, leukopenia, hemolytic anemia, and allograft dysfunction. Infections from CMV are seen more often with the use of polyclonal antilymphocyte preparations; CMV infection is seen less often with the newer, humanized monoclonal antibodies basiliximab and daclizumab. At most transplant centers, antibody titers (IgG and IgM) for CMV are drawn on both the donor and the recipient before transplantation. If the donor is IgG-positive for CMV and the recipient is negative, we administer intravenous ganciclovir for the first 14 days after transplantation, followed by oral ganciclovir (or valganciclovir) for an additional 3 months. If the recipient is CMV IgG–seropositive at the time of transplantation, we prescribe 3 months of oral ganciclovir (or valganciclovir). If both donor and recipient are seronegative for CMV, no prophylaxis is administered. In the case of suspected infection, intravenous ganciclovir is given and is quite effective, although relapses can occur. We use the CMV antigenemia test for pp65 antigen for detection of active CMV infection. Although CMV infection is most likely to be primary in infant transplantation, one must also be alert to the fact that reactivation of a previous latent infection can also occur. As a result, CMV must be in the differential diagnosis of a transplant patient with a fever. CMV infection after the initial 6 months posttransplantation is much less common.

Over the past decade, posttransplant issues related to VZV infection have declined, mainly related to mandatory use of Varivax in most healthy children and all children prior to transplantation if they do not demonstrate immunity by naturally acquired infection or prior vaccination. We have postponed LD transplantation in a few young children to allow immunity to develop after vaccination or, if necessary, revaccination with Varivax. Primary infection with this virus can be very severe, leading to pneumonitis, encephalitis, hepatitis with hepatic failure, and disseminated intravascular coagulation. For the few remaining patients who were seronegative at the time of transplantation and who could not be immunized with Varivax, VZ immunoglobulin (VZIG) should be given within the first 72 hours after an exposure to chickenpox. It is effective in attenuating the disease in 75 percent of cases, yet there have been reports of death in children who have received VZIG at the appropriate time.[108,109]

In the event of a suspicious rash possibly indicating VZV infection, immunofluorescence antibody tests of the lesion(s) are sent and treatment with intravenous acyclovir (1500 mg/m^2/day) or ganciclovir (5 mg/kg per dose, adjusted for kidney dysfunction) is started. Also, the immunosuppression doses are altered; azathioprine, mycophenolate mofetil (MMF), or rapamycin are usually held during the acute infection, as the presence of these drugs 3 days into the infection has been associated with a higher mortality risk.[110] It has also been shown in the liver transplant literature that when higher cyclosporine doses (15 to 26 mg/kg/day) are used, higher morbidity and mortality have been seen, in comparison with the use of low-dose cyclosporine (7.1 to 13.7 mg/kg/day).[111] This has led some to speculate that the intensity of the immunosuppression at the time of exposure can influence the severity of primary VZV infection.[86]

The infectious complications of infant transplantation were reported by Najarian et al.[3] They found that 15 of 75 infants developed a UTI at some point during follow-up. This high frequency of UTIs appears to be potentially unique to the infant. It should be remembered though that roughly 30 to 50 percent of infants who reach ESRD may have some degree of bladder dysfunction, which would increase the risk of UTI. With regard to viral etiology, the same center reported two infants dying from viral respiratory infections, including one infant with respiratory syncytial virus. Varicella occurred in 17 of their 75 infants. Treatment included stopping the azathioprine and administering intravenous acyclovir. Patients exposed to chickenpox were passively immunized with VZIG. This treatment plan resulted in no mortality and no episodes of rejection. Also of note is that there were five episodes of sepsis and four deaths in splenectomized patients. No episodes of sepsis have been reported by that center since splenectomy at the time of transplant was abandoned.

Since most infants and children have not been exposed to EBV before transplantation, primary EBV infection, as well as the posttransplant lymphoproliferative disease (PTLD) that is related to EBV, will often be problematic, even well beyond the first year after transplantation.[112] Treatment for patients with PTLD includes reduction of immunosuppression, antiviral antibiotics, and, for some, chemotherapy and/or specific anti–B-cell antibodies. Routine EBV surveillance has been recommended for EBV-naive patients at risk, but it is unclear whether clinicians should alter immunosuppression for asymptomatic patients whose viral load becomes positive.[113]

Provided that MMR vaccine has been administered before transplantation with documentation of positive titers, we rarely see posttransplant complications related to measles, mumps, or rubella infection.

Hypertension can occur in the posttransplant patient quite commonly. NAPRTCS reported an incidence of 72 percent of transplanted children on antihypertensive medication 1 month after transplant, which fell to 53 percent at 30 months.[2] The mechanism for hypertension in the transplant patient includes intrinsic causes, such as acute or chronic rejection, in addition to disease recurrence. Extrinsic causes include renal artery stenosis, medication effects from corticosteroids and cyclosporine, and hypertension from the native kidneys (renin-mediated) if they are still present.[114]

Immunosuppression Protocols

The majority of current immunosuppression protocols for children after kidney transplantation include the use of monoclonal antibodies in the immediate postoperative period in addition to oral maintenance immunosuppression.[115] Two interleukin-2–receptor monoclonal antibodies, currently in use, have been approved by the U.S. Food and Drug Administration: basiliximab (Simulect; Novartis Pharmaceuticals, East Hanover, NJ) and daclizumab (Zenapax; Roche Pharmaceuticals, Nutley, NJ), each with its own dosing schedule. Other available antibodies include polyclonal preparations such as the antithymocyte globulin preparations ATGAM (Upjohn Company, Kalamazoo, MI) and Thymoglobulin (Genzyme Corporation, Cambridge, MA). The oldest monoclonal preparation, OKT3 (Ortho Biotech, Raritan, NJ), a monoclonal antibody to the CD3 complex on mature T cells, is rarely used now as induction therapy in children. Ettenger et al. have reviewed the subject in great detail.[116] One major advantage of this approach lies in providing a rejection-free period during the first month posttransplant to allow the graft to begin functioning. It also provides a window of opportunity to study the pharmacokinetics of the oral immunosuppressives, thus keeping the patient protected from rejection while the optimal doses of these maintenance immunosuppressants are being learned. This is very important in infants, who are known to metabolize cyclosporine and tacrolimus more rapidly, making their trough levels difficult to predict early on.

Induction immunosuppression, by providing "background" immunosuppression, allows the transplant nephrologist to delay the institution of cyclosporine or tacrolimus. This is important in infancy, because the incidence of primary nonfunction may be higher in these patients and can be increased further by afferent arteriolar vasoconstrictive effect of calcineurin inhibitors. Strong support for the use of this strategy for CAD transplant is given in this review because it is reported that this change in immunosuppression strategy after analysis by a Cox Proportional Hazards Model was shown to have had a bigger influence on the improvement of pediatric CAD renal transplant at UCLA than had the effect of donor age. Despite the use of sequential immunosuppression, breakthrough allograft rejection during polyclonal induction can occur and has been reported in the infant with subtherapeutic cyclosporine levels.[117]

During the late 1990s, with the advent of the newer oral immunosuppressive medications and the humanized monoclonal antilymphocyte preparations, a rationale for trying to minimize glucocorticosteroids and their many potential complications was promoted. Sarwal et al. at Stanford piloted a protocol of complete steroid avoidance in children. They showed that superior patient as well as graft survival could be achieved with a regimen of tacrolimus, MMF, and extended use of daclizumab.[118] With follow-up periods up to 41 months and using protocol biopsies to monitor for rejection and drug toxicity, overall patient and graft survival were 98 percent. Hypertension was uncommon and linear growth was excellent as compared with steroid-treated controls. Despite the use of tacrolimus, no new cases of diabetes mellitus developed. And thus the stage has been set for larger, multicenter trials of steroid-free regimens in children. Currently, our immunosuppression regimen for kidney transplants at Northwestern University/Children's Memorial Hospital consists of three doses of intravenous methylprednisolone (10 mg/kg during the transplant procedure, 5 mg/kg on day 1 after surgery, and 2.5 mg/kg on day 2 after surgery), and two doses of Simulect (10 or 20 mg during the transplant surgery and 10 or 20 mg on day 4 after surgery). In addition, oral tacrolimus is given at a dose of 0.1 mg/kg every 12 hours, with the dose adjusted to achieve a 12-hour trough level of 8 to 10 ng/mL and oral sirolimus at a dose of 3 mg/m^2 once daily with the dose adjusted to achieve a 24-hour trough level of 10 to 15 ng/mL. We generally substitute the use of MMF for sirolimus in patients with glomerular disease as the cause of their ESRD, at a dose of 500 mg/m^2 every 12 hours orally or intravenously. We no longer use oral prednisone for routine immunosuppression in the low-risk patient. In the face of delayed graft function, the institution of tacrolimus is delayed and both sirolimus and MMF are used to prevent acute rejection. Failure to achieve satisfactory graft function by 10 to 14 days necessitates a kidney biopsy to rule out superimposed rejection.[90]

Identification and Treatment of Allograft Rejection

Acute cellular rejection may be a difficult diagnosis to make, especially in an infant that has received an adult kidney, since much tissue injury must occur before the serum creatinine begins to rise owing to the relatively large kidney mass present. Clinical clues in the infant include new-onset or worsening hypertension, fever, irritability, and, less commonly, a rising serum creatinine level.[119] Allograft tenderness is seen less frequently since the advent of calcineurin inhibitors, cyclosporine, and tacrolimus; as a result, the other clinical clues, mentioned above, are most relied on, with the most sensitive likely to be hypertension. The "gold standard" for the diagnosis is percutaneous kidney biopsy looking for the presence of lymphocytic interstitial infiltrate with tubulitis.[120] It should be noted, though, that a study by Matas et al. showed that 12 of 50 asymptomatic transplant patients biopsied prior to discharge from the hospital showed acute interstitial infiltrate, and 5 of these 12 (41 percent) never went on to show clinical evidence of rejection.[120] Nonetheless, the biopsy, which is performed using an 18-gauge needle under sedation and local anesthesia, is still used to decide whether or not to institute antirejection treatment, because it is the most specific means of diagnosis available.

Our first-line treatment for mild to moderate tubulointerstitial rejection is pulse methylprednisolone therapy at a dose of 10 mg/kg given intravenously on 3 consecutive days. Serum creatinine and urine output are followed closely, in addition to looking for improvement of the hypertension. The elevated blood pressure secondary to acute rejection, unlike nearly all other causes of hypertension, responds dramatically to steroids, so this is a very useful clinical sign. Fever, on the other hand, can be blunted by the anti-inflammatory effects of steroids, making it a less reliable clinical sign to follow. We treat moderate to severe acute cellular rejection with pulse methylprednisolone therapy, as noted above, in conjunction with a 7- to 10-day course of Thymoglobulin at a dose of 1.5 mg/kg/day. Humoral (vascular) rejection or rejection episodes refractory to corticosteroids (about one-third of cases) are treated with a 7- to 10-day course of Thymoglobulin at a dose of 1.5 mg/kg/day.

Posttransplantation Growth in the Infant

The primary reason to perform kidney transplantation in children is that it provides an excellent opportunity to optimize growth while normalizing the lifestyle of the patient and family. Factors in transplantation that correlate with optimal growth include excellent graft function and minimal or no steroid therapy. Acute allograft rejection, then, can be a setback to the goal of achieving optimum growth in children, since both a diminution of renal function and accompanying high-dose corticosteroid treatment can hamper the process of catch-up growth. Recurrent rejection episodes are additive when it comes to growth inhibition.

As stated earlier, most growth occurs in the first or second year of life. Brain volume increases more than twofold in the first 2 years of life, achieving about 80 percent its total size.[10] Linear growth, too, occurs at a rapid rate in the first few years of life. A newborn infant will double in length by age 4; 50 percent of this growth occurs during the first year of life, when the mean growth velocity is 25 cm/year. Infants can lose 0.6 height standard deviation score (SDS)/month during the first 6 months of life as a result of poor individual growth in comparison with their rapidly growing peers. One can see, then, how the development of renal failure in the first 2 years of life can have a major impact on long-term growth and development; moreover, the age of onset of renal failure is the key determinant to severity of growth impairment, with the youngest children being the most affected.[121]

At the University of Minnesota, 30 children who underwent a successful kidney transplant in the first 2 years of life were evaluated; neurologic improvement was found to be significant in the majority of these.[122] The study concluded that "renal transplantation in young children with chronic renal failure is often associated with significant improvements in cognitive and psychomotor function, as well as improved cephalic growth." In the more recent era, the combination of improved care prior to transplant along with improved allograft survival in the infant should result in an even better outcome.

The best method for measuring the success of posttransplant growth is not universally agreed on. Some measure final adult height when it is attained, whereas others follow the growth velocity or height SDSs ("z score"). Nonetheless, since the majority of children enter renal transplantation with some evidence of growth retardation, it is generally expected that these patients will achieve an acceleration in growth velocity above that expected for age, so as to attain catch-up growth. Harmon and Jabs reviewed the factors that are most influential in posttransplant growth.[123] Age at the time of transplant was deemed important, as had been reported previously.[124,125] Younger patients were more capable of achieving accelerated growth rates than were older children and adolescents.

Immunosuppressive regimens have also been found to affect posttransplant growth. The use of alternate-day steroids has been shown to be beneficial to growth when compared with daily steroid administration.[126,127] Initial reports of growth with complete avoidance of steroids have been very encouraging,[118] but a report of 36 pediatric kidney transplant patients withdrawn from steroids in an attempt to reduce cardiovascular risk factors indicates that steroid withdrawal may not always be successful. In all, 22 of 36 patients experienced an acute rejection episode at a mean of 14 months, with graft loss from chronic rejection occurring in 3 patients.[128] If a substantially higher risk of rejection occurs with steroid withdrawal, this will result in worsening of growth potential due to diminished graft function and overall increased steroid dosage.

Growth in patients on calcineurin inhibitors has been shown to be better than that in those who were previously immunosuppressed on azathioprine and prednisone. Although the exact mechanism is not known, it is believed to be a combination of the steroid-sparing effect and the overall improved long-term graft function that results from a lower incidence of rejection.[129]

Allograft function further affects growth. Earlier work by Jabs et al. found an elevated creatinine in 8 of 11 of their patients not growing well posttransplant compared with only 3 of 14 of those who were growing well.[130] An elevated creatinine ranged between 1.5 and 2.0 mg/dL in this study. While growth is seen in pretransplant, predialysis patients with GFRs in the range of 10 to 15 mL/min/1.73 m^2, it is unclear why slight decreases in GFR in the transplant population can have such a negative effect on growth. Ettenger et al. also noted that those children who grew well posttransplant were below 9 years of age, were on minimal corticosteroid doses (<0.25 mg/kg/day of prednisone), and had calculated GFR >90 mL/min/1.73 m^2.[103] Additional factors that appeared to be linked to posttransplant growth are "endocrinologic factors." Harmon and Jabs state that the declining growth velocity and delayed secondary sexual characteristics in posttransplant patients entering early adolescence can be attributed to low nocturnal growth hormone and gonadotropin secretion.[130] This has led to the use of rhGH treatment in selected patients. In a recent publication of a randomized controlled trial on the use of rhGH in stable kidney transplant recipients, Fine and colleagues showed a significant increase in both linear growth and improvement in height SDS z-score in patients receiving rhGH as compared with controls. Growth velocity averaged 10.1 cm in pubertal patients in comparison to 3.9 cm in controls. In prepubertal patients on rhGH, average growth was 8.1 cm, vs. 3.7 for controls. Furthermore, there was no difference in graft function between treated and untreated patients during the study, nor were there differences in adverse effects, including episodes of rejection.[131]

Thus endocrinologic factors, the immunosuppressive regimen and the function of the graft each appear to be important components to posttransplant growth in infants. The fact that younger patients are more successful at achieving posttransplant catch-up growth makes the transplantation of the very young and rapidly growing infant even more desirable. If the objective is for the patient to be metabolically normal with excellent growth posttransplant, selecting a living donor organ and providing adequate immunosuppression would seem to offer the best chance of excellent allograft function. Also, if steroid dosage is negatively correlated with growth, using an immunosuppression regimen that would minimize or avoid steroids seems equally important.

Early infant transplantation differed substantially from that of the modern era. Bilateral nephrectomies were almost universal in all infant transplants; in addition, the children often underwent splenectomy for immunosuppressive purposes. Nephrectomies are much less common now, and pretransplant splenectomy was abandoned in 1984 after no long-term benefit on graft survival was demonstrated.[132] The immunosuppressive regimen began with prednisone and azathioprine in addition to methylprednisolone given intravenously for 3 days postoperatively and Minnesota antilymphoblast globulin (ALG) intravenously for 14 days postoperatively. Now the calcineurin inhibitors, cyclosporine or tacrolimus, are used to prevent rejection. Mycophenolate or sirolimus has replaced azathioprine. Humanized monoclonal antibodies have replaced Minnesota ALG. Low-dose steroids or no-steroid regimens are gaining popularity. Donor-specific blood transfusions were used in the mid-1980s but were stopped due to increased antigen sensitization of the recipient. Most important, a great number of CAD transplants in small infants came from donors below 6 years of age; as previously stated, due to much better CAD allograft survival when adult kidneys are used, small kidneys are rarely utilized in transplantation today.

One can see how studies that span a decade or more, while providing nice follow-up results, are difficult to use in predicting the potential outcome of an infant transplanted today. No longer will the infant undergo a splenectomy, receive donor-specific blood transfusions, or receive a renal allograft from a young donor. Further, the infant will now receive aggressive immunosuppression including calcineurin inhibitors, newer oral agents such as MMF or sirolimus, and newer antilymphocyte preparations.

SUMMARY

Kidney failure in infancy has a large impact on the growth and development of these metabolically active patients. Meticulous attention to the correction of acidosis, anemia, and renal osteodystrophy, while also maintaining aggressive nutrition, can blunt these adverse effects of uremia. Patients with anuric renal failure or congenital nephrotic syndrome with subsequent nephrectomy will require some form of dialysis in order to keep them metabolically stable while aggressive nutrition is maintained. Complications from both PD and HD exist, but PD is usually well tolerated by most infants and preferred by most families.

In patients with high-output (polyuric) renal failure, preemptive renal transplantation should be considered. Experience with infant transplantation spans decades in some centers, and, in experienced centers, the results with LD transplants in infants equal those in adolescent children and adults. The data with CAD transplantation from centers using adult donor kidneys and sequential immunosuppression give very encouraging results as well. Multicenter studies that cover several years often report disappointing

results for infant CAD kidney transplantation; however, data on the use of CAD infant kidneys—associated with a higher incidence of thrombosis and primary nonfunction—often represent a large part of any given study. Thus, the initial, disappointing long-term results for CAD infant transplant were misleading. While CAD kidneys have not yet been shown to be equivalent to LD transplants in infants, one should still seriously consider an adult CAD kidney transplant with the use of sequential immunosuppression if an LD is unavailable and long-term dialysis is the other option.

While complications—including hypertension, infection, and death—exist in all forms of RRT, the mode that allows the patient and family to function most normally is that of kidney transplantation. Of course, the management of transplant patients, especially infants, can be very challenging; therefore each individual center must use the modality with which it is most comfortable. If long-term dialysis appears imminent in a center with minimal transplant experience, a referral to a transplant center that is comfortable caring for infant transplants seems best for the long-term interest of the patient and family.

REFERENCES

1. Murray JE, Merrill JP, Harrison JH. Kidney transplantation between seven pairs of identical twins. *Ann Surg* 1958;148: 343.
2. McEnery PT, Stablein DM, Arbus G, et al. Renal transplantation in children. A report of the North American Pediatric Renal Transplantation Cooperative Study. *N Engl J Med* 1992;326:1727–1732.
3. Najarian JS, Frey DJ, Matas AJ, et al. Renal transplantation in infants. *Ann Surg* 1990;212:353–366.
4. Salusky IB, Von Lilien T, Anchondo M, et al. Experience with continuous cycling peritoneal dialysis during the first year of life. *Pediatr Nephrol* 1987;1:172–175.
5. Kohaut EC, Whelchel J, Waldo FB, et al. Aggressive therapy of infants with renal failure. *Pediatr Nephrol* 1987;1: 150–153.
6. Briscoe DM, Kim MS, Lillehei C, et al. Outcome of renal transplantation in children less than two years of age. *Kidney Int* 1992;42:657–662.
7. Alexander SR, Sullivan EK, Harmon WE, et al. Maintenance dialysis in North American children and adolescents: a preliminary report. *Kidney Int* 1993;44:S104–S109.
8. U.S. Renal Data System (USRDS). ESRD in children. In: *USRDS 1993 Annual Data Report*. Bethesda, MD: The National Institutes of Health, National Institute of Diabetes and Digestive and Kidney Disease, 1993;105(4):69–81.
9. Mahan JD, Mauer SM, Sibley RK, et al. Congenital nephrotic syndrome: evolution of medical management and results of renal transplantation. *J Pediatr* 1984;105: 549–557.
10. Wassner SJ, Baum M. Conservative management of chronic renal insufficiency. In: Barratt TM, Avner ED, Harmon WE

eds. *Pediatric Nephrology,* 4th ed. Baltimore: Williams & Wilkins, 1999:1155–1182.

11. Sedman AB. Aluminum toxicity of childhood. *Pediatr Nephrol* 1992;6:383–393.

12. Sedman AB, Miller NL, Warady BA, et al. Aluminum loading in children with chronic renal failure. *Kidney Int* 1984; 26:201–204.

13. Wassner SJ. The role of nutrition in the care of children with renal insufficiency. *Pediatr Clin North Am* 1982;29: 973–991.

14. Rizzoni G, Basso T, Setari M. Growth in children with chronic renal failure on conservative treatment. *Kidney Int* 1984;26:52–58.

15. Parekh RS, Flynn JT, Smoyer WE, et al. Improved growth in young children with severe chronic renal insufficiency who use specified nutritional therapy. *J Am Soc Nephrol* 2001;12: 2418–2426.

16. Van Dyck M, Sidler S, Proesmans W. Chronic renal failure in infants: effect of strict conservative treatment on growth. *Eur J Pediatr* 1998;157:759–762.

17. Ledermann SE, Spitz L, Moloney J, et al. Gastrostomy feeding in infants and children on peritoneal dialysis. *Pediatr Nephrol* 2002;17:246–250.

18. Ramage IJ, Geary DF, Harvey E, et al. Efficacy of gastrostomy feeding in infants and older children receiving chronic peritoneal dialysis. *Perit Dial Int* 1999;19:231–236.

19. Brewer ED. Pediatric experience with intradialytic parenteral nutrition and supplemental tube feeding. *Am J Kidney Dis* 1999; 33:205–207.

20. Davies BW, Watson AR, Coleman JE, et al. Do gastrostomies close spontaneously? A review of the fate of gastrostomies following successful renal transplantation in children. *Pediatr Surg Int* 2001;17:326–328.

21. Dabbagh S, Fassinger N, Fleischmann L. Effect of recombinant human erythropoietin (EPO) on nutrition and growth in children on dialysis (D). *Perit Dial Int* 1993;13:S86.

22. Brandt JR, Avner ED, Hickman RO, Watkins SL. Safety and efficacy of erythropoietin in children with chronic renal failure. *Pediatr Nephrol* 1999;13:143–147.

23. Lerner G, Kale AS, Warady BA, et al. Pharmacokinetics of darbopoetin alfa in pediatric patients with chronic kidney disease. *Pediatr Nephrol* 2002;17:933–937.

24. Morgan HE, Gautam M, Geary DF. Maintenance intravenous iron therapy in pediatric hemodialysis patients. *Pediatr Nephrol* 2001;16:779–783.

25. Sherbotie JR, Flynn JT, Bunchman TE. Indications, results, and complications of tacrolimus conversion in isolated pediatric renal transplantation. Presented at the 3rd International Congress on Pediatric Transplantation. Boston, July 8–10, 1998. *Pediatr Transplant* 1998;2(1) abstr #113:59.

26. Alexander SR. Pediatric uses of recombinant human erythropoietin: the outlook in 1991. *Am J Kidney Dis* 1991;28: 42–53.

27. Salusky IB, Ramires JA, Goodman WG. Recent advances in the management of renal osteodystrophy in children. *Curr Opin Nephrol Hypertens* 1993;2:580–587.

28. Kohaut EC. Growth in children treated with continuous ambulatory peritoneal dialysis. *Int J Pediatr Nephrol* 1983;4: 93–98.

29. McConnell S, Sedman AB, Bunchman TE. Growth and PTH activity in the pediatric peritoneal dialysis population. *Perit Dial Int* 1994;14:S40.

30. Blum WF, Ranke MB, Kietzmann, et al. Growth hormone resistance and inhibition of somatomedin activity by excess of insulin-like growth factor binding protein in uraemia. *Pediatr Nephrol* 1991;5:539–544.

31. Powell DR, Liu F, Baker B, et al. Characterization of insulin-like growth factor binding protein-3 in chronic renal failure serum. *Pediatr Res* 1993;33:136–143.

32. Fine RN, Kohaut EC, Brown D, et al. Growth after recombinant human growth hormone treatment in children with chronic renal failure: report of a multicenter randomized double-blind placebo-controlled study. *J Pediatr* 1994;124: 374–382.

33. Pryde PG, Sedman AS, Nugent CE, et al. Angiotensin-converting enzyme inhibitor fetopathy. *J Am Soc Nephrol* 1993; 3:1575–1582.

34. McGraw ME, Haka-Ikse K. Neurologic-development sequelae of chronic renal failure in infancy. *J Pediatr* 1985;106: 579.

35. Polinksy MS, Kaiser BA, Stover JB, et al. Neurologic development of children with severe chronic renal failure from infancy. *Pediatr Nephrol* 1987;1:157–165.

36. Winick M, Rosso P. Head circumference and cellular growth of the brain in normal and marasmic children. *J Pediatr* 1969;74:774–775.

37. Pryor HB, Thelander H. Abnormally small head size and intellect in children. *J Pediatr* 1968;73:593–598.

38. Rotundo A, Nevins TE, Lipton M, et al. Progressive encephalopathy in children with chronic renal insufficiency in infancy. *Kidney Int* 1982;21:486–491.

39. Warady BA, Kriley M, Lovell H, et al. Growth and development of infants with end-stage renal disease receiving long-term peritoneal dialysis. *J Pediatr* 1988;112:714–719.

40. Fennell RS, Fennell EB, Carter RL, et al. A longitudinal study of the cognitive function of children and renal failure. *Pediatr Nephrol* 1990;4:11–15.

41. Fennell RS, Fennell EB, Carter RL, et al. Association between renal function and cognition in childhood chronic renal failure. *Pediatr Nephrol* 1990;4:16–20.

42. Warady BA, Belden B, Kohaut E. Neurodevelopmental outcome of children initiating peritoneal dialysis in early infancy. *Pediatr Nephrol* 1999;13:759–765.

43. Qvist E, Pihko H, Fageruud P, et al. Neurodevelopmental outcome in high-risk patients after renal transplantation in early childhood. *Pediatr Transplant* 2002;6:53–62.

44. Madden SJ, Ledermann SE, Guerrero-Blanco M, et al. Cognitive and psychosocial outcome of infants dialyzed in infancy. *Child Care Health Dev* 2003;29:55–61.

45. Warady BA, Morgenstern BZ, Alexander SR. Peritoneal dialysis. In: Avner ED, Harmon WE, Niaudet P, eds. *Pediatric Nephrology,* 5th ed. Philadelphia: Lippincott, Williams & Wilkins; 2004:1375–1394.

46. Baum M, Powell D, Calvin S, et al. Continuous ambulatory peritoneal dialysis in children. *N Engl J Med* 1982;307: 1537–1542.

47. Salusky IB, Lucullo L, Nelson P, et al. Continuous ambulatory peritoneal dialysis in children. *Pediatr Clin North Am* 1982;29:1005–1013.

48. Watson AR. Stress and burden of care in families with children commencing renal replacement therapy. *Adv Perit Dial* 1997; 13:300–304.

49. Bromberg JS, Baliga PR. Renal transplantation in a noncompliant patient. *N Engl J Med* 1994;330:371.

50. Reddingius RE, Schroder CH, Monnens LAH. Intraperitoneal administration of recombinant human erythropoietin in children on continuous ambulatory peritoneal dialysis. *Eur J Pediatr* 1992;151:540–542.

51. Dulaney JT, Hatch FE Jr. Peritoneal dialysis and loss of proteins: a review. *Kidney Int* 1984;26:253–262.

52. Brewer ED, Holmes S, Tealey J. Initiation and maintenance of growth in infants with end stage renal disease (ESRD) managed with chronic peritoneal dialysis (CPD) and nasogastric tube (NG) feeding. *Kidney Int* 1986;29:230.

53. Valentini RP, Mudge NA, Bunchman TE. Dialysis modality comparison of IGFBP-3 removal in children: could this have a potential growth benefit? *Adv Perit Dial* 1994;10:327–330.

54. Stone MM, Fonkalsrud EW, Salusky IB, et al. Surgical management of peritoneal dialysis catheters in children: five-year experience with 1,800 patient-month follow-up. *J Pediatr Surg* 1986;21:1177–1181.

55. Paulson WD, Bock GH, Nelson AP, et al. Hyponatremia in the very young chronic peritoneal dialysis patient. *Am J Kidney Dis* 1989;14:196–199.

56. Drachman R, Schlesinger M, Shapira H, et al. The immune status of uraemic children/adolescents with chronic renal failure and renal replacement therapy. *Pediatr Nephrol* 1989;3:305–308.

57. Hisano S, Miyazaki C, Hatae K, et al. Immune status of children on continuous ambulatory peritoneal dialysis. *Pediatr Nephrol* 1992;6:179–181.

58. Moxey-Mims MM, Preston K, Fivush B, et al. Heptavax-B in pediatric dialysis patients: effect of systemic lupus erythematosus. *Pediatr Nephrol* 1990;4:171–173.

59. Fivush BA, Case B, Warady BA, et al. Defective antibody response to *Hemophilus Influenzae* type b immunization in children receiving peritoneal dialysis. *Pediatr Nephrol* 1993;7:548–550.

60. Schulman SL, Deforest A, Kaiser BA, et al. Response to measles-mumps-rubella vaccine in children on dialysis. *Pediatr Nephrol* 1992;6:187–189.

61. Fivush BA, Case B, May MW, et al. Hypogammaglobulinemia in children undergoing continuous ambulatory peritoneal dialysis. *Pediatr Nephrol* 1989;3:186–188.

62. Katz A, Kashtan CE, Greenberg LJ, et al. Hypogammaglobulinemia in uremic infants receiving peritoneal dialysis. *J Pediatr* 1990;117:258–261.

63. Giacchino F, Quarello F, Pellerey M, et al. Continuous ambulatory peritoneal dialysis improves immunodeficiency in uremic patients. *Nephron* 1983;35:209–210.

64. Neu AM, Lederman HM, Fivush BA. Hypogammaglobulinemia and fatal sepsis in an infant maintained on peritoneal dialysis. *Pediatr Nephrol* 1993;7:455–456.

65. Schroder CH, de Jong MCJW, Monnens LAH. Group B streptococcus: an unusual cause of severe peritonitis in young children treated with continuous ambulatory peritoneal dialysis. *Am J Kidney Dis* 1991;27:231–232.

66. Holtta TM, Ronnholm KA, Jalanko H, et al. Peritoneal dialysis in children under 5 years of age. *Perit Dial Int* 1997; 17:573–580.

67. Ledermann SE, Scanes ME, Fernando ON, et al. Long-term outcome of peritoneal dialysis in infants. *J Pediatr* 2000; 136:24–29.

68. Donckerwolcke R, Bunchman T. Hemodialysis in infants and small children. *Pediatr Nephrol* 1994;8:103–106.

69. Knight F, Gorynski L, Bentson M, et al. Hemodialysis of the infant or small child with chronic renal failure. *ANNA J* 1993;20:315–323.

70. Mahan JD, Mauer SM, Nevins TE. The Hickman catheter. A new haemodialysis access device for infants and small children. *Kidney Int* 1983;24:318–319.

71. Bunchman T, Gardner J, Kershaw D, et al. Vascular access for hemodialysis or CVVH(D) in infants and children. *Dial Transplant* 1994;23:314–318.

72. Jenkins RD, Kuhn RJ, Funk JE. Clinical implications of catheter variability on neonatal continuous hemofiltration. *ASAIO Trans* 1988;34:108–111.

73. Geary DF, Gajaria M, Fryer-Keene S, et al. Low dose and heparin-free hemodialysis in children. *Pediatr Nephrol* 1991;5:220–224.

74. Bunchman TE. Chronic dialysis in the infant less than 1 year of age (review). *Pediatr Nephrol* 1995;9(suppl):S18–22.

75. Potter DE, San Luis E, Wipfler JE, et al. Comparison of continuous ambulatory peritoneal dialysis and hemodialysis in children. *Kidney Int* 1986;19:S11–S14.

76. Al-Hermi BE, Al-Saran K, Seeker D, et al. Hemodialysis for end-stage renal disease in children weighing less than 10 kg. *Pediatr Nephrol* 1999; 13:401–403.

77. Shroff R, Wright E, Ledermann S, et al. Chronic hemodialysis in infants and children under 2 years of age. *Pediatr Nephrol* 2003;18:378–383.

78. Grimm PC, Ettenger R. Pediatric renal transplantation. *Adv Pediatr* 1992;39:441–493.

79. Nevins TE, Danielson G. Prior dialysis does not affect the outcome of pediatric renal transplantation. *Pediatr Nephrol* 1991;5:211–214.

80. Flom LS, Reisman EM, Donovan JM, et al. Favorable experience with pre-emptive renal transplantation in children. *Pediatr Nephrol* 1992;6:258–261.

81. Fine R, Tejani A, Sullivan EK. Pre-emptive renal transplantation in children: report of the North American Pediatric Renal Transplant Cooperative Study (NAPRTCS). *Clin Transplant* 1994;8:474–478.

82. Mange KC, Joffe MM, Feldman HI. Effect of the use or nonuse of long-term dialysis on the subsequent survival of renal transplants from living donors. *N Engl J Med* 2001;344:726–731.

83. Najarian JS, Almond PS, Gillingham KJ, et al. Renal transplantation in the first five years of life. *Kidney Int* 1993; 44(suppl):40–44.

84. Burns MW, Watkins SL, Mitchell ME, et al. Treatment of bladder dysfunction in children with end-stage renal disease. *J Pediatr Surg* 1992;27:170–174.

85. *Report of the Committee on Infectious Diseases. Varicella-Zoster Infections.* Elk Grove Village, IL: American Academy of Pediatrics, 2003.

86. Lynfield R, Herrin JT, Rubin RH. Varicella in pediatric renal transplant recipients. *Pediatrics* 1992;90:216–220.

87. Gershon AA. Immunizations for pediatric transplant patients. *Kidney Int* 1993;44:S87–S90.

88. Plotkin SA, Starr SE, Friedman HM, et al. Vaccines for the prevention of human cytomegalovirus infection. *Rev Infect Dis* 1990;7:S827–S838.

89. Najarian JS, Almond PS, Mauer M, et al. Renal transplantation in the first year of life: the treatment of choice for infants with end-stage renal disease. *J Am Soc Nephrol* 1992;2(suppl 3):S228–S233.

90. Bunchman T, Ham J, Sedman A, et al. Superior allograft survival in pediatric renal transplant recipients. *Transplant Proc* 1994;26:24–25.

91. Arbus GS, Rochon J, Thompson D. Survival of cadaveric renal transplant grafts from young donors and in young recipients. *Pediatr Nephrol* 1991;5:152–157.

92. Najarian JS, Chavers BM, McHugh LE, et al. 20 years or more of follow-up of living kidney donors. *Lancet* 1992; 340:807–810.

93. Evans E, Ettenger RB. Immune response in pediatric renal transplantation. In: Tejani AH, Fine RN eds. *Pediatric Renal Transplantation.* New York: Wiley-Liss, 1994: 17–21.

94. Cerilli J, Evans WE, Sotos JF. Renal transplantation in infants and children. *Transplant Proc* 1972;4:633–636.

95. Miller LC, Bock GH, Lum CT, et al. Transplantation of adult kidney into the very small child: long-term outcome. *J Pediatr* 1982;100:675–680.

96. Nevins TE. Transplantation in infants less than 1 year of age. *Pediatr Nephrol* 1987;1:154–156.

97. So SKS, Chang P, Najarian JS, et al. Growth and development in infants after renal transplantation. *J Pediatr* 1987; 110:343–350.

98. Fine RN. Growth after renal transplantation in children. *J Pediatr* 1987;110:414–416.

99. Ettenger RB, Rosenthal JT, Marik J, et al. Successful cadaveric renal transplantation in infants and young children. *Transplant Proc* 1989;21:1707–1708.

100. McLorie GA, Geary DF, Balfe JW, et al. The azotemic infant. Management options. *Dial Pediatr Urol* 1988;11:1–8.

101. Harmon WE, Alexander SR, Tejani A, et al. The effect of donor age on graft survival in pediatric cadaver renal transplant recipients: a report of the North American Pediatric Renal Transplant Cooperative Study. *Transplantation* 1992; 54:232–237.

102. Bunchman T, Kershaw D, Merion R, et al. T cell subset analysis by flow cytometry during MALG induction for pediatric renal transplantation. *Transplantation* 1993;55: 1190–1193.

103. Ettenger RB, Blifeld C, Prince H, et al. The pediatric nephrologist's dilemma: growth after renal transplantation and in interaction with age as a possible immunologic variable. *J Pediatr* 1987;111:1022–1025.

104. Bunchman TE, Fryd DS, Sibley RK, et al. Manifestations of renal allograft rejection in small children receiving adult kidneys. *Pediatr Nephrol* 1990;4:255–258.

105. Ettenger RB. Children are different: the challenges of pediatric renal transplantation. *Am J Kidney Dis* 1992;20: 668–672.

106. Carlier M, Squifflet JP, Pirson Y, et al. Maximal hydration during anesthesia increases pulmonary arterial pressures and improves early function of human renal transplants. *Transplantation* 1982;34:201–204.

107. Harmon WE, Stablein D, Alexander SR, et al. Graft thrombosis in pediatric renal transplant recipients. *Transplantation* 1991;51:406–412.

108. Rubin RH. Infectious disease complications in renal transplantation. *Kidney Int* 1993;44:221–236.

109. Rubin RH, Tolkoff-Rubin NE. Opportunistic infections in renal allograft recipients. *Transplant Proc* 1988;20: S12–S18.

110. Feldhoff CM, Balfour HH, Simmons RL, et al. Varicella in children with renal transplants. *J Pediatr* 1981;98:25–31.

111. McGregor RS, Zitelli BJ, Urbach AH, et al. Varicella in pediatric orthotopic liver transplant recipients. *Pediatrics* 1989;83:256–261.

112. Qu L, Green M, Webber S, et al. Epstein-Barr virus gene expression in the peripheral blood of transplant recipients with chronic circulating viral loads. *Transplantation* 1998;66: 1641–1644.

113. Green M, Webber SA. EBV viral load monitoring: unanswered questions. *Am J Transplant* 2002;2:894–895.

114. Curtis JJ. Distinguishing the causes of post-transplantation hypertension. *Pediatr Nephrol* 1991;5:108–111.

115. North American Pediatric Renal Transplant Cooperative Study (NAPRTCS). *2003 Annual Report.* Sec. 3, p. 2.

116. Ettenger R, Marik J, Rosenthal JT. Sequential therapy in pediatric cadaveric renal transplantation: a critical analysis. *J Am Soc Nephrol* 1992;2:S304–S311.

117. Bunchman T, Kershaw D, Merion R, et al. OKT3 reversal of biopsy proven allograft rejection occurring during MALG induction in the pediatric renal recipient. *Clin Transplant* 1993;7:219–222.

118. Sarwal MM, Vidhun JR, Alexander SR, et al. Continued superior outcomes with modification and lengthened follow-up of a steroid-avoidance pilot with extended daclizumab induction in pediatric renal transplantation. *Transplantation* 2003;76:1331–1339.

119. Bunchman T, Mauer S. What is the best way to diagnose renal allograft rejection in the small child? *Pediatr Nephrol* 1990;4:218.

120. Matas AJ, Sibley R, Mauer SM, et al. Pre-discharge, post-transplant kidney biopsy does not predict rejection. *J Surg Res* 1982;32:269–274.

121. Fine RN. Growth in children with renal insufficiency. In: Nissenson AR, Fine RN, Gentile DE, eds. *Clinical Dialysis,* 2d ed. Norwalk, CT: Appleton & Lange, 1990:667–675.

122. Davis ID, Chang PN, Nevins TE. Successful renal transplantation accelerates development in young uremic children. *Pediatrics* 1990;86:594–600.

123. Harmon WE, Jabs K. Factors affecting growth after renal transplantation. *J Am Soc Nephrol* 1992;2:S295–S303.

124. Inglefinger JR, Grupe WE, Harmon WE, et al. Growth acceleration following renal transplantation in children less than 7 years of age. *Pediatrics* 1981;68:255–259.

125. Rees L, Greene A, Adlard P. Growth and endocrine function after renal transplantation. *Arch Dis Child* 1988;63: 1326–1332.

126. McEnery PT. Growth and development of children with renal transplantation use of alternate-day steroid therapy. *J Pediatr* 1973;83:806–814.

127. Broyer M, Guest G, Gagnadoux MF. Growth rate in children receiving alternate-day corticosteroid treatment after kidney transplantation. *J Pediatr* 1992;120:721–725.

128. Ingulli E, Sharma V, Singh A, et al. Steroid withdrawal, rejection and the mixed lymphocyte reaction in children after transplantation. *Kidney Int* 1993;44:S36–S39.

129. Offner G, Hoyer PF, Juppner H, et al. Somatic growth after kidney transplantation, beneficial effect of cyclosporine in comparison with conventional immunosuppression. *Am J Dis Child* 1987;141:541–546.

130. Jabs KL, Van Dop C, Harmon WE. Endocrinologic evaluation of children who grow poorly following renal transplantation. *Transplantation* 1990;49:71–79.

131. Fine RN, Stablein D, Cohen AH, et al. Recombinant human growth hormone post-renal transplantation in children: a randomized controlled study of the NAPRTCS. *Kidney Int* 2002;62:688–696.

132. Sutherland DE, Fryd DS, So SK, et al. Long-term effect of splenectomy versus no splenectomy in renal transplant patients. Re-analysis of a randomized prospective study. *Transplantation* 1984;38:619–624.

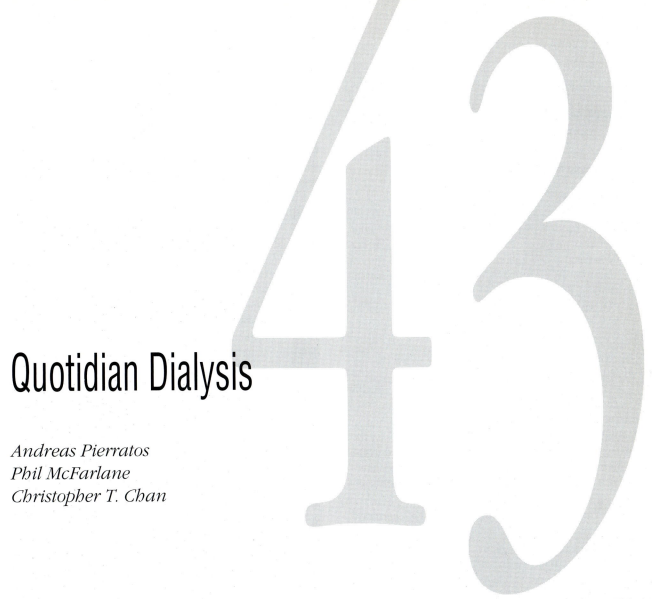

Quotidian Dialysis

Andreas Pierratos
Phil McFarlane
Christopher T. Chan

The recent interest in daily hemodialysis was born out of the impasse in the effort to improve survival and quality of life in patients with end-stage renal disease (ESRD). During the early years of hemodialysis, long once-a-week dialysis sessions were the rule, following which twice- and then thrice-weekly sessions were implemented. Inefficient dialyzers meant treatments lasted 8 hours or more. Patients were often trained to perform dialysis in the home, as a method of containing costs, so that more of them could be offered treatment. Government funding of dialysis costs through the 1960s and '70s eased access to in-center hemodialysis units, and the use of home hemodialysis began to diminish.[1] Improvements in technology and misinterpretation of the results of the National Cooperative Dialysis Study (NCDS) led to a progressive shortening of duration of hemodialysis treatments.

Despite the technological improvements, the annual mortality rate among patients on dialysis remains at about 20 percent.[2] One premise has related this high mortality to poor clearance of uremic toxins, a situation that should im-

prove with more aggressive dialysis techniques. This hypothesis was tested in the HEMO study,[3] a prospective randomized controlled study that failed to show a positive effect on patient survival when dialysis dose (but not dialysis time) was increased from a per-treatment Kt/V of 1.32 to 1.71 in a thrice-weekly regimen. Similarly, no decrease in mortality was seen in the ADEMEX study, with peritoneal dialysis doses greater than a weekly Kt/V of 1.7.[4] While providing more dialysis within conventional hemodialysis and peritoneal dialysis prescriptions has not reduced mortality, intensive hemodialysis by less conventional techniques has been shown to improve many patient outcomes. Reports have demonstrated decreased cardiovascular morbidity, improved blood pressure (BP) and anemia control, and higher quality of life and survival by using alternative hemodialysis schedules or techniques.[5] These less conventional methods include long intermittent hemodialysis, short daily hemodialysis, long nightly hemodialysis, and the use of convective techniques in the form of hemofiltration and hemodiafiltration. Many of these techniques are performed in the home rather than the in-center setting. Techniques including new-generation sorbents[6] and the use of live tubular cells as part of the bioartificial kidney[7] have also attracted interest. In this chapter we discuss the effect of daily dialysis on patient outcomes.

Long Intermittent Hemodialysis

Several dialysis centers have never discarded the long 8-hour dialysis treatments performed during the genesis of hemodialysis. The dialysis unit with the largest experience in this regard is in Tassin, France, where a 75 percent 10-year patient survival in a cohort of 876 patients has been reported.[8] Despite the early biases with regard to patient selection criteria, the mortality rates among the more recent patient cohorts continue to be only half those reported by the USRDS. Long intermittent hemodialysis is characterized by excellent BP control, which is presumably achieved by a decrease in extracellular fluid volume through ultrafiltration and sodium restriction.[9] Interestingly, despite the improvement in BP control, left ventricular hypertrophy is still present in 76 percent of these patients.[10,11] Patients on long intermittent hemodialysis have not been spared dialysis-related amyloidosis.[12] This may be partially related to the cuprophan dialyzers and acetate-based dialysate used in the early cohorts. Phosphate control is improved on long intermittent hemodialysis, but phosphate binders are still often needed.

In the United States, more than 300 patients currently receive long in-center or home nocturnal treatments either thrice a week or every other night.[13] This form of dialysis strives to achieve some of the benefits of long frequent treatments at a lower cost, while providing potentially more convenient scheduling at the center.

Home Hemodialysis

Home hemodialysis was the dominant dialysis modality in the 1970s, with more than 40 percent of the patients in the United States being dialyzed at home.[1] Although there are no well-designed studies comparing the outcomes between home and in-center hemodialysis, there is unanimous support for this treatment, which provides a high level of patient independence and rehabilitation[14] and possibly lower mortality at a low cost.[15] Studies on home hemodialysis suffer from the unavoidable patient selection biases toward those who are healthier, younger, and more motivated. The current shortage of nurses specializing in dialysis in many countries and reports of cost containment with home hemodialysis have also made home hemodialysis more attractive.[16] Long intermittent home hemodialysis at night was introduced by Shaldon in the 1960s.[17] More frequent home treatments are rising in popularity based on reported clinical outcome improvements.

DAILY (QUOTIDIAN) HEMODIALYSIS

Daily hemodialysis is practiced on average six times a week. The short daily form lasts for an average of 2 to 2.5 hours at maximal blood and dialysate flow rates and is practiced in center or at home. The long nightly version is practiced mainly at home for an average of 8 hours using lower blood and dialysate flows.

Terminology

Although there is no consensus on terminology, the term *quotidian hemodialysis* designates daily dialysis, with *hemeral* referring to daytime dialysis and *nocturnal* to the long nightly version. The term *short daily hemodialysis* is in widespread use, as is *daily nocturnal home hemodialysis*. The term *intensive hemodialysis* has been proposed to describe collectively all the methods that offer either longer duration or higher frequency than conventional hemodialysis.[18]

History of Daily Hemodialysis

The first publication on daily hemodialysis, by DePalma, appeared in 1969.[19] Several attempts to use daily hemodialysis in the United States were terminated for financial or logistical reasons, but all the research groups reported improved quality of life, BP, and anemia control.[20] Buoncristiani's group and others in Italy continued to use short daily hemodialysis and have reported extensively on their more than 20 years of experience with this method.[21,22] The international experience of the early era of daily hemodialysis, including mainly Italian data, has been reviewed by Woods.[23] Twardowski demonstrated that daily hemodialysis had significantly improved a variety of clinical and biochemical parameters. His recent efforts as well as support by industry were instrumental in reviving interest in daily hemodialysis.[24,25] In 1994, Uldall reported experience from the use of quotidian nocturnal home hemodialysis 6 to 7 nights a week.[26] The use of quotidian hemodialysis and the relevant publications have increased significantly over the last 5 years. A more detailed history of quotidian hemodialysis is available elsewhere.[27] Although hemofiltration and hemodiafiltration were pioneered by Henderson in the 1980s, their use in outpatients has been mostly limited to Europe.[28,29] Recently, technological improvements have led to publications on the use of daily hemodiafiltration both in center and at home.[30,31]

Method

Both short daily and nocturnal hemodialysis can be carried out using conventional hemodialysis machines. Recently several machines were modified or designed de novo to facilitate daily home hemodialysis. Most of their new features aim to simplify the machine's operation so that patient training is easier, or to add unique features that are useful for short or long home hemodialysis.[32–38] These features include mobile flat screens, fewer alarms, easier or automated setup, capability for remote monitoring, low dialysate flow, ultrapure dialysate, in situ dialyzer reuse, use of hemoperfusion techniques, or use of batch dialysate or sorbent cartridges. Flow of blood and dialysate are kept at a maximum during short daily hemodialysis to maximize efficiency. Blood flow during quotidian nocturnal hemodialysis is 200 to 400 mL/min (typically about 250 mL/min) and dialysate flow 100 to 500 mL/min (typically about 300 mL/min).[39] No sodium or ultrafiltration ramping is necessary on quotidian hemodialysis. Anticoagulation during hemodialysis is similar to that in conventional hemodialysis. No data exist on whether high-flux dialyzers or ultrapure dialysate [less than 0.1 colony-forming unit (CFU) per milliliter of bacteria and less than 0.03 endotoxin units (EU) per milliliter of endotoxin] should be used.

The composition of the dialysate used for short daily hemodialysis is similar to that for conventional hemodialysis. For quotidian nocturnal hemodialysis, dialysate usually has a lower bicarbonate level (typically 30 meq/L) and a higher calcium (typically 3.2 meq/L or 1.6 mmol/L); most patients also require phosphate supplementation (typically 1.50 mg/dL or 0.50 mmol/L). Adjustment of calcium concentration is often achieved by having the patient add calcium chloride powder at prescribed volumes to the acid concentrate (7 mL of powder in a 4-L acid concentrate jug increases final dialysate calcium by about 0.5 meq/L or 0.25 mmol/L).[39] In the absence of a commercially available phosphate additive, sodium phosphate is added in the form of oral Fleet or a Fleet enema into either the "acid-" or the bicarbonate-containing dialysate (30 mL of Fleet enema into 4 L of "acid concentrate" provides a final dialysate phosphate of about 1.2 mg/dL or 0.4 mmol/L).[40] The low pH of the acid concentrate prevents the precipitation of calcium and phosphate.[41]

Blood Access. The use of native arteriovenous (AV) fistulas is encouraged for both forms of quotidian hemodialysis. Synthetic grafts as well as central venous catheters can be used in both methods. Some centers use the "buttonhole" technique, where cannulation occurs repeatedly at the same site, allowing a subcutaneous tract composed of scar tissue to develop between the skin and the access. Although their use is not mandatory, noncutting needles, which are guided by the tract into the fistula, are said to be associated with a lower incidence of blood leak. Anecdotal reports of easier cannulation and greater patient comfort have increased the popularity of the buttonhole technique. As accurate placement of the needle is facilitated when the person inserting the needles is familiar with the access, this technique has proven popular among home and self-care hemodialysis patients who perform their own cannulation.[42] Meticulous attention to antisepsis and scab removal is needed in using the buttonhole technique.

Nocturnal hemodialysis requires extra safety precautions. They include the following: (1) The use of preperforated central venous catheter caps so that dialysis is performed without catheter cap removal, therefore minimizing the risk of air embolism (e.g., Interlink); (2) A nondisposable, locking box to prevent accidental separation of the blood tubing and catheter; (3) A moisture sensor (such as a conventional enuresis alarm) taped to the fistula needle sites to alert the user to a possible blood leak or needle dislodgment; and (4) Floor moisture sensors close to the dialysis machines to alert the user to possible blood or dialysate leaks.[39,43] The single-needle system reduces the dialysis dose provided by quotidian nocturnal hemodialysis minimally, but it may increase safety in the event of accidental needle dislodgment and may increase patient comfort and improve access survival by decreasing the number of cannulations. Quotidian nocturnal hemodialysis programs should consider using single-needle systems for these reasons.

Live Monitoring. Several dialysis centers practice live remote monitoring of the patients on quotidian nocturnal hemodialysis.[43–45] This is achieved by a telephone or Internet connection, with the latter preferred when long-distance telephone charges are applicable. Centralized monitoring of large geographic areas improves cost-effectiveness. An observer responds to unattended alarms or incorrect machine settings by calling the patient. If the patient does not answer the phone call, then the observer can arrange for emergency dispatch of an ambulance. Continuous monitoring of vital signs may be desirable but has not yet been developed. The incremental safety (and therefore necessity) of remote monitoring has not been established. Anecdotal reports suggest that some patients are reassured by remote monitoring, especially during the first few months of nocturnal dialysis, and monitoring can also help collect data on dialysis characteristics and compliance. Patients at several centers perform home nocturnal hemodialysis without monitoring, with nothing untoward reported to date. Although in most programs the presence of a partner for nocturnal hemodialysis has been required, in others either a partner or remote monitoring is required.

Patient Selection and Training

The demographic characteristics of patients who have selected quotidian hemodialysis have tended to fall into two groups. The first group includes those patients selected by their dialysis teams because of conditions such as unstable hemodynamics during dialysis, uncontrolled hypertension, congestive heart failure, ascites, malnutrition, or intractable uremia. The second group includes those who selected quotidian treatments themselves, typically in order to improve quality of life or to have free time to work. The first group tends to consist of older patients who have recently started dialysis and who have multiple significant comorbid conditions. The second group consists of younger patients who have been on dialysis for several years and who tend to be free of comorbid conditions, especially diabetes and cardiovascular disease. This bimodal population introduces difficulty in studying clinical outcomes. There is no medical contraindication for quotidian dialysis in center or at home except for contraindications to systemic heparinization on quotidian nocturnal hemodialysis. Ability and willingness to be trained as well as adequate housing are the only prerequisites for training for home quotidian hemodialysis. Cardiovascular instability is an indication for quotidian dialysis rather than a contraindication for enrollment. Either the patient or a helper (usually a family member) is trained to perform the dialysis at home. The length of training can be as short as 1 to 2 weeks for patients previously performing self-care hemodialysis, but it typically runs for 5 to 6 weeks in previously untrained individuals. Training is usually performed three times a week, concurrent with the patient's dialysis treatments. For nocturnal hemodialysis, some centers have trainees demonstrate their readiness by performing one or more overnight treatments while supervised at the training center.

Solute Removal

How best to measure adequacy of uremic solute removal with intensive hemodialysis is still a matter of debate. The early positive results reported by Buoncristiani suggest that despite a Kt/V of only 0.26 per treatment, quotidian hemodialysis is associated with improved quality of life and BP control.[21] Furthermore, patient mortality during the initial years on dialysis is similar for peritoneal and hemodialysis, despite the lower weekly Kt/V provided by CAPD.[46] This has led to the assumption that dialysis administered daily or continuously offers advantages over intermittent dialysis delivering the same Kt/V. Several new instruments have been developed to measure dialysis dose across different dialysis techniques and levels of residual kidney function. The renal urea clearance (EKR) proposed by Casino and Lopez is equal to the amount of urea clearance provided by native renal function—that is, the amount required to produce a serum urea concentration equal to the time-averaged concentration (TAC) of urea achieved on dialysis.[47] The normalized Kt/V proposed by Depner represents the Kt/V of a hypothetical solute that diffuses more slowly than urea across the dialysis membrane or intercompartmental barriers.[48] This measure favors intensive dialysis, since the removal of such a solute increases with dialysis time and frequency. Gotch has proposed the standard Kt/V (stdKt/V) that

is calculated based on the midweek predialysis urea.[49] Since steady-state urea on CAPD and predialysis urea on conventional hemodialysis are similar when these methods are delivered at doses suggested by the Dialysis Outcomes Quality Initiative (DOQI) guidelines, the stdKt/V is about 2.0 per week for both methods. Daily hemodialysis for the same number of hours per week as conventional hemodialysis results in lower predialysis urea values and so offers a higher stdKt/V, at about 3.0.[50] Using this rationale, in order to provide a weekly stdKt/V of only 2, the daily dose on short daily hemodialysis can be decreased to an equilibrated Kt/V (eKt/V) of 0.38 per treatment (less than half of the required dose of 1.05 on conventional hemodialysis) or a single Kt/V of 0.53 to 0.56 (less that half of the required 1.2 on conventional hemodialysis but reflecting the higher postdialysis urea rebound on shorter dialysis). The stdKt/V on quotidian nocturnal hemodialysis is about 5.0, as this method offers both long and frequent sessions.[50,51] The use of stdKt/V has been extended to the measurement of middle molecules.[52] How well these measures correlate with clinical outcomes remains to be determined.

Convective techniques, including hemofiltration and hemodiafiltration, offer higher removal of higher-molecular-weight solutes,[53] and measures of urea kinetics may not accurately determine the adequacy of dialysis with these methods. Indeed, the Kt/V offered by hemofiltration at affordable rates of infusion of sterile replacement solution is lower than that of conventional hemodialysis. This is not the case with hemodiafiltration, which also provides diffusive solute transport. The use of daily hemofiltration was recently introduced at doses based on the stdKt/V. The use of about 15 L of replacement solution daily for 6 days a week in an average-size patient provides a stdKt/V of about 2.0 per week, which is similar to that of conventional hemodialysis but lower than short daily hemodialysis of equal weekly duration.[31]

Increased clearance of middle molecules has been associated with better patient survival.[54,55] The length of dialysis treatments largely determines middle-molecule removal. Daily dialysis permits frequent equilibration of solute level with less rebound and thus provides better middle-molecule removal. This increase is modest if the measurement is based on the TAC of the solute, as in the calculation of EKR,[51] but it is significant when it is based on the predialysis concentration of the solute, as in the case of stdKt/V.[56] Middle-molecule removal is increased significantly by quotidian nocturnal hemodialysis irrespective of the calculation method, since both time and frequency increase.[51,56,57] Hemofiltration increases the removal of middle molecules due to the solvent drag effect; thus short daily hemofiltration is more effective at removing middle molecules than short daily hemodialysis despite lower small-molecule removal.[52] The effects of these differences on clinical outcomes needs further investigation. The weekly dialysate beta$_2$-microglobulin mass increased fourfold, from 127 to 585 mg, after the conversion from conventional to quotidian nocturnal hemodialysis. Serum beta$_2$-microglobulin levels decreased from 27.2 to 13.7 mg/dL in 9 months.[58] Similarly, serum beta$_2$ microglobulin levels decreased on daily hemodiafiltration.[30]

Advanced glycation end products have been reported to decrease upon conversion from conventional to short and long daily hemodialysis.[59,60] Elevated homocysteine levels have been associated with increased risk of cardiovascular disease and are elevated in patients on dialysis. Homocysteine levels are reported to be lower (by about about 6 μmol/L) in patients on quotidian nocturnal hemodialysis vs. those on conventional hemodialysis.[61] While short daily hemodialysis also reduces homocysteine levels, quotidian nocturnal hemodialysis appears to reduce these levels even further.[62] Protein-bound molecules are not removed easily by dialysis, but they appear to be cleared more efficiently on quotidian hemodialysis. For example, the predialysis levels of indole-3-acetic and acid indoxyl sulfate were significantly lower on short daily hemodialysis than on conventional hemodialysis.[59]

OUTCOMES

Health Ecomomics and Quality of Life

Health Economics. The cost of in-center hemodialysis is estimated to be between $50,000 and $100,000 per patient-year (all costs in this chapter have been converted to 2003 U.S. dollars), which approaches the limit that society will accept for a life-sustaining therapy.[63] These costs are driven by the need for expensive equipment and consumables, the requirement for repeated longitudinal treatments, and the need for specialized health care professionals. Dialysis programs increase hospital expenses through additional administrative overhead, inpatient admissions, and diagnostic investigations. Comorbid conditions such as anemia and cardiovascular disease contribute to high costs for medications and physician services. In most developing countries, these costs are prohibitive and death due to ESRD is common.[64–67]

Costs could be constrained by restricting access to dialysis or by reducing the quality of dialysis; however, these methods are generally unpalatable.[68] Alternatively, new forms of dialysis could reduce costs by improving patient health, in hope of reducing costs such as medications and hospital admissions, which are influenced primarily by patient characteristics. Another strategy would be to reduce the cost of items primarily influenced by the type of dialysis (such as staffing, overhead, and consumable costs). McFarlane et al. prospectively compared costs for a group of 33 home quotidian nocturnal hemodialysis patients to those for a demographically similar group of 23 conventional in-cen-

ter hemodialysis patients.[69] Kroeker et al. prospectively compared costs for 10 home short daily hemodialysis patients, 12 quotidian nocturnal hemodialysis patients, and 22 patients on conventional hemodialysis in center to retrospectively collected costs for in-center hemodialysis during the previous year.[70] Using a similar design, Ting et al. reported on 22 patients converted to short daily hemodialysis (20 in center, 2 home-based).[71] Finally, Mohr et al. used a decision-analysis model to estimate costs on conventional in-center hemodialysis, home quotidian nocturnal hemodialysis, home short daily hemodialysis, and in-center short daily hemodialysis.[72]

Reducing Costs by Improving Patient Outcomes. The treatment of medical events requiring hospitalization can be very costly. In the McFarlane and Ting studies, there was a trend toward fewer hospital admissions and reduced costs for hospitalization in the quotidian groups. Ting et al. reported a significant reduction in hospital admissions after conversion to quotidian hemodialysis in a larger group of patients.[73] In the Kroeker study, these costs fell after conversion to quotidian dialysis, but they rose in those remaining on conventional in-center hemodialysis. The Mohr model determined that hospital costs for all forms of quotidian hemodialysis were less than for in-center conventional hemodialysis. Indeed, this model predicted that 80 percent of the overall cost savings of daily dialysis related to reductions in hospital admissions (Table 43–1).

Another marker of the impact of comorbid conditions is the use of cardiovascular medications and human recombinant erythropoietin (rHuEPO). In the McFarlane study, there was a trend toward lower medication costs, with significant reductions in the costs of rHuEPO and cardiovascular medications. There were similar trends in the Kroeker and Ting studies. The Mohr model also predicted lower costs for rHuEPO and antihypertensive agents for the quotidian hemodialysis groups.

These studies suggest that improving patient health through quotidian hemodialysis can lower total health care costs by reducing the cost of hospital admissions and medications.

Reducing Costs by Reducing Fixed Modality Costs. In developed countries, staffing costs are universally the largest dialysis cost category, contributing between one-quarter and one-third of total health care costs for in-center conventional hemodialysis.[74] In the McFarlane study, staffing costs were half as much for home quotidian nocturnal hemodialysis than in-center conventional hemodialysis, while in the Kroeker study, staffing costs were about six times higher for in-center conventional hemodialysis than for home quotidian nocturnal hemodialysis or home short daily hemodialysis. These reductions have additional benefits, as the lack of hemodialysis nurses has limited expansion of dialysis pro-

TABLE 43–1. SUMMARY OF COSTS FROM SELECTED STUDIES

McFarlane et al.

	IHD[1]	HNHD[2]
Staffing	$17,656	$8,765*
Dialysis materials	$5,259	$13,273*
Medications	$9,642	$7,179
Admissions/consultations	$5,593	$960
Overhead/support	$9,934	$3,339*
Other	$7,100	$11,628
Total	**$55,184**	**$45,144***

Kroeker et al.

	HNHD[2]	HSDHD[3]	IHD control[6]
Staffing	$3,380	$3,720	$20,171
Dialysis materials	$15,271	$15,591	$7,674
Medications	$16,792	$13,398	$14,055
Admissions/consultations	$3,031	$1,281	$2,688
Overhead/support	$7,128	$6,756	$2,726
Other	$11,202	$10,642	$8,202
Change from previous year	–$13,306	–$7,465	$2,339
Total	**$56,804**	**$51,388**	**$55,516**

Ting et al.

	SDH[7] vs. IHD[1]
Extra supply cost/year	–$2,750
Extra labor cost/year	–$619
EPO savings/year	$5,685
Antihypertensive savings/year	$397
Hospitalization cost reduction/year	$2,514
Total Savings/year	**$5,227**

Mohr et al.

	IHD[1]	HNHD[2]	HSDHD[3]	ISHDH[4]
Dialysis	$23,296	$26,500	$26,131	$28,473
Hospitalization	$28,966	$16,517	$16,517	$16,517
EPO	$6,902	$4,068	$4,068	$4,068
Antihypertensive medications	$493	$247	$247	$247
Other	$24,652	$23,789	$23,789	$25,638
Total	**$84,309**	**$71,121**	**$70,752**	**$74,943**

[1]IHD = conventional in-center hemodialysis, [2]HNHD = home nocturnal hemodialysis, [3]HSDHD = home short daily hemodialys, [4]ISHDH = in-center short daily hemodialysis, [5]IHD retro = conventional in-center hemodialysis costs calculated retrospectively in year prior to study, [6]IHD control = costs for patients remaining on conventional in-center hemodialysis during study period, [7]SDH = short daily hemodialysis (20 in-center, 2 home)
*p<.05

grams in many jurisdictions. Overhead costs are also reduced in home-based programs (Table 43–1).[69,75,76]

Cost savings in staffing and overhead are important in offsetting expected cost increases in other areas, as doubling the frequency of dialysis necessitates a doubling of the cost of consumables. In the McFarlane study, the costs of dialysis materials were significantly higher for home quotidian nocturnal hemodialysis. The Kroeker study confirmed the predicted doubling of consumable costs for quo-

tidian dialysis. In the Ting study, materials and staffing costs were estimated to be about $2700 higher per patient-year.

Capital equipment costs are also expected to be significantly higher when dialysis is performed in the home. Hemodialysis machines in an in-center unit are typically shared among six or more patients, with water-treatment equipment shared among all patients. Home-based programs require separate hemodialysis machines and water-treatment equipment for each participant. In the McFarlane study, capital costs for equipment were significantly higher for home quotidian nocturnal hemodialysis—a finding seen in studies of home conventional hemodialysis.[75,76]

These studies suggest that the use of quotidian hemodialysis doubles the cost of dialysis consumables, and home-based hemodialysis programs substantially increase per-patient capital equipment costs. Home quotidian hemodialysis programs can lower staffing and overhead costs. Whether this is true for in-center programs is less clear, although it would be reasonable to expect that in-center quotidian dialysis would not result in the same savings in staffing and overhead seen for home-based programs.

Total Costs of Health Care. The total cost of health care for in-center conventional hemodialysis is consistently higher than that for quotidian hemodialysis. In the McFarlane study, the total cost of health care was about $10,000 less per patient-year in the group receiving home quotidian nocturnal hemodialysis. In the Kroeker study, the total cost of health care fell in the home quotidian nocturnal hemodialysis and home short daily hemodialysis groups, but it rose in the group that remained on in-center conventional hemodialysis. Ting estimated a cost-savings of about $5200 per patient year for in-center short daily hemodialysis. The Mohr model predicted that in-center conventional hemodialysis would be the most expensive modality, followed by in-center short daily and home quotidian nocturnal, with the least expensive option being home short daily hemodialysis (Table 43–1).

These studies suggest that the greater costs of consumables associated with high dialysis frequency and increased capital costs associated with home-based therapies can be overcome by cost savings in modality-specific areas, such as staffing and overhead, and patient-specific areas, such as medications and hospital admissions. On balance, total health care costs for quotidian hemodialysis are expected to be lower than those for conventional in-center hemodialysis. Indeed, even when the study perspective is restricted to costs borne at the level of the hemodialysis unit (staffing, overhead, consumables, and capital), home quotidian hemodialysis should be less expensive than conventional in-center hemodialysis.[69]

QUALITY OF LIFE

The quality of life reported for patients performing in-center hemodialysis is among the worst reported for chronic illnesses.[77] Studies have measured quality of life in hemodialysis patients using disease-specific measurements, disease-independent instruments, utility measures, and instruments unique to hemodialysis. The use of a variety of assessment tools allows us to examine overall quality of life as well as to determine which specific aspects of a person's life have been affected by quotidian hemodialysis.

Utility Scores

Utility scores estimate overall quality of life by assessing a patient's preference between health states. Utility is often graded on a scale between 0 (a quality of life equivalent to death) and 1 (the best quality of life imaginable).[78] Utility scores are the preferred outcome measure in health economics and are used to calculate quality-adjusted life years (QALYs) in cost-utility studies.[79] Patients receiving conventional hemodialysis typically report utility scores of about 0.5, which represents a quality of life worse than that in patients who suffer from blindness or paraplegia (Fig. 43–1).[77] In a subset of the McFarlane study[80] and in a study by Heidenheim et al. that analyzed the same population examined in the Kroeker study,[81] mean utility scores for patients receiving home quotidian hemodialysis were higher than those seen in patients on conventional hemodialysis. Indeed, the quotidian groups had utility scores similar to historically reported values following kidney transplantation. This is supported by anecdotal reports of home quotidian nocturnal hemodialysis patients removing themselves from transplant waiting lists, presumably as they had no expectation of incremental benefit from transplantation. Heidenheim also reported that individuals receiving quotidian hemodialysis retrospectively rated their utility on IHD as much worse than their experience while receiving intensive hemodialysis.

Disease-Independent Measures

Other studies have attempted to quantify the effect of intensive dialysis by using tools suitable for many disease states (Table 43–2). These scales can identify the quality-of-life domains that have contributed to improvements in overall quality of life. Brissenden et al. reported that in 18 patients converted to home quotidian nocturnal hemodialysis, significant improvements were seen in the Sickness Impact Profile (SIP) and Short Form 36 (SF-36) scores.[82] Levels of depression fell in this group, as measured by the Beck Depression Index. Kooistra et al. found that SF-36 scores improved in 13 patients after conversion from in-center conventional hemodialysis to home short daily hemodialysis, primarily driven by improvements in energy.[83] In the same study, Nottingham Health Index scores improved with home short daily hemodialysis, as the result of improvements in physical functioning and mental health. In the Heidenheim study, SF-36 scores in both physical and mental functioning were improved in patients converted to home short daily hemodialysis but not in those converted to home

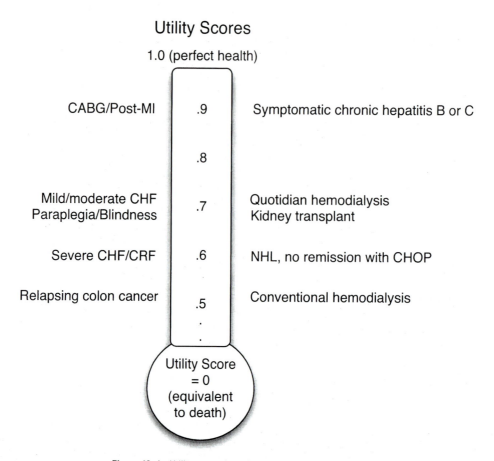

Figure 43–1. Utility scores in various chronic medical conditions.

quotidian nocturnal hemodialysis or those who remained on in-center conventional hemodialysis.

Disease-Dependent and Hemodialysis-Specific Measures

Using a renal disease–specific tool, Heidenheim reported a reduction in the number and severity of dialysis-related symptoms as well as a dramatic reduction in time to recover from dialysis in quotidian hemodialysis patients.[81] Ting et al. have reported that KDQOL scores improve with conversion to home short daily hemodialysis, with significant changes seen in almost every quality-of-life category.[73]

The Effect of Quotidian Hemodialysis on Costs and Quality of Life: A Summary

These trials suggest that quotidian hemodialysis is cost-neutral or cost-saving relative to conventional in-center hemodialysis. Overall quality of life is improved by quotidian dialysis, typically by improving a wide range of symptoms that affect physical and social functioning. This suggests that quotidian hemodialysis is economically "dominant"

relative to conventional in-center hemodialysis, improving outcomes while reducing costs. However, the evidence to support this conclusion has limitations. In some studies, small sample sizes led to instability in costing and quality-of-life estimates, and the strength of conclusions based on these data is limited by the lack of statistical significance of the results. Modeling of the costs of a new technology often requires analysis of unpublished data—a difficulty that the Mohr study shares. It is difficult to quantify the independent effects of quotidian dialysis from patient case-mix bias in many of these studies. Finally, patients performing quotidian hemodialysis often have different demographic profiles and comorbidities than the average in-center hemodialysis patient, and the generalizability of these results to the broader in-center conventional hemodialysis population is unclear. Despite their limitations, these studies are encouraging and lead to an expectation that quotidian hemodialysis can be performed without significant increases in total health care costs. While this has been established for home-based therapies, these conclusions are less firm for in-center quotidian hemodialysis. These cost savings should be accompanied by quality-of-life improvements in most pa-

TABLE 43–2. A SUMMARY OF QUALITY OF LIFE MEASUREMENTS FROM SELECTED STUDIES OF QUOTIDIAN HEMODIALYSIS[a]

Utility scores				
McFarlane et al.		IHD	HNHD	
		0.52	0.77	
Heidenheim et al.		HNHD	HSDHD	IHD
		0.78	0.84	0.70
Disease-independent measures				
Brissenden et al.	**SF-36**	IHD	HNHD	
	Social functioning	54.2	79.2	
	Physical functioning	60.6	69.0	
	Role physical	39.2	36.1	
	SIP			
	Total	14.0	9.5	
	Beck Depression Index			
	Total	8.5	6.0	
Kooistra et al.		IHD	HSDHD	
	Nottingham Health Profile			
	Energy	45.1	18.1	
	RAND-36			
	Physical functioning	14.0	9.5	
	Mental health	72.3	78.8	
Disease-dependent/hemodialysis-specific measures				
Ting et al.	**KD-QOL**	IHD	HSDHD	
	Health survey[b]	42.8	56.3	
	ESRD-specific survey[c]	59.3	70.4	
	Well-being during dialysis	72.3	87.5	
	Well-being after dialysis	56.4	72.7	
Heidenheim et al.		HNHD	HSDHD	IHD
	No dialysis symptoms	2.9	3.1	4.1
	Recovery time (minutes)	4.3	16.0	442.1
	No disease symptoms	4.7	4.8	7.3

IHD, conventional in center hemodialysis; HNHD, home nocturnal hemodialysis; HSDHD, home short daily hemodialysis.

[a]All differences reached statistical significance for at least one time point in study.

[b]Significant improvements in physical functioning, physical role, general health, emotional well-being, emotion role, social functioning, and energy.

[c]Significant improvement is symptoms/problem list, effects and burden of kidney disease, cognitive function, quality of social interaction, sexual function and sleep

tients. Future research should help clarify the impact of quotidian hemodialysis on costs for in-center therapies and the effect on costs and quality of life in more diverse patient populations.

CARDIOVASCULAR OUTCOMES

Cardiovascular disease continues to be the leading cause of morbidity and mortality in patients with ESRD. Thus far, modest increases in thrice-weekly hemodialysis dosing have not reduced the burden of cardiovascular disease.[3] In contrast, frequent hemodialysis in the forms of short daily hemodialysis and quotidian nocturnal hemodialysis has demonstrated improvements in cardiovascular outcomes.

Blood Pressure and Left Ventricular Geometry

BP control is superior with intensive hemodialysis; however, emerging data suggest that the mechanisms underlying the BP-lowering effect of short daily hemodialysis and nocturnal hemodialysis may differ. In a prospective crossover study involving short daily hemodialysis, Fagugli et al. describe improvements in BP control and a fall in antihypertensive use, but left ventricular mass index (LVMI)—a potent adverse prognosticator—also decreased.[84] These investigators proposed that a decrease in the control of extracellular fluid volume could be an important contributing factor to the reduction of BP and LVMI. The nocturnal hemodialysis experience has uniformly confirmed the dramatic BP–lowering effect of this modality.[39,43,85] Chan et al. reported restoration of normal BP in 28 NHD patients followed for 3 years after conversion from conventional to nocturnal hemodialysis. LVMI also decreased significantly, from 147 to 122 g/m^2. A similar control cohort did not demonstrate such improvements.[86] Unlike the short daily hemodialysis reports, the data did not indicate a change in the nadir of extracellular fluid volume, suggesting that other potential explanations are needed to explain the antihypertensive effect of nocturnal hemodialysis. Indeed, Nesrallah et al. recently reported the London (Ontario) experience, showing that both short daily hemodialysis and nocturnal hemodialysis resulted in normalization of BP.[87] However, these investigators found that extracellular fluid control was critical only in the short daily hemodialysis cohort. Taken together, the current available data suggest that short daily hemodialysis lowers BP by improving extracellular fluid control, whereas nocturnal hemodialysis may improve BP control via additional mechanisms, such as enhanced removal or decreased production of neurohormonal substances, as addressed below.

Other Cardiovascular Changes

In addition to the described changes in BP and LVMI, quotidian nocturnal hemodialysis has also been associated with other cardiovascular effects. The impact of nocturnal hemodialysis on impaired left ventricular systolic function was described in six ESRD patients with diminished ejection fraction (< 40 percent).[88] In addition to normalization of BP, these patients experienced a marked increase in left ventricular ejection fraction (from 28 to 41 percent) after conversion to quotidian nocturnal hemodialysis. A case report demonstrated a restoration of peripheral vascular flow to the lower extremities with nocturnal hemodialysis.[89]

MECHANISTIC ANALYSES

Recent studies have provided important insights into the mechanisms by which frequent dialysis improves BP and cardiovascular regulation.

Studies of Quotidian Nocturnal Hemodialysis

In a prospective cohort study, changes in hemodynamics as well as in neurohormonal and vascular responsiveness were followed in 18 ESRD patients before and after conversion to nocturnal hemodialysis.[90] The nocturnal hemodialysis cohort had a dramatic lowering of BP without alterations in stroke volume or cardiac output. Total peripheral resistance (TPR) fell significantly, from 1967 to 1499 $dyne.s.cm^{-5}$, suggesting that the hypotensive effect of nocturnal hemodialysis is mediated through a reduction in an elevated TPR rather than a fall in the intravascular volume. Our group assessed endothelial function in this patient cohort by measuring brachial artery responsiveness to reactive hyperemia (a measure of endothelium-dependent vasodilation) and responsiveness to nitroglycerin (a measure of endothelium-independent vasodilation).[90] Brachial artery response to hyperemia increased significantly, from –2.7 percent on conventional hemodialysis to 4.7 percent after 1 month of nocturnal hemodialysis and to 8.0 percent after 2 months. The endothelium-independent response improved similarly over the same time period. These observations are the first to suggest a sustained time-dependent improvement in vascular responsiveness with nocturnal hemodialysis.

Our data suggest that nocturnal hemodialysis patients have a fundamentally different hemodynamic state as compared to conventionally dialyzed individuals. Indeed, a review of the first 15 nocturnal hemodialysis patients who underwent renal transplantation added further evidence to our hypothesis. In comparison to a similar control cohort, our patient population had similar renal allograft outcomes up to 24 months. However, there was a substantial worsening of BP in the nocturnally dialyzed patients after renal transplantation, whereas conventional hemodialysis patients had an improvement in BP control.[91]

Decreased heart rate variability, a measure of autonomic modulation, has been correlated with cardiovascular mortality in healthy individuals and following myocardial infarction.[92] Patients with ESRD have increased sympathetic activity as well as decreased heart rate variability, findings that correlate with mortality.[93] Conversion from conventional to quotidian nocturnal hemodialysis was found to be associated with increased heart rate variability

during sleep.[94] How this affects clinical outcomes is yet to be determined.

Other Daily Hemodialysis Studies

Zilch et al. found a decrease in sympathetic activity on short daily hemodialysis.[95] A decrease in brain natriuretic peptide (BNP) on short daily hemodialysis was reported by Odar-Cederlof et al.[96] The serum levels of this neurohormone have been found to correlate with mortality in the ESRD population.[97]

rHuEPO DOSE AND ANEMIA CONTROL

Anemia is associated with poor uremia control and is an established cardiovascular risk factor in patients with ESRD. There have been conflicting reports of the impact of intensive hemodialysis on anemia management. Most groups described a fall in rHuEPO requirements and an increase in hemoglobin concentrations.[23,73] However, negative results have also been reported.[83] Woods et al. reviewed results from 72 ESRD patients undergoing short daily dialysis and concluded that conversion to this modality is associated with a rise in the patients' hematocrit by 3 percentage points.[23] Recent data reported by Ting et al. in a cohort of ESRD patients with high comorbidity who converted from conventional hemodialysis to short daily dialysis indicated a fall in the rHuEPO requirement by 45 percent with an increase in hemoglobin concentrations.[73]

Since much controversy surrounds the impact of iron administration, we conducted a controlled cohort study to test the hypothesis that augmentation of solute clearance by nocturnal hemodialysis would improve anemia management.[98] Our analysis included 63 nocturnal hemodialysis patients and 32 on self-care dialysis. There were no differences in baseline iron indices between the two groups. After conversion to nocturnal hemodialysis, there was a substantial increase in hemoglobin concentrations with a fall in rHuEPO requirements. In contrast, the control cohort did not reflect such changes.

The enhancement of solute clearance may also improve anemia management. Further prospective studies are needed to delineate the mechanisms and clinical impact of intensive hemodialysis on anemia control and responsiveness to rHuEPO.

Nutrition

Nutritional parameters of patients on dialysis correlate with morbidity and mortality.[99] Serum albumin concentration increases with protein and calorie intake and can decrease in the presence of inflammation.[100] It has been a consistent observation that patients who converted to daily hemodialysis experienced improved appetite and weight gain. Galland et al. reported an average of 2.7 kg of weight gain in a series of 10 patients 1 year after conversion from conventional to quotidian hemodialysis.[101] In 48 patients followed at Humber River Regional Hospital for an average of 24.5 months, body weight increased significantly (from 77.8 to 80.3 kg, $p = 0.001$). There was no change in the already normal serum albumin in these patients.[39] Galland et al. also reported a significant increase in serum albumin (from 38.5 to 41.3 g/L, $p = 0.016$); however, Kooistra et al.[83] did not find an increase in albumin 6 months after a similar conversion in 13 patients, nor did Ting et al. after the conversion of patients with significant comorbidities.[73] In a prospective study, Spanner et al. reported that serum albumin rose in 11 patients receiving short daily hemodialysis but, after 9 months, fell in 12 patients receiving quotidian nocturnal hemodialysis. These patients had an increase in the normalized protein equivalent of total nitrogen appearance (nPNA) when compared to baseline values, and the quotidian patients had higher nPNA values than 21 control patients receiving conventional hemodialysis.[62] These trends reached statistical significance in the short daily patients but not in the nocturnal hemodialysis patients.

Raj et al. described that, while serum essential and nonessential amino acids increased in 11 patients after conversion to quotidian nocturnal hemodialysis, some abnormalities of amino acids consistent with uremia persisted.[102] Despite daily amino acid losses of more than 10 g into the dialysate, the total body nitrogen as measured by in vivo neutron-activation analysis did not reveal a decline in a group of 24 patients followed while on quotidian nocturnal hemodialysis for 15.7 months.[103] In summary, many nutritional parameters are positively affected by intensive hemodialysis; however, this effect appears to be blunted or absent in patients with significant comorbid conditions. Future work should examine prospectively the impact of intensive hemodialysis on nutritional parameters in larger groups of patients.

Mineral Metabolism

Disorders of mineral metabolism are responsible for significant morbidity and mortality in patients with ESRD. Hyperphosphatemia and an elevated calcium-phosphorus product can contribute to cardiovascular disease in these patients. The independent role of hypercalcemia is less clear.[104] Dietetic restrictions imposed on patients aiming to control hyperphosphatemia can lead to inadequate protein intake. Although the molecular weight of phosphate is low, it is removed by hemodialysis less efficiently than urea, due to its slow mobilization from the intracellular compartment. An early decrease in serum phosphate during hemodialysis, which rebounds prior to and after the end of dialysis, is consistent with this notion.[105] High-flux dialyzers and the convective process can increase phosphate removal; however,

the main determinant of phosphate removal is dialysis duration. Frequency of dialysis also increases phosphate removal, since it allows for daily equilibration of the serum levels, therefore restoring the blood to dialysate gradient.[57] The effect of the different forms of quotidian dialysis on phosphate control is as follows:

Short Daily Hemodialysis. Most of the studies have reported minimal decrease in serum phosphate or phosphate binders unless dialysis time was longer than 2 hours.[73,83,10] Measurement of phosphate in dialysate suggests that phosphate removal increases on short daily hemodialysis, but an increase in protein intake results in no net effect on serum phosphate.[107] No significant changes in PTH levels have been reported.

Quotidian Nocturnal Hemodialysis. The long, frequent dialysis sessions associated with quotidian nocturnal hemodialysis double phosphate removal, allowing discontinuation of phosphate binders and increased dietary phosphate intake.[108] Indeed, in more than 50 percent of patients, complete dietary liberalization does not result in sufficient phosphate intake, so that phosphate must be added to the dialysate.[43,10] Normalization of serum phosphate typically results in normalization of the calcium-phosphorus product and allows a safe increase in the dialysate calcium, which can result in a higher serum calcium and lower PTH levels without the use of vitamin D analogues.[109] The amount of phosphate added to the dialysate can increase significantly in cases of bone repair, during pregnancy, or after suppression of PTH. Tumoral calcinosis resolved in one patient after conversion to quotidian nocturnal hemodialysis.[110]

Patients on quotidian nocturnal hemodialysis may be in negative calcium balance, as they typically no longer receive calcium-containing phosphate binders while facing calcium losses during ultrafiltration.[198,111] Dialysate calcium has to be high enough that the serum calcium rises during dialysis. Intermittent measurement of PTH and alkaline phosphatase levels as well bone densitometry are helpful in individualizing dialysate calcium needs. An increase in PTH or alkaline phosphatase signifies inadequate levels of dialysate calcium. Dialysate calcium levels can be adjusted by the addition of powdered calcium chloride into the acid concentrate until the desired pre- and postdialysis calcium and PTH levels are achieved. By following this approach in our center in 58 patients over 7 years, the average dialysate calcium was 1.63 ± 0.10 mmol/L, serum pre- and postdialysis calcium was 2.4 and 2.68, and phosphorus was 1.23 and 0.87 mmol/L, respectively.[109] PTH levels declined from 580 ± 590 to 228 ± 295 pg/mL. However, these calcium levels may be too high, as bone biopsies in 15 patients revealed a high prevalence of adynamic bone disease.[109] The role of vitamin D analogues in patients on quotidian nocturnal hemodialysis is unknown.

Sleep

Sleep disorders such as sleep apnea, periodic limb movement, and daytime sleepiness are highly prevalent in ESRD patients.[112] Sleep apnea is associated with daytime sleepiness and increased cardiovascular morbidity and mortality.[113] It is present in 50 to 70 percent of ESRD patients and does not improve with conventional hemodialysis or CAPD.[112] Of 14 patients tested prior to nocturnal hemodialysis training, 8 had sleep apnea (57 percent), which had previously been recognized in only 1 patient. Upon conversion to quotidian nocturnal hemodialysis, sleep apnea improved significantly in all but the patient with preexisting sleep apnea. This was associated with an increase in the minimal oxygen saturation.[114] The prevalence of daytime sleepiness in 24 patients on conventional hemodialysis was 54 percent, but it did not change after conversion to quotidian nocturnal hemodialysis.[115] Similarly, there was no improvement in the frequency of periodic limb movements. There are no data on the effects of short daily hemodialysis on sleep disorders.

Patient Survival

Data on patient survival on quotidian hemodialysis are inadequate. In 1999, Woods reported an 80 percent 5-year patient survival on short daily hemodialysis using accessible data.[23]

Daily Hemofiltration

Hemofiltration and hemodiafiltration were described in the 1970s[116] and found to provide better removal of middle molecules through convective solute transfer, better hemodynamic tolerance and BP control. and possibly lower mortality.[117–119] However, the need to infuse a high volume of sterile replacement solution imposed technical and financial demands that prevented the widespread use of these methods. Despite the higher rate of middle-molecule removal and decline of the postdialysis serum levels of beta$_2$ microglobulin, the predialysis levels were unaffected by thrice-weekly hemodiafiltration.[120] In contrast, improved phosphate control has been reported through the use of thrice-weekly hemodiafiltration.[121] Recent technological improvements have allowed the cost-effective on-line production of replacement solution, although the technical complexity of the equipment remains a barrier for home use.[122] There is only limited use of quotidian hemodiafiltration or hemofiltration, with the former recently used in the

in-center setting and the latter at home, using preprepared sterile replacement solution.[30,31] Lower predialysis serum beta$_2$ microglobulin has been reported with quotidian hemodiafiltration.[30] Early clinical results from the use of short daily hemofiltration are encouraging and are similar to the results obtained through the use of short daily hemodialysis, although no incremental benefits have been identified.

Comparison of the Modalities

The choice of the dialysis modality is based on the advantages of the specific method, patient needs, expertise of the dialysis facility, and preference of the patients and care providers. Another significant factor in the choice is the cost of the modality and the structure of the reimbursement system, which affect on the financial sustainability of a modality to dialysis providers and the industry at large. Technological improvements can increase utilization of a modality; in turn, the anticipated utilization of a dialysis method affects further investment in research and development.

At this point there are no adequate studies comparing the various forms of intensive hemodialysis. The main choices are (1) long intermittent hemodialysis performed every second day on either a hemeral or nocturnal schedule and delivered either at home or in center, (2) short daily hemodialysis at home or in center, (3) quotidian nocturnal hemodialysis at home, and (4) short daily hemodiafiltration at home or in center. Quotidian nocturnal hemodialysis is the closest to native kidney function and provides the highest clearance of both small and large molecules while offering the best hemodynamic profile. Other advantages are excellent phosphate control and improvement of sleep apnea. These advantages are to be weighed against the potential for deficiency syndromes, long exposure to dialysis membranes, and safety concerns at night. After almost 10 years of utilizing this modality, no evidence of a negative impact on these issues has been identified.

The only study comparing short daily hemodialysis to quotidian nocturnal hemodialysis was published recently[123]—a prospective nonrandomized study of 11 patients on short daily hemodialysis, 12 patients on nocturnal hemodialysis, and controls on conventional hemodialysis followed for 5 to 36 months. The study confirmed the higher dose delivered with nocturnal hemodialysis as well as better phosphate control. It confirmed improvements in quality of life and BP control for both modalities when compared with conventional hemodialysis. It raised the possibility of better nutritional outcomes on short daily vs. nocturnal hemodialysis. In view of the small number of patients involved and the lack of patient randomization, these questions must be addressed by other studies. There are no studies comparing long intermittent hemodialysis to quotidian hemodialysis.

The main advantage of long intermittent hemodialysis is its favorable financial profile as well as the known improved hemodynamic benefits and increased middle-molecule removal. Hemofiltration has the added advantage of better removal of middle molecules, which may lead to better outcomes. More studies are awaited with interest.

Penetration/Obstacles/The Future

Although no accurate information is available, there are likely about 1000 patients on quotidian hemodialysis. About 400 patients have been trained for home quotidian nocturnal hemodialysis in Canada, the United States, The Netherlands, Australia, Sweden, Germany, Denmark, and elsewhere. The main obstacle to the utilization of quotidian hemodialysis is the unfavorable reimbursement structure. In most countries, the dialysis provider is burdened with increased costs arising from the frequency of the method, but the fiscal benefits in the form of decreased hospitalization rates and decreased medication costs benefit the payer, not the provider. Furthermore, in the United States, the decrease in the utilization of some intravenous medications when quotidian dialysis is used, including rHuEPO and vitamin D analogues, both of which create profits for dialysis centers and decrease the profit margin of the providers, creating a disincentive for adoption of quotidian hemodialysis. For dialysis centers in which the reimbursement structure is based on a capitated system or where the expense of dialysis is paid out of a global hospital budget, quotidian hemodialysis can provide overall cost savings.[124] The favorable financial profile of quotidian hemodialysis is based on the relatively low ratio of the cost of consumables to the cost of labor in developed nations. In countries with higher consumable/labor cost ratios, the quotidian hemodialysis cost can be prohibitive.

The second significant obstacle to the increased utilization of quotidian hemodialysis is related to patients' willingness and ability to perform home hemodialysis. Increasing average age and comorbidity is associated with a decreased ability to be trained. Furthermore, the culture in the dialysis units often does not promote patient self-reliance. This, in combination with the complexity of current hemodialysis machines, decreases the eligibility of patients to a speculated level of about 20 percent. The use of in-center intensive dialysis modalities is obviously not affected by these factors, and the failure to utilize them is related to potentially increased expenses and lack of awareness of their benefits of the methods.

More data collected from randomized controlled studies are needed to improve the reimbursement rates for dialysis and convince payers that the provision of quotidian hemodialysis is warranted.[125] The National Institutes of Health in collaboration with the Centers for Medicare and Medicaid services (CMS) have funded pilot studies in three centers.[126] They will compare prospectively short and nocturnal hemodialysis to conventional hemodialysis. The results of these studies (expected in 2008) may be used to launch randomized controlled studies in the future. A quotidian hemodialysis registry currently in the last stages of development will also be useful in collecting data from many centers and providing pilot data for further studies.[127] In the meantime, the increase in utilization of the methods will be relatively slow and the use of every-other-night hemodialysis should be considered.

CONCLUSION

Despite the lack of prospective randomized controlled studies on quotidian hemodialysis, existing studies consistently demonstrate that quotidian hemodialysis in both short and long forms provides improvement in quality of life, blood pressure control, phosphate control, and likely anemia control as well as improved nutrition. Provided that a solution is found to the reimbursement problem, through either increase in the rates or restructuring of the reimbursement system, quotidian dialysis is likely to become a more prevalent choice in the treatment of ESRD patients. The role of hemofiltration may also grow. These methods, along with every other nightlong hemodialysis modality, will provide revitalization of home hemodialysis, bringing the benefits of increased patient independence and social and vocational rehabilitation to more patients while also providing a solution to the nursing shortage now prevalent in many countries. Studies of all aspects of quotidian hemodialysis are necessary to increase our understanding of the methods and also to provide the data necessary for their appropriate reimbursement.

REFERENCES

1. Blagg CR. A brief history of home hemodialysis. *Adv Renal Replace Ther* 1996;3(2):99–105.
2. USRDS: The United States Renal Data System: overall hospitalization and mortality. *Am J Kidney Dis* 2003;42 (6 suppl 5):S136–S140.
3. Eknoyan G, Beck GJ, Cheung AK, et al. Effect of dialysis dose and membrane flux in maintenance hemodialysis. *N Engl J Med* 2002;347(25):2010–2019.
4. Paniagua R, Amato D, Vonesh E, et al. Effects of increased peritoneal clearances on mortality rates in peritoneal dialysis: ADEMEX, a prospective, randomized, controlled trial. *J Am Soc Nephrol* 2002;13(5):1307–1320.
5. Pierratos A. Daily hemodialysis: why the renewed interest? (see comments). *Am J Kidney Dis* 1998;32(6 suppl 4): S76– S82.

6. Winchester JF. Sorbent hemoperfusion in end-stage renal disease: an in-depth review. *Adv Renal Replace Ther* 2002; 9(1):19–25.

7. Fissell WH, Lou L, Abrishami S, et al. Bioartificial kidney ameliorates gram-negative bacteria-induced septic shock in uremic animals. *J Am Soc Nephrol* 2003;14(2):454–461.

8. Laurent G, Charra B. The results of an 8 h thrice weekly haemodialysis schedule. *Nephrol Dial Transplant* 1998; 13(suppl 6):125–131.

9. Charra B, Calemard E, Cuche M, Laurent G. Control of hypertension and prolonged survival on maintenance hemodialysis. *Nephron* 1983;33(2):96–99.

10. Covic A, Goldsmith DJ, Georgescu G, et al. Echocardiographic findings in long-term, long-hour hemodialysis patients. *Clin Nephrol* 1996;45(2):104–110.

11. Huting J, Kramer W, Charra B, et al. Asymmetric septal hypertrophy and left atrial dilatation in patients with end-stage renal disease on long-term hemodialysis. *Clin Nephrol* 1989;32(6):276–283.

12. Laurent G, Calemard E, Charra B. Dialysis related amyloidosis. *Kidney Int Suppl* 1988;24:S32–S34.

13. Kurella M, Hung A, Tichy M, et al. Intermittent nocturnal in-center hemodialysis: UCSF-Mt Zion experience. *J Am Soc Nephrol* 2002;13:410A.

14. Oberley ET, Schatell DR. Home hemodialysis: survival, quality of life, and rehabilitation. *Adv Renal Replace Ther* 1996;3(2):147–153.

15. Woods JD, Port FK, Stannard D, et al. Comparison of mortality with home hemodialysis and center hemodialysis: a national study. *Kidney Int* 1996;49(5):1464–1470.

16. National Institute for Clinical Excellence. The clinical and cost effectiveness of home compared with hospital haemodialysis for patients with end-stage renal failure. http://www.nice.org.uk/pdf/HvH_full_guidance.pdf 2002.

17. Shaldon S. Independence in maintenance haemodialysis. *Lancet* 1968;1(7541):520.

18. Chertow GM. "Wishing don't make it so"—Why we need a randomized clinical trial of high-intensity hemodialysis. *J Am Soc Nephrol* 2001;12(12):2850–2853.

19. DePalma JR, Pecker EA, Maxwell MH. A new automatic coil dialyser system for "daily" dialysis. *Proc EDTA* 1969;6: 26–34.

20. Snyder D, Louis BM, Gorfien P, Mordujovich J. Clinical experience with long-term brief, "daily" haemodialysis. *Proc EDTA* 1975;11:128–135.

21. Buoncristiani U, Quintaliani G, Cozzari M, et al. Daily dialysis: long-term clinical metabolic results. *Kidney Int* 1988;24:S137–S140.

22. Bonomini V, Mioli V, Albertazzi A, Scolari P. Daily-dialysis programme: indications and results. *Nephrol Dial Transplant* 1998;13(11):2774–2777.

23. Woods JD, Port FK, Orzol S, et al. Clinical and biochemical correlates of starting "daily" hemodialysis. *Kidney Int* 1999; 55(6):2467–2476.

24. Twardowski ZJ. Effect of long term increase in the frequency and/or prolongation of dialysis duration on certain clinical manifestations and results of laboratory investigations in patients with chronic renal failure. *Acta Med Pol* 1975;16:31–44.

25. Twardowski ZJ. Daily dialysis: is this a reasonable option for the new millennium? *Nephrol Dial Transplant* 2001; 16(7):1321–1324.

26. Uldall PR, Francoeur R, Ouwendyk M. Simplified nocturnal home hemodialysis (SNHHD). A new approach to renal replacement therapy. *J Am Soc Nephrol* 1994;5:428.

27. Kjellstrand CM, Ing T. Daily hemodialysis: history and revival of a superior dialysis method. *ASAIO J* 1998;44(3): 117–122.

28. Henderson LW, Ford C, Colton CK, et al. Uremic blood cleansing by diafiltration using a hollow fiber ultrafilter. *Trans Am Soc Artif Intern Organs* 1970;16:107–112.

29. Henderson LW. The beginning of clinical hemofiltration: a personal account. *ASAIO J* 2003;49(5):513–517.

30. Maduell F, Navarro V, Torregrosa E, et al. Change from three times a week on-line hemodiafiltration to short daily on-line hemodiafiltration. *Kidney Int* 2003;64(1):305–313.

31. Zimmerman DL, Swedko PJ, Posen GA, Burns KD. Daily hemofiltration with a simplified method of delivery. *ASAIO J* 2003;49(4):426–429.

32. Twardowski ZJ. PHD: the technological solution for daily haemodialysis? *Nephrol Dial Transplant* 2003;18(1):19–23.

33. Ledebo I, Fredin R. The Gambro system for home daily dialysis. *Semin Dial* 2004;17(2):162–163.

34. Kelly TD. Baxter aurora dialysis system. *Semin Dial* 2004;17(2):154–155

35. Schlaeper C, Diaz-Buxo JA. The Fresenius medical care home hemodialysis system. *Semin Dial* 2004;17(2): 159–161.

36. Ash SR. The Allient dialysis system. *Semin Dial* 2004; 17(2):164–166.

37. Trewin E. Bellco formula domus home care system. *Semin Dial* 2004;17(2):156–158.

38. Clark WR, Turk JE. The NxStage system one. *Semin Dial* 2004;17(2):167–170.

39. Pierratos A, Ouwendyk M, Francoeur R, et al. Nocturnal hemodialysis: three-year experience (see comments). *J Am Soc Nephrol* 1998;9(5):859–868.

40. Yu AW, Soundararajan R, Nawab ZM, et al. Raising plasma phosphorus levels by phosphorus-enriched, bicarbonate-containing dialysate in hemodialysis patients. *Artif Organs* 1992;16(4):414–416.

41. Ing TS, Yu AW, Agrawal B, et al. Increasing plasma phosphorus values by enriching with phosphorus the "acid concentrate" of a bicarbonate-buffered dialysate delivery system. *Int J Artif Organs* 1992;15(12):701–703.

42. Twardowski Z, Kubara H. Different sites versus constant sites of needle insertion into arteriovenous fistulas for treatment by repeated dialysis. *Dial Transplant* 1979;8:978–980.

43. Pierratos A. Nocturnal home haemodialysis: an update on a 5-year experience. *Nephrol Dial Transplant* 1999;14(12): 2835–2840.

44. Hoy CD. Remote monitoring of daily nocturnal hemodialysis. *Hemodial Int* 2001;4:8–12.

45. Heidenheim AP, Leitch R, Kortas C, Lindsay RM. Patient monitoring in the London daily/nocturnal hemodialysis study. *Am J Kidney Dis* 2003;42(1 suppl):61–65.

46. Fenton SS, Schaubel DE, Desmeules M, et al. Hemodialysis versus peritoneal dialysis: a comparison of adjusted mortal-

ity rates (see comments). *Am J Kidney Dis* 1997;30(3): 334–342.

47. Casino FG, Lopez T. The equivalent renal urea clearance: a new parameter to assess dialysis dose. *Nephrol Dial Transplant* 1996;11(8):1574–1581.

48. Depner TA. Daily hemodialysis efficiency: an analysis of solute kinetics. *Adv Renal Replace Ther* 2001;8(4):227–235.

49. Gotch FA. The current place of urea kinetic modelling with respect to different dialysis modalities. *Nephrol Dial Transplant* 1998;13(suppl 6):10–14.

50. Suri R, Depner TA, Blake PG, et al. Adequacy of quotidian hemodialysis. *Am J Kidney Dis* 2003;42(1 suppl):42–48.

51. Clark WR, Leypoldt JK, Henderson LW, et al. Quantifying the effect of changes in the hemodialysis prescription on effective solute removal with a mathematical model. *J Am Soc Nephrol* 1999;10(3):601–609.

52. Leypoldt JK, Jaber BL, Lysaght MJ, et al. Kinetics and dosing predictions for daily haemofiltration. *Nephrol Dial Transplant* 2003;18(4):769–776.

53. Leypoldt JK. Solute fluxes in different treatment modalities. *Nephrol Dial Transplant* 2000;15(suppl 1):3–9.

54. Leypoldt JK, Cheung AK, Carroll CE, et al. Effect of dialysis membranes and middle molecule removal on chronic hemodialysis patient survival. *Am J Kidney Dis* 1999;33(2): 349–355.

55. Cheung AK, Levin NW, Greene T, et al. Effects of high-flux hemodialysis on clinical outcomes: results of the HEMO Study. *J Am Soc Nephrol* 2003;14(12):3251–3263.

56. Goldfarb-Rumyantzev AS, Cheung AK, Leypoldt JK. Computer simulation of small-solute and middle-molecule removal during short daily and long thrice-weekly hemodialysis. *Am J Kidney Dis* 2002;40(6):1211–1218.

57. Pierratos A. Effect of therapy time and frequency on effective solute removal. *Semin Dial* 2001;14(4):284–288.

58. Raj DS, Ouwendyk M, Francoeur R, Pierratos A. Beta(2)-microglobulin kinetics in nocturnal haemodialysis. *Nephrol Dial Transplant* 2000;15(1):58–64.

59. Floridi A, Antolini F, Galli F, et al. Daily haemodialysis improves indices of protein glycation. *Nephrol Dial Transplant* 2002;17(5):871–878.

60. Cacho C, Erhard P, Priester A, et al. Nocturnal dialysis reduces serum pentosidine in patients with ESRD. *Perit Dial Int* 2001;21(suppl 1):S61.

61. Friedman AN, Bostom AG, Levey AS, et al. Plasma total homocysteine levels among patients undergoing nocturnal versus standard hemodialysis. *J Am Soc Nephrol* 2002;13(1): 265–268.

62. Spanner E, Suri R, Heidenheim AP, Lindsay RM. The impact of quotidian hemodialysis on nutrition. *Am J Kidney Dis* 2003;42(1 suppl):30–35.

63. Laupacis A, Feeny D, Detsky AS, Tugwell PX. How attractive does a new technology have to be to warrant adoption and utilization? Tentative guidelines for using clinical and economic evaluations (see comments). *CMAJ* 1992;146 (4):473–481.

64. Cheng IK. Peritoneal dialysis in Asia. *Perit Dial Int* 1996;16(suppl 1):S381–S385.

65. Rao M, Juneja R, Shirly RB, Jacob CK. Haemodialysis for end-stage renal disease in Southern India—a perspective from a tertiary referral care centre (news). *Nephrol Dial Transplant* 1998;13(10):2494–2500.

66. Mittal S, Kher V, Gulati S, et al. Chronic renal failure in India. *Renal Failure* 1997;19(6):763–770.

67. Barton EN, Williams W, Morgan AG, Burden RP. A prospective study of ward referrals for renal disease at a Jamaican and a United Kingdom hospital. *West Indian Med J* 1996;45(4):110–112.

68. McFarlane PA, Mendelssohn DC. A call to arms: economic barriers to optimal dialysis care. *Perit Dial Int* 2000;20(1): 7–12.

69. McFarlane PA, Pierratos A, Redelmeier DA. Cost savings of home nocturnal versus conventional in-center hemodialysis. *Kidney Int* 2002;62(6):2216–2222.

70. Kroeker A, Clark WF, Heidenheim AP, et al. An operating cost comparison between conventional and home quotidian hemodialysis. *Am J Kidney Dis* 2003;42(1 Suppl):49–55.

71. Ting G, Carrie B, Freitas T, Zarghamee S. Global ESRD costs associated with a short daily hemodialysis program in the United States. *Home Hemodial Int* 1999;3:41–44.

72. Mohr PE, Neumann PJ, Franco SJ, et al. The case for daily dialysis: its impact on costs and quality of life. *Am J Kidney Dis* 2001;37(4):777–789.

73. Ting GO, Kjellstrand C, Freitas T, et al. Long-term study of high-comorbidity ESRD patients converted from conventional to short daily hemodialysis. *Am J Kidney Dis* 2003; 42(5):1020–1035.

74. McFarlane PA. Reducing hemodialysis costs: conventional and quotidian home hemodialysis in Canada. *Semin Dial* 2004;17(2):118–124.

75. Lee H, Manns B, Taub K, et al. Cost analysis of ongoing care of patients with end-stage renal disease: the impact of dialysis modality and dialysis access. *Am J Kidney Dis* 2002;40(3):611–622.

76. Goeree R, Manalich J, Grootendorst P, et al. Cost analysis of dialysis treatments for end-stage renal disease (ESRD). *Clin Invest Med* 1995;18(6):455–464.

77. Bell CM, Chapman RH, Stone PW, et al. An off-the-shelf help list: a comprehensive catalog of preference scores from published cost-utility analyses. *Med Decision Making* 2001; 21(4):288–294.

78. Drummond MF, O'Brien BJ, Stoddart GL, Torrance GW. *Methods for the Economic Evaluation of Health Care Programmes*, 2d ed. Oxford, UK: Oxford University Press, 1997.

79. Russell LB, Gold MR, Siegel JE, et al. The role of cost-effectiveness analysis in health and medicine. Panel on Cost-Effectiveness in Health and Medicine (comment). *JAMA* 1996;276(14):1172–1177.

80. McFarlane PA, Bayoumi AM, Pierratos A, Redelmeier DA. The quality of life and cost utility of home nocturnal and conventional in-center hemodialysis. *Kidney Int* 2003;64(3): 1004–1011.

81. Heidenheim AP, Muirhead N, Moist L, Lindsay RM. Patient quality of life on quotidian hemodialysis. *Am J Kidney Dis* 2003;42(1 suppl):36–41.

82. Brissenden JE, Pierratos A, Ouwendyk M, Roscoe JM. Improvements in quality of life with nocturnal hemodialysis. *J Am Soc Nephrol* 1998;9:168A.

83. Kooistra MP, Vos J, Koomans HA, Vos PF. Daily home haemodialysis in The Netherlands: effects on metabolic control, haemodynamics, and quality of life. *Nephrol Dial Transplant* 1998;13(11):2853–2860.

84. Fagugli RM, Reboldi G, Quintaliani G, et al. Short daily hemodialysis: blood pressure control and left ventricular mass reduction in hypertensive hemodialysis patients. *Am J Kidney Dis* 2001;38(2):371–376.

85. Lockridge RSJ, Albert J, Andrerson H, et al. Nightly home hemodialysis: fifteen months of experience in Lynchburg, Virginia. *Home Hemodial Int* 1999;3:23–28.

86. Chan CT, Floras JS, Miller JA, et al. Regression of left ventricular hypertrophy after conversion to nocturnal hemodialysis. *Kidney Int* 2002;61(6):2235–2239.

87. Nesrallah G, Suri R, Moist L, et al. Volume control and blood pressure management in patients undergoing quotidian hemodialysis. *Am J Kidney Dis* 2003;42(1 suppl):13–17.

88. Chan C, Floras JS, Miller JA, Pierratos A. Improvement in ejection fraction by nocturnal haemodialysis in end-stage renal failure patients with coexisting heart failure. *Nephrol Dial Transplant* 2002;17(8):1518–1521.

89. Chan CT, Mardirossian S, Faratro R, Richardson RM. Improvement in lower-extremity peripheral arterial disease by nocturnal hemodialysis. *Am J Kidney Dis* 2003;41(1):225–229.

90. Chan CT, Harvey PJ, Picton P, et al. Short-term blood pressure, noradrenergic, and vascular effects of nocturnal home hemodialysis. *Hypertension* 2003;42(5):925–931.

91. McCormick BB, Pierratos A, Fenton S, et al. Review of clinical outcomes in nocturnal haemodialysis patients after renal transplantation. *Nephrol Dial Transplant* 2004;19(3):714–719.

92. Tsuji H, Larson MG, Venditti FJ Jr, et al. Impact of reduced heart rate variability on risk for cardiac events. The Framingham Heart Study. *Circulation* 1996;94(11):2850–2855.

93. Fukuta H, Hayano J, Ishihara S, et al. Prognostic value of heart rate variability in patients with end-stage renal disease on chronic haemodialysis. *Nephrol Dial Transplant* 2003;18(2):318–325.

94. Chan CT, Hanly P, Gabor J, et al. Impact of nocturnal hemodialysis on the variability of heart rate and duration of hypoxemia during sleep. *Kidney Int* 2004;65(2):661–665.

95. Zilch O, Vos PF, Oey LP, et al. Daily dialysis reduces peripheral vascular resistance and sympathetic activity. *J Am Soc Nephrol* 2001;12:280A.

96. Odar-Cederlof IE, Bjellerup P, Juhlin-Dannfelt A, et al. Brain natriuretic peptide (BNP) in plasma reflects left ventricular (LV) dysfunction in hemodialysis (HD) patients and decreases with daily dialysis. *J Am Soc Nephrol* 2001;12:404A.

97. Odar-Cederlof I, Ericsson F, Theodorsson E, Kjellstrand CM. Neuropeptide-Y and atrial natriuretic peptide as prognostic markers in patients on hemodialysis. *ASAIO J* 2003;49(1):74–80.

98. Schwartz D, Pierratos A, Richardson RMA, et al. Impact of nocturnal home hemodialysis on anemia management in patients with end-stage renal disease. *J Am Soc Nephrol* 2003;14:498A.

99. Lowrie EG, Lew NL. Death risk in hemodialysis patients: the predictive value of commonly measured variables and an evaluation of death rate differences between facilities. *Am J Kidney Dis* 1990;15(5):458–482.

100. Kaysen GA, Dubin JA, Muller HG, et al. Relationships among inflammation nutrition and physiologic mechanisms establishing albumin levels in hemodialysis patients. *Kidney Int* 2002;61(6):2240–2249.

101. Galland R, Traeger J, Arkouche W, et al. Short daily hemodialysis rapidly improves nutritional status in hemodialysis patients. *Kidney Int* 2001;60(4):1555–1560.

102. Raj DS, Ouwendyk M, Francoeur R, Pierratos A. Plasma amino acid profile on nocturnal hemodialysis. *Blood Purif* 2000;18(2):97–102.

103. Pierratos A, Ouwendyk M, Rassi M. Total Body nitrogen increases on nocturnal hemodialysis. *J Am Soc Nephrol* 1999;10:299A.

104. Block GA, Hulbert-Shearon TE, Levin NW, Port FK. Association of serum phosphorus and calcium x phosphate product with mortality risk in chronic hemodialysis patients: a national study. *Am J Kidney Dis* 1998;31(4):607–617.

105. DeSoi CA, Umans JG. Phosphate kinetics during high-flux hemodialysis. *J Am Soc Nephrol* 1993;4(5):1214–1218.

106. Chan CT, Murali K, Ilumin M, Richardson RMA. Improvement in phosphate control with short daily in–center hemodialysis (SDHD). *J Am Soc Nephrol* 2001;12:262A.

107. Traeger J, Galland R, Ferrier ML, Delawari E. Optimal control of phosphatemia by short daily hemodialysis. *J Am Soc Nephrol* 2002;13:410A–411A.

108. Mucsi I, Hercz G, Uldall R, et al. Control of serum phosphate without any phosphate binders in patients treated with nocturnal hemodialysis. *Kidney Int* 1998;53(5):1399–1404.

109. Pierratos A, Hercz G, Sherrard DJ, et al. Calcium, phosphorus metabolism and bone pathology on long term nocturnal hemodialysis. *J Am Soc Nephrol* 2001;12:274A.

110. Kim SJ, Goldstein M, Szabo T, Pierratos A. Resolution of massive uremic tumoral calcinosis with daily nocturnal home hemodialysis. *Am J Kidney Dis* 2003;41(3):E12.

111. Al Hejaili F, Kortas C, Leitch R, et al. Nocturnal but not short hours quotidian hemodialysis requires an elevated dialysate calcium concentration. *J Am Nephrol* 2003;14(9):2322–2328.

112. Parker KP. Sleep disturbances in dialysis patients. *Sleep Med Rev* 2003;7(2):131–143.

113. Hung J, Whitford EG, Parsons RW, Hillman DR. Association of sleep apnoea with myocardial infarction in men. *Lancet* 1990;336(8710):261–264.

114. Hanly PJ, Pierratos A. Improvement of sleep apnea in patients with chronic renal failure who undergo nocturnal hemodialysis. *N Engl J Med* 2001;344(2):102–107.

115. Hanly PJ, Gabor JY, Chan C, Pierratos A. Daytime sleepiness in patients with CRF: impact of nocturnal hemodialysis. *Am J Kidney Dis* 2003;41(2):403–410.

116. Henderson LW, Silverstein ME, Ford CA, Lysaght MJ. Clinical response to maintenance hemodiafiltration. *Kidney Int Suppl* 1975;(2):58–63.

117. Altieri P, Sorba G, Bolasco P, et al. Predilution haemofiltration—the Second Sardinian Multicentre Study: comparisons

between haemofiltration and haemodialysis during identical Kt/V and session times in a long-term cross-over study. *Nephrol Dial Transplant* 2001;16(6):1207–1213.

118. Baldamus CA, Quellhorst E. Outcome of long-term hemofiltration. *Kidney Int Suppl* 1985;17:S41–S46.

119. Locatelli F, Marcelli D, Conte F, et al. Comparison of mortality in ESRD patients on convective and diffusive extracorporeal treatments. The Registro Lombardo Dialisi E Trapianto. *Kidney Int* 1999;55(1):286–293.

120. Ward RA, Schmidt B, Hullin J, et al. A comparison of online hemodiafiltration and high-flux hemodialysis: a prospective clinical study. *J Am Soc Nephrol* 2000;11(12): 2344–2350.

121. Minutolo R, Bellizzi V, Cioffi M, et al. Postdialytic rebound of serum phosphorus: pathogenetic and clinical insights. *J Am Soc Nephrol* 2002;13(4):1046–1054.

122. Ledebo I. On-line hemodiafiltration: technique and therapy. *Adv Renal Replace Ther* 1999;6(2):195–208.

123. Lindsay RM. Introduction. *Am J Kidney Dis* 2003; 42 (1 suppl):3–4.

124. Hannah RG. The role of managed care in daily dialysis. *ASAIO J* 2001;47(5):462–463.

125. Briggs JP. Evidence-based medicine in the dialysis unit: a few lessons from the USRDS and from the NCDS and HEMO trials. *Semin Dial* 2004;17(2):136–141.

126. NIH. Frequent Hemodialysis Clinical Trials. http://grants1.nih.gov/grants/guide/rfa-files/RFA-DK-03–005.html. 2003.

127. Nesrallah G, Moist L, Awaraji C, Lindsay RL. An international registry to compare quotidian dialysis regimens with conventional thrice-weekly hemodialysis: why, how, and potential pitfalls. *Semin Dial* 2004;17(2):131–135.

Hemodialysis Access in Children

Walter S. Andrews

Peritoneal dialysis tends to be the preferred dialysis modality for children. However, hemodialysis is still an important component of the management of end-stage renal disease (ESRD) in children. This is especially true in situations when peritoneal dialysis is either not feasible or impractical. Some of the indications for the usage of hemodialysis over peritoneal dialysis would include anatomic problems, such as the presence of an ileostomy or an ureterocutaneostomy; chronic pulmonary disease; recent abdominal surgery; leaking peritoneal dialysis catheter; or severe colitis. Other possible indications for hemodialysis could include concern about the ability of the family to manage peritoneal dialysis or the peritoneal catheter, or patient or family preference for hemodialysis.

In the latest review of the North American Pediatrics Renal Transplant Cooperative Study (NAPRTCS)(2003),[1] 40 percent of the patients who were started on renal replacement therapy were started on hemodialysis. As in peritoneal dialysis, the long-term Achilles heel of hemodialysis has been the creation of a stable vascular access.

This chapter reviews different types of hemodialysis access and their use in children. It must be pointed out, however, that the data on the use of these different types of hemodialysis access in children are relatively few. When possible, aggregate data are given; but in some areas, due to the lack of data, single-center reports are reviewed.

Three predominant types of vascular access are utilized in children: the hemodialysis vascular access catheter, the autogenous arteriovenous (AV) fistula, and the AV graft, which can be constructed from a variety of different materials. These different types of access are discussed in detail, along with their associated benefits and potential complications.

HEMODIALYSIS VASCULAR ACCESS CATHETERS

Many types of hemodialysis access catheters are available on the market. They are either uncuffed or cuffed: meaning that there is either the presence or absence of a woven Dacron cuff on the catheter. The purpose of the cuff is to provide a tissue seal around the catheter to prevent ascending bacterial infections. The catheters are also divided into double-lumen fixed catheters, double-lumen split catheters

(Ash Split Cath, MEDCOMP, Harleysville, PA), and the Tesio catheter system (two separate single-lumen catheters, which are used for the arterial and venous access, respectively).

Uncuffed Catheters

Uncuffed double-lumen fixed catheters are generally used for acute hemodialysis. These catheters come in a variety of sizes (7, 9, and 11.5F) to accommodate different patients. The absence of a cuff allows these catheters to be put in percutaneously, requiring only local anesthesia with or without intravenous sedation. It is not unusual for these catheters to be placed in the pediatric intensive care unit in children requiring acute renal replacement therapy.

Unfortunately, the operational life of these catheters is relatively short, usually due to infectious or thrombotic complications. There is little literature regarding the use of uncuffed catheters in children. Goldstein et al. reviewed the outcomes of 80 catheters placed acutely in 23 pediatric patients.[2] The median survival of the uncuffed catheters was 31 days and their 2-month actuarial survival was 48 percent. In this series, the majority of uncuffed catheters (39 percent) were removed electively. The most common complication leading to uncuffed catheter removal was catheter kinking (36 percent). Eight percent of the uncuffed catheters were lost due to infection, making for a catheter infection rate of 0.58 catheters per patient-year.

Cuffed Catheters

Cuffed catheters are the most common type used for more permanent hemodialysis access. In a review of the 1994 NAPRTCS database, Bunchman noted that 36 percent of the children were maintained on hemodialysis; at that time, cuffed catheters were utilized in 63 percent of the patients.[3] Of these catheters, 82 percent were in the subclavian vein, 12 percent in the internal jugular vein, and 6 percent in the femoral vein. On rereviewing these data, one finds that not much has changed (Fig. 44–1).[1] Still, the majority of children are undergoing hemodialysis via a cuffed catheter (79.2 percent). Slightly fewer catheters were placed in the subclavian position (63 percent) and significantly more in the internal jugular position (32 percent). There was no change in the percentage of catheters placed in the femoral position (4 percent). The major complications associated with cuffed catheters are infection, thrombosis, and kinking or trauma to the catheter.

Infection rates associated with pediatric catheters are reported variously in either infections per patient-year or infectious episodes per 1000 catheter days. In children, the catheter infection rates have been reported to be 0.46 infec-

HEMODIALYSIS ACCESS*

	N (2315)	% (100)
External Percutaneous Catheter	1833	79.2
Subclavian vein	1151	
Jugular vein	591	
Femoral vein	80	
Single lumen	61	
Double lumen	1761	
External Arteriovenous Shunt	7	0.3
Internal Arteriovenous Fistula	274	11.8
Internal Arteriovenous Graft	201	8.7
Autologous vein	7	
Bovine graft		1
PTFE graft	185	
Other graft	4	

*Twenty-four HD courses had missing values.

Figure 44–1. Types of pediatric vascular access noted in the 2003 NAPRTCS review. (From NAPRTCS.[1] With permission.)

tions per patient-year or 1.1 to 1.6 infections per 1000 catheter days.[2,4-6] These figures compare favorably with the reported adult catheter infection rates of between 0.26 and 1.23 catheter infections per year or 0.29 vs. 3.36 catheter infections per 1000 catheter days.[7-9] The most common infecting organism is *Staphylococcus*.[5,10]

Treatment of a catheter infection starts with antibiotics, but antibiotics alone have yielded a catheter salvage rate of less than 20 percent.[10] Besides systemic antibiotic treatment, such a catheter can be salvaged by removing it and exchanging it over a guidewire for a new catheter. In the absence of a tunnel-site infection, exchange of a cuffed catheter over a guidewire was able to increase the 1-year catheter survival rates from 27 to 92 percent.[6] Several adult series report successful catheter salvage using an exchange over a guidewire for both infection and thrombosis. With this aggressive approach, a significant improvement in catheter survival rates has been noticed, from 54 percent at 1 year to 75 percent at 4 years.[11-15] Despite these optimistic outcomes, cuffed catheters carry a substantially higher risk of infection than other types of hemodialysis access. Using a relative risk scale with AV fistulas as 1, cuffed hemodialysis catheters carry a relative risk of 7.6.[10] This increased risk of infection must always be kept in mind in selecting a cuffed catheter for long-term hemodialysis access.

Thrombosis rates for cuffed catheters are reported to run between 1.88 and 2.2 episodes per 1000 catheter days.[2,16] These catheters again can be salvaged by a variety of techniques, including catheter exchange over a guidewire, thrombolytic therapy, or catheter stripping for the removal of an obstructing fibrin sheath. This last technique is performed by the interventional radiologist.

Another problem associated with long-term catheter usage is stenosis or thrombosis of the vessel through which the catheter has been placed. For this reason, several authors now feel that the subclavian route for the insertion of a dialysis catheter is no longer acceptable and that only the internal jugular vein should be utilized.[11] Stenosis or thrombosis of the subclavian vein renders that extremity unusable for later construction of an AV fistula or AV graft, thereby eliminating a potential site for hemodialysis access.

The Tesio catheter system is unique in that it uses two separate catheters for the arterial and venous limbs as opposed to a single catheter with two lumens. The data on the Tesio catheter are somewhat better than those reported for standard double-lumen catheters. In a study by Sheth et al., a median catheter survival of 322 days for the Tesio catheter system vs. 91 days for a dual-lumen catheter system was noted.[17] This translated to a 1-year actuarial survival rate for the Tesio catheter at 46 vs. 0 percent for the double-lumen catheters.[2,18] The Tesio system also had a lower catheter infection rate of only 1 episode per 20 catheter months.

In summary, our current approach for the placement of a cuffed hemodialysis catheter is the internal jugular vein. At present, we are using the Ash catheter (Figs. 44–2 and 44–3). This catheter combines the ease of insertion of a single-lumen catheter with the benefit of two separate catheters in the vascular system. The catheters are carefully monitored for any infectious or thrombotic complications. If these occur, they are best treated with intravenous antibiotic therapy (for infection) followed by catheter exchange over a guidewire. With these techniques, it appears very reasonable that catheters should be able to function for at least a year in the pediatric population.

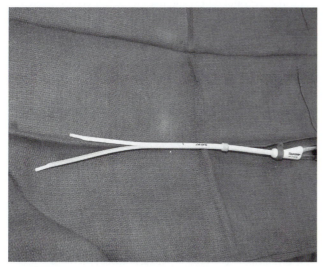

Figure 44–2. Ash split catheter. (Courtesy of MEDCOMP, Harleysville, PA.)

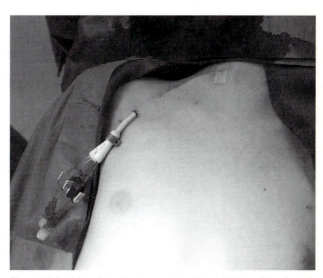

Figure 44–3. Ash catheter in place entering the right internal jugular vein and exiting on the anterior chest wall.

NONMECHANICAL-ACCESS THROMBOSIS

One of the most common reasons for loss of any form of hemodialysis access is thrombosis. The reasons for thrombosis vary widely depending on the access type. With hemodialysis catheters, the reason for thrombosis usually includes the presence of the fibrin sheath or of clot within the catheter. With AV fistulas, it is usually because of either arterial inflow or venous outflow stenosis; in patients with AV grafts, the most common reason is intimal hypertrophy on the venous side of the graft at the graft-vein junction. However, there has always been the concern that hemodialysis patients can be "hypercoagulable." A variety of conditions can cause a hypercoagulable state. Among the chemicals and antibodies that have been implicated in causing a hypercoagulable state are homocysteine, and anticardiolipin, antiphospholipid, and anti–heparin platelet factor IV antibodies.

Hyperhomocystinemia has been identified as a risk factor in arterial and venous thrombotic events.[19–21] Hyperhomocystinemia is also noted to be prevalent in the dialysis-dependent ESRD population.[22] The question then becomes is it possible that hyperhomocystinemia can potentially have an influence on dialysis access thrombosis? Shemin et al. found an independent association between plasma total homocysteine levels and the risk for access thrombosis.[23] However, a study by Hojs et al. noted no significant differences in total homocysteine concentrations between thrombosis prone and non–thrombosis prone dialysis patients.[24] These findings were similar to the findings of Manns et al. and Tamura et al., who again found no significant difference in the plasma homocysteine concentrations between thrombosis-prone and control dialysis groups.[25,26] Manns et al. studied 118 patients, among whom 30 percent had episodes of vascular access thrombosis.[26] Again, when mean plasma homocysteine levels were measured, there was no difference in levels between those patients who had at least one documented episode of vascular access thrombosis and those who had no such episodes.

Whereas there seems to be some uncertainty as to the contribution of homocysteine to vascular access thrombosis, the literature appears to favor the concept that hyperhomocystinemia is not a direct contributor to vascular access thrombosis. The treatment for hyperhomocystinemia is high-dosage folic acid. Whereas such a regimen has been shown to decrease homocysteine levels, there are no data showing a concomitant drop in the rate of vascular access thrombosis.

Anticardiolipin antibodies have also been associated with thrombotic events.[27–29] Valeri et al. looked for the presence of anticardiolipin antibodies prospectively in 230 dialysis patients.[30] They found that patients with elevated anticardiolipin antibodies who also had AV grafts tended to have shorter mean and median graft survival times. They also felt that the risk of thrombosis with elevated anticardiolipin antibody levels was independent of the increased risk of thrombosis associated with an AV graft alone. Their findings were supported by a study by Sallam et al.,[31] who found, in children between the ages of 5 and 18 years, a very strong association between positive anticardiolipin antibodies and thrombosis of AV fistulas. A total of 70 percent of patients with positive anticardiolipin antibodies were found to have had a thrombosis of their vascular access. Haviv et al. also found a positive correlation between elevated anticardiolipin antibodies and recurrent AV access occlusions.[32] Manns et al., looking at anticardiolipin antibody status, found that none of their patients had an elevated anticardiolipin antibody level, including those with vascular access thrombosis.[26] Therefore they concluded that high titers of anticardiolipin antibody were not an important predisposing factor to the development of graft thrombosis.

Again, there are data in the literature both for and against the utility of looking for elevated anticardiolipin antibody levels as a potential risk factor for vascular access thrombosis. The current recommendations for treatment of an elevated anticardiolipin antibody level include low-molecular-weight heparin or oral warfarin. Since neither of these treatment modalities is totally benign, they should generally not be used until a patient has had an episode of graft thrombosis.

Another potential condition of hypercoagulability that has been evaluated is the presence of anti–heparin platelet factor IV antibodies. These were investigated by O'Shey et al. in their hemodialysis population.[33] In their group, only 1 percent of the patients tested weekly proved to be positive for the anti–heparin platelet factor IV antibody, and none had a significant history of AV thrombosis or thrombocy-topenia. The authors therefore concluded that the prevalence of anti–heparin platelet factor IV antibodies was probably low in hemodialysis patients and therefore was not a significant risk factor for graft thrombosis.

AV FISTULAS AND AV GRAFTS IN CHILDREN

The AV fistula has been utilized in children for a number of years. In 1973, Boyer et al. reported a 54 percent success rate of radiocephalic fistula in children who weighed less than 20 kg.[34] This weight range was extended down to children who weighed less than 10 kg by Bourquelot et al., who reported creating successful distal AV fistulas using a microsurgical technique.[35] This technique was then picked up by a variety of authors and by 1984 some were reporting a 100 percent patency rate in association with the microsurgical technique in children weighing less than 20 kg.[36] Bagolin et al. reviewed their 11-year experience, between 1985 and 1994, with AV fistulas in children.[37] They noted a primary patency rate of 89 percent in children who weighed less than 15 kg and a 90 percent patency rate in children who weighed more than 15 kg. At 4 years after AV fistula replacement, the patency rate was 70 percent in patients who weighed more than 15 kg and 57 percent in those who weighed less than 15 kg. These authors found early complications in 9 percent of their 90 patients. This included mostly thrombosis of the AV fistula and a hematoma at the operative site. Both these complications were treated successfully by surgical intervention. They found late complications in 26 percent of their patients, which included thrombosis and severe stenosis at the anastomotic site. They strongly proposed the use of microsurgical techniques in creation of the AV fistula by using 8 to 10-0 sutures in creation of the AV fistula and using an operative microscope. They also recommended the use of the upper-arm ischemia technique, where the arm is exsanguinated and a tourniquet is applied during creation of the AV fistula. In this way, there is no spasm of the artery because no clamps or vessel loops are utilized and the anastomosis is created in a bloodless field.[38]

Lumsden et al. reported their experience with hemodialysis access in 24 children between 1985 and 1992.[16] They utilized a variety of techniques for establishing access, including 15 AV fistulas, 37 expanded polytetrafluoroethylene (ePTFE) bridge grafts, 9 bovine AV bridge grafts, and 29 chronic central venous catheters. Their mean fistula patency rate was 6.2 ± 10.2 months; one-third of the fistulas failed to mature enough to be used.

In their upper extremity ePTFE grafts, Lumsden et al. found a mean functional patency of 11 ± 11.1 months; but in their groin loops, their primary patency was only 4.1 ± 5 months. In their ePTFE group, there were eight graft infections, which all resulted in graft loss. The ePTFE grafts required numerous thrombectomies as well as patch angioplasties for outflow of stenosis. The thrombectomies and repair of outflow obstructions extended the patency of the ePTFE grafts to 10.5 ± 17 months.

In their chronic indwelling venous hemodialysis catheters, Lumsden et al. note that the mean duration of dialysis was 8.1 ± 6.9 weeks. The catheter failures were due to a combination of catheter infections and thrombosis. They note that each patient had multiple different dialysis access procedures and that the mean dialysis time provided by each type of dialysis access was only 7.3 months.

Overall, the recommendations of Lumsden et al. were to use central venous dialysis catheters for children weighing less than 20 kg, especially in those who could be transplanted within 6 to 12 months. In older children or children weighing more than than 30 kg, they recommend primary AV fistulas first; only if these failed would they go to ePTFE grafts. They advocate the use of hemodialysis catheters in smaller children due to their decreased success rates with AV fistulas in this population. They also recommended that if a Brescia-Cimino fistula is not feasible, their second choice would be a fistula from the brachial artery to the cephalic vein in children weighing more than than 20 kg. They emphasize the fact that a native AV fistula takes time to mature and therefore is not suitable for patients who require immediate access for hemodialysis. In their series, even though they had a mean patency rate of 11 months, they felt that their ePTFE bridge grafts functioned poorly in children who weighed less than 30 kg, and these grafts often required multiple revisions. They also strongly discouraged the use of ePTFE grafts in the lower extremities secondary to poor patency and a potential damage to the iliac veins, thereby making future transplantation much more difficult.

Brittinger et al. reviewed their experience with 784 access procedures that were done over 20 years in children between 2 and 18 years of age.[39] The vast majority of these procedures (63 percent) were AV fistulas created in the wrist. Their preference was to begin at the wrist with an end-to-side anastomosis between the radial artery and the cephalic vein. They felt that the side-to-side fistula in the wrist led to very high shunt flow rates with a subsequent 30 percent incidence of steal syndrome in the wrist. If the wrist was not suitable, their second choice was a fistula in the upper arm or antecubital fossa from the brachial artery to the cephalic vein. If the cephalic vein was not suitable, then they moved to the basilic vein. However, they recommend a two-step procedure, where the fistula between the brachial artery and the basilic vein is created initially, followed, in 10 days, by a transposition of the basilic vein from its usual deep position to a subcutaneous position to make it accessible for dialysis.

Expanded PTFE grafts were used in 13 percent of their accesses. A majority of the grafts placed by Brittinger et al. were thigh grafts in younger children (2 to 10 years of age)

and then arm grafts in the group 15 to 18 years of age. They recommend using grafts between 6 and 7 mm to prevent high shunt flows. As far as graft technique, they recommend the forearm loop graft if the upper extremity is going to be utilized. They extend the arterial portion of the loop across the elbow to be a straight part of the brachial artery. They then anastomose the venous portion to either the basilic or cephalic vein above the elbow. They also recommend this loop type of graft over using a straight graft between the brachial artery and the axillary vein. They advocate the loop because the most common problem with grafts is venous outflow stenosis secondary to intimal hyperplasia. If the venous anastomosis is lower in the arm, the graft can usually be salvaged by either a patch graft or an interposition graft bridging the stenotic lesion. This is very difficult to do if the venous portion of the graft is in the axilla.

Brittinger et al. also advocate thigh grafts as a suitable alternative in small children. They report that their experience with thigh grafts was very acceptable, with 12-month complication-free function rates between 50 and 75 percent, depending on the age group, vs. 69 percent for their upper arm grafts.

When Brittinger et al. reviewed their complications, overall their most common complication was intimal hyperplasia, which caused stenosis in one-third of their patients. This was corrected by either creating another anastomosis between the artery and vein distal to the stenotic lesion or using a bypass graft around the stenotic lesion. They also stated the second most common cause of problems with their fistulas or grafts was repeated needle punctures in the same area of the graft or fistula (22 percent). They felt that this was not a major problem in AV fistulas, and the short stenotic segments that occur because of this usually can be treated with a patch angioplasty. However, in the case of AV grafts, repeated cannulations in the same area can cause false aneurysms, which can then become infected and ultimately lead to graft demise. In this situation, they again recommend bypassing these aneurysms. They feel that an infected false aneurysm is a high-level surgical urgency and must be removed, followed by bypass of that portion of the graft.

Brittinger et al. report that infection was fairly rare and usually easily treated in autogenous access types. In prosthetic grafts, however, infection is a severe complication for both the graft and the patient. Mortalities have been reported in those patients where systemic infection is associated with the infected graft.[40,41] In general, if an infection occurs within weeks of graft placement, the entire graft must almost always be removed. If the graft has been in place for some time and is well integrated into the tissue, then the infected segment can often be removed and a bypass graft placed. However, if the patient has severe systemic sepsis or if the sepsis does not resolve after removal of the infected portion of the graft, the entire graft must be removed.

HEMODIALYSIS ACCESS MONITORING

The most significant problem leading to graft or fistula failure is stenosis of the fistula. Such stenosis can occur either in the arterial limb, at the arterial venous anastomosis itself, or in the venous limb of the graft. The premise has been that early detection of this stenosis prior to thrombosis can then lead to either a surgical or interventional radiologic approach that could correct the stenosis before the fistula thromboses.

In a recent publication, the National Kidney Foundation–Kidney Disease Outcomes Quality Initiative (NKF-K/DOQI) has recommended that the measurement of access flow (Qa) is the preferred method of surveillance of both AV fistulas and ePTFE grafts.[42] Garland et al. reviewed a variety of techniques to determine Qa.[43] These included ultrasound dilution, measurements of differential conductivity between arterial and venous flows, thermodilution techniques, and hemodilution techniques.[44] These investigators concluded that the ultrasound dilution technique was the current "gold standard" for measurement of Qa. The NKF-K/DOQI recommendations are that the Qa measurements be performed on AV fistulas and AV grafts monthly and that a significant stenosis is defined is > 50 percent reduction in normal vessel diameter associated with hemodynamic, functional, or clinical abnormalities. Their suggestions are that an access with a Qa of less than 600 mL/min or less than a 1000 mL/min that is decreased by more than 25 percent over 4 months should be referred for a fistulogram.[42] Garland et al. point out that multiple studies do support a correlation between low Qa and eventual graft thrombosis.[45–47]

In an attempt to determine whether the above parameters were in fact useful in predicting graft failure, Lumsden et al. did a randomized study utilizing prophylactic balloon angioplasty in ePTFE grafts that showed decreased flows followed by a fistulogram that showed a > 50 percent stenosis.[48] Interestingly, their study showed no advantage to prophylactic angioplasty in preventing graft thrombosis. However, they did not evaluate Qa postprocedure to see whether, in fact, there was an improvement.[48] Two subsequent studies have shown that if the postangioplasty flow was not increased to within 20 percent of the preangioplasty flow or if the increase in postangioplasty flow was less than 50 percent, these grafts had significantly less survival and potentially should warrant surgical intervention.[49,50]

On the basis of these data, it seems reasonable that vascular accesses should be screened routinely. If a problem is detected, a fistulogram should be performed; if a stenosis is discovered, the patient should undergo interventional radiologic treatment. This approach has been shown to be cost-effective and it significantly prolongs vascular access patency.

Goldstein et al. evaluated the NKF-K/DOQI information and applied them to a pediatric population.[51] In this study they adapted the NKF-K/DOQI Qa flow recommendations to children by correcting the flow measurements to 1.73 m[2]. They noted that no patient with a Qa flow rate of > 700 mL/min/1.73 m[2] developed thrombosis within 30 days of their ultrasound dilution flow measurement, whereas patients with a Qa of < 600 mL/min/1.73 m[2] developed thrombosis within 1 week after measurement.

Dynamic venous pressure monitoring has been reported as a technique commonly used to monitor vascular access in children on hemodialysis.[52,53] However, there have been some studies suggesting that venous pressure monitoring may be at best a late predictor of access malfunction or, at worst, no predictor at all. Chand et al., using venous pressure monitors in a study of 10 children, found that monitoring of dynamic venous pressure was of no value in predicting access stenosis or thrombosis.[54]

Treatment for vascular access stenosis has either been surgical revision of the fistula or an interventional radiologic approach using percutaneous angioplasty. There are several articles in the literature on adults suggesting the benefits of percutaneous angioplasty. Lahoche et al. looked at the use of percutaneous angioplasty to treat AV fistula stenosis in children.[55] In a review of 46 children, they found a stenosis rate of approximately 25 percent. These stenoses were incurred anywhere between 1 and 60 months after the creation of the fistula. They occurred in the artery, at the AV anastomosis, and most commonly in the venous limb. The authors quote a 100 percent success rate using balloon angioplasty for the venous stenosis, albeit up to three procedures were required to achieve this. In order to be successful, they note that the balloon had to be of adequate diameter to ensure elimination of the wrist at the stenosis and also that high-pressure inflation (>10 bars) must be used to prevent recurrence. In their series, no AV fistula was damaged and subsequent dialysis sessions were performed as scheduled.

Another complication that can arise with vascular access grafts and which can be very debilitating is the steal syndrome. The placement of a vascular access results in a high-flow, low-resistance circuit. If the resistance in the circuit is low enough, blood can be "stolen" from the distal arterial circulation, resulting in diminished peripheral arterial blood flow. Fortunately, collateral circulation is usually sufficient to prevent the development of this problem; however, ischemic symptoms can develop in between 1 to 8 percent of patients after AV fistula creation.[56,57] The symptoms include rest pain, paresthesias, or gangrene of the extremity. On physical examination, one can find diminished peripheral pulses, pallor, or evidence of sensory or motor neuropathy. Confirmation of the problem is provided by digital plethysmography looking for a diminution of the amplitude of the digital waveforms distal to the fistula as compared to other extremities. Occlusion of the fistula with subsequent normalization of the digital waveform confirms the presence of a steal syndrome. Treatment is usually either AV fistula ligation, which obviously results in the total loss of the fistula, or a method to constrict the flow through the fistula, usually by placing a band around it. This band increases the resistance within the fistula, thereby increasing the distal arterial flow. This technique, however, can be difficult because a band that is too tight will lead to fistula loss and one that is too loose will not result in adequate distal flow, thereby failing to relieve the symptoms. Another approach to this problem is the technique of distal revascularization with interval ligation (DRIL) to improve peripheral circulation. In this procedure, an arterial bypass graft is placed that bypasses the AV anastomosis. The artery immediately distal to the fistula is then ligated. Therefore flow to the distal artery is via the bypass graft. Wixon et al. report excellent success with this procedure, with no loss of AV fistulas.[58]

Most of the studies that have been done in evaluating long-term success of vascular access have been compiled in adults. As noted above, there are very few data on vascular access, especially AV fistulas and AV grafts, in children. The adult population is distinctly different from the pediatric population because of factors that tend to be present in much higher proportions in the adult population, such as diabetes, advanced age, and obesity. Reddan et al., in an analysis of the data from the ESRD Core Indicator/CMP Project, evaluated over 8700 patients as a representative sample of the adult hemodialysis population.[59] Interestingly, their conclusions paralleled those derived from studies in children. They recommended that an autologus AV fistula should be established in preference to an AV graft and that less than 10 percent of maintenance hemodialysis patients should be chronically dialyzed using percutaneously placed catheters. They feel that an AV fistula should be attempted in at least 50 percent of hemodialysis patients and should be the vascular access for at least 40 percent of patients who are on hemodialysis.

In summary, keeping in mind the latest UNOS initiatives to transplant young children early if hemodialysis access is necessary, a percutaneously placed dialysis catheter with aggressive management of any complications should be an adequate access for a period of 1 year. If, however, the patient is potentially going to be listed for more than 1 year, a native AV fistula should be established starting at the wrist. AV grafts should be employed only in situations where a native AV fistula cannot be created. AV fistulas and AV grafts should have their Qa serially monitored, and any decrease in flow should be followed by a fistulogram. If a problem is found, it should be treated with either percutaneous angioplasty or direct surgical intervention. A workup for a hypercoagulable state is warranted in the situation of recurrent access thrombosis.

REFERENCES

1. North American Pediatrics Renal Transplant Cooperative Study. *2003 Annual Report.* Rockville MD: NAPRTCS, 2003.
2. Goldstein SL, Macierowski CT, Jabs K. Hemodialysis catheter survival and complications in children and adolescents. *Pediatr Nephrol* 1997;11(1):74–77.
3. Bunchman TE. Pediatric hemodialysis: lessons from the past, ideas for the future. *Kidney Int Suppl* 1996;53:S64–S67.
4. Vathada M et al. Complications of hemodialysis catheters in children. *Dial Transplant* 1994;23:240–247.
5. Rovner M et al. Comparisoin of cuffed v. uncuffed catheters for extracorporeal therapy in pediatric patients. *Dial Transplant* 1992;21:513–522.
6. Sharma A et al. Survival and complications of cuffed catheters in children on chronic hemodialysis. *Pediatr Nephrol* 1999;13(3):245–248.
7. Moss AH et al. Use of a silicone dual-lumen catheter with a Dacron cuff as a long-term vascular access for hemodialysis patients. *Am J Kidney Dis* 1990;16(3):211–215.
8. Swartz RD et al. Successful use of cuffed central venous hemodialysis catheters inserted percutaneously. *J Am Soc Nephrol* 1994;4(9):1719–1725.
9. McDowell DE et al. Percutaneously placed dual-lumen silicone catheters for long-term hemodialysis: use of a silicone dual-lumen catheter with a Dacron cuff as a long-term vascular access for hemodialysis patients. *Am Surg* 1993;59 (9):569–573.
10. Butterly DW, Schwab SJ. Catheter access for hemodialysis: an overview. *Semin Dial* 2001;14(6):411–415.
11. Akoh JA. Use of permanent dual lumen catheters for long-term haemodialysis. *Int Surg* 1999;84(2):171–175.
12. Carlisle EJ et al. Septicemia in long-term jugular hemodialysis catheters; eradicating infection by changing the catheter over a guidewire. *Int J Artif Organs* 1991;14(3):150–153.
13. Shaffer D. Catheter-related sepsis complicating long-term, tunnelled central venous dialysis catheters: management by guidewire exchange. *Am J Kidney Dis* 1995;25(4):593–596.
14. Robinson D, Suhocki P, Schwab SJ. Treatment of infected tunneled venous access hemodialysis catheters with guidewire exchange. *Kidney Int* 1998;53(6):1792–1794.
15. Bethard G. Management of bacteria associated with tunnel-cuffed hemodialysis catheters. *JASN* 1999;10:1045–1049.
16. Lumsden AB et al. Hemodialysis access in the pediatric patient population. *Am J Surg* 1994;168(2):197–201.
17. Sheth, RD et al. Successful use of Tesio catheters in pediatric patients receiving chronic hemodialysis. *Am J Kidney Dis* 2001;38(3):553–539.
18. Lerner GR et al. Chronic dialysis in children and adolescents. The 1996 annual report of the North American Pediatric Renal Transplant Cooperative Study. *Pediatr Nephrol* 1999; 13(5):404–417.
19. Fermo I et al. Prevalence of moderate hyperhomocysteinemia in patients with early-onset venous and arterial occlusive disease. *Ann Intern Med* 1995;123(10):747–753.
20. den Heijer M et al. Is hyperhomocysteinaemia a risk factor for recurrent venous thrombosis? *Lancet* 1995;345(8954): 882–885.

21. Petri M et al. Plasma homocysteine as a risk factor for atherothrombotic events in systemic lupus erythematosus. *Lancet* 1996;348(9035):1120–1124.

22. Bostom AG, Lathrop L. Hyperhomocysteinemia in end-stage renal disease: prevalence, etiology, and potential relationship to arteriosclerotic outcomes. *Kidney Int* 1997;52(1):10–20.

23. Shemin D et al. Plasma total homocysteine and hemodialysis access thrombosis: a prospective study. *J Am Soc Nephrol* 1999;10(5):1095–1099.

24. Hojs R et al. Homocysteine and vascular access thrombosis in hemodialysis patients. *Renal Failure* 2002;24(2):215–222.

25. Tamura T, Bergman SM, Morgan SL. Homocysteine, B vitamins, and vascular-access thrombosis in patients treated with hemodialysis. *Am J Kidney Dis* 1998;32(3):475–481.

26. Manns BJ et al. Hyperhomocysteinemia, anticardiolipin antibody status, and risk for vascular access thrombosis in hemodialysis patients. *Kidney Int* 1999;55(1):315–320.

27. Loizou S et al. Measurement of anti-cardiolipin antibodies by an enzyme-linked immunosorbent assay (ELISA): standardization and quantitation of results. *Clin Exp Immunol* 1985; 62(3):738–745.

28. Harris EN et al. Anticardiolipin antibodies: detection by radioimmunoassay and association with thrombosis in systemic lupus erythematosus. *Lancet* 1983;2(8361):1211–1214.

29. Harris EN et al. Thrombosis, recurrent fetal loss, and thrombocytopenia. Predictive value of the anticardiolipin antibody test. *Arch Intern Med* 1986;146(11):2153–2156.

30. Valeri A, Joseph R, Radhakrishnan J. A large prospective survey of anti-cardiolipin antibodies in chronic hemodialysis patients. *Clin Nephrol* 1999;51(2):116–121.

31. Sallam S et al. Anticardiolipin antibodies in children on chronic haemodialysis. *Nephrol Dial Transplant* 1994;9(9): 1292–1294.

32. Haviv YS. Association of anticardiolipin antibodies with vascular access occlusion in hemodialysis patients: cause or effect? *Nephron* 2000;86(4):447–454.

33. O'Shea SI et al. Frequency of anti-heparin-platelet factor 4 antibodies in hemodialysis patients and correlation with recurrent vascular access thrombosis. *Am J Hematol* 2002; 69(1):72–73.

34. Broyer M et al. [Bypass and arteriovenous fistula for chronic hemodialysis in children]. *Arch Fr Pediatr* 1973;30(2): 145–161.

35. Bourquelot P, Wolfeler L, Lamy L. Microsurgery for haemodialysis distal arteriovenous fistulae in children weighing less than 10 kg. *Proc Eur Dial Transplant Assoc* 1981;18: 537–541.

36. Yazbeck S, O'Regan S. Microsurgery for Brescia-Cimino fistula construction in pediatric patients. *Nephron* 1984;38(3): 209–212.

37. Bagolan P et al. A ten-year experience of Brescia-Cimino arteriovenous fistula in children: technical evolution and refinements. *J Vasc Surg* 1998;27(4):640–644.

38. Bourquelot PD. Preventive haemostasis with an inflatable tourniquet for microsurgical distal arteriovenous fistulas for haemodialysis. *Microsurgery* 1993;14(7):462–463.

39. Brittinger WD et al. Vascular access for hemodialysis in children. *Pediatr Nephrol* 1997;11(1):87–95.

40. Nghiem DD, Schulak JA, Corry RJ. Management of the infected hemodialysis access grafts. *Trans Am Soc Artif Intern Organs* 1983;29:360–362.

41. Ditzel A, Wilkins S, Cohen J, The management of infected arterial venous ePTFE grafts. *Dial Transplant* 1998;17: 422–425.

42. III. NKF-K/DOQI Clinical Practice Guidelines for Vascular Access: update 2000. *Am J Kidney Dis* 2001;37(1 suppl 1):S137–S181.

43. Garland JS, Moist LM, Lindsay RM. Are hemodialysis access flow measurements by ultrasound dilution the standard of care for access surveillance? *Adv Renal Replace Ther* 2002;9(2):91–98.

44. Krivitski NM. Theory and validation of access flow measurement by dilution technique during hemodialysis. *Kidney Int* 1995;48(1):244–250.

45. May RE et al. Predictive measures of vascular access thrombosis: a prospective study. *Kidney Int* 1997;52(6):1656–1662.

46. Lok CE et al. Reducing vascular access morbidity: a comparative trial of two vascular access monitoring strategies. *Nephrol Dial Transplant* 2003;18(6):1174–1180.

47. Moist L, Elliot J, Kribs J. Predictive measures of AV graft stenosis compared to angiography: a prospective longitudinal study. *J Am Soc Nephrol* 1999;10:213a.

48. Lumsden AB et al. Prophylactic balloon angioplasty fails to prolong the patency of expanded polytetrafluoroethylene arteriovenous grafts: results of a prospective randomized study. *J Vasc Surg* 1997;26(3):382–390; discussion 390–392.

49. Schwab SJ et al. Hemodialysis arteriovenous access: detection of stenosis and response to treatment by vascular access blood flow. *Kidney Int* 2001;59(1):358–362.

50. Faiyaz R, Zuckerman D, Alspauga J. Increase in vascular access blood flow following venous angioplasty determines PTFE graft survival. *J Am Soc Nephrol* 2001;12:288a.

51. Goldstein SL et al. Proactive monitoring of pediatric hemodialysis vascular access: effects of ultrasound dilution on thrombosis rates. *Kidney Int* 2002;62(1):272–275.

52. Depner TA. Techniques for prospective detection of venous stenosis. *Adv Renal Replace Ther* 1994;1(2):119–130.

53. Levy SS, Sherman RA, Nosher JL. Value of clinical screening for detection of asymptomatic hemodialysis vascular access stenoses. *Angiology* 1992;43(5):421–424.

54. Chand DH, Poe SA, Strife CF. Venous pressure monitoring does not accurately predict access failure in children. *Pediatr Nephrol* 2002;17(9):765–769.

55. Lahoche, A et al. Percutaneous angioplasty of arteriovenous (Brescia-Cimino) fistulae in children. *Pediatr Nephrol* 1997; 11(4):468–472.

56. Zibari GB et al, Complications from permanent hemodialysis vascular access. *Surgery* 1988;104(4):681–686.

57. Odland MD et al. Management of dialysis-associated steal syndrome complicating upper extremity arteriovenous fistulas: use of intraoperative digital photoplethysmography. *Surgery* 1991;110(4):664–669; discussion 669–370.

58. Wixon CL, Hughes JD, Mills JL. Understanding strategies for the treatment of ischemic steal syndrome after hemodialysis access. *J Am Coll Surg* 2000;191(3):301–310.

59. Reddan, D et al. National profile of practice patterns for hemodialysis vascular access in the United States. *J Am Soc Nephrol* 2002;13(8):2117–2124.

Surgical Issues in Pediatric Peritoneal Dialysis

Walter S. Andrews

Peritoneal dialysis (PD) has become the predominant dialytic modality for children with end-stage renal disease (ESRD). This is especially true for children who acquire ESRD during the first decade of life.[1] According to the North American Pediatric Renal Transplant Cooperative Study (NAPRTCS) annual report from 2003, of the 5800 patients who were registered within the study and receiving dialysis, 60 percent percent were receiving PD.[2] The reason for the selection of PD in children has been its ability to greatly reduce the need for dietary restrictions, its simplicity of operation, the lack of a need for routine blood access, and the ability to allow the child to attend school while undergoing dialysis.[3]

However, in order for there to be successful PD, there must be successful peritoneal access. This chapter explores the different types and techniques for peritoneal access in children. There are many different catheter and surgical insertion techniques and also some lessons to learned from the literature that hopefully can decrease the complications associated with PD.

ACCESS TYPES

A variety of different PD catheters have been developed over time. These include various combinations of intraperitoneal and extraperitoneal cuffs, catheter disks, and various catheter configurations, all of which were designed to improve dialysate inflow and outflow and to minimize leaks and infections at the catheter-peritoneal and catheter-skin interfaces.

In the 2003 NAPRTCS data, 93 percent of patients had either a Tenckhoff straight catheter (29 percent) or a Tenckhoff curled catheter (63 percent).[2] The curled Tenckhoff catheter was also reported as being the most commonly used pediatric catheter (88 percent usage) in the 1995 survey of the Pediatric Peritoneal Dialysis Study Consortia (PPDSC).[4] The presumed advantages of coiled catheters over the original straight catheters include the following: (1) better separation between the abdominal wall and the bowel, (2) the curl design makes more side holes available for inflow and outflow, (3) the curl design causes less inflow pain, (4) there is less tendency for a curled catheter to migrate, (5) such catheters are less prone to omental wrapping, and (6) they are potentially less traumatic to the bowel. The 2003 NAPRTCS data report no difference in peritonitis rates with different catheter types[2] (Fig. 45–1). However, definite data proving these presumed advantages are currently lacking.[5]

The next issue is whether to include one or two Dacron cuffs on the catheter. If a single-cuff catheter is used, it is recommended that the cuff be positioned between the rectus sheaths in the rectus muscle. In one series, this decreased the incidence of subsequent peritonitis by about 37 percent when compared to subcutaneous placement of the deep cuff.[6] When a second cuff was added, there were initial reports of problems with its cutaneous extrusion.[7,8] There are no recent reports describing the incidence of distal cuff extrusion with double-cuffed catheters in children; however, two series from 1986 and 1998 reported a distal cuff extrusion rate of 8 percent.[9,10] This caused a swing back to single-cuff catheters, as seen in the 2003 NAPRTCS data, where 56 percent of the patients had a single-cuff catheter and 43 percent had a double-cuff catheter.[2] However, some data suggest that single-cuff catheters are associated with a higher incidence of exit-site infections and peritonitis.[11] Lewis et al. compared the incidence of catheter infections in children with single- and double-cuff peritoneal catheters. There was a significant decrease in infections in the double-cuff group.[12] A similar conclusion was drawn by Warady et al.; they reported a lower incidence of peritonitis in double-cuff catheters (1 per 15.4 patient-months) compared to single cuff catheters (1 per 12.6 patient-months). The 2003 NAPRTCS data shows a longer time to first peritonitis in the two-cuff catheter group[2] (Fig. 45–2).

The next catheter variable depends on the type of bend that the catheter takes after it leaves the peritoneal cavity. The original Tenckhoff catheter was a totally straight catheter. Since then the swan-neck catheter has been developed, which has an inverted U-shaped arc (170 to 180 degrees) between the deep and superficial cuffs. The purpose of this arc is to (1) allow the catheter to exit the skin in a downward-pointing direction and (2) to allow the curled end of the catheter to enter the abdomen in an unstressed condition, thereby decreasing the chance of its migration out of the pelvis. A modification of this catheter type is the swan-neck presternal catheter. The major difference between it and the standard swan-neck catheter is that the presternal catheter has a very long subcutaneous portion. The catheter usually exits over the anterior chest wall. This catheter is utilized when it is necessary to make the exit site remote from the abdomen, as in patients with stomas. Warchol et al. noted that the use of this type of catheter resulted in an exit-site infection rate of 1 per 162 patient-months, as compared to the reported pediatric PD catheter exit-site infection rate of 1 per 25 to 71 patient-months.[13]

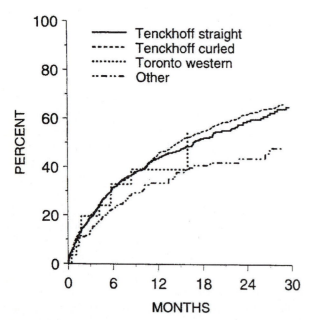

Figure 45–1. Comparison between different types of intraperitoneal catheter configurations and the time to the development of the first episode of peritonitis. These curves are not significantly different. [Adapted from North American Pediatric Renal Transplant Cooperative Study (NAPRTCS). *2003 Annual Report.* Rockville MD: EMMES Corp., 2003, with permission.]

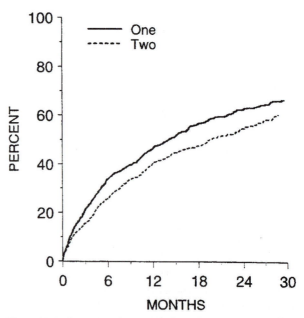

Figure 45–2. Comparison between single- and double-cuffed catheters and the time to the development of the first episode of peritonitis. [Adapted from North American Pediatric Renal Transplant Cooperative Study (NAPRTCS). *2003 Annual Report.* Rockville MD: EMMES Corp., 2003, with permission.]

Open Technique

The best open technique utilizes an incision over the rectus muscle, which is split in the direction of its fibers. The posterior sheath is then opened longitudinally. The catheter is threaded over a stiffening wire to allow its placement deep in the pelvis. The posterior sheath is closed and the inner cuff fixed to the posterior sheath as part of this closure. The internal cuff is then positioned within the rectus muscle and the anterior sheath closed tightly around the catheter with a second purse-string suture around the catheter cuff at the level of the anterior rectus sheath. The catheter is then tunneled out to the skin.

The advantage of this technique is the ability to directly visualize the placement of the catheter into the pelvis. In addition, the open technique easily allows the simultaneous performance of an omentectomy.

The major problem with this technique is the necessity for a significant incision in the peritoneum. For optimal dialysis performance, this technique usually requires a 2-week rest period between the time of catheter insertion and the initiation of dialysis. This allows for healing of the peritoneal incision and incorporation of the cuff into the peritoneum and posterior sheath.

Laparoscopic Technique

With the development of laparoscopy, techniques have been developed that allow the percutaneous placement of a PD catheter under direct vision. The advantage of the laparoscopic technique is that it allows the use of a much smaller peritoneal incision, thereby decreasing the chance of dialysate leak.

We currently use a modification of the technique first described by Daschner et al.[25]

Prophylactic antibiotics are administered to all patients prior to surgery. Under general anesthesia, a vertical incision is made in the umbilicus and the umbilical fascia is sharply incised. Using blunt dissection, the peritoneum is entered and, depending on the child's size, either a 3- or 5-mm port is placed. A corresponding 3- or 5-mm laparoscope is then inserted and the abdomen insufflated. The insertion site of the PD catheter is then determined such that the exit site is downward-pointing and either above the belt line or diaper area (infants) or, in very large children, below the belt line. If the patient has the potential for a gastrostomy in the future, the catheter exit site is positioned on the right-hand side of the abdomen. Otherwise, the catheter is placed on the left-hand side of the abdomen to avoid any interference with the future transplant incision. The peritoneal entrance site is positioned so that the inner catheter cuff will be located between both sheaths of the rectus muscle. At this point, either a 3- or 5-mm instrument is inserted through a stab wound at the marked catheter exit site. If an omentectomy is to be performed, a second 3- to 5-mm port

is then inserted at the marked entrance site of the catheter. The omentum can then be removed by the use of electrocautery and/or clips. We feel that a complete omentectomy is not absolutely necessary as long as the majority of the omentum is removed.

After the omentectomy has been performed, a guidewire is inserted into the abdomen via the entrance-site port. The port is then removed and the skin incision enlarged to approximately 1 cm. Using a peel-away sheath technique, a 20F sheath is inserted into the abdomen over the guidewire (Fig. 45–6). The PD catheter is then placed on a stiffener and inserted into the pelvis under direct vision. Pneumoperitoneum is maintained by pushing the proximal cuff of the PD catheter into the sheath, thereby preventing gas loss. Once the catheter has been positioned in the pelvis, the sheath is removed (Fig. 45–7). As the sheath is being removed, the inner cuff is positioned to lie between the anterior and posterior portions of the rectus sheath. The inner cuff is then fixed to the anterior rectus sheath with a purse-string suture. Care is taken to make sure that the innermost portion of the cuff does not project into the peritoneum (Fig. 45–8).

The peritoneum is also carefully inspected for any evidence of any indirect hernias. If these are identified, they are fixed after the PD catheter has been inserted.

The camera and all ports are then removed and the umbilical fascia is repaired.

At the previously marked exit site of the catheter, using either the previous 20F sheath dilator or a tendon passer, a deep subcutaneous tunnel is created between the catheter exit and entrance sites. The catheter is then pulled through the tunnel, positioning the proximal cuff so that it is at least 2 cm from the exit site. At this point, fibrin sealant is injected around the proximal cuff site at the level of the anterior rectus sheath and also down the tunnel between the proximal and distal cuffs. We feel that this helps to ensure a leak-free closure. The entrance site of the catheter is then

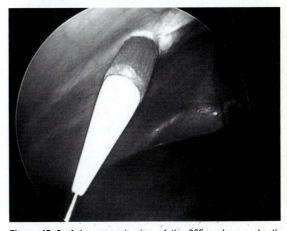

Figure 45–6. A laparoscopic view of the 20F peel-away sheath being inserted into the peritoneum over a guidewire.

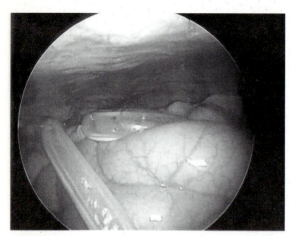

Figure 45–7. A laparoscopic view of the PD catheter, which lies positioned in the pelvis. The catheter is sitting between the bowel and the anterior abdominal wall.

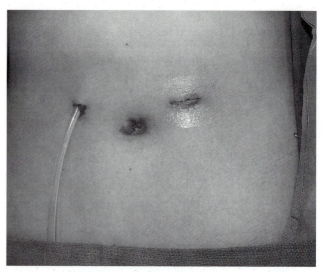

Figure 45–9. The abdomen after the laparoscopic insertion of the PD catheter. The catheter has a downward-facing exit site, a swan-neck curve, and a small insertion site on the left side. The umbilical port site has been closed.

closed in two layers. The exit site of the catheter is dressed, and no fixation suture is used at the exit site (Fig. 45–9).

POSTIMPLANTATION CARE

The exit site of the catheter, since it is not occlusive, is a major potential source for infection after PD catheter placement. One approach to deal with this problem was reported by Moncrief and Popovich.[26] They leave the external portion of the catheter coiled underneath the skin. After 2 weeks, when both cuffs have had an opportunity to undergo tissue incorporation, the patient is brought back to the operating room and the external component of the catheter is exteriorized. Twardowski et al. have described another approach to catheter management.[27–29] Initially, the exit site should be only covered with several layers of sterile gauze.

Some oozing from the exit site is common and the gauze can wick this away from the skin. An occlusive dressing should *not* be used. Occlusive dressings tend to trap fluid at the exit site, allowing for bacterial growth and subsequent infection. Second, trauma to the exit site, usually from repeated catheter motion, must be minimized. Therefore dressing changes should be done no more than once a week. After the exit site is colonized by bacteria (weeks 2 and 3), more frequent dressing changes are required. In addition, specially trained staff should optimally do the dressing changes. This allows a consistent aseptic technique to be followed.[30] The patient should also avoid submerging the exit site in water during the healing process to avoid colonization of the site with water-borne contaminants.

TIMING OF CATHETER USE

Some controversy exists as to whether the catheter should be used immediately or a period of time should elapse prior to use. The 1998 ISPD catheter guidelines recommended a dialysis-free period of 10 to 15 days after a catheter insertion.[18] This is supported by a study by Remes et al., who recommended a 10-day waiting period prior to starting dialysis. Another study, by Patel et al., compares immediate vs. delayed (an average of 20 days) catheter use.[31] They noted an increased incidence of dialysate leaks in the immediate-use group but also a disconcerting increase in exit-site infections, tunnel infections, and peritonitis in the delayed-use group. Unfortunately, their study is both retrospective and nonrandomized. This may have led to some investigator bias in selecting which patients should have delayed vs. im-

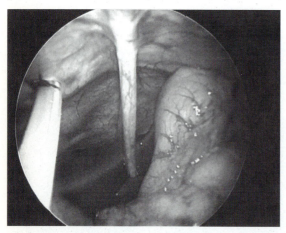

Figure 45–8. A laparoscopic view of the PD catheter (left), showing it leaving the peritoneal cavity. Note that the inner cuff is not visible within the peritoneal cavity.

mediate catheter use. It does, however, suggest that a randomized study should be done to evaluate this question.

MECHANICAL COMPLICATIONS

Mechanical complications are generally felt to be the second most common reason (after infection) for catheter failure. These complications include obstruction of the catheter by omentum, migration of the catheter out of the pelvis, and blockage of the catheter by fibrin or clots. The issue of obstruction by omentum has been previously reviewed. Migration of the catheter out of the pelvis can lead to either poor dialysate inflow or outflow or increased pain with dialysis. One approach to repositioning the catheter is the use of interventional radiology. This involves using a guidewire to move the catheter back to a workable position in the abdomen. With this technique, Savader et al. reported that they were able to obtain a durable patency rate of 50 percent in those patients who had an early catheter malposition (less than 30 days) and a durable patency rate of 82 percent with late malpositions (greater than 30 days).[32]

Our center has used a laparoscopic approach to reposition catheters. In patients who have had no previous abdominal procedures besides the Tenckhoff catheter, we create a pneumoperitoneum by insufflating through the malpositioned PD catheter. Once pneumoperitoneum is achieved, a 3-mm port is placed in the left upper quadrant and a 3-mm laparoscope inserted. A stab wound is then made in the right upper quadrant and a 3-mm grasper is inserted. The catheter is then manipulated under direct vision and repositioned back into the pelvis. Any adhesions encountered during the repositioning of the catheter are now lysed. In addition, we have used this technique to free catheters that have become encased in adhesions. These adhesions can be lysed laparoscopically; this technique avoids a large incision in the peritoneum, thus allowing a quick return to dialysis.

Tissue plasminogen activator (t-PA) has been shown to be very effective in unblocking catheters occluded by fibrin or blood clot. Approximately 2 mg of t-PA is reconstituted in 40 mL of normal saline and instilled in the catheter for 1 hour. This resulted in a restoration of patency in 57 percent of the catheters.[33,34]

EXIT-SITE INFECTION, TUNNEL INFECTION, AND PERITONITIS

Exit-site and tunnel infections are a significant cause of catheter failure if these infections cannot be controlled. In a review of the North American Pediatric Renal Transplant Cooperative Study data from 1992 to 1997, the incidence of exit-site/tunnel infections increased from 11 percent at 30 days after catheter insertion to 30 percent by 1 year.[11] The

associated peritonitis rate was 1 per 13.2 patient-months. By regression analysis, the independent risk factors related to peritonitis were black race, single-cuffed catheters, and upward-pointing exit sites. Traditionally, infected catheters would have to be removed if the infections could not be eradicated. However, a study by Wu et al. describes a technique where the intraperitoneal portion of the dialysis catheter could be preserved and only the external ,infected portion of the catheter excised.[35] This was accomplished by cutting down on the entrance site of the catheter into the peritoneum. This part of the catheter is usually uninvolved by an exit-site or tunnel infection. At this point the catheter is divided just above the internal cuff and a new external portion with a new external cuff is then glued in place and passed out to the skin via a separate tunnel. The infected external portion of the catheter is then removed.

Wu et al. reported 26 catheter revisions in 23 patients with 100 percent resolution of the infections and without any interruption of PD. To date, we have not had to utilize this technique, but certainly it would be worth considering in the case of those patients who would tolerate an interruption of PD only with difficulty.

If, however, the catheter is irrevocably infected and must be removed, an important decision must be made. Should the catheter be removed and a new PD catheter inserted immediately, or should it merely be removed and a new catheter inserted later? Fredensborg et al. reported a review of 58 episodes of PD catheter infections that required PD catheter replacement. The patients were divided into two groups, one for removal and immediate reimplantation and another for delayed implantation (1 to 30 days, average 14 days).[36] They noted no differences between these groups with respect to time to first infection after the PD catheter replacement or subsequent loss of the reinserted catheter due to infection. This is also consistent with other studies. We therefore advocate simultaneous removal and replacement of the PD catheter rather than delayed catheter replacement.

TIMING OF CATHETER REMOVAL AFTER KIDNEY TRANSPLANTATION

Several studies have looked at the timing of the removal of the PD catheter after successful renal transplantation. Both studies noted that there was no significant early increase in catheter infections after kidney transplantation if the PD catheters were left in place despite the fact that they were not being used and the patients were immunosuppressed.[37,38] In the Andreetta (Italian Registry) study,[37] catheters were left in place for an average of 8 to 10 weeks after transplant. In the Arbeiter study,[38] an increased incidence of catheter infections after the first posttransplant month was noted. They also noted that the majority of complications that would require the use of the catheter occurred within the first month.

For this reason, they say that the peritoneal catheter can be safely left in place for a month, after which it should be removed if it is no longer needed.

COMPLICATIONS WITH PD CATHETER REMOVAL

An interesting short report by Korzets et al. makes the case that the removal of a PD catheter can be associated with significant complications.[39] In their series of 40 catheter removals, 10 had complications (25 percent) and 8 of these required further surgical intervention. Half of their complications were related to bleeding. Their usual technique was to remove the PD catheters under local anesthesia, which they felt contributed significantly to their complication rate. They also make a strong case against using traction as the removal technique because of the complications of a retained cuff and subsequent infection. The removal of a PD catheter is a real operation that requires strict attention to detail to prevent annoying but potentially significant complications that could require a return to the operating room.

REFERENCES

1. Warady BA, Bunchman TE. An update on peritoneal dialysis and hemodialysis in the pediatric population. *Curr Opin Pediatr* 1996;8(2):135–140.

2. North American Pediatric Renal Transplant Cooperative Study (NAPRTCS). *2003 Annual Report.* Rockville MD: EMMES Corp, 2003.

3. Salusky IB, Holloway M. Selection of peritoneal dialysis for pediatric patients. *Perit Dial Int* 1997;17(suppl 3):S35–S37.

4. Neu AM, Kohaut EC, Warady BA. Current approach to peritoneal access in North American children: a report of the Pediatric Peritoneal Dialysis Study Consortium. *Adv Perit Dial* 1995;11:289–292.

5. Gokal R et al. Peritoneal catheters and exit-site practices toward optimum peritoneal access: 1998 update. (Official report from the International Society for Peritoneal Dialysis.) *Perit Dial Int* 1998;18(1):11–33.

6. Lewis M et al. Routine omentectomy is not required in children undergoing chronic peritoneal dialysis. *Adv Perit Dial* 1995;11:293–295.

7. Alexander SR, Tank ES. Surgical aspects of continuous ambulatory peritoneal dialysis in infants, children and adolescents. *J Urol* 1982;127(3):501–504.

8. Vigneau A, Hardy B, Balfe J. Chronic peritoneal catheter in children: one or two dacron cuffs(letter)? *Perit Dial Bull* 1981;1:151.

9. Stone MM et al. Surgical management of peritoneal dialysis catheters in children: five-year experience with 1,800 patient-month follow-up. *J Pediatr Surg* 1986;21(12):1177–1181.

10. Rinaldi S et al. The Italian Registry of Pediatric Chronic Peritoneal Dialysis: a ten-year experience with chronic peritoneal dialysis catheters. *Perit Dial Int* 1998;18(1):71–74.

11. Furth SL et al. Peritoneal dialysis catheter infections and peritonitis in children: a report of the North American Pediatric Renal Transplant Cooperative Study. *Pediatr Nephrol* 2000;15(3–4): 179–182.

12. Lewis MA et al. A comparison of double-cuffed with single-cuffed Tenckhoff catheters in the prevention of infection in pediatric patients. *Adv Perit Dial* 1997;13:274–276.

13. Warchol S, Roszkowska-Blaim M, Sieniawska M. Swan neck presternal peritoneal dialysis catheter: five-year experience in children. *Perit Dial Int* 1998;18(2):183–187.

14. Warady BA et al. Renal transplantation, chronic dialysis, and chronic renal insufficiency in children and adolescents. The 1995 Annual Report of the North American Pediatric Renal Transplant Cooperative Study. *Pediatr Nephrol* 1997;11(1): 49–64.

15. Chadha V et al. Chest wall peritoneal dialysis catheter placement in infants with a colostomy. *Adv Perit Dial* 2000;16: 318–320.

16. Remes J et al. Five years of surgical experience with peritoneal dialysis. *Acta Chir Belg* 1998;98(2):66–70.

17. Conlin MJ, Tank ES. Minimizing surgical problems of peritoneal dialysis in children. *J Urol* 1995;154(2 Pt 2):917–919.

18. Harvey EA. Peritoneal access in children. *Perit Dial Int* 2001; 21(suppl 3):S218–s222.

19. Sardegna KM, Beck AM, Strife CF. Evaluation of perioperative antibiotics at the time of dialysis catheter placement. *Pediatr Nephrol* 1998;12(2):149–152.

20. Warady BA. Peritoneal dialysis catheter related infections in children. *Pediatr Infect Dis J* 1998;17(12):1165–1166.

21. Reissman P et al. Placement of a peritoneal dialysis catheter with routine omentectomy—does it prevent obstruction of the catheter? *Eur J Surg* 1998;164(9):703–707.

22. Pumford N, Cassey J, Uttley WS. Omentectomy with peritoneal catheter placement in acute renal failure. *Nephron* 1994;68(3):327–328.

23. Sojo E et al. Is fibrin glue useful in preventing dialysate leakage in children on CAPD? Preliminary results of a prospective randomized study. *Adv Perit Dial* 1997;13:277–280.

24. Popovich RP, Moncrief JW, Decherd JF, et al. The definition of a novel portable-wearable equilibrium peritoneal technique. *Abstr Am Soc Artif Intern Organs* 1976;5(64).

25. Daschner M et al. Laparoscopic Tenckhoff catheter implantation in children. *Perit Dial Int* 2002;22(1):22–26.

26. Moncrief JW, Popovich RP. Moncrief-Popovich catheter: implantation technique and clinical results. *Perit Dial Int* 1994; 14(suppl 3):S56–S58.

27. Twardowski ZJ, Prowant BF. Exit-site healing post catheter implantation. *Perit Dial Int* 1996;16(suppl 3):S51–S70.

28. Twardowski ZJ, Prowant BF. Exit-site study methods and results. *Perit Dial Int* 1996;16(suppl 3):S6–S31.

29. Twardowski ZJ, Prowant BF. Classification of normal and diseased exit sites. *Perit Dial Int* 1996; 16(suppl 3):S32–S50.

30. Jones LL, Tweedy L, Warady BA. The impact of exit-site care and catheter design on the incidence of catheter-related infections. *Adv Perit Dial* 1995;11:302–305.

31. Patel UD, Mottes TA, Flynn JT. Delayed compared with immediate use of peritoneal catheter in pediatric peritoneal dialysis. *Adv Perit Dial* 2001;17:253–259.

32. Savader SJ et al. Guide wire directed manipulation of malfunctioning peritoneal dialysis catheters: a critical analysis. *J Vasc Interv Radiol* 1997;8(6):957–963.

33. Shea M, Hmiel SP, Beck AM. Use of tissue plasminogen activator for thrombolysis in occluded peritoneal dialysis catheters in children. *Adv Perit Dial* 2001;17:249–252.

34. Sakarcan A, Stallworth JR. Tissue plasminogen activator for occluded peritoneal dialysis catheter. *Pediatr Nephrol* 2002; 17(3):155–156.

35. Wu YM et al. Surgical management of refractory exit-site/tunnel infection of Tenckhoff catheter: technical innovations of partial replantation Partial replantation of Tenckhoff catheters to treat intractable exit-site/tunnel infection. *Perit Dial Int* 1999;19(5):451–454.

36. Fredensborg BB et al. Reinsertion of PD catheters during PD-related infections performed either simultaneously or after an intervening period. *Perit Dial Int* 1995;15(8):374–378.

37. Andreetta B et al. Complications linked to chronic peritoneal dialysis in children after kidney transplantation: experience of the Italian Registry of Pediatric Chronic Peritoneal Dialysis. *Perit Dial Int* 1996;16(suppl 1):S570–S573.

38. Arbeiter K et al. Timing of peritoneal dialysis catheter removal after pediatric renal transplantation. *Perit Dial Int* 2001;21(5):467–470.

39. Korzets Z et al. Early postoperative complications of removal of Tenckhoff peritoneal dialysis catheter. *Perit Dial Int* 2000; 20(6):789–791.

Renal Osteodystrophy in Pediatric Patients

Cheryl P. Sanchez

Linear growth impairment and bone deformities are disabling complications associated with chronic renal failure in young and growing children. Despite improvements in the management of children with kidney disease, their growth remains suboptimal. In the most recent North American Pediatric Cooperative Study (NAPRTCS) data, the baseline standard deviation score for height (H-SDS) remains low, at −1.64 in children undergoing chronic dialysis therapy and −1.4 in pediatric patients with chronic renal insufficiency.[1,2] Thus, early diagnosis and prompt intervention in growing children are of utmost importance to avoid permanent disabling skeletal complications. The ultimate goal of early treatment in children afflicted with growth retardation secondary to chronic renal failure is to optimize the quality of life in these patients, so they will become productive adults.

Renal osteodystrophy encompasses the spectrum of high-turnover to low-turnover bone lesions, and these histologic lesions may change in response to various treatment modalities. This chapter summarizes the major factors that contribute to the pathogenesis of renal bone disease, clinical presentation in pediatric patients, diagnostic tests available, and the therapeutic interventions currently utilized in the management of bone disease in children with chronic renal failure.

PATHOGENESIS OF RENAL BONE DISEASE

Development of High-Turnover Bone (Secondary Hyperparathyroidism)

Although several factors may contribute to the development of bone disease in chronic renal failure, the initial events that trigger the development of secondary hyperparathyroidism are still unclear today. Several studies have shown that secondary hyperparathyroidism occurs early in the course of chronic renal failure. Reichel and colleagues have demonstrated the presence of elevated parathyroid hormone (PTH) levels in 30 percent of adult patients with calculated glomerular filtration rate (GFR) between 60 to 90 mL/min per 1.73 m^2.[3] In addition, Malluche and coworkers have shown histologic features associated with secondary hyperparathyroidism in adult patients with chronic renal insufficiency.[4]

Hypocalcemia and Retention of Phosphorus. Early studies have demonstrated that hyperphosphatemia plays an important role in the development of secondary hyperparathyroidism in chronic renal failure. Elevated serum phosphorus levels have been associated with hypocalcemia, inhibition of the enzyme 1α-hydroxylase, and direct stimulation of PTH secretion without changes in calcium and calcitriol levels.[5,6] Early experiments by Slatopolsky and colleagues have demonstrated that phosphorus has direct posttranscriptional effects on PTH synthesis and secretion.[7] In addition, Moallem and coworkers have described a marked increase in PTH mRNA expression through posttranscriptional events in the parathyroid glands of rats fed a hypocalcemic diet.[8] Phosphorus directly regulates PTH secretion, gene expression, and cell proliferation.[5,9,10] Direct intravenous phosphorus infusion increased PTH levels independent of serum calcium levels in mongrel dogs with normal renal function.[11] The underlying mechanisms of the direct action of phosphorus on the parathyroid gland are unclear, although a role for a possible phosphorus sensor needs to be evaluated. Tatsumi and colleagues have proposed that a Na$^+$-dependent phosphate cotransporter in the cell membrane of the parathyroid cell may act as a phosphate sensor.[12] Almaden et al. have proposed that elevated levels of extracellular phosphate may regulate PTH secretion through the phospholipase A$_2$-arachidonic acid pathway.[10]

Recent studies have suggested that phosphatonins may play a role in the overall balance of phosphorus independent of calcium, parathyroid hormone, and calcitriol regulation. Phosphatonins are circulating humoral factors that were discovered through studies in pathologic conditions associated with phosphate-wasting disorders such as X-linked hypophosphatemic rickets and tumor-induced osteomalacia.[13] Intraperitoneal FGF23 administration in normal mice induced phosphaturia accompanied by a decline in serum phosphate levels without changes in calcium and PTH concentrations.[13] In adult patients with varying degrees of renal failure, serum levels of FGF23 increased with a decline in renal function.[14] The exact mechanism by which FGF23 participates in phosphate homeostasis is still unknown; however, Larsson and colleagues have proposed that the elevated serum levels of FGF23 in renal failure may be due to decreased renal clearance or an increase in production as a response to alterations in phosphorus load.[14]

Several reports have demonstrated that the maintenance of adult patients on chronic dialysis therapy with serum phosphorus levels greater than 6.5 mg/dL was associ-

ated with an increase in cardiovascular mortality risk and worsening of the effects of coronary atherosclerosis.[15,16] Goodman and coworkers have described that in patients less than 20 years old, coronary artery calcification was not evident when measured using electron-beam computed tomography (EBCT) (Fig. 46–1); however, the coronary artery calcification score nearly doubled in patients who underwent repeat EBCT scanning after a mean period of 20 months of follow-up.[17] Serum phosphorus level, calcium-phosphorus ion product, and the daily dose of calcium intake were much higher in patients who had elevated coronary artery calcification scores, and these patients were on chronic dialysis therapy longer.[17] Similar findings have been reported by Oh and colleagues in 39 patients with end-stage renal disease (ESRD) aged 19 to 39 years with childhood-onset chronic renal failure who were being treated with dialysis.[18] Thus, the use of calcium salts as phosphate-binding agents, especially in young pediatric patients with chronic renal failure, should be done judiciously and monitored closely in order to prevent the development of coronary artery calcifications when these patients reach adulthood.

Alterations in Calcitriol [1,25-(OH)$_2$D$_3$] Synthesis. Serum calcitriol levels begin to decline early in the course of chronic renal failure. Uremic plasma contains various small molecular substances, including guanidinosuccinic acid (GSA), which lower calcitriol production by directly inhibiting renal 1α-hydroxylase activity and partially diminish the binding affinity of the vitamin D receptor (VDR) to its target genes, leading to a reduction in the biological action of calcitriol.[19] There is increasing evidence that, in renal failure, calcitriol affects the parathyroid gland directly through its actions on the VDR independent of changes in serum calcium or phosphorus levels.[20]

Martinez and colleagues have demonstrated low serum calcitriol levels in adult patients with calculated glomerular

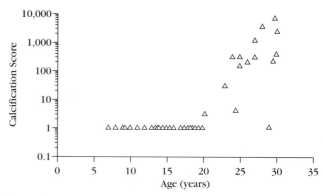

Figure 46–1. Coronary artery calcification scores in children and young adult dialysis patients according to age. The coronary artery calcifications scores were obtained using electron-beam computed tomography. The *y* axis is logarithmic. (Adapted from Goodman et al.[17] with permission).

filtration rates below 80 mL/min.[21] In addition, Portale and collaborators have reported that serum calcitriol levels declined by 40 percent in children with mean GFRs of approximately 32 ± 4 mL/min/1.73 m^2 (Fig. 46–2).[22] Subnormal levels of calcitriol can lead to diminished intestinal calcium absorption, hypocalcemia, and the development of secondary hyperparathyroidism.[23]

Changes in PTH Synthesis and Metabolism. In renal failure, there is a reduction in the plasma clearance of PTH and its various peptide fragments, leading to the accumulation of C-terminal fragments in the blood. The N-terminal mediates most of the actions of PTH by activating the type I PTH receptor. The initial stimulus for the development of secondary hyperparathyroidism in renal failure is still unclear. Elevations in serum PTH levels occur in incipient renal failure even with normal serum phosphorus and calcium levels.[4] Malluche and colleagues have demonstrated histologic evidence of hyperparathyroid bone disease in adult patients with mild chronic renal failure accompanied by normal or elevated PTH carboxy-terminal fragments.[24] Skeletal changes associated with increases in serum PTH carboxy-terminal fragments were also reported by Norman and coworkers in children with renal function between 50 to 75 percent of normal.[25] In earlier stages of renal failure, the parathyroid gland undergoes generalized diffuse hyperplasia, but it is not unusual to detect nodular areas within the same gland; these nodular areas have lower expression of VDR that may lead to poor response to calcitriol therapy.[26]

The persistent oversecretion of PTH in chronic renal failure may also be secondary to alterations in the sensitivity of the parathyroid gland to calcium. The parathyroid cells express a cell-surface calcium-sensing receptor that participates in the regulation of PTH secretion.[27] The set point for PTH release in parathyroid cells obtained from the parathyroid gland of patients with advanced secondary hy-

perparathyroidism is higher than that of patients with normal renal function.[28] In contrast, Ramirez and colleagues have shown that the calculated set point in children undergoing dialysis therapy did not differ from that of normal volunteers.[29] The same findings were reported by Messa and coworkers in predialysis adult patients with chronic renal failure.[30] The downregulation of the calcium-sensing receptor has been shown in the hyperplastic nodular parathyroid gland obtained from patients with severe secondary hyperparathyroidism.[31] It was previously thought that restoring the expression of the calcium-sensing receptor might contribute to the arrest of parathyroid gland hyperplasia; however, Ritter et al. have reported that the upregulation of the calcium receptor in rats with renal failure fed low phosphorus diet is a late event and is not involved in the arrest of parathyroid gland hyperplasia.[32]

The majority of the recent investigations and current guidelines in the diagnosis and management of secondary hyperparathyroidism are based almost exclusively on PTH measurements obtained using the first-generation immunometric assays. The current recommendation is to maintain the serum "intact" PTH levels within three to four times the upper limits of normal in children on chronic dialysis therapy, especially during vitamin D therapy to prevent the development of adynamic bone.[33] Serum intact PTH levels above 200 pg/mL and serum calcium below 10 mg/dL are 100 percent specific and 85 percent predictive for high-turnover bone disease, whereas intact PTH levels below 150 pg/mL and serum calcium greater than 10 mg/dL were 92 percent specific for distinguishing patients with adynamic bone disease (Fig. 46–3).[33] Quarles and coworkers have demonstrated that serum intact PTH levels about 165 pg/mL were associated with normal rates of bone formation, intact PTH levels above 180 pg/mL had histologic evidence of increased bone formation and peritrabecular fibrosis, and intact PTH levels greater than 500 pg/mL showed

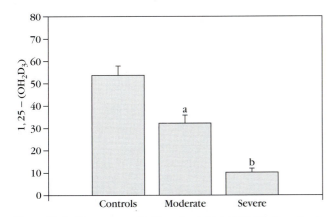

Figure 46–2. Plasma concentrations of calcitriol (1,25-dihydroxyvitamin D$_3$) in children with normal renal function (controls) and in children with moderate and severe chronic renal failure; a <0.002 vs. controls, b <0.001 vs. controls. (Modified from Portale et al.[22] with permission.)

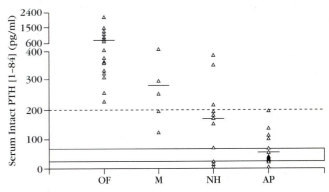

Figure 46–3. Serum intact PTH levels according to histologic subtype of bone disease in pediatric patients undergoing peritoneal dialysis. Abbreviations: OF, osteitis fibrosa; M, mild lesions of secondary hyperparathyroidism; AP, adynamic or aplastic bone; NH, normal bone histology. Solid lines represent the upper and lower limits of the assay for PTH. (Adapted from Salusky et al.[33] with permission.)

osteosclerosis in adult patients undergoing chronic dialysis therapy.[34] Slatopolsky and colleagues have demonstrated that maintaining higher serum intact PTH levels may overestimate the overall degree of secondary hyperparathyroidism, since most of these assays measure both the intact hormone (1–84) and the biologically inactive 7–84 fragment.[35]

There is limited information describing the relationship between bone histomorphometric variables and the "whole" PTH(1–84) level measured with the second-generation parathyroid hormone assays. Serum whole PTH concentration using the second-generation immunoassay is approximately 30 to 60 percent lower than PTH determined using the first-generation tests[36-38]; a high degree of correlation was also demonstrated between these two PTH assays (Fig. 46–4).[36,38,39,40] Most of the bone biopsy data currently available have been generated using the first-generation PTH immunoassay or other older radioimmunoassays in adult and pediatric patients treated with chronic dialysis therapy. Only a few studies have been done so far to evaluate bone biopsy information using the second-generation "whole" PTH assay. Monier-Faugere and coworkers demonstrated that the ratio of PTH(1–84)/C-PTH fragments predicted high- or low-turnover bone disease in 51 adult patients on dialysis.[41] More recent studies however, in both children and adult patients on dialysis therapy, showed that the ratio between the "whole" PTH and the 7–84 fragments did not differ in those with high- or low-turnover renal osteodystrophy.[37,38]

There is very little information on the relationship between the first- or second-generation PTH immunoassays and bone histology in predialysis patients with chronic renal failure. In 15 children with moderate chronic renal failure, the prevalent skeletal histologic finding was normal bone formation in 60 percent of patients; 27 percent had lesions of secondary hyperparathyroidism and 13 percent had osteomalacia.[42] The average serum intact PTH level in children with normal bone formation was 70 ± 30 pg/mL; it was 234 ± 177 pg/mL in children with secondary hyper-

parathyroidism and 88 ±80 pg/mL in children with osteomalacia. Although, the current recommendation is to maintain the serum intact PTH levels three to four times the upper limits of normal in patients undergoing chronic dialysis therapy, very mild elevations of PTH levels may be associated with histologic lesions of secondary hyperparathyroidism in children and adult patients with mild to moderate chronic renal failure.[42,43] Waller and colleagues have reported that pediatric patients with a mean GFR of 22 mL/min/1.73 m² had significant improvements in growth (H-SDS) when the intact PTH levels were maintained within the upper range of normal (Fig. 46–5).[44] Until more studies are available, serum intact PTH levels in patients with mild to moderate chronic renal failure who are not yet on dialysis therapy should probably be maintained within the appropriate normal limits.

Abnormalities in the growth-plate cartilage have been demonstrated in rats with chronic renal failure and secondary hyperparathyroidism, including downregulation of the PTH/PTHrP receptor, alterations in collagen metabolism, changes in the width and architecture of the growth plate, and decreased insulin-like growth factor I (IGF-I) expression (Fig. 46–6).[45,46] The rate of longitudinal growth was significantly diminished in uremic rats with both mild and advanced secondary hyperparathyroidism as compared to animals given an ad libitum diet.[45]

Skeletal Resistance to the Calcemic Actions of the Parathyroid Hormone. The precise mechanisms by which the calcemic actions of PTH are blunted in patients with chronic renal failure and secondary hyperparathyroidism are still unknown, but several factors may play significant roles, including reduction in VDR and calcium-sensing receptor expression in the parathyroid gland, elevated serum phosphorus

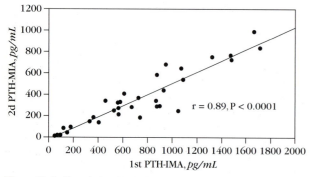

Figure 46–4. The relationship between serum intact parathyroid hormone levels assessed using the first-generation assay (intact, x axis) and the second-generation assay (whole, y axis). (Adapted from Salusky et al.[38] with permission.)

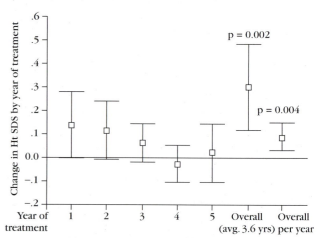

Figure 46–5. Changes in standard deviations scores for height (H-SDS) in children with chronic renal failure obtained yearly during the study period (error bars represent 95 percent confidence intervals). The overall mean H-SDS for the entire study period and values obtained yearly are shown in the last two data points. From Waller et al.[44] with permission.)

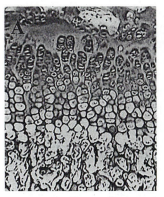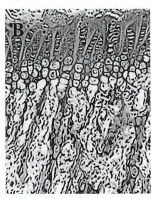

Figure 46–6. The growth-plate cartilage in 5/6 nephrectomized rats with mild (*A*) and severe (*B*) secondary hyperparathyroidism. Note the lower height of the growth plate and the distortion of its architecture in animals with advanced secondary hyperparathyroidism (*B*).

levels, desensitization of various receptors involved in PTH metabolism, and alterations in vitamin D synthesis and degradation. Because of skeletal resistance, the current recommendation is to keep circulating "intact" PTH levels at approximately three to four times the upper limits of normal in order to maintain normal bone turnover in patients undergoing chronic dialysis (Table 46–1). In chronic renal failure, the presence of circulating elevated levels of the biologically inactive 7–84 PTH fragments may explain the need for higher levels of intact PTH to prevent the development of adynamic bone, especially during vitamin D therapy.[35] When given to rats with normal renal function, the 7–84 PTH fragment decreased the calcemic response to PTH (1–84) by 94 percent, decreased phosphaturic response by 50.2 percent,[35] and lowered the rate of bone formation in thyroparathyroidectomized rats.[47] The current recommendation of maintaining a higher target serum PTH level, however, may not be satisfactory in the long run, since the parathyroid gland continues to function above normal; this can lead to parathyroid gland hyperplasia and hypertrophy and eventually progression to nodular hyperplasia, which may be difficult to control.

Contributions of Metabolic Acidosis. Acid and base balance has complex effects on calcium and phosphorus metabo-

TABLE 46–1. TARGET "INTACT" PTH LEVELS ACCORDING TO THE STAGE OF CHRONIC KIDNEY DISEASE

Chronic Kidney Disease Stage	GFR Range (mL/min/1.73 m^2)	Target "Intact" PTH Levels (pg/mL)
3	30–59	35–70
4	15–29	70–110
5	<15 or dialysis	150–300

SOURCE: National Kidney Foundation DOQI Guidelines Clinical Practice Guidelines for Bone Metabolism and Disease in Chronic Kidney Disease. *Am J Kidney Dis* 2003;42: S21–S28, with permission.[83]

lism. Metabolic acidosis promotes bone demineralization by continuous net efflux of calcium to buffer the protons leading to negative calcium balance in renal failure.[48,49] In addition, metabolic acidosis causes movement of inorganic phosphorus from the nonextracellular compartment to the extracellular fluid, thus worsening hyperphosphatemia and increasing PTH levels (Fig. 46–7).[50,51] Several studies have demonstrated that correction of metabolic acidosis leads to a significant reduction of serum PTH levels and restores parathyroid gland sensitivity to changes in serum calcium in dialysis patients.[48,52] Furthermore, correction of metabolic acidosis in adult patients with moderate renal failure increased serum calcitriol levels without any changes in serum calcium or phosphorus levels.[53] The exact mechanisms are unknown, but many cell functions are pH-dependent, and there is a possibility that metabolic acidosis may alter receptor binding to calcium. Growth impairment, decreased bone formation, changes in the growth-plate cartilage, and dysfunction of the growth hormone and insulin growth factor I (IGF-I) system have been demonstrated in the young acidotic rat.[54] Thus the control of metabolic acidosis may be of significant value in the treatment and management of bone disease in children with chronic renal failure.

Development of Low-Turnover Bone

Secondary to the availability of vitamin D, increase in calcium intake, and adequate control of dietary phosphorus, the prevalence of osteomalacia has declined in children with renal failure. Low-turnover bone associated with aluminum toxicity was seldom reported in the 1990s because of the judicious use of aluminum-containing phosphate binders and the increased use of calcium salts. Conversely, high calcium intake to bind dietary phosphorus, aggressive use of vitamin D therapy to control secondary hyperparathyroidism, and the use of higher-calcium dialysate may have contributed to the increased prevalence of adynamic or aplastic bone in children.[55,56] Histologic findings of low to normal bone formation rate and low osteoblast

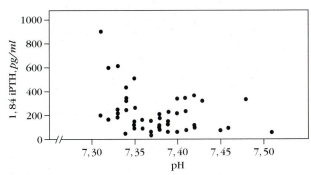

Figure 46–7. Correlation between metabolic acidosis and serum intact PTH levels in patients with chronic renal failure. From Ritz et al.[50] with permission.)

and osteoclast number are usually accompanied by biochemical findings of low PTH levels, low serum alkaline phosphatase, and, at times, the development of hypercalcemia in adynamic bone. The clinical implications of adynamic bone require further investigation in children; however, a decline in linear growth has been demonstrated after 12 months of high-dose intermittent calcitriol therapy in prepubertal pediatric patients on peritoneal dialysis.[57]

CLINICAL SIGNS AND SYMPTOMS

Growth Retardation

A substantial proportion of pediatric patients with chronic renal failure are growth-retarded, especially very young children, who have the greatest potential for linear growth during infancy and early childhood. In the 1996 NAPRTCS report, the mean height in children less than 5 years of age with chronic renal insufficiency was below the third percentile for age and sex, H-SDS was less than –1.9.[58] Five years later, the H-SDS for infants less than 24 months of age remained at –1.8; for children between 2 to 5 years of age, the H-SDS, at –1.77 was not improved. The height deficit was worst in young children who were undergoing dialysis therapy.[1] In addition, there was no improvement in H-SDS from baseline to final adult height in children who underwent renal transplantation during childhood.[59] Linear growth is affected by multiple factors, including nutrition, metabolic acidosis, bone disease, growth hormone, and IGF-I. Growth velocity is maximal in infancy, and the magnitude of growth loss is greatest during this time period; therefore any intervention should be instituted early in order to maximize recovery in longitudinal growth. Nutritional requirements must be optimized and growth patterns be monitored very closely in very young children. In pubertal children, a delay in growth spurt has been reported, possibly due to alterations in regulation of the gonadotrophic hormones.

Van Dyck and colleagues have reported that despite adequate caloric intake and correction of metabolic abnormalities, a decline in H-SDS was still demonstrated in infants with chronic renal failure with GFRs below 25 mL/min/1.73 m² (Fig. 46–8).[60] Such findings may be explained in part by alterations in the regulation of growth hormone and IGF-I-dependent processes. Several investigators have demonstrated a decline in hepatic IGF-I production and growth-plate IGF-I expression in nephrectomized rats.[45,61] Despite normal serum levels of IGF-I, there is considerable reduction in IGF-I availability due to the accumulation of various IGF-binding proteins, particularly IGF-binding protein-3 fragments secondary to a decline in renal clearance.[62] Experimental studies performed by Schaefer and colleagues have demonstrated dysregulation in the he-

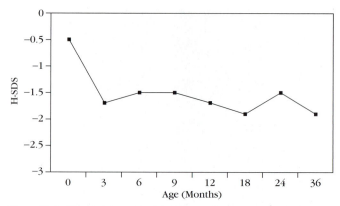

Figure 46–8. Mean height standard deviation scores for height (H-SDS) in children with chronic renal failure followed from infancy and managed conservatively with sodium bicarbonate, vitamin D, and adequate caloric intake. (Modified from Van Dyck et al.[60] with permission.)

patic JAK-STAT signaling pathway for growth hormone activation in uremic rats; these changes were accompanied by overexpression of the inhibitor proteins SOCs (suppressor of cytokine signaling).[63]

Skeletal Deformities

Chronic renal failure has been associated with the development of various skeletal abnormalities. Barrett and colleagues have reported that genu valgum was the most common skeletal disorder in more than 60 percent of children with chronic renal failure who had radiographic evidence of renal osteodystrophy.[64] Genu valgum is a combination of slippage of the distal femoral epiphysis and changes in the proximal tibial lateral growth plate.[65] The nature of the skeletal deformity in pediatric patients with chronic renal failure is somewhat relative to the age of onset of renal failure. Children who are less than 3 years old may exhibit exaggeration of the physiologic varus alignment of the lower extremity, whereas older children may show an accentuated valgus deformity.[66] In addition to genu valgum, other skeletal deformities reported in children with chronic renal failure include stress fractures, genu varum, ankle varum and valgum, bowing of long bones, pes equinovarus, osteonecrosis, epiphysiolysis, scoliosis, and coxa vara. Radiographic features associated with vitamin D–dependent rickets have been demonstrated in young children, including metaphyseal widening of the wrist (Fig. 46–9) and ankle, craniotabes, and rachitic rosary. Pathologic or stress fractures may arise if the bones remain bowed and weak (Fig. 46–10). Possible correction and improvement of the skeletal abnormalities may occur if optimal metabolic control is attained during the period of rapid growth; however, surgical correction may still be required.

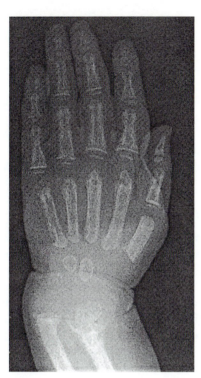

Figure 46–9. Subperiosteal resorption in the phalanges of a child maintained on peritoneal dialysis with severe secondary hyperparathyroidism. There is loss of cortical margins with extensive cortical tunneling of all the metacarpals and phalanges. Note the frayed appearance of the ulna and radius, widening of the wrist, and poor skeletal mineralization.

Slipped Capital Femoral Epiphysis (SCFE)

Hip abnormalities can occur early in very young children with chronic renal failure (Fig. 46–11). Oppenheim and colleagues have demonstrated that the prevalence of SCFE has declined over the last 20 years, probably due to improvement in the management of secondary hyperparathyroidism, better metabolic control, and closer monitoring of these children.[67] The slip location in chronic renal failure has been described as metaphyseal. Early histologic studies performed by Krempien and colleagues have demonstrated that the metaphysis adjacent to the growth plate was poorly trabeculated and inadequately vascularized, and that the metaphyseal cortex was thinned by endosteal and subperiosteal resorption.[68] In the growth-plate cartilage, there was a dense fibrous band between the chondrocytes and the metaphysis, providing a plane of slippage.[69] Thus, epiphyseal slipping in children with chronic renal failure can be a net result of poorly controlled advanced secondary hyperparathyroidism. The upper and lower femoral epiphyses are usually affected in preschool children and the upper femoral and/or the distal radial or ulnar epiphyses are often involved in older children.[69]

Surgical correction has been controversial in the management of SCFE in children with chronic renal failure because of the possibility of surgery-induced avascular necro-

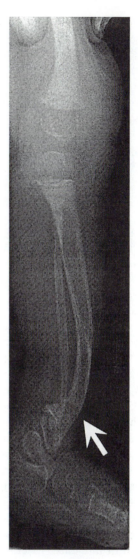

Figure 46–10. Severe concave posterior bowing of the distal tibia and fibula with flaring of the metaphyses and very irregular cortical margins. The arrow denotes a stress or insufficiency fracture.

sis and premature femoral physeal closure, resulting in leg-length discrepancy.[67] Recent reports, however, have demonstrated that surgical pin fixation may be helpful to prevent further slip progression, with minimal complications.[67]

Bone Pain

Skeletal pain may be a nonspecific finding in children with chronic renal failure. Bone pain has been described mostly in patients with low-turnover bone or adynamic bone with or without an associated elevated level of aluminum.[70] Children complaining of pain should be evaluated thoroughly for the presence of stress fracture or slipped epiphyses. Clinical symptoms can vary from nonspecific pain, limping, or problems with weight bearing.[64]

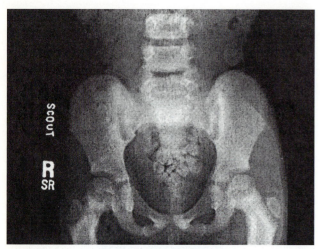

Figure 46–11. Cupping and sclerosis of bilateral femoral metaphyses with widening of the physes of the femoral heads and at the bilateral sacroiliac joints.

Myopathy

Muscle involvement in uremia remains one of the limitations for full rehabilitation of patients with chronic renal failure, especially in those maintained on chronic dialysis. Severe muscle involvement can include muscle wasting, diffuse pain, weakness, numbness, and contracture of the extremities. The exact etiology for the myopathy described in renal failure is still unclear; however, several factors have been reported that may contribute to muscle pain and weakness in uremic patients, including rapid fluid removal, electrolyte imbalance, and the presence of calcific uremic arteriolopathy (CUA).[71] There are currently no tests to evaluate muscular involvement in uremia. Electromyograms, nerve conduction studies, and serum levels of muscle enzymes do not show specific findings. Muscle biopsy may show severe atrophy without any inflammation and the presence of calcification of small and medium sized vessels.[71] Improvement in muscle strength has been reported after vitamin D therapy or parathyroidectomy.[72]

Extraskeletal Calcification

Calciphylaxis was first described in an adult patient with renal failure in 1968. Milliner and colleagues reported the presence of soft tissue calcification in autopsies of approximately 60 percent of children who had undergone dialysis therapy.[73] The most frequent sites of deposition were blood vessels, lungs, kidney, myocardium, coronary artery, central nervous system, and gastric mucosa.[73] Coronary artery calcification scores greater than tenfold normal were found in 92 percent of young adult dialysis patients 19 to 39 years of age.[18] Using EBCT, Goodman and associates found that dialysis patients below 20 years of age had no evidence of coronary artery calcification, but it was already detected in 14 of 16 patients who were between 20 to 30 years of age.[17] The prevalence of mineral deposition was higher in patients who had onset of chronic renal failure at a young age; treatment with some form of vitamin D, particularly calcitriol; elevated calcium-phosphorus product; high phosphorus levels; and large doses of calcium salt intake. A large study has reported an increase in cardiovascular morbidity and mortality in adult dialysis patients with serum phosphorus levels greater than 6.5 mg/dL and calcium-phosphorus product higher than 72 mg^2/dL^2.[74]

Dental Problems

There is limited information on the oral manifestations of bone disease in children with chronic renal failure. In some case reports, skeletal lesions associated with the development of severe secondary hyperparathyroidism ("brown tumors") have been demonstrated, leading to facial deformity and jaw enlargement.[75–77] Other bone changes include the loss of lamina dura and tooth demineralization.[78] Children should be evaluated early and followed closely by a pediatric dentist.

DIAGNOSTIC EVALUATION

Biochemical Parameters

Calcium. Hypocalcemia is a frequent finding in patients with chronic renal failure. Fractional intestinal absorption of calcium decreased progressively in adult patients, associated with the decline in their renal function.[79] Several etiologic factors may account for the low serum calcium levels in renal failure, including poor nutrition, inadequate production of calcitriol, or hyperphosphatemia. Calcium per se, through its actions on the calcium receptor, directly regulates parathyroid hormone gene expression and synthesis. Nephrectomized rats fed a low-calcium diet had a tenfold increase in PTH mRNA levels.[8] Hypercalcemia has been reported in patients with adynamic bone, aluminum-related bone disease, or secondary hyperparathyroidism—also in those receiving vitamin D therapy, undergoing prolonged immobilization, and receiving calcium salts as phosphate-binding agents. In patients with adynamic bone, hypercalcemic episodes occur due to the skeleton's inability to incorporate an acute calcium load either from increased calcium intake, vitamin D therapy, or the use of high-calcium dialysis fluid.[80]

Phosphorus. Hyperphosphatemia is prevalent among patients with chronic renal failure. Multiple clinical studies have demonstrated that chronic elevations of serum levels of phosphorus were associated with an increase in cardiovascular morbidity in adult patients on dialysis. The clinical implications of these findings require further evaluation in children with chronic renal failure. Serum phosphorus concentration varies widely in children and is age-dependent. Phosphorus levels should be maintained between 5.0 and 7.5 mg/dL in infants and between 4 and 5.5 mg/dL in older children.[81] Hypophosphatemia occurs infrequently in children with chronic renal failure and is usually seen in patients with some form of tubular problem, e.g., cystinosis or Fanconi's syndrome.

Parathyroid Hormone. The development of a PTH assay that can precisely measure the active fragments of the PTH in chronic renal failure has been challenging. The first-generation commercial PTH assay (Intact PTH assay) measures both the 1–84 molecule and the 7–84 N-truncated PTH fragments that accumulate in renal failure. Serum levels of the non-PTH(1–84) increased with the decline in GFR: 21 percent in healthy volunteers, 32 percent in patients with GFR below 30 mL/min/1.73 m², and 50 percent in dialysis patients, with PTH(1–84) making up the difference.[82] The ratio of the 1–84 to 7–84 levels measured using the Intact assay declined only when the GFR was below 30 mL/min/1.73 m². As shown in earlier experiments, the 7–84 biologically inactive PTH fragments antagonize the calcemic effects of the PTH and may contribute to the skeletal resistance reported in dialysis patients with secondary hyperparathyroidism.[35]

Most bone biopsy studies performed within the last decade have been correlated with serum PTH levels measured with the first-generation PTH assay. Using these histologic studies, the current recommendation is to maintain the serum Intact PTH levels three to four times the upper limits of normal (150 to 300 pg/mL) in dialysis patients to prevent the development of adynamic bone (see Table 46–1).[33,83] Comparisons between the first-generation (Intact) and second generation (Whole) PTH assays have been performed in children with chronic renal failure and those who are undergoing dialysis. Although the Intact PTH levels are approximately 40 to 50 percent higher that the Whole PTH levels, there was good correlation between the bone formation rate calculated from bone biopsy specimens and the serum PTH levels measured using the Intact and Whole PTH assays.[38] Furthermore, normal bone formation rates were associated with a mean serum PTH level of 196 ±180 pg/mL (Intact PTH) and 126 ± 165 pg/mL (Whole PTH), thus reinforcing earlier recommendations of maintaining serum PTH levels within three to four times the upper limit of normal for both assays.[38] Subnormal rates of bone formation were associated with serum PTH levels that were maintained at two times the upper limit of normal.[38] Further studies are required to evaluate the use of the ratio PTH(1–84)/PTH (7–84) fragments as a good predictor of bone turnover in patients with chronic renal failure.[37–41]

Recommended target levels for serum PTH using the first-generation assay in adult patients with chronic renal failure have been published by the National Kidney Foundation Kidney Disease Outcomes Quality Initiative (DOQI) (Table 46–1).

Alkaline Phosphatase. The use of total alkaline phosphatase as a marker for osteoblastic activity has been reported as a poor predictor, compared to PTH, of bone histology in chronic renal failure. The introduction of the newer immunoassay to measure bone-specific alkaline phosphatase may be a better marker in evaluating bone turnover in patients with renal failure. The bone isoenzyme is specifically derived from osteoblasts expressed during the maturation and early mineralization phase.[84] Bone alkaline phosphatase levels correlated with height velocity, intact PTH, and trabecular bone mineral density in 90 pediatric patients with chronic renal failure managed conservatively, undergoing dialysis, and after renal transplantation.[85] Total serum alkaline phosphatase levels above 250 IU/L were 96 percent specific and 55 percent sensitive in predicting bone lesions associated with secondary hyperparathyroidism, whereas levels below 200 IU/L were 100 percent sensitive and 58 percent specific for predicting lesions of adynamic bone.[33]

Aluminum. Monitoring of serum aluminum levels is done infrequently in dialysis centers due to a significant decline in the use of aluminum as a phosphate-binding agent. Plasma aluminum levels reflect more recent exposure and do not measure aluminum tissue deposition. Aluminum toxicity can manifest as encephalopathy, anemia, and osteomalacia. Bone biopsy specimens with aluminum staining greater than 15 to 25 percent and an increase in plasma aluminum level greater than 50 μg/L following a deferoxamine (DFO) infusion test are diagnostic.

Radiographic Presentation

The most common radiographic finding is the presence of subperiosteal resorption in the cortical bone (see Fig. 46–9). Intensive cortical resorptive lesions are most likely to occur in the distal ends of the ulna and radius, the neck of the humerus, the phalanges, the medial border of the humerus, at the upper areas of tibia and fibula, at the ends of the clavicles, and in the pelvic bones. Widening or fraying of the radiolucent zone in the region of the growth plate, called growth-zone or rachitic lesions, can be demonstrated in a plain radiograph in patients with secondary hyperparathyroidism (see Fig. 46–10). Rickets seen in the context of renal osteodystrophy differs morphologically from lesions demonstrated in the vitamin D–deficiency state. Progressive bowing of the tibia or femur may lead to recurrent stress or pathologic fractures (see Fig. 46–10). Bone age determinations, according to Greulich and Pyle, are often below normal relative to the patient's chronological age.

Bone Mineral Density Measurements

Measurements of bone mass are widely used for diagnosis of osteoporosis and identify patients at risk for developing fractures. Using dual-energy x-ray absorptiometry (DEXA) to evaluate bone mass in adult patients who had ESRD as children, Groothoff and colleagues demonstrated a significant decline in bone mineral density measurements in the lumbar spine and femoral neck.[86] More than 50 percent of the patients had bone mineral density Z scores below –2.5, while 61.4 percent were growth-retarded, 36.8 percent had symptoms of bone disease, and 17.8 percent were disabled by some form of bone disease.[86] Although DEXA is commonly used to assess bone mass, results in children with chronic renal failure may not be accurate, since most of these patients have growth impairment and therefore smaller bones. In addition, DEXA measurements do not differentiate between cortical and cancellous bone.

Recently, the technique of using quantitative ultrasound (QUS) has been utilized to assess bone mass in the calcaneal, tibial, and phalangeal bones in patients with chronic renal failure. Advantages of this technique include lack of radiation exposure, portability, low cost, and short time required for the test. There was a decline in bone mineral density in both predialysis and dialysis children measured using quantitative ultrasound; the bone mineral density values did not change with progressive decline in renal function.[87]

Measurements to differentiate between cortical and cancellous bone can be obtained using quantitative computed tomography (QCT). This technique has been applied to measure bone mineral density using the appendicular skeleton (peripheral QCT). Lima and coworkers have reported that cortical bone mineral density declined and trabecular bone mass increased in 21 pediatric patients on peritoneal dialysis.[88] In children with adynamic bone, the trabecular bone mass was much lower and the cortical bone density was higher than in those with high-turnover bone lesions.[88] The implications of these findings in predicting future fracture risk in pediatric patients with chronic renal failure are still unclear. In adult dialysis patients, Taal and colleagues have reported that the presence of osteoporosis or osteopenia increased mortality risk by approximately 3.3 to 4.3-fold.[89]

Bone Scintigraphy

Bone scans have limited use in the diagnosis and follow-up of children with chronic renal failure. Various bone scanning agents can be used with technetium–99, including diphosphonates and dimercaptosuccinic acid (DMSA). Ratios of lumbar vertebra/soft tissue uptake were reported to decline after vitamin D therapy in adult patients on hemodialysis.[90] Abnormal scans have been shown in approximately 83 percent of adult dialysis patients with histologic evidence of bone disease, whereas only 46 percent such cases were detected using radiographic studies.[91] Using bone scintigraphy, soft tissue calcifications have been demonstrated in various organs, including the lungs and the viscera in children with chronic renal failure.[73,92]

Bone Biopsy

Bone histomophometry remains the "gold standard" for the diagnosis of the different types of bone disease in patients with chronic renal failure. The bone biopsy procedure has been demonstrated to be well tolerated and safe in children. To evaluate the rate of bone formation, tetracycline (or other forms) is usually administered at a dose of 15 mg/kg/day in two to three doses for 2 consecutive days 7 to 14 days apart.[93] For children below 8 years of age, the dose of tetracycline is kept below 10 mg/kg/day to avoid toxicity. The indications for bone biopsy in children include unexplained hypercalcemia associated with low PTH levels or prior to parathyroidectomy, suspicion of aluminum-related bone disease, and assessment of therapeutic response.

Osteitis fibrosa remains the predominant histologic finding in children with ESRD,[33,94] although recent reports by Ziolkowska and colleagues have demonstrated a higher number of children with adynamic bone, especially in patients maintained on CAPD and receiving some form of vitamin D therapy and calcium salt.[56] The histologic findings associated with high-turnover bone include an increase in the rate of bone formation, increase in osteoclast and osteoblast numbers, and presence of peritrabecular fibrosis in the metaphysis. In osteomalacia, there is an excess amount of osteoid or unmineralized bone and a low rate of bone formation. The osteoid seams are usually wide and may have lamellations, accompanied by a decrease in number and activity of both osteoclasts and osteoblasts. Histochemical staining for aluminum should be performed in all bone biopsy specimens, especially in the presence of low-turnover bone. An adynamic or aplastic bone lesion is characterized by a low number of osteoclasts or osteoblasts, few osteoid seams, absence of peritrabecular fibrosis, diminished to absent tetracycline label, subnormal rate of bone formation, and absence of aluminum staining. A mixed lesion of renal osteodystrophy is characterized by a combination of histologic features of both osteitis fibrosa and osteomalacia; this may represent a transition between these skeletal lesions.

PREVENTION AND TREATMENT

The severity of skeletal complications associated with chronic renal failure and secondary hyperparathyroidism is greatest in very young children; thus therapy in the prevention of these disabling bone complications should be optimal in this age group. The primary goal of treatment in children with secondary hyperparathyroidism is to maintain serum PTH levels that correspond to a normal rate of skeletal remodeling, so as to promote growth in these young patients.

Control of Hyperphosphatemia and Maintaining Normocalcemia

It is essential to follow the total caloric intake and growth in infants and children with chronic renal failure. Caloric supplementation is not unusual in this patient population and is usually administered orally, by a nasogastric or gastrostomy tube if the daily intake does not meet the recommended nutritional requirement for age. The Food and Nutrition Board of the Institute of Medicine has made recommendations regarding phosphorus intake in a pediatric patient with normal renal function: 100 mg/day from 0 to 6 months, 275 mg/day from age 7 to 12 months, 460 mg/day from age 1 to 3 years, 500 mg/day from age 4 to 8 years, and 1250 mg/day from age 9 to 18 years.[81] The maximum amount of phosphorus that is tolerated by children has been reported as 3000 mg/day in those between 1 and 8 years of age and 4000 mg/day in those between 9 and 18 years of age.[81] Serum phosphorus levels must be maintained within age-appropriate normal limits. The normal range for serum phosphorus in infants is between 5 and 7.5 mg/dL; in older children, it is between 4 and 5.5 mg/dL; and in adults, it is between 2.5 and 4.5 mg/dL. Phosphorus is widely distributed in animal proteins, some vegetables, cereals, dairy products, and soda. Daily phosphorus intake is usually limited in children with progressive renal failure so as to prevent the development of secondary hyperparathyroidism, since removal of phosphorus by dialysis is usually inadequate. Peritoneal dialysis removes approximately 240 to 440 mg/day, and 600 mg is cleared by hemodialysis. Thus, conventional dialysis therapy alone is unable to adequately lower serum phosphorus levels; however, nocturnal hemodialysis therapy performed six to seven times a week has been reported to decrease serum phosphorus levels by 50 percent more than conventional hemodialysis, secondary to longer duration and increased frequency.[95] Nocturnal hemodialysis is not yet performed in pediatric patients, and the technique may not be feasible in them, particularly in very young children and infants.

Dietary phosphorus restriction is an integral part in the management of hyperphosphatemia in patients with chronic renal failure. Previous clinical studies have demonstrated that phosphorus restriction in children with moderate chronic renal failure lowered PTH levels and increase serum calcitriol levels in the presence of normal serum calcium levels.[96,97] Dietary phosphorus restriction of approximately 600 to 1000 mg/day is usually prescribed in patients with chronic renal failure so as to prevent and lessen the severity of secondary hyperparathyroidism, but the food becomes unpalatable to most children and may lead to inadequate caloric intake. Compliance with dietary phosphorus restriction is difficult to achieve in most patients, so phosphate-binding agents to reduce intestinal phosphorus absorption have been utilized.

Approximately 15 to 20 years ago, aluminum-containing agents were used to lower serum phosphorus levels in patients with chronic renal failure. Several studies, however, have shown that aluminum accumulates in the blood and in several tissues, leading to aluminum toxicity in the skeleton, brain, and other organs.[98–100] Salusky and coworkers have reported that even limited amounts of aluminum administered to very young patients undergoing dialysis therapy were associated with a measurable risk of aluminum accumulation and tissue toxicity[99]; thus the administration of these agents should be avoided in pediatric patients.

Calcium-containing salts are the most common agents currently used to lower serum phosphorus levels and maintain normocalcemia. Schaefer and colleagues have demonstrated equivalent effectiveness in controlling hyperphosphatemia between calcium carbonate and calcium acetate[101]; calcium salts containing citrate should be avoided in patients with renal failure. Calcium carbonate is usually started at doses between 200 and 500 mg of elemental calcium and should be taken with meals or snacks. Dosages vary widely and are adjusted according to target serum calcium and phosphorus levels, depending on the patient's age. High doses of calcium carbonate alone were as effective as calcitriol in the control of elevated serum parathyroid hormone levels in adult patients with mild secondary hyperparathyroidism maintained on chronic hemodialysis therapy (Fig. 46–12).[102]

In pediatric patients, serum calcium levels should be maintained between 8.5 and 10.5 mg/dL.[81] Calcium retention is relatively low in toddlers; it increases with puberty, but there are only a few studies available about the calcium requirements before the onset of puberty. The 1997 recom-

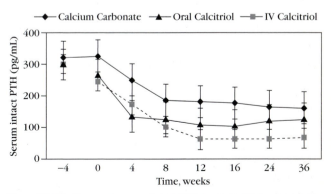

Figure 46–12. Changes in serum intact PTH levels (1–84) in response to treatment with calcium carbonate (◆), daily oral calcitriol (▲), and intermittent intravenous calcitriol (■). (p = NS when controlled for the initial PTH levels). (Modified from Indridason and Quarles,[102] with permission.)

mendation of the Food and Nutrition Board of the Institute of Medicine for calcium intake in the pediatric population are as follows: 210 mg/day for age 0 to 6 months, 270 mg/day for 7 to 12 months, 500 mg/day for 1 to 2 years, 800 mg/day for 3 to 8 years, and 1300 mg/day for 9 to 18 years.[81] The maximum tolerable amount for calcium intake is 2500 mg/day in children between 1 and 18 years of age.[81]

With the widespread use of calcium salts, problems with hypercalcemia have been reported frequently, especially when calcium is used concurrently with vitamin D therapy.[55,103] This issue is especially important in adult patients with chronic renal failure because of problems associated with vascular calcification.[17,104] Although studies have shown increased cardiovascular mortality risk in adult patients with persistently higher phosphorus levels and elevated calcium x phosphorus product, the implications of these findings in children with chronic renal failure are still unclear. Goodman and colleagues have shown that the coronary calcification score measured using EBCT was not significantly elevated in patients less than 20 years old[17]; however, pediatric patients may carry a heavier calcium burden as they grow into adulthood.

With the concurrent use of vitamin D and calcium salts as a phosphate binder, the use of a low-calcium dialysate concentration at 2.5 meq/L has been shown to be beneficial in preventing hypercalcemia.[105,106] After 12 months of low-calcium dialysis, however, serum intact PTH levels rose and induced a negative calcium loss in adult patients on hemodialysis.[107]

To avoid complications associated with the intake of high doses of calcium salts, a newer agent, sevelamer hydrochloride—a tasteless, odorless calcium- and aluminum-free polymer that binds phosphorus in the gastrointestinal tract through ion exchange and hydrogen binding—may prove to be a safe and effective phosphate-binding agent in adult and pediatric patients with chronic renal failure.[108,109] Previous studies have demonstrated that sevelamer hydrochloride lowered serum phosphorus and PTH levels without any decrement in serum calcium levels.[110] In addition, there was a considerable reduction in low-density lipoprotein (LDL) and increase in high-density lipoprotein (HDL) levels; this may be beneficial in patients with renal failure by lowering the cardiovascular risk related to dyslipidemia.[110] To control hyperphosphatemia in pediatric patients on continuous cycling peritoneal dialysis, the dose of sevelamer hydrochloride used was 163 ± 46 mg/kg or 6700 ± 2400 mg/day without any associated changes in serum calcium, bicarbonate, cholesterol, HDL, or LDL.[108] Further studies are required to prove its efficacy and tolerability in the pediatric population, including the reported metabolic acidosis that occurred in adult patients during the treatment period[111]; this may have a significant impact particularly on growth if used in the long-term treatment of hyperphosphatemia in children.

In addition to sevelamer hydrochloride, there are other phosphate-binding agents in various stages of development, including iron-containing compounds, colestimide, lanthanum carbonate, and magnesium salts.[112–116] Lanthanum carbonate is a rare earth element, a noncalcium, nonaluminum phosphate binder with minimal gastrointestinal absorption (0.00003 percent) and low oral bioavailability compared to aluminum.[116] Oral doses between 750 to 3000 mg/day were well tolerated and effective in lowering serum phosphorus levels in 126 adult dialysis patients, with few adverse events.[116] Colestimide is a calcium- and aluminum-free phosphate binder that is widely used for the treatment of hypercholesterolemia; its chemical structure is similar to that of sevelamer hydrochloride.[114] Currently, there are no pediatric studies available to evaluate the efficacy and safety of these phosphate-binding agents in children.

Aluminum-containing agents are effective phosphate binders; however, adverse complications associated with long-term therapy—including encephalopathy, anemia, and bone disease—have limited its use in patients with chronic renal failure. Plasma aluminum levels have been used to monitor toxicity in children, but blood levels may not reflect the total aluminum burden in the body. Despite recommended doses, aluminum staining in the bone and a rise in plasma level after DFO infusion have been reported.[99] In cases of severe hyperphosphatemia (e.g., tumor lysis syndrome), aluminum may be given for short period of time (less than 4 weeks); doses should not exceed 30 mg/kg/day in children, and should not be administered concurrently with any form of citrate.[117,118]

Vitamin D Therapy

Calcitriol [$1,25\text{-}(OH)_2D_3$], introduced in the 1970s, has been demonstrated to be effective in the reduction of serum PTH levels in adult patients requiring dialysis therapy, whether given daily or intermittently, by the intravenous, oral, or intraperitoneal route.[119–122] Calcitriol lowers PTH gene transcription, decreases parathyroid cell proliferation, and increases the expression of VDR and calcium-sensing receptor in the parathyroid gland.[31,123,124] Although calcitriol has favorable effects on the parathyroid gland and the skeleton in secondary hyperparathyroidism, there is substantial evidence that calcitriol directly increases gastrointestinal absorption of calcium and phosphorus, which may lead to the undesirable complications related to hyperphosphatemia and hypercalcemia.[72,125] Thus, during the last decade, a wide variety of vitamin D analogues have been developed to retain the desirable effects of calcitriol for the treatment of secondary hyperparathyroidism and lessen the likelihood of increasing serum calcium and phosphorus levels in patients with chronic renal failure.

Vitamin D Therapy in Chronic Renal Failure. The primary aim in the use of vitamin D therapy for the treatment of secondary hyperparathyroidism in children with mild to moderate chronic renal failure is to protect the growing skeleton against the consequences of progressive renal failure and to prevent parathyroid gland hyperplasia without adversely affecting renal function. There are a limited number of pediatric clinical reports over the last 30 years in the use of calcitriol and other vitamin D analogues in the management of renal bone disease in children. Radiographic and histologic improvement of skeletal lesions associated with secondary hyperparathyroidism have been reported after treatment with daily doses of various vitamin D analogues, including calcitriol [1,25-$(OH)_2D_3$], alfacalcidol [1α-$(OH)_2D_3$], dihydrotachysterol [DHT_2], and calcifediol [25-$(OH)D_2$] in children with moderate to severe chronic renal failure.[126–132] There have been reports of hypercalcemia and deterioration of renal function in some children and adult patients undergoing treatment with vitamin D analogues, especially with the use of calcitriol.[133,134]

Most of the studies performed in children with moderate to severe chronic renal failure reported the use of vitamin D analogues on a daily basis. Ardissino and colleagues have demonstrated that calcitriol significantly lowered serum PTH levels, whether given daily or intermittently (twice per week), in children with chronic renal failure (Fig. 46–13).[135] The decline in serum PTH levels was associated with an increase in serum calcium and serum phosphorus levels; changes in skeletal histology were not evaluated in this study.[135] In adult patients with mild to moderate renal failure, the use of daily calcitriol, 0.125 to 0.5 µg, led to the resolution of histologic features associated with secondary hyperparathyroidism and significantly decreased PTH lev-

els[136–141]; however, hypercalcemia occurred in some patients who were taking aluminum compounds or calcium-containing salts as phosphate-binding agents.

Overall, early treatment with daily doses of oral calcitriol in patients with mild to moderate chronic renal failure has been reported to improve linear growth in children, suppress PTH levels, and improve histologic lesions of secondary hyperparathyroidism. Treatment with vitamin D should be initiated when serum PTH levels are above the target ranges (see Table 46–1). Pediatric patients can be started with doses between 0.125 to 0.25 µg daily and gradually titrated to achieve the target PTH levels. Serum PTH levels, calcium, and phosphorus must be monitored monthly in very young children and every 3 months once the serum levels are stable. Elevations in serum calcium and deterioration of renal function should be taken into consideration when patients with mild to moderate renal failure are being treated with doses greater than 0.5 µg daily.

Vitamin D Therapy in Dialysis Patients. Current management of secondary hyperparathyroidism relies predominantly on the use of calcium-containing salts as phosphate binding agents and the use of oral, intravenous, or intraperitoneal vitamin D sterols to control excess PTH secretion in patients on maintenance dialysis therapy. Early studies have suggested that high doses of calcitriol given intravenously three times weekly (intermittent or pulse) may be more effective in preventing parathyroid gland hyperplasia compared to daily oral therapy.[142] Despite differences in the route of administration, studies performed by Moe and colleagues have shown that the serum concentration of calcitriol given

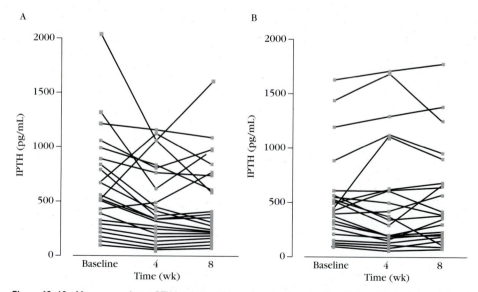

Figure 46–13. Mean serum intact PTH levels in children treated with daily (*A*) and intermittent (*B*) doses of oral calcitriol during the 8-week study period. The weekly dose is equivalent in both groups. The gray lines represent individual response and the black lines the mean change for each group. *$p < 0.03$, **$p < 0.02$ versus baseline PTH levels. (From Ardissino et al.[135] with permission.)

daily or intermittently (pulse) was equivalent 12 hours after a single dose in adult patients undergoing peritoneal dialysis with moderate secondary hyperparathyroidism.[122] In addition, the rate of decline of the serum PTH levels measured by immunoradiometric assay was similar in both groups.[122]

There are only a few studies in children undergoing dialysis therapy treated with daily calcitriol or other vitamin D analogues. Most of these reports demonstrated minor improvements in bone histology or radiographic findings of secondary hyperparathyroidism if calcitriol was given in higher doses and administered concurrently with some form of calcium supplementation either to control serum phosphorus or correct hypocalcemia.[143–145] In contrast to these findings, several studies in children did not show any histologic or radiographic improvements despite considerable reduction in serum PTH levels and increase in serum calcium levels during daily calcitriol or calcifediol therapy.[93,146–148] However, it is unclear what serum PTH levels correlated with histologic or radiographic improvement in these studies, since the PTH levels were measured with various PTH assays and therefore are not consistent.

Intermittent or pulse therapy with vitamin D analogues has generated interest because of the progression of osteitis fibrosa and failure to decrease the size of the parathyroid gland with daily calcitriol therapy. There are only a few pediatric studies available that utilize intermittent vitamin D therapy, and most of these reports relied mostly on descriptions of the biochemical changes and not on the alterations occurring in the skeleton. Intermittent or pulse therapy may be considered when serum PTH levels exceed 500 pg/mL. Patients can be started at 0.5 to 1.0 μg per dose given either orally, intravenously, or intraperitoneally three times weekly and adjusted according to target PTH levels (see Table 46–1). Intact PTH levels should be maintained within the target level and vitamin D dose adjusted when the PTH level is below 300 pg/mL so as to prevent the development of adynamic bone. Salusky and coworkers have shown that there were bone histologic improvements in 46 children undergoing peritoneal dialysis with moderate to severe secondary hyperparathyroidism treated with equivalent doses of either intraperitoneal or oral pulse calcitriol.[149] Similar findings were described by Goodman and colleagues in 14 children that received 12 months of intermittent calcitriol therapy at a dose of 1.25 μg three times weekly who were also being dialyzed with 3.5 meq/L of calcium and given calcium carbonate as the phosphate binder.[55] Concurrent with the significant decline in the rate of bone formation, there was a progressive reduction in serum intact PTH levels from 850 ± 380 to 150 ± 170 pg/mL, increase in serum calcium levels, and diminution in alkaline phosphatase levels.[55] There is little information on the implications of adynamic bone in children with chronic renal failure; however, a significant reduction in linear growth has been demonstrated in 16 prepubertal children who developed adynamic

bone after 12 months of high-dose intermittent calcitriol therapy.[57] In contrast, a recent study by Schmitt and colleagues reported that 12 months of daily or intermittent calcitriol therapy did not significantly affect longitudinal growth in prepubertal children with chronic renal failure.[150] The differences in findings are probably due to the lower calcitriol dose used in the study by Schmitt and colleagues to control secondary hyperparathyroidism, since these patients had not started dialysis therapy and the presence of skeletal resistance may not be significant. Although pulse calcitriol therapy maybe effective in PTH suppression and improvement of osteitis fibrosa in children with moderate to severe secondary hyperparathyroidism, episodes of hypercalcemia and hyperphosphatemia have increased, necessitating reduction and sometimes withdrawal of calcitriol; such episodes are usually seen in patients who are dialyzed against a higher calcium bath and are using calcium salts to control hyperphosphatemia.

In adult dialysis patients, intermittent therapy with calcitriol and other less calcemic vitamin D analogues—including paracalcitol [19-nor-1,25(OH)$_2$D$_2$], oxacalcitriol [22-oxa-1α,25(OH)$_2$D$_3$], and doxercalciferol [1α-(OH)D$_2$]—has been reported to be effective in the control of secondary hyperparathyroidism.[151–156] Although less commonly reported in patients treated with paracalcitol and doxercalciferol, hypercalcemia, hyperphosphatemia, and an elevated calcium x phosphorus product have been demonstrated in some adult patients undergoing chronic dialysis therapy.[154,155] There are currently no published studies or treatment guidelines in the use of the less calcemic vitamin D analogues in pediatric patients with chronic renal failure. In addition, there is very little information available in the use of the second-generation PTH assay during treatment with other vitamin D analogues.

Adequate control of secondary hyperparathyroidism must be ensured prior to growth hormone therapy. Recombinant human growth hormone has been demonstrated to increase serum PTH and phosphate levels in children with chronic renal failure. Growth hormone therapy must be discontinued if serum PTH levels continue to rise and restarted only if the PTH levels fall within the target PTH level. Although concomitant vitamin D therapy may blunt the effects of growth hormone in renal failure,[157] control of secondary hyperparathyroidism is extremely important in children who are candidates for growth hormone treatment.

Treatment with Calcimimetic Compounds

Calcimimetic agents are novel compounds that lower the threshold for activation of the calcium-sensing receptor by extracellular calcium ions, thereby lowering the set point for calcium-regulated PTH release and rendering parathyroid cells more sensitive to the inhibitory actions of calcium. These compounds are especially useful in the treatment of patients with secondary hyperparathyroidism whose serum calcium levels are already elevated and in whom vitamin D therapy may exacerbate problems of hypercalcemia and hyperphosphatemia. In addition, calcimimetic agents can also be used to achieve daily intermittent or sustained decreases in serum PTH levels; these plasma oscillations of PTH levels have been demonstrated to favorably increase bone mass in some types of osteoporosis in humans and in animals,[158,159] and to increase longitudinal growth in uremic rats independent of treatment with calcitriol.[160] The second-generation calcimimetic agent AMG 073 has been demonstrated to significantly lower PTH levels by 26 percent independent of serum calcitriol levels and decreased calcium x phosphorus product, with minimal problems of hypocalcemia after 12 weeks of therapy in adult patients maintained on hemodialysis.[161,162] The use of calcimimetic agents is quite promising; it represents an innovative therapeutic approach and provides an additional option in the management of children with secondary hyperparathyroidism. Currently, there are no published data on the use and safety of calcimimetic agents in children with renal failure. Calcium-sensing receptors are present in the hypertrophic chondrocytes of the growth-plate cartilage, hence the use of any agent that may modify or possibly block the actions of this receptor may affect growth, especially in very young children.[163]

Parathyroidectomy

Overall, the number of patients who develop advanced secondary hyperparathyroidism necessitating surgical parathyroidectomy has steadily declined over the years with the availability of the various vitamin D analogues and better control of hyperphosphatemia. Parathyroid gland hyperplasia characterized by marked elevations of PTH and osteitis fibrosa on bone biopsy usually results from poorly controlled secondary hyperparathyroidism. Currently, clinical indications for surgical parathyroidectomy include hypercalcemia and hyperphosphatemia associated with very elevated serum levels of circulating PTH unresponsive to medical therapy, progressive extraskeletal calcifications, persistent bone pain, multiple and recurrent fractures, and appearance of calciphylaxis. Ethanol injection into the parathyroid gland as an alternative to surgical parathyroidectomy has been performed in some Japanese patients,[164,165] but this procedure is not widely performed elsewhere. If possible, prior to parathyroidectomy, patients should undergo a bone biopsy procedure in order to exclude aluminum-related bone disease, which can worsen after the surgery. The quick parathyroid hormone assay (QPTH) has been developed over the last 10 years and has gained widespread acceptance among surgeons as an intraoperative adjunct to localize hypersecreting parathyroid glands and measure changes in circulating serum PTH levels.[166]

Most of the patients undergoing parathyroidectomy for severe secondary hyperparathyroidism will develop postoperative hypocalcemia, called "hungry bone syndrome," due to the rapid skeletal uptake of calcium. Intravenous calcium should be started once serum calcium levels are below normal (less than 8.5 mg/dL) and may be required 24 to 48 hours after parathyroidectomy. Calcium supplementation should be started once patients are able to tolerate taking oral medications. Vitamin D therapy (preferably calcitriol) should be given 24 hours preoperatively and should be continued postparathyroidectomy to enhance the gastrointestinal absorption of calcium. Concurrent postoperative hypophosphatemia is usually not treated unless the serum levels are below 2 mg/dL.

Corrrection of Metabolic Acidosis

The presence of metabolic acidosis has been associated with a reduction in bone mineralization, lower serum calcitriol levels, and alterations in the sensitivity of the parathyroid gland to minute changes in serum calcium concentrations.[52–54] Treatment with any available base, such as sodium citrate or sodium bicarbonate, should be implemented to normalize the serum bicarbonate and restore serum pH to normal. It is imperative, however, to make sure that patients are able to handle the extra sodium from these medications and to avoid drugs or any food item that may contain aluminum, especially in using citrate. Early studies have shown that citrate enhances the gastrointestinal absorption of aluminum, leading to aluminum toxicity in patients with chronic renal failure.[118]

CONCLUSION

Our understanding of secondary hyperparathyroidism and renal bone disease has increased over the years, but the clinical strategies that are currently employed to prevent the development of bone disease in children are still evolving. In the management of children with chronic renal failure, hypocalcemia should be corrected early, age-appropriate serum phosphorus levels must be achieved, metabolic acidosis must be treated, and serum intact PTH levels must be maintained within the recommended target ranges. The primary aim in the early treatment of secondary hyperparathyroidism in children with chronic renal failure is to protect the young skeleton against the effects of progressive renal failure and prevent the development of parathyroid gland hyperplasia.

ACKNOWLEDGMENT

Supported in part by USPHS grant no. NIDDK 56688–01 and by funds from the UW Department of Pediatrics Research Funds.

REFERENCES

1. Seikaly MG, Ho PL, Emmett L, et al. Chronic renal insufficiency in children: the 2001 Annual Report of the NAPRTCS. *Pediatr Nephrol* 2003;18:796–804.

2. Neu AM, Ho PLM, McDonald RA, et al. Chronic dialysis in children and adolescents: the 2001 NAPRTCS Annual Report. *Pediatr Nephrol* 2001;17:656–663.

3. Reichel H, Deibert B, Scmidt-Gayk H, et al. Calcium metabolism in early chronic renal failure: implications for the pathogenesis of hyperparathyroidism. *Nephrol Dial Transplant* 1991;6:162–169.

4. Malluche HH, Ritz E, Lange HP, et al. Bone histology in incipient and advanced renal failure. *Kidney Int* 1976;9:355–362.

5. Naveh-Many T, Rahamimov R, Livni N, et al. Parathyroid cell proliferation in normal and chronic renal failure rats. *J Clin Invest* 1995;96:1786–1793.

6. Denda M, Finch J, Slatopolsky E. Phosphorus accelerates the development of parathyroid hyperplasia and secondary hyperparathyroidism in rats with renal failure. *Am J Kidney Dis* 1996;28:596–602.

7. Slatopolsky E, Delmez JA. Pathogenesis of secondary hyperparathyroidism. *Am J Kidney Dis* 1994;23:229–236.

8. Moallem E, Kilav R, Silver J, et al. RNA-protein binding and post-transcriptional regulation of parathyroid hormone gene expression by calcium and phosphate. *J Biol Chem* 1998;273:5253–5259.

9. Slatopolsky E, Finch J, Denda M, et al. Phosphorus restriction prevents parathyroid gland growth. *J Clin Invest* 1996;97:2534–2540.

10. Almaden Y, Canalejo A, Ballesteros E, et al. Effect of high extracellular phosphate concentration on arachidonic acid production by parathyroid tissue in vitro. *J Am Soc Nephrol* 2000;11:1712–1718.

11. Estepa JC, Aguilera-Tejero E, Lopez I, et al. Effect of phosphate on parathyroid hormone secretion in vivo. *J Bone Miner Res* 1999;14:1848–1854.

12. Tatsumi S, Segawa H, Morita K, et al. Molecular cloning and hormonal regulation of Pit-1, a sodium-dependent phosphate cotransporter from rat parathyroid glands. *Endocrinology* 1998;139:1692–1699.

13. Schiavi SC, Kumar R. The phosphatonin pathway: new insights in phosphate homeostasis. *Kidney Int* 2004;65:1–14.

14. Larsson T, Nisbeth U, Ljunggren O, et al. Circulating concentration of FGF-23 increases as renal function declines in patients with chronic kidney disease, but does not change in response to variation in phosphate intake in healthy volunteers. *Kidney Int* 2003;64:2272–2279.

15. Block G, Port F. Re-evaluation of risks associated with hyperphosphatemia and hyperparathyroidism in dialysis patients: recommendations for a change in management. *Am J Kidney Dis* 2000;35:1226–1237.

16. Ganesh SK, Stack AG, Levin NW, et al. Association of elevated serum Po_4, Ca X Po_4 product, and parathyroid hormone with cardiac mortality risk in chronic hemodialysis patients. *J Am Soc Nephrol* 2001;12:2131–2138.

17. Goodman WG, Goldin J, Kuizon B, et al. coronary artery calcification in young adults with end-stage renal disease who are undergoing dialysis. *N Engl J Med* 2000;342:1478–1483.

18. Oh J, Wunsch R, Turzer M, et al. Advanced coronary and carotid arteriopathy in young adults with childhood-onset chronic renal failure. *Circulation* 2002;106:100–105.

19. Hsu CH, Patel SR. Uremic plasma contains factors inhibiting 1α-hydroxylase activity. *J Am Soc Nephrol* 1992;3:947–952.

20. Korkor AB. Reduced binding of [3h]1,25-dihydroxyvitamin D_3 in the parathyroid glands of patients with renal failure. *J Clin Invest* 1987;316:25.

21. Martinez I, Saracho R, Montenegro J, et al. A deficit of calcitriol synthesis may not be the initial factor in the pathogenesis of secondary hyperparathyroidism. *Nephrol Dial Transplant* 1996;11(suppl 3):22–28.

22. Portale AA, Booth BE, Tsai HC, et al. reduced plasma concentration of 1,25-dihydroxyvitamin D in children with moderate renal insufficiency. *Kidney Int* 1982;21:627–632.

23. Pitts TO, Piraino BH, Mitro R, et al. Hyperparathyroidism and 1,25-dihydroxyvitamin d deficiency in mild, moderate, and severe renal failure. *J Clin Endocrinol Metab* 1988;67:876–881.

24. Malluche HH, Faugere M-C. Renal bone disease 1990: an unmet challenge for the nephrologist. *Kidney Int* 1990;38:193–211.

25. Norman M, Mazur AT, Borden S, et al. Early diagnosis of juvenile renal osteodystrophy. *J Pediatr* 1980;97(2):226–232.

26. Fukuda N, Tanaka H, Tominaga Y, et al. Decreased 1,25-dihydroxyvitamin D_3 receptor density is associated with a more severe form of parathyroid hyperplasia in chronic uremic patients. *J Clin Invest* 1993;92:1436–1443.

27. Brown EM, Gamba G, Riccardi D, et al. Cloning and characterization of an extracellular Ca^{2+}-sensing receptor from bovine parathyroid. *Nature* 1993;366:575–580.

28. Brown EM, Wilson RE, Eastman RC, et al. Abnormal regulation of parathyroid hormone release by calcium in secondary hyperparathyroidism due to chronic renal failure. *J Clin Endocrinol Metab* 1982;54:172–179.

29. Ramirez JA, Goodman WG, Gornbein J, et al. Direct in vivo comparison of calcium-regulated parathyroid hormone secretion in normal volunteers and patients with secondary hyperparathyroidism. *J Clin Endocrinol Metab* 1993;76:1489–1494.

30. Messa P, Vallone C, Mioni G, et al. Direct in vivo assessment of parathyroid hormone-calcium relationship curve in renal patients. *Kidney Int* 1994;46:1713–1720.

31. Yano S, Sugimoto T, Tsukamoto T, et al. Association of Decreased calcium-sensing receptor expression with proliferation of parathyroid cells in secondary hyperparathyroidism. *Kidney Int* 2000;58:1980–1986.

32. Ritter CS, Martin DR, Lu Y, et al. Reversal of secondary hyperparathyroidism by phosphate restriction restores parathyroid calcium-sensing receptor expression and function. *J Bone Miner Res* 2002;17:2206–2213.

33. Salusky IB, Ramirez JA, Oppenheim W, et al. Biochemical markers of renal osteodystrophy in pediatric patients undergoing CAPD/CCPD. *Kidney Int* 1994;45:253–258.

34. Quarles LD, Lobaugh B, Murphy G. Intact Parathyroid hormone overestimates the presence and severity of parathyroid-mediated osseous abnormalities in uremia. *J Clin Endocrinol Metab* 1992;75:145–150.

35. Slatopolsky E, Finch J, Clay P, et al. A novel mechanism for skeletal resistance in uremia. *Kidney Int* 2000;58:753–761.

36. Salomon R, Charbit M, Gagnadoux M-F, et al. High serum levels of a non-(1–84) parathyroid hormone (PTH) fragment in pediatric hemodialysis patients. *Pediatr Nephrol* 2001;16:1011–1014.

37. Coen G, Bonucci E, Ballanti P, et al. PTH1–84 and PTH (7–84) in the noninvasive diagnosis of renal bone disease. *Am J Kidney Dis* 2002;40:348–354.

38. Salusky IB, Goodman WG, Kuizon BD, et al. Similar predictive value of bone turnover using the first- and second-generation immunometric PTH assays in pediatric patients treated with peritoneal dialysis. *Kidney Int* 2003;63:1801–1808.

39. Reichel H, Esser A, Roth H-J, et al. Influence of PTH assay methodology on differential diagnosis of renal bone disease. *Nephrol Dial Transplant* 2003;18:759–768.

40. Waller S, Reynolds A, Ridout D, et al. Parathyroid hormone and its fragments in children with chronic renal failure. *Pediatr Nephrol* 2003;18:1242–1248.

41. Monier-Faugere M-C, Geng Z, Mawad H, et al. Improved assessment of bone turnover by the PTH (1–84)/large C-PTH fragments ratio in ESRD patients. *Kidney Int* 2001;60:1460–1468.

42. Salem M, Sanchez C, Kuizon B, et al. Renal bone diseases in children with chronic renal failure. *J Am Soc Nephrol* 1998;9:549A.

43. Hamdy NAT, Kanis JA, Beneton MNC, et al. Effect of alfacalcidol on natural course of renal bone disease in mild to moderate renal failure. *Br Med J* 1995;310:358–361.

44. Waller S, Ledermann S, Trompeter R, et al. Catch-up growth with normal parathyroid hormone levels in chronic renal failure. *Pediatr Nephrol* 2003;18:1236–1241.

45. Sanchez C, He Y, Leiferman E, et al. Bone elongation in rats with renal failure and mild or advanced secondary hyperparathyroidism. *Kidney Int* 2004;65(5):1740–1748.

46. Cobo A, Carbajo E, Santos F, et al. Morphometry of uremic rat growth plate. *Miner Electrolyte Metab* 1996;22:192–195.

47. Langub MC, Monier-Faugere M-C, Wang G, et al. Administration of PTH-(7–84) antagonizes the effects of PTH-(1–84) on bone in rats with moderate renal failure. *Endocrinology* 2003;144:1135–1138.

48. Graham KA, Hoenich NA, Tarbit M, et al. Correction of acidosis in hemodialysis patients increases the sensitivity of the parathyroid glands to calcium. *J Am Soc Nephrol* 1997;8:627–631.

49. Bushinsky DA. Net calcium efflux from live bone during chronic metabolic, but not respiratory acidosis. *Am J Physiol* 1989;265:836–842.

50. Ritz E, Matthias S, Seidel A, et al. Disturbed calcium metabolism in renal failure-pathogenesis and therapeutic strategies. *Kidney Int* 1992;42:S37–S42.

51. Barsotti G, Lazzeri M, Cristofano C, et al. The role of metabolic acidosis in causing uremic hyperphosphatemia. *Miner Electrolyte Metab* 1986;12:103–106.

52. Movilli E, Zani R, Carli O, et al. Direct effect of the correction of acidosis on plasma parathyroid hormone concentrations, calcium and phosphate in hemodialysis patients: a prospective study. *Nephron* 2001;87:257–262.

53. Lu KC, Lin SH, Yu FC, et al. Influence of metabolic acidosis on serum $1,25(OH)_2D_3$ levels in chronic renal failure. *Miner Electrolyte Metab* 1995;21:398–402.

54. Carbajo E, Lopez JM, Santos F, et al. Histologic and dynamic changes induced by chronic metabolic acidosis in the rat growth plate. *J Am Soc Nephrol* 2001;12:1228–1234.

55. Goodman WG, Ramirez JA, Belin TR, et al. Development of adynamic bone in patients with secondary hyperparathyroidism after intermittent calcitriol therapy. *Kidney Int* 1994;46:1160–1166.

56. Ziolkowska H, Paniczyk-Tomaszewska M, Debinski A, et al. Bone biopsy results and serum bone turnover parameters in uremic children. *Acta Pediatr* 2000;89:666–671.

57. Kuizon BD, Goodman WG, Juppner H, et al. Diminished linear growth during intermittent calcitriol therapy in children undergoing CCPD. *Kidney Int* 1998;53:205–211.

58. Fivush BA, Jabs K, Neu AM, et al. Chronic renal insufficiency in children and adolescents: the 1996 annual report of NAPRCTS. *Pediatr Nephrol* 1998;12:328–337.

59. Fine RN, Ho M, Tejani A. The contribution of renal transplantation to final adult height: a report of the North American Pediatric Renal Transplant Cooperative Study (NAPRTCS). *Pediatr Nephrol* 16:951–1056.

60. Van Dyck M, Bilem N, Proesmans W. Conservative treatment for chronic renal failure from birth: a 3-year follow-up study. *Pediatr Nephrol* 1999;13:865–869.

61. Tonshoff B, Powell DR, Zhao D, et al. Decreased hepatic insulin-like growth factor (IGF)-I and increased IGF binding protein-1 and -2 gene expression in experimental uremia. *Endocrinology* 1997;128:938–946.

62. Tonshoff B, Blum WF, Wingen A-M, et al. Serum insulin-like growth factors (IGFs) and IGF binding proteins 1,2, and 3 in children with chronic renal failure: relationship to height and glomerular filtration rate. *J Clin Endocrinol Metab* 1995;80:2684–2691.

63. Schaefer F, Chen Y, Tsao T, et al. Impaired JAK-STAT signal transduction contributes to growth hormone resistance in chronic uremia. *J Clin Invest* 2001;108:467–475.

64. Barrett IR, Papadimitriou DG. Skeletal disorders in children with renal failure. *J Pediatr Orthop* 1996;16:264–272.

65. Oppenheim WL, Shayestehfar S, Salusky IB. Tibial physeal changes in renal osteodystrophy: lateral Blount's disease. *J Pediatr Orthop* 1992;12:774–779.

66. Davids JR, Fisher R, Lum G, et al. Angular deformity of the lower extremity in children with renal osteodystrophy. *J Pediatr Orthop* 1992;12:291–299.

67. Oppenheim W, Bowen R, McDonough P, et al. Outcome of slipped capital femoral epiphysis in renal osteodystrophy. *J Pediatr Orthop* 2003;23:169–174.

68. Krempien B, Mehls O, Ritz E. Morphological studies on the pathogenesis of epiphyseal slipping in uremic children. *Virchows Archiv A Path Anat Histol* 1974;362:129–143.

69. Mehls O, Ritz E, Krempien B, et al. Slipped epiphyses in renal osteodystrophy. *Arch Dis Child* 1975;50:545–554.

70. Sherrard DJ, Hercz G, Pei Y, et al. The aplastic form of renal osteodystrophy. *Nephrol Dial Transplant* 1996;11(suppl 3): 29–31.

71. Kunis C, Markowitz G, Liu-Jarin X, et al. Painful myopathy and end-stage renal disease. *Am J Kidney Dis* 2001;37: 1098–1094.

72. Henderson RG, Ledingham JGG, Oliver DO, et al. Effects of 1,25-dihydrocholecalciferol on calcium absorption, muscle weakness, and bone disease in chronic renal failure. *Lancet* 1974;2(7871):14–7.

73. Milliner DS, Zinsmeister AR, Liberman E, et al. Soft tissue calcification in pediatric patients with end-stage renal disease. *Kidney Int* 1990;38:931–936.

74. Block GA, Hulbert-Shearon TE, Levin NW, et al. Association of serum phosphorus and calcium x phosphate product with mortality risk in chronic hemodialysis patients: a national study. *Am J Kidney Dis* 1998;31:607–617.

75. Phelps K, Bansal M, Twersky J. Jaw enlargement complicating secondary hyperparathyroidism in three hemodialysis patients. *Clin Nephrol* 1994;41:173–179.

76. Catizone L, Casolino D, Santoro A, et al. An unusual manifestation of renal osteodystrophy. *Nephron* 1984;37: 133–136.

77. Shanmugham M, Alhady S. Hyperparathyroidism with osteitis fibrosa cystica in the maxilla. *J Laryngol Otol* 1984;98:417–420.

78. Antonelli J, Hottel T. Oral manifestations of renal osteodystrophy: case report and review of the literature. *Spec Care Dentist* 2003;23:28–34.

79. Malluche H, Ritz E, Werner E, et al. Long-term administration of vitamin D steroles in incipient and advanced renal failure: effect on bone histology. *Clin Nephrol* 1978;10: 219–228.

80. Kurz P, Monier-Faugere M-C, Bognar B, et al. Evidence for abnormal calcium homeostasis in patients with adynamic bone disease. *Kidney Int* 1994;46:855–861.

81. Food and Nutrition Board, National Institute of Medicine. *Dietary Reference Intakes for Calcium, Phosphorus, Magnesium, Vitamins, Fluoride.* Washington, DC: National Academy of Sciences, 1997.

82. Brossard J, Lepage R, Cardinal H, et al. Influence of glomerular filtration rate on non (1–84) Parathyroid hormone (PTH) detected by intact PTH assays. *Clin Chem* 2000;46:647–703.

83. National Kidney Foundation. DOQI guidelines, clinical practice guidelines for bone metabolism and disease in chronic kidney disease. *Am J Kidney Dis* 2003:42(suppl 3): S12–S28.

84. Stein GS, Lian JB, Owen TA. Relationship of cell growth to the regulation of tissue-specific gene expression during osteoblast differentiation. *FASEB J* 1990;4:3111–3123.

85. Behnke B, Kemper M, Kruse H, et al. Bone alkaline phosphatase in children with chronic renal failure. *Nephrol Dial Transplant* 1998;13:662–667.

86. Groothoff JW, Offringa M, Eck-Smit BLFV, et al. Severe Bone Disease and Low Bone Mineral Density after Juvenile Renal Failure. *Kidney Int* 2003;63:266–275.

87. Pluskiewicz W, Adamczyk P, Drozdzowska B, et al. Skeletal Status in Children and Adolescents with Chronic Renal Failure before Onset of Dialysis or on Dialysis. *Osteoporosis International* 2003;14:283–288.

88. Lima EM, Goodman WG, Kuizon BD, et al. Bone Density Measurements in Pediatric Patients with Renal Osteodystrophy. *Pediatr Nephrol* 18:554–559.

89. Taal MW, Roe S, Masud T, et al. Total Hip Bone Mass Predicts Survival in Chronic Hemodialysis Patients. *Kidney Int* 2003;63:1116–1120.

90. Sarikaya A, Sen S, Hacimahmutoglu S, et al. 99mTc(V)-DMSA scintigraphy in monitoring the response of bone disease to vitamin D_3 therapy in renal osteodystrophy. *Ann Nucl Med* 2002;16:19–23.

91. de Graaf P, Schicht I, Pauwels E, et al. Bone Scintigraphy in Renal Osteodystrophy. *J Nuclear Med* 1978;19:1289–1296.

92. Drachman R, Baillet G, Gagnadoux M, et al. Pulmonary Calcifications in Children on Dialysis. *Nephron* 1986;44: 46–50.

93. Salusky IB, Coburn JW, Brill J, et al. Bone disease in pediatric patients undergoing dialysis with CAPD or CCPD. *Kidney Int* 1988;33:975–982.

94. Mathias R, Salusky IB, Harmon W, et al. Renal bone disease in pediatric and young adult patients on hemodialysis in a children's hospital. *J Am Soc Nephrol* 1993;3:1938–1946.

95. Mucsi I, Hercz G, Uldall R, et al. Control of serum phosphorus without any phosphate binders in patients treated with nocturnal hemodialysis. *Kidney Int* 1998;53:527–531.

96. Portale AA, Booth BE, Halloran BP, et al. Effect of dietary phosphorus on circulating concentrations of 1,25-dihydroxyvitamin and immunoreactive parathyroid hormone in children with moderate renal insufficiency. *J Clin Invest* 1984;73:1580–1589.

97. McCrory WW, Gertner JM, Burke FM, et al. Effects of dietary phosphate restriction in children with chronic renal failure. *J Pediatr* 1987;111:410–412.

98. Andreoli SP, Bergstein JM and Sherrard DJ: Aluminum intoxication from aluminum-containing phosphate binders in children with azotemia not undergoing dialysis. *N Engl J Med* 1984;310:1079–1084.

99. Salusky IB, Foley J, Nelson P, et al. Aluminum accumulation during treatment with aluminum hydroxide and dialysis in children and young adults with chronic renal disease. *N Engl J Med* 1991;324:527–531.

100. Coburn JW, Norris KC. Diagnosis of aluminum-related bone disease and treatment of aluminum toxicity with deferoxamine. *Semin Nephrol* 1986;6:12–21.

101. Schaefer K, Scheer J, Asmus G, et al. The treatment of uremic hyperphosphatemia with calcium acetate and calcium carbonate: a comparative study. *Nephrol Dial Transplant* 1991;6:170–175.

102. Indridason OS and Quarles LD. Comparison of treatments for mild secondary hyperparathyroidism in hemodialysis patients. Durham Renal Osteodystrophy Study Group. *Kidney Int* 2000;57:282–292.

103. Andreoli SP, Dunson JW, Bergstein JM. Calcium carbonate is an effective phosphorus binder in children with chronic renal failure. *Am J Kidney Dis* 1987;9:206–210.

104. Block GA. Prevalence and clinical consequences of elevated ca x p product in hemodialysis patients. *Clin Nephrol* 2000;54:318–324.

105. Weinrich T, Passlick-Deetjen J, Ritz E. Low dialysate calcium in continuous ambulatory peritoneal dialysis: a randomized controlled multicenter trial. *Am J Kidney Dis* 1995; 25:452–460.

106. Johnson DW, Rigby RJ, McIntyre HD, et al. A randomized trial comparing 1.25 Mmol/L calcium dialysate to 1.75 Mmol/L calcium dialysate in CAPD Patients. *Nephrol Dial Transplant* 1996;11:88–93.

107. Fernandez E, Borras M, Pais B, et al. Low-calcium dialysate stimulates parathormone secretion and its long-term use worsens secondary hyperparathyroidism. *J Am Soc Nephrol* 1995;6:132–135.

108. Mahdavi H, Kuizon B, Gales B, et al. Sevelamer hydrochloride: an effective phosphate binder in dialyzed children. *Pediatr Nephrol* 2003;18:1260–1264.

109. Slatopolsky EA, Burke SK, Dillon MA: Renagel, a nonabsorbed calcium- and aluminum-free phosphate binder, lowers serum phosphorus and parathyroid hormone. *Kidney Int* 1999;55:299–307.

110. Chertow GM, Burke SK, Dillon MA, et al. Long-term effects of sevelamer hydrochloride on the calcium x phosphate product and lipid profile of hemodialysis patients. *Nephrol Dial Transplant* 1999;14:2907–2914.

111. Chertow GM, Burke SK, Lazarus JM, et al. Poly[allylamine hydrochloride] (Renagel): a noncalcemic phosphate binder for the treatment of hyperphosphatemia in chronic renal failure. *Am J Kidney Dis* 1997;29:66–71.

112. Hsu CH, Patel SR, Young EW. New phosphate binding agents: ferric compounds. *J Am Soc Nephrol* 1999;10:1274–1280.

113. Hergesell O and Ritz E: Stabilized polynuclear iron hydroxide is an efficient oral phosphate binder in uraemic patients. *Nephrol Dial Transplant* 1999;14:863–867.

114. Date T, Shigematsu T, Kawashita Y, et al. Colestimide can be used as a phosphate binder to treat uraemia in end-stage renal disease patients. *Nephrol Dial Transplant* 2003;18:90iii–93iii.

115. Delmez JA, Kelber J, Norword KY, et al. Magnesium carbonate as a phosphate binder: a prospective, controlled, cross-over study. *Kidney Int* 1996;49:163–167.

116. Joy M, Finn W. Randomized, double-blind, placebo-controlled, dose-titration, phase III study assessing the efficacy and tolerability of lanthanum carbonate: a new phosphate binder for the treatment of hyperphosphatemia. *Am J Kid Dis* 2003;42:96–107.

117. Winney RJ, Cowie JF, Robson JS. Role of plasma aluminum in the detection and prevention of aluminum toxicity. *Kidney Int* 1986;18:S91–S95.

118. Molitoris BA, Froment DH, Mackenzie TA, et al. Citrate: a major factor in the toxicity of orally administered aluminum compounds. *Kidney Int* 1989;36:949–953.

119. Cannella G, Bonucci E, Rolla D, et al. Evidence of healing of secondary hyperparathyroidism in chronically hemodialyzed uremic patients treated with long-term intravenous calcitriol. *Kidney Int* 1994;46:1124–1132.

120. Delmez JA, Dougan CS, Gearing BK, et al. The effects of intraperitoneal calcitriol on calcium and parathyroid hormone. *Kidney Int* 1987;31:795–799.

121. Dunlay R, Rodriguez M, Felsenfeld AJ, et al. Direct inhibitory effect of calcitriol on parathyroid function (sigmoidal curve) in dialysis. *Kidney Int* 1989;36:1093–1098.

122. Moe SM, Kraus MA, Gassensmith CM, et al. safety and efficacy of pulse and daily calcitriol in patients on CAPD: a Randomized trial. *Nephrol Dial Transplant* 1998;13: 1234–1241.

123. Denda M, Finch J, Brown AJ, et al. 1,25-Dihydroxyvitamin D_3 and 22-oxacalcitriol prevent the decrease in vitamin D receptor content in the parathyroid glands of uremic rats. *Kidney Int* 1996;50:34–39.

124. Naveh-Many T, Marx R, Keshet E, et al. Regulation of 1,25-dihydroxyvitamin D_3 receptor gene expression by 1,25-dihydroxyvitamin D_3 in the parathyroid in vivo. *J Clin Invest* 1990;86:1968–1975.

125. Peacock M, Gallagher JC, Nordin BEC. Action of 1α-hydroxyvitamin D_3 on calcium absorption and bone resorption in man. *Lancet* 1974;1(7854):385–389.

126. Chesney RW, Moorthy AV, Eisman JA, et al. Increased growth after long-term oral 1a,25-vitamin D_3 in childhood renal osteodystrophy. *N Engl J Med* 1978;298:238–242.

127. Chan JCM, Kodroff MB, Landwehr DM. Effects of 1,25-dihydroxyvitamin D_3 on renal function, mineral balance, and growth in children with severe chronic renal failure. *Pediatrics* 1981;68:559–571.

128. Hymes LC, Warshaw BL. Vitamin D replacement therapy and renal function. *Am J Dis Child* 1984;138:1125–1128.

129. Kanis JA. The use of Alfacalcidol in the prevention of bone disease in early renal failure. *Nephrol Dial Transplant* 1995;10:23–28.

130. Langman CB, Mazur AT, Baron R, et al. 25-Hydroxyvitamin D3 (Calcifediol) therapy of juvenile renal osteodystrophy: beneficial effect on linear growth velocity. *J Pediatr* 1982; 100:815–820.

131. Trachtman H, Gauthier B. Parenteral calcitriol for treatment of severe renal osteodystrophy in children with chronic renal insufficiency. *J Pediatr* 1987;110:966–970.

132. Eke FU, Winterborn MH. Effect of low dose 1α-hydroxycholecalciferol on glomerular filtration rate in moderate renal failure. *Arch Dis Child* 1983;58:810–813.

133. Christiansen C, Rodbro P, Christensen MS, et al. Is 1,25-dihydroxy-cholecalciferol harmful to renal function in patients with chronic renal failure? *Clin Endocrinol* 1981;15: 229–236.

134. Tougaard L, Sorensen E, Brochner-Mortensen J, et al. Controlled trial of 1α-hydrocholecalciferol in chronic renal failure. *Lancet* 1976;1:1044–1047.

135. Ardissino G, Schmitt CP, Testa S, et al. Calcitriol pulse therapy is not more effective than daily calcitriol therapy in controlling secondary hyperparathyroidism in children with chronic renal failure. *Pediatr Nephrol* 2000;14:664–668.

136. Bianchi ML, Colantonio G, Campanini F, et al. Calcitriol and calcium carbonate therapy in early chronic renal failure. *Nephrol Dial Transplant* 1994;9:1595–1599.

137. Ritz E, Kuster S, Schmidt-Gayk H, et al. Low-dose calcitriol prevents the rise in 1,84 iPTH without affecting serum calcium and phosphate in patients with moderate renal failure (Prospective Placebo-Controlled Multicentre Trial). *Nephrol Dial Transplant* 1995;10:2228–2234.

138. Baker LRI, Abrams SML, Roe CJ, et al. 1,25(OH)$_2$D$_3$ administration in moderate renal failure: a prospective double-blind trial. *Kidney Int* 1989;35:661–669.

139. Coen G, Mazzaferro S, Bonucci E, et al. Treatment of secondary hyperparathyroidism of predialysis chronic renal failure with low doses of $1,25(OH)_2D_3$: humoral and histomorphometric results. *Miner Electrolyte Metab* 1986;12: 375–382.

140. Nordal KP, Dahl E. Low dose calcitriol versus placebo in patients with predialysis chronic renal failure. *J Clin Endocrinol Metab* 1988;67:929–936.

141. Nielsen HE, Romer FK, Melsen F, et al. 1α-Hydroxyvitamin D_3 treatment of nondialyzed patients with chronic renal failure. Effects on bone, mineral metabolism and kidney function. *Clin Nephrol* 1980;13:103–108.

142. Slatopolsky E, Weerts C, Thielan J, et al. Marked suppression of secondary hyperparathyroidism by intravenous administration of 1,25-dihydroxycholecalciferol in uremic patients. *J Clin Invest* 1984;74:2136–2143.

143. Potter DE, Wilson CJ, Ozonoff MB. Hyperparathyroid bone disease in children undergoing long-term hemodialysis; treatment with vitamin D. *J Pediatr* 1974;85:60–66.

144. Paunier L, Salusky IB, Slatopolsky E, et al. Renal osteodystrosphy in children undergoing continuous ambulatory peritoneal dialysis. *Pediatr Res* 1984;18:742–747.

145. Hodson EM, Evans RA, Dunstan CR, et al. Treatment of childhood renal osteodystrophy with calcitriol or ergocalciferol. *Clin Nephrol* 1985;24:192–200.

146. Hewitt IK, Stefanidis C, Reilly BJ, et al. Renal osteodystrophy in children undergoing continuous ambulatory peritoneal dialysis. *J Pediatr* 1983;103:729–734.

147. Jones CL, Vieth R, Spino M, et al. Comparisons between oral and intraperitoneal 1,25-dihydroxyvitamin D_3 therapy in children treated with peritoneal dialysis. *Clin Nephrol* 1994;42:44–49.

148. Witmer G, Margolis A, Fontaine O, et al. Effects of 25-hydroxycholecalciferol on bone lesions of children with terminal renal failure. *Kidney Int* 1976;10:395–408.

149. Salusky IB, Kuizon BD, Belin TR, et al. Intermittent calcitriol therapy in secondary hyperparathyroidism: a comparison between oral and intraperitoneal administration. *Kidney Int* 1998;54:907–914.

150. Schmitt CP, Ardissino G, Testa S, et al. Growth in children with chronic renal failure on intermittent versus daily calcitriol. *Pediatr Nephrol* 2003;18:440–444.

151. Quarles LD, Yohay DA, Carroll BA, et al. Prospective trial of pulse oral versus intravenous calcitriol treatment of hyperparathyroidism in ESRD. *Kidney Int* 1994;45: 1710–1721.

152. Tsukamoto Y, Hanaoka M, Matsuo T, et al. Effect of 22-oxacalcitriol on bone histology of hemodialyzed patients with severe secondary hyperparathyroidism. *Am J Kidney Dis* 2000;35:458–464.

153. Kinugasa E, Akizawa T, Takahashi J, et al. Effects of 1,25-dihydroxy-22-oxavitamin D_3 on parathyroid gland function in haemodialysis patients with secondary hyperparathyroidism. *Nephrol Dial Transplant* 2002;17:20–27.

154. Martin KJ, Gonzalez EA, Gellens M, et al. 19-nor-1-α25-dihydroxyvitamin D_2 (Paracalcitol) safely and effectively reduces the levels of intact parathyroid hormone in patients on hemodialysis. *J Am Soc Nephrol* 1998;9:1427–1432.

155. Tan AU Jr, Levine BS, Mazess RB, et al. Effective suppression of parathyroid hormone by 1α-hydroxyvitamin D_2 in hemodialysis patients with moderate to severe secondary hyperparathyroidism. *Kidney Int* 1997;51:317–323.

156. Frazao JM, Elangovan L, Maung HM, et al. Intermittent doxercalciferol (1-α-hydroxyvitamin D_2) therapy for secondary hyperparathyroidism. *Am J Kidney Dis* 2000;36: 550–561.

157. Sanchez CP, Salusky IB, Kuizon BD, et al. Growth of long bones in renal failure: roles of hyperparathyroidism, growth hormone and calcitriol. *Kidney Int* 1998;54:1879–1887.

158. Ishii H, Wada M, Furuya Y, et al. Daily intermittent decreases in serum levels of parathyroid hormone have an anabolic-like action on the bones of uremic rats with low-turnover bone and osteomalacia. *Bone* 2000;26:175–182.

159. Lane NE, Sanchez S, Modin GW, et al. Parathyroid hormone treatment can reverse corticosteroid-induced osteoporosis. Results of a randomized controlled clinical trial. *J Clin Invest* 1998;102:1627–1633.

160. Schmitt CP, Hessing S, Oh J, et al. Intermittent administration of parathyroid hormone (1–37) improves growth and bone mineral density in uremic rats. *Kidney Int* 2000;57: 1484–1492.

161. Lindberg JS, Moe SM, Goodman WG, et al. The calcimimetic AMG 073 reduces parathyroid hormone and calcium x phosphorus in secondary hyperparathyroidism. *Kidney Int* 2003;63:248–254.

162. Goodman WG, Hladik GA, Turner SA, et al. The calcimimetic agent AMG 073 lowers plasma parathyroid hormone levels in hemodialysis patients with secondary hyperparathyroidism. *J Am Soc Nephrol* 2002;13:1017–1024.

163. Chang W, Tu C, Chen T-H, et al. Expression and signal transduction of calcium-sensing receptors in cartilage and bone. *Endocrinology* 1999;140:5883–5893.

164. Kakuta T, Fukagawa M, Fujisaki T, et al. Prognosis of parathyroid function after successful percutaneous ethanol injection therapy guided by color Doppler flow mapping in chronic dialysis patients. *Am J Kidney Dis* 1999;33: 1091–1099.

165. Kitaoka M, Fukagawa M, Ogata E, et al. Reduction of Functioning parathyroid cell mass by ethanol injection in chronic dialysis patients. *Kidney Int* 1994;46:1110–1117.

166. Carneiro DM, Solorzano CC, Nader MC, et al. Comparison of intraoperative IPTH assay (QPTH): criteria in guiding parathyroidectomy: which criterion is the most accurate? *Surgery* 2003;134:973–981.

Management of Anemia in Pediatric Patients

Larry A. Greenbaum

Anemia is a common problem in children with chronic kidney disease (CKD); it is almost universal in children with end-stage renal disease (ESRD). While recombinant human erythropoietin (rHuEPO) has revolutionized the treatment of anemia in children with CKD, anemia management remains challenging. Many children are still anemic due to iron deficiency, inadequate rHuEPO dosing, blood loss, acute or chronic inflammation, secondary hyperparathyroidism, and nutritional deficiencies. There are many unanswered questions, including the optimal target hemoglobin (Hb), the best approach for correcting iron deficiency, and the role of darbepoetin alpha in treating the anemia of CKD in children.

This chapter briefly reviews the pathophysiology of anemia in CKD. Chapter 26 provides a more detailed review of this topic. The remainder of this chapter focuses on the epidemiology, clinical evaluation, and treatment of anemia in children with CKD. While it cites adult studies, there is an emphasis on the pediatric literature. Chapter 26 provides a more comprehensive review of the adult literature. There are European[1] and American [National Kidney Foundation Kidney Disease Outcome Quality Initiative (NKF-K/DOQI) guidelines][2] recommendations for the management of anemia in CKD.

PATHOPHYSIOLOGY OF ANEMIA

A variety of factors contribute to the anemia in CKD (Table 47–1). The dramatic improvement in anemia with rHuEPO emphasizes the central role of erythropoietin deficiency in the pathophysiology of the anemia in CKD. Yet the continued presence of anemia, despite the availability of rHuEPO, underscores the multifactorial etiology of the anemia in children with CKD.

TABLE 47–1. CAUSES OF ANEMIA IN CHRONIC KIDNEY DISEASE

Erythropoietin deficiency
Blood loss
Hemolysis
Bone marrow suppression
Iron deficiency
Inadequate dialysis
Malnutrition
Chronic or acute inflammation
Infection
Hyperparathyroidism
B_{12} or folate deficiency
Aluminum toxicity
Carnitine deficiency
Medications (e.g., ACE inhibitors)
Systemic disease
  Hemoglobinopathy
  Hypothyroidism
  Systemic lupus erythematosus

Erythropoietin Deficiency

During CKD, damage to the kidneys leads to a decrease in erythropoietin production. In both pediatric[3,4] and adult[5] patients with CKD, erythropoietin levels are inappropriately low for the degree of anemia. The level of glomerular filtration rate (GFR) at which anemia develops varies between patients, partially due to the nature of the underlying kidney disease. In one study, significant anemia in children was noted only when the GFR was less than 20 mL/min/1.73m^2.[4] In another study, a GFR less than 35 mL/min/1.73m^2 was the cutoff for anemia.[3]

Blood Loss

Excessive blood loss contributes to anemia and iron deficiency (see below) in CKD. Sources of blood loss include phlebotomy, blood lost in the dialyzer and tubing during hemodialysis (HD),[6–9] gastrointestinal losses,[8] and increased menstrual bleeding due to the acquired defect in platelet function of CKD. Intestinal blood loss is higher in children receiving HD than in other children with CKD.[8]

Decreased Red Blood Cell Survival

The life span of red blood cells (RBCs) is decreased in adults[10,11] and children[8] with CKD. There is an increase in the osmotic fragility of RBCs in patients receiving HD.[12] Decreased red cell survival may be partially due to carnitine deficiency (see below)[13] and a direct consequence of erythropoietin deficiency, since there is evidence of increased red cell survival in CKD patients after starting rHuEPO.[14]

Bone-Marrow Suppression

Serum from children with CKD directly suppresses the production of RBCs in vitro.[3] The specific inhibitory substances have not been definitively identified.

Dialysis appears to effectively remove some of these molecules. In one study, the initiation of HD led to an increase in hematocrit despite a decrease in endogenous erythropoietin levels.[15] Moreover, as described below, increased dose of dialysis appears to have a beneficial effect on RBC production, allowing for decreased dosing of rHuEPO.[16–19]

Iron Deficiency

Iron deficiency is an important cause of anemia in patients with CKD. A variety of factors are responsible for iron deficiency in children with CKD (Table 47–2).

The increase in RBC synthesis that occurs when using rHuEPO frequently depletes iron stores. In a number of studies of rHuEPO, use of intravenous iron was necessary, despite the routine use of oral iron, in order to correct acquired iron deficiency.[20–22]

In one study of older children, a serum transferrin saturation (TSAT) less than 20 percent was an independent predictor of anemia after multiple regression.[23] However, serum ferritin level was not predictive of anemia.[23]

Inadequate Dialysis

In adult dialysis patients, there is evidence that inadequate dialysis contributes to anemia and that an increase in dialysis adequacy has a beneficial effect on anemia.[16–19] Moreover, there is an inverse relationship between dialysis adequacy and rHuEPO dosing.[24,25] There is limited published information in the pediatric population. In a study of 12- to 17-year-old HD patients, the children with Hb less than 11 g/dL had a slightly lower Kt/V (1.53 vs. 1.46), but dialysis adequacy did not predict anemia in the multiple regression analysis.[23] The lack of effect of dialysis adequacy on anemia may be partially explained by the high overall Kt/V in this patient population.[23] The salutary effect of increased dialysis dose on anemia in adults included patients with an initial Kt/V lower than the NKF-K/DOQI target of 1.2.[16,17]

TABLE 47–2. CAUSES OF IRON DEFICIENCY IN CHILDREN WITH CHRONIC KIDNEY DISEASE

Blood loss
  Phlebotomy
  Hemodialysis
  Menses
  Gastrointestinal
Dietary iron deficiency
Poor absorption of enteral iron
Iron depletion during rHuEPO therapy

KEY: rHuEPO = recombinant human erythropoietin.

Malnutrition

Malnutrition may be another factor contributing to anemia in CKD. In a retrospective study in adults, two surrogates of nutritional status, albumin and creatinine, predicted Hb concentration.[16] Another study showed a direct relationship between serum albumin and hematocrit in adult HD patients.[17] In one pediatric study, low albumin was one predictor of anemia.[23]

There are multiple possible mechanisms to explain the relationship between malnutrition and anemia. Generalized malnutrition may be a marker for nutritional iron deficiency. Alternatively, other nutrients that influence the production of RBCs or RBC survival may be deficient. Another possible mechanism is the relationship between markers of malnutrition and markers of inflammation.[26] For example, serum albumin and serum C-reactive protein are inversely related in studies of adult dialysis patients.[27] As described below, inflammation is another mechanism of resistance to rHuEPO. It is possible that inflammation causes malnutrition, and this directly causes resistance to rHuEPO. An alternative explanation is that inflammation directly causes rHuEPO resistance, and that malnutrition is a surrogate marker of inflammation.

Inflammation and Infection

Acute and chronic inflammation are well-known causes of decreased RBC synthesis.[28] Inflammation is one of the mechanisms of the anemia of chronic disease[29] and of the decreased erythropoiesis that occurs during infection.[30] Inflammation and decreased RBC synthesis also occur after surgical procedures.[31]

Markers of inflammation are commonly increased in dialysis patients.[26,32] There are a variety of putative mechanisms. Surgical procedures and acute infections are more common in patients receiving dialysis. The impaired immune system in uremia may lead to an increase in nonspecific inflammation.[28] CKD patients may have underlying systemic diseases, such as systemic lupus erythematosus (SLE) or Wegener's granulomatosis. The HD procedure may induce inflammation via complement activation, direct activation of inflammatory cells by the dialysis membrane, and diffusion of endotoxin into the patient from the dialysate.[26,33]

A variety of studies in adults have shown an inverse relationship between rHuEPO dose and markers of inflammation.[27,32,34] HD patients with a serum C-reactive protein (CRP) level greater than 20 mg/L received 80 percent more rHuEPO than patients with a CRP level below 20 mg/L.[27] Infection delays the response to rHuEPO therapy.[22] While CRP is the most commonly studied marker of inflammation in dialysis patients, there are studies examining other markers of inflammation. In one study, multiple regression showed that interleukin 6 (IL-6) was a better predictor of rHuEPO dose than CRP.[33]

One postulated mechanism for the effect of inflammation on RBC production is an inflammatory block, a condition where body stores of iron are adequate but there is ineffective delivery of iron to the bone marrow. This prevents erythropoiesis even in the presence of sufficient erythropoietin. Inflammation may cause an inflammatory block via sequestration of iron in ferritin, which increases during inflammation, and the reticuloendothelial system, which is activated during inflammation and takes up iron.[28] Findings may include high CRP levels, resistance to rHuEPO, high serum ferritin levels, and low levels of serum iron and TSAT.[27] The inflammatory block in CKD patients is analogous to the anemia that occurs in a variety of chronic diseases.[29]

Along with an inflammatory block, enteral iron absorption is decreased in patients with CKD and elevated CRP levels.[35] Moreover, there is evidence that cytokines produced during inflammation have a direct suppressive effect on the production of RBCs.[36,37] Inflammation in dialysis patients is also associated with malnutrition,[32] which, as described previously, is another putative mechanism of anemia.

Given the role of inflammation, it has been hypothesized that use of a more biocompatible dialyzer might increase patient responsiveness to rHuEPO. Nevertheless, two randomized studies in adults have not shown any beneficial effect of more biocompatible dialyzers on anemia or rHuEPO dosing.[18,38] In contrast, in a randomized study investigating the effect of ultrapure dialysate on inflammation and use of rHuEPO, patients that used ultrapure dialysate had decreased levels of CRP and IL-6 and a sustained reduction in their dose of rHuEPO.[33]

Hyperparathyroidism

Hyperparathyroidism may affect production of RBCs. This has been observed in both primary hyperparathyroidism[39] and in the secondary hyperparathyroidism due to CKD.[40,41] In one adult study, patients who required high doses of rHuEPO had higher parathyroid hormone (PTH) levels and more bone marrow fibrosis on bone biopsy.[42] Patients with primary[39] or secondary hyperparathyroidism[40,41] have an increase in hematocrit after parathyroidectomy.

B$_{12}$ or Folate Deficiency

Patient with CKD may rarely develop a megaloblastic anemia due to folate or B$_{12}$ deficiency.[43,44] Poor nutritional intake and dialytic losses may predispose CKD patients to deficiencies of these water-soluble vitamins. There is some evidence that routine folate supplementation improves the response to rHuEPO even in the absence of low serum levels of folic acid.[45] Others have questioned the need for routine folate supplementation in HD patients.[46–49]

Aluminum Toxicity

Aluminum overload may cause a microcytic anemia in patients with CKD.[50,51] In the pre-rHuEPO era, treatment of aluminum overload with deferoxamine resulted in an increased Hb in patients on dialysis.[52] In one study, elevated aluminum levels were associated with a decreased initial response to rHuEPO but did not affect maintenance dose requirements.[53] Because of the recognition of the dangers of aluminum-containing phosphate binders,[54–56] aluminum overload is currently an uncommon cause of anemia in children with CKD.

Carnitine Deficiency

Carnitine deficiency may occur in CKD, principally due to removal of carnitine by dialysis, although decreased dietary intake and endogenous synthesis may also contribute.[57] In addition, renal carnitine losses are increased in patients with Fanconi's syndrome.[58,59] Carnitine deficiency may decrease RBC survival by reducing the strength of the RBC membrane.[13,57] There are some studies suggesting that intravenous carnitine can reduce rHuEPO dose requirements in adults receiving HD,[13,60] but there is disagreement regarding the strength of the available evidence.[2,57] One pediatric study showed an increase in the hematocrit with intravenous L-carnitine in two patients.[61] Oral carnitine should not be used in dialysis patients because of concerns regarding toxic metabolites.[57] The role of intravenous carnitine in pediatric HD patients requires further study.

Medications

A variety of medications can inhibit erythropoiesis. Angiotensin-converting enzyme (ACE) inhibitors are especially pertinent in CKD patients because of their widespread use. There is evidence that ACE inhibitors may blunt the response to rHuEPO,[62–64] although other studies have not found such an effect.[65,66]

EPIDEMIOLOGY OF ANEMIA

Despite the availability of rHuEPO, anemia remains common in both adults and children. Anemia is especially common in adult predialysis patients.[67] In the United States, less than 23 percent of adults had a hematocrit greater than 33 percent at initiation dialysis in 1999.[68] Nevertheless, only 28 percent of these patients were receiving rHuEPO.[68]

The 2003 report of the North American Pediatric Renal Transplant Cooperative Study (NAPRTCS) has data on pediatric dialysis patients from 1992–2002.[69] Forty-eight percent of patients who received rHuEPO during the first month of dialysis had a hematocrit of greater or equal to 33 percent at 6 months after initiation of dialysis. A hematocrit of 33 percent or greater was present at 6 months in 43 percent in patients who started rHuEPO after 1 month of dialysis and was present in only 33 percent of patients who did not receive rHuEPO during the first 6 months of dialysis.[69]

A recent study focused on patients between 12 and 17 years of age who were receiving HD in the United States during 2000. Thirty-seven percent of the patients had an Hb less than 11 g/dL. Multiple regression showed that dialyzing less than 6 months, a low serum albumin, and a mean TSAT less than 20 percent were significant predictors of anemia.[23]

More recent data are available from the 2002 annual report from the Centers for Medicare and Medicaid.[70] These data are from the United States between October and December 2001. Among HD patients below 18 years of age, the mean Hb was 11.2 g/dL, with a standard deviation of 1.6 g/dL. Thirty-eight percent of the patients had a mean Hb below 11 g/dL, despite the fact that 97 percent of the patients were receiving rHuEPO. The percentage of patients with a mean Hb below 11 g/dL decreased in both 2000 and 2001, possibly reflecting both an increase in prescribed rHuEPO dosing and the percentage of patients prescribed intravenous iron. In univariate analysis, risk factors for an Hb below 11 g/dL were dialysis for less than 6 months, mean Kt/V <1.2, a low serum albumin, and use of a catheter for vascular access.[70]

CLINICAL EFFECTS OF ANEMIA

Anemia causes many of the clinical consequences of CKD (Table 47–3). There is evidence that anemia increases mortality in adults, perhaps through its deleterious cardiovascular effects. In addition, correction of anemia ameliorates a wide variety of systemic symptoms in adults and children. Finally, there is some evidence that correction of anemia may slow the progression of predialysis CKD to ESRD.[71]

TABLE 47–3. CLINICAL EFFECTS OF ANEMIA

Cardiovascular
    Left ventricular hypertrophy
Systemic
    Fatigue
    Depression
    Decreased quality of life
    Sleep disturbances
    Decreased exercise tolerance
    Impaired cognitive function
    Loss of appetite

Mortality

Studies in adult dialysis patients have shown an association between anemia and mortality.[16,72,73] In a large retrospective study, an Hb below 8 g/dL was associated with a twofold increase risk of death, but there was no improvement in mortality with an Hb above 11 g/dL.[16] This suggests that mortality is affected only by severe anemia. In contrast, other retrospective studies showed an improvement in mortality[74] and decreased hospitalizations[75] when the hematocrit was between 33 and 36 percent vs. less than 33 percent.

The current NKF-K/DOQI target Hb is 11 to 12 g/dL. A number of studies have examined the beneficial effect of a higher target Hb in adult dialysis patients. In one randomized study of high-risk HD patients, there was no benefit in targeting a hematocrit in the normal range.[76] In fact, the study was stopped early because there were more deaths in the group targeted to a hematocrit of 42 percent compared to the group targeted to a hematocrit of 30 percent. In contrast, a retrospective multivariate analysis showed a decrease in hospitalization rates in patients with a hematocrit more than 36 percent; mortality rates were not different when compared to patients with a hematocrit of 33 to 36 percent.[77] There are no pediatric studies that address the relationship between anemia in CKD and mortality.

Cardiovascular Disease

Cardiovascular disease is the leading cause of mortality in adults[78] and children[79] receiving dialysis. Anemia appears to be a significant risk factor for cardiovascular morbidity in adults with CKD.[72,80–83] Treatment of anemia with rHuEPO has beneficial cardiovascular effects in adults receiving dialysis[84,85] and in the predialysis population.[86] There may be additional cardiovascular advantages to normalizing a patient's Hb.[87]

There are a few pediatric studies addressing this issue. In a group of children receiving dialysis, treatment of anemia with rHuEPO partially corrected the elevated cardiac index in 6 months and produced a significant reduction in left ventricular mass index by 12 months.[88] In a study by Mitsnefes and coworkers,[89] children with severe left ventricular hypertrophy (LVH) had significantly lower Hb values than children without LVH. However, anemia did not predict LVH in the final multiple regression model.[89]

Systemic Symptoms

Anemia causes a variety of systemic symptoms in CKD (see Table 47–3). There is significant overlap with uremic symptoms, emphasizing the importance of correcting anemia before attributing some of these findings to uremia. Because of the overlap with uremic symptoms, most studies on the systemic effects of anemia in CKD have evaluated the results of correcting anemia with rHuEPO.

The clinical trials in adults of rHuEPO demonstrated improvement in many systemic symptoms. In a phase III trial, which compared baseline and follow-up results, there were statistically significant improvements in a variety of outcomes, including functional ability, sleep and eating behavior, energy and activity level, health status, well-being, psychological affect, sex life, and happiness.[90] Similar results were seen in a study that randomized predialysis patients with anemia to rHuEPO or no treatment.[91]

In a study of adults with underlying cardiovascular disease, patients treated with rHuEPO were randomized to a target Hb of 10 or 13.5 g/dL. The group with a higher target had improvements in fatigue, depression, and relationships.[85] In another study, patients were randomized to placebo, low-target Hb (9.5 to 11 g/dL) or high-target Hb (11.5 to 13 g/dL). Compared to placebo, patients treated with rHuEPO had improvement in scores for fatigue, physical symptoms, relationships, depression, and distance walked in the stress test, but there were no differences in the two different target Hb groups.[92]

Other studies of the effect of rHuEPO have shown improvement in exercise duration,[20,93] energy levels,[94] cognitive function,[95] social functioning,[96] oxygen consumption,[20] and work capacity.[94] A normal target Hb may result in further improvement in quality-of-life scores[87] and cognitive function.[97]

Correction of anemia with rHuEPO probably has similar beneficial effects in children, but studies are limited. There is ample evidence for the deleterious effects of anemia on child development.[98] When rHuEPO was given to a group of children receiving HD, there was improvement in quality of life, exercise tolerance, and ventilatory aerobic threshold.[99] Quality of life also improved in another study.[100] One study of rHuEPO in children showed a statistically significant increase in the Wechsler intelligence score.[101] Another study has shown an improvement in appetite.[102] In a group of children receiving peritoneal dialysis (PD), rHuEPO therapy produced significant improvements in peak oxygen consumption and treadmill time during exercise testing.[103] There does not appear to be a beneficial effect of anemia correction on the growth retardation of CKD.[104,105]

CLINICAL EVALUATION OF ANEMIA

Initial Evaluation

Most children with CKD do not need an extensive evaluation for the etiology of their anemia. Inadequate erythropoietin production is the usual explanation, and most children are treated empirically with rHuEPO unless there are specific findings that suggest an alternative cause (Table 47–4).

TABLE 47–4. INDICATIONS FOR ADDITIONAL EVALUATION IN CHILDREN WITH CHRONIC KIDNEY DISEASE AND ANEMIA

Indication	Response
Macrocytosis	Consider B$_{12}$ or folate deficiency unless due to brisk reticulocytosis
Decreased platelets and/or white blood cells	Consider malignancy, acute infection or medications
History of using aluminum-containing phosphate binders or other symptoms of aluminum overload	Consider aluminum toxicity
Anemia despite adequate reticulocytosis	Consider excessive blood loss or hemolysis
Microcytosis	Consider iron deficiency, hemoglobinopathy, or inflammation
Iron deficiency prior to starting rHuEPO[a]	Evaluate for causes of iron deficiency (see Table 47–2)

[a]Recombinant human erythropoietin.

Other ominous etiologies of anemia, such as significant gastrointestinal bleeding or occult malignancies, are less common in children than adults with CKD.

The initial evaluation of children with CKD and anemia should include a complete blood count, reticulocyte count, ferritin, iron, total iron-binding capacity (TIBC), and a TSAT. A cost-effectiveness analysis in adults argues against routine screening for aluminum overload or deficiencies of folate or B$_{12}$.[106] Erythropoietin deficiency causes a normocytic anemia; macrocytosis or microcytosis should lead to consideration of other etiologies (see Table 47–4). A low mean corpuscular volume (MCV) occurs with iron deficiency, thalassemia, and in up to 50 percent of patients with the anemia of chronic disease. A high MCV suggests the possibility of B$_{12}$ or folate deficiency. Concomitant depression of white cells or platelets raises the specter of malignancy, although an isolated low white blood cell count may be due to a transient viral infection or a medication. SLE may cause depression of the white blood cell count or platelet count or an autoimmune Coombs-positive hemolytic anemia. Erythropoietin deficiency causes an inappropriately low reticulocyte count; the presence of an adequate reticulocytosis suggests alternative explanations, such as blood loss or hemolysis.

Iron deficiency is common in children with CKD even prior to starting rHuEPO. There are a variety of explanations for iron deficiency in children with CKD (see Table 47–2). All children with CKD should be queried about gastrointestinal blood loss and, when appropriate, menstrual losses. A more aggressive workup (e.g., testing stool for occult blood or endoscopy) is appropriate in children with severe unexplained iron deficiency prior to receiving rHuEPO. Along with low serum ferritin and TSAT, children with severe iron deficiency typically have a low MCV.

The principal reason for evaluating the ferritin and TSAT is to establish a baseline, since iron deficiency is likely to develop during treatment with rHuEPO. In addition, while all patients starting on rHuEPO should receive oral iron supplementation unless iron overload is present, iron deficiency prior to starting rHuEPO may significantly attenuate the response to therapy. Such patients are candidates for intravenous iron (see below).

Chronic Monitoring

Routine monitoring in children with anemia due to CKD includes periodic assessment of Hb and iron stores (discussed below). The MCV is routinely monitored along with the Hb. The development of macrocytosis in a patient after starting rHuEPO is usually due to the expected reticulocytosis; an increasing Hb, arguing against a nutritional deficiency anemia, supports this explanation. Iron overload may also cause an increased MCV.[107] The development of microcytosis is usually due to iron deficiency.

A decrease in Hb and an increase in rHuEPO dose requirements are expected during acute infections[30,108] or after surgical procedures.[31] Dose requirements increase following blood loss that causes a fall in Hb; this persists until the Hb returns to the target range. Depleted iron stores are the usual explanation for a poor response to rHuEPO. As discussed below, some children have a functional iron deficiency and may respond to intravenous iron even though the ferritin and TSAT are not low. Additional evaluation is indicated in children who have an unexplained increase in rHuEPO dose requirement, need unexpectedly large doses of rHuEPO, or have a decreasing Hb.

A reticulocyte count is the usual first step in evaluating unexplained anemia or an excessive rHuEPO requirement. An appropriately elevated reticulocyte count argues that the patient is anemic due to blood loss or hemolysis. Blood loss is also suggested by minimal changes in ferritin and TSAT despite the use of multiple doses of intravenous iron. The child should then have stool tested for occult blood; an evaluation for hemolysis may also be appropriate [e.g., Coombs test, bilirubin, haptoglobin, lactate dehydrogenase (LDH)]. Inadequate reticulocytosis suggests that there is a defect in red cell production. This may be due to poor compliance or technique failure in the patient receiving home rHuEPO injections. There may be a readily identifiable explanation, such as severe secondary hyperparathyroidism. Alternatively, additional testing may be necessary. A serum aluminum level is an appropriate test in the child with a history of using aluminum-containing phosphate binders. One of the most common causes of a poor response to rHuEPO is an inflammatory block due to acute or chronic inflammation. An elevated CRP supports this diagnosis.[27,28,34] Other testing, depending on the patient, may include a serum carnitine level and serum levels of folate and B$_{12}$. Refractory anemia with no identifiable explanation should be evaluated by a hematologist.[2]

TREATMENT OF ANEMIA

Replacement of deficient erythropoietin production, using either rHuEPO or darbepoetin alpha, is necessary in most children with ESRD and many children with predialysis CKD. In addition, almost all patients treated with erythropoietin require oral or intravenous iron. When possible, other underlying causes of anemia should be corrected (see Table 47–1). Blood transfusion should be used only when a patient with significant anemia has symptoms that will reverse with transfusion.

There is evidence that use of a fixed algorithm for administration and dose adjustment of rHuEPO and iron may increase the percentage of patients that achieve a target Hb[109] or decrease the dose requirements for rHuEPO.[110] Unfortunately, the optimal algorithm, in either adults or children, has not been determined.

Target Hemoglobin

A target Hb must be defined for each patient. The NKF-K/DOQI recommends a target Hb of 11 to 12 g/dL.[2] This is based on adult literature suggesting that most of the benefits of rHuEPO are achieved when the Hb reaches 11 g/dL. As detailed above, there is evidence for increased benefit with a higher target Hb but also some concern regarding increased mortality in one large randomized study. Nevertheless, other important considerations are the high cost of rHuEPO and the lack of Medicare reimbursement for a higher target Hb.

There are no data on the ideal target Hb in children. Most children in the United States have a target Hb of 11 to 12 g/dL, per the NKF-K/DOQI guidelines.[2] Yet there are clearly children who should have a higher target Hb (e.g., a child with cyanotic heart disease) or a lower target (e.g., a child with sickle cell disease).

Hemoglobin Monitoring

The preference for Hb monitoring over hematocrit is based on the greater consistency of Hb measurements.[2] In children receiving HD, blood samples should be taken immediately prior to dialysis.

The frequency of Hb monitoring depends on the patient. Children who are on a stable dose of rHuEPO and within their target Hb can have an Hb performed as infrequently as monthly if they are receiving dialysis and even less often if they are at the predialysis stage. After starting rHuEPO or after a dosing change, an Hb should be obtained every 1 to 2 weeks until the Hb has stabilized within the target range.

Recombinant Human Erythropoietin

Most children receiving dialysis are treated with rHuEPO. Among the children summarized in the 2003 NAPRTCS report, 88 percent received rHuEPO during the first month of dialysis; this increased to 95 percent 2 years after starting dialysis. Initial use was less common in children receiving PD than in those on HD (86 vs. 92 percent); but 2 years after dialysis initiation, use of rHuEPO was 95 and 96 percent in children receiving PD and HD, respectively.[69]

Efficacy

Initial studies in adult HD patients demonstrated the dramatic effectiveness of intravenous rHuEPO in correcting the anemia of CKD.[111–113] Similar results were obtained using subcutaneous rHuEPO in predialysis patients[94,114,115] and patients receiving PD.[20–22]

A number of studies have reported on the effectiveness of rHuEPO in pediatric patients,[99–101,103,116–127] including one placebo-controlled trial.[102] The designs and results of these studies are summarized in Table 47–5.

Pharmacokinetics

The pharmacokinetics of rHuEPO has been studied in children and adults with CKD. There are clear differences based on the route of administration, with less complete absorption of subcutaneous rHuEPO but a significantly longer half-life when compared to intravenous administration (Table 47–6). In adult studies, bioavailability of subcutaneous rHuEPO ranges from 21.5 to 44 percent.[128–131] For intravenous dosing, there is evidence that the half-life of rHuEPO increases as the dose increases.[132]

A number of studies have examined the pharmacokinetics of rHuEPO in children (see Table 47–6).[117,133–136] The volume of distribution of intravenous rHuEPO is approximately equivalent to the plasma volume.[133–135] In a study of patients from 9 to 16 years of age, the pharmacokinetics of subcutaneous and intravenous rHuEPO were compared.[134] Subcutaneous rHuEPO concentration peaked at a mean of 10 hours and 40 percent was absorbed. The mean rHuEPO half-life was 5.6 hours for intravenous dosing and 21.1 hours for subcutaneous dosing.[134] Braun and colleagues studied subcutaneous administration in patients between 7 to 20 years of age with various stages of CKD.[135] The peak concentration was reached at a mean of 14.3 hours and the mean half-life was also 14.3 hours. There were no significant differences in the pharmacokinetic data between young and old patients or predialysis and ESRD patients.[135] Another study compared the pharmacokinetics of subcutaneous rHuEPO in children receiving PD and in predialysis patients.[136] The half-lives were comparable (13.3 hours in predialysis patients and 13.5 hours in PD patients), but the

TABLE 47–5. PEDIATRIC STUDIES OF RECOMBINANT HUMAN ERYTHROPOIETIN

Study Design (reference)[a]	Outcome
PD patients treated with 450 U/kg/week (three doses); dose frequency reduced when reached target (Sinai-Trieman et al.[116])	Good response; 4/5 patients on 150 U/kg/week maintenance.
HD patients treated with 75 U/kg/week; dose doubled every 2 weeks as needed (Montini et al.[99])	Good response.
HD patients treated with 300–450 U/kg/week (Rigden et al.[127])	Good response.
PD patients treated with 300 U/kg/week (one dose; intravenous) (Offner et al.[118])	Good response; maintenance dose was 100 U/kg/week.
PD patients treated with 150 U/kg/week (3 doses/week) (Ongkingco et al.[120])	Rapid correction in all patients.
HD patients treated with 40–100 U/kg/week (3 doses/week) and PD patients treated with 300 U/kg/week (1 dose/week) (Scigalla[119])	Median dose at 12 months was 138 U/kg/week. (Children <5 years required a median dose of 321 U/kg/week.)
PD patients treated with 100 U/kg/week (2 doses/week) (Warady et al.[103])	Good response; dose decreased to maintain target Hb.
HD patients treated with 150 U/kg/week (3 doses); dose changed by 25 U/kg/week (Campos and Garin[121])	Effective correction of anemia with a mean dose of 187 U/kg/week. Maintenance doses were 142, 108 and 145 Us/kg/week at 3, 6, and 9 months, respectively.
PD patients treated with 50 U/kg/week divided into 2 doses. Dose increased by 50 U/kg/week every 4 weeks if needed (Montini et al.[117])	Achieved target Hb at a mean dose of 102 U/kg/week. Mean dose subsequently decreased.
Predialysis patients treated with an initial dose of 150 U/kg/week (1 dose) (Scharer et al.[122])	All reached target Hb. Mean dose when on maintenance rHuEPO was 133 U/kg/week.
PD patients treated with 100 or 120 U/kg/week (2 or 3 injections) to achieve normal hematocrit; dose doubled if inadequate response (Aufricht et al.[123])	Median dose to achieve target was 120 U/kg/week. Maintenance dose ~2/3 of highest weekly dose.
CKD patients treated with 150 U/kg/week (3 doses/week) IV (HD patients) or SC (others); dose (30 U/kg/week) and interval adjusted (Jabs et al.[102])	Good response. Mean weekly dose requirements: HD (155 U), PD (91 U); PD < 5 years (128 U); PD 5–14 years (82 U); PD 15–17 years (81 U).
HD patients started on 75 U/kg/week (intravenous 2–3 times/week); dose titrated by 75 U/kg/week (Van Damme-Lombaerts et al.[100])	81% achieved target Hb. Median maintenance dose was 225 U/kg/week in children <30 kg and 107 U/kg/week in children >30 kg. Concluded that 150 U/kg/week a more appropriate starting dose.
Predialysis, HD and PD patients treated with an initial dose of 100 U/kg/week (2 doses/week) (Burke et al.[101])	19/22 reached target Hb. Maintenance dose was 45–125 U/kg/week (1 dose/week).
PD patients treated with either 50 U/kg/week (1 dose/week) or 150 U/kg/week (3 doses/week) (Yalcinkaya et al.[124])	Correction more rapid with higher dose, but more likely to develop hypertension.
HD and PD patients received a fixed dose or rHuEPO (50 U/kg SC per week) (Sieniawska et al.[126])	Good response in PD patients and poor response in HD patients.
Randomized patients to 150 U/kg/week (1 dose) or 450 U/kg/week (3 doses) using IV administration (HD patients) or SC administration (PD and predialysis patients). Dose decreased after reach target (Brandt et al.[125])	Higher percentage of high dose group reached target Hb (95 vs. 66%). HD patients required a higher maintenance dose (243 U/kg/week) than PD (155 U/kg/week) or predialysis patients (143 U/kg/week).

KEY: HD, hemodialysis; PD, peritoneal dialysis; rHuEPO, recombinant human erythropoietin; IV, intravenous; SC, subcutaneous
[a]Dosing in PD and predialysis patients is SC unless specifically stated.

TABLE 47–6. HALF-LIFE[a] OF rHuEPO AND DARBEPOETIN ALPHA IN PEDIATRIC AND ADULT PATIENTS

Medication	Pediatric	Adult
rHuEPO		
IV	5.6 ± 3 hours[134]	7.9 ± 4.2 hours[129]
	7.5 ± 0.9 hours[133]	4.5 ± 0.9 hours[130]
		5.4 ± 1.7 hours[131]
		8.2 hours[128]
SC	21.1 ± 4.5 hours[134]	24.4 ± 27 hours[129]
	14.3 ± 7 hours[135]	25 ± 12 hours[130]
	25.2 hours[117]	
Darbepoetin alpha		
IV	22.1 ± 4.8 hours[167]	25.3 ± 7.3 hours[166]
SC	42.8 ± 23 hours[167]	48.8 ± 12.7 hours[166]

[a]Mean ± standard deviation.

volume of distribution and drug clearance were higher in the children receiving PD.[136]

In adult[128,129] and pediatric[134] studies, the bioavailability of intraperitoneal rHuEPO was significantly lower than that of subcutaneous rHuEPO. In one pediatric study, administration of rHuEPO with a small volume of dialysate resulted in a significant improvement in the bioavailability of intraperitoneal rHuEPO.[137] Nevertheless, few children receive intraperitoneal dosing.[69]

Dosing

Individualized Dose Requirements. In an initial study of rHuEPO, there was more than a 40-fold difference in dose per kilogram even though the patient population was confined to adults receiving HD.[113] A similar variation in dosing has subsequently been seen in other adult[21] and pediatric studies.[69,70] A number of factors influence the dose of rHuEPO needed to achieve the target Hb (Table 47–7).

Intravenous vs. Subcutaneous Dosing. Because of its longer half-life, subcutaneous rHuEPO is more effective than intravenous rHuEPO in adult HD patients, permitting lower doses to achieve the same target Hb.[138–142] In a nonrandomized observational study, children receiving HD were given less rHuEPO when they were treated with subcutaneous dosing instead of intravenous dosing.[70]

As described in the 2003 NAPRTCS report, 96 percent of PD patients received subcutaneous rHuEPO and 87 percent of HD patients received intravenous therapy.[69] Despite the NFK-K/DOQI recommendation to use subcutaneous dosing in all patients,[2] there is reluctance to subject pediatric patients to additional injections, especially since many are already receiving daily injections of recombinant human growth hormone. This is confirmed by United States data from children receiving HD in 2001: 93 percent received intravenous rHuEPO.[70] Nevertheless, this may change over time, especially given the NKF-K/DOQI recommendations[2] and the data suggesting that once-weekly subcutaneous rHuEPO may be a satisfactory alternative to thrice-weekly injections.[143,144]

When children receive intravenous dosing, it is important to inject rHuEPO via the blood lines. Use of the venous drip chamber may result in reduced drug delivery due to "trapping" of rHuEPO, although this appears to be somewhat machine-dependent.[145]

PD vs. HD. Children receiving PD require less rHuEPO than children receiving HD even when both groups receive rHuEPO subcutaneously.[126] This is presumably due mainly to blood loss during HD, although other factors may contribute. The high use of intravenous rHuEPO dosing in HD patients likely further increases the difference in dose requirements that has been seen in other pediatric studies.[102,125]

Dosing Intervals. Frequency of intravenous dosing is usually thrice weekly in HD patients because patients receive rHuEPO at the time of dialysis. This optimizes the cost-ef-

TABLE 47–7. FACTORS INFLUENCING ERYTHROPOIETIN DOSING

Route of administration
Mode of dialysis
Initial and target hemoglobin
Endogenous erythropoietin
Patient's age
Dosing frequency
Presence of other causes of anemia (see Table 47–1)

fectiveness of intravenous rHuEPO since, due to its short half-life, more frequent dosing minimizes the amount of time with subtherapeutic levels. HD patients who receive subcutaneous dosing may receive less frequent dosing, principally to reduce the number of injections. In fact, there is evidence that weekly subcutaneous dosing in HD patients does not increase the need for rHuEPO when compared to twice- or thrice-weekly dosing.[143,144] Less frequent intravenous injections are sometimes adequate in children who require very low doses of rHuEPO, usually due to production of endogenous erythropoietin.

Most children receiving PD do not receive thrice-weekly injections of rHuEPO.[69] Weekly injections are most common, although twice-weekly injections are also common, and a small percentage receives less frequent injections.[69]

Dose Requirements. There are many variables affecting the required dose of rHuEPO in children with ESRD (see Table 47–7). The amount of blood loss from HD, blood draws and other sources increases the need for rHuEPO. Blood draws can be especially problematic in the youngest patients because they often need more frequent monitoring, and the relative losses per kilogram of body weight tend to be higher. As detailed above, route and frequency of administration heavily influence the effectiveness of a given weekly dose of rHuEPO. Concurrent causes of poor response to rHuEPO—such as iron deficiency, inflammation, or hyperparathyroidism—often result in higher doses. Finally, residual renal production of erythropoietin can decrease the need for rHuEPO.

Pediatric experience with dosing rHuEPO is summarized in Table 47–5. A wide variety of doses have been effective in pediatric patients. Average dose requirements are higher in children receiving HD.[102] When analyzed, the dosing requirements of younger children are significantly higher than those of older children.[102,119]

In the 2003 NAPRTCS report, the average dose of rHuEPO was about 200 U/kg/week in children more than 12 years old. The average dose was slightly higher in children between 6 and 12 years old. Among the children less than 6 years old, the average dose was closer to 300 U/kg/week, albeit with considerable variability over time. The higher dosing in the younger children occurred despite the higher frequency of PD in this population. The average dose of rHuEPO in children receiving PD was less than that in children receiving HD.[69]

The increased dosing needs of rHuEPO in younger patients are even more dramatic when only HD patients are analyzed. While children between 10 to 17 years of age required slightly more than 300 U/kg/week, the 5 to 9 years age group required about 450 U/kg/week and the 0–4 years age group received an average of over 700 U/kg/week.[70]

There are many possible explanations for the higher dosing needs of younger children. These may include increased relative blood loss during HD or due to phlebotomy, less aggressive treatment of iron deficiency, and differences in the pharmacokinetics of rHuEPO in younger children. There is no evidence for different dosing needs of rHuEPO in children based on gender or race.[69]

Dose Adjustments. Frequent dose adjustments are typically necessary in patients receiving rHuEPO.[146] This is probably related to variation in factors that cause anemia (see Table 47–1) and that influence dosing of rHuEPO (see Table 47–7). In addition, more active erythropoiesis is needed to increase a patient's Hb. Hence, the dose that patients need to increase their Hb level into the target range is often more than the dose needed to maintain a stable Hb.[112,113,147] Patients may need higher doses of rHuEPO at the start of therapy or after a decrease in Hb due to blood loss or a transient illness.

Dosing Recommendations in Children

Initiation with rHuEPO. The NKF-K/DOQI guidelines recommend a starting dose of rHuEPO of 80 to 120 U/kg/week in adults receiving subcutaneous dosing and 120 to 180 U/kg/week in adults receiving intravenous dosing.[2] In children receiving PD or in predialysis patients, an appropriate starting dose for subcutaneous rHuEPO is 100 U/kg/week divided into two subcutaneous doses. Children less than 5 years of age are likely to need a higher dose; a starting dose of 150 U/kg/week may be appropriate in such patients, especially if severe anemia (Hb < 8 g/dL) is present. For children receiving HD and intravenous rHuEPO dosing, a starting dose of 150 U/kg/week divided into three doses is reasonable, again with the caveat that higher doses are likely necessary in children below 5 years of age. A starting dose of 200 to 250 U/kg/week may be more appropriate in such patients, especially if there is concomitant severe anemia.

For children receiving subcutaneous dosing, the site of injection should be rotated.[2] The discomfort of subcutaneous dosing can be reduced[148] by utilizing the multidose vial, which contains the local anesthetic benzyl alcohol as a preservative. In children who are using a single-use vial, adding bacteriostatic saline, which contains benzyl alcohol, to the rHuEPO in a 1:1 ratio can decrease injection-site pain.

Changing Route of Administration of rHuEPO. On initiating HD, most children are converted to intravenous dosing of rHuEPO, which should then almost always be given thrice weekly. Based on adult studies,[138–140] NKF-K/DOQI recommends increasing the total weekly dose by 50 percent when a patient changes from subcutaneous to intravenous dosing. Similarly, patients changing from intravenous dosing to subcutaneous dosing should have their weekly dose decreased by 33 percent.[2] However, most pediatric patients who convert between intravenous and subcutaneous dosing are also changing dialysis modality. Given the higher needs for rHuEPO in children on HD,[69] patients changing to intravenous dosing because they are initiating HD may need an additional increase in their dose. In children below age 10 and certainly those below age 5, rHuEPO dosing requirements during HD are very high.[70] This suggests that these patients may need an increase in their rHuEPO dose after beginning HD irrespective of any change in route of administration. Young children should have careful monitoring of their Hb when initiating HD, so that the dose of rHuEPO can be increased further if necessary. Even in older children, there is extreme variability in the dose requirements when converting to intravenous dosing; dose requirements may increase or decrease. The ability to treat iron deficiency more aggressively in children receiving HD (see below) may result in a decrease in rHuEPO requirements.

Dose Adjustments. The goal of rHuEPO therapy is to maintain the patient's Hb within a desired target range. Overly rapid increases in Hb can be associated with hypertension and should be avoided. In patients with an Hb below the target, the goal is to increase the Hb by 1 to 2 g/dL per month. Figure 47–1 presents one algorithm for adjusting rHuEPO dosing.

Complications

Side effects of rHuEPO may be due to a direct reaction to the medication or a consequence of its intended action, correction of anemia. An increase in blood pressure has been observed in a number of studies.[20,21,92,113,114] Patients may therefore require increased doses of antihypertensive medications.[20,92,113] If uncontrolled, the increase in blood pressure may lead to seizures.[113] An increase in blood pressure after starting rHuEPO therapy has also been seen in pediatric studies.[102,117,120,121,125] This appears to be more common in children who receive higher doses of rHuEPO and have a consequent more rapid increase in Hb.[124]

The mechanism of hypertension during rHuEPO therapy is the subject of continued speculation.[149] The concept that hypertension is a consequence of increased RBC mass has been questioned.[150] A direct effect of rHuEPO on endothelin production has been seen in some studies.[151,152] There is also evidence for an effect of rHuEPO on intracellular calcium and nitric oxide.[153]

There are some studies suggesting an increase in vascular access clotting with rHuEPO therapy in adults receiving HD,[92,154] presumably due to the increase in hematocrit, which increases blood viscosity and partially corrects the platelet dysfunction associated with uremia. Moreover, in a study where patients were randomized to achieve a hematocrit of either 42 or 30 percent, there was more access clot-

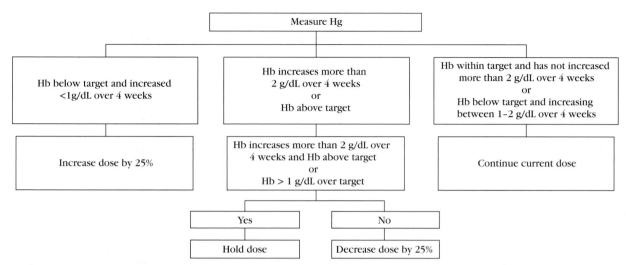

Figure 47–1. Dose adjustment strategy for children receiving rHuEPO or darbepoetin alpha. In some instances, especially for patients on subcutaneous dosing, the dose frequency may be reduced instead of or in addition to decreasing the weekly dose by 25 percent.

ting in the group assigned to the higher hematocrit.[76] In contrast, other studies have not shown a detrimental effect on vascular access.[113,155] In addition, the introduction of rHuEPO has not led to an increase in pulmonary embolisms.[156]

The increase in hematocrit from rHuEPO may theoretically have an adverse effect on dialytic clearance due to the decrease in plasma volume as the hematocrit increases. In one study, there were statistically significant increases in serum creatinine, phosphate, and potassium following correction of severe anemia by rHuEPO.[113] BUN did not increase, presumably because urea diffuses readily from RBCs during dialysis.[157] One pediatric study found a small, statistically insignificant increase in potassium.[125] Minor changes in dialysis prescription were necessary in a group of patients who had a large change in Hb.[24] Overall, the change in dialytic clearance is relatively small and is not felt to be clinically significant.[1,2]

Iron deficiency may develop in adults[113] and children[102,120,121,125] treated with rHuEPO. This is secondary to iron utilization for RBC synthesis. Hence, unless iron overload is present, all patients treated with rHuEPO should receive iron supplementation and be screened for iron deficiency before and during therapy (see below).

The initial studies of rHuEPO tended to have more significant adverse effects from correcting anemia. This is because the enrolled population was severely anemic and the increase in Hb was often quite dramatic. This emphasizes the importance of increased vigilance for adverse effects when patients who are severely anemic receive rHuEPO. In addition, this is the rationale for decreasing the dose of rHuEPO in patients who have an Hb below target but an overly rapid increase in Hb (see above).

A rare complication of rHuEPO is the development of antierythropoietin antibodies.[158,159] These antibodies neu-

tralize both endogenous erythropoietin and rHuEPO, resulting in RBC aplasia.

DARBEPOETIN ALPHA

While rHuEPO is effective at correcting the anemia of ESRD, the need for frequent injections is taxing for children and their parents. Darbepoetin alpha (Aranesp) was genetically engineered to have a longer half-life than rHuEPO, permitting less frequent administration.

Efficacy

There are no efficacy data in children, but darbepoetin alpha has been extensively compared to rHuEPO in adults with CKD. Two studies have randomized dialysis patients to either continue rHuEPO or switch to darbepoetin alpha.[160,161] Dosing intervals were increased in the darbepoetin alpha group. Patients receiving twice- or thrice-weekly rHuEPO were given darbepoetin alpha weekly. Patients receiving weekly rHuEPO received darbepoetin alpha every other week. There were no significant differences in change of Hb from baseline, Hb variance or Hb instability when the rHuEPO groups were compared with the darbepoetin alpha groups.[160,161]

Other studies have focused on predialysis patients who were rHuEPO-naive. A large multicenter study randomized rHuEPO-naive predialysis patients to subcutaneous dosing of either twice-weekly rHuEPO or once-weekly darbepoetin alpha, with dose titration to achieve a target Hb.[147] There were no significant differences in the percentage of patients who achieved the target Hb or the amount of time required to reach the target level. Suranyi and colleagues studied rHuEPO naive predialysis patients.[162] Darbepoetin alpha was given every 2 weeks and target Hb levels were achieved in a median time of 5 weeks. In another study of predialysis patients, dosing of darbepoetin alpha every 2 weeks resulted in achievement of target Hb in a mean of 6 weeks.[163]

One study has evaluated converting adults receiving darbepoetin alpha every other week to a dosing schedule of every 4 weeks.[164] The patients were initially converted to every-3-week dosing; 91 percent maintained a stable Hb and were eligible for every-4-week dosing. Among the patients who were placed on every-4-week dosing, 83 percent maintained a stable Hb. There was no change in the mean weekly darbepoetin alpha dose when the patients were on every-3-week dosing and only a 2.2 percent increase when the patients were switched to every-4-week dosing.

Pharmacokinetics

Studies on erythropoietin have shown that its half-life is directly related to the amount of protein glycosylation.[165] Darbepoetin alpha was genetically engineered by changing five amino acids in the sequence of rHuEPO. This created two new glycosylation sites, increasing the number of N-linked carbohydrate addition sites from three to five. Studies in adult patients have shown that darbepoetin alpha has a longer half-life than rHuEPO (see Table 47–6). In a comparison of intravenous administration, darbepoetin alpha had a half-life of 23.5 hours versus 8.5 hours for rHuEPO.[166] In contrast to the approximately threefold increase in half-life with intravenous administration, there was a twofold increase with subcutaneous administration: a half-life of 24 hours with rHuEPO and 48.8 hours with darbepoetin alpha.[166]

One study has evaluated the half-life of darbepoetin alpha in 12 pediatric patients with CKD.[167] Most of the patients (9) were receiving HD, but another patient (1) was receiving PD and others (2) were not yet receiving dialysis. Each patient received one dose of darbepoetin alpha (0.5 μg/kg) intravenously and subcutaneously. The half-life of darbepoetin alpha with intravenous administration was 22.1 hours (SD = 4.5 hours). The half-life was 42.8 hours (SD = 4.8 hours) with subcutaneous administration. These results are comparable to those of the similarly designed study in adults.[166] The pharmacokinetics were similar to the adult study except for increased bioavailability (54 vs. 37 percent) and an earlier T_{max} (36 vs. 54 hours) in the pediatric patients when darbepoetin alpha was administered subcutaneously.[166,167] Hence, darbepoetin alpha may be absorbed more rapidly in pediatric patients.[167] More rapid absorption was also seen in pediatric studies of rHuEPO.[134]

Dosing

Based on protein mass, 1 μg of darbepoetin alpha is equivalent to 200 U of rHuEPO. This ratio has been used in converting patients from rHuEPO to darbepoetin alpha in a

number of clinical studies.[160,161] It has also been used in randomizing rHuEPO-naive predialysis patients to rHuEPO or darbepoetin alpha.[147] Nevertheless, the dose of darbepoetin alpha recommended by the manufacturer in converting patients from rHuEPO to darbepoetin alpha is not a direct conversion based on the ratio of 1 μg darbepoetin alpha to 200 U rHuEPO (Table 47–8). The recommended conversion ratios are based on an analysis of the dose-conversion clinical trials.[168] This analysis indicates that proportionally less darbepoetin alpha was needed in patients who began the trial on higher doses of rHuEPO.[168] Thus, patients who are on higher doses of rHuEPO need less darbepoetin alpha than the ratio of 1 μg to 200 U would suggest. There is no clear explanation for this observation. One postulated mechanism is a greater increase in efficacy with high doses of darbepoetin alpha than with high doses of rHuEPO.[168] Alternatively, there may simply be a "regression to the mean" in patients who were on higher doses of rHuEPO. The patients on high doses of rHuEPO may have had a transient explanation for their high prestudy rHuEPO requirement (e.g., iron deficiency or inflammation) that subsequently resolved, thus decreasing their need for darbepoetin alpha during the study.

While Table 47–8 is a useful starting point, the dose-conversion studies suggest that there is a great deal of variation in the ultimate dose of darbepoetin alpha required by a patient after conversion from rHuEPO.[168] This is expected, given that doses of rHuEPO[146] and darbepoetin alpha[160,161] tend to vary over time. It is also important to remember that these recommendations are based on decreasing the dosing frequency in converting to darbepoetin alpha. Animal studies indicate that the relative potency of darbepoetin alpha compared to rHuEPO increases significantly if it is administered using the same dosing intervals as rHuEPO.[165] For example, weekly dosing used with rHuEPO should become every-other-week dosing with darbepoetin alpha. Conversion from weekly rHuEPO to weekly darbepoetin alpha may require a different dosing table.

TABLE 47–8. STARTING DOSE OF DARBEPOETIN ALPHA BASED ON PREVIOUS DOSING OF RECOMBINANT HUMAN ERYTHROPOIETIN (rHuEPO)[a]

Previous Weekly rHuEPO Dose (U/week)	Weekly Darbepoetin Alpha Dose (μg/week)
<2,500	6.25
2,500–4,999	12.5
5,000–10,999	25
11,000–17,999	40
18,000–33,999	60
34,000–89,999	100
≥90,000	200

[a]Table based on manufacturer's recommendations.

Dosing of darbepoetin alpha is somewhat dictated by the available preparations of this drug (Table 47–9). While rHuEPO is available in both single- and multidose vials, darbepoetin alpha is available only in single-dose vials. Drug that is not used from a single-dose vial must often be discarded, resulting in considerable unnecessary expense. Thus, initial dose selection is often based on the available preparations. Moreover, dose changes are less likely to be based on an absolute percentage dose change (e.g., 25 percent), as is done with rHuEPO. Rather, to minimize the wasting of medication, dose changes are partially influenced by the preparations available.

The lack of a multidose vial for darbepoetin alpha is especially problematic for pediatric dosing. First, many small pediatric patients are likely to need less than the 25 µg in the smallest available single-dose vial. This results in wasting of the unused medication. Second, pediatric patients may not tolerate the discomfort of 1-mL injections or may require multiple injections in order to tolerate the full 1-mL volume of the single-dose vial. The availability of darbepoetin alpha in more concentrated single-dose prefilled syringes is a useful alternative, but these preparations are available only at the higher end of the dosing scale (see Table 47–9). Thus, in order to minimize the number and volume of injections, it may be preferable to dose darbepoetin alpha every 3 to 4 weeks in some children. This would hopefully allow more patients to utilize the more concentrated single-dose prefilled syringes.

The route of administration appears to have less effect with darbepoetin alpha than with rHuEPO. Intravenous administration requires higher doses than subcutaneous administration of rHuEPO.[138–140] In contrast, one study suggests no such difference with darbepoetin alpha.[160] This may be because the half-life of intravenous darbepoetin alpha is approximately three times that of intravenous rHuEPO, but there is only a twofold increase in half-life when subcutaneous darbepoetin alpha is compared to subcutaneous rHuEPO (see Table 47–6). Thus, the proportional increase in half-life is less with subcutaneous darbepoetin alpha than with intravenous darbepoetin alpha. Moreover, like rHuEPO, not all of subcutaneous darbepoetin alpha is absorbed. The increase in bioavailability with intravenous darbepoetin alpha may compensate for the shorter half-life.

Studies of darbepoetin alpha as used in adults have not directly compared different starting doses. In one study of predialysis patients, the starting dose was 0.45 µg/kg weekly.[147] The median dose when the target Hb was achieved was 0.46 µg/kg, but the median dose after 24 weeks was 0.34 µg/kg.[147] Two studies of predialysis patients used a starting dose of 0.75 µg/kg every other week, and the median dose at achievement of the target Hb was 60 µg in both studies.[162,163]

Dosing Recommendations in Children

There are no published data on dosing of darbepoetin alpha in pediatric patients. These recommendations are extrapolated from adult data and pediatric experience with rHuEPO.

Converting from rHuEPO. Recommendations for converting patients from rHuEPO to darbepoetin alpha based on adult data are presented in Table 47–8. Patients who were receiving rHuEPO twice or thrice weekly should receive darbepoetin alpha weekly, and patients who were receiving weekly rHuEPO should receive darbepoetin alpha every other week.

Initiation with Darbepoetin Alpha. In older pediatric patients (>5 years), a starting dose of 0.45 µg/kg should be given weekly. Alternatively, the starting dose could be increased to 0.75 µg/kg and given every 2 weeks. Given the observation that children below 6 years of age often require higher doses of rHuEPO, darbepoetin alpha should be initiated weekly in this population, with a starting dose of 0.45 to 0.60 µg/kg. Every-2-weeks dosing at initiation could be considered in such patients if their Hb is only mildly below target. In contrast, given the lack of experience with darbepoetin alpha, any child with a level of anemia that is close to requiring a blood transfusion should be started on rHuEPO until more experience with darbepoetin alpha becomes available. Conversion to darbepoetin alpha can be considered once the patient has reached his or her target Hb.

Dose Adjustments. As occurs with rHuEPO,[146] frequent dose adjustments of darbepoetin alpha are often necessary, especially when one is trying to keep Hb levels within a narrow target range.[160,161] Many patients will require lower doses after their Hb reaches the target range. Moreover, decreased dosing frequency is generally desirable in order to minimize the number of injections. The protocol for dose adjustment for rHuEPO can be applied to darbepoetin alpha (see Fig. 47–1), with the caveat that rounding doses based on the available preparations (see Table 47–9) can avoid excessive wasting of the medication. Nevertheless, excessive rounding is not appropriate; some patients will need to discard some of their medication. Table 47–10 presents one system for dose adjustment.

TABLE 47–9. AVAILABLE PREPARATIONS OF DARBEPOETIN ALPHA

25 µg	40 µg	60 µg[a]	100 µg[a]	150 µg[a]	200 µg[a]	300 µg[a]	500 µg

[a]Preparations that are available in low volumes (0.3 to 0.6 mL, depending on the dose). The other preparations are available only in 1-mL doses.

TABLE 47–10. DOSE ADJUSTMENT TABLE FOR DARBEPOETIN ALPHA[a]

6.25	10	15	20	30	40	50	60	80	100	130	150	200

[a]Doses are in micrograms. The dose to the left of the current dose should be used for dose decreases and the dose to the right of the current dose for dose increases.

Dosing frequency of darbepoetin alpha can be gradually reduced from weekly to every other week to every 3 weeks to every 4 weeks. Not all patients will tolerate decreased dosing frequency, especially beyond every 3 weeks. The dosing frequency can be reduced whenever the patient has an Hb level that would normally mandate decreasing the dose. The total weekly dose should remain the same. Alternatively, the dosing frequency can be reduced in patients who are on a stable darbepoetin alpha dose and have an Hb in the target range. The total weekly dose should remain the same. Consideration should be given to increasing the dosing frequency if a patient requires more than one dosing increase, especially if the total weekly dose is relatively high. In such cases, the total weekly dose should remain the same.

Complications

Side-effect profiles have been similar in studies comparing intravenous darbepoetin alpha with intravenous rHuEPO.[160,161] In one study, there was a statistically significant increase in pruritus in the group receiving darbepoetin alpha.[160] When these drugs are administered subcutaneously, injection-site pain appears to be more common with darbepoetin alpha. There have been no documented cases of antibodies developing to darbepoetin alpha, despite screening for such antibodies in both adult[147,160–162] and pediatric studies.[167]

The longer half-life of darbepoetin alpha compared to rHuEPO raises the theoretical concern that overly rapid increases in Hb or prolonged high Hb concentrations may be more likely with darbepoetin alpha. This was evaluated in clinical studies and no difference between darbepoetin alpha and rHuEPO was detected.[147]

Monitoring Iron Stores

Serum ferritin and TSAT are currently the most widely used tests for monitoring iron stores. A variety of other tests, such as soluble transferrin receptor,[169] percentage of hypochromic RBCs,[170] and erythrocyte zinc protoporphyrin[171] have been evaluated, but none of these are readily available in the United States. TSAT and serum ferritin should be tested at initiation of rHuEPO and monthly until the patient achieves the target Hb. Subsequent monitoring should occur at least every 3 months.[2] Children receiving intravenous iron doses of more than 10 mg/kg or more than 500 mg should have a delay of at least 2 weeks before serum iron parameters are

checked. A delay of at least 1 week is appropriate for intravenous iron doses of more than 2 mg/kg or more than 100 mg.[172]

Diagnosis of Iron Deficiency

There are two "gold standards" for diagnosing iron deficiency in patients with CKD. The first is bone marrow assessment of iron stores, a test that is impractical on a routine basis. The second is the response to intravenous iron. An increase in Hb or a decrease in rHuEPO dose after receiving intravenous iron suggests that the patient was iron-deficient. The second definition is not perfect—the "response" to intravenous iron may be coincidental or the patient may not respond for other reasons—but it is the most widely used gold standard in clinical research and clinical practice.

The traditional criterion for iron deficiency, the combination of a low serum ferritin and a low TSAT, are not applicable in patients with CKD. The serum ferritin is especially problematic because ferritin is an acute-phase reactant, and it is therefore often elevated in CKD patients because of infection and nonspecific inflammation. Moreover, treatment of rHuEPO can induce functional iron deficiency. This occurs because the high rate of RBC synthesis depletes the readily available iron, even though total body iron stores may be adequate. Patients with functional iron deficiency due to rapid erythropoiesis may have a normal ferritin but a low TSAT. Often the ferritin level decreases in these patients yet remains in the normal range; it is therefore not as useful a predictor of iron deficiency as the TSAT. This has been shown in adults.[173,174] A normal ferritin does not exclude iron deficiency in children with CKD.[175,176]

Although a normal or elevated serum ferritin does not exclude iron deficiency, a low serum ferritin is a specific predictor of iron deficiency in adults[177,178] and children[121,179] with CKD. There is some debate over the definition of a "low" serum ferritin, with sensitivity increasing and specificity decreasing as the cutoff increases. In one study, a serum ferritin below 200 ng/mL was very specific for iron deficiency.[178] No studies have evaluated the specificity of different cutoff values for ferritin for identifying iron deficiency in children with CKD. The NKF-K/DOQI recommends treating all patients with a serum ferritin below 100 ng/mL for iron deficiency.[2]

A TSAT below 20 percent has been widely used as a criterion for iron deficiency in patients with CKD. In one pediatric study, it was highly specific in identifying iron deficiency.[176] The NKF-K/DOQI recommends treating all patients with a TSAT <20 percent for iron deficiency.[2] Yet, there are clearly patients with a TSAT above 20 percent who respond to intravenous iron.[180] Like ferritin, the predictive value of the TSAT for iron deficiency can be influenced by factors other than iron stores. For example, hypoproteinemia, as may occur in malnutrition or nephrotic syndrome, can lead to a decrease in the serum transferrin. Adults with CKD and a serum transferrin less than 150 mg/dL may have iron deficiency despite a TSAT greater than 20 percent.[178] Patients with a serum ferritin below 100 ng/mL or a TSAT <20 percent should be treated for iron deficiency. Nevertheless, there are clearly patients who do not meet this definition of iron deficiency and will still respond to intravenous iron.[180] The NKF-K/DOQI therefore recommends a trial of intravenous iron in CKD patients who are unable to reach their target Hb or who require large doses of rHuEPO to maintain their Hb as long as the serum ferritin level is less than 800 ng/mL and the TSAT is less than 50 percent.[2]

A TSAT below 20 percent and a serum ferritin above 100 ng/mL suggests functional iron deficiency, as described above. This same scenario can also occur with an inflammatory block, a condition where inflammation prevents effective delivery of iron for erythropoiesis (see the preceding discussion of inflammation). Clinical signs of infection, a low serum iron, an elevated CRP, an increasing ferritin, and a poor response to intravenous iron support a diagnosis of an inflammatory block.

Iron

After erythropoietin deficiency, iron deficiency is the leading cause of anemia in children with CKD. Treatment of iron deficiency often allows achievement of the target Hb with a lower dose of rHuEPO. Iron therapy should not be given to patients who have iron overload, which is most commonly defined as a ferritin greater than 800 ng/mL or a TSAT >50 percent.

Oral Iron. Only a small percentage of oral iron is absorbed, thus limiting its efficacy in patients who have high iron requirements due to blood loss, such as children receiving HD.[8] Moreover, problems with gastric irritation and constipation may limit compliance.[181]

There is an upregulation in oral iron absorption in dialysis patients who have a low serum ferritin[182,183] or decreased marrow iron stores.[184] The enhancement of erythropoiesis from administration of rHuEPO may[183] or may not[185] increase iron absorption in HD patients who have adequate levels of ferritin. HD patients have decreased absorption of oral iron when compared to normal controls[186]; inflammation, as measured by CRP levels, may further decrease iron absorption.[35]

Oral iron absorption improves when the dose is not given with food,[183,187] so iron should be given either 1 hour before a meal or 2 hours after a meal. Children should receive a dose of 3 to 4 mg/kg/day of elemental iron (with a maximum dose of 150 to 300 mg/day). Oral iron should not be given to HD patients who are receiving maintenance dosing of intravenous iron.

Oral iron may be adequate therapy in many children who have yet to begin dialysis or who are receiving PD. In adults[188,189] and children[175,176] receiving HD, oral iron is often not sufficient to correct absolute or functional iron deficiency.

Intravenous Iron. Given the limitations of oral iron and the high incidence of iron deficiency in dialysis patients, intravenous iron is frequently utilized in adults and children with CKD. During a 3-month period in 2001, 68 percent of children in the United States receiving HD were prescribed intravenous iron.[70] Yet 35 percent of patients with a TSAT below 20 percent and a ferritin below 100 ng/mL did not receive any intravenous iron during this same period.[70] The overall percentage of children receiving intravenous iron has increased; only 53 percent received intravenous iron in 1999.[70]

There are currently four intravenous iron preparations available in the United States: iron dextran (INFeD or Dexferrum); sodium ferric gluconate conjugate in sucrose, hence referred to as iron gluconate (Ferrlecit); and iron sucrose (Venofer). The European Pediatric Peritoneal Dialysis Working Group recommends not using iron dextran due to concerns about life-threatening anaphylactic reactions (see below).[190]

Efficacy. A large number of studies in adults have demonstrated the efficacy of intravenous iron in correcting iron deficiency, improving Hb levels, and reducing rHuEPO dosing requirements.[188,191-195] There are limited pediatric data; four published studies, all showing a positive effect of intravenous iron, are summarized in Table 47–11.[175,176,196,197]

There are a few studies comparing the efficacy of maintenance vs. intermittent need-based dosing of intravenous iron in HD patients. Maintenance protocols may decrease rHuEPO dose requirements in adults[172] and children.[197] This is presumably secondary to the transient iron deficiency that may occur with a need-based approach. An additional factor may be more efficient use of iron for RBC synthesis when intravenous iron is given in regular, small doses as opposed to large bolus doses.[198] With small doses, less iron may be trapped in the reticuloendothelial system, where it becomes unavailable for RBC synthesis.

Acute Dosing. The goal of acute dosing is to normalize the serum ferritin and the TSAT. In some cases, an acute dose may be used as a trial of intravenous iron in a patient with normal iron studies, but a poor response to rHuEPO. In adult HD patients, studies suggest that a total dose of 1000

TABLE 47–11. PEDIATRIC STUDIES OF INTRAVENOUS IRON

Study Design (reference)	Outcome[a]
HD patients received 1 mg/kg/week of iron gluconate for 3 months. (Tebrock et al.[175])	Hb increased from 7.8 to 9.2 g/dL; ferritin increased from 200 to 395 mg/dL. rHuEPO dose decreased from 6500 U to 6150 U.
HD patients with iron deficiency received 4 mg/kg (maximum of 100 mg) of iron dextran during 10 consecutive dialysis sessions. (Greenbaum et al.[176])	rHuEPO dose decreased from 3784 U to 2115 U. Hematocrit increased from 31.8 to 35%.
HD, predialysis and renal transplant patients received various doses and courses of iron gluconate. (Yorgin et al.[196])	Hematocrit increased from 30.3 to 36.4%. rHuEPO dose decreased from 251.5 to 100.7 U/kg/week.
HD patients received 2 mg/kg iron sucrose weekly if not iron overloaded; they received 7 mg/kg x 1 if iron-deficient. (Morgan et al.[197])	Treated patients required less rHuEPO (74 U/kg/week) than historical controls (194 U/kg/week).

KEY: HD, hemodialysis; PD, peritoneal dialysis; rHuEPO, recombinant human erythropoietin; Hb, hemoglobin.
[a]Outcome results are expressed as mean values.

mg of iron is appropriate,[2] since smaller doses are not as effective.[194] The same dose has been used in older children with good results.[176]

Acute dosing is usually given over multiple sessions in patients receiving HD; 1000 mg of either iron gluconate or iron sucrose cannot be given during one HD session. The specific iron preparation dictates the number of doses and size of the dose. Iron gluconate, which comes in 62.5-mg vials, is usually given in 125-mg doses during eight consecutive dialysis sessions.[194] Iron sucrose (100-mg vials)[199,200] and iron dextran (50-mg vials) are usually given in 100-mg doses over 10 consecutive dialysis sessions, although higher individual doses of iron dextran can be used.[201]

For CKD patients not receiving HD, intravenous iron is effective,[195,202] but dosing is less convenient because of the lack of intravenous access. Single doses of iron dextran have ranged from 200 to 1000 mg, with administration over 1 to 6 hours, depending on the dose.[195,203,204] Alternatively, patients have had a good response to weekly or monthly infusions of 100- or 200-mg doses of iron sucrose, although one study suggests that the rate of infusion of the 200-mg dose must be decreased to minimize side effects.[202,205] Iron sucrose doses of 300 mg given over 2 hours appears to be well tolerated. Doses of iron sucrose as high as 500 mg have been given,[206,207] but the infusion time must be extended to avoid side effects.[208] In children, one study reported administration of doses of 7 mg/kg of iron sucrose, with a maximum dose of 200 mg.[197]

Iron gluconate in doses of 250 mg over 60 or 90 minutes, were well tolerated.[209,210] There is limited experience with higher single doses of iron gluconate.[209] In children,

one study reported administration of doses ranging from 1.5 to 8.8 mg/kg, with the child receiving the highest dose having a significant adverse event.[196]

Chronic Dosing. Acute dosing is effective in correcting iron deficiency, but, especially in HD patients, there is a risk of ongoing episodes of iron deficiency due to continued blood loss. This has led to more frequent use of chronic intravenous iron protocols in adults receiving HD, potentially producing a decrease in rHuEPO dose requirements.[188,193,211] In one pediatric study, 1 mg/kg of iron gluconate for 12 weeks led to a significant increase in Hb.[175] In another pediatric study, chronic intravenous iron sucrose [2 mg/kg (max = 200 mg) weekly] produced a significant reduction in the dosing of rHuEPO.[197]

Dosing Recommendations in Children. All patients should receive a test dose prior to receiving iron dextran because of the risk of an anaphylactic reaction (see below); a physician should be present. Test doses should be based on patient weight: <10 kg (10 mg), 10 to 20 kg (15 mg), and >20 kg (25 mg). Iron dextran should generally be avoided, given its potential for life-threatening side effects. Test doses are not necessary for iron sucrose or iron gluconate.

In children receiving HD, the total acute dose of intravenous iron should be approximately 25 mg/kg, up to a maximum dose of 1000 mg. This dose is typically divided over 8 to 12 dialysis sessions, with dosing designed to minimize wasting of drug (Tables 47–12 and 47–13). Acute doses are given when the patient has a TSAT below 20 percent, a ferritin below 100 ng/mL, or functional iron deficiency is suspected. Intravenous iron should not be given when the TSAT is greater than 50 percent or the serum ferritin is more than 800 ng/mL. Maintenance intravenous iron in children receiving HD should be started at about 1 mg/kg/week, usually given as a once-per-week dose. The maintenance dose is titrated to keep the TSAT between 20 and 50 percent and the ferritin between 100 and 800 ng/mL. For children receiving PD or those who have not yet begun dialysis, the goal is usually to minimize the need for intravenous line placement by maximizing the dose given during a single infusion. The maximum dose of iron gluconate is 4

TABLE 47–12. ACUTE DOSING OF IRON GLUCONATE IN PEDIATRIC PATIENTS RECEIVING HEMODIALYSIS

Weight	Iron Gluconate Dose[a]
<25 kg	2.5 mg/kg/dose x 10 doses
25–29 kg	62.5 mg/dose x 10 doses
30–39 kg	62.5 mg/dose x 12 doses
≥40 kg	125 mg/dose x 8 doses[b]

[a]Infuse over at least 10 minutes unless noted.
[b]Patients between 40 and 50 kg should receive their dose over at least 1 hour.

TABLE 47–13. ACUTE DOSING OF IRON SUCROSE IN PEDIATRIC PATIENTS RECEIVING HEMODIALYSIS

Weight	Iron Sucrose Dose
<25 kg	4 mg/kg/dose x 7 doses[a]
25–29 kg	100 mg/dose x 8 doses[a]
30–34 kg	100 mg/dose x 9 doses[b]
≥35 kg	100 mg/dose x 10 doses[b]

[a]Infuse over at least 1 hour.
[b]Infuse over at least 15 minutes (may give by intravenous push over at least 5 minutes if total dose is less than 3 mg/kg).

mg/kg (250 mg if the patient weighs >60 kg), which should be given over at least 90 minutes. The maximum dose of iron sucrose is 8 mg/kg (500 mg if the patient weighs >60 kg), which should be given over 4 hours.

Complications. There are some complications of intravenous iron that are specific to the particular preparation. Iron dextran may cause an acute, potentially fatal anaphylactic reaction.[212–214] These reactions appear to be more common with DexFerrum than with INFeD.[214] Iron sucrose[215] and iron gluconate[194,216] have a safer side-effect profile. Children[196] and adults[194,199,215] who have had anaphylactic reactions to iron dextran have tolerated these other iron preparations. This has led to questions regarding the continued appropriateness of using iron dextran.[190,217,218] In addition to anaphylaxis, high doses of iron dextran may cause patients to develop arthralgias and myalgias.[219]

There are reports of laboratory findings and clinical symptoms that may be due to acute iron toxicity during the use of iron sucrose and iron gluconate.[220, 221] This effect is related to the dose and infusion rate[202, 222] and is presumably secondary to the rapid release of free iron. Symptoms with iron gluconate have included loin pain, hypotension, emesis, and paresthesias.[222] Side effects of iron sucrose have included rash, flushing and hypotension, which was rapidly reversible.[223] These side effects limit the maximum single dose of these compounds when compared to iron dextran, which releases iron at a slower rate. One pediatric patient appeared to have such a reaction when he was given 5.4 mg/kg of iron gluconate.[196]

Iron overload is a potential complication of all forms of intravenous iron therapy; careful monitoring should prevent it. Nevertheless, 14 percent of U.S. pediatric HD patients had a ferritin concentration greater than 800 ng/mL in 2001.[70] There is concern that current protocols for intravenous iron may lead to increasing problems with iron overload.[224] Aggressive rHuEPO therapy and phlebotomy can be used to treat severe iron overload if it develops.[225] Transient iron overload has been seen in children receiving maintenance intravenous iron.[197]

Intravenous iron may increase the risk of infection. Sequestration of iron, which is essential for bacterial growth, is a defense against infection.[226] Iron overload predisposes HD patients to infection,[227] and correction of iron overload improves neutrophil function.[228] Intravenous iron in HD patients has a negative effect on neutrophil function.[229,230] Yet serum ferritin was not a predictor of infection in patients on HD,[231] and a multivariate analysis did not find a relationship between intravenous iron and infection, although there was a trend toward more infections among those patients who received large amounts of intravenous iron vs. those who received lower doses.[232] Given this potential complication, intravenous iron should be discontinued in patients with acute infections.[1]

REFERENCES

1. Working Party for European Best Practice Guidelines for the Management of Anaemia in Patients with Chronic Renal Failure. European best practice guidelines for the management of anaemia in patients with chronic renal failure. *Nephrol Dial Transplant* 1999;14:S1.
2. National Kidney Foundation. NKF-K/DOQI clinical practice guidelines for anemia of chronic kidney disease. *Am J Kidney Dis* 2001;37:S182.
3. McGonigle RJ, Boineau FG, Beckman B, et al. Erythropoietin and inhibitors of in vitro erythropoiesis in the development of anemia in children with renal disease. *J Lab Clin Med* 1985;105:449.
4. Chandra M, Clemons GK, McVicar MI. Relation of serum erythropoietin levels to renal excretory function: evidence for lowered set point for erythropoietin production in chronic renal failure. *J Pediatr* 1988;113:1015.
5. Caro J, Brown S, Miller O, et al. Erythropoietin levels in uremic nephric and anephric patients. *J Lab Clin Med* 1979; 93:449.
6. Lindsay RM, Burton JA, Edward N, et al. Dialyzer blood loss. *Clin Nephrol* 1973;1:29.
7. Lindsay RM, Burton JA, King P, et al. The measurement of dialyzer blood loss. *Clin Nephrol* 1973;1:24.
8. Muller-Wiefel DE, Sinn H, Gilli G, et al. Hemolysis and blood loss in children with chronic renal failure. *Clin Nephrol* 1977;8:481.
9. Longnecker RE, Goffinet JA, Hendler ED. Blood loss during maintenance hemodialysis. *Trans Am Soc Artif Intern Organs* 1974;20A:135.
10. Eschbach JW Jr, Funk D, Adamson J, et al. Erythropoiesis in patients with renal failure undergoing chronic dialysis. *N Engl J Med* 1967;276:653.
11. Kominami N, Lowrie EG, Ianhez LE, et al. The effect of total nephrectomy on hematopoiesis in patients undergoing chronic hemodialysis. *J Lab Clin Med* 1971;78:524.
12. Wu SG, Jeng FR, Wei SY, et al. Red blood cell osmotic fragility in chronically hemodialyzed patients. *Nephron* 1998;78:28.
13. Kletzmayr J, Mayer G, Legenstein E, et al. Anemia and carnitine supplementation in hemodialyzed patients. *Kidney Int* 1999;69(suppl):S93.

14. Polenakovic M, Sikole A. Is erythropoietin a survival factor for red blood cells? *J Am Soc Nephrol* 1996;7:1178.

15. Radtke HW, Frei U, Erbes PM, et al. Improving anemia by hemodialysis: effect of serum erythropoietin. *Kidney Int* 1980;17:382.

16. Madore F, Lowrie EG, Brugnara C, et al. Anemia in hemodialysis patients: variables affecting this outcome predictor. *J Am Soc Nephrol* 1997;8:1921.

17. Ifudu O, Feldman J, Friedman EA. The intensity of hemodialysis and the response to erythropoietin in patients with end-stage renal disease. *N Engl J Med* 1996;334:420.

18. Richardson D, Lindley E, Bartlett C, et al. A randomized, controlled study of the consequences of hemodialysis membrane composition on erythropoietic response. *Am J Kidney Dis* 2003;42:551.

19. Ifudu O, Friedman EA. Effect of increased hemodialysis dose on endogenous erythropoietin production in end-stage renal disease. *Nephron* 1998;79:50.

20. Macdougall IC, Davies ME, Hutton RD, et al. The treatment of renal anaemia in CAPD patients with recombinant human erythropoietin. *Nephrol Dial Transplant* 1990;5:950.

21. Nissenson AR, Korbet S, Faber M, et al. Multicenter trial of erythropoietin in patients on peritoneal dialysis. *J Am Soc Nephrol* 1995;5:1517.

22. Barany P, Clyne N, Hylander B, et al. Subcutaneous epoetin beta in renal anemia: an open multicenter dose titration study of patients on continuous peritoneal dialysis. *Perit Dial Int* 1995;15:54.

23. Frankenfield DL, Neu AM, Warady BA, et al. Anemia in pediatric hemodialysis patients: Results from the 2001 ESRD Clinical Performance Measures Project. *Kidney Int* 2003;64:1120.

24. Paganini EP, Abdulhadi MH, Garcia J, et al. Recombinant human erythropoietin correction of anemia. Dialysis efficiency, waste retention, and chronic dose variables. *ASAIO Trans* 1989;35:513.

25. Movilli E, Cancarini GC, Zani R, et al. Adequacy of dialysis reduces the doses of recombinant erythropoietin independently from the use of biocompatible membranes in haemodialysis patients. *Nephrol Dial Transplant* 2001;16:111.

26. Kalantar-Zadeh K, Ikizler TA, Block G, et al. Malnutrition-inflammation complex syndrome in dialysis patients: Causes and consequences. *Am J Kidney Dis* 2003;42:864.

27. Barany P, Divino Filho JC, Bergstrom J. High C-reactive protein is a strong predictor of resistance to erythropoietin in hemodialysis patients. *Am J Kidney Dis* 1997;29:565.

28. Barany P. Inflammation, serum C-reactive protein, and erythropoietin resistance. *Nephrol Dial Transplant* 2001;16:224.

29. Krantz SB. Pathogenesis and treatment of the anemia of chronic disease. *Am J Med Sci* 1994;307:353.

30. Muirhead N, Hodsman AB. Occult infection and resistance of anaemia to rHuEPO therapy in renal failure. *Nephrol Dial Transplant* 1990;5:232.

31. van Iperen CE, Kraaijenhagen RJ, Biesma DH, et al. Iron metabolism and erythropoiesis after surgery. *Br J Surg* 1998;85:41.

32. Owen WF, Lowrie EG. C-reactive protein as an outcome predictor for maintenance hemodialysis patients. *Kidney Int* 1998;54:627.

33. Sitter T, Bergner A, Schiffl H. Dialysate related cytokine induction and response to recombinant human erythropoietin in haemodialysis patients. *Nephrol Dial Transplant* 2000;15:1207.

34. Gunnell J, Yeun JY, Depner TA, et al. Acute-phase response predicts erythropoietin resistance in hemodialysis and peritoneal dialysis patients. *Am J Kidney Dis* 1999;33:63.

35. Kooistra MP, Niemantsverdriet EC, van Es A, et al. Iron absorption in erythropoietin-treated haemodialysis patients: effects of iron availability, inflammation and aluminium. *Nephrol Dial Transplant* 1998;13:82.

36. Allen DA, Breen C, Yaqoob MM, et al. Inhibition of CFU-E colony formation in uremic patients with inflammatory disease: role of IFN-gamma and TNF-alpha. *J Investig Med* 1999;47:204.

37. Goicoechea M, Martin J, de Sequera P, et al. Role of cytokines in the response to erythropoietin in hemodialysis patients. *Kidney Int* 1998;54:1337.

38. Locatelli F, Andrulli S, Pecchini F, et al. Effect of high-flux dialysis on the anaemia of haemodialysis patients. *Nephrol Dial Transplant* 2000;15:1399.

39. Boxer M, Ellman L, Geller R, et al. Anemia in primary hyperparathyroidism. *Arch Intern Med* 137:588.

40. Zingraff J, Drueke T, Marie P, et al. Anemia and secondary hyperparathyroidism. *Arch Intern Med* 1978;138:1650.

41. Barbour GL: Effect of parathyroidectomy on anemia in chronic renal failure. *Arch Intern Med* 139:889.

42. Rao DS, Shih MS, Mohini R. Effect of serum parathyroid hormone and bone marrow fibrosis on the response to erythropoietin in uremia. *N Engl J Med* 1993;328:171.

43. Hampers CL, Streiff R, Nathan DG, et al. Megaloblastic hematopoiesis in uremia and in patients on long-term hemodialysis. *N Engl J Med* 1967;276:551.

44. Zachee P, Chew SL, Daelemans R, et al. Erythropoietin resistance due to vitamin B12 deficiency. Case report and retrospective analysis of B12 levels after erythropoietin treatment. *Am J Nephrol* 1992;12:188.

45. Pronai W, Riegler-Keil M, Silberbauer K, et al. Folic acid supplementation improves erythropoietin response. *Nephron* 1995;71:395.

46. Ono K, Hisasue Y. Is folate supplementation necessary in hemodialysis patients on erythropoietin therapy. *Clin Nephrol* 1992;38:290.

47. Bamonti-Catena F, Buccianti G, Porcella A, et al. Folate measurements in patients on regular hemodialysis treatment. *Am J Kidney Dis* 1999;33:492.

48. Lee EY, Kim JS, Lee HJ, et al. Do dialysis patients need extra folate supplementation? *Adv Perit Dial* 1999;15:247.

49. Westhuyzen J, Matherson K, Tracey R, et al. Effect of withdrawal of folic acid supplementation in maintenance hemodialysis patients. *Clin Nephrol* 1993;40:96.

50. Kaiser L, Schwartz KA.: Aluminum-induced anemia. *Am J Kidney Dis* 1985;6:348.

51. Yuan B, Klein MH, Contiguglia RS, et al. The role of aluminum in the pathogenesis of anemia in an outpatient hemodialysis population. *Renal Failure* 1989;11:91.

52. Bia MJ, Cooper K, Schnall S, et al. Aluminum induced anemia: pathogenesis and treatment in patients on chronic hemodialysis. *Kidney Int* 1989;36:852.

53. Muirhead N, Hodsman AB, Hollomby DJ, et al. The role of aluminium and parathyroid hormone in erythropoietin resistance in haemodialysis patients. *Nephrol Dial Transplant* 1991;6:342.

54. Sedman AB, Miller NL, Warady BA, et al. Aluminum loading in children with chronic renal failure. *Kidney Int* 1984; 26:201.

55. Salusky IB, Coburn JW, Paunier L, et al. Role of aluminum hydroxide in raising serum aluminum levels in children undergoing continuous ambulatory peritoneal dialysis. *J Pediatr* 1984;105:717.

56. Andreoli SP, Bergstein JM, Sherrard DJ. Aluminum intoxication from aluminum-containing phosphate binders in children with azotemia not undergoing dialysis. *N Engl J Med* 1984;310:1079.

57. Eknoyan G, Latos D, Lindberg J. Practice recommendations for the use of L-carnitine in dialysis-related carnitine disorder National Kidney Foundation Carnitine Consensus Conference. *Am J Kidney Dis* 2003;41:868.

58. Gahl WA, Bernardini I, Dalakas M, et al. Oral carnitine therapy in children with cystinosis and renal Fanconi syndrome. *J Clin Invest* 1988;81:549.

59. Bernardini I, Rizzo WB, Dalakas M, et al. Plasma and muscle free carnitine deficiency due to renal Fanconi syndrome. *J Clin Invest* 1985;75:1124.

60. Labonia WD. L-carnitine effects on anemia in hemodialyzed patients treated with erythropoietin. *Am J Kidney Dis* 1995;26:757.

61. Berard E, Iordache A. Effect of low doses of L-carnitine on the response to recombinant human erythropoietin in hemodialyzed children: about two cases. *Nephron* 1992;62: 368.

62. Dhondt AW, Vanholder RC, Ringoir SM. Angiotensin-converting enzyme inhibitors and higher erythropoietin requirement in chronic haemodialysis patients. *Nephrol Dial Transplant* 1995;10:2107.

63. Albitar S, Genin R, Fen-Chong M, et al. High dose enalapril impairs the response to erythropoietin treatment in haemodialysis patients. *Nephrol Dial Transplant* 1998;13: 1206.

64. Erturk S, Nergizoglu G, Ates K, et al. The impact of withdrawing ACE inhibitors on erythropoietin responsiveness and left ventricular hypertrophy in haemodialysis patients. *Nephrol Dial Transplant* 1999;14:1912.

65. Abu-Alfa AK, Cruz D, Perazella MA, et al. ACE inhibitors do not induce recombinant human erythropoietin resistance in hemodialysis patients. *Am J Kidney Dis* 2000;35:1076.

66. Sanchez JA: ACE inhibitors do not decrease rHuEPO response in patients with end-stage renal failure. *Nephrol Dial Transplant* 1995;10:1476.

67. Kazmi WH, Kausz AT, Khan S, et al. Anemia: an early complication of chronic renal insufficiency. *Am J Kidney Dis* 2001;38:803.

68. Obrador GT, Roberts T, St Peter WL, et al. Trends in anemia at initiation of dialysis in the United States. *Kidney Int* 2001; 60:1875.

69. Ho M, Stablein DM. *North American Pediatric Renal Transplant Cooperative Study (NAPRTCS) Annual Report.* Rockville, MD: 2003.

70. Centers for Medicare & Medicaid Services. 2002 annual report, end stage renal disease clinical performance measures project. *Am J Kidney Dis* 2003;42:S1.

71. Kuriyama S, Tomonari H, Yoshida H, et al. Reversal of anemia by erythropoietin therapy retards the progression of chronic renal failure, especially in nondiabetic patients. *Nephron* 1997;77:176.

72. Foley RN, Parfrey PS, Harnett JD, et al. The impact of anemia on cardiomyopathy, morbidity, and mortality in end-stage renal disease. *Am J Kidney Dis* 1996;28:53.

73. Collins AJ, Ma JZ, Ebben J. Impact of hematocrit on morbidity and mortality. *Semin Nephrol* 2000;20:345.

74. Ma JZ, Ebben J, Xia H, et al. Hematocrit level and associated mortality in hemodialysis patients. *J Am Soc Nephrol* 1999;10:610.

75. Xia H, Ebben J, Ma JZ, et al. Hematocrit levels and hospitalization risks in hemodialysis patients. *J Am Soc Nephrol* 1999;10:1309.

76. Besarab A, Bolton WK, Browne JK, et al. The effects of normal as compared with low hematocrit values in patients with cardiac disease who are receiving hemodialysis and epoetin. *N Engl J Med* 1998;339:584.

77. Collins AJ, Li S, St Peter W, et al. Death, hospitalization, and economic associations among incident hemodialysis patients with hematocrit values of 36 to 39%. *J Am Soc Nephrol* 2001;12:2465.

78. U.S. Renal Data System. *USRDS 2000 Annual Data Report.* Bethesda, MD: The National Institutes of Health, National Institute of Diabetes and Digestive and Kidney Diseases, June 2000.

79. Chavers BM, Li S, Collins AJ, et al. Cardiovascular disease in pediatric chronic dialysis patients. *Kidney Int* 2002; 62:648.

80. Silberberg JS, Rahal DP, Patton DR, et al. Role of anemia in the pathogenesis of left ventricular hypertrophy in end-stage renal disease. *Am J Cardiol* 1989;64:222.

81. Levin A, Singer J, Thompson CR, et al. Prevalent left ventricular hypertrophy in the predialysis population: identifying opportunities for intervention. *Am J Kidney Dis* 1995; 27:347.

82. Levin A, Thompson CR, Ethier J, et al. Left ventricular mass index increase in early renal disease: impact of decline in hemoglobin. *Am J Kidney Dis* 1999;34:125.

83. Levin A, Foley RN. Cardiovascular disease in chronic renal insufficiency. *Am J Kidney Dis* 2000;36:S24.

84. Silberberg J, Racine N, Barre P, et al. Regression of left ventricular hypertrophy in dialysis patients following correction of anemia with recombinant human erythropoietin. *Can J Cardiol* 1990;6:1.

85. Foley RN, Parfrey PS, Morgan J, et al. Effect of hemoglobin levels in hemodialysis patients with asymptomatic cardiomyopathy. *Kidney Int* 2000;58:1325.

86. Besarab A, Levin A. Defining a renal anemia management period. *Am J Kidney Dis* 2000;36:S13.

87. McMahon LP, Mason K, Skinner SL, et al. Effects of haemoglobin normalization on quality of life and cardiovas-

cular parameters in end-stage renal failure. *Nephrol Dial Transplant* 2000;15:1425.

88. Morris KP, Skinner JR, Hunter S, et al. Cardiovascular abnormalities in end stage renal failure: the effect of anaemia or uraemia? *Arch Dis Child* 1994;71:119.

89. Mitsnefes MM, Daniels SR, Schwartz SM, et al. Severe left ventricular hypertrophy in pediatric dialysis: prevalence and predictors. *Pediatr Nephrol* 2000;14:898.

90. Evans RW, Rader B, Manninen DL. The quality of life of hemodialysis recipients treated with recombinant human erythropoietin. Cooperative Multicenter EPO Clinical Trial Group. *JAMA* 1990;263:825.

91. Revicki DA, Brown RE, Feeny DH, et al. Health-related quality of life associated with recombinant human erythropoietin therapy for predialysis chronic renal disease patients. *Am J Kidney Dis* 1995;25:548.

92. Canadian Erythropoietin Study Group. Association between recombinant human erythropoietin and quality of life and exercise capacity of patients receiving haemodialysis. *BMJ* 1990;300:573.

93. Clyne N, Jogestrand T. Effect of erythropoietin treatment on physical exercise capacity and on renal function in predialytic uremic patients. *Nephron* 1992;60:390.

94. The US Recombinant Erythropoietin Predialysis Study Group. Double-blind, placebo-controlled study of the therapeutic use of recombinant human erythropoietin for anemia associated with chronic renal failure in predialysis patients. *Am J Kidney Dis* 1991;18:50.

95. Marsh JT, Brown WS, Wolcott D, et al. rHuEPO treatment improves brain and cognitive function of anemic dialysis patients. *Kidney Int* 1991;39:155.

96. Beusterien KM, Nissenson AR, Port FK, et al. The effects of recombinant human erythropoietin on functional health and well-being in chronic dialysis patients. *J Am Soc Nephrol* 1996;7:763.

97. Pickett JL, Theberge DC, Brown WS, et al. Normalizing hematocrit in dialysis patients improves brain function. *Am J Kidney Dis* 1999;33:1122.

98. Walter T, De Andraca I, Chadud P, et al. Iron deficiency anemia: adverse effects on infant psychomotor development. *Pediatrics* 1989;84:7.

99. Montini G, Zacchello G, Baraldi E, et al. Benefits and risks of anemia correction with recombinant human erythropoietin in children maintained by hemodialysis. *J Pediatr* 1990; 117:556.

100. Van Damme-Lombaerts R, Broyer M, Businger J, et al. A study of recombinant human erythropoietin in the treatment of anaemia of chronic renal failure in children on haemodialysis. *Pediatr Nephrol* 1994;8:338.

101. Burke JR. Low-dose subcutaneous recombinant erythropoietin in children with chronic renal failure. Australian and New Zealand Paediatric Nephrology Association. *Pediatr Nephrol* 1995;9:558.

102. Jabs K, Alexander S, McCabe D, et al. Primary results from the U.S. multicenter pediatric recombinant erythropoietin (EPO) study. *J Am Soc Nephrol* 1994;5:546.

103. Warady BA, Sabath RJ, Smith CA, et al. Recombinant human erythropoietin therapy in pediatric patients receiving long-term peritoneal dialysis. *Pediatr Nephrol* 1991;5:718.

104. Scigalla P, Bonzel KE, Bulla M, et al. Therapy of renal anemia with recombinant human erythropoietin in children with end-stage renal disease. *Contrib Nephrol* 1989;76:227.

105. Jabs K. The effects of recombinant human erythropoietin on growth and nutritional status. *Pediatr Nephrol* 1996; 10:324.

106. Hutchinson FN, Jones WJ. A cost-effectiveness analysis of anemia screening before erythropoietin in patients with end-stage renal disease. *Am J Kidney Dis* 1997;29:651.

107. Gokal R, Weatherall DJ, Bunch C. Iron induced increase in red cell size in haemodialysis patients. *Q J Med* 1979;48: 393.

108. Hymes LC, Hawthorne SM, Clowers BM. Impaired response to recombinant erythropoietin therapy in children with peritonitis. *Dial Transplant* 1994;23:462.

109. Patterson P, Allon M. Prospective evaluation of an anemia treatment algorithm in hemodialysis patients. *Am J Kidney Dis* 1998;32:635.

110. Brimble KS, Rabbat CG, McKenna P, et al. Protocolized anemia management with erythropoietin in hemodialysis patients: a randomized controlled trial. *J Am Soc Nephrol* 2003;14:2654.

111. Winearls CG, Oliver DO, Pippard MJ, et al. Effect of human erythropoietin derived from recombinant DNA on the anaemia of patients maintained by chronic haemodialysis. *Lancet* 1986;2:1175.

112. Eschbach JW, Egrie JC, Downing MR, et al. Correction of the anemia of end-stage renal disease with recombinant human erythropoietin. Results of a combined phase I and II clinical trial. *N Engl J Med* 1987;316:73.

113. Eschbach JW, Abdulhadi MH, Browne JK, et al. Recombinant human erythropoietin in anemic patients with end-stage renal disease. Results of a phase III multicenter clinical trial. *Ann Intern Med* 1989;111:992.

114. Eschbach JW, Kelly MR, Haley NR, et al. Treatment of the anemia of progressive renal failure with recombinant human erythropoietin. *N Engl J Med* 1989;321:158.

115. Watson AJ, Gimenez LF, Cotton S, et al. Treatment of the anemia of chronic renal failure with subcutaneous recombinant human erythropoietin. *Am J Med* 1990;89:432.

116. Sinai-Trieman L, Salusky IB, Fine RN. Use of subcutaneous recombinant human erythropoietin in children undergoing continuous cycling peritoneal dialysis. *J Pediatr* 1989;114: 550.

117. Montini G, Zacchello G, Perfumo F, et al. Pharmacokinetics and hematologic response to subcutaneous administration of recombinant human erythropoietin in children undergoing long-term peritoneal dialysis: a multicenter study. *J Pediatr* 1993;122:297.

118. Offner G, Hoyer PF, Latta K, et al. One year's experience with recombinant erythropoietin in children undergoing continuous ambulatory or cycling peritoneal dialysis. *Pediatr Nephrol* 1990;4:498.

119. Scigalla P. Effect of recombinant human erythropoietin treatment on renal anemia and body growth of children with end-stage renal disease. The European Multicenter Study Group. *Contrib Nephrol* 1991;88:201.

120. Ongkingco JR, Ruley EJ, Turner ME. Use of low-dose subcutaneous recombinant human erythropoietin in end-stage

renal disease: experience with children receiving continuous cycling peritoneal dialysis. *Am J Kidney Dis* 1991;18:446.

121. Campos A, Garin EH. Therapy of renal anemia in children and adolescents with recombinant human erythropoietin (rHuEPO). *Clin Pediatr (Phila)* 1992;31:94.

122. Scharer K, Klare B, Braun A, et al. Treatment of renal anemia by subcutaneous erythropoietin in children with preterminal chronic renal failure. *Acta Paediatr* 1993;82:953.

123. Aufricht C, Balzar E, Steger H, et al. Subcutaneous recombinant human erythropoietin in children with renal anemia on continuous ambulatory peritoneal dialysis. *Acta Paediatr* 1993;82:959.

124. Yalcinkaya F, Tumer N, Cakar N, et al. Low-dose erythropoietin is effective and safe in children on continuous ambulatory peritoneal dialysis. *Pediatr Nephrol* 1997;11:350.

125. Brandt JR, Avner ED, Hickman RO, et al. Safety and efficacy of erythropoietin in children with chronic renal failure. *Pediatr Nephrol* 1999;13:143.

126. Sieniawska M, Roszkowska-Blaim M. Recombinant human erythropoietin dosage in children undergoing hemodialysis and continuous ambulatory peritoneal dialysis. *Pediatr Nephrol* 1997;11:628.

127. Rigden SP, Montini G, Morris M, et al. Recombinant human erythropoietin therapy in children maintained by haemodialysis. *Pediatr Nephrol* 1990;4:618.

128. Macdougall IC, Roberts DE, Neubert P, et al. Pharmacokinetics of recombinant human erythropoietin in patients on continuous ambulatory peritoneal dialysis. *Lancet* 1989;1:425.

129. Ateshkadi A, Johnson CA, Oxton LL, et al. Pharmacokinetics of intraperitoneal, intravenous, and subcutaneous recombinant human erythropoietin in patients on continuous ambulatory peritoneal dialysis. *Am J Kidney Dis* 1993;21:635.

130. Salmonson T, Danielson BG, Wikstrom B. The pharmacokinetics of recombinant human erythropoietin after intravenous and subcutaneous administration to healthy subjects. *Br J Clin Pharmacol* 1990;29:709.

131. Brockmoller J, Kochling J, Weber W, et al. The pharmacokinetics and pharmacodynamics of recombinant human erythropoietin in haemodialysis patients. *Br J Clin Pharmacol* 1992;34:499.

132. Flaharty KK, Grimm AM, Vlasses PH. Epoetin: human recombinant erythropoietin. *Clin Pharm* 1989;8:769.

133. Jabs K, Grant JR, Harmon W, et al. Pharmacokinetics of Epoetin alfa (rHuEpo) in pediatric hemodialysis (HD) patients (abstr). *J Am Soc Nephrol* 1991;2:380.

134. Evans JH, Brocklebank JT, Bowmer CJ, et al. Pharmacokinetics of recombinant human erythropoietin in children with renal failure. *Nephrol Dial Transplant* 1991;6:709.

135. Braun A, Ding R, Seidel C, et al. Pharmacokinetics of recombinant human erythropoietin applied subcutaneously to children with chronic renal failure. *Pediatr Nephrol* 1993;7:61.

136. Cakar N, Ekim M, Tumer N, et al. Pharmacokinetics of recombinant human erythropoietin in children with chronic renal failure. *Int Urol Nephrol* 1997;29:377.

137. Reddingius RE, Schroder CH, Koster AM, et al. Pharmacokinetics of recombinant human erythropoietin in children treated with continuous ambulatory peritoneal dialysis. *Eur J Pediatr* 1994;153:850.

138. Besarab A, Flaharty KK, Erslev AJ, et al. Clinical pharmacology and economics of recombinant human erythropoietin in end-stage renal disease: the case for subcutaneous administration. *J Am Soc Nephrol* 1992;2:1405.

139. Horl WH. Optimal route of administration of erythropoietin in chronic renal failure patients: intravenous versus subcutaneous. *Acta Haematol* 1992;87:16.

140. Kaufman JS, Reda DJ, Fye CL, et al. Subcutaneous compared with intravenous epoetin in patients receiving hemodialysis. Department of Veterans Affairs Cooperative Study Group on Erythropoietin in Hemodialysis Patients. *N Engl J Med* 1998;339:578.

141. Paganini EP, Eschbach JW, Lazarus JM, et al. Intravenous versus subcutaneous dosing of epoetin alfa in hemodialysis patients. *Am J Kidney Dis* 1995;26:331.

142. Parker KP, Mitch WE, Stivelman JC, et al. Safety and efficacy of low-dose subcutaneous erythropoietin in hemodialysis patients. *J Am Soc Nephrol* 1997;8:288.

143. Lago M, Perez-Garcia R, Garcia de Vinuesa MS, et al. Efficiency of once-weekly subcutaneous administration of recombinant human erythropoietin versus three times a week administration in hemodialysis patients. *Nephron* 1996;72:723.

144. Weiss LG, Clyne N, Divino Fihlho J, et al. The efficacy of once weekly compared with two or three times weekly subcutaneous epoetin beta: results from a randomized controlled multicentre trial. Swedish Study Group. *Nephrol Dial Transplant* 2000;15:2014.

145. Petersen J, Kang MS, Yeh I: The site of injection affects erythropoietin levels during dialysis. *ASAIO J* 1996;42:263.

146. Uehlinger DE, Gotch FA, Sheiner LB. A pharmacodynamic model of erythropoietin therapy for uremic anemia. *Clin Pharmacol Ther* 1992;51:76.

147. Locatelli F, Olivares J, Walker R, et al. Novel erythropoiesis stimulating protein for treatment of anemia in chronic renal insufficiency. *Kidney Int* 2001;60:741.

148. St Peter WL, Lewis MJ, Macres MG. Pain comparison after subcutaneous administration of single-dose formulation versus multidose formulation of epogen in hemodialysis patients. *Am J Kidney Dis* 1998;32:470.

149. Vaziri ND. Mechanism of erythropoietin-induced hypertension. *Am J Kidney Dis* 1999;33:821.

150. Kaupke CJ, Kim S, Vaziri ND. Effect of erythrocyte mass on arterial blood pressure in dialysis patients receiving maintenance erythropoietin therapy. *J Am Soc Nephrol* 1994;4:1874.

151. Kang DH, Yoon KI, Han DS. Acute effects of recombinant human erythropoietin on plasma levels of proendothelin-1 and endothelin-1 in haemodialysis patients. *Nephrol Dial Transplant* 1998;13:2877.

152. Rodrigue ME, Moreau C, Lariviere R, et al. Relationship between eicosanoids and endothelin-1 in the pathogenesis of erythropoietin-induced hypertension in uremic rats. *J Cardiovasc Pharmacol* 2003;41:388.

153. Ni Z, Wang XQ, Vaziri ND. Nitric oxide metabolism in erythropoietin-induced hypertension: effect of calcium channel blockade. *Hypertension* 1998;32:724.

154. Bahlmann J, Schoter KH, Scigalla P, et al. Morbidity and mortality in hemodialysis patients with and without erythropoietin treatment: a controlled study. *Contrib Nephrol* 1991; 88:90.

155. De Marchi S, Cecchin E, Falleti E, et al. Long-term effects of erythropoietin therapy on fistula stenosis and plasma concentrations of PDGF and MCP-1 in hemodialysis patients. *J Am Soc Nephrol* 1997;8:1147.

156. Wiesholzer M, Kitzwogerer M, Harm F, et al. Prevalence of preterminal pulmonary thromboembolism among patients on maintenance hemodialysis treatment before and after introduction of recombinant erythropoietin. *Am J Kidney Dis* 1999;33:702.

157. Cheung AK, Alford MF, Wilson MM, et al. Urea movement across erythrocyte membrane during artificial kidney treatment. *Kidney Int* 1983;23:866.

158. Peces R, de la Torre M, Alcazar R, et al. Antibodies against recombinant human erythropoietin in a patient with erythropoietin-resistant anemia. *N Engl J Med* 1996;335:523.

159. Casadevall N, Nataf J, Viron B, et al. Pure red-cell aplasia and antierythropoietin antibodies in patients treated with recombinant erythropoietin. *N Engl J Med* 2003;346:469.

160. Vanrenterghem Y, Barany P, Mann JF, et al. Randomized trial of darbepoetin alfa for treatment of renal anemia at a reduced dose frequency compared with rHuEPO in dialysis patients. *Kidney Int* 2002;62:2167.

161. Nissenson AR, Swan SK, Lindberg JS, et al. Randomized, controlled trial of darbepoetin alfa for the treatment of anemia in hemodialysis patients. *Am J Kidney Dis* 2002;40: 110.

162. Suranyi MG, Lindberg JS, Navarro J, et al. Treatment of anemia with darbepoetin alfa administered de novo once every other week in chronic kidney disease. *Am J Nephrol* 2003;23:106.

163. Toto RD, Navarro J, Roger S, et al. Aranesp (darbepoetin alfa) administered once every other week treats anemia in patients with chronic kidney disease (CKD) not receiving renal replacement therapy. *J Am Soc Nephrol* 2002;13:635A.

164. Walker R. Aranesp (darbepoetin alfa) administered at a reduced frequency of once every 4 weeks (Q4W) maintains hemoglobin levels in patients with chronic kidney disease (CKD) receiving dialysis. Paper presented at National Kidney Foundation Clinical Nephrology Meeting, 2003.

165. Egrie JC, Browne JK. Development and characterization of novel erythropoiesis stimulating protein (NESP). *Nephrol Dial Transplant* 2001;16:3.

166. Macdougall IC, Gray SJ, Elston O, et al. Pharmacokinetics of novel erythropoiesis stimulating protein compared with epoetin alfa in dialysis patients. *J Am Soc Nephrol* 1999;10: 2392.

167. Lerner G, Kale AS, Warady BA, et al. Pharmacokinetics of darbepoetin alfa in pediatric patients with chronic kidney disease. *Pediatr Nephrol* 2002;17:933.

168. Scott SD. Dose conversion from recombinant human erythropoietin to darbepoetin alfa: recommendations from clinical studies. *Pharmacotherapy* 2002;22:160S.

169. Daschner M, Mehls O, Schaefer F. Soluble transferrin receptor is correlated with erythropoietin sensitivity in dialysis patients. *Clin Nephrol* 1999;52:246.

170. Richardson D, Bartlett C, Will EJ. Optimizing erythropoietin therapy in hemodialysis patients. *Am J Kidney Dis* 2001;38:109.

171. Fishbane S, Lynn RI. The utility of zinc protoporphyrin for predicting the need for intravenous iron therapy in hemodialysis patients. *Am J Kidney Dis* 1995;25:426.

172. Besarab A, Kaiser JW, Frinak S. A study of parenteral iron regimens in hemodialysis patients. *Am J Kidney Dis* 1999; 34:21.

173. Kooistra MP, van Es A, Struyvenberg A, et al. Iron metabolism in patients with the anaemia of end-stage renal disease during treatment with recombinant human erythropoietin. *Br J Haematol* 1991;79:634.

174. Fishbane S, Lynn RI: The efficacy of iron dextran for the treatment of iron deficiency in hemodialysis patients. *Clin Nephrol* 1995;44:238.

175. Tenbrock K, Muller-Berghaus J, Michalk D, et al. Intravenous iron treatment of renal anemia in children on hemodialysis. *Pediatr Nephrol* 1999;13:580.

176. Greenbaum LA, Pan CG, Caley C, et al. Intravenous iron dextran and erythropoietin use in pediatric hemodialysis patients. *Pediatr Nephrol* 2000;14:908.

177. Allegra V, Mengozzi G, Vasile A. Iron deficiency in maintenance hemodialysis patients: assessment of diagnosis criteria and of three different iron treatments. *Nephron* 1991;57: 175.

178. Kalantar-Zadeh K, Hoffken B, Wunsch H, et al. Diagnosis of iron deficiency anemia in renal failure patients during the post-erythropoietin era. *Am J Kidney Dis* 1995;26:292.

179. Morris KP, Watson S, Reid MM, et al. Assessing iron status in children with chronic renal failure on erythropoietin: which measurements should we use? *Pediatr Nephrol* 1994; 8:51.

180. Fishbane S, Kowalski EA, Imbriano LJ, et al. The evaluation of iron status in hemodialysis patients. *J Am Soc Nephrol* 1996;7:2654.

181. Cook JD, Carriaga M, Kahn SG, et al. Gastric delivery system for iron supplementation. *Lancet* 1990;335:1136.

182. Eschbach JW, Cook JD, Scribner BH, et al. Iron balance in hemodialysis patients. *Ann Intern Med* 1977;87:710.

183. Skikne BS, Cook JD. Effect of enhanced erythropoiesis on iron absorption. *J Lab Clin Med* 1992;120:746.

184. Milman N. Iron absorption measured by whole body counting and the relation to marrow iron stores in chronic uremia. *Clin Nephrol* 1982;17:77.

185. Donnelly SM, Posen GA, Ali MA. Oral iron absorption in hemodialysis patients treated with erythropoietin. *Clin Invest Med* 1991;14:271.

186. Goch J, Birgegard G, Danielson BG, et al. Iron absorption in patients with chronic uremia on maintenance hemodialysis and in healthy volunteers measured with a simple oral iron load test. *Nephron* 1996;73:403.

187. Piraio-Biroli G, Bothwell TH, Finch CA. Iron absorption II. The absorption of radioiron administered with a standard meal in man. *J Lab Clin Med* 1958;51:24.

188. Fishbane S, Frei GL, Maesaka J. Reduction in recombinant human erythropoietin doses by the use of chronic intravenous iron supplementation. *Am J Kidney Dis* 1995; 26:41.

189. Macdougall IC, Tucker B, Thompson J, et al. A randomized controlled study of iron supplementation in patients treated with erythropoietin. *Kidney Int* 1996;50:1694.

190. Schroder CH. The management of anemia in pediatric peritoneal dialysis patients. *Pediatr Nephrol* 2003;18:805.

191. Nyvad O, Danielsen H, Madsen S. Intravenous iron-sucrose complex to reduce epoetin demand in dialysis patients. *Lancet* 1994;344:1305.

192. Sunder-Plassmann G, Horl WH. Importance of iron supply for erythropoietin therapy. *Nephrol Dial Transplant* 1995;10:2070.

193. Taylor JE, Peat N, Porter C, et al. Regular low-dose intravenous iron therapy improves response to erythropoietin in haemodialysis patients. *Nephrol Dial Transplant* 1996;11:1079.

194. Nissenson AR, Lindsay RM, Swan S, et al. Sodium ferric gluconate complex in sucrose is safe and effective in hemodialysis patients: North American Clinical Trial. *Am J Kidney Dis* 1999;33:471.

195. Ahsan N. Intravenous infusion of total dose iron is superior to oral iron in treatment of anemia in peritoneal dialysis patients: a single center comparative study. *J Am Soc Nephrol* 1998;9:664.

196. Yorgin PD, Belson A, Sarwal M, et al. Sodium ferric gluconate therapy in renal transplant and renal failure patients. *Pediatr Nephrol* 2000;15:171.

197. Morgan HE, Gautam M, Geary DF. Maintenance intravenous iron therapy in pediatric hemodialysis patients. *Pediatr Nephrol* 2001;16:779.

198. Bolanos L, Castro P, Falcon TG, et al. Continuous intravenous sodium ferric gluconate improves efficacy in the maintenance phase of rHuEPO administration in hemodialysis patients. *Am J Nephrol* 2002;22:67.

199. Van Wyck DB, Cavallo G, Spinowitz BS, et al. Safety and efficacy of iron sucrose in patients sensitive to iron dextran: North American clinical trial. *Am J Kidney Dis* 2000;36:88.

200. Charytan C, Levin N, Al-Saloum M, et al. Efficacy and safety of iron sucrose for iron deficiency in patients with dialysis-associated anemia: North American clinical trial. *Am J Kidney Dis* 2001;37:300.

201. Auerbach M, Winchester J, Wahab A, et al. A randomized trial of three iron dextran infusion methods for anemia in EPO-treated dialysis patients. *Am J Kidney Dis* 1998;31:81.

202. Vychytil A, Haag-Weber M. Iron status and iron supplementation in peritoneal dialysis patients. *Kidney Int* 1999;69(suppl):S71.

203. Anuradha S, Singh NP, Agarwal SK. Total dose infusion iron dextran therapy in predialysis chronic renal failure patients. *Renal Failure* 2002;24:307.

204. Dahdah K, Patrie JT, Bolton WK. Intravenous iron dextran treatment in predialysis patients with chronic renal failure. *Am J Kidney Dis* 2000;36:775.

205. Silverberg DS, Blum M, Agbaria Z, et al. The effect of i.v. iron alone or in combination with low-dose erythropoietin in the rapid correction of anemia of chronic renal failure in the predialysis period. *Clin Nephrol* 2001;55:212.

206. Domrongkitchaiporn S, Jirakranont B, Atamasrikul K, et al. Indices of iron status in continuous ambulatory peritoneal dialysis patients. *Am J Kidney Dis* 1999;34:29.

207. Prakash S, Walele A, Dimkovic N, et al. Experience with a large dose (500 mg) of intravenous iron dextran and iron saccharate in peritoneal dialysis patients. *Perit Dial Int* 2001;21:290.

208. Chandler G, Harchowal J, Macdougall IC. Intravenous iron sucrose: establishing a safe dose. *Am J Kidney Dis* 2001;38:988.

209. Folkert VW, Michael B, Agarwal R, et al. Chronic use of sodium ferric gluconate complex in hemodialysis patients: safety of higher-dose (> or =250 mg) administration. *Am J Kidney Dis* 2003;41:651.

210. Javier AM. Weekly administration of high-dose sodium ferric gluconate is safe and effective in peritoneal dialysis patients. *ANNA J* 2002;29:183.

211. Besarab A, Amin N, Ahsan M, et al. Optimization of epoetin therapy with intravenous iron therapy in hemodialysis patients. *J Am Soc Nephrol* 2000;11:530.

212. Hamstra RD, Block MH, Schocket AL. Intravenous iron dextran in clinical medicine. *JAMA* 1980;243:1726.

213. Faich G, Strobos J. Sodium ferric gluconate complex in sucrose: safer intravenous iron therapy than iron dextrans. *Am J Kidney Dis* 1999;33:464.

214. Fletes R, Lazarus JM, Gage J, et al. Suspected iron dextran-related adverse drug events in hemodialysis patients. *Am J Kidney Dis* 2001;37:743.

215. Coyne DW, Adkinson NF, Nissenson AR, et al. Sodium ferric gluconate complex in hemodialysis patients. II. Adverse reactions in iron dextran-sensitive and dextran-tolerant patients. *Kidney Int* 2003;63:217.

216. Michael B, Coyne DW, Fishbane S, et al. Sodium ferric gluconate complex in hemodialysis patients: adverse reactions compared to placebo and iron dextran. *Kidney Int* 2003;61:1830.

217. Lewis MJ, Swan SK.: The generation of non-dextran intravenous iron: is iron dextran obsolete? *Seminars in Dialysis* 2000;13:9.

218. Horl WH. Should we still use iron dextran in hemodialysis patients? *Am J Kidney Dis* 2001;37:859.

219. Auerbach M, Chaudhry M, Goldman H, et al. Value of methylprednisolone in prevention of the arthralgia-myalgia syndrome associated with the total dose infusion of iron dextran: a double blind randomized trial. *J Lab Clin Med* 1998;131:257.

220. Zanen AL, Adriaansen HJ, van Bommel EF, et al. "Oversaturation" of transferrin after intravenous ferric gluconate (Ferrlecit) in haemodialysis patients. *Nephrol Dial Transplant* 1996;11:820.

221. Sunder-Plassmann G, Horl WH. Safety of intravenous injection of iron saccharate in haemodialysis patients. *Nephrol Dial Transplant* 1996;11:1797.

222. Pascual J, Teruel JL, Liano F, et al. Serious adverse reactions after intravenous ferric gluconate. *Nephrol Dial Transplant* 1992;7:271.

223. Hoigne R, Breymann C, Kunzi UP, et al. Parenteral iron therapy: problems and possible solutions. *Schweiz Med Wochenschr* 1998;128:528.

224. Kirschbaum B. Serial ferritin concentrations in hemodialysis patients receiving intravenous iron. *Clin Nephrol* 2002;57:452.

225. Lazarus JM, Hakim RM, Newell J. Recombinant human erythropoietin and phlebotomy in the treatment of iron overload in chronic hemodialysis patients. *Am J Kidney Dis* 1990;16:101.

226. Weinberg ED.: Iron withholding: a defense against infection and neoplasia. *Physiol Rev* 1984;64:65.

227. Seifert A, von Herrath D, Schaefer K. Iron overload, but not treatment with desferrioxamine favours the development of septicemia in patients on maintenance hemodialysis. *Q J Med* 1987;65:1015.

228. Boelaert JR, Cantinieaux BF, Hariga CF, et al. Recombinant erythropoietin reverses polymorphonuclear granulocyte dysfunction in iron-overloaded dialysis patients. *Nephrol Dial Transplant* 1990;5:504.

229. Patruta SI, Edlinger R, Sunder-Plassmann G, et al. Neutrophil impairment associated with iron therapy in hemodialysis patients with functional iron deficiency. *J Am Soc Nephrol* 1998;9:655.

230. Deicher R, Ziai F, Cohen G, et al. High-dose parenteral iron sucrose depresses neutrophil intracellular killing capacity. *Kidney Int* 2003;64:728.

231. Hoen B, Kessler M, Hestin D, et al. Risk factors for bacterial infections in chronic haemodialysis adult patients: a multicentre prospective survey. *Nephrol Dial Transplant* 1995;10:377.

232. Hoen B, Paul-Dauphin A, Kessler M. Intravenous iron administration does not significantly increase the risk of bacteremia in chronic hemodialysis patients. *Clin Nephrol* 2002;57:457.

Index

NOTE: Page numbers followed by *f* indicate figures; those followed by *t* indicate tables.